Study Guide for

# Pharmacology and the Nursing Process

## Seventh Edition

**Linda Lane Lilley, RN, PhD**
**Shelly Rainforth Collins, PharmD**
**Julie S. Snyder, MSN, RN-BC**

*Study Guide prepared by*

**Julie S. Snyder, MSN, RN-BC**
Adjunct Faculty
School of Nursing
Old Dominion University
Norfolk, Virginia

*Student Study Tips by*

**Diane Savoca**
Coordinator of Student Transition
St. Louis Community College at Florissant Valley
St. Louis, Missouri

MOSBY

3251 Riverport Lane
St. Louis, Missouri 63043

STUDY GUIDE FOR PHARMACOLOGY
AND THE NURSING PROCESS, SEVENTH EDITION

ISBN: 978-0-323-09129-9

**Notices**

Knowledge and best practice in this field are constantly changing. As new research and experience broaden our understanding, changes in research methods, professional practices, or medical treatment may become necessary.

Practitioners and researchers must always rely on their own experience and knowledge in evaluating and using any information, methods, compounds, or experiments described herein. In using such information or methods they should be mindful of their own safety and the safety of others, including parties for whom they have a professional responsibility.

With respect to any drug or pharmaceutical products identified, readers are advised to check the most current information provided (i) on procedures featured or (ii) by the manufacturer of each product to be administered, to verify the recommended dose or formula, the method and duration of administration, and contraindications. It is the responsibility of practitioners, relying on their own experience and knowledge of their patients, to make diagnoses, to determine dosages and the best treatment for each individual patient, and to take all appropriate safety precautions.

To the fullest extent of the law, neither the Publisher nor the authors, contributors, or editors, assume any liability for any injury and/or damage to persons or property as a matter of products liability, negligence or otherwise, or from any use or operation of any methods, products, instructions, or ideas contained in the material herein.

**International Standard Book Number 978-0-323-09129-9**

*Executive Content Strategist:* Lee Henderson
*Content Development Specialist:* Jacqueline Twomey
*Book Production Manager:* Jeffrey Patterson
*Project Manager:* Clay Broeker
*Publishing Services:* Lisa Hernandez

Printed in the United States of America

Last digit is the print number: 9 8 7 6 5 4 3 2

Working together to grow
libraries in developing countries

www.elsevier.com | www.bookaid.org | www.sabre.org

ELSEVIER   BOOK AID International   Sabre Foundation

# Contents

Student Study Tips . . . . . . . . . . . . . . . . . . . . . . . . . . . . . . . . . . . . . . . . . . . . . . . .1

**Chapter 1**     The Nursing Process and Drug Therapy . . . . . . . . . . . . . . . . . . . . . . . . . .21
**Chapter 2**     Pharmacologic Principles. . . . . . . . . . . . . . . . . . . . . . . . . . . . . . . . . . . . .23
**Chapter 3**     Lifespan Considerations. . . . . . . . . . . . . . . . . . . . . . . . . . . . . . . . . . . . . .27
**Chapter 4**     Cultural, Legal, and Ethical Considerations . . . . . . . . . . . . . . . . . . . . .29
**Chapter 5**     Medication Errors: Preventing and Responding . . . . . . . . . . . . . . . . .33
**Chapter 6**     Patient Education and Drug Therapy. . . . . . . . . . . . . . . . . . . . . . . . . . .35
**Chapter 7**     Over-the-Counter Drugs and Herbal and Dietary Supplements . . . .37
**Chapter 8**     Gene Therapy and Pharmacogenomics . . . . . . . . . . . . . . . . . . . . . . . .41
**Chapter 9**     Photo Atlas of Drug Administration . . . . . . . . . . . . . . . . . . . . . . . . . .43
**Chapter 10**    Analgesic Drugs. . . . . . . . . . . . . . . . . . . . . . . . . . . . . . . . . . . . . . . . . . .47
**Chapter 11**    General and Local Anesthetics. . . . . . . . . . . . . . . . . . . . . . . . . . . . . . . .51
**Chapter 12**    Central Nervous System Depressants and Muscle Relaxants . . . . . . .53
**Chapter 13**    Central Nervous System Stimulants and Related Drugs . . . . . . . . . . .55
**Chapter 14**    Antiepileptic Drugs . . . . . . . . . . . . . . . . . . . . . . . . . . . . . . . . . . . . . . .57
**Chapter 15**    Antiparkinson Drugs . . . . . . . . . . . . . . . . . . . . . . . . . . . . . . . . . . . . . .61
**Chapter 16**    Psychotherapeutic Drugs . . . . . . . . . . . . . . . . . . . . . . . . . . . . . . . . . . .63
**Chapter 17**    Substance Abuse . . . . . . . . . . . . . . . . . . . . . . . . . . . . . . . . . . . . . . . . . .67
**Chapter 18**    Adrenergic Drugs. . . . . . . . . . . . . . . . . . . . . . . . . . . . . . . . . . . . . . . . . .69
**Chapter 19**    Adrenergic-Blocking Drugs. . . . . . . . . . . . . . . . . . . . . . . . . . . . . . . . . .71
**Chapter 20**    Cholinergic Drugs . . . . . . . . . . . . . . . . . . . . . . . . . . . . . . . . . . . . . . . .73
**Chapter 21**    Cholinergic-Blocking Drugs . . . . . . . . . . . . . . . . . . . . . . . . . . . . . . . . .75
**Chapter 22**    Antihypertensive Drugs . . . . . . . . . . . . . . . . . . . . . . . . . . . . . . . . . . . .77
**Chapter 23**    Antianginal Drugs . . . . . . . . . . . . . . . . . . . . . . . . . . . . . . . . . . . . . . . .81
**Chapter 24**    Heart Failure Drugs . . . . . . . . . . . . . . . . . . . . . . . . . . . . . . . . . . . . . . .83
**Chapter 25**    Antidysrhythmic Drugs . . . . . . . . . . . . . . . . . . . . . . . . . . . . . . . . . . . .85
**Chapter 26**    Coagulation Modifier Drugs . . . . . . . . . . . . . . . . . . . . . . . . . . . . . . . .87
**Chapter 27**    Antilipemic Drugs . . . . . . . . . . . . . . . . . . . . . . . . . . . . . . . . . . . . . . . .91
**Chapter 28**    Diuretic Drugs . . . . . . . . . . . . . . . . . . . . . . . . . . . . . . . . . . . . . . . . . . .93
**Chapter 29**    Fluids and Electrolytes. . . . . . . . . . . . . . . . . . . . . . . . . . . . . . . . . . . . .97
**Chapter 30**    Pituitary Drugs. . . . . . . . . . . . . . . . . . . . . . . . . . . . . . . . . . . . . . . . . . .99
**Chapter 31**    Thyroid and Antithyroid Drugs . . . . . . . . . . . . . . . . . . . . . . . . . . . . .101
**Chapter 32**    Antidiabetic Drugs. . . . . . . . . . . . . . . . . . . . . . . . . . . . . . . . . . . . . . .105
**Chapter 33**    Adrenal Drugs . . . . . . . . . . . . . . . . . . . . . . . . . . . . . . . . . . . . . . . . . .107
**Chapter 34**    Women's Health Drugs . . . . . . . . . . . . . . . . . . . . . . . . . . . . . . . . . . .109
**Chapter 35**    Men's Health Drugs. . . . . . . . . . . . . . . . . . . . . . . . . . . . . . . . . . . . . .113
**Chapter 36**    Antihistamines, Decongestants, Antitussives, and Expectorants. . . .115
**Chapter 37**    Respiratory Drugs . . . . . . . . . . . . . . . . . . . . . . . . . . . . . . . . . . . . . . .117
**Chapter 38**    Antibiotics Part 1 . . . . . . . . . . . . . . . . . . . . . . . . . . . . . . . . . . . . . . . .119

**Chapter 39**   Antibiotics Part 2 . . . . . . . . . . . . . . . . . . . . . . . . . . . . . . . . . . . . . . . . . . . . . . . . . . . . . . . . . . .123

**Chapter 40**   Antiviral Drugs . . . . . . . . . . . . . . . . . . . . . . . . . . . . . . . . . . . . . . . . . . . . . . . . . . . . . . . . . . . . .125

**Chapter 41**   Antitubercular Drugs . . . . . . . . . . . . . . . . . . . . . . . . . . . . . . . . . . . . . . . . . . . . . . . . . . . . . . . .127

**Chapter 42**   Antifungal Drugs . . . . . . . . . . . . . . . . . . . . . . . . . . . . . . . . . . . . . . . . . . . . . . . . . . . . . . . . . . . .129

**Chapter 43**   Antimalarial, Antiprotozoal, and Anthelmintic Drugs. . . . . . . . . . . . . . . . . . . . . . . . . . . . . .131

**Chapter 44**   Antiinflammatory and Antigout Drugs . . . . . . . . . . . . . . . . . . . . . . . . . . . . . . . . . . . . . . . . . .133

**Chapter 45**   Antineoplastic Drugs Part 1: Cancer Overview and Cell Cycle–Specific Drugs . . . . . . . . . . . . . . . . . .135

**Chapter 46**   Antineoplastic Drugs Part 2: Cell Cycle–Nonspecific and Miscellaneous Drugs. . . . . . . . . . . . . . . . .139

**Chapter 47**   Biologic Response–Modifying and Antirheumatic Drugs. . . . . . . . . . . . . . . . . . . . . . . . . . . . .141

**Chapter 48**   Immunosuppressant Drugs. . . . . . . . . . . . . . . . . . . . . . . . . . . . . . . . . . . . . . . . . . . . . . . . . . . . .143

**Chapter 49**   Immunizing Drugs and Biochemical Terrorism. . . . . . . . . . . . . . . . . . . . . . . . . . . . . . . . . . . .145

**Chapter 50**   Acid-Controlling Drugs. . . . . . . . . . . . . . . . . . . . . . . . . . . . . . . . . . . . . . . . . . . . . . . . . . . . . . .149

**Chapter 51**   Bowel Disorder Drugs . . . . . . . . . . . . . . . . . . . . . . . . . . . . . . . . . . . . . . . . . . . . . . . . . . . . . . . .151

**Chapter 52**   Antiemetic and Antinausea Drugs . . . . . . . . . . . . . . . . . . . . . . . . . . . . . . . . . . . . . . . . . . . . . .155

**Chapter 53**   Vitamins and Minerals. . . . . . . . . . . . . . . . . . . . . . . . . . . . . . . . . . . . . . . . . . . . . . . . . . . . . . . .157

**Chapter 54**   Anemia Drugs . . . . . . . . . . . . . . . . . . . . . . . . . . . . . . . . . . . . . . . . . . . . . . . . . . . . . . . . . . . . . .159

**Chapter 55**   Nutritional Supplements . . . . . . . . . . . . . . . . . . . . . . . . . . . . . . . . . . . . . . . . . . . . . . . . . . . . . .161

**Chapter 56**   Dermatologic Drugs. . . . . . . . . . . . . . . . . . . . . . . . . . . . . . . . . . . . . . . . . . . . . . . . . . . . . . . . . .165

**Chapter 57**   Ophthalmic Drugs . . . . . . . . . . . . . . . . . . . . . . . . . . . . . . . . . . . . . . . . . . . . . . . . . . . . . . . . . . .167

**Chapter 58**   Otic Drugs . . . . . . . . . . . . . . . . . . . . . . . . . . . . . . . . . . . . . . . . . . . . . . . . . . . . . . . . . . . . . . . . .169

Overview of Dosage Calculations . . . . . . . . . . . . . . . . . . . . . . . . . . . . . . . . . . . . . . . . . . . . . .171

Answer Key . . . . . . . . . . . . . . . . . . . . . . . . . . . . . . . . . . . . . . . . . . . . . . . . . . . . . . . . . . . . . . . .195

# Student Study Tips

## CHOOSE TO MANAGE YOUR TIME

Time and money have much in common. They can be spent, saved, invested, given away, stolen, and wasted. The big difference between these two commodities is that you can earn more money. Your time is limited. Learn to manage your time now and the quality of your life will increase because you will have more time to do what you enjoy.

You may not enjoy studying. What you want is to be a nurse, and studying is one choice that will get you what you want. Being a nurse will bring you the satisfaction that you need. I, for one, am very thankful that you have made this decision. The world needs dedicated skilled nurses. To meet this need, you must make the decision to manage your time effectively.

## Establish Goals and Create Action Plans

One key to time management is having clear goals and an action plan to accomplish these goals. This is more than saying, "I want to be a nurse" or "I want to ace my pharmacology midterm." It is a decision to spend time now to get clarity and direction so that you will have more time later to relax. The following guidelines can help you get what you want.

### Guidelines for Setting Goals

There are some basic guidelines to follow when setting goals:

- **Be realistic**. The goal must be something that you can reasonably expect to accomplish. A goal of scoring 100% on each and every unit test is not realistic, but a goal of scoring 85% or better is.
- **Be specific.** Goals must set out exactly what needs to be done. Do not simply state, "I will study for the exam." Specify how many hours, what days, and what times you will study. The more specific the goal statement, the easier it is to establish a plan, complete that plan, and thus achieve the goal set.
- **Establish a time limit.** Specify a time limit for completing each step in the plan and an overall deadline for accomplishing the goal.

- **Make the goal and actions measurable.** State the goal and each step in the plan for achieving it in a way that will enable you to measure your progress toward completion.

The following is an example of how this goal and action process works: You have a chapter test a week from today. The test will cover approximately 45 pages of text material, and there are 40 specific pharmacologic terms you must know. In addition, you have been given about 20 pages of supplementary handouts in class. What will you do in the next 7 days to prepare for this test?

*Goal Statement:*
**I will study to make a good grade on this exam.**
This is a poor goal statement because it is not specific, sets no time limits, and offers no real way to measure progress. The intent is good, but the implementation of such a vague goal is usually poor.

*Revision 1:*
**I will spend 2 hours a day studying for the next chapter test in order to get at least an 80% score.**
This is a better goal statement. If one assumes that 2 hours per day is realistic, then the goal is more specific, the grade goal is measurable, and there is a time limit of sorts. This goal statement might be good enough, but it could still be improved.

*Final Version:*
**I will spend 2 hours per day, from 2:30 to 4:30 PM, for the next 7 days studying for the chapter test in order to score at least 80%.**
This is what is needed. This version states how much time, when, how many days, and for what purpose. Setting clear goals helps you get started and serves as a motivator to keep you working.

### Guidelines for Action Statements

A goal, no matter how well stated, is not enough. There must be action statements to help you make day-to-day progress toward meeting the goal. The guidelines that apply to defining your goal also apply to establishing the action statements—they should be realistic, specific, measurable, and time-limited. They spell out what is going to be done day to day. Here are three examples of good action statements for the sample goal:

- I will master six pharmacology terms each day.
- I will spend from 2:30 to 3:00 PM each day reviewing class handouts.
- I will review 10 pages of text material from 3:00 to 4:00 PM each day.

These examples should give you a good idea of how to go about developing a clear goal and a set of actions to carry out to achieve that goal.

## Organize Tasks and Create Schedules

It takes time to make time. It is your choice. Either you set your schedule or others will do it for you. It is 2:30 PM. The phone rings and friends want you to go out or your boss wants you to work overtime or your sister wants you to watch the kids. When you have an action plan and a schedule, your choices are clear. This is the time you scheduled to review class handouts. Can you reschedule this review or do you want to keep this promise you have made to yourself to accomplish your goal? No matter what you decide, you have maintained control over your time.

Your goals and action plans are the foundation for your time management. The next key is to organize tasks and create schedules.

### Guidelines for Organizing Tasks

1. Divide tasks into three categories:
   a. Jobs that **have to be done,** such as going to class, going to work, eating, and getting adequate rest. These jobs are the easiest to accomplish because the consequences of not doing them are serious. If you do not go to class, failure is almost a sure thing. If you do not go to work, soon there will be no paycheck. The consequences of not eating or sleeping are obvious.
   b. Jobs that **should be done,** such as studying, paying bills, cleaning the house, and all of those other necessary but unpleasant tasks that are part of life. The "should-be-done" jobs are the most difficult to accomplish because they are the jobs that are all too easy to put off doing. These are also the jobs for which time management skills are most essential.
   c. Things that you **want to do.** These include all of the fun things that provide pleasure and escape from the routines of class, study, and work. Most of us are very successful at finding time to do what we want to do, even when there is a sizable backlog of "should-be-done" chores waiting. This choice can lead to procrastination

and stress. The important things are maintaining balance and staying focused on your goals.

2. Prioritize items in your **"have-to-be-done" category** based on your physical and mental health needs. Examine the consequences of not doing these activities. If you can live without doing an activity, then it is not a need.

3. Prioritize your **"should-be-done" category** based on your physical and mental health needs. Examine the consequences of not doing these activities. Can you accomplish your established goals without doing a given activity? If so, then it is not a need.

4. Prioritize your **"want-to-do" category.** Some recreational time is absolutely essential in any effective time management system. "Want-to-do" activities can often be used as incentives for completing what should be done.

5. Use incentives to accomplish what you should do. For each person the rewards will be different. Spend a little time determining what will work for you. It might be watching your favorite reality show, prime time drama, or comedy show; going to the movie theater to see a new release; reading a book for pleasure; or just spending some time with family or friends.

### Guidelines for Creating Workable Schedules

You will need three types of schedule: **master, weekly,** and **daily.**

Start by developing a **master schedule** table on your computer that has seven columns and 15 to 17 rows. The columns are the days in the week and the rows are the hours in the day. The left-hand column will represent Sunday and the far right will be Saturday. Start at the top of each column with the time you usually get up in the morning and end each column with the time you usually go to bed. A typical master schedule might begin at 6 AM and end at 11 PM.

Once the blank schedule sheet is prepared, the next step is to fill in those hours that correspond to the activities you have to do. These are the hours others control, and the activities are those that occur at the same hour, on the same day or days, and for several weeks or longer. For example, the semester's schedule of classes is the first set of activities to enter into the master schedule. Other activities such as work, travel, worship services, and any other regular activities also belong in the master schedule.

The master schedule should contain only those recurring activities that cannot be done at any other time. Activities such as doing the laundry, watching television, and shopping should not be included, because the time when you do them is more flexible. The idea behind compiling the master schedule is to establish those times of the day that are "spent" and therefore cannot be used for any other activities. The empty blocks that remain represent the time you have to do everything else. Figure 1-1 shows a sample master schedule.

Creating a master schedule takes no more than half an hour, and it will generally serve you for an entire semester. The only reason to compile a new master schedule is that a significant schedule change has occurred. You may get a new work assignment or your nursing practicum site may change and require an additional 15 or 20 minutes of travel time. Then a new master schedule should be drawn up to accommodate the increase in time that is now necessary. Once the master schedule is completed, make four or five copies of it. These copies will be used to prepare the detailed weekly schedule.

Next, move on to developing your weekly schedule. The master schedule helps you identify the time you have available to complete the "should-be-done" and "want-to-do" task lists. The weekly schedule is more complex. It is intended to help you plan for study, recreation, family time, and all of those other activities that you want to fit into a typical week. To prepare the detailed weekly

schedule, take one of the copies you made of the master schedule and begin to fill in activities in the open blocks of time. The first blocks of time you should assign are the most important ones for any student—study time. This is what time management is all about—scheduling the needed hours for study (Figure 1-2).

**When filling in study hours, consider these important factors:**

- **Amount of planned study time.** There is an old rule pertaining to study time, and even though it is an old rule, it is still a very good guideline. The rule is to plan 2 hours of study time for each 1 hour spent in class. For example, a three-credit-hour course meets 3 hours per week, so you need to plan 6 hours of study time per week for this course. Remember, this is a general rule. Some courses will not actually require as much time as you allot, whereas others will require more. The reason for beginning a semester with this approach is simple. It is easy to find things to do with time you do not need for study, but once a semester is underway, it can be very difficult to find additional study time. If you do not plan enough study time at the beginning, you will soon find yourself in a constant battle to keep up. The result is frustration, anxiety, and a sense of impending doom—feelings you do not need when you want to perform at your very best.

- **Personal prime time.** Do you wake up early, ready to charge forward, but find it difficult to be productive after 10 PM? Do you do your best work in the afternoon and early evening and prefer to sleep until

|  | SUN | MON | TUES | WED | THUR | FRI | SAT |
|---|---|---|---|---|---|---|---|
| 7:00 | | GET UP | | GET UP | | GET UP | |
| 8:00 | | TRAVEL | | TRAVEL | | TRAVEL | |
| 9:00 | GET UP | CLASS | | CLASS | | CLASS | |
| 10:00 | CHURCH | CLASS | TRAVEL | CLASS | TRAVEL | CLASS | |
| 11:00 | CHURCH | | PRACTICUM | | PRACTICUM | | |
| 12:00 | | CLASS | PRACTICUM | CLASS | PRACTICUM | | |
| 1:00 | | | PRACTICUM | | PRACTICUM | | |
| 2:00 | | PERSONAL | PRACTICUM | | PRACTICUM | | |
| 3:00 | | PERSONAL | | | | | |
| 4:00 | | AEROBICS | | AEROBICS | | AEROBICS | |
| 5:00 | | | | | | | |
| 6:00 | | DINNER | DINNER | DINNER | DINNER | DINNER | |
| 7:00 | | | | | | | FUN |
| 8:00 | | | | | | | FUN |
| 9:00 | | | | | | | FUN |
| 10:00 | | | | | | | FUN |
| 11:00 | BEDTIME | BEDTIME | BEDTIME | BEDTIME | BEDTIME | BEDTIME | FUN |

**Figure 1-1.** The master schedule. This is an essential first step in managing time effectively.

| | SUN | MON | TUES | WED | THUR | FRI | SAT |
|---|---|---|---|---|---|---|---|
| 7:00 | | GET UP | | GET UP | | GET UP | |
| 8:00 | | TRAVEL | | TRAVEL | | TRAVEL | |
| 9:00 | GET UP | CLASS | STUDY | CLASS | STUDY | CLASS | |
| 10:00 | CHURCH | CLASS | TRAVEL | CLASS | TRAVEL | CLASS | STUDY |
| 11:00 | CHURCH | LUNCH | PRACTICUM | LUNCH | PRACTICUM | LUNCH | STUDY |
| 12:00 | | CLASS | PRACTICUM | CLASS | PRACTICUM | | PERSONAL |
| 1:00 | | STUDY | PRACTICUM | STUDY | PRACTICUM | STUDY | PERSONAL |
| 2:00 | FREE | STUDY | PRACTICUM | STUDY | PRACTICUM | STUDY | PERSONAL |
| 3:00 | | | TRAVEL | | TRAVEL | | |
| 4:00 | | AEROBICS | | AEROBICS | | AEROBICS | |
| 5:00 | | | | | | | |
| 6:00 | | DINNER | DINNER | DINNER | DINNER | DINNER | |
| 7:00 | STUDY | STUDY | STUDY | STUDY | STUDY | STUDY | FUN |
| 8:00 | STUDY | | STUDY | | STUDY | | FUN |
| 9:00 | STUDY | REVIEW | REVIEW | REVIEW | REVIEW | | FUN |
| 10:00 | | | | | | | FUN |
| 11:00 | BEDTIME | BEDTIME | BEDTIME | BEDTIME | BEDTIME | BEDTIME | FUN |

**Figure 1-2.** The detailed weekly schedule. Study times should be filled in first.

10 AM? Are you a night owl? Answers to these questions will reveal your prime time, those times of the day when your ability to concentrate is at its best and you can accomplish the most. These are the times you want to use for study. It is not always possible, because of class and work schedules, to schedule all study time in your prime hours, but it is essential that those hours be used for study as much as possible. It would be foolish to plan to study your toughest material between 9 and 11 PM when you know that is a time when just reading the daily paper is a challenge.

- **Study hours for specific courses and general study hours.** The reason for scheduling both general and specific study times is that the study demands of different courses vary from day to day and week to week. For instance, you will need some hours of study every week to master new material, terms, and concepts in pharmacology, but the study time demands will increase in the days just before exams, midterms, and project due dates. The hours set aside for specific courses are for accomplishing the day-to-day study demands; the unassigned study hours are for meeting the changing demands posed by these special circumstances. These unassigned study hours also let you meet unexpected demands. No matter how carefully you plan your time, something will happen to prevent you from using the time block you had set aside for learning.

Be patient and evaluate what works for you. It usually takes two or three attempts over a period of 3 weeks to arrive at a detailed schedule that works well

for you. There is a tendency on the first attempt to try to schedule some important activity for every waking hour. Ultimately such a schedule will make you feel as though there is no time for fun. Determine what is not working for you and make appropriate adjustments. Each week your schedule will come closer to being realistic and effective. The need to evaluate and revise is the reason for making several copies of the master schedule. Or you may want to use an electronic calendar. It saves time in the revision process, and saving time is, after all, what time management is all about.

Your last scheduling activity is to create **daily schedules and lists.** No matter how carefully and thoughtfully you prepare the detailed weekly schedule, it cannot include all the tasks you will face. You will have small tasks, infrequent tasks, and unexpected tasks that will need to be added to your schedule. Each day as you think of things you want or need to do the next day, write them down. Carry a small notebook that will fit into a pocket or purse. Many cell phones have a list and/or calendar feature. Once a day, review the list and set priorities for the next day.

**Consider the following when setting priorities:**

- **There are only 24 hours in each day.** Be realistic about what you are able to accomplish. Do not plan to review three chapters of text material on a day when you know there will not be enough time to cover more than half of one chapter.
- **Not everything is important.** Rank your tasks as A, B, or C, with A being the most important and C being the least important. Then go about completing

your As. Procrastinating about your B and C lists is not a sin. For example, going to the dry cleaner is critical if the outfit you must wear tomorrow is there, but if you do not absolutely have to have that outfit tomorrow, then the trip to the dry cleaner is a low priority and can be postponed to another day. Then it will be on your A list.

- **Rewriting to-do lists can steal your time.** You may want to make one weekly list and mark the tasks as A, B, or C. Put only A tasks on your daily to-do list. If you have extra time you can look at your weekly list. Or you can keep your tasks on note cards and then each day stack them in priority order.
- **Planning your route can save you time.** Look at the small tasks listed, such as picking up milk and dog food, dropping off dry cleaning, and going to the bank. Not only plan to do those errands, but also think about the order in which they should be done. Planning your route so that it completes a circle from home to the cleaners to the grocery store to the bank to home will be much more time-efficient than going from home to the grocery store, back home, then to the cleaners, back home, then to the bank, and finally back home again.
- **As you complete a job on the daily list, cross it off.** Crossing it off tells you that you are making progress and motivates you to move to the next item on the list. If not every item is crossed off, remember that tomorrow is another day. Celebrate what you did get done and create a plan for tomorrow that will help you accomplish your goals.
- **Remember your goals and planned action steps.** When unexpected daily tasks push them onto the B list, be sure to revise your plan to get back onto your time line. Put planning on your A list.
- **Waiting time can be a gift.** Small blocks of time are often lost or wasted because it does not seem as though anything significant could be accomplished during them. If you learn to use these small blocks effectively, you can free up larger blocks for more time-consuming or fun tasks. If a class ends 10 minutes early or if you are waiting for your ride, use the time for study. Take advantage of such "found" time to review five vocabulary terms, rework a set of class notes, or preview the next five pages of assigned reading. Using the odd minutes in the day to your advantage can really help you achieve your goals as a student.

Your time is a valuable resource for you to manage or to waste. The choice is yours. Stop for a few minutes and think over the previous strategies on how to manage your time: establishing goals and creating action plans, organizing tasks, and creating schedules. Which of these strategies will you choose to apply?

# CHOOSE TO USE YOUR RESOURCES

This Study Guide is one of the resources that will help you be successful in this course. When you choose to apply these study tips, they will help you to be successful in all of your course work. Three other resources are your textbook, your instructor, and your classmates.

## Your Textbook

The authors of your textbook have taken great care in organizing the information provided in a manner that will assist your learning. Each part starts with study skills tips that build on the tips that are presented in the Study Guide. At the beginning of each chapter, you will find specific objectives describing what you are expected to know and be able to do as a result of studying each chapter. Each chapter also contains a list of key terms. Take 10 minutes right now to perform a survey of your textbook so that you know what to expect over the term of this course. Look for chapter titles and Key Points. Later in this Study Guide you will find tips for mastering your textbook.

## Your Instructor

Some students look at their instructor in awe. She or he is so smart and has so much experience. This is true, but he or she is also a teacher who cares about pharmacology and your learning. Your instructor wants to hear your questions because this demonstrates that you are interested in learning and you are actively engaged with the material in your textbook and lectures. The instructor is an expert on the content and the type of tests that will be given in the class. Ask questions about what will be covered on a test and the type of questions you can expect. Office hours are designed to make your instructor available to you. Choose to get your money's worth and use them!

## Your Classmates

We all have different learning styles, strengths, and perspectives on the course material. Participating in a study group can be a valuable addition to your nursing school experience. These groups can be a fun way to learn. Teaching others helps us to learn and aids in organizing the course material. A study group is made up of students who are in the same class and who want to learn by discussing the course material. There are guidelines for organizing successful study groups.

1. Carefully **select members** for your group.
   - Choose students who have **abilities and motivation** similar to your own. Socializing and gossiping can eat up valuable study time. Noncommitted and underprepared classmates can be a drain.

- Look for students who have a **common time to meet.**
- Select classmates who have **different learning styles** from yours. They might understand the reading material or lecture material better than you. They may be able to draw a diagram that will help your learning.
- Find students who have good communication skills—people who know how to listen, ask good questions, and explain concepts.

2. Clarify the **group's purpose and expectations.**
   - Where and when will you meet?
   - How often will you meet? How long will the meetings be?
   - How much individual preparation between meetings is expected?
   - Can family members, children, or other students come to the meetings?
3. **Exchange names, phone numbers, addresses, and e-mail addresses.** Have a plan in case of emergencies.
4. **Plan an agenda** for each meeting.
   - Put the date and goal for the session on the top.
   - List the activities that will help you accomplish the goal.
   - At the end of the study session, list the results of your efforts and set the date and time for your next session.
   - Make assignments for the next session.

There are also some useful strategies to follow:

1. Exchange lecture notes and discuss content for clarity and completeness.
2. Divide up difficult reading material and develop a lesson to teach the information to each other.
3. Quiz each other by turning objectives at the beginning of each chapter into questions.
4. Use the Critical Thinking and Application and Case Study sections in this Study Guide as a basis for discussions.
5. Create and take your own practice tests. Discuss the results.
6. Develop flash cards that review key vocabulary terms.

This list could go on and on. Work with your group to design the strategy that works for you. Each study group you work with will be different.

Often in career programs like those in nursing, medical, and law schools, the course study group will turn into a learning group. **Learning groups may meet over several semesters even when the members are not taking the same classes.** Learning groups help you to prepare for licensing examinations, laboratory work, clinics, or practicum experiences. They focus on understanding and application in the field.

## CHOOSE TO DEVELOP YOUR VOCABULARY

Participating in study groups and learning groups is an asset when you are working to develop a new vocabulary. Every specialty or discipline has its own language that must be learned for full mastery to occur. When you learn vocabulary with a group, you can hear others using the terms and they start to become real to you. Courses such as this one on pharmacology contain extremely complex material, and terminology is a major component of that complexity. As you learn to integrate this vocabulary into your discussions of the discipline, it will seem less like a foreign language. In technologic, scientific, and medical areas, mastering the vocabulary can make the difference between being successful and struggling constantly to understand the ideas and concepts being presented. It is therefore helpful to adopt some strategies that can make the process of vocabulary development easier and more effective. Working with a study group is one strategy, but there are several more.

### Use Dictionaries

You must have a good current desk reference dictionary. *Current* means the most recent edition of whatever dictionary you choose. A dictionary published 10 or 15 years ago may contain most of what you need, but unless there have been periodic revisions, as shown on the copyright page, it is almost certain to lack some information, and this may cause you problems. A desk reference dictionary is a hard-bound dictionary and not a condensed or paperback version. Paperbacks are convenient to carry around, but to get the dictionary to this convenient size, some words have been omitted and some definitions have been shortened. This is not what you want. You need the most complete and current edition you can find and afford.

You may or may not need a medical dictionary. You will probably have access to one or more at your college or departmental library. The best way to decide whether you need to invest in such a specialized dictionary is to ask your instructor for his or her advice.

### Reference the Key Terms

As soon as you look at any of the chapters in this text, you will discover the key terms. This list contains the terms and definitions the authors consider essential for a full understanding of the material. The key terms will not necessarily contain every term that is unfamiliar to you. (This is why you need a good dictionary.) You can begin the process of mastering vocabulary by paying particular attention to the key terms.

### Create Flash Cards

Obtain a supply of note cards. Pick the size that best accommodates your handwriting style and size. If 5" × 7" cards do not fit into your notebook, purse, or book bag and this discourages you from carrying them around with you, then use 3" × 5" cards. Remember, the flash cards these become are one of the best things you can study on the run.

> Hypercholesterolemia, a condition in which greater-than-normal amounts of cholesterol..

## Use What You Know

When you encounter an unfamiliar word, do not automatically assume that you have no idea what it means. Use the knowledge you have already acquired in other nursing courses and throughout your life.

For instance, *psychotherapeutic* appears in the chapter title for Chapter 16. Your first reaction may be that you do not know what this term means. By using what you know, however, you may be able to make an educated guess as to the meaning of the word without consulting either the text glossary or a dictionary.

This is how you make that educated guess. Consider that the first part of the word is *psycho.* By this point in your career as a student, you know that *psycho* refers to the mind. This is a good start. Now consider the next part of the word. The meaning of *therapeutic* may or may not be evident to you, but it should remind you of a simpler word, *therapy,* which is the treatment used to cure or alleviate an illness or condition. Put *mind* and *treatment* together, and it would seem that *psychotherapeutic* must refer to the treatment of mental problems.

Note that this is an educated guess. It may not be a perfect definition, but it will give you a basis for acquiring a fuller understanding when the term is defined in the glossary or introduced and defined in the text of the chapter. A sentence in Chapter 16 confirms that this educated guess is very close to the actual meaning: "The treatment of mental disorders is called *psychotherapeutics.*" Using this approach to analyzing the meaning of a word not only confirms that you have a basic understanding of the word but also cultivates a mental link between what you know and the more specific definition provided in the text. Words and their meanings learned in this way are usually easier to grasp and easier to retain. Unfortunately, this technique will not work with some of the terms

used in pharmacology because they are so specialized and specific to the field. This calls for the use of other techniques.

## Learn the Standard Abbreviations

Make sure as you read that you pay attention to the "shorthand" used. For example, in Chapter 12, the abbreviation *CNS* is used repeatedly. The first time it is presented, the author identifies it as standing for *central nervous system* by putting the abbreviation in parentheses after the term. Thereafter, the abbreviation is used in lieu of the long term. The same thing is done for *REM* in this chapter. It is essential that you learn these abbreviations and recall each, not as a set of meaningless letters but as a key term that must be mastered.

### *Establish Relationships*

REM is an abbreviation for *rapid eye movement,* and this term refers to a particular stage of sleep. Chapter 12 deals with CNS depressants. Relating REM to the focus of this chapter will help you remember that CNS depressants are used to influence sleep. The idea is to establish a clear relationship between the terms used and the ideas presented. Words should not be learned in isolation from the material; otherwise, you may know a lot of words and their meanings but not be able to relate them to ideas and content. *On tests, you are not likely to be asked just to repeat memorized definitions.* Instead, you will be asked to integrate these meanings into your answers to questions about nursing practices and applications.

Another important way of relating words to meanings is to link the meanings of closely related terms. The words *hypnotic* and *sedative* are good examples of this. In looking at the meanings in the list of key terms, you will find that each refers to a certain class of drugs. Both classes of drugs influence the CNS, but the drugs in each have a somewhat different effect. It is useful to start with the understanding that both affect the CNS but then to appreciate how the terms relate to each other. Sedatives inhibit the CNS but do not cause sleep; hypnotics at low dosages have the same effect, but at higher dosages they may induce sleep. In this learning method, you learn meanings by looking at the general similarities and then at the specific differences between terms. In doing this, you have learned both words and should never have any problems relating the words to their meanings.

## CHOOSE TO TAKE EFFECTIVE LECTURE NOTES

## Why Take Notes?

The primary reason for taking notes is to help your memory. It is impossible to remember everything that is said during a 1- to 2-hour lecture. The very act of writing something down helps strengthen learning and memory. In addition, note-taking helps to focus attention on the lecture. It is very easy to take mental vacations during a lecture; note-taking helps keep you involved.

## Note-Taking Problems

1. **Selectivity** is the biggest challenge. How do you know what is really important?
2. **Unfamiliar vocabulary** causes confusion. This is particularly true in a course heavy in technical, medical, and pharmaceutical terminology such as this one.
3. Hard-to-read or even **illegible handwriting** is frustrating.
4. It is **difficult to listen and write at the same time.** It splits one's focus and often gets in the way of understanding.

## Note-Taking Solutions

1. Realize that note-takers are made, not born. You can learn to be more effective as both a note-taker and note-user, but **this requires some practice** and a willingness to adopt new techniques.
2. **Use the vocabulary development** strategies previously discussed so that you will have a better understanding of the lecture material.
3. **Note-taking is a five-stage process** that is spread out over the days and weeks between lectures and the time when you are reviewing your notes in preparation for a test.

### Stage 1: Be Prepared

Note-taking begins before the lecture. Read assigned material before class. This provides you with the background needed to listen intelligently to the lecture and to be selective when taking notes. You will have less unfamiliar vocabulary. The lecture will bring the textbook content to life for you.

Go to class a few minutes early and review your notes from the previous lecture. This will help warm up your brain so it will be ready to receive new information.

### Stage 2: Active Listening

Taking quality class notes requires active listening. This is one of the most challenging aspects of being a good note-taker. It requires an awareness of both the lecturer's language and his or her nonverbal style. You have to pay attention not only to what is said, the verbal aspect, but also to the visual, nonverbal, aspect of the presentation.

Active listening requires selectivity. If you spend the lecture time trying to write down every word, you will not be able to listen to and therefore grasp the ideas. Focus on the most important ideas, terms, and facts to be recorded for later review. Writing less and listening more is a good rule to follow for note-taking.

Learn to listen for key words and phrases. These vary with the subject content and with the individual lecturer, so there is no way to provide a single, definitive list of them. However, there are some verbal signals (words) that will give you clues that the lecturer is about to give important information:

- Sequence words—*first, second, next, then, last, finally*
- Contrast words—*but, however, on the other hand*
- Importance words—*significant, key, main, main point, most important*

The use of words and phrases such as these is the lecturer's way of signaling the relative importance and progression of certain facts and ideas. As important as these words are, however, it is also necessary to be aware of the volume, tone, and pace of delivery. Some instructors will slow down or repeat ideas that are important. Other instructors may speak louder and point into the air to emphasize a point. Get to know your instructor's style and you will be able to anticipate what will be on the test. Of course, if the instructor says, "One of the most important drugs in the treatment of …," then you should immediately know that what follows is an important point for your notes. The instructor has even told you it is important. As you practice active listening and observing in the lecture environment, you will find that your ability to discern the important ideas will improve.

Stages 1 and 2 are preparation for the real work that goes on in the last three stages.

### Stage 3: In-Class Note-Taking

The split-page note format requires a change in the way you set up your notepaper. In this method, each sheet is divided into two parts by drawing a line down the full length of the page to create a left-hand column that is 2½ to 3 inches in width and a right-hand column that is 5½ to 6 inches in width. The right-hand column should be used for taking class notes. (The function of the left-hand column will be explained in the description of Stages 4 and 5.)

There is no magic formula for note-taking. Simply take the best notes you can. Remember, notes are personal. Do not judge your notes against those of other classmates. Some will take a lot of notes, and others with a different background and expectations will take far fewer notes. The key point is to do what works for you. When what you are doing stops working, then try another strategy.

Here are some tips for taking effective lecture notes that may make the process easier and more effective for you:

- **Write in your own words** most of the time. Writing ideas in your own style will make them easier to learn and remember.
- **Leave space** between main points. When you sense that the lecturer has moved to a new idea, leave a couple of lines blank on your notepaper. That way, if the lecturer returns to this point later, you will have room to add further notes. Even if there is no need for additional notes, the blank lines will help you see the organization of the ideas and the relationship between them. This space can also be used to add information from the textbook.
- Indicate **direct cues** from the lecturer, such as "This will be on the test," "This is a difficult concept," or even "Know this." Put a star or a check in your notes so you will remember to study this information when preparing for the test.
- Be especially aware of the **visual presentation.** This consists of information written on the chalkboard or presented using an overhead projector, slide projector, PowerPoint display, or other electronic display. Many lecturers outline key points on the chalkboard as a means of staying focused on the points they want to cover. Use this information to help you stay equally focused. Electronic displays are often chosen because the ideas can best be understood when they are presented visually.
- The **repetition** of certain points is the single most useful tip that they are really important. When an idea, term, or fact is important, the lecturer will almost certainly repeat it. For instance, the lecturer will introduce a new term, define it, give a couple of examples to clarify the definition, and finally redefine the term. This repetition is a signal that it is very important for you to learn the information.
- Be alert for **questions directed to the class.** These questions are another way the speaker stresses important information and are also a way for him or her to find out how well the students have understood what has been said. Such questions are thus also cues that certain information is important.
- Be **actively involved** in what is going on in class. This means being willing to respond to a question directed to the class. It also means asking questions when things are not clear. Do not feel that because no-one else is asking questions, you are the only person who does not understand something. It is highly probable that there are others who are just as confused. Your objective in class is to understand the lecture and record key ideas in your notes so that you can study effectively. Questions are not dumb if they relate to the material being presented.

## Stage 4: Out-of-Class Reworking

The notes you take in class are only one part of the effective study of lecture material. Out-of-class reworking of these notes is critical, and this is where the left-hand column of your notepaper comes into use. Ideally, this reworking should be done immediately after the class ends, but this is not always possible. It must be done within 24 hours, however, to get full benefit from this strategy. Reworking class notes will not take more than 10 to 15 minutes to complete, but it will save you hours of study time later on.

The following is the recommended method for reworking your class notes:

- **Read over the class notes.** Look for major topics, key ideas, terms, and the organization pattern. At this point you are not trying to remember everything you got from the lecture. You are looking for places where your notes are incomplete or confusing. If you read your notes soon after the lecture, you will be able to clarify points or add missing material because most of what was said will still be fresh in your mind. If you wait until the next day (or worse, the next week), what is now only confusing will by then be a complete mystery. Taking the time to read your notes over soon after you take them will save much time and frustration later on.
- **Write topic heads for lecture segments** in the empty left-hand column of your notes. As you read your notes, identify the major topics that were discussed. For example, look at Chapter 11 in the text. The chapter title tells you that it is about general and local anesthetics, but the information does not stop there. Further topics are discussed and divided into subgroups. Headings are necessary to break down very complex material into understandable blocks. You should be doing the same thing with your notes. Limit your labels to three to five words. You are not trying to rewrite class notes but to make the organization of the ideas crystal-clear. Sometimes the notes

on the chalkboard or PowerPoint slide will provide the labels for you. Sometimes the labels will be included in a lesson outline furnished by the instructor. Often, however, you will have to compose your own labels. With practice you will develop this skill. Keep at it. These labels are an essential aspect of the final stage of this note-taking method.

- **List vocabulary.** The left-hand column is also a great place to put content-specific vocabulary. Look again at Chapter 11. Notice that there is a list of key terms for that chapter. This is provided so that you can immediately begin to focus on the content-specific vocabulary you will have to master for that chapter. You can create your own personal list of the terms used in the lecture. As you read over your notes, each time you encounter terms from the text or new terms introduced in the lecture, note the word in the left-hand column. Doing this will help you learn the needed vocabulary.
- **Expand.** Often during a lecture, you will only have time to write fragments of information. These may be meaningful at the time you write them but can be confusing later. Therefore, as you read your notes, fill in those places where there may be such gaps; otherwise, what was a small problem will become a big one later on. It will not take long, and it will pay off. You may use the left-hand column or the lines that you left blank for adding such information.

**Remember: The reworking must be done the same day as the lecture for it to be efficient and productive.** The longer the interval between the lecture and this reworking, the greater the likelihood of forgetting. When you read notes the same day as the lecture, you will be able to recall almost everything said. The reworking process will only take 10 minutes or so to complete, but it will pay off in a significantly improved set of class notes. Of equal importance is the fact that the reworking process is preparation for the final, critical stage in the note-taking process.

## Stage 5: Frequent, Active Review

Notes, no matter how good, need to be **studied early and often.** Learning and memory depend on rehearsal, or review, and this must be an active process. Rereading notes will improve your understanding and memory somewhat, but there is a technique you can use that will accomplish much more. This technique will help you to be an active learner and encourage frequent rehearsal. It is also efficient because it will only take you 10 to 15 minutes to completely review 2 or 3 days' worth of class notes.

**When to Review**   The first review of your notes should be performed within 2 days of the lecture. If the lecture has taken place on Monday, your review should occur on Tuesday or Wednesday. Do not wait more than 2 days. Studies have repeatedly shown that we forget nearly 50% of what we learn in the first 24 hours after we learn it. The reworking process will slow the forgetting process, but it will not stop it. The longer you wait to review your notes, the more time it will take and the more difficult it will be when you finally do it.

When to do a second, third, or any additional reviews depends on the success of the previous review. Review each day until you find that you remember and understand 80% or more of the material (you have to be the judge). When this is accomplished, the next review can wait for 3 or 4 days. If you find that after the first review you recall or understand only 70% of the material (an average amount), then the next review should occur within 2 or 3 days. If the amount you remember is less than 70%, you should review the material the next day. You must assess your own performance on each review to determine how soon to schedule another review. There are no hard and fast rules for this. A good review does not mean you have mastered the material forever, and what you remember clearly at one review may be the very thing you forget the next time around. **The only rule is to review frequently.** By doing this you will be well-prepared for quizzes, tests, or any other measure of your learning.

**How to Review**   To review your notes, **cover the right-hand column** (class notes) with a blank sheet of paper. Look at the topics, vocabulary, and further notes that you added to the left-hand column during the reworking process. These will serve as your study guide for review. Look at the first topic heading you have written. It might be something like "Hypnotics." Turn that heading into one or more questions. What are hypnotics? When are they used? What are the side effects? Are there patients for whom hypnotics are inappropriate? Ask these questions aloud; do not just think them. **Framing questions orally is what makes this review active.** Now that you have asked a question, the next step is obvious. Answer it without looking at the covered notes. Say the answer aloud. This oral question-and-answer process forces you to state the information in your own words and style. In addition, you are relying on more faculties in your learning than just the visual one of rereading. You are speaking and listening, which is more active than just looking at the words. **Recall is strongly enhanced when you express the information in your own words.**

Another benefit of this review process is that it **helps identify what you do not know.** If you ask a question and find yourself struggling to respond, then it will be clear that this is something you have not yet mastered. When this happens, uncover the class notes pertaining to that topic and read what is needed. Sometimes only three or four words will be needed to trigger recall. When this happens, immediately cover the notes and resume your oral response. Sometimes you will have to read a large portion of the notes to trigger your memory. The reading is now focused on material that you have clearly identified as unknown. This means that your review time will be much more productive. Instead of reading everything known and unknown, you will now be concentrating on reinforcing the known material and studying the unknown. **The best way to prepare for a test is to take a test.** By using the question-and-answer model, you are creating and taking your own test. You may discover that many of the questions you asked yourself also appear in some form on the classroom test covering that same material. If you have already answered the question several times for yourself, it will be easy to answer it on the test.

**Two-Page Split-Note Variation**   There is a variation of the split-page notepaper format that some students find works better for them. If you find that the 6-inch-wide right-hand column is too narrow for taking class notes, simply take your class notes on the right-hand page in your notebook and use the left-hand page for the reworking process. This allows more room for the charts, diagrams, or complex formulas that are often part of the lecture material in courses such as pharmacology. This two-page method will also allow you to incorporate text notes. To do this, divide the left-hand page into two columns of equal width. Use the right-hand column for the reworking of class notes and the left-hand column for text notes on the same topic.

**On-the-Run Action**   Record the information you find to be most difficult to remember on 3" × 5" cards and carry them with you in your pocket or purse. When you are waiting in traffic or for an appointment, just pull out the cards and review again. This "found" time may add points to your test scores that you have lost in the past.

## CHOOSE TO MASTER YOUR TEXTBOOKS

Many students find themselves falling asleep while reading their textbooks. Text material can be long, complex, sometimes confusing, and often highly technical. It can seem as though the more you read, the more there is to learn and the less you understand. Close the book and everything you have just read evaporates from your memory. If you feel like this, just remember—you are not alone. Every student feels this way. However, there are effective ways to maximize your learning and memory and maybe even reduce the time it takes to do this.

Many different study systems have been devised to aid in the mastery of textbook material, and each has worked for some students. The model presented here is a combination of the best elements of this multitude of systems and the best one for dealing with the subject matter in this pharmacology text.

Getting the most from a lecture requires active listening. The same active process applies to the reading of a textbook. Several techniques promote active reading. A good study system such as the PURR method presented in the textbook is one part of the process, but a good study system can be enhanced by reading with a pencil. Making text notations will help you concentrate and also make future review of the material more productive.

There are three notation systems:

- Highlighting-underlining
- Marginal notation
- Written text notes

Each of these notation systems has certain advantages and disadvantages. No single one will work perfectly all the time. Just as you must use different techniques to meet the different needs of your patients, you also need to use different techniques of text notation to meet the different needs you have as a learner. First, though, let's discuss two general guidelines that apply to the different systems of text notation.

## General Guidelines

1. **Read first.** Before you begin to make any text notations, you must first read the material. The objective of text notations is to identify the important ideas, facts, and terms just as this is the objective of listening during a lecture. If you attempt to mark text while reading it for the first time, everything will seem important and you will find yourself making far too many notations or highlighting far too much material.

2. **Be selective.** Be very selective. The objective of text notation is much like that of taking notes during a lecture—to pick out the important ideas for immediate learning and for future review. If you have ever looked at a used textbook, you are sure to have seen that the previous owner has highlighted nearly every line on some pages. Excessive marking means the reader was not discerning the important ideas

as he or she was reading. If you are taking separate handwritten notes, you should **limit what you write down** to the major headings and subheadings, important and unfamiliar vocabulary, and no more than two sentences of personal notes for each paragraph. The object is not to rewrite the chapter but to distill the important information. If you are highlighting, limit the material marked to no more than 20% to 25% of the total material. This is not to say that you must impose this limit on every paragraph, but it should be an overall goal.

## Text Notation Systems

### Text Conventions

As you read and prepare for making text notations, be aware of certain conventions used throughout the text. These help the reader focus on what the authors consider important. By now you have noticed the use of headings in this study tips chapter. Look back at some of them and you will also notice that they are styled differently— some are all capitals; others have only the first letter of each word capitalized. These represent main topics and subtopics. Now look at a chapter in your text. Examine the way headings and boldfacing draw your eyes to certain words, phrases, and portions of the page. These are text conventions provided by the authors to help you understand the organization of the material and the relationships within the text content. Other text conventions that you should note are numbered lists, bulleted lists, special display material, and the like.

### Language Conventions

Another important aspect of text notation is to become language-sensitive. In a class lecture, when you hear a professor say, for instance, "One of the most important anesthetics is…," the words *most important* are a direct cue that this is a significant point for your notes. The same type of cueing often occurs in the text. The authors want to make certain that their important ideas are communicated to you, the reader. Because the authors cannot speak to you face to face, however, they must rely on a certain written style to get important points across. This means that you must become aware of that style so that you can identify these important ideas. For example, in a sentence saying "The main use of opioids is to alleviate moderate to severe pain," the phrase *main use* is the author's way of telling you not only what is coming but also what you should be taking note of.

Pay attention if a paragraph begins with the phrase "The most significant effects…" Whenever an author uses words or phrases such as these, it tells you that something important is being discussed. When you highlight text, phrases such as *most important, main use,* and *most significant* are the cues you should look for to help iden-

tify the most important information. The combination of text conventions and language conventions helps make the reading and marking of text more successful.

### How to Highlight and Underline

Text marking is done to help in future review. This means that text marking is a personal process and should be used to point out only the most important information. The previous two sections on conventions gave you some concrete ideas on what to mark in your textbook. The main point is **read before you mark.**

It is essential that you read meaningful blocks of text before you do any marking. A meaningful block may be as little as a single paragraph but never less. It may be as much as an entire chapter. In a text such as *Pharmacology and the Nursing Process,* in which the material is highly technical and challenging, it is unlikely that you will want to read more than a section of the chapter at a time before going back to highlight.

Look at Chapter 12. The first paragraph mentions the boldfaced terms *sedatives* and *hypnotics.* As you read this paragraph the first time, do not mark anything. Instead **read for a general understanding of the content.** After this, go to the beginning of the section about Sleep and note the following language conventions: *two basic elements, different stages, summarized,* and *is known as.* These are all words and phrases that point out important information that should be highlighted. You may not actually need to highlight all of the information flagged by these words and phrases. Some of it is probably already familiar to you because of earlier courses you have taken or earlier chapters you have read in this text. Avoid highlighting information you have already mastered.

## Review

### When

How soon after you have done some form of text notation should you review what you have highlighted? Ideally review should begin within 24 to 48 hours after the initial learning has occurred. Psychologists have studied learning, memory, and forgetting and have found that we forget approximately 50% of what we learn after the first day or two. Therefore, the sooner you begin to review, the easier it is to move learning from short-term memory (quickly learned and quickly forgotten) to long-term memory.

### How

The process for reviewing any text notations follows the same general principles that apply to lecture notes. The intent is to make your review an active process in which real learning takes place. For example, if you have written questions in the text's margins, try to answer these questions without rereading the text. If you are able to answer the question to your satisfaction, then move on to the next question. If you have highlighted terms and definitions, cover the definition and try to define the term without looking at the text. If you are able to do this, you have effectively moved material into long-term memory. If you cannot define the term, then read the text definition. As you read, think about the meaning and think about strategies you might use to help you remember the term and definition the next time. You will find additional memory strategies in the later section on studying for exams. The key is always to focus on being an active learner.

### How Often

How often you review is a personal matter. The best way to judge is to be aware of your success, or lack of it, in the current review session. If you do very well at recalling information, then you can probably wait 3 to 4 days for the next review. If the review goes okay, then the next session should take place within 2 days. If you find yourself reviewing your own notations with little understanding and limited memory, then the next review should take place the following day. Each time you review, it will get easier and faster, and as you practice this approach to reviewing your text notations, you will gradually acquire a good sense of how often you need to review to maintain mastery of the material.

## CHOOSE TO PASS EXAMS

You can pass your exams by **applying the recommendations and strategies** offered in this section. Start by following the dozen basic rules of exam success.

## Rules for Success on Exams

1. Accept your anxiety as normal. Tests are important, both in the short-term, from the standpoint of grades and successful completion of this course, and also in the long-term, from the standpoint of completing the program and getting your degree and eventually the job you want. This fact can cause stress.

2. Reduce your stress by **studying often, not long.** The most important rule in preparing for exams is simple—spend at least 15 minutes every day (Saturdays, Sundays, and holidays included) in reviewing the "old" material. The more time you can find for this each day, the better, but spend at least 15 minutes. This one action will do more to reduce test anxiety than anything else you do. The more time you devote to reviewing past material learned, the more confident you will feel about your knowledge of the topic. This confidence will accompany you into the classroom on the exam day, and it will help you get the test score you want and of which you are capable. Just remember—**start the review process on the first day of the semester** and do some review every single day until the final exam.

3. Balance your review time between your lecture notes, textbook notes or highlighting, and any handouts you may have been given.

4. Ask your instructor about the exam. If he or she says the test is mostly on the lecture, then you may want to spend more time reviewing your class notes. Ask about the type of questions that will be on the exam. Will the test consist entirely of multiple-choice questions? Will it have true-or-false items? Will there be matching, short-answer, or essay questions? You should not study any differently for a multiple-choice exam than you should for a short-answer or essay exam. However, knowing the type or types of questions that will be on the test will help you develop a strategy for quizzing yourself.

5. Work with your study group to create practice tests. For example, if you know the test will consist of multiple-choice questions, then as you do your review, think of the kinds of questions you would ask if you were composing the test. Consider what would be a good question, what would be the right answer, and what would be other answers that would appear right but would in fact be incorrect.

6. Take the practice tests in each chapter and on the Evolve website for the text. Practice writing out the answers of short-answer or essay questions. **The best way to prepare for a test is to take one.**

7. **Study wisely, not hard.** Use the study strategies offered in this guide so you can save time and be able to get a good night's sleep the night before your exam. Cramming is not smart, and it is hard work that increases stress while reducing learning. When you cram, your mind is more likely to go blank during a test. When you cram, the information is in your short-term memory so you will need to relearn it before a comprehensive exam. Relearning takes more time. The stress caused by cramming may interfere with your sleep. Your brain needs sleep to function at its best.

8. Prepare for exams when and where you are most alert and able to concentrate. **Use your personal prime time,** which was discussed earlier in the time management section. If you are most alert at night, study at night. If you are most alert at 2 AM, study in the early morning hours. Study where you can focus your attention and avoid distractions. This may be in the library or in a quiet corner of your home. The key point is to keep on doing what is working for you. If you are distracted or falling asleep, you may want to change when and where you are studying.

9. **Relax the last hour before an exam.** Your brain needs some recovery time to function effectively.

10. Survey the test before you start answering the questions. Plan how to complete the exam in the time allowed. Read the directions carefully and answer the questions you know for sure first.

11. Before turning in the exam, make sure that you have answered all of the questions. If you are to fill in the boxes on an answer sheet that will be read electronically, be sure you have put only one answer per line and that you have answered each question. If you must make a correction, be sure to erase carefully and thoroughly.

12. Celebrate your success. Congratulate yourself for choosing to pass your exam by applying the exam preparation and exam-taking skills that have been proven to work.

## Strategies for Reviewing Class Notes

Look at your class notes. If you have been using the split-page model described earlier, you have made your own topic headings in the left-hand column beside the class notes. Cover the class notes and turn each heading into one or more questions. Think carefully about the answers and then answer aloud. By answering questions aloud, you are forcing yourself to think about what you know and organizing that knowledge in the way that is most meaningful to you. If you can answer your questions, then you have demonstrated that you know the material, and there is no immediate need to reread that section of notes. If you cannot answer one of your questions, then you know you need to review that material more intensively. Uncover the notes and read the pertinent ones. You are now using your review time effectively, because instead of just rereading everything, which invites boredom—or, worse yet, daydreaming—the rereading is directed at the material of which you are unsure. The result is more efficient use of your time and more effective learning.

## Strategies for Reviewing the Textbook

The technique you used for studying your class notes will also work for studying text material. As mentioned, in this book the authors have provided you with a variety of features that can help enormously. First, look at the objectives at the beginning of each chapter to be studied. Even if you have been assigned only small portions of the chapter, it is important to consider the objectives for the chapter as a whole. Ask yourself whether you have met these objectives. This is a quick way of assessing how much review may be necessary. If you feel confident that you have accomplished most of the objectives, then the review should go quickly. If you feel uncertain about many of them, then the review is going to take more time.

The next task is to consider the topic headings and language conventions. Use them in the same way as you have used the labels in your notes. Turn them into questions and answer these questions aloud. If you can answer them, then there is no need to reread. If you cannot, then you will need to reread the pertinent text.

Again, this way of reviewing is focusing your time and energy mostly where it is needed—on the material you have not yet mastered. Each time you review the text (or class notes), the sections of material you reread may differ. This is to be expected. You cannot remember everything forever, but if you spend time each day doing this type of review, you will remember more and for longer periods of time.

## Strategies for Reviewing Terminology

One aspect of nursing that can seem overwhelming is the terminology. It is highly technical and specialized. Learning it poses the same kind of challenge as learning a foreign language. In fact, it almost is a foreign language. However, for the concepts and ideas to be mastered, the terms must be mastered. One of the best ways to go about doing this is to use a technique you probably learned in grade school—flash cards. Put each term on one side of a 3" × 5" note card and the definition or other essential information about the term on the back. Group together cards containing terms that have common word elements (e.g., terms beginning with *cardio-*) or that concern common concepts (e.g., terms to do with renal function). The more relationships you can establish among words, the easier it will be to learn and remember them.

### *On-the-Run Action*

Get in the habit of carrying a deck of 10 to 15 of these cards with you. When you have a few minutes, review as many cards as time allows. Sometimes start with the term side of the card and try to recall what is written on the back. Other times look at the definition on the back of the card and try to recall the term. Do not focus exclusively on term-to-definition learning because you may be given definitions or some variation on the exam and be asked to provide the terms.

## Exam Time

This is it. The culmination of all your work—lectures, notes, flash cards, textbook reading, and handouts. **It is time to relax.** Test anxiety interferes with test performance. If you have put to use the learning techniques described in this chapter, you are ready for the exam. You have mastered the material, and you can do well on the exam. If you continue to experience test anxiety in spite of preparing thoroughly for the exam, it might be a good idea to visit a professional counselor on your campus.

Avoid cramming and remain confident in the learning techniques you have chosen to apply. This can usually control normal nervousness. Besides these learning techniques, however, techniques are also available for dealing with the various types of exam questions, and these are discussed in this section. None of these strategies can guarantee a 10-point jump in your test score. Only the degree to which you have mastered the material can make that sort of difference. However, each of the strategies described in this section may help you answer one or two questions correctly that you might otherwise have missed. **These test-taking strategies are not intended to replace regular study** and mastery; however, they are intended to enhance your test performance. If you use these strategies, you will see a positive gain in your test performance.

When the teacher passes out the exam, all your work and preparation are about to pay off, but do not just leap into the test. Take a couple of minutes to put yourself in a frame of mind for doing well on the test. At this point, you have a perfect test score—you have not answered any questions incorrectly yet. It is likely that you will get some answers wrong, but do not start out by making mistakes that cost you points that you should not have lost.

**First, look over the entire test.** Do not read it, but turn the pages and look at a question here and a question there. How many items are there on the test? Are all the questions of one type, or is there a mixture of types? Knowing in advance the length of the test and the types of questions helps you plan your strategy for taking the test.

**Second, read the directions.** This is the first opportunity you have to make a mistake that could cost points. Some directions for true-or-false questions may ask you to correct the statement and make it true. Others may ask you to justify your answer. When you respond with just a T or an F, you have lost important points because you did not read the directions.

**Third, create a plan to complete the test in the time allowed.** For example, if the test has 50 multiple-choice questions and the time limit is 40 minutes, then you know you will have to average a little better than one item per minute. Obviously you will need to allocate more time to essay questions if they are on the exam. Plan to glance at your watch or the classroom clock occasionally during the exam to make sure you are not losing time or going too quickly. Pace yourself. If you are answering questions quickly and are confident that the answers are right, do not worry about being ahead of schedule. If you spend too much time on individual questions, you may try to decide the answers to the last questions quickly, and this increases your chances of making errors. Planning a strategy for finishing the test within the time allowed helps you maintain a sharp focus on the task and enables you to do the best job possible.

**Fourth, start answering the questions.** If the test consists of only one type of question, then start with the first question. However, if the test has multiple-choice, true-or-false, and short-essay questions, for example, you must decide where it is best for you to start. If you find essay questions easy to do, then perhaps you should start with these. There is no reason you have to begin with the multiple-choice questions. On the other hand, if you find essay questions a challenge, then do not start with them. Begin the test in a way that will give you confidence.

## Tips for Answering the Questions

- Start with the first question or with those types of questions you feel most confident answering. Wherever you choose to start, there is a strategy you can use that can improve your test performance.
- Read the question carefully, and if you know the answer, indicate it and move on to the next question. If you cannot immediately think of the answer, give it a few seconds of thought. If the answer comes, indicate it and move on. If the answer still does not come or if the question is confusing, then skip to the next question.
- In the first pass through the exam, answer what you know and skip what you do not know. Answering the questions you are sure of increases your confidence and saves time. This is buying you time to devote to the questions with which you have more difficulty.
- Notice that the subjects of the questions on a particular exam are related, that the answers to questions you have skipped may be provided by other questions on the test, or that a later question may trigger recall of the correct answer. Skipping questions of which you are unsure offers one more opportunity to get the correct answer.
- After you have gone through the entire test completing the questions to which you are confident you know the answers, go back to the items you skipped. First check the time, however, so you know how much time you have left to answer these questions. On this second pass through the exam, you will often be surprised at how many questions you now can answer that drew a complete blank before.
- Answer every question. A question without an answer is the same as a wrong answer. *Go ahead and guess.* You have studied for the test and you know the material well. You are not making a random

guess based on no information. You are guessing based on what you have learned and your best assessment of the question.

■ When you have answered all the questions on a page, put a check in the upper right corner of this page. Avoid going back and second-guessing yourself. There is nothing worse than changing right answers to wrong ones. Have confidence in your own knowledge and let go of the test. If you are the first person to complete a test but are sure of what you did, then turn it in. At the same time, do not let what others in the class are doing affect your test strategy. If you are the last person to turn the test in, it does not mean you know less than those who were faster. It simply means that you are a careful, thoughtful test-taker.

## Strategies for Specific Types of Questions

For each type of question there are particular strategies you can use that can help prevent incorrect responses. Many times students miss questions not because of a lack of information but because of a poor strategy. Sometimes the error stems from misreading a question, for instance, overlooking a key word such as *not*, or from choosing an answer that does not quite fit the question asked. Errors like these can be costly. Expect to find some questions on a test to which you do not remember the answer or that are worded in a confusing way. A perfect test score is a great goal, but be realistic and accept the fact that perfect scores may be few and far between. At the same time, do not lose points because of careless and preventable errors.

### *Strategy for Multiple-Choice Questions*

Multiple-choice questions can be challenging, because students think that they will recognize the right answer when they see it or that the right answer will somehow stand out from the other choices. This is a dangerous misconception. The more carefully the question is constructed, the more each of the choices will seem like the correct response. The successful student can do several things to improve performance on multiple-choice questions.

Before the strategies for analyzing multiple-choice questions are discussed, it is important to understand each part of a question and its purpose. There are three parts to a multiple-choice question: stem, distractors, and the correct choice.

First, there is the **question stem.** This is the complete question that one or more of the response choices will answer.

EXAMPLE:
*If excessive amounts of water-soluble vitamins are ingested, what usually happens?*

Notice that this could just as easily be a short-answer question. In this case, the stem is a complete sentence that should be answered by one of the response choices. The stem can also be an incomplete statement that one or more of the response choices completes correctly.

EXAMPLE:
*The likelihood that a drug will have therapeutic effects increases dramatically when:*

This statement is incomplete, and you must pick out the response choice that best completes it.

The second part of multiple-choice questions is the **distractors.** These are the response choices that do not best answer or complete the stem. They are known as *distractors* because that is their purpose, to distract you from the best choice. Good distractors are usually very similar to the **best choice.** If you have not studied enough, a good distractor will be a very tempting choice, but you must reduce the allure of distractors.

The third and final part of all multiple-choice questions is the best choice. This is the choice you want to pick. Notice that it is the "best" choice. In many multiple-choice questions there may be more than one response choice that appears to answer the stem, and the differences between the responses may be slight. Your task is therefore to identify the option that **best** answers the stem, not necessarily the only right choice.

**Recall** The most reliable way to ensure that you select the correct response to a multiple-choice question is to recall it. Depend on your learning and memory to furnish the answer to the question. To do this, read the stem, and then *stop!* Do not look at the response options yet. Try to recall what you know and, based on this, what you would give as the answer. After you have taken a few seconds to do this, then look at all of the choices and select the one that most nearly matches the answer you recalled. It is important that you consider all the choices and not just choose the first option that seems to fit the answer you recall. Remember the distractors. Choice B may look okay, but choice D may be worded in a way that makes D a slightly better choice. If you do not weigh all the choices, you are not maximizing your chances of correctly answering each question.

Once you have decided on an answer, there is one more important step before you mark it. Look at the stem again. Does your choice answer the question that was asked? If the question stem asks "why," be sure the response you have chosen is a reason. If the question stem is singular, then be sure the option is singular, and the same for plural stems and plural responses. Many times, checking to make sure that the choice makes sense in relation to the stem will reveal the correct answer.

This is the most reliable technique to use for answering multiple-choice questions. If you do this for every multiple-choice question on the test, your accuracy rate will be very high, and you will not need any further strategy. Unfortunately, however, recall does not always work, and when it does not, there are some additional strategies you can apply to improve your chances of picking the correct answer.

**Recognition and Elimination**   Read each of the answer options carefully. Usually at least one of them will be clearly wrong. Eliminate this one from consideration. Now you have reduced the number of response choices by one and improved the odds. Continue to analyze the options. If you can eliminate one more choice in a four-option question, you have reduced the odds to 50/50, the same as the odds of correct random guessing for true-or-false questions. There are still some strategies that will help you pick the best choice. In addition, while you are eliminating the wrong choices, recall often occurs. One of the options may serve as a trigger that causes you to remember what a few seconds ago had seemed completely forgotten.

**Look-Alike Answers**   After you have eliminated one or more choices, you may discover that two of the options are very similar. This can be very helpful, because it may mean that one of these look-alike answers is the best choice and the other is a very good distractor. Test both of these options against the stem. Ask yourself which one completes the incomplete statement grammatically and which one answers the question more fully and completely. The option that best completes or answers the stem is the one you should choose. Here, too, pause for a few seconds, give your brain time to reflect, and recall may occur.

**Absolutes**   The presence of absolute words and phrases can also help you determine the correct answer to a multiple-choice item. If an answer choice contains an absolute (e.g., *none, never, must, cannot*), be very cautious. Remember that there are not many things in this world that are absolute, and in an area as complex as pharmacology, an absolute in an option may be reason to eliminate it from consideration as the best choice. This is

only a guideline and should not be taken to be true 100% of the time; however, it can help you reduce the number of choices.

All of these strategies can help you analyze the response choices so that you have the best possible chance of selecting the correct choice. When you are ready to mark the answer, keep in mind that the final step is always to test your response against the stem.

If, after you have tried all of these strategies, you find yourself still unable to choose a response, there is one final strategy. Ask the instructor for clarification of the question. There is nothing to lose by asking and everything to gain. The worst that can happen is that the instructor will tell you that he or she cannot answer your question. The best that can happen is that the instructor will rephrase the question in a way that resolves the problem for you.

When asking for such clarification, try to phrase your question in a way that encourages a response. Do not simply state that you do not understand the question. This is generally not the approach that invites an answer. If you are having trouble with a term in the stem or response choices, ask for a definition. If there is a phrase that is unclear or a response choice that is confusing, ask for clarification. Anything you do to make your question more specific increases the likelihood that the instructor will answer it.

After all other avenues have been exhausted, remember the final rule. **Never leave a question unanswered.** Even if answering is no more than an educated guess on your part, go ahead and mark an answer. You might be right, but if you leave it blank, you will certainly be wrong and lose precious points.

### Strategy for Short-Answer and Essay Questions

Notice that this strategy applies to both short-answer and essay questions. Both types of questions require careful thought and planning before you write an answer. It is helpful to get into the habit of regarding short-answer questions as short-essay questions. Too often students lose points on short-answer questions by being too brief. A short answer should usually consist of three or four sentences, but frequently students interpret "short answer" to mean four or five words.

Start answering these questions by analyzing the question carefully and then framing a response that will fully answer it. Assume that the reader—in this case, the course instructor—does not know anything and that you have to explain it all. Short-answer and essay questions require you to show what you know. Do not assume that the instructor can read your mind or read between the lines of your response to discern what you knew but did not include. It is better to have a little more than was needed in your answer than not enough. Extra information will not hurt, but missing information will always cost points. Once again, remember that the idea is to gain a point here and there throughout the test, which will result in a higher score and a better grade for the course.

## Two Key Issues

1. In writing answers to short-answer and essay questions, it is essential to answer exactly the question that is asked. This means that you must understand the question before you do any writing. Unlike with true-or-false and multiple-choice questions, which you should try to answer using every possible strategy before seeking help, with these questions you should ask for help before doing anything. The first opportunity you have to lose points in an essay question occurs with the first reading of the question. If you misread the question, you may write an excellent answer but not the right one. Such a mistake can be costly.

2. A good answer must be organized so that it is clear and logical to the reader. Do not read a question and start writing down whatever ideas spring to mind. Spend a minute or two thinking and planning the structure of the answer so that your ideas are clearly stated and the supporting details relate directly to each idea. Your instructor, the reader, will have a difficult time grading your essay if he or she has to read it two or three times to figure out what you were trying to say. Organization and clarity of expression really pay off in essay exams.

## Five Steps to Good Essay Answers

1. **Read the questions carefully.** As was discussed earlier, misreading the question can result in a high-quality answer that does not address the question asked. Read and think about the question's major focus. Do not jump on the first familiar phrase or term and start writing without further thought.

2. **Decide on an approach.** Telling you to read the question carefully is good advice, but without some strategy to apply to the reading it might be difficult advice to carry out. Here is a strategy to help you read carefully and begin to plan your answer. Look at the question as you read, and identify the words and phrases that tell you what to do. Some standard "what-to-do" words and phrases are used consistently in essay questions, such as *discuss, compare, contrast, explain, tell why,* and *analyze.* Circle each of these words or phrases as you read the question. The second part of the decision step is to underline what you are to write about. This circling and underlining will force a careful reading of the question and help you begin the process of organizing the answer. The sample question that follows is marked to show the circle and underline strategy.

SAMPLE QUESTION:

(Discuss) the <u>ways</u> in which <u>pediatric and elderly patients</u> are <u>alike</u> in <u>determining appropriate dosage</u>. (Explain) why <u>adult dosage</u> may be <u>inappropriate</u> and the <u>dangers</u> in <u>using adult dosage</u> in these special populations.

3. **Compile a brief written outline.** Before you start writing your answer, take a few minutes to organize the points you want to cover. This should not be an elaborate outline with Roman numerals, capital letters, and Arabic numbers, but rather a quick sketch of the question and the points you want to make in the answer. The circle-and-underline step described earlier will help make this easy to do.

SAMPLE OUTLINE[1]:

Discuss
- Pediatric and elderly patients' similarity with regard to drug dosage
  - Body weight factor
  - Organ function

Explain
- Reasons adult dosage inappropriate
  - Drugs not tested on pediatric and elderly population
- Dangers of adult dosage
  - Possible organ damage
  - Increased absorption and possible side effects

Sketching out an outline like this will organize your ideas, speed your writing, and ensure that you are answering the question asked.

4. **Write an answer.** With the question analyzed and a quick outline in place, it is time to put your answer on paper. The basic structure of an exam essay or answer to a short-answer question is the same as that for an in-class composition on an assigned topic. Every rule on which composition teachers insist for writing assignments should be followed in writing essay answers.

Any answer of more than four or five sentences should follow the basic three-part essay structure of introduction, body, and conclusion.

The **introduction** should be only one or two sentences long. It tells the reader what you are going to present in your answer. There is a relatively simple way to write an essay introduction. State the question positively and add a few words that show the main points you intend to make in your answer.

---

[1]This is a model of the process of the Decision and Outline Steps. It is not to be viewed as an accurate outline of pharmacologic content

SAMPLE INTRODUCTION:

*Pediatric and elderly patients have a number of similarities that must be considered in determining drug dosage. Two of the most important are body weight and organ function, and these factors can make adult dosages inappropriate for these two populations.*

These two sentences tell the reader exactly what you plan to discuss. From this point on, it becomes your task to explain why those two are important and how they affect drug dosage. You have told the reader what to expect, and you have begun to organize your answer.

The **body** is the most important part of any essay answer. In it you want to state the ideas, concepts, and points that you believe answer the question. These should be stated clearly and positively. Do not ramble on trying to cover all the possible variations that might fit into an answer. Decide on the most important, most significant points you have to make. Then state them and support and explain with relevant details that show how and why your points answer the question. For short-answer questions where three to five sentences are expected, drop the introduction and conclusion, and put all of your energy into a clear, concise body.

For the **conclusion,** there should be a concluding sentence or two to let the reader know that you have finished. Like the introduction, it should be brief and direct. Restate the question, and summarize the key points made in your answer.

SAMPLE CONCLUSION:

*It is evident that elderly and pediatric patients are very similar in their responses to drug dosages. Clearly the factors of body weight and organ function will play a major role in determining the appropriate dosages for these two groups.*

5. **Read the answer.** The writing has been completed. Before you turn in the paper, take another minute or two and read over what you have written. Look for errors that would make the reader pause, question what you have said, or be unable to read a word or phrase. Sometimes the mind works much faster than the pen, and a word or phrase is left out in writing. Use a caret (^) and insert the word or phrase where it belongs. If your writing got a little sloppy and a word is hard to read, cross it out and print it clearly right above. Proofreading and correcting small errors like these will make the answer easier to read and understand. Anything that contributes to the overall quality of an answer will influence the grade in a positive manner. You will not have time to rewrite an answer, but you should correct obvious errors.

## Strategy for True-or-False Questions

True-or-false items outwardly appear to be fairly simple. After all, the statement is either true or false. The odds of answering correctly are 50/50, and if all else fails, a coin toss can decide the issue. Appearances are deceiving, however, and true-or-false questions can be very challenging to answer. Good test strategy should be applied to answer all types of questions, because the object is to get the best score you can, and this represents the total points for all correct answers.

**Read the Question**  Reading the question may seem like such an obvious part of all test-taking strategies that it may appear absurd even to be told to do this. If you do not pay careful attention to the wording of true-or-false statements, however, then you are increasing the odds of making an otherwise avoidable error. Take the time to read and understand the statement. Read it all the way through to the end. Do not jump to conclusions based on half of the statement.

**Assume That the Statement Is True**  As you read each true-or-false statement, begin with the assumption that the statement is true. The idea behind this strategy is that it will cause you to read the statement carefully, which will result in your choosing the correct answer. This approach to reading the statement makes the reading an active process, because you are then reading to confirm the truth in the statement. You will be analyzing the statement as you read, looking for any information that would contradict or change the statement from true to false. You will also be choosing your answer as you read rather than waiting to the end to decide whether the statement was true or false. Obviously not every statement will be true, but this step makes you a much more thoughtful reader, and that encourages better test performance.

Remember one other important rule when analyzing true-or-false statements. **If any part of the statement is false, then the entire statement is false.** There may be only one altered word or prefix (such as *un-* or *anti-*) that changes a statement from true to false, but that is all that is required.

**Strategies for Analysis**  Sometimes, no matter how carefully you have read the question, the answer is not immediately obvious. When that happens, there are a number of strategies you can use to analyze the question. Using these strategies will not guarantee that you will get the correct answer, but they will often help you see something about the statement you might have overlooked and assist you in identifying the correct answer.

**Absolutes and Qualifiers**    Absolutes are words such as *none, never, all,* or *always.* These words mean that there are absolutely no exceptions to the statement. For instance, the statement "All birds fly" means just that. Every bird, past, present, and future, has flown or does fly. If there is or has been just one bird that has not flown or does not fly, then the statement is false. "All" in this statement is an absolute. True-or-false statements that contain such absolutes are usually false. In an area as complex as pharmacology, it is unlikely that there are many absolutes. If you are struggling with a question that has you stumped, look for absolute words. They may help you determine the answer.

On the other hand, there are words that suggest the possibility of exceptions. Such words or phrases are called *qualifiers*; examples of these are *some, possibly, in most cases,* and *will generally.* "Most birds can fly" is an example of a qualified statement. The word *most* tells you that some not precisely specified number of all birds can fly. This makes it more probable that the statement is true.

**Stated in the Negative**    A true-or-false statement that is rendered in the negative can be very difficult to answer. To draw on the earlier example, "It is not true that all birds can fly" is such a statement. The word *not* in this statement can make it much more complex to read and answer. There is a relatively simple way to deal with this type of statement. Read it as though the negative were not included, so that it becomes "It is true that all

birds can fly." This statement is clearly false. Because the word *not* reverses the meaning of the statement, this makes the statement "It is not true that all birds can fly" true. Simply put, if the statement is true without the negative, then it becomes false with the negative. Similarly, if it is false without the negative, then it is true with the negative.

**Strings**    A string is a true-or-false statement that requires careful attention. It is a statement that contains a list of several words or phrases, but often one or more of the words or phrases is false. It is easy to read the statement and see that the first two or three words or phrases are true but then to overlook the one that is incorrect, with the consequence that you mark the answer as true when it is actually false. An example of a string is "Many warm-weather crops, such as tomatoes, can be grown year-round in southern California, southern Florida, South America, and South Dakota." As you read this statement, it is easy to be lured by the words *southern* and *South* into thinking that the statement is true without noting the fact that South Dakota is a northern state with fairly harsh winters and that there are parts of South America where the climate is very cold. The statement is false, but the string can trick you into thinking that the statement is true.

These strategies for analyzing true-or-false items can help you increase the number of correct answers, but they are not intended to replace study and learning. The best way to perform well on any test is to know the answers based on your own learning. When the answer does not immediately come to mind, however, apply these strategies. Although they will not necessarily lead to a 10-point difference in your score, they may help you add 2 points to your score. Better scores mean better course grades, and of course, this results in improved self-confidence and improved chances of success.

## CONCLUSION
Remember: These study tips are only as valuable as you make them!

# CHAPTER 1

# The Nursing Process and Drug Therapy

## Chapter Review and NCLEX® Examination Preparation

**Select the best answer for each question.**

1. Which phase of the nursing process requires the nurse to establish a comprehensive baseline of data concerning a particular patient?
   a. Assessment
   b. Planning
   c. Implementation
   d. Evaluation

2. The nurse monitors the fulfillment of goals, and may revise them, during which phase of the nursing process?
   a. Assessment
   b. Planning
   c. Implementation
   d. Evaluation

3. The nurse prepares and administers prescribed medications during which phase of the nursing process?
   a. Assessment
   b. Planning
   c. Implementation
   d. Evaluation

4. When developing a plan of care, which nursing action ensures the goal statement is patient-centered?
   a. Considering family input
   b. Involving the patient
   c. Developing the goal first, and then sharing it with the patient
   d. Including the physician

5. The nurse includes which information as part of a complete medication profile? *(Select all that apply.)*
   a. Use of "street" drugs
   b. Current laboratory work
   c. History of surgeries
   d. Use of alcohol
   e. Use of herbal products
   f. Family history

6. During which phase of the nursing process does the nurse prioritize the nursing diagnoses?
   a. Assessment
   b. Planning
   c. Implementation
   d. Evaluation

7. The nurse is preparing to administer morning doses of medications to a patient and has just checked the patient's name on the identification band. The patient has stated his name. Which is the nurse's next appropriate action?
   a. Administer the medications.
   b. Ask the patient's wife to verify the patient's identity.
   c. Ask the patient to verify his date of birth.
   d. Check the chart for the patient's date of birth.

8. The nurse is administering a medication and the order reads: Give 250 mcg PO now. The tablets in the medication dispensing cabinet are in milligram strength. What is the right dose of the drug in milligrams? _____

9. The nurse is administering a medication and the order reads: Give 0.125 mg PO now. The tablets in the medication dispensing cabinet are in microgram strength. What is the right dose of the drug in micrograms? _____

10. Place the steps of the nursing process in order, with (1) being the first step and (5) being the last step.
    _____ a. Implementation
    _____ b. Planning
    _____ c. Evaluation
    _____ d. Assessment
    _____ e. Formulation of nursing diagnoses

# Critical Thinking and Application

**Answer the following questions on a separate sheet of paper.**

11. Below is a list of data gathered during an assessment of Ms. B., a young woman visiting an outpatient clinic with what she describes as "maybe an ulcer." Label each item as either objective data (O) or subjective data (S).

   _____ Ms. B. tells the nurse that she smokes a pack of cigarettes a day.

   _____ She is 5 feet 5 inches tall and weighs 135 pounds.

   _____ The nurse finds that Ms. B.'s pulse rate is 68 beats/min and her blood pressure is 128/72 mm Hg.

   _____ Her stool was tested for occult blood by a laboratory technician; the results were negative.

   _____ Ms. B. says that she does not experience nausea, but she reports pain and heartburn, especially after eating popcorn—something she and her husband have always done while watching TV before bedtime.

   _____ She experiences occasional increases in stomach pain, a "feeling of heat" in her abdomen and chest at night when she lies down, and increased incidents of heartburn.

12. Identify the "Six Rights" of drug administration and specify ways to ensure that each of these rights is addressed.

13. The following items will help in reviewing the nursing process:

Data are collected during the (a) _____ phase of the nursing process.

Data can be classified as (b) _____ or (c) _____.

To formulate the nursing diagnosis, the nurse must first (d) _____ the information collected.

The planning phase includes identification of (e) _____ and (f) _____.

The (g) _____ phase consists of carrying out the nursing care plan.

The (h) _____ phase is ongoing and includes monitoring the patient's response to medication and determining the status of goals.

14. During a busy night shift, the nurse notices a medication order that reads: "Give amoxicillin, 500 mg PO three times a day." What is the most important thing the nurse must check before giving this medication to the patient?

# Case Study

**Read the scenario and answer the following questions on a separate sheet of paper.**

A 75-year-old woman has been admitted to the hospital due to nausea and vomiting. She also has a diagnosis of hepatitis C. She says she stopped drinking 3 years ago but has had increasing problems with peripheral edema and shortness of breath and has had trouble getting out of bed or a chair by herself. Laboratory results show that her liver enzyme levels are slightly elevated; her sodium and potassium levels are decreased. Her blood pressure is 160/98 mm Hg, her pulse rate is 98 beats/min, and her respiratory rate is 24 breaths/min. She is afebrile and states that she is having slight abdominal pain.

1. From the brief facts given, what information will be important to consider when obtaining a medication profile?

2. From the nursing diagnoses in Box 1-3, choose at least two current and two "risk for" nursing diagnoses for this patient. How would you determine the priority of the nursing diagnoses?

3. The physician wrote the following drug order:

*November 4, 2013*

*Give Lasix now.*

             *Charles Simmons, MD*

| Patient's Name: Jane Dow    F    Age: 75 |
| Medical Record No: 1234567    Date of Birth: 1/16/38 |

What elements, if any, are missing from the medication order? What will you do next?

4. After the order is clarified, the pharmacy sends up furosemide (Lasix), 80-mg tablets, but the patient is unable to swallow them because of her nausea. Your colleague suggests giving the furosemide to her as an intravenous injection. What will you do next?

5. After the patient receives the dose of furosemide, what will you do?

CHAPTER 2

# Pharmacologic Principles

## Chapter Review and NCLEX® Examination Preparation

**Select the best answer for each question.**

1. Number the following drug forms in order of speed of dissolution and absorption, with (1) being the fastest and (5) being the slowest:
   _____ a. Capsules
   _____ b. Enteric-coated tablets
   _____ c. Elixirs
   _____ d. Powders
   _____ e. Orally disintegrating tablets

2. When considering the various routes of drug elimination, the nurse is aware that elimination occurs mainly by which routes?
   a. Renal tubules and skin
   b. Skin and lungs
   c. Bowel and renal tubules
   d. Lungs and gastrointestinal tract

3. The nurse is aware that excessive drug dosages, impaired metabolism, or inadequate excretion may result in which drug effect?
   a. Tolerance
   b. Cumulative effect
   c. Incompatibility
   d. Antagonistic effect

4. Drug half-life is defined as the amount of time required for 50% of a drug to:
   a. be absorbed by the body.
   b. reach a therapeutic level.
   c. exert a response.
   d. be removed by the body.

5. The nurse recognizes that drugs given by which route will be altered by the first-pass effect? *(Select all that apply.)*
   a. Oral
   b. Sublingual
   c. Subcutaneous
   d. Intravenous
   e. Rectal

6. If a drug binds with an enzyme and thereby prevents the enzyme from binding to its normal target cell, it will produce which effect?
   a. Receptor interaction
   b. Enzyme affinity
   c. Enzyme interaction
   d. Nonspecific interaction

7. The nurse is reviewing a list of a patient's medications, and notes that one of the drugs is known to have a low therapeutic index. Which statement accurately explains this concept?
   a. The difference between a therapeutic dose and toxic dose is large.
   b. The difference between a therapeutic dose and toxic dose is small.
   c. The dose needed to reach a therapeutic level is small.
   d. The drug has only a slight chance of being effective.

8. The nurse prepares to obtain a patient's blood sample from a central line for a drug level that is to be drawn just before that medication's next dose. What is the timing of this blood draw known as?
   a. Half-life
   b. Therapeutic level
   c. Peak level
   d. Trough level

9. A drug has a half-life of 4 hours. If at 0800 the drug level is measured as 200 mg/L, at what time would the drug level be 50 mg/L? _____

**Match each field of study with the corresponding job description of a person working in that field.**

10. _____ Pharmaceutics

11. _____ Pharmacokinetics

12. _____ Pharmacodynamics

13. _____ Pharmacogenomics

14. _____ Pharmacotherapeutics

15. _____ Pharmacognosy

16. _____ Toxicology

17. _____ Pharmacoeconomics

a. Lisa is researching botanical and zoologic sources of drugs to treat multiple sclerosis. She is part of a university research team that is currently experimenting with varying the biochemical composition and therapeutic effects of several possible new drugs.

b. Jeffrey works for a pharmaceutical corporation. One of its new drugs looks very promising, and Jeffrey's company is experimenting with dosage forms for this investigational new drug. He is responsible for measuring the relationship between the physiochemical properties of the dosage form and the clinical therapeutic response.

c. Micah is performing a cost-benefit analysis to compare the effectiveness of two blood pressure medications for a health insurance company.

d. Devon researches various poisons and is particularly concerned with the detection and treatment of the effects of drugs and other chemicals in certain mammals.

e. Diane and Phil have spent the last 3 years gathering family histories, legal case reports, and current clinical data to identify possible genetic factors that influence individuals' responses to meperidine and related drugs.

f. David works on a study that is gathering data on the use of two different drugs for the treatment of rheumatoid arthritis.

g. Leslie's laboratory monitors drug distribution rates between various body compartments, from absorption through excretion. Recently, her laboratory was able to suggest a positive change in the dosage regimen for an injectable drug, bringing her firm a prestigious award.

h. Gregory's research unit recently recommended two new contraindications for the use of a newly marketed drug after discovering previously unknown biochemical and physiologic interactions of this drug with another unrelated drug.

## Critical Thinking and Application

**Answer the following questions on a separate sheet of paper.**

18. Mr. C. is to receive a drug that can be given by injection, either intramuscularly or subcutaneously. Mr. C.'s condition dictates that the drug needs to be absorbed quickly. Which route of administration will the prescriber order? How can the nurse further increase absorption?

19. Ms. D. had a thyroidectomy four years ago, and has been taking the thyroid hormone levothyroxine (Synthroid) since the surgery. She visits her primary care provider for periodic labwork to check her hormone levels. This is an example of which type of drug therapy: acute, maintenance, supplemental, or palliative? Explain your answer.

20. E.S. has a prescription for an extended-release, enteric-coated tablet. The next day, his wife calls to ask about crushing the tablet. "He just cannot swallow that big pill." What is the nurse's best answer?

## Case Study

**Read the scenario and answer the following questions on a separate sheet of paper.**

A 65-year-old man with liver cirrhosis is admitted to the medical-surgical unit with nausea and vomiting. He also has a diagnosis of heart failure. You note that his serum albumin (protein) level is low. The physician has written admission orders, and you are trying to make the patient comfortable. He is to take nothing by mouth except for clear liquids. An intravenous infusion of dextrose 5% in water at 50 mL/hr has been ordered, and the nurses have had difficulty inserting his intravenous (IV) line.

1. One of the drugs ordered is known to reach a maximum level in the body of 200 mg/L and has a half-life of 2 hours. If this maximum level of 200 mg/L is reached at 4 PM, then what will the drug's level in the body be at 10 PM?

2. Describe how factors identified in the patient's history would affect the following:
   a. Absorption
   b. Distribution
   c. Metabolism
   d. Excretion

3. Placement of a peripherally inserted central catheter is ordered. The physician writes an order for a dose of an IVPB antibiotic to be given as soon as IV access is established. What is the reason for this order?

4. This patient is also receiving digoxin (Lanoxin) for heart failure. This drug is known to have a low therapeutic index. Explain this concept, and what will be done to monitor it.

# CHAPTER 3

# Lifespan Considerations

## Chapter Review and NCLEX® Examination Preparation

**Select the best answer for each question.**

1. Which physiologic factor is most responsible for the differences in the pharmacokinetic and pharmacodynamic behavior of drugs in neonates and adults?
   a. Infant's stature
   b. Infant's smaller weight
   c. Immaturity of neonatal organs
   d. Adult's longer exposure to toxins

2. A woman who has just discovered that she is pregnant is asking the nurse about taking medications. The nurse keeps in mind that the greatest risk for drug-induced developmental defects occurs during which trimester of pregnancy?
   a. First
   b. Second
   c. Third
   d. The risk is the same throughout pregnancy.

3. Most drug references provide recommended pediatric dosages based on which of the following?
   a. Total body water content
   b. Fat-to-lean mass ratio
   c. Height
   d. Body weight

4. The nurse recognizes that drug dosages in older adults are based on which factor(s)?
   a. More on age than on height or weight
   b. On body weight and organ function
   c. On the total body water content
   d. On the strength of the drug

5. When giving medications to older adults, the nurse will keep in mind the changes that occur due to aging. Which statements regarding changes in the older patient are true? *(Select all that apply.)*
   a. Fat content is increased.
   b. Gastric pH is less acidic because of reduced hydrochloric acid production.
   c. Protein albumin binding sites are reduced because of decreased serum protein.
   d. Total body water content increases as body composition changes.
   e. The absorptive surface area of the gastrointestinal tract is increased due to flattening and blunting of the villi.

6. A child is to receive a medication that is dosed as 8 mg/kg. The child weighs 40 kg. What is the dose of medication that the nurse will administer to this child? _____

7. A toddler is to receive a daily dose of digoxin (Lanoxin) 2 mcg/kg/day IV. The toddler weighs 23 pounds. Calculate the amount of medication in milligrams that the toddler will receive.

   _____

8. The medication in Question 7 is available in a vial of 0.1 mg/mL. Calculate how much solution the nurse will draw up into the syringe, and then mark the syringe with your answer. _____

**Match each pregnancy safety category with its corresponding description.**

9. _____ Category A

10. _____ Category B

11. _____ Category C

12. _____ Category D

13. _____ Category X

a. Possible fetal risk in humans is reported; however, consideration of potential benefit versus risk may, in selected cases, warrant use of these drugs in pregnant women.

b. Studies indicate no risk to animal fetuses; information for humans is not available.

c. Fetal abnormalities are reported, and positive evidence of fetal risk in humans is available from animal and/or human studies.

d. Studies indicate no risk to the human fetus.

e. Adverse effects are reported in animal fetuses; information for humans is not available.

## Critical Thinking and Application

**Answer the following questions on a separate sheet of paper.**

14. The nurse works at a community clinic frequented by a number of older patients. Mrs. M. comes to the clinic complaining of dizziness and nausea. As the nurse takes her medication history, she shows the nurse her "pill box." Inside the nurse sees almost a dozen different pills, all to be taken at noon. How could this happen? How could she possibly need so many medications at the same time?

15. The physician confirms that Mrs. M.'s "new symptoms," as she refers to them, are a result of polypharmacy. She protests, telling the nurse, "Honey, I've got news for the doctor. I've had to take lots of drugs at the same time all my life. It never bothered me before. Why would it now when I'm even more used to it?" Explain at least three physiologic changes that occur with aging and the way in which these changes affect pharmacokinetics and pharmacodynamics.

16. A 14-year-old girl has been diagnosed with type 1 diabetes mellitus, and the nurse is preparing to teach her how to test her own blood glucose levels with a glucometer. Describe some strategies that would be effective for this teaching session.

## Case Study

**Read the scenario and answer the following questions on a separate sheet of paper.**

You are performing telephone triage in a pediatric clinic. A mother calls about her 28-month-old toddler, who has had chickenpox for 2 days. She wants to give aspirin because the toddler's fever is 101° F (38.3° C) but is unsure because her toddler "hates to take pills."

1. Should the mother use aspirin for this fever? Refer to Chapter 44 as needed for developmental considerations for the use of aspirin.

2. The mother states that her husband is going to the drugstore for some medicine. What advice will you give her regarding the dosage form of an antipyretic for her toddler?

3. When the husband returns from the store, he shows the mother the bottle of generic acetaminophen liquid suspension formula for children that was recommended by the store's pharmacist. He wonders, though, why the pharmacist would need to know the toddler's weight before suggesting this medication. Explain.

4. The toddler receives a dose of 1 teaspoon per the directions for a child of his weight of 28 pounds. Later, when his 5-year-old sister needs a dose, she receives 1.5 teaspoons because she weighs 45 pounds. If the drug contains 160 mg per teaspoon, then how many milligrams of medication did the 5-year-old child receive in her dose?

5. What should the parents look for when evaluating the children's response to a dose of acetaminophen?

# CHAPTER 4

# Cultural, Legal, and Ethical Considerations

## Chapter Review and NCLEX® Examination Preparation

**Select the best answer for each question.**

1. When reviewing drug classifications, the nurse knows that drugs classified as category C-I, which are to be dispensed "only with an approved protocol," include which drugs?
   a. Codeine, cocaine, and meperidine (Demerol)
   b. Heroin, LSD, and marijuana
   c. Phenobarbital, chloral hydrate, and benzodiazepines
   d. Cough preparations and diarrhea-control drugs

2. When a health care provider is writing a prescription for a drug, he or she is not permitted to mark a refill on the prescription if the drug falls into which category?
   a. C-II
   b. C-III
   c. C-IV
   d. C-V

3. The nurse is aware that the ethical principle of "Do no harm" is known by which name?
   a. Autonomy
   b. Beneficence
   c. Confidentiality
   d. Nonmaleficence

4. Which legal act required drug manufacturers to establish the safety and efficacy of a new drug before its approval for use?
   a. Federal Food and Drugs Act of 1906
   b. Federal Food, Drug, and Cosmetic Act of 1938
   c. Kefauver-Harris Amendment of 1962
   d. Durham-Humphrey Amendment of 1951

5. Which is the correct definition for *placebo*?
   a. An investigational drug used in a new drug study
   b. An inert substance that is not a drug
   c. A legend drug that requires a prescription
   d. A substance that is not approved as a drug but is used as an herbal product

6. The nurse is performing an admission assessment. Which finding is considered part of the cultural assessment?
   a. The patient uses aspirin as needed for pain.
   b. The patient has a history of hypertension.
   c. The patient is allergic to shellfish.
   d. The patient does not eat pork products for religious reasons.

7. While reviewing a newsletter about medications, the nurse notices that one drug has a new black box warning from the Food and Drug Administration (FDA). What does this warning entail? *(Select all that apply.)*
   a. The drug is about to be recalled by the FDA.
   b. Serious adverse effects have been reported with the use of this drug.
   c. The drug can still be prescribed, but the warning is present to make sure that the prescriber is aware of the potential risks.
   d. The drug manufacturer has refused to recall the medication, despite documented problems.
   e. The drug cannot be prescribed.

8. The nurse is assessing an unresponsive patient when a visitor enters the room. The visitor asks, "Oh, what happened to him? He was fine yesterday!" Which is the most appropriate response from the nurse?
   a. "Sorry, but I am not allowed to tell you."
   b. "He had a stroke yesterday while in church, and there is little hope for him to recover."
   c. "You will need to speak to his physician about his condition."
   d. "Before I can give any information about him, I need to ask who you are. Let's go outside the room and talk."

9. The nurse is to administer ranitidine (Zantac) 150 mg IV. The available medication is ranitidine 25 mg/mL. How many milliliters will the nurse administer?

10. Mark the syringe with the amount of medication the nurse will draw up for Question 9.

**Match each investigational drug study phase with its corresponding description.**

11. _____ Phase I

12. _____ Phase II

13. _____ Phase III

14. _____ Phase IV

a. A study using small numbers of volunteers who have the disease or disorder that the drug is meant to diagnose or treat. Subjects are monitored for drug effectiveness and adverse effects.

b. Postmarketing studies conducted by drug companies to obtain further proof of the drug's therapeutic and adverse effects.

c. A study that involves a large number of patients at research centers designed to monitor for infrequent adverse effects and to identify any associated risks. Double-blind, placebo-controlled studies eliminate patient and researcher bias.

d. A study that uses small numbers of healthy volunteers, as opposed to volunteers with the target ailment, to determine dosage range and pharmacokinetics.

**Match each cultural group with its corresponding cultural practice.**

15. _____ Asian

16. _____ Hispanic

17. _____ Native American

18. _____ African American

a. Some may seek a balance between the body and mind through the use of "cold" remedies or foods for "hot" illnesses, and vice versa.

b. Some may use folk medicine, protective bracelets, and laying on of hands.

c. Some believe that opposing forces lead to illness or health, depending on which force is dominant in the individual and whether the forces are balanced. Balance produces healthy states.

d. Some believe in the need for a balance among body, mind, and environment to maintain health and harmony with nature.

## Critical Thinking and Application

**Answer the following questions on a separate sheet of paper.**

19. During morning report, a nurse has been asked to work on a transplant unit for the day. The nurse has personal objections to working on that unit for religious reasons. What is the best course of action for the nurse in this situation?

20. Identify a cultural group in the area in which you live, and explore the health belief practices for that group.
    a. Are there any barriers to adequate health care?
    b. What is the attitude toward Western medicines and health treatments?
    c. What questions should you ask in your cultural assessment?

## Case Study

**Read the scenario and answer the following questions on a separate sheet of paper.**

You work in an outpatient treatment clinic for patients with human immunodeficiency virus (HIV) infection. During a recent staff meeting, the medical director discussed a new drug that has shown good results in clinical trials in another country. This drug has not yet been tested in the United States. She stated that she hopes to start clinical trials of that drug in the HIV clinic.

The following week, you are asked to start a new drug regimen for four patients with HIV infection. One of the drugs is new to you, and when you ask about it, the medical director replies, "Oh, that's the new drug I mentioned last week! One of my colleagues in that country sent me some samples, so we're going to try it here. The Food and Drug Administration has already started trials here in the United States. We will be comparing how these four patients do compared with four other patients who are in the same stages of HIV infection. The patients won't even know about this change."

1. Should you give the drugs as requested? If not, what needs be done to correct the situation?

2. What ethical principle(s) guide your decision?

3. One of the potential study patients, brought in by his brother, seems reluctant to answer questions and says he "doesn't need any drugs." Upon further questioning, you find out that he would prefer to take some home remedies that his mother has made for him. How will you handle this situation?

4. When you meet with potential study patients, several mention that they fear others will find out about their illness if they participate in the study. What will you tell these patients?

# CHAPTER 5

# Medication Errors: Preventing and Responding

## Chapter Review and NCLEX® Examination Preparation

**Provide the best answer for each question.**

1. A(n) _____ is defined as any preventable adverse drug event that involves inappropriate medication use by a patient or health care professional. It may or may not cause harm to the patient.

2. A(n) _____ reaction is defined as any abnormal and unexpected response to a medication, other than an allergic reaction, that is peculiar to an individual patient.

3. A(n) _____ is an immunologic reaction resulting from an unusual sensitivity of a patient to a particular medication.

4. A(n) _____ is a type of adverse drug event that is defined as any unexpected, unintended, or excessive response to a medication given at therapeutic dosages.

5. A(n) _____ is an undesirable occurrence related to administration of or failure to administer a prescribed medication.

6. True or false: High-alert medications are involved in more errors than other drugs. Explain your answer.

7. True or false: All adverse drug events are caused by medication errors. Explain your answer.

8. Identify six ways to avoid medication errors.

9. Name at least four of the classes of medications that are considered "high-alert" drugs.

10. The National Coordinating Council for Medication Error Reporting and Prevention recommends that certain terms be written out in full instead of being abbreviated. Write out the full meaning of each abbreviated word or phrase that appears in bold in the following list.

| | |
|---|---|
| Digoxin 125 **mcg** PO now | |
| Lasix 40 mg IV **qd** | |
| **d/c** all meds | |
| NPH insulin 12 **u** subcut every morning before breakfast | |
| Floxin Otic 1 **gtt AD** bid | |
| Lactulose 30 mL PO **q.o.d.** | |

11. The medication order reads: "Metoprolol 25 mg PO twice a day for high blood pressure. Hold if systolic blood pressure is less than 95 mm Hg." Today the pharmacy supplied 50-mg tablets because there were no 25-mg tablets in stock.
    a. How many tablets will the nurse administer per dose? _____
    b. The nurse gives the patient the entire tablet. How many milligrams does the patient receive? _____
    c. What will the nurse do next? _____

12. The order reads: "Give levothyroxine (Synthroid) 50 mcg PO every morning." Which of these correctly depicts the dose in milligrams?
    a. .05 mg
    b. 0.05 mg
    c. 0.050 mg
    d. 50000 mg

13. The order reads: "Give furosemide 50 mg per gastrostomy tube every morning." The medication is available in liquid form, 10 mg/1 mL. Calculate how much medication the nurse will administer.

_____

14. Mark the medication cup with the answer you obtained for Question 13.

## Case Study

**Read the scenario and answer the following questions on a separate sheet of paper.**

A nursing student discovers that she has given her patient two aspirin tablets instead of the one-tablet daily dose that was ordered for antiplatelet effects. She is upset and talks to her fellow students, who tell her to keep quiet about it. "One extra aspirin won't hurt your patient," they tell her.

1. What should the nursing student do first? Describe other appropriate actions after this.

2. How could the student have prevented this error?

3. Should the patient be told about it? Explain your answer.

4. If the patient was not hurt by this incident, then is it considered a medication error? Explain.

5. The student has decided to inform her instructor. The instructor helps the student complete a hospital incident report, and a report to the U.S. Pharmacopeia Medication Errors Reporting Program (USPMERP). Explain the reason for this report. Will the student's name be reported to the USPMERP?

# CHAPTER 6

# Patient Education and Drug Therapy

## Chapter Review and NCLEX® Examination Preparation

**Select the best answer for each question.**

1.  A nurse is preparing for an education session on safe medication administration. Which is the best example of a learning activity that involves the cognitive domain?
    a.  Teaching a patient how to self-administer nasal spray
    b.  Teaching a patient how to measure the pulse before taking digoxin
    c.  Discussing which foods to avoid while taking oral anticoagulants
    d.  Teaching a family member how to give an injection

2.  The nurse is developing a discharge plan regarding a patient's medications. When is the most ideal time to begin discharge planning?
    a.  When family members are present
    b.  Just before the patient leaves the hospital
    c.  When the patient has been medicated for pain
    d.  As soon as possible when the patient is ready

3.  The nurse is providing discharge teaching for a patient who has a new colostomy following a partial colectomy. The patient is very upset and anxious because of the colostomy. Which statement about this level of anxiety is true?
    a.  It may be an obstacle to learning at this time.
    b.  It means that a family member needs to be taught instead of the patient.
    c.  It will have no effect on the patient's ability to learn.
    d.  It may result in the patient having an increased motivation to learn.

4.  A nurse has completed an education session on self-administration of insulin injections. Which statement(s) describe(s) successful learning in the affective domain? *(Select all that apply.)*
    a.  The patient states, "I am feeling more confident about insulin self-injection."
    b.  The patient states, "It is important to check my blood sugar before I take the insulin."
    c.  The patient states, "Insulin works to lower my blood sugar levels."
    d.  The patient measures the correct amount of insulin in the syringe for the injection.
    e.  The patient injects himself with insulin using the correct technique.

5.  A patient has been instructed to take 25 mg of diphenhydramine (Benadryl) oral syrup twice a day as treatment for a severe case of poison ivy. The medication comes in a bottle that contains 12.5 mg/5 mL. The nurse will be teaching the patient how to measure a dose of the medication. How many milliliters will the nurse measure for each dose?

    _____

6.  During a teaching session, the nurse demonstrates how to draw up insulin into a syringe. The patient then provides a return demonstration and draws up 17 units of insulin. Mark on the syringe the correct dose of 17 units.

## Critical Thinking and Application

**Answer the following questions on a separate sheet of paper.**

7. The nurse is to present information regarding antihypertensive drug therapy to two patients, a 40-year-old and a 78-year-old. Describe the differences in interventions the nurse would use in his or her teaching strategies related to possible alterations in thought processes and sensory-perceptual status in these two patients.

8. The nurse is to present information to a young mother on how to help her 8-year-old child use a metered-dose inhaler. Neither the mother nor her child speaks English. Discuss strategies the nurse will use in developing a teaching plan for them.

9. The patient has been taking oral hypoglycemics for 1 month, and her blood glucose readings are still very high. On assessment, the nurse discovers a possible reason for these high readings. Develop a nursing diagnosis for this patient based on the following:
   a. The patient says that no one has ever told her about required dietary restrictions.
   b. The patient tells the nurse that she only takes the medication if she feels ill.

10. Develop a measurable goal and specific outcome criteria related to teaching a patient about the medication therapy for transdermal nitroglycerin patches. Refer to Chapter 23 as needed.

11. Develop a patient teaching plan for a 55-year-old patient who will be receiving warfarin (Coumadin) therapy after discharge. Refer to Chapter 26 in the text for information. Include the following:
   a. Assessment—the objective and subjective data that would be needed
   b. Nursing diagnosis
   c. Planning—a measurable goal and outcome criteria
   d. Implementation—specific educational strategies
   e. Evaluation—means for validating that learning has occurred

## Case Study

**Read the scenario and answer the following questions on a separate sheet of paper.**

A 77-year-old male, accompanied by his wife, visits the office for a 3-month checkup. He has been treated for hypertension and has a history of angina. While in the office, he pulls a small bottle of sublingual nitroglycerin tablets from his pants pocket and states, "I never go anywhere without these." He says he "gets along okay" with his medicines at home and that it "doesn't hurt anything" if he misses a day or two of his medications. His blood pressure today is 130/92 mm Hg, pulse rate is 88 beats/min, and respiratory rate is 12 breaths/min. Previously, his blood pressure readings have been 160/98, 152/92, and 148/94 mm Hg.

After the patient is evaluated by the physician, new medication orders are written as follows:
- hydrochlorothiazide (HCTZ), 25-mg tablet, once a day
- potassium chloride (K-Dur), 20-mEq tablet, once a day
- diltiazem (Cardizem), 60-mg tablet, three times a day
- lansoprazole (Prevacid), 15-mg capsule, before breakfast and dinner
- nitroglycerin sublingual tablets, as needed for chest pain

1. Based on your assessment, what nursing diagnosis would you suggest for this situation?

2. State a goal and outcome criteria for your nursing diagnosis.

3. Describe the teaching strategies you would use when teaching this patient about how to take his medications correctly.

4. How would you evaluate the effectiveness of the education process in this situation?

# CHAPTER 7

# Over-the-Counter Drugs and Herbal and Dietary Supplements

## Critical Thinking Crossword

**Each statement refers to an herbal product that is described in this text. For reference, see the list of Safety: Herbal Therapies and Dietary Supplements boxes on the inside back cover of your text.**

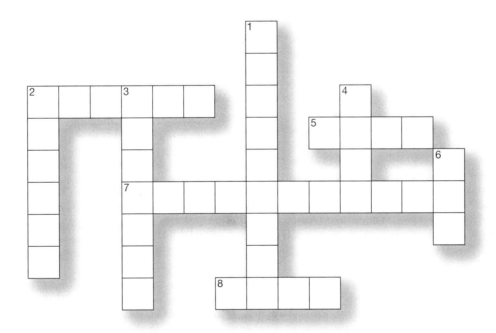

**Across**

2. Used for relief of nausea and vomiting induced by cancer chemotherapy, morning sickness, and motion sickness.
5. Both the seed and the oil of this plant are used to reduce high cholesterol levels.
7. Used to relieve the symptoms of benign prostatic hyperplasia (two words).
8. Used to help promote relaxation or sleep. However, prolonged use may cause yellow discoloration of nails and skin and a risk of liver toxicity.

**Down**

1. Used for its immunostimulant effect to reduce cold symptoms and recovery time when taken early in the illness.
2. The dried leaf of this plant is used by some to prevent organic brain syndrome.
3. Has been used for over 5000 years to improve physical endurance and concentration and reduce stress.
4. The topical application of this plant has been known for years to aid in wound healing.
6. Used by women for relief of menopause symptoms, as an alternative to hormonal therapy.

# Chapter Review and NCLEX® Examination Preparation

**Select the best answer for each question.**

1. Which drug classes are commonly used as over-the-counter (OTC) remedies? *(Select all that apply.)*
   a. Nonsteroidal antiinflammatory drugs
   b. Cold remedies
   c. Antibiotics
   d. Smoking deterrent systems
   e. Antihypertensive drugs
   f. Histamine 2 ($H_2$) blockers

2. The nurse is reviewing drug therapy with over-the-counter (OTC) medications. Which is an advantage of OTC remedies?
   a. Third-party health insurance payers usually cover the costs.
   b. Patients can feel better faster when self-medicating.
   c. There are fewer drug interactions.
   d. Patients can self-treat minor ailments and reduce physician visits.

3. A patient is discussing his wish to use herbal products instead of medications and exclaims, "They work! The government tests them!" How will the nurse respond?
   a. "The U.S. Food and Drug Administration enforces standards of herbal product quality and safety."
   b. "The U.S. Food and Drug Administration requires the manufacturers of herbal products to prove that the herbals are effective."
   c. "The U.S. government sets standards for quality control of herbal products."
   d. "In the U.S., herbal products are classified as dietary supplements and do not undergo testing for effectiveness."

4. A patient is asking about taking omega-3 fatty acids to reduce his cholesterol levels because he has a family history of coronary artery disease. Which nursing diagnosis is most appropriate for this patient?
   a. Noncompliance
   b. Readiness for enhanced self-health management
   c. Decreased cardiac output
   d. Risk for constipation

5. The nurse is admitting a patient who has a diagnosis of right lower lobe pneumonia. Upon assessment, the nurse learns that the patient is wearing an herbal pack on her chest. What will the nurse do first?
   a. Remove the pack immediately.
   b. Report the pack to the physician.
   c. Ask the patient about the herbal pack.
   d. Document the presence of the herbal pack.

6. A construction worker is treating himself with acetaminophen after an injury on the job. After 2 days, he comes to the urgent care facility because he thinks his hand is broken. He tells the nurse that he has been taking two "extra-strength" acetaminophen tablets six times a day but he still has pain. Each tablet is 500 mg. How many milligrams per day has he taken? _____

7. Is there a concern regarding the construction worker's acetaminophen intake (see Question 6)? Explain your answer. _____

8. A patient is taking paroxetine (Paxil), a selective serotonin reuptake inhibitor (SSRI), as part of treatment for depression. The patient tells the nurse that he has taken herbal products in the past and shows a list to the nurse. Which herbal product, if taken by the patient who is taking an SSRI, would cause an interaction?
   a. Garlic
   b. Echinacea
   c. St. John's wort
   d. Saw palmetto

9. During a clinic visit for a yearly examination, a patient asks the nurse about medications to take for heartburn. The patient shows the nurse the medication bottles that she had in her medicine cabinet. Which of these would be appropriate to use for the patient's heartburn, after checking for contraindications and other drug interactions? *(Select all that apply.)*
   a. chlorpheniramine maleate (Chlor-Trimeton)
   b. famotidine (Pepcid AC)
   c. clotrimazole (Lotrimin)
   d. orlistat (Allī)
   e. omeprazole (Prilosec OTC)

## Critical Thinking and Application

**Answer the following questions on a separate sheet of paper.**

10. Review the Safety: Herbal Therapies and Dietary Supplements boxes for garlic, ginger, ginseng, flax, saw palmetto, ginkgo, and valerian in the appropriate chapters. (To help you locate these boxes, see the list inside the back cover of your textbook.) Which of these herbal products may have serious interactions with anticoagulants such as warfarin (Coumadin) and heparin?

11. List the types of individuals who may have more frequent adverse reactions to OTC drugs.

12. A patient tells the nurse that he has had diarrhea for over 3 weeks and has been self-treating it at home with over-the-counter (OTC) drugs. "I thought it was something that I ate and that it would go away, but it didn't," he says. He states he feels tired and weak, and the nurse notes that he shows some signs of dehydration. What concerns are there, if any, with this patient's self-treatment with OTC medications?

13. Identify an OTC product or herbal or dietary supplement that you (or a family member) take and review the indications, drug interactions, contraindications, and adverse effects. Did you find any concerns?

## Case Study

**Read the scenario and answer the following questions on a separate sheet of paper. You may need to refer to the list of Safety: Herbal Therapies and Dietary Supplements boxes on the inside back cover of your textbook.**

A 30-year-old woman is in the clinic for her yearly gynecologic checkup. She is not pregnant but would like to have children soon and states that she and her husband are trying to conceive. She says that she is "very concerned" about her health, and watches her diet and exercises regularly to stay in shape. She has a family history of heart disease but no other health concerns. Her physical assessment reveals no abnormalities or health problems.

On her medical history sheet, she writes that she takes several drug and herbal products as follows:

- Echinacea, from September to March, to prevent the flu
- Adult aspirin, one tablet every day, to prevent a heart attack
- Garlic tablets twice a day for her heart
- Kava tea, as needed for relaxation
- One glass of red wine with dinner
- Valerian capsules for sleep, as needed (usually three or four times a week)

1. Does the patient's regimen of drugs and herbal products pose any risk for drug or herbal interactions?

2. Do any of these products have a potential for problems if used long-term?

3. Will you focus on any specific information when taking the patient's history or performing an assessment, given that she is using these drugs and herbal products?

4. She tells you that she thinks the herbal products are "safe" because the government would not allow them to be sold if they were not. Is this true?

5. What would you emphasize when teaching her about the use of herbal products and OTC drugs?

# CHAPTER 8

# Gene Therapy and Pharmacogenomics

## Chapter Review and NCLEX® Examination Preparation

**Match each definition with its corresponding term. (Note: Not all terms will be used.)**

1. _____ A structure in the nucleus that contains a thread of DNA which transmits genetic information

2. _____ A term for all of the chromosomal material within a cell

3. _____ The biologic unit of heredity

4. _____ The complete set of genetic material of any organism

5. _____ The study of genomes, including the way genes and their products work in both health and disease

a. Allele
b. Gene
c. Genome
d. Genomics
e. Genetics
f. Chromatin
g. Chromosome

**Select the best answer for each question.**

6. The nurse is reviewing concepts of gene therapy. Which statements correctly describe a possible approach to gene therapy? *(Select all that apply.)*
   a. Replacing a mutated gene with a healthy copy of the gene
   b. Preventing an immature gene from growing into a mature gene
   c. Inactivating a mutated gene that is functioning improperly
   d. Introducing a new gene into the body to help fight a disease
   e. Causing the body to produce new genes

7. The nurse is explaining concepts of ethical issues related to gene therapy in the United States. Which statement is correct?
   a. The U.S. Food and Drug Administration approves all human clinical gene therapy trials.
   b. Gene therapy research poses little risk to the subjects who participate in studies.
   c. Eugenics is currently part of gene therapy research in the United States.
   d. Gene therapy is exempt from approval by an institutional review board.

## Critical Thinking and Application

**Answer the following questions on a separate sheet of paper.**

8. Describe the concept of eugenics as related to gene therapy in the United States.

9. What is recombinant DNA? Give an example of how this technology is useful in pharmacology.

10. A patient asks the nurse, "I read something about gene therapy. Has it been approved in the United States for routine treatment of disease?" How will the nurse answer the patient?

11. During a health history interview before a scheduled surgery, a patient tells the nurse, "Everyone in my family has had a bad reaction to pain medicines. Do you think I will also?" What is the most important action for the nurse at this time? How will the nurse answer this patient?

12. A patient's sister is visiting the patient, who is recovering from breast cancer surgery. As the sister leaves, she takes the nurse aside and asks, "I need to know something. I know they did genetic testing. Does she have the type of breast cancer that is genetic?" How will the nurse answer the patient's sister? Explain your answer.

## Case Study

**Read the scenario and answer the following questions on a separate sheet of paper.**

Dale, a 32-year-old construction worker, fell off a roof 2 months ago and, as a result, needs to have surgery on his ankle. The nurse is preparing him for the surgery and begins the admission process. During the interview, Dale mentions that he is a bit nervous because his cousin had surgery and had a "terrible reaction" to the medications.

1. Is this information about his cousin significant? Explain.

2. What further questions will the nurse ask?

3. When obtaining a genetic history, how many generations back should the nurse ask about?

4. What will be done about Dale's surgery?

# CHAPTER 9

# Photo Atlas of Drug Administration

## Chapter Review and NCLEX® Examination Preparation

**Select the best answer for each question.**

1. The nurse is preparing to give an intradermal injection, and will perform which action?
   a. Massage the site lightly after the injection.
   b. Have the patient massage the site until the pain diminishes.
   c. Avoid massaging the site.
   d. Apply heat to the site after the injection.

2. When giving a medication via intravenous push, how will the nurse correctly occlude the intravenous line?
   a. By pinching or clamping the tubing just above the injection port
   b. By pinching the tubing at least 2 inches above the injection port
   c. By folding the tubing just below the injection port
   d. It is not necessary to occlude the tubing for this procedure.

3. The nurse is adding more than one medication to a solution. What action is most important at this time?
   a. Use an equal volume of each medication.
   b. Assess the two drugs for compatibility.
   c. Add the drugs at least 1 hour apart.
   d. Use the same needle for both medications.

4. When administering oral medications, the nurse will follow which correct procedure?
   a. If a patient cannot swallow medications, crush all the medications together and administer with applesauce.
   b. Give oral medications with meals to avoid gastrointestinal upset.
   c. Stay with the patient until each medication has been swallowed.
   d. Give all medications on an empty stomach to facilitate absorption.

5. After administering eardrops, which action by the nurse is correct?
   a. Press a cotton ball firmly into the ear canal.
   b. Have the patient sit up and tilt the head for 2 to 3 minutes.
   c. Gently massage the tragus of the ear.
   d. Have the patient remain in the side-lying position for 20 minutes.

6. Which position is correct when the nurse administers nasal drops for the frontal or maxillary sinuses?
   a. Tilt the patient's head backward and facing toward the left side.
   b. Tilt the patient's head back over the edge of the bed with the head turned toward the side treated.
   c. Place a pillow under the patient's shoulders and tilt the head back.
   d. Tilt the patient's head to the side opposite the side treated.

7. Which action by the nurse is most correct when administering drugs via a nasogastric tube?
   a. Allow the fluid to flow via gravity.
   b. Use gentle but consistent pressure when forcing the fluid into the tube.
   c. Shake the tube gently to facilitate the movement of fluid in the tube.
   d. Confirm placement of the tube after the medication is given.

8. The nurse is preparing to give a Z-track intramuscular injection. This technique is indicated in which situation?
   a. When there is insufficient muscle mass in the landmarked area
   b. Whenever massaging the area after medication administration is contraindicated
   c. With medications that are known to be irritating, painful, and/or staining to tissues
   d. With any injection that is given into the dorsogluteal muscle

9. When giving sublingual medications, the nurse recalls that medications given by this route have which advantage?
   a. They are immediately absorbed.
   b. They are excreted rapidly.
   c. They are metabolized immediately.
   d. They are distributed equally.

10. The prochlorperazine (Compazine) rectal suppository is twice the strength of what has actually been ordered. Which is the nurse's best action?
   a. Cut the suppository in half.
   b. Call the physician for clarification.
   c. Administer another type of suppository.
   d. Instruct the patient to retain the suppository for only 5 minutes.

11. During medication administration, which will the nurse consider to be a contraindication to the administration of rectal suppositories?
   a. Vomiting
   b. Fever
   c. Constipation
   d. Rectal bleeding

12. The nurse will apply a transdermal patch to a site that is:
   a. over a bone.
   b. nonhairy.
   c. moist.
   d. within a skinfold.

13. What is important for the nurse to teach the patient about the instillation of nasal drops?
   a. Clear the nasal passages by blowing the nose gently before administering the medication.
   b. Clear the nasal passages by blowing the nose gently after administering the medication.
   c. Sit in a semi-Fowler's position for 5 minutes after the instillation of the medication.
   d. Place the nose dropper approximately ½ inch into the nostril when instilling drops.

14. Which interventions are correct regarding the administration of ophthalmic medications? *(Select all that apply.)*
   a. Have the patient look upward while instilling the medication.
   b. Instill the prescribed number of drops into the conjunctival sac.
   c. Have the patient close his or her eyes tightly after the drop has been instilled.
   d. Apply gentle pressure to the patient's nasolacrimal duct for 30 to 60 seconds after instilling the drops.
   e. Apply ointment to the conjunctival sac starting at the outer canthus and working toward the inner canthus.

15. When withdrawing insulin from a vial, the nurse needs to remove 14 units for the medication dosage. How much air will the nurse inject into the vial before removing the medication? Mark the syringe with your answer.

16. A 2-month-old needs to receive pain medication after surgery. The order reads: "Give morphine sulfate, 0.05 mg/kg IV now." The infant weighs 10.5 pounds. Calculate the number of milligrams the infant will receive. Round to hundredths. _____

17. Referring to your answer for Question 16, calculate how many milliliters of medication the nurse will draw up, and indicate the amount on the syringe below. The medication comes in a vial of 0.5 mg/mL. _____

## Critical Thinking and Application

**Answer the following questions on a separate sheet of paper.**

18. Describe how to assess injection sites for each of the following:
    a. Subcutaneous injections
    b. Intramuscular injections
    c. Intradermal injections

19. Describe the proper technique of needle insertion for each of the following:
    a. Subcutaneous injections
    b. Intramuscular injections
    c. Intradermal injections

20. You are administering an intramuscular injection to your patient. After the needle enters the site, you grasp the lower end of the syringe barrel with your nondominant hand and slowly pull back on the plunger to aspirate the drug. Blood appears in the syringe. What is the best action at this time?

21. You are preparing an oral liquid medication for a patient. How does the usual procedure change when the volume of medication required is less than 5 mL?

22. A patient has been given a new inhaler that contains 100 doses of medication. The order specifies that the patient is to take "one puff four times a day." How many days will this inhaler last before it becomes empty?

## Case Study

**Read the scenario and answer the following questions on a separate sheet of paper.**

A mother comes to a family practice office with her 2-year-old daughter and 8-month-old son. She is planning a trip abroad and needs to obtain immunizations for herself and her children before she leaves.

1. The mother and the infant each need to be given an intramuscular immunization. Describe the differences in choosing sites and giving an intramuscular injection to the mother and the infant.

2. The 2-year-old daughter has an ear infection and the physician has prescribed eardrops. What will you teach the mother about giving these eardrops to her daughter?

3. Two days later, the mother brings the infant back to the office because he has developed a high fever. You prepare to give the infant a liquid oral antipyretic and note that the dose is 2 mL. How do you measure this medication?

4. The mother wants to add the medication to the baby's bottle. What is the best method for administering the liquid medication to the infant?

# CHAPTER 10

# Analgesic Drugs

## Critical Thinking Crossword

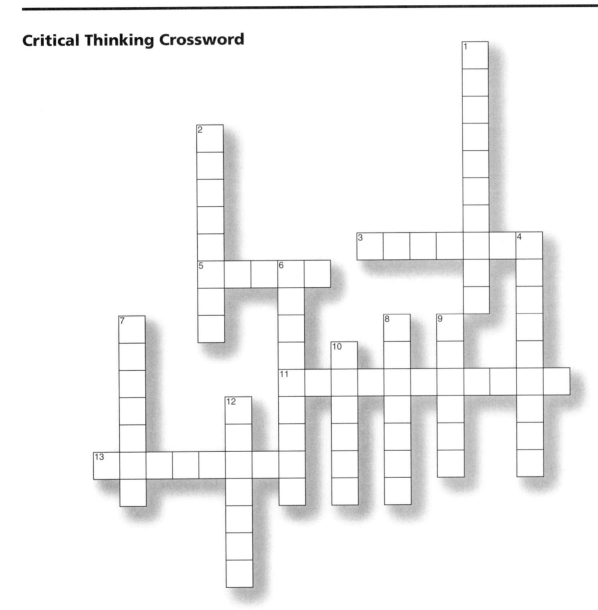

**Across**

3. Any drug that binds to a receptor and causes a response has _____ properties.
5. Mrs. M. had breast reduction surgery yesterday and is complaining of pain around her incisions. Mrs. M. is experiencing _____ pain.
11. Mrs. G. is experiencing pain and itching due to a severe case of poison ivy on the skin of her arms and legs. She is experiencing _____ pain.
13. Mr. E. paces the floor all night, holding his side. The pain is so severe that he is nauseated. His wife brings him to the emergency department, where it is quickly discovered that Mr. E. has a kidney stone. The type of pain he has been experiencing is _____ pain.

**Down**

1. Mr. D.'s drug binds to a receptor, but the drug prevents, or blocks, a response. He is taking a drug with _____ properties.
2. When a second drug is given with a primary analgesic to enhance the analgesic effect, the second drug is being used as a(n) _____ drug.
4. Mr. P. is receiving an opioid around the clock for late-stage cancer pain. Lately, he has found that the pain medication is not working as well as it did a week ago. This is an example of opioid _____.
6. The level of stimulus needed to produce a painful sensation is referred to as the *pain* _____.
7. Mr. J. twisted his ankle in a friendly basketball game with his peers after work. His wife brings him to the urgent care center several hours later because of the pain. Mr. J. is probably experiencing _____ pain.
8. Mrs. H. has experienced back pain "for years." She says that it is worse in the late afternoon and at night but that "really, even when it lessens somewhat, it is there all the time in some form." Mrs. H. is experiencing _____ pain.
9. Mr. R. is brought to the emergency department in severe pain. The emergency department team recognizes the need to immediately bring the pain under some control. After assessing that it is not contraindicated, the attending physician initiates administration of a very strong pain reliever. This is no doubt a(n) _____ analgesic.
10. This word is often used interchangeably with the term *opioid*.
12. Ms. T. is taking a drug that binds to part of a receptor and causes effects that are not as strong as those of a pure agonist. She is taking a(n) _____ agonist.

## Chapter Review and NCLEX® Examination Preparation

**Select the best answer for each question.**

1. During a marathon, a runner had to drop out after 16 miles because of severe muscle spasms. Which type of pain is the runner experiencing?
   a. Chronic pain
   b. Somatic pain
   c. Visceral pain
   d. Superficial pain

2. A young man has been taken to the emergency department because of a suspected overdose of morphine tablets. The nurse prepares to administer which drug?
   a. atropine
   b. meperedine (Demerol)
   c. flumazenil (Romazicon)
   d. naloxone (Narcan)

3. An anticonvulsant drug has been ordered as part of a patient's pain management program. The nurse explains to the patient that the purpose of the anticonvulsant is to:
   a. produce sleep.
   b. prevent seizures.
   c. relieve neuropathic pain.
   d. reduce anxiety.

4. Moderate to severe pain is best treated with which of these medications?
   a. acetaminophen (Tylenol)
   b. naloxone (Narcan)
   c. alprazolam (Xanax)
   d. fentanyl (Duragesic)

5. The nurse is preparing to administer an opioid analgesic. Which factors should be assessed before the dose is given? *(Select all that apply.)*
   a. Blood clotting times
   b. The level of pain rated on a scale
   c. Prior analgesic use (time, type, amount, and effectiveness)
   d. Dietary history
   e. Allergies

6. A patient visits the clinic, complaining of severe knee pain. He states that he twisted his knee last week and has been self-medicating with an old prescription of Percocet and extra-strength acetaminophen (Tylenol). He tells the nurse that he takes "two of the Tylenols four times a day, and two Percocets twice a day." The Percocet contains acetaminophen 325 mg and oxycodone 5 mg; the extra-strength acetaminophen contains 500 mg per tablet. How much acetaminophen has he taken per day, and is this a concern? Explain your answer.

7. A postoperative patient is complaining of pain at a level of 7 on a 1–10 scale. The nurse checks the medication administration sheet and sees that the patient can receive morphine oral solution (Roxanol) 6 mg PO every 4 hours, and the patient has not had a dose for 8 hours. The medication comes in a 5-mL unit dose container that is labeled 10 mg/5 mL. How many milliliters will the nurse administer to the patient? _____

8. A patient is to receive fentanyl (Sublimaze) 60 mcg IV stat. The drug is available in vials that contain 50 mcg/mL. How many milliliters will the nurse administer for this dose? _____

9. Mark the syringe with the answer you obtained for Question 8.

**Match each type of pain with its corresponding description.**

10. _____ Acute pain

11. _____ Chronic pain

12. _____ Somatic pain

13. _____ Visceral pain

14. _____ Superficial pain

15. _____ Vascular pain

16. _____ Neuropathic pain

17. _____ Phantom pain

18. _____ Central pain

a. Pain that is thought to account for most migraine headaches
b. Pain that relates to a body part that has been removed
c. Pain that originates from the skin or mucous membranes
d. Pain that occurs with tumors, trauma, or inflammation of the brain
e. Persistent or recurring pain that is often difficult to treat
f. Pain that is sudden and usually subsides when treated
g. Pain that originates from the organs or smooth muscles
h. Pain that originates from the skeletal muscles, ligaments, or joints
i. Pain that results from injury or damage to the peripheral nerve fibers

## Case Study

**Read the scenario and answer the following questions on a separate sheet of paper.**

A 58-year-old woman has been admitted for a total abdominal hysterectomy. That evening she asks for pain medication. Upon assessment, you find that she rates her pain level as an "8" on a scale from 1–10 and states that her pain is located mainly in the immediate area around her incision. You prepare to give her an intravenous dose of morphine sulfate.

1. What type of pain is she experiencing?

2. Within an hour of receiving the morphine, the patient complains that her skin feels "itchy" but she cannot see any hives. What do you tell her?

3. What serious adverse effect is possible if she receives too much morphine sulfate? What, if anything, can be given to treat this?

4. The next day, she is ready to be discharged home. Her physician writes a prescription for hydrocodone/acetaminophen (Vicodin). The patient sees the generic label and asks why the medication contains Tylenol. Explain the purpose of the acetaminophen (Tylenol) in this medication and for her pain treatment.

# CHAPTER 11

# General and Local Anesthetics

## Chapter Review and NCLEX® Examination Preparation

**Match each term with its corresponding definition or description.**

1. _____ A type of anesthetic that is applied directly to the skin and mucous membranes.

2. _____ A commonly used, long-acting, nondepolarizing neuromuscular blocking drug (NMBD).

3. _____ The term for anesthetic drugs that alter the central nervous system (CNS), resulting in loss of consciousness and deep muscle relaxation.

4. _____ A type of anesthetic drug that reduces pain sensations at the level of the peripheral nerves.

5. _____ Drugs used in combination with anesthetics for anesthesia initiation (induction), sedation, reduction of anxiety, and amnesia.

6. _____ The term for drugs that depress the CNS; used for surgical procedures.

7. _____ The practice of using combinations of drugs to produce general anesthesia rather than using a single drug.

8. _____ An anticholinergic drug given preoperatively to dry secretions.

9. _____ Generic name for the drug that is most often used for moderate sedation procedures.

10 _____ The only depolarizing neuromuscular blocking drug (NMBD) available; used for endotracheal intubation.

a. Anesthetics
b. Midazolam
c. Atropine
d. Adjunctive
e. Local
f. Topical
g. Pancuronium
h. Succinylcholine
i. Balanced
j. General

**Select the best answer for each question.**

11. Which drug classes are used as adjunctive drugs with anesthesia? *(Select all that apply.)*
    a. Sedative-hypnotics
    b. Anticonvulsants
    c. Anticholinergics
    d. Inhaled gas
    e. Opioid analgesics

12. While assisting with a procedure in the emergency department, the nurse prepares lidocaine (Xylocaine) for use with which type of anesthesia?
    a. Moderate sedation
    b. Infiltration
    c. Intravenous
    d. General

13. The nurse monitoring a patient after surgery keeps in mind that the primary concern with use of a neuromuscular blocking drug is which adverse effect?
    a. Respiratory arrest
    b. Headache
    c. Bradycardia
    d. Hypertension

14. To decrease the possibility of a headache after spinal anesthesia, the nurse will provide which instruction to the patient?
    a. Sit in high Fowler's position.
    b. Maintain strict bedrest.
    c. Limit fluids.
    d. Ambulate in the hall several times a day.

15. The nurse is reviewing a policy for local anesthesia. Local anesthesia is indicated for which procedure(s)? *(Select all that apply.)*
    a. Cardioversions
    b. Suturing a skin laceration
    c. Diagnostic procedures
    d. Long-duration surgery
    e. Dental procedures

16. A patient who has just returned from surgery has suddenly developed a severe elevation in body temperature. The nurse recognizes that this change may indicate which condition?
    a. A normal temperature change after surgery
    b. Malignant hypertension
    c. Malignant hyperthermia
    d. Fever

17. During a procedure, the nurse is monitoring a patient who has received dexmedetomidine (Precedex) for moderate sedation. The nurse will observe for which potential adverse effect?
    a. Respiratory depression
    b. Tachycardia
    c. Dizziness
    d. Hypotension

18. A patient is receiving a neuromuscular blocking drug. Indicate the order in which the following areas become paralyzed once this drug is given (1 = first, 3 = last).
    _____  a. Limbs, neck, trunk muscles
    _____  b. Intercostal muscles and diaphragm
    _____  c. Small, rapidly moving muscles, such as those of the fingers and eyes

19. A patient has an order to receive atropine sulfate, 0.4 mg IM, as a preoperative medication. The vial contains atropine sulfate, 1 mg/mL. How many milliliters of medication will the nurse draw up for this injection? _____

20. In preparation for a colonoscopy, a patient is to receive midazolam (Versed), 0.05 mg IV push over 2 minutes. The medication comes in a strength of 1 mg/mL. How much medication will the nurse draw up into the syringe for this dose?

    _____

## Critical Thinking and Application

**Answer the following questions on a separate sheet of paper.**

21. Henry is a student nurse who has assisted the nurse anesthetist in surgery on prior occasions. Today, however, he is nervous because it is a child who will undergo general anesthesia. Why might this make Henry more nervous than usual?

22. Mr. S. is being administered a neuromuscular blocking drug while he is receiving mechanical ventilation. What is the most important thing the nurse needs to remember when working with him during this therapy?

23. Mrs. E. will undergo cardioversion this afternoon, and the nurse anesthetist has explained to her that she will not be asleep but that she will not remember the procedure. Mrs. E. asks, "How can this be?" What is the nurse anesthetist's explanation?

24. A patient is in the emergency department because he accidentally put a nail into his arm with a nail gun. The emergency provider requests "lidocaine with epinephrine," but the only type available in the supply cart is "plain" lidocaine. What is the difference, and why does it matter which one is used?

## Case Study

**Read the scenario and answer the following questions on a separate sheet of paper.**

You are a nursing student, and today you are assigned to an observation day in the operating room, with a certified registered nurse anesthetist (CRNA) as your contact for the day. The first case is a patient undergoing a right lower lung lobectomy due to lung cancer. The patient has a history of paraplegia from an old automobile accident. The patient's blood pressure has been maintained at 120/72 mm Hg, and the pulse has ranged from 100 to 110 beats/min during the surgery. The patient's body temperature has lowered to 96.2° F (35.7° C) after surgery. The patient's respirations have been maintained by ventilator.

1. Before the surgery, the CRNA explained that the patient will undergo "balanced anesthesia." What is meant by this term?

2. What is the purpose of administering the drug succinylcholine (Anectine) during anesthesia?

3. As your patient goes to the postanesthesia care unit (PACU), the CRNA asks you to monitor for signs of succinylcholine toxicity. Why would this be of concern at this time?

4. What can be done if the patient has received too much succinylcholine?

5. Another patient is undergoing a procedure performed using local anesthesia. Are there advantages of this type of anesthesia over general anesthesia?

6. In the PACU, what are the main concerns of the nurse monitoring the patient recovering from anesthesia?

# CHAPTER 12

# Central Nervous System Depressants and Muscle Relaxants

## Chapter Review and NCLEX® Examination Preparation

**Select the best answer for each question.**

1. When reviewing actions of drugs, the nurse recognizes that a hypnotic is a drug that performs which action?
   a. Produces sleep
   b. Stops seizures
   c. Prevents nausea and vomiting
   d. Relieves pain

2. A patient who has been taking a benzodiazepine for 5 weeks has been instructed to stop the medication. Which instruction will the nurse provide to the patient on how to discontinue the medication?
   a. Stop taking the drug immediately.
   b. Plan a gradual reduction in dosage.
   c. Overlap this medication with another drug.
   d. Take the medication every other day for a number of weeks.

3. A patient will be undergoing a brief surgical procedure to obtain a biopsy from a superficial mass on his arm. The nurse expects that which type of barbiturate will be used at this time?
   a. Ultrashort
   b. Short
   c. Intermediate
   d. Long

4. While monitoring a patient who took an overdose of barbiturates, the nurse keeps in mind that the cause of death would be which of these?
   a. Tachycardia
   b. Hypertension
   c. Dyspnea
   d. Respiratory arrest

5. A patient with back muscle spasms is being treated with a skeletal muscle relaxant. In order to ensure that these drugs are most effective, the nurse will make sure what other treatment is ordered?
   a. Benzodiazepines
   b. Moist heat
   c. Physical therapy
   d. Aspirin

6. The nurse is providing care for a patient who has accidentally taken an overdose of benzodiazepines. Which drug would be used to treat this patient?
   a. methamphetamine
   b. flumazenil (Romazicon)
   c. epinephrine
   d. naloxone (Narcan)

7. A patient will be receiving the barbiturate phenobarbital as part of treatment for seizures. The nurse assesses the patient's current list of medications. Which medication(s) is/are known to cause interactions with barbiturates? (*Select all that apply.*)
   a. Benzodiazepines
   b. Proton pump inhibitors
   c. Oral contraceptives
   d. Anticoagulants
   e. Monoamine oxidase inhibitors (MAOIs)

8. A child will be receiving PO midazolam (Versed) as preoperative sedation. The child weighs 33 pounds. The dose ordered is 0.5 mg/kg, and the medication is available as a syrup, with a concentration of 2 mg/mL.
   a. What will be the dosage for this child?

   _____

   b. How much is the PO dose for this child in milliliters? _____

9. A patient is to receive diazepam (Valium) 10 mg twice a day via a PEG tube. The medication comes in a liquid, with a concentration of 5 mg/5 mL. How many milliliters will the nurse administer with each dose? _____

10. Mark the medication cup with the amount of medication the nurse will administer for Question 9.

## Critical Thinking and Application

**Answer the following questions on a separate sheet of paper.**

11. A 19-year-old college freshman is brought into the emergency department with a suspected barbiturate overdose. What symptoms would you expect to see? How is overdose treated?

12. Jackie is taking benzodiazepines to treat her insomnia. Today she visits your clinic and states that she is going to Europe for 2 months and wants a prescription that will allow her to take enough medication along for her entire stay. The physician declines. She is a little insulted and asks you why the physician refused her request. "Does my doctor think I'm an addict or something?" What do you explain to her? What other options are possible for her?

13. Mrs. A., who is 81 years of age, weighs significantly more than her 47-year-old daughter, yet she is given a lower dosage of a benzodiazepine for insomnia of a similar degree. Explain the rationale for the lower dose.

14. You have been asked to take a patient history for William, who will be given a benzodiazepine.
    a. What conditions or disorders will you ask about?
    b. What drug intake will you be most concerned about?
    c. What if William were an infant? A great-grandfather? Would this additional information matter? Why or why not?

15. Mr. P. is recovering from an automobile accident and has received a prescription for cyclobenzaprine for painful muscle spasms.
    a. What patient teaching will he need about this medication?
    b. What other measures should be included in addition to this drug therapy?

## Case Study

**Read the scenario and answer the following questions on a separate sheet of paper.**

A 54-year-old woman has had problems with insomnia "off and on for a few years" and has tried over-the-counter medications, herbal remedies, and prescription drugs. She likes to drink a glass of wine each night before going to bed. Today she is visiting the clinic for a checkup and asks for a prescription for secobarbital (Seconal) because that was the last drug she tried several years ago. The physician prescribes zaleplon (Sonata) instead. She says she can't understand why the doctor won't refill her prescription for Seconal.

1. Why did the physician change her prescription?

2. What are the consequences of long-term use of barbiturates?

3. What interactions should she be cautioned about while she is taking zaleplon?

4. What other patient teaching is important for this patient?

# CHAPTER 13

# Central Nervous System Stimulants and Related Drugs

## Chapter Review and NCLEX® Examination Preparation

**Select the best answer for each question.**

1. The nurse is reviewing a patient's medication administration record. Which best describes a common use for doxapram (Dopram)?
   a. To control increased respiration caused by other drugs
   b. To treat drug-induced respiratory depression
   c. To treat postoperative respiratory excitation
   d. To stimulate respirations in patients with a head injury

2. The nurse is administering a stimulant drug. Which are results of stimulation of the central nervous system (CNS) by these drugs? *(Select all that apply.)*
   a. Increased fatigue
   b. Decreased drowsiness
   c. Increased respiration
   d. Bradycardia
   e. Euphoria

3. A patient has asked for a cup of coffee. The nurse keeps in mind that patients with a history of which condition need to avoid caffeine?
   a. Cardiac dysrhythmias
   b. Asthma
   c. Diabetes mellitus
   d. Gallbladder disease

4. The physician has ordered orlistat (Xenical). The nurse recognizes that this drug is used to treat which condition?
   a. Anorexia
   b. Malnutrition
   c. Narcolepsy
   d. Obesity

5. When a child is taking drugs for attention deficit hyperactivity disorder (ADHD), what will the nurse instruct the caregivers to closely monitor in the child?
   a. Blood glucose levels
   b. Physical growth, especially weight
   c. Grades at school
   d. Respiratory rates

6. A patient with migraine headaches is being evaluated. One potential treatment is ergotamine tablets. The nurse notes that the patient has the following conditions. Which would be a contraindication to the use of ergotamine? *(Select all that apply.)*
   a. Asthma
   b. Hypertension
   c. Glaucoma
   d. Diabetes mellitus
   e. Coronary heart disease

7. A patient will be taking sumatriptan (Imitrex) as part of treatment for migraine headaches. Before beginning therapy, the nurse reviews the patient's current list of medications. Which medications may have an interaction with sumatriptan? *(Select all that apply.)*
   a. Opioids
   b. Ergot alkaloids
   c. Selective serotonin reuptake inhibitors (SSRIs)
   d. Monoamine oxidase inhibitors (MAOIs)
   e. Nonsteroidal antiinflammatory drugs (NSAIDs)

8. A child will be taking amphetamine/dextroamphetamine (Adderall) for ADHD. He weighs 88 pounds, and the initial dose ordered is 2.5 mg/kg daily. How many milligrams will the nurse administer with each dose? _____

9. The medication order reads: "Give doxapram (Dopram) 0.5 mg/kg IV STAT." The patient weighs 165 pounds. How much medication will the patient receive? _____

## Critical Thinking and Application

**Answer the following questions on a separate sheet of paper.**

10. Stacey, age 35, reports that she falls asleep unexpectedly at work, in class, and even while singing in her city's choir.
    a. Which condition might Stacey have?
    b. What might be the drug of choice for Stacey?
    c. Describe the therapeutic effects of such drugs.
    d. Draw up a patient teaching plan for Stacey. Offer guidelines for substances she might be wise to avoid.

11. Five-year-old Jeffrey is taking atomoxetine (Strattera) for ADHD. What specific precautions must be taken with children who are taking ADHD drugs? Why?

12. What nutritional counseling is needed for patients taking orlistat (Xenical)?

13. Sadie experiences migraine headaches about four times a year and has a new prescription for a serotonin receptor agonist. She tells you that she hopes that the medication will prevent her "awful headaches." What is the best response to Sadie's comments?

14. George, a 14-year-old student, has been taking a medication for ADHD for 6 months. At today's follow-up visit, the physician suggests that George take a "drug holiday" on the weekends and during the school's spring break. Explain the reasoning behind drug holidays.

## Case Study

**Read the scenario and answer the following questions on a separate sheet of paper.**

Nancy, a 44-year-old accountant, has had an increasing number of headaches in the past year. When she has these headaches, she often is nauseated and vomits. She has been to her physician, who has ordered several diagnostic tests. As a result, Nancy has been diagnosed with migraine headaches and will be given a prescription for a serotonin receptor agonist.

1. How do serotonin receptor agonists work in the treatment of migraine headaches?

2. What dosage form(s) would be helpful for Nancy's situation?

3. If the physician decides to write a prescription for sumatriptan (Imitrex), Nancy's history should be assessed for which conditions?

4. What foods may be associated with the development of migraine headaches?

5. What else should be included in the treatment regimen for Nancy's migraine headaches?

CHAPTER 14

# Antiepileptic Drugs

## Critical Thinking Crossword

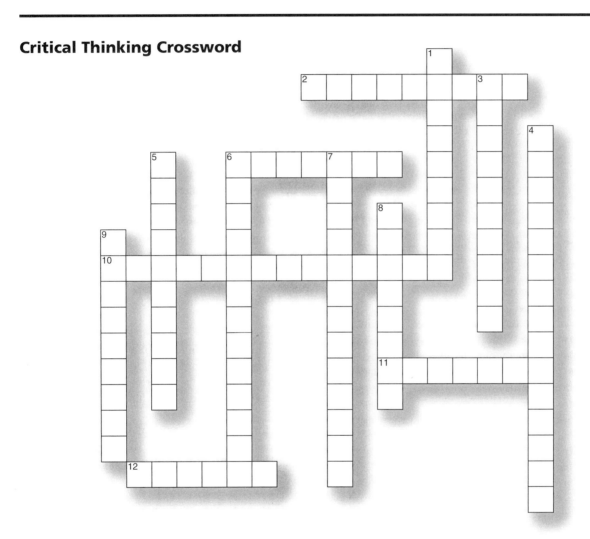

**Across**

2. Status epilepticus is considered a life-threatening medical _____.
6. A type of epilepsy with an unknown cause
10. A potential adverse effect of valproic acid
11. A brief episode of abnormal electrical activity in the nerve cells of the brain
12. Intravenously administered antiepileptic drugs are given _____ to avoid serious adverse effects.

**Down**

1. A type of epilepsy with a distinct cause
3. An involuntary spasmodic contraction of voluntary muscles throughout the body

4. This class of drugs is one of the first-line drugs used to treat status epilepticus.
5. Another term for 6 Across
6. A barbiturate used primarily to control tonic-clonic and partial seizures
7. The metabolic process that occurs when the metabolism of a drug increases over time, which leads to lower-than-expected drug concentrations
8. Recurrent episodes of convulsive seizures
9. Generic name of a first-line antiepileptic drug, which can cause gingival hyperplasia with long-term use

# Chapter Review and NCLEX® Examination Preparation

**Select the best answer for each question.**

1. A patient has been taking antiepileptic drugs for a year. The nurse is reviewing his recent history and will monitor for which condition that may develop during this time?
   a. Loss of appetite
   b. Jaundice
   c. Weight loss
   d. Suicidal thoughts or behavior

2. A patient is experiencing a seizure that has lasted for several minutes and he has not regained consciousness. The nurse recognizes that this is a life-threatening emergency known as:
   a. status epilepticus.
   b. tonic-clonic convulsion.
   c. epilepsy.
   d. secondary epilepsy.

3. The nurse is giving an intravenous dose of phenytoin (Dilantin). Which guidelines will the nurse follow for administration? *(Select all that apply.)*
   a. Inject phenytoin quickly.
   b. Inject phenytoin slowly.
   c. The injection of phenytoin is followed by an injection of sterile saline.
   d. Do not infuse phenytoin continuously.
   e. Mix the phenytoin with $D_5W$ (5% dextrose and water) for the infusion.

4. The nurse is administering phenobarbital (Luminal) and will monitor the patient for which possible adverse effect?
   a. Constipation
   b. Gingival hyperplasia
   c. Drowsiness
   d. Dysrhythmias

5. A patient has been admitted to the emergency department with status epilepticus. The nurse knows that which of these drugs is considered the drug of choice for this condition?
   a. phenobarbital (Luminal)
   b. diazepam (Valium)
   c. valproic acid
   d. phenytoin (Dilantin)

6. A patient who is experiencing neuropathic pain tells the nurse that the physician is going to start him on a new medication that is generally used to treat seizures. The nurse anticipates that which drug will be ordered?
   a. phenobarbital (Luminal)
   b. phenytoin (Dilantin)
   c. gabapentin (Neurontin)
   d. tiagabine (Gabitril)

7. Phenytoin (Dilantin) is prescribed for a patient. The nurse checks the patient's current list of medications and notes that interactions may occur with which drugs or drug classes? *(Select all that apply.)*
   a. Proton pump inhibitors
   b. warfarin (Coumadin)
   c. Sulfonamide antibiotics
   d. Corticosteroids
   e. Oral contraceptives

8. A patient is unable to take oral medications and has received a loading dose of phenytoin (Dilantin) intravenously. The orders call for him to receive phenytoin 5 mg/kg/day in three divided doses. The medication comes in a vial with 50 mg/mL. The patient weighs 90 kg.
   a. How many milligrams will the patient receive each day? For each dose? _____
   b. How many milliliters of medication will be drawn up for each dose? _____

9. Indicate on the syringe the amount of medication the nurse will draw up for each dose of the medication in Question 8.

## Critical Thinking and Application

**Answer the following questions on a separate sheet of paper.**

10. What is meant by *autoinduction* in a drug? Identify at least one antiepileptic drug that undergoes autoinduction.

11. Jeremy, an 8-year-old boy, has resisted his oral doses of topiramate (Topamax), which has made compliance with the drug regimen difficult. His mother calls and says that she has found a way to get him to take it: she crushes the tablet and sprinkles it on flavored gelatin. She is delighted. How will the nurse respond?

12. Rosie, a 24-year-old paralegal, has been on antiepileptic drugs for several years, with her seizures well controlled with the drug therapy. She is in the clinic for an annual checkup and tells the nurse, "I want to stop all my medicines because we want to have a baby. I've always read that these drugs are unsafe for the unborn baby. What do I need to do?" What is the nurse's best response?

## Case Study

**Read the scenario and answer the following questions on a separate sheet of paper.**

Four-year-old Mattie has started preschool. Today the teacher called Mattie's mother to tell her that she noticed that Mattie seems to have a problem with "daydreaming." She explained that Mattie seemed inattentive during group work and was staring out into space several times a day. She was also worried because she saw Mattie's eyes move back and forth rapidly during these episodes. These "spells" lasted a minute or two, and then Mattie seemed fine. The mother has brought Mattie to the pediatric office to have her checked. The health care provider suspects that Mattie is experiencing a type of seizure disorder and has ordered some diagnostic testing.

1. What type of seizure is Mattie experiencing?

2. Mattie's mother is given a prescription for a liquid antiepileptic drug for Mattie. What is important to teach the mother regarding administration of this type of medication?

3. What will the nurse teach Mattie's mother to monitor for during Mattie's drug therapy with this medication?

4. After a year, Mattie's mother is pleased that the seizures have "disappeared" and wants to take Mattie off the medication. What is the best response in this situation by the nurse?

# CHAPTER 15

# Antiparkinson Drugs

## Chapter Review and NCLEX® Examination Preparation

Select the best answer for each question.

1. A patient with Parkinson's disease has difficulty performing voluntary movements. What is the correct term for this symptom?
   a. Akinesia
   b. Dyskinesia
   c. Chorea
   d. Dystonia

2. Which drug may be used early in the treatment of Parkinson's disease but eventually loses effectiveness and must be replaced by another drug?
   a. amantadine (Symmetrel)
   b. levodopa (Larodopa)
   c. selegiline (Eldepryl)
   d. tolcapone (Tasmar)

3. Which drug may be used prophylactically to delay the development of the debilitation of Parkinson's disease for up to 18 years?
   a. levodopa (Larodopa)
   b. benztropine (Cogentin)
   c. carbidopa (Lodosyn)
   d. selegiline (Eldepryl)

4. A patient who is newly diagnosed with Parkinson's disease and beginning medication therapy with entacapone (Comtan), a COMT inhibitor, asks the nurse, "How soon will improvement occur?" What is the nurse's best response?
   a. "That varies from patient to patient."
   b. "You should discuss that with your physician."
   c. "You should notice a difference in a few days."
   d. "It may take several weeks before you notice any degree of improvement."

5. A patient asks the nurse why a second drug is given with his drugs for Parkinson's disease. The nurse notes that this drug, an anticholinergic, is given to control or minimize which symptoms? *(Select all that apply.)*
   a. Drooling
   b. Constipation
   c. Muscle rigidity
   d. Bradykinesia
   e. Dry mouth

6. The nurse is providing teaching on COMT inhibitors to a patient with a new prescription. The nurse will be sure to educate the patient on the possibility of which adverse effect?
   a. Dizziness
   b. Urine discoloration
   c. Leg edema
   d. Visual changes

7. Carbidopa-levodopa (Sinemet) is prescribed for a patient with Parkinson's disease. The nurse will inform the patient of which possible adverse effects? *(Select all that apply.)*
   a. Palpitations
   b. Insomnia
   c. Hypotension
   d. Urinary frequency
   e. GI distress

8. The medication order reads: "Give benztropine (Cogentin) 2.5 mg PO every morning." The medication is available in 1-mg tablets. How many tablets will the nurse administer? _____

## Critical Thinking and Application

**Answer the following questions on a separate sheet of paper.**

9. Mr. H. is about to have levodopa added to his carbidopa treatment regimen.
   a. Why must dopamine be administered in the form of levodopa?
   b. What problems are avoided when carbidopa is given with levodopa?
   c. How does the carbidopa work when given with levodopa?

10. Mrs. R., a 35-year-old new mother, has experienced slowing movements, cogwheel rigidity, and pill-rolling tremor. She has been diagnosed with Parkinson's disease, a somewhat rare occurrence in someone her age. In addition to the usual history questions, what must the nurse ask in anticipation of dopaminergic therapy in Mrs. R.'s specific situation?

11. Jane, age 45, is taking benztropine in addition to a dopaminergic drug for Parkinson's disease. Her 76-year-old neighbor comments that he cannot take benztropine because it is too risky for him. Jane calls and asks why this is not a concern in her case. What do you say?

12. Explain the difference between the concepts of the "on-off phenomenon" and the "wearing off phenomenon."

## Case Study

**Read the scenario and answer the following questions on a separate sheet of paper.**

Alexander, a 54-year-old man, has been diagnosed with Parkinson's disease and is about to start drug therapy. His symptoms are mild, yet he has some akinesia that interferes with his ability to type at work. The physician explains that Alexander may have to take a variety of drugs as the disease progresses.

1. What is the underlying pathologic defect in Parkinson's disease?

2. What is the aim of drug therapy for Parkinson's disease?

3. The first drugs prescribed for Alexander are amantadine (Symmetrel) along with levodopa-carbidopa (Sinemet CR). What is the purpose of taking the amantadine at this time?

4. The physician tells Alexander that the amantadine may be helpful in the early stages but will need to be changed at a later date. Why is this true?

5. How does the carbidopa affect the "on-off phenomenon" that may occur with the use of levodopa?

# CHAPTER 16

# Psychotherapeutic Drugs

## Chapter Review and NCLEX® Examination Preparation

**Select the best answer for each question.**

1. The nurse is administering the antipsychotic drug clozapine (Clozaril) and should monitor the patient for what long-term problem(s) associated with this drug? *(Select all that apply.)*
   a. Mood swings
   b. Agranulocytosis
   c. Weight gain
   d. Photosensitivity
   e. Increased appetite

2. During therapy for depression with a selective serotonin reuptake inhibitor (SSRI), it is most important for the nurse to instruct the family to monitor for which adverse effect?
   a. Suicidal thoughts
   b. Visual disturbances
   c. Tardive dyskinesia
   d. Bleeding tendencies

3. The wife of a patient who has started taking antidepressant therapy asks, "How long will it take for him to feel better?" What is the nurse's best response?
   a. "Well, depression rarely responds to medication therapy."
   b. "He should be feeling better in a few days."
   c. "It may take 4 to 6 weeks before you see an improvement."
   d. "You may not see any effects for several months."

4. When administering certain antipsychotic drugs, the nurse monitors for extrapyramidal effects such as: *(Select all that apply.)*
   a. tremors.
   b. elation and a sense of well-being.
   c. painful muscle spasms.
   d. motor restlessness.
   e. bradycardia.

5. The nurse instructs a patient who is undergoing therapy with monoamine oxidase inhibitors (MAOIs) to avoid tyramine-containing foods. What medical emergency may occur if the patient eats these foods while taking MAOIs?
   a. Gastric hemorrhage
   b. Toxic shock
   c. Cardiac arrest
   d. Hypertensive crisis

6. A patient has been taking antipsychotic medication for years, and his wife has noticed that he has had some new physical symptoms. She describes him as having odd facial movements, sticking out his tongue, and having movements of his arms that he cannot seem to control. The nurse suspects that the patient is exhibiting signs of which condition?
   a. Hypomania
   b. Serotonin syndrome
   c. Tardive dyskinesia
   d. Neuroleptic malignant syndrome

7. A patient will be receiving benztropine (Cogentin) 1.5 mg PO daily. The medication comes in 0.5-mg tablets. How many tablets will the nurse administer per dose? _____

8. A patient is to receive lithium carbonate, 1800 mg/day in two divided doses. The medication is available in 300-mg capsules. How many milligrams of lithium will the patient receive for each dose? How many capsules per dose?

   _____

**Match each term with its corresponding definition or description.**

9. _____   buspirone (BuSpar)

10. _____   tyramine

11. _____   tricyclics

12. _____   psychosis

13. _____   mania

14. _____   diazepam (Valium)

15. _____   amitriptyline (Elavil)

16. _____   risperidone (Risperdal)

17. _____   benzodiazepines

18. _____   lithium (Eskalith)

19. _____   anxiety

20. _____   affective disorders

21. _____   depression

22. _____   bipolar affective disorder

23. _____   extrapyramidal

a. The unpleasant state of mind in which real or imagined dangers are anticipated and/or exaggerated

b. A state characterized by an expansive emotional state (including symptoms of extreme excitement and elation) and hyperactivity

c. A group of psychotropic drugs prescribed to alleviate anxiety

d. Emotional disorders characterized by changes in mood

e. A major psychologic disorder characterized by episodes of mania or hypomania, cycling with depression

f. Patients taking MAOIs need to be taught to avoid foods that contain this substance.

g. An older class of antidepressant drugs

h. An abnormal emotional state characterized by exaggerated feelings of sadness, melancholy, and worthlessness out of proportion to reality

i. A long-acting benzodiazepine

j. The most widely used tricyclic antidepressant

k. An atypical antipsychotic drug used to treat schizophrenia

l. A non-benzodiazepine drug used to treat anxiety

m. Term for the symptoms/adverse effects that often occur with antipsychotic medications

n. Medication used to treat mania

o. A type of serious mental illness that can take several different forms and is associated with being truly out of touch with reality

## Critical Thinking and Application

**Answer the following questions on a separate sheet of paper.**

24. Carl, a 26-year-old unemployed electrician, is brought to the emergency department by his sister. He is extremely drowsy and confused, and his breathing is slow and shallow. The sister tells you that Carl has been seeing a psychiatrist for his "anxiety" and had a prescription for "nerve pills."
    a. What do you suspect might be wrong with Carl?
    b. How will he likely be treated?

25. Mr. D., a 49-year-old restaurant owner, has been prescribed the MAOI phenelzine (Nardil). After the physician leaves the room but before you have a chance to discuss Mr. D.'s medication regimen with him, he turns to his wife and says, "I'm sure this medicine will work. Let's have a bottle of wine tonight to celebrate our anniversary."
    a. What teaching is necessary in this situation?
    b. A few weeks later, Mr. D. is brought to the emergency department with a severe headache, stiff neck, sweating, and elevated blood pressure. His wife says his symptoms started a few minutes after they ate at their favorite restaurant. What is wrong with Mr. D., and what has probably caused it?

26. Beth has been diagnosed with depression. Why might the physician prescribe a second-generation antidepressant instead of a first-generation antidepressant?

27. A young adult has been admitted to the emergency department with a suspected overdose of a tricyclic antidepressant. The physicians are monitoring his cardiac status closely. Why is this?

## Case Study

**Read the scenario and answer the following questions on a separate sheet of paper.**

Gene, a 38-year-old businessman, mentions during a checkup that he has felt very anxious and upset over the past few months. He discusses the pressures of his business and states that he has had trouble sleeping at night, which makes him more irritable. Lately he has been very worried over a contract proposal presentation that will take place in a few months. The physician gives him a prescription for alprazolam (Xanax), 0.25 mg three times a day.

1. Gene is concerned about potential adverse effects of this medication. What will you tell him?

2. What other measures will be taken for Gene at this time?

3. After 3 months, Gene is back in the office for a follow-up appointment. He is upset because a friend told him about another friend who was taking that same medication but died due to an overdose. Gene wants to stop taking the alprazolam immediately. Is this recommended? If not, why not?

4. What are the symptoms of alprazolam overdose, and what is the antidote, if any?

5. Six months later, Gene is no longer taking alprazolam but comes back to the office because he still feels anxious. The physician gives him a prescription for buspirone (BuSpar), 15 mg twice a day. Gene questions why he is given a different drug. What are the advantages, if any, of taking buspirone instead of alprazolam?

# CHAPTER 17

# Substance Abuse

## Chapter Review and NCLEX® Examination Preparation

**Match each drug with its corresponding description.**

1. _____ cocaine

2. _____ ecstasy

3. _____ flumazenil (Romazicon)

4. _____ heroin

5. _____ disulfiram (Antabuse)

6. _____ nicotine

7. _____ naltrexone (ReVia)

8. _____ bupropion (Zyban)

9. _____ methamphetamine

10. _____ "roofies"

a. A nicotine-free treatment for nicotine dependence
b. Known as the "date rape" drug
c. This substance is commonly manufactured from the over-the-counter decongestant pseudoephedrine.
d. The addictive chemical in tobacco products
e. An opioid that is injected by "mainlining" or "skin popping"
f. Used to antagonize the action of benzodiazepines and reverse sedation
g. Used to deter the use of alcohol during alcohol abuse treatment
h. A stimulant that is either "snorted" through the nasal passages or injected intravenously
i. A stimulant that is popular at "raves" with college-age students
j. An opioid antagonist used for opioid abuse or dependence

**Select the best answer for each question.**

11. A patient who has been taking disulfiram (Antabuse) therapy for 3 months has been off the therapy for 2 days. He decides to go out with friends to have a beer. What effects may he experience? *(Select all that apply.)*
    a. Diaphoresis
    b. Diarrhea
    c. Vomiting
    d. Euphoria
    e. Drowsiness
    f. Facial flushing

12. During an information session about drug abuse, the nurse relates that the most common drug effect(s) that lead to abuse of opioids include:
    a. hallucinations.
    b. sleep.
    c. stimulation.
    d. relaxation and euphoria.

13. The nurse is assisting a patient who is experiencing opioid withdrawal and anticipates the possible use of which medications? *(Select all that apply.)*
    a. disulfiram (Antabuse)
    b. clonidine (Catapres)
    c. methadone
    d. bupropion (Zyban)
    e. naltrexone (ReVia)

14. When teaching a patient about drug interactions, the nurse is aware that combining benzodiazepines with ethanol or barbiturates may lead to death due to:
    a. cardiac dysrhythmia.
    b. convulsions.
    c. respiratory arrest.
    d. stroke.

15. A patient with a known history of chronic excessive ingestion of ethanol has developed memory problems and comes to the health clinic with hard-to-believe stories of what has happened to him. The nurse recognizes that these symptoms are associated with which disorder?
    a. Cerebrovascular accident
    b. Korsakoff's psychosis
    c. Narcolepsy
    d. Bipolar disorder

16. A patient is to receive flumazenil (Romazicon), 0.2 mg, IV push over 30 seconds as initial treatment for a possible benzodiazepine overdose. The medication is available in a 0.1 mg/mL vial. How many milliliters of medication will the nurse draw up into the syringe for this dose? _____

## Critical Thinking and Application

**Answer the following questions on a separate sheet of paper.**

17. Describe how nicotine is used to ease withdrawal from nicotine use. Compare the use of bupropion (Zyban) and varenicline (Chantix) in smoking cessation programs.

18. How is medication therapy different for mild, moderate, and severe alcohol withdrawal?

19. A woman brings her teenage daughter into the emergency department. The teen is lethargic, dizzy, and has been vomiting. While the teen is being examined and stabilized, the mother tells the nurse that her daughter told her that she and her friends used cough syrup to get high. The mother states, "How could cough syrup do this?" What is the nurse's best answer?

20. Explain why the decongestant pseudoephedrine is restricted.

## Case Study

**Read the scenario and answer the following questions on a separate sheet of paper.**

A 19-year-old male, Mr. C., is admitted to the emergency department after he collapsed at a fraternity party. The paramedics state that there were beer-drinking contests at the party, and it is unknown how much Mr. C. had to drink. His friend says that Mr. C. was upset over breaking up with a girlfriend and he was worried about how heavily Mr. C. has been drinking in the past 2 weeks.

Mr. C. is semiconscious but unable to answer questions coherently, and his speech is slurred. His blood pressure is 100/58 mm Hg, his pulse rate is 110 beats/min, and his breathing is heavy with a respiratory rate of 16 breaths/min. He vomited on the way to the hospital.

1. Is ethanol considered a central nervous system stimulant or depressant?

2. What are the effects of severe alcoholic intoxication on the cardiovascular and respiratory systems?

3. The patient is admitted to the medical unit for observation. For what will you observe at this time?

4. The next evening, Mr. C. is more alert but still unsteady in his gait. He says he wants to go home, but you notice fine tremors of his hands. Should he be discharged at this time? Explain.

5. If Mr. C. continues the pattern of heavy drinking, what effects could the chronic ingestion of ethanol have on his body?

# CHAPTER 18

# Adrenergic Drugs

## Chapter Review and NCLEX® Examination Preparation

**Select the best answer for each question.**

1. What is another name for an adrenergic drug?
   a. Anticholinergic drug
   b. Parasympathetic drug
   c. Central nervous system drug
   d. Sympathomimetic drug

2. The nurse is administering an adrenergic drug and will monitor for which possible effect?
   a. Hypotension
   b. Increased heart rate
   c. Decreased respiratory rate
   d. Urinary retention

3. The nurse is aware that adrenergic drugs may be used to treat which conditions? *(Select all that apply.)*
   a. Asthma
   b. Open-angle glaucoma
   c. Hypertension
   d. Nasal congestion
   e. Seizures
   f. Nausea and vomiting

4. A woman who is allergic to bees has just been stung while out in her garden. She reaches for her bee-sting kit, which would most likely contain which drug?
   a. epinephrine (EpiPen)
   b. phenylephrine (Neo-Synephrine)
   c. formoterol (Perforomist)
   d. norepinephrine (Levophed)

5. A 13-year-old girl was diagnosed with asthma 2 years ago. Today her physician wants to start her on salmeterol (Serevent) administered via inhaler. The nurse needs to remember to include which statement when teaching the girl and her family about this drug?
   a. "It should be taken at the first sign of an asthma attack."
   b. "The dosage is two puffs every 4 hours or any time needed for asthma attacks."
   c. "This inhaler is for prevention of asthma attacks, not for an acute attack."
   d. "Be sure to take your steroid inhaler first."

6. The nurse is reviewing the medication orders of a newly admitted patient who has an infusion of the adrenergic drug dopamine. Which of these drugs or drug classes, if also given to the patient, may cause an interaction? *(Select all that apply.)*
   a. Tricyclic antidepressants
   b. Monoamine oxidase inhibitors (MAOIs)
   c. Anticoagulants
   d. Corticosteroids
   e. Antihistamines

7. An infant is having an allergic reaction and is to receive two doses of epinephrine 10 mcg/kg subcutaneously. The infant weighs 11 pounds. How many micrograms of medication will the infant receive with each dose? _____

8. The nurse is to administer epinephrine 0.5 mg subcutaneously. The ampule contains 1 mL of medication and is labeled "Epinephrine 1:1000." How many milliliters of epinephrine will the nurse give?

   _____

9. Mark the syringe with the amount of medication the nurse will draw up for Question 8.

## Critical Thinking and Application

**Answer the following questions on a separate sheet of paper.**

10. The mother of 3-year-old Kyle is giving him phenylephrine (Neo-Synephrine) drops as a nasal decongestant.
    a. How does this medication help with nasal congestion?
    b. Kyle's mother comes back to the clinic and complains that after a week his congestion is worse, not better. What possible explanation can the nurse offer?

11. Mr. D., who has had a history of problems with a hormonal imbalance, has been admitted for septic shock, and the physician prescribes dopamine. However, the nurse double-checks the patient's history before administering the drug. What condition may be a contraindication to dopamine?

12. Mr. G. and Mr. C. are both on dopamine infusions. Mr. G.'s infusion is being administered at a low rate, and Mr. C.'s at a high rate. Why might these infusion rates be different?

13. A patient in the intensive care unit has received too high a dose of epinephrine. The nurse will monitor for what effects? What will the nurse expect to do for this patient?

14. Greg, a 49-year-old construction worker, is in the urgent care center for treatment of a leg laceration. Just after a dose of intravenous penicillin is started, he begins to wheeze and says, "Oh, I just remembered. I'm allergic to penicillin!"
    a. What is happening?
    b. What will the nurse do first?
    c. What drug will be given in this situation?

## Case Study

**Read the scenario and answer the following questions on a separate sheet of paper.**

Sixteen-year-old Maureen, who plays soccer on her high school team, has been treated for asthma for a year. Her symptoms have been controlled with an inhaled steroid and occasional use of an albuterol metered-dose inhaler. This afternoon, though, her mother brings her into the urgent care center because Maureen has had trouble "getting her breath" after a particularly rough game. Maureen complains of a feeling of "tightness" in her chest and wants to sit up. She appears anxious and has a nonproductive cough. Her respiratory rate is 28 breaths/min, and her peak expiratory flow is 70% of normal. Chest auscultation reveals a short inspiratory period with prolonged expiratory wheezes in both lungs.

1. The physician orders albuterol (Ventolin) to be given through a nebulizer. What should you assess before giving this medication? During and after administration?

2. Why is the albuterol given via inhalation rather than orally?

3. After the nebulizer medication treatment is completed, Maureen complains of feeling "shaky and jittery." What do you tell her?

4. The physician gives Maureen a prescription for a salmeterol (Serevent) inhaler. What is important to teach Maureen and her mother about this medication?

# CHAPTER 19

# Adrenergic-Blocking Drugs

## Chapter Review and NCLEX® Examination Preparation

**Select the best answer for each question.**

1. Adrenergic blockade at the alpha-adrenergic receptors leads to which of the following effects? *(Select all that apply.)*
   a. Vasodilation
   b. Decreased blood pressure
   c. Increased blood pressure
   d. Constriction of the pupil
   e. Tachycardia

2. The nurse discovers that the intravenous infusion of a patient who has been receiving an intravenous vasopressor has infiltrated. The nurse will expect which drug to be used to reverse the effects of the vasopressor in the infiltrated area?
   a. phentolamine (Regitine)
   b. prazosin (Minipress)
   c. epinephrine (Adrenalin)
   d. metoprolol (Lopressor)

3. A patient has a new prescription for a beta blocker as part of treatment for hypertension. The nurse is reviewing the patient's current medications and notes that there may be a concern regarding interactions with which medication?
   a. Thyroid hormone supplement
   b. Antibiotic for a sinus infection
   c. Oral hypoglycemic for type 2 diabetes mellitus
   d. Oral contraceptive

4. A patient has been given an alpha-blocker as treatment for benign prostatic hyperplasia. Which instruction is important to include when the nurse is teaching him about the effects of this medication?
   a. Avoid foods and drinks that contain caffeine.
   b. Change to sitting or standing positions slowly to avoid a sudden drop in blood pressure.
   c. Watch for weight loss of 2 pounds within a week.
   d. Take extra supplements of calcium.

5. A patient who has been taking a beta blocker for 6 months tells the nurse during a follow-up visit that she wants to stop taking this medication. She is wondering if there is any problem with stopping the medication today. What is the nurse's best response?
   a. "No, there are no ill effects if this medication is stopped."
   b. "There should be only minimal effects if you stop this medication."
   c. "You may experience orthostatic hypotension if you stop this medication abruptly."
   d. "If you stop this medication suddenly, there is a possibility you may experience chest pain or rebound hypertension."

6. A patient has been taking tamsulosin (Flomax) for about a year. During today's office visit, he asks the physician about taking a drug for erectile dysfunction. How does the nurse expect the physician to respond?
   a. "These drugs are safe to take together."
   b. "You can take them together, but the dosage of the Flomax will need to be reduced."
   c. "Taking these two drugs together may lead to dangerously low blood pressure."
   d. "You will be able to try taking these two drugs together, but watch for side effects."

7. An admission order reads, "Start IV of 0.9% normal saline and infuse 1 L over the next 12 hours." The nurse will set the infusion pump to what rate?

   _____

8. A patient is to receive labetalol (Trandate) 20 mg IV push over 10 minutes, STAT. The medication is available in a vial that contains 5 mg/mL. How many milliliters will the nurse administer for this dose?

   _____

## Critical Thinking and Application

**Answer the following questions on a separate sheet of paper.**

9. Mrs. W., a patient on a cardiac step-down unit, is receiving a dopamine intravenous infusion. When the nurse first comes on the late-night shift, Mrs. W. seems just fine. However, the next time the nurse checks on her, the intravenous line has dislodged and the infusion has infiltrated. What could happen as a result? Is this serious? What treatment will the nurse expect to see ordered? Describe the procedure and provide the rationale.

10. Mr. C. has had a myocardial infarction (MI). He is told that he will be prescribed a "cardioprotective drug." He asks the nurse to explain. How can some beta blockers be said to "protect" the heart?

11. Ms. M. has been prescribed a beta blocker. She is about to be released from the hospital, but first her nurse gives her instructions about taking her apical pulse for 1 full minute, as well as her blood pressure. Why? What should she be looking for? Is there anything she should be instructed to report to her physician?

12. Mr. S., a 78-year-old widower, has a new prescription for tamsulosin (Flomax) because of a new diagnosis of benign prostatic hyperplasia. What concern, if any, is there with this drug? What teaching will he need?

## Case Study

**Read the scenario and answer the following questions on a separate sheet of paper.**

Bruce, a 58-year-old accountant, is in the hospital after having an MI. The physician has told him that damage to his heart was minimal and the patient has started post-MI rehabilitation and education. In addition to the MI, he has had asthma for years that has been managed poorly. The physician discusses starting Bruce on a beta blocker to "protect his heart" and gives him a prescription for atenolol (Tenormin).

1. What type of beta blocker is appropriate for Bruce, and why?

2. Discuss how atenolol helps in this situation.

3. What adverse effects will you teach Bruce to expect when taking this medication?

4. At his 3-month checkup, Bruce tells you that he wants to stop taking this medication. Should this medication be stopped abruptly? What do you think may be the reason that Bruce wants to stop taking the atenolol?

# CHAPTER 20

# Cholinergic Drugs

## Chapter Review and NCLEX® Examination Preparation

**Match each definition with its corresponding term. (Note: Not all terms will be used.)**

1. _____ Antidote for overdose of a cholinergic drug

2. _____ Cholinergic drugs that act by making more acetylcholine (ACh) available at the receptor site, thus allowing ACh to bind to and stimulate the receptor

3. _____ Cholinergic drugs that bind to cholinergic receptors and activate them

4. _____ Receptors located postsynaptically in the effector organs (smooth muscle, cardiac muscle, glands) supplied by the parasympathetic fibers

5. _____ Receptors located in the ganglia of the parasympathetic nervous system (PSNS) and the sympathetic nervous system (SNS)

6. _____ A description of the action of the PSNS

7. _____ The neurotransmitter responsible for the transmission of nerve impulses to the effector cells in the PSNS

8. _____ The enzyme responsible for breaking down ACh

a. Cholinesterase
b. Muscarinic
c. Catecholamine
d. "Fight or flight"
e. "Rest and digest"
f. Direct-acting cholinergic drugs
g. Indirect-acting cholinergic drugs
h. Atropine
i. Acetylcholine
j. Nicotinic

**Select the best answer for each question.**

9. The desired effects of cholinergic drugs come from stimulation of which receptors?
   a. Cholinergic
   b. Nicotinic
   c. Muscarinic
   d. Ganglionic

10. The undesirable effects of cholinergic drugs come from stimulation of which receptors?
   a. Cholinergic
   b. Nicotinic
   c. Muscarinic
   d. Ganglionic

11. The patient mentions bethanechol (Urecholine) when asked about his medication history. The nurse recognizes that this drug is used for the treatment of which condition?
   a. Diarrhea
   b. Urinary retention
   c. Urinary incontinence
   d. Bladder spasms

12. When caring for a patient with a diagnosis of myasthenia gravis, the nurse can expect to see which drug ordered for the symptomatic treatment of this disease?
   a. bethanechol (Urecholine)
   b. tacrine (Cognex)
   c. donepezil (Aricept)
   d. pyridostigmine (Mestinon)

13. A 62-year-old woman has started taking donepezil (Aricept) for early-stage Alzheimer's disease. Her daughter expresses relief that "there is finally a pill to cure Alzheimer's disease." What is the nurse's best response?
   a. "She can expect reversal of symptoms within a few days."
   b. "The dosage will need to be increased if no improvement is noted."
   c. "This drug may help to improve symptoms, but it is not intended as a cure."
   d. "Yes, it has been a great help for many patients."

14. A patient has received an inadvertent overdose of a cholinergic drug. The nurse will monitor for which early signs of a cholinergic crisis? *(Select all that apply.)*
    a. Dry mouth
    b. Salivation
    c. Flushing of the skin
    d. Abdominal cramps
    e. Constipation
    f. Dyspnea

15. The nurse will prepare to give which drug to a patient who is experiencing a cholinergic crisis?
    a. atropine
    b. tacrine (Cognex)
    c. donepezil (Aricept)
    d. physostigmine (Antilirium)

16. The nurse is monitoring a patient who has been receiving bethanechol (Urecholine) after abdominal surgery. Which of these are therapeutic outcomes for this medication? *(Select all that apply.)*
    a. Decreased heart rate
    b. Passage of flatus
    c. Decreased temperature
    d. A bowel movement
    e. Decreased respiratory secretions

17. An intravenous piggyback medication is ordered to infuse over 1 hour. The volume of the medication bag is 100 mL; the tubing drop factor is 10 gtt/mL. What is the rate for a gravity infusion of this medication? _____

18. The order reads: "Give pyridostigmine (Mestinon) 0.25 mg/kg IV now." The patient weighs 235 pounds. How many milligrams of medication will the patient receive? *(Record answer using one decimal place.)* _____

## Critical Thinking and Application

**Answer the following questions on a separate sheet of paper.**

19. List the effects of cholinergic poisoning by using the acronym SLUDGE.

20. Mrs. S. has recently had abdominal surgery, and she is resting well except that she is unable to void her urine. She has some distension in her lower abdomen over the symphysis pubis.
    a. What is likely to be the drug of choice?
    b. Mrs. S. is still unable to void her urine. Her urinary retention worsens and becomes painful, and she begins to exhibit signs of a renal stone, which is confirmed by radiography. How much can the physician increase her dosage?

21. Mr. K. has been determined to have a high potential for a negative reaction to the cholinergic prescribed to him. However, his physician believes that the potential benefits are worth the risk.
    a. The nurse will closely monitor Mr. K. for what reaction?
    b. In addition to close monitoring, what else can the nurse do to prepare?

22. Ms. B. has recently been diagnosed with myasthenia gravis and is taking medication for the treatment of symptoms associated with the disease. She asks the nurse, "How much success can I expect?"
    a. How should the nurse respond?
    b. What kind of negative effects should Mrs. B. report to her physician?

## Case Study

**Read the scenario and answer the following questions on a separate sheet of paper.**

Arthur, a 68-year-old retired banker, has been diagnosed with early-stage Alzheimer's disease. He has remained active in his church and likes to golf every week. He is in the office today with his son and is asking about the "new drugs that are available to reverse Alzheimer's disease." The son is concerned because Arthur was diagnosed with Parkinson's disease 6 months ago, but it has been controlled well with medications.

1. What drugs are available to "reverse Alzheimer's disease?" Explain.

2. The physician is considering either galantamine (Razadyne) or rivastigmine (Exelon) for Arthur. Is there anything in his history that may influence the choice of medication?

3. Describe the different mechanisms of action of direct-acting and indirect-acting cholinergic-blocking drugs.

4. Arthur is given a prescription for rivastigmine. What are the possible adverse effects, and what should he and his son be told regarding ways to manage these adverse effects?

5. A few months later, Arthur's son reports that Arthur has trouble swallowing tablets. What is a possible solution to this problem?

# CHAPTER 21

# Cholinergic-Blocking Drugs

## Chapter Review and NCLEX® Examination Preparation

**Select the best answer for each question.**

1. Before giving an anticholinergic drug, the nurse will check the patient's history for which conditions? *(Select all that apply.)*
   a. Glaucoma
   b. Osteoporosis
   c. Acute asthma
   d. Thyroid disease
   e. Diabetes mellitus
   f. Benign prostatic hyperplasia

2. The nurse will monitor for which adverse effects of anticholinergic drugs? *(Select all that apply.)*
   a. Dilated pupils
   b. Constricted pupils
   c. Dry mouth
   d. Urinary retention
   e. Urinary frequency
   f. Diarrhea

3. In reviewing the medication orders for a newly admitted patient, the nurse recognizes that which is an indication for atropine sulfate?
   a. Myasthenia gravis
   b. Reduction of secretions preoperatively
   c. Tachycardia due to sinoatrial node defects
   d. Narrow-angle glaucoma

4. During patient teaching for a 70-year-old man who will be taking an anticholinergic drug, the nurse will reinforce that this medication places the patient at higher risk for which problem?
   a. Angina
   b. Fluid overload
   c. Heatstroke
   d. Hypothermia

5. A 28-year-old woman is preparing to take a cruise and has asked for a prescription drug to prevent motion sickness. The physician orders scopolamine transdermal patches (Transderm-Scōp). The nurse will include which statement when teaching the patient about this drug?
   a. "The patch can be applied anywhere on the upper body."
   b. "Apply the patch 4 to 5 hours before travel."
   c. "Apply the patch just before boarding the ship."
   d. "Be sure to change the patch daily."

6. A patient has a new prescription for tolterodine (Detrol). Which condition, if present, would make it necessary to reduce the usual dosage of this drug?
   a. Coronary artery disease
   b. Diabetes mellitus
   c. Hypertension
   d. Cirrhosis of the liver

7. The preoperative orders read, "Give atropine 0.6 mg IV push, 30 minutes before the procedure." The medication comes in a 1 mg/mL vial. How much medication will the nurse administer? _____

8. A 14-month-old toddler is in the preoperative area, and the order reads: "Give glycopyrrolate (Robinul) 4 mcg/kg IV now." The toddler weighs 22 pounds.
   a. How many micrograms of medication will the toddler receive for this dose? _____
   b. The medication is available in a vial that contains 0.2 mg/mL. How many milliliters will the nurse draw up into the syringe for this dose?
   _____

## Critical Thinking and Application

**Answer the following questions on a separate sheet of paper.**

9. A patient is given atropine sulfate before surgery. Describe how this drug is helpful during the perioperative period. What other drug can be used for this purpose?

10. Mr. M. is brought into the emergency department with an overdose of a cholinergic blocker. He is still conscious.
    a. Describe how Mr. M. will be treated.
    b. How will the nurse respond if Mr. M. begins having hallucinations related to the overdose?

11. Mr. H. is taking dicyclomine (Bentyl) for irritable bowel syndrome. He calls the clinic and tells the nurse that he would like to get his doctor's permission to take an antihistamine for his cold. What drug interactions might he expect?

12. How does atropine work in the following situations?
    a. A patient is experiencing severe bradycardia, with a heart rate of 38 beats/min, and he is losing consciousness.
    b. A crop duster pilot has been exposed to an organophosphate insecticide in an industrial accident.

## Case Study

**Read the scenario and answer the following questions on a separate sheet of paper.**

Mrs. W., age 63, is in the outpatient clinic today for a physical. During history-taking, she admits to having a "terrible problem" with her bladder. She describes having sudden urges to urinate and is "ashamed to say" that, at times, she has lost control of her bladder. She has had no other health issues except for "some eye problems" off and on for the past year. The provider is considering starting Mrs. W. on tolterodine (Detrol).

1. What are the contraindications for this medication? Are there any potential concerns given Mrs. W.'s history?

2. What are the advantages of using tolterodine rather than other drugs with similar actions?

3. Mrs. W. enjoys working outside in her yard. What special precautions does she need to take?

4. After a week of therapy, she calls the clinic to complain of a dry mouth. She said she didn't think this was supposed to happen with this drug. What advice do you give to her?

# CHAPTER 22

# Antihypertensive Drugs

## Critical Thinking Crossword

### Across

1. High blood pressure associated with renal, pulmonary, endocrine, and vascular diseases is known as _____ hypertension.
5. Another term for 3 Down
7. A common adverse effect of adrenergic drugs involving a sudden drop in blood pressure when patients change position is known as _____ hypotension.
8. These drugs are used in the management of hypertensive emergencies.

### Down

2. Another term for 3 Down
3. Elevated systemic arterial pressure for which no cause can be found is known as _____ hypertension.
4. The primary effect of these drugs is to decrease plasma and extracellular fluid volumes.
6. Drugs that are often used as first-line drugs in the treatment of both heart failure and hypertension are known by the acronym _____ inhibitors.

# Chapter Review and NCLEX® Examination Preparation

**Select the best answer for each question.**

1. A 46-year-old man has been taking clonidine for 5 months. For the last 2 months, his blood pressure has been normal. During this office visit, he tells the nurse that he would like to stop taking the drug. What is the nurse's best response?
   a. "I'm sure the doctor will stop it—your blood pressure is normal now."
   b. "Your doctor will probably have you stop taking the drug for a month, and then we'll see how you do."
   c. "This drug should not be stopped suddenly; let's talk to your doctor."
   d. "It's likely that you can stop the drug if you exercise and avoid salty foods."

2. When administering angiotensin-converting enzyme (ACE) inhibitors, the nurse keeps in mind that which are possible adverse effects? *(Select all that apply.)*
   a. Diarrhea
   b. Fatigue
   c. Restlessness
   d. Headaches
   e. A dry cough
   f. Tremors

3. A patient with type 2 diabetes mellitus has developed hypertension. What is the blood pressure goal for this patient?
   a. Less than 110/80 mm Hg
   b. Less than 130/80 mm Hg
   c. Less than 130/84 mm Hg
   d. Less than 140/90 mm Hg

4. A patient is being treated for a hypertensive emergency. The nurse expects which drug to be used?
   a. sodium nitroprusside (Nitropress)
   b. losartan (Cozaar)
   c. captopril (Capoten)
   d. prazosin (Minipress)

5. A patient in her eighth month of pregnancy has preeclampsia. Her blood pressure is 210/100 mm Hg this morning. This type of hypertension is classified as which of the following?
   a. Primary
   b. Idiopathic
   c. Essential
   d. Secondary

6. A beta$_1$ blocker is prescribed for a patient with heart failure and hypertension. Which adverse effects, if present, may indicate a serious problem is developing while the patient is on this medication? *(Select all that apply.)*
   a. Edema
   b. Nightmares
   c. Shortness of breath
   d. Nervousness
   e. Constipation

7. The order reads, "Give captopril 25 mg PO every 8 hours." The available tablets are 12.5-mg strength. How many tablets will the nurse administer per dose? _____

8. The order reads, "Give enalapril (Vasotec) 5 mg IV push over 5 minutes now." The medication is available in a vial with the strength of 1.25 mg/mL. How many milliliters will the nurse administer for this dose? _____

# Critical Thinking and Application

**Answer the following questions on a separate sheet of paper.**

9. Mr. Q., 61 years of age, comes to the emergency department with symptoms of a severe hypertensive emergency. The emergency department resident on call initiates therapy with sodium nitroprusside (Nitropress). The patient is transferred to the intensive care unit and monitored. Hours later, his blood pressure falls to 100/60 mm Hg, and he is lethargic and complaining of feeling dizzy. What will the nurse do?

10. Indicate which ACE inhibitor would be best for the following patients. Explain your answers.
    a. Irene, who has liver dysfunction, has high blood pressure, and is seriously ill
    b. Kory, who has a history of poor adherence to his medication regimen

11. Mr. B. will be starting prazosin (Minipress) for hypertension. What will he be taught before he takes even the first dose of this medication?

12. White and African-American patients are known to respond differently to antihypertensive agents.
    a. Which antihypertensives are considered more effective in white patients than in African-American patients?
    b. Which antihypertensives are considered more effective in African-American patients than in white patients?

## Case Study

**Read the scenario and answer the following questions on a separate sheet of paper.**

John, a 44-year-old African-American man, has been seen twice in the last month for "blood pressure problems." At the first visit, his blood pressure was 144/90 mm Hg; at the second visit, his blood pressure was 154/96 mm Hg. The provider is preparing to start antihypertensive therapy. John has no other medical conditions.

1. What initial drug therapy would be appropriate for him? What factors are considered when choosing which drug to use?

2. John tells you that he hopes this medication will not "slow him down" because he likes to "jump out of bed and get started" with his day. What teaching will you provide for him to help him adjust to his blood pressure medication?

3. John also mentions that he likes to go the gym three times a week and visit with his friends in the sauna after a good workout. What teaching will you emphasize for this patient?

CHAPTER 23

# Antianginal Drugs

## Chapter Review and NCLEX® Examination Preparation

**Select the best answer for each question.**

1. What is the purpose of antianginal drug therapy?
   a. To increase myocardial oxygen demand
   b. To increase blood flow to peripheral arteries
   c. To increase blood flow to ischemic cardiac muscle
   d. To decrease blood flow to ischemic cardiac muscle

2. The nurse will teach a patient who will be taking nitroglycerin (Nitrostat) about which common adverse effect of this drug?
   a. Blurred vision
   b. Dizziness
   c. Headache
   d. Weakness

3. The nurse is reviewing dosage forms of nitroglycerin (Nitrostat). This drug can be given by which routes? *(Select all that apply.)*
   a. Continuous intravenous drip
   b. Intravenous bolus
   c. Sublingual spray
   d. Oral dosage forms
   e. Topical ointment
   f. Rectal suppository

4. For a patient using transdermal nitroglycerin patches, the nurse knows that the prescriber will order which procedure for preventing tolerance?
   a. Leave the old patch on for 2 hours when applying a new patch.
   b. Apply a new patch every other day.
   c. Leave the patch off for 24 hours once a week.
   d. Remove the patch at night for 8 hours and then apply a new patch in the morning.

5. Patients who are taking beta blockers for angina need to be taught which information?
   a. These drugs are for long-term prevention of angina episodes.
   b. These drugs must be taken as soon as angina pain occurs.
   c. These drugs will be discontinued if dizziness is experienced.
   d. These drugs need to be carried with the patient at all times in case angina occurs.

6. A patient with coronary artery spasms will be most effectively treated with which type of antianginal medication?
   a. Beta blockers
   b. Calcium channel blockers
   c. Nitrates
   d. Nitrites

7. During his morning walk, a man begins to experience chest pain. He sits down and takes one nitroglycerin sublingual tablet. After 5 minutes, the chest pain is worsening. What action would be the priority in this situation?
   a. Call 911 (emergency medical services).
   b. Take another nitroglycerin tablet.
   c. Take two more nitroglycerin tablets at the same time.
   d. Sit quietly to wait for the pain to subside.

8. The order reads "Give isosorbide dinitrate (Dilatrate-SR) 80 mg twice a day." The medication is available in 40-mg capsules. How many capsules will the patient receive for each dose?

---

## Critical Thinking and Application

**Answer the following questions on a separate sheet of paper.**

9. The order reads "Nitroglycerin transdermal patch, 0.2 mg/hr; apply one patch in the morning and remove every evening at 10 PM." The pharmacy has supplied a transdermal patch that supplies 0.4 mg/hr. What will the nurse do in order to administer this drug?

10. The nurse is playing racquetball at a community center when he notices a commotion at a gathering of senior citizens in a nearby room. The nurse rushes in to find a man lying unconscious on the floor. Several people say that he is having a "heart attack." One man hands the nurse a pill bottle and asks, "Would it help to give him one of my heart pills?" A woman agrees, saying, "Yes! Can't you put it under his tongue?" The nurse sees that the medication bottle is labeled Isordil (isosorbide dinitrate). What does the nurse know about this medication and what needs to be done next?

11. Ms. V. is a 70-year-old patient seen in the emergency department for a laceration to her thumb. During the assessment, Ms. V. tells the nurse that she has been "tired and depressed" and has been having "nightmares" since her physician prescribed heart medicine for her angina. Which drug does the nurse suspect Ms. V. is taking and why?

12. During a home visit with Theresa, she shows the nurse a journal entry describing the duration, time of onset, and severity of a recent angina attack. She reports no adverse effects to her nitroglycerin and shows the nurse where she keeps the tablets—in a clear plastic pillbox on the kitchen windowsill. What will the nurse discuss with Theresa?

## Case Study

**Read the scenario and answer the following questions on a separate sheet of paper.**

While playing handball, 59-year-old Gideon experiences chest pain. He has had angina before and has sublingual nitroglycerin (Nitro-Bid) in his gym bag.

1. What type of angina is he experiencing?

2. What should he do to treat this episode of angina?

3. After Gideon takes the nitroglycerin tablet, the chest pain does not subside. He wants his handball partner to drive him to the hospital. Is this appropriate? Explain your answer.

4. Other than nitroglycerin, which class of drugs is typically used for this type of angina?

# CHAPTER 24

# Heart Failure Drugs

## Chapter Review and NCLEX® Examination Preparation

**Select the best answer for each question.**

1. As part of treatment for early heart failure, a patient is started on an angiotensin-converting enzyme (ACE) inhibitor. The nurse will monitor the patient's laboratory work for which potential effect?
   a. Agranulocytosis
   b. Proteinuria
   c. Hyperkalemia
   d. Hypoglycemia

2. Before giving oral digoxin (Lanoxin), the nurse discovers that the patient's radial pulse is 52 beats/min. What will be the nurse's next action?
   a. Give the dose.
   b. Delay the dose until later.
   c. Hold the dose and notify the physician.
   d. Check the apical pulse for 1 minute.

3. Which statement regarding digoxin therapy and potassium levels is correct?
   a. Low potassium levels increase the chance of digoxin toxicity.
   b. High potassium levels increase the chance of digoxin toxicity.
   c. Digoxin reduces the excretion of potassium in the kidneys.
   d. Digoxin promotes the excretion of potassium in the kidneys.

4. When infusing milrinone (Primacor), the nurse will keep which consideration in mind?
   a. The patient must be monitored for hyperkalemia.
   b. The patient's cardiac status must be monitored closely.
   c. The drug may cause reddish discoloration of the extremities.
   d. Hypertension is the primary effect seen with excessive doses.

5. When caring for a patient who is taking digoxin, the nurse will monitor for which signs and symptoms of toxicity? *(Select all that apply.)*
   a. Anorexia
   b. Diarrhea
   c. Visual changes
   d. Nausea and vomiting
   e. Headache
   f. Bradycardia

6. A patient who has heart failure will be started on an oral ACE inhibitor. While monitoring the patient's response to this drug therapy, which laboratory tests would be a priority? *(Select all that apply.)*
   a. White blood cell count
   b. Platelet count
   c. Serum potassium level
   d. Serum magnesium level
   e. Creatinine level
   f. Blood urea nitrogen (BUN)

7. A patient is to receive an initial dose of digoxin (Lanoxin), 0.5 mg IV push, followed by an oral maintenance dose of 0.25 mg PO daily, starting the next day. The medication is available in ampules that contain 0.25 mg/mL. How many milliliters will he receive for the IV dose? _____

8.  Mark the syringe with the correct amount of digoxin the patient will receive for the IV dose in Question 7.

9.  Convert the 0.25-mg dose to micrograms. _____

## Critical Thinking and Application

**Answer the following questions on a separate sheet of paper.**

10. The nurse is caring for Mrs. C., who is undergoing cardiac glycoside therapy. She begins to vomit and complains of a headache and fatigue. Diagnostic studies reveal short episodes of ventricular tachycardia on the ECG and a serum potassium level of 6 mEq/L. What action might the nurse expect to be taken?

11. Explain the limitations of nesiritide (Natrecor) therapy for heart failure.

12. While monitoring Mr. F. after oral digoxin (Lanoxin) administration, the nurse notes increased urinary output, decreased dyspnea and fatigue, and constipation. Mr. F. complains that if he were allowed to eat bran as often as he used to, he wouldn't be constipated. What do the nurse's findings indicate? How will the nurse response to Mr. F.?

13. Mr. M. is experiencing heart failure that has not responded well to diuretic and digoxin therapy. The physician changes his medication to milrinone.
    a.  What effect does milrinone have on cardiac muscle contractility and the blood vessels?
    b.  What advantage does this phosphodiesterase inhibitor have over the cardiac glycosides?
    c.  What is the primary adverse effect of milrinone?

## Case Study

**Read the scenario and answer the following questions on a separate sheet of paper.**

A 68-year-old woman is admitted to the hospital with a diagnosis of mild left-sided heart failure. At rest she is comfortable, but she has noticed that she has symptoms when she tries to get dressed or do simple housework. She becomes short of breath with activity, tires easily but cannot sleep at night, and feels "generally irritable." She also has diffuse bilateral crackles that do not clear with coughing and a third heart sound. She has slight pedal edema. The physician has ordered therapy with intravenous digoxin (Lanoxin).

1.  Digoxin has several effects. Explain the meaning of each of the following:
    a.  Positive inotropic effect
    b.  Negative chronotropic effect
    c.  Negative dromotropic effect

2.  As a result of these effects, what would you expect to see with regard to each of the following?
    a.  Stroke volume
    b.  Venous blood pressure and vein engorgement
    c.  Coronary circulation
    d.  Diuresis

3.  After 3 days of therapy, the patient complains of feeling nauseated and has no appetite. She also wonders why the lights are so bright and blurry. Her radial pulse rate is 52 beats/min. When you check the results of her laboratory work, you note that her digoxin level from that morning is 3.5 ng/mL. What will you do?

# CHAPTER 25

# Antidysrhythmic Drugs

## Chapter Review and NCLEX® Examination Preparation

**Select the best answer for each question.**

1. The nurse notes in the patient's medication history that the patient is receiving a lidocaine infusion. Based on this finding, the nurse interprets that the patient has which disorder?
   a. Atrial fibrillation
   b. Bradycardia
   c. Complete heart block
   d. Ventricular dysrhythmias

2. When monitoring a patient who is taking quinidine (Quinidex), the nurse recognizes that possible adverse effects of this drug include which of these conditions? *(Select all that apply.)*
   a. Weakness
   b. Tachycardia
   c. Gastrointestinal upset
   d. Tinnitus
   e. Ventricular ectopic beats

3. The nurse is administering amiodarone (Cordarone) and should monitor for which potential adverse effect?
   a. Pulmonary toxicity
   b. Hypertension
   c. Urinary retention
   d. Constipation

4. A patient is about to receive a dose of verapamil (Calan). The nurse notes that this medication is used to treat which condition?
   a. Cardiac asystole
   b. Heart block
   c. Ventricular dysrhythmia, including premature ventricular contraction
   d. Recurrent paroxysmal supraventricular tachycardia (PSVT)

5. A patient is experiencing a rapid dysrhythmia, and the nurse is preparing to administer adenosine (Adenocard). Which is the correct administration technique for this drug?
   a. It should be given as a fast intravenous push.
   b. It should be given intravenously, slowly, over at least 5 minutes.
   c. It should be taken with food or milk.
   d. It should be given as an intravenous drip infusion.

6. If a drug has a prodysrhythmic effect, then the nurse must monitor the patient for which effect?
   a. Decreased heart rate
   b. New dysrhythmias
   c. A decrease in dysrhythmias
   d. Reduced blood pressure

7. A patient will be starting therapy with quinidine (Quinidex). Which of these drugs, if also on the patient's medication list, may cause a potential drug interaction? *(Select all that apply.)*
   a. cimetidine (Tagamet)
   b. amiodarone (Cordarone)
   c. digoxin (Lanoxin)
   d. warfarin (Coumadin)
   e. erythromycin (Erythrocin)

8. A patient with sustained ventricular tachycardia will be receiving a lidocaine infusion following a bolus dose. The order reads, "Give a bolus of 1.5 mg/kg, then start a drip at 2 mg/min." The lidocaine is available as 20 mg/mL, and the patient weighs 220 pounds. How many milligrams of lidocaine will be given in the bolus dose? _____

9. A patient is to receive adenosine (Adenocard) as initial treatment for PSVT. The dose is 6 mg IV push. The medication is available in a vial that contains 3 mg/mL. How many milliliters will the nurse draw up into the syringe for this dose? _____

10. Match the site to its correct intrinsic rate.
    _____ a. Sinoatrial node
    _____ b. Atrioventricular node
    _____ c. Purkinje fibers
    (1) 40 to 60 beats/min
    (2) 40 or fewer beats/min
    (3) 60 to 100 beats/min

# Critical Thinking and Application

**Answer the following questions on a separate sheet of paper.**

11. Mr. K., who has been diagnosed with hypertension, is hospitalized after a myocardial infarction (MI).
    a. To reduce the risk of sudden cardiac death in Mr. K., the physician prescribes a drug from which class? Why?
    b. How would a history of asthma in Mr. K. affect the drug choice?

12. Mr. N. has a life-threatening ventricular tachycardia that has been resistant to treatment. What drug will the nurse expect to be used and what precautions are necessary with this drug?

13. Mr. M. is a 50-year-old schoolteacher being treated with lidocaine after an MI.
    a. He is very upset and says that he hates injections; he wants to know why he can't just take a pill. What will the nurse tell him?
    b. If Mr. M. has a history of cirrhosis, how would the dosage of the lidocaine be affected?

14. Alicia calls the health clinic complaining of diarrhea and lightheadedness. She says she cannot remember whether she took her quinidine (Quinidex) yesterday and wants to know whether she should take two doses today, especially because she is feeling so bad. What will the nurse tell Alicia?

# Case Study

**Read the scenario and answer the following questions on a separate sheet of paper.**

Jack, age 39, has a new prescription for verapamil (Calan) as part of his treatment for occasional PSVT. This is the first time he has taken this medication. He states he has no previous history of heart problems but that he does smoke one pack of cigarettes a day.

1. How do calcium channel blockers such as verapamil work?

2. What therapeutic effects are expected?

3. What may be a concern regarding his health history?

4. After 4 months of therapy, Jack experiences dizziness, dyspnea, and a very rapid heart rate and is taken to the emergency department. He is diagnosed with sustained PSVT, and intravenous diltiazem (Cardizem) does not help. What drug may be tried next?

# CHAPTER 26

# Coagulation Modifier Drugs

## Chapter Review and NCLEX® Examination Preparation

**Match each definition with its corresponding term. (Note: Not all terms will be used; terms may be used more than once.)**

1. _____ A drug that prevents the lysis of fibrin, thereby promoting clot formation

2. _____ The termination of bleeding by mechanical or chemical means

3. _____ A substance that prevents platelet plugs from forming

4. _____ The general term for a drug that dissolves thrombi

5. _____ The general term for a substance that prevents or delays coagulation of the blood

6. _____ A laboratory test used to measure the effectiveness of heparin therapy

7. _____ Two tests used to monitor the effects of drug therapy with warfarin sodium

8. _____ A standardized measure of the degree of coagulation achieved by drug therapy with warfarin sodium

9. _____ A substance that reverses the effect of heparin

10. _____ A substance that reverses the effect of warfarin sodium

11. _____ A pharmaceutically available tissue plasminogen activator (tPA) that is created through recombinant DNA techniques

12. _____ A blood clot that dislodges and travels through the bloodstream

a. prothrombin time (PT)
b. activated partial thromboplastin time (aPTT)
c. International Normalized Ratio (INR)
d. rivaroxaban (Xarelto)
e. alteplase (Activase)
f. thrombus

g. embolus
h. vitamin K
i. protamine sulfate
j. antiplatelet drug
k. antifibrinolytic
l. thrombolytic drug
m. anticoagulant
n. hemostasis

**Select the best answer for each question.**

13. The nurse is reviewing the use of anticoagulants. Anticoagulant therapy is appropriate for which conditions? *(Select all that apply.)*
    a. Atrial fibrillation
    b. Thrombocytopenia
    c. Myocardial infarction
    d. Presence of mechanical heart valve
    e. Aneurysm
    f. Leukemia

14. During teaching of a patient who will be taking warfarin sodium (Coumadin) at home, which statement by the nurse is correct regarding over-the-counter drug use?
    a. "Choose nonsteroidal antiinflammatory drugs as needed for pain relief."
    b. "Aspirin products may result in increased bleeding."
    c. "Vitamin E therapy is recommended to improve the effect of the warfarin."
    d. "Mineral oil is the laxative of choice while taking anticoagulants."

15. A patient is at risk for a stroke. Which drug is recommended to prevent platelet aggregation for stroke prevention by the American Stroke Society?
    a. aspirin
    b. warfarin sodium (Coumadin)
    c. heparin
    d. alteplase (Activase)

16. When administering subcutaneous heparin, the nurse will remember to perform which action?
    a. Use the same sites for injection to reduce trauma.
    b. Use a 1-inch needle for subcutaneous injections.
    c. Inject the medication without aspirating for blood return.
    d. Massage the site after the injection to increase absorption.

17. During thrombolytic therapy, the nurse monitors for bleeding. Which symptoms may indicate a serious bleeding problem? *(Select all that apply.)*
    a. Hypertension
    b. Hypotension
    c. Decreased level of consciousness
    d. Increased pulse rate
    e. Restlessness

18. Which drug is most often used for deep vein thrombosis (DVT) prevention after major orthopedic surgery, even after the patient has gone home?
    a. Antiplatelet drugs, such as aspirin
    b. Adenosine diphosphate (ADP) inhibitors, such as clopidogrel (Plavix)
    c. Anticoagulants, such as warfarin sodium (Coumadin)
    d. Low-molecular–weight heparins, such as enoxaparin (Lovenox)

19. The nurse is preparing a patient's morning medications and, upon reviewing the list of drugs, notes that the patient is to receive heparin 5,000 units and enoxaparin (Lovenox), both subcutaneously. What is the nurse's priority action at this time?
    a. Administer the drugs in separate sites.
    b. Hold the drugs and clarify the order with the prescriber.
    c. Administer the enoxaparin and hold the heparin.
    d. Check the patient's aPTT.

20. A patient is to receive a bolus dose of heparin 8,000 units via IV push. The vial contains heparin 10,000 units per mL. How many milliliters of medication will the nurse draw up to administer the ordered dose?_____

21. A patient who weighs 165 pounds is to receive daily doses of fondaparinux (Arixtra). According to the dosage chart for the drug below, how many milligrams will this patient receive per dose?_____

| Patient weight less than 50 kg | 5 mg daily |
| Patient weight 50-100 kg | 7.5 mg daily |
| Patient weight over 100 kg | 10 mg daily |

## Critical Thinking and Application

**Answer the following questions on a separate sheet of paper.**

22. The nurse is preparing to administer a new order of enoxaparin (Lovenox) to a patient. Upon checking the patient, the nurse notes that the patient has an epidural catheter. What is the priority action of the nurse at this time?

23. During cardiopulmonary bypass for heart surgery, Mr. J. was intentionally given a large dose of heparin. The surgeon then determines that the effects of the heparin need to be reversed quickly.
    a. How will this be done?
    b. How will the amount of antidote be determined?
    c. What is the most commonly used test for determining the effects of heparin therapy?

24. A patient is experiencing warfarin toxicity from accidentally taking too many warfarin tablets.
    a. What will be used as an antidote?
    b. How will the dose of the antidote be determined?
    c. After 4 days, the patient requires anticoagulation again. What drug will be ordered?

25. Following surgery, Mr. T. has a chest tube in place. The site has been bleeding excessively. What type of drug might the physician prescribe in this situation and why?

26. William, a 38-year-old writer who has von Willebrand's disease, has undergone emergency surgery after an automobile accident. What drug is used in the management of bleeding in patients like William? What is its effect?

27. Tobias has been given alteplase (Activase) during his treatment for acute myocardial infarction. A few minutes later, Tobias suffers a reinfarction. What drug does the nurse expect Tobias to receive now?

28. Ursula, an inpatient on the nurse's unit, is on anticoagulant therapy. The nurse enters her room to find that she is restless and confused.
    a. Why are these findings significant?
    b. What other problems might the nurse expect to find?
    c. What will the nurse do?

29. Sara is receiving subcutaneous heparin 5,000 units twice a day for DVT prevention. Will her anticoagulation be monitored by laboratory work? Explain.

## Case Study

**Read the scenario and answer the following questions on a separate sheet of paper.**

After experiencing transient ischemic attacks, Doug has been started on clopidogrel (Plavix). He has had a history of atherosclerotic heart disease and has had problems with peptic ulcer disease.

1. He asks, "Why am I taking this fancy medicine? Why can't I just take an aspirin a day, like they say on television?" What do you tell him?

2. What should he be taught to report to his health care provider while he is taking this drug?

3. What precautions should he follow while he is taking this drug?

4. What herbal products should he avoid while he is taking this drug?

# CHAPTER 27

# Antilipemic Drugs

## Chapter Review and NCLEX® Examination Preparation

**Select the best answer for each question.**

1. Patients taking cholestyramine (Questran) may experience which adverse effects?
   a. Blurred vision and photophobia
   b. Drowsiness and difficulty concentrating
   c. Diarrhea and abdominal cramps
   d. Belching and bloating

2. The nurse will instruct the patient who is taking antilipemic drugs about which dietary measures? *(Select all that apply.)*
   a. Taking supplements of fat-soluble vitamins
   b. Taking supplements of B vitamins
   c. Increasing fluid intake
   d. Choosing foods that are lower in cholesterol and saturated fats
   e. Increasing the intake of raw vegetables, fruit, and bran

3. In reviewing the history of a newly admitted cardiac patient, the nurse knows that the patient would have a contraindication to antilipemic therapy if which condition is present?
   a. Liver disease
   b. Renal disease
   c. Coronary artery disease
   d. Diabetes mellitus

4. A woman is being screened in the cardiac clinic for risk factors for coronary artery disease. Which would be considered a negative (favorable) risk factor for her?
   a. High-density lipoprotein (HDL) cholesterol level of 30 mg/dL
   b. HDL cholesterol level of 75 mg/dL
   c. Low-density lipoprotein (LDL) level of 25 mg/dL
   d. History of diabetes mellitus

5. A patient who has started taking niacin complains that he "hates the side effects." Which statement by the nurse is most appropriate?
   a. "You will soon build up tolerance to these side effects."
   b. "You need to take the niacin on an empty stomach."
   c. "You can take the niacin every other day if the side effects are bothersome."
   d. "Try taking a small dose of ibuprofen (Advil) 30 minutes before taking the niacin."

6. A patient asks, "What is considered the 'good cholesterol?'" How will the nurse answer?
   a. Very low-density lipoprotein (VLDL)
   b. LDL
   c. HDL
   d. Triglycerides

7. The nurse is preparing to administer a newly ordered statin drug to a patient, and is reviewing the patient's list of current medications. Which medications may cause an interaction with the statin drug? *(Select all that apply.)*
   a. warfarin (Coumadin)
   b. metformin (Glucophage)
   c. erythromycin (Erythrocin)
   d. cyclosporine (Gengraf)
   e. gemfibrozil (Lopid)

8. The medication order reads, "Give lovastatin (Mevacor) 30 mg daily at bedtime, PO." The medication is available in 20-mg tablets. How many tablets will the nurse administer to the patient?

   _____

9. A patient is to receive niacin (Niaspan), 1.5 g/day in 2 divided doses. The medication is available in 250-mg extended-release tablets. How many milligrams will the patient receive for each dose? How many tablets per dose? _____

## Critical Thinking and Application

**Answer the following questions on a separate sheet of paper.**

10. For each of the following drugs, name the antilipemic category and briefly describe how the drug lowers lipid levels.
    a.   gemfibrozil (Lopid)
    b.   niacin
    c.   lovastatin (Mevacor)
    d.   cholestyramine (Questran)

11. Mr. H. is a 46-year-old business executive who travels frequently. He is slightly overweight "from all that room service," but he did quit smoking 6 years ago. He has no history of coronary heart disease (CHD), nor family history of CHD. During a routine checkup, Mr. H. is found to have an LDL cholesterol level of 170 mg/dL. He says, "I'm a busy man! Just give me some pills. I've got a plane to catch!" Will the physician prescribe an antilipemic for Mr. H.? Explain your answer.

12. Mrs. K. has been treated with cholestyramine (Questran) for type IIa hyperlipidemia for the past 2 months. She tells the nurse that she "can't stand being so irregular" and that she has developed another "embarrassing problem" as well. What does the nurse suspect is wrong with Mrs. K., and how can the nurse help her?

13. Justus is a 55-year-old attorney being treated with lovastatin (Mevacor) for his hyperlipidemia. His current health status includes mild hypertension and a peptic ulcer. The nurse knows that niacin is frequently prescribed as an adjunct to other antilipemic drugs. Would niacin be helpful for Justus? Explain your answer.

14. You are visiting Mrs. N., a homebound patient who is being treated for hyperlipidemia and hypertension. During your visit, Mrs. N. takes her antihypertensive medication and then begins to mix her dose of cholestyramine into a glass of orange juice. What patient teaching does Mrs. N. require?

## Case Study

**Read the scenario and answer the following questions on a separate sheet of paper.**

Mr. M. has been diagnosed with type IIa hyperlipidemia and has been given a prescription for atorvastatin (Lipitor). He acts thrilled with the news, and says, "Great! Now I don't have to worry about watching my diet because I'm on this medicine!"

1. Is he right? What type of dietary guidelines should he follow while on this therapy?

2. What therapeutic effects do you hope to see as a result of his taking this medication?

3. After 2 months of therapy, you note that his liver enzyme levels are slightly elevated. Is this a concern? What other laboratory values will be monitored while Mr. M. is taking atorvastatin?

4. Mr. M. calls the office to complain about some muscle pain. He thought he had pulled a muscle during a tennis match, but the pain has not lessened in 3 days. Is this a concern?

# CHAPTER 28

# Diuretic Drugs

## Chapter Review and NCLEX® Examination Preparation

**Match each term with its corresponding definition.**

1. _____ Diuretics

2. _____ Potassium-sparing diuretics

3. _____ Loop of Henle

4. _____ Osmotic diuretics

5. _____ Thiazides

6. _____ Ascites

7. _____ CAIs

8. _____ Loop diuretics

9. _____ Nephron

10. _____ GFR

a. Potent diuretics that act along the ascending limb of the loop of Henle; furosemide is an example
b. Abbreviation for the term that describes a gauge of how well the kidneys are functioning as filters
c. A general term for drugs that accelerate the rate of urine formation
d. The main structural unit of the kidney
e. Part of the kidney structure located between the proximal and distal convoluted tubules
f. Diuretics that result in the diuresis of sodium and water and the retention of potassium; spironolactone is an example
g. Diuretics that act on the distal convoluted tubule, where they inhibit sodium and water resorption; hydrochlorothiazide (HCTZ) is an example
h. Abbreviation for a class of diuretics that inhibit the enzyme carbonic anhydrase; acetazolamide is an example
i. Drugs that induce diuresis by increasing the osmotic pressure of the glomerular filtrate, which results in rapid diuresis; mannitol is an example
j. An abnormal intraperitoneal accumulation of fluid

**Select the best answer for each question.**

11. Which are indications for the use of diuretics? *(Select all that apply.)*
    a. To increase urine output
    b. To reduce uric acid levels
    c. To treat hypertension
    d. To treat open-angle glaucoma
    e. To treat edema associated with heart failure

12. When providing patient teaching to a patient who is taking a potassium-sparing diuretic such as spironolactone (Aldactone), the nurse will include which dietary guidelines?
    a. There are no dietary restrictions with this medication.
    b. The patient needs to consume foods high in potassium, such as bananas and orange juice.
    c. The patient needs to avoid excessive intake of foods high in potassium.
    d. The patient needs to drink 1 to 2 liters of fluid per day.

13. When teaching a patient about diuretic therapy, which would the nurse indicate as the best time of day to take these medications?
    a. Morning
    b. Midday
    c. Bedtime
    d. Time of day does not matter.

14. When monitoring a patient for hypokalemia related to diuretic use, the nurse looks for which possible symptoms?
    a. Nausea, vomiting, and anorexia
    b. Diarrhea and abdominal pain
    c. Orthostatic hypotension
    d. Muscle weakness and lethargy

15. A patient with severe heart failure has been started on therapy with a carbonic anhydrase inhibitor (CAI), but the nurse mentions that this medication may be stopped in a few days. What is the reason for this short treatment?
    a. CAIs are not the first choice for treatment of heart failure.
    b. Metabolic acidosis develops in 2 to 4 days after therapy is started.
    c. It is expected that CAIs will dramatically reduce the fluid overload related to heart failure.
    d. Allergic reactions to CAIs are common.

16. A patient has a new order for daily doses of spironolactone (Aldactone). Which condition, if present, may be a contraindication to this drug therapy? *(Select all that apply.)*
    a. Heart failure
    b. Renal failure
    c. Diabetes mellitus
    d. Deep vein thrombosis
    e. Hyperkalemia

17. A patient is to receive furosemide (Lasix) 120 mg every morning via PEG tube. The medication is available in a liquid form, 40 mg/5 mL. Mark on the medication cup how many milliliters the patient will receive for this dose.

18. A patient is to receive 30 g of mannitol (Osmitrol) intravenously. The medication on hand is mannitol 20% in a 500-mL bag. How many milliliters will the patient receive? _____

## Critical Thinking and Application

**Answer the following questions on a separate sheet of paper.**

19. Ms. A. is a 62-year-old retired teacher who is being treated for diabetes and open-angle glaucoma. The health care provider has prescribed a diuretic as an adjunct drug in the management of Ms. A.'s glaucoma.
    a. Which diuretic drug was probably prescribed?
    b. What undesirable effect of the drug does the provider need to consider?

20. The nurse is about to administer mannitol (Osmitrol) to Arthur, who is in early acute renal failure.
    a. What is the significance of Arthur's renal blood flow and glomerular filtration in this situation?
    b. By what means will the nurse administer the mannitol? What special guidelines will be followed?
    c. Arthur later complains of a headache and chills. Should the mannitol therapy be ended? Explain your answer.

21. Mr. F. has been admitted for treatment of ascites. He also has some renal impairment and a history of heavy drinking.
    a. Which diuretic drug will the nurse expect to be administered to Mr. F.?
    b. What monitoring will be performed frequently? Why?

22. Brendan, a 39-year-old bricklayer, is taking a thiazide diuretic for hypertension. During a follow-up visit, he tells the nurse that he thinks the drug is affecting his "love life."
    a. To what adverse effect of thiazide therapy is Brendan probably referring?
    b. While the nurse is talking, she notices a package of licorice in Brendan's coat pocket. He tells her that he eats the candy "for energy," especially because he has been feeling so tired the past couple of days. What will the nurse tell Brendan?

23. The nurse receives a call from Mrs. H., who recently started diuretic therapy for hypertension. Mrs. H. is concerned because her neighbor, who also takes medication for hypertension, has told her not to eat a lot of bananas or other foods containing potassium. "But you told me to eat foods high in potassium," Mrs. H. says to the nurse, "What's going on?" What will the nurse respond to Mrs. H.?

24. Mrs. P. will be started on diuretic therapy for hypertension, but she also has moderate renal failure. Which diuretic—a loop diuretic or a thiazide diuretic—would be more effective for Mrs. P.? Explain your answer.

## Case Study

**Read the scenario and answer the following questions on a separate sheet of paper.**

Lily has been taking furosemide (Lasix) for 3 months as part of her treatment for heart failure. At this time, she is complaining that she is feeling tired and has muscle weakness and no appetite; her blood pressure is 100/50 mm Hg.

1. What do her symptoms suggest? How did this happen?

2. What dietary measures could she have taken to prevent this problem?

The physician switches her medication to spironolactone (Aldactone).

3. How does this drug differ from furosemide?

4. You will check for what drug interactions before she begins taking the spironolactone?

# CHAPTER 29

# Fluids and Electrolytes

## Chapter Review and NCLEX® Examination Preparation

**Select the best answer for each question.**

1. Which are common uses of crystalloids? *(Select all that apply.)*
   a. Fluid replacement
   b. Promotion of urinary flow
   c. Transport of oxygen to cells
   d. Replacement of electrolytes
   e. As maintenance fluids
   f. Replacement of clotting factors

2. The intravenous order for a newly admitted patient calls for "Normal saline to run at 100 mL/hr." The nurse will choose which concentration of normal saline?
   a. 0.33%
   b. 0.45%
   c. 0.9%
   d. 3.0%

3. A patient has been admitted with severe dehydration after working outside on a very hot day. The nurse expects which intravenous product to be ordered?
   a. Albumin
   b. Hetastarch
   c. Fresh frozen plasma
   d. 0.9% sodium chloride

4. When giving intravenous potassium, which is important for the nurse to remember?
   a. Intravenous doses are preferred over oral dosage forms.
   b. Intravenous solutions should contain at least 50 mEq/L.
   c. Potassium must always be given in diluted form.
   d. It is given by slow intravenous bolus.

5. The nurse monitors for which signs of a possible transfusion reaction when a patient is receiving blood products?
   a. Subnormal temperature and hypertension
   b. Apprehension, restlessness, fever, and chills
   c. Decreased pulse and respirations and fever
   d. Headache, nausea, and lethargy

6. A patient with a blood disorder needs a replacement product that contains clotting factors. The nurse expects which product to be given?
   a. Albumin
   b. Fresh frozen plasma
   c. Packed red blood cells
   d. 0.9 % normal saline

7. A patient is receiving conivaptan (Vaprisol). Which of these are appropriate actions by the nurse?
   a. Administer the drug by slow IV push over 10 minutes.
   b. Report serum sodium levels of 149 mEq/L.
   c. Monitor for hyperkalemia.
   d. Implement measures to prevent constipation.

8. The following IV is to be given: 1000 mL $D_5W$ with 20 mEq potassium chloride (KCl) over the next 24 hours. The tubing drop factor is 15.
   a. At what rate will the KCl be administered?

   _____

   b. What will the gtt/min be? _____

9. An IVPB antibiotic needs to infuse over 30 minutes. The IVPB bag contains 50 mL. Calculate the setting for the infusion pump. _____

## Critical Thinking and Application

**Answer the following questions on a separate sheet of paper.**

10. Name advantages and disadvantages of using crystalloids to replace fluid in patients with dehydration.

11. Some fluids are known as *oxygen-carrying resuscitation fluids*.
    a. Which class of fluids is given this designation?
    b. Why are these fluids able to carry oxygen?
    c. Why is their origin a potential problem for a recipient?

12. Tanya, a 16-year-old student, is brought to the clinic by her mother, who says that Tanya has been on "some sort of fad diet." The mother is concerned because Tanya is tired and weak. During the nurse's assessment, Tanya admits that she has been using laxatives and eating very little during the past few weeks. Her sodium level is 136 mEq/L, and her potassium level is 2.8 mEq/L. What electrolyte imbalance is Tanya probably experiencing? How can it be corrected?

13. Mr. S., a 45-year-old mail carrier, has come to the emergency department sweating profusely and complaining of stomach cramps and diarrhea. He says that he has been "miserable" from the heat the past few days. His serum sodium level is 128 mEq/L.
    a. What electrolyte imbalance does the patient have?
    b. The health care provider prescribes oral sodium tablets. What adverse effect of sodium may be of special concern for Mr. S.?

14. Victor is receiving a transfusion of a blood product.
    a. The nurse observes Victor, knowing that an adverse reaction to the transfusion may be manifested by what signs and symptoms?
    b. Victor's wife is crying and says, "People get AIDS from transfusions. What happens if Victor gets AIDS?" What will the nurse tell her?
    c. Forty-five minutes after the transfusion was started, Victor is restless and his pulse rate has increased. Explain the nurse's next actions, including the priority action.

## Case Study

**Read the scenario and answer the following questions on a separate sheet of paper.**

An older man was admitted to the unit with hypoproteinemia caused by chronic malnutrition. You note that he has some edema over his body, and his total protein level is 4.8 g/dL.

1. What is the relationship between his serum total protein level and the edema you have noted?

2. You are preparing to give him 1 unit of 5% albumin. How does albumin work in this situation?

3. What advantages does albumin have over crystalloids in this situation?

4. You will monitor for what adverse effects while he is receiving albumin?

# CHAPTER 30

# Pituitary Drugs

## Chapter Review and NCLEX® Examination Preparation

1. Complete the following table.

| Hormone | Function | Mimicking Drug(s) |
|---------|----------|-------------------|
| Adrenocorticotropic hormone (ACTH, corticotropin) | Targets adrenal gland; mediates adaptation to stressors; promotes synthesis of the following three hormones:<br>a. | b. |
| Growth hormone | c. | d. |
| e. | Increases water resorption in distal tubules and collecting duct of nephron; concentrates urine; potent vasoconstrictor | f. |
| Oxytocin | g. | h. |

Select the best answer for each question.

2. When administering vasopressin, which is the priority vital sign for the nurse to monitor?
   a. Temperature
   b. Pulse
   c. Respirations
   d. Blood pressure

3. A nurse is administering octreotide (Sandostatin) to a patient who has a metastatic carcinoid tumor. The patient asks about the purpose of this drug. What is the nurse's best response?
   a. "This drug helps to reduce the size of your tumor."
   b. "This drug works to prevent the spread of your tumor."
   c. "This drug helps to control the flushing and diarrhea that you are experiencing."
   d. "This drug reduces the nausea and vomiting you are having from the chemotherapy."

4. Which nursing diagnosis is most appropriate for a patient who is receiving a pituitary drug?
   a. Constipation
   b. Disturbed body image
   c. Impaired physical mobility
   d. Impaired skin integrity

5. The nurse will instruct a patient taking desmopressin acetate as a nasal spray for the treatment of diabetes insipidus to perform which action to obtain maximum benefit from the drug?
   a. Clear the nasal passages before spraying the medication.
   b. Blow his nose after taking the medication.
   c. Take an over-the-counter preparation to control mucus if nasal congestion occurs.
   d. Press on the pump once to prime it before delivering the dose.

6. During vasopressin therapy, which is the priority nursing action?
   a. Check blood glucose levels regularly.
   b. Monitor the electrocardiogram for changes.
   c. Monitor the IV site for signs of infiltration.
   d. Watch for hyperthermia.

7. When assessing a patient who is receiving octreotide (Sandostatin) therapy, the nurse will closely monitor which assessment finding?
   a. Blood glucose levels
   b. Pulse
   c. Weight
   d. Serum potassium levels

8. A child who weighs 44 pounds and is experiencing growth failure is to receive growth hormone therapy. The dosage ordered is 0.3 mg/kg per week, to be given as a series of one injection per day for 6 days.
   a. What is the total dose per week that this child will receive? _____
   b. What is the dose per injection? _____

9. The order reads: "Give octreotide (Sandostatin) 50 mcg IV bid." The medication is available in a strength of 0.1 mg/mL. How many milliliters will the nurse draw up for this dose? Indicate your answer on the syringe.

## Critical Thinking and Application

**Answer the following questions on a separate sheet of paper.**

10. The nurse has recently begun working in a specialized endocrinology clinic. Her first patient, Patricia, a second-grader, is not growing at the expected rate. The physician has determined that Patricia is a candidate for somatropin therapy. What will be emphasized when the nurse is teaching her parents about giving this drug?

11. A patient is being assessed for possible adrenocortical insufficiency. The physician orders a dose of cosyntropin (Cortrosyn). The patient, upon hearing that he will be receiving an injection, states "Oh, good! The doctor has already found something to cure me!" How will the nurse respond?

## Case Study

**Read the scenario and answer the following questions on a separate sheet of paper.**

Mr. C. has been experiencing severe thirst, which he reports "makes me go to the bathroom all the time, it seems." He is also dehydrated, despite the large amounts of water he has been drinking. He is diagnosed with diabetes insipidus.

1. What two drugs may be used to treat diabetes insipidus?

2. What are the possible cautions to the use of these drugs?

3. The physician decides that Mr. C. should do well with vasopressin (Pitressin) therapy. Indicate how you would describe the treatment and its therapeutic effects (that is, how it mimics the natural hormone) to the patient.

4. Following your explanation, Mr. C. says, "Okay, okay, but what does it do for me?" Explain the physical improvements Mr. C. should be able to see.

# CHAPTER 31

# Thyroid and Antithyroid Drugs

## Critical Thinking Crossword

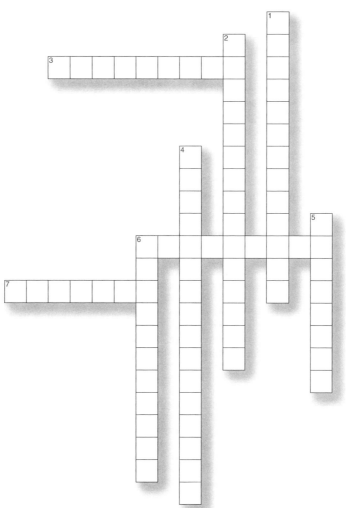

**Across**

3. The type of hypothyroidism that results from insufficient secretion of thyroid-stimulating hormone (TSH) from the pituitary gland
6. The principal thyroid hormone that influences the metabolic rate
7. The type of hypothyroidism that is due to the inability of the thyroid gland to perform a function

**Down**

1. The most commonly prescribed synthetic thyroid hormone
2. Excessive secretion of thyroid hormones
4. A drug used to treat hyperthyroidism
5. The type of hypothyroidism that stems from reduced secretion of thyrotropin-releasing hormone from the hypothalamus
6. Another name for TSH

# Chapter Review and NCLEX® Examination Preparation

**Select the best answer for each question.**

1. A patient who is beginning therapy with levothyroxine (Synthroid) asks the nurse when the medication will start working. What is the nurse's best answer?
   a. Immediately
   b. Within a few days
   c. Within a few weeks
   d. Within a few months

2. A patient wants to switch brands of levothyroxine (Synthroid). What is the nurse's best response?
   a. "If you do this, you should reduce the dosage of your current brand before starting the new one."
   b. "Levothyroxine has been standardized, so there is only one brand."
   c. "It shouldn't matter if you switch brands; they are all very much the same."
   d. "You should check with your provider before switching brands."

3. Patient teaching for a patient taking antithyroid medication will include the need to avoid which foods?
   a. Soy products and seafood
   b. Bananas and oranges
   c. Dairy products
   d. Processed meats and cheese

4. Which information needs to be included in the nurse's teaching of patients taking thyroid medications? *(Select all that apply.)*
   a. Keeping a log or journal of individual responses and a graph of pulse rate, weight, and mood would be helpful.
   b. The medication will be discontinued if the adverse effects become too strong.
   c. The medication needs to be taken at the same time every day.
   d. Nervousness, irritability, and insomnia may be a result of a dosage that is too high.
   e. Take thyroid replacement drugs after meals.

5. A patient is scheduled for a radioactive isotope study. The scheduling nurse notes that he takes levothyroxine (Levothroid) daily. Which medication order needs to be made before the radioactive isotope study is scheduled?
   a. Continue to take the levothyroxine as ordered.
   b. Do not take the levothyroxine on the morning of the test.
   c. Stop the levothyroxine about 4 weeks before the test.
   d. Reduce the levothyroxine dosage by one-half 1 week before the test.

6. The nurse has been providing patient education regarding thyroid hormone replacement therapy. Which statement by the patient reflects a need for further teaching?
   a. "I will take this pill in the mornings."
   b. "Sometimes this medicine can make my heart skip beats, but that's a normal side effect."
   c. "I need to take this pill on an empty stomach, and wait about 30 to 60 minutes before eating."
   d. "I will be sure to go to the clinic to have my thyroid levels tested regularly."

7. Levothyroxine (Synthroid) 88 mcg PO is ordered. What is 88 mcg expressed as mg?

   _____

8. The order reads, "Give levothyroxine (Synthroid) 150 mcg IV now." The vial of medication, once reconstituted, contains 0.1 mg/mL. How many milliliters will the nurse draw up for this dose?

   _____

# Critical Thinking and Application

**Answer the following questions on a separate sheet of paper.**

9. Mrs. W., age 43, comes into the clinic complaining of hair loss, lethargy, and constipation. "I just can't eat anything," she says. As the nurse takes her blood pressure, he notices that her skin feels thickened. She also seems to have a lump in her neck. The primary care provider makes a diagnosis of hypothyroidism. Suggest several possible appropriate medications. Which of those is generally preferred? Why?

10. After undergoing a thyroidectomy as treatment for a thyroid tumor that turned out to be benign, Rebecca is given a prescription for levothyroxine (Levothroid). "I thought I would be cured after this surgery!" she exclaimed. "Why do I have to take a pill every day?" What will the nurse explain to Rebecca?

11. The nurse is examining changes in a medication administration record after new orders were written. One new medication order reads, "levothyroxine (Levothroid), 200 mg, once a day." The nurse suspects an error. What is wrong with this order?

12. Rory, age 32, has been given a prescription for propylthiouracil (PTU) as part of treatment for Graves' disease. What laboratory tests are important to assess before she begins this medication?

## Case Study

**Read the scenario and answer the following questions on a separate sheet of paper.**

Goldie, a 38-year-old teacher, has come to the clinic complaining of having "no energy or appetite" and yet her weight has increased by 15 pounds in the last month. You note that her hair is thin and her skin is dull. Laboratory work reveals an elevated level of thyroid stimulating hormone (TSH). A diagnosis of hypothyroidism is made.

1. What medication do you expect to be ordered for Goldie?

2. Explain the concept of "euthyroid" as it would relate to Goldie's condition.

3. One month after therapy has begun, Goldie calls the office to complain that she "can't sleep at all" since she started taking the medication. She says she tries to take it at the same time every morning but often forgets and takes it at dinnertime. What teaching, if any, does she need to help her with this problem?

# CHAPTER 32

# Antidiabetic Drugs

## Chapter Review and NCLEX® Examination Preparation

**Select the best answer for each question.**

1. When administering insulin, the nurse must keep in mind that which is the most immediate and serious adverse effect of insulin therapy?
   a. Hyperglycemia
   b. Hypoglycemia
   c. Bradycardia
   d. Orthostatic hypotension

2. A dose of long-acting insulin has been ordered for bedtime for a diabetic patient. The nurse expects to give which type of insulin?
   a. Regular
   b. Lispro
   c. NPH
   d. Glargine

3. A patient is to be placed on an insulin drip to control his high blood glucose levels. The nurse knows that the type of insulin that would be used for this intravenous infusion would be which of these?
   a. Regular
   b. Lispro
   c. NPH
   d. Glargine

4. While monitoring a patient who is receiving insulin therapy, the nurse observes for which signs of hypoglycemia?
   a. Decreased pulse and respiratory rates and flushed skin
   b. Increased pulse rate and a fruity, acetone breath odor
   c. Irritability, sweating, and confusion
   d. Increased urine output and edema

5. When will the nurse administer the drug acarbose (Precose)?
   a. With the first bite of a meal
   b. 15 minutes before a meal
   c. 30 minutes before a meal
   d. 1 hour after eating

6. A patient taking glipizide (Glucotrol) asks the nurse, "How does my insulin pill work, anyway?" Which information will the nurse provide to the patient regarding the mechanism of action of glipizide?
   a. "It increases insulin production."
   b. "It helps the body use insulin."
   c. "It decreases the amount of glucose made by the liver."
   d. "It decreases the amount of glucose the body takes in from food."

7. The nurse is reviewing the history of a patient who will be taking the amylin mimetic drug pramlintide (Symlin). Which condition is a contraindication to the use of this drug?
   a. Hypertension
   b. Coronary artery disease
   c. Hypothyroidism
   d. Gastroparesis

8. The nurse will monitor for significant interactions if sitagliptin (Januvia) is given with which of these?
   a. Corticosteroids
   b. Sulfonylureas
   c. Thyroid drugs
   d. Nonsteroidal antiinflammatory drugs

9. The sliding-scale insulin order reads, "Do bedside glucose testing before meals. For glucose results over 150 mg/dL, give regular (Humulin R) insulin, 1 unit for every 20 mg/dL over 150 mg/dL." If the blood glucose level is 238 mg/dL, the patient will receive _____ unit(s) of insulin.

10. A patient will be receiving NPH insulin 30 units combined with 7 units of regular insulin. Mark the insulin syringe at the line that indicates the combined dose of insulin.

## Critical Thinking and Application

**Answer the following questions on a separate sheet of paper.**

11. What is the mechanism of action of each drug?
    a. pramlintide (Symlin)
    b. metformin (Glucophage)

12. Alice occasionally experiences hypoglycemia as a result of her diabetes drug therapy.
    a. The nurse will teach Alice about what signs and symptoms of hypoglycemia?
    b. The nurse knows that one of the early signs of hypoglycemia is irritability. Why is this true?
    c. If Alice experiences hypoglycemia at home, what are the treatment options?

13. The newly graduated nurse is preparing a dose of Novolin-R insulin to administer to a patient.
    a. Before the nurse administers the medication, how will the nurse's co-worker verify the order?
    b. After examining the syringe, the nurse's co-worker tells the graduate nurse that the syringe must be discarded because the insulin is cloudy. The new graduate states, "Insulin is supposed to look this way." Who is right, the new nurse or the co-worker?
    c. The nurse examines the vial. A date on the label indicates that it has been on the shelf in this room for 2 months. Is this a problem?

14. Mrs. F. is 5 feet tall and weighs 180 pounds. During a routine physical, laboratory studies indicate an elevated fasting blood glucose level and a hemoglobin A1C level of 6.6%. The nurse's assessment of Mrs. F. reveals that she is a smoker with mild hypertension. The physician suspects type 2 diabetes. What initial treatment is indicated for Mrs. F.? Explain your answer.

15. Dennis takes glipizide (Glucotrol). He comes to the emergency department late one Sunday evening complaining that he feels weak, he vomited earlier, he has a headache, and his face "feels hot." You note that Dennis has profound flushing and is sweating.
    a. What do Dennis's signs and symptoms indicate?
    b. What will you assess immediately?
    c. What may have caused this?

16. A patient who has been taking metformin (Glucophage) for type 2 diabetes mellitus needs to have a radiology exam with contrast dye. What is the nurse's best action regarding the metformin?

17. For each symptom listed below, specify whether it is associated with hyperglycemia or hypoglycemia.
    a. Irritability
    b. Fatigue
    c. Polydipsia
    d. Tremors
    e. Sweating

## Case Study

**Read the scenario and answer the following questions on a separate sheet of paper.**

The physician is planning to prescribe glipizide (Glucotrol) for Mr. D., a 50-year-old financial advisor with a history of renal failure and type 2 diabetes. In particular, Mr. D. requires treatment for the short-term elevation in blood glucose level that occurs after he eats.

1. Are there specific guidelines for when this drug needs to be taken?

2. At a visit 3 months later, during a blood draw for fasting lab work, Mr. D. tells the nurse, "I've been good for the past few days, so I'm sure my fasting levels are okay. But thankfully the doctor won't know how I've been sneaking snacks." What laboratory test will be ordered to monitor Mr. D.'s diabetes, and what will this test indicate?

3. A few weeks later, Mr. D. comes down with gastroenteritis. He is vomiting and has been unable to eat all day. What should he do, and why?

# CHAPTER 33

# Adrenal Drugs

## Chapter Review and NCLEX® Examination Preparation

**Select the best answer for each question.**

1. A 50-year-old man has been taking prednisone (Deltasone) as part of treatment for bronchitis. He notices that the dosage of the medication decreases. During a follow-up office visit, he asks the nurse why he must continue the medication and why he cannot just stop taking it now that he feels better. What is the rationale behind the tapering dosages?
   a. Sudden discontinuation of this medication may result in adrenal insufficiency.
   b. The patient would experience withdrawal symptoms if the drug were discontinued abruptly.
   c. Cushing's syndrome may develop as a reaction to a sudden drop in serum cortisone levels.
   d. Once the symptoms have started to disappear, lower dosages are needed.

2. The nurse is reviewing the use of oral glucocorticoids. Which of these is the preferred oral glucocorticoid for antiinflammatory or immunosuppressant purposes?
   a. fludrocortisone (Florinef)
   b. dexamethasone (generic)
   c. prednisone (Deltasone)
   d. hydrocortisone (Solu-Cortef)

3. When monitoring a patient who is taking corticosteroids, the nurse observes for which adverse effects? *(Select all that apply.)*
   a. Fragile skin
   b. Hyperglycemia
   c. Nervousness
   d. Hypotension
   e. Weight loss
   f. Drowsiness

4. A patient has Cushing's syndrome. The nurse expects which drug to be used to inhibit the function of the adrenal cortex in the treatment of this syndrome?
   a. dexamethasone (generic)
   b. aminoglutethimide (Cytadren)
   c. hydrocortisone (Solu-Cortef)
   d. fludrocortisone (Florinef)

5. A patient who has been taking corticosteroids has developed a "moon face" and facial redness, and has many bruises on her arms. Which of these is the most appropriate nursing diagnosis?
   a. Risk for infection
   b. Imbalanced nutrition: Less than body requirements
   c. Deficient fluid volume
   d. Disturbed body image

6. Because corticosteroids may cause sodium retention, the nurse will closely monitor patients with which condition when administering corticosteroids?
   a. Diabetes mellitus
   b. Seizure disorders
   c. Heart failure
   d. Hyperthyroidism

7. The nurse is administering aminoglutethimide to a patient, and will monitor for which adverse effects? *(Select all that apply.)*
   a. Constipation
   b. Dizziness
   c. Anorexia
   d. Hypertension
   e. Lethargy

8. The order reads, "Give dexamethasone 1.5 mg, twice a day." The medication is available in 3-mg tablets. How many tablets will the nurse give for each dose?

   _____

9. An infant is to receive methylprednisolone (Solu-Medrol) 0.5 mg/kg IV every 6 hours. The infant weighs 14 pounds. How many milligrams of medication will this infant receive per dose? *(Record answer using one decimal place.)* _____

## Critical Thinking and Application

**Answer the following questions on a separate sheet of paper.**

10. Ms. R., a 30-year-old hospital receptionist, is receiving glucocorticoid therapy after a kidney transplant. The nurse is reviewing her drug regimen with her when she says that she frequently uses aspirin or ibuprofen to treat problems like headaches or menstrual cramps. She also mentions that she enjoys walking for exercise and likes to visit sick children on the hospital's pediatric ward when she has time. What issues will the nurse discuss with Ms. R.?

11. Peter has developed a severe skin rash after a camping trip. The health care provider is planning to prescribe prednisone (Deltasone). The nursing assessment reveals that Peter has type 1 diabetes.
    a. Does that finding affect Peter's treatment? Explain your answer.
    b. To help minimize gastrointestinal effects, what advice will the nurse have for someone taking an oral form of a systemic glucocorticoid?

12. The nurse is watching a student nurse prepare to apply a topical glucocorticoid to a patient's skin rash. After donning gloves, she places some of the medication on her finger. Should the nurse intervene, or is the student nurse doing fine so far? What other consideration is involved in determining the technique for applying a topical drug?

13. Nina has been prescribed a steroid drug delivered via inhaler. What special instructions will the nurse give her?

## Case Study

**Read the scenario and answer the following questions on a separate sheet of paper.**

Julie is in the urgent care center because of an exacerbation of asthma. She is usually able to control it with inhaled bronchodilators, but the physician decides to give her a short course of prednisone (Deltasone) in a dose that started high and then tapered down over 2 weeks.

1. Why is the dose tapered instead of just discontinued after a week?

2. Julie is taking prednisone for only two weeks. What are potential effects of long-term therapy, such as therapy for a month or more?

3. Julie tells the nurse that she takes an oral contraceptive and that she often uses ibuprofen (Advil) for her aches and pains. What concerns are there about drug interactions? Explain your answer.

4. What time of day will she take this drug? Explain.

# CHAPTER 34

# Women's Health Drugs

## Chapter Review and NCLEX® Examination Preparation

**Select the best answer for each question.**

1. When reviewing the health history of a patient who wants to begin taking oral contraceptives, the nurse recalls that which conditions are contraindications to this drug therapy? *(Select all that apply.)*
   a. Multiple sclerosis
   b. Pregnancy
   c. Thrombophlebitic disorders
   d. Hypothyroidism
   e. Estrogen-dependent cancers

2. When the nurse is teaching patients about postmenopausal estrogen replacement therapy, which statement is correct?
   a. "The smallest dose that is effective will be prescribed."
   b. "Oral forms should be taken on an empty stomach for best absorption."
   c. "Estrogen therapy should be long-term to prevent menopausal symptoms."
   d. "If estrogen is taken, supplemental calcium will not be needed."

3. When combination oral contraceptives are given to provide postcoital emergency contraception, the nurse must remember which fact?
   a. They are not effective if the woman is already pregnant.
   b. They should be taken within 12 hours of unprotected intercourse.
   c. They are given in one dose.
   d. They are intended to terminate pregnancy.

4. When reviewing an order for dinoprostone cervical gel (Prepidil), the nurse recalls that this drug is used for which purpose?
   a. To induce abortion during the third trimester
   b. To improve cervical ripening near term for labor induction
   c. To soften the cervix in women who are experiencing infertility problems
   d. To reduce postpartum uterine atony and hemorrhage

5. A pregnant woman is experiencing contractions. The nurse remembers that pharmacologic measures to stop contractions are used during which timeframe?
   a. Before the 20th week of gestation
   b. Between the 20th and 37th weeks
   c. After the 37th week
   d. At any time during the pregnancy if delivery is not desired

6. What patient teaching is appropriate for a patient taking alendronate (Fosamax)? *(Select all that apply.)*
   a. Take with food.
   b. Take at night just before going to bed.
   c. Take with an 8-oz glass of water.
   d. Take with a sip of water.
   e. Take first thing in the morning upon arising.
   f. Do not lie down for at least 30 minutes after taking.

7. A patient is beginning a new prescription of raloxifene (Evista). The nurse will teach the patient to expect which potential adverse effects? *(Select all that apply.)*
   a. Leg cramps
   b. Loss of appetite
   c. Diarrhea
   d. Hot flashes
   e. Drowsiness

8. The patient is to receive medroxyprogesterone (Depo-Provera) 500 mg weekly on Mondays for four weeks. The medication is available in vials of 400 mg/mL. How many milliliters will the nurse administer with each injection? *(Record answer using one decimal place.)* _____

Mark the syringe with the correct amount the nurse will draw up for this injection.

9. A patient is to receive megestrol (Megace) 400 mg each morning as an appetite stimulant. The medication is available in an oral suspension with a concentration of 40 mg/mL. How many milliliters will the nurse administer for this dose? _____

## Critical Thinking and Application

**Answer the following questions on a separate sheet of paper.**

10. Isabelle is a 48-year-old woman exhibiting symptoms of menopause. Assessment of Isabelle reveals a history of depression and mild arthritis.
    a. What will the nurse need to ask Isabelle and why?
    b. The health care provider decides to prescribe estrogen therapy. At this time, what does the nurse know about the dose and the length of time it will be administered?

11. Ms. K., age 25, has type 2 diabetes that is controlled by oral medications. She is at the clinic today because her menstrual periods have ceased. The nurse practitioner has decided to prescribe a hormonal drug.
    a. Which drug will the nurse practitioner likely prescribe?
    b. How will this hormone therapy potentially affect Ms. K.'s diabetes? What will she need to do?

12. Jacklyn receives a prescription for norethindrone and ethinyl estradiol (Ortho-Novum) for birth control. At a follow-up visit 4 months later, she tells the nurse practitioner, "I'm really messing up. I take the pills for 3 weeks, but when I'm off them for a week, sometimes I don't remember to start again!"
    a. What might the nurse practitioner suggest to help Jacklyn?

    b. Jacklyn then expresses concern that her menstrual bleeding, now that she is taking birth control pills, is "nothing compared with what it used to be." She asks the nurse practitioner whether she is okay. What will the nurse practitioner tell Jacklyn?

13. Ms. J., a sales associate in a bookstore, is being treated for fertility problems. She is currently on a drug regimen that includes human chorionic gonadotropin and clomiphene (Clomid). Why is she taking two fertility drugs?

14. Mrs. I. has been taking estrogen therapy for several weeks. During a routine checkup, she tells the nurse that she has not been able to quit smoking yet. She also mentions that she is going to Aruba for a vacation the next month. What patient teaching does Mrs. I. require?

15. Mrs. S., age 33, comes in for her yearly gynecologic examination, and the provider recommends alendronate (Fosamax), 5 mg daily. Mrs. S. experienced early menopause last year and asks the nurse, "Why did my doctor wait until now to start me on estrogen? I didn't need it before." What will the nurse explain about the purpose of this medication?

16. Mr. G. is receiving 400 mg of megestrol (Megace). This drug is a progestin, a female hormone. Why is a male patient receiving this medication?

## Case Study

**Read the scenario and answer the following questions on a separate sheet of paper.**

J.Q., age 24, has decided that she wants to try oral birth control, and is in the nurse practitioner's office today for an evaluation. During the health history, she tells the nurse that she has never used oral contraceptives but that she is currently sexually active. She also states that she takes no other medications or herbal products. After a physical assessment, the nurse practitioner prescribes norethindrone and ethinyl estradiol (Ortho-Novum 7/7/7) oral contraceptive.

1. What laboratory test is most important to check before J.Q. starts the oral contraceptive?

2. The nurse needs to assess for what other potential risk factors before J.Q. begins the oral contraceptive?

3. After 6 months, J.Q. calls the office and states, "I forgot to take my birth control pills for 3 days in a row. What do I do now?"

# CHAPTER 35

# Men's Health Drugs

## Chapter Review and NCLEX® Examination Preparation

**Select the best answer for each question.**

1. A 19-year-old college football player asks a nurse about taking steroids to help him "beef up" his muscles. Which statement is true?
   a. There should be no problems as long as he does not exceed the recommended dosage.
   b. Long-term use may cause a life-threatening liver condition.
   c. He would need to be careful to watch for excessive weight loss.
   d. These drugs also tend to increase the male's sperm count.

2. In which situations would androgens be prescribed for a woman? *(Select all that apply.)*
   a. Development of secondary sex characteristics
   b. Fibrocystic breast disease
   c. Ovarian cancer
   d. Treatment of endometriosis
   e. Postmenopausal osteoporosis prevention
   f. Inoperable breast cancer

3. A patient will be receiving testosterone therapy for male hypogonadism and has a new prescription for transdermal testosterone (Testoderm). The nurse needs to include which teaching about the use of this medication?
   a. Apply the patch only to the scrotum.
   b. Apply the patch to the chest, back, or shoulders.
   c. If the adverse effects become bothersome, the patient should stop using the patch.
   d. The patch should be applied to a different area of the upper body each day.

4. Before a patient begins therapy with finasteride (Proscar), the nurse should make sure that which laboratory test has been performed?
   a. Blood glucose level
   b. Complete blood count
   c. Urinalysis
   d. Prostate-specific antigen (PSA) level

5. A patient is taking finasteride (Proscar) for the treatment of benign prostatic hyperplasia. His wife, who is 3 months pregnant, is worried about the adverse effects that may occur with this drug. Which statement by the nurse is the most important at this time?
   a. "Gastric upset may be reduced if he takes this drug on an empty stomach."
   b. "He should notice therapeutic effects of increased libido and erection within 1 month."
   c. "This medication should not even be handled by pregnant women because it may harm the fetus."
   d. "He may experience transient hair loss while taking this medication."

6. A male patient wants to know if there are any drugs that can be used for baldness. The nurse knows that which drug, in low dosages, is used for androgenetic alopecia in men?
   a. finasteride (Propecia)
   b. vardenafil (Levitra)
   c. danazol (Danocrine)
   d. oxandrolone (Oxandrin)

7. A patient has asked for a new prescription for sildenafil (Viagra), an erectile dysfunction drug. As the nurse reviews his current medications, which drug, if taken by the patient, would cause a significant interaction?
   a. warfarin (Coumadin), an oral anticoagulant
   b. amoxicillin (Amoxil), an antibiotic
   c. esomeprazole (Nexium), a proton pump inhibitor
   d. isosorbide dinitrate (Isordil), a nitrate

8. A patient has a new prescription for finasteride (Proscar). The nurse will instruct the patient about which potential adverse effects? *(Select all that apply.)*
   a. Loss of erection
   b. Gynecomastia
   c. Headaches
   d. Increased libido
   e. Ejaculatory dysfunction

9. A patient is to receive testosterone cypionate (Depo-Testosterone) 300 mg every 2 weeks as an intramuscular injection. The medication is available in two strengths: 100 mg/mL and 200 mg/mL.
   a. Which is the most appropriate strength?
   
   _____
   
   b. How many milliliters will the nurse administer per injection? _____

## Critical Thinking and Application

**Answer the following questions on a separate sheet of paper.**

10. Mr. M. is being treated for hypogonadism. He has been taking intramuscular injections of testosterone cypionate (Depo-Testosterone) but has complained about the pain caused by the injections. Today he will be switched to an oral dosage form. He expects to get "testosterone pills." However, the nurse remembers the poor performance of the drug when given via that route, and she tells him that it will probably not be testosterone itself.
    a. Mr. M. is skeptical of switching drugs and asks for more information. Explain specifically why oral testosterone does not work well.
    b. What does the nurse predict Mr. M. will receive instead?
    c. Discuss potential contraindications that might apply to this patient.

11. Mr. M. is prescribed methyltestosterone buccally. He reports that he gets "tired" of waiting for the buccal tablet to dissolve and asks whether he can swallow or chew it, at least after it is mostly dissolved.
    a. If Mr. M. lets most of the tablet dissolve on its own, is it acceptable to compromise, for the sake of patient compliance, by letting him chew or swallow the rest?
    b. "And while we're on the subject," Mr. M. says, "I'm going on a fishing trip next week. I'd like not to have to bother with the pills. Can we work something out so that I stop temporarily and pick back up with the treatment as soon as I get back?" What is the best answer for Mr. M.?

12. Mr. H. has been prescribed finasteride (Proscar) for his benign prostatic hyperplasia. He asks, "How does it work?" The nurse explains that it will cause his prostate to decrease in size and alleviate discomfort. He is concerned about taking this new drug. What are the most important things for the nurse to include in his patient teaching plan?

13. Compare the application methods for the following forms of testosterone: Testoderm patch, Androderm patch, and AndroGel.

## Case Study

**Read the scenario and answer the following questions on a separate sheet of paper.**

Mr. E., age 72, has asked the physician for "help with a private matter." He tells the health care provider that he would like to try Viagra, "that drug that helps with a certain problem."

1. What assessment findings may contraindicate the use of sildenafil (Viagra) by Mr. E.?

2. If he is a candidate for therapy with Viagra, what patient teaching should he receive?

3. What concerns would there be about his liver function? About his vision?

4. When should he take this medication?

# CHAPTER 36

# Antihistamines, Decongestants, Antitussives, and Expectorants

## Chapter Review and NCLEX® Examination Preparation

**Select the best answer for each question.**

1. The nurse who is providing patient teaching about antihistamine use will include which information? *(Select all that apply.)*
   a. Antihistamines are best tolerated when taken with meals.
   b. The patient can chew gum if he or she experiences dry mouth.
   c. Drowsiness is a frequent side effect of antihistamines.
   d. Over-the-counter medications are generally safe to use with antihistamines.
   e. The patient should avoid drinking alcoholic beverages while on these drugs.

2. A patient asks the nurse about the newer antihistamines. He wants one that does not cause drowsiness. Which of these drugs is appropriate?
   a. loratadine (Claritin)
   b. diphenhydramine (Benadryl)
   c. dimenhydrinate (Dramamine)
   d. meclizine (Antivert)

3. Which drugs are considered first-line drugs for the treatment of nasal congestion? *(Select all that apply.)*
   a. Antihistamines such as diphenhydramine
   b. Decongestants such as naphazoline
   c. Antitussives such as dextromethorphan
   d. Expectorants such as guaifenesin
   e. Inhaled corticosteroids such as beclomethasone

4. When giving an antitussive, the nurse remembers that they are used primarily for what reason?
   a. To relieve nasal congestion
   b. To thin secretions to ease removal of excessive secretions
   c. To stop the cough reflex when the cough is nonproductive
   d. To suppress productive and nonproductive coughs

5. The nurse is administering an expectorant and will provide which teaching?
   a. Avoid fluids for 30 to 35 minutes after the dose.
   b. Drink extra fluids, unless contraindicated, to aid in expectoration of sputum.
   c. Avoid driving or operating heavy machinery while taking this medication.
   d. Expect secretions to become thicker.

6. A patient has been self-medicating with diphenhydramine (Benadryl) to help her sleep. She calls the clinic nurse to ask, "Why do I feel so tired during the day after I take this pill? I get a good night's sleep!" Which statement by the nurse is correct?
   a. "You are probably getting too much sleep."
   b. "You are taking too much of the drug."
   c. "This drug is not really meant to help people sleep."
   d. "This drug often causes a 'hangover effect' during the day after taking it."

7. A patient is asking about taking an antihistamine for springtime allergies. The nurse assesses for contraindications to antihistamine therapy. Which of these conditions, if present, would be a contraindication? *(Select all that apply.)*
   a. Type 2 diabetes mellitus
   b. Benign prostatic hyperplasia
   c. Hyperthyroidism
   d. Narrow-angle glaucoma
   e. Asthma

8. A patient is to receive guaifenesin, 300 mg, via his nasogastric tube. The available medication is syrup, 100 mg/5 mL.

   a. How many milliliters will the nurse administer?

   _____

   b. Mark the medication cup with your answer.

9. A 5-year-old child is to receive a one-time dose of diphenhydramine (Benadryl), 6.25 mg PO. The medication is available in a liquid syrup form with a concentration of 12.5 mg/5 mL. How many milliliters will the nurse administer for this dose?

   _____

## Critical Thinking and Application

**Answer the following questions on a separate sheet of paper.**

10. Mrs. L. was seen in the office several days ago with a common cold. She has been on decongestant therapy with naphazoline nasal spray (Privine) since that time. Today she calls to say, "I thought I was getting over this, but suddenly my nose is more stuffed up than ever." Does Mrs. L. possibly need a stronger dosage of the decongestant? Explain your answer.

11. Keith has been using a topical nasal decongestant for the past few days. He calls the health care provider's office to report that he is feeling nervous and dizzy and that his heart seems to be racing. What might be the cause of Keith's symptoms?

12. How does benzonatate (Tessalon Perles) differ from other antitussive drugs in its mechanism of action? In its drug interaction profile?

13. One day the nurse encounters her neighbor Irene as she is returning home from work. Irene is on her way to the drugstore, she tells the nurse, because she has been experiencing a nonproductive cough and wants to get a cough medicine "to loosen things up." The nurse recalls that Irene mentioned a few months ago that she has problems with her thyroid. How should the nurse respond to Irene's comment? Explain your answer.

14. Lisa is a 5-year-old patient who has bronchitis accompanied by a nonproductive cough. The provider has prescribed Robitussin DM for the cough. Lisa's father tells the nurse that his 11-year-old son was prescribed Robitussin A-C several months earlier for a severe cough. He asks whether his son's cough medicine would help Lisa because "there's plenty left in the bottle." What will the nurse tell him?

15. Britney gave birth recently and is breastfeeding her baby. She calls the pediatrician's office because she wants to take an over-the-counter antihistamine for her allergies. "It's okay now that I've given birth, right?" What is the nurse's best answer?

## Case Study

**Read the scenario and answer the following questions on a separate sheet of paper.**

James, a 35-year-old electrician, is seen in the emergency department with a rash on his arms and hands that appeared after he was working in his yard. You suspect that the physician will prescribe topical diphenhydramine (Benadryl), but during the nursing assessment, James tells you that he has diabetes.

1. How does James's diabetes affect his possible treatment with diphenhydramine?

2. If James does receive a topical diphenhydramine preparation, what other drug might be found in combination with it?

The topical medication did not help his rash, and James has been switched to oral diphenhydramine. He tells you that he expects to return to work tomorrow and hopes this medication "does the trick."

3. What cautions, if any, should James be aware of while taking this medication?

4. Are there any concerns with drug interactions?

# CHAPTER 37

# Respiratory Drugs

## Chapter Review and NCLEX® Examination Preparation

**Select the best answer for each of the following.**

1. The nurse is teaching a group of patients about the use of bronchodilators. It is important to remind them that using bronchodilators too frequently may cause which adverse effects? *(Select all that apply.)*
   a. Blurred vision
   b. Increased heart rate
   c. Decreased heart rate
   d. Nausea
   e. Nervousness
   f. Tremors

2. For patients taking a leukotriene receptor antagonist, the nurse should include which information in the patient teaching?
   a. If a dose is missed, the patient may take a double dose to maintain blood levels.
   b. The patient should gargle or rinse the mouth after using the inhaler.
   c. The medication should be taken at the first sign of bronchospasm.
   d. Improvement should be seen within a week of use.

3. Which drug acts by blocking leukotrienes, thus reducing inflammation in the lungs?
   a. cromolyn (Intal)
   b. montelukast (Singulair)
   c. theophylline (Elixophyllin)
   d. albuterol (Proventil)

4. A patient is experiencing status asthmaticus. The nurse will prepare to administer which drug first?
   a. epinephrine
   b. methylprednisolone (Solu-Medrol)
   c. cromolyn (Intal)
   d. montelukast (Singulair)

5. When a patient is taking parenteral xanthine derivatives such as aminophylline, the nurse should monitor for which adverse effect?
   a. Decreased respirations
   b. Hypotension
   c. Tachycardia
   d. Hypoglycemia

6. A patient who has asthma may be prescribed which type of inhaled drug for its antiinflammatory effects?
   a. Corticosteroid
   b. Anticholinergic
   c. Xanthine derivative
   d. Beta adrenergic

7. A patient is to receive a new prescription for an ipratropium (Atrovent) inhaler. The nurse will assess for which potential contraindications? *(Select all that apply.)*
   a. Allergy to soy lecithin
   b. Allergy to peanuts
   c. Allergy to iodine products
   d. Hypertension
   e. Seizure disorders

8. A patient has a new prescription for a Combivent (ipratropium bromide/albuterol sulfate) metered-dose inhaler. The patient is to take two puffs, four times a day. The inhaler contains 200 "puffs." In how many days should the patient replace the inhaler? _____

9. A 6-year-old child is to receive albuterol (Proventil) 0.2 mg/kg PO two times a day. The child weighs 40 pounds. How many milligrams will the child receive per dose? *(Record answer using one decimal place.)*

   _____

# Critical Thinking and Application

**Answer the following questions on a separate sheet of paper.**

10. Tom, a 70-year-old retiree who smoked for 40 years, has been diagnosed with chronic obstructive pulmonary disease (COPD); the treatment regimen prescribed includes theophylline (Theo-Dur). After a few weeks, Tom tells the nurse that he is experiencing nausea and "bad heartburn at night." The laboratory studies show the level of theophylline in his blood to be 30 mcg/mL. What might be wrong with Tom, and how can it be corrected?

11. Sylvia has come to the clinic today complaining of nausea, palpitations, and anxiety. She says that her heart feels "as if it's going to fly out of my chest." Physical examination confirms an increased heart rate. Sylvia's records indicate that she has asthma for which she uses an albuterol inhaler. When asked about the inhaler, she states that she uses it "whenever I feel short of breath." What is causing Sylvia's complaints?

12. Mrs. V., a 65-year-old office manager, has arthritis, glaucoma, and emphysema. The health care provider is planning treatment for her emphysema.
    a. What three types of drugs might be considered for treatment of COPD?
    b. What factor must the provider keep in mind when determining the best drug for Mrs. V.?

13. Several months ago, the physician prescribed an orally administered corticosteroid for Mr. Z., who has chronic bronchial asthma.
    a. What are the disadvantages of administering the corticosteroids orally? Is there an alternative route?
    b. Today the physician adds beclomethasone dipropionate (Beclovent) to Mr. Z.'s drug regimen and also reduces the dosage of the oral corticosteroid. Why was the oral corticosteroid not discontinued?

14. Alice has been treated for asthma for several months and has the following inhalers: albuterol (Proventil) and fluticasone (Flovent). Which one should she choose if she experiences an asthma attack? Explain your answer.

15. Justin calls the nurse at the office because he experiences "palpitations and a racing heart" every morning after breakfast. He is taking theophylline (Theo-Dur) as part of his treatment for asthma. Upon questioning, he states that he has been drinking an extra cup of coffee in the morning "to get going" because his coughing has kept him from sleeping well. What could be his problem?

# Case Study

**Read the scenario and answer the following questions on a separate sheet of paper.**

Jennie has been treated for adult-onset asthma for 3 years. She has been doing fairly well with her inhalers, but today she receives a prescription for montelukast (Singulair), one 10-mg tablet daily.

1. How does this medication differ from the corticosteroids that are used to reduce inflammation?

2. Jennie says, "I hope this medicine works better than the other one I took when I had an asthma attack." How will you reply?

3. Jennie takes ibuprofen (Advil) on occasion for arthritic pain. How do you advise Jennie regarding taking over-the-counter drugs with montelukast?

4. After 3 months, Jennie stops taking the montelukast. She says, "My symptoms are better, and I don't want to take medicine unless I need it." Is this appropriate?

# CHAPTER 38

# Antibiotics Part 1

## Critical Thinking Crossword

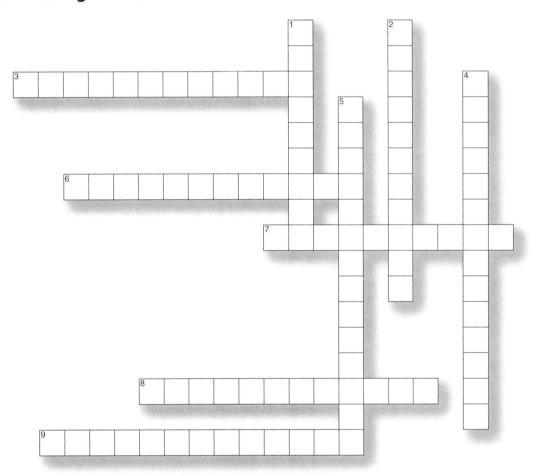

### Across

3. Antibiotics taken before exposure to an infectious organism in an effort to prevent the development of infection
6. This class of antibiotics may cause tooth discoloration in children under age 8.
7. Anaphylactic reactions are common with this class of antibiotics.
8. Antibiotics that kill bacteria
9. There is a chance of cross-reactivity between this class of antibiotics and the class in 7 Across.

### Down

1. The classification for the drug erythromycin
2. This class of antibiotics is commonly used for urinary tract infections.
4. Antibiotics that inhibit the growth of bacteria
5. An infection that occurs during antimicrobial treatment for another infection and involves overgrowth of a nonsusceptible organism

## Chapter Review and NCLEX® Examination Preparation

**Select the best answer for each question.**

1. The nurse is reviewing the drugs ordered for a patient. A drug interaction occurs between penicillins and which drugs? *(Select all that apply.)*
   a. Alcohol
   b. Oral contraceptives
   c. Digoxin
   d. Nonsteroidal antiinflammatory drugs
   e. Warfarin
   f. Anticonvulsants

2. Which intervention is important for the nurse to perform before beginning antibiotic therapy?
   a. Obtain a specimen for culture and sensitivity.
   b. Give with an antacid to reduce gastrointestinal (GI) upset.
   c. Monitor for adverse effects.
   d. Restrict oral fluids.

3. The nurse will instruct a patient who is receiving a tetracycline antibiotic to take it using which guideline?
   a. It needs to be taken with milk.
   b. It needs to be taken with 8 oz of water.
   c. It needs to be taken 30 minutes before iron preparations are taken.
   d. An antacid should also be taken to decrease GI discomfort.

4. A patient is to receive antibiotic therapy with a cephalosporin. When assessing the patient's drug history, the nurse recognizes that an allergy to which drug class may be a possible contraindication to cephalosporin therapy?
   a. Cardiac glycosides
   b. Thiazide diuretics
   c. Penicillins
   d. Macrolides

5. When asked about drug allergies, a patient says, "I can't take sulfa drugs because I'm allergic to them." Which question will the nurse ask next?
   a. "Do you have any other drug allergies?"
   b. "Who prescribed that drug for you?"
   c. "How long ago did this happen?"
   d. "What happened when you took the sulfa drug?"

6. Which statement accurately describes the action of antiseptics?
   a. They are used to kill organisms on nonliving objects.
   b. They are used to kill organisms on living tissue.
   c. They are used to sterilize equipment.
   d. They are used to inhibit the growth of organisms on living tissue.

7. During a class on health care–associated infections, the nurse shares several facts about these infections. Which statements about health care–associated infections are true? *(Select all that apply.)*
   a. They are contracted in the home or community.
   b. They are contracted in a hospital or institution.
   c. They are more difficult to treat.
   d. The organisms that cause these infections are more virulent.
   e. The infection is incubating at the time of admission.

8. A patient is to receive 2 million units of penicillin G potassium per day, every 6 hours in IV piggyback doses. The medication is available in vials of 1 million units/50 mL, and each dose needs to be mixed in 50 mL of $D_5W$. How many milliliters will the nurse draw up for each IV piggyback dose?

   _____

9. A patient is to receive medication through a feeding tube. The order reads, "Give amoxicillin 250 mg per feeding tube every 8 hours." When reconstituted, the concentration of the medication is 125 mg/5 mL. How many milliliters will the nurse give per dose?

   _____

## Critical Thinking and Application

**Answer the following questions on a separate sheet of paper.**

10. A patient is receiving imipenem/cilastatin (Primaxin) and asks the nurse, "Why does that medicine bag have two names listed? Am I receiving two drugs?" What is the best explanation for the patient?

11. Mr. R., a 50-year-old banker, is scheduled for colon surgery tomorrow. The surgeon is planning to administer a prophylactic antibiotic. What drug is frequently used for this purpose, and why?

12. Sean is a 19-year-old college freshman who has been diagnosed with gonorrhea. The provider has prescribed doxycycline therapy. During the nursing assessment, Sean discusses his diet, which includes "lots of meat, milk, and veggies." Sean also tells the nurse that he jogs frequently and is a member of the tennis team.
    a. In addition to instruction about sexually transmitted infections, what patient teaching about the medication does Sean require?
    b. A few days later, Sean calls and complains of an upset stomach and diarrhea. What does the nurse suspect might be wrong with Sean?

13. Sandra has bronchitis and has been taking an antibiotic for 1 week. She calls the nurse and complains of severe genital itching and a whitish discharge in her vaginal area. What has happened, and what caused it?

## Case Study

**Read the scenario and answer the following questions on a separate sheet of paper.**

A 78-year-old patient admitted to the hospital with a stroke 2 days earlier has developed a urinary tract infection. His Foley catheter is draining urine that is cloudy and dark yellowish-orange with a strong odor. He is receiving an intravenous heparin infusion and has a history of type 2 diabetes. The physician orders co-trimoxazole (Bactrim).

1. What will the nurse assess before giving this medication?

2. Are there any potential drug interactions?

3. Why was this particular antibiotic chosen?

4. Is this antibiotic bactericidal or bacteriostatic? Explain.

# CHAPTER 39

# Antibiotics Part 2

## Chapter Review and NCLEX® Examination Preparation

**Select the best answer for each question.**

1. When patients are receiving aminoglycosides, the nurse must monitor for tinnitus and dizziness, which may indicate which problem?
   a. Cardiotoxicity
   b. Hepatotoxicity
   c. Ototoxicity
   d. Nephrotoxicity

2. A patient is being prepared for colon surgery and will be receiving neomycin tablets during the day before surgery. He asks the nurse why he needs to take this medicine before he even has surgery. What is the nurse's best response?
   a. "This medicine helps to clear out your bowels before surgery."
   b. "It helps to reduce the number of bacteria in your intestines before surgery."
   c. "It is given to sterilize your bowel before surgery."
   d. "It is given to prevent an infection after surgery."

3. A patient has been admitted to the unit with a stage IV pressure ulcer. After 2 days, the wound culture results come back positive for methicillin-resistant *Staphylococcus aureus* (MRSA). The nurse knows that the drug of choice for the treatment of MRSA infection is which drug?
   a. vancomycin (Vancocin)
   b. gentamicin (Garamycin)
   c. ciprofloxacin (Cipro)
   d. colistimethate (Coly-Mycin)

4. A patient who is receiving vancomycin (Vancocin) therapy needs to notify the nurse immediately if which effects are noted? *(Select all that apply.)*
   a. Ringing in the ears
   b. Dizziness
   c. Hearing loss
   d. Flushing of the face
   e. Nausea

5. After an infusion of colistimethate (Coly-Mycin), the nurse will report to the prescriber if the patient complains of which adverse effects? *(Select all that apply.)*
   a. Numbness
   b. Vertigo
   c. Upset stomach
   d. Insomnia
   e. Dizziness

6. The nurse is reviewing the list of medications for a patient who will be starting antibiotic therapy with an aminoglycoside. Which medication, if present, may present a potential interaction with the aminoglycoside? *(Select all that apply.)*
   a. metoprolol (Lopressor), a beta blocker
   b. furosemide (Lasix), a loop diuretic
   c. warfarin (Coumadin), an oral anticoagulant
   d. vancomycin (Vancocin), an antibiotic
   e. levothyroxine (Synthroid), a thyroid hormone

7. A patient will be taking oral neomycin before having bowel surgery. The order reads, "Give 1 g per hour for 4 doses PO." The patient cannot swallow pills, so an oral solution has been ordered. The solution is 125 mg/5 mL. How many milliliters will the nurse give for each 1-g dose? _____

8. The order reads, "Give colistimethate (Coly-Mycin) 2.5 mg/kg/day IVPB. Infuse over 5 minutes." The patient weighs 165 pounds. How many milligrams will the patient receive per dose? *(Record answer using one decimal place.)* _____

## Critical Thinking and Application

**Answer the following questions on a separate sheet of paper.**

9. Angie has a severe infection and is receiving an aminoglycoside once a day. She says, "They tell me I have a terrible infection. Why am I not getting the antibiotic more than once a day? I don't understand!" What will the nurse tell her?

10. Explain the concept of "trough" levels during aminoglycoside therapy and the way in which renal function is monitored.

11. Greg has been taking amiodarone (Cordarone) for a heart rhythm problem. He has developed an infection from an open wound, and the sensitivity report indicates that levofloxacin (Levaquin) is the best choice to fight this infection. Are there any concerns?

12. Nitrofurantoin (Macrodantin) has been ordered for a patient who has a severe urinary tract infection caused by *Escherichia coli*. Explain why this drug is used for this type of infection.

## Case Study

**Read the scenario and answer the following questions on a separate sheet of paper.**

Virgil has been admitted to your unit and placed on aminoglycoside therapy as part of treatment for a urinary tract infection with *Pseudomonas*. He is 65 years old, awake and alert, but anxious about his problem and wants to "hurry up and get better."

1. For which two serious toxicities will you monitor, what are their symptoms, and how can they be prevented?

2. The physician adds penicillin to Virgil's drug regimen. Explain the reason for this.

3. Virgil's "trough" aminoglycoside level is 3.0 mcg/mL, and his serum creatinine level is increased from 2 days earlier. Are these results a concern? What will you do? Explain.

# CHAPTER 40

# Antiviral Drugs

## Chapter Review and NCLEX® Examination Preparation

**Select the best answer for each question.**

1. The nurse is administering acyclovir (Zovirax) and recalls that it is considered the drug of choice for treatment of which viral infection?
   a. Cytomegalovirus (CMV)
   b. Human immunodeficiency virus (HIV)
   c. Respiratory syncytial virus (RSV)
   d. Varicella-zoster virus (VZV)

2. When administering ganciclovir (Cytovene), the nurse keeps in mind that the main dose-limiting toxicity for this drug is which condition?
   a. Renal failure
   b. Gastrointestinal disturbances
   c. Peripheral neuropathy
   d. Bone marrow suppression

3. When reviewing the health history of a patient who is to receive foscarnet (Foscavir), the nurse knows that which condition would be a contraindication to its use?
   a. Renal failure
   b. CMV retinitis
   c. Asthma
   d. Immunosuppression

4. When reviewing the use of amantadine (Symmetrel), the nurse expects that the drug would be used most appropriately in which patient?
   a. A 29-year-old man who tests positive for HIV
   b. A 22-year-old woman who is in her eighth month of pregnancy and tests positive for HIV
   c. A heart transplant patient who has influenza A
   d. Older adult patients who require prophylaxis for influenza B

5. A patient calls the clinic nurse to ask for oseltamivir (Tamiflu) "because I was exposed to the flu over the weekend at a family reunion." The nurse knows that Tamiflu is indicated for which condition? *(Select all that apply.)*
   a. Prevention of infection after exposure to influenza virus types A and B
   b. Reduction of the duration of influenza in adults
   c. Treatment of topical herpes simplex virus infections
   d. Reduction of the severity of shingles symptoms
   e. Treatment of lower respiratory tract infections caused by respiratory syncytial virus

6. The nurse is preparing to administer the aerosol form of ribavirin. Which condition is a contraindication to the drug?
   a. Asthma
   b. Pregnancy
   c. Hypertension
   d. Type 2 diabetes

7. The order reads, "Give acyclovir, 0.25 g IVPB now." The medication comes in a vial that contains 1000 mg. The label reads, "Add 20 mL of diluent for a solution that contains 50 mg/mL." The medication will be added to 100 mL $D_5W$ for IV piggyback infusion. How many milliliters of reconstituted medication will the nurse add to the 100-mL bag for infusion?

   _____

8. The order for a 1-year-old child reads, "Give amantadine (Symmetrel) 4.4 mg/kg/day in 2 divided doses." The child weighs 22 pounds. How many milligrams will the child receive per dose?

   _____

## Critical Thinking and Application

**Answer the following questions on a separate sheet of paper.**

9. Amy is 12 weeks into her pregnancy when she discovers that she is HIV-positive. Amy is very upset and says, "I won't live long enough to have this baby. We're both going to die." Is it possible to treat Amy and/or the fetus? Explain your answer.

10. Bailey, a 53-year-old teacher, has shingles.
    a. What drug will the nurse expect the physician to prescribe?
    b. Several months later, Bailey calls the office to say that her symptoms have returned. What action will the nurse expect to be taken now?

11. Brenda, age 2 years, has bronchopneumonia caused by respiratory syncytial virus (RSV).
    a. What antiviral drug is used to treat RSV?
    b. Brenda's mother wonders whether the treatment will be completed before Brenda's birthday, which is 2 weeks away. What will the nurse tell her?

12. A 25-year-old man has acquired immunodeficiency syndrome (AIDS). He was treated with zidovudine (Retrovir) for several months, but now the physician has switched him to didanosine powder (Videx). What frequently is the reason that patients are switched from zidovudine to another anti-HIV drug?

13. The nurse overhears a co-worker explaining to a student nurse the procedure for administering acyclovir intravenously. "After the acyclovir is diluted in sterile water," the co-worker says, "we'll administer this over at least an hour." Should the nurse intervene? Explain your answer.

14. Stacy has had flu symptoms for 4 days and feels miserable. She calls the nurse practitioner in the clinic to ask for "that medicine, Tamiflu, that is supposed to make the flu symptoms better." Will Stacy receive this medication at this time? Explain your answer.

15. Matt has had an organ transplant. What antiviral drug may be used, even though he does not have a viral infection at this time?

## Case Study

**Read the scenario and answer the following questions on a separate sheet of paper.**

Mr. C., a 30-year-old stockbroker, has been diagnosed with genital herpes simplex type 2 (HSV-2) infection. The health care provider has prescribed topical acyclovir (Zovirax).

1. What patient teaching do you provide to Mr. C. regarding administration of this drug?

2. Mr. C. asks you how long it will take for the acyclovir to cure his herpes. What is your reply?

3. What else will you discuss with Mr. C., who is sexually active?

4. HSV-2 is closely related to which other viruses?

# CHAPTER 41

# Antitubercular Drugs

## Chapter Review and NCLEX® Examination Preparation

**Select the best answer for each question.**

1. A patient will be receiving long-term isoniazid (INH) therapy. What laboratory tests are most important for the nurse to monitor during therapy?
   a. Liver enzyme levels
   b. Hematocrit and hemoglobin level
   c. Creatinine level
   d. Platelet count

2. The nurse should include which information in the teaching plan for a patient who is taking isoniazid (INH)?
   a. Urine and saliva may be reddish-orange.
   b. Pyridoxine (vitamin $B_6$) may be needed to prevent neurotoxicity.
   c. Injection sites should be rotated daily.
   d. The medication should be taken with an antacid to reduce gastric distress.

3. Patients who are in the initial period of treatment for tuberculosis need to be taught to perform which procedures? *(Select all that apply.)*
   a. Wash their hands and cover their mouths when coughing or sneezing to reduce the spread of tuberculosis.
   b. Throw away dirty tissues in the proper receptacle.
   c. Be sure to get adequate rest, nutrition, and relaxation.
   d. Skip medication doses occasionally if gastric distress occurs.
   e. Avoid all visitors until symptoms improve.

4. A patient newly diagnosed with tuberculosis asks the nurse how long he will need to take "all this medicine." The nurse replies that drug therapy for active tuberculosis may need to last how long?
   a. 6 months
   b. 12 months
   c. 24 months
   d. A lifetime

5. The nurse is explaining antitubercular therapy to a patient. The patient asks, "Why do I have to take so many different medications?" What is the nurse's best response?
   a. "It helps to prevent the tuberculosis from becoming resistant to the drugs."
   b. "It makes sure that the disease is cured."
   c. "These medications will reduce symptoms immediately."
   d. "You will have fewer side effects."

6. The nurse is reviewing the medication list of a patient who has been newly diagnosed with tuberculosis and will be taking rifampin (Rifadin). Which class of drugs, if taken with the rifampin, may cause increased metabolism? *(Select all that apply.)*
   a. Beta blockers
   b. Proton pump inhibitors
   c. Selective serotonin reuptake inhibitors
   d. Oral anticoagulants
   e. Oral antidiabetic drugs

7. The patient is to receive isoniazid (INH) 0.3 g daily. The medication is available as 100-mg tablets. How many tablets will the nurse administer per dose?

   _____

8. The patient has new orders for pyrazinamide, 30 mg/kg/day. The patient weighs 132 pounds. How many milligrams will the patient receive per day? Is this dosage safe? _____

## Critical Thinking and Application

**Answer the following questions on a separate sheet of paper.**

9. Diane, a 33-year-old proofreader, has been prescribed prophylactic isoniazid (INH) treatment.
   a. What laboratory studies should be performed before the start of therapy? Why?
   b. After Diane has taken isoniazid for 2 months, the physician significantly reduces her dosage of the drug. Why might that be?

10. Ms. I. is undergoing antitubercular therapy that includes streptomycin and rifampin.
    a. How is streptomycin administered?
    b. Ms. I. takes an oral contraceptive. Is that a concern given Ms. I.'s antitubercular therapy? Explain your answer.

11. Why would an eye examination be performed before instituting antitubercular therapy?

12. Mr. F. is on antitubercular therapy. During his first follow-up visit, he is evasive when the nurse asks him about his compliance with his therapy regimen. He does tell the nurse that he has been very busy lately, entertaining various clients "at everything from cocktail parties to big sit-down dinners."
    a. What issues will the nurse discuss with Mr. F.?
    b. Several weeks later, Mr. F. returns for another follow-up visit. On examination, the nurse sees no apparent signs of the tuberculosis. How can Mr. F.'s therapeutic response be confirmed?

13. Frannie is a homeless 68-year-old woman who lives in a shelter some of the time. She was diagnosed at the community health clinic with tuberculosis and antitubercular therapy has been instituted.
    a. What patient education issues are of particular concern in Frannie's case?
    b. Frannie is staying at the shelter and seems to be handling her medication regimen well, but one day she comes by the clinic to tell the nurse that she is afraid the medication may be bad for her. "Whenever I go to the bathroom, everything is reddish-orange," she says. What do you suspect is going on and what do you tell Frannie?

## Case Study

**Read the scenario and answer the following questions on a separate sheet of paper.**

George, a 73-year-old retired plant foreman, has been diagnosed with tuberculosis. Nursing assessment reveals a history of gout and diabetes. He also has a history of heavy drinking.

1. What considerations will the physician keep in mind when deciding on a first-line drug for George?

2. George tells you that he has been told that he has a "liver problem." His medical record mentions that he is a slow acetylator. How does this affect his therapy?

3. How will his history of "heavy drinking" affect his therapy?

4. You instruct George about taking vitamin $B_6$ along with the isoniazid (INH) therapy. When he asks you why this is necessary, what will you tell him?

# CHAPTER 42

# Antifungal Drugs

## Chapter Review and NCLEX® Examination Preparation

**Match each definition with the corresponding term.**

1. _____ Single-celled fungi that reproduce by budding

2. _____ One of the major chemical groups of antifungal drugs; includes amphotericin B and nystatin

3. _____ A very large, diverse group of eukaryotic, thallus-forming microorganisms that requires an external carbon source

4. _____ Another of the major groups of antifungal drugs; includes ketoconazole

5. _____ A term for fungal infection of the mouth

6. _____ One of the older antifungal drugs that acts by preventing susceptible fungi from reproducing

7. _____ The drug of choice for many severe, systemic fungal infections; also, the oldest antifungal drug

8. _____ An antifungal drug commonly used to treat candidal diaper rash

9. _____ An infection caused by fungi

10. _____ Multicellular fungi characterized by long, branching filaments called *hyphae*, which entwine to form a mycelium

a. Thrush
b. Molds
c. griseofulvin
d. Mycosis
e. Polyenes
f. Fungi
g. Imidazoles
h. amphotericin B
i. nystatin
j. Yeast

**Select the best answer for each question.**

11. An infant has thrush. The nurse expects to administer which drug for the treatment of thrush?
    a. amphotericin B (Fungizone)
    b. fluconazole (Diflucan)
    c. nystatin (Mycostatin)
    d. miconazole (Monistat)

12. During an infusion of amphotericin B, the nurse monitors for which adverse effects? *(Select all that apply.)*
    a. Nausea
    b. Fever
    c. Malaise
    d. Constipation
    e. Chills
    f. Hypertension

13. A patient calls the gynecologic clinic because she has begun to menstruate while taking vaginal cream for a vaginal infection. She asks the nurse, "What should I do about taking this vaginal medicine right now?" Which is the nurse's best response?
    a. "You need to stop the medication until the menstrual flow has stopped."
    b. "Just take the medication at night only."
    c. "You should stop the medication for 3 days, then start it again."
    d. "It's okay to continue to take the medication."

14. A patient will be receiving a one-dose treatment for vaginal candidiasis. The nurse expects to administer which drug?
    a. ketoconazole (Nizoral)
    b. fluconazole (Diflucan)
    c. griseofulvin
    d. terbinafine (Lamisil)

15. The nurse is administering an antifungal drug to a patient who has a severe systemic fungal infection. Which drug is most appropriate for this patient?
    a. amphotericin B (Fungizone)
    b. fluconazole (Diflucan)
    c. griseofulvin
    d. flucytosine

16. The nurse is administering a new order for amphotericin B (Fungizone) and reviews the patient's current medications. Which medications, if also ordered, may cause an interaction with the amphotericin B? *(Select all that apply.)*
    a. digoxin (Lanoxin), a cardiac glycoside
    b. metoprolol (Lopressor), a beta blocker
    c. warfarin (Coumadin), an oral anticoagulant
    d. levothyroxine (Synthroid), a hormone replacement
    e. hydrochlorothiazide, a thiazide diuretic

17. The order reads, "Give amphotericin B (Fungizone) 20 mg in 300 mL D$_5$W over 6 hours." The nurse will set the infusion pump to what rate? _____

18. A patient is to receive voriconazole (Vfend) as follows: 6 mg/kg q12h × 2 doses, then change to 4 mg/kg q12h. The patient weighs 242 pounds. How much will the patient receive for each 6 mg/kg dose? The 4 mg/kg dose? _____

## Critical Thinking and Application

**Answer the following questions on a separate sheet of paper.**

19. Mr. K. has cryptococcal meningitis, and the physician has prescribed fluconazole (Diflucan).
    a. Why did the physician choose this drug rather than one of the other -azole antifungals?
    b. The results of Mr. K.'s cerebrospinal fluid culture eventually come back negative. When he hears the good news, he says, "Great! I'm tired of taking this medicine." What will be the nurse's response?

20. The physician is planning intravenous amphotericin B (Fungizone) therapy for James.
    a. What guidelines will the nurse follow in administering the drug?
    b. What adverse effects will the nurse expect James to experience?
    c. Should the nurse stop the infusion if those effects occur? Explain your answer.

21. Chrissie has a prescription for nystatin oral troches to treat thrush. After a few days, she calls the nurse practitioner to report that her mouth is not better. "I've been chewing them slowly every time I take one. I don't understand why it's not working!" she says. What is the nurse's response?

22. David has a severe fungal infection and the physician has prescribed a lipid formulation of amphotericin B (Fungizone). Why was this formulation ordered, and what are the advantages and disadvantages?

## Case Study

**Read the scenario and answer the following questions on a separate sheet of paper.**

Sally has pneumonia with invasive aspergillosis. She has been treated for 2 weeks without showing much improvement and the physician is considering starting voriconazole (Vfend) therapy. Sally is also receiving a medication for treatment of a cardiac dysrhythmia.

1. What is the reason for starting voriconazole therapy now rather than earlier?

2. What consideration may arise depending on the cardiac medication she is taking?

3. What needs to be monitored while she is taking voriconazole?

# CHAPTER 43

# Antimalarial, Antiprotozoal, and Anthelmintic Drugs

## Chapter Review and NCLEX® Examination Preparation

**Select the best answer for each question.**

1. Before beginning antiprotozoal therapy, the nurse will assess for which possible contraindications?
   a. Underlying renal or liver disease and pregnancy
   b. Porphyria and glucose-6-phosphate dehydrogenase (G6PD) deficiency
   c. Glaucoma, cataracts, anemia, and petechiae
   d. Constipation, gastritis, and lactose intolerance

2. The nurse will warn the patient taking metronidazole (Flagyl) about which possible adverse effect? *(Select all that apply.)*
   a. Reddish-orange urine
   b. Anorexia
   c. Cough
   d. Weakness
   e. Headache
   f. A metallic taste in the mouth

3. A patient is taking quinine therapy for malaria. The prescriber has decided to add a sulfonamide or tetracycline drug along with the quinine. When the nurse gives the patient the prescription for this new medication, the patient is upset about having to take "another pill." What is the nurse's best explanation for the second drug?
   a. "The antibiotic treats bacterial infections that accompany malaria."
   b. "The antibiotic reduces the severe adverse effects of quinine."
   c. "The antibiotic will help the quinine to work more effectively against the malaria."
   d. "The antibiotic therapy is also needed to kill the parasite that causes malaria."

4. Which drugs are used mainly for the management of *Pneumocystis jirovecii* (formerly *Pneumocystis carinii*) pneumonia? *(Select all that apply.)*
   a. metronidazole (Flagyl)
   b. pentamidine (NebuPent)
   c. ivermectin (Stromectol)
   d. pyrantel (Antiminth)
   e. atovaquone (Mepron)

5. The nurse is reviewing anthelmintic therapy. Which statement is true regarding anthelmintic therapy?
   a. The medication can be stopped once symptoms disappear.
   b. Anthelmintics are more effective in their parenteral forms.
   c. Anthelmintics are broad in their actions and can be substituted easily for one another if a given medication is not well-tolerated.
   d. Specific anthelmintic drugs are used to target specific organisms.

6. The nurse is reviewing the medication list of a patient with a new prescription for mefloquine (Lariam). Which drugs may have an interaction with the mefloquine? *(Select all that apply.)*
   a. Beta blockers
   b. Antidiabetic drugs
   c. Calcium channel blockers
   d. Proton pump inhibitors
   e. Thiazide diuretics

7. A patient with *Pneumocystis jirovecii* pneumonia will be receiving pentamidine (NebuPent) intravenously. The order reads, "Give 4 mg/kg/day once daily." The medication comes in a 300-mg vial and is to be reconstituted with 5 mL of sterile water, with a resulting concentration of 60 mg/mL. The dose will then be added to a 100-mL bag of $D_5W$ for the infusion. The patient weighs 154 pounds. What is the dose for this patient and how many milliliters of medication will the nurse add to the infusion bag? *(Record answer using one decimal place.)*

8. A patient is to receive mefloquine (Lariam) 1250 mg in a single dose for treatment of malaria. The medication is available in 250-mg tablets. How many tablets will the patient receive?

---

## Critical Thinking and Application

**Answer the following questions on a separate sheet of paper.**

9. Professor H. has just returned from a research sabbatical in Africa where she did not adequately protect herself from mosquito exposure; thus, she has contracted malaria. What kind of parasite causes malaria? Which drug is recommended if the parasite is in the exoerythrocytic phase of development? What exactly is the exoerythrocytic phase?

10. Professor H.'s nurse practitioner would like to prescribe the drug identified in the answer to Question 9. The patient will be assessed for which contraindications?

11. Professor H.'s husband, who accompanied her on her trip, has even more recently begun to develop signs of malaria. He is given chloroquine (Aralen), a 4-aminoquinoline derivative. Unlike his wife, however, Mr. H. sees no diminishing of his symptoms. His strain of malaria appears to be chloroquine-resistant. What alternative(s) will the nurse practitioner suggest for Mr. H.?

12. The medical clinic has a full waiting room this morning. Patient A is being seen for an intestinal disorder that he acquired after swimming in a local lake. Patient B has acquired immunodeficiency syndrome (AIDS) and is showing early signs of pneumonia. Patient C is being treated and evaluated on a regular basis for a sexually transmitted infection. Here's your challenge: All three patients have something in common in terms of the causes of their disorders. Describe what that could be. Second, based on that commonality, predict what disorder, of those discussed in this chapter, each patient may have. (Hint: One patient has giardiasis.) Third, select the drugs you feel the physician is likely to prescribe for each patient.

## Case Study

**Read the scenario and answer the following questions on a separate sheet of paper.**

Sandra, age 15, has been diagnosed with an infestation of intestinal roundworms, specifically ascariasis, after a visit to another country. You are preparing to medicate her with pyrantel (Pin-X).

1. How is this infestation diagnosed?

2. What are the contraindications to therapy with pyrantel?

3. The recommended dosage for pyrantel is 11 mg/kg, up to a maximum of 1 g, in a one-time dose. If Sandra weighs 57 kg, what dose will she receive?

4. What are expected adverse effects of this medication?

# CHAPTER 44

# Antiinflammatory and Antigout Drugs

## Chapter Review and NCLEX® Examination Preparation

**Select the best answer for each question.**

1. When teaching a patient about the common adverse effects of therapy with nonsteroidal antiinflammatory drugs (NSAIDs), the nurse will mention which possible adverse effect?
   a. Dizziness
   b. Heartburn
   c. Palpitations
   d. Diarrhea

2. A 13-year-old patient has the flu, and her mother is concerned about her fever of 103° F (39.4° C). Which of these medications will the prescriber suggest the mother use to treat the teen's fever?
   a. aspirin
   b. acetaminophen (Tylenol)
   c. indomethacin (Indocin)
   d. ketorolac (Toradol)

3. A patient is receiving treatment with allopurinol (Zyloprim) for an acute flare-up of gout. Which statements will the nurse include during patient teaching? *(Select all that apply.)*
   a. "Be sure to avoid alcohol and caffeine."
   b. "Take the medication with meals to prevent stomach problems."
   c. "You need to take this medication on an empty stomach to improve absorption."
   d. "You need to increase fluid intake to up to 3 liters per day."
   e. "Call your provider immediately if you note any skin rashes or abnormalities."

4. When reviewing the health history of a patient who is to receive NSAID therapy, the nurse keeps in mind that contraindications for the use of these drugs include which condition?
   a. Pericarditis
   b. Osteoarthritis
   c. Bleeding disorders
   d. Juvenile rheumatoid arthritis

5. The nurse is reviewing the use of the COX-2 inhibitor celecoxib (Celebrex). Which conditions are indications for celecoxib? *(Select all that apply.)*
   a. Osteoarthritis
   b. Prevention of thrombotic events
   c. Rheumatoid arthritis
   d. Primary dysmenorrhea
   e. Fever reduction

6. The nurse is reviewing a patient's medications and sees an order for ketorolac (Toradol). This drug is ordered for which condition?
   a. Fever
   b. Mild pain
   c. Moderate to severe acute pain
   d. Long-term chronic pain conditions

7. A child is to receive celecoxib (Celebrex) as part of treatment for juvenile rheumatoid arthritis. The dose ordered is 100 mg twice daily PO. The child weighs 33 pounds. According to the text, the dosing chart for pediatric administration of celecoxib is:

| Less than 25 kg | 50 mg twice daily PO |
| More than 25 kg | 100 mg twice daily PO |

Is the ordered dose appropriate for this child? Explain your answer.

8. The order reads, "Give ketorolac (Toradol) 20 mg IV every 6 hours as needed for pain." The medication is available in a concentration of 15 mg/mL. How much will the nurse draw up for each dose? Mark the syringe to indicate your answer. *(Record answer using one decimal place.)*

## Critical Thinking and Application

**Answer the following questions on a separate sheet of paper.**

9. Ms. B. is brought into the emergency department with severe tinnitus, hearing loss, and some confusion. On examination the nurse discovers that the patient's blood glucose level is 52 mg/dL. Her husband tells you that she had been experiencing back pain and has been using "a lot of aspirin" over the past few weeks. What do her symptoms and history suggest? Explain your answer.

10. Mr. C. comes to the emergency department with symptoms that are similar to Ms. B.'s but not as extensive. He is experiencing drowsiness, lethargy, and disorientation, and had a seizure while en route to the hospital. His girlfriend tells the nurse that she noticed an empty bottle of ibuprofen (Advil) by his bed when she found him. What do his symptoms and history suggest? What would the nurse expect if the situation were allowed to progress?

11. Mr. H. has come to the clinic complaining of a severe flare-up of his gout. He tells the nurse that he does not take his medicine on a regular basis because it "kills" his stomach. He also says that he hates to take medicine but hates the gout more. He has a prescription for allopurinol (Zyloprim) and a follow-up appointment for next month. What patient teaching does Mr. H. need?

12. Eileen has had arthritic joint pain for months and her current pain management regimen has been less than successful. During a checkup today, she tells the nurse that she has heard of a drug, Toradol, which "works wonders." She wants to try it for "a couple of months" to see if it can help her.
    a. What will the nurse tell her?
    b. What could happen if Eileen takes the ketorolac (Toradol) on a long-term basis?

13. Your neighbor calls you over to "check out this aspirin bottle" that she found in her medicine cabinet. It has a strong vinegary odor. She wants to know if she can still take it for her headaches. What will you tell her?

14. Randy has a history of hypertension and coronary artery disease. Today he is being evaluated for acute gout, and the prescriber is considering febuxostat (Uloric). Are there any concerns, based on Randy's history, if he takes this drug for gout? Explain your answer.

## Case Study

**Read the scenario and answer the following questions on a separate sheet of paper.**

Sadie has been taking indomethacin (Indocin) as part of therapy for osteoarthritis, but lately has noticed that it has been less effective. Her provider has decided to try celecoxib (Celebrex). Sadie has a history of hepatitis (15 years earlier).

1. What advantages might there be to treatment with celecoxib rather than indomethacin?

2. What potential adverse effects will you warn Sadie about before she takes this medication? What should she report?

3. What allergies are important to assess before Sadie takes this medication?

4. She asks you if she can drink her usual glass of wine each evening while taking this medication. What will you tell her?

# CHAPTER 45

# Antineoplastic Drugs Part 1: Cancer Overview and Cell Cycle–Specific Drugs

## Critical Thinking Crossword

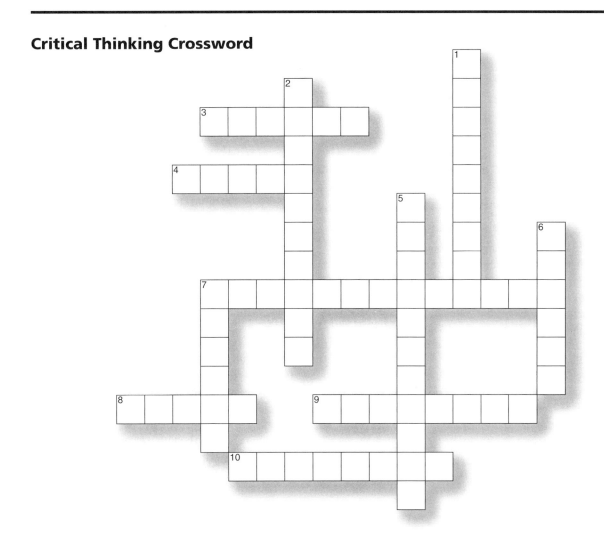

**Across**

3. Mr. H. is told that his cancer has metastasized. His physician explains to him that this means it has _____ to other areas of his body.

4. Your patient is receiving methotrexate. Your instructor asks for a full description of its mechanism of action, so you explain that it will inhibit dihydrofolic reductase from converting _____ acid to a reduced folate, and thus ultimately prevent the synthesis of DNA and cell reproduction. The result, you explain, is that the cell will die.

7. Mr. B. has just undergone a series of chemotherapeutic treatments when it is discovered that the antineoplastic drug has leaked into surrounding tissues; in other words, _____ of the drug has occurred.

8. Mr. C. is very interested in his chemotherapy process. As you are discussing a drug's action, he hears you use the term _____, and he asks you what it means. You explain that this is the point at which the lowest neutrophil count occurs after administration of a chemotherapy agent that causes bone marrow suppression.

9. Ms. F. has been given her first chemotherapy treatment. However, it soon becomes apparent that the adverse effects she is experiencing prevent her from being given dosages that will be high enough to be effective. These are dose-_____ adverse effects.
10. Ms. H. has a hematologic malignancy. Her bone marrow is being rapidly replaced with leukemic blasts; she also has abnormal numbers (and forms) of immature white blood cells in her circulation, and even her lymph nodes, spleen, and liver are being infiltrated. Ms. H.'s type of cancer is known as _____.

**Down**

1. Ms. P. had a biopsy performed on the same day that Ms. L. (6 Down) did. When her biopsy specimen is analyzed, however, the results are the opposite of Ms. L.'s; that is, her lump is considered _____.
2. Mr. K. has been treated with methotrexate for its folate-antagonistic properties. Now, however, he seems to be experiencing a toxicity reaction. The treatment he will receive will be _____ rescue.
5. Mr. G. is receiving chemotherapy with a drug that is considered cytotoxic during any phase of the cellular growth cycle. This drug is known as cell cycle–_____.
6. Ms. L. recently underwent biopsy of a lump near her breast. Several days later, her physician calls and tells her that the lump is noncancerous and therefore is not an immediate threat to life. She is relieved to hear, then, that it is _____.
7. Mr. Y.'s physician is not surprised to find that Mr. Y. has nausea and vomiting; the methotrexate therapy is displaying a strong _____ potential in this patient.

## Chapter Review and NCLEX® Examination Preparation

**Select the best answer for each question.**

1. When administering antineoplastic drugs, the nurse needs to keep in mind that the general adverse effects of these drugs include: *(Select all that apply.)*
   a. bone marrow suppression.
   b. infertility.
   c. diarrhea.
   d. urinary retention.
   e. nausea and vomiting.
   f. stomatitis.

2. A patient will be receiving chemotherapy with paclitaxel (Taxol). What will the nurse expect to do along with administering this drug?
   a. Administer platelet infusions.
   b. Provide acetaminophen (Tylenol) as needed.
   c. Keep the patient on "nothing-by-mouth" status because of expected nausea and vomiting.
   d. Premedicate with a steroid, $H_2$ receptor antagonist, and antihistamine.

3. As the nurse is preparing to give the patient chemotherapy, the patient asks the nurse why more than one drug is used. The nurse will explain that combinations of chemotherapeutic drugs are used to:
   a. reduce drug resistance.
   b. reduce the incidence of adverse effects.
   c. decrease the cost of treatment.
   d. reduce treatment time.

4. If extravasation of an antineoplastic drug occurs, what will the nurse do first?
   a. Remove the intravenous catheter immediately.
   b. Stop the drug infusion without removing the intravenous catheter.
   c. Aspirate residual drug or blood from the tube if possible.
   d. Administer the appropriate antidote.

5. During chemotherapy, the nurse will monitor the patient for which symptoms of stomatitis?
   a. Indigestion and heartburn
   b. Severe vomiting and anorexia
   c. Pain or soreness of the mouth
   d. Diarrhea and perianal irritation

6. A patient is receiving leucovorin as part of his chemotherapy regimen. The nurse expects that the patient is receiving which antineoplastic drug?
   a. cladribine (Leustatin)
   b. fluorouracil (Adrucil)
   c. vincristine (Vincasar PFS)
   d. methotrexate (Trexall)

7. The nurse is monitoring a patient who has developed thrombocytopenia after two rounds of chemotherapy. Which signs or symptoms will the nurse look for in this patient? *(Select all that apply.)*
   a. Bruising
   b. Increased fatigue
   c. Ulcerations on mucous membranes inside the mouth
   d. Temperature above 100.5° F (38.1° C)
   e. Increased bleeding from venipunctures

8. A patient will be receiving daily doses of asparaginase (Elspar). The order is for 200 units/kg/day up to 40,000 units per dose IV. The patient weighs 275 pounds. How many units will the patient receive per dose? Is this dose within the safe limit?

   _____

9. A patient will be receiving chemotherapy with IV cladribine (Leustatin). The order reads, "Give 0.09 mg/kg each day for 7 days." The medication is to be added to 500 mL of normal saline and is available in a 1-mg/mL solution. The patient weighs 200 pounds.
   a. How many mg is each daily dose? _(Record answer using one decimal place.)_ _____
   b. How many milliliters of medication will be added to each infusion? _____

## Case Study

**Read the scenario and answer the following questions on a separate sheet of paper.**

Allen, a 40-year-old physician, has been diagnosed with acute lymphocytic leukemia and will be receiving chemotherapy with methotrexate (Trexall). He is scheduled to receive his first treatment today.

1. What is methotrexate's classification, and how does it work?

2. What laboratory test results should be checked before he receives this medication?

3. Allen tells you that he often has problems with ankle pain from an old injury and takes ibuprofen (Motrin) for pain relief. Is this a concern?

4. What other medications may be given along with the methotrexate chemotherapy and why?

# CHAPTER 46

# Antineoplastic Drugs Part 2: Cell Cycle–Nonspecific and Miscellaneous Drugs

## Chapter Review and NCLEX® Examination Preparation

**Select the best answer for each question.**

1. While hanging a new infusion bag of a chemotherapy drug, the nurse accidentally spills a small amount of solution on the floor. What is the nurse's best action?
   a. Let it dry, then mop the floor.
   b. Wipe the area with a paper towel.
   c. Use a spill kit to clean the area.
   d. Ask the housekeeping department to wipe the floor.

2. The nurse is reviewing the medication list for a patient who will be receiving mitotane (Lysodren) treatments. A drug from which class would cause the most concern if administered along with the mitotane?
   a. Benzodiazepine
   b. Thyroid replacement hormone
   c. Insulin
   d. Beta blocker

3. A patient receiving chemotherapy for a testicular tumor complains of hearing a "loud ringing sound" in his ears. The nurse expects what to happen next regarding the chemotherapy?
   a. It will continue as ordered.
   b. It will be stopped until the patient's hearing is evaluated.
   c. It will be withheld for a day, then resumed.
   d. It will be stopped until renal studies are performed.

4. When teaching a patient who is receiving outpatient chemotherapy about potential problems, the nurse needs to mention signs and symptoms of an oncologic emergency, which include which of the following? *(Select all that apply.)*
   a. Swollen tongue
   b. Alopecia
   c. Blood in the urine
   d. Nausea and vomiting
   e. Temperature of 100.5° F (38.1° C) or higher
   f. Chills

5. The nurse monitors very closely for signs of renal toxicity when which of these antineoplastic drugs is given?
   a. doxorubicin (Adriamycin)
   b. cisplatin (Platinol)
   c. bevacizumab (Avastin)
   d. mitotane (Lysodren)

6. A patient who has cancer is to receive a course of chemotherapy with doxorubicin (Adriamycin). Which coexisting condition will require very close monitoring while the patient is taking this drug?
   a. Hypertension
   b. Diabetes mellitus
   c. Gout
   d. Cardiomyopathy

7. A patient will be receiving mitotane (Lysodren), and the nurse is reviewing the patient's medication list for potential interactions. Which drugs may interact with mitotane? *(Select all that apply.)*
   a. digoxin (Lanoxin)
   b. warfarin (Coumadin)
   c. phenytoin (Dilantin)
   d. glucophage (Metformin)
   e. spironolactone (Aldactone)

8. The orders read, "Administer normal saline, 3 L, over 24 hours, beginning 12 hours before the cisplatin chemotherapy begins." The nurse will program the infusion pump to deliver the normal saline at what rate? _____

9. A patient will be receiving cisplatin chemotherapy. The order reads, "Give 100 mg/m² in 1000 mL $D_5W$ over 22 hours." The nurse will program the infusion pump to deliver the infusion at what rate?

   _____

## Critical Thinking and Application

**Answer the following questions on a separate sheet of paper.**

10. Describe the concept of cytoprotection and provide at least two examples of how this may be accomplished during chemotherapy.

11. Mrs. S. has been receiving bleomycin to treat a lung tumor, and lately she has been experiencing increased difficulty breathing. She tells the nurse, "I guess this cancer is getting worse. The medicine is not working." Will the nurse agree, or is there another possible concern?

12. During a busy evening shift, an oncologist tells the nurse that he wants to start Mrs. N.'s chemotherapy immediately. The oncologist asks the nurse to mix the drug as soon as possible and start the infusion. Should the nurse do this? Explain your answer.

13. Mr. G., who had been receiving an infusion of mechlorethamine (Mustargen), has an infiltrated intravenous site. He wants the nurse to pull out the intravenous line immediately because "it hurts so much." What will the nurse do? How will this extravasation be treated?

## Case Study

**Read the scenario and answer the following questions on a separate sheet of paper.**

Dottie, age 63, has been diagnosed with mid-stage ovarian cancer and will be receiving chemotherapy with cisplatin (Platinol) after surgery. She is understandably anxious about the therapy but says she wants to "beat the cancer."

1. Cisplatin is associated with three main toxicities. Describe each one.

2. Before Dottie receives the therapy, what will be assessed?

3. During therapy, Dottie complains of an "odd tingling" in her toes. Is this a concern? Explain.

4. Dottie tells you that she'd rather "drink nothing" when she is feeling nauseated. Is this a concern? Explain what you need to teach her about fluids.

# CHAPTER 47

# Biologic Response–Modifying and Antirheumatic Drugs

## Chapter Review and NCLEX® Examination Preparation

**Match each definition with its corresponding term. (Note: Not all terms will be used.)**

1. _____ A type of cytokine that promotes resistance to viral infection in uninfected cells

2. _____ Cytokines that regulate the growth, differentiation, and function of bone marrow stem cells

3. _____ Cytokines that are produced by sensitized T lymphocytes upon contact with antigen particles

4. _____ An immunoglobulin that binds to antigens to form a special complex

5. _____ A substance that is recognized as foreign by the body's immune system

6. _____ Leukocytes of the cell-mediated immune system

7. _____ Leukocytes of the humoral immune system

a. Colony-stimulating factors
b. Antibody
c. B lymphocytes (B cells)
d. T lymphocytes (T cells)
e. Interferons
f. Lymphokine-activated killer cells
g. Lymphokines
h. Antigen
i. Memory cells

**Select the best answer for each question.**

8. While teaching a patient about the possible adverse effects of the interferons, the nurse should mention which effects? *(Select all that apply.)*
   a. Myalgia
   b. Fever
   c. Diarrhea
   d. Fatigue
   e. Chills
   f. Dizziness

9. A patient is starting therapy with adalimumab (Humira) after a course of therapy with methotrexate (Trexall) failed to improve the patient's condition. The nurse recognizes that this patient is being treated for which condition?
   a. Advanced-stage cancer
   b. Multiple sclerosis
   c. Severe rheumatoid arthritis
   d. Systemic lupus erythematosus

10. A patient will be starting therapy with etanercept (Enbrel) as part of treatment for severe rheumatoid arthritis. Which conditions, if present, may be a contraindication for this drug? *(Select all that apply.)*
    a. Latex allergy
    b. Active bacterial infection
    c. Diabetes mellitus
    d. Latent tuberculosis
    e. Acute hepatitis B
    f. Peanut allergy

11. The order reads, "Give oprelvekin (Neumega) 50 mcg/kg daily for 14 days subcut. The medication comes in a strength of 5 mg/mL once reconstituted. The patient weighs 110 pounds.
    a. How many milligrams will the patient receive per dose? _____
    b. How many milliliters will the nurse draw up into the syringe for this dose? Mark the syringe with your answer.

12. A patient is to receive 400 mcg of filgrastim (Neupogen) subcut daily for 1 week. The vial contains 480 mcg/1.6 mL. How many milliliters will the nurse draw up into the syringe for the dose? _____

## Critical Thinking and Application

**Answer the following questions on a separate sheet of paper.**

13. Sonja is to receive interferon therapy as part of the treatment for cancer. Sonja is very athletic and participates in sports activities on a regular basis. The oncologist explains that there is a dose-limiting adverse effect of this type of drug that may have a huge effect on her daily activities. What is this adverse effect, and how will it concern Sonja?

14. Trevor is receiving chemotherapy as part of his treatment for Hodgkin's disease. As he begins therapy, he tells the nurse, "I've seen those commercials about the drugs that increase your white blood cell count. Can't I start taking one of them now to keep my counts from getting so low?" What are the drugs he is referring to, and how will the nurse answer?

15. Brittany has a history of thrombocytopenia, and the results of today's laboratory work have indicated a critically low platelet count. She has received 2 units of platelets, and the oncologist has decided to give her a medication to improve her platelet counts. What drug will be given, how will it be given, and what concerns are there while her platelet count is so low?

16. Dustin will be receiving treatments with methotrexate (Trexall) for severe rheumatoid arthritis. The nurse is reviewing the medication administration record (MAR) and sees the following transcribed order, "methotrexate, 7.5 mg per day PO." What will be the nurse's next action?

## Case Study

**Read the scenario and answer the following questions on a separate sheet of paper.**

Donna, a 62-year-old florist, is in the hospital because of severe dehydration after her second round of chemotherapy for ovarian cancer. At this time, the laboratory results revealed a critically low platelet count, and the oncologist has ordered a transfusion of 3 units of platelets. However, Donna states that she cannot accept the platelet transfusion because of her religious convictions. As a result, there are orders to begin therapy with oprelvekin (Neumega).

1. What is the classification of oprelvekin?

2. What laboratory test results will you monitor while she is taking this medication and why?

3. Donna asks, "I am worried about bleeding. When can this drug be started, and how long will I have to take it?" What will you explain to Donna about how this drug is given?

4. What patient teaching is important while Donna is taking this drug?

# CHAPTER 48

# Immunosuppressant Drugs

## Chapter Review and NCLEX® Examination Preparation

**Select the best answer for each question.**

1. When monitoring patients on immunosuppressant therapy, the nurse must keep in mind that the major risk factor for patients taking these drugs is which condition?
   a. Severe hypotension with potential renal failure
   b. Increased susceptibility to opportunistic infections
   c. Decreased platelet aggregation
   d. Increased bleeding tendencies

2. A patient is experiencing rejection of a transplanted organ. The nurse expects which drug to be given to manage this?
   a. azathioprine (Imuran)
   b. cyclosporine (Sandimmune)
   c. muromonab-CD3 (Orthoclone OKT3)
   d. glatiramer acetate (Copaxone)

3. The nurse is discussing drug therapy with cyclosporine (Sandimmune). Which food product inhibits metabolism enzymes and possibly increases the activity of cyclosporine?
   a. Dairy products
   b. Orange juice
   c. Grapefruit juice
   d. Red wines

4. When teaching patients who are taking oral doses of immunosuppressants, how will the nurse instruct the patient to take the medication?
   a. With food to minimize gastrointestinal upset
   b. On an empty stomach to increase absorption rate
   c. Only when adverse effects are tolerable
   d. Mixed with water only

5. The nurse providing teaching for patients taking immunosuppressants will include which information? *(Select all that apply.)*
   a. The mouth and tongue should be inspected carefully for white patches.
   b. Allergic reactions to these drugs are rare.
   c. Patients should avoid crowds to minimize the risk of infection.
   d. Patients should report any fever, sore throat, chills, or joint pain.
   e. Patients should take oral forms with food to avoid gastrointestinal upset.

6. Which drugs are indicated for the treatment of multiple sclerosis? *(Select all that apply.)*
   a. glatiramer acetate (Copaxone)
   b. azathioprine (Imuran)
   c. basiliximab (Simulect)
   d. daclizumab (Zenapax)
   e. fingolimod (Gilenya)

7. A patient will be taking cyclosporine (Sandimmune) after transplant surgery. Which of these are potential adverse effects of cyclosporine therapy? *(Select all that apply.)*
   a. Hypertension
   b. Fever
   c. Nephrotoxicity
   d. Fluid retention
   e. Hypotension
   f. Post-transplant diabetes mellitus

8. The order reads, "Give mycophenolate mofetil (CellCept) 1 g PO twice daily." The capsules are available in 250-mg strength. How many capsules will the patient receive per dose? _____

9. A patient is about to undergo transplant surgery and will be receiving a preoperative dose of cyclosporine (Sandimmune) 8 hours before the surgery. The ordered dose is "cyclosporine, 6 mg/kg/dose, IV, give 8 hours preoperatively." The patient weighs 275 pounds. The medication is available as 50 mg/mL.
   a. The dose for this patient is how many milligrams? _____
   b. How many milliliters will the nurse administer for this dose? _____

## Critical Thinking and Application

**Answer the following questions on a separate sheet of paper.**

10. Mrs. F. is about to undergo kidney transplant surgery. The physician plans for her to start taking daclizumab (Zenapax).
    a. Mrs. F. asks the nurse why she is taking this medication. How will the nurse answer?
    b. Three days before her surgery, an oral antifungal drug is added to Mrs. F.'s regimen. "Why do I have to take this, too?" she asks. How will the nurse answer?

11. A patient on cyclosporine (Neoral) therapy is convinced that the cyclosporine is upsetting his stomach. What can be done to alleviate this problem?

12. A hospitalized patient has asked the nurse to mix the doses of cyclosporine in his disposable Styrofoam cup with milk before he drinks it. What will the nurse do?

13. Tess has had a renal transplant. She is being given muromonab-CD3 (Orthoclone OKT3) intravenously, 5 mg/day in a single bolus. On the second day, she begins to exhibit chest pain, dyspnea, and wheezing. What is happening? What does the nurse need to do at this time? What can be ordered to reduce these problems?

14. John has relapsing-remitting multiple sclerosis and is in the hospital because of an acute exacerbation. The physician talks to him about a "different type" of therapy with an immunosuppressant drug. What drug will be used, and how can it help John?

## Case Study

**Read the scenario and answer the following questions on a separate sheet of paper.**

Mr. K. had renal transplant surgery 6 months ago and so far has had no problems with organ rejection. He is taking cyclosporine (Sandimmune) in a maintenance dose. He wants to go back to work and is in for a checkup before approval is given for a return to his job.

1. He asks if he will have to continue the cyclosporine. What is your response?

2. He complains of difficulty swallowing, and as you examine his mouth, you look for signs of oral candidiasis. What findings would indicate that he has this condition?

3. After 2 weeks at work, Mr. K. calls to report that he has the flu. He has a sore throat, chills, and achy joints, and he is very tired. What is your advice?

4. Mr. K. tells you that his job sometimes requires him to travel to remote areas of the world. What concerns are there with vaccinations, if any?

# CHAPTER 49

# Immunizing Drugs and Biochemical Terrorism

## Chapter Review and NCLEX® Examination Preparation

1.  Complete the following chart by filling in all missing information.

| Drug | Active or Passive? | Purpose |
|---|---|---|
| a. | b. | Herpes zoster prevention (over age 60) |
| Hib | c. | d. |
| e. | Active | Hepatitis B prophylaxis |
| f. | g. | Postpartum antibody suppression |
| BCG vaccine | h. | i. |
| DTaP | j. | k. |
| Tetanus immunoglobulin | l. | m. |
| Td | n. | o. |

**Select the best answer for each question.**

2. The immunity that is passed from a mother to her nursing infant through antibodies in breast milk is known as which type of immunity?
   a. Artificially acquired passive immunity
   b. Naturally acquired passive immunity
   c. Active immunity
   d. Genetic immunity

3. Which substance contains microorganisms that trigger the formation of antibodies against specific pathogens?
   a. Antivenin
   b. Serum
   c. Toxoid
   d. Vaccine

4. When reviewing various immunizing drugs, the nurse recalls that some products provide long-lasting immunity against a particular pathogen. Which is an example of this type of product?
   a. Poliovirus vaccine
   b. Tetanus immune globulin
   c. $Rh_o(D)$ immune globulin
   d. Black widow spider antivenin

5. The nurse is preparing to give a second dose of DTaP vaccine to a 6-month-old infant. The infant's mother tells the nurse that the last time he received this vaccination, the injection site on his leg became warm and slightly reddened. Which is the nurse's best action?
   a. Explain that these effects can be expected and give the medication.
   b. Give half the prescribed dose this week and the other half next week if tolerated well.
   c. Skip the dose and notify the physician.
   d. Wait 6 months and then administer the dose.

6. A nurse has been stuck by a used needle while starting an intravenous line. Which preparation is used as prophylaxis against disease after exposure to blood and body fluids?
   a. Hib vaccine
   b. $Rh_o(D)$ immune globulin
   c. Hepatitis B immune globulin
   d. Hepatitis antitoxin

7. The nurse is providing patient teaching to a 24-year-old woman regarding the human papillomavirus (HPV) vaccine. Which statement by the woman indicates that more teaching is needed? *(Select all that apply.)*
   a. "This vaccine only takes one injection."
   b. "I need to have this vaccine before I turn 26."
   c. "It is safe to take this vaccine if I am pregnant."
   d. "This vaccination prevents the virus that commonly causes genital warts."
   e. "My 13-year-old sister should take this vaccine, too."

8. A newborn will be receiving her first dose of hepatitis B vaccine (inactivated). The dose is 5 mcg IM at birth, then again at 1 month and 6 months. Five mcg is equivalent to how many mg? _____

9. A 7-month-old infant will be receiving influenza virus vaccine (Fluzone), 0.25 mL IM. Mark the correct dose on the syringe.

## Critical Thinking and Application

**Answer the following questions on a separate sheet of paper.**

10. Emily, age 25, has stepped on a rusty piece of metal, and will be receiving a tetanus booster after the wound is cleansed and stitched. Her last tetanus booster, a Td, was 10 years ago. Which booster is she likely to receive today? Explain your answer.

11. Jim, a cabinetmaker, is cut by a woodworking tool and comes to the clinic for stitches. When the nurse asks him about his tetanus vaccination history, he says, "I have no idea when my last tetanus shot was—I thought once I had all the shots for school that I was set for life! Surely I don't need any more." What will the nurse explain to Jim?

12. Mrs. T., an 82-year-old widow, is in the office for a follow-up appointment to evaluate her emphysema. The physician recommends that she have an influenza virus vaccine. As the nurse prepares the injection, Mrs. T. says, "I had a flu shot last year—why do I need another one this year?" What is the nurse's explanation to her?

13. Mr. S. brings his toddler, Carl, in for a 12-month well-child checkup. Before the nurse gives the measles-mumps-rubella (MMR) vaccine injection, what adverse effects will she tell Mr. S. to watch for in Carl's response to the immunization? What can be done to relieve these adverse effects?

14. There have been news reports about anthrax threats. Your neighbor is worried and asks you which type of anthrax is the most deadly. What does he mean by "which type," and what is the answer to his question?

15. Paul has received several immunizations in preparation for an overseas trip. He expected to feel some soreness at the injection sites, but the next morning he wakes up with swelling of the face and tongue, difficulty breathing, shortness of breath, nausea and vomiting, and a fever of 102° F (38.9° C). What is happening, and what should he do?

## Case Study

**Read the scenario and answer the following questions on a separate sheet of paper.**

You are volunteering at a local animal shelter and helping to care for a sick dog that has just been admitted. During the examination, the dog nipped both you and the veterinarian. A little later, the veterinarian tells you that she fears that the dog has rabies and that both of you have been exposed. The veterinarian tells you that she has received a vaccine for rabies, but that you will need to be vaccinated immediately.

1. Is rabies a virus or a bacteria?

2. Did the vaccine the veterinarian received previously give her active or passive immunization? Explain.

3. Will the vaccine you receive give you active or passive immunization? Explain why this particular type of vaccine is preferred in your situation.

# CHAPTER 50

# Acid-Controlling Drugs

## Chapter Review and NCLEX® Examination Preparation

**Match each definition with its corresponding term. (Note: Not all terms will be used; some definitions may have more than one answer; some terms may be used more than once.)**

1. _____ Drugs known as *H₂ blockers* that reduce acid secretion in the stomach

2. _____ Drugs that block all acid secretion in the stomach

3. _____ Generic name for a cytoprotective drug

4. _____ The cells responsible for producing and secreting hydrochloric acid in the stomach

5. _____ A type of antacid that can cause diarrhea

6. _____ Antacids that have constipating effects

7. _____ The cause of many peptic ulcers

8. _____ Drugs used to relieve the painful symptoms associated with gas

9. _____ A type of antacid that may contribute to the development of kidney stones

10. _____ A highly soluble antacid form with a quick onset but short duration of action

a. Aluminum-containing antacids
b. Calcium-containing antacids
c. Magnesium-containing antacids
d. Antiflatulents
e. Proton pump inhibitors
f. *Helicobacter pylori*
g. Sodium bicarbonate
h. Histamine type 2 receptor antagonists
i. Sucralfate
j. Chief cells
k. Parietal cells

**Select the best answer for each question.**

11. A patient with renal failure wants to take an antacid for "sour stomach." The nurse needs to consider that some antacids may be dangerous when taken by patients with renal failure and will recommend which type of antacid?
    a. Activated charcoal
    b. Aluminum-containing antacids
    c. Calcium-containing antacids
    d. Magnesium-containing antacids

12. A patient with peptic ulcer disease will be starting medication therapy. He tells the nurse that he smokes and wonders if that will affect his treatment. Which is the nurse's best response?
    a. "Smoking has no effect on these medications."
    b. "The actions of antacids are less potent when you smoke."
    c. "Smoking has been shown to decrease the effectiveness of H₂ blockers."
    d. "Smoking has been shown to increase the adverse effects of H₂ blockers."

13. Which drug class would be used as first-line therapy for gastroesophageal reflux disease (GERD) that has not responded to customary medical treatment?
    a. H₂ blockers
    b. Antacids
    c. Mucosal protectants
    d. Proton pump inhibitors

14. The nurse is administering a proton pump inhibitor during morning medication rounds. Which statements about proton pump inhibitors are true? *(Select all that apply.)*
    a. They should be taken 1 hour before antacids.
    b. They should be taken 30 to 60 minutes before meals.
    c. They should be taken with meals.
    d. They are part of the treatment of patients with *H. pylori* infections.
    e. There are very few adverse effects with these drugs.

15. A pregnant woman asks the nurse about taking an antacid for indigestion. What is the nurse's best response?
    a. "You won't be allowed to take an antacid while you are pregnant."
    b. "Let's check with your obstetrician to see what is recommended."
    c. "Go ahead and use an aluminum-based antacid."
    d. "Sodium bicarbonate would be the safest choice."

16. A patient is to receive cimetidine (Tagamet), 300 mg IVPB twice a day. The medication is available in a concentration of 150 mg/mL. How many milliliters will the nurse draw up to prepare for the IVPB dose?

_____

17. The patient is to receive pantoprazole (Protonix) 40 mg, mixed in 100 mL of D₅W over 30 minutes, IV. The nurse will set the infusion pump to what rate?

_____

## Critical Thinking and Application

**Answer the following questions on a separate sheet of paper.**

18. A neighbor, Mr. M., comes over to get advice on antacids. He says he has taken Maalox "for years" for indigestion, but it is no longer helping. He asks the nurse, "Can you recommend another antacid or one of those expensive, fancy pills that the pharmacy sells? Or should I just take baking soda?" How will the nurse respond?

19. Mrs. K. is advised to take omeprazole (Prilosec) capsules to treat her severe case of GERD; nothing else has worked. Develop a patient teaching plan that will instruct Mrs. K. about how to take this medication.

20. Mr. A. has called to ask which antacid he should take. He has been to the store and is confused by the great variety on the shelves. He says he needs something for "occasional heartburn" when he eats something too spicy. He has a history of heart failure and is taking antihypertensive drugs. What type of antacid should he take and what other instructions will he need?

21. Mr. S. is taking enteric-coated aspirin for mild arthritis symptoms. He tells the nurse that he plans to take the aspirin with his favorite antacid, Maalox, because he does not want any stomach problems. What will the nurse tell him?

22. The nurse is caring for a patient who has been transferred to the step-down unit after spending a week in the intensive care unit after a myocardial infarction. The nurse notices that the patient's medication list includes a proton pump inhibitor, but there is no mention of any GI disorders on his chart. What is the reason for this medication?

## Case Study

**Read the scenario and answer the following questions on a separate sheet of paper.**

Edna, age 78, has been self-treating with antacids for "heartburn" for 6 months. After an upper gastrointestinal tract endoscopy, she has been diagnosed with GERD. The decision has been made to start treatment with cimetidine (Tagamet). Edna has been generally healthy except for a history of asthma. She says that she does not smoke but that she enjoys going to a bingo session every Saturday for a few hours where there is smoking, beer, and pizza.

1. When Edna sees the prescription for cimetidine, she asks, "Why do I need a prescription? I can buy this over the counter!" What will you say in reply?

2. How will the cimetidine help her GERD?

3. What cautions, if any, are associated with the use of cimetidine?

4. Will staying in a smoke-filled room affect her therapy? Explain.

# CHAPTER 51

# Bowel Disorder Drugs

## Critical Thinking Crossword

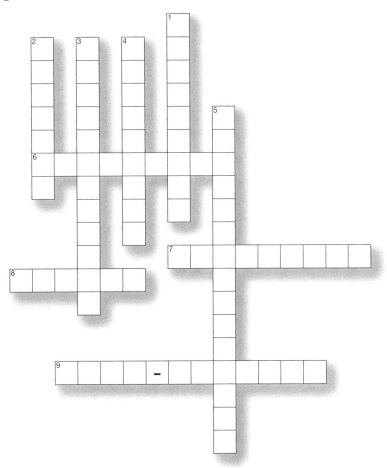

**Across**

6. A type of laxative that softens the stool
7. Another word for intestinal flora modifier
8. One type of laxative that increases osmotic pressure in the small intestine, increasing water content and resulting in distention
9. Laxatives that absorb water into the intestine, increasing the volume and distending the bowel (two words)

**Down**

1. Antidiarrheal drug that acts by coating the walls of the gastrointestinal tract, and binding to causative bacteria or toxin to allow elimination via the stool
2. These drugs decrease bowel motility
3. Another type of laxative that increases fecal water content in the large intestine, resulting in distention, increased peristalsis, and evacuation
4. A laxative that stimulates the nerves that supply the intestine, which results in increased peristalsis
5. Antidiarrheal drug that acts by decreasing peristalsis and muscular tone of the intestine, thus slowing the movement of substances through the gastrointestinal tract

## Chapter Review and NCLEX® Examination Preparation

**Select the best answer for each question.**

1. The nurse is reviewing the use of bismuth subsalicylate (Pepto-Bismol). This medication would be the most appropriate choice for which patient?
   a. A 7-year-old child who has chickenpox
   b. A 23-year-old woman who has severe abdominal pain
   c. A 45-year-old man who is complaining of constipation
   d. A 58-year-old man who developed diarrhea after traveling out of the country

2. The nurse will teach a patient who is self-treating with bismuth subsalicylate (Pepto-Bismol) to avoid which drug because of the possibility of toxicity?
   a. aspirin
   b. acetaminophen (Tylenol)
   c. calcium supplements
   d. vitamin tablets

3. A patient asks for an over-the-counter medication that will provide rapid relief of constipation. After ruling out possible contraindications, which drug would be most appropriate?
   a. psyllium (Metamucil)
   b. methylcellulose (Citrucel)
   c. docusate sodium (Colace)
   d. magnesium hydroxide (Milk of Magnesia)

4. A patient has been given PEG-3350 in a solution of polyethylene glycol (GoLYTELY) as preparation for a colonoscopy. He started having diarrhea after about 45 minutes. Two hours later, he tells the nurse that "the diarrhea has not stopped yet." What will the nurse do?
   a. Give the patient an antidiarrheal drug, such as loperamide (Lomotil).
   b. Give the patient another dose of the GoLYTELY to finish cleansing his bowel.
   c. Remind the patient that it may take up to 4 hours to completely evacuate the bowel.
   d. Report this to the physician immediately.

5. A 79-year-old woman visits the clinic today and tells the nurse that her "bowels just aren't right." She wants advice on the best laxative to take so that she can have a bowel movement every day. Which is an appropriate response by the nurse? *(Select all that apply.)*
   a. "A normal bowel pattern does not necessarily mean that you will have a bowel movement every day."
   b. "Try taking Metamucil with sips of water."
   c. "You can try taking Milk of Magnesia every other day—it's a mild laxative."
   d. "Let's talk about increasing fluids and fiber in your diet."
   e. "Mineral oil would be safe for long-term use if needed."

6. A patient has been taking alosetron (Lotronex) for 3 weeks as part of treatment for irritable bowel syndrome. Today she calls the clinic to report that she has been experiencing constipation. The nurse will expect which priority action to be taken?
   a. The dosage will be increased by 1 mg.
   b. The patient will be told to take a bulk-forming laxative.
   c. The patient will be given Milk of Magnesia to relieve the constipation quickly.
   d. The drug will be discontinued immediately.

7. The order for a child with severe diarrhea reads: Give diphenoxylate with atropine (Lomotil) 0.3 mg/kg/day in 4 divided doses. The medication is available in an oral solution with a concentration of 2.5 mg/5 mL. The child weighs 44 pounds.
   a. How many milligrams will the child receive per dose? _____
   b. How many milliliters will the child receive per dose? _____

8. The order for a child reads: "Give lactulose (Chronulac) 5 g, PO daily after breakfast." The medication is available as an oral solution in a unit-dose package that contains 10 g/15 mL. How many mL will the nurse administer per dose?

   _____

## Critical Thinking and Application

**Answer the following questions on a separate sheet of paper.**

9. Anna has called the health clinic in a panic. She says that she has been taking Pepto-Bismol for diarrhea and noticed this morning that her tongue "is a funny color." She asks, "Have I overdosed on this stuff? What should I do?" What will the nurse tell Anna?

10. Mrs. B. is a 65-year-old retiree with osteoporosis and narrow-angle glaucoma. She has recently developed diarrhea and the physician is considering antidiarrheal therapy. Mrs. B. tells the nurse that her husband recently "had a bout of diarrhea" for which he took Donnatal. Mrs. B. wonders whether Donnatal would help in her case. What will the nurse tell her?

11. Hillary has come to the physician's office complaining of constipation. During the nurse's assessment, Hillary mentions that she recently started graduate school and has not had time lately to keep up her usual exercise regimen and that her diet "is a disaster." She says that, on some days, all she has time to do is grab a milkshake or cheese and crackers at the student center. She also tells the nurse that she has been taking antacids for "heartburn." What might be causing Hillary's constipation?

12. Ira, age 45, has chronic constipation.
    a. What are the advantages of bulk-forming laxatives in treating Ira's problem?
    b. The provider prescribes psyllium. What instructions will the nurse give Ira regarding its administration?

13. Drake is a 5-year-old boy with constipation. The family nurse practitioner has suggested the use of glycerin suppositories.
    a. Why is glycerin a good choice for Drake?
    b. The parents will monitor for what adverse effects?

## Case Study

**Read the scenario and answer the following questions on a separate sheet of paper.**

Charles, age 54, recently completed a 2-week course of antibiotic therapy for pneumonia. He is now experiencing severe diarrhea.

1. What is the probable cause of his diarrhea?

2. What antidiarrheal product is indicated for Charles?

3. How does it work?

4. Is it considered a drug or a dietary supplement? Explain.

# CHAPTER 52

# Antiemetic and Antinausea Drugs

## Chapter Review and NCLEX® Examination Preparation

**Select the best answer for each question.**

1. The nurse is giving medication to reduce nausea. Which antiemetic drug class is known to cause drying of secretions and drowsiness when given? *(Select all that apply.)*
   a. Antihistamines
   b. Antidopaminergic drugs
   c. Serotonin blockers
   d. Tetrahydrocannabinoids
   e. Anticholinergics

2. A nurse is reviewing chemotherapy with a newly hired nurse on the oncology unit. Which antinausea drug or drug class is indicated for preventing chemotherapy-induced nausea and vomiting? *(Select all that apply.)*
   a. Antihistamines
   b. Antidopaminergic drugs
   c. Serotonin blockers
   d. Phosphorated carbohydrate solution (Emetrol)
   e. Tetrahydrocannabinoids

3. When reviewing the drugs used for nausea and vomiting, the nurse recalls that which drug is a synthetic derivative of the major active substance in marijuana?
   a. ondansetron (Zofran)
   b. metoclopramide (Reglan)
   c. prochlorperazine (Compazine)
   d. dronabinol (Marinol)

4. A patient is undergoing chemotherapy. When giving antiemetics, the nurse will remember that these drugs are most effective against nausea when given at which time?
   a. Before meals
   b. At bedtime
   c. Before the chemotherapy begins
   d. Just after the chemotherapy begins

5. When giving dronabinol (Marinol) to a patient with acquired immunodeficiency syndrome (AIDS), the nurse knows that this drug may also have what therapeutic effect in addition to reducing nausea?
   a. Euphoria
   b. Enhanced appetite
   c. Reduced pain
   d. Enhanced sleep

6. A patient calls in to the clinic to ask for something for his upset stomach. He admits to "eating a lot of food that's bad for me" the night before and wants something to help him to feel better. The nurse expects which drug will be most appropriate for this patient?
   a. metoclopramide (Reglan)
   b. prochlorperazine (Compazine)
   c. aprepitant (Emend)
   d. phosphorated carbohydrate solution (Emetrol)

7. A mother discovers that her child has eaten half a bottle of children's multivitamins. Which is the appropriate first action in this situation?
   a. Give one dose of syrup of ipecac.
   b. Take the child to the pediatric clinic.
   c. Call the national poison control hotline for instructions.
   d. Call 911 for emergency transport to a hospital.

8.  The order reads: "Give prochlorperazine (Compazine) 10 mg IM every 4 hours as needed for nausea. Maximum of 4 doses/day." The medication is available in an ampule that contains 5 mg/mL. Mark the syringe with the amount the nurse will administer for each dose.

9.  A patient is about to receive his first chemotherapy treatment with a drug that is known to cause nausea and vomiting. One of the premedication orders reads, "Give ondansetron (Zofran) PO 24 mg one-half hour before chemotherapy begins." The medication is ordered in a syrup that contains 4 mg/5 mL because the patient does not like to take pills. How many milliliters of medication will the nurse administer for this dose? _____

## Critical Thinking and Application

**Answer the following questions on a separate sheet of paper.**

10. Petra has gastroesophageal reflux disease, and the health care provider has ordered oral metoclopramide (Reglan), four times a day for 2 weeks.
    a.  What instructions will the nurse give Petra regarding administration of the medication?
    b.  A few days later, Petra calls to say that she thinks the medication is "too strong." She also mentions that her evening routine includes "a couple of glasses of wine." What will the nurse tell Petra?

11. Nellie has been prescribed prochlorperazine (Compazine) via an intramuscular injection. She is on "nothing-by-mouth" status and has no intravenous access at this time. The nurse is preparing the injection when Nellie says, "I hate shots. Can't I just take it by mouth?" What alternatives are there for this drug, and what will the nurse do?

12. Chuck, age 33, is in a later stage of AIDS. He has lost much weight and has no appetite. His physician has prescribed dronabinol (Marinol). When Chuck finds out that this medication is derived from marijuana, he becomes very upset. "Why is the doctor giving me pot?" he asks. What will the nurse explain?

## Case Study

**Read the scenario and answer the following questions on a separate sheet of paper.**

Mr. O. is preparing for his second course of chemotherapy as part of treatment for leukemia. One of the chemotherapy premedications is ondansetron (Zofran). His chemotherapy will last daily for 1 week.

1.  What are potential contraindications to the use of ondansetron?

2.  Mr. O. tells you that when he is at home, he still has nausea, and is puzzled because "I take the medicine for nausea as soon as I feel nauseated." How will you address his comments?

3.  One day Mr. O. complains to you that he gets a headache every time the ondansetron is administered. What should you do?

# CHAPTER 53

# Vitamins and Minerals

## Chapter Review and NCLEX® Examination Preparation

**Match each definition with the corresponding term.**

1. _____ Specialized protein that catalyzes biochemical reactions

2. _____ A condition that results from a deficiency of cyanocobalamin

3. _____ A nonprotein substance that combines with a protein molecule to form an active enzyme

4. _____ A condition caused by a vitamin D deficiency that is characterized by soft, pliable bones

5. _____ An inorganic substance that, when ingested, attaches to enzymes or other organic molecules

6. _____ An organic compound essential in small quantities for normal physiologic and metabolic functioning of the body

7. _____ A condition resulting from an ascorbic acid deficiency

8. _____ An essential organic compound that can be dissolved and stored in the liver and fatty tissues

9. _____ Biologically active chemicals that make up vitamin E compounds

10. _____ A disease of the peripheral nerves caused by a dietary deficiency of thiamine

11. _____ An essential organic compound that can be dissolved in water but is not stored in the body for long periods of time

12. _____ A disease resulting from a niacin deficiency or a metabolic defect that interferes with the conversion of tryptophan to niacin

a. Beriberi
b. Coenzyme
c. Enzyme
d. Fat-soluble vitamin
e. Mineral
f. Pellagra
g. Pernicious anemia
h. Rickets
i. Scurvy
j. Tocopherols
k. Vitamin
l. Water-soluble vitamin

**Select the best answer for each question.**

13. When giving vitamins, the nurse needs to remember that certain vitamins can be toxic if consumed in excess amounts. These include which vitamins? *(Select all that apply.)*
    a. Vitamin A
    b. Vitamin C
    c. Niacin
    d. Vitamin D
    e. Vitamin K
    f. Folic acid

14. A patient believes that taking megadoses of vitamin C is healthy. What should the nurse tell the patient about megadoses of vitamin C?
    a. They are usually nontoxic because vitamin C is water-soluble.
    b. They can produce nausea, vomiting, headache, and abdominal cramps.
    c. Megadoses of vitamin C can lead to scurvylike symptoms.
    d. They may cause dangerous heart dysrhythmias.

15. A patient has ingested an excessive amount of water-soluble vitamins. The nurse expects what to happen?
    a. The body will store them in muscle and fat tissue until needed.
    b. They are stored in the liver until needed.
    c. They circulate in the blood, bound to proteins, until needed.
    d. Excess amounts are excreted in the urine.

16. When reviewing the diet of a patient who has a calcium deficiency, the nurse recalls that efficient absorption of calcium in the diet requires adequate amounts of which substance?
    a. Magnesium
    b. Intrinsic factor
    c. Coenzymes
    d. Vitamin D

17. A patient is to receive one liter of $D_5W$ with one ampule of multivitamins over the next 10 hours. The nurse will set the infusion pump at what rate for this IV infusion? _____

18. The order reads, "Give vitamin K (Aqua-MEPHYTON) 2 mg subcutaneously now." The patient is a child, age 5 years. The medication is available in an ampule, 1 mg/0.5 mL. How many milliliters will the nurse draw up for the injection?

    _____

## Critical Thinking and Application

**Answer the following questions on a separate sheet of paper.**

19. After Mr. W. is treated for colitis with a broad-spectrum antibiotic, he begins to show signs of hypoprothrombinemia caused by vitamin K deficiency. How did this happen, and how will he receive supplements?

20. Mrs. S. has developed vitamin D deficiency as a result of long-term use of lubricant laxatives. She is advised to take supplements for her vitamin D deficiency. However, her health care provider also advises her to get vitamin D through more natural sources. Explain the "natural sources" of vitamin D.

21. Ms. E. has recently undergone an ileal resection and is experiencing some signs of malabsorption. When routine laboratory tests are performed, the nurse discovers that she is mildly anemic.
    a. What type of anemia does the nurse expect?
    b. What about her condition is contributing to this deficiency?
    c. How is this condition treated?

22. Mr. G. is hospitalized with severe hypocalcemia and will be receiving intravenous calcium. What are the safety concerns when giving intravenous calcium?

## Case Study

**Read the scenario and answer the following questions on a separate sheet of paper.**

A patient with a long history of alcoholism has been admitted to the intensive care unit with an irregular cardiac rhythm and increased confusion. His magnesium level is noted to be 1.2 mg/dL, so he was placed on an intravenous magnesium infusion.

1. What is the normal serum magnesium level?

2. What is your priority when assessing the patient during intravenous magnesium infusion?

3. Twelve hours later, you note that the patient's respirations are 10 breaths/minute, and his Achilles tendon reflexes are diminished. What will you do next?

4. What is the antidote for magnesium toxicity?

# CHAPTER 54

# Anemia Drugs

## Chapter Review and NCLEX® Examination Preparation

**Select the best answer for each question.**

1. Three days after beginning therapy with oral iron tablets, a patient calls the office. "I'm very worried because my bowel movements are black!" What will the nurse do?
   a. Instruct the patient to stop the iron tablets for a week.
   b. Instruct the patient to take the tablets every other day instead of daily.
   c. Ask the patient to come into the office for a checkup.
   d. Explain to the patient that this is an expected effect of the medication.

2. A patient will be taking an oral iron preparation. Which of these are possible adverse effects? *(Select all that apply.)*
   a. Dizziness
   b. Nausea
   c. Vomiting
   d. Drowsiness
   e. Orthostatic hypotension
   f. Stomach cramps

3. The nurse is preparing to administer folic acid. What occurs if folic acid is given to treat anemia without determining the underlying cause of the anemia?
   a. Erythropoiesis is inhibited.
   b. Excessive levels of folic acid may accumulate, causing toxicity.
   c. The symptoms of pernicious anemia may be masked, delaying treatment.
   d. Intestinal intrinsic factor is destroyed.

4. A patient is about to receive folic acid supplementation. The nurse knows that indications for folic acid supplementation include which of the following? *(Select all that apply.)*
   a. Iron-deficiency anemia
   b. Tropical sprue
   c. Prevention of fetal neural tube defects
   d. Pernicious anemia
   e. Hemolytic anemia

5. When teaching a patient about oral iron preparations, the nurse will include which instructions? *(Select all that apply.)*
   a. Mix the liquid iron preparations with antacids to reduce gastrointestinal distress.
   b. Take the iron with meals if gastrointestinal distress occurs.
   c. Liquid forms should be taken through a straw to avoid discoloration of tooth enamel.
   d. Oral forms should be taken with juice or water, not milk.
   e. Iron products will turn the stools black.

6. A patient will be receiving darbepoetin (Aranesp) as part of treatment for post-chemotherapy bone marrow suppression. Which finding is a contraindication to darbepoetin therapy?
   a. Pulse rate 100 beats/minute
   b. Blood pressure 128/79 mm Hg
   c. Hemoglobin level 11 g/dL
   d. White blood cell count 7,000/mm$^3$

7. The nurse is preparing to give iron sucrose (Venofer) to a 58-year-old patient, and will monitor for which common adverse effect?
   a. Hypotension
   b. Dyspnea
   c. Itching
   d. Cramps

8. A patient will be receiving epoetin alfa (Epogen) 150 units/kg, subcutaneously, three times a week. The patient weighs 110 pounds. The medication is available in a concentration of 10,000 units/mL. How many milliliters will the nurse administer for each dose? Mark the syringe with your answer. *(Record answer using two decimal places.)*

9. A 5-year-old child who is receiving hemodialysis is to receive 8 doses of sodium ferric gluconate (Ferrlecit) 1.5 mg/kg IV, with future dialysis sessions. The child weighs 38 pounds. How many milligrams is each dose? *(Record answer using a whole number.)* _____

## Critical Thinking and Application

**Answer the following questions on a separate sheet of paper.**

10. Mr. P. is prescribed intramuscular iron dextran. However, before the nurse can give him his first injection, the pharmacist suggests that she give him a smaller dose of 25 mg first. Why does the pharmacist suggest this? How should intramuscular iron dextran be administered?

11. Mrs. S. will be taking iron for treatment of anemia, and her provider instructed her to take it with orange juice. She asks the nurse for an explanation of this. What will the nurse tell her?

12. What are the advantages of receiving ferric gluconate (Ferrlecit) or iron sucrose (Venofer) injections instead of iron dextran?

13. Connie, age 58, is in the hospital because of extreme weakness. She has a history of chronic renal failure, and there is a new order for epoetin alfa (Epogen). What laboratory results are monitored during epoetin therapy, and why?

## Case Study

**Read the scenario and answer the following questions on a separate sheet of paper.**

Maureen has been given ferrous fumarate (Femiron) capsules with instructions to take two capsules twice a day as part of her treatment for iron-deficiency anemia.

1. She asks you if she can take this drug with meals. What is your answer?

2. What else will you warn her to expect with this medication?

3. After a week, Maureen calls you because she does not like to swallow capsules. She says that her mother has iron tablets that are labeled ferrous sulfate. She wants to know if she can take those tablets instead. What do you tell her?

4. Because Maureen does not like the capsules, her iron preparation has been switched to an oral liquid suspension. While you are teaching her how to give herself the correct dosage, what else is important for you to tell her about liquid iron preparations?

CHAPTER 55

# Nutritional Supplements

## Critical Thinking Crossword

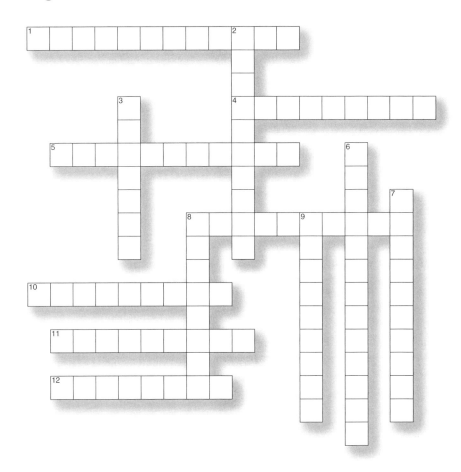

**Across**

1. Mr. G. is receiving an oral antibiotic when it is determined that he is going to need nutritional supplementation as well. However, you are concerned that the nutritional supplement will decrease the absorption of this drug because of high gastric acid content or prolonged emptying time. What is the generic name of this antibiotic?

4. Ms. C. needs amino acids in nutritional supplements. The main use, or primary role, of amino acids is protein synthesis, or _____.

5. Mr. H. is about to receive a _____, in which a feeding tube will be surgically inserted directly into his stomach.

8. Mrs. P. is worried about her husband, who has postsurgical nausea. She sees that his roommate is receiving total parenteral nutrition (TPN) and asks "Can't you do that for my husband, just while he's so nauseated?" TPN, you explain, is to be used only when enteral support is impossible or when the gastrointestinal tract's _____ or functional capacity is insufficient.

10. Ms. D. comes to the clinic when a cut on her hand "just won't heal up." She also says that as long as she is here, she would like to report symptoms of hair loss and a scaly rash on her skin. She wants a prescription for her skin problem, but the provider says, "There's something more going on here." After

performing some lab work, it is found that Ms. D. also has a decreased platelet level and some evidence of possible fatty liver. The provider states that Ms. D. has essential _____ (two words) deficiency.

11. Mr. J. is having trouble eating, which has resulted in an inadequate intake of dietary amino acids. His provider explains that he needs nutritional supplementation through enteral nutrition to ensure that he gets enough of these amino acids, because they cannot be produced by his own body. Mr. J. is suffering from a deficiency of _____ amino acids.

12. Mr. C., a college sophomore, takes a great deal of interest in the supplementary nutritional product he is receiving and asks to read the label. He says, "There are some amino acids missing from this. Why aren't you giving me all of them?" You explain that some amino acids, all but eight, are manufactured in the body, using _____ sources.

**Down**

2. When Ms. C. (from 4 Across) asks why she needs amino acid supplemental feedings, you explain that amino acids promote growth and help with wound healing. One of the principal ways they do so is by reducing or slowing the breakdown of proteins, or _____.

3. Mr. and Mrs. R. drink Ensure to meet a few extra nutritional needs they have experienced with aging. Their nephew recently had surgery, and while recovering, he received nasogastric delivery of a modular formulation to supplement a polymeric feeding formulation he needed. When their grandson was an infant, his parents supplemented his breast-feeding with an infant nutritional formulation. Each member of the R. clan discussed here has received some form of _____ nutrition.

6. The amino acids in 8 Down are _____ amino acids.

7. You are explaining to Mrs. N.'s family that the parenteral nutritional supplementation you are about to start will help her by bypassing the entire gastrointestinal system, eliminating the need for absorption, _____, and excretion.

8. The nursing student is reviewing amino acids, and is trying to recall the two amino acids that are not produced in large enough quantities during infancy and childhood. One of these is histidine; the other one is _____.

9. Mr. K. has been receiving peripheral parenteral nutrition. During an assessment, you note that his vein becomes inflamed. What problem is this?

## Chapter Review and NCLEX® Examination Preparation

**Select the best answer for each question.**

1. The nurse is assessing a patient who is receiving a peripheral parenteral nutrition (PPN) infusion. The maximum concentration of dextrose in PPN infusions is which percentage?
   a. 10%
   b. 20%
   c. 50%
   d. 100%

2. A patient has a need for a nutritional supplement that contains complex nutrients derived from proteins, carbohydrates, and fat. However, this patient is lactose-intolerant. The nurse knows that which product would be most suitable for this patient?
   a. Casec
   b. Polycose
   c. Ensure
   d. Vivonex

3. When monitoring a patient who is receiving TPN through a central line, the nurse will observe for which complications? *(Select all that apply.)*
   a. Pneumothorax
   b. Aspiration
   c. Hyperglycemia
   d. Infection
   e. Air embolus

4. A patient who is just starting to take enteral nutritional supplements will be taught by the nurse to expect which most common adverse effect?
   a. Anorexia
   b. Constipation
   c. Diarrhea
   d. Flatulence

5. When reviewing a patient's need for nutritional supplementation, the nurse remembers that PPN is most appropriate for which type of patient?
   a. Patients who will receive parenteral nutrition for less than 2 weeks
   b. Patients who will receive parenteral nutrition for more than 2 weeks
   c. Patients with severe nutritional problems
   d. Patients who wish to reduce their weight

6. A patient with type 1 diabetes mellitus will be receiving enteral nutrition for 4 months after surgery. Which of these nutritional solutions is most appropriate for this patient?
   a. Jevity
   b. Polycose
   c. Ensure
   d. Glucerna

7. A patient will be receiving TPN. The first bag is to infuse at 50 mL/hour for 4 hours, then 75 mL/hour for 4 hours, then at 100 mL/hour thereafter. What is the intravenous intake for the TPN over the first 12 hours of the infusion? _____

8. A patient is receiving a PEG tube feeding of Glucerna at 70 mL/hour via a feeding pump. What will be the PEG tube intake over a 24-hour period?

   _____

## Critical Thinking and Application

**Answer the following questions on a separate sheet of paper.**

9. Ms. S. is receiving an enteral feeding through a PEG tube.
   a. What symptoms would she develop if she were lactose-intolerant?
   b. Her tube feeding rate is 50 mL/hr. After 24 hours, you note that the residual amount is 120 mL. What is the nurse's priority action?

10. Mr. R., who is on TPN therapy, has a weak pulse, hypertension, tachycardia, and decreased urine output. He seems somewhat confused, and the nurse finds that he now has pitting edema in his ankles. What is happening, and what are the priority actions of the nurse?

## Case Study

**Read the scenario and answer the following questions on a separate sheet of paper.**

You are caring for Mrs. T., who is receiving peripheral parenteral nutrition (PPN) through an intravenous (IV) line in her right forearm. Your assessment shows that bag No. 3 is infusing at 100 mL/hr via an infusion pump, and the bag has about 300 mL remaining. The site is intact without redness or swelling.

1. Two hours later, Mrs. T. calls you because she accidentally pulled the IV line out of her arm. The remaining 100 mL of PPN has spilled on the floor. You have tried to reinsert the IV line but have not had success yet. What could occur if you cannot restart the infusion?

2. At last, the IV line has been reinserted, but you then discover that bag No. 4 has not yet been ordered from the pharmacy. What will you hang until PPN bag No. 4 is ready?

3. What else will you monitor while Mrs. T. is receiving PPN?

CHAPTER 56

# Dermatologic Drugs

## Chapter Review and NCLEX® Examination Preparation

**Select the best answer for each question.**

1. Which statement accurately describes antifungal therapy for topical infections?
   a. The length of treatment required to eradicate the organism may be from several weeks to as long as a year.
   b. Antifungal therapy works best when the affected area is exposed to sunlight.
   c. Oral drugs are the preferred drugs for treating topical fungal infections.
   d. Antifungal therapy is palliative only; fungi are rarely eradicated from topical areas.

2. When instructing a patient on how to use miconazole (Monistat) vaginal cream for vaginal yeast infections, the nurse will keep in mind that this medication will be given in which manner?
   a. Insert once every other day at bedtime for 1 week.
   b. Insert once daily at bedtime for 7 consecutive days.
   c. A one-time dose is administered in the morning.
   d. Insert every night at bedtime until symptoms stop.

3. A patient has a painful sunburn that covers a large area of her body and has asked the nurse for "something to make it feel better." The nurse keeps in mind that which formulation of topical medication will be easiest to use to cover this large area?
   a. Aerosol spray
   b. Gel
   c. Oil
   d. Cream

4. A patient needs a medication that has excellent emollient properties. Because she works as a swimming coach, the medication prescribed should not wash off when it comes in contact with water. If each has the same healing properties, which formulation would be the best for this patient?
   a. Aerosol spray
   b. Oil
   c. Gel
   d. Cream

5. The nurse is administering topical antiviral drugs. Which statements about these drugs are true? *(Select all that apply.)*
   a. Common adverse effects include stinging, itching, and rash.
   b. Topically applied acyclovir (Zovirax) does not cure viral skin infections but does seem to decrease the healing time and pain.
   c. Topically applied acyclovir can cure viral skin infections if applied as soon as symptoms appear.
   d. Antiviral drugs are applied topically for the treatment of both initial and recurrent herpes simplex infections.
   e. Topical antiviral drugs are used more often than systemic antiviral drugs for the treatment of viral skin conditions.

6. A 22-year-old woman is taking isotretinoin (Amnesteem) as part of the treatment for severe cystic acne. Which statement about isotretinoin therapy is true?
   a. This drug reduces acne by causing skin peeling.
   b. Its use is contraindicated if she is allergic to erythromycin.
   c. She will need to apply it twice a day to her face after washing her face thoroughly.
   d. She will need to use two forms of birth control while taking this medication.

7. Before using povidone-iodine (Betadine) solution to prepare skin for surgery, the nurse will ask the patient about allergies to which substance?
   a. Shellfish
   b. Penicillin
   c. Mercury
   d. Milk

8. A patient will be receiving fluorouracil (Efudex) cream as part of treatment for basal cell carcinoma of skin on her nose. The nurse will instruct the patient about which possible adverse effects? *(Select all that apply.)*
   a. Swelling
   b. Scaling
   c. Pallor
   d. Burning
   e. Tenderness

9. The order for a patient who has a severely infected skin wound reads, "Administer clindamycin (Cleocin) 300 mg diluted in 50 mL 0.9% NS IVPB every 6 hours. Infuse over 30 minutes." When calculating the rate for this IVPB, the nurse will set the infusion pump to what rate?

   _____

10. A patient will be receiving intravenous amphotericin B (Fungizone) for a severe fungal infection that has not responded to other medications. The order reads, "75 mg in 1000 mL D$_5$W to infuse over 6 hours." The nurse will set the infusion pump to what rate?

    _____

## Critical Thinking and Application

**Answer the following questions on a separate sheet of paper.**

11. Mr. M. has a topical skin infection. He is prescribed clindamycin (Cleocin T). He has never used this drug before. What assessments are important before the nurse administers this drug?

12. The nurse is getting ready to apply topical erythromycin to a patient's skin rash. The affected area of the skin is not oozing or even moist, but the nurse wears gloves. Why?

13. Mr. L.'s two children brought "something" home from school, and within a day, he had "it" too. He tells the nurse that he has applied lindane (Kwell) to everyone's scalp, but he has come to the clinic to have his children and himself checked because he is not confident that he has "taken care of things properly." For what are Mr. L. and his children being treated? Describe for him the basic steps in using lindane. What other measures does he need to take?

14. A newly admitted patient has a stage III pressure ulcer that shows areas of exudate along with areas of healed granulation tissue. The orders for wound care include application of cadexomer iodine (Iodosorb). Explain what needs to be assessed before applying this medication and its purpose in wound care.

15. A patient with an infected pressure ulcer that contains an area of eschar needs to have the area surgically débrided, but instead the physician orders collagenase (Santyl) treatment of the wound. What could be the reason for this order instead of surgery and what is the purpose of this medication?

## Case Study

**Read the scenario and answer the following questions on a separate sheet of paper.**

Judy is in the clinic today because she burned her arm last evening while frying chicken. She has a second-degree burn over a 5-inch area of her forearm. She did not apply anything to it overnight, and the wound is reddened and peeling.

1. The physician instructs you to apply silver sulfadiazine (Silvadene) cream to the site. What needs to be done before the cream is applied?

2. You instruct Judy that the area will need to be kept covered. Why is this necessary?

3. Do you need to wear gloves when applying this cream? Explain.

4. Are there any adverse effects associated with this medication?

# CHAPTER 57

# Ophthalmic Drugs

## Chapter Review and NCLEX® Examination Preparation

**Match each definition with the corresponding term. (Note: Not all terms will be used.)**

1. _____ Adjustment of the lens of the eye for variations in distance

2. _____ Inflammation of the eyelids

3. _____ The clear, watery fluid that circulates in the anterior and posterior chambers of the eye

4. _____ An abnormal condition of the lens of the eye, characterized by loss of transparency

5. _____ Paralysis of the ciliary muscles, which prevents accommodation of the lens for variations in distance

6. _____ Excessive intraocular pressure caused by obstruction of the outflow of aqueous humor

7. _____ The mucous membrane that lines the eyelids and the exposed anterior surface of the eye

8. _____ Drugs that constrict the pupil

9. _____ The vascular middle layer of the eye, containing the iris, ciliary body, and choroid

10. _____ Drugs that dilate the pupil

a. Cycloplegia
b. Conjunctiva
c. Accommodation
d. Glaucoma
e. Mydriatics
f. Miotics
g. Uvea
h. Blepharitis
i. Vitreous humor
j. Aqueous humor
k. Cataract

**Select the best answer for each question.**

11. When reviewing the medical record of a patient with a new order for a carbonic anhydrase inhibitor, the nurse knows that which condition would be a potential problem for a patient taking this drug?
    a. Glaucoma
    b. Ocular hypertension
    c. Allergy to sulfa drugs
    d. Allergy to penicillin

12. During an ophthalmic procedure, the patient receives ophthalmic acetylcholine. The nurse is aware that which effect is the purpose of administering this drug?
    a. To produce mydriasis for ophthalmic examination
    b. To produce immediate miosis during ophthalmic surgery
    c. To cause cycloplegia to allow for measurement of intraocular pressure
    d. To provide topical anesthesia during ophthalmic surgery

13. When giving latanoprost (Xalatan) eyedrops, the nurse will advise the patient of which possible adverse effects?
    a. Temporary eye color changes, from light eye colors to brown
    b. Permanent eye color changes, from light eye colors to brown
    c. Photosensitivity
    d. Bradycardia and hypotension

14. A patient has come to the emergency department with an eye injury. After fluorescein (AK-Fluor) is applied, the physician sees an area with a green halo. This indicates which condition?
    a. A corneal defect
    b. A conjunctival lesion
    c. The presence of a hard contact lens
    d. A foreign object

15. When applying ophthalmic drugs, the nurse will follow which instructions? *(Select all that apply.)*
    a. Apply drops directly onto the cornea.
    b. Apply drops into the conjunctival sac.
    c. Apply pressure to the inner canthus for 1 minute after medication administration.
    d. Apply ointments in a thin layer.
    e. Avoid touching the eye with the tip of the medication dropper.

16. A newborn infant is about to receive medication that prevents gonorrheal eye infection. The nurse will prepare to administer which drug?
    a. dexamethasone (Maxidex) ointment
    b. gentamicin (Genoptic) solution
    c. erythromycin ointment
    d. sulfacetamide (Cetamide) solution

17. A patient will be receiving acetazolamide (Diamox), 250 mg PO four times a day, as part of treatment for glaucoma. The tablets are available in 125-mg strength. How many tablets will the patient receive per dose? _____

18. A patient has an order for an IV to infuse at 75 mL/hour. The IV will infuse by gravity drip; the administration set delivers 15 gtt/mL. What is the gtt/min that the nurse will need to use for this infusion?
_____

## Critical Thinking and Application

**Answer the following questions on a separate sheet of paper.**

19. Jonathan has blue eyes; Julie has brown eyes. Why would the drug effects of the miotics on the iris be less pronounced in Julie?

20. Mrs. N., a 60-year-old librarian, has open-angle glaucoma. The ophthalmologist prescribes dipivefrin (Propine).
    a. Why might the physician have chosen that drug over epinephrine?
    b. What effects will the nurse tell Mrs. N. to expect when first taking dipivefrin?
    c. Will the nurse expect any serious reactions to the drug? Explain your answer.

21. The ophthalmologist prescribes a beta-adrenergic blocker for Ned, who has ocular hypertension. Ned experiences what he calls "an allergic reaction" to the drug, and the physician changes Ned's medication to another beta-blocking drug, timolol (Timoptic). Because both of these drugs are beta-adrenergic blockers and Ned had a reaction to the first drug, why would the physician simply switch Ned to another drug in the same category?

22. The nurse is preparing to administer sulfacetamide to Tony, a patient with an eye infection.
    a. Why will the nurse cleanse Tony's eye before administering the medication?
    b. Before using the sulfacetamide, the nurse examines it and then throws the solution away and orders another container of sulfacetamide. Why did the nurse do that?

23. Louisa has an inflammatory disorder of the eye for which the nurse practitioner has prescribed a topical ophthalmic nonsteroidal antiinflammatory drug (NSAID). Why was an NSAID chosen over a corticosteroid?

24. Ms. L. has been prescribed ophthalmic corticosteroid drops for an inflammation of her eye. The next day she calls the clinic and tells the nurse, "These drops sting so much when I use them that I can't even put in my contacts." What is the priority when the nurse responds to her statement?

25. The nurse is administering medications to a patient. The patient is due to receive both latanoprost (Xalatan) eyedrops and pilocarpine (Pilocar) eye gel at the same time. Which drug needs to be given first? Explain your answer.

## Case Study

**Read the scenario and answer the following questions on a separate sheet of paper.**

Mr. W., age 72, has developed a bacterial ocular infection and has a prescription for erythromycin ocular ointment. You are teaching him how to self-administer the medication.

1. How will this drug be administered?

2. You will educate Mr. W. about what safety precautions to take after he receives a dose of this medication?

3. After receiving the first dose, Mr. W. complains that the medication "burns and stings." What will you say to Mr. W. about this?

4. Mr. W. tells you, "I have some eyedrops from a few months ago when I had some allergy problems. I am sure they will help me now. Can I take them with this ointment?" What is your best response?

# CHAPTER 58

# Otic Drugs

## Chapter Review and NCLEX® Examination Preparation

**Select the best answer for each question.**

1. When assessing for otitis media, the nurse remembers that common symptoms of this condition include which of the following? *(Select all that apply.)*
   a. Pain
   b. Malaise
   c. Ear drainage
   d. Hearing loss
   e. Fever

2. A patient with a severe middle ear infection will generally require treatment with which type of drug?
   a. Topical steroids
   b. Systemic steroids
   c. Topical antibiotics
   d. Systemic antibiotics

3. An older adult patient has a buildup of cerumen in his left ear. The nurse expects that this patient will receive which type of drug for this problem?
   a. Antifungal
   b. Wax emulsifier
   c. Steroid
   d. Local analgesic

4. Before giving eardrops, the nurse checks for potential contraindications to the use of otic preparations, such as which of these conditions?
   a. Eardrum perforation
   b. Infection
   c. Presence of cerumen
   d. Mastoiditis

5. A child has a case of otitis media. The nurse knows that otitis media in children is usually preceded by:
   a. participation on a swim team.
   b. injury with a foreign object.
   c. upper respiratory tract infection.
   d. mastoiditis.

6. A child with an ear infection will be receiving amoxicillin (Amoxil) suspension PO. The order reads: "Give 125 mg (5 mL) three times a day PO." The child weighs 11 kg.
   a. How many milligrams of medication will this child receive in 24 hours? _____
   b. The safe dosage range of the medication is 20 to 40 mg/kg/day. What is the safe range (in milligrams) for this child? _____
   c. Is the ordered dose within the safe range?

   _____
   d. Mark on the medication cup how many milliliters the patient will receive for this dose.

## Critical Thinking and Application

**Answer the following questions on a separate sheet of paper.**

7. A patient calls the clinic complaining of severe pain in and drainage from his left ear. He also says he "had a little mishap" on his motorcycle yesterday. What will the nurse tell him?

8. Why are antiinfective otic drugs frequently combined with steroids?

9. André, a 30-year-old teacher, has an ear infection and a new prescription for eardrops.
   a. What might be done before he takes the eardrops?
   b. What safety measures are important to inform André about regarding self-administration of the eardrops?

10. Mrs. F., a 52-year-old office manager, has come to the clinic today complaining of a painful, "itchy" left ear. The physician's assistant diagnoses an infection of the external auditory canal and prescribes eardrop medication that contains a combination of polymyxin B and hydrocortisone.
    a. What is the advantage of using a product containing hydrocortisone?
    b. What would be a contraindication to Mrs. F.'s use of these eardrops?

11. Why do so many otic combination products contain local anesthetic drugs?

12. Ben, a 2-year-old toddler, attends day care, and his brother Drew is a 6-year-old kindergartener. They both require otic drugs for ear infections.
    a. What instructions will the nurse give the boys' parents regarding instillation of the drops?
    b. A few days after they are first seen, the boys' mother brings them back for a follow-up visit. Ben and Drew do not seem to be in pain and there is no redness or swelling in either child's ears. What does this mean?

13. During a home visit, the nurse observes Esther's husband preparing her eardrops. He puts a glass of water in the microwave, saying that he will soak the bottle of eardrops in hot water to warm them up.
    a. Why is this a concern?
    b. Immediately after her husband instills the drops, Esther sits up and asks whether they are now doing everything right. What will the nurse tell her?

14. A 4-year-old child will be receiving oral amoxicillin suspension for treatment for otitis media. The nurse gives the prescription to the child's mother, and asks her if she has any questions. The mother states, "Just to make sure, I will pour this liquid into his ears, correct? And I can stop it when his symptoms go away, right?" What is the priority when answering her questions?

## Case Study

**Read the scenario and answer the following questions on a separate sheet of paper.**

Mark, who is 45 years old, comes to the office complaining of a "heavy" feeling in his left ear, with slight pain and decreased hearing. When you walk into the examination room, you find Mark inserting a cotton-tipped applicator into his ear "to scratch it."

1. What is a possible reason for his symptoms?

2. What can be done to address this problem?

3. You give Mark a container of carbamide peroxide (Debrox) drops. Before you continue, he asks you how many times a day he needs to take this medication and whether he can take it with meals. How is this medication given?

4. Why is there a combination of carbamide peroxide and glycerin in the Debrox?

# Overview of Dosage Calculations

There are many important aspects to consider when performing dosage calculations, but probably the most important one is common sense. If a drug dose calculation does not seem right, then most likely it is not. The administration of drugs to patients is a shared responsibility among the patient, prescriber, pharmacist, and nurse. All those involved have a moral, ethical, and legal responsibility to ensure that the administration takes place in a safe and effective way. There are many checks and balances in the system to guarantee that this happens. The necessary basic calculations involved in the safe and accurate administration of medications to patients are described in this section.

Calculating drug doses is one small part of the overall process of pharmacologic therapy. Before you actually calculate a drug dose, you must follow many steps. The nurse will evaluate the patient and the prescribed medication for the following "rights": right patient, right drug, right dose, right time, and right route. In addition, the nurse must document correctly after the drug is given. Other principles to follow to decrease the likelihood of mistakes are to calculate doses systematically and to perform calculations consistently time after time so that the process becomes easier with each calculation.

It also helps to have a peer check your calculations, especially if the dose seems unusual or the math is very difficult. Make use of a calculator to help you with the arithmetic. Remember that common sense should prevail. If a calculation shows that you are to give 25 mg of digoxin and the strongest strength is 0.25 mg, common sense tells you that the patient should not be given 100 pills, especially since drug dosage forms are usually manufactured with the most commonly prescribed dosages in mind.

You must have basic arithmetic skills before beginning. The following basic principles may need to be reviewed:

- Basic multiplication
- Basic division
- Roman numerals
- Fractions (reducing to lowest terms, addition, subtraction, multiplication, division, mixed numbers)
- Decimals (addition, subtraction, multiplication, division)
- Ratios and percentages (changing a fraction to a percentage, changing a ratio to a percentage)
- Solving for $x$ in a simple equation

## RULES TO REMEMBER
- Before calculating a drug dose for a particular patient, you must first convert all units of measure to a SINGLE unit of measure, if this has not already been done. For example, do NOT attempt to guess a dosage if the drug is ordered in grains but the drug label is in milligrams. The best approach is to convert to the units of measure used on the drug label. You may have to convert the patient's weight from pounds to kilograms if the medication is ordered to be given per kilogram of weight.
- **Rounding**. Always round your answers to the nearest dose that is measurable, after verifying that the dose is correct for that patient.
  - If a tablet is scored, you may round to the nearest half tablet.
    **Example:** 1.8 tablets, give 2 tablets
    1.2 tablets, give 1 tablet
  - If a tablet is unscored, call the pharmacy. It is very difficult to cut an unscored tablet accurately. Remember that enteric-coated, sustained-release, or extended-release formulations cannot be cut or crushed!
  - Recheck your calculations if the dose is more than 1 or 2 tablets.

Disclaimer: Please note that the drugs and dosages within this chapter are examples for educational purposes only; please refer to appropriate drug resources for dosage information.

- To round liquids, look at the equipment you plan to use. Some syringes are marked in tenths or hundredths of a milliliter. Larger syringes are marked in 0.2-mL increments. Tuberculin syringes are marked in hundredths. For liquid medications, NEVER round up to the nearest WHOLE number. If the answer is 1.8 mL, DO NOT round up to 2 mL. Rounding up in these situations may lead to overdosing. However, if you are using an electronic infusion pump, you will probably need to round to the nearest whole number.
- To round to the nearest tenth, look at the hundredths column. If it is 0.5 or more, round UP to the next tenth (using one decimal place).

  **Example:**  To round to the nearest tenth (using one decimal place):

  1.78 or 1.75, round to 1.8

  1.32 or 1.34, round to 1.3
- A syringe calibrated in hundredths permits more exact measurement of small dosages. To round to the nearest hundredth, look at the thousandth column. If it is 0.005 or more, round UP to the next hundredth (using two decimal places).

  **Example:**  To round to the nearest hundredth (using two decimal places):

  1.847, round to 1.85

  1.653, round to 1.65
- NOTE: Never round liquid medications to the nearest whole number. If the answer is 1.6 mL, DO NOT round up to 2 mL! Such increases may lead to overdoses.
- PEDIATRIC DOSES are rounded to the TENTHS place, not whole numbers. Rounding to whole numbers may lead to overdoses.

- ■ **Leading Zeros.** Always insert a zero (0) in front of decimals when the number is less than a whole number. This draws attention to the decimal and avoids potential errors.

  **Example:**  0.05 is CORRECT.

  .05 is NOT correct.
- ■ **Trailing Zeroes.** Never place a lone zero after a decimal point. If the decimal is not noticed, a dangerous dosage error may occur.

  **Example:**  3 is CORRECT.

  3.0 is NOT correct and may be mistaken for 30.
- ■ **Labeling.** Always label your answers with the appropriate unit. If the problem asked for a number of tablets, write "tablets." If you are to give an injection, use "mL." Heparin and insulin, however, use "units" instead of "mg" or "mcg." Problems using an intravenous infusion pump are always asking for mL/hr. THINK about what the question is asking and then label your answer appropriately.
- ■ **Common Sense.** Use common sense! Drug companies typically formulate medications that are close to the usual doses and medications that can provide the ordered dose with one or two tablets. If your answer indicates that you need to give 60 mL intramuscularly, CHECK IT AGAIN! Remember, you can only give 2 to 3 mL intramuscularly, depending on institution policies, so a dosage of 60 mL would be inappropriate.

## INTERPRETING MEDICATION LABELS

Medication labels contain a great amount of information—much of it in small print. The drug manufacturer prints some labels; others are prepared by pharmacy technicians or pharmacists for institutional use. The most important information follows:

- ■ Generic name—the first letter is usually lowercase; this is the name used by all companies that produce the drug
- ■ Trade, brand, or proprietary name—the first letter is usually capitalized; this name is used only by the manufacturer of the drug and may be followed by the "®" symbol
- ■ Unit dose per milliliter, per tablet, per capsule, and so on
- ■ Total amount in the container
- ■ Route(s)
- ■ Directions for preparation, if needed
- ■ Directions for storage
- ■ Expiration date

Other information, such as a specification for adult or pediatric use, may be noted on the label.

**Example:**

Generic name:                          ciprofloxacin hydrochloride
Trade name:                            Cipro
Unit dose:                             750 mg per tablet
Total amount in container:             50 tablets
Route:                                 (It is assumed that tablets are oral route.)

**For the following labels, identify the information requested:**

1.

Generic name: _____

Trade name: _____

Unit dose: _____

Total amount in container: _____

Route: _____

2.

Generic name: _____

Trade name: _____

Unit dose: _____

Total amount in container: _____

Route: _____

3.

NDC 0009-0626-02    10 ml Vial

**Depo-Provera®**
Sterile Aqueous Suspension
sterile medroxyprogesterone
acetate suspension, USP

**400 mg per ml**

For intramuscular use only
Caution: Federal law prohibits
dispensing without prescription.

**Upjohn**

See package insert for complete
product information.
Shake vigorously immediately before
each use.
Store at controlled room temperature
15°-30° C (59°-86° F)
Each ml contains: Medroxyprogesterone
acetate, 400 mg.
Also, polyethylene glycol 3350, 20.3 mg;
sodium sulfate anhydrous, 11 mg;
myristyl-gamma picolinium chloride,
1.69 mg added as preservative. When
necessary, pH was adjusted with sodium
hydroxide and/or hydrochloric acid.
813 273 000

The Upjohn Company
Kalamazoo, Michigan 49001, USA

Generic name: _____

Trade name: _____

Unit dose: _____

Total amount in container: _____

Route: _____

4.

Single-Dose Vial    For IV or IM use
Contains Benzyl Alcohol as a Preservative
See package insert for complete
product information.
Per 2 mL (when mixed):
* hydrocortisone sodium succinate equiv.
to hydrocortisone, 250 mg. Protect
solution from light. Discard after 3 days.

814 070 205   Reconstituted ...........

The Upjohn Company
Kalamazoo, MI 49001, USA

2 mL Act-O-Vial®    NDC 0009-0909-08

**Solu-Cortef®** Sterile Powder
hydrocortisone sodium succinate
for injection, USP

**250 mg***

Generic name: _____

Trade name: _____

Unit dose: _____

Total amount in container: _____

Route: _____

## SECTION I: BASIC CONVERSIONS USING RATIO AND PROPORTION

There is more than one way to calculate dosages; the examples in this guide use the principle of ratio and proportion to calculate how much medication to give. A proportion is a way of stating a relationship of equality between two ratios. Ratio and proportion problems can be used to calculate ONE of the numbers in the equation if it is not known. The simple rule to use is this:

*The product of the outside terms equals the product of the inside terms.*

If one of the terms is not known, it is designated as *x*. The problem is then set up to solve for *x*.

**Example:**
The problem "1 : 100 :: 4 : *x*" actually means:
"The relationship of 1 to 100 is the same as the relationship of 4 to *x*." The *x* is unknown.

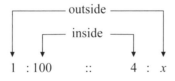

1 and *x* are the "outsides"; 100 and 4 are the "insides." To solve for *x*, multiply the "outsides" ($1 \times x$) together, multiply the "insides" ($100 \times 4$) together, and form an equation:

$(1 \times x) = (100 \times 4)$
$1x = 400$
$x = 400$

**Proof:** You may prove your equation as follows: Insert the answer for *x* in the original equation, then solve.

1 × 400 = 400 (outsides)
100 × 4 = 400 (insides)
400 = 400; the answer for *x* is correct.

### Example:
5 : 25 :: 15 : *x*

Multiply the "outsides" and the "insides" and form an equation; then solve for *x*.
(5 × *x*) = (25 × 15)
5*x* = 375
*x* = 375/5
*x* = 75

### Proof:
5 × 75 = 375
25 × 15 = 375
375 = 375

The following chart provides a few common equivalents used in pharmacology. These equivalents are then used in ratio and proportion problems to calculate appropriate dosages.

## BASIC EQUIVALENTS

| Metric Equivalents | Other Equivalents |
|---|---|
| **Weight**<br>1 mg (milligram) = 1000 mcg (micrograms)<br>1 g (gram) = 1000 mg (milligrams)<br>1 kg (kilogram) = 1000 g (grams) | **Weight**<br>1 gr (grain) = 60 mg (milligrams)<br>1 g (gram) = 1000 mg = gr xv (15 grains)<br>  (approximately)<br>1 kg (kilogram) = 2.2 lb (pounds) |
| **Volume**<br>1000 mL (milliliters) = 1 L (liter) | **Volume**<br>1 oz (ounce) = 30 mL (milliliters)<br>1 tsp (teaspoon) = 5 mL<br>1 tbsp (tablespoon) = 15 mL<br>2 tbsp = 30 mL |

To find basic equivalents from one unit of measure to another, use the ratio and proportion approach.

**Example 1:** The drug dosage is 500 mg. You have scored tablets on hand that are 1 g each. How many tablets will you give?

You have *grams* on hand. You need to change the *milligrams* needed to the equivalent grams on hand.

Find the proper equivalents:
Equivalent: 1 g = 1000 mg
Next, set up the ratio and proportion equation.
On the LEFT side, put the ratio that you ***know***: 1 g is 1000 mg
On the RIGHT side, put the ratio that you ***want to know***: How many g (*x*) is 500 mg?

***Know***          ***Want to Know***
1 g : 1000 mg :: *x* g : 500 mg

Solve for *x*: (1 × 500) = (1000 × *x*); 500 = 1000*x*; *x* = 500/1000; *x* = 0.5
You will give 0.5 (half) of the 1-g tablet, which equals 500 mg.

To double-check your answer, substitute your answer for the *x* and solve. The "outsides" should equal the "insides."
$1 \times 500 = 500$; $1000 \times 0.5 = 500$; $500 = 500$

**Example 2:** Cough syrup, 45 mL, is ordered. The cough syrup comes in a 2-oz bottle. How many oz do you give?
You have 2 oz on hand. You need to give 45 mL.
Equivalent: 1 oz = 30 mL

*Know:* 1 oz is 30 mL; *want to know:* How many oz is 45 mL?

*Know*          *Want to Know*
1 oz : 30 mL :: *x* oz : 45 mL

$(1 \times 45) = (30 \times x)$; $45 = 30x$; $x = 45/30 = 1.5$ oz = 45 mL
**Proof:** $1 \times 45 = 45$; $30 \times 1.5 = 45$; $45 = 45$

**Example 3:** Mabel weighs 122 lb. How many kilograms does she weigh?
Equivalent: 1 kg = 2.2 lb

*Know*          *Want to Know*
1 kg : 2.2 lb :: *x* kg : 122 lb

$(1 \times 122) = (2.2 \times x)$; $122 = 2.2x$; $122/2.2 = x$; $x = 55.45$ lb; round off to tenths: 55.5 lb
**Proof:** $1 \times 122 = 122$; $2.2 \times 55.45 = 121.99$ (rounds to 122)

**Example 4:** You have an injectable solution that is 50-mg strength. How many mcg are in 50 mg?
Equivalent: 1 mg = 1000 mcg

*Know*          *Want to Know*
1 mg : 1000 mcg :: 50 mg : *x* mcg

$(1 \times x) = (1000 \times 50)$; $1x = 50,000$; $x = 50,000$; therefore 50 mg = 50,000 mcg
**Proof:** $1 \times 50,000 = 50,000$; $1000 \times 50 = 50,000$

**Example 5:** Elixir is ordered as follows: "Give 2 tsp PO now." How many mL will you give?
Equivalent: 1 tsp = 5 mL

*Know*          *Want to Know*
1 tsp : 5 mL :: 2 tsp : *x* mL

$(1 \times x) = (5 \times 2)$; $1x = 10$; $x = 10$ mL
**Proof:** $1 \times 10 = 10$; $5 \times 2 = 10$; $10 = 10$
So, give 10 mL to equal 2 tsp.

**Example 6:** You have an injection that delivers 75 mcg. How many mg does it deliver?
Equivalent: 1 mg = 1000 mcg

*Know*          *Want to Know*
1 mg : 1000 mcg :: *x* mg : 75 mcg

$(1 \times 75) = (1000 \times x)$; $75 = 1000x$; $x = 75/1000$; $x = 0.075$
So, 75 mcg = 0.075 mg. (Don't forget the leading zero!)
**Proof:** $1 \times 75 = 75$; $1000 \times 0.075 = 75$; $75 = 75$

## PRACTICE PROBLEMS

**Calculate the following conversions.**

1. 600 mg = _____ mcg
2. 1500 mg = _____ mcg
3. 5000 mcg = _____ mg
4. 5 g = _____ mg
5. 2.5 g = _____ mg
6. 900 mg = _____ g
7. 8 kg = _____ g
8. 750 mL = _____ L
9. 975 L = _____ mL
10. 500 mL = _____ L

11. gr xvi = _____ mg
12. 90 mg = _____ gr
13. 4 tsp = _____ mL
14. 60 mL = _____ tsp
15. 90 mL = _____ tbsp
16. 3 oz = _____ mL
17. 6 mL = _____ oz
18. 90 kg = _____ lb
19. 150 lb = _____ kg
20. 11 kg = _____ lb

## SECTION II: CALCULATING ORAL DOSES

To calculate oral dosages of medications, use the same ratio and proportion procedures described in Section I. Label all terms, and check your answers by proving them.

The first step in doing medication dosage calculation problems is examining the order and the medication on hand. The units for both the order and the medicine on hand MUST be the same units (e.g., mg, mL). If they are not the same, then a conversion must first be done to change the ordered dose to the same units as the medication on hand.

Remember these rules:

- NEVER substitute one form of a medication for another, even if the dosage amount is the same. Parenteral forms of oral drugs are not equivalent, and the resulting drug effects might be dangerous.
- Do not forget to place a zero in front of a decimal point (e.g., 0.75 mg). It reminds you that the number is a decimal, not a whole number.
- Convert the drug ordered to the units of the drug at hand.
- Place what you have on hand (what you know)—information from the label—on the LEFT side of the equation.
- Place what is ordered (what you want to know) on the RIGHT side of the equation.
- Solve the equation as described in Section I.
- ALWAYS label the units of your answer (tablets, capsules, mL, etc.).
- Consult the pharmacist before splitting a tablet. Enteric-coated tablets and most capsules must not be broken.

**Example 1:** The prescription reads, "Give 500 mg PO." The unit dose is 250 mg/tablet. How many tablets will you give?

**Ordered:** 500 mg        **Unit dose:** 250 mg/tablet
**NOTE:** Units match (mg).

*Know*        *Want to Know*
250 mg : 1 tablet :: 500 mg : $x$ tablet

$(250 \times x) = (1 \times 500)$; $250x = 500$; $x = 500/250 = 2$
**Answer:** Give 2 tablets.
**Proof:** $250 \times 2 = 500$; $1 \times 500 = 500$; $500 = 500$

**Example 2:** The order is to give 175 mg. The tablets on hand are 350-mg scored tablets. How many tablets will you give?

**Ordered:** 175 mg        **Unit dose:** 350 mg/tablet
**NOTE:** Units match (mg).

*Know*                *Want to Know*
350 mg : 1 tablet :: 175 mg : *x* tablet

$(350 \times x) = (1 \times 175); 350x = 175; x = 175/350 = 0.5$
**Answer:** Give 0.5 tablet (one-half of the scored tablet).
**Proof:** $350 \times 0.5 = 175; 1 \times 175 = 175; 175 = 175$

**Example 3:** You are asked to administer 100 mg of a drug. You have 0.05-g tablets on hand. How many tablets will you give?

**Ordered:** 100 mg        **Unit dose:** 0.05 g/tablet
**NOTE:** Units do not match (mg and g).
**First:** Calculate: 100 mg = *x* g (equivalent: 1 g = 1000 mg)

*Know*            *Want to Know*
1 g : 1000 mg :: *x* g : 100 mg

$(1 \times 100) = (1000 \times x); 100 = 1000x; x = 100/1000 = 0.1$
100 mg = 0.1 g
Now that you have the ordered dose and the dose on hand in the same units, you can complete the problem.

**Ordered:** 0.1 g (100 mg)      **Unit dose:** 0.05 g/tablet

*Know*            *Want to Know*
0.05 g : 1 tablet :: 0.1 g : *x* tablet

$(0.05 \times x) = (1 \times 0.1); 0.05\, x = 0.1; x \times 0.1/0.05 = 2$
**Answer:** Give 2 tablets.
**Proof:** $0.05 \times 2 = 0.1; 1 \times 0.1 = 0.1; 0.1 = 0.1$

**Example 4:** You are instructed to give 0.5 g of a drug. You have 250-mg tablets on hand. How many tablets will you give?

**Ordered:** 0.5 g          **Unit dose:** 250 mg/tablet
**NOTE:** Units do not match (g and mg).
**First:** Calculate: 0.5 g = *x* mg (equivalent: 1 g = 1000 mg)

*Know*            *Want to Know*
1 g : 1000 mg :: 0.5 g : *x* mg

$(1 \times x) = (1000 \times 0.5); 1x = 500; x = 500$
0.5 g = 500 mg
Now that you have the ordered dose and the dose on hand in the same units, you can complete the problem.

**Ordered:** 500 mg (0.5 g)  **Unit dose:** 250 mg/tablet

*Know*                *Want to Know*
250 mg : 1 tablet :: 500 mg : *x* tablet

$(250 \times x) = (1 \times 500); 250x = 500; x = 500/250 = 2$
**Answer:** Give 2 tablets.
**Proof:** $250 \times 2 = 500; 1 \times 500 = 500; 500 = 500$

**Example 5:** You are to administer 200 mg of guaifenesin (Robitussin) syrup. You have a bottle labeled 100 mg/5 mL. How many mL will you give?
**Ordered:** 200 mg          **Unit dose:** 100 mg/5 mL
**NOTE:** Units match (mg).

***Know***          ***Want to Know***
100 mg : 5 mL :: 200 mg : $x$ mL

$(100 \times x) = (5 \times 200)$; $100x = 1000$; $x = 1000/100 = 10$
**Answer:** Give 10 mL.
**Proof:** $100 \times 10 = 1000$; $5 \times 200 = 1000$; $1000 = 1000$

## PRACTICE PROBLEMS

**Perform the following calculations.**

1. Dose ordered: ascorbic acid 0.5 g PO
   Dose on hand: 500-mg tablets
   How many tablets will you give? _____

2. Dose ordered: digoxin (Lanoxin) 0.5 mg PO
   Dose on hand: 250-mcg tablets
   How many tablets will you give? _____

3. Dose ordered: 0.15 g PO
   Dose on hand: 300-mg tablets
   How many tablets will you give? _____

4. Dose ordered: diphenhydramine (Benadryl) syrup 50 mg PO
   Dose on hand: syrup 12.5 mg/5 mL
   How many milliliters will you give? _____

5. Dose ordered: 600 mg PO
   Dose on hand: gr v tablets
   How many tablets will you give? _____

6. Dose ordered: cefaclor (Ceclor) 0.1 g PO
   Dose on hand: oral suspension 125 mg/5 mL
   How many milliliters will you give? _____

7. Dose ordered: zidovudine (Retrovir) 0.3 g PO
   Dose on hand: 100-mg capsules
   How many capsules will you give? _____

8. Dose ordered: potassium chloride liquid 30 mEq PO
   Dose on hand: 20 mEq/15 mL
   How many milliliters will you give? _____

9. Dose ordered: 0.15 g PO
   Dose on hand: 50-mg capsules
   How many capsules will you give? _____

10. Dose ordered: 2 g PO
    Dose on hand: 500-mg tablets
    How many tablets will you give? _____

## SECTION III: RECONSTITUTING MEDICATIONS

Many parenteral medications come in powder or crystal form and must be reconstituted by the addition of a diluent to create a liquid form before administration. Instructions for dissolving medications can be found in the literature that accompanies the medication or on the medication label. In most facilities, the pharmacy department has taken over the task of reconstituting medications. However, there are still instances where you may be required to reconstitute a drug and then draw up the proper dose for parenteral use. Medications for IV use that need to be reconstituted are sent with delivery systems that match 50- or 100-mL IV bags, and reconstitution occurs as the nurse prepares the medication for use. Some medications for intramuscular administration also need to be reconstituted before use. Following are examples of those instances in which nurses will be reconstituting medications before use.

As an example, the instructions may read:

*Add 1.2 mL normal saline to make 2 mL of reconstituted solution that yields 100 mg/mL.*

This tells the nurse that the medication takes up 0.8 mL of space: 1.2 mL + 0.8 mL = 2 mL of medication solution. The label of the medication container will tell the nurse how many units, grams, milligrams, or micrograms are in each milliliter of the reconstituted drug. In this example, the dose on hand, after reconstitution, is 100 mg/mL.

Remember these concepts:

- Read all instructions for reconstitution before doing anything! Be sure to ask the pharmacist if you have any questions.
- When reconstituting medications, be certain to use the exact type of diluent indicated, and add the exact amount of diluent as directed. Substitutions or inaccurate amounts of diluent can inactivate the medication or alter the concentration, thus altering the dose received by the patient.
- If the container is a multiple-dose vial, the nurse who reconstitutes the medication must put the date, time, amount of diluent used, and his or her initials on the label. Follow the facility's policy for multiple-dose vials.
- Many solutions are unstable after being reconstituted. Be sure to follow the directions on the label for proper storage of reconstituted medications. Follow the facility's policy for labeling the reconstituted solution.
- Make note of the time limit or expiration date for the reconstituted medication. Do not use the medication after it has expired.
- Ratio solutions indicate the number of grams of the medication per total milliliters of solution. For example, a medication that is designated 1:1000 has 1 g of medication per 1000 mL of solution.

**In order to avoid overdosing, it is essential that the nurse choose the correct ratio solution!**

- Percentage (%) solutions indicate the number of grams of the medication per 100 mL of solution. For example, a medication that is designated 10% has 10 g of drug per 100 mL of solution.
- COMPARE: "1:1000" indicates 1 g per 1000 mL
  "10%" indicates 10 g per 100 mL

**As you calculate parenteral dosages:**

- If the amount is greater than 1 mL, round $x$ (the amount to be given) to tenths and use a 3-mL syringe to measure it.
- Small (less than 0.5 mL, or pediatric) dosages are rounded to hundredths and measured in a tuberculin syringe. The tuberculin syringe is calibrated in 0.01-mL increments.
- THINK! For adults, the maximum volume of an IM injection is usually 3 mL. (Facility policies regarding the maximum volume of an IM injection may vary.) Sometimes the dose might have to be given in two divided doses; for example, a dose of 4 mL IM would usually be divided into two 2-mL doses. However, if your calculations yield an unusual number, such as 10 mL IM, look over your calculation and repeat your math! Double-check your calculations with a peer.

**Always remember to note the route ordered. IM doses and IV doses are NOT always the same amount and the drug formulations may differ. Confusing the route may have fatal results.**

**Example 1:** You receive an order for morphine 12 mg IM. The medication vial reads: 10 mg/mL. How much morphine would you give?
Does this medication require reconstitution?
Would you use a 3-mL or a tuberculin syringe to measure this drug?

**Ordered:** 12 mg          **Unit dose:** 10 mg/mL

*Know*          *Want to Know*
10 mg : 1 mL :: 12 mg : $x$ mL

$(10 \times x) = (1 \times 12)$; $10x = 12$; $x = 12/10 = 1.2$
**Answer:** 1.2 mL measured in a 3-mL syringe. This medication does not require reconstitution.
**Proof:** $10 \times 1.2 = 12$; $1 \times 12 = 12$

**Example 2:** The ordered dose is 2.5 mg IV.

How much medication would you give?
Does this medication require reconstitution?
Would you use a 3-mL or a tuberculin syringe to measure this drug?

**Ordered:** 2.5 mg          **Unit dose:** 10 mg/1 mL

*Know*          *Want to Know*
10 mg : 1 mL :: 2.5 mg : $x$ mL

$(10 \times x) = (1 \times 2.5)$; $10x = 2.5$; $x = 2.5/10 = 0.25$
**Answer:** 0.25 mL measured in a tuberculin syringe. Reconstitution is not needed.
**Proof:** $10 \times 0.25 = 2.5$; $1 \times 2.5 = 2.5$; $2.5 = 2.5$

**Example 3:** You receive an order for penicillin G potassium 400,000 units IM.

Which dilution would you choose for the ordered dose?
How much penicillin G potassium would you give?
Would you use a 3-mL or a tuberculin syringe to measure this drug?

**Ordered:** 400,000 units    **Unit dose:** Choosing the 1.8 mL diluent amount, unit dose is 500,000 units/mL.

*Know*               *Want to Know*
500,000 units : 1 mL :: 400,000 : $x$ mL

$(500,000 \times x) = (1 \times 400,000)$; $500,000x = 400,000$; $x = 400,000/500,000 = 0.8$
**Answer:** 0.8 mL measured in either a 3-mL or tuberculin syringe.
**Proof:** $500,000 \times 0.8 = 400,000$; $1 \times 400,000 = 400,000$; $400,000 = 400,000$

**NOTE:** Choose the concentration that is close to the ordered dose. Choosing the 1.8 mL diluent amount allows for the injection amount to be small yet easily measured. If you had chosen the 10 mL diluent amount, the injection would have been 4 mL; choosing the 20 mL diluent would have made the injection amount 8 mL. Because of the volume limits for IM injections, both would have required at least two separate injections!

**Example 4:** You receive an order for epinephrine 0.6 mg subcut. The medication label reads:

> 1 mL ampule
> Epinephrine 1:1000
> For subcut or IM use

What is the dose on hand?
How much epinephrine would you give?
Would you use a 3-mL or a tuberculin syringe to measure the drug?

**First:** Figure the dose on hand.
1:1000 = 1 g in 1000 mL = 1000 mg in 1000 mL = 1 mg in 1 mL
Then complete the problem:

**Ordered:** 0.6 mg        **Unit dose:** 1 mg/mL

**Know**        **Want to Know**
1 mg : 1 mL :: 0.6 mg : $x$ mL

$(1 \times x) = (1 \times 0.6)$; $1x = 0.6$; $x = 0.6$
**Answer:** 0.6 mL measured in either a 3-mL or tuberculin syringe.
**Proof:** $1 \times 0.6 = 0.6$; $1 \times 0.6 = 0.6$; $0.6 = 0.6$

**Example 5:** Calcium gluconate 5 g IV push over 5 minutes.

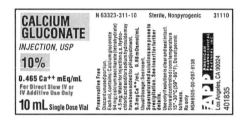

What is the dose on hand?
How much calcium gluconate would you give?
**First:** Figure the dose on hand.
10% = 10 g in 100 mL = 0.1 g per 1 mL
Then complete the problem:

**Ordered:** 5 g        **Unit dose:** 0.1 g/mL

**Know**        **Want to Know**
0.1 g : 1 mL :: 5 g : $x$ mL

$(0.1 \times x) = (1 \times 5)$; $0.1x = 5$; $x = 5/0.1$; $x = 50$
**Answer:** 50 mL
**Proof:** $0.1 \times 50 = 5$; $1 \times 5 = 5$; $5 = 5$

## PRACTICE PROBLEMS

**Perform the following calculations.**

1.  Dose ordered: thiamine 200 mg IV
    On hand: 10-mL vial, 100 mg/mL
    How much will you give? _____

2.  Dose ordered: gentamicin (Garamycin) 60 mg IM
    On hand: 40 mg/mL
    How much will you give? _____

3.  Dose ordered: heparin 8000 units subcut
    On hand: 1-mL vial, 10,000 units/mL
    How much will you give? _____

4.  Dose ordered: medication 750 mg IV
    On hand: 1-g vial
    Instructions for reconstitution: Add 1.5 mL sterile water. Reconstituted solution will contain approximately 500 mg medication solution per mL.
    How much will you give? _____

5.  Dose ordered: ampicillin 500 mg IV
    On hand: 1-g vial powder for injection
    The reconstituted solution contains 125 mg/5 mL.
    How much will you give? _____

6. Dose ordered: penicillin G potassium 300,000 units IM

   On hand: 1,000,000-units vial

   Instructions for reconstitution: Using only sterile water, add 9.6 mL to provide 100,000 units/mL, or 4.6 mL to provide 200,000 units/mL.

   Which concentration would you choose for this dose? _____

   How much will you give? _____

7. Dose ordered: epinephrine 750 mcg subcut

   On hand: 1:1000

   How much will you give? _____

8. Dose ordered: medication 0.2 mg IVPB

   On hand: 1:5000

   How much will you give? _____

9. Dose ordered: calcium chloride 900 mg IVPB

   On hand: calcium chloride 10% vial. How much will you give? _____

10. Dose ordered: magnesium sulfate 4 g IVPB

    On hand: magnesium sulfate 50% vial

    How much will you give? _____

## SECTION IV: PEDIATRIC CALCULATIONS

Doses used in pediatric patients must differ from those used in adults. The most common method for calculating doses for pediatric patients is weight-based (i.e., mg/kg). In some cases, dosages may be calculated using body surface area (BSA) calculations.

## Body Surface Area Calculations

The BSA is a common method used to calculate therapeutic pediatric dosages. It requires the use of a chart called a *West nomogram* (see Figure 3-1 in your text) that converts weight to square meters ($m^2$) of BSA. The average adult is assumed to weigh 140 lb and have a BSA of 1.73 $m^2$. The BSA may be used to calculate the pediatric dose of certain medications.

- For a child of normal height and weight, find the $m^2$ for that weight on the shaded area of the nomogram chart.

  **Example:** Using Figure 3-1 in your text, find the BSA for a child who weighs 40 lb and is 38 inches tall (normal height for her weight). According to the nomogram, the BSA for 40 lb is 0.74 $m^2$.

- For a child who is underweight or overweight, the BSA is indicated at the point where a straight line connecting the height and weight intersects the unshaded surface area (SA) column.

  **Example:** Using Figure 3-1, find the BSA for a child who weighs 25 lb and has a height of 30 inches (underweight). According to the nomogram, the BSA for this child is 0.51 $m^2$.

There are two types of BSA problems.

1. The first type involves medications for which the literature provides recommended dosages in $m^2$.

**STEP 1:** Check the order, and look up the recommended dose.

The order is for 15 mg PO.

The literature states that 40 mg/$m^2$ is safe for children.

**STEP 2:** Determine child's height and weight. Then consult the appropriate nomogram to obtain the BSA in $m^2$. This child weighs 22 lb and has a normal height of 70 cm. The BSA is approximately 0.46 $m^2$.

**STEP 3:** Calculate the recommended mg/$m^2$ dose (from the literature) using ratio and proportion. Then, for a safety check, compare it with the dose ordered.

For this calculation, what you know is the literature's recommendation (40 mg/$m^2$). What you want to know is the milligrams per the child's BSA (which is 0.46 $m^2$).

***Know***        ***Want to Know***

40 mg : 1 $m^2$ :: $x$ mg : 0.46 $m^2$

$(40 \times 0.46) = (1 \times x)$; $18.4 = 1x$; $x = 18.4$ (Pediatric doses are rounded to tenths place; do not round to whole numbers.)

**Answer:** 18.4 mg is the safe dose limit.

**Decision:** The order for 15 mg is safe.

## Practice:

The medication ordered is 100 mg.

**STEP 1:** The literature recommends 50 mg/m$^2$ for children.

**STEP 2:** The child weighs 10 lb and has a normal height for his weight. The BSA is 0.27 m$^2$.

**STEP 3:** Calculate the dose for this child's BSA:

*Know*       *Want to Know*
50 mg : 1 m$^2$ :: $x$ mg : 0.27 m$^2$

$(50 \times 0.27) = (1 \times x)$; $13.5 = 1x$; $x = 13.5$ (Pediatric doses are rounded to tenths place; do not round to whole numbers.)
**Answer:** 13.5 mg is the safe dose limit.
**Decision:** The order for 15 mg exceeds the safe dose limit and therefore is NOT safe. Notify the physician.

2. The second type of BSA involves situations when a recommended dose is cited in the literature for adults but not for children.

**STEP 1:** Determine the BSA (m$^2$) of the child by dividing the adult dose by 1.73 m$^2$ (the average adult's BSA).

**STEP 2:** Multiply the result by the average adult dose.

$$\frac{\text{Child's BSA (m}^2)}{\text{Average adult's BSA}} \times \text{Average adult dose of drug} = \text{Estimated child's dose}$$

**Example:** A 6-lb child has a BSA of 0.20 m$^2$, and the average adult dose of a drug is 300 mg. What would be the estimated safe dose for a child?

$$\frac{0.20 \text{ m}^2}{1.73 \text{ m}^2} \times 300 \text{ mg} = 34.68 \text{ mg}$$

**Answer:** 34.7 mg is the estimated safe dose for this child. (Round to tenths place for pediatric doses.)

## Practice:

The average adult dose for a medication is 20 mg. The child has a BSA of 0.6 m$^2$. What would be the estimated safe dose for a child?

$$\frac{0.60 \text{ m}^2}{1.73 \text{ m}^2} \times 20 \text{ mg} = 6.94 \text{ mg}$$

**Answer:** 6.9 mg is the estimated safe dose for this child. (Round to tenths place for pediatric doses.)

## Weight-Based Calculations

When calculating the proper dose according to weight, STEP 1 involves changing the weight from pounds to kilograms (if necessary).

- Be careful when converting ounces and pounds to kilograms. First, ounces must be converted to part of a pound (by dividing the ounces by 16). Remember, 16 ounces = 1 pound. Therefore 8 oz does not convert to 0.8 lb! Convert 8 ounces to pounds by dividing by 16: 8/16 = 0.5; 8 oz = 0.5 lb.
- Once you have converted ounces to pounds, then add the ounces to the pounds. For example, 10 lb 8 oz would equal 10.5 lb. You are now ready to convert pounds to kilograms.
- Remember: 1 kg = 2.2 lb. To convert 10.5 lb to kilograms, divide the pounds by 2.2.
- 1 kg : 2.2 lb :: $x$ kg : 10.5 lb; $(1 \times 10.5) = (2.2 \times x)$; $10.5 = 2.2x$; $x = 10.5/2.2 = 4.8$ kg (rounded to tenths)
- DO NOT round pediatric weights to whole numbers!
- Once you have converted the child's weight to kg, you are ready for STEP 2.

**STEP 2** involves calculating the therapeutic dosage ranges for a child based on his or her weight. The nurse uses the child's weight (in kilograms) to calculate the low and high acceptable doses for that medication. This will give a range of dosage that this child could receive for this medication.

**STEP 3** involves THINKING and comparing the ordered dose with the therapeutic dosage range that was calculated for that child. If the ordered dose is under or over the calculated therapeutic dosage range, then do not give the medication and notify the physician.

- **STEP 1:** Convert the child's weight from pounds to kilograms.
- **STEP 2:** Calculate therapeutic dose range (low and high).
- **STEP 3:** (1) Is the ordered dose safe (does not exceed the dosage range)?
    (2) Is the ordered dose therapeutic (falling within the recommended dosage range, not too low)?

**Example 1:** The ordered dose is 50 mg acetaminophen (Tylenol). The infant weighs 15 lb. The therapeutic dosage range for acetaminophen is 10 to 15 mg/kg/dose.

**STEP 1:** Convert pounds to kilograms by dividing 15 by 2.2.
15/2.2 = 6.82; 15 lb = 6.8 kg (Round pediatric weights to tenths, not to whole numbers.)

**STEP 2:** Calculate the therapeutic dosage range for this infant based on his weight.
Low dose: 10 mg/kg/dose × 6.8 kg = 68 mg/dose (note that the "kg" cancel out).
High dose: 15 mg/kg/dose × 6.8 kg = 102 mg/dose (note that the "kg" cancel out).
The therapeutic dosage range for this infant is 68 to 102 mg/dose for acetaminophen.

**STEP 3:** Compare the ordered dose with the therapeutic dosage range calculated in STEP 2.
**Answer:** The ordered dose of 50 mg is not therapeutic because it falls under the low recommended dose.

**Question:** If the doctor orders 110 mg of acetaminophen for this infant, would that be a safe and therapeutic dose?
**Answer:** No, it would neither be safe nor therapeutic because it is higher than 102 mg.

**Example 2:** The ordered dose is amoxicillin (Amoxil) 275 mg q 8 hr PO. The patient weighs 35 lb. The therapeutic dosage range for amoxicillin is 20 to 40 mg/kg/24 hr in divided doses.

**STEP 1:** Convert pounds to kilograms by dividing 35 by 2.2.
35/2.2 = 15.9; 35 lb = 15.9 kg

**STEP 2:** Calculate the therapeutic dosage range for this child based on his weight.
Low dose: 20 mg/kg/24 hr × 15.9 kg = 318 mg/24 hr
High dose: 40 mg/kg/24 hr × 15.9 kg = 636 mg/24 hr

**NOTE:** These ranges are for 24 hours! The dosage is every 8 hours, so dividing 24 hours by 8 tells us that there will be 3 doses within 24 hours. To figure out the single dosage for the low and high ranges, divide each 24-hour dose by 3:

318 mg/24 hr divided by 3 doses = 106 mg/dose
636 mg/24 hr divided by 3 doses = 212 mg/dose

**Answer:** The safe range for a single dose of amoxicillin for this child is 106 to 212 mg/dose. (An alternate way to figure a single dose is to calculate the amount of medication the ordered dose would provide in 24 hours. In this example, knowing there are three doses given every 8 hours in a 24-hour period, multiplying the dose ordered by 3 would yield the ordered dose for 24 hours: 275 mg × 3 doses = 825 mg/24 hr.)

**STEP 3:** Is the ordered dose of 275 mg therapeutic for this child?
**Answer:** No, the ordered dose of 275 mg exceeds the therapeutic dosage range for this patient. Consult the physician. (Note also that the calculated 24-hour dose of 825 mg/24 hr exceeds the high range of 636 mg/24 hr calculated for this child.)

Many pediatric medications come in several concentrations. It is ESSENTIAL to use the correct concentration of medication to ensure accurate dosage and prevent accidental underdosage or overdosage.

**Example:** Acetaminophen comes in many forms, including:
    elixir, 160 mg/5 mL
    liquid suspension, 160 mg/5 mL, 500 mg/5 mL, 500 mg/15 mL
    chewable tablet, 80 mg/tablet
    tablet, 325 or 500 mg/tablet
    orally disintegrating tablet, 80 or 160 mg/tablet
    suppository, 120, 325, or 650 mg
(NOTE: The infant drops concentration of 80 mg/0.8 mL has been removed from the market.)

A 4-month-old infant weighs 13 lb and has a fever of 101.5° F (38.6° C). What would be the therapeutic dosage range of acetaminophen this infant could receive? The recommended range is 10 to 15 mg/kg/dose.

**STEP 1:** 13 lb = 5.9 kg

**STEP 2:** Low dose: 10 mg/kg/dose × 5.9 = 59 mg/dose
High dose: 15 mg/kg/dose × 5.9 = 88.5 mg/dose
**Answer:** The therapeutic dosage range for this infant is 59 to 88.5 mg/dose.
Referring to the forms of acetaminophen listed above, which form would you choose if this infant was to receive a 60-mg dose?
**Answer:** Choose the elixir, 160 mg/5 mL, and administer 1.9 mL with a calibrated oral syringe or dropper. (160 mg : 5 mL :: 60 mg : $x$; $x$ = 1.875, which rounds to 1.9 mL)

**STEP 3:** Is the ordered dose of 60 mg therapeutic for this infant?
**Answer:** Yes, the 60-mg dose falls within the 59 to 88.5 mg/dose range for this infant.

Choose the medication form that is manufactured for infants and children. The infant cannot take tablets; suppositories are not the first choice unless the infant cannot take oral medications. Rectal doses may be a little higher than oral doses, and cutting suppositories in half is not recommended because the medication may not be distributed evenly within the suppository. NOTE: Most liquid medication packages for infants and children have specific instructions for dosing and include the specific dropper to use for measuring liquids.

## PRACTICE PROBLEMS

**Perform the following calculations.**

1.  Your 6-year-old patient weighs 40 lb. Morphine sulfate via continuous infusion is ordered at 1 mg/hr. The therapeutic dosage range for continuous intravenous infusion is 0.025 to 2.6 mg/kg/hr.
    a.  What are the low and high doses for this child? _____
    b.  Is the ordered dose within a safe and therapeutic range? _____

2.  A 5-year-old child weighs 33 lb. Ibuprofen is ordered at 120 mg PO q 8 hr. The therapeutic dosage range is 5 to 10 mg/kg/dose q 6 hr to q 8 hr, and the maximum dose is 40 mg/kg/24 hr.
    a.  What are the low and high doses for this child? _____
    b.  What is the maximum amount this child can receive in 24 hours? _____
    c.  Is the ordered dose within a safe and therapeutic range? _____

3.  A 10-year-old patient weighs 70 lb. Ceftazidime is ordered at 1.7 g q 8 hr IV. The therapeutic dosage range is 100 to 150 mg/kg/24 hr (divided q 8 hr IV).
    a.  What are the low and high doses for this child in 24 hours? _____
    b.  What are the low and high doses for this child per individual dose? _____
    c.  Is the ordered dose within a safe and therapeutic range? _____

4.  Your patient weighs 15 lb. The medication ordered is 150 mcg bid. The therapeutic dosage range of the medication is 0.02 to 0.05 mg/kg/day.
    a.  What are the low and high doses for this child in 24 hours? _____
    b.  What are the low and high doses for this child per individual dose? _____
    c.  Is the ordered dose within a safe and therapeutic range? _____

5.  A child weighs 34 lb. The medication ordered is 30 mg IM preoperatively. The therapeutic dosage range is 1 to 2.2 mg/kg.
    a.  What are the low and high doses for this child per individual dose? _____
    b.  Is the ordered dose within a safe and therapeutic range? _____

6.  For a child weighing 50 lb, medication is ordered at 0.2 mg daily IV. The therapeutic dosage range is 4 to 5 mcg/kg/day.
    a.  What are the low and high doses for this child per individual dose? _____
    b.  Is the ordered dose within a safe and therapeutic range? _____

## SECTION V: BASIC INTRAVENOUS CALCULATIONS

Intravenous (IV) fluids and medications are given over a designated period of time. For instance, the order may read:

*Give 1000 mL normal saline over 8 hours IV.*

For IVs that infuse with an infusion pump, the milliliters per hour is calculated (mL/hr).

For IVs that infuse by gravity, the rate at which an IV is given is measured in terms of drops per minute (gtt/min).

To calculate mL/hr and gtt/min, we need to consider what the order contains and what equipment is used. In order to calculate drops per minute, we need to know the drop factor of the IV tubing. The size of the drops delivered per milliliter can vary with different types of tubing. The drop factor of a certain tubing set is printed on the packaging label.

Adding to the above order:

*The drop factor for the IV tubing is 15 gtt/mL.*

The order now reads:

*Give 1000 mL normal saline over 8 hours IV. The drop factor is 15 gtt/mL.*

**STEP 1:** Calculate milliliters per hour.

We know that 1000 mL is to infuse over 8 hours. We want to know how much is to infuse over 1 hour. Set up the equation:

***Know***        ***Want to Know***
1000 mL : 8 hr :: $x$ mL : 1 hr

$(1000 \times 1) = (8 \times x)$; $1000 = 8x$; $x = 8/1000$; $x = 125$ mL/hr

**Rate:** To give 1000 mL normal saline over 8 hours, give 125 mL/hr for 8 hours.

*A quick way to determine the hourly rate is to divide the TOTAL VOLUME by the TOTAL TIME (if the time is in hours): 1000 mL × 8 hr = 125 mL/hr.*

**STEP 2:** Calculate the gtt/min.

To set up a gravity IV drip, further calculations are needed. To ensure the proper rate, one must count the drops per minute (gtt/min).

We know the rate is 125 mL/hr and the drop factor is 15 gtt/mL. Since we need to change from hours to minutes, another equivalent we'll need is 60 min = 1 hr.

When mL/hr is known, the formula for calculating gtt/min is as follows:

$$\frac{\text{drop factor (gtt/mL)}}{\text{time (min)}} \times \text{hourly rate (mL/hr)}$$

Plugging in what we know:

$$\frac{15 \text{ gtt/mL*}}{60 \text{ min/hr}} \times 125/\text{hr} = x \text{ gtt/min}$$

*To make it easier to calculate, reduce the 15/60 fraction to 1/4 before multiplying by 125.

$1/4 \times 125 = 125/4 = 31.25$ (round mL/hr to whole numbers)

**Answer:** 31 gtt/min for a gravity drip

**Points to remember:**

- The drop factor varies per IV tubing set manufacturer. It can range from 10 to 60 gtt/mL.
- Infusion sets that deliver 60 gtt/mL are called *microdrips*.
- **STEP 1:** To calculate mL/hr, divide the TOTAL VOLUME by the TOTAL TIME (in hours).
- **STEP 2:** To calculate gtt/min when the hourly rate is known, use the formula:

$$\frac{\text{drop factor (gtt/mL)}}{\text{time (min)}} \times \text{hourly rate (mL/hr)}$$

- THINK! If you are using an infusion pump, you need to calculate milliliters per hour.
- THINK! Round off your answer to the nearest whole number. You cannot count a partial drop! Also, electronic infusion pumps will usually use the nearest whole number in mL. (Exceptions to this may occur in critical care or pediatric settings.)

**Example 1:** The order reads "200 mL to be infused for 1 hr." If the drop factor is 15 gtt/mL, how many gtt/min will be given?
*Start at STEP 1 or STEP 2?*
Start at STEP 1. You need to know the hourly rate in mL/hr.

**STEP 1:** Calculate mL/hr. Divide total volume by the total time (in hours).
200 mL over 1 hr = 200 mL/hr.

**STEP 2:** Calculate gtt/min using the formula:

$$\frac{\text{drop factor}}{\text{time (min)}} \times \text{hourly rate} = 15/60 \times 200 = 1/4 \times 200 = 50$$

**Answer:** 50 gtt/min

**Example 2:** The order is for 1000 mL to infuse at 150 mL/hr. The drop factor is 20 gtt/mL. How many gtt/min will be given?
*Start at STEP 1 or STEP 2?*
Start at STEP 2. The hourly rate, 150 mL/hr, has been given.

**STEP 2:** Calculate gtt/min using the formula:

$$\frac{\text{drop factor}}{\text{time (min)}} \times \text{hourly rate} = 20/60 \times 150 = 1/3 \times 150 = 50$$

**Answer:** 50 gtt/min

**Example 3:** You receive an order for 200 mL to be infused for 90 minutes. You have a microdrip set (60 gtt/mL). How many gtt/min will be given?
*Start at STEP 1 or STEP 2?*
Start at STEP 1. Calculate the hourly rate. Remember, 60 min = 1 hr.

**STEP 1:** Calculate mL/hr.

*Know*              *Want to Know*
200 mL : 90 min :: $x$ mL : 60 min

$(200 \times 60) - (90 \times x)$; $12,000 - 90x$; $x - 12,000/90$ $x - 133.33$
**Rate:** 133 mL/hr (Round to nearest whole number.)

**STEP 2:** Calculate gtt/min using the formula:

$$\frac{\text{drop factor}}{\text{time (min)}} \times \text{hourly rate} = 60/60 \times 133 = 133$$

**Answer:** 133 gtt/min

Shortcut: For microdrips, when the drip factor is 60 and the time is 60 minutes, the "60s" cancel out to "1" and the result is that the ordered mL/hr = the gtt/min.

## PRACTICE PROBLEMS

**Calculate the following, and prove your answers.**

1. Give 1000 mL lactated Ringer's solution over 6 hours. The drop factor is 15 gtt/mL.
   *Start at STEP 1 or STEP 2?*
   a. mL/hr: _____
   b. gtt/min: _____

2. Infuse 600 mL blood over 3 hours. The blood administration set has a drop factor of 10 gtt/mL.
   *Start at STEP 1 or STEP 2?*
   a. mL/hr: _____
   b. gtt/min: _____

3. Infuse 1000 mL normal saline over 12 hours, using tubing with a drop factor of 15 gtt/mL.
   *Start at STEP 1 or STEP 2?*
   a. mL/hr: _____
   b. gtt/min: _____

4. Infuse 200 mL $D_5NS$ over 2 hours using a microdrip set.
   *Start at STEP 1 or STEP 2?*
   a. mL/hr: _____
   b. gtt/min: _____
   c. What is the drop factor? _____

5. Infuse $D_5W$ at 75 mL/hr. The drop factor is 10 gtt/mL.
   *Start at STEP 1 or STEP 2?*
   gtt/min: _____

6. Infuse $D_5W$ at 75 mL/hr. The drop factor is 15 gtt/mL.
   *Start at STEP 1 or STEP 2?*
   gtt/min: _____

7. Infuse $D_5W$ at 75 mL/hr. The drop factor is 20 gtt/mL.
   *Start at STEP 1 or STEP 2?*
   gtt/min: _____

8. After looking at your answers for Questions 5, 6, and 7, what observation can you make about the relationship between the drop factor and the resulting gtt/min?

9. Give 50 mL of an antibiotic over 30 minutes. You will be using an infusion pump.
   *Start at STEP 1 or STEP 2?*
   a. mL/hr: _____
   b. gtt/min: _____
   c. Do you need to calculate both mL/hr and gtt/min for this situation? _____

10. Infuse 500 mL normal saline over 4 hours, using tubing with a drop factor of 60 gtt/mL.
    *Start at STEP 1 or STEP 2?*
    a. mL/hr: _____
    b. gtt/min: _____

## PRACTICE QUIZ

**Convert the following.**

1. 750 mcg   =   _____ mg

2. 8 g   =   _____ mg

3. 250 lb   =   _____ kg

4. 75 kg   =   _____ lb

5. 3 tsp   =   _____ mL

6. gr x   =   _____ mg

**Calculate the following, and prove your answers.**

7. Dose ordered: indomethacin (Indocin) (oral suspension) 50 mg qid
   Dose on hand: Oral suspension 25 mg/5 mL
   How much would you give per dose? _____

8. Dose ordered: procainamide (Pronestyl) 0.5 g q 4 hr PO
   Dose on hand: 500-mg tablets
   How much would you give per dose? _____

9. Dose ordered: phenytoin (Dilantin) 100 mg IV now
   Dose on hand: 5-mL ampule labeled "50 mg/mL"
   How much would you give per dose? _____

10. Dose ordered: lidocaine (Xylocaine) 50 mg IV now
    Dose on hand: lidocaine 1% in 5-mL ampule
    How much would you give? _____

11. Dose ordered: epinephrine 0.25 mg subcut now
    Dose on hand: epinephrine 1:1000 ampule
    How much would you give? _____

12. Dose ordered: heparin 15,000 units IV bolus
    Dose on hand: heparin 10,000 units/mL (5-mL vial)
    How much would you give? _____

13. Dose ordered: furosemide (Lasix) 50 mg PO daily
    Dose on hand: furosemide oral solution, 10 mg/mL
    Child's weight: 22 lb
    Therapeutic dosage range: 1 to 6 mg/kg/day in doses divided every 12 hours
    a. What is the safe and therapeutic range for this child (specify both per day and per dose)?
       _____
    b. Is the ordered dose safe and therapeutic?
       _____

14. Ordered: Infuse normal saline 500 mL over 8 hours. The tubing drop factor is 15.
    a. What is the rate of the IV? _____
    b. What is the gtt/min? _____

15. Ordered: $D_5$1/2NS to infuse at 50 mL/hr via an infusion pump.
    a. How will this be administered—mL/hr or gtt/min? _____
    b. What is the rate? _____

16. Ordered: 1000 mL $D_5$W to infuse over 24 hours. The tubing drop factor is 60.
    a. What is the rate of the IV? _____
    b. What is the gtt/min? _____

17. Ordered: ticarcillin 500 mg IM q 6 hr
    Dose on hand: Medication powder for injection (See label.)

a. How much does this vial contain? _____
b. How much will you give for each dose? _____

18. Ordered: penicillin G 500,000 units IV q 6 hr

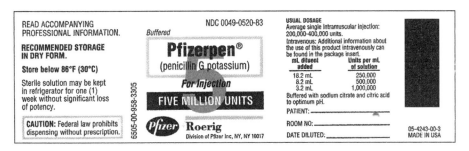

a. What concentration should you choose? _____
b. How much diluent should you add to the vial to obtain this concentration? _____
c. How much medication will you give? _____
d. How do you label the vial? _____

19. A child weighs 31 lb.
    Dose ordered: cefazolin 225 mg IV piggyback q 6 hr
    Dose on hand: See label.
    Maximum safe dose: 25-100 mg/kg/day, divided every 6 hours.

a. How much would you give for this dose? _____
b. What is the maximum safe dose for this child in 24 hours? Per dose? _____
c. How much total medication will this child receive in 24 hours? _____
d. Is the ordered dose within a safe and therapeutic range? _____

20. Dose ordered: digoxin (Lanoxin) 125 mcg daily
    Dose on hand: Pediatric elixir 0.05 mg/mL
    How much would you give? _____

21.

    Dose ordered: octreotide acetate (Sandostatin) 0.025 mg IV bolus now
    Dose on hand: See label.
    How much would you give for this dose? _____

22.

    Dose ordered: cimetidine (Tagamet) 800 mg PO at bedtime
    Dose on hand: See label.
    How much would you give for this dose? _____

23.

    Dose ordered: captopril (Capoten) 6.25 mg PO three times/day
    Dose on hand: See label.
    How much would you give for each dose? _____

24.

Dose ordered: heparin 15,000 IV push now
Dose on hand: See label.
How much would you give for this dose? _____

25.

Dose ordered: atropine 0.4 mg IM now
Dose on hand: See label.
How much would you give for this dose? _____

# Answer Key

---

## CHAPTER 1
## The Nursing Process and Drug Therapy

### Chapter Review and NCLEX® Examination Preparation/Critical Thinking and Application

1. a
2. d
3. c
4. b
5. a, d, e
6. b
7. c
8. 0.25 mg (See Overview of Dosage Calculations, Section I.)
9. 125 mcg (See Overview of Dosage Calculations, Section I.)
10. 1 = d; 2 = e; 3 = b; 4 = a; 5 = c
11. S, O, O, O, S, S
12. Answers may vary slightly with each one but should include the following:
    - *Right drug*: Compare drug orders and medication labels. Consider whether the drug is appropriate for that patient. Obtain information about the patient's medical history and a thorough, updated medication history, including over-the-counter medications taken.
    - *Right dose*: Check the order and the label on the medication, and check the "rights" at least three times before administering the medication. Recheck the math calculations for dosages and contact the physician when clarification is needed. Check the dose and confirm that it is appropriate for the patient's age and size, and also check the prescribed dose against the available drug stocks and against the normal dosage range.
    - *Right time*: Assess for a conflict between the pharmacokinetic and pharmacodynamic properties of the drugs prescribed and the patient's lifestyle and likelihood of compliance.
    - *Right route*: Never assume the route of administration or change it; always check with the physician or prescriber.
    - *Right patient*: Check the patient's identity before administering a medication. Ask for the patient's name, and check the identification band or brace-

let to confirm the patient's name, identification number, and allergies. The Joint Commission requires the use of two patient identifiers, such as name and birthday, Social Security number, or medical record number.
    - *Right documentation*: Record the date and time of medication administration, name of medication, dose, route, and site of administration. Don't forget to document the patient's response to the medication.
13. a. assessment
    b. objective
    c. subjective
    d. analyze
    e. goals
    f. outcome criteria
    g. implementation
    h. evaluation
14. The nurse must be sure to question the patient for any allergies, especially drug allergies, before giving this medication. If an allergy is present, question the patient about the type of reaction that occurred, and do not give the medication until the order is clarified with the prescriber.

### Case Study

1. See the discussion in Chapter 1 of the textbook under Assessment. Important points include the following:
    - Use of prescription and over-the-counter medications
    - Use of home remedies, herbal treatments, vitamins
    - Intake of alcohol, tobacco, caffeine
    - Current or prior use of street drugs
    - Health history
    - Family history
    - Allergies
2. Answers will vary but may include the following:
    - Activity intolerance
    - Acute pain
    - Deficient knowledge
    - Fatigue
    - Ineffective breathing pattern
    - Ineffective health maintenance

- Ineffective therapeutic regimen management
- Nausea
- Risk for aspiration
- Risk for impaired liver function
- Risk for injury
- Risk for falls

Prioritization will depend on the nursing diagnoses chosen but are developed with the patient's input. Often, actual diagnoses are prioritized before risk diagnoses.

3. The medication order is missing the route of delivery and the dose amount. Contact the physician to clarify the incomplete order.

4. Once again, contact the physician and never change the medication route without an order.

5. After administering any drug, evaluate the patient's response to the drug therapy. In this case, monitoring intake and output, monitoring vital signs, and watching for orthostatic blood pressure changes would be important.

# CHAPTER 2
## Pharmacologic Principles

### Chapter Review and NCLEX® Examination Preparation/Critical Thinking and Application

1. 1 = e; 2 = c; 3 = d; 4 = a; 5 = b
2. c
3. b
4. d
5. a, e
6. c
7. b
8. d
9. 1600
10. b
11. g
12. h
13. e
14. f
15. a
16. d
17. c
18. Because muscles have a greater blood supply than the skin, drugs injected intramuscularly are typically absorbed faster than those injected subcutaneously. Absorption can be increased by applying heat to the injection site or by massaging the injection site, which increases the blood flow to the area and thus enhances absorption.
19. This is an example of supplemental therapy—drug therapy that supplies the body with a substance needed to maintain normal function.

20. Extended-release oral dosage forms must not be crushed, as this could cause accelerated release of drug from the dosage form and possible toxicity. Enteric-coated tablets also are not recommended for crushing. This would cause disruption of the tablet coating designed to protect the stomach lining from the local effects of the drug and/or protect the drug from being prematurely disrupted by stomach acid.

### Case Study

1. Half-life is the time it takes for one-half of the original amount of a drug in the body to be eliminated and is a measure of the rate at which drugs are excreted by the body. If the half-life is 2 hours, then in this example, the drug levels would be as follows:
   4 PM = 200 mg/L
   6 PM = 100 mg/L
   8 PM = 50 mg/L
   10 PM = 25 mg/L

2. a. He has nausea and vomiting and cannot take medications by mouth. His medications will need to be given parenterally.
   b. Because of his decreased serum albumin level, a smaller amount of drugs that are usually protein bound will be bound to protein, and as a result, more free drug will be circulating and the duration of drug action may be increased. In addition, his heart failure may result in decreased cardiac output and thus decreased distribution.
   c. His liver failure will result in decreased metabolism of drugs, which increases the chance for drug toxicities if the drugs accumulate in his body.
   d. Because his liver may not be able to effectively metabolize drugs and convert them to water-soluble compounds, excretion through the kidneys may be decreased. This would also contribute to drug accumulation.

3. This situation illustrates prophylactic therapy to *prevent* illness or other undesirable outcome. Prophylactic intravenous antibiotic therapy may be used to prevent infection during a high-risk surgery or procedure, such as placement of the peripherally inserted central catheter.

4. Therapeutic index is the ratio between the toxic and therapeutic concentrations of a drug. A low therapeutic index means that the difference between a therapeutically active dose and a toxic dose is small. As a result, the drug has a greater likelihood of causing an adverse reaction. The nurse should monitor the patient's response carefully when a drug has a low therapeutic index by looking for signs and symptoms of toxicity as well as ensuring that drug levels are checked periodically.

## CHAPTER 3
## Lifespan Considerations

### Chapter Review and NCLEX® Examination Preparation/Critical Thinking and Application

1. c
2. a
3. d
4. b
5. a, b, c
6. 320 mg (See Overview of Dosage Calculations, Section IV.)
7. 0.021 mg (23 pounds = 10.5 kg; 2 mcg × 10.5 kg = 21 mcg = 0.021 mg)
8. 0.21 mL

9. d
10. b
11. e
12. a
13. c
14. Keep in mind that older patients take a greater proportion of both prescription and over-the-counter (OTC) medications, and they commonly take multiple medications on a daily basis. In addition, older adults also have more chronic diseases than younger people. They may see several different specialists, each of whom may prescribe a different set of medications. In addition, some patients self-administer OTC products to ease the discomfort of even more ailments. This use of multiple mediations is called *polypharmacy.*
15. Drawing on the information in Table 3-3: Physiologic Changes in the Elderly Patient, a variety of physiologic changes affecting the cardiovascular, gastrointestinal, hepatic, and renal systems may be described.
16. It would be important to prepare her in advance for the teaching session. Let her know what to expect, and include her parent, if possible, in the teaching session. It is also important to allow her time to express her feelings about this new diagnosis and the need to test her own blood glucose levels. Allow her to make choices when appropriate (i.e., choosing a glucometer with a special color). After demonstrating the procedure, encourage her participation and allow for return demonstration.

### Case Study

1. Children and teenagers should not take aspirin to treat chickenpox or flulike symptoms because Reye's syndrome—a rare but serious illness—has been associated with aspirin use at these ages. It is important to check for precautions when giving any medication to children.
2. If the toddler does not like or cannot take pills, have the parent ask the pharmacist for a liquid form of the medication, which may be flavored and better accepted by the child than a pill. Some pediatric medications also come in quick-dissolving oral tablets or films.
3. Most OTC preparations for children have dosages based on the child's weight. The most common dosage calculation method for children is the milligrams per kilogram formula. However, for OTC preparations, the manufacturer will convert kilograms to pounds to make dosing by the parents easier.
4. The 5-year-old child received 240 mg (at 160 mg/tsp, 1.5 tsp = 240 mg).
5. The parents should monitor the children's fevers—the expected response is that the fevers will go down. In addition, because the medication also has analgesic effects, signs of discomfort may decrease. The parents should also monitor for any adverse effects of the medication or worsening of the children's illnesses.

## CHAPTER 4
## Cultural, Legal, and Ethical Considerations

### Chapter Review and NCLEX® Examination Preparation/Critical Thinking and Application

1. b
2. a
3. d
4. c
5. b
6. d
7. b, c
8. d
9. 6 mL
10.

11. d
12. a
13. c
14. b
15. c
16. a
17. d
18. b
19. The nurse also has the right to refuse to participate in any treatment or aspect of a patient's care that

violates the nurse's personal ethical principles. However, this must be done without deserting the patient, and in some facilities the nurse may be transferred to another patient care assignment only if the nurse manager or nurse supervisor approves the transfer. The nurse needs to discuss the situation with the immediate supervisor, and hopefully another solution can be reached. The nurse must always remember, however, that the ANA *Code of Ethics* and professional responsibility and accountability require the nurse to provide nonjudgmental nursing care from the start of the patient's treatment until the time of the patient's discharge.

20. Answers will vary depending on the group identified.
    a. Barriers may include language, poverty, access, pride, and beliefs regarding medical practices.
    b. Attitudes will vary depending on the group identified.
    c. Questions may include the following topics: health beliefs and practices, past use of medicine, folk remedies, home remedies, use of over-the-counter drugs and treatments, usual responses to illness, responsiveness to medical treatments, religious practices and beliefs, and dietary habits.

**Case Study**

1. You should not give the drugs until it is established that the study has been reviewed by an institutional review board and that the patient has given informed consent. As a professional, the nurse has the responsibility to provide safe nursing care and it is within the nurse's realm of practice to provide information and assist the patient facing decisions regarding health care. The nurse also has the right to refuse to participate in any treatment or aspect of a patient's care that violates personal ethical principles.

2. Principles include the following:
   • Autonomy—the patient's right to self-determination. The nurse supports this by ensuring informed consent.
   • Beneficence—the duty to do good. Will the patient be best served by this course of action?
   • Nonmaleficence—the duty to do no harm.
   • Veracity—the duty to tell the truth, especially with regard to investigational drugs and informed consent.

3. Some patients believe strongly in using home remedies instead of medications. Sometimes these remedies can be integrated into HIV treatment. You should assess and consider health beliefs and practices at the beginning of the therapeutic relationship. Because the patient believes drugs are not needed, the nurse has a duty to provide education so that the patient has the knowledge needed in order to make a sound judgment.

4. The issue of confidentiality should be discussed. The researchers have a duty to respect privileged information about a patient. Measures that the researchers will use to ensure the confidentiality of participants should be discussed.

# CHAPTER 5
## Medication Errors: Preventing and Responding

**Chapter Review and NCLEX® Examination Preparation/Critical Thinking and Application**

1. medication error
2. idiosyncratic
3. allergic reaction
4. adverse drug reaction (ADR)
5. adverse drug event (ADE)
6. False. High-alert medications are not necessarily involved in more errors than other drugs. However, the potential for patient harm is higher with these medications.
7. False. Adverse drug events include medication errors and adverse drug reactions.
8. To avoid medication errors: Follow the Six Rights! Carefully read all drug labels and confirm the Six Rights of medication administration. Repeat a verbal order and spell the drug name out loud. Never assume a route of administration; if an order is unclear or incomplete, clarify the order with the prescriber. Always read the label three times and check the medication order before administering the medication. See the textbook for other possible answers.
9. Refer to Box 5-1: Examples of High-Alert Medications.
10. Digoxin 125 micrograms PO now
    Lasix 40 mg IV daily (every day)
    Discontinue all meds
    NPH insulin 12 units subcut every morning before breakfast
    Floxin Otic 1 drop right ear bid
    Lactulose 30 mL PO every other day
11. a. One-half of a 50-mg tablet. (See Overview of Dosage Calculations, Section II.)
    b. A 50-mg dose, which is a double dose.
    c. Because this medication can have an effect on the patient's blood pressure and heart rate, the nurse will immediately check and record the patient's vital signs and caution the patient about getting out of bed without help. The patient's physician will be notified, and the patient must be monitored frequently throughout the day. In addition to telling the patient about the double dose, the nurse will need to follow facility protocol for reporting a medication error, which would include completing a U.S. Pharmacopeia Medication Er-

rors Reporting Program (USPMERP) report for the national database.

12. b

13. 5 mL

14.

### Case Study

1. The nursing student needs to inform her instructor of the error immediately. Then together they need to monitor the patient's response and follow the institution's procedure for reporting a medication error. Reporting medication errors is a professional and ethical responsibility.

2. By checking the Six Rights before giving this medication. In this situation, she missed the right dose. In addition, if the student had understood the rationale for the medication (i.e., the low dose needed for antiplatelet therapy), then she may have avoided this error. One must be knowledgeable about medications and the rationale for their use in a particular patient before administering them.

3. According to Chapter 5, the recommendation is that the patient be told of the error both as ethical practice and because of the legal implications.

4. Yes. A medication error is defined as "any preventable adverse drug event involving inappropriate medication use by a patient or health care professional." It may or may not cause harm to the patient.

5. The USPMERP exists to gather and disseminate safety information regarding medications. By reporting this error, the student contributes to the USPMERP database of medication errors and their causes. This service is confidential.

## CHAPTER 6
## Patient Education and Drug Therapy

### Chapter Review and NCLEX® Examination Preparation/Critical Thinking and Application

1. c
2. d
3. a
4. a, b
5. 10 mL per dose (See Overview of Dosage Calculations, Section II.)

6.

7. Refer to the information in Chapter 22 for specific information about antihypertensive drug therapy. In addition, Table 6-1 provides information relevant to the development of teaching strategies for the 78-year-old patient.

8. Refer to Box 6-1. Ideally, a health care professional who speaks the mother's language should do the teaching. It is essential that an interpreter be found so that questions from the mother can be answered adequately. Other strategies include using pictures and illustrations and demonstrating by example. In addition, the patient needs to be provided with detailed written instructions in her native language.

9. a. Answers will vary, but the nursing diagnosis addresses Deficient knowledge.
   b. Answers will vary, but the nursing diagnosis addresses Noncompliance or Ineffective health maintenance.

10. Answers will vary, but an example would be:
    Goal: Patient demonstrates correct technique for application of the transdermal nitroglycerin patch.
    Outcome criteria: Patient applies patch to a clean, nonhairy area of the skin, and rotates application sites.

11. Teaching plans will vary somewhat in format, but each should contain the following information:
    a. Some of the assessment items listed in the text in the section Assessment of Learning Needs Related to Drug Therapy.
    b. Deficient knowledge.
    c. A measurable goal with outcome criteria related to the nursing diagnosis.
    d. Specific educational strategies for providing the information needed.
    e. Specific questions designed to validate whether learning has occurred.

### Case Study

1. Both "Deficient knowledge" and "Noncompliance" are possible answers. In this case, "Deficient knowledge" is probably the most correct, because this nursing diagnosis exists when the patient has a lack of or limited understanding about his or her medications. For example, as you will read in Chapter 23, nitroglycerin tablets should not be stored in one's pants pockets because the body heat may destroy the active compounds in the tablets. In addition, the patient was not aware of the importance of not missing doses of antihypertensive medication. Noncompliance exists when the patient does not take the medication as directed or at all, and the data collected

indicate that the patient's condition has recurred or has not resolved. In this case, his blood pressure has improved from previous readings, despite what he has said about taking his medications.

2. Answers may vary. A goal for the nursing diagnosis of "Deficient knowledge" in this case may be the following: "The patient self-administers his prescribed medications on schedule without missing doses." Outcome criteria may include the following: "The patient is able to describe the schedule of medications ordered." "The patient is able to state the rationale for consistent dosing of antihypertensive medications." "The patient is able to state the proper storage and administration of sublingual nitroglycerin tablets." "The patient is able to identify potential side effects of the prescribed medications and knows when to report them."

3. Again, answers may vary. Refer to Box 6-1. Suggestions include the following:
   • A teaching session regarding medication administration needs to be held with both the patient and his wife in attendance. If necessary, find out whether they have any children or neighbors nearby who may be able to assist with medications as needed.
   • Assist the patient in developing a daily time calendar for taking the medications prescribed.
   • Suggest the use of a daily or weekly pill container that can assist in reminding when doses are due. If necessary, a neighbor or the patient's son or daughter can come over periodically to fill this container.
   • Discuss and provide written literature on the purposes and side effects of each medication ordered and on other important issues regarding these medications.

4. Confirm whether learning has occurred by asking the patient and his wife questions related to the teaching session. Assess their understanding of the time calendar and the concept of using pill containers. Follow-up can be accomplished via telephone as needed, and a return visit to review medications can be scheduled. In addition, the patient must keep return appointments to the office so that the therapeutic outcomes of the drug therapy (i.e., blood pressure readings) can be measured.

# CHAPTER 7
## Over-the-Counter Drugs and Herbal and Dietary Supplements

### Critical Thinking Crossword Puzzle
*Across*
2. Ginger
5. Flax

7. Saw palmetto
8. Kava
*Down*
1. Echinacea
2. Gingko
3. Ginseng
4. Aloe
6. Soy

### Chapter Review and NCLEX® Examination Preparation/Critical Thinking and Application
1. a, b, d, f
2. d
3. d
4. b
5. c
6. 6,000 mg total per day
7. YES, there is a concern! Acetaminophen doses must not exceed a total of 3 grams per day, and hepatic toxicity may occur with excessive doses.
8. c
9. b, e
10. Garlic, ginger, ginkgo, ginseng, flax, and valerian
11. Older adults; children; patients with single and/or multiple acute and chronic illnesses; patients who are frail or in poor health; patients who are debilitated and nutritionally deficient; and those with suppressed immune systems. In addition, those who have a history of renal, hepatic, cardiac, or vascular disorders may have problems with over-the-counter (OTC) medications.
12. Normally, OTC medications are used only for short-term treatment of common minor illnesses. Having diarrhea for 3 weeks puts the patient at risk for dehydration. In addition, delaying an evaluation of the cause of the diarrhea also delays the opportunity to treat what could be a serious illness or disease.
13. Answers will vary.

### Case Study
1. The aspirin and garlic tablets may interfere with platelet and clotting functions. If the wine is taken with the kava and/or valerian, central nervous system depression may occur.
2. The Food and Drug Administration (FDA) has issued a warning about the use of kava and possible liver toxicity. Also, tolerance may develop in patients who use echinacea for longer than 8 weeks.
3. Because she is trying to conceive, she needs to consider the fact that the herbal drugs have not been tested or proved safe for use in pregnancy. Also, aspirin use is contraindicated in pregnancy because of its antiplatelet effects.
4. Herbal products are not required by the FDA to be proven safe or effective. They are classified as dietary supplements and are not subject to the same

rules as are drugs. Therefore, the patient must receive adequate information about the herbal products, including their risks, side effects, and possible benefits.

5. Many patients believe that if a product is "natural" then it is safe. Discuss each product with the patient, and instruct the patient about possible contraindications, safe use, frequency of dosing, specifics about how to take the product, and the way to monitor for both therapeutic effects and complications or toxic effects.

# CHAPTER 8
## Gene Therapy and Pharmacogenomics

### Chapter Review and NCLEX® Examination Preparation/Critical Thinking and Application

1. g
2. f
3. b
4. c
5. d
6. a, c, d
7. a
8. A major ethical issue related to gene therapy is that of eugenics. *Eugenics* is the intentional selection before birth of genotypes that are considered more desirable than others. For similar reasons, the prospect of being able to manipulate genes in human *germ cells* (sperm and eggs), at a preembryonic stage, is also a potential ethical hazard of gene therapy. Theoretically, even cosmetic modifications could be attempted by using such techniques as a part of routine family planning. Because of ethical concerns such as these, U.S. gene therapy research is limited to somatic cells only. Gene therapy in *germ-line* (reproductive) cells is currently not approved for funding by the National Institutes of Health.
9. Recombinant DNA is DNA that has been artificially synthesized or modified in a laboratory setting. This technology is used to make recombinant forms of drugs such as hormones, vaccines, and antitoxins. An example of this technology is the alteration of the *Escherichia coli* genome so that these bacteria manufacture a recombinant form of human insulin.
10. The general goal of gene therapy is to transfer to the patient exogenous genes that will either provide a temporary substitute for, or initiate permanent changes in, the patient's own genetic functioning to treat a given disease. Although hundreds of gene therapy clinical trials have been approved by the U.S. Food and Drug Administration (FDA), no gene therapy to date has been approved for routine treatment of disease. Gene therapy techniques are being studied for the treatment of acquired illnesses such as cancer, heart disease, and diabetes.

11. This patient's comment is a clue to a potential genetic issue. An unusual or other-than-expected reaction to a drug in family members might point to a difference in the patient's ability to metabolize certain drugs. It is essential that the nurse investigate this comment further and obtain details about what has happened with the family members, how they reacted to the surgery, and the outcomes. This information will need to be communicated to the patient's surgeon and anesthesiologist. The nurse will tell the patient that while there is no way to predict how he will respond to medication, measures will be taken to ensure his safety.
12. Maintaining privacy and confidentiality is of utmost importance during genetic testing and counseling. The patient is the one who decides whether to include or exclude any family members from the discussion and from knowledge of the results of genetic testing. Nurses must protect against improper disclosure of information to other family members, friends of the family, other health care providers, and insurance providers. The nurse will tell the patient's sister that only the patient is able to share that information.

### Case Study

1. This information about Dale's cousin may be significant! An unusual or other-than-expected reaction to a drug in family members may point to a difference in the patient's ability to metabolize certain drugs. Genetic factors may alter a patient's metabolism of a particular drug, resulting in either increased or decreased drug action.
2. The nurse will ask about the type of medication Dale's cousin received, the type of surgery, and obtain details about the reaction that occurred, as well as the treatment. The nurse will also ask if any other family members have had unusual reactions to drugs, and whether Dale himself has had any problems.
3. The family history needs to cover at least three generations and include the current and past health status of each family member.
4. The surgeon and anesthesiologist will work to adjust the planned drug therapy for Dale's surgery according to the genetic variation that has been identified. In addition, during surgery, the patient will be monitored closely for any unusual responses.

# CHAPTER 9
## Photo Atlas of Drug Administration

### Chapter Review and NCLEX® Examination Preparation/Critical Thinking and Application

1. c
2. a
3. b
4. c
5. c
6. b
7. a
8. c
9. a
10. b
11. d
12. b
13. a
14. a, b, d
15. 14 units

16. 0.24 mg
17. 0.48 mL

18. a. Palpate sites for masses or tenderness and assess the amount of subcutaneous tissue.
    b. Note the integrity and size of the muscle and palpate for tenderness.
    c. Note any lesions or discoloration of the forearm.
19. See the descriptions under textbook Figure 9-38 for each type of injection.
20. Remove the needle and ensure that the site is not bleeding. Discard the medication and syringe, draw up new medication, and repeat the procedure in a different location.
21. Rather than pouring it into a medication cup, draw small volumes of liquid medications into a calibrated oral syringe.
22. 100 divided by 4 (4 puffs/day) would equal 25 days.

### Case Study

1. For the adult, the ventrogluteal site is the preferred injection site; however, immunizations are often given in the deltoid muscle because of the small volume size. If the adult is of average size, choose a needle that is 1 1/2 inches long and 21- to 25-gauge and insert the needle at a 90-degree angle. For the infant, the preferred site is the vastus lateralis muscle. The needle must be of the correct length to ensure that it reaches muscle tissue, not the subcutaneous layer.
2. For an infant or child younger than 3 years of age, pull the pinna of the ear down and back before the drops are administered. Direct the drops along the sides of the ear rather than directly onto the eardrum. Take the drops out of refrigeration about an hour before administering them. The mother needs to stay with her child and ensure that the child lies on her side for 5 to 10 minutes. Gentle massage of the tragus area of the ear with her finger will help distribute the medication down the ear canal.
3. Liquid medication doses under 5 mL must be drawn up in a calibrated oral syringe. A medicine cup does not provide accurate measurements for small doses under 5 mL.
4. Liquids are usually ordered because infants cannot swallow pills or capsules. Do not add the medication to a bottle of formula. The infant may refuse the feeding or may not drink all of the bottle and, as a result, would not get the entire dosage of medication. A plastic disposable oral dosing syringe is recommended for measuring small doses of liquid medications. Position the infant so that the head is slightly elevated. Place the plastic dropper or syringe inside the infant's mouth, beside the tongue, and administer the liquid in small amounts while allowing the infant to swallow each time. Take great care to prevent aspiration. A crying infant can easily aspirate medication.

# CHAPTER 10
## Analgesic Drugs

### Critical Thinking Crossword
*Across*
3. Agonist
5. Acute
11. Superficial
13. Visceral

*Down*
1. Antagonist
2. Adjuvant
4. Tolerance
6. Threshold
7. Somatic
8. Chronic
9. Opioid
10. Opiate
12. Partial

### Chapter Review and NCLEX® Examination Preparation
1. b
2. d

3. c
4. d
5. b, c, e
6. Based on the patient's statements, he was taking a total of 5300 mg of acetaminophen per day! (Two Percocets twice a day equals 1300 mg; two extra-strength acetaminophens four times a day equal 4000 mg). YES, this is a concern, because the standard maximum daily dose for acetaminophen is 3000 mg per day. He is at risk for liver damage.
7. 3 mL (See Overview of Dosage Calculations, Section II.)
8. 1.2 mL (See Overview of Dosage Calculations, Section II.)
9.

10. f
11. e
12. h
13. g
14. c
15. a
16. i
17. b
18. d

## Case Study

1. Superficial pain, which originates from the skin or mucous membranes.
2. All opioids cause some histamine release. It is thought that this histamine release is responsible for many of the unwanted side effects, such as itching.
3. The most serious side effect of opioids is central nervous system depression, which may lead to respiratory depression. Naloxone (Narcan), an opioid reversal drug, may have to be administered to reverse severe respiratory depression.
4. The use of a nonopioid analgesic with an opioid is known as *adjuvant analgesic therapy*. This allows the use of smaller doses of opioids, which accomplishes two important functions. First, it diminishes some of the side effects that are seen with higher doses of opioids, such as respiratory depression, constipation, and urinary retention. Second, it approaches the pain stimulus by another mechanism of action and has a resulting synergistic beneficial effect in reducing the pain.

## CHAPTER 11
## General and Local Anesthetics

### Chapter Review and NCLEX® Examination Preparation/Critical Thinking and Application

1. f
2. g
3. j
4. e
5. d
6. a
7. i
8. c
9. b
10. h
11. a, c, e
12. b
13. a
14. b
15. b, c, e
16. c
17. d
18. 1 = c; 2 = a; 3 = b
19. 0.4 mL (See Overview of Dosage Calculations, Section III.)
20. 0.05 mL (See Overview of Dosage Calculations, Section III.)
21. Pediatric patients are more susceptible to problems such as central nervous system depression, toxicity, atelectasis, pneumonia, and cardiac abnormalities because their hepatic, cardiac, respiratory, and renal systems are not fully developed or fully functional.
22. These drugs cause paralysis of the respiratory muscles. The nurse will need to monitor the mechanical ventilation closely because if the ventilator does not work, the patient will not be able to breathe on his own. Emergency resuscitation equipment must be kept nearby. In addition, these drugs do not cause sedation, and the patient is still able to hear and feel. Most facilities have protocols for sedation during the use of these drugs. However, it is important to remain professional at all times and to take the time to reassure the patient and orient him to his surroundings, what noises mean, and what procedures are going to be done to him. Remind the family that he is still able to hear what is said.
23. She will be given a combination of intravenous medications that will produce analgesia and also amnesia of the procedure, but she will still be alert enough to breathe on her own and follow verbal directions as needed. In some cases, local anesthesia will be used to enhance patient comfort. This type of sedation is called *moderate (*or *procedural,* or *conscious) seda-*

*tion*; it is associated with fewer complications and a shorter recovery time than general anesthesia.

24. Yes, there is a difference. Lidocaine with epinephrine is used when the vasoconstriction effects of epinephrine are needed. The vasoconstriction confines the anesthetic (lidocaine) to the local area of injection, and also acts to reduce bleeding. The two types of lidocaine are not interchangeable.

## Case Study

1. In balanced anesthesia, minimal doses of a combination of anesthetic drugs (both intravenous and inhaled) are given to achieve the desired level of anesthesia for the surgical procedure. Adjunctive drugs may also be used and commonly include sedative-hypnotics, narcotics, and neuromuscular blocking drugs (NMBDs) (depolarizing drugs such as succinylcholine and the nondepolarizing or competitive drugs such as pancuronium or d-tubocurarine). Combining several different drugs makes it possible for general anesthesia to be accomplished with smaller amounts of anesthetic gases and thereby reduces the side effects.

2. The main therapeutic use of the NMBD succinylcholine is to maintain controlled ventilation during surgical procedures. When respiratory muscles are paralyzed by NMBDs, mechanical ventilation is easier because the body's drive to control respirations is eliminated by the drug; this allows the ventilator to have total control of the respirations.

3. Multiple medical conditions (listed in Box 11-4) can predispose an individual to toxicity. These conditions increase the sensitivity of an individual to NMBDs and prolong their effects. Because the patient's temperature has decreased, hypothermia may lead to an increased sensitivity to the medication. In addition, the history of paraplegia is another condition that may predispose this patient to toxicity.

4. Anticholinesterase drugs such as neostigmine, pyridostigmine, and edrophonium are antidotes and are used to reverse muscle paralysis.

5. Local anesthesia is most commonly used in settings in which loss of consciousness, whole-body relaxation, and loss of responsiveness are either unnecessary or unwanted. A lower incidence of toxic effects is associated with the use of local anesthetics, because very little of these drugs is absorbed systemically.

6. Regardless of the type of anesthesia a patient is receiving, one of the most important nursing considerations during this time is close and frequent observation of the patient and all body systems, with specific attention to the ABCs of care (airway, breathing, and circulation) and vital signs. Resuscitative equipment, as well as any drug antidote, should be kept nearby in case of cardiorespiratory distress

or arrest. Other nursing actions include monitoring all aspects of body functions, instituting safety measures, and implementing the physician's orders.

## CHAPTER 12
## Central Nervous System Depressants and Muscle Relaxants

### Chapter Review and NCLEX® Examination Preparation/Critical Thinking and Application

1. a
2. b
3. a
4. d
5. c
6. b
7. a, c, d, e
8. a. 7.5 mg
   b. 3.75 mL (See Overview of Dosage Calculations, Section IV.)
9. 10 mL
10.

11. An overdose of barbiturates produces CNS depression ranging from sleep to profound coma and death. Respiratory depression progresses to Cheyne-Stokes respirations, hypoventilation, and cyanosis. Patients often have cold, clammy skin or are hypothermic, and later they can exhibit fever, areflexia, tachycardia, and hypotension. The priority of care would be to maintain the ABCs (airway, breathing, and circulation), especially respirations, because respiratory depression is likely. There is no antidote for barbiturate overdose.

12. These drugs can be taken for insomnia only if their use is limited to the short-term (less than 2 to 4 weeks). With long-term use, rebound insomnia and severe withdrawal can develop. If Jackie needs to take something to help her sleep while she is on her trip, the nonbenzodiazepine hypnotics may be an option; and, of course, you could provide patient teaching on nonpharmacologic methods to aid sleep.

13. Benzodiazepines can create a significant fall hazard in elderly patients and the lowest effective dose must be used in this patient population.

14. a. Ask about allergies, central nervous system (CNS) disorders, sleep disorders, diabetes, addictive disorders, personality disorders, thyroid conditions, and renal and liver function.

b. Alcohol and CNS depressants, but also all prescribed or over-the-counter medications and herbal products used.

c. The patient's age matters, because these drugs have increased effects in older persons and small children.

15. a. Patient teaching should include information about potential side effects and potential drug interactions. In addition, safety measures to prevent injury stemming from decreased sensorium must be emphasized.

b. These medications are most effective when used in conjunction with rest and physical therapy.

## Case Study

1. Barbiturates are considered controlled substances because of the potential for misuse and the severe effects that result if they are not used appropriately. Other hypnotic drugs are now used because they have fewer side effects and are safer than the older barbiturates. Barbiturates are no longer recommended for insomnia.

2. Barbiturates are habit-forming; they have a low therapeutic index; and severe withdrawal effects may occur when the medication is stopped. Other drugs are now recommended for treatment of insomnia.

3. Other CNS depressants, especially alcohol, should be avoided. There may also be an additive effect when the herbal products kava or valerian are used.

4. Zaleplon is indicated for the short-term treatment of insomnia; it is not approved for long-term use. It has a very short half-life, so the patient should be taught that if sleep difficulties include early awakenings, a dose can be taken as long as it is at least 4 hours before the patient must arise. In addition, the patient should explore other nonpharmacologic options for the treatment of insomnia and try to find the cause of the sleep problems. See Box 12-1 for information on nonpharmacologic measures to promote sleep.

# CHAPTER 13
## Central Nervous System Stimulants and Related Drugs

### Chapter Review and NCLEX® Examination Preparation/Critical Thinking and Application

1. b
2. b, c, e
3. a
4. d
5. b
6. b, c, e
7. b, c, d
8. 100 mg (See Overview of Dosage Calculations, Section IV.)

9. 37.5 mg (See Overview of Dosage Calculations, Section IV.)

10. a. Stacey probably has narcolepsy.

b. Methylphenidate (an amphetamine) or modafinil (a nonamphetamine) may be ordered.

c. These drugs boost mental alertness, increase motor activity, and diminish the patient's sense of fatigue by stimulating the cerebral cortex and possibly the reticular activating system.

d. Stacey should avoid other central nervous system stimulants, in particular caffeine-containing products (e.g., coffee, tea, colas, and chocolate). She should check with her physician before taking any over-the-counter drug or herbal product, and she should not consume any substance that contains alcohol. In addition, she should keep a journal to document her response to the medication.

11. Weight loss due to anorexia is associated with these drugs, and so it is important to monitor for weight gain or loss in children who are taking drugs for attention deficit hyperactivity disorder. Height and weight should be measured and recorded before therapy is initiated, and growth rate should be plotted during therapy. Nutritional status should be assessed, with attention to daily dietary intake as well as the amount eaten before drug therapy and after therapy is initiated.

12. With orlistat, patients need to watch dietary fat intake. Restricting the intake of fat to less than 30% of total caloric intake may help decrease the occurrence of gastrointestinal side effects. Supplementation with fat-soluble vitamins may be indicated.

13. These drugs work to reduce the severity of the headaches but do not prevent headaches.

14. Specialists sometimes recommend periodic "drug holidays" (e.g., 1 day per week without medication) to diminish the addictive tendencies of the stimulant drugs. School-aged children often do not take these drugs on weekends and school vacations.

## Case Study

1. Serotonin receptor agonists work by stimulating 5-HT1 receptors in the brain; this stimulation results in constriction of dilated blood vessels in the brain and decreased release of inflammatory neuropeptides.

2. Orally administered medications may not be tolerated because of the nausea and vomiting that often accompany the headaches. Alternative formulations such as subcutaneous self-injections, sublingual forms, and nasal sprays are advantageous. They also typically have a more rapid onset of action, producing relief in some patients in 10 to 15 minutes compared with 1 to 2 hours with tablets.

3. Use of sumatriptan is contraindicated in patients with drug allergy and the presence of serious cardiovascular disease, because of the vasoconstrictive potential of these medications.

4. Foods containing tyramine should be avoided, because tyramine is known to precipitate severe headaches. Tyramine-containing foods include beer, wine, aged cheese, food additives, preservatives, artificial sweeteners, chocolate, and caffeine.

5. Keeping a journal of the occurrence of headaches, precipitating factors, and response to drug therapy is also encouraged so that the patient's progress and response to drug therapy can be followed.

# CHAPTER 14
## Antiepileptic Drugs

### Critical Thinking Crossword
*Across*
2. Emergency
6. Primary
10. Hepatotoxicity
11. Seizure
12. Slowly

*Down*
1. Secondary
3. Convulsion
4. Benzodiazepines
5. Idiopathic
6. Phenobarbital
7. Autoinduction
8. Epilepsy
9. Phenytoin

### Chapter Review and NCLEX® Examination Preparation/Critical Thinking and Application
1. d
2. a
3. b, c, d
4. c
5. b
6. c
7. a, b, c
8. a. 450 mg per day; 150 mg per dose
   b. 3 mL per dose
9.

10. Carbamazepine undergoes autoinduction, the process by which the metabolism of a drug increases over time, which leads to lower-than-expected drug concentrations.

11. Jeremy's mother needs to be told that topiramate must be taken whole, not crushed, broken in half, or chewed. It does have a very bitter taste and seems to be better tolerated when taken with food. She can still give it with gelatin, as long as the dosage form remains whole.

12. While it is true that pregnancy is a common contraindication to antiepileptic drugs, the prescriber will consider the risks to the mother and infant of untreated maternal epilepsy and the increased risks for seizure activity. The newer-generation antiepileptic drugs appear to be safer in pregnancy than the traditional drugs; many women take these drugs throughout their pregnancies. However, women with epilepsy need to be monitored closely by both an obstetrician and a neurologist during pregnancy. Birth defects in infants of epileptic mothers are higher than normal, regardless of whether the mother was receiving drug therapy.

### Case Study
1. The signs and symptoms that Mattie is experiencing are typical of absence seizures. These are most often seen in children.

2. She needs to be sure to measure the dose carefully with an exact graduated device or oral syringe, rather than using a household teaspoon, and to give the medication at the same time daily. She needs to report excessive sedation, confusion, lethargy, or decreased movement. See the Patient Teaching Tips in your textbook for more information.

3. Encourage her to keep a journal to record Mattie's signs and symptoms before, during, and after any seizure activity to measure the therapeutic effectiveness of the medication.

4. A therapeutic response to antiepileptic drugs does not mean that the patient has been cured of the seizures but only that seizure activity is decreased or absent. Further evaluation will be needed before a decision is made to stop the medication. Treatment may need to last for years or may be lifelong.

# CHAPTER 15
## Antiparkinson Drugs

### Chapter Review and NCLEX® Examination Preparation/Critical Thinking and Application
1. b
2. a
3. d
4. c
5. a, c
6. b
7. a, c, e
8. 2.5 tablets

9.  a. Dopamine must be given in this form because exogenously administered dopamine cannot pass through the blood-brain barrier; levodopa can.

    b. The addition of carbidopa avoids the high peripheral levels of dopamine and unwanted side effects induced by the very large dosages of levodopa necessary when the drug is given alone.

    c. Carbidopa does not cross the blood-brain barrier and thus prevents levodopa breakdown in the periphery. This, in turn, allows levodopa to reach and cross the blood-brain barrier. Once in the brain, the levodopa is then broken down to dopamine, which can be used directly.

10. The nurse must ask whether Mrs. R. is lactating; if so, use of amantadine is contraindicated. In addition, pregnancy may be a contraindication to many antiparkinsonian drugs.

11. Older patients, especially men with benign prostatic hyperplasia, are at risk for urinary retention. Jane's neighbor may or may not have that condition, but his age is a major factor. Jane's age is not a concern at this time. This drug may also cause palpitations.

12. The "on-off phenomenon" occurs because of rapid swings in the patient's response to levodopa. The result is worsening of the disease when too little dopamine is present, or dyskinesias when too much is present. In contrast, the "wearing-off phenomenon" occurs when antiparkinson's disease medications begin to lose their effectiveness, despite maximal dosing, as the disease progresses.

## Case Study

1.  The primary cause of Parkinson's disease is an imbalance in the two neurotransmitters dopamine and acetylcholine (ACh) in the basal ganglia of the brain. This imbalance is caused by a failure of the nerve terminals in the substantia nigra to produce dopamine, which acts in the basal ganglia to control body movements. A correct balance between dopamine and ACh is needed for the proper regulation of posture, muscle tone, and voluntary movement. The deficiency of dopamine can also lead to excessive ACh activity because of the lack of dopamine's normal balancing effect. Symptoms of Parkinson's disease do not appear until approximately 80% of the dopamine store in the substantia nigra of the basal ganglia has been depleted.

2.  Drug therapy is aimed at increasing the levels of dopamine at the remaining functioning nerve terminals. It is also aimed at blocking the effects of ACh and slowing the progression of the disease.

3.  Amantadine causes the release of dopamine from nerve endings that are still intact. The result is higher levels of dopamine in the central nervous system.

4.  It is most effective in the early stages of Parkinson's disease, but as the disease progresses and the number of functioning nerves diminishes, amantadine's effect is also reduced. Amantadine is usually effective for only 6 to 12 months.

5.  Patients with Parkinson's disease often experience rapid swings in response to levodopa; this fluctuating response is known as the "on-off phenomenon." This phenomenon is seen in patients who take levodopa for a long time. Such patients may experience periods when they have good control ("on" time) and periods when they have bad control or breakthrough Parkinson's disease ("off" time). Carbidopa is a peripheral decarboxylase inhibitor that does not cross the blood-brain barrier. As a result, carbidopa is able to prevent levodopa from breaking down in the periphery and allows more levodopa to reach and cross the blood-brain barrier. Levodopa-carbidopa combinations, such as Sinemet CR, may help decrease the "off" time.

## CHAPTER 16
### Psychotherapeutic Drugs

### Chapter Review and NCLEX® Examination Preparation/Critical Thinking and Application

1.  b, c, e
2.  a
3.  c
4.  a, c, d
5.  d
6.  c
7.  3 tablets (See Overview of Dosage Calculations, Section II.)
8.  900 mg; 3 capsules (See Overview of Dosage Calculations, Section II.)
9.  l
10. f
11. g
12. o
13. b
14. i
15. j
16. k
17. c
18. n
19. a
20. d
21. h
22. e
23. m
24. a. Carl may have taken an overdose of the benzodiazepine.

    b. If an overdose of the benzodiazepine is suspected, flumazenil (Romazicon) may be given to reverse the effect of the benzodiazepine overdose. The treatment for benzodiazepine overdose is generally supportive.

25. a. Mr. D. needs to be aware of the foods and drinks, including red wine, that he can no longer have because they contain tyramine.
    b. It appears that Mr. D. may have inadvertently ingested something containing tyramine, which has caused a hypertensive crisis.
26. Second-generation antidepressants offer an advantage over other antidepressants because they have fewer and less severe side effects.
27. If the antidepressant taken is a first-generation (tricyclic) antidepressant, excessive dosages could result in lethal cardiac dysrhythmias as well as seizures. These dysrhythmias are responsible for most of the deaths due to tricyclic antidepressant overdoses.

**Case Study**

1. See Table 16-2 for potential adverse effects of benzodiazepines. Most are related to their effects on the central nervous system. Patient teaching includes warning the patient to avoid driving or operating heavy equipment or machinery until he becomes accustomed to the side effects of the medication. In addition, measures should be taken to avoid orthostatic hypotension. Finally, he should avoid alcohol and other central nervous system depressants while taking this medication.
2. If he is experiencing life-altering anxiety, then he should also consider obtaining psychotherapy to assist him at this time.
3. Benzodiazepines are potentially habit-forming and addictive, with possible withdrawal symptoms such as anxiety, panic attacks, convulsions, nausea, and vomiting. The medication should not be withdrawn abruptly. Patients should always be advised to take the medication as directed and never to stop taking the medicine abruptly. Benzodiazepines should be withdrawn gradually.
4. There is a potential for benzodiazepines to cause serious life-threatening toxicities, but when taken alone in normal dosages in otherwise healthy patients, they are very safe and effective anxiolytics. When they are taken with other sedating medications or with alcohol, however, life-threatening respiratory depression or arrest can occur. An overdose of benzodiazepines may result in one or more of the following symptoms: somnolence, confusion, coma, and respiratory depression. Overdose may be treated with the benzodiazepine-specific antidote flumazenil (Romazicon) or administration of activated charcoal.
5. Buspirone has the advantages of being both nonsedating and non–habit-forming compared with the benzodiazepines.

# CHAPTER 17
## Substance Abuse

### Chapter Review and NCLEX® Examination Preparation/Critical Thinking and Application

1. h
2. i
3. f
4. e
5. g
6. d
7. j
8. a
9. c
10. b
11. a, c, f
12. d
13. b, c, e
14. c
15. b
16. 2 mL (See Overview of Dosage Calculations, Section IV.)
17. The nicotine transdermal system (patch) and nicotine polacrilex (gum) can be used to supply nicotine without the carcinogens in tobacco. The patches provide a stepwise reduction in delivery and work by gradually reducing the nicotine dose over time. With the gum, rapid chewing releases an immediate dose of nicotine, but this dose is about half of what the average smoker receives from one cigarette, and the onset of action is longer than with smoking. Therefore, the reinforcement and self-reward effects of smoking are minimized. Zyban is a sustained-release form of the antidepressant bupropion and was the first nicotine-free prescription medicine used to treat nicotine dependence. Varenicline (Chantix) both activates and antagonizes the *alpha-4-beta-2* nicotinic receptors in the brain. This effect provides some stimulation to nicotine receptors, while also reducing the pleasurable effects of nicotine from smoking. This drug has demonstrated greater efficacy than bupropion.
18. Benzodiazepines are used for all three levels of ethanol withdrawal. Lower dosages are used for mild symptoms and higher dosages are needed for severe withdrawal. The oral route is preferred; however, it is often necessary to use the intravenous route for patients experiencing severe withdrawal. Patients who are experiencing severe withdrawal often require monitoring in an intensive care unit for cardiac and respiratory function, fluid and nutrition replacement, vital signs, and mental status. Restraints are indicated for a patient who is confused or agitated to protect the patient from self-harm and to protect others (delirium tremens can be a terrifying and life-threatening state). Thiamine administration, hydra-

tion, and magnesium replacement may be indicated depending on the severity of the withdrawal state.

19. Dextromethorphan is an ingredient in several over-the-counter products, including Robitussin DM cough syrup and Mucinex DM tablets. Some adolescents have discovered that taking dextromethorphan in large amounts leads to a "high" that is accompanied by hallucinations. The hallucinations have been documented to be similar to those associated with the street drug phencyclidine (PCP). In addition, it has been found that teens who abuse dextromethorphan may also abuse other drugs such as lysergic acid diethylamide (LSD), PCP, ecstasy, and inhalants. The hazardous short- or long-term effects that may occur with these drugs include nausea, hot flashes, reduced mental status, dizziness, seizures, loss of coordination and balance, brain damage, and death.

20. Methamphetamine is a chemical class of amphetamine, but it has a much stronger effect on the CNS than the other classes of amphetamine. Crystallized methamphetamine, known as *ice, crystal,* or *crystal meth,* is a smokable and more powerful form of the drug. The over-the-counter (OTC) decongestant pseudoephedrine is commonly used to synthesize methamphetamine in secret drug laboratories, often in private homes. This practice has led to dramatic increases in the abuse of this drug. In 2005, the Combat Methamphetamine Epidemic Act required restricted retail sales of all nonprescription drug products containing pseudoephedrine. Specific restrictions include allowing sales only from *behind* the pharmacy counter, requiring photo identification and electronic or paper recordkeeping of purchasers (which must remain on file for 2 years), and setting maximum allowable amount (in grams) of pseudoephedrine that can be sold per consumer per month.

**Case Study**

1. Ethanol is a central nervous system depressant.
2. Acute severe alcoholic intoxication may cause cardiovascular depression, and long-term excessive use has largely irreversible effects on the heart. Moderate amounts may either stimulate or depress respiration, but large amounts produce lethal respiratory depression.
3. First, you should monitor the patient's respiratory and cardiovascular status and prevent injury from falling or aspiration from vomiting. In addition, you should be alert to the patient's behavior and mental status to identify changes in his condition. Withdrawal from alcohol can lead to serious conditions such as delirium tremens. Careful assessment of vital signs and mental status is imperative at this time, because early withdrawal symptoms may be an increase in blood pressure and pulse with an altered mental status.

4. Mr. C. should stay in the hospital for observation for and possible treatment of delirium tremens, which may begin with tremors and agitation and progress to hallucinations and sometimes death. See Box 17-6 for information on treatment of ethanol withdrawal.
5. Chronic excessive ingestion of ethanol is directly associated with several serious mental and neurologic disorders. Nutritional and vitamin B deficiencies can occur, which result in conditions such as Wernicke's encephalopathy, Korsakoff's psychosis, polyneuritis, and nicotinic acid deficiency encephalopathy. Seizures may also occur. In addition, long-term ingestion of ethanol may result in alcoholic hepatitis or liver cirrhosis.

# CHAPTER 18
## Adrenergic Drugs

### Chapter Review and NCLEX® Examination Preparation/Critical Thinking and Application

1. d
2. b
3. a, b, d
4. a
5. c
6. a, b, e
7. 50 mcg per dose (See Overview of Dosage Calculations, Section IV.)
8. 0.5 mL (See Overview of Dosage Calculations, Section III.)
9.

10. a. The alpha-adrenergic activity of this drug causes vasoconstriction in the nasal mucosa. This produces shrinkage of the mucosa and promotes easier nasal breathing.
    b. Perhaps she administered the spray too often. Excessive use of nasal decongestants can lead to greater congestion because of a rebound phenomenon.
11. Use of the drug is contraindicated in patients who have a tumor that secretes catecholamines, such as a pheochromocytoma.
12. The action of dopamine depends on the dosage. At low dosages, it can dilate blood vessels in the brain, heart, kidneys, and mesentery, increasing blood flow to these areas. Increased renal flow may help remove excess fluid volume. At higher infusion rates, dopamine can improve contractility and cardiac output.
13. The toxic effects of adrenergic drugs are mainly an extension of their common adverse effects, such as

seizures, hypotension or hypertension, dysrhythmias, and other effects, but the two most life-threatening toxic effects involve the central nervous system and cardiovascular system. Seizures can be managed effectively with diazepam. An extreme elevation in blood pressure poses the risk of hemorrhage in the brain and elsewhere in the body. To lower the blood pressure quickly, a rapid-acting beta-adrenergic blocking drug can be used to reverse the adrenergic effects. Most of the adrenergic drugs have very short half-lives; therefore, their effects are relatively short-lived. Stopping the drug should quickly cause the toxic symptoms to subside. The treatment of overdoses often focuses on treating the symptoms and supporting the patient's respiratory and cardiac functions.

14. a. He is probably having an anaphylactic reaction to the penicillin.
    b. First, the nurse must stop the medication! Then she will have someone else notify the physician while she stays with the patient to monitor and support the ABCs (airway, breathing, and circulation).
    c. Epinephrine is the drug of choice for anaphylactic reactions.

**Case Study**
1. Before giving this medication, you should assess for hypersensitivity to albuterol and assess breath sounds and vital signs (blood pressure, pulse rate, respiratory rate) to obtain a baseline for comparative purposes. Because this medication may cause tachycardia and cardiac dysrhythmias, the patient's pulse rate and rhythm should be monitored during the treatment. Afterward, you should assess the patient's vital signs and breath sounds again, and assess for therapeutic response to the medication.
2. The onset of inhaled albuterol is almost immediate; it would take more time for orally administered albuterol to be absorbed and to become effective. Therefore, the inhaled form will take effect faster than the oral form.
3. These are expected side effects of the albuterol and will soon wear off.
4. Salmeterol is indicated for asthma and prevention of bronchospasms in patients who may need long-term maintenance therapy for their asthma. Patients should be taught that salmeterol is not to be used for relief of acute symptoms, and education about its dosing is important. Dosing of salmeterol is usually 1 puff twice daily 12 hours apart for maintenance. For prevention of exercise-induced asthma, the recommendation is 2 puffs 1/2 to 1 hour before exercise and no additional dosing for 12 hours. If Maureen is still taking the inhaled steroid, then the bronchodilator should be taken first, and she should

wait approximately 5 minutes before using the steroid inhaler. The patient will need to rinse her mouth with warm water after taking the inhaled corticosteroid. All equipment should be cleaned regularly.

# CHAPTER 19
## Adrenergic-Blocking Drugs

**Chapter Review and NCLEX® Examination Preparation/Critical Thinking and Application**
1. a, b, d
2. a
3. c
4. b
5. d
6. c
7. 83 mL per hour (See Overview of Dosage Calculations, Section V.)
8. 4 mL
9. Extravasation can cause vasoconstriction and ultimately tissue death (necrosis). If the vasoconstriction is not reversed quickly, the whole limb can be lost. Phentolamine, an alpha blocker, can reverse this potent vasoconstriction and restore blood flow to the ischemic, vasoconstricted area. When phentolamine is injected subcutaneously in a circular fashion around the extravasation site, it causes alpha-adrenergic receptor blockade and vasodilation. This in turn increases blood flow to the ischemic tissue and thus prevents permanent damage.
10. Some beta blockers are considered cardioprotective because they inhibit stimulation by the circulating catecholamines that were released during muscle damage, such as that caused by a myocardial infarction. When a beta blocker occupies their receptors, the circulating catecholamines cannot bind to their receptors. Thus, the beta blockers "protect" the heart from being stimulated by these catecholamines, which would only further increase the heart rate and the contractile force, and thereby increase myocardial oxygen demand.
11. She should take her apical pulse for 1 full minute and monitor her blood pressure because cardiac depression can occur with these drugs. If her systolic blood pressure decreases to lower than 100 mm Hg or her pulse decreases to fewer than 60 beats/min, she needs to contact her physician. She should also report any weight gain, especially 2 pounds or more in a 24-hour period or 5 pounds or more in a week, as well as any weakness, shortness of breath, or edema.
12. A common problem with the alpha blockers such as tamsulosin is that when patients first start taking these drugs, they may experience lightheadedness and orthostatic hypotension. Patients usually

quickly develop a tolerance to this effect. He should be taught to take care when standing up to prevent falling if he gets lightheaded; taking the first dose at bedtime may help. In addition, other adverse effects of blurred vision, dizziness, and drowsiness may lead to injuries if he should fall. Special care must be taken for safety until he knows how he responds to the medication.

**Case Study**

1. Nonselective beta blockers (which block both beta$_1$ and beta$_2$ receptors) may precipitate bradycardia and hypotension; their use is contraindicated in asthma. Therefore, if the patient has heart disease as well as respiratory disease, a beta$_1$ blocker, or "cardiose-lective" drug, would be very beneficial because it would not produce constriction or increased airway resistance as would beta$_2$ blockers.

2. When a beta blocker is given, it occupies receptors and prevents circulating catecholamines (which are released when a myocardial infarction occurs) from binding to these receptors. The beta blocker thus prevents stimulation of the heart by these catechol-amines, which would further increase heart rate, contractile force, and myocardial oxygen demand. In addition, cardioselective beta$_1$ blockers such as atenolol block the beta$_1$-adrenergic receptors on the surface of the heart. This reduces myocardial stimu-lation, which in turn reduces heart rate, slows con-duction through the atrioventricular node, prolongs sinoatrial node recovery, and decreases myocardial oxygen demand by decreasing myocardial contrac-tile force (contractility).

3. Table 19-4 lists beta blocker–induced adverse ef-fects. Patient teaching will include instructions to monitor the apical pulse for 1 full minute and moni-tor blood pressure because of the cardiac depression that can occur, and to notify the physician if systolic blood pressure decreases to lower than 100 mm Hg or pulse decreases to fewer than 60 beats/min. In addition, patients need to report any weight gain, especially a gain of 2 pounds or more in a 24-hour period or 5 pounds or more in a week, as well as any weakness, shortness of breath, and edema. These symptoms may indicate the onset of heart failure. The patient should also be taught about orthostatic changes and cautioned to rise slowly when getting up to avoid syncope. For other teaching points, see Patient Teaching Tips in the text.

4. Make sure that patients are weaned off these medica-tions slowly, if this is indicated, because of the pos-sible rebound hypertension or chest pain that rapid withdrawal can precipitate. Beta blockers may cause impotence, which may be the reason Bruce wants to stop the medication, but the nurse needs to ask Bruce about his reason for wanting to stop atenolol.

# CHAPTER 20
## Cholinergic Drugs

**Chapter Review and NCLEX® Examination Preparation/Critical Thinking and Application**

1. h
2. g
3. f
4. b
5. j
6. e
7. i
8. a
9. c
10. b
11. b
12. d
13. c
14. b, c, d, f
15. a
16. b, d
17. 17 gtt/min (16.7 rounds to 17) (See Overview of Dosage Calculations, Section V.)
18. 26.7 mg (See Overview of Dosage Calculations, Section IV.)
19. SLUDGE stands for *S*alivation, *L*acrimation, *U*rinary incontinence, *D*iarrhea, *G*astrointestinal cramps, and *E*mesis.
20. a. Bethanechol (Urecholine) is the drug of choice.
    b. None. Bethanechol use is contraindicated in pa-tients with a genitourinary obstruction. The drug will be discontinued immediately.
21. a. Cholinergic crisis
    b. Ensure that atropine, the antidote, is readily avail-able.
22. a. She should experience less eyelid drooping (pto-sis), less double vision (diplopia), less difficulty swallowing and chewing, and/or less weakness.
    b. She needs to report any increased muscle weak-ness, abdominal cramps, diarrhea, or difficulty breathing.

**Case Study**

1. There are no "cures" for Alzheimer's disease, but there are several drugs available for management of symptoms. Their use can sometimes yield enough improvement in a patient's mental status to make a noticeable improvement in the quality of life for patients as well as caregivers and family members. However, individual response to these medications does vary from patient to patient. Available drugs include donepezil (Aricept), tacrine (Cognex), galan-tamine (Razadyne, Reminyl), rivastigmine (Exelon), and memantine (Namenda).

2. Rivastigmine is also approved for treating dementia that is associated with Parkinson's disease.

3. Direct-acting cholinergic agonists bind to cholinergic receptors and activate them. Indirect-acting cholinergic agonists act by making more acetylcholine (ACh) available at the receptor site. As a result, ACh binds to and stimulates the receptors. It does this by inhibiting the action of cholinesterase, the enzyme responsible for breaking down ACh.

4. Adverse effects of rivastigmine include dizziness, headache, nausea and vomiting, diarrhea, and anorexia (loss of appetite). Administering this drug with meals helps decrease the gastrointestinal side effects, although absorption may also be decreased. Patients who become dizzy with the therapy must be assisted with ambulation. Doses are titrated carefully to help minimize adverse effects.

5. Rivastigmine is also available in rapid orally disintegrating tablets, which may be easier for Arthur to take.

# CHAPTER 21
## Cholinergic-Blocking Drugs

### Chapter Review and NCLEX® Examination Preparation/Critical Thinking and Application

1. a, c, f
2. a, c, d
3. b
4. c
5. b
6. d
7. 0.6 mL
8. a. 40 mcg (See Overview of Dosage Calculations, Section IV.)
   b. 0.2 mL
9. Atropine sulfate is used preoperatively to reduce salivation and excessive secretions in the respiratory and gastrointestinal tracts. Glycopyrrolate (Robinul) is also used for this purpose.
10. a. Initially, Mr. M. will be treated with hospitalization and close, continuous monitoring (including continuous electrocardiographic monitoring). Fluid therapy and other standard measures used to treat shock are instituted as needed. Activated charcoal may be effective in removing the drug that has not yet been absorbed.
    b. In the case of hallucinations, physostigmine has proven helpful, although its use as an antidote for cholinergic blocker overdose is controversial because it has the potential to produce severe adverse effects such as seizures and cardiac asystole, and is usually reserved for the treatment of patients who show extreme delirium or agitation or who could inflict injury upon themselves.

11. Antihistamines can have additive effects with cholinergic blockers, resulting in increased anticholinergic effects.

12. a. In the treatment of symptomatic bradycardia, higher dosages of atropine result in an increase in heart rate because of the cholinergic-blocking effects on the heart's conduction system. Atropine blocks the inhibitory vagal (cholinergic) effects on the pacemaker cells of the sinoatrial and atrioventricular nodes, which will hopefully lead to an increased heart rate due to unopposed sympathetic stimulation.
    b. Atropine has a therapeutic effect in cases of exposure to organophosphate insecticides because it blocks cholinergic receptors.

### Case Study

1. Tolterodine should not be used in patients with narrow-angle glaucoma or urinary retention. If patients have a history of decreased liver function or are taking drugs that inhibit cytochrome P-450 enzyme 3A4, the tolterodine dose will be reduced. Mrs. W.'s "eye problems" need to be evaluated further to rule out glaucoma.

2. Tolterodine appears to be associated with a much lower incidence of dry mouth. This may be due to tolterodine's specificity for the bladder as opposed to the salivary glands.

3. When these cholinergic-blocking drugs are used to treat urinary incontinence, the inability to sweat or perspire should be managed with an increase in fluids and avoidance of extreme heat. Mrs. W. needs to avoid overheating when working outside.

4. Although this drug may be associated with a lower incidence of dry mouth, it may still cause this unpleasant side effect because it is a cholinergic-blocking drug. Dry mouth may be managed best by drinking adequate fluids, chewing gum, performing frequent mouth care, sucking on sugar-free hard candy, and using saliva substitute products.

# CHAPTER 22
## Antihypertensive Drugs

### Critical Thinking Crossword
*Across*
1. Secondary
5. Idiopathic
7. Orthostatic
8. Vasodilators
*Down*
2. Essential
3. Primary
4. Diuretics
6. ACE

## Chapter Review and NCLEX® Examination Preparation/Critical Thinking and Application

1. c
2. b, d, e
3. b
4. a
5. d
6. a, c
7. 2 tablets per dose (See Overview of Dosage Calculations, Section II.)
8. 4 mL (See Overview of Dosage Calculations, Section V.)
9. Because nitroprusside has a very short half-life (10 minutes), the nurse will first discontinue the infusion. Treatment for the hypotension is supportive; pressor drugs can be given to raise the blood pressure quickly if necessary.
10. a. Captopril is probably best for Irene. In critically ill patients, a drug with a short half-life (such as captopril) is better, because if problems arise, they will be short-lived. Also, Irene has liver dysfunction, so captopril has an advantage because it is not a prodrug (a prodrug is inactive in its initial form and must be biotransformed in the liver to its active form to be effective).
    b. Because of his history of poor adherence, Kory would benefit from a drug with a long half-life and long duration of action, which he would need to take only once a day. Therefore, one of the newer ACE inhibitors—benazepril, fosinopril, lisinopril, quinapril, or ramipril—would be best.
11. There is a first-dose effect with prazosin. This means that the patient will experience a considerable drop in blood pressure after taking the first dose, so he needs to take it if he will be lying down for a while or before bedtime and arise slowly. This effect decreases with time or with a reduction in the dosage, as ordered by the physician.
12. a. Beta blockers and ACE inhibitors
    b. Calcium channel blockers and diuretics

## Case Study

1. Initial drug therapy would include thiazide-type diuretics. Other drugs that may also be started include ACE inhibitors, angiotensin II receptor blockers, beta blockers, calcium channel blockers, or a combination. Because John is African American, calcium channel blockers and diuretics would most likely be chosen over beta blockers and ACE inhibitors.
2. Teach him about the possibility of orthostatic hypotension and instruct him to change positions slowly—especially after stooping or bending over or when rising from supine or sitting to standing.
3. Exercise is an important part of a healthy lifestyle. However, emphasize the importance of safety and the need to avoid excessive exercise, hot climates,

saunas, hot tubs, and hot environments. Heat may precipitate vasodilation and lead to worsening of hypotension with the risk of fainting and injury to himself.

# CHAPTER 23
## Antianginal Drugs

## Chapter Review and NCLEX® Examination Preparation/Critical Thinking and Application

1. c
2. c
3. a, c, d, e
4. d
5. a
6. b
7. a
8. 2 capsules
9. DO NOT cut the patch in half! The nurse needs to call the pharmacy to obtain the correct dosage of the transdermal patch, one that delivers 0.2 mg/hr.
10. The nurse will call 911 and assist the patient until the ambulance arrives. The nurse will check the "ABCs" and administer CPR if it becomes necessary. At this time, the nurse does not know the man's condition, and certainly cannot administer someone else's medication to him. Isordil is available in a sublingual form, but the nurse cannot administer one person's medication to another person, especially to someone with an undetermined condition.
11. Ms. V. might be taking a beta blocker. Fatigue and lethargy are the most common patient complaints with the use of beta blockers, and mental depression can be exacerbated, particularly in older adults. Also, one of the central nervous system adverse effects of beta blockers is the occurrence of unusual dreams.
12. Theresa has a good start, but she also needs to include in her journal a description of the activity she was performing at the time her angina occurred and the number of tablets she had to take before the pain subsided. Also, she must keep the tablets in an airtight, dark glass bottle away from sunlight, because the active ingredient in nitroglycerin is easily destroyed. The fact that she had no adverse effects such as headache may indicate that the drug is no longer active and needs to be replaced.

## Case Study

1. Chronic stable angina, also known as *classic* or *effort angina*, can be triggered by either exertion or stress (cold temperature or emotions).
2. When experiencing an acute anginal attack, he needs to stop his activity and lie down immediately, take 1 sublingual tablet as soon as possible after the pain begins, remain calm, and rest.

3. If he obtains no relief after taking 1 sublingual tablet, his handball partner should call 911 immediately and have emergency response personnel take him to the hospital. The emergency response team would be better equipped to help him if further complications (such as a myocardial infarction) occur. The patient can take 1 more tablet, while awaiting emergency care, and a third tablet 5 minutes later, but no more than three tablets total.

4. Beta blockers are most effective in the treatment of typical exertional angina.

# CHAPTER 24
## Heart Failure Drugs

### Chapter Review and NCLEX® Examination Preparation/Critical Thinking and Application

1. c
2. d
3. a
4. b
5. a, c, d, e, f
6. c, e, f
7. 2 mL
8.

9. 250 mcg
10. Vomiting, headache, fatigue, and dysrhythmia are adverse effects of cardiac glycosides. The presence of a serum potassium level of more than 5 mEq/L, along with these symptoms, means that administration of digoxin immune Fab is indicated for the treatment of severe digoxin toxicity.

11. At this time, nesiritide is generally used in the intensive care setting as a final effort to treat severe, life-threatening heart failure, often in combination with several other cardiostimulatory medications. It is no longer recommended as a first-line drug for heart failure. Instead, it is recommended that its use be strictly limited to treatment of patients with acutely decompensated heart failure who have dyspnea at rest. It should not be used to replace diuretics and should not be used repetitively or to improve renal function.

12. Increased urinary output and decreased dyspnea and fatigue are therapeutic effects of digoxin. The constipation needs to be assessed. Mr. F. should not consume large amounts of bran or other foods high in fiber because the bran will bind to the digitalis and make less of the drug available for absorption.

13. a. Milrinone increases the force of contraction (positive inotropic effect) and relaxes the blood vessels (vasodilation), causing a reduction in afterload, or the force against which the heart must pump to eject its volume.
    b. Phosphodiesterase inhibitors have a wider therapeutic window than digoxin.
    c. Ventricular cardiac dysrhythmias

**Case Study**

1. Positive inotropic effect: Increases myocardial contractility
   Negative chronotropic effect: Decreases heart rate
   Negative dromotropic effect: Slows the conduction of electrical impulses in the heart

2. Effects on:
   • Stroke volume: Increased
   • Venous blood pressure and vein engorgement: Decreased
   • Coronary circulation: Increased
   • Diuresis: Increased due to improved circulation

3. First, complete your assessment by checking her apical pulse, heart and lung sounds, and blood pressure. In addition, check her potassium level, because low levels of potassium may lead to digoxin toxicity. If you have not yet given the digoxin dose, hold it and call the physician immediately. Monitor her for signs of digoxin toxicity, especially dangerous dysrhythmias. The digoxin level of 3.5 ng/mL is above the therapeutic range.

# CHAPTER 25
## Antidysrhythmic Drugs

### Chapter Review and NCLEX® Examination Preparation/Critical Thinking and Application

1. d
2. c, d, e
3. a
4. d
5. a
6. b
7. b, c, e
8. 150 mg
9. 2 mL
10. a, (3); b, (1); c, (2)
11. a. Class II antidysrhythmics, or beta blockers, are indicated because they have been shown to significantly reduce the incidence of sudden cardiac death after myocardial infarction.
    b. If Mr. K. had asthma, cardioselective beta blockers would be indicated. Noncardioselective beta blockers block not only the beta$_1$-adrenergic receptors in the heart, but also the beta$_2$-adrenergic receptors in the lungs. As a result, preexisting asthma could be worsened if a noncardioselective beta blocker is administered.

12. Amiodarone is indicated for the management of life-threatening ventricular tachycardia or ventricular fibrillation that is resistant to other drug therapy. Although it is very effective, amiodarone can penetrate and concentrate in the adipose tissue of any organ in the body, where it may have unwanted effects. It may cause either hypothyroidism or hyperthyroidism, corneal microdeposits, pulmonary toxicity (which is fatal in about 10% of patients), and even dysrhythmias. Amiodarone has a very long half-life and the side effects may take months to subside.

13. a. Lidocaine must be injected intramuscularly or intravenously; when lidocaine is taken orally, the liver converts most of it to inactive metabolites.

    b. Lidocaine is extensively metabolized in the liver. For patients in liver failure or with a history of cirrhosis, a dosage reduction of 50% is recommended.

14. Alicia should not double up on her medication. The physician needs to be contacted about the missed dose and about Alicia's symptoms of diarrhea and lightheadedness, which are adverse effects of the quinidine.

**Case Study**

1. Calcium channel blockers block the slow inward flow of calcium ions into the slow (calcium) channels in cardiac conduction tissue. The conduction effects of these drugs are limited to the atria and the AV node, where conduction is prolonged and the tissues are made more refractory to stimulation. As a result, they reduce the incidence of paroxysmal supraventricular tachycardia (PSVT). These drugs have little effect on the ventricular tissues.

2. Prevention or reduction of supraventricular rhythms

3. Calcium channel blockers are contraindicated in the presence of pulmonary congestion. A further assessment of his respiratory status must be performed before the medication is started.

4. The physician may prescribe adenosine (Adenocard), which is useful for the treatment of PSVT that has failed to respond to verapamil.

# CHAPTER 26
# Coagulation Modifier Drugs

## Chapter Review and NCLEX® Examination Preparation/Critical Thinking and Application

1. k
2. n
3. j
4. l
5. m
6. b
7. a, c
8. c
9. i
10. h
11. e
12. g
13. a, c, d
14. b
15. a
16. c
17. b, c, d, e
18. d
19. b
20. 0.8 mL
21. 7.5 mg (patient weighs 75 kg)
22. Low-molecular–weight heparins (LMWHs) such as enoxaparin are contraindicated in patients with an indwelling epidural catheter. The medication can be given 2 hours after the epidural is removed. This is very important for nurses to remember, because giving an LMWH with an epidural has been associated with epidural hematoma.

23. a. The anticoagulant effects of heparin can be reversed with protamine sulfate.

    b. In general, 1 mg of protamine sulfate can reverse the effects of 100 units of heparin.

    c. The activated partial thromboplastin time (aPTT) is the test most commonly used.

24. a. Vitamin K

    b. Current recommendations are to use the lowest amount of vitamin K possible, based on the clinical situation.

    c. After the use of vitamin K for warfarin toxicity, warfarin resistance will occur for up to 7 days; thus the patient cannot be anticoagulated by warfarin during this period. In such cases, either heparin or an LMWH may need to be added to provide adequate anticoagulation if necessary.

25. The physician will probably prescribe one of the antifibrinolytic drugs, which are used to stop excessive oozing from surgical sites, such as chest tubes.

26. Desmopressin is used in patients with type I von Willebrand's disease; it increases the levels of clotting factor VIII.

27. The alteplase can be readministered because it has a very short half-life of 5 minutes. Because of its short half-life, it is given along with heparin to prevent reocclusion of the infarcted blood vessel.

28. a. They are possible indications of bleeding problems related to the anticoagulation therapy.

    b. Ursula might also be exhibiting a change in pulse rate or rhythm, blood pressure, or level of consciousness.

    c. The nurse will notify the physician immediately. She must not administer any other anticoagulants; if Ursula is receiving a continuous infusion of an anticoagulant, she must stop the infusion. The nurse will take Ursula's vital signs and stay with her. She will prepare to administer the appropriate antidote.

29. Heparin is commonly used for DVT prophylaxis in a dose of 5000 units two or three times a day given subcutaneously, and does not need to be monitored when used for prophylaxis.

**Case Study**

1. Use of aspirin is contraindicated in the presence of peptic ulcer disease. Doug has been started on the clopidogrel therapy to reduce the risk of stroke.

2. He should be taught to watch for signs of abnormal bleeding and should immediately report any of the following signs and symptoms to the health care provider: respiratory difficulty, back pain, skin rash, evidence of gastrointestinal bleeding, any other bleeding abnormality, diarrhea, acute severe headache, and change in vision (blurred vision or loss of vision).

3. He needs to take measures to prevent bleeding, such as using a soft toothbrush and an electric razor, and should take great care when trimming his nails, gardening, and participating in rough or contact sports. He needs to take precautions to protect himself from injury and subsequent bleeding or bruising, which can be extremely dangerous while he is taking antiplatelet drugs.

4. Herbal products that contain St. John's wort, garlic, ginger, ginseng, and ginkgo should be avoided because they have anticoagulant properties.

# CHAPTER 27
## Antilipemic Drugs

### Chapter Review and NCLEX® Examination Preparation/Critical Thinking and Application

1. d
2. a, c, d, e
3. a
4. b
5. d
6. c
7. a, c, d, e
8. 1.5 tablets
9. 750 mg per dose; 3 tablets per dose
10. a. Fibric acid derivative—it is believed that these drugs work by activating the lipoprotein lipase, an enzyme responsible for the breakdown of cholesterol.
    b. Lipid-lowering drug and vitamin—exact mechanism unknown; beneficial effects are believed to be related to its ability to inhibit lipolysis in adipose tissue, decrease esterification of triglycerides in the liver, and increase the activity of lipase.
    c. HMG–CoA reductase inhibitor—reduces blood cholesterol by decreasing the rate of cholesterol production.
    d. Bile acid sequestrant—binds bile, preventing the resorption of the bile acids from the small intestine. The insoluble bile acid and resin (drug) complex that is formed is excreted in the feces.

11. Unless Mr. H. has additional risk factors, his high level of low-density lipoprotein (LDL) cholesterol alone does not warrant drug therapy at this time. He will be recommended for dietary therapy with an LDL goal of less than 160 mg/dL. All reasonable nonpharmacologic means of controlling Mr. H.'s LDL level need to be tried and found to fail before he is given drug therapy. Mr. H. needs to find time in his busy schedule to exercise and eat more wisely. See Table 27-3.

12. Mrs. K. is probably experiencing constipation and either belching or increased flatulence associated with cholestyramine use (she may also be experiencing heartburn, nausea, and bloating). Mrs. K. requires extra patient teaching and support to help her maintain compliance with the drug therapy; she should be assured that these adverse effects will probably diminish over time.

13. No. Justus is not a candidate for niacin therapy because niacin use is contraindicated in patients with peptic ulcer. Also, when niacin is taken with an HMG–CoA reductase inhibitor, the likelihood of myopathy development is greatly increased, although it is not uncommon to see these drugs used together.

14. Mrs. N. must take her antihypertensive and cholestyramine (Questran) at different times of the day because the bile acid sequestrant may interfere significantly with the absorption of other drugs taken at the same time. All other drugs should be taken at least 1 hour before or 4 to 6 hours after the administration of antilipemics.

**Case Study**

1. No, he is not right. Dietary measures are a part of antilipemic therapy. Nonpharmacologic measures include consumption of a low-fat, low-cholesterol diet; supervised, moderate exercise; weight loss; cessation of smoking and drinking; and relaxation therapy.

2. This drug is used primarily to lower total and LDL cholesterol levels as well as triglyceride levels; it has been shown to raise the HDL level as well.

3. Elevations in liver enzyme levels may also occur, and the patient will be monitored for excessive elevations, which may indicate the need for alternative drug therapy. In addition, total cholesterol level, LDL/HDL ratio, and triglyceride levels need to be monitored to evaluate therapeutic effect.

4. Myopathy (muscle pain) is an uncommon but clinically important side effect that may occur in some patients taking statins. It may progress to a serious condition known as *rhabdomyolysis* in which the breakdown of muscle protein occurs, leading to myoglobinuria and possible renal damage. Patients receiving statin therapy need to be taught to report unexplained muscle pain to their health care provider immediately.

# CHAPTER 28
## Diuretic Drugs

### Chapter Review and NCLEX® Examination Preparation/Critical Thinking and Application

1. c
2. f
3. e
4. i
5. g
6. j
7. h
8. a
9. d
10. b
11. a, c, d, e
12. c
13. a
14. d
15. b
16. b, e
17. 15 mL

18. 150 mL (hint: 20% indicates 20 g per 100 mL)

$$\frac{20 \text{ g}}{100 \text{ mL}} = \frac{30 \text{ g}}{x \text{ mL}}$$

(20 g)(x mL) = (100 mL)(30 g); 20x = 3000;
x = 150 mL
(See Overview of Dosage Calculations, Section III.)

19. a. Ms. A. was probably prescribed a carbonic anhydrase inhibitor (CAI).
    b. An undesirable effect of the CAIs is that they elevate the blood glucose level, causing glycosuria in diabetic patients. They may also interact with some oral antidiabetic drugs.

20. a. For mannitol to be effective in treating acute renal failure, enough renal blood flow and glomerular filtration must exist to enable the drug to reach the tubules.
    b. Mannitol is always administered intravenously through a filter, because it can crystallize when exposed to low temperatures (which is more likely to occur when concentrations exceed 15%). In addition, inspect the fluid container visually for precipitants.
    c. Arthur's headache and chills are probably side effects of the mannitol therapy. At this time the therapy should be continued, but Arthur needs to be monitored for the development of more serious adverse effects.

21. a. Mr. F. will probably be prescribed spironolactone in high doses; this drug is used often for the treatment of ascites associated with cirrhosis of the liver.
    b. His serum potassium level will need to be monitored frequently because he has impaired renal function. The spironolactone may cause hyperkalemia.

22. a. Impotence and decreased libido are among the side effects of thiazide. Brendan is possibly experiencing these effects.
    b. He needs to stop eating licorice, because its consumption can lead to an additive hypokalemia in patients taking thiazide. Brendan's fatigue may be the result of severe hypokalemia and will be evaluated.

23. It is likely that Mrs. H.'s neighbor was prescribed one of the potassium-sparing diuretics and thus was not instructed to eat additional potassium-rich foods. Mrs. H. needs to follow the dietary recommendations provided for her, not for her neighbor.

24. Loop diuretics have a distinct advantage over thiazide diuretics in that their diuretic action continues even when creatinine clearance decreases below 25 mL/min. This means that even when kidney function diminishes, loop diuretics can still work. As renal function decreases, the efficacy of thiazides diminishes, because delivery of the drug to the site of activity is impaired. Thiazides are not to be used if creatinine clearance is less than 30 to 50 mL/min. Normal creatinine clearance is 125 mL/min, depending on age of the patient. However, metolazone remains effective to a creatinine clearance of 10 mL/min, and thus can be used in cases of renal failure.

### Case Study

1. These symptoms suggest hypokalemia. Furosemide causes potassium to be excreted along with sodium and water.
2. She could have eaten foods high in potassium, including bananas, oranges, apricots, dates, raisins, broccoli, green beans, potatoes, tomatoes, meats, fish, wheat bread, and legumes.
3. Spironolactone is a potassium-sparing diuretic; it causes sodium and water to be excreted, but potassium is retained.

4. The use of ACE inhibitors or potassium supplements in combination with potassium-sparing diuretics can result in hyperkalemia. When taken together, lithium and potassium-sparing diuretics can result in lithium toxicity. The use of nonsteroidal antiinflammatory drugs with potassium-sparing diuretics can reduce the effectiveness of the diuretics.

# CHAPTER 29
# Fluids and Electrolytes

## Chapter Review and NCLEX® Examination Preparation/Critical Thinking and Application

1. a, b, d, e
2. c
3. d
4. c
5. b
6. b
7. b
8. a. 42 mL/hour
   b. 11 gtt/min (rounded up from 10.5) (See the Overview of Dosage Calculations, Section V.)
9. 100 mL/hour (50 mL : 0.5 hr :: x mL : 1 hr; x = 100 mL/hr)
10. **Advantages:** Crystalloids are less expensive than colloids and blood products for replacing fluids and better for emergency short-term plasma volume expansion. They also promote urinary flow. They do not carry the risk of transmission of viral diseases or anaphylaxis and do not promote bleeding.
    **Disadvantages:** The fluids can leak out of the plasma into the tissues and cells, which results in edema (such as peripheral edema or pulmonary edema). They may dilute plasma proteins, resulting in lower colloid oncotic pressure (COP), and dilute erythrocyte concentration, resulting in decreased oxygen tension. Large volumes are needed to be effective, but prolonged infusions and administration of large volumes may worsen acidosis or alkalosis. Lastly, their effects are relatively short-lived compared with those of colloids.
11. a. Blood products
    b. They are the only fluids that contain hemoglobin.
    c. They are natural products that require human donors, which means that they can be incompatible with a recipient's immune system. These products can also transmit pathogens from the donor to the recipient.
12. Tanya is exhibiting early symptoms of hypokalemia. Initial treatment will include potassium supplements, either IV or oral, until the laboratory results return to normal. At home, she needs to eat foods high in potassium, such as bananas, oranges, apricots, dates, raisins, broccoli, green beans, potatoes, tomatoes, meats, fish, wheat bread, and legumes. In addition, she will need therapy to address her eating disorder issues.
13. a. Hyponatremia
    b. Vomiting is a possible adverse effect of oral administration of sodium chloride; if vomiting occurs, he needs to be careful about monitoring for further fluid and electrolyte loss.
14. a. Signs of transfusion reaction include apprehension, restlessness, flushed skin, increased pulse and respiration rate, dyspnea, rash, joint or lower back pain, swelling, fever and chills, nausea, weakness, and jaundice.
    b. Although it is possible for pathogens such as that causing acquired immunodeficiency syndrome (AIDS) to be transmitted via blood products, reassure Victor's wife that techniques are now used that have drastically reduced the incidence of such problems.
    c. Victor's restlessness and increased pulse are signs of a reaction to the blood product. The nurse will stop the transfusion immediately, and change the infusion to normal saline. The nurse will stay with Victor and assess his vital signs, and have another nurse notify the physician immediately; the facility's protocol for transfusion reactions will be followed.

## Case Study

1. The normal total protein level is in the range of 7.4 g/dL. If the level drops below 5.3 g/dL, the colloid oncotic pressure (COP) becomes less than the hydrostatic pressure, and fluid shifts into the tissues, which results in edema.
2. The albumin will increase the COP and move fluid from outside the blood vessels to inside the blood vessels, thus reducing the edema.
3. Colloids such as albumin are the choice for this patient. Crystalloids can leak out of the plasma into the tissues and cells, resulting in edema anywhere in the body. Crystalloids also dilute the proteins in the plasma, further reducing the COP. Finally, crystalloids are more likely to cause edema because of the larger volumes needed to achieve the desired clinical effect. Colloids reduce edema and expand plasma volume by pulling fluid from the extravascular space into the blood vessels.
4. Colloids can alter the coagulation system, which results in impaired coagulation and possibly bleeding. They have no oxygen-carrying ability and contain no clotting factors, and they may also dilute the plasma protein concentration, which may impair the function of platelets.

# CHAPTER 30
## Pituitary Drugs

### Chapter Review and NCLEX® Examination Preparation/Critical Thinking and Application

1.  a. Glucocorticoids, mineralocorticoids, androgens
    b. Cosyntropin
    c. Regulates anabolic processes related to growth and adaptation to stressors; promotes skeletal and muscle growth; increases protein synthesis; increases liver glycogenolysis; increases fat mobilization
    d. Somatropin and somatrem
    e. Antidiuretic hormone
    f. Vasopressin and desmopressin
    g. Promotes uterine contractions
    h. Pitocin
2.  d
3.  c
4.  b
5.  a
6.  c
7.  a
8.  a. Total dose per week for this child (44 lb = 20 kg) is 6 mg
    b. Dose per injection (6 daily injections) = 1 mg per dose per day for 6 days
9.  0.5 mL

10. In addition to information about proper subcutaneous injection techniques, the teaching plan needs to include a reminder of the dosage form and amount and the importance of compliance with therapy, as well as keeping the follow-up appointments. The nurse will show the parents how to keep a journal of Patricia's growth measurements.
11. Cosyntropin (Cortrosyn) is used for the diagnosis of adrenocortical insufficiency, not for treatment. Once a diagnosis is made, the actual drug treatment generally involves replacement hormonal therapy using drug forms of the deficient corticosteroid hormones.

### Case Study
1. Vasopressin or desmopressin
2. Vasopressin should be given cautiously in patients with migraine headaches, seizures, cardiovascular disease, renal disease, and asthma.
3. Treatment will be injections, either intramuscular or subcutaneous, two to four times a day. This drug therapy will increase water resorption in the distal tubules and collecting ducts of the nephron, performing all the physiologic functions of antidiuretic hormone. As a result, water excretion is diminished.

4. Therapy should eliminate his severe thirst and decrease his urinary output.

# CHAPTER 31
## Thyroid and Antithyroid Drugs

### Critical Thinking Crossword
*Across*
3. Secondary
6. Thyroxine
7. Primary
*Down*
1. Levothyroxine
2. Hyperthyroidism
4. Propylthiouracil
5. Tertiary
6. Thyrotropin

### Chapter Review and NCLEX® Examination Preparation/Critical Thinking and Application
1. c
2. d
3. a
4. a, c, d
5. c
6. b
7. 0.088 mg
8. 1.5 mL
9. Mrs. W. probably has hypothyroidism, which may result in the formation of a goiter, an enlargement of the thyroid gland resulting from its overstimulation by elevated levels of thyroid-stimulating hormone. She may benefit from one of the thyroid drugs, including thyroid, levothyroxine, liothyronine, or liotrix. Levothyroxine is generally preferred because, as a chemically pure formulation of 100% thyroxine, its hormonal content is standardized; therefore, its effect is predictable.
10. Surgery to remove all or part of the thyroid gland is an effective way to treat hyperthyroidism, but as a result, lifelong hormone replacement is normally required.
11. There are two errors. (1) Levothyroxine is dosed in micrograms. A common medication error is to write the intended dose in milligrams instead of micrograms. If not caught, this error would result in a thousandfold overdose. Doses higher than 200 **mcg** must be questioned in case this error occurred. (2) The route is not written. This drug would be administered PO.
12. The most damaging or serious adverse effects of propylthiouracil (PTU) medications are liver and bone marrow toxicity. Therefore, it is important to assess liver function studies as well as a complete blood count (white blood cells, red blood cells, platelets).

In addition, PTU is rated as a pregnancy category D drug; a pregnancy test will be needed.

## Case Study

1. Her symptoms suggest hypothyroidism, and a thyroid replacement hormone, such as levothyroxine, would be indicated for this condition.
2. The thyroid preparations are given to replace what the thyroid gland cannot itself produce to achieve normal thyroid levels, known as a "euthyroid" condition.
3. Thyroid preparations need to be taken at the same time every day to maintain constant blood levels. Taking the medication in the morning will help reduce problems with insomnia, which may result when the medication is taken later in the day or in the evening.

# CHAPTER 32
# Antidiabetic Drugs

## Chapter Review and NCLEX® Examination Preparation/Critical Thinking and Application

1. b
2. d
3. a
4. c
5. a
6. a
7. d
8. b
9. 4 units ($238 - 150 = 88 \div 20 = 4.4$). (Answer is 4, because 20 divides into 88 four whole times. The "left-over" 8 does not add up to 20, so it does not count toward the insulin dose.)
10. 37 units

11. a. Pramlintide, an incretin mimetic, given by subcutaneous injection, works by mimicking the action of the natural pancreatic hormone amylin. Amylin is secreted along with insulin in response to food intake and influences postmeal glucose levels by slowing gastric emptying, suppressing glucagon secretion (which reduces the liver's glucose output), and increases the sense of satiety. As a result, blood glucose levels are reduced.
    b. Metformin works primarily by inhibiting hepatic glucose production and increasing the sensitivity of peripheral tissue to insulin, thus lowering blood glucose levels.
12. a. Confusion, irritability, tremor, and sweating

b. The brain needs a constant amount of glucose to function; thus the central nervous system manifestations of hypoglycemia (such as irritability and confusion) are often the first to appear.
    c. In the conscious person, oral forms of glucose are used, such as rapidly dissolving buccal tablets or semisolid gel forms designed for rapid mucosal absorption. She could also try corn syrup, honey, fruit juice, a nondiet soft drink, or a small snack such as crackers or half a sandwich.
13. a. The graduate nurse will check the order at least three times and then have another licensed nurse check the prepared injection to be sure it is in accordance with the prescriber's order. These second checks may vary with facilities.
    b. The graduate nurse's co-worker. Novolin-R is regular insulin, and regular insulin is clear.
    c. If left at room temperature, the insulin in the vial must be discarded after 1 month.
14. Mrs. F. needs to make some significant lifestyle changes. She must stop smoking, lose weight, and exercise regularly, which will help with both the high blood glucose level and the hypertension. The American Diabetes Association also recommends that, in addition to lifestyle changes, the oral biguanide drug metformin (Glucophage) be started as initial therapy for lowering blood glucose levels.
15. a. Disulfiram-type reaction
    b. In addition to assessing vital signs, assess his blood glucose level immediately.
    c. Dennis may have been drinking alcohol. Sulfonylureas may interact with alcohol in a way that is similar to the interaction with disulfiram, which is used to deter alcohol ingestion in people with chronic alcoholism. This *disulfiram-type* reaction includes vomiting and hypertension. In addition, the alcohol taken with the sulfonylurea may enhance the action of the antidiabetic drug, causing increased hypoglycemia.
16. If the patient receiving metformin is to undergo diagnostic studies with contrast dye, the prescriber will need to discontinue the drug on the day of the test and restart it 48 hours after the tests. It may be necessary to reevaluate the patient's renal status.
17. a. Hypoglycemia
    b. Hyperglycemia
    c. Hyperglycemia
    d. Hypoglycemia
    e. Hypoglycemia

## Case Study

1. Glipizide works best if given 30 minutes before meals. This allows the timing of the insulin secretion induced by the glipizide to correspond with the elevation in blood glucose level induced by the meal

in much the same way as endogenous insulin levels are raised in a person without diabetes. Its effect is much like the body's normal response to meals, and will help to keep the blood glucose levels from becoming too high.

2. To provide a picture of the patient's adherence to the therapy regimen for the previous several months, a hemoglobin A1C is measured. This value reflects how well the patient has been doing with diet and drug therapy.

3. Mr. D. should contact his provider immediately. He may require a change in his diabetic treatment while he is sick, because vomiting and inability to eat can cause a change in his blood glucose levels. If he is unable to eat and yet takes the glipizide, he is at risk for experiencing severe hypoglycemia.

## CHAPTER 33
## Adrenal Drugs

### Chapter Review and NCLEX® Examination Preparation/Critical Thinking and Application

1. a
2. c
3. a, b, c
4. b
5. d
6. c
7. b, c, e
8. 1/2 tablet
9. 3.2 mg per dose
10. Ms. R.'s glucocorticoid can interact with aspirin and other nonsteroidal antiinflammatory drugs (NSAIDs), producing additive effects and increasing the chance of gastric ulcer development. Also, she must avoid people with infections, because her own immune system is suppressed. The children in the hospital may have infections. In addition, she needs to report any fever, increased weakness and lethargy, or sore throat.
11. a. The use of systemic glucocorticoids with antidiabetic drugs may reduce the hypoglycemic effect of those drugs. Determine a baseline blood glucose level, and monitor Peter for any problems.
    b. Oral dosage forms must be taken with milk or food to minimize gastrointestinal upset. Another option is for the provider to order a histamine-2 receptor antagonist or proton pump inhibitors to prevent ulcer formation (glucocorticoids may cause gastric ulcers). Patients must be instructed not to take the drug with alcohol, aspirin, or other NSAIDs to minimize gastric irritation and the chance for gastric bleeding.

12. The nurse should intervene. The student nurse needs to wear clean (nonsterile) gloves when applying the medication with a sterile tongue depressor or cotton-tipped applicator if the skin is intact. If the skin is not intact, a sterile technique should be used.

13. In addition to routine teaching about metered-dose inhaler administration technique, the nurse will instruct Nina to rinse out her mouth with lukewarm water after each use of the inhaler to prevent the development of an oral fungal infection.

### Case Study

1. One very important point about corticosteroids is that they must not be stopped abruptly. These drugs require a tapering of the daily dose, because the administration of these drugs causes the endogenous (body's own) production of the hormones to stop. This is referred to as *HPA* or *adrenal suppression*. This suppression places the patient at risk of developing hypoadrenal crisis (shock, circulatory collapse) in times of increased stress (i.e., surgery, trauma). Tapering of daily doses allows the HPA axis the time to recover and to start stimulating the normal production of the endogenous hormones.

2. Short- or long-term therapy may cause steroid psychosis. In addition, long-term effects cause cushingoid symptoms, including moon face, weight gain, muscle wasting, and increased deposition of fat in the trunk area, leading to truncal obesity. (See Table 33-4.)

3. Oral contraceptives may increase the half-life of adrenal drugs. The prescriber will consider this when establishing the dose. She needs to be instructed not to use the nonsteroidal antiinflammatory drug ibuprofen while taking the prednisone because taking these drugs together may cause additive GI effects and an increased chance of gastric ulcer development.

4. The best time is early in the morning (6:00 AM to 9:00 AM) because this follows the normal diurnal pattern of endogenous corticosteroid secretion and results in the least amount of adrenal suppression.

## CHAPTER 34
## Women's Health Drugs

### Chapter Review and NCLEX® Examination Preparation/Critical Thinking and Application

1. b, c, e
2. a
3. a
4. b
5. b
6. c, e, f
7. a, d

8.  1.3 mL (1.25 rounds to 1.3)

9.  10 mL
10. a. The nurse will ask Isabelle if she is taking medication for her depression. Estrogen therapy is indicated for the symptoms of menopause, but the use of estrogen with a tricyclic antidepressant may result in toxicity of the latter drug.
    b. The smallest dose of estrogen that alleviates the symptoms is used for the shortest possible time.
11. a. The nurse practitioner will probably prescribe medroxyprogesterone, which is indicated for treatment of secondary amenorrhea.
    b. The progestin may cause a decrease in glucose tolerance when given with antidiabetic drugs. Ms. K. will need to carefully monitor her blood glucose levels.
12. a. Perhaps Jacklyn's prescription could be switched to a 28-day form of Ortho-Novum, which is taken for all 28 days of the menstrual cycle rather than for 3 weeks with 1 week off.
    b. One of the benefits of oral contraceptive use is decreased blood loss during menstruation.
13. These drugs work to promote fertility in two different ways. Clomiphene is given to cause ovarian follicle maturation. Choriogonadotropin alfa is then given to stimulate the rupture of the mature follicles and to develop the corpus luteum, which supports early pregnancy.
14. Mrs. I. needs to know that smoking can diminish the therapeutic effects of the estrogen she is taking and add to the risk of thrombosis. Also, she should be cautioned to wear sunscreen while in Aruba, because estrogen makes the skin more susceptible to sunburn.
15. Mrs. S. is assuming that the medication is estrogen therapy. Alendronate (Fosamax) is indicated to prevent osteoporosis in postmenopausal women. The nurse will need to explain to her that it is a nonestrogen, nonhormonal medication used for prevention of bone loss in the postmenopausal period.
16. Megestrol is used in the management of anorexia, cachexia, or unexplained substantial weight loss in patients with acquired immunodeficiency syndrome (AIDS). In addition, it may be used to stimulate appetite and promote weight gain in patients (male or female) with cancer.

**Case Study**

1.  It is essential to perform a pregnancy test to rule out pregnancy before J.Q. begins the oral contraceptive.
2.  Smoking would increase J.Q.'s risk for thromboembolic events if she begins oral contraceptives that contain estrogen. In addition, the smoking may reduce the estrogenic effects. In addition, assess for

a history of thromboembolic events such as myocardial infarction, venous thrombosis, pulmonary embolism, or stroke.

3.  Oral contraceptive hormones must be taken at the same time every day and exactly as prescribed. If one dose is missed, advise the patient to take the dose as soon as it is remembered; however, if it is close to the next dose time, advise the patient not to double up and to use a backup form of contraception in these situations. Provide more specific instructions regarding the omission of more than one pill and/or 1 day's dose depending on the specific oral contraceptive drug prescribed.

# CHAPTER 35
## Men's Health Drugs

### Chapter Review and NCLEX® Examination Preparation/Critical Thinking and Application

1.  b
2.  b, d, f
3.  a
4.  d
5.  c
6.  a
7.  d
8.  a, b, e
9.  a. The nurse should use the 200 mg/mL strength. Using the 100 mg/mL strength would require 3 mL, which may require two separate injections.
    b. The nurse will administer 1.5 mL of the 200 mg/mL strength.
10. a. Testosterone's poor performance in the oral dosage form is due to the fact that most of a dose is metabolized and destroyed by the liver before it can reach the circulation.
    b. Methyltestosterone (Android) and fluoxymesterone (Halotestin) are both testosterone derivatives that are effective when given orally, or buccally with the methyltestosterone.
    c. With either drug, contraindications that could apply to Mr. M. include significant cardiac, hepatic, or renal disease; male breast cancer; genital bleeding; or prostate cancer.
11. a. No. The manufacturer's guidelines suggest that the patient not swallow, chew, or eat the buccal tablet but that it be completely absorbed in the mouth. The part of the drug that is swallowed will not reach the intended site of action because of heavy first-pass metabolism.
    b. Patients taking any hormone-related drug should never abruptly stop the drug. The prescriber may consider whether a transdermal form is suitable for Mr. M.
12. With finasteride, education about the drug's therapeutic effects as well as adverse effects should be

provided at the patient's educational level. Female family members, significant others, and caregivers who are pregnant or of childbearing age should be educated about the need to avoid exposure during handling of this drug, including *not* touching any broken or crushed tablets, which could result in exposure to the drug and the risk of teratogenic effects. Wearing gloves is recommended. Finasteride may be given orally without regard to meals. It should be protected from exposure to light and heat.

13. The Testoderm patch is applied only to the scrotal skin. The skin should be clean, dry scrotal skin that has been shaved for optimal skin contact. These patches are replaced every day. Androderm patches should be applied to clean, dry skin on the back, abdomen, upper arms, or thighs; the scrotum and bony areas (shoulder, hip) should be avoided. These patches are often ordered to be changed every 7 days. AndroGel is applied to the shoulders, arms, or abdominal skin daily.

### Case Study

1. Sildenafil (Viagra) is contraindicated in patients with cardiovascular disorders and is contraindicated if the patient is taking nitrates because of the potential for severe hypotensive effects.

2. Headache, flushing, and dyspepsia are the most common adverse effects reported. Priapism, an abnormally prolonged penile erection, is a rare occurrence but if it occurs, it is a medical emergency and he needs to seek care immediately. In addition, he should report any visual changes immediately.

3. Older individuals experience declining liver function, so drugs may not be metabolized as effectively as when they were younger. A decreased dosage of sildenafil is generally indicated for patients over 65 years of age and for those with liver or renal impairment. In addition, there have been reports of vision loss in men who have been taking this class of drugs.

4. Sildenafil should be taken 1 hour before intercourse and no more than once a day.

## CHAPTER 36
## Antihistamines, Decongestants, Antitussives, and Expectorants

### Chapter Review and NCLEX® Examination Preparation/Critical Thinking and Application

1. a, b, c, e
2. a
3. b, e
4. c
5. b
6. d
7. b, d, e

8. a. 15 mL (See Overview of Dosage Calculations, Section II.)
   b.

9. 2.5 mL
10. No. Mrs. L. is likely experiencing rebound congestion caused by sustained use of the naphazoline for several days.
11. Keith is exhibiting symptoms of the cardiovascular effects that can occur when a topically applied adrenergic nasal decongestant is absorbed into the bloodstream. Usually the amount absorbed is too small to cause systemic effects at normal dosages. Excessive dosages of these medications, however, are more likely to cause systemic effects elsewhere in the body. These may include cardiovascular effects such as hypertension and palpitations and CNS effects such as headache, nervousness, and dizziness. These systemic effects are the result of alpha-adrenergic stimulation of the heart, blood vessels, and CNS.
12. Benzonatate's mechanism of action is entirely different from that of the other drugs. It suppresses the cough reflex by numbing the stretch receptors, which keeps the cough reflex from being stimulated in the medulla. It is associated with fewer drug interactions than the opioid antitussives and dextromethorphan.
13. The nurse will ask Irene whether she is taking any thyroid medication or whether she has cardiac disease, glaucoma, or hypertension. A drug interaction can occur if she takes dextromethorphan (an antitussive) with an antithyroid drug. The other conditions listed are contraindications. Irene should call her health care provider before she goes to the drugstore.
14. First, Lisa's brother received Robitussin A-C, an opioid antitussive containing codeine, for his cough. Lisa has been prescribed Robitussin, an expectorant, for her nonproductive cough associated with bronchitis. Second, even if the two children were prescribed the same drug, Lisa is only 5 years old and requires a smaller dosage than her brother. Prescription medications should not be shared among family members.
15. Antihistamines should generally be used with caution in lactating mothers. The decision will be made by weighing the drug's potential effect on the baby versus the need for her to take the medication.

### Case Study

1. James's diabetes should not affect his treatment.

2. The topical diphenhydramine might come in combination with a drug such as calamine, camphor, or zinc oxide.

3. He should be informed that taking any of the sedating antihistamines may cause drowsiness, and so he should be instructed to avoid driving or operating heavy machinery should these side effects occur or until he knows how he responds to the medication.

4. James should also be informed not to consume alcohol or take other central nervous system depressants because they may interact with the diphenhydramine to exacerbate drowsiness and sedation.

# CHAPTER 37
## Respiratory Drugs

### Chapter Review and NCLEX® Examination Preparation/Critical Thinking and Application
1. b, d, e, f
2. d
3. b
4. a
5. c
6. a
7. a, b
8. After 25 days (8 puffs per day, divided into 200 doses)
9. 3.6 mg
10. Tom is exhibiting some side effects of theophylline therapy, and the level in his blood is too high (the common therapeutic range for theophylline is a blood level of 10 to 20 mcg/dL). It is likely that the dosage will be decreased.
11. Sylvia is exhibiting dose-related adverse effects of the albuterol. If Sylvia is now using the albuterol more frequently as a rescue inhaler, the health care provider will need to review and adjust her medication regimen.
12. a. Anticholinergics, corticosteroids, and beta agonists
    b. Of concern is Mrs. V.'s glaucoma. Anticholinergics are to be used cautiously in patients with acute narrow-angle glaucoma.
13. a. The disadvantage of administering the corticosteroids orally is that they can then lead to systemic effects, such as increased susceptibility to infection, fluid and electrolyte disturbances, endocrine effects, dermatologic effects, and nervous system effects. They can also interact with other systemically administered drugs. The advantage of administering corticosteroids by inhalation is that they are delivered directly to the site of action—the lungs. This generally limits, but does not completely prevent, systemic effects.
    b. The use of an inhaled corticosteroid frequently allows for a reduction in the daily dose of the

systemic corticosteroid. This reduction should be gradual to prevent Addisonian crisis due to suppression of the adrenal gland.

14. The albuterol is a beta agonist that can be used to treat acute bronchospasms. The fluticasone is a corticosteroid and is not effective for acute bronchospasm. Fluticasone is useful for long-term management of asthma and works to reduce inflammation.

15. He needs to be reminded to avoid foods and beverages that contain caffeine (e.g., chocolate, coffee, cola, cocoa, tea), because their consumption can exacerbate CNS stimulation.

### Case Study
1. Montelukast, a leukotriene receptor antagonist, works to reduce the inflammatory response in the lungs but does not have the adverse effects that corticosteroids have.
2. Leukotriene receptor antagonists are primarily used for prophylaxis and chronic management of asthma and are not appropriate for treatment of acute asthma attacks; however, they should decrease the frequency of the attacks.
3. You should tell Jennie that she needs to check with her health care provider before taking any over-the-counter medications.
4. These drugs should be taken every night on a continuous schedule, even if symptoms improve.

# CHAPTER 38
## Antibiotics Part 1

### Critical Thinking Crossword
*Across*
3. Prophylactic
6. Tetracycline
7. Penicillin
8. Bactericidal
9. Cephalosporin
*Down*
1. Macrolide
2. Sulfonamide
4. Bacteriostatic
5. Superinfection

### Chapter Review and NCLEX® Examination Preparation/Critical Thinking and Application
1. b, d, e
2. a
3. b
4. c
5. d
6. d
7. b, c, d
8. 25 mL per dose. Each dose will contain 500,000 units (every 6 hours will be 4 doses per day; divide 2 million units per day by 4 to get 500,000 units per

dose). (See Overview of Dosage Calculations, Section III.)

9. 10 mL

10. Imipenem/cilastatin (Primaxin) does contain two drugs, but one of the drugs (cilastatin) works to prevent the antibiotic (imipenem) from being destroyed by bacterial enzymes that can make the antibiotic ineffective.

11. Cefoxitin (Mefoxin) is frequently used in patients undergoing abdominal surgeries because it can effectively kill intestinal bacteria, including anaerobic bacteria.

12. a. Sean must not take the doxycycline with milk because that can result in a significant reduction in the absorption of the drug. Also, Sean needs to be aware that tetracyclines can cause photosensitivity; he needs to avoid direct exposure to sunlight and use sunscreen and/or protective clothing.

    b. The diarrhea is probably the result of alteration of the intestinal flora caused by the drug therapy.

13. She is experiencing a superinfection because the antibiotics she has been taking for her bronchitis have reduced the normal vaginal bacterial flora, and the yeast that is usually kept in balance by this normal flora has an opportunity to grow and cause an infection.

## Case Study

1. He needs to be assessed for renal problems and blood dyscrasias. Also, the use of co-trimoxazole is contraindicated in cases of known drug allergy to sulfonamides or chemically related drugs such as sulfonylureas (used for diabetes), thiazide and loop diuretics, and carbonic anhydrase inhibitors.

2. If he is taking a sulfonylurea for his type 2 diabetes, close monitoring is needed, because sulfonamides can potentiate the hypoglycemic effects of sulfonylureas in patients with diabetes. In addition, although he is currently receiving intravenous heparin and not warfarin, he may be switched to oral anticoagulants soon, so keep in mind that sulfonamides can potentiate the anticoagulant effects of warfarin and lead to hemorrhage.

3. These antibiotics achieve very high concentrations in the kidneys, through which they are eliminated. Therefore, they are primarily used in the treatment of urinary tract infections.

4. Sulfonamides do not actually destroy bacteria but inhibit their growth. For this reason, they are considered bacteriostatic antibiotics. Bactericidal antibiotics kill bacteria.

# CHAPTER 39
## Antibiotics Part 2

### Chapter Review and NCLEX® Examination Preparation/Critical Thinking and Application

1. c

2. b

3. a

4. a, b, c

5. a, b, e

6. b, c, d

7. 40 mL (See Overview of Dosage Calculations, Section II.)

8. 187.5 mg

9. The current practice is once-a-day aminoglycoside dosing. The nurse can tell her that studies have shown that once-daily dosing provides a sufficient plasma drug concentration to kill bacteria and also has either an equal or lower risk of toxicity compared with multiple daily dosing. Hopefully this type of dosing will be safer and more effective for her.

10. A blood sample for measurement of "trough" level is drawn at least 8-12 hours after completion of dose administration. The therapeutic goal is a trough level at or below 1 mcg/mL. If the trough level is above 2 mcg/mL, then the patient is at greater risk for ototoxicity and nephrotoxicity. Trough levels are normally monitored initially then once every 5 to 7 days until the drug therapy is discontinued. The patient's serum creatinine level will also be measured at least every 3 days as an index of renal function, and drug dosages will be adjusted as needed for any changes in renal function.

11. Yes. In patients who receive amiodarone therapy, dangerous cardiac dysrhythmias are more likely to occur when quinolones are taken. Hopefully another drug besides levofloxacin has shown effectiveness against the bacteria that is causing his infection.

12. Nitrofurantoin is used primarily to treat urinary tract infections because it is renally excreted and concentrates in the urine.

## Case Study

1. Ototoxicity and nephrotoxicity. Symptoms of ototoxicity include dizziness, tinnitus, and hearing loss. Symptoms of nephrotoxicity include urinary casts, proteinuria, and increased blood urea nitrogen and serum creatinine levels. Monitoring the drug's trough levels as well as renal function studies can help prevent those toxicities.

2. The aminoglycosides and penicillins are often used together because they have a synergistic effect; that is, the combined effect of the two drugs is greater than that of either drug alone.

3. Yes, there is a concern! The desired trough level is 1 mcg/mL, so a level of 3 mcg/mL could mean that he is receiving a dose that is too high. The increased serum creatinine level is also a concern because it could be an indication of impaired renal function. The physician must be notified immediately and doses of the aminoglycoside withheld until the physician responds.

# CHAPTER 40
## Antiviral Drugs

### Chapter Review and NCLEX® Examination Preparation/Critical Thinking and Application

1. d
2. d
3. a
4. c
5. a, b
6. b
7. 5 mL
8. 22 mg
9. Yes. Zidovudine, one of the few anti–human immunodeficiency virus (HIV) drugs known to prolong patient survival, can be used for maternal and fetal treatment. During the pregnancy, Amy can receive the oral form of the drug. During labor she can receive the drug intravenously. Drug therapy for the infant can begin within 12 hours of delivery and continue for 6 weeks.
10. a. Acyclovir (Zovirax) is indicated for herpes zoster (shingles).
    b. Bailey will be treated with acyclovir again; it is the drug of choice for treatment of both initial and recurrent episodes of shingles.
11. a. Ribavirin is used to treat infections caused by respiratory syncytial virus.
    b. Yes. Brenda's treatment will last at least 3 days but not longer than 7 days.
12. The patient may be experiencing zidovudine's major dose-limiting adverse effect, which is bone marrow suppression.
13. No. The nurse's co-worker is doing fine. Acyclovir administered by intravenous infusion is first diluted in the solution recommended by the manufacturer and is administered slowly over at least 1 hour to prevent renal damage.
14. No. Therapy with oseltamivir (Tamiflu) needs to begin within 2 days of the onset of influenza. It is probably too late for this medication to be effective for Stacy.
15. Ganciclovir may be administered to *prevent* cytomegalovirus (CMV) disease (generalized infection) in high-risk patients, such as those receiving organ transplants.

### Case Study

1. Mr. C. needs to use a glove when applying topical acyclovir (Zovirax) to the affected area, which should be kept clean and dry. Also, he should not use any other creams or ointments on the area.
2. Mr. C.'s herpes infection cannot be "cured," although the acyclovir will help to manage the symptoms.
3. Stress the importance of treatment for Mr. C. and his sexual partner, and discuss with him how to prevent transmission of the virus.

4. There are several viruses in the *Herpesviridae* family, including herpes simplex type 1 (HSV-1), which causes mucocutaneous herpes—usually blisters around the mouth; varicella-zoster virus (herpes simplex type 3, or HSV-3), which causes both chickenpox and shingles; herpesvirus type 4 (also called Epstein-Barr virus or EBV); and herpesvirus type 8, which is believed by some to cause Kaposi's sarcoma, a cancer associated with acquired immunodeficiency syndrome (AIDS).

# CHAPTER 41
## Antitubercular Drugs

### Chapter Review and NCLEX® Examination Preparation/Critical Thinking and Application

1. a
2. b
3. a, b, c
4. c
5. a
6. a, d, e
7. 3 tablets (See Overview of Dosage Calculations, Sections I and II.)
8. 1800 mg; yes, maximum dose is 2 grams (2000 mg)
9. a. Liver function studies should be performed because isoniazid can cause hepatic impairment. In addition, an eye examination is important because the drug may cause visual disturbances.
    b. Diane may be a slow acetylator. Acetylation, the process by which isoniazid is metabolized in the liver, requires certain enzymes to break down the isoniazid. In slow acetylators, who have a genetic deficiency of these enzymes, the isoniazid accumulates. The dosage of isoniazid may need to be adjusted downward in these patients.
10. a. Streptomycin is administered intramuscularly, deep into a large muscle mass, and the sites are rotated.
    b. Although it may not be a concern in terms of Ms. I.'s streptomycin therapy, oral contraceptives become ineffective when given with rifampin. If rifampin is part of her therapy, Ms. I. should switch to another form of birth control.
11. A thorough eye examination may be called for before therapy is initiated, because ethambutol can cause a decrease in visual acuity resulting from optic neuritis, which is also a contraindication to the use of ethambutol. In addition, isoniazid may cause optic neuritis and visual disturbances.
12. a. Mr. F. needs to know that his compliance with therapy is essential for achieving a cure. Although he is keeping his follow-up appointments, Mr. F. also needs to take his medication as ordered. He should be warned not to consume alcohol,

because the antitubercular drugs may cause liver toxicity, and he should be encouraged to take care of himself by ensuring adequate nutrition, rest, and relaxation.

b. The therapeutic response can be confirmed by results of laboratory studies (sputum culture and sensitivity tests) and chest radiographic findings.

13. a. Frannie, like all patients taking antitubercular drugs, needs to be compliant with the therapy regimen and keep her follow-up appointments. She should be reminded that she can spread the disease (during the initial period of the illness); she should wash her hands frequently and cover her mouth when coughing or sneezing. Frannie also needs adequate nutrition and rest.

b. It is likely that Frannie is on rifampin therapy. She should be told that her urine, stool, saliva, sputum, sweat, and tears may become red-orange-brown in color and that this is an effect of rifampin therapy.

## Case Study

1. George's gout is a consideration; pyrazinamide can cause hyperuricemia, so gout or flare-ups of gout can occur in susceptible patients. His diabetes is a concern too; ethambutol should be used cautiously in patients with diabetes. A baseline hearing test should be performed if streptomycin is considered, because this drug may cause ototoxicity. In addition, liver function studies are needed because his heavy alcohol use may have caused liver damage.

2. An individual with a genetic deficiency of the liver enzymes that metabolize drugs can be classified as a "slow acetylator." When isoniazid is taken by slow acetylators, the drug accumulates because there are not enough of the enzymes to break down the isoniazid. As a result, the dosage of isoniazid may need to be reduced.

3. Results of liver function studies should be assessed carefully before therapy is initiated, because some drugs (isoniazid, pyrazinamide) are hepatotoxic. Liver function test results should be monitored closely during therapy as well.

4. Isoniazid can cause a pyridoxine (vitamin $B_6$) deficiency. Patients should take pyridoxine as prescribed by the physician to prevent some of the neurologic effects of vitamin $B_6$ deficiency such as numbness and tingling of the extremities (peripheral neuritis).

## CHAPTER 42
## Antifungal Drugs

### Chapter Review and NCLEX® Examination Preparation/Critical Thinking and Application

1. j
2. e
3. f
4. g
5. a
6. c
7. h
8. i
9. d
10. b
11. c
12. a, b, c, e
13. d
14. b
15. a
16. a, e
17. 50 mL/hour (See Overview of Dosage Calculations, Section V.)
18. 660 mg; 440 mg
19. a. Fluconazole (Diflucan), unlike itraconazole and other azoles, can pass into the cerebrospinal fluid, which makes it useful in the treatment of cryptococcal meningitis.

b. Unfortunately, Mr. K. will need to remain on the medication (at a reduced dosage) for 10 to 12 weeks after the negative results on his cerebrospinal fluid culture.

20. a. The amphotericin B needs to be diluted according to the manufacturer's guidelines and administered using an infusion pump. The nurse must not use solutions that are cloudy or that have visible precipitates. Prior to administration, the nurse will check for an order to premedicate the patient with an antiemetic, antihistamine, antipyretic, and/or corticosteroid to prevent or minimize infusion-related reactions.

b. The nurse will monitor closely for expected adverse effects such as cardiac dysrhythmias, visual disturbances, paresthesias (numbness or tingling of the hands or feet), respiratory difficulty, pain, fever, chills, and nausea.

c. No, unless a severe reaction occurs (e.g., exacerbation of adverse effects or a decline in vital signs). To decrease the severity of expected adverse effects, the patient may be pretreated with an antipyretic (e.g., acetaminophen), antihistamines, and antiemetics.

21. Nystatin oral troches or lozenges are to be dissolved slowly and completely in the mouth for the best effects and should not be chewed or swallowed. Chrissie needs a review of how to use this medication.

22. Lipid formulations of amphotericin B have been developed in an attempt to decrease the incidence of its adverse effects and increase its efficacy. The disadvantage is that they are more expensive than conventional amphotericin B.

**Case Study**

1. Voriconazole is used to treat major fungal infections in patients who do not tolerate or respond to other antifungal drugs. The physician probably tried other drugs first.
2. Use of voriconazole is contraindicated in patients taking other drugs that are metabolized by cytochrome P-450 enzyme 3A4 (e.g., quinidine) because of the risk of inducing serious cardiac dysrhythmias.
3. Careful cardiac monitoring is needed if Sally is also taking quinidine while taking this antifungal drug.

# CHAPTER 43
## Antimalarial, Antiprotozoal, and Anthelmintic Drugs

**Chapter Review and NCLEX® Examination Preparation/Critical Thinking and Application**

1. a
2. b, c, d, e
3. c
4. b, e
5. d
6. a, c
7. The dose is 280 mg (4 mg/kg × 70 kg); the nurse will draw up 4.7 mL of the diluted solution for the infusion. (See Overview of Dosage Calculations, Section III.)
8. 5 tablets
9. Malaria is caused by Plasmodium organisms. During the asexual stage of the Plasmodium life cycle, which occurs in the human host, the parasite resides for a while outside the erythrocyte; this is called the *exoerythrocytic phase*. The most effective drug for eradicating the parasite during this phase is primaquine.
10. Before primaquine is administered, Professor H. will be given a pregnancy test. This is a pregnancy category C drug, so the nurse will need to know if certain precautions are needed in Professor H.'s case. She will also be assessed for hypersensitivity, and any disease states that cause granulocytopenia (rheumatoid arthritis, systemic lupus erythematosus). In addition, primaquine must be used with caution in patients with methemoglobinemia, porphyria, methemoglobin reductase deficiency, and glucose-6-phosphate dehydrogenase (G6PD) deficiency.
11. Mefloquine is indicated for the treatment of chloroquine-resistant malaria. Quinine, an older drug, may also be used. Quinine can be used alone but is more commonly given in combination with pyrimethamine, a sulfonamide, or a tetracycline (such as doxycycline).
12. Each of these three patients has a protozoal infection. The patient with the intestinal disorder has giardiasis. The patient with acquired immunodeficiency syndrome (AIDS) has pneumocystosis. The patient with the sexually transmitted infection has trichomoniasis. See Table 43-3 for specific drugs used to treat these diseases.

**Case Study**

1. Intestinal roundworms are diagnosed based on symptoms and examination of stool specimens.
2. Contraindications include allergy to the medication and pregnancy. Even though she is only 15 years of age, she will be assessed for possible pregnancy before this medication is given. In addition, her liver function test results will be assessed, because use of pyrantel is contraindicated in patients with liver disease.
3. Based on her weight of 57 kg, the dose for her would be 627 mg (11 mg × 57 kg).
4. Adverse effects of pyrantel therapy include headache, dizziness, insomnia, and skin rashes, as well as anorexia, cramps, diarrhea, nausea, and vomiting.

# CHAPTER 44
## Antiinflammatory and Antigout Drugs

**Chapter Review and NCLEX® Examination Preparation/Critical Thinking and Application**

1. b
2. b
3. a, b, d, e
4. c
5. a, c, d
6. c
7. No. The child weighs 15 kg, and the appropriate dose for that weight is 50 mg PO twice daily, not 100 mg.
8. 1.3 mL

9. Chronic salicylate intoxication, which occurs as a result of either high dosages or prolonged therapy with high dosages of aspirin.
10. Mr. C. has an acute overdose of a nonsalicylate nonsteroidal antiinflammatory drug (NSAID). If the condition progresses, symptoms can include intense headache, dizziness, cerebral edema, cardiac arrest, and even death in extreme cases.

11. Mr. H. needs to know that compliance with the entire medical regimen is important for the success of his treatment for gout. Allopurinol needs to be taken with meals to help prevent the occurrence of gastrointestinal symptoms such as nausea, vomiting, and anorexia. Increase fluids to 3 liters per day, and hazardous activities must be avoided if dizziness or drowsiness occurs with the medication. Also, alcohol and caffeine need to be avoided, because these drugs will increase uric acid levels and decrease the levels of allopurinol.

12. a. Ketorolac (Toradol) is indicated for the short-term management (up to 5 days) of moderate to severe acute pain that requires analgesia at the opioid level. It is not indicated for treatment of minor or chronic painful conditions.

    b. The main adverse effects of ketorolac (Toradol) include renal impairment, gastrointestinal pain, dyspepsia, and nausea. These problems limit the length of time that the medication can be used.

13. The vinegary odor means that the aspirin has experienced some chemical breakdown, and she should not use it! She needs to discard it safely and purchase a new bottle.

14. Febuxostat is indicated for the treatment of acute gout but may pose a risk of cardiovascular events. Randy's history of hypertension and coronary artery disease may be of concern.

## Case Study

1. The specific COX-2 selectivity of these drugs allows them to control the inflammation and pain without producing some of the toxicity associated with NSAID therapy.

2. The most common adverse effects include fatigue, dizziness, lower extremity edema, hypertension, dyspepsia, nausea, heartburn, and epigastric discomfort. Any stomach pain, unusual bleeding, or blood in vomit or stool must be reported to the physician immediately. Chest pain, palpitations, and any gastrointestinal problems need to be reported as well.

3. Celecoxib is not used in patients with known sulfa allergy.

4. She needs to avoid alcohol and aspirin while taking this medication and told to check with her provider before taking any over-the-counter medications.

# CHAPTER 45
## Antineoplastic Drugs Part 1: Cancer Overview and Cell Cycle–Specific Drugs

### Critical Thinking Crossword
*Across*
3. Spread
4. Folic

7. Extravasation
8. Nadir
9. Limiting
10. Leukemia
*Down*
1. Malignant
2. Leucovorin
5. Nonspecific
6. Benign
7. Emetic

## Chapter Review and NCLEX® Examination Preparation
1. a, b, c, e, f
2. d
3. a
4. b
5. c
6. d
7. a, e
8. 25,000 units; yes
9. a. 8.2 mg
   b. 8.2 mL

## Case Study

1. Methotrexate is an antimetabolite—specifically, a folate antagonist. It inhibits the action of an enzyme that is responsible for converting folic acid to a substance used by the cell to synthesize DNA for cell reproduction. As a result, the cell dies.

2. Laboratory test results should be checked for white blood cell and red blood cell counts, hemoglobin level and hematocrit, platelet counts, and renal and liver function studies.

3. The concurrent administration of nonsteroidal antiinflammatory drugs (NSAIDs) and methotrexate may lead to possible reduced renal elimination of methotrexate with potentially fatal hematologic and GI toxicity. Allen should be instructed to avoid all NSAIDs, including aspirin, while taking methotrexate.

4. Antiemetic therapy will be needed to decrease nausea and vomiting. Leucovorin may be used to protect the patient from potentially fatal bone marrow suppression, a toxic effect of methotrexate.

# CHAPTER 46
## Antineoplastic Drugs Part 2: Cell Cycle–Nonspecific and Miscellaneous Drugs

### Chapter Review and NCLEX® Examination Preparation/Critical Thinking and Application
1. c
2. a
3. b

4. a, c, e, f
5. b
6. d
7. b, c, e
8. 125 mL/hr
9. 46 mL/hr (rounded up from 45.5) (See Overview of Dosage Calculations, Section V.)
10. Cytoprotective drugs help to reduce the toxicity of various antineoplastics. As a result, the adverse effects may be reduced so increased dosages of the antineoplastic medication may be tolerated, which allows greater cancer cell kill. Examples include:
    - Amifostine (Ethyol), used during therapy with cisplatin to reduce renal toxicity
    - Dexrazoxane (Zinecard), used during therapy with doxorubicin to reduce cardiac toxicity
11. The nurse will not agree. The nurse recognizes that the most likely cause of the patient's respiratory problems is the development of pulmonary toxicity (pulmonary fibrosis and pneumonitis) secondary to therapy with bleomycin.
12. No! In most facilities, institutional guidelines direct that the pharmacy department mix these drugs. Special requirements must be met for the safety of those working with these drugs, including the use of a laminar airflow hood and appropriate personal protection equipment (such as gown, mask, and gloves). It would not be safe for the nurse or for those around the nurse to mix the chemotherapy drug on the nursing unit.
13. The nurse will stop the infusion immediately but won't pull out the intravenous catheter quite yet. The physician must be notified immediately, and the nurse will expect to receive orders to treat this extravasation of mechlorethamine by injecting a solution of 10% sodium thiosulfate and sterile water (see Table 46-2) through the existing line into the extravasated site (then remove the line) as well as multiple subcutaneous injections into the site. Over the next few hours, the patient will receive repeated subcutaneous injections into the area, and cold compresses will be applied to the site.

**Case Study**

1. Nephrotoxicity (possible damage to the kidneys), peripheral neuropathy (possible damage to peripheral nerves), and ototoxicity (possible damage to hearing and vestibular function).
2. Baseline renal studies need to be performed, because this drug is highly nephrotoxic. If Dottie is receiving any other drugs that are potentially nephrotoxic (such as aminoglycoside therapy), dosage changes will need to be considered. If she has gout, concurrent use of cisplatin may result in hyperuricemia or worsening of the gout. Baseline auditory studies are needed, as well as baseline liver function studies and

measurement of white blood cell count, hemoglobin level, hematocrit, and platelet level, because of the anticipated bone marrow suppression.
3. Because peripheral neuropathies may occur, numbness, tingling, or pain in the extremities must be reported to the physician immediately to prevent complications and enhance comfort.
4. Yes, this is a concern, because dehydration while taking cisplatin may lead to renal damage. Patients who are at home after treatment with this drug need to be reminded of the importance of hydration and need to be told to contact the physician if they experience dry mucous membranes, very dark amber urine, or little or no urinary output, or vomiting of large amounts over a period of 8 hours or less. It may be a challenge, but she needs to try to take in 3000 mL of fluid per day to prevent dehydration.

# CHAPTER 47
## Biologic Response–Modifying and Antirheumatic Drugs

**Chapter Review and NCLEX® Examination Preparation/Critical Thinking and Application**

1. e
2. a
3. g
4. b
5. h
6. d
7. c
8. a, b, c, d, e
9. c
10. a, b, d, e
11. a. 2.5 mg
    b. 0.5 mL

12. 1.3 mL (See Overview of Dosage Calculations, Section III.)
13. The major dose-limiting side effect of interferons is fatigue. Patients taking high dosages become so exhausted that they are often confined to bed. Sonja needs to know this before she starts the therapy.
14. Colony-stimulating factors (CSFs) such as filgrastim (Neupogen), pegfilgrastim (Neulasta), and sargramostim (Leukine) can be given for chemotherapy-induced leukopenia. These drugs should be administered 24 hours after the chemotherapy drugs have been given, because the myelosuppressive effects of the chemotherapy drugs tend to cancel out the therapeutic benefits of the CSFs.
15. She will receive oprelvekin (Neumega), which is given via subcutaneous injections daily for up to 21 days. Because she has severe thrombocytopenia,

however, the nurse must be careful to prevent excessive bleeding and bruising at the injection sites and to teach Brittany measures to reduce bleeding risks.

16. Methotrexate is given *weekly*, not daily! The nurse needs to clarify and correct this mistranscribed order. It is very important to note that the drug is given once per week, not once per day. Serious medication errors, including deaths, have occurred when the drug is given daily instead of once a week.

**Case Study**

1. Oprelvekin has a dual classification as both an interleukin (interleukin-11 [IL-11]) and hematopoietic drug.
2. A complete blood count will be monitored, specifically to note the platelet counts, to monitor the therapeutic effects of the oprelvekin, and to watch for decreasing levels of hemoglobin/hematocrit, which may indicate that blood loss is occurring.
3. Treatment may be ordered to begin within 6 to 24 hours after completion of antineoplastic therapy. She will receive daily subcutaneous dosing for up to 21 days. The injection sites will be rotated in areas including the thigh, abdomen, hip, and upper arm.
4. Donna will need teaching about ways to reduce risk of bleeding, such as using a soft toothbrush, not flossing her teeth, and not using a razor if she shaves her underarms or legs. In addition, she needs to be aware that any cuts or wounds, including injection sites, may bleed longer. Direct pressure should be applied to control bleeding. The site will require close monitoring until bleeding has stopped. She needs to report any abnormal bleeding from her gums, nose, or in her stool or urine to her physician immediately.

# CHAPTER 48
## Immunosuppressant Drugs

**Chapter Review and NCLEX® Examination Preparation/Critical Thinking and Application**

1. b
2. c
3. c
4. a
5. a, c, d, e
6. a, e
7. a, c, f
8. 4 capsules
9. a. 750 mg for this dose
   b. 15 mL (See Overview of Dosage Calculations, Section II.)
10. a. Daclizumab can help prevent organ rejection. If Mrs. F.'s immune system cannot recognize the new kidney as foreign, it will not mount an immune response against it. This promotes success of the transplant.

b. The antifungal drug is added several days before surgery as prophylaxis for oral candidiasis.
11. Encourage the patient to take the drug with meals or mixed with chocolate milk, milk, or orange juice to prevent stomach upset.
12. Styrofoam containers or cups should be avoided, because the drug has been found to adhere to the inside wall of such containers. The nurse needs to find a glass or cup that is not made of Styrofoam. Once the drug is mixed, the patient needs to drink it immediately.
13. Tess is experiencing symptoms consistent with adverse effects of muromonab-CD3. The nurse will need to monitor her closely for signs of fluid retention and pulmonary edema as well as for an allergy-like reaction known as *cytokine release syndrome*, which can be severe. Patients are often premedicated with corticosteroids (e.g., intravenous methylprednisolone) in an effort to avoid or alleviate this problem.
14. Fingliod (Gilenya) and glatiramer acetate (Copaxone) are immunosuppressants that are indicated for reduction of the frequency of relapses (exacerbations) in a type of multiple sclerosis known as *relapsing-remitting multiple sclerosis.*

**Case Study**

1. Yes, immunosuppressant therapy will be lifelong.
2. White patches on the tongue, mucous membranes, and oral pharynx would be indicative of candidiasis.
3. Mr. K. needs to be seen by a physician immediately. These symptoms could indicate that he has a severe infection.
4. Patients taking immunosuppressant drugs need to avoid live vaccines because of the immunosuppressant therapy. There may be a risk of an infection developing due to the administration of a live vaccine to a person with lowered immunity.

# CHAPTER 49
## Immunizing Drugs and Biochemical Terrorism

**Chapter Review and NCLEX® Examination Preparation/Critical Thinking and Application**

1. a. Zoster vaccine (Zostavax)
   b. Active
   c. Active
   d. *Haemophilus influenzae* type b prophylaxis
   e. Hepatitis B virus vaccine (inactivated)
   f. $Rh_o$(D) immunoglobulin (RhoGAM)
   g. Passive
   h. Active
   i. Tuberculosis prophylaxis
   j. Active

    k. Diphtheria, tetanus, and pertussis prophylaxis, pediatric

    l. Passive

    m. Postexposure passive tetanus prophylaxis

    n. Active

    o. Diphtheria and tetanus prophylaxis (pediatric [over age 7] and adult)

2. b
3. d
4. a
5. a
6. c
7. a, c
8. 0.005 mg (See Overview of Dosage Calculations, Section I.)
9.

10. She will most likely receive the DTaP (diphtheria, tetanus, and acellular pertussis vaccine [Adacel]). With the recent increase in cases of pertussis, the DTaP is recommended for adults in place of the Td, which lacks the pertussis component.

11. Sometimes, after vaccination, the levels of antibodies against a particular pathogen decline over time and a second dose of the vaccine is given to restore the antibody titers to a level that can protect the person against the infection. This second dose is referred to as a *booster shot.*

12. Each year a new influenza vaccine is developed that contains three influenza virus strains that represent the strains most likely to circulate in the United States in the upcoming winter. The vaccination from the previous year may not be effective for the influenza virus strains occurring in the current year.

13. Carl may experience localized swelling, redness, discomfort, and warmth at the injection site. Acetaminophen and rest are recommended for the relief of these side effects, and application of warm compresses to the injection site may also help ease some of the discomfort.

14. There are three types of anthrax based on the routes of inoculation: cutaneous, inhalational, and gastrointestinal. Of the three, anthrax contracted by inhalation of the bacterial spores is the most deadly and has a mortality rate of more than 80%.

15. Paul is experiencing more than the expected adverse effects of his vaccinations. He is probably experiencing "serum sickness," which may occur after repeated injections of equine-derived immunizing drugs. Because his symptoms may indicate respiratory impairment, he needs to be taken to the hospital for evaluation and monitoring; he needs to call 911 rather than try to drive himself to the hospital. He may receive analgesics, antihistamines, epinephrine, and/or corticosteroids to treat this reaction.

**Case Study**

1. Rabies is a very potent virus.

2. Those at high risk for rabies exposure, such as veterinarians, will receive the rabies virus vaccine (Imovax, RabAvert) as preexposure prophylaxis, followed by booster shots every 2 to 5 years based on blood titers. This is a type of active immunization.

3. You will receive drugs that give both active and passive immunization. Postexposure prophylaxis consists of injections of the rabies virus vaccine (see the answer to Question 2) and also rabies immune globulin (Imogam Rabies-HT). Because rabies can progress so rapidly, the body does not have time to mount an adequate immune defense—death occurs before it can do so. The passive immunization confers a temporary protection that is usually sufficient to keep the invading organism from causing death, even though it does not stimulate an antibody response. The active immunization you receive will stimulate an antibody response.

# CHAPTER 50
## Acid-Controlling Drugs

**Chapter Review and NCLEX® Examination Preparation/Critical Thinking and Application**

1. h
2. e
3. i
4. k
5. c
6. a, b
7. f
8. d
9. b
10. g
11. b
12. c
13. d
14. b, d, e
15. b
16. 2 mL
17. 200 mL/hr (See Overview of Dosage Calculations, Section V.)
18. You need to let him know that long-term self-medication with antacids may mask symptoms of serious underlying diseases. He needs to be evaluated for possible bleeding ulcer or even a malignancy, but you may not want to scare him with those possibilities! If his current self-treatment is no longer working, he needs a medical evaluation. Advise him not to take the baking soda but to instead see his provider.
19. Omeprazole must be taken 30 to 60 minutes before meals, and the capsule must be taken whole, not

crushed, opened, or chewed. Omeprazole may also be given with antacids, if ordered.

20. Patients with heart failure or hypertension need to use antacids that are low in sodium. Suggest an aluminum-based antacid. Instruct patients to take the antacid alone, not at the same time as other medications (unless specifically instructed to do so), because the antacid will interfere with the absorption of the other medications. Antacids should be taken 1 hour before or 1 to 2 hours after other medications. If symptoms continue or worsen, consult the health care provider.

21. Antacids may promote premature dissolving of the enteric coating; if the coating is destroyed early in the stomach, gastrointestinal upset may occur. He needs to take the aspirin tablets with food, not with antacids.

22. Stress ulcer prophylaxis (or therapy to prevent severe GI damage) is undertaken in almost every critically ill patient in an intensive care unit (ICU) and for many patients on general medical surgical units.

## Case Study

1. Although histamine-2 ($H_2$) antagonists are available over the counter, the dose of the over-the-counter preparation will not be the same strength as the usual dose of the prescription formulation.

2. The drug effects of the $H_2$ blockers are limited to specific blocking actions on the parietal cells of the gastric glands in the stomach. As a result, hydrogen ion production is decreased, which leads to an increase in the pH of the stomach (i.e., decreased stomach acid).

3. Use of $H_2$ receptor antagonists is contraindicated in patients with known drug allergy or impaired renal function or liver disease. Cautious use is recommended in patients who are confused, disoriented, or older. Interactions may occur with drugs that have a narrow therapeutic range. Caution must be used if she is taking theophylline for her asthma. Patients requiring these medications must avoid aspirin and other nonsteroidal antiinflammatory drugs, alcohol, and caffeine because of their ulcerogenic or gastrointestinal tract–irritating effects.

4. Smoking has been shown to decrease the effectiveness of $H_2$ blockers because the absorption of $H_2$ antagonists is impaired in individuals who smoke. Hopefully if she herself is not smoking, this will not be a problem for her, but spending several hours in a smoke-filled room may have an effect. Also, the beer and possibly spicy pizza may aggravate the underlying condition.

# CHAPTER 51
## Bowel Disorder Drugs

### Critical Thinking Crossword
*Across*
6. Emollient
7. Probiotic
8. Saline
9. Bulk-forming
*Down*
1. Adsorbent
2. Opiates
3. Hyperosmotic
4. Stimulant
5. Anticholinergic

### Chapter Review and NCLEX® Examination Preparation/Critical Thinking and Application
1. d
2. a
3. d
4. c
5. a, d
6. d
7. a. 1.5 mg per dose (6 mg per day)
   b. 3 mL per dose
8. 7.5 mL (See Overview of Dosage Calculations, Section II.)
9. Darkening of the tongue or stool is a temporary and harmless side effect associated with the use of bismuth subsalicylate (Pepto-Bismol).
10. Use of the belladonna alkaloid preparations, such as Donnatal, are contraindicated in patients with narrow-angle glaucoma. She should not use this drug.
11. Several factors may be causing Hillary's constipation: lack of proper exercise, poor diet (which might involve inadequate roughage and an excess of dairy products), use of aluminum-containing antacids, and stress.
12. a. The bulk-forming laxatives tend to produce normal stools, have few systemic effects, and are among the safest available.
    b. Ira needs to mix the medication with at least 6 to 8 oz of fluid and drink it immediately. He should never take it dry.
13. a. Because glycerin is very mild, it is often used in children.
    b. Abdominal bloating and rectal irritation

### Case Study
1. Antibiotic therapy destroys the balance of normal flora in the intestines, and diarrhea-causing bacteria proliferate.

2. *Lactobacillus acidophilus,* a probiotic, is indicated for diarrhea caused by antibiotic treatment that has destroyed the normal intestinal flora.

3. Supplying *Lactobacillus acidophilus* bacteria helps restore the balance of normal flora and suppress the growth of diarrhea-causing bacteria.

4. It is considered a dietary supplement. It is often used to treat uncomplicated diarrhea, although this is an off-label use (not approved by the Food and Drug Administration).

# CHAPTER 52
## Antiemetic and Antinausea Drugs

### Chapter Review and NCLEX® Examination Preparation/Critical Thinking and Application

1. a, b, d, e
2. c, e
3. d
4. c
5. b
6. d
7. c
8. 2 mL

9. 30 mL (See Overview of Dosage Calculations, Section II.)

10. a. Petra should take the metoclopramide 30 minutes before meals and at bedtime.
    b. Combining metoclopramide with alcohol can result in additive CNS depression. Petra needs to be instructed not to take the medication with alcohol.

11. This drug comes in oral, intramuscular, intravenous, and rectal forms, but because she was on "nothing-by-mouth" status and has no intravenous access, the intramuscular route was ordered. The nurse can call Nellie's health care provider to obtain an order for an alternate route but cannot change the route without an order, because the dosage may also be different.

12. Dronabinol is a synthetic derivative of the major active substance in marijuana. The nurse explains to him that it is used to stimulate appetite and weight gain in patients with acquired immunodeficiency syndrome (AIDS).

### Case Study

1. The only listed contraindication is drug allergy.
2. Antiemetics are often administered before a chemotherapy drug is given, frequently 1/2 to 3 hours before treatment.
3. The headache is caused by the ondansetron and can be relieved with acetaminophen.

# CHAPTER 53
## Vitamins and Minerals

### Chapter Review and NCLEX® Examination Preparation/Critical Thinking and Application

1. c
2. g
3. b
4. h
5. e
6. k
7. i
8. d
9. j
10. a
11. l
12. f
13. a, d, e
14. b
15. d
16. d
17. 100 mL/hour
18. 1 mL (See Overview of Dosage Calculations, Section III.)
19. Broad-spectrum antibiotics can inhibit the intestinal flora, which provide the body with vitamin $K_2$. As a result, a deficiency may occur. Vitamin K can be given either orally or by injection in adults.
20. Dietary sources of vitamin D include fish oils, salmon, sardines, and herring; fortified milk, bread, and cereals; and animal livers, tuna, eggs, and butter. In addition, vitamin D is synthesized in the skin through exposure to ultraviolet radiation (sunshine).
21. a. Pernicious anemia
    b. The absorption of cyanocobalamin (vitamin $B_{12}$, or extrinsic factor) requires the presence of intrinsic factor, which is a glycoprotein secreted by gastric parietal cells. Once the binding takes place, the complex is absorbed in the small intestine. Because an ileal resection removes a portion of the small intestine, malabsorption of cyanocobalamin can occur.
    c. Cyanocobalamin injections are used to treat pernicious anemia caused by a lack of intrinsic factor.
22. To avoid venous irritation, give intravenous calcium via an intravenous infusion pump and with proper dilution. Giving intravenous calcium too rapidly may precipitate severe hypercalcemia with subsequent cardiac irregularities, delirium, and coma. Administer intravenous calcium slowly, as ordered, and within the manufacturer guidelines (e.g., usually less than 1 mL/min). Patients need to remain recumbent for 15 minutes after the infusion to prevent further problems. Should extravasation of the intravenous calcium solution occur, discontinue the infusion

immediately but leave the intravenous catheter in place for antidote administration. The prescriber may then order an injection of 1% procaine and/or other antidotes or fluids to reduce vasospasm at the site and dilute the irritating effects of calcium on surrounding tissue. However, follow all facility policies and procedural guidelines and/or manufacturer insert information as deemed appropriate.

### Case Study

1. Normal serum magnesium levels are 1.7 to 2.2 mg/dL.
2. During intravenous magnesium infusion, monitor the patient's ECG and vital signs, and rate patellar or knee-jerk reflexes. Impaired reflexes are used as an indication of drug-related CNS depressant effects. CNS depression may quickly lead to respiratory and/or cardiac depression; thus perform frequent monitoring. Document the infusion and infusion site, and record each set of vital sign measurements and ratings of reflexes appropriately. Other signs that require immediate attention are confusion, irregular heart rhythm, cramping, unusual fatigue, lightheadedness, and dizziness.
3. Contact the prescriber immediately, stop the infusion, and monitor the patient.
4. Calcium gluconate must be readily accessible for use as an antidote to magnesium toxicity.

## CHAPTER 54
## Anemia Drugs

### Chapter Review and NCLEX® Examination Preparation/Critical Thinking and Application
1. d
2. b, c, f
3. c
4. b, c
5. b, c, d, e
6. c
7. a
8. 0.75 mL

9. 26 mg (rounded up from 25.9) (See Overview of Dosage Calculations, Section III.)
10. Anyone who is about to receive a first dose of iron dextran is at risk for fatal anaphylaxis. Because of this, a test dose of 25 mg of iron dextran should be administered by the chosen route and appropriate method. An anaphylactic reaction may occur within a few moments, although waiting at least 1 hour before giving the rest of the initial dose is recommended. Intramuscular iron is to be administered

deep in a large muscle mass using a Z-track method and a 23-gauge, 1 1/2-inch needle.
11. The orange juice contains ascorbic acid (vitamin C), which enhances the absorption of iron.
12. The risk of anaphylaxis for both drugs is much less than with iron dextran, and a test dose is not required.
13. Hemoglobin level and hematocrit are to be monitored carefully. If therapy is not halted when the target hemoglobin level of 12 g/dL is reached or if the hemoglobin level and hematocrit rise too quickly, hypertension and seizures can result.

### Case Study

1. Oral forms should be taken with juice, preferably orange juice, or water (but not antacids or milk) between meals for maximal absorption. Should gastrointestinal distress occur, however, the iron can be taken with meals.
2. Remind her that use of any iron product will cause the stools to turn black.
3. You should tell her that one iron product cannot be substituted for another because each product contains different forms of the iron salt in different amounts.
4. Liquid oral forms of iron are to be diluted per the manufacturer's instructions and taken through a plastic straw to avoid discoloration of tooth enamel.

## CHAPTER 55
## Nutritional Supplements

### Critical Thinking Crossword
*Across*
1. Erythromycin
4. Anabolism
5. Gastrostomy
8. Absorptive
10. Fatty acid
11. Essential
12. Nitrogen
*Down*
2. Catabolism
3. Enteral
6. Semiessential
7. Metabolism
8. Arginine
9. Phlebitis

### Chapter Review and NCLEX® Examination Preparation/Critical Thinking and Application
1. a
2. c
3. a, c, d, e
4. c

5. a
6. d
7. 900 mL
8. 1680 mL over 24 hours
9. a. Patients who suffer from this condition experience cramping, diarrhea, abdominal bloating, and flatulence with the ingestion of lactose. In this case, lactose-free solutions need to be used.
   b. The residual should not be more than 2 hours' worth of feeding—in this case, no more than 100 mL. You need to return the aspirate, put the feeding on hold, elevate the head of the bed, and notify the provider.
10. Mr. R. is showing signs of fluid overload. The nurse should first reduce the infusion rate, remain with the patient and continue to assess his vital signs, and have another nurse notify the physician immediately.

**Case Study**

1. If peripheral (or total) parenteral nutrition is discontinued abruptly, rebound hypoglycemia may occur because the pancreas has not had time to adjust to the reduced blood glucose levels. Hypoglycemia is manifested by cold, clammy skin; dizziness; tachycardia; and tingling of the extremities.
2. To prevent hypoglycemia, hang a solution of 5% to 10% glucose to infuse until bag No. 4 is ready. (Some institutions may use up to 12.5% solutions of glucose.) You also need to call to make sure the pharmacy is preparing the infusion bag.
3. During this infusion, her blood glucose levels need to be monitored on a regular basis. You will assess for signs of both hyperglycemia and hypoglycemia, signs of infection, and signs of fluid overload.

# CHAPTER 56
## Dermatologic Drugs

**Chapter Review and NCLEX® Examination Preparation/Critical Thinking and Application**

1. a
2. b
3. a
4. b
5. a, b, d
6. d
7. a
8. a, b, d, e
9. 100 mL/hour
10. 167 mL/hour (See Overview of Dosage Calculations, Section V.)
11. The nurse will first ask Mr. M. about any allergies to other forms of drugs. If he has an allergy to a particular antibacterial drug, that drug should not be used topically either. If culture and sensitivity testing

is to be carried out, the nurse must be sure to collect the specimen before the first application of the antibacterial drug.
12. Gloves are used not only to prevent contamination from the patient's secretions but also to prevent absorption of the medication through the skin of the person applying the medication.
13. Mr. L. and his children are being treated for head lice. Tell him the following:
"Leave the shampoo on for 4 minutes, then rinse and dry the hair. Then use a nit comb to remove nits (eggs) from the hair shafts." Other measures he needs to take include decontaminating the clothing and personal articles of the infested people. All clothing, linens, stuffed toys, and so on must be washed in hot, soapy water or dry-cleaned.
14. Assess the patient for allergy to iodine. Cadexomer iodine (Iodosorb) is used to chemically débride the wound by absorbing exudates. It is not harmful to viable cells, but it does stain tissue.
15. It is possible that the patient is not a candidate for surgery at this time or is taking anticoagulants, which could cause the area to bleed excessively if surgical débridement is performed. The prescribed medication selectively removes necrotic tissue without harming normal tissue and can be used on infected wounds.

**Case Study**

1. Assess Judy's allergies, especially any allergies to sulfonamide drugs. This cream is to be applied only to areas that have been cleansed and débrided. The wound bed may need to be débrided before the cream can be applied.
2. The dressing helps keep the medication at the intended site and provides protection to the wound. In addition, it keeps the cream from soiling the clothing.
3. Yes! You need to wear gloves to prevent contamination of the medication and avoid exposure to Judy's wound secretions. The cream needs to be applied with a sterile, gloved hand.
4. The adverse effects of silver sulfadiazine are similar to those of other topical drugs and include pain, burning, and itching.

# CHAPTER 57
## Ophthalmic Drugs

**Chapter Review and NCLEX® Examination Preparation/Critical Thinking and Application**

1. c
2. h
3. j
4. k

5. a
6. d
7. b
8. f
9. g
10. e
11. c
12. b
13. b
14. d
15. b, c, d, e
16. c
17. 2 tablets
18. 19 gtt/min (See Overview of Dosage Calculations, Section V.)
19. The effect is less pronounced in individuals with dark eyes (brown or hazel), because pigment absorbs the drugs, thus reducing therapeutic effects; dark eyes have more pigment than light eyes (blue).
20. a. Dipivefrin (Propine), a prodrug of epinephrine, has better lipophilicity than epinephrine and can penetrate into the anterior chamber of the eye. It is 4 to 11 times more potent than epinephrine in reducing intraocular pressure. In addition, it is less likely to have systemic adverse effects.
    b. Burning, eye pain, and lacrimation may occur at first, but these usually subside over time.
    c. No. Systemic effects are rare; they include cardiovascular effects and possibly headaches and faintness.
21. Ned may have had an allergic reaction to a preservative, such as benzalkonium chloride, in the first drug that was tried. Timolol is available in a preservative-free product.
22. a. Purulent drainage or exudate would inhibit the product's effectiveness.
    b. The solution must have been cloudy; in that case, it needs to be discarded—only clear solutions should be administered.
23. The nonsteroidal antiinflammatory drugs are considered less toxic, and they are preferred over the corticosteroids as initial topical therapy for inflammation.
24. Stinging is normal after instillation of the drops. It is important to inform Ms. L. that she should not wear her contact lenses while taking this medication. The lenses may lead to further irritation.
25. The eyedrops need to be administered first, and then the pilocarpine gel at least 5 minutes after the drops are administered.

## Case Study

1. The ointment should be applied to the conjunctival sac, not directly onto the cornea or eyeball, moving from the inner canthus to the outer edge of the eye. Excess medication can be removed with a tissue, but he should not rub his eyes. See Chapter 9 for specific instructions.
2. Ointments may cause a temporary blurriness to the vision because of the film that bathes over the eye. This film will decrease once absorbed, and vision should become clearer. He will need to be careful and prevent falling if his vision is blurry. In addition, he should not touch the tip of the medication container to his eye or to his fingers in order to prevent contamination of the medication.
3. Burning and stinging are common but transient effects of ophthalmic antimicrobial drugs, and they should subside shortly.
4. He should *not* take this medication! It is most likely contaminated, and is not ordered for his current problem. In addition, if the drops were a corticosteroid, there could be immunosuppressive effects, which may interfere with the antimicrobial's action.

# CHAPTER 58
# Otic Drugs

## Chapter Review and NCLEX® Examination Preparation/Critical Thinking and Application

1. a, b, d, e
2. d
3. b
4. a
5. c
6. a. 375 mg
   b. Low range (20 mg/kg): 220 mg; high range (40 mg/kg): 440 mg
   c. Yes, 375 mg is in the range of 220 and 440 mg. (See Overview of Dosage Calculations, Section III.)
   d.

7. The patient needs medical care immediately. His symptoms may be indicative of head trauma.
8. To take advantage of the steroidal antiinflammatory, antipruritic, and antiallergic drug effects.
9. a. Clean the ear, remove all cerumen by irrigation, and ensure that the dropper is clean. The drops also need to be at room temperature.
   b. He might become dizzy, so he needs to be supine when the drops are instilled.
10. a. The hydrocortisone will help reduce the inflammation and itching associated with the infection.
    b. A drug hypersensitivity or a perforated eardrum

11. Many ear disorders involve pain and inflammation; the anesthetic effect of the local anesthetic drugs makes them beneficial in treating these conditions by reducing the discomfort associated with ear disorders.

12. a. The instructions are different for each boy. Hold the pinna up and back during instillation of eardrops in children older than 3 years of age, like Drew. For children 3 years of age or younger, like Ben, gently pull the pinna down and back.
    b. Reduced pain, redness, and swelling are therapeutic effects of the medication.

13. a. Esther's husband should warm the eardrops to body temperature by holding the bottle under warm running water, not by soaking it in hot water—especially because he needs to be careful not to let water get into the bottle or damage the label.
    b. Esther must not sit up right away. She needs to lie down on the side opposite the side of the affected ear for about 5 minutes after the drug is instilled. As an alternative, she can gently insert a small cotton ball into the ear canal to keep the drug in place, but the cotton ball should not be forced into the ear canal.

14. It is essential that the mother knows the correct route for the medication! Systemic antibiotics, such as liquid amoxicillin, are often used to treat otitis media. The nurse will explain to the child's mother that this drug is to be swallowed (oral) and demonstrate how to measure the correct dose after gently shaking the suspension. The nurse will emphasize that this drug is NOT to go into the child's ears. Lastly, the nurse will discuss what to expect regarding symptom improvement, and when to return to the clinic if symptoms do not improve.

### Case Study

1. Mark probably has an impaction of earwax in his ear canal. Such a buildup can cause pain and temporary deafness.

2. Teach Mark not to insert anything into his ear canal. He will need to know how to clean his ears properly and how to use cerumen removal drugs. You may need to irrigate his ear canals before medication therapy is started.

3. This medication is given as otic (ear) drops. He will need to follow the manufacturer's recommendations for administration. He needs to lie on the side opposite of the affected ear for about 5 minutes after instillation of the drug. A small cotton ball may be inserted gently into the ear canal to keep the drug there, but it must not be forced or jammed down into the ear canal. When administering the drops, he needs to pull the pinna of his ear up and back.

4. The carbamide peroxide will slowly release hydrogen peroxide and oxygen, and this effervescent effect will mechanically act to loosen the cerumen. In addition, the glycerin will soften the cerumen, making it easier to remove.

## OVERVIEW OF DOSAGE CALCULATIONS
### Introduction

**Interpreting Medication Labels**

1. Generic name:      rifampin
   Trade name:        Rifadin
   Unit dose:         300-mg capsules
   Total in container: 30 capsules
   Route:             oral (It is assumed that capsules and tablets are oral route.)

2. Generic name:      amoxicillin
   Trade name:        Amoxil
   Unit dose:         125 mg per 5 mL
   Total in container: 100 mL (when reconstituted)
   Route:             oral

3. Generic name:      medroxyprogesterone acetate suspension
   Trade name:        Depo-Provera
   Unit dose:         400 mg per mL
   Total in container: 10 mL
   Route:             intramuscular use only

4. Generic name:      hydrocortisone sodium succinate
   Trade name:        Solu-Cortef
   Unit dose:         250 mg
   Total in container: 250 mg per 2 mL (when mixed)
   Route:             intravenous or intramuscular

## Section I

**Basic Conversions Using Ratio and Proportion**

1. 600,000 mcg
2. 1,500,000 mcg
3. 5 mg
4. 5000 mg
5. 2500 mg
6. 0.9 g *(Don't forget the leading zero.)*
7. 8000 g
8. 0.75 L *(Don't forget the leading zero.)*
9. 975,000 mL
10. 0.5 L *(Don't forget the leading zero.)*
11. 960 mg
12. 1.5 gr
13. 20 mL

14. 12 tsp
15. 6 tbsp
16. 90 mL
17. 0.2 oz *(Don't forget the leading zero.)*
18. 198 lb
19. 68.2 kg *(rounded to tenths)*
20. 24.2 lb

## Section II

### Calculating Oral Doses

1. 1 tablet
   0.5 g = 500 mg; each tablet is 500 mg; therefore 1 tablet is needed
2. 2 tablets
   0.5 mg = 500 mcg;
   250 mcg : 1 tablet :: 500 mcg : $x$ tablet
   Proof: $250 \times 2 = 500$; $1 \times 500 = 500$
3. 0.5 tablet
   0.15 g = 150 mg;
   300 mg : 1 tablet :: 150 mg : $x$ tablet
   Proof: $300 \times 0.5 = 150$; $1 \times 150 = 150$
4. 20 mL
   12.5 mg : 5 mL :: 50 mg : $x$ mL
   Proof: $12.5 \times 20 = 250$; $5 \times 50 = 250$
5. 2 tablets
   600 mg = gr x; gr v : 1 tablet :: gr x : $x$ tablet
   Proof: gr v $\times$ 2 = gr x; $1 \times$ gr x = gr x
   NOTE: With this problem, since most are more familiar with metric doses, you may convert the dose on hand, gr v, to 300 mg. Then set up your problem:
   300 mg : 1 tab :: 600 mg : $x$
6. 4 mL
   0.1 g = 100 mg; 125 mg : 5 mL :: 100 mg : $x$ mL
   Proof: $125 \times 4 = 500$; $5 \times 100 = 500$
7. 3 capsules
   0.3 g = 300 mg;
   100 mg : 1 tablet :: 300 mg : $x$
   Proof: $100 \times 3 = 300$; $1 \times 300 = 300$
8. 22.5 mL
   20 mEq : 15 mL :: 30 mEq : $x$
   Proof: $20 \times 22.5 = 450$; $15 \times 30 = 450$
9. 3 capsules
   0.15 g = 150 mg;
   50 mg : 1 capsule :: 150 mg : $x$
   Proof: $50 \times 3 = 150$; $1 \times 150 = 150$
10. 4 tablets
    2 g = 2000 mg;
    500 mg : 1 tablet :: 2000 mg : $x$
    Proof: $500 \times 4 = 2000$; $1 \times 2000 = 2000$

## Section III

### Reconstituting Medications

1. 2 mL
   100 mg : 1 mL :: 200 mg : $x$
   Proof: $100 \times 2 = 200$; $1 \times 200 = 200$
2. 1.5 mL
   40 mg : 1 mL :: 60 mg : $x$
   Proof: $40 \times 1.5 = 60$; $1 \times 60 = 60$
3. 0.8 mL
   10,000 units : 1 mL :: 8000 units : $x$
   Proof: $10,000 \times 0.8 = 8000$; $1 \times 8000 = 8000$
4. 1.5 mL
   500 mg : 1 mL :: 750 mg : $x$
   Proof: $500 \times 1.5 = 750$; $1 \times 750 = 750$
5. 20 mL
   125 mg : 5 mL :: 500 mg : $x$
   Proof: $125 \times 20 = 2500$; $5 \times 500 = 2500$
6. Choose the concentration using 4.6-mL diluent. Using the 9.6-mL diluent would necessitate giving 3 mL intramuscularly versus 1.5 mL using the 4.6-mL diluent.
   1.5 mL
   200,000 units : 1 mL :: 300,000 units : $x$ mL
   Proof: $200,000 \times 1.5 = 300,000$; $1 \times 300,000 = 300,000$
7. 0.75 mL
   First: Convert mcg to mg : 750 mcg = 0.75 mg
   1:1000 indicates 1 g in 1000 mL, or 1000 mg in 1000 mL, or 1 mg/mL.
   1 mg : 1 mL :: 0.75 mg : $x$
   Proof: $1 \times 0.75 = 0.75$; $1 \times 0.75 = 0.75$
8. 1 mL
   NOTE: 1:5000 indicates 1 g in 5000 mL, or 1000 mg in 5000 mL, or 0.2 mg/mL.
   0.2 mg : 1 mL :: 0.2 mg : $x$
   Proof: $0.2 \times 1 = 0.2$; $1 \times 0.2 = 0.2$
9. 9 mL
   NOTE: 10% indicates 10 g per 100 mL, or 0.1 g/mL. Need to ensure units that are alike: 900 mg = 0.9 g
   0.1 g : 1 mL :: 0.9 g : $x$
   Proof: $0.1 \times 9 = 0.9$; $1 \times 0.9 = 0.9$
10. 8 mL
    NOTE: 50% indicates 50 g per 100 mL, or 0.5 g/mL.
    0.5 g = 1 mL :: 4 g : $x$
    Proof: $0.5 \times 8 = 4$; $1 \times 4 = 4$

## Section IV

### Pediatric Calculations

1. a. 0.46 to 47.3 mg/hr
   40 lb = 18.2 kg
   Low dose: 0.025 mg/kg/hr $\times$ 18.2 kg = 0.455, rounded to 0.46 mg/hr
   High dose: 2.6 mg/kg/hr $\times$ 18.2 kg = 47.32, rounded to 47.3 mg/hr

b. Yes, the ordered dose of 1 mg/hr falls within the safe range for this child.

2. a. 75 to 150 mg/dose
   33 lb = 15 kg
   Low dose: 5 mg/kg/dose × 15 kg = 75 mg/dose
   High dose: 10 mg/kg/dose × 15 kg = 150 mg/dose
   b. 600 mg (40 mg × 15 kg = 600 mg/kg/24 hr)
   c. Yes, the ordered dose of 120 mg falls within the safe and therapeutic range for this child.

3. a. 3180 to 4770 mg/24 hr
   70 lb = 31.8 kg
   Low dose: 100 mg/kg/24 hr × 31.8 kg = 3180 mg/24 hr
   High dose: 150 mg/kg/24 hr × 31.8 kg = 4770 mg/24 hr
   b. 1060 to 1590 mg/dose
   Three doses in 24 hours; 3180 ÷ 3 = 1060 mg/dose; 4770 ÷ 3 = 1590 mg/dose
   c. No. 1.7 g = 1700 mg, which exceeds the safe dosage range for this drug for this child. (Did you remember to convert g to mg?)

4. a. 0.14 to 0.34 mg/day
   15 lb = 6.8 kg
   Low dose: 0.02 mg/kg/day × 6.8 kg = 0.136 rounded to 0.14 mg/day
   High dose: 0.05 mg/kg/day × 6.8 kg = 0.34 mg/day
   b. 0.07 to 0.17 mg/dose
   "bid" doses are given twice in 24 hours. 0.14 ÷ 2 = 0.07 mg/dose; 0.36 ÷ 2 = 0.17 mg/dose
   c. Yes, 150 mcg = 0.15 mg, which falls within the safe and therapeutic dosage range for this child. (Did you remember to convert mcg to mg?)

5. a. 15.5 to 34.1 mg/kg/dose
   34 lb = 15.5 kg
   Low dose: 1 mg/kg/dose × 15.5 kg = 15.5 mg/dose
   High dose: 2.2 mg/kg/dose × 15.5 kg = 34.1 mg/dose
   b. Yes, the ordered dose of 30 mg is within the safe and therapeutic dose range for this child.

6. a. 90.8 to 113.5 mcg/kg/day
   50 lb = 22.7 kg
   Low dose: 4 mcg/kg/day × 22.7 kg = 90.8 mcg/day
   High dose: 5 mcg/kg/day × 22.7 kg = 113.5 mcg/day
   b. No. The ordered dose, 0.2 mg = 200 mcg, which exceeds the safe and therapeutic dosage range for this child. (Did you remember to convert mcg to mg?)

## Section V

### Basic Intravenous Calculations

1. Start at STEP 1. You need to calculate the hourly rate.
   a. 167 mL/hr
   1000 mL :: 6 hr :: $x$ : 1 hr
   $(1000 × 1) = (6 × x)$; $1000 = 6x$;
   $x = 1000/6 = 166.66$ (Round to nearest whole number.)
   Proof: $1000 × 1 = 1000$; $6 × 167 = 1002$ (slight difference due to previous rounding)
   (Alternate method: 1000 mL ÷ 6 hr = 166.67 or 167 mL/hr)
   b. 42 gtt/min (Round to nearest whole number.)
   STEP 2:
   $\frac{\text{drop factor}}{\text{time (min)}}$ × hourly rate = 15/60 × 167 = 1/4 × 200 = 41.75 (rounded to nearest whole number)

2. Start at STEP 1. You need to calculate the hourly rate.
   a. 200 mL/hr
   600 mL : 3 hr :: $x$ : 1 hr
   $(600 × 1) = (3 × x)$; $600 = 3x$;
   $x = 600/3 = 200$
   Proof: $600 × 1 = 600$; $3 × 200 = 600$
   (Alternate method: 600 mL ÷ 3 hr = 200 mL/hr)
   b. 33 gtt/min (Round to nearest whole number.)
   STEP 2:
   $\frac{\text{drop factor}}{\text{time (min)}}$ × hourly rate = 10/60 × 200 = 1/6 × 200 = 33.33 (rounded to nearest whole number)

3. Start at STEP 1. You need to calculate the hourly rate.
   a. 83 mL/hr
   1000 mL : 12 hr :: $x$ : 1 hr
   $(1000 × 1) = (12 × x)$; $1000 = 12x$; $x = 1000/12 = 83.33$ (Round to nearest whole number.)
   Proof: $1000 × 1 = 1000$; $12 × 83 = 996$ (slight difference due to previous rounding)
   (Alternate method: 1000 mL ÷ 12 hr = 83.33 or 83 mL/hr)
   b. 21 gtt/min (Round to nearest whole number.)
   STEP 2:
   $\frac{\text{drop factor}}{\text{time (min)}}$ × hourly rate = 15/60 × 83 = 1/4 × 83 = 20.75 (rounded to nearest whole number)

4. Start at STEP 1. You need to calculate the hourly rate.
   a. 100 mL/hr
   200 mL : 2 hr :: $x$ : 1 hr
   $(200 × 1) = (2 × x)$; $200 = 2x$; $x = 200/2 = 100$
   Proof: $200 × 1 = 200$; $2 × 100 = 200$
   (Alternate method: 200 mL ÷ 2 hr = 100 mL/hr)

b. 100 gtt/min
STEP 2:
$$\frac{\text{drop factor}}{\text{time (min)}} \times \text{hourly rate} = 60/60 \times 100 = 1 \times 100 = 100$$

c. The drop factor for microdrip tubing is 60 gtt/mL.

5. Start at STEP 2. The hourly rate has been provided (75 mL/hr).
13 gtt/min (Round to nearest whole number.)
STEP 2:
$$\frac{\text{drop factor}}{\text{time (min)}} \times \text{hourly rate} = 10/60 \times 75 = 1/4 \times 75 = 12.75 \text{ (rounded to nearest whole number)}$$

6. Start at STEP 2. The hourly rate has been provided (75 mL/hr).
19 gtt/min (Round to nearest whole number.)
STEP 2:
$$\frac{\text{drop factor}}{\text{time (min)}} \times \text{hourly rate} = 15/60 \times 75 = 1/4 \times 75 = 18.75 \text{ (rounded to nearest whole number)}$$

7. Start at STEP 2. The hourly rate has been provided (75 mL/hr).
25 gtt/min
STEP 2:
$$\frac{\text{drop factor}}{\text{time (min)}} \times \text{hourly rate} = 20/60 \times 75 = 1/3 \times 75 = 25 \text{ (rounded to nearest whole number)}$$

8. As the drop factor increases, the gtt/min also increases.

9. a. 100 mL/hr
b. and c. Since the infusion pump delivers in mL/hr, it is unnecessary to calculate gtt/min.
Start at STEP 1. You need to calculate the hourly rate. Remember, 30 min = 0.5 hr.
50 mL : 0.5 hr :: $x$ mL : 1 hr
$(50 \times 1) = (0.5 \times x)$; $50 = 0.5x$;
$x = 50/0.5 = 100$
Proof: $50 \times 1 = 50$; $0.5 \times 100 = 50$
(Alternate method: 50 mL ÷ 0.5 hr = 100 mL/hr)

10. Start at STEP 1. You need to calculate the hourly rate.
a. 125 mL/hr
500 mL : 4 hr :: $x$ : 1 hr
$(500 \times 1) = (4 \times x)$; $500 = 4x$;
$x = 500/4 = 125$
Proof: $500 \times 1 = 500$; $4 \times 125 = 500$
(Alternate method: 500 mL ÷ 4 hr = 125 mL/hr)
b. 125 gtt/min
STEP 2:
$$\frac{\text{drop factor}}{\text{time (min)}} \times \text{hourly rate} = 60/60 \times 125 = 1 \times 125 = 125 \text{ (rounded to nearest whole number)}$$

## Practice Quiz

1. 0.75 mg
1000 mcg : 1 mg :: 750 mcg : $x$ mg
Proof: $1000 \times 0.75 = 750$; $1 \times 750 = 750$
2. 8000 mg
1 g : 1000 mg :: 8 g : $x$ mg
Proof: $1 \times 8000 = 8000$; $1000 \times 8 = 8000$
3. 113.6 kg
1 kg : 2.2 lb :: $x$ kg : 250 lb
Proof: $1 \times 250 = 250$; $2.2 \times 113.6 = 249.92$ (rounds to 250)
4. 165 lb
1 kg : 2.2 lb :: 75 kg : $x$ lb
Proof: $1 \times 165 = 165$; $2.2 \times 75 = 165$
5. 15 mL
1 tsp : 5 mL :: 3 tsp : $x$ mL
Proof: $1 \times 15 = 15$; $5 \times 3 = 15$
6. 600 mg
gr i (1) : 60 mg :: gr x (10) : $x$ mg
Proof: 1 (gr i) $\times 600 = 600$; $60 \times 10$ (gr x) $= 600$
7. 10 mL
25 mg : 5 mL :: 50 mg : $x$ mL
Proof: $25 \times 10 = 250$; $5 \times 50 = 250$
8. 1 tablet
STEP 1: Convert g to mg : 0.5 g = 500 mg
500 mg : 1 tablet :: 500 mg : $x$ tablet
Proof: $500 \times 1 = 500$; $1 \times 500 = 500$
9. 2 mL
50 mg : 1 mL :: 100 mg : $x$ mL
Proof: $50 \times 2 = 100$; $1 \times 100 = 100$
10. 5 mL
1% indicates 1 g in 100 mL, which equals 1000 mg/100 mL, or 10 mg/1 mL.
10 mg : 1 mL :: 50 mg : $x$ mL
Proof: $10 \times 5 = 50$; $1 \times 50 = 50$
11. 0.25 mL
1:1000 indicates 1 g in 1000 mL, which equals 1000 mg/1000 mL, or 1 mg/mL.
1 mg : 1 mL :: 0.25 mg : $x$ mL
Proof: $1 \times 0.25 = 0.25$; $1 \times 0.25 = 0.25$
12. 1.5 mL
10,000 units: 1 mL :: 15,000 units: $x$ mL
Proof: $10,000 \times 1.5 = 15,000$; $1 \times 15,000 = 15,000$
13. a. 10 to 60 mg/day; 5 to 30 mg/dose (divided every 12 hours)
b. No, the dose of 50 mg exceeds the safe and therapeutic dosage range for this child.
22 lb = 10 kg
Low range: 1mg/kg/day × 10 kg = 10 mg/day (divided every 12 hours)
High range: 6 mg/kg/day × 10 kg = 60 mg/day (divided every 12 hours)
14. a. 63 mL/hr
500 mL ÷ 8 hr = 62.5 (rounded to 63 mL/hr)

b. 16 gtt/min

$$\frac{\text{drop factor}}{\text{time (min)}} \times \text{ hourly rate} = 15/60 \times 63 =$$
$$1/4 \times 63 = 15.75 \text{ (rounded to nearest whole number)}$$

15. a. Infusion pumps deliver mL/hr.
    b. 50 mL/hr (as stated in the question)

16. a. 42 mL/hr
    1000 mL ÷ 24 hr = 41.67 (rounded to 42 mL/hr)
    b. 42 gtt/min (Remember that if the drop factor is 60, the rate is the same as the gtt/min.)

$$\frac{\text{drop factor}}{\text{time (min)}} \times \text{ hourly rate} = 60/60 \times 42 =$$
$$1 \times 42 \text{ gtt/min}$$

17. a. 1 g (1000 mg)
    b. 1.3 mL
    1000 mg : 2.6 mL :: 500 mg : $x$ mL
    Proof: 1000 × 1.3 = 1300; 2.6 × 500 = 1300

18. a. 500,000 units/mL
    b. 8.2 mL
    c. 1 mL (concentration is 500,000 units per 1 mL)
    d. Label the multidose vial with the date, time, amount of diluent used, and user's initials.

19. a. 1 mL (when reconstituted, each mL contains 225 mg)
    b. 31 lb = 14.1 kg; 14.1 kg × 100 mg/kg/day = 1410 mg/kg/day (maximum dose in 24 hours)
    1410 mg/kg/day divided into 4 doses = 352.5 mg/dose every 6 hours (for the maximum dose range)

c. 225 mg/dose × 4 doses/24 hours = 900 mg/24 hours
d. Yes
   The ordered dose of 900 mg/24 hours does not exceed the 1410 maximum dose.

20. 2.5 mL
    125 mcg = 0.125 mg
    0.05 mg : 1 mL :: 0.125 mg : $x$ mg
    Proof: 0.05 × 2.5 = 0.125 × 1 = 0.125

21. 0.25 mL
    0.025 mg = 25 mcg
    100 mcg : 1 mL :: 25 mcg : $x$ mL
    Proof: 100 × 0.25 = 25 × 1 = 25

22. 13.3 mL
    300 mg : 5 mL :: 800 mg : $x$ mL
    Proof: 300 × 13.3 = 3990; 800 × 5 = 4000. *(Remember, you had to round the dose to 13.3, therefore 3990 will not be exactly the same as 4000.)*

23. One-half of a tablet
    12.5 mg : 1 tablet :: 6.25 mg : $x$ tablet
    Proof: 12.5 × 0.5 = 6.25; 6.25 × 1 = 6.25

24. 0.75 mL
    20,000 units : 1 mL :: 15,000 units : $x$ mL
    Proof: 20,000 × 0.75 = 15,000; 15,000 × 1 = 15,000

25. 4 mL
    0.1 mg : 1 mL :: 0.4 mg : $x$ mL
    Proof: 0.1 × 4 = 0.4; 0.4 × 1 = 0.4

# Notes

# Notes

# BRIEF CONTENTS

**PART 1: PHARMACOLOGY BASICS,  1**

Study Skills Tips: Introduction to Study Skills Concepts, PURR, and Pharmacology Basics

1   The Nursing Process and Drug Therapy,  6
2   Pharmacologic Principles,  17
3   Lifespan Considerations,  37
4   Cultural, Legal, and Ethical Considerations,  50
5   Medication Errors: Preventing and Responding,  64
6   Patient Education and Drug Therapy,  74
7   Over-the-Counter Drugs and Herbal and Dietary Supplements,  84
8   Gene Therapy and Pharmacogenomics,  94
9   Photo Atlas of Drug Administration,  102

**PART 2: DRUGS AFFECTING THE CENTRAL NERVOUS SYSTEM,  137**

Study Skills Tips: Vocabulary, Text Notation, and Language Conventions

10   Analgesic Drugs,  139
11   General and Local Anesthetics,  169
12   Central Nervous System Depressants and Muscle Relaxants,  188
13   Central Nervous System Stimulants and Related Drugs,  203
14   Antiepileptic Drugs,  219
15   Antiparkinson Drugs,  237
16   Psychotherapeutic Drugs,  253
17   Substance Abuse,  281

**PART 3: DRUGS AFFECTING THE AUTONOMIC NERVOUS SYSTEM,  296**

Study Skills Tips: PURR Application and Study Groups

18   Adrenergic Drugs,  298
19   Adrenergic-Blocking Drugs,  312
20   Cholinergic Drugs,  324
21   Cholinergic-Blocking Drugs,  334

**PART 4: DRUGS AFFECTING THE CARDIOVASCULAR AND RENAL SYSTEMS,  343**

Study Skills Tips: Linking Learning and Text Notation

22   Antihypertensive Drugs,  347
23   Antianginal Drugs,  368
24   Heart Failure Drugs,  382
25   Antidysrhythmic Drugs,  396
26   Coagulation Modifier Drugs,  418
27   Antilipemic Drugs,  443
28   Diuretic Drugs,  459
29   Fluids and Electrolytes,  473

**PART 5: DRUGS AFFECTING THE ENDOCRINE SYSTEM,  491**

Study Skills Tips: Questioning Strategy

30   Pituitary Drugs,  493
31   Thyroid and Antithyroid Drugs,  501
32   Antidiabetic Drugs,  510
33   Adrenal Drugs,  533
34   Women's Health Drugs,  543
35   Men's Health Drugs,  564

**PART 6: DRUGS AFFECTING THE RESPIRATORY SYSTEM,  573**

Study Skills Tips: Study on the Run and PURR

36   Antihistamines, Decongestants, Antitussives, and Expectorants,  575
37   Respiratory Drugs,  588

**PART 7: ANTIINFECTIVE AND ANTIINFLAMMATORY DRUGS,  607**

Study Skills Tips: Nursing Process, Assessment, Nursing Diagnoses, and Evaluation

38   Antibiotics Part 1,  609
39   Antibiotics Part 2,  633
40   Antiviral Drugs,  650
41   Antitubercular Drugs,  672
42   Antifungal Drugs,  682
43   Antimalarial, Antiprotozoal, and Anthelmintic Drugs,  692
44   Antiinflammatory and Antigout Drugs,  706

**PART 8: IMMUNE AND BIOLOGIC MODIFIERS AND CHEMOTHERAPEUTIC DRUGS,  720**

Study Skills Tips: Manage Time, Evaluate Prior Performance, Anticipate the Test, and Plan for Distributed Study

45   Antineoplastic Drugs Part 1: Cancer Overview and Cell Cycle–Specific Drugs,  722
46   Antineoplastic Drugs Part 2: Cell Cycle–Nonspecific and Miscellaneous Drugs,  748
47   Biologic Response–Modifying and Antirheumatic Drugs,  762
48   Immunosuppressant Drugs,  784
49   Immunizing Drugs and Biochemical Terrorism,  795

**PART 9: DRUGS AFFECTING THE GASTROINTESTINAL SYSTEM AND NUTRITION,  813**

Study Skills Tips: Active Questioning, What Are the Right Questions, Kinds of Questions, and Questioning Application

50   Acid-Controlling Drugs,  815
51   Bowel Disorder Drugs,  829
52   Antiemetic and Antinausea Drugs,  844
53   Vitamins and Minerals,  856
54   Anemia Drugs,  877
55   Nutritional Supplements,  888

**PART 10: DERMATOLOGIC, OPHTHALMIC, AND OTIC DRUGS,  899**

Study Skills Tips: Time Management, PURR, and Repeat the Steps

56   Dermatologic Drugs,  901
57   Ophthalmic Drugs,  916
58   Otic Drugs,  937

Appendix: Pharmaceutical Abbreviations,  943

Case Study Photo Credits,  944

Index,  945

### Linda Lane Lilley, RN, PhD

Linda Lilley received her diploma from Norfolk General School of Nursing, BSN from the University of Virginia, Master of Science (Nursing) from Old Dominion University, and PhD in Nursing from George Mason University. As an Associate Professor Emeritus and University Professor at Old Dominion University, her teaching experience in nursing education spans over 25 years, including almost 20 years at Old Dominion. Linda's teaching expertise includes drug therapy and the nursing process, adult nursing, physical assessment, fundamentals in nursing, oncology nursing, nursing theory, and trends in health care. The awarding of the University's most prestigious title of University Professor reflects her teaching excellence as a tenured faculty member. She has also been a two-time university nominee for the State Council of Higher Education in Virginia award for excellence in teaching, service, and scholarship. Linda received the 2012 Distinguished Nursing Alumni Award from Old Dominion University School of Nursing for her "continued work on the successful pharmacology textbook published by Elsevier" and to recognize her "extraordinary work and the impact [the book] has had on baccalaureate education." While at Old Dominion University, Linda mentored and taught undergraduate and graduate students as well as registered nurses returning for their BSN. Linda authored the MED ERRORS column for the *American Journal of Nursing* between 1994 and 1999 as well as numerous other peer-reviewed, published articles in professional nursing journals. Since retirement in 2005, Linda has continued to be active in nursing, serving as a member on dissertation committees with the College of Health Sciences and maintaining membership and involvement in numerous professional and academic organizations. Dr. Lilley has served as a consultant with school nurses in the city of Virginia Beach, a member on the City of Virginia Beach's Health Advisory Board, and currently a member of the City of Virginia Beach's Community Health Advisory Board and the Youth Community Action Team (YCAT). Linda also served as an appointed member on the national advisory panel on medication errors prevention with the U.S. Pharmacopeia in Rockville, Maryland. She continues to educate nursing students and professional nurses about drug therapy and the nursing process and speaks on the topics of drug therapy, safe medication use, humor and healing, and grief and loss.

### Shelly Rainforth Collins, PharmD

Shelly Rainforth Collins received her Doctor of Pharmacy degree from the University of Nebraska, College of Pharmacy in 1985, with High Distinction. She then completed a clinical pharmacy residency at Memorial Medical Center of Long Beach in Long Beach California. She worked as a pediatric clinical pharmacist (neonatal specialist) at Memorial Medical Center before moving to Mobile, Alabama. She was the Assistant Director of Clinical Pharmacy Services at Mobile Infirmary Medical Center. She currently serves as the Clinical Pharmacy Specialist/Coordinator of Clinical Pharmacy Services at Chesapeake Regional Medical Center in Chesapeake, Virginia. Her practice focuses on developing and implementing clinical pharmacy services as well as medication safety and Joint Commission medication management standards and national patient safety goals. She also works as staff pharmacist at Chesapeake Regional Medical Center. She is president of Drug Information Consultants, a business offering consultation and expert witness review for attorneys on medical malpractice cases. Shelly was awarded the Clinical Pharmacist of the Year Award in 2007 from the Virginia Society of Healthsystem Pharmacists. She led a multidisciplinary team that won the Clinical Achievement of the Year Award from George Mason University School of Public Health in 2007 for promoting safety with narcotics in patients with sleep apnea; this program has also received national recognition. She was awarded the Service Excellence Award from Chesapeake Regional Medical Center. Shelly's professional affiliations include the American Society of Healthsystem Pharmacists and the Virginia Society of Healthsystem Pharmacists.

### Julie S. Snyder, MSN, RN-BC

Julie Snyder received her diploma from Norfolk General Hospital School of Nursing and her BSN and MSN from Old Dominion University. After working in medical-surgical nursing, she worked in nursing staff development and community education. After 8 years, she transferred to the academic setting and has since taught fundamentals of nursing, pharmacology, physical assessment, gerontologic nursing, and adult medical-surgical nursing. She has been certified by the ANCC in Nursing Continuing Education and Staff Development and currently holds ANCC certification in Medical-Surgical Nursing. She is a member of Sigma Theta Tau International and was inducted into Phi Kappi Phi as Outstanding Alumni for Old Dominion University. She has worked for Elsevier as a reviewer and ancillary writer since 1997. Julie's professional service has included serving on the Virginia Nurses' Association Continuing Education Committee, serving as Educational Development Committee chair for the Epsilon Chi chapter of Sigma Theta Tau, serving as an item writer for the ANCC, working with a regional hospital educators' group, and serving as a consultant on various projects for local hospital education departments.

# Pharmacology
## and the
# Nursing Process

## 7th
### EDITION

**Linda Lane Lilley, RN, PhD**
Associate Professor Emeritus
School of Nursing
Old Dominion University
Norfolk, Virginia

**Shelly Rainforth Collins, PharmD**
Clinical Pharmacy Specialist
Coordinator of Clinical Pharmacy Services
Chesapeake Regional Medical Center
Chesapeake, Virginia
President
Drug Information Consultants
Chesapeake, Virginia

**Julie S. Snyder, MSN, RN-BC**
Adjunct Faculty
School of Nursing
Old Dominion University
Norfolk, Virginia

*With Study Skills Tips by*
**Diane Savoca**
Coordinator of Student Transition
St. Louis Community College at Florissant Valley
St. Louis, Missouri

ELSEVIER

3251 Riverport Lane
St. Louis, Missouri 63043

---

**Notices**

Knowledge and best practice in this field are constantly changing. As new research and experience broaden our understanding, changes in research methods, professional practices, or medical treatment may become necessary.

Practitioners and researchers must always rely on their own experience and knowledge in evaluating and using any information, methods, compounds, or experiments described herein. In using such information or methods they should be mindful of their own safety and the safety of others, including parties for whom they have a professional responsibility.

With respect to any drug or pharmaceutical products identified, readers are advised to check the most current information provided (i) on procedures featured or (ii) by the manufacturer of each product to be administered, to verify the recommended dose or formula, the method and duration of administration, and contraindications. It is the responsibility of practitioners, relying on their own experience and knowledge of their patients, to make diagnoses, to determine dosages and the best treatment for each individual patient, and to take all appropriate safety precautions.

To the fullest extent of the law, neither the Publisher nor the authors, contributors, or editors, assume any liability for any injury and/or damage to persons or property as a matter of products liability, negligence or otherwise, or from any use or operation of any methods, products, instructions, or ideas contained in the material herein.

---

**Library of Congress Cataloging-in-Publication Data**
Lilley, Linda Lane.
    Pharmacology and the nursing process/Linda Lane Lilley, Shelly Rainforth Collins, Julie S. Snyder; with study skills tips by Diane Savoca. -- 7th ed.
        p. ; cm.
    Rev. ed. of: Pharmacology and the nursing process/Linda Lane Lilley ... [et al.]. 6th ed. c2011.
    Includes bibliographical references and index.
    ISBN 978-0-323-08789-6 (pbk. : alk. paper)
    I. Collins, Shelly Rainforth. II. Snyder, Julie S. III. Savoca, Diane. IV. Pharmacology and the nursing process. V. Title.
    [DNLM: 1.  Pharmacology--Nurses' Instruction. 2.  Drug Therapy--Nurses' Instruction. 3.  Pharmaceutical Preparations--administration & dosage--Nurses' Instruction. QV 4]
    LC classification  not assigned
    615'.1--dc23                                                                2012036416

*Executive Content Strategist*: Lee Henderson
*Content Development Specialist*: Jacqueline Twomey
*Publishing Services Manager*: Jeff Patterson
*Senior Project Manager*: Clay S. Broeker
*Designer*: Amy Buxton

Printed in Canada

Last digit is the print number:  9  8  7  6  5  4  3  2  1

## Critical Thinking and Prioritization Questions

**Julie S. Snyder, MSN, RN-BC**
Adjunct Faculty
School of Nursing
Old Dominion University
Norfolk, Virginia

## Key Points—Downloadable

**Peggy Slota, DNP, RN, FAAN**
Associate Professor
Director, DNP and Graduate Nursing Leadership Programs
Carlow University School of Nursing
Pittsburgh, Pennsylvania

## PowerPoint® Slides

**Valerie Baker, ACNS, BC**
Assistant Professor
Villa Maria School of Nursing
Morosky College of Health Professions and Sciences
Gannon University
Erie, Pennsylvania

## Review Questions for the NCLEX® Examination

**Stephanie C. Butkus, MS, RN**
Associate Professor
Division of Nursing
Kettering College
Kettering, Ohio

## TEACH® for Nurses Lesson Plans

**Sharon Souter, RN, PhD, CNE**
Dean and Professor
College of Nursing
University of Mary Hardin-Baylor
Belton, Texas

## Test Bank

**Julie S. Snyder, MSN, RN-BC**
Adjunct Faculty
School of Nursing
Old Dominion University
Norfolk, Virginia

## Unfolding Case Studies

**Donna D. Ignatavicius, MS, RN, ANEF**
Speaker and Curriculum Consultant for Academic Nursing Programs
Founder, Boot Camp for Nurse Educators®
President, DI Associates, Inc.
Placitas, New Mexico

**Jennifer D. Powers, MSN, FNP-BC, RN**
Assistant Professor
National University Nevada
Henderson, Nevada

# REVIEWERS

Now in its seventh edition, *Pharmacology and the Nursing Process* provides the most current and clinically relevant nursing pharmacology content in a visually appealing, understandable, and practical format. The accessible size, clear writing style, and full-color design of *Pharmacology and the Nursing Process* are ideal for today's busy nursing student. The book not only presents drug information that the nursing student needs to know but also provides information on what the professional nurse may encounter during drug administration in a variety of health care settings, including accounts of real-life medication errors and tips for avoiding those errors. Edition after edition, the book has become increasingly inviting and engaging for the adult learner to read and study. Features that help set the book apart include:

- A focus on the role of prioritization in nursing care
- A strong focus on drug classes to help students acquire a better knowledge of how various drug classes work in the body, allowing them to apply this knowledge to individual drugs
- Ease of readability to make this difficult content more understandable
- Integrated study skills content that helps students understand and learn the particularly demanding subject of pharmacology while also equipping them with tools that they can use in other courses and as lifelong learners who are building an evidence-based practice.

The use of color has continued to complement the text by making the book more engaging for nursing students. Color is used throughout to:

- Highlight important content
- Illustrate how drugs work in the body in numerous anatomic and drug process color illustrations
- Improve the visual appearance of the content to make it more engaging and appealing to today's more visually sophisticated reader

We believe that the use of color and other visual engagement devices in these ways significantly improves students' involvement and understanding of pharmacology.

For this edition, the author team has focused even more closely on providing the most "need-to-know" information, enhancing readability, and emphasizing the nursing process and prioritization throughout. Many of the updates for this edition are in response to actual questions posed by students.

Sharing the goal of creating a nursing pharmacology textbook that is not only academically rigorous but also practical and easy to use, the authors bring together a unique combination of experience. The author team is comprised of an Associate Professor Emeritus with a PhD in nursing and more than 25 years of teaching experience, a clinical pharmacist with a PharmD and 28 years of experience in hospital pharmacy practice, and a nursing clinical instructor who holds a Master of Science in Nursing degree and has 25 years of teaching experience.

## ORGANIZATION

This book includes 58 chapters presented in 10 parts, organized by body system. The 9 "concepts" chapters in Part 1 lay a solid foundation for the subsequent drug units and address the following topics:

- The nursing process and drug therapy
- Pharmacologic principles
- Lifespan considerations related to pharmacology
- Cultural, legal, and ethical considerations
- Preventing and responding to medication errors
- Patient education and drug therapy
- Over-the-counter drugs and herbal and dietary supplements
- Gene therapy and pharmacogenomics
- Drug administration techniques, including more than 100 drawings and photographs

Parts 2 through 10 present pharmacology and nursing management in a time-tested body systems/drug function framework. This approach facilitates learning by grouping functionally related drugs and drug groups. It provides an effective means of integrating the content into medical-surgical/adult health nursing courses or for teaching pharmacology in a separate course.

The 49 drug chapters in these 9 Parts constitute the main portion of the book. Drugs are presented in a consistent format with an emphasis on drug classes and key similarities and differences among the drugs in each class. Each chapter is subdivided into two discussions, beginning with (1) a brief overview of anatomy, physiology, and pathophysiology and a complete discussion of pharmacology, followed by (2) a comprehensive yet succinct application of the nursing process.

Pharmacology is presented for each drug group in a consistent format:

- Mechanism of Action and Drug Effects
- Indications
- Contraindications
- Adverse Effects (often including Toxicity and Management of Overdose)
- Interactions
- Dosages

Drug class discussions conclude with specially highlighted Drug Profiles—brief narrative "capsules" of individual drugs in the class or group, including Pharmacokinetics tables for each drug. Key drugs (prototypical drugs within a class) are identified throughout with a ♦ symbol for easy identification.

The pharmacology section is followed by a Nursing Process discussion that relates to the entire drug group. This nursing content is covered in the following, familiar nursing process format:

- Assessment
- Nursing Diagnoses
- Planning (including Goals and Outcome Criteria)
- Implementation
- Evaluation

At the end of each Nursing Process section is a Patient Teaching Tips box that summarizes key points for nursing students and/or practicing nurses to include in the education of patients about their medications. These boxes focus on teaching how the drugs work, possible interactions, adverse effects, and other information related to the safe and effective use of the drug(s). The role of the nurse as patient educator and advocate continues to grow in importance in professional practice, so there is emphasis on this key content in each chapter in this edition.

Additionally, each Part begins with a Study Skills Tips section that presents a study skills topic and relates it to the unit being discussed. Topics include time management, note taking, studying, test taking, and others. This unique feature is intended to aid students who find pharmacology difficult and to provide a tool that may prove beneficial throughout their nursing school careers. This arrangement of content can be especially helpful to faculty who teach pharmacology through an integrated approach because it helps the student identify key content and concepts.

## NEW TO THIS EDITION

To further improve the hallmark readability and user-friendliness of *Pharmacology and the Nursing Process*, each line of the text has been edited for this edition with a special focus on an active, direct-address writing style. This refreshing and engaging writing style helps students navigate more easily through the textbook and thus the difficult subject of pharmacology and the nursing process.

The seventh edition of *Pharmacology and the Nursing Process* also features an enhanced focus on "need-to-know" content. The information on drug adverse effects has been streamlined to reflect only the most common and most serious adverse effects rather than listing all reported adverse effects. These adverse effects are also now listed in order of those most commonly seen. Another area that has been reduced for an optimized focus is that of drug dosages; only those dosages that are seen in most common indications are included in the text and tables. (For other dosages, the student should refer to an up-to-date drug handbook or drug reference.) This need-to-know approach to drug indications and adverse effects is crucial in helping the adult learner focus on the most essential content needed for safe drug administration.

It is important to remember that although this textbook provides all of the need-to-know *pharmacology* content that students will need for an entry level of practice, it is first and foremost a *nursing* textbook rather than a pharmacology textbook, with a strong emphasis on the nursing process and professional nursing practice. Nursing care related to the specifics of drug therapy has been further prioritized in this edition by numbering the nursing diagnoses and corresponding goals and outcome criteria in the coverage of the planning phase of the nursing process. The section on implementation also offers all of the most essential information, followed by a section on the evaluation of therapeutic and adverse effects. These changes highlight the significance of the nursing process as a foundation in drug therapy while helping the student to make strong cognitive connections among nursing diagnoses, goals, and outcome criteria.

This edition also integrates the six Quality and Safety Education for Nurses (QSEN) competencies. Funded by the Robert Wood Johnson Foundation, the QSEN project has the overall goal of addressing the challenge of preparing future nurses with knowledge, skills, and attitudes needed to continually improve the quality and safety of healthcare systems. The QSEN competencies are together aimed at reducing the 1.9 million drug-related hospitalizations seen in the United States at the outset of the initiative. Leading the integration of QSEN competencies into prelicensure nursing pharmacology textbooks, *Pharmacology and the Nursing Process* addresses the safety and quality competencies through the following special boxes:

- Evidence-Based Practice
- Patient-Centered Care: Cultural Implications
- Patient-Centered Care: Lifespan Considerations for the Elderly Patient
- Patient-Centered Care: Lifespan Considerations for the Pediatric Patient
- Safety: Herbal Therapies and Dietary Supplements
- Safety: Laboratory Values Related to Drug Therapy
- Safety and Quality Improvement: Preventing Medication Errors
- Teamwork and Collaboration: Legal and Ethical Principles
- Teamwork and Collaboration: Pharmacokinetic Bridge to Nursing Practice

The QSEN initiative is also highlighted in the new *TEACH for Nurses* Lesson Plans provided for this edition (see Supplemental Resources).

The pharmacology and nursing content in each of the 58 chapters has been thoroughly revised and critically reviewed by nursing instructors, practicing nurses, and a PharmD to reflect the latest drug information and nursing content. Key updates include:

- A more effectively organized classification of psychotherapeutic drugs in Chapter 16 into 3 subcategories: (1) anxiolytics, (2) mood stabilizers and antidepressants, and (3) antipsychotic drugs
- The most recent evidence-based guidelines on management of diabetes mellitus in Chapter 32, with an emphasis on new diabetes drugs
- The most recent evidence-based guidelines on the treatment of rheumatoid arthritis in Chapter 47
- Revision of Chapter 48 on immunosuppressant drugs to provide an emphasis on transplant therapy
- Revised NCLEX® Examination Review Questions at the end of each chapter, including alternate-item format and new dosage calculation questions

## ADDITIONAL TEACHING/LEARNING FEATURES

The book also includes a variety of innovative teaching/learning features that prepare the student for important content to be covered in each chapter and encourage review and reinforcement of that content. Chapter-opener features include the following:

- Learning Objectives
- List of Evolve Resources available to students

- Summary of Drug Profiles in the chapter, with page number references
- Key terms with definitions and page number references (key terms being in bold blue type throughout the narrative to emphasize this essential terminology)
  The following features appear at the end of each chapter:
- Patient Teaching Tips related to drug therapy
- Key Points boxes summarizing important chapter content
- NCLEX® Examination Review Questions, with answers provided upside-down at the bottom of the section for quick and easy review

  In addition to the special boxes listed previously, other special features that appear throughout the text include:
- Case Studies, with answer guidelines provided on the Evolve website
- Dosages tables listing generic and trade names, pharmacologic class, usual dosage ranges, and indications for the drugs

  For a more comprehensive listing of the special features, please see the inside back cover of the book.

## SUPPLEMENTAL RESOURCES

A comprehensive ancillary package is available to students and instructors using classroom quantities of *Pharmacology and the Nursing Process*. The following supplemental resources have been thoroughly revised for this edition and can significantly assist teaching and learning of pharmacology:

### Study Guide

The carefully prepared student workbook—written by one of the textbook authors for careful alignment with the content and focus of the book—includes the following:

- Student Study Tips that reinforce the Study Skills in the text and provide a "how to" guide to applying test-taking strategies
- Worksheets for each chapter, with NCLEX®-style questions (now with more application-based, alternate-item, and dosage calculation questions), critical thinking and application questions, and other activities
- Case Studies followed by related critical thinking questions
- An updated Overview of Dosage Calculations with helpful tips for calculating doses, sample drug labels, practice problems, and a quiz
- Answers to all questions (provided in the back of the book) to facilitate self-study

### Evolve Website

Located at http://evolve.elsevier.com/Lilley/, the Evolve website for this book includes the following:

#### For students:

- More than 550 NCLEX® Examination Review Questions
- Critical Thinking and Prioritization Questions with answer guidelines
- 35 state-of-the-art animations
- Printable, expanded Key Points for each chapter
- Printable IV Therapy and Medication Safety Checklists

- Content Updates
- Answers to Case Studies from the book

#### For instructors:

- NEW *TEACH for Nurses* Lesson Plans that focus on the most important content from each chapter and provide innovative strategies for student engagement and learning. These new Lesson Plans include strategies for integrating nursing curriculum standards (QSEN, concept-based learning, and the BSN essentials), links to all relevant student and instructor resources, and an original instructor-only Case Study in each chapter.
- ExamView Test Bank that features more than 800 NCLEX® Examination–format test questions (100 new, including alternate-item questions) with text page references, rationales, and answers coded for NCLEX® Client Needs category, nursing process step, and cognitive level (new and old Bloom's taxonomy). The robust ExamView testing application, provided at no cost to faculty, allows instructors to create new tests; edit, add, and delete test questions; sort questions by NCLEX® Client Needs category, cognitive level, and nursing process step; and administer and grade tests online, with automated scoring and gradebook functionality.
- PowerPoint Lecture Slides consisting of more than 2100 customizable text slides for instructors to use in lectures. The presentations include new Unfolding Case Studies and applicable illustrations from the book's Image Collection. Audience Response System Questions (three or more discussion-oriented questions per chapter for use with i>Clicker and other systems) are folded into these presentations.
- An Image Collection with approximately 220 full-color images from the book for instructors to use in lectures
- Access to all student resources listed above

### Pharmacology Online

Pharmacology Online for *Pharmacology and the Nursing Process*, seventh edition (ISBN: 978-0-323-09167-1), is a dynamic, unit-by-unit online course that includes interactive self-study modules, a collection of interactive learning activities, and a media-rich library of supplemental resources.

- *Self-Study Modules* go beyond the basic principles of pharmacology, with animations and NCLEX® Examination–style questions to help students assess their understanding of pharmacology concepts.
- *Interactive Case Studies* immerse students in true-to-life scenarios that require them to make important choices in patient care and patient teaching.
- *"Roadside Assistance"* Video Clips use humor and analogy in a uniquely fun and engaging way to teach key concepts.
- Interactive Learning Activities, Discussion Questions, Practice Quizzes for the NCLEX® Examination, and more are also included.

## ACKNOWLEDGMENTS

This book truly has been a collaborative effort. We wish to thank the instructors who provided input on an ongoing basis throughout the development of the previous editions.

We thank Lee Henderson and Jackie Twomey for taking on the Lilley text as a new project. Having spent six editions with the editorial team from St. Louis, we had our anxieties about the switch to the Philadelphia team, but it has been a smooth and very productive transition. Lee and Jackie's guidance, attention to detail, and support have been much appreciated, and their suggestions for improving readability and organization of content helped to make the seventh edition better than ever. Thanks for their patience and nurturing manner! We thank Kristin Geen and Jamie Horn for their contributions and support throughout the fourth, fifth, and sixth editions. We are also grateful to Jeff Patterson and Clay Broeker for very capably guiding the project through to publication. Diane Savoca lent her study skills expertise and has updated the unique and appropriate Study Skills features for students; for her collaboration, we are most grateful. Finally, we thank Joe Albanese for his contributions to the first edition of the book, Bob Aucker for his contributions to the first three editions, and Scott Harrington for contributions through the sixth edition.

Linda thanks her daughter Karen for her unwavering and constant support. Long hours and time spent researching and writing has preempted time with family, but Karen has always understood. Linda wishes to dedicate this book to Karen Leanne Lilley Harris as she remains her inspiration and encouragement for all professional and personal endeavors and accomplishments. The memory of Linda's parents, John and Thelma Lane, who passed away during the fourth edition, and in-laws J.C. and Mary Anne Lilley, who passed away during the fifth and sixth editions, has continued to provide inspiration and a sense of pride in all her work. Students and graduates of Old Dominion University School of Nursing have been eager to provide feedback and support, beginning with the class of 1990 and continuing through the class of 2005. Without their participation, the book would not have been so user-friendly and helpful to students beginning the study of drug therapy. Linda attributes her successes and accomplishments to a strong sense of purpose, faith, and family and an appreciation for the light-hearted side of life. To Jibby Baucom, Linda offers many thanks, because without her recommendation to Mosby, Inc., the book would never have been developed. Robin Carter, Kristin Geen, Jamie Horn, Lee Henderson, and Jackie Twomey have been constant resources and more than just editors with Elsevier; they have been sources of strength and encouragement. Their excellent work ethic, positivity, and calming natures will be forever appreciated. The fifth through seventh editions have also involved Clay Broeker, who has been a tremendous resource with production issues; his contributions to this edition have been strong and forward-thinking. Elsevier has shared some of its best employees with Linda beginning with the first day of the first edition; for that, Linda is most thankful.

Shelly would like to dedicate this edition to the memory of her mother, Rogene Rainforth, who passed away in July of 2011. It was because of her inspiration and steadfast love that Shelly has succeeded both personally and professionally. To Shelly's father, Charles Rainforth of Hastings, Nebraska, your strength, compassion, optimism, pride, and love never cease to amaze. Shelly would like to thank her daughter Kristin Collins for her patience and understanding. You are her source of pride, accomplishment, and inspiration. It has been such a joy watching you grow into the beautiful young woman you are today. Your future students will be inspired by your grace. Shelly would also like to thank Linda Lilley, Julie Snyder, Lee Henderson, and Jackie Twomey for the opportunity to be part of this wonderful book; it is truly an honor to be associated with all of you. To the pharmacy staff at Chesapeake Regional Medical Center, Shelly is proud not only to call you her colleagues, but also her friends. Shelly also thanks the pharmacists at Long Beach Memorial Medical Center, for the knowledge you imparted during her residency training. Finally, to Shelly's nephew and new pharmacist, Chris Rainforth, welcome to the profession!

Julie wishes to dedicate this edition to her husband Jonathan. He has been a steadfast and loving supporter over the years. Julie also thanks her daughter Emily Martin; son-in-law Randy Martin; and her parents Willis and Jean Simmons, for their unfailing support and encouragement. They were all patient despite the long hours working on revisions. The pharmacists at Chesapeake Regional Medical Center have always been great resources, as have the staff nurses who work alongside our students in the clinical settings. Thanks also to Rick Brady and Chesapeake Regional Medical Center for their previous assistance with the photo shoot for the Photo Atlas of Drug Administration. This support and the encouragement of family, friends, and colleagues are vital to projects like this. Thanks also to Lee Henderson and Jackie Twomey at Elsevier for providing the support needed to keep this project on track. Julie is grateful to the St. Louis Elsevier team of Kristin Geen and Jamie Horn for guidance and support during the previous editions. Thanks also to Shelly Rainforth Collins for her clinical insight. Deep appreciation goes to Dr. Linda L. Lilley for her unfailing encouragement, mentoring, and friendship over the years. Dr. Lilley is a fine example of a nurse and nurse educator, and her joy in teaching is always evident. Thanks also to each student who has provided feedback and comments on the text and study aids. Most importantly, Julie gives thanks to God, our source of hope and strength. Finally, to those who teach, although your work may seem to go unnoticed or unappreciated, your impact will always be remembered in the accomplishments of your students. Your inspiration and motivation shape the future.

## WE WELCOME YOUR FEEDBACK

We always welcome comments from instructors and students who use this book so that we may continue to make improvements and be responsive to your needs in future editions. Please send any comments you may have for us to the attention of the publisher at lee.henderson@elsevier.com.

**Linda Lane Lilley, RN, PhD**
**Shelly Rainforth Collins, PharmD**
**Julie S. Snyder, MSN, RN-BC**

# Pharmacology Basics

## INTRODUCTION TO STUDY SKILLS CONCEPTS

What to study? When to study? How much to study? How to study? In the best of worlds, every student would have all the skills necessary to be effective in all academic areas. Unfortunately, many students do not know how to study effectively or have developed techniques that work well in some circumstances but not in others. The purpose of the Study Skills Tips is to introduce you to the steps to follow in learning text and maintaining focus on the appropriate material. This section also offers some specific examples for selected chapters in Part 1 to help you apply the study techniques and strategies discussed here.

Extensive discussion of study skills, including how to manage time, take lecture notes, master the text, prepare for and take examinations, establish effective study groups, and develop vocabulary are presented in the Study Guide that accompanies this text. These tools are important to any student, but they become even more valuable for students in challenging technical areas such as nursing and pharmacology. The techniques described here and in the Study Guide will not necessarily make learning easy, but they will help you achieve your goals as a student.

## PURR

*PURR* is a handy mnemonic device representing a four-step process that will lead to mastery of material. These steps are as follows:
- Prepare
- Understand
- Rehearse
- Review

The PURR approach has positive and negative aspects. The negative aspect is that it requires you to go through every chapter four times. The good news is that you will not actually *read* the chapter four times. You will only *go through* it four times. Only one of those times consists of a slow, careful, intensive reading. The other trips through the chapter are much quicker. The first time you go through the chapter, it should take only 5 or 10 minutes. Each time you go through the chapter, you are processing the information in distinctly different ways. The PURR approach will enhance your learning, and if you use it from the first assignment on, you will find that it takes you less time than you were spending before you adopted the PURR approach to learn what you need.

## Prepare

Reading the text, like any complex process, is not something to dive into without thought and planning. *Pharmacology and the Nursing Process* is organized to help you learn the material, but you have to take advantage of what the authors have done for you to facilitate this. Preparing to read means setting goals and objectives for your own learning, but the tools you need to help you do this are already in place. Look at the opening pages of any chapter in the text, and you will see a standard structure.

Every chapter begins with a **title.** Learn to use the title as the first step in preparing to learn. Chapter 4 is entitled "Cultural, Legal, and Ethical Considerations." This instantly identifies what the chapter is about. Do not start reading immediately; instead think about the title for a few seconds. Are there any unfamiliar terms? If  your answer is "No," great. If it is "Yes," then you already have some focus for your reading, because you know you will need to learn the unfamiliar terms and their meanings.

The next feature of every chapter is the **objectives.** You need objectives for learning, and the authors have anticipated this. Read the objectives actively. Do not just look at the words; think about the objectives. Ask yourself the following questions: What do I already know about this material? How do these objectives relate to earlier assignments? How do they relate to objectives the instructor has given? The chapter objectives identify things you should be able to do after you have read the material. Do not wait until you have read the chapter to start trying to respond. *Prepare* means getting the brain engaged from the beginning. Studying the chapter objectives establishes a direction and purpose for your reading. This will enable you to maintain concentration and focus while you read.

Another feature in the opening pages of each chapter is the **key terms.** This is one of the most valuable tools the authors have provided. They know that there are many terms to learn and are giving you a head start on learning them. Spend a few minutes with the glossary. Notice the terms that are also used in the chapter objectives and are bolded in the text. Go back and look at the objectives, and think about what you have learned from the glossary. As you study the glossary, look for shared root words, prefixes, or suffixes. If words share such common word elements, these words also have a shared meaning. Learning the meaning of common word elements can simplify the whole process of learning vocabulary. Perhaps you remember in elementary school being told to "look for the little words in the big word." This is essentially the same technique—one that worked then and one that will work now.

Now make a quick pass through the chapter or the assigned pages from the chapter. Focus on the text conventions, which are described later in this chapter. Look for anything that stands out in the chapter, such as boldfaced text, boxed material, and tables. This provides a quick overview of the chapter, which will make the next steps in the PURR process much more effective and efficient.

The **chapter headings** show the major points to be covered. Study them and notice the major headings (topics) and the subordinate headings (subtopics). They essentially provide a picture of the chapter, and using this picture is a fundamental step in preparing to read. As you read through the chapter headings, turn the topics and subtopics into a series of questions that you want to be able to answer when you finish reading. Think about the objectives and how these headings relate to them. Finally, in the headings devoted to specific classes of drugs, notice that there are elements that are common to every class. The last two headings are always "Implementation" and "Evaluation." This tells you that these are two common elements that you will be expected to know at the end of every chapter. The minutes you spend *preparing* will pay off in a big way when you start to read.

Preparing makes the whole approach to learning an active one. It may not make the chapters the most exciting reading you will ever do, but it will help you accomplish your personal learning objectives as well as those set by the authors.

### On-the-Run Action

Preparing is great to do during "found" time. It should not take more than 5 or 10 minutes. Time between classes, time spent waiting for the coffee water to boil, or any other small block of time that usually just slips away can be used to accomplish this step.

### Understand

Now read the assignment. Go to your desk, the library, or wherever you have chosen for serious study. Reading the assignment is where all of your preparation pays off. If you did the *Prepare* step earlier in the day, it is not a bad idea to spend a minute or two going through the chapter features again to get your focus. As you read the assignment, remember the chapter objectives and notice the chapter headings in the body of the chapter. As you read, rephrase the chapter headings as questions to help keep you focused on the task at hand. Because this is the first time you are really focusing on the concepts and the details, this is not the time to do any text notations. Read and, as you read, think. Terms from the key terms are repeated, and their meanings are often expanded and clarified in the body of the text. Pay attention to these terms as you read. Think about what they mean and how you would define them to someone else. Read for meaning. Read to *understand.* Do not read just to get to the end of the assignment. That is a passive action. Ask yourself questions. Analyze, respond, and react as you read.

Often, reading assignments are too long to be read with complete understanding in one session. If you find that your concentration is flagging or you do not remember anything you read on the previous page, it is time to take a break. All too often students have only one objective—to finish the assignment. You might be able to force yourself to continue reading, but you will not learn much. Mark your place and take a 5- or 10-minute break. Take a walk, read the daily comic strips, get a soda or a cup of coffee, and then go back to reading. When you come back to the assignment, spend the first 3 or 4 minutes reviewing. Look back at the previous chapter heading and think about what you were reading before the break. The chapter can be broken down into many small reading sessions, but it is critical that you not lose sight of the chapter as a whole. Spending these minutes in review may seem like time that could be better spent continuing with the reading, but this fast review will save time in the long run.

There is no quick way to read a chapter. You will not find an "on-the-run action" for this step because it cannot be done this way. However, if you do the *Prepare* step first, you will be surprised at how much more easily you get the reading done and how much more learning you have achieved in the process.

## Rehearse

Rehearsing is the third step. It starts the process of consolidating your learning and establishing a basis for long-term memory. Rehearsal accomplishes two things. First, it helps you find out what you understand from the reading. Knowing what you know is really important. Second, it identifies what you do not understand, and this may be an even more important benefit. Knowing what you do not know before it comes to light during an examination is critical.

### How to Rehearse

Everything you do in the *Prepare* and *Understand* steps comes into play in the *Rehearse* step. Rehearsal should begin with the features at the top of the chapter. Open the text to the beginning of the chapter. Start with the chapter title, and begin to quiz yourself on what you have read. Compose three or four questions pertaining to the chapter title, and then try to answer them to your satisfaction. The questions you ask yourself should be both literal (asking for specific information presented in the chapter) and interpretive (testing your comprehension of concepts and relationships). An example of a literal question using the Chapter 4 title might be, "What are the definitions of *cultural, legal,* and *ethical?*" This question would help you determine whether you can satisfactorily define these terms in your own words. Asking and answering questions such as this always serves to move learning from short-term to long-term memory. Literal questions are very important to help you grasp the factual information and terminology contained in the reading assignment. However, it is also necessary to ask questions that stimulate thought about the concepts and the relationships between the facts and concepts presented in the chapter. An example of an interpretive question regarding the Chapter 4 title might be, "What are the most important *cultural, legal,* and *ethical* concepts pertaining to the use of drugs?" Sometimes you will find that, even though

the question is interpretive, the authors have anticipated the question and the text does contain the direct answer to your question. Other times you will need to formulate your own response by pulling together bits and pieces of information from the entire reading assignment.

Once you have exhausted the question potential for the chapter title, move on to the chapter objectives. Use the same process here. Rephrase the objectives as questions, and try to answer them. Remember that the object of rehearsal is to reinforce what you have learned and to identify areas where you need to spend additional time (review).

Go to the key terms. Cover the definitions, and try to define each term in your own words. Another method is to cover the term and, on the basis of the definition, name the term. Do not just memorize the definition, because you may find the information presented differently on an examination, and you will then be unable to respond.

Now proceed to the chapter or assigned pages. The chapter headings are the main tools for rehearsal. Apply the same question-and-answer technique used for the title and objectives to test what you may already know about the chapter content. Turn the headings into questions, and answer them. Look at the text for boldfaced and italicized items, lists, and other text conventions. These too can become the basis for questions. The tables and diagrams should also be used for this purpose. Keep in mind the importance of asking both literal and interpretive questions. Some of the questions you ask yourself should also tie different topic headings together. Ask yourself how topic A relates to topic B.

As you proceed through the chapter, do not worry if you cannot answer the questions you ask. As stated earlier, one of the goals of the rehearsal process is to identify what you need to spend more time on. If you can give no response to a particular question, put a mark in the margin of the pertinent place in the text to remind yourself to come back and spend more time on this material, but move on at this point. Rehearsal should be a relatively quick procedure. Once you become accustomed to using the PURR method, it should take no more than 15 or 20 minutes to rehearse 15 pages after completing the *Prepare* and *Understand* steps.

As you reach the end of the chapter, skim the *Implementation* and *Evaluation* sections. Make sure that the relationship between these sections and the information in the rest of the chapter is clear. If you have questions or concerns, note them in the margins and ask your instructor to clarify these points. Although the objective is to master the chapter content as an independent learner, sometimes it is essential to ask questions of the instructor to facilitate the process.

### When to Rehearse

Ideally rehearsal should take place almost immediately after you finish reading the material. Take a 10- to 15-minute break, and then start the process. The longer the gap between reading and rehearsal, the more you will forget and the longer it will take to rehearse. If you are breaking down a reading assignment into smaller segments, do the rehearsal for each segment before you begin reading the new material. This helps maintain the sense of continuity in the chapter. This seems like a lot of work to do in a study session, but with practice it will go quickly and you will be pleasantly surprised at the quality and quantity of your learning.

## Review

*Review* is the fourth and final step in the PURR process, and it is an essential step. No matter how well you have learned material in the preceding steps, forgetting will always occur. Reviewing is the only way to store what you have learned in long-term memory. The good news is that, using the PURR approach, the review can be done for small segments of material and can be accomplished relatively quickly.

### How to Review

The basic review process is essentially the same as the rehearsal process, with some limited rereading as the only difference. When you cannot immediately answer a question, read the pertinent material again. *This does not mean you should read the entire chapter again.* Often the answer to the question will pop into your mind after you have read only a few lines. When this happens, stop reading and go back to responding to your question. The idea is to reread only as much material as is necessary to make the answer clear. One or two words or one or two sentences may trigger personal recall, but it may also take two or three paragraphs for this to happen.

### How Often to Review

How many times should you review material in this way? This actually depends on many factors, such as the difficulty of the material, the length of the assignment, and your personal background. Only you can determine how often you need to review, but there are some guidelines that will help you decide this for yourself.

First, consider the difficulty of the material. If it is very complex, contains many new terms and difficult concepts, and seems difficult to grasp, then you should review very frequently. On the other hand, if the material is straightforward and you are able to relate it well to what you have already learned, then less frequent reviews will serve to keep the material in your memory.

Second, consider how well the review went. If you had difficulty answering many questions to your satisfaction or had to do a lot of rereading, you should schedule another review soon (a day or two later at most).

The success of each review session should be used to help you determine when to schedule another session. The review step is a means of monitoring the success of the learning process. If reviews go well, limited rereading is necessary, and you are able to give clear answers to your questions, then you can wait several days (4 or 5) before reviewing this material again. A mediocre review, more extensive rereading, and poor answers

indicate that you should let only 2 or 3 days go by before reviewing the material again. If the review goes very poorly, you should plan to review the material again the next day. It is up to you to judge the success of each review and to decide how often you need to review. The nice thing about PURR is that it enables you to monitor your success and to regulate the learning process easily.

### Techniques for Rehearsal and Review

Both rehearsal and review foster active learning, which helps you maintain interest in the material and strengthens your memory. For these benefits to occur, it is essential that the review and rehearsal processes be done orally. Talking to yourself is one way to accomplish this, but working with a study group is another and sometimes more interesting way to rehearse and review. Strategies for establishing and maintaining effective study groups can be found in the Study Guide that accompanies this text. You can find a short overview in the introduction to Part 3 of this text. Study groups are not for everyone. The key is to do what works for you. If studying alone produces the results you want, then continue. If not, you may want to try a study group.

When you ask questions and give your answers out loud, this forces you to think about the material. It helps you organize it and translate it into your own words. The object is not to memorize everything you have read but to understand and be able to explain it. Eventually you will need to answer questions on an examination. Framing questions as a part of the learning process is a way to anticipate examination questions. The more questions you ask yourself during study time, the more likely some of the questions on the examination will be ones you have asked yourself. When you work with a study group, you have several brains anticipating test questions. Further, by doing the rehearsal and review orally, you will find it easier to recall the answers during the examination, because this oral model requires more than just remembering seeing the material; you will actually be able to hear the rehearsed answers in your mind. As stated earlier, another advantage of performing the rehearsal and review processes orally is that it helps to identify what needs further study. When your oral answer is fragmentary, contains many "uhs," and is really disorganized, then you know that you need to devote more time to learning the given term, fact, or concept.

The PURR system may seem like a lot of work at first. The idea of going through a chapter four times understandably seems daunting. Add to this the need for several review sessions, and the first reaction is likely to be, "This won't work" or "I don't have time to do this." Don't take that attitude. This system does work. It cultivates interest, aids concentration, fosters mastery of the material, and ensures long-term memory for the material, which is important not just for doing well on examinations but also for doing well as a nurse, when the safe care of patients is at stake. The PURR system will work if you use it. It may take 3 or 4 weeks to get comfortable with the system, but if you keep at it, pretty soon it will become a good habit. After a while, you will not be able to imagine studying in any other way.

Like all study systems, the PURR method is a model. As you use it, you may discover ways of changing it that work better for you. That is okay. Do not hesitate to make adjustments that better suit your learning style and strategies. Just remember as you start out that *Preparation, Understanding, Rehearsal,* and *Review* are solid learning principles and cannot be ignored.

Study skills tips are included on the pages at the beginning of each part of the book. These hints are directly applied to the content found within the chapters of the following unit.

## PHARMACOLOGY BASICS

### Prepare

As you begin to work with individual chapters, consider how the first step in the PURR system can be used to help you set a purpose and become an active learner.

### Chapter 1 Objectives

Consider Objective 1 of Chapter 1: "List the five phases of the nursing process." Now turn the objective into a question: What are the five phases of the nursing process? Now move to Objective 2 and make it a question: What are the components of the assessment process for patients receiving medications, including collection and analysis of subjective and objective data? You might recognize that this question relates to Objective 1 because assessment is one phase of the nursing process. By putting Objective 2 into question format, you will begin to expand the focus of the first objective, and you will begin to concentrate on active learning with a clear purpose.

When you begin to read Chapter 1, you will discover that the five phases of the nursing process are repeated as topic headings, and you have the Objective 2 question on which to focus your reading. Begin now to develop the habit of applying this strategy to the objectives in every chapter assigned before you begin to read. Remember to look at the chapter headings at this point as well. It is amazing how much can be learned by using the text structures provided.

### Vocabulary Development

Turn to Chapter 2. Objective 1 makes an important point: "Define the common terms used in pharmacology." Success depends heavily on knowledge of the "language." The objective makes it clear that this chapter contains a number of terms that the author views as important to be mastered. This is only Chapter 2, and now is the time to begin to apply yourself to mastering the language of this content. Look at the key terms. There are seven terms that share the common element *pharmaco.* Although each of these seven words has a different meaning, the words have something in common. *Pharmaco* is an example of a group word. No matter what prefixes, group

words, and/or suffixes are added to it, a part of the meaning of any word containing *pharmaco* will be "drug" or "medicine." Look up a word containing *pharmaco* in any dictionary, and you will find that its definition pertains to "drug" or "medicine" in some way. Although you probably already knew that, it is always beneficial to start working on a new technique with something that is familiar. Look at four of the words that begin with *pharmaco,* and consider the rest of the word:

dynamics        genomics        gnosy        kinetics

What does each of these word parts mean? The meaning of *pharmacodynamics* is simply the combination of the meanings of *pharmaco* and *dynamics.* The definition, according to the key terms, begins "the study of the biochemical and physiologic interactions of drugs." You could simply memorize this definition, which would seem to accomplish Objective 1. However, memorization does not always equal understanding. Try another approach. What does *dynamics* mean? Think about the word, and relate it to your own experience and background. It appears to deal with movement or action. If you look it up in the dictionary, all the meanings given seem to relate in some fashion to the idea of motion and/or action. A simplistic definition of *pharmacodynamics* would be "drugs in action." Certainly this is not a technical or medical definition, but it contributes a great deal to an understanding of the definition provided in the glossary. This is the object of learning vocabulary. Do not memorize words without understanding. Apply a little thought, and relate the term and definition in a way that makes the meaning personal for you. When you do that, you will find that you understand the glossary definition better, and your ability to retain the meaning will be significantly improved. This means that the test item asking you to select the definition for *pharmacodynamics* from a list of similar definitions will be much easier to answer, because you will remember action and movement and look for the choice that best represents that concept.

Apply this same strategy to the word part *genomics.* Once you know what genomics means, you must determine how to connect that to the meaning in the text. After you have the definitions for *gnosy* and *kinetics,* you can apply the same procedure. When you have done this with all four word parts, you will discover that you will not need to spend a great amount of time trying to memorize esoteric definitions. You will have personalized the meanings. These meanings will stay with you much more readily than those learned by rote memorization. By the way, do you know what *biochemical* and *physiologic* mean? These terms are used in the definition of *pharmacodynamics.* You need to know what they mean to fully understand *pharmacodynamics.*

# The Nursing Process and Drug Therapy

## OBJECTIVES

When you reach the end of this chapter, you will be able to do the following:

1  List the five phases of the nursing process.
2  Identify the components of the assessment process for patients receiving medications, including collection and analysis of subjective and objective data.
3  Discuss the process of formulating nursing diagnoses for patients receiving medications.
4  Identify goals and outcome criteria for patients receiving medications.
5  Discuss the evaluation process as it relates to the administration of medications and as reflected by goals and outcome criteria.

6  Develop a nursing care plan that is based on the nursing process as it relates to medication administration.
7  Briefly discuss the "Six Rights" associated with safe medication administration.
8  Discuss the professional responsibility and standards of practice for the professional nurse as related to the medication administration process.
9  Discuss the additional rights associated with safe medication administration.

## KEY TERMS

**Compliance** Implementation or fulfillment of a prescriber's or caregiver's prescribed course of treatment or therapeutic plan by a patient. Use of *compliance* versus *adherence* in this textbook is supportive of the terms used in the current listing of NANDA-I nursing diagnoses. (p. 8)

**Goals** Statements that are time specific and describe generally what is to be accomplished to address a specific nursing diagnosis. (p. 7)

**Medication error** Any preventable adverse drug event involving inappropriate medication use by a patient or health care professional; it may or may not cause the patient harm. (p. 15)

**Noncompliance** An informed decision on the part of the patient not to adhere to or follow a therapeutic plan or suggestion. Use of *noncompliance* versus *nonadherence* in this

textbook is supportive of the terms used in the current listing of NANDA-I nursing diagnoses. (p. 9)

**Nursing process** An organizational framework for the practice of nursing. It encompasses all steps taken by the nurse in caring for a patient: assessment, nursing diagnoses, planning (with goals and outcome criteria), implementation of the plan (with patient teaching), and evaluation. (p. 7)

**Outcome criteria** Descriptions of specific patient behaviors or responses that demonstrate meeting of or achievement of goals related to each nursing diagnosis. These statements, as with goals, are verifiable, framed in behavioral terms, measurable, and time specific. Outcome criteria are considered to be specific, whereas goals are broad. (p. 7)

**Prescriber** Any health care professional licensed by the appropriate regulatory board to prescribe medications. (p. 8)

## OVERVIEW OF THE NURSING PROCESS

The nursing process is a well-established, research-supported framework for professional nursing practice. It is a flexible, adaptable, and adjustable five-step process consisting of assessment, nursing diagnoses, planning (including establishment of goals and outcome criteria), implementation (including patient education), and evaluation. As such, the nursing process ensures the delivery of thorough, individualized, and quality nursing care to patients, regardless of age, gender, medical diagnosis, or setting. Through use of the nursing process combined with knowledge and skills, the professional nurse will be able to develop effective solutions to meet patient's needs. The nursing process is usually discussed in nursing courses and/or textbooks that deal with the fundamentals of nursing practice, nursing theory, physical assessment, adult or pediatric nursing, and other nursing specialty areas. However, because of the importance of the nursing process in the care of patients, the process in all of its five phases is described in each chapter as it relates to specific drug groups or classifications.

Critical thinking is a major part of the nursing process and involves the use of the mind and thought processes to gather information and then develop conclusions, make decisions, draw inferences, and reflect upon all aspects of patient care. The elements of the nursing process address the physical, emotional, spiritual, sexual, financial, cultural, and cognitive aspects of a patient. Attention to these many aspects allows a more holistic approach to patient care. For example, a cardiologist may focus on cardiac functioning and pathology, a physical therapist on movement, and a chaplain on the spiritual aspects of patient care. However, it is the professional nurse who thinks critically about, processes, and incorporates all of these aspects and points of information about the patient and then uses this information to develop and coordinate patient care. Therefore, the nursing process remains a central process and framework for nursing care. Box 1-1 provides guidelines for nursing care planning related to drug therapy and the nursing process.

## ASSESSMENT

During the initial assessment phase of the nursing process, data are collected, reviewed, and analyzed. Performing a comprehensive assessment allows you to formulate a nursing diagnosis related to the patient's needs—for the purposes of this textbook, specifically needs related to drug administration. Information about the patient may come from a variety of sources, including the patient; the patient's family, caregiver, or significant other; and the patient's chart. Methods of data collection include interviewing, direct and indirect questioning, observation, medical records review, head-to-toe physical examination, and a nursing assessment. Data are categorized into objective and subjective data. Objective data may be defined as any information gathered through the senses or that which is seen, heard, felt, or smelled. Objective data may also be obtained from a nursing physical assessment; nursing history; past and present medical history; results of laboratory tests, diagnostic studies, or procedures; measurement of vital signs, weight, and height; and medication profile. Medication profiles include, but are not limited to, the following information: any and all drug use; use of home or folk remedies and herbal and/or homeopathic treatments, plant or animal extracts, and dietary supplements; intake of alcohol, tobacco, and caffeine; current or past history of illegal drug use; use of over-the-counter (OTC) medications (e.g., aspirin, acetaminophen, vitamins, laxatives, cold preparations, sinus medications, antacids, acid reducers, antidiarrheals, minerals, elements); use of hormonal drugs (e.g., testosterone, estrogens, progestins, oral contraceptives); past and present health history and associated drug regimen(s); family history and racial, ethnic, and/or cultural attributes with attention to specific or different responses to medications as well as any unusual individual responses; and growth and developmental stage (e.g., Erikson's developmental tasks) and issues related to the patient's age and medication regimen. A holistic nursing assessment includes gathering of data about the whole individual, including physical/emotional realms, religious preference, health beliefs, sociocultural characteristics, race, ethnicity, lifestyle, stressors, socioeconomic status, educational level, motor skills, cognitive ability, support systems, lifestyle, and use of any alternative and complementary therapies. Subjective data include information shared through the spoken word by any reliable source, such as the patient, spouse, family member, significant other, and/or caregiver.

Assessment about the specific drug is also important and involves the collection of specific information about prescribed, OTC, and herbal/complementary/alternative therapeutic drug use, with attention to the drug's action; signs and symptoms of allergic reaction; adverse effects; dosages and routes of administration; contraindications; drug incompatibilities; drug-drug, drug-food, and drug–laboratory test interactions; and toxicities and available antidotes. Nursing pharmacology textbooks provide a more nursing-specific knowledge base regarding drug therapy as related to the nursing process. Use of current references or those dated within the last 3 years is highly recommended. Some examples of authoritative sources include the *Physicians' Desk Reference, Mosby's Drug Consult,* drug manufacturers' inserts, drug handbooks, and/or licensed pharmacists. Reliable online resources include, but are not limited to, the U.S. Pharmacopeia (USP) (http://www.usp.org), U.S. Food and Drug Administration (http://www.fda.gov), and http://www.WebMD.com. Other online resources are cited throughout this textbook.

Gather additional data about the patient and a given drug by asking these simple questions: What is the patient's oral intake? Tolerance of fluids? Swallowing ability for pills, tablets, capsules, and liquids? If there is difficulty swallowing, what is the degree of difficulty and are there solutions to the problem, such as use of thickening agents with fluids or use of other dosage forms? What are the results of laboratory and other diagnostic tests related to organ functioning and drug therapy? What do renal function studies (e.g., blood urea nitrogen level, serum creatinine level) show? What are the results of hepatic function tests (e.g., total protein level, serum levels of bilirubin, alkaline phosphatase,

## BOX 1-1    GUIDELINES FOR NURSING CARE PLANNING

This sample presents useful information for developing a nursing process–focused care plan for patients receiving medications. Brief listings and discussions of what must be contained in each phase of the nursing process are included. This sample may be used as a template for formatting nursing care plans in a variety of patient care situations/settings.

### Assessment
#### Objective Data
Objective data include information available through the senses, such as what is seen, felt, heard, and smelled. Among the sources of data are the chart, laboratory test results, reports of diagnostic procedures, physical assessment, and examination findings. Examples of specific data are age, height, weight, allergies, medication profile, and health history.

#### Subjective Data
Subjective data include all spoken information shared by the patient, such as complaints, problems, or stated needs (e.g., patient complains of "dizziness, headache, vomiting, and feeling hot for 10 days").

### Nursing Diagnoses
Once the assessment phase has been completed, the nurse analyzes objective and subjective data about the patient and the drug and formulates nursing diagnoses. The following is an example of a nursing diagnosis statement: "Deficient knowledge related to lack of experience with medication regimen and second-grade reading level as an adult as evidenced by inability to perform a return demonstration and inability to state adverse effects to report to the prescriber." This statement of the nursing diagnosis can be broken down into three parts, as follows:

- Part 1—"Deficient knowledge." This is the statement of the human response of the patient to illness, injury, medications, or significant change. This can be an actual response, an increased risk, or an opportunity to improve the patient's health status. The nursing diagnosis related to knowledge may be identified as either deficient or readiness for enhanced (knowledge).
- Part 2—"Related to lack of experience with medication regimen and second-grade reading level as an adult." This portion of the statement identifies factors related to the response; it often includes multiple factors with some degree of connection between them. The nursing diagnosis statement does not necessarily claim that there is a cause-and-effect link between these factors and the response, only that there is a connection.

- Part 3—"As evidenced by inability to perform a return demonstration and inability to state adverse effects to report to the prescriber." This statement lists clues, cues, evidence, and/or data that support the nurse's claim that the nursing diagnosis is accurate.

Nursing diagnoses are prioritized in order of criticality based on patient needs or problems. The ABCs of care (*a*irway, *b*reathing, and *c*irculation) are often used as a basis for prioritization. Prioritizing always begins with the most important, significant, or critical need of the patient. Nursing diagnoses that involve actual responses are always ranked above nursing diagnoses that involve only risks.

### Planning: Goals and Outcome Criteria
The planning phase includes the identification of goals and outcome criteria, provides time frames, and is patient oriented. Goals are objective, realistic, and measurable patient-centered statements with time frames and are broad, whereas outcome criteria are more specific descriptions of patient goals.

### Implementation
In the implementation phase, the nurse intervenes on behalf of the patient to address specific patient problems and needs. This is done through independent nursing actions; collaborative activities such as physical therapy, occupational therapy, and music therapy; and implementation of medical orders. Family, significant others, and caregivers assist in carrying out this phase of the nursing care plan. Specific interventions that relate to particular drugs (e.g., giving a particular cardiac drug only after monitoring the patient's pulse and blood pressure), nonpharmacologic interventions that enhance the therapeutic effects of medications, and patient education are major components of the implementation phase. See the previous text discussion of the nursing process for more information on nursing interventions.

### Evaluation
Evaluation is the part of the nursing process that includes monitoring whether patient goals and outcome criteria related to the nursing diagnoses are met. Monitoring includes observing for therapeutic effects of drug treatment as well as for adverse effects and toxicity. Many indicators are used to monitor these aspects of drug therapy as well as the results of appropriately related nonpharmacologic interventions. If the goals and outcome criteria are met, the nursing care plan may or may not be revised to include new nursing diagnoses; such changes are made only if appropriate. If goals and outcome criteria are not met, revisions are made to the entire nursing care plan with further evaluation.

---

creatinine phosphokinase, other liver enzymes)? What are the patient's white blood cell and red blood cell counts? Hemoglobin and hematocrit levels? Current as well as past health status and presence of illness? What are the patient's experiences with use of any drug regimen? What has been the patient's relationship with health care professionals and/or experiences with previous therapeutic regimens? What are current and past values for blood pressure, pulse rate, temperature, and respiratory rate? What medications is the patient currently taking, and how is the patient taking and tolerating them? Are there issues of compliance? Any use of folk medicines or folk remedies? What is the patient's understanding of the medication? Are there any age-related concerns? If patients are not reliable historians, family members, significant others, and/or caregivers may provide answers to these questions.

It is worth mentioning that there is often discussion about the difference between the terms *compliance* and *adherence*. Both of these terms, though not to be used interchangeably, are used to describe the extent to which patients take medications as prescribed. Often the term *adherence* is perceived as implying more collaboration and active role between patients and their providers (see Key Terms definition of *compliance*). Once assessment of the patient and the drug has been completed, the specific prescription or medication order (from any prescriber) must be checked for the following six elements: (1) patient's name, (2) date the drug order was written, (3) name of drug(s), (4) drug dosage amount and frequency, (5) route of administration, and (6) prescriber's signature.

It is also important during assessment to consider the traditional, nontraditional, expanded, and collaborative roles of the nurse. Physicians and dentists are no longer the only practitioners legally able to prescribe and write medication orders. Nurse practitioners and physician assistants have gained the professional privilege of legally prescribing medications. Remain current on legal regulations as well as specific state nurse practice acts and standards of care.

## Analysis of Data

Once data about the patient and drug have been collected and reviewed, critically analyze and synthesize the information. Verify all information and document appropriately, and it is at this point that the sum of the information about the patient and drug are used in the development of nursing diagnoses.

### CASE STUDY

#### The Nursing Process and Pharmacology

 Dollie, a 27-year-old social worker, is visiting the clinic today for a physical examination. She states that she and her husband want to "start a family," but she has not had a physical for several years. She was told when she was 22 years of age that she had "anemia" and was given iron tablets, but Dollie states that she has not taken them for years. She said she "felt better" and did not think she needed them. She denies any use of tobacco and illegal drugs; she states that she may have a drink with dinner once or twice a month. She uses tea tree oil on her face twice a day to reduce acne breakouts. She denies using any other drugs.

1. What other questions does the nurse need to ask during this assessment phase?
2. After laboratory work is performed, Dollie is told that she is slightly anemic. The prescriber recommends that she resume taking iron supplements as well as folic acid. She is willing to try again and says that she is "all about doing what's right to stay healthy and become a mother." What nursing diagnoses would be appropriate at this time?
3. Dollie is given a prescription that reads as follows: "Ferrous sulfate 325 mg, PO for anemia." When she goes to the pharmacy, the pharmacist tells her that the prescription is incomplete. What is missing? What should be done?
4. After 4 weeks, Dollie's latest laboratory results indicate that she still has anemia. However, Dollie states, "I feel so much better that I'm planning to stop taking the iron tablets. I hate to take medicine." How should the nurse handle this?

For answers, see http://evolve.elsevier.com/Lilley.

## NURSING DIAGNOSES

Nursing diagnoses are developed by professional nurses and are used as a means of communicating and sharing information about the patient and the patient experience. Nursing diagnoses are the result of critical thinking, creativity, and accurate collection of data regarding the patient as well as the drug. Nursing diagnoses related to drug therapy will most likely grow out of data associated with the following: deficient knowledge; risk for injury; noncompliance; and various disturbances, deficits, excesses, impairments in bodily functions, and/or other problems or concerns as related to drug therapy. The development and classification of nursing diagnoses has been carried out by the North American Nursing Diagnosis Association International (NANDA-I) (formerly NANDA). NANDA-I is the formal organization recognized by professional nursing groups (e.g., the American Nurses Association [ANA]). NANDA-I is considered to be the major contributor to the development of nursing knowledge and the leading authority (on nursing diagnoses). The purpose of NANDA-I is to increase the visibility

### BOX 1-2 A BRIEF LOOK AT NANDA AND THE NURSING PROCESS

The North American Nursing Diagnosis Association International (NANDA-I) (formerly NANDA) fulfills the following roles: (1) increases the visibility of nursing's contribution to patient care, (2) develops, refines, and classifies information and phenomena related to professional nursing practice, (3) provides a working organization for the development of evidence-based nursing diagnoses, and (4) supports the improvement of quality nursing care through evidence-based practice and access to a global network of professional nurses. In 1987, NANDA and the American Nurses Association endorsed a framework for establishing nursing diagnoses, and in 1990 *Nursing Diagnoses* became the official journal of NANDA. In 2001 and 2003, NANDA modified and updated the listing of nursing diagnoses, but nursing diagnoses continued to be submitted for consideration by the Ad Hoc Research Committee of NANDA. This period resulted in changes such as replacement of the phrase *potential for* with *risk for.* The terms *impaired, deficient, ineffective, decreased, increased,* and *imbalanced* replaced the outdated terms *altered* and *alteration,* although the outdated terms may still be in use. In 2002, NANDA changed its name to NANDA-I ("I" for international) to reflect the organization's global reach. In 2007-2008, there were 188 nursing diagnoses (up from 172) with changes to defining characteristics and related or risk factors. There were also some 15 newly approved nursing diagnoses. More changes occurred in the 2009-2011 version of NANDA-I's *Nursing Diagnoses: Definitions and Classifications,* with 21 new, 9 revised, and 6 retired nursing diagnoses. Most current is the *2012-2014 NANDA-I Approved Nursing Diagnoses.* There are 23 new, 33 revised, and 2 retired nursing diagnoses. Other changes are discussed in the 2012-2014 NANDA-I *Nursing Diagnoses: Definitions and Classifications.*

of nursing's contribution to the care of patients and to further develop, refine, and classify the information and phenomena related to nurses and professional nursing practice. In 2000, a classification system was adopted with a taxonomy including 13 domains divided into 106 classes and over 150 nursing diagnoses. Using this system, the nurse was able to choose a nursing diagnosis from the established list and individualize the nursing care plan. The 2009-2011 NANDA approved nursing diagnoses included many changes with revisions, as well as several new diagnoses and a listing of retired nursing diagnoses. The newest list, 2012-2014 NANDA-I approved nursing diagnoses, are still characterized with domains and classes but also with changes that include several new and revised nursing diagnoses or diagnoses with a key word changed. See Box 1-2 for more information about the 2012-2014 NANDA approved nursing diagnoses.

Formulation of nursing diagnoses is usually a three-step process with nursing diagnoses stated as follows: Part one of the statement is the human response of the patient to illness, injury, or significant change. This response can be an actual problem, an increased risk of developing a problem, or an opportunity or intent to improve the patient's health. Part two of the nursing diagnosis statement identifies the factor(s) related to the response, with more than one factor often named. The nursing diagnosis statement does not necessarily claim a cause-and-effect link between these factors and the response; it indicates only that there is a connection between them. Part three of the nursing diagnosis statement contains a listing of clues, cues, evidence, or other data that support the nurse's claim that this diagnosis is accurate. Tips for writing nursing diagnoses include

## BOX 1-3 CURRENT NANDA-I–APPROVED NURSING DIAGNOSES MOST RELEVANT TO DRUG THERAPY

Activity intolerance (and risk for)
Adverse reaction to iodinated contrast media, risk for*
Airway clearance, ineffective
Allergy response, latex (and risk for)
Aspiration, risk for
Bleeding, risk for
Body image, disturbed
Body temperature, risk for imbalanced
Breathing pattern, ineffective
Cardiac output, decreased
Caregiver role strain (and risk for)
Comfort, impaired (and readiness for enhanced)
Communication, readiness for enhanced
Confusion (acute, chronic, or risk for acute)
Constipation (perceived and risk for)
Coping (defensive, ineffective, and readiness for enhanced)
Death anxiety†
Decision-making, readiness for enhanced
Diarrhea
Electrolyte imbalance, risk for
Falls, risk for
Fatigue
Fear
Fluid volume, deficient (and excess, risk for deficient, and risk for imbalanced)
Gas exchange, impaired
Growth and development, delayed
Health maintenance, ineffective
Home maintenance, impaired
Health-seeking behaviors±
Human dignity, risk for compromised
Hyperthermia
Hypothermia
Immunization status, readiness for enhanced
Incontinence (functional urinary, overflow urinary, reflex urinary, stress urinary, urge urinary, risk for urge urinary)
Infection, risk for
Injury, risk for
Insomnia

Knowledge (deficient, readiness for enhanced)
Latex allergy response, risk for*
Lifestyle, sedentary
Liver function, risk for impaired
Loneliness, risk for
Memory, impaired
Mobility (impaired bed, impaired physical, impaired wheelchair)
Nausea
Noncompliance
Nutrition, imbalanced (less than body requirements, more than body requirements, risk for imbalanced, readiness for enhanced)
Oral mucous membrane, impaired
Pain (acute, chronic)
Peripheral neurovascular dysfunction, risk for
Poisoning, risk for
Powerlessness (and risk for)
Self-care deficit (bathing, dressing)†
Self-esteem, chronic low (and risk for)*
Self-esteem, low (situational, risk for situational)
Self-health management (ineffective and readiness for enhanced)†
Sensory perception, disturbed±
Sexual dysfunction
Sexuality pattern, ineffective
Skin integrity, impaired (and risk for)
Sleep deprivation
Sleep pattern, disturbed
Stress overload
Suicide, risk for
Surgical recovery, delayed
Swallowing, impaired
Therapeutic regimen management, ineffective family
Tissue integrity, impaired
Tissue perfusion (risk for decreased cardiac, risk for ineffective cerebral, risk for ineffective peripheral)†
Urinary elimination (impaired, readiness for enhanced)
Urinary retention
Verbal communication, impaired†
Walking, impaired

From *Nursing diagnoses: definitions and classification 20012-2014.* Copyright © 2012, 1994-2012 by NANDA International. Used by arrangement with Wiley-Blackwell Publishing, a company of John Wiley & Sons.
*New nursing diagnosis.
†Revised nursing diagnoses or diagnoses in which a key word has changed.
±Retired nursing diagnoses.
*NANDA-I,* North American Nursing Diagnosis Association.

the following: begin with a statement of a human response; connect the first part of the statement or the human response with the second part, the cause, using the phrase "related to"; be sure that the first two parts are not restatements of one another; include several factors in the second part of the statement, such as associated factors, if appropriate; select a cause for the second part of the statement that can be changed by nursing interventions; avoid negative wording or language; and, finally, list clues or cues that led to the nursing diagnosis in the third part of the statement, which may also include more defining characteristics (e.g., "as evidenced by"). A listing of NANDA-approved nursing diagnoses (2012-2014) most relevant to drug therapy

is provided in Box 1-3. These nursing diagnoses, as well as all other phases of the nursing process, will be presented in the chapters that follow because the nursing process provides the framework of practice for all professional nurses and is also used to organize the nursing sections of this textbook.

## PLANNING

After data are collected and nursing diagnoses are formulated, the planning phase begins; this includes identification of goals and outcome criteria. The major purposes of the planning phase are to prioritize the nursing diagnoses and specify goals and outcome criteria, including the time frame for their achievement. The planning phase provides time to obtain special equipment for interventions, review the possible procedures or techniques to be used, and gather information for oneself (the nurse) or for the patient. This step leads to the provision of safe care if professional judgment is combined with the acquisition of knowledge about the patient and the medications to be given.

## Goals and Outcome Criteria

Goals are objective, measurable, and realistic, with an established time period for achievement of the outcomes, which are specifically stated in the outcome criteria. Patient goals reflect expected and measurable changes in behavior through nursing care and are developed in collaboration with the patient. Patient goals developed in the planning phase of the nursing process are behavior based and may be categorized into physiologic, psychological, spiritual, sexual, cognitive, motor, and/or other domains.

Outcome criteria are concrete descriptions of patient goals. They are patient focused, succinct, and well thought out. Outcome criteria also include expectations for behavior indicating something that can be changed and with a specific time frame or deadline. The ultimate aim of these criteria is the safe and effective administration of medications. Outcome criteria also reflect each nursing diagnosis and serve as a guide to the implementation phase of the nursing process. Formulation of outcome criteria begins with the analysis of the judgments made about patient data and subsequent nursing diagnoses and ends with the development of a nursing care plan. Outcome criteria provide a standard for measuring movement toward goals. With regard to medication administration, these outcomes may address special storage and handling techniques, administration procedures, equipment needed, drug interactions, adverse effects, and contraindications. In this textbook, specific time frames are *not* provided in each chapter's nursing process section because patient care is individualized in every situation.

## IMPLEMENTATION

Implementation is guided by the preceding phases of the nursing process (i.e., assessment, nursing diagnoses, and planning). Implementation requires constant communication and collaboration with the patient and with members of the health care team involved in the patient's care, as well as with any family members, significant others, or other caregivers. Implementation consists of initiation and completion of specific nursing actions as defined by nursing diagnoses, goals, and outcome criteria. Implementation of nursing actions may be independent, collaborative, or dependent upon a prescriber's order. Statements of interventions include frequency, specific instructions, and any other pertinent information. With medication administration, you need to know and understand all of the information about the patient and about each medication prescribed (see assessment questions). In years past, nurses adhered to the "Five Rights" of medication administration: right drug, right dose, right time, right route, and right patient. However, continued support exists for referring to "Six Rights" of medication administration

with the addition of "right documentation." The Six Rights are discussed in detail in the next section. These "rights" of medication administration have been identified as basic standards of care as related to drug therapy. However, even implementation of the Six Rights does not reflect the complexity of the role of the professional nurse because they focus more on the individual/patient than on the system as a whole or the entire medication administration process beginning with the prescriber's order. Viewed from an individual/patient focus, there are additional rights (or entitlements) to be considered when administering medications. These include the right to:

- Patient safety, ensured by use of the correct procedures, equipment, and techniques of medication administration and documentation
- Individualized, holistic, accurate, and complete patient education
- Double-checking and constant analysis of the system (i.e., the process of drug administration including all personnel involved, such as the prescriber, the nurse, the nursing unit, and the pharmacy department, as well as patient education)
- Proper drug storage
- Accurate calculation and preparation of the dose of medication and proper use of all types of medication delivery systems
- Careful checking of the transcription of medication orders
- Accurate use of the various routes of administration and awareness of the specific implications of their use
- Close consideration of special situations (e.g., patient difficulty in swallowing, use of a nasogastric tube, unconsciousness of the patient, advanced patient age)
- Implementation of all appropriate measures to prevent and report medication errors

## Six Rights of Medication Administration
### Right Drug

The "right drug" begins with the registered nurse's valid license to practice. Some states allow currently licensed practical nurses to administer medications with specific guidelines. The registered nurse is responsible for checking all medication orders and/or prescriptions. To ensure that the correct drug is given, you must check the specific medication order against the medication label or profile three times before giving the medication. Conduct the first check of the right drug/drug name while you prepare the medication for administration. At this time, consider whether the drug is appropriate for the patient and, if doubt exists or an error is deemed possible, contact the prescriber and/pharmacist immediately. It is also appropriate at this time to note the drug's indication and be aware that a drug may have multiple indications, including off-label use and non–FDA-approved indications. In this textbook, each particular drug is discussed in the chapter that deals with its main indication, but the drug may also be cross-referenced in other chapters if it has multiple uses.

All medication orders or prescriptions are required by law to be signed by the prescriber involved in the patient's care. If a verbal order is given, the prescriber must sign the order within 24 hours or as per facility protocol. Verbal and/or telephone

**EVIDENCE-BASED PRACTICE**

## *Improving Retention, Confidence, and Competence of New Graduate Nurses: A 10-Year Longitudinal Study*

### Review

In 1999, the Children's Hospital Los Angeles (CHLA) found that despite efforts and monies to support their internship for new graduate nurses, they continued to experience a high turnover rate: 36% of new graduates hired were leaving in less than 12 months, and 56% were leaving within 2 years. The vicious cycle of hiring, educating, and rehiring resulted in negative influences on nursing and patient care. With key nursing leaders from CHLA, the next 10 years were spent trying to find improved ways to attract new graduates into the profession and the hospital. Aggressive development, evaluation, and ideas for improvement led to a RN residency program with results of positive outcomes for hospitals, new graduates, and patient care. A model for successful "recruiting, engaging, and retaining new graduate nurses" was a beneficial outcome for CHLA and the nursing profession.

### Type of Evidence

Development of the Versant RN residency program (1999) began as a 1-year pilot study with approximately 700 hours of guided clinical experience for each new graduate nurse with a one-on-one preceptor. Additionally, a mentor was assigned for each new graduate, and debriefing and self-care sessions to discuss practice issues and subsequent strategies were held. These hours of clinical included other experiences in other areas/departments of the hospital with approximately 225 hours of didactic time with corresponding hands-on skills training sessions. The pilot study's goals were to help with transition of the new graduate to the role of the professional RN; increase level of self-confidence; and provide competent, safe, and quality care while also increasing retention of new graduates within the organization. Development of the RN residency was initially treated as a basic research effort and all those who participated (organizations) had to obtain institutional review board approval prior to implementing the program. As the programs were initiated throughout the country in various hospital settings, research continued. In 2009, there were 10 years of evidence-based outcomes with support of the success of the RN residency program. At this 10-year time period, Versant moved the residency program out of traditional research status. However, data collection protocols are still intact and continue to be followed with confidentiality of responses in the measurement instruments and evaluations.

Measures used to evaluate the pilot study included self-report and observation instruments with previously established reliability and validity. Demographic and evaluation instruments were also developed for the pilot. Additional measurements included the Slater Nursing Competencies Rating Scale (Wandelt and Stewart, 1975). After completion of the pilot study, several other hospitals in California had participated. By July 2003, 118 new graduates had completed the residency program at these sites. With the increase in programs, CHLA created Versant in 2004 and then launched a web-based management system, Voyager, to provide access to the residency curriculum, measurement instruments, and other information for individual residents related to competency achievement and goal progression.

### Results of the Study

Results of the residency program indicated that graduates who were hired had equal or better results on all concept outcome measures. Concepts measured included, but were not limited to, the following: competency, satisfaction, confidence, empowerment/autonomy/role dissonance, group cohesion/organizational commitment, and turnover intent. Results of the pilot study indicated that the graduates hired in the residency program had equal or better results on all measures. The pilot study then continued forward with 56 graduates. There was also modification of measurement instruments and use of a new competency rating scale (see Slater Nursing Competencies Rating Scale). Data analysis performed on the Versant National Database included various statistics including data reduction, correlation matrix analysis, descriptive statistics for demographics, and regression analysis.

Following the pilot study, more pediatric hospitals in California participated and results indicated that the program was appropriate for use in other hospitals. Furthermore, to make this happen at a national level, it was maintained that a business model with an easy method of collecting/accessing/sharing data and information needed to be developed and implemented. CHLA created Versant and then launched a web-based management system (see Type of Evidence). At the end of the 10-year mark, over 6000 new graduates had completed the Versant RN residency. Participants were from small rural hospitals to large health care systems.

### Link of Evidence to Nursing Practice

After collection of data over a 10-year period and reflection back on the research, there are definite actions needed (not only on an individual level but on an organizational level) to achieve positive, successful outcomes in an RN residency program. Some of these outcomes include defining a set of standards based upon competencies that are outcome validated; teaching to those same standards; monitoring as well as managing the individual and organizational adherence to those standards; and use of quantitative as well as qualitative outcome measures to objectively evaluate the successful performance of competencies in the new graduate. Key characteristics identified in a successful RN residency program include standardization, evidence-based content/curriculum, clinical immersion, support systems (e.g., preceptors and/or experts), accountability, communication, consistent and precise evaluations, individual and organization-wide commitment, a management system for performance and outcomes, research and development, continuous outcome-driven program improvement, and a delivery system with structured framework for managing an RN residency program at an individual hospital setting or at a health care system. This fascinating study and its results support the need for a clinical immersion program for new graduate nurses. The authors recommend that an 18-week program be implemented with dedicated preceptors and extensive follow-up of the RN residents. The results also support the need for mentoring, ongoing support and guidance throughout the first year of practice for the RN resident. Further studies of significance to nursing practice included the need for additional structural supportive components throughout the first year as well as development of further evaluation and coaching strategies to help everyone focus on the residents and long-term success in nursing.

Reference: Ulrich B, Krozek C, Early S, et al: Improving retention, confidence, and competence of new graduate nurses: results from a 10-year longitudinal database, *Nurs Econ* 28(6):363-375, 2010.

orders are often used in emergencies and time-sensitive patient care situations. To be sure that the right drug is given, information about the patient and drug (see previous discussion of the assessment phase) must be obtained to make certain that all variables and data have been considered. Approved, current authoritative references (see earlier discussion) are the reliable sources of information about prescribed drugs. Avoid relying upon the knowledge of peers as this is unsafe nursing practice.

Remain current in your knowledge of generic (nonproprietary) drug names as well as trade names (proprietary name that is registered by a specific drug manufacturer); however, use of the drug's generic name is now preferred in clinical practice to reduce the risk of medication errors. A single drug often has numerous trade names, and drugs in different classes may have similarly spelled names, increasing the possibility of medication errors. Therefore, when it comes to the "right drug" phase of the medication administration process, use of a drug's generic name is recommended to help avoid a medication error and enhance patient safety. (See Chapter 2 for more information on the naming of drugs).

If there are questions about the medication order at any time during the medication administration process, contact the prescriber for clarification. Never make any assumptions when it comes to drug administration, and, as previously emphasized in this chapter, confirm at least three times the right drug, right dose, right time, right route, right patient, and right documentation before giving the medication.

## Right Dose

Whenever a medication is ordered, a dosage is identified from the prescriber's order. Always check the dose and confirm that it is appropriate for the patient's age and size. Also, check the prescribed dose against the available drug stocks and against the normal dosage range. Recheck all mathematical calculations, and pay careful attention to decimal points, the misplacement of which could lead to a tenfold or even greater overdose. Leading zeros, or zeros placed before a decimal point, are allowed, but trailing zeros, or zeros following the decimal point, are to be avoided. For example, 0.2 mg is allowed, but 2.0 mg is not acceptable, because it could easily be mistaken for 20 mg, especially with unclear penmanship. Patient variables (e.g., vital signs, age, gender, weight, height) require careful assessment because of the need for dosage adjustments in response to specific parameters. Pediatric and elderly patients are more sensitive to medications than younger and middle-age adult patients; thus, use extra caution with drug dosage amounts for these patients.

---

### ⚡ SAFETY AND QUALITY IMPROVEMENT: PREVENTING MEDICATION ERRORS

#### Right Dose?

The nurse is reviewing the orders for a newly admitted patient. One order reads: "Tylenol, 2 tablets PO, every 4 hours as needed for pain or fever."

The pharmacist calls to clarify this order, saying, "The dose is not clear." What does the pharmacist mean by this? The order says "2 tablets." Isn't that the dose?

NO! If you look up Tylenol (acetaminophen) in a drug resource book, you will see that Tylenol tablets are available in strengths of both 325 mg and 500 mg. The order is missing the "right dose" and needs to be clarified. *Never* assume the dose of a medication order!

---

## Right Time

Each health care agency or institution has a policy regarding routine medication administration times; therefore, always check this policy. However, when giving a medication at the prescribed time, you may be confronted with a conflict between the timing suggested by the prescriber and specific pharmacokinetic or pharmacodynamic drug properties, concurrent drug therapy, dietary influences, laboratory and/or diagnostic testing, and specific patient variables. For example, the prescribed right time for administration of antihypertensive drugs may be four times a day, but for an active, professional 42-year-old male patient working 14 hours a

day, taking a medication four times daily may not be feasible, and this regimen may lead to noncompliance and subsequent complications. Appropriate actions include contacting the prescriber and inquiring about the possibility of prescribing another drug with a different dosing frequency (e.g., once or twice daily).

For routine medication orders, give the medications no more than ½ hour before or after the actual time specified in the prescriber's order (i.e., if a medication is ordered to be given at 0900 every morning, you may give it at any time between 0830 and 0930); the exception is medications designated to be given stat (immediately), which you must administer within ½ hour of the time the order is written. Assess and follow the hospital or facility policy and procedure for any other specific information concerning the "½ hour before or after" rule. For medication orders with the annotation "prn" (*pro re nata*, or "as required"), you must give the medication at special times and under certain circumstances. For example, an analgesic is ordered every 4 to 6 hours *prn* for pain; after one dose of the medication, the patient complains of pain. After assessment, intervention with another dose of analgesic would occur, but only 4 to 6 hours after the previous dose. In addition, because of the increasing incidence of medication errors related to the use of abbreviations, many prescribers are using the wording "as required" or "as needed" instead of the abbreviation "prn." Military time is used when medication and other orders are written into a patient's chart (Table 1-1).

---

### TABLE 1-1  CONVERSION OF STANDARD TIME TO MILITARY TIME

| STANDARD TIME | MILITARY TIME |
|---|---|
| 1 AM | 0100 |
| 2 AM | 0200 |
| 3 AM | 0300 |
| 4 AM | 0400 |
| 5 AM | 0500 |
| 6 AM | 0600 |
| 7 AM | 0700 |
| 8 AM | 0800 |
| 9 AM | 0900 |
| 10 AM | 1000 |
| 11 AM | 1100 |
| 12 PM (noon) | 1200 |
| 1 PM | 1300 |
| 2 PM | 1400 |
| 3 PM | 1500 |
| 4 PM | 1600 |
| 5 PM | 1700 |
| 6 PM | 1800 |
| 7 PM | 1900 |
| 8 PM | 2000 |
| 9 PM | 2100 |
| 10 PM | 2200 |
| 11 PM | 2300 |
| 12 AM (midnight) | 2400 |

Nursing judgment may lead to some variations in timing, and you must document any change and the rationale for the change. If medications are ordered to be given once every day, twice daily, three times daily, or even four times daily, the times of administration may be changed if it is not harmful to the patient or if the medication or the patient's condition does not require adherence to an exact schedule, but only if the change is approved by the prescriber. For example, suppose that an antacid is ordered to be given three times daily at 0900, 1300, and 1700, but the nurse has misread the order and gives the first dose at 1100. Depending on the hospital or facility policy, the medication, and the patient's condition, such an occurrence may not be considered an error, because the dosing may be changed once the prescriber is contacted, so that the drug is given at 1100, 1500, and 1900 without harm to the patient and without incident to the nurse. If this were an antihypertensive medication, the patient's condition and well-being could be greatly compromised by one missed or late dose. Thus, falling behind in dosing times is not to be taken lightly or ignored. Never underestimate the effect of a change in the dosing or timing of medication, because one missed dose of certain medications can be life threatening.

Other factors must be considered in determining the right time, such as multiple-drug therapy, drug-drug or drug-food compatibility, scheduling of diagnostic studies, bioavailability of the drug (e.g., the need for consistent timing of doses around the clock to maintain blood levels), drug actions, and any biorhythm effects such as occur with steroids. It is also critical to patient safety to avoid using abbreviations for *any* component of a drug order (i.e., dose, time, route). Spell out *all* terms (e.g., *three times daily* instead of *tid*) in their entirety. Be careful to write out all words and abbreviations, because the possibility of miscommunication or misinterpretation poses a risk to the patient.

## Right Route

As previously stated, you must know the particulars about each medication before administering it to ensure that the right drug, dose, and route are being used. A complete medication order includes the route of administration. If a medication order does not include the route, be sure to ask the prescriber to clarify it. Never *assume* the route of administration.

## Right Patient

Checking the patient's identity before giving each medication dose is critical to the patient's safety. Ask the patient to state his or her name, and then check the patient's identification band to confirm the patient's name, identification number, age, and allergies. With pediatric patients, the parents and/or legal guardians are often the ones who identify the patient for the purpose of administration of prescribed medications. With newborns and in labor and delivery situations, the mother and baby have identification bracelets with matching numbers, which must be checked before giving medications. With elderly patients or patients with altered sensorium or level of consciousness, asking the patient his or her name or having the patient state his or her name is neither realistic nor safe. Therefore, checking

the identification band against the medication profile, medication order, or other treatment or service orders is crucial to avoid errors. In 2008, The Joint Commission released National Patient Safety Goals for patient care. These goals emphasize the use of two identifiers when providing care, treatment, or services to patients. To meet these goals, The Joint Commission recommends that the patient be identified "reliably" and also that the service or treatment (e.g., medication administration) be matched to that individual. The Joint Commission's statement of National Patient Safety Goals indicates that the two identifiers may be in the same location, such as on a wristband. In fact, it is patient-specific information that is the identifier. Acceptable identifiers include the patient's name, an assigned identification number, a telephone number, or other patient-specific identifier. Armbands are commonly used in the acute care setting and may serve as one identifier, with the other one being date of birth, Social Security number, or home address.

## Right Documentation

Documentation of information related to medication administration is crucial to patient safety. Recording patient observations and nursing actions has always been an important ethical responsibility, but now it is becoming a major medical-legal consideration as well. Because of its significance in professional nursing practice, correct documentation is becoming known as the "sixth right" of medication administration. Always assess the patient's chart for the presence of the following information: date and time of medication administration, name of medication, dose, route, and site of administration. Documentation of drug action may also be made in the regularly scheduled assessments for changes in symptoms the patient is experiencing, adverse effects, toxicity, and any other drug-related physical and/or psychological symptoms. Documentation must also reflect any improvement in the patient's condition, symptoms, or disease process as well as no change or a lack of improvement. You must not only document these observations, but report them to the prescriber promptly in keeping with your critical thinking and judgment. Document any teaching, as well as an assessment of the degree of understanding exhibited by the patient. Other information that needs documentation includes the following: (1) if a drug is *not* administered with the reason why and any actions taken, (2) refusal of a medication with information about the reason for refusal, if possible; if a medication is refused, respect the patient's right (to refuse), determine the reason, take appropriate action including notifying the prescriber, and revise the nursing care plan; never return unwrapped medication to a container, and discard according to agency policy; if wrapper remains intact, return medication to the pharmacy and revise the nursing care plan as needed; (3) actual time of drug administration; and (4) data regarding clinical observations and treatment of the patient if a medication error has occurred. If there is a medication error, complete an incident report with the entire event, surrounding circumstances, therapeutic response, adverse effects, and notification of the prescriber described in detail. However, do not record completion of an incident report in the medical chart.

## Medication Errors

When the Six Rights (and other rights) of drug administration are discussed, medication errors must be considered. Medication errors are a major problem for all of health care, regardless of the setting. The National Coordinating Council for Medication Error Reporting and Prevention defines a medication error as any *preventable* event that may cause or lead to inappropriate medication use or patient harm while the medication is in the control of the health care professional, patient, or consumer. Such events may be related to professional practice, health care products, procedures, or systems, including prescribing; order communication; product labeling, packaging, and nomenclature; compounding; dispensing; distribution; administration; education; monitoring; and use (http://www.nccmerp.org/about MedErrors.html). Both patient-related and system-related factors must always be considered when the medication administration process and the prevention of medication errors are being examined. See Chapter 5 for further discussion of medication errors and their prevention.

## EVALUATION

Evaluation occurs after the nursing care plan has been implemented. It is systematic, ongoing, and a dynamic phase of the nursing process as related to drug therapy. It includes monitoring the fulfillment of goals and outcome criteria, as well as monitoring the patient's therapeutic response to the drug and its adverse effects and toxic effects. Documentation is also a very important component of evaluation and consists of clear, concise, abbreviation-free charting that records information related to goals and outcome criteria as well as information related to any aspect of the medication administration process, including therapeutic effects versus adverse effects or toxic effects of medications (see the Teamwork and Collaboration: Legal and Ethical Principles box).

Evaluation also includes monitoring the implementation of standards of care. Several standards are in place to help in the evaluation of outcomes of care, such as those established by state nurse practice acts and by The Joint Commission.

### TEAMWORK AND COLLABORATION: LEGAL AND ETHICAL PRINCIPLES

#### Charting Don'ts

- Don't record staffing problems (don't mention them in a patient's chart, but instead talk with the nurse manager and/or other appropriate personnel).
- Don't record a peer's conflicts, such as charting possible disputes between a patient and a nurse.
- Don't mention the term *incident report* in charting. These reports are confidential and filed separately. Chart only the facts of the medication error or incident and appropriate actions taken.
- Don't use the following terms: *by mistake, by accident, accidentally, unintentional,* or *miscalculated.*
- Don't chart anything but facts.
- Don't chart casual conversations with peers, prescribers, or other members of the health care team.
- Don't use abbreviations. Some agencies or facilities may still keep a list of approved abbreviations, but overall their use is discouraged.
- Don't use negative language!

Modified from Institute for Safe Medication Practices: *ISMP Medication Safety Alert,* Huntingdon Valley, PA, February 20, 2003, The Institute; and InjuryBoard.com: Medication and prescription errors, available at http://www.injuryboard.com.

Guidelines for nursing services policies and procedures are established by The Joint Commission. There are even specific standards regarding medication administration to protect both the patient and the nurse. The ANA *Code of Ethics* and Patient Rights statement are also used in establishing and evaluating standards of care.

In summary, the nursing process is an ongoing and constantly evolving process (see Box 1-1). The nursing process, as it relates to drug therapy, involves the way in which a nurse gathers, analyzes, organizes, provides, and acts upon data about the patient within the context of prudent nursing care and standards of care. The nurse's ability to make astute assessments, formulate sound nursing diagnoses, establish goals and outcome criteria, correctly administer drugs, and continually evaluate patients' responses to drugs increases with additional experience and knowledge.

## KEY POINTS

- The nursing process is an ongoing, constantly changing and evolving framework for professional nursing practice. It may be applied to all facets of nursing care, including medication administration.
- The phases of the nursing process include assessment; development of nursing diagnoses; planning, with establishment of goals and outcome criteria; implementation, including patient education; and evaluation.
- Nursing diagnoses are formulated based on objective and subjective data and help to drive the nursing care plan. Nursing diagnoses have been developed through a formal process conducted by NANDA-I and are constantly updated and revised. Safe, therapeutic, and effective medication

administration is a major responsibility of professional nurses as they apply the nursing process to the care of their patients.
- Nurses are responsible for safe and prudent decision-making in the nursing care of their patients, including the provision of drug therapy; in accomplishing this task, they attend to the Six Rights and adhere to legal and ethical standards related to medication administration and documentation. There are additional rights related to drug administration. These rights deserve worthy consideration before initiation of the medication administration process. Observance of all of these rights enhances patient safety and helps avoid medication errors.

# NCLEX® EXAMINATION REVIEW QUESTIONS

1  An 86-year-old patient is being discharged to home on digitalis therapy and has very little information regarding the medication. Which statement best reflects a realistic outcome of patient teaching activities?
   a  The patient and patient's daughter will state the proper way to take the drug.
   b  The nurse will provide teaching about the drug's adverse effects.
   c  The patient will state all the symptoms of digitalis toxicity.
   d  The patient will call the prescriber if adverse effects occur.

2  A patient has a new prescription for a blood pressure medication that may cause him to feel dizzy during the first few days of therapy. Which is the best nursing diagnosis for this situation?
   a  Activity intolerance
   b  Risk for injury
   c  Disturbed body image
   d  Self-care deficit

3  A patient's chart includes an order that reads as follows: "Lanoxin 250 mcg once daily at 0900." Which action by the nurse is correct?
   a  The nurse gives the drug via the transdermal route.
   b  The nurse gives the drug orally.
   c  The nurse gives the drug intravenously.
   d  The nurse contacts the prescriber to clarify the dosage route.

4  The nurse is compiling a drug history for a patient. Which question from the nurse will obtain the most information from the patient?
   a  "Do you depend on sleeping pills to get to sleep?"
   b  "Do you have a family history of heart disease?"
   c  "When you have pain, what do you do to relieve it?"
   d  "What childhood diseases did you have?"

5  A 77-year-old man who has been diagnosed with an upper respiratory tract infection tells the nurse that he is allergic to penicillin. Which is the most appropriate response by the nurse?
   a  "That's to be expected—lots of people are allergic to penicillin."
   b  "This allergy is not of major concern because the drug is given so commonly."
   c  "What type of reaction did you have when you took penicillin?"
   d  "Drug allergies don't usually occur in older individuals because they have built up resistance."

6  The nurse is preparing a care plan for a patient who has been newly diagnosed with type 2 diabetes mellitus. Put into correct order the steps of the nursing process, with 1 being the first step and 5 being the last step.
   a  Implementation
   b  Planning
   c  Assessment
   d  Evaluation
   e  Nursing diagnoses

7  The nurse is reviewing new medication orders that have been written for a newly admitted patient. The nurse will need to clarify which orders? *Select all that apply.*
   a  Metformin (Glucophage) 1000 mg PO twice a day
   b  Sitagliptin (Januvia) 50 mg daily
   c  Simvastatin (Zocor) 20 mg PO every evening
   d  Irbesartan (Avapro) 300 mg PO once a day
   e  Docusate (Colace) as needed for constipation

1. a, 2. b, 3. d, 4. c, 5. c, 6. a = 4, b = 3, c = 1, d = 5, e = 2, 7. b, e

For Critical Thinking and Prioritization Questions, see http://evolve.elsevier.com/Lilley

# Pharmacologic Principles

## OBJECTIVES

When you reach the end of this chapter, you will be able to do the following:

1. Define the common terms used in pharmacology (see Key Terms).
2. Understand the general concepts such as pharmaceutics, pharmacokinetics, and pharmacodynamics and their application in drug therapy and the nursing process.
3. Demonstrate an understanding of the various drug dosage forms as related to drug therapy and the nursing process.
4. Discuss the relevance of the four aspects of pharmacokinetics (absorption, distribution, metabolism, excretion) to professional nursing practice as related to drug therapy for a variety of patients and health care settings.
5. Discuss the use of natural drug sources in the development of new drugs.
6. Develop a nursing care plan that takes into account general pharmacologic principles, specifically pharmacokinetic principles, as they relate to the nursing process.

## KEY TERMS

**Additive effects** Drug interactions in which the effect of a combination of two or more drugs with similar actions is equivalent to the sum of the individual effects of the same drugs given alone. For example, 1 + 1 = 2 (compare with synergistic effects). (p. 33)

**Adverse drug event** Any undesirable occurrence related to administering or failing to administer a prescribed medication. (p. 33)

**Adverse drug reaction** Any unexpected, unintended, undesired, or excessive response to a medication given at therapeutic dosages (as opposed to overdose). (p. 34)

**Adverse effects** A general term for any undesirable effects that are a direct response to one or more drugs. (p. 31)

**Agonist** A drug that binds to and stimulates the activity of one or more receptors in the body. (p. 30)

**Allergic reaction** An immunologic hypersensitivity reaction resulting from the unusual sensitivity of a patient to a particular medication; a type of adverse drug event. (p. 34)

**Antagonist** A drug that binds to and inhibits the activity of one or more receptors in the body. Antagonists are also called *inhibitors*. (p. 30)

**Antagonistic effects** Drug interactions in which the effect of a combination of two or more drugs is less than the sum of the individual effects of the same drugs given alone (1 + 1 equals less than 2); it is usually caused by an antagonizing (blocking or reducing) effect of one drug on another. (p. 33)

**Bioavailability** A measure of the extent of drug absorption for a given drug and route (from 0% to 100%). (p. 22)

**Biotransformation** One or more biochemical reactions involving a parent drug. Biotransformation occurs mainly in the liver and produces a metabolite that is either inactive or active. Also known as *metabolism*. (p. 27)

## KEY TERMS—cont'd

**Blood-brain barrier** The barrier system that restricts the passage of various chemicals and microscopic entities (e.g., bacteria, viruses) between the bloodstream and the central nervous system. It still allows for the passage of essential substances such as oxygen. (p. 27)

**Chemical name** The name that describes the chemical composition and molecular structure of a drug. (p. 19)

**Contraindication** Any condition, especially one related to a disease state or patient characteristic, including current or recent drug therapy, that renders a particular form of treatment improper or undesirable. (p. 31)

**Cytochrome P-450** The general name for a large class of enzymes that play a significant role in drug metabolism and drug interactions. (p. 27)

**Dependence** A state in which there is a compulsive or chronic need, as for a drug. (p. 32)

**Dissolution** The process by which solid forms of drugs disintegrate in the gastrointestinal tract and become soluble before being absorbed into the circulation. (p. 21)

**Drug** Any chemical that affects the physiologic processes of a living organism. (p. 19)

**Drug actions** The processes involved in the interaction between a drug and body cells (e.g., the action of a drug on a receptor protein); also called *mechanism of action.* (p. 20)

**Drug classification** A method of grouping drugs; may be based on structure or therapeutic use. (p. 20)

**Drug effects** The physiologic reactions of the body to a drug. They can be therapeutic or toxic and describe how the body is affected as a whole by the drug. The terms *onset, peak,* and *duration* are used to describe drug effects (most often referring to therapeutic effects). (p. 29)

**Drug-induced teratogenesis** The development of congenital anomalies or defects in the developing fetus caused by the toxic effects of drugs. (p. 35)

**Drug interaction** Alteration in the pharmacologic or pharmacokinetic activity of a given drug caused by the presence of one or more additional drugs; it is usually related to effects on the enzymes required for metabolism of the involved drugs. (p. 32)

**Duration of action** The length of time the concentration of a drug in the blood or tissues is sufficient to elicit a response. (p. 29)

**Enzymes** Protein molecules that catalyze one or more of a variety of biochemical reactions, including those related to the body's physiologic processes as well as those related to drug metabolism. (p. 30)

**First-pass effect** The initial metabolism in the liver of a drug absorbed from the gastrointestinal tract before the drug reaches systemic circulation through the bloodstream. (p. 22)

**Generic name** The name given to a drug by the United States Adopted Names Council. Also called the *nonproprietary name.* The generic name is much shorter and simpler than the chemical name and is not protected by trademark. (p. 19)

**Glucose-6-phosphate dehydrogenase (G6PD) deficiency** A hereditary condition in which red blood cells break down when the body is exposed to certain drugs. (p. 34)

**Half-life** In pharmacokinetics, the time required for half of an administered dose of drug to be eliminated by the body, or the time it takes for the blood level of a drug to be reduced by 50% (also called *elimination half-life*). (p. 29)

**Idiosyncratic reaction** An abnormal and unexpected response to a medication, other than an allergic reaction, that is peculiar to an individual patient. (p. 34)

**Incompatibility** The characteristic that causes two parenteral drugs or solutions to undergo a reaction when mixed or given together that results in the chemical deterioration of at least one of the drugs. (p. 33)

**Intraarterial** Within an artery (e.g., intraarterial injection). (p. 23)

**Intraarticular** Within a joint (e.g., intraarticular injection). (p. 23)

**Intrathecal** Within a sheath (e.g., the theca of the spinal cord, as in an intrathecal injection into the subarachnoid space). (p. 23)

**Medication error** Any preventable adverse drug event (see above) involving inappropriate medication use by a patient or health care professional; it may or may not cause patient harm. (p. 33)

**Medication use process** The prescribing, dispensing, and administering of medications, and the monitoring of their effects. (p. 33)

**Metabolite** A chemical form of a drug that is the product of one or more biochemical (metabolic) reactions involving the parent drug (see later). Active metabolites are those that have pharmacologic activity of their own, even if the parent drug is inactive (see *prodrug*). Inactive metabolites lack pharmacologic activity and are simply drug waste products awaiting excretion from the body (e.g., via the urinary, gastrointestinal, or respiratory tract). (p. 34)

**Onset of action** The time required for a drug to elicit a therapeutic response after dosing. (p. 29)

**Parent drug** The chemical form of a drug that is administered before it is metabolized by the body's biochemical reactions into its active or inactive metabolites (see *metabolite*). A parent drug that is not pharmacologically active itself is called a *prodrug.* A prodrug is then metabolized to pharmacologically active metabolites. (p. 22)

**Peak effect** The time required for a drug to reach its maximum therapeutic response in the body. (p. 29)

**Peak level** The maximum concentration of a drug in the body after administration, usually measured in a blood sample for therapeutic drug monitoring. (p. 30)

**Pharmaceutics** The science of preparing and dispensing drugs, including dosage form design. (p. 20)

**Pharmacodynamics** The study of the biochemical and physiologic interactions of drugs at their sites of activity. It examines the physicochemical properties of drugs and their pharmacologic interactions with body receptors. (p. 20)

**Pharmacoeconomics** The study of economic factors impacting the cost of drug therapy. (p. 20)

**Pharmacogenomics** The study of the influence of genetic factors on drug response, including the nature of genetic aberrations that result in the absence, overabundance, or insufficiency of drug-metabolizing enzymes (also called *pharmacogenomics;* see Chapter 8). (p. 34)

**Pharmacognosy** The study of drugs that are obtained from natural plant and animal sources. (p. 20)

**Pharmacokinetics** The study of what happens to a drug from the time it is put into the body until the parent drug and all metabolites have left the body. Pharmacokinetics represent the drug absorption into, distribution and metabolism within, and excretion from the body. (p. 20)

**Pharmacology** The broadest term for the study or science of drugs. (p. 19)

**Pharmacotherapeutics** The treatment of pathologic conditions through the use of drugs. (p. 20)

**Prodrug** An inactive drug dosage form that is converted to an active metabolite by various biochemical reactions once it is inside the body. (p. 27)

**Receptor** A molecular structure within or on the outer surface of a cell. Receptors bind specific substances (e.g., drug molecules), and one or more corresponding cellular effects (drug actions) occurs as a result of this drug-receptor interaction. (p. 30)

**Steady state** The physiologic state in which the amount of drug removed via elimination is equal to the amount of drug absorbed with each dose. (p. 29)

**Substrates** Substances (e.g., drugs or natural biochemicals in the body) on which an enzyme acts. (p. 27)

**Synergistic effects** Drug interactions in which the effect of a combination of two or more drugs with similar actions is greater than the sum of the individual effects of the same drugs given alone. For example, 1 + 1 is greater than 2 (compare with *additive effects*). (p. 33)

**Therapeutic drug monitoring** The process of measuring drug levels to identify a patient's drug exposure and to allow adjustment of dosages with the goals of maximizing therapeutic effects and minimizing toxicity. (p. 30)

**Therapeutic effect** The desired or intended effect of a particular medication. (p. 30)

**Therapeutic index** The ratio between the toxic and therapeutic concentrations of a drug. (p. 32)

**Tolerance** Reduced response to a drug after prolonged use. (p. 32)

**Toxic** The quality of being poisonous (i.e., injurious to health or dangerous to life). (p. 20)

**Toxicity** The condition of producing adverse bodily effects due to poisonous qualities. (p. 30)

**Toxicology** The study of poisons, including toxic drug effects, and applicable treatments. (p. 20)

**Trade name** The commercial name given to a drug product by its manufacturer; also called the *proprietary name.* (p. 19)

**Trough level** The lowest concentration of drug reached in the body after it falls from its peak level, usually measured in a blood sample for therapeutic drug monitoring. (p. 30)

## OVERVIEW

Any chemical that affects the physiologic processes of a living organism can broadly be defined as a drug. The study or science of drugs is known as pharmacology. Pharmacology encompasses a variety of topics, including the following:

- Absorption
- Biochemical effects
- Biotransformation (metabolism)
- Distribution
- Drug history
- Drug origin
- Excretion
- Mechanisms of action
- Physical and chemical properties
- Physical effects
- Drug receptor mechanisms
- Therapeutic (beneficial) effects
- Toxic (harmful) effects

Pharmacology includes the following several subspecialty areas: *pharmaceutics, pharmacokinetics, pharmacodynamics, pharmacogenomics (pharmacogenetics), pharmacoeconomics, pharmacotherapeutics, pharmacognosy,* and *toxicology.* Knowledge of pharmacology enables the nurse to better understand how drugs affect humans. Without understanding basic pharmacologic principles, the nurse cannot fully appreciate the therapeutic benefits and potential toxicity of drugs.

Throughout the process of its development, a drug will acquire at least three different names. The chemical name describes the drug's chemical composition and molecular structure. The generic name, or nonproprietary name, is often much shorter and simpler than the chemical name. The generic name is used in most official drug compendiums to list drugs. The trade name, or proprietary name, is the drug's registered trademark, and indicates that its commercial use is restricted to the owner of the patent for the drug (Figure 2-1). The patent owner is usually the manufacturer of the drug. Trade names are generally created by the manufacturer with marketability in mind. For this reason, they are usually shorter and easier to pronounce and remember than generic drug names. The *patent life* of a newly discovered drug molecule is normally 17 years. This is the length of time from patent approval until patent expiration. Because the research processes for new drug development normally require about 10 years, a drug manufacturer generally has the remaining 7 years for sales profits before patent expiration. A significant amount of these profits serves to offset the multimillion-dollar costs for research and development of the drug.

After the patent for a given drug expires, other manufacturers may legally begin to manufacture *generic* drugs with the same

**FIGURE 2-1** Chemical structure of the common analgesic ibuprofen and the chemical, generic, and trade names for the drug.

active ingredient. At this point, the drug price usually decreases substantially. Due to the high cost of drugs, many institutions have implemented programs in which one drug in a class of several drugs is chosen as the preferred agent, even though the drugs do not have the same active ingredients. This is called *therapeutic equivalence.* Before one drug can be therapeutically substituted for another, the drugs must have been proven to have the same therapeutic effect in the body.

Drugs are grouped together based on their similar properties. This is known as a drug classification. Drugs can be classified by their structure (e.g., beta-adrenergic blockers) or by their therapeutic use (e.g., antibiotics, antihypertensives, antidepressants). Within the broad classification, each class may have subclasses; for example, penicillins are a subclass within the group of antibiotics and beta-adrenergic blockers are a subclass within the group of antihypertensives.

Three basic areas of pharmacology—*pharmaceutics, pharmacokinetics,* and *pharmacodynamics*—describe the relationship between the dose of a drug given to a patient and the activity of that drug in treating the patient's disorder. Pharmaceutics is the study of how various dosage forms influence the way in which the drug affects the body. Pharmacokinetics is the study of what the body does to the drug. Pharmacokinetics involves the processes of absorption, distribution, metabolism, and excretion. Pharmacodynamics, on the other hand, is the study of what the drug does to the body. Pharmacodynamics involves drug-receptor relationships. Figure 2-2 illustrates the three phases of drug activity, starting with the pharmaceutical phase, proceeding to the pharmacokinetic phase, and finishing with the pharmacodynamic phase.

Pharmacotherapeutics (also called therapeutics) focuses on the clinical use of drugs to prevent and treat diseases. It defines the principles of drug actions—the cellular processes that change in response to the presence of drug molecules. Some drug mechanisms of action are more clearly understood than others. Drugs are categorized into pharmacologic classes according to their physiologic functions (e.g., beta-adrenergic blockers) and primary disease states treated (e.g., anticonvulsants, antiinfectives). The U.S. Food and Drug Administration (FDA) regulates the approval and clinical use of all drugs in the United States, including the requirement of an expiration date on all drugs. This textbook focuses almost exclusively on current FDA-approved indications for the drugs discussed in each chapter and on drugs that are currently available in the United States at the time of this writing. Only FDA-approved indications are permitted to be described in the manufacturer's

**FIGURE 2-2** Phases of drug activity. (From McKenry LM, Tessier E, Hogan M: *Mosby's pharmacology in nursing,* ed 22, St Louis, 2006, Mosby.)

written information, or labeling, for a given drug product. At times, prescribers may elect to use drugs for non–FDA-approved indications. This is known as *off-label prescribing* and often requires seasoned clinical judgment on the part of the prescriber. Evolving over time in clinical practice, previously off-label indications often become FDA-approved indications for a given drug.

The study of the adverse effects of drugs and other chemicals on living systems is known as toxicology. Toxic effects are often an extension of a drug's therapeutic action. Therefore, toxicology frequently involves overlapping principles of both pharmacotherapy and toxicology. The study of natural (versus synthetic) drug sources (i.e., plants, animals, minerals) is called pharmacognosy. Pharmacoeconomics focuses on the economic aspects of drug therapy.

**TABLE 2-1  DRUG ABSORPTION OF VARIOUS ORAL PREPARATIONS**

| | |
|---|---|
| Oral disintegration, buccal tablets, and oral soluble wafers | Fastest |
| Liquids, elixirs, and syrups | |
| Suspension solutions | |
| Powders | |
| Capsules | |
| Tablets | |
| Coated tablets | |
| Enteric-coated tablets | Slowest |

**TABLE 2-2  DOSAGE FORMS**

| ROUTE | FORMS |
|---|---|
| Enteral | Tablets, capsules, oral soluble wafers, pills, timed-release capsules, timed-release tablets, elixirs, suspensions, syrups, emulsions, solutions, lozenges or troches, rectal suppositories, sublingual or buccal tablets |
| Parenteral | Injectable forms, solutions, suspensions, emulsions, powders for reconstitution |
| Topical | Aerosols, ointments, creams, pastes, powders, solutions, foams, gels, transdermal patches, inhalers, rectal and vaginal suppositories |

In summary, pharmacology is a very dynamic science that incorporates several different disciplines. Traditionally, chemistry has been seen as the primary basis of pharmacology, but pharmacology also relies heavily on physiology and biology.

## PHARMACEUTICS

Different drug dosage forms have different pharmaceutical properties. Dosage form determines the rate at which drug dissolution (dissolving of solid dosage forms and their absorption, e.g., from gastrointestinal [GI] tract fluids) occurs. A drug to be ingested orally may be in either a solid form (tablet, capsule, or powder) or a liquid form (solution or suspension). Table 2-1 lists various oral drug preparations and the relative rate at which they are absorbed. Oral drugs that are liquids (e.g., elixirs, syrups) are already dissolved and are usually absorbed more quickly than solid dosage forms. Enteric-coated tablets, on the other hand, have a coating that prevents them from being broken down in the acidic pH environment of the stomach and therefore are not absorbed until they reach the higher (more alkaline) pH of the intestines. This pharmaceutical property results in slower dissolution and therefore slower absorption.

Particle size within a tablet or capsule can make different dosage forms of the same drug dissolve at different rates, become absorbed at different rates, and thus have different times to onset of action. An example is the difference between micronized glyburide and nonmicronized glyburide. Micronized glyburide reaches a maximum concentration peak faster than does the nonmicronized formulation. Dosage form design for injectable drugs tends to be more straightforward than that for oral dosage forms. However, some injections are carefully formulated to reduce drug toxicity (e.g., liposomal amphotericin B).

Combination dosage forms contain multiple drugs in one dose. Examples of these combination forms include the cholesterol and antihypertensive medications atorvastatin/amlodipine tablets called Caduet and bacitracin/neomycin/polymyxin B/hydrocortisone ointment (generic). There are large numbers of such combination dosage forms; key examples are cited in the various chapters of this book.

A variety of dosage forms exist to provide both accurate and convenient drug delivery systems (Table 2-2). These delivery systems are designed to achieve a desired therapeutic response with minimal adverse effects. Many dosage forms have been developed to encourage patient adherence with the medication regimen. Extended-release tablets and capsules release drug molecules in the patient's GI tract over a prolonged period of time. This ultimately prolongs drug absorption as well as duration of action. This is the opposite of immediate-release dosage forms, which release all of the active ingredient immediately upon dissolution in the GI tract. Extended-release dosage forms are normally easily identified by various capital letter abbreviations attached to their names. Examples of this nomenclature are SR (slow release or sustained release), SA (sustained action), CR (controlled release), XL (extended length), and XT (extended time). Convenience of administration correlates strongly with patient adherence, because these forms often require fewer daily doses. Extended-release oral dosage forms must not be crushed, as this could cause accelerated release of drug from the dosage form and possible toxicity. Enteric-coated tablets also are not recommended for crushing. This would cause disruption of the tablet coating designed to protect the stomach lining from the local effects of the drug and/or protect the drug from being prematurely disrupted by stomach acid. The ability to crush a tablet or open a capsule can facilitate drug administration when patients are unable or unwilling to swallow a tablet or capsule and also when medications need to be given through an enteral feeding tube. Capsules, powder, or liquid contents can often be added to soft foods such as applesauce or pudding, or dissolved in a beverage. Granules contained in capsules are usually for extended drug release and normally should not be crushed or chewed by the patient. However, they can often be swallowed when sprinkled on one of the soft foods. Consultation with a pharmacist, reading the product literature, or use of other suitable source is necessary if any question exists as to whether a drug can be crushed or mixed with specific food or beverages.

An increasingly popular dosage form is drug products that dissolve in the mouth and are absorbed through the oral mucosa. These include orally disintegrating tablets as well as thin wafers that also dissolve in the mouth. Depending on the specific drug product, the dosage form may dissolve on the tongue, under the tongue, or in the buccal (cheek) pocket.

The specific characteristics of various dosage forms have a large impact on how and to what extent the drug is absorbed. For a drug to work at a specific site in the body, either it must be applied directly at the site in an active form or it must have a way of getting to that site. Oral dosage forms rely on gastric and intestinal enzymes and pH environments to break the medication down into particles that are small enough to be absorbed into the circulation. Once absorbed through the mucosa of the stomach or intestines, the drug is then transported to the site of action by blood or lymph.

Many topically applied dosage forms work directly on the surface of the skin. Once the drug is applied, it is already in a form that allows it to act immediately. However, with other topical dosage forms, the skin acts as a barrier through which the drug must pass to get into the circulation; once there, the drug is then carried to its site of action (e.g., fentanyl transdermal patch for pain).

Dosage forms that are administered via injection are called *parenteral* forms. They must have certain characteristics to be safe and effective. The arteries and veins that carry drugs throughout the body can easily be damaged if the drug is too concentrated or corrosive. The pH of injections must be very similar to that of the blood for these drugs to be administered safely. Parenteral dosage forms that are injected intravenously are immediately placed into solution in the bloodstream and do not have to be dissolved in the body. Therefore, 100% absorption is assumed to occur immediately upon intravenous injection.

## PHARMACOKINETICS

A drug's time to onset of action, time to peak effect, and duration of action are all characteristics defined by pharmacokinetics. Pharmacokinetics is the study of what happens to a drug from the time it is put into the body until the parent drug and all metabolites have left the body. Thus, drug absorption into, distribution and metabolism within, and excretion from the body represent the combined focus of pharmacokinetics.

### Absorption

Absorption is the movement of a drug from its site of administration into the bloodstream for distribution to the tissues. Bioavailability is the term used to express the extent of drug absorption. For example, a drug that is absorbed from the intestine must first pass through the liver before it reaches the systemic circulation. If a large proportion of a drug is chemically changed into inactive metabolites in the liver, then a much smaller amount of drug will pass into the circulation (i.e., will be bioavailable). Such a drug is said to have a high first-pass effect (e.g., oral nitrates). First-pass effect reduces the bioavailability of the drug to less than 100%. Many drugs administered by mouth have a bioavailability of less than 100%, whereas drugs administered by the intravenous route are 100% bioavailable. If two medications have the same bioavailability and same concentration of active ingredient, they are said to be bioequivalent (e.g., a brand-name drug and the same generic drug).

Various factors affect the rate of drug absorption. How a drug is administered, or its route of administration, affects the rate and extent of absorption of that drug. Although a number of dosage formulations are available for delivering medications, they can all be categorized into three basic routes of administration: enteral (GI tract), parenteral, and topical.

### Enteral Route

In enteral drug administration, the drug is absorbed into the systemic circulation through the mucosa of the stomach and/or small or large intestine. The rate of absorption can be altered by many factors. Orally administered drugs are absorbed from the intestinal lumen into the blood system and transported to the liver. Once the drug is in the liver, hepatic enzyme systems metabolize it, and the remaining active ingredients are passed into the general circulation. Many factors can alter the absorption of drugs, including acid changes within the stomach, absorption changes in the intestines, and the presence or absence of food and fluid. Various factors that affect the acidity of the stomach include the time of day; the age of the patient; and the presence and types of medications (e.g., $H_2$ blockers or proton pump inhibitors [see Chapter 50]), foods, or beverages. Enteric-coating is designed to protect the stomach by having drug dissolution and absorption occur in the intestines. Taking an enteric-coated medication with a large amount food may cause it to be dissolved by acidic stomach contents and thus reduce intestinal drug absorption and negate the coating's stomach-protective properties. Anticholinergic drugs slow GI transit time (or the time it takes for substances in the stomach to be dissolved for eventual transport to and absorption from the intestines). This may reduce the amount of drug absorption and therapeutic effect for acid-susceptible drugs that become broken down by stomach acids. The presence of food may enhance the absorption of some fat-soluble drugs or of drugs that are more easily broken down in an acidic environment.

Drug absorption may also be altered in patients who have had portions of the small intestine removed because of disease. This is known as *short bowel syndrome.* Similarly, bariatric weight loss surgery reduces the size of the stomach. As a result, medication absorption can be altered, because stomach contents are delivered to the intestines more rapidly than usual after such surgery. This is called *gastric dumping*. Examples of drugs to be taken on an empty stomach and those to be taken with food are provided in Box 2-1. The stomach and small intestine are highly vascularized. When blood flow to this area is decreased, absorption may also be decreased. Sepsis and exercise are examples of circumstances under which blood flow to the GI tract is often reduced. In both cases, blood tends to be routed to the heart and other vital organs. In the case of exercise, it is also routed to the skeletal muscles.

Rectally administered drugs are often given for systemic effects (e.g., antinausea, analgesia, antipyretic effects), but they are also used to treat disease within the rectum or adjacent bowel (e.g., antiinflammatory ointment for hemorrhoids, corticosteroid enemas for colitis). In the latter case, rectal administration may also be thought of as a *topical* route of drug administration.

*Sublingual and Buccal Routes.* Drugs administered by the *sublingual* route are absorbed into the highly vascularized tissue under the tongue—the oral mucosa. Sublingual nitroglycerin is an example. Sublingually administered drugs are absorbed rapidly because the area under the tongue has a large blood supply. These drugs bypass the liver and yet are systemically bioavailable. The same applies for drugs administered by the *buccal route* (the oral mucosa between the cheek and the gum). Through these routes, drugs such as nitroglycerin are absorbed rapidly into the bloodstream and delivered to their site of action (e.g., coronary arteries).

## Parenteral Route

The parenteral route is the fastest route by which a drug can be absorbed, followed by the enteral and topical routes. *Parenteral* is a general term meaning any route of administration other than the GI tract. It most commonly refers to injection. Intravenous injection delivers the drug directly into the circulation, where it is distributed with the blood throughout the body. Drugs given by intramuscular injection and subcutaneous injection are absorbed more slowly than those given intravenously. These drug formulations are usually absorbed over a period of several hours; however, some are specially formulated to be released over days, weeks, or months.

Drugs can be injected intradermally, subcutaneously, *intraarterially*, intramuscularly, *intrathecally*, intraarticularly, or intravenously. Physicians, or advanced practice nurses, usually give intraarterial, intrathecal, or intraarticular injections. Medications given by the parenteral route have the advantage of bypassing the first-pass effect of the liver. Parenteral administration offers an alternative route of delivery for medications that cannot be given orally and poses fewer obstacles to absorption. However, drugs that are administered by the parenteral route must still be absorbed into cells and tissues before they can exert their pharmacologic effect (Table 2-3).

## ⚡ SAFETY AND QUALITY IMPROVEMENT: PREVENTING MEDICATION ERRORS

### *Does IV = PO?*

The prescriber writes an order for "Lasix 80 mg IV STAT × 1 dose" for a patient who is short of breath with pulmonary edema. When the nurse goes to give the drug, only the PO form is immediately available. Someone must go to the pharmacy to pick up the IV dose. Another nurse says, "Go ahead and give the pill. He needs it fast. It's all the same!" But is it?

Remember, the oral forms of medications must be processed through the gastrointestinal tract, absorbed through the small intestines, and undergo the first-pass effect in the liver before the drug can reach the intended site of action. However, IV forms are injected directly into the circulation and can act almost immediately because the first-pass effect is bypassed. The time until onset of action for the PO form is 30 to 60 minutes; for the IV form, this time is *5 minutes*. This patient is in respiratory distress, and the immediate effect of the diuretic is desired. In addition, because of the first-pass effect, the available amount of orally administered drug that actually reaches the site of action would be less than the available amount of intravenously administered drug. Therefore, IV does NOT equal PO! Never change the route of administration of a medication; if questions come up, always check with the prescriber.

*Subcutaneous, Intradermal, and Intramuscular Routes.* Injections into the fatty subcutaneous tissues under the dermal layer of skin are referred to as *subcutaneous* injections. Injections under the more superficial skin layers immediately underneath the epidermal layer of skin and into the dermal layer are known as *intradermal* injections. Injections given into the muscle beneath the subcutaneous fatty tissue are referred to as *intramuscular* injections. Muscles have a greater blood supply than does the skin; therefore, drugs injected intramuscularly are typically absorbed faster than drugs injected subcutaneously. Absorption from either of these sites may be increased by applying heat to the injection site or by massaging the site. Both methods increase blood flow to the area, thereby enhancing drug absorption. In contrast, the presence of cold, hypotension, or poor peripheral blood flow compromises the circulation, reducing drug activity by reducing drug delivery to the tissues. Most intramuscularly injected drugs are absorbed over several hours. However, specially formulated long-acting intramuscular dosage forms called *depot drugs* have been designed for slow absorption over a period of several days to a few months or longer. The intramuscular corticosteroid known as *methylprednisolone acetate* can provide antiinflammatory effects for several weeks. The intramuscular contraceptive medroxyprogesterone acetate normally prevents pregnancy for 3 months per dose.

## TABLE 2-3    ROUTES OF ADMINISTRATION AND RELATED NURSING CONSIDERATIONS

| ROUTE | ADVANTAGES | DISADVANTAGES | NURSING CONSIDERATIONS |
|---|---|---|---|
| Intravenous (IV) | Provides rapid onset (drug delivered immediately to bloodstream); allows more direct control of drug level in blood; gives option of larger fluid volume, therefore diluting irritating drugs; avoids first-pass metabolism | Higher cost; inconvenience (e.g., not self-administered); irreversibility of drug action in most cases and inability to retrieve medication; risk of fluid overload; greater likelihood of infection; possibility of embolism | Continuous intravenous infusions require frequent monitoring to be sure that the correct volume and amount are administered and that the drug reaches safe, therapeutic blood levels. Intravenous drugs and solutions must be checked for compatibilities. Intravenous sites are to be monitored for redness, swelling, heat, and drainage—all indicative of complications, such as thrombophlebitis. If intermittent intravenous infusions are used, clearing or flushing of the line with normal saline before and after is generally indicated to keep the intravenous site patent and minimize incompatibilities. |
| Intramuscular (IM); subcutaneous | Intramuscular injections are good for poorly soluble drugs, which are often given in "depot" preparation form and are then absorbed over a prolonged period; onsets of action differ depending on route. | Discomfort of injection; inconvenience; bruising; slower onset of action compared to intravenous, although quicker than oral in most situations | Using landmarks to identify correct intramuscular and subcutaneous sites is always required and recommended as a nursing standard of care. For adults, the intramuscular site of choice is the ventral gluteal muscle with use of a 1½-inch (sometimes 1-inch in very thin or emaciated patients) and 20- to 25-gauge needle for aqueous solutions and 18- to 25-gauge needle for viscous or oil-based solutions. Subcutaneous injections are recommended to be given at a 90-degree angle with a proper size syringe and needle (½- to ⅝-inch); in emaciated or very thin patients, the subcutaneous angle is at 45 degrees. Subcutaneous injections require a 26- to 30-gauge, ½-inch needle inserted at a 90-degree angle. Selection of correct size of syringe and needle is key to safe administration by these routes and is based on thorough assessment of the patient as well as the characteristics of the drug. |
| Oral | Usually easier, more convenient, and less expensive; safer than injection, dosing more likely to be reversible in cases of accidental ingestion (e.g., through induction of emesis, administration of activated charcoal) | Variable absorption; inactivation of some drugs by stomach acid and/or pH; problems with first-pass effect or presystemic metabolism; greater dependence of drug action on patient variables | Enteral routes include oral administration and involve a variety of dosage forms (e.g., liquids, solutions, tablets, and enteric-coated pills or tablets). Some medications are recommended to be taken with food, while others are recommended not to be taken with food; it is also suggested that oral dosage forms of drugs be taken with at least 6 to 8 oz of fluid, such as water. Other factors to consider include other medicines being taken at the same time and concurrent use of dairy products or antacids. If oral forms are given via nasogastric tube or gastrostomy tube, tube placement in stomach must be assessed prior to giving the medication and the patient's head is to remain elevated; flushing the nasogastric tube with at least 30 to 60 mL of water before and after the drug has been given is recommended to help maintain tube patency and prevent clogging. |
| Sublingual, buccal (subtypes of oral, but more parenteral than enteral) | Absorbed more rapidly from oral mucosa and leads to more rapid onset of action; avoids breakdown of drug by stomach acid; avoids first-pass metabolism because gastric absorption is bypassed | Patients may swallow pill instead of keeping under tongue until dissolved; pills often smaller to handle | Drugs given via the sublingual route are to be placed under the tongue; once dissolved, the drug may be swallowed. When using the buccal route, medication is placed between the cheek and gum. Both of these dosage forms are relatively nonirritating; the drug usually is without flavor and water-soluble. |
| Rectal | Provides relatively rapid absorption; good alternative when oral route not feasible; useful for local or systemic drug delivery; usually leads to mixed first-pass and non–first-pass metabolism | Possible discomfort and embarrassment to patient; often higher cost than oral route | Absorption via this route is erratic and unpredictable, but it provides a safe alternative when nausea or vomiting prevents oral dosing of drugs. The patient must be placed on his or her left side so that the normal anatomy of the colon allows safe and effective insertion of the rectal dosage form. Suppositories are inserted using a gloved hand and/or gloved index finger and water-soluble lubricant. Drug must be administered exactly as ordered. |
| Topical | Delivers medication directly to affected area; decreases likelihood of systemic drug effects | Sometimes awkward to self-administer (e.g., eyedrops); can be messy; usually higher cost than oral route | Most dermatologic drugs are given via topical route in form of a solution, ointment, spray, or drops. Maximal absorption of topical drugs is enhanced with skin that is clean and free of debris; if measurement of ointment is necessary—such as with topical nitroglycerin—application must be done carefully and per instructions (e.g., apply 1 inch of ointment). Gloves help minimize cross-contamination and prevent absorption of drug into the nurse's own skin. If the patient's skin is not intact, sterile technique is needed. |

## TABLE 2-3   ROUTES OF ADMINISTRATION AND RELATED NURSING CONSIDERATIONS—cont'd

| ROUTE | ADVANTAGES | DISADVANTAGES | NURSING CONSIDERATIONS |
|---|---|---|---|
| Transdermal (subtype of topical) | Provides relatively constant rate of drug absorption; one patch can last 1 to 7 days, depending on drug; avoids first-pass metabolism | Rate of absorption can be affected by excessive perspiration and body temperature; patch may peel off; cost is higher; used patches must be disposed of safely | Transdermal drugs should be placed on alternating sites and on a clean, nonhairy, nonirritated area, and only after the previously applied patch has been removed and that area cleansed and dried. Transdermal drugs generally come in a single-dose, adhesive-backed drug application system. |
| Inhalational | Provides rapid absorption; drug delivered directly to lung tissues where most of these drugs exert their actions | Rate of absorption can be too rapid, increasing the risk of exaggerated drug effects; requires more patient education for self-administration; some patients may have difficulty with administration technique | Inhaled medications are to be used exactly as prescribed and with clean equipment. Instructions need to be given to the patient/family/caregiver regarding medications to be used as well as the proper use, storage, and safe-keeping of inhalers, spacers, and nebulizers. Chapter 9 describes and shows how medications are inhaled. |

NOTE: For more information on avoiding the use of abbreviations associated with dosage routes, dosage amounts, dosage frequency, and drug names, as well as the use of symbols, please visit www.ismp.org.

## Topical Route

The topical route of drug administration involves application of medications to various body surfaces. Several topical drug delivery systems exist. Topically administered drugs can be applied to the skin, eyes, ears, nose, lungs, rectum, or vagina. Topical application delivers a uniform amount of drug over a longer period, but the effects of the drug are usually slower in their onset and more prolonged in their duration of action as compared to oral or parenteral administration. This can be a problem if the patient begins to experience adverse effects from the drug and a considerable amount of drug has already been absorbed. All topical routes of drug administration avoid first-pass effects of the liver, with the exception of rectal administration. Because the rectum is part of the GI tract, some drug will be absorbed into the capillaries that feed the portal vein to the liver. However, some drugs will also be absorbed locally into perirectal tissues. Therefore, rectally administered drugs are said to have a mixed first-pass and non–first-pass absorption and metabolism. Box 2-2 lists the various drug routes and indicates whether they are associated with first-pass effects in the liver.

Ointments, gels, and creams are common types of topically administered drugs. Examples include sunscreens, antibiotics, and nitroglycerin ointment. The drawback to their use is that their systemic absorption is often erratic and unreliable. Generally, these medications are used for local effects, but some are used for systemic effects (e.g., nitroglycerin ointment for maintenance treatment of angina). Topically applied drugs can also be used in the treatment of various illnesses of the eyes, ears, and sinuses. Eye, ear, and nose drops are administered primarily for local effects, whereas nasal sprays may be used for both systemic and local effects (e.g., oxymetazoline for nasal sinus congestion, sumatriptan for migraine headaches). Vaginal medications may also be given for systemic effects (e.g., progestational hormone therapy with progesterone vaginal suppositories) but are more commonly used for local effects (e.g., treatment of vaginal yeast infection with miconazole [Monistat] vaginal cream).

### BOX 2-2   DRUG ROUTES AND FIRST-PASS EFFECTS

| First-Pass Routes | Non–First-Pass Routes |
|---|---|
| Hepatic arterial | Aural (instilled into the ear) |
| Oral | Buccal |
| Portal venous | Inhaled |
| Rectal* | Intraarterial |
| | Intramuscular |
| | Intranasal |
| | Intraocular |
| | Intravaginal |
| | Intravenous |
| | Subcutaneous |
| | Sublingual |
| | Transdermal |

*Leads to both first-pass and non–first-pass effects.

**Transdermal Route.** Transdermal drug delivery through adhesive patches is an elaborate topical route of drug administration that is commonly used for systemic drug effects. Some examples of drugs administered by this route are fentanyl (for pain), nitroglycerin (for angina), nicotine (for smoking cessation), estrogen (for menopausal symptoms), and clonidine (for hypertension). Transdermal patches are usually designed to deliver a constant amount of drug per unit of time for a specified time period. For example, a nitroglycerin patch may deliver 0.1 or 0.2 mg/hr over 24 hours, whereas a fentanyl patch may deliver 25 to 100 mcg/hr over a 72-hour period. This route is suitable for patients who cannot tolerate oral administration and provides a practical and convenient method for drug delivery.

**Inhaled Route.** Inhalation is another type of topical drug administration. Inhaled drugs are delivered to the lungs as micrometer-sized drug particles. This small drug size is necessary for the drug to be transported to the small air sacs within the lungs (alveoli). Once the small particles of drug are in the alveoli, drug absorption is fairly rapid. Many pulmonary and

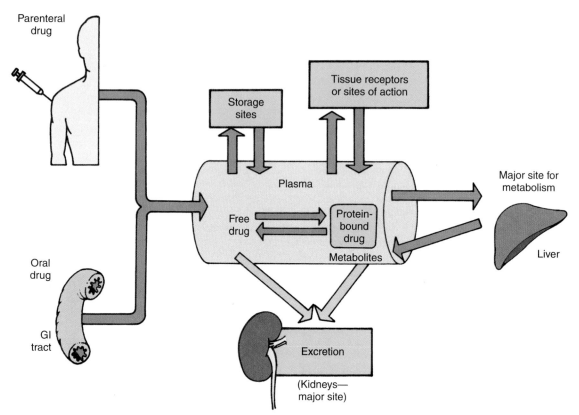

FIGURE 2-3 Drug transport in the body. *GI*, Gastrointestinal. (From McKenry LM, Salerno E: *Mosby's pharmacology in nursing*, ed 19, St Louis, 1995, Mosby.)

other types of diseases can be treated with such topically applied (inhaled) drugs. Examples of inhaled drugs are albuterol, which is used to treat bronchial constriction in individuals with asthma, and fluticasone, which is used for antiinflammatory purposes in patients with asthma and allergies.

## Distribution

Distribution refers to the transport of a drug by the bloodstream to its site of action (Figure 2-3). Drugs are distributed first to those areas with extensive blood supply. Areas of rapid distribution include the heart, liver, kidneys, and brain. Areas of slower distribution include muscle, skin, and fat. Once a drug enters the bloodstream (circulation), it is distributed throughout the body. At this point, it is also starting to be eliminated by the organs that metabolize and excrete drugs—primarily the liver and the kidneys. Only drug molecules that are not bound to plasma proteins can freely distribute to *extravascular* tissue (outside the blood vessels) to reach their site of action. If a drug is bound to plasma proteins, the drug-protein complex is generally too large to pass through the walls of blood capillaries into tissues (Figure 2-4). Albumin is the most common blood protein and carries the majority of protein-bound drug molecules. If a given drug binds to albumin, then there is only a limited amount of drug that is *not* bound. This unbound portion is pharmacologically active and is considered "free" drug, whereas "bound" drug is pharmacologically inactive. Certain conditions that cause low albumin levels, such as extensive burns and malnourished states, result in a

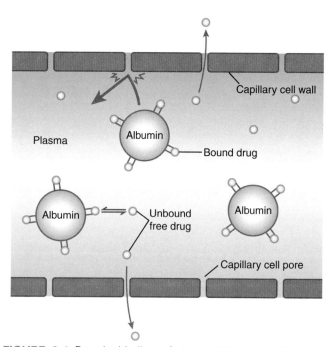

FIGURE 2-4 Protein binding of drugs. Albumin is the most prevalent protein in plasma and the most important of the proteins to which drugs bind. Only unbound (free) drug molecules can leave the vascular system. Bound molecules are too large to fit through the pores in the capillary wall.

larger fraction of free (unbound and active) drug. This can raise the risk of drug toxicity.

When an individual is taking two medications that are highly protein bound, the medications may compete for binding sites on the albumin molecule. Because of this competition, there is more free, unbound drug. This can lead to an unpredictable drug response called a *drug-drug interaction*. A drug-drug interaction occurs when the presence of one drug decreases or increases the actions of another drug that is administered concurrently (i.e., given at the same time).

A theoretical volume, called the *volume of distribution*, is sometimes used to describe the various areas in which drugs may be distributed. These areas, or *compartments*, may be the blood *(intravascular space)*, total body water, body fat, or other body tissues and organs. Typically a drug that is highly water-soluble (hydrophilic) will have a smaller volume of distribution and high blood concentrations. In contrast, fat-soluble drugs (lipophilic) have a larger volume of distribution and low blood concentrations. There are some sites in the body into which it may be very difficult to distribute a drug. These sites typically either have a poor blood supply (e.g., bone) or have physiologic barriers that make it difficult for drugs to pass through (e.g., the brain due to the blood-brain barrier).

## Metabolism

Metabolism is also referred to as biotransformation. It involves the biochemical alteration of a drug into an inactive metabolite, a more soluble compound, a more potent active metabolite (as in the conversion of an inactive prodrug to its active form), or a less active metabolite. Metabolism is the next step after absorption and distribution. The organ most responsible for the metabolism of drugs is the liver. Other metabolic tissues include skeletal muscle, kidneys, lungs, plasma, and intestinal mucosa.

Hepatic metabolism involves the activity of a very large class of enzymes known as cytochrome P-450 enzymes (or simply P-450 enzymes), also known as *microsomal* enzymes. These enzymes control a variety of reactions that aid in the metabolism of medications. They are largely targeted at lipid-soluble *(nonpolar* [no charge]) drugs (also known as *lipophilic* ["fat loving"]), which are typically very difficult to eliminate. These include the majority of medications. Those medications with water-soluble (polar or *hydrophilic* ["water loving"]) molecules may be more easily metabolized by simpler chemical reactions such as hydrolysis. Some of the chemical reactions by which the liver can metabolize drugs are listed in Table 2-4. Drug molecules that are the metabolic targets of specific enzymes are said to be substrates for those enzymes. Specific P-450 enzymes are identified by standardized number and letter designations. Some of the most common P-450 enzymes and their corresponding drug substrates are listed in Table 2-5. The P-450 system is one of the most important systems that influence drug-drug interactions. The list of drugs that are metabolized by the P-450 enzyme system is constantly changing as new drugs are introduced into the market. For further information, see websites such as http://www.medicine.iupui.edu/flockhart/table.htm and http://www.nursinglink.com/training/articles/320-clinically-significant-drug-interaction-with-the-cytochrome-p450-enzyme-system.

| TABLE 2-4 | MECHANISMS OF BIOTRANSFORMATION | |
|---|---|---|
| **TYPE OF BIOTRANSFORMATION** | **MECHANISM** | **RESULT** |
| Oxidation Reduction Hydrolysis | Chemical reactions | Increase polarity of chemical, making it more water-soluble and more easily excreted. This often results in a loss of pharmacologic activity. |
| Conjugation (e.g., glucuronidation, glycination, sulfation, methylation, alkylation) | Combination with another substance (e.g., glucuronide, glycine, sulfate, methyl groups, alkyl groups) | Forms a less toxic product with less activity. |

| TABLE 2-5 | COMMON LIVER CYTOCHROME P-450 ENZYMES AND CORRESPONDING DRUG SUBSTRATES |
|---|---|
| **ENZYME** | **COMMON DRUG SUBSTRATES** |
| 1A2 | acetaminophen, caffeine, theophylline, warfarin |
| 2C9 | ibuprofen, phenytoin |
| 2C19 | diazepam, naproxen, omeprazole, propranolol |
| 2D6 | codeine, fluoxetine, hydrocodone, metoprolol, oxycodone, paroxetine, risperidone, tricyclic antidepressants |
| 2E1 | acetaminophen, ethanol |
| 3A4 | acetaminophen, amiodarone, cyclosporine, diltiazem, ethinyl estradiol, indinavir, lidocaine, macrolides, progesterone, spironolactone, sulfamethoxazole, testosterone, verapamil |

The biotransformation capabilities of the liver can vary considerably from patient to patient. The various factors that can alter the biotransformation include genetics, diseases, and the concurrent use of other medications (Table 2-6).

Many drugs can inhibit drug-metabolizing enzymes and are called *enzyme inhibitors*. Decreases or delays in drug metabolism result in the accumulation of the drug and prolongation of the effects of the drug, which can lead to drug toxicity. In contrast, some drugs can stimulate drug metabolism and are called *enzyme inducers*. This can cause decreased pharmacologic effects. This often occurs with the repeated administration of certain drugs that stimulate the formation of new microsomal enzymes.

## Excretion

Excretion is the elimination of drugs from the body. Whether they are parent compounds or active or inactive metabolites, all drugs must eventually be removed from the body. The primary organ responsible for this elimination is the kidney. Two other organs that play an important role in the excretion of drugs are the liver and the bowel. Most drugs are metabolized in the liver by various mechanisms. Therefore, by the time most drugs

## TABLE 2-6 EXAMPLES OF CONDITIONS AND DRUGS THAT AFFECT DRUG METABOLISM

| | | DRUG METABOLISM | |
| --- | --- | --- | --- |
| CATEGORY | EXAMPLE | INCREASED | DECREASED |
| Diseases | Cardiovascular dysfunction | | X |
| | Renal insufficiency | | X |
| Conditions | Starvation | | X |
| | Obstructive jaundice | | X |
| | Genetic constitution | | |
| |   Fast acetylator | X | |
| |   Slow acetylator | | X |
| Drugs | Barbiturates | X | |
| | rifampin (P-450 inducer) | X | |
| | phenytoin (P-450 inducer) | X | |
| | ketoconazole (P-450 inhibitor) | | X |

reach the kidneys, they have undergone extensive biotransformation, and only a relatively small fraction of the original drug is excreted as the original compound. Other drugs may bypass hepatic metabolism and reach the kidneys in their original form. Drugs that have been metabolized by the liver become more polar and water-soluble. This makes their elimination by the kidneys much easier, because the urinary tract is water-based. The kidneys themselves are also capable of metabolizing various drugs, although usually to a lesser extent than the liver.

The actual act of renal excretion is accomplished through *glomerular filtration, active tubular reabsorption,* and *active tubular secretion.* Free (unbound) water-soluble drugs and metabolites go through passive glomerular filtration. Many substances present in the nephrons go through active reabsorption and are taken back up into the systemic circulation and transported away from the kidney. This process is an attempt by the body to retain needed substances. Some substances may also be secreted into the nephron from the vasculature surrounding it. The processes of filtration, reabsorption, and secretion for urinary elimination are shown in Figure 2-5.

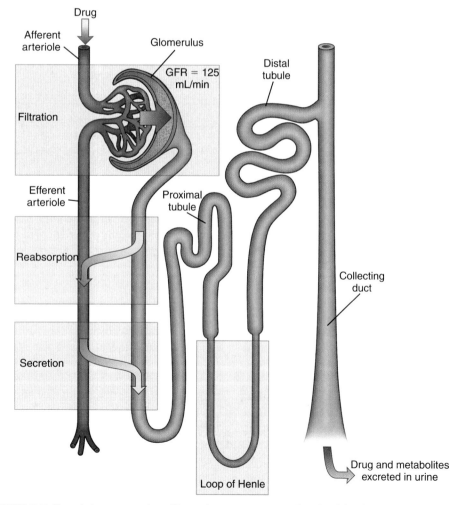

**FIGURE 2-5** Renal drug excretion. The primary processes involved in drug excretion and the approximate location where these processes take place in the kidney are illustrated. *GFR,* Glomerular filtration rate.

The excretion of drugs by the intestines is another route of elimination. This process is referred to as *biliary excretion.* Drugs that are eliminated by this route are taken up by the liver, released into the bile, and eliminated in the feces. Once certain drugs, such as fat-soluble drugs, are in the bile, they may be reabsorbed into the bloodstream, returned to the liver, and again secreted into the bile. This process is called *enterohepatic recirculation.* Enterohepatically recirculated drugs persist in the body for much longer periods. Less common routes of elimination are the lungs and the sweat, salivary, and mammary glands.

## Half-Life

Another pharmacokinetic variable is the half-life of the drug. By definition, the half-life is the time required for one-half (50%) of a given drug to be removed from the body. It is a measure of the rate at which the drug is eliminated from the body. For instance, if the peak level of a particular drug is 100 mg/L and the measured drug level is 50 mg/L in 8 hours, then the estimated half-life of that drug is 8 hours. The concept of drug half-life viewed from several different perspectives is shown in Table 2-7.

| TABLE 2-7 | EXAMPLE OF DRUG HALF-LIFE VIEWED FROM DIFFERENT PERSPECTIVES | | | | | |
|---|---|---|---|---|---|---|
| **METRIC** | **CHANGING VALUES** | | | | | |
| Hours after peak concentration | 0 | 8 | 16 | 24 | 32 | 40 |
| Drug concentration (mg/L) | 100 (peak) | 50 | 25 | 12.5 | 6.25 | 3.125 (trough) |
| Number of half-lives | 0 | 1 | 2 | 3 | 4 | 5 |
| Percentage of drug removed | 0 | 50 | 75 | 88 | 94 | 97 |

After about five half-lives, most drugs are considered to be effectively removed from the body. At that time approximately 97% of the drug has been eliminated, and what little amount remains is usually too small to have either therapeutic or toxic effects.

The concept of half-life is clinically useful for determining when steady state will be reached in a patient taking a particular drug. Steady state refers to the physiologic state in which the amount of drug removed via elimination (e.g., renal clearance) is equal to the amount of drug absorbed with each dose. This physiologic plateau phenomenon typically occurs after four to five half-lives of administered drug. Therefore, if a drug has an extremely long half-life, it will take much longer for the drug to reach steady-state blood levels. Once steady-state blood levels have been reached, there are consistent levels of drug in the body that correlate with maximum therapeutic benefits.

## Onset, Peak, and Duration

The pharmacokinetic terms *absorption, distribution, metabolism,* and *excretion* are all used to describe the movement of drugs through the body. Drug actions are the processes involved in the interaction between a drug and a cell (e.g., a drug's action on a receptor). In contrast, drug effects are the physiologic reactions of the body to the drug. The terms *onset, peak, duration,* and *trough* are used to describe drug effects. *Peak* and *trough* are also used to describe drug concentrations, which are usually measured from blood samples.

A drug's onset of action is the time required for the drug to elicit a therapeutic response. A drug's peak effect is the time required for a drug to reach its maximum therapeutic response. Physiologically, this corresponds to increasing drug concentrations at the site of action. The duration of action of a drug is the length of time that the drug concentration is sufficient (without more doses) to elicit a therapeutic response. These concepts are illustrated in Figure 2-6.

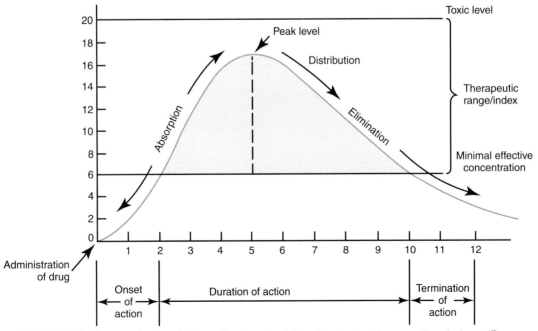

**FIGURE 2-6** Characteristics of drug effect and relationship to the therapeutic window. (From McKenry LM, Tessier E, Hogan M: *Mosby's pharmacology in nursing,* ed 22, St Louis, 2006, Mosby.)

The length of time until the onset and peak of action and the duration of action play an important part in determining the peak level (highest blood level) and trough level (lowest blood level) of a drug. If the peak blood level is too high, then drug toxicity may occur. The toxicity may be mild, such as intensification of the effects of the given drug (e.g., excessive sedation resulting from overdose of a drug with sedative properties). However, it can also be severe (e.g., damage to vital organs due to excessive drug exposure). If the trough blood level is too low, then the drug may not be at therapeutic levels to produce a response. (A common example is antibiotic drug therapy with aminoglycoside antibiotics [see Chapter 39]). In therapeutic drug monitoring, peak (highest) and trough (lowest) values are measured to verify adequate drug exposure, maximize therapeutic effects, and minimize drug toxicity. This monitoring is often carried out by a clinical pharmacist working with other members of the health care team.

## PHARMACODYNAMICS

Pharmacodynamics is concerned with the mechanisms of drug action in living tissues. Drug-induced changes in normal physiologic functions are explained by the principles of pharmacodynamics. A positive change in a faulty physiologic system is called a therapeutic effect of a drug. Such an effect is the goal of drug therapy. Understanding the pharmacodynamic characteristics of a drug can aid in assessing the drug's therapeutic effect.

### Mechanism of Action

Drugs can produce actions (therapeutic effects) in several ways. The effects of a particular drug depend on the characteristics of the cells or tissue targeted by the drug. Once the drug is at the site of action, it can modify (increase or decrease) the rate at which that cell or tissue functions, or it can modify the strength of function of that cell or tissue. A drug cannot, however, cause a cell or tissue to perform a function that is not part of its natural physiology.

Drugs can exert their actions in three basic ways: through receptors, enzymes, and *nonselective interactions*. It should also be noted that not all mechanisms of action have been identified for all drugs. Thus, a drug may be said to have an unknown or unclear mechanism of action, even though it has observable therapeutic effects in the body.

### Receptor Interactions

A receptor can be defined as a reactive site on the surface or inside of a cell. If the mechanism of action of a drug involves a receptor interaction, then the molecular structure of the drug is critical. Drug-receptor interaction is the joining of the drug molecule with a reactive site on the surface of a cell or tissue. Most commonly, this site is a protein structure within the cell membrane. Once a drug binds to and interacts with the receptor, a pharmacologic response is produced (Figure 2-7). The degree to which a drug attaches to and binds with a receptor is called its *affinity*. The drug with the best "fit" and strongest affinity for the receptor will elicit the greatest response from the cell or tissue. A drug becomes bound to the receptor through the formation of chemical bonds between the receptor on the

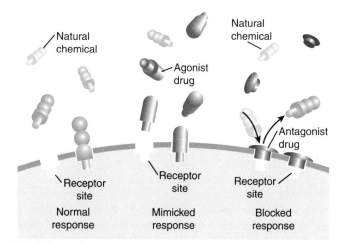

**FIGURE 2-7** Drugs act by forming a chemical bond with specific receptor sites, similar to a key and lock. The better the "fit," the better the response. Drugs with complete attachment and response are called *agonists*. Drugs that attach but do not elicit a response are called *antagonists*.

| TABLE 2-8 | DRUG-RECEPTOR INTERACTIONS |
|---|---|
| **DRUG TYPE** | **ACTION** |
| Agonist | Drug binds to the receptor; there is a response. |
| Partial agonist (agonist-antagonist) | Drug binds to the receptor; the response is diminished compared with that elicited by an agonist. |
| Antagonist | Drug binds to the receptor; there is no response. Drug prevents binding of agonists. |
| Competitive antagonist | Drug competes with the agonist for binding to the receptor. If it binds, there is no response. |
| Noncompetitive antagonist | Drug combines with different parts of the receptor and inactivates it; agonist then has no effect. |

cell and the active site on the drug molecule. Drugs interact with receptors in different ways either to elicit or to block a physiologic response. Table 2-8 describes the different types of drug-receptor interaction.

### Enzyme Interactions

Enzymes are the substances that catalyze nearly every biochemical reaction in a cell. Drugs can produce effects by interacting with these enzyme systems. For a drug to alter a physiologic response in this way, it may either inhibit (more common) or enhance (less common) the action of a specific enzyme. This process is called *selective interaction*. Drug-enzyme interaction occurs when the drug chemically binds to an enzyme molecule in such a way that it alters (inhibits or enhances) the enzyme's interaction with its normal target molecules in the body.

### Nonselective Interactions

Drugs with nonspecific mechanisms of action do not interact with receptors or enzymes. Instead, their main targets are cell membranes and various cellular processes such as metabolic activities. These drugs can either physically interfere with or chemically alter cellular structures or processes. Some cancer drugs and antibiotics have this mechanism of action. By incorporating themselves into the normal metabolic process, they cause a defect in the final product or state. This defect may be an improperly formed cell wall that results in cell death through cell lysis, or it may be the lack of a necessary energy substrate, which leads to cell starvation and death.

## PHARMACOTHERAPEUTICS

Before drug therapy is initiated, an end point or expected outcome of therapy needs to be established. This desired therapeutic outcome is patient-specific, established in collaboration with the patient, and, if appropriate, determined with other members of the health care team. Outcomes need to be clearly defined and must be either measurable or observable by monitoring. Outcome goals must be realistic and prioritized so that drug therapy begins with interventions that are essential to the patient's well-being. Examples include curing a disease, eliminating or reducing a preexisting symptom, arresting or slowing a disease process, preventing a disease or other unwanted condition, or otherwise improving quality of life. These goals and outcomes are not the same as nursing goals and outcomes. See Chapter 1 for a more specific discussion of the nursing process.

Patient therapy assessment is the process by which a practitioner integrates his or her knowledge of medical and drug-related facts with information about a specific patient's medical and social history. Items to be considered in the assessment are drugs currently used (prescription, over-the-counter, herbal, and illicit or street drugs), pregnancy and breastfeeding status, and concurrent illnesses that could contraindicate initiation of a given medication. A contraindication for a medication is any patient condition, especially a disease state, that makes the use of the given medication dangerous for the patient. Careful attention to this assessment process helps to ensure an optimal therapeutic plan. The implementation of a treatment plan can involve several types and combinations of therapies. The type of therapy can be categorized as *acute, maintenance, supplemental* (or *replacement*), *palliative, supportive, prophylactic,* or *empiric.*

### Acute Therapy

Acute therapy often involves more intensive drug treatment and is implemented in the acutely ill (those with rapid onset of illness) or the critically ill. It is often needed to sustain life or treat disease. Examples are the administration of vasopressors to maintain blood pressure and cardiac output after open heart surgery, the use of volume expanders for a patient who is in shock, and intensive chemotherapy for a patient with newly diagnosed cancer.

### Maintenance Therapy

Maintenance therapy does not eradicate problems the patient may already have but will prevent progression of a disease or condition. It is used for the treatment of chronic illnesses such as hypertension. In the latter case, maintenance therapy maintains the patient's blood pressure within given limits, which prevents certain end-organ damage. Another example of maintenance therapy is the use of oral contraceptives for birth control.

### Supplemental Therapy

Supplemental (or replacement) therapy supplies the body with a substance needed to maintain normal function. This substance may be needed either because it cannot be made by the body or because it is produced in insufficient quantity. Examples are the administration of insulin to diabetic patients and of iron to patients with iron-deficiency anemia.

### Palliative Therapy

The goal of palliative therapy is to make the patient as comfortable as possible. Palliative therapy focuses on providing patients with relief from the symptoms, pain, and stress of a serious illness. The goal is to improve quality of life for both the patient and the family. It is typically used in the end stages of an illness when attempts at curative therapy have failed; however, it can be provided along with curative treatment. Examples are the use of high-dose opioid analgesics to relieve pain in the final stages of cancer.

### Supportive Therapy

Supportive therapy maintains the integrity of body functions while the patient is recovering from illness or trauma. Examples are provision of fluids and electrolytes to prevent dehydration in a patient with influenza who is vomiting and has diarrhea, and administration of fluids, volume expanders, or blood products to a patient who has lost blood during surgery.

### Prophylactic Therapy and Empiric Therapy

Prophylactic therapy is drug therapy provided to *prevent* illness or other undesirable outcome during *planned* events. A common example is the use of preoperative antibiotic therapy for surgical procedures. The antibiotic is given before the incision is made, so that the antibiotic can kill any potential pathogens. Another example is the administration of disease-specific vaccines to individuals traveling to geographic areas where a given disease is known to be endemic.

Empiric therapy is based on clinical probabilities. It involves drug administration when a certain pathologic condition has an uncertain but high likelihood of occurrence based on the patient's initial presenting symptoms. A common example is use of antibiotics active against the organism most commonly associated with a specific infection before the results of the culture and sensitivity reports are available.

### Monitoring

Once the appropriate therapy has been implemented, the effectiveness of the therapy—that is, the clinical response of the patient to the treatment—must be evaluated. Evaluating the clinical response requires familiarity with both the drug's intended therapeutic action (beneficial effects) and its unintended possible adverse effects (predictable adverse drug reactions). Examples of monitoring include observing for the therapeutic effect of reduced blood pressure following administration of antihypertensive drugs and observing for the toxic effect of leukopenia after administering antineoplastic (cancer chemotherapy) drugs. Another example is performing a pain assessment after giving pain medication. It should be noted that this text generally highlights only the most common adverse effects of a given drug; however, the drug may have many other less commonly reported adverse effects. Always keep in mind that patients may sometimes experience less common and less readily identifiable adverse drug effects. Consult comprehensive references, pharmacists, or poison and drug information center staff when there is uncertainty regarding adverse effects that a patient may be experiencing.

All drugs are potentially toxic and can have cumulative effects. Recognizing these toxic effects and knowing their manifestations are integral components of the monitoring process. A drug can accumulate when it is absorbed more quickly than it is eliminated or when it is administered before the previous dose has been metabolized or cleared from the body. Knowledge of the organs responsible for metabolizing and eliminating a drug combined with knowledge of how a particular drug is metabolized and excreted enables the nurse to anticipate problems and treat them appropriately if they occur.

### Therapeutic Index

The ratio of a drug's toxic level to the level that provides therapeutic benefits is referred to as the drug's therapeutic index. The safety of a particular drug therapy is determined by this index. A low therapeutic index means that the difference between a therapeutically active dose and a toxic dose is small. A drug with a low therapeutic index has a greater likelihood than other drugs of causing an adverse reaction, and therefore its use requires closer monitoring. Examples of such drugs are warfarin and digoxin. In contrast, a drug with a high therapeutic index, such as amoxicillin, is rarely associated with overdose events.

### Drug Concentration

All drugs reach a certain concentration in the blood. Drug concentrations can be an important tool for evaluating the clinical response to drug therapy. Certain drug levels are associated with therapeutic responses, whereas other drug levels are associated with toxic effects. Toxic drug levels are typically seen when the body's normal mechanisms for metabolizing and excreting drugs are compromised. This commonly occurs when liver and kidney functions are impaired or when the liver or kidneys are immature (as in neonates). Dosage adjustments should be made in these patients to appropriately accommodate their impaired metabolism and excretion.

### Patient's Condition

Another patient-specific factor to be considered is the patient's concurrent diseases or other medical conditions. A patient's response to a drug may vary greatly depending on physiologic and psychological demands. Disease of any kind, infection, cardiovascular function, and GI function are just a few of the physiologic elements that can alter a patient's therapeutic response. Stress, depression, and anxiety can also be important psychological factors affecting response.

### Tolerance and Dependence

To provide optimal drug therapy, it is important to understand and differentiate between tolerance and dependence. Tolerance

| TABLE 2-9 | COMMON FOOD AND DRUG INTERACTIONS | |
|---|---|---|
| **FOOD** | **DRUG (CATEGORY)** | **RESULT** |
| Leafy green vegetables | warfarin (anticoagulant) | Decreased anticoagulant effect from warfarin |
| Dairy products | tetracycline, levofloxacin, ciprofloxacin, moxifloxacin (antibiotics) | Chemical binding of the drug leading to decreased effect and treatment failures |
| Grapefruit juice | amiodarone (antidysrhythmic), buspirone (antianxiety), carbamazepine (antiseizure), cyclosporine, tacrolimus (immunosuppressants), felodipine, nifedipine, nimodipine, nisoldipine (calcium channel blockers), simvastatin, atorvastatin (anticholesterol drugs) | Decreased metabolism of drugs and increased effects |
| Aged cheese, wine | Monoamine oxidase inhibitors | Hypertensive crisis |

is a decreasing response to repeated drug doses. Dependence is a physiologic or psychological need for a drug. *Physical dependence* is the physiologic need for a drug to avoid physical withdrawal symptoms (e.g., tachycardia in an opioid-addicted patient). *Psychological dependence* is also known as *addiction* and is the obsessive desire for the euphoric effects of a drug. Addiction typically involves the recreational use of various drugs such as benzodiazepines, opioids, and amphetamines. See Chapter 17 for further discussion of dependence and addiction.

### Interactions

Drugs may interact with other drugs, with foods, or with agents administered as part of laboratory tests. Knowledge of drug interactions is vital for the appropriate monitoring of drug therapy. The more drugs a patient receives, the more likely that a drug interaction will occur. This is especially true in older adults, who typically have an increased sensitivity to drug effects and are receiving several medications. In addition, over-the-counter medications and herbal therapies can interact significantly with prescribed medications. Food also can interact significantly with certain drugs. See Table 2-9 for the most common food and drug interactions.

Alteration of the action of one drug by another is referred to as drug interaction. A drug interaction can either increase or decrease the actions of one or both of the involved drugs. Drug interactions can be either beneficial or harmful. Numerous drug interactions can occur and have been reported. Please note that only those drug interactions that are considered to be significant with at least a good probability of occurring and/or those that require dosage/therapy adjustment are discussed in this textbook. An authoritative resource may be used as a means of exploring all possible drug interactions.

Concurrently administered drugs may interact with each other and alter the pharmacokinetics of one another during any

## TABLE 2-10   EXAMPLES OF DRUG INTERACTIONS AND THEIR EFFECTS ON PHARMACOKINETICS

| PHARMACOKINETIC PHASE | DRUG COMBINATION | MECHANISM | RESULT |
|---|---|---|---|
| Absorption | Antacid with levofloxacin | Antacids bind to the levofloxacin preventing adequate absorption | Decreased effectiveness of levofloxacin, resulting from decreased blood levels (harmful) |
| Distribution | warfarin with amiodarone | Both drugs compete for protein-binding sites | Higher levels of free (unbound) warfarin and amiodarone, which increases actions of both drugs (harmful) |
| Metabolism | erythromycin with cyclosporine | Both drugs compete for the same hepatic enzymes | Decreased metabolism of cyclosporine, possibly resulting in toxic levels of cyclosporine (harmful) |
| Excretion | amoxicillin with probenecid | Inhibits the secretion of amoxicillin into the kidneys | Elevation and prolongation of plasma levels of amoxicillin (can be beneficial) |

of the four phases of pharmacokinetics: absorption, distribution, metabolism, or excretion. Table 2-10 provides examples of drug interactions during each of these phases. Most commonly, drug interactions occur when there is competition between two drugs for metabolizing enzymes, such as the cytochrome P-450 enzymes listed in Table 2-5. As a result, the speed of metabolism of one or both drugs may be enhanced or reduced. This change in metabolism of one or both drugs can lead to subtherapeutic or toxic drug actions.

Many terms are used to categorize drug interactions. When two drugs with similar actions are given together, they can have additive effects (1 + 1 = 2). Examples are the many combinations of analgesic products, such as antihistamine and opioid combinations (e.g., promethazine and codeine) for treatment of cold symptoms, and acetaminophen and opioid combinations (e.g., acetaminophen and oxycodone) for treatment of pain. Often drugs are used together for their additive effects so that smaller doses of each drug can be given.

Synergistic effects occur when two drugs administered together interact in such a way that their combined effects are greater than the sum of the effects for each drug given alone (1 + 1 = greater than 2). The combination of hydrochlorothiazide with lisinopril for the treatment of hypertension is an example.

Antagonistic effects are said to occur when the combination of two drugs results in drug effects that are less than the sum of the effects for each drug given separately (1 + 1 = less than 2). An example of this type of interaction occurs when the antibiotic ciprofloxacin is given simultaneously with antacids, vitamins, iron, or dairy products. These drugs reduce the absorption of ciprofloxacin and lead to decreased effectiveness of the antibiotic.

Incompatibility is a term most commonly used to describe parenteral drugs. Drug incompatibility occurs when two parenteral drugs or solutions are mixed together and the result is a chemical deterioration of one or both of the drugs or the formation of a physical precipitate. The combination of two such drugs usually produces a precipitate, haziness, or color change in the solution. Before administering any intravenous medication, the nurse must always inspect the bag for precipitate. If the solution appears cloudy or if visible flecks are seen, the bag must be discarded and not given to the patient. An example of incompatible drugs is the combination of parenteral furosemide and heparin.

## Adverse Drug Events

The recognition of the potential hazards and detrimental effects of medication use is a topic that continues to receive much attention in the literature. This focus has contributed to an increasing body of knowledge regarding this topic as well as the development of new terminology. Health care institutions are under increasing pressure to develop effective strategies for preventing adverse effects of drugs.

Adverse drug event (ADE) is a broad term for any undesirable occurrence involving medications. A similarly broad term also seen in the literature is *drug misadventure.* Patient outcomes associated with adverse drug events vary from no effects to mild discomfort to life-threatening complications, permanent disability, disfigurement, or death. Adverse drug events can be preventable (see discussion of medication errors later in Chapter 5) or nonpreventable. Fortunately, many adverse drug events result in no measurable patient harm. Adverse drug events can be both external and internal. The most common causes of adverse drug events *external* to the patient are errors by caregivers (both professional and nonprofessional) and malfunctioning of equipment (e.g., intravenous infusion pumps). An adverse drug event can be internal, or *patient induced,* such as when a patient fails to take medication as prescribed or drinks alcoholic beverages that he or she was advised not to consume while taking a given medication. An impending adverse drug event that is noticed before it actually occurs is considered a *potential* adverse drug event (and appropriate steps must be taken to avoid such a "near miss" in the future). A less common situation, but one still worth mentioning, is an *adverse drug withdrawal event.* This is an adverse outcome associated with discontinuation of drug therapy, such as hypertension caused by abruptly discontinuing blood pressure medication or return of infection caused by stopping antibiotic therapy too soon.

The two most common broad categories of adverse drug event are medication errors and adverse drug reactions. A medication error is a preventable situation in which there is a compromise in the "Six Rights" of medication use: *right drug, right dose, right time, right route, right patient,* and *right documentation.* Medication errors are more common than adverse drug reactions. Medication errors occur during the *prescribing, dispensing, administering,* or *monitoring* of drug therapy. These four phases are collectively known as the medication use process. See Chapter 5 for further discussion of medication errors.

An adverse drug reaction (ADR) (see Chapter 5) is any reaction to a drug that is unexpected and undesirable and occurs at therapeutic drug dosages. Adverse drug reactions may or may not be caused by medication errors. Adverse drug reactions may result in hospital admission, prolongation of hospital stay, change in drug therapy, initiation of supportive treatment, or complication of a patient's disease state. Adverse drug reactions are caused by processes inside the patient's body. They may or may not be preventable, depending on the situation. Mild adverse drug reactions (e.g., *drug adverse effects*—see later in the chapter) usually do not require a change in the patient's drug therapy or other interventions. More severe adverse drug reactions, however, are likely to require changes to a patient's drug regimen. Severe adverse drug reactions can be permanently or significantly disabling, life threatening, or fatal. They may require or prolong hospitalization, lead to organ damage (e.g., to the liver, kidneys, bone marrow, skin), cause congenital anomalies, or require specific interventions to prevent permanent impairment or tissue damage.

Adverse drug reactions that are specific to particular drug groups are discussed in the corresponding drug chapters in this book. Four general categories are discussed here: pharmacologic reaction, hypersensitivity (allergic) reaction, idiosyncratic reaction, and drug interaction.

A pharmacologic reaction is an extension of the drug's normal effects in the body. For example, a drug that is used to lower blood pressure in a patient causes a pharmacologic adverse drug reaction when it lowers the blood pressure to the point at which the patient becomes unconscious.

Pharmacologic reactions that result in adverse effects are predictable, well-known adverse drug reactions resulting in minor or no changes in patient management. They have predictable frequency and intensity, and their occurrence is related to the dose. They also usually resolve upon discontinuation of drug therapy.

An allergic reaction (also known as a *hypersensitivity reaction*) involves the patient's immune system. Immune system proteins known as *immunoglobulins* (see Chapters 48 and 49) recognize the drug molecule, its metabolite(s), or another ingredient in a drug formulation as a dangerous foreign substance. At this point, an *immune response* may occur in which immunoglobulin proteins bind to the drug substance in an attempt to neutralize the drug. Various chemical mediators, such as *histamine,* as well as *cytokines* and other inflammatory substances (e.g., *prostaglandins* [see Chapter 44]) usually are released during this process. This response can result in reactions ranging from mild reactions such as skin erythema or mild rash to severe, even life-threatening reactions such as constriction of bronchial airways and tachycardia.

It can be assumed throughout this textbook that use of any drug is contraindicated if the patient has a known allergy to that specific drug product. Allergy information may be reported by the patient as part of his or her history or may be observed by health care personnel during a patient encounter. In either case, every effort must be made to document as fully as possible the name of the drug product and the degree and details of the adverse reaction that occurred. For example: "Penicillin; skin rash, pruritus" or "Penicillin; urticaria and anaphylactic shock requiring emergency intervention."

In more extreme cases of disease or injury (e.g., cancer, snakebite), it may be deemed reasonable to administer a given drug *in spite of* a reported allergic or other adverse reaction. In such cases, the patient will likely be premedicated with additional medications (e.g., acetaminophen [Tylenol], diphenhydramine [Benadryl], prednisone) as an attempt to control any adverse reactions that may occur.

An idiosyncratic reaction is not the result of a known pharmacologic property of a drug or of a patient allergy, but instead occurs unexpectedly in a particular patient. Such a reaction is a genetically determined abnormal response to normal dosages of a drug. The study of such traits, which are solely revealed by drug administration, is called pharmacogenomics (see Chapter 8). Idiosyncratic drug reactions are usually caused by a deficiency or excess of drug-metabolizing enzymes. Many pharmacogenomic disorders exist. An example is glucose-6-phosphate dehydrogenase (G6PD) deficiency. This disease affects approximately 100 million people. People who lack proper levels of G6PD have idiosyncratic reactions to a wide range of drugs. There are more than 80 variations of the disease, and all produce some degree of drug-induced hemolysis. Drugs that are capable of inducing hemolysis in such patients are listed in Box 2-3.

The final type of adverse drug reaction is due to drug interaction. As described earlier, drug interaction occurs when the presence of two (or more) drugs in the body produces an unwanted effect. This unwanted effect can result when one drug either enhances or reduces the effects of another drug. Some drug interactions are intentional and beneficial (see Table 2-10). However, most clinically significant drug interactions

---

### ⊕ PATIENT-CENTERED CARE: CULTURAL IMPLICATIONS

#### *Glucose-6-Phosphate Dehydrogenase Deficiency*

Glucose-6-phosphate dehydrogenase (G6PD) is an enzyme found in abundant amounts in the tissues of most individuals. It reduces the risk of hemolysis of red blood cells when they are exposed to oxidizing drugs such as aspirin. Approximately 13% of African-American men and 20% of African-American women carry the gene that results in G6PD deficiency. Approximately 14% of Sardinians and more than 50% of the Kurdish Jewish population also show G6PD deficiencies. When exposed to drugs such as sulfonamides, antimalarials, and aspirin, patients with this deficiency may suffer life-threatening hemolysis of the red blood cells, whereas individuals with adequate quantities of the enzyme have no problems in taking these drugs.

---

### BOX 2-3 DRUGS TO AVOID IN PATIENTS WITH GLUCOSE-6-PHOSPHATE DEHYDROGENASE DEFICIENCY

| | |
|---|---|
| Aspirin | Probenecid |
| Nitrofurantoin | Sulfonamides |
| Primaquine | |

are harmful. Drug interactions specific to particular drugs are discussed in detail in the chapters dealing with those drugs.

## Other Drug Effects

Other drug-related effects that must be considered during drug therapy are teratogenic, mutagenic, and carcinogenic effects. These can result in devastating patient outcomes and may be prevented in many instances by appropriate monitoring.

Teratogenic effects of drugs or other chemicals result in structural defects in the fetus. Compounds that produce such effects are called *teratogens*. Prenatal development involves a delicate program of interrelated embryologic events. Any significant disruption in this process of *embryogenesis* can have a teratogenic effect. Drugs that are capable of crossing the placenta can cause drug-induced teratogenesis. Drugs administered during pregnancy can produce different types of congenital anomalies. The period during which the fetus is most vulnerable to teratogenic effects begins with the third week of development and usually ends after the third month. Chapter 3 describes the FDA safety classification for drugs used by pregnant women.

Mutagenic effects are permanent changes in the genetic composition of living organisms and consist of alterations in chromosome structure, the number of chromosomes, or the genetic code of the deoxyribonucleic acid (DNA) molecule. Drugs that are capable of inducing mutations are called *mutagens*. Radiation, viruses, chemicals (e.g., industrial chemicals such as benzene), and drugs can all act as mutagenic agents in humans. Drugs that affect genetic processes are active primarily during cell reproduction (mitosis).

Carcinogenic effects are the cancer-causing effects of drugs, other chemicals, radiation, and viruses. Agents that produce such effects are called *carcinogens*. Some exogenous causes of cancer are listed in Box 2-4.

## PHARMACOGNOSY

The source of all early drugs was nature, and the study of these natural drug sources (plants and animals) is called *pharmacognosy*. Although many drugs in current use are synthetically derived, most were first isolated in nature. The four main sources for drugs are plants, animals, minerals, and laboratory synthesis. Plants provide many weak acids and weak bases (alkaloids) that are very useful and potent drugs. Alkaloids are more common, including atropine (belladonna plant), caffeine (coffee bean), and nicotine (tobacco leaf). Animals are the source of many hormone drugs. Conjugated estrogens are derived from the urine of pregnant mares, hence the drug trade name Premarin. *Equine* is the term used for any horse-derived drug. Insulin comes from two sources: pigs (porcine) and humans. Human insulin is now far more commonly used than animal insulins thanks to the use of recombinant DNA techniques. Heparin is another commonly used drug that is derived from pigs (porcine heparin). Some common mineral sources of currently used drugs are salicylic acid, aluminum hydroxide, and sodium chloride.

## PHARMACOECONOMICS

*Pharmacoeconomics* is the study of the economic factors influencing the cost of drug therapy. One example is performing a *cost-benefit analysis* of one antibiotic versus another when competing drugs are considered for inclusion in a hospital formulary. Such studies typically examine treatment outcomes data (e.g., how many patients recovered and how soon) in relation to the comparative total costs of treatment with the drugs in question.

## TOXICOLOGY

The study of poisons and unwanted responses to both drugs and other chemicals is known as *toxicology*. Toxicology is the science of the adverse effects of chemicals on living organisms. Clinical toxicology deals specifically with the care of the poisoned patient. Poisoning can result from a variety of causes, ranging from drug overdose to ingestion of household cleaning agents to snakebite. Poison control centers are health care institutions equipped with sufficient personnel and information resources to recommend appropriate treatment for the poisoned patient.

Effective treatment of the poisoned patient is based on a system of priorities, the first of which is to preserve the patient's vital functions by maintaining the airway, ventilation, and circulation. The second priority is to prevent absorption of the toxic substance and/or speed its elimination from the body using one or more of the variety of clinical methods available. Several common poisons and their specific antidotes are listed in Table 2-11.

| TABLE 2-11 | COMMON POISONS AND THEIR ANTIDOTES* | |
|---|---|
| **SUBSTANCE** | **ANTIDOTE** |
| Acetaminophen | Acetylcysteine |
| Organophosphates (e.g., insecticides) | Atropine |
| Tricyclic antidepressants, quinidine | Sodium bicarbonate |
| Calcium channel blockers | Intravenous calcium |
| Iron salts | Deferoxamine |
| Digoxin and other cardiac glycosides | Digoxin antibodies |
| Ethylene glycol (e.g., automotive antifreeze solution), methanol | Ethanol (same as alcohol used for drinking), given intravenously |
| Benzodiazepines | Flumazenil |
| Beta blockers | Glucagon |
| Opiates, opioid drugs | Naloxone |
| Carbon monoxide (by inhalation) | Oxygen (at high concentration), known as bariatric therapy |

*These and other antidotes are discussed throughout this textbook where applicable.

| BOX 2-4 | EXOGENOUS CAUSES OF CANCER | |
|---|---|
| Dietary customs | Environmental pollution |
| Drug abuse | Food-processing procedures |
| Carcinogenic drugs | Food production procedures |
| Workplace chemicals | Oncogenic viruses |
| Radiation | Smoking |

## SUMMARY

A thorough understanding of the pharmacologic principles of pharmacokinetics, pharmacodynamics, pharmacotherapeutics, and toxicology is essential in drug therapy and to safe, quality nursing practice. Medications may be very helpful in treating disease, but unless the nurse has an adequate, up-to-date knowledge base and clinical skills and engages in critical thinking and good decision-making, any treatment may become harmful. Application of pharmacologic principles enables the nurse to provide safe and effective drug therapy while always acting on behalf of the patient and respecting the patient's rights. Nursing considerations associated with various routes of drug administration are summarized in Table 2-3.

## KEY POINTS

- The following definitions related to drug therapy are important to remember: *pharmacology*—the study or science of drugs; *pharmacokinetics*—the study of drug distribution among various body compartments after a drug has entered the body, including the phases of absorption, distribution, metabolism, and excretion; *pharmaceutics*—the science of dosage form design.
- The nurse's role in drug therapy and the nursing process is more than just the memorization of the names of drugs, their uses, and associated interventions. It involves a thorough comprehension of all aspects of pharmaceutics, pharmacokinetics, and pharmacodynamics and the sound application of this drug knowledge to a variety of clinical situations. See Chapter 1 for further discussion of drug therapy as it relates to the nursing process.
- Drug actions are related to the pharmacologic, pharmaceutical, pharmacokinetic, and pharmacodynamic properties of a given medication, and each of these has a specific influence on the overall effects produced by the drug in a patient.
- Selection of the route of administration is based on patient variables and the specific characteristics of a drug.
- Nursing considerations vary depending on the drug as well as the route of administration.

## NCLEX® EXAMINATION REVIEW QUESTIONS

1 An elderly woman took a prescription medicine to help her to sleep; however, she felt restless all night and did not sleep at all. The nurse recognizes that this woman has experienced which type of reaction or effect?
   a Allergic reaction
   b Idiosyncratic reaction
   c Mutagenic effect
   d Synergistic effect

2 While caring for a patient with cirrhosis or hepatitis, the nurse knows that abnormalities in which phase of pharmacokinetics may occur?
   a Absorption
   b Distribution
   c Metabolism
   d Excretion

3 A patient who has advanced cancer is receiving opioid medications around the clock to "keep him comfortable" as he nears the end of his life. Which term best describes this type of therapy?
   a Palliative therapy
   b Maintenance therapy
   c Supportive therapy
   d Supplemental therapy

4 The nurse is giving medications to a patient in heart failure. The intravenous route is chosen instead of the intramuscular route. The nurse knows that the factor that most influences the decision about which route to use is the patient's
   a altered biliary function.
   b increased glomerular filtration.
   c reduced liver metabolism.
   d diminished circulation.

5 A patient has just received a prescription for an enteric-coated stool softener. When teaching the patient, the nurse should include which statement?
   a "Take the tablet with 2 to 3 ounces of orange juice."
   b "Avoid taking all other medications with any enteric-coated tablet."
   c "Crush the tablet before swallowing if you have problems with swallowing."
   d "Be sure to swallow the tablet whole without chewing it."

6 Each statement describes a phase of pharmacokinetics. Put the statements in order, with 1 indicating the phase that occurs first and 4 indicating the phase that occurs last.
   a Enzymes in the liver transform the drug into an inactive metabolite.
   b Drug metabolites are secreted through passive glomerular filtration into the renal tubules.
   c A drug binds to the plasma protein albumin and circulates through the body.
   d A drug moves from the intestinal lumen into the mesenteric blood system.

7 A drug that delivers 500 mg has a half-life of 4 hours. How many milligrams of drug will remain in the body after 1 half-life?

1. b, 2. c, 3. a, 4. d, 5. d, 6. a = 3, b = 4, c = 2, d = 1, 7. 250 mg

For Critical Thinking and Prioritization Questions, see http://evolve.elsevier.com/Lilley.

# Lifespan Considerations

## OBJECTIVES

When you reach the end of this chapter, you will be able to do the following:

1  Discuss the influences of the patient's age on the effects of drugs and drug responses.
2  Identify drug-related concerns during pregnancy and lactation and provide an explanation of the physiologic basis for these concerns.
3  Summarize the impact of age-related physiologic changes on the pharmacokinetic aspects of drug therapy.
4  Explain how these age-related changes in pharmacokinetics influence various drug effects and drug responses across the lifespan.

5  Provide several examples of how age affects the absorption, distribution, metabolism, and excretion of drugs.
6  Calculate a drug dose for a pediatric patient using the various formulas available.
7  Identify the importance of a body surface area nomogram for drug calculations in pediatric patients.
8  Develop a nursing care plan for drug therapy and the nursing process that takes into account lifespan considerations.

## KEY TERMS

**Active transport** The active (energy-requiring) movement of a substance between different tissues via pumping mechanisms contained within cell membranes. (p. 38)

**Diffusion** The passive movement of a substance (e.g., a drug) between different tissues from areas of higher concentration to areas of lower concentration. (Compare with *active transport*.) (p. 38)

**Elderly** Pertaining to a person who is 65 years of age or older. (Note: Some sources consider "elderly" to be 55 years of age or older.) (p. 42)

**Neonate** Pertaining to a person younger than 1 month of age; newborn infant. (p. 38)

**Nomogram** A graphic tool for estimating drug dosages using various body measurements. (p. 40)

**Pediatric** Pertaining to a person who is 12 years of age or younger. (p. 39)

**Polypharmacy** The use of many different drugs concurrently in treating a patient, who often has several health problems. (p. 42)

From the beginning to the end of life, the human body changes in many ways. These changes have a dramatic effect on the four phases of pharmacokinetics—drug absorption, distribution, metabolism, and excretion. Newborn, pediatric, and elderly patients each have special needs. Drug therapy at the two ends of the spectrum of life is more likely to result in adverse effects and toxicity. This is especially true if certain basic principles are not understood and followed. Fortunately, response to drug therapy changes in a predictable manner in younger and older patients. Knowing the effect that age has on the pharmacokinetic characteristics of drugs helps predict these changes.

Most experience with drugs and pharmacology has been gained from the adult population. The majority of drug studies have focused on the population between 13 and 65 years of age. It has been estimated that 75% of currently approved drugs lack U.S. Food and Drug Administration (FDA) approval for pediatric use and therefore lack specific dosage guidelines for neonates and children. Fortunately, many excellent pediatric drug dosage books are available. Most drugs are effective in younger and older patients, but drugs often behave very differently in patients at the opposite ends of the age spectrum. It is vitally important from the standpoint of safe and effective drug administration to understand what these differences are and how to adjust for them.

## DRUG THERAPY DURING PREGNANCY

A fetus is exposed to many of the same substances as the mother, including any drugs that she takes—prescription, nonprescription, or street drugs. The first trimester of pregnancy is generally the period of greatest danger of drug-induced developmental defects.

Transfer of both drugs and nutrients to the fetus occurs primarily by diffusion across the placenta, although not all drugs cross the placenta. Recall from chemistry that diffusion is a passive process based on differences in concentration between different tissues. Active transport requires the expenditure of energy and often involves some sort of cell-surface protein pump. The factors that contribute to the safety or potential harm of drug therapy during pregnancy can be broadly broken down into three areas: drug properties, fetal gestational age, and maternal factors.

Drug properties that impact drug transfer to the fetus include the drug's chemistry, dosage, and concurrently administered drugs. Examples of relevant chemical properties include molecular weight, protein binding, lipid solubility, and chemical structure. Important drug dosage variables include dose and duration of therapy.

Fetal gestational age is an important factor in determining the potential for harmful drug effects to the fetus. The fetus is at greatest risk for drug-induced developmental defects during the first trimester of pregnancy. During this period, the fetus undergoes rapid cell proliferation. Skeleton, muscles, limbs, and visceral organs are developing at their most rapid rate. Self-treatment of minor illness is strongly discouraged anytime during pregnancy, but especially during the first trimester. Gestational age is also important in determining when a drug can most easily cross the placenta to the fetus. During the last trimester, the greatest percentage of maternally absorbed drug gets to the fetus.

Maternal factors also play a role in determining drug effects on the fetus. Any change in the mother's physiology can affect the amount of drug to which the fetus may be exposed. Maternal kidney and liver function affect drug metabolism and excretion. Impairment in either kidney or liver function may result in higher drug levels and/or prolonged drug exposure, and thus increased fetal transfer. Maternal genotype may also affect how certain drugs are metabolized (pharmacogenetics). The lack of certain enzyme systems may result in adverse drug effects to the fetus when the mother is exposed to a drug that is normally metabolized by the given enzyme.

Although exposure of the fetus to drugs is most detrimental during the first trimester, drug transfer to the fetus is more likely during the last trimester. This is the result of enhanced blood flow to the fetus, increased fetal surface area, and increased amount of free drug in the mother's circulation.

It is important to use drugs judiciously during pregnancy; however, there are certain situations that require their use. Without drug therapy, maternal conditions such as hypertension, epilepsy, diabetes, and infection could seriously endanger both the mother and the fetus, and the potential for harm far outweighs the risks of appropriate drug therapy.

The FDA classifies drugs according to their safety for use during pregnancy. This system of drug classification is based primarily on animal studies and limited human studies. This is due in part to ethical dilemmas surrounding the study of potential adverse effects on fetuses. We have learned from several unfortunate mistakes, such as the maternal use of thalidomide, which causes birth defects, and diethylstilbestrol (DES), which causes a high incidence of gynecologic malignancy in female offspring. The most widely used index of potential fetal risk of drugs is the FDA's pregnancy safety category system. The five safety categories are described in Table 3-1. The FDA is in the process of changing the pregnancy categories; however, the information is not yet published at the time of this writing. The information will be posted on http://evolve.elsevier.com/Lilley once it becomes available.

## DRUG THERAPY DURING BREASTFEEDING

Breastfed infants are at risk for exposure to drugs consumed by the mother. A wide variety of drugs easily cross from the mother's circulation into the breast milk and subsequently to the breastfeeding infant. Drug properties similar to those discussed in the previous section influence the exposure of infants to drugs via breastfeeding. The primary drug characteristics that increase the likelihood of drug transfer via breastfeeding include fat solubility, low molecular weight, nonionization, and high concentration.

Fortunately, breast milk is not the primary route for maternal drug excretion. Drug levels in breast milk are usually lower than those in the maternal circulation. The actual amount of exposure depends largely on the volume of milk consumed. The ultimate decision as to whether a breastfeeding mother takes a particular drug depends on the risk/benefit ratio. The risks of drug transfer to the infant in relation to the benefits of continuing breastfeeding and the therapeutic benefits to the mother must be considered on a case-by-case basis.

## TABLE 3-1 PREGNANCY SAFETY CATEGORIES

| CATEGORY | DESCRIPTION |
| --- | --- |
| Category A | Studies indicate no risk to the human fetus. |
| Category B | Studies indicate no risk to the animal fetus; information for humans is not available. |
| Category C | Adverse effects reported in the animal fetus; information for humans is not available. |
| Category D | Possible fetal risk in humans has been reported; however, in selected cases consideration of the potential benefit versus risk may warrant use of these drugs in pregnant women. |
| Category X | Fetal abnormalities have been reported, and positive evidence of fetal risk in humans is available from animal and/or human studies. These drugs are not be used in pregnant women. |

## TABLE 3-2 CLASSIFICATION OF YOUNG PATIENTS

| AGE RANGE | CLASSIFICATION |
| --- | --- |
| Younger than 38 weeks' gestation | Premature or preterm infant |
| Younger than 1 month | Neonate or newborn infant |
| 1 month up to 1 year | Infant |
| 1 year up to 12 years | Child |

NOTE: The meaning of the term *pediatric* may vary with the individual drug and clinical situation. Often the maximum age for a pediatric patient may be identified as 16 years of age. Consult manufacturer's guidelines for specific dosing information.

## CONSIDERATIONS FOR NEONATAL AND PEDIATRIC PATIENTS

Pediatric patients are defined based on age. A *neonate* is defined as between birth and 1 month of age. An *infant* is between 1 and 12 months of age, and a *child* is between 1 and 12 years of age. The age ranges that correspond to the various terms applied to pediatric patients are shown in Table 3-2.

### Physiology and Pharmacokinetics

Pediatric patients handle drugs much differently than adult patients, based primarily on the immaturity of vital organs. In both neonates and older pediatric patients, anatomic structures and physiologic systems and functions are still in the process of developing. The Patient-Centered Care: Lifespan Considerations for the Pediatric Patient box on this page lists those physiologic factors that alter the pharmacokinetic properties of drugs in young patients.

### Pharmacodynamics

Drug actions (or pharmacodynamics) are altered in young patients, and the maturity of various organs determines how drugs act in the body. Certain drugs may be more toxic, whereas others may be less toxic. The sensitivity of receptor sites may also vary with age; thus, higher or lower dosages may be required depending on the drug. In addition, rapidly developing tissues

## PATIENT-CENTERED CARE: LIFESPAN CONSIDERATIONS FOR THE PEDIATRIC PATIENT

### Pharmacokinetic Changes in the Neonate and Pediatric Patient

**Absorption**
- Gastric pH is less acidic because acid-producing cells in the stomach are immature until approximately 1 to 2 years of age.
- Gastric emptying is slowed because of slow or irregular peristalsis.
- First-pass elimination by the liver is reduced because of the immaturity of the liver and reduced levels of microsomal enzymes.
- Intramuscular absorption is faster and irregular.

**Distribution**
- Total body water is 70% to 80% in full-term infants, 85% in premature newborns, and 64% in children 1 to 12 years of age.
- Fat content is lower in young patients because of greater total body water.
- Protein binding is decreased because of decreased production of protein by the immature liver.
- More drugs enter the brain because of an immature blood-brain barrier.

**Metabolism**
- Levels of microsomal enzymes are decreased because the immature liver has not yet started producing enough.
- Older children may have increased metabolism and require higher dosages once hepatic enzymes are produced.
- Many variables affect metabolism in premature infants, infants, and children, including the status of liver enzyme production, genetic differences, and substances to which the mother was exposed during pregnancy.

**Excretion**
- Glomerular filtration rate and tubular secretion and resorption are all decreased in young patients because of kidney immaturity.
- Perfusion to the kidneys may be decreased, which results in reduced renal function, concentrating ability, and excretion of drugs.

may be more sensitive to certain drugs, and therefore smaller dosages may be required. Certain drugs are contraindicated during the growth years. For instance, tetracycline may permanently discolor a young person's teeth; corticosteroids may suppress growth when given systemically (but not when delivered via asthma inhalers, for example); and quinolone antibiotics may damage cartilage.

### Dosage Calculations for Pediatric Patients

Most drugs have not been sufficiently investigated to ensure their safety and effectiveness in children. In spite of this, there are numerous excellent pediatric dosage references. Because pediatric patients (especially premature infants and neonates) have small bodies and immature organs, they are very susceptible to drug interactions, toxicity, and unusual drug responses. Pediatric patients require different dosage calculations than do adults. Characteristics of pediatric patients that have a significant effect on dosage include the following:

- Skin is thinner and more permeable.
- Stomach lacks acid to kill bacteria.
- Lungs have weaker mucous barriers.

- Body temperature is less well regulated, and dehydration occurs easily.
- Liver and kidneys are immature, and, therefore, drug metabolism and excretion are impaired.

Many formulas for pediatric dosage calculation have been used throughout the years. Formulas involving age, weight, and body surface area (BSA) are most commonly employed as the basis for calculations. BSA-based formulas are the most accurate of these dosage formulas.

To use the BSA method, the nurse needs the following information:

- Drug order with drug name, dose, route, time, and frequency
- Information regarding available dosage forms

- Pediatric patient's height in centimeters (cm) and weight in kilograms (kg)
- BSA nomogram for children (e.g., West nomogram, shown in Figure 3-1)
- Recommended adult drug dosage

The West nomogram (see Figure 3-1) uses a child's height and weight to determine the child's BSA. This information is then inserted into the BSA formula to obtain a drug dosage for a specific pediatric patient. Consider the following examples:

$$\frac{\text{BSA of adult}}{\text{BSA of child}} \times \text{adult dose} = \text{estimated child's dose}$$

**FIGURE 3-1** West nomogram for infants and children. S.A., Surface area. (Modified from data by Boyd E, West CD. In Kliegman RM, Stanton BF, St. Geme III JW, et al, editors: *Nelson textbook of pediatrics*, ed 19, Philadelphia, 2011, Saunders.)

$$\text{BSA of child} (m^2) \times \frac{\text{manufacturer's recommended dose}}{m^2} = \text{estimated child's dose}$$

Calculating the dosage according to the body weight is the most commonly used method today. Most drug references recommend dosages based on milligrams per kilogram of body weight. The following information is needed to calculate the pediatric dosage:
- Drug order (as discussed previously)
- Pediatric patient's weight in kilograms (1 kilogram = 2.2 pounds) (For example, a 10-lb baby weighs 4.5 kg; divide the number of pounds by 2.2 to determine kilograms.)
- Pediatric dosage as per manufacturer or drug formulary guidelines
- Information regarding available dosage forms

When using either of the previous methods, you must do the following to ensure the correct pediatric dose:
- Determine the pediatric patient's weight in kilograms.
- Use a current drug reference to determine the usual dosage range per 24 hours in milligrams (mg) per kilogram (kg). It must be noted that some drugs are stated as mg/kg/dose.
- Determine the dose parameters by multiplying the weight by the minimum and maximum daily doses of the drug (the safe range).
- Determine the total amount of the drug to administer per dose and per day.
- Compare the drug dosage prescribed with the calculated safe range.
- If the drug dosage raises any concerns or varies from the safe range, contact the health care provider or prescriber immediately and do not give the drug!

A common source of medication error and potential toxicity is confusing pounds with kilograms. Unless otherwise noted, the child's weight is to be given in kilograms, not pounds. Take great care to ensure that the correct weight is reported to the prescriber. In calculating pediatric dosages, the factor of organ maturity must always be considered along with BSA, age, and weight. When all of these physical developmental factors are

## PATIENT-CENTERED CARE: LIFESPAN CONSIDERATIONS FOR THE PEDIATRIC PATIENT

### Age-Related Considerations for Medication Administration from Infancy to Adolescence

**General Interventions**
- Always come prepared for the procedure (e.g., prepare for injections with needleless syringe, and gather all needed equipment).
- Ask the parent and/or child (if age-appropriate) if the parent will remain for the procedure (for in-hospital administration).
- Assess for comfort methods that are appropriate before and after drug administration.

**Infants**
- While maintaining safe and secure positioning of the infant (e.g., with parent holding, rocking, cuddling, soothing), perform the procedure (e.g., injection) swiftly and safely.
- Allow self-comforting measures as age-appropriate (e.g., use of pacifier, fingers in mouth, self-movement).

**Toddlers**
- Offer a brief, concrete explanation of the procedure but with realistic expectations of the child's actual understanding of the information. Parents, caregivers, or other legal guardians must be part of the process. Hold the child securely while administering the medication.
- Accept aggressive behavior as a healthy response, but only within reasonable limits.
- Provide comfort measures immediately after the procedure (e.g., touching, holding).
- Help the child understand the treatment and his or her feelings through puppet play or play with stuffed animals or hospital equipment such as empty, needleless syringes.
- Provide for healthy ways to release aggression such as age-appropriate supervised playtime.

**Preschoolers**
- Offer a brief, concrete explanation of the procedure at the patient's level and with the parent or caregiver present.

- Provide comfort measures after the procedure (e.g., touching, holding).
- Identify and accept aggressive responses and provide age-appropriate outlets.
- Make use of magical thinking (e.g., using ointments or "special medicines" to make discomfort go away).
- Note that the role of the parent in providing comfort and understanding is very important.

**School-Age Children**
- Explain the procedure, allowing for some control over body and situation.
- Provide comfort measures.
- Explore feelings and concepts through the use of therapeutic play. Art may be used to help the patient express fears. Use of age-appropriate books and realistic hospital equipment may also be helpful.
- Set appropriate behavior limits (e.g., okay to cry or scream, but not to bite).
- Provide activities for releasing aggression and anger.
- Use the opportunity to teach about the relationship between receiving medication and body function and structure (e.g., what a seizure is and how medication helps prevent the seizure).
- Offer the complete picture (e.g., need to take medication, relax with deep breaths; medication will help prevent pain).

**Adolescents**
- Prepare the patient in advance for the procedure but without scare tactics.
- Allow for expression in a way that does not cause losing face, such as giving the adolescent time alone after the procedure (e.g., once a seizure is controlled) and giving the adolescent time to discuss his or her feelings.
- Explore with the adolescent any current concepts of self, hospitalization, and illness, and correct any misconceptions.
- Encourage self-expression, individuality, and self-care.
- Encourage participation in procedures as appropriate.

Modified from McKenry LM, Salerno E: *Mosby's pharmacology in nursing*, ed 22, St Louis, 2006, Mosby; Blaber M: Related to nursing intervention in pain. Newington's Children's Hospital manual for global pediatric nursing assessment (unpublished manuscript).

considered and doses are calculated correctly, the likelihood of safe and effective drug administration is increased. Emotional developmental considerations must also be a part of the decision-making process in drug therapy for pediatric patients (see the Patient-Centered Care: Lifespan Considerations for the Pediatric Patient box on p. 41).

## CONSIDERATIONS FOR ELDERLY PATIENTS

Due to the decline in organ function that occurs with advancing age, elderly patients handle drugs physiologically differently than adult patients. Drug therapy in the elderly is more likely to result in adverse effects and toxicity.

In this textbook, the word *elderly* is used instead of the word *geriatric*; however, these terms are synonymous. An elderly patient is defined as a person who is 65 years of age or older. This segment of the population is growing at a dramatic pace (see the Patient-Centered Care: Lifespan Considerations for the Elderly Patient box on this page). At the beginning of the twentieth century, the elderly constituted a mere 4% of the total population. At that time, more people died of infections than of chronic illnesses such as heart disease, cancer, and diabetes. As medical and health care technology has advanced, so has the ability to prolong life. This has resulted in a growing population of older adults. Today patients older than 65 years of age constitute 13% of the population. Life expectancy is currently approximately 78.1 years, and it is estimated that 20% of the population will be 65 years of age or older by 2030. These trends are expected to continue as new disease prevention and treatment methods are developed.

### PATIENT-CENTERED CARE: LIFESPAN CONSIDERATIONS FOR THE ELDERLY PATIENT

*Percentage of Population Older than Age 65*

| YEAR | PERCENTAGE OLDER THAN AGE 65 |
|------|------------------------------|
| 1900 | 4% |
| 2000 | 12% |
| 2020 | 20% |

### Issues in Clinical Drug Use in the Elderly

The elderly population consumes a larger proportion of all medications than other population groups, taking 30% of all prescription drugs and over 40% of over-the-counter drugs. At any given time, the average elderly patient takes four or five prescription drugs as well as two over-the-counter medications, which can increase the risk of drug interactions. Commonly prescribed drugs for the elderly include antihypertensives, beta blockers, diuretics, insulin, and potassium supplements. The most commonly used over-the-counter drugs are analgesics, laxatives, and nonsteroidal anti-inflammatory drugs (NSAIDs). Elderly patients, especially those of certain ethnicities, may use various folk remedies of unknown composition that are unfamiliar to their health care providers.

Not only do elderly patients consume a greater proportion of prescription and over-the-counter medications, they commonly take multiple medications on a daily basis. About 1 in 3 elderly patients take more than 8 different drugs each day, with many taking 15 or more. One reason for the use of multiple medications is the more frequent occurrence of chronic diseases and the multiple drug options available for treatment. More than 80% of patients taking eight or more drugs have one or more chronic illnesses. More complicated medication regimens predispose elderly patients to self-medication errors, especially those with reduced visual acuity and manual dexterity. Such sensory and motor deficits can be particularly problematic when elderly patients split their own tablets. The practice of pill splitting occurs commonly for financial reasons, because lower- and higher-strength tablets often have similar costs. Furthermore, some insurance companies require tablet splitting for this reason. Other factors that may contribute to medication errors in the elderly include lack of adequate patient education and understanding of their drug regimens, and use of multiple prescribers and multiple pharmacies. In this age of medical specialization, patients may see several prescribers for their many illnesses. Because of this, it is very important for the patient to use only one pharmacy so that monitoring for drug interactions and duplicate therapy can occur.

Elderly patients are hospitalized frequently due to adverse drug reactions. Many people, including the elderly, use complementary and alternative medicines such as herbal remedies and dietary supplements, which can interact with prescription drugs. The simultaneous use of multiple medications is called polypharmacy. As the number of medications a person takes increases, so does the risk of drug interaction. For example, the chance of a drug interaction is approximately 6% for a patient receiving two medications. This risk rises dramatically as the number of drugs the patient is taking increases. For a patient taking five medications, the chance of a drug interaction is 50%, and for those taking 10 or more medications, the chance is 100%.

Some drugs may be given specifically to counteract the adverse effects of other drugs (e.g., a potassium supplement to counteract the potassium loss caused by certain diuretic medications), which is one example of what is known as the *prescribing cascade*. Sometimes it is difficult to distinguish adverse drug effects from disease symptoms. Although such prescribing is sometimes appropriate, it also increases the potential for more adverse drug events (including drug interactions, hospitalization or prolonged hospital stays, hip fractures secondary to drug-induced falls, addiction risk, anorexia, confusion, urinary retention, and fatigue). Recognizing polypharmacy and taking steps to reduce it whenever possible by decreasing the number and/or dosages of drugs taken can significantly reduce the incidence of adverse outcomes. Appropriate drug doses for elderly patients may sometimes be one-half to two-thirds of the standard adult dose. As a general rule, dosing for the elderly should follow the admonition, "Start low and go slow," which means to start with the lowest possible dose (often less than an average adult dose) and increase the dose slowly, based on patient response.

Another important issue is noncompliance, or nonadherence, with prescribed medication regimens. Drug nonadherence is reported to occur in roughly 40% of elderly patients and is associated with increased rates of hospitalization. Some patients want to adhere to their medication regimen but truly cannot

| TABLE 3-3 | PHYSIOLOGIC CHANGES IN THE ELDERLY PATIENT |
|---|---|
| **SYSTEM** | **PHYSIOLOGIC CHANGE** |
| Cardiovascular | ↓ Cardiac output = ↓ absorption and distribution |
| | ↓ Blood flow = ↓ absorption and distribution |
| Gastrointestinal | ↑ pH (alkaline gastric secretions) = altered absorption |
| | ↓ Peristalsis = delayed gastric emptying |
| Hepatic | ↓ Enzyme production = ↓ metabolism |
| | ↓ Blood flow = ↓ metabolism |
| Renal | ↓ Blood flow = ↓ excretion |
| | ↓ Function = ↓ excretion |
| | ↓ Glomerular filtration rate = ↓ excretion |

afford the medicine. Patients in this situation need to be referred to a health care social worker or their prescriber. Many drug companies offer patient assistance for expensive medications.

## Physiologic Changes

Physiologic changes associated with aging affect the action of many drugs. As the body ages, the functioning of several organ systems slowly declines. The collective physiologic changes associated with the aging process have a major effect on the disposition and action of drugs. Table 3-3 lists some of the body systems most affected by the aging process.

The sensitivity of the elderly patient to many drugs requires careful monitoring and dosage adjustment. The criteria for drug dosages in older adults must include consideration of body weight and organ functioning, with emphasis on liver, renal, cardiovascular, and central nervous system function (similar to the criteria for pediatric dosages). With aging, there is a general decrease in body weight.

Changes in drug molecule receptors in the body can make a patient more or less sensitive to certain medications. For example, elderly patients commonly have increased sensitivity to central nervous system depressant medications (e.g., anxiolytics, tricyclic antidepressants) because of reduced integrity of the blood-brain barrier.

It is important to monitor the results of laboratory tests that have been ordered for elderly patients. These values serve as a gauge of organ function. The most important organs from the standpoint of the breakdown and elimination of drugs are the liver and the kidneys. Kidney function is assessed by measuring serum creatinine and blood urea nitrogen levels. Creatinine is a byproduct of muscle metabolism. Because muscle mass declines with age, the serum creatinine level may provide a misleading index of renal function. For example, a frail elderly female may have a reported serum creatinine value that is lower than normal, and this may lead one to falsely think that her renal function is normal. In actuality, because this patient has limited muscle mass, she cannot produce creatinine. The seasoned clinician knows that renal function declines with age and that this value alone does not give an accurate estimate of renal function. The most accurate way to determine creatinine clearance is by collecting a patient's urine for 24 hours. This test is quite cumbersome, however, and is not used very often. Fortunately, several equations exist that allow pharmacists and prescribers to

accurately assess renal function in the elderly. Frequency of testing for renal function is often dictated by the degree of renal dysfunction and the type of medications being prescribed or used.

Liver function is assessed by testing the blood for liver enzymes such as aspartate aminotransferase (AST) and alanine aminotransferase (ALT). These laboratory values can help in assessing the ability to metabolize and eliminate medications and can aid in anticipating the risk of toxicity and/or drug accumulation. Laboratory assessments need to be conducted at least annually, both for preventive health monitoring and for screening for possible toxic effects of drug therapy. Such assessments may be indicated more frequently (e.g., every 1, 3, or 6 months) in those patients requiring higher-risk drug regimens.

## Pharmacokinetics

The pharmacokinetic phases of absorption, distribution, metabolism, and excretion (see Chapter 2) may be different in the older adult than in the younger adult. Awareness of these differences helps ensure appropriate administration of drugs and monitoring of elderly patients. The Patient-Centered Care: Lifespan Considerations for the Elderly Patient box on this page lists the four pharmacokinetic phases and summarizes how they are altered by the aging process.

### PATIENT-CENTERED CARE: LIFESPAN CONSIDERATIONS FOR THE ELDERLY PATIENT

#### *Pharmacokinetic Changes*

**Absorption**
- Gastric pH is less acidic because of a gradual reduction in the production of hydrochloric acid in the stomach.
- Gastric emptying is slowed because of a decline in smooth muscle tone and motor activity.
- Movement throughout the gastrointestinal tract is slower because of decreased muscle tone and motor activity.
- Blood flow to the gastrointestinal tract is reduced by 40% to 50% because of decreased cardiac output and decreased perfusion.
- The absorptive surface area is decreased because the aging process blunts and flattens villi.

**Distribution**
- In adults 40 to 60 years of age, total body water is 55% in males and 47% in females; in those older than 60 years of age, total body water is 52% in males and 46% in females.
- Fat content is increased because of decreased lean body mass.
- Protein (albumin) binding sites are reduced because of decreased production of proteins by the aging liver and reduced protein intake.

**Metabolism**
- The levels of microsomal enzymes are decreased because the capacity of the aging liver to produce them is reduced.
- Liver blood flow is reduced by approximately 1.5% per year after 25 years of age, which decreases hepatic metabolism.

**Excretion**
- Glomerular filtration rate is decreased by 40% to 50%, primarily because of decreased blood flow.
- The number of intact nephrons is decreased.

## Absorption

Absorption in the older person can be altered by many mechanisms. Advancing age results in reduced absorption of both dietary nutrients and drugs. Several physiologic changes account for this reduction in absorption. Elderly patients have a gradual reduction in the ability of the stomach to produce hydrochloric acid, which results in a decrease in gastric acidity and may alter the absorption of some drugs. In addition, the combination of decreased cardiac output and advancing atherosclerosis results in a general reduction in the flow of blood to major organs, including the stomach. By 65 years of age, there is an approximately 50% reduction in blood flow to the gastrointestinal (GI) tract. Absorption, whether of nutrient or drug, is dependent on good blood supply to the stomach and intestines. The absorptive surface area of an elderly person's GI tract is often reduced, thus decreasing drug absorption.

GI motility is important for moving substances out of the stomach and also for moving them throughout the GI tract. Muscle tone and motor activity in the GI tract are reduced in older adults. This often results in constipation, for which older adults frequently take laxatives. This use of laxatives may accelerate GI motility enough to actually reduce the absorption of drugs.

## Distribution

The distribution of medications throughout the body is also different in older adults. There seems to be a gradual reduction in the total body water content with aging. Therefore, the concentrations of highly water-soluble (hydrophilic) drugs may be higher in elderly patients because they have less body water in which the drugs can be diluted. The composition of the body also changes with aging, with a decrease in lean muscle mass and an increase in body fat. In both men and women, there is an approximately 20% reduction in muscle mass between 25 and 65 years of age and a corresponding 20% increase in body fat. Fat-soluble or lipophilic drugs, such as hypnotics and sedatives, are primarily distributed to fatty tissues and may result in prolonged drug actions and/or toxicity.

Elderly patients may have reduced protein concentrations, due in large part to reduced liver function. Reduced dietary intake and/or poor GI protein absorption can cause nutritional deficiencies and reduced blood protein levels. Regardless of the cause, the result is a reduced number of protein-binding sites for highly protein-bound drugs. This results in higher levels of unbound (active) drug in the blood. Remember that only drugs not bound to proteins are active. Therefore, the effects of highly protein-bound drugs may be enhanced if their dosages are not adjusted to accommodate any reduced serum albumin concentrations. Some highly protein-bound drugs include warfarin and phenytoin.

## Metabolism

Metabolism declines with advancing age. The transformation of active drugs into inactive metabolites is primarily performed by the liver. The liver loses mass with age and slowly loses its ability to metabolize drugs effectively due to reduced production of microsomal (cytochrome P-450) enzymes. There is also a reduction in blood flow to the liver because of reduced cardiac output and atherosclerosis. A reduction in the hepatic blood flow of approximately 1.5% per year occurs after 25 years of age. All of these factors contribute to prolonging the half-life of many drugs (e.g., warfarin), which can potentially result in drug accumulation if serum drug levels are not closely monitored.

## Excretion

Renal function declines in roughly two-thirds of elderly patients. A reduction in the glomerular filtration rate of 40% to 50%, combined with a reduction in cardiac output leading to reduced renal perfusion, can result in delayed drug excretion and therefore drug accumulation. This is especially true for drugs with a low therapeutic index such as digoxin. Renal function needs to be monitored frequently. Appropriate dose and interval adjustments may be determined based on the results of renal and liver function studies as well as the presence of therapeutic levels of the drug in the serum. If a decrease in renal and liver function is known, adjust the dosage so that drug accumulation and toxicity may be avoided or minimized.

## Problematic Medications for the Elderly

Certain classes of drugs are more likely to cause problems in elderly patients because of many of the physiologic alterations and pharmacokinetic changes already discussed. Table 3-4 lists some of the more common medications that are problematic. Some drugs to be avoided in the elderly have been identified by various professional organizations such as the American Nurses Association as well as by various other authoritative sources. Since the 1990s, a very effective tool, the Beers criteria, has been used to identify drugs that may be inappropriately prescribed, ineffective, or cause adverse drug reactions in elderly patients (see the Evidence-Based Practice box on p. 45). The Beers criteria are very useful and help determine risk-associated situations for the elderly and specific drugs that may be problematic.

## NURSING PROCESS

## ASSESSMENT

Before any medication is administered to a pediatric patient, obtain a health history and medication history with assistance from the parent, caregiver, or legal guardian. The following are some areas to be included:

- Age
- Age-related concerns about organ functioning
- Age-related fears
- Allergies to drugs and food
- Baseline values for vital signs
- Head-to-toe physical assessment findings
- Height in feet/inches and centimeters
- Weight in kilograms and pounds
- Level of growth and development and related developmental tasks

## TABLE 3-4 MEDICATIONS AND CONDITIONS REQUIRING SPECIAL CONSIDERATIONS IN THE ELDERLY PATIENT

| MEDICATION | COMMON COMPLICATIONS |
|---|---|
| Analgesics | |
|   Opioids | Confusion, constipation, urinary retention, nausea, vomiting, respiratory depression, falls |
|   Nonsteroidal antiinflammatory drugs (NSAIDs) | Edema, nausea, gastric ulceration, bleeding, renal toxicity |
| Anticoagulants (heparin, warfarin) | Major and minor bleeding episodes, many drug interactions, dietary interactions |
| Anticholinergics | Blurred vision, dry mouth, constipation, confusion, urinary retention, tachycardia |
| Antidepressants | Sedation and strong anticholinergic adverse effects (see above) |
| Antihypertensives | Nausea, hypotension, diarrhea, bradycardia, heart failure, impotence |
| Cardiac glycosides (e.g., digoxin) | Visual disorders, nausea, diarrhea, dysrhythmias, hallucinations, decreased appetite, weight loss |
| Central nervous system (CNS) depressants (muscle relaxants, opioids) | Sedation, weakness, dry mouth, confusion, urinary retention, ataxia |
| Sedatives and hypnotics | Confusion, daytime sedation, ataxia, lethargy, increased risk of falls |
| Thiazide diuretics | Electrolyte imbalance, rashes, fatigue, leg cramps, dehydration |

| CONDITION | DRUGS REQUIRING SPECIAL CAUTION AND MONITORING |
|---|---|
| Bladder flow obstruction | Anticholinergics, antihistamines, decongestants, antidepressants |
| Clotting disorders | NSAIDs, aspirin, antiplatelet drugs |
| Chronic constipation | Calcium channel blockers, tricyclic antidepressants, anticholinergics |
| Chronic obstructive pulmonary disease | Long-acting sedatives or hypnotics, narcotics, beta blockers |
| Heart failure and hypertension | Sodium, decongestants, amphetamines, over-the-counter cold products |
| Insomnia | Decongestants, bronchodilators, monoamine oxidase inhibitors |
| Parkinson's disease | Antipsychotics, phenothiazines |
| Syncope, falls | Sedatives, hypnotics, opioids, CNS depressants, muscle relaxants, antidepressants, antihypertensives |

## EVIDENCE-BASED PRACTICE

### Update on Application of the Beers Criteria for Prevention of Adverse Drug Events in Older Adults

**Review**

In 1991, a panel of experts led by Mark H. Beers, MD, identified a list of "potentially inappropriate medications" (PIM) for use in individuals 65 years of age and older. These criteria were intended for use with nursing home residents and then were expanded and revised to include all settings of geriatric care. The specific aim of the project was to predict adverse drug reactions (ADRs) in this age group. The Beers Criteria were updated in 1997 and 2002 and provided a listing of drugs and drug classes to be avoided in the elderly. The criteria also identified disease states considered to be contraindications for some drugs. In 2005, research was conducted to confirm the relationship between PIM prescribing, as defined by Beers Criteria, and the occurrence of ADRs in elderly patients treated at outpatient clinics. In 2012, a list of medications was identified and classified into three categories: (1) potentially inappropriate medications and classes to avoid in the older adult, (2) potentially inappropriate medications and classes to avoid in older adults with certain diseases and syndromes, and (3) medications to be used with caution in older adults

**Type of Evidence**

The 2012 Beers Criteria were considered greatly improved because of the inclusion of important updates to the previous list of medications. Additionally, there was consideration of the challenges of assisting and guiding clinicians in avoiding certain drugs in older adults and/or the need for cautious use. The quality of the criteria was also improved by: (1) application of an evidence-based approach, (2) support of the American Geriatrics Society (AGS) in conjunction with an interdisciplinary panel of experts in geriatric care and pharmacotherapy, (3) use of a time-tested method for developing care guidelines while using the Institute of Medicine's standards for evidence/transparency as an important benchmark, and, (4) an extensive review of more than 2000 high-quality research studies about prescription medications for this age group.

**Results of Study**

Fifty-three medications/medication classes were included in the 2012 AGS Beers Criteria. There was a list of 34 medications and types of medications labeled as "potentially inappropriate", 14 common health problems with associated medications that were also potentially inappropriate, and 14 types of potentially inappropriate drugs to be used only with caution—all with older adults. Nineteen medications/medication classes were dropped from the 2003 list. The update allows thoughtful application of the Criteria for closer monitoring of drug use, application and interventions to decrease adverse drug events in older adults, and better patient outcomes.

**Link of Evidence to Nursing Practice**

These Criteria are improved and provide a much needed update for drugs to avoid and use with caution in older adults. They also increase awareness of inappropriate medication use in this age group and may also be integrated into electronic health records. With the support of the AGS, the Criteria will continue to develop over time and will continue to help improve the health of older adults.

Data from American Geriatrics Society 2012 Beers Criteria Update Expert Panel: American Geriatrics Society updated Beers Criteria for potentially inappropriate medication use in older adults, *J Am Geriatr Soc* 60(4):616-631, 2012; Fick DM, Semla TP: 2012 American Geriatrics Society Beers Criteria: new year, new criteria, new perspective, *J Am Geriatr Soc* 60(4):614-615, 2012.

- Medical and medication history (including adverse drug reactions); current medications, related dosage forms, and routes; patient's tolerance of the forms and/or routes
- State of anxiety of the patient and/or family members or caregiver
- Use of prescription and over-the-counter medications in the home setting
- Usual method of medication administration, such as use of a calibrated spoon or needleless syringe
- Usual response to medications
- Motor and cognitive responses and their age-appropriateness
- Resources available to the patient and family

In addition, check and recheck the prescriber's orders because there is no room for error when administering medications to pediatric patients—or any patients for that matter. Carefully perform medication dosage calculations, and check several times for accuracy. Calculations for dosages take into account a variety of information and variables that may affect patient response, and use of body surface area (BSA) formulas and body weight formulas (milligrams per kilogram) are recommended. In addition to an assessment of the patient, an assessment of the drug and related information is needed, focusing specifically on the drug's purpose, dosage ranges, routes of administration, cautions, and contraindications. The saying that pediatric patients are just "small adults" is incorrect, because in pediatric patients every organ is anatomically and physiologically immature and not fully functioning. As pediatric patients grow older, their BSA and weight are still lower, so extreme caution is continually needed when giving them medications. Immature organ and system development will influence pharmacokinetics and thus affect the way the pediatric patient responds to a drug. Organ function may be determined through laboratory testing. The following studies may be ordered by the prescriber before beginning drug therapy as well as during and after drug therapy: hepatic and renal function studies, red blood cell and white blood cell counts, and measurement of hemoglobin and hematocrit levels and serum protein levels.

Assessment data to be gathered for the elderly patient may include the following:
- Age
- Allergies to drugs and food
- Dietary habits
- Sensory, visual, hearing, cognitive, and motor-skill deficits
- Financial status and any limitations
- List of all health-related care providers, including physicians, dentists, optometrists and ophthalmologists, podiatrists, and alternative medicine health care practitioners such as osteopathic physicians, chiropractors, and nurse practitioners
- Past and present medical history
- Listing of medications, past and present, including prescription drugs, over-the-counter medications, herbals, nutritional supplements, vitamins, and home remedies
- Existence of polypharmacy (the use of more than one medication)
- Self-medication practices

- Laboratory test results, especially those indicative of renal and liver function
- History of smoking and use of alcohol with notation of amount, frequency, and years of use
- Risk situations related to drug therapy identified by the Beers criteria (see the Evidence-Based Practice box on p. 45)

One way to collect data about the various medications or drugs being taken by the elderly is to obtain the information from the patient and/or caregiver using the brown-bag technique. This is an effective means of identifying various drugs the patient is taking, regardless of the patient's age, and may be used in conjunction with a complete review of the patient's medical history or record. The brown-bag technique requires the patient/caregiver to place all medications used in a bag and bring them to the health care provider. All medications need to be brought in their original containers. A list of medications with generic names, dosages, routes of administration, and frequencies is then compiled. This list of medications is then compared with what is prescribed to what the patient states he or she is actually taking. Medication reconciliation procedures are performed in health care facilities when assessing and tracking medications taken by the patient (see Chapter 5). In addition, the patient's insight into his or her medical problems is a very beneficial piece of information in developing a plan of care. It is also important for the nurse to realize that although elderly patients may be able to provide the required information themselves, many may be confused or poorly informed about their medications and/or health condition. In such cases, consult with a more reliable historian, such as a significant other, family member, or caregiver. Elderly patients may also have sensory deficits that require the nurse to speak slowly, loudly, and clearly while facing the patient.

With the elderly patient—as with a patient of any age—thoroughly assess support systems and the patient's ability to take medications safely. Whenever possible with the elderly, health care providers/prescribers need to opt for a nonpharmacologic approach to treatment first, if appropriate. Other data to collect include information about acute or chronic illnesses, nutritional problems, cardiac problems, respiratory illnesses, and GI tract disorders. Laboratory tests related to lifespan considerations that are often ordered include hemoglobin and hematocrit levels, red blood cell and white blood cell counts, blood urea nitrogen level, serum and urine creatinine levels, urine specific gravity, serum electrolyte levels, and protein and serum albumin levels.

## NURSING DIAGNOSES

1. Imbalanced nutrition, less than body requirements, related to the impact of age and drug therapy and possible adverse effects
2. Deficient knowledge related to information about drugs and their adverse effects or about when to contact the prescriber
3. Risk for injury related to adverse effects of medications or to the method of drug administration
4. Risk for injury related to idiosyncratic reactions to drugs due to age-related drug sensitivity

## PATIENT-CENTERED CARE: LIFESPAN CONSIDERATIONS FOR THE ELDERLY PATIENT

### A Brief Look at the Sixth Leading Cause of Death in the United States: Alzheimer's Disease

- In 2011, approximately 5.4 million Americans were identified as having Alzheimer's disease with nearly 4% of these individuals with early onset Alzheimer's (affecting people younger than age 65).,
- Alzheimer's is the sixth leading cause of death in the United States. It is the only cause of death among the top 10 in the United States that cannot be prevented, cured, or slowed.
- Alzheimer's mortality rate is on the rise and deaths due to Alzheimer's disease have increased approximately 66% during the years 2000 to 2008.
- Alzheimer's disease is the most common cause of dementia and accounts for approximately 50% to 80% of cases. Early clinical symptoms include difficulty remembering names and recent events as well as apathy and depression. Later clinical symptoms include impaired judgment, confusion, behavioral changes, and difficulty swallowing/speaking and walking.
- The pathology associated with Alzheimer's disease is a disruption of brain cells in specific regions involved in the formulation of new memories. Other difficulties are experienced as damage spreads. Warning signs include memory loss that is disruptive to activities of daily living; challenges in problem solving, leading to difficulty in completing the most familiar of tasks at home, work, or even at leisure; confusion to time and place; trouble with spatial

relationships; and difficulty understanding visual images. For a more complete listing of the symptoms of Alzheimer's disease, refer to the 2011 Alzheimer's Disease Facts and Figures (Alzheimer's Association, 2011, available at www.alz.org).
- Alzheimer's disease is ultimately fatal.
- Advancing age is the greatest risk factor. Most of the individuals with Alzheimer's are age 65 or older, and the likelihood doubles about every 5 years after age 65. After the age of 85, the risk is almost 50%.
- Another important risk factor is family history, with an increased likelihood of developing the disease in those who have a parent, brother, sister, or child with Alzheimer's.
- New criteria and guidelines for diagnosing Alzheimer's were published in 2011 recommending that the disease be considered one with three stages beginning well before the development of symptoms. Hallmark abnormalities include deposits of protein fragment beta-amyloid (plaques) and twisted strands of the protein tau (tangles) as well as evidence of nerve cell damage and death in the brain.
- Latinos and African Americans, in the United States, have higher rates of vascular disease and so, as such, may also be at greater risk of developing Alzheimer's.

Data from Alzheimer's Association: 2011 Alzheimer's disease facts and figures, available at http://www.alz.org.

## PLANNING

### GOALS

1. Patient (caregiver, parent, or legal guardian) states measures to enhance nutritional status due to age- and drug-related factors, as well as any adverse drug effects on everyday nutrition.
2. Patient (caregiver, parent, or legal guardian) states the importance of adhering to the prescribed drug therapy (or takes medication as prescribed with assistance).
3. Patient contacts the prescriber when appropriate, such as when unusual effects occur during drug therapy.
4. Patient (caregiver, parent, or legal guardian) identifies ways to minimize complications, adverse effects, reactions, and injury to self associated with the therapeutic medication regimen.

### OUTCOME CRITERIA

1. Patient (caregiver, parent, or legal guardian) lists recommended caloric and protein intake as well as examples of all the major food groups with the assistance of nutritional consultation.
   - Patient (caregiver, parent, or legal guardian) identifies when to contact the prescriber if nausea, vomiting, loss of appetite, diarrhea, constipation, or other problems arise during medication therapy.
2. Patient (caregiver, parent, or legal guardian) states rationale for medication as well as importance in the timing, dosage, and duration of therapy and is able to identify what the specific medication looks like.
   - Patient (caregiver, parent, or legal guardian) describes intended therapeutic effects of the medication(s), such as improvement in condition with decrease in symptoms and with limited adverse effects.

- Patient (caregiver, parent, or legal guardian) demonstrates safe method of self- or assisted medication administration, such as use of a week-long pill mechanism with day of week and associated times, and has all medications safely labeled.
- Patient (caregiver, parent, or legal guardian) follows instructions specific to the route of administration for the medication ordered, while also demonstrating (if appropriate) techniques, such as special application of an ointment as prescribed, measuring and taking liquid medication, and taking medication with proper food/fluids, for the duration of treatment.
3. Patient (caregiver, parent, or legal guardian) lists all unintended adverse effects and possible toxicity associated with medication regimen while also stating when to contact health care provider such as occurrence of fever, pain, vomiting, rash, diarrhea, difficulty breathing, and/or worsening of condition being treated.
4. Patient (caregiver, legal guardian, or parent) reports safe medication administration upon return appointment after beginning prescribed therapy.
   - Patient (caregiver, legal guardian, or parent) minimizes adverse effects and danger to self by taking medication(s) as prescribed, at the right time, with right dosing, and with attention to intake of proper amount of fluids (4 to 6 oz of water with oral dosages) and with or without food, as indicated while remaining cognitive of safety measures appropriate to specific drug regimen.

## IMPLEMENTATION

It is always important to emphasize and practice the Six Rights of medication administration (see Chapter 1) and follow the prescriber's order and/or medication instructions. Check all drugs three times against the Six Rights and the prescriber's order before the drug is given to the patient. This usually applies for acute care and long-term care inpatient and outpatient situations. For the *pediatric* patient, some specific nursing actions are as follows: (1) If needed, mix medications in a substance or fluid other than essential foods (e.g., milk, orange juice, or cereal) because the child may develop a dislike for the essential food item(s). Instead, find a liquid or food item that may be used to make the medication(s) taste better. Sherbet or flavored ice cream is often used. Only resort to this intervention if the patient cannot swallow the dosage form or if the taste needs to be made more palatable. (2) Do not add drug(s) to fluid in a cup or bottle because the amount of drug consumed would then be impossible to calculate if the entire amount of fluid is not consumed. (3) Always document special techniques of drug administration so that others involved in the patient's care may benefit from the suggestion. For example, if the child takes an unpleasant-tasting pill, liquid, or tablet after eating a frozen popsicle, then this information would be valuable to another caregiver. (4) Unless contraindicated, add small amounts of water or fluids to elixirs to enhance the child's tolerance of the medication. Remember that it is essential for the child to take the entire volume, so remain cautious with this practice and only use an amount of fluid mixture that you know the child will tolerate. (5) Avoid using the word *candy* in place of the word *drug* or *medication*. Medications must be called *medicines* and their dangers made known to children. Taking medications is no game, and children must understand this for their own safety! (6) Keep all medications out of the reach of children of all ages. Be sure that parents and other family members in the same household understand this and request child-protective lids or tops for their medications. Childproof locks or closures may also be used on cabinets holding medications. (7) Inquire about how the child usually takes medication (e.g., preference of liquid versus pill or tablet dosage forms) and whether there are any helpful hints from the family/caregiver that may be helpful. See the Patient-Centered Care: Lifespan Considerations for the Pediatric Patient box on p. 41 for further information on medication administration beginning with infancy through adolescence. For more information about dosage calculations for medication administration in pediatric patients, an online site providing examples and programs to help with pediatric drug dosage calculations is available at http://www.testandcalc.com and http://www.mapharm.com/dosage_calc.htm.

Encourage *elderly* patients to take medications as directed and not to discontinue them or double up on doses unless recommended or ordered to do so by their health care provider/prescriber. The patient or caregiver must understand the treatment- and/or medication-related instructions, especially those related to safety measures, such as keeping all medications out of the reach of children. Transdermal patches provide a different challenge in that if they fall off onto the floor or bedding, a child or infant in that environment may have accidental exposure to the effects of the medication. Serious adverse reactions have been reported concerning the accidental adhering of a transdermal patch to a child/infant while crawling or playing on the floor/carpet. Toxic and even fatal reactions may occur depending on the medication and dosage. Provide written and oral instructions concerning the drug name, action, purpose, dosage, time of administration, route, adverse effects, safety of administration, storage, interactions, and any cautions about or contraindications to its use. Remember that simple is always best! Always try to find ways to make the patient's therapeutic regimen easy to understand. Always be alert to polypharmacy, and be sure the patient or caregiver understands the dangers of multiple drug use. Patient education may prove to be helpful in preventing and/or minimizing problems associated with polypharmacy. If a nurse advocate or a nurse practitioner with prescription privileges has the opportunity to review the patient's chart, simplified written instructions must be provided with the purpose of the drug, how to best take the medication(s), and a list of drug interactions and adverse effects. Information must be provided in bold, large print. Among the specific interventions that have proved to be helpful in promoting medication safety in the elderly is the use of the Beers criteria (see the Evidence-Based Practice box on p. 45). These criteria provide a systematic way of identifying prescription medications that are potentially harmful to elderly patients. The prescriber and nurse must constantly remember that clinical judgment and knowledge base are important in making critical decisions about a patient's care and drug therapy. In addition, keeping abreast of evidence-based nursing, such as application of the Beers criteria, is important for the nurse to remain current in clinical nursing practice. Specific guidelines for medication administration by various routes are presented in detail in the photo atlas in Chapter 9.

In summary, drug therapy across the lifespan must be well thought out, with full consideration to the patient's age, gender, cultural background, ethnicity, medical history, and medication profile. When all phases of the nursing process and the specific lifespan considerations discussed in this chapter are included, there is a better chance of decreasing adverse effects, reducing risks to the patient, and increasing drug safety.

## CASE STUDY

### *Polypharmacy and the Elderly*

R.M., a 77-year-old retired librarian, sees several physician specialists for a variety of health problems. She uses the pharmacy at a large discount store but also has prescriptions filled at a nearby pharmacy, which she uses when she does not feel like going into the larger store. Her medication list is as follows:

Thiazide diuretic, prescribed for peripheral edema

Potassium tablets, prescribed to prevent hypokalemia

Beta blocker, prescribed for hypertension

Warfarin, taken every evening because of a history of deep vein thrombosis

Thyroid replacement hormone because of a history of hypothyroidism

Multivitamin tablet for seniors

1. What medications may cause problems for R.M.? Explain your answer.
2. What measures can be taken to reduce these problems?

   R.M. visits the pharmacy to pick up some medications for a cold. She has chosen a popular over-the-counter decongestant, an antihistamine preparation, and a nonsteroidal antiinflammatory drug for her "aches and pains."
3. Should she use these medications? If not, what advice would you give to her about choosing over-the-counter medications?

For answers, see http://evolve.elsevier.com/Lilley.

# EVALUATION

When dealing with lifespan issues as related to drug therapy, observation and monitoring for therapeutic effects as well as adverse effects is critical to safe and effective therapy. You must know the patient's profile and history as well as information about the drug. The drug's purpose, specific use in the patient, simply stated actions, dose, frequency of dosing, adverse effects, cautions, and contraindications need to be listed and kept available at all times. This information will allow more comprehensive monitoring of drug therapy, regardless of the age of the patient.

## KEY POINTS

- There are many age-related pharmacokinetic effects that lead to dramatic differences in drug absorption, distribution, metabolism, and excretion in the young and the elderly. At one end of the lifespan is the pediatric patient, and at the other end is the elderly patient, both of whom are very sensitive to the effects of drugs.
- Most common dosage calculations use the milligrams per kilogram formula related to age; however, BSA is also used in drug calculations, and organ maturity is considered. It is important for the nurse to know that many elements besides the mathematical calculation itself contribute to safe dosage calculations. Safety must remain the first priority and concern with consideration of the Six Rights of medication administration (see Chapter 1).
- The percentage of the population older than 65 years of age continues to grow, and polypharmacy remains a concern with the increasing number of elderly patients. A current list of all medications and drug allergies must be on their person or with their family/caregiver at all times.
- Your responsibility is to act as a patient advocate as well as to be informed about growth and developmental principles and the effects of various drugs during the lifespan and in various phases of illness.

## NCLEX® EXAMINATION REVIEW QUESTIONS

1 The nurse is reviewing factors that influence pharmacokinetics in the neonatal patient. Which factor puts the neonatal patient at risk with regard to drug therapy?
   a Immature renal system
   b Hyperperistalsis in the GI tract
   c Irregular temperature regulation
   d Smaller circulatory capacity

2 The physiologic differences in the pediatric patient compared with the adult patient affect the amount of drug needed to produce a therapeutic effect. The nurse is aware that one of the main differences is that infants have
   a increased protein in circulation.
   b fat composition lower than 0.001%.
   c more muscular body composition.
   d water composition of approximately 75%.

3 While teaching a 76-year-old patient about the adverse effects of his medications, the nurse encourages him to keep a journal of the adverse effects he experiences. This intervention is important for the elderly patient because of which alterations in pharmacokinetics?
   a Increased renal excretion of protein-bound drugs
   b More alkaline gastric pH, resulting in more adverse effects
   c Decreased blood flow to the liver, resulting in altered metabolism
   d Less adipose tissue to store fat-soluble drugs

4 When the nurse is reviewing a list of medications taken by an 88-year-old patient, the patient says, "I get dizzy when I stand up." She also states that she has nearly fainted "a time or two" in the afternoons. Her systolic blood pressure drops 15 points when she stands up. Which type of medication may be responsible for these effects?
   a NSAIDs
   b Cardiac glycosides
   c Anticoagulants
   d Antihypertensives

5 A pregnant patient who is at 32 weeks' gestation has a cold and calls the office to ask about taking an over-the-counter medication that is rated as pregnancy category A. Which answer by the nurse is correct?
   a "This drug causes problems in the human fetus, so you should not take this medication."
   b "This drug may cause problems in the human fetus, but nothing has been proven in clinical trials. It is best not to take this medication."
   c "This drug has not caused problems in animals, but no testing has been done in humans. It is probably safe to take."
   d "Studies indicate that there is no risk to the human fetus, so it is okay to take this medication as directed if you need it."

6 The nurse is preparing to administer an injection to a preschool-age child. Which approaches are appropriate for this age group? (Select all that apply.)
   a Explain to the child in advance about the injection.
   b Provide a brief, concrete explanation about the injection.
   c Encourage participation in the procedure.
   d Make use of magical thinking.
   e Provide comfort measures after the injection.

7 The nurse is preparing to give an oral dose of acetaminophen (Tylenol) to a child who weighs 12 kg. The dose is 15 mg/kg. How many milligrams will the nurse administer for this dose?

*1. a, 2. d, 3. c, 4. d, 5. d, 6. b, d, e, 7. 180 mg*

For Critical Thinking and Prioritization Questions, see http://evolve.elsevier.com/Lilley.

# Cultural, Legal, and Ethical Considerations

## OBJECTIVES

When you reach the end of this chapter, you will be able to do the following:

1. Discuss the various cultural factors that may influence an individual's response to medications.
2. Identify various cultural phenomena affecting health care and use of medications.
3. List the drugs that are more commonly associated with variations in response due to cultural and racial/ethnic factors.
4. Briefly discuss the important components of drug legislation at the state and federal levels.
5. Provide examples of how drug legislation impacts drug therapy, professional nursing practice, and the nursing process.
6. Discuss the various categories of controlled substances, and give specific drug examples in each category.
7. Identify the process involved in the development of new drugs, including the investigational new drug application, the phases of investigational drug studies, and the process for obtaining informed consent.
8. Discuss the nurse's role in the development of new and investigational drugs and the informed consent process.
9. Discuss the ethical principles and how they apply to pharmacology and the nursing process.
10. Identify the ethical principles involved in making an ethical decision.
11. Develop a nursing care plan that addresses the cultural, legal, and ethical care of patients with a specific focus on drug therapy and the nursing process.

## KEY TERMS

**Bias** Any systematic error in a measurement process. One common effort to avoid bias in research studies involves the use of blinded study designs (see later). (p. 57)

**Black box warning** A type of warning that appears in a drug's prescribing information and is required by the U.S. Food and Drug Administration (FDA) to alert prescribers of serious adverse events that have occurred with the given drug. (p. 57)

**Blinded investigational drug study** A research design in which the subjects are purposely unaware of whether the substance they are administered is the drug under study or a placebo. This method serves to minimize bias on the part of research subjects in reporting their body's responses to investigational drugs. (p. 57)

**Controlled substances** Any drugs listed on one of the "schedules" of the Controlled Substance Act (also called *scheduled drugs*). (p. 55)

**Culture** The customary beliefs, social forms, and material traits of a racial, religious, or social group. (p. 51)

**Double-blind investigational drug study** A research design in which both the investigator(s) and the subjects are purposely unaware of whether the substance administered to a given subject is the drug under study or a placebo. This method minimizes bias on the part of both the investigator and the subject. (p. 57)

**Drug polymorphism** Variation in response to a drug because of a patient's age, gender, size, and/or body composition. (p. 52)

**Ethics**  The rules of conduct recognized in respect to a particular class of human actions or a particular group. (p. 59)

**Ethnicity**  Relating to or characteristics of a human group having racial, religious, language, and other traits in common. (p. 51)

**Ethnopharmacology**  The study of the effect of ethnicity on drug responses, specifically drug absorption, metabolism, distribution, and excretion (i.e., pharmacokinetics; see Chapter 2) as well as the study of genetic variations to drugs (i.e., pharmacogenetics). (p. 51)

**Expedited drug approval**  Acceleration of the usual investigational new drug approval process by the FDA and pharmaceutical companies, usually for drugs used to treat life-threatening diseases. (p. 55)

**Health Insurance Portability and Accountability Act (HIPAA)**  An act that protects health insurance coverage for workers and their families when they change jobs. It also protects patient information. If confidentiality of a patient is breached, severe fines may be imposed. (p. 54)

**Informed consent**  Written permission obtained from a patient consenting to a specific procedure (e.g., receiving an investigational drug), after the patient has been given information regarding the procedure deemed necessary for him or her to make a sound or "informed" decision. (p. 56)

**Investigational new drug (IND)**  A drug not yet approved for marketing by the FDA but available for use in experiments to determine its safety and efficacy. (p. 56)

**Investigational new drug application**  An application that must be submitted to the FDA before a drug can be studied in humans. (p. 56)

**Legend drugs**  Another name for prescription drugs. (p. 55)

**Malpractice**  A special type of negligence or the failure of a professional and/or individual with specialized education and training to act in a reasonable and prudent way. (p. 58)

**Narcotic**  A legal term established under the Harrison Narcotic Act of 1914. It originally applied to drugs that produced insensibility or stupor, especially the opioids (e.g., morphine, heroin). The term is currently used in clinical settings to refer to any medically administered controlled substance and in legal settings to refer to any illicit or "street" drug. (p. 55)

**Negligence**  The failure to act in a reasonable and prudent manner or failure of the nurse to give the care that a reasonably prudent (cautious) nurse would render or use under similar circumstances. (p. 58)

**Orphan drugs**  A special category of drugs that have been identified to help treat patients with rare diseases. (p. 55)

**Over-the-counter drugs**  Drugs available to consumers without a prescription. Also called nonprescription drugs. (p. 53)

**Placebo**  An inactive (inert) substance (e.g., saline, distilled water, starch, sugar) that is not a drug but is formulated to resemble a drug for research purposes. (p. 57)

**Race**  Descendants of a common ancestor; a tribe, family, or people believed to belong to the same lineage. (p. 51)

## CULTURAL CONSIDERATIONS

The United States is a very culturally diverse nation as evidenced by its constantly and rapidly changing demographics. Minority groups, being approximately one third of the U.S. population, are expected to become the majority by 2042 and will represent 54% of the nation's population by 2050. That is, the combined population of all groups except non-Hispanic, single-race whites is projected to be approximately 235 million out of a total U.S. population of 439 million in 2050. The non-Hispanic, single-race white population is projected to be only slightly larger in 2050 (at about 203 million) than in 2010. It is predicted that nearly one in three U.S. residents will be Hispanic by 2050. The African-American population is projected to increase from 41 million (about 14%) to about 66 million (or 15%) by 2050. The Asian population is projected to increase from 15 million to about 40 million, rising from a current 5.1% to 9.2% of the total. Of the remaining racial groups, Native Americans and Alaska Natives are projected to increase in number from 4.9 million to 8.6 million (or from 1.6% to 2% of the total population). The population of Native Hawaiians and other Pacific Islanders is expected to more than double, from 1.1 million to 2.6 million. The number of people who identify themselves as being of two or more races is projected to more than triple, from about 5 million to 16 million.

The field of ethnopharmacology provides an expanding body of knowledge for understanding the specific impact of cultural factors on patient drug response. It is hampered, however, by the lack of clarity in terms such as race, ethnicity, and culture. For example, although some researchers have used the term *Hispanic* to encompass geographic groups as diverse as Puerto Ricans, Mexicans, and Peruvians, other researchers have used it to denote a specific racial group. It is impossible to know a patient's genotype by either physical appearance or health care history.

It is essential to be up to date in your knowledge of the nursing process and understanding of the art and science of professional nursing practice. Cultural assessment needs to be part of the assessment phase of the nursing process. Acknowledgment and acceptance of the influences of a patient's cultural beliefs, values, and customs is necessary to promote optimal health and wellness. Some relevant practices are discussed in the Patient-Centered Care: Cultural Implications box on p. 52.

### Influence of Ethnicity and Genetics on Drug Response

The concept of polymorphism is critical to an understanding of how the same drug may result in very different responses in different individuals. For example, why does a Chinese patient

## ⊕ PATIENT-CENTERED CARE: CULTURAL IMPLICATIONS

### A Brief Review of Common Practices among Selected Cultural Groups

| CULTURAL GROUP | COMMON HEALTH BELIEFS AND ALTERNATIVE HEALERS | VERBAL AND NONVERBAL COMMUNICATION; TOUCH/TIME | FAMILY | BIOLOGIC VARIATIONS |
|---|---|---|---|---|
| African | Practice folk medicine; employ "root doctors" as healers; spiritualist<br>Use herbs, oils, and roots | Asking personal questions of someone met for the first time seen as intrusive and not proper<br>Direct eye contact seen as rude<br>Present oriented | Have close extended family ties<br>Women play important key role in making health care decisions | Keloid formation, sickle cell anemia, lactose intolerance, skin color |
| Asian | Believe in traditional medicine; hot and cold foods; herbs/teas/soups; use of acupuncturist, acupressurist, and herbalist | High respect of others, especially of individuals in positions of authority<br>Not usually comfortable with custom of shaking hands with those of opposite sex<br>Present oriented | Have close extended family ties; family needs more important than individual needs | Many drug interactions, lactose intolerance, skin color, thalassemia |
| Hispanic | View health as a result of good luck and living right; see illness as a result of doing a bad deed<br>Heat, cold, and herbs used as remedies<br>Use curandero, spiritualist | Expressing negative feelings seen as impolite<br>Avoiding eye contact seen as respectful and attentive<br>Touching acceptable between two persons in conversation | Have close extended family ties; all family members involved in health care decisions | Lactose intolerance, skin color |
| Native American | Believe in harmony with nature and ill spirits causing disease<br>Use medicine man | Speak in low tone of voice<br>Light touch of a person's hand is preferred versus a firm handshake as a greeting<br>Present oriented | Have close extended family ties; emphasis on family | Lactose intolerance, skin color, cleft uvula problems |

Data from Bhui K, Dinos S: Health beliefs and culture: Essential considerations for outcome measurement, *Dis Manag Health Out* 16(6):411-419, 2008; Giger JN, Davidhizar RE: *Transcultural nursing: assessment and intervention*, ed 4, St Louis, 2004, Mosby.

require lower dosages of an antianxiety drug than a white patient? Why does an African-American patient respond differently to antihypertensives than a white patient? Drug polymorphism refers to the effect of a patient's age, gender, size, body composition, and other characteristics on the pharmacokinetics of specific drugs. Factors contributing to drug polymorphism may be categorized into environmental factors (e.g., diet and nutritional status), cultural factors, and genetic (inherited) factors.

Medication response depends greatly on the level of the patient's compliance with the therapy regimen. Yet compliance may vary depending on the patient's cultural beliefs, experiences with medications, personal expectations, family expectations and influence, and level of education. Compliance is not the only issue, however. Prescribers must also be aware that some patients use alternative therapies, such as herbal and homeopathic remedies, that can inhibit or accelerate drug metabolism and therefore alter a drug's response.

Environmental and economic factors (e.g., diet) can contribute to drug response. For example, a diet high in fat has been documented to increase the absorption of the drug griseofulvin (an antifungal drug). Malnutrition with deficiencies in protein, vitamins, and minerals may modify the functioning of metabolic enzymes, which may alter the body's ability to absorb or eliminate a medication.

Historically, most clinical drug trials were conducted using white men, often college students, as research subjects. However, there are data that demonstrate the impact of genetic factors on drug *pharmacokinetics* and drug *pharmacodynamics* or drug response (see Chapter 8). Some individuals of European and African descent are known to be *slow acetylators*. This means that their bodies attach acetyl groups to drug molecules at a relatively slow rate, which results in elevated drug concentrations. This situation may warrant lower drug dosages. A classic example of a drug whose metabolism is affected by this characteristic is the antituberculosis drug isoniazid. In contrast, some patients of Japanese and Inuit descent are more rapid acetylators and metabolize drugs more quickly, which predisposes the patient to subtherapeutic drug concentrations and may require higher drug dosages.

Levels of the cytochrome P-450 enzymes (see Chapter 2) are also known to vary between ethnic groups. This has effects on the ability to metabolize many drugs. Most psychotropic drugs (see Chapter 16) are metabolized in the liver in a two-phase process. Cytochrome P-450 enzymes often control phase I of the hepatic metabolism of both antidepressants and antipsychotic drugs. This can affect plasma drug levels, and therefore the intensity of drug response, at different doses. Groups of Asian patients have been shown to be "poor metabolizers" of these drugs and often require lower dosages to achieve desired therapeutic effects. In contrast, white patients are more likely to be classified as "ultrarapid metabolizers" and may require higher drug dosages.

Variations are also reported between ethnic groups in the occurrence of adverse effects. For example, African American patients taking lithium may need to be monitored more closely for symptoms of drug toxicity, because serum drug levels may be higher than in white patients given the same dosage. Likewise, Japanese and Taiwanese patients may require lower dosages of lithium. For the treatment of hypertension, thiazide diuretics appear to be more effective in African Americans than in whites. Several additional examples of racial and ethnic differences in drug response are outlined in the Patient-Centered Care: Cultural Implications box below.

### ⊕ PATIENT CENTERED-CARE: CULTURAL IMPLICATIONS

**Examples of Varying Drug Responses in Different Racial or Ethnic Groups**

| RACIAL OR ETHNIC GROUP | DRUG CLASSIFICATION | RESPONSE |
|---|---|---|
| African Americans | Antihypertensive drugs | African Americans respond better to diuretics than to beta blockers and angiotensin-converting enzyme inhibitors. African Americans respond less effectively to beta blockers. African Americans respond best to calcium channel blockers, especially diltiazem. African Americans respond less effectively to single-drug therapy. |
| Asians and Hispanics | Antipsychotic and antianxiety drugs | Asians need lower dosages of certain drugs such as haloperidol. Asians and Hispanics respond better to lower dosages of antidepressants. Chinese require lower dosages of antipsychotics. Japanese require lower dosages of antimanic drugs. |

NOTE: The comparison group for all responses is whites.

Individuals throughout the world share common views and beliefs regarding health practices and medication use. However, specific cultural influences, beliefs, and practices do exist. Awareness of cultural differences is critical for the care of patients because of the constantly changing U.S. demographics. As a result of these changes, attending to each patient's cultural background helps to ensure safe and quality nursing care, including medication administration.

For example, some African Americans have health beliefs and practices that include an emphasis on proper diet and rest; the use of herbal teas, laxatives, protective bracelets; and the use of folk medicine, prayer, and the "laying on of hands." Reliance on various home remedies can also be an important component of their health practices. Some Asian-American patients, especially

the Chinese, believe in the concepts of *yin* and *yang*. Yin and yang are opposing forces that lead to illness or health, depending on which force is dominant in the individual and whether the forces are balanced. Balance produces healthy states. Other common health practices of Asian Americans include use of acupuncture, herbal remedies, and heat. All such beliefs and practices need to be considered—especially when the patient values their use more highly than the use of medications. Many of these beliefs are strongly grounded in religion. The Asian and Pacific Islander racial/ethnic group also includes Thais, Vietnamese, Filipinos, Koreans, and Japanese, among others.

Some Native Americans believe in preserving harmony with nature or keeping a balance between the body and mind and the environment to maintain health. Ill spirits are seen as the cause of disease. The traditional healer for this culture is the medicine man, and treatments vary from massage and application of heat to acts of purification. Some individuals of Hispanic descent view health as a result of good luck and living right and illness as a result of bad luck or committing a bad deed. To restore health, these individuals seek a balance between the body and mind through the use of cold remedies or foods for "hot" illnesses (of blood or yellow bile) and hot remedies for "cold" illnesses (of phlegm or black bile). Hispanics may use a variety of religious rituals for healing (e.g., lighting of candles), which may also be practiced by adherents of other religions and/or belief systems. It is very important to remember that these beliefs vary from patient to patient; therefore, consult with the patient rather than assume that the patient holds certain beliefs because he or she belongs to a certain ethnic group.

Barriers to adequate health care for the culturally diverse U.S. patient population include language, poverty, access, pride, and beliefs regarding medical practices. Medications may have a different meaning to different cultures, as would any form of medical treatment. Therefore, before any medication is administered, complete a thorough cultural assessment. This assessment includes questions regarding the following:

- Languages spoken, written, and understood; need for an interpreter
- Health beliefs and practices
- Past uses of medicine
- Use of herbal treatments, folk remedies, home remedies, or supplements
- Use of over-the-counter drugs
- Usual responses to illness
- Responsiveness to medical treatment
- Religious practices and beliefs (e.g., many Christian Scientists believe in taking no medications at all)
- Support from the patient's cultural community that may provide resources or assistance as needed, such as religious connections, leaders, family members, or friends
- Dietary habits

## Cultural Nursing Considerations and Drug Therapy

It is important to be knowledgeable about drugs that may elicit varied responses in culturally diverse patients or those from different racial/ethnic groups. Varied responses may include differences in therapeutic dosages and adverse effects, so that some patients may have therapeutic responses at lower dosages than are typically recommended. For example, in Hispanic individuals taking traditional antipsychotics, symptoms may be managed effectively at lower dosages than the usual recommended dosage range.

Another aspect of cultural care as it relates to drug therapy is the recognition that patterns of communication may differ based on a patient's race or ethnicity. Communication also includes the use of language, tone, volume, as well as spatial distancing, touch, eye contact, greetings, and naming format. It is important to assess (see Box 4-3) and apply these aspects of cultural and racial/ethnic variations to patient care and to drug therapy and the nursing process. One specific example of cultural diversity is the use of verb tense; some languages, such as the Chinese language, do not have numerous verb tenses as compared to the English language. Therefore, very precise instructions must be included in patient education about medication(s) and how to best and safely take them. Avoiding the use of contractions such as *can't, won't,* and *don't* is important with patients from other countries to prevent confusion. Instead, use of *cannot, will not,* and *do not* is recommended to improve understanding.

## LEGAL CONSIDERATIONS

Prescription drug use is vital to treating and preventing illness. However, due to safety reasons, its use is regulated by several different agencies, including the Food and Drug Administration (FDA), The Drug Enforcement Agency (DEA), and individual state laws. Traditionally, only medical doctors (M.D.) and doctors of osteopathy (D.O.) had the privilege of prescribing medications. Dentists and podiatrists are also allowed to prescribe medications so long as it is within the scope of their practice. In some states, other health care professionals may also prescribe, including licensed physician's assistants (P.A.s) and advanced practice registered nurses (APRNs).

As the number and complexity of prescriptions continue to increase and technology continually changes, so do the laws regarding their use. With the ever-changing role of the professional nurse and other members of the health care team and with the increasing pace of technologic advances, each role becomes more complex. Even more autonomy has been gained by the professional nurse over his or her nursing practice. With this increasing autonomy comes greater liability and legal accountability; therefore, the professional nurse must be aware and duly consider this responsibility as he or she practices. Specific laws and regulations are discussed later and in the nursing process section of this chapter.

## U.S. Drug and Related Legislation

Until the beginning of the twentieth century there were no federal rules and regulations in the United States to protect consumers from the dangers of medications. The various legislative interventions that have occurred have often been prompted by large-scale serious adverse drug reactions. One example is the sulfanilamide tragedy of 1937. Over 100 deaths occurred in the United States when people ingested a diethylene glycol solution of sulfanilamide that had been marketed as a therapeutic drug. Diethylene glycol is a component of automobile antifreeze solution, and the drug containing it was never tested for its toxicity. Another prominent example is the thalidomide tragedy that occurred in Europe between the 1940s and 1960s. Many pregnant women who took this sedative-hypnotic drug gave birth to seriously deformed infants.

A recent and significant piece of legislation is the Health Insurance Portability and Accountability Act (HIPAA) of 1996. HIPAA requires all health care providers, health insurance and life insurance companies, public health authorities, employers, and schools to maintain patient privacy regarding protected health information. Protected health information includes any individually identifying information such as patients' health conditions, account numbers, prescription numbers, medications, and payment information. Such information can be oral and/or recorded in any paper or electronic form. The primary purpose of federal legislation is to ensure the safety and efficacy of new drugs and, in the case of HIPAA, to protect patient confidentiality. Table 4-1 provides a timeline summary of major U.S. drug legislation.

## New Drug Development

Research into and development of new drugs is an ongoing process. The pharmaceutical manufacturing industry is a multibillion-dollar industry. Pharmaceutical companies must continuously develop new and better drugs to maintain a competitive edge. The research required for the development of these new drugs may take several years. Hundreds of substances are isolated that never make it to market. Once a potentially beneficial drug has been identified, the pharmaceutical company must follow a very regulated, systematic process before the drug can be sold on the open market. This highly sophisticated process is regulated and carefully monitored by the Food and Drug Administration (FDA). The primary purpose of the FDA is to protect the patient and ensure drug effectiveness.

This U.S. system of drug research and development is one of the most stringent in the world. It was developed out of concern for patient safety and drug efficacy. Much time, funding, and documentation are required to ensure that these two very important objectives are met. Many drugs are marketed and used in foreign countries long before they receive approval for use in the United States. Drug-related calamities are more likely to be avoided by this more stringent drug approval system. The thalidomide tragedy mentioned earlier in the chapter, which resulted from the use of a drug that was marketed in Europe but not in the United States, is an illustrative example. A balance must be achieved between making new lifesaving therapies available and protecting consumers from potential drug-induced adverse effects. Historically, the FDA has had less regulatory authority over vitamin, herbal, and homeopathic preparations because they are designated as dietary supplements rather than drugs. In 1994, Congress passed the Dietary Supplement Health and Education Act, which requires manufacturers of such products at least to ensure their safety (although not necessarily their efficacy) and prohibits them from making any

## TABLE 4-1   SUMMARY OF MAJOR U.S. DRUG AND RELATED LEGISLATION

| NAME OF LEGISLATION (YEAR) | PROVISIONS/COMMENTS |
|---|---|
| Federal Food and Drugs Act (FFDA, 1906) | Required drug manufacturers to list on the drug product label the presence of dangerous and possibly addicting substances; recognized the *U.S. Pharmacopeia* and *National Formulary* as printed references standards for drugs |
| Sherley Amendment (1912) to FFDA | Prohibited fraudulent claims for drug products |
| Harrison Narcotic Act (1914) | Established the legal term narcotic and regulated the manufacture and sale of habit-forming drugs |
| Federal Food, Drug, and Cosmetic Act (FFDCA,1938; amendment to FFDA) | Required drug manufacturers to provide data proving drug safety with FDA review; established the investigational new drug application process (prompted by sulfanilamide elixir tragedy) |
| Durham-Humphrey Amendment (1951) to FFDCA | Established legend drugs or prescription drugs; drug labels must carry the legend, "Caution—Federal law prohibits dispensing without a prescription" |
| Kefauver-Harris Amendments (1962) to FFDCA | Required manufacturers to demonstrate both therapeutic efficacy *and* safety of new drugs (prompted by thalidomide tragedy) |
| Controlled Substance Act (1970) | Established "schedules" for controlled substances (Tables 4-2 and 4-3); promoted drug addiction education, research, and treatment |
| Orphan Drug Act (1983) | Enabled the FDA to promote research and marketing of orphan drugs used to treat rare diseases |
| Accelerated Drug Review Regulations (1991) | Enabled faster approval by the FDA of drugs to treat life-threatening illnesses (prompted by HIV/AIDS epidemic) |
| Health Insurance Portability and Accountability Act (1996) | More commonly known by its acronym, *HIPAA;* officially required all health-related organizations as well as schools to maintain privacy of protected health information |
| Medicare Prescription Drug Improvement and Modernization Act (2003) | More commonly known as *Medicare Part D;* provides seniors and disabled persons with an insurance benefit program for prescription drugs; the cost of medications is shared by the patient and the federal government |

*AIDS,* Acquired immunodeficiency syndrome; *FDA,* Food and Drug Administration; *HIV,* human immunodeficiency virus.

unsubstantiated claims in the product labeling. For example, a product label may read "For depression" but cannot read "Known to cure depression." Reliable, objective information about these kinds of products is limited but is growing as more formal research studies are conducted. In 1998, Congress established the National Center for Complementary and Alternative Medicine as a new branch of the National Institutes of Health. The function of this center is to conduct rigorous scientific studies of alternative medical treatments and to publish the data from such studies. Consumer demand for alternative medicine products continues to drive this process. Patients must exercise caution in using such products and to communicate regularly with their health care providers regarding their use.

### U.S. Food and Drug Administration Drug Approval Process

The FDA is responsible for approving drugs for clinical safety and efficacy before they are brought to the market. There are stringent steps, each of which may take years, that must be completed before the drug can be approved. The FDA has made certain lifesaving investigational drug therapies available sooner than usual by offering an expedited drug approval process, also known as "fast track" approval. Acquired Immune Deficiency Syndrome (AIDS) was the first major public health crisis for which the FDA began granting expedited drug approval. This process allowed pharmaceutical manufacturers to shorten the approval process and allowed prescribers to give medications that showed promise during early phase I and phase II clinical trials to qualified patients with AIDS. In such cases, when a trial continues to show favorable results, the overall process of drug approval is hastened. The concept of expedited drug approval became controversial after the FDA-initiated

## TABLE 4-2   CONTROLLED SUBSTANCES: SCHEDULE CATEGORIES

| SCHEDULE | ABUSE POTENTIAL | MEDICAL USE | DEPENDENCY POTENTIAL |
|---|---|---|---|
| C-I | High | None | Severe physical and psychological |
| C-II | High | Accepted | Severe physical and psychological |
| C-III | Less than C-II | Accepted | Moderate to low physical or high psychological |
| C-IV | Less than C-III | Accepted | Limited physical or psychological |
| C-V | Less than C-IV | Accepted | Limited physical or psychological |

manufacturer recall of the antiinflammatory drug rofecoxib (Vioxx) in 2004. This recall followed multiple case reports of severe cardiovascular events, including fatalities, associated with the use of this drug. Evidence then emerged suggesting that the FDA had granted approval for this drug without receiving the requisite safety data from its manufacturer. This unfortunate example has reduced the number of drugs approved via the expedited approval process. More information and specific drugs approved under this fast-track process can be found at http://www.fda.gov.

The drug approval process is quite complex and prolonged. It normally begins with *preclinical* testing phases, which include *in vitro* studies (using tissue samples and cell cultures) and animal studies. *Clinical* (human) studies follow the preclinical phase. There are four clinical phases. The drug is put on the

**TABLE 4-3** **CONTROLLED SUBSTANCES: CATEGORIES, DISPENSING RESTRICTIONS, AND EXAMPLES**

| SCHEDULE | DISPENSING RESTRICTIONS | EXAMPLES |
|---|---|---|
| C-I | Only with approved protocol | Heroin, lysergic acid diethylamide (LSD), marijuana, mescaline, peyote, psilocybin, and methaqualone |
| C-II | Written prescription only* No prescription refills Container must have warning label | Codeine, cocaine, hydromorphone, meperidine, morphine, methadone, secobarbital, pentobarbital, oxycodone, amphetamine, methylphenidate, and others |
| C-III | Written or oral prescription that expires in 6 months No more than five refills in a 6-month period Container must have warning label | Codeine with selected other medications (e.g., acetaminophen), hydrocodone, pentobarbital rectal suppositories, and dihydrocodeine combination products |
| C-IV | Written or oral prescription that expires in 6 months No more than five refills in a 6-month period Container must have warning label | Phenobarbital, chloral hydrate, meprobamate, benzodiazepines (e.g., diazepam, temazepam, lorazepam), dextropropoxyphene, pentazocine, and others |
| C-V | Written prescription or over the counter (varies with state law) | Medications generally for relief of coughs or diarrhea containing limited quantities of certain opioid controlled substances |

*Legally permitted to be telephoned in for major emergencies only. If telephoned in, written prescription is required within 72 hours.

market after phase III is completed if an investigational new drug application submitted by the manufacturer is approved by the FDA. The collective goal of these phases is to provide information on the safety, toxicity, efficacy, potency, bioavailability, and purity of the new drug.

## Preclinical Investigational Drug Studies

Current medical ethics still require that all new drugs undergo laboratory testing using both *in vitro* (cell or tissue) and animal studies before any testing in human subjects can be done. *In vitro* studies include testing of the response of various types of mammalian (including human) cells and tissues to different concentrations of the investigational drug. Various types of cells and tissues used for this purpose are collected from living or dead animal or human subjects (e.g., surgical or autopsy specimens). *In vitro* studies help researchers to determine early on if a substance might be too toxic for human patients. Many prospective new drugs are ruled out for human use during this

preclinical phase of drug testing. However, a small percentage of the many drugs tested in this manner are referred for further clinical testing in human subjects.

## Four Clinical Phases of Investigational Drug Studies

Before any testing on humans begins, the subjects must provide informed consent, and it must be documented. Informed consent involves the careful explanation to the human test patient or *research subject* of the purpose of the study, the procedures to be used, the possible benefits, and the risks involved. This explanation is followed by written documentation on a *consent form*. The informed consent document, or consent form, must be written in a language understood by the patient and must be dated and signed by the patient and at least one witness. Informed consent is always voluntary. By law, informed consent must be obtained more than a given number of days or hours before certain procedures are performed and must always be obtained when the patient is fully mentally competent. The informed consent process may be carried out by a nurse or other health care professional, depending on how a given study is designed.

Medical ethics dictate that participants in experimental drug studies be informed volunteers and not be coerced to participate in any way. Therefore, informed consent must be obtained from all patients (or their legal guardians) before they can be enrolled in an investigational new drug (IND) study. Some patients may have unrealistic expectations of the IND's usefulness. Often they have the misconception that because an investigational drug is new it must automatically be better than existing forms of therapy. Other volunteers may be reluctant to enter the study because they think they will be treated as "guinea pigs." Whatever the circumstances of the study, the research subjects must be informed of all potential hazards as well as the possible benefits of the new therapy. It must be stressed to all patients that involvement in IND studies is voluntary and that any individual can either decline to participate or quit the study at any time without affecting the delivery of any previously agreed-upon health care services.

*Phase I.* Phase I studies usually involve small numbers of healthy subjects rather than those who have the disease or ailment that the new drug is intended to treat. An exception might be a study involving a very toxic drug used to treat a life-threatening illness. In this case, the only study subjects might be those who already have the illness and for whom other viable treatment options may not be available. The purpose of phase I studies is to determine the optimal dosage range and the pharmacokinetics of the drug (i.e., absorption, distribution, metabolism, and excretion) and to ascertain if further testing is needed. Blood tests, urinalyses, assessments of vital signs, and specific monitoring tests are also performed.

*Phase II.* Phase II studies involve small numbers of volunteers who have the disease or ailment that the drug is designed to diagnose or treat. Study participants are closely monitored to determine the drug's effectiveness and identify any adverse effects. Therapeutic dosage ranges are refined during this phase. If no serious adverse effects occur, the study can progress to phase III.

*Phase III.* Phase III studies involve large numbers of patients who are followed by medical research centers and other types of health care entities. The patients may be treated at the center itself or may be spread over a wider geographic area. The purpose of this larger sample size is to provide information about infrequent or rare adverse effects that may not yet have been observed during previous smaller studies. Information obtained during this clinical phase helps identify any risks associated with the new drug. To enhance objectivity, many studies are designed to incorporate a placebo. A placebo is an inert substance that is not a drug (e.g., normal saline). Placebos are given to a portion of the research subjects to separate out the real benefits of the investigational drug from the apparent benefits arising out of researcher or subject bias regarding expected or desired results of the drug therapy. A study incorporating a placebo is called a *placebo-controlled study*. If the study subject does not know whether the drug he or she is administered is a placebo or the investigational drug, but the investigator does know, the study is referred to as a blinded investigational drug study. In most studies, neither the research staff nor the subjects being tested know which subjects are being given the real drug and which are receiving the placebo. This further enhances the objectivity of the study results and is known as a double-blind investigational drug study because both the researcher and the subject are "blinded" to the actual identity of the substance administered to a given subject. Both drug and placebo dosage forms given to patients often look identical except for a secret code that appears on the medication itself and/or its container. At the completion of the study, this code is revealed or broken to determine which study patients received the drug and which were given the placebo. The code can also be broken before study completion by the principle investigator in the event of a clinical emergency that requires a determination of what substance individual patients received.

The three objectives of phase III studies are to establish the drug's clinical effectiveness, safety, and dosage range. After phase III is completed, the FDA receives a report from the manufacturer, at which time the drug company submits a new drug application (NDA). The approval of the application paves the way for the pharmaceutical company to market the new drug exclusively until the patent for the drug molecule expires. This is normally 17 years after discovery of the molecule and includes the 10- to 12-year period generally required to complete drug research. Therefore, a new drug manufacturer typically has 5 to 7 years after drug marketing to recoup research costs, which are usually in the hundreds of millions of dollars for a single drug.

*Phase IV.* Phase IV studies are postmarketing studies voluntarily conducted by pharmaceutical companies to obtain further proof of the therapeutic and adverse effects of the new drug. However, these studies may be mandated by the FDA. Data from such studies are usually gathered for at least 2 years after the drug's release. Often these studies compare the safety and efficacy of the new drug with that of another drug in the same therapeutic category. An example would be a comparison of a new nonsteroidal antiinflammatory drug with ibuprofen in the treatment of osteoarthritis. Some medications make it through all phases of clinical trials without causing any problems among study patients. However, when they are used in the larger general population, severe adverse effects may appear for the first time. If a pattern of

severe reactions to a newly marketed drug begins to emerge, the FDA may request that the manufacturer of the drug issue a black box warning or a voluntary recall. A black box warning indicates that serious adverse effects have been reported with the drug. The drug can still be prescribed; however, the prescriber must be aware of the potential risk (see Table 4-1). In the rare occasion that the drug manufacturer refuses to recall the medication, and if the number and/or severity of reactions reaches a certain level, then the FDA may seek court action to condemn the product and allow it to be seized by legal authorities. Such an action, in effect, becomes an involuntary recall on behalf of the manufacturer. There are three designated classes of drug recall based on FDA response to postmarketing data for a given drug:

- **Class I:** The most serious type of recall—use of the drug product carries a reasonable probability of serious adverse health effects or death.
- **Class II:** Less severe—use of the drug product may result in temporary or medically reversible health effects, but the probability of lasting major adverse health effects is low.
- **Class III:** Least severe—use of the drug product is not likely to result in any significant health problems.

Notification by the FDA of a drug recall or drug warnings may be in the form of press releases, website announcements (http://www.fda.gov), or letters to health professionals. Such FDA items provide the latest information when a drug has newly identified hazards. The FDA has a voluntary program called MedWatch in which professionals are encouraged to report any adverse events seen with newly approved drugs. Information can be found at www.fda.gov/medwatch. Drug information of this kind is continually evolving as new events are observed and reported by clinicians and patients. Recommended actions change with time, so use the most current information available along with sound clinical judgment.

## Legal Nursing Considerations and Drug Therapy

State and federal legislation dictate the boundaries for professional nursing practice. Standards of care and nurse practice acts identify the definition of the scope and role of the professional nurse (Box 4-1). Nurse practice acts further define/identify: (1) the scope of nursing practice, (2) expanded nursing roles, (3) educational requirements for nurses, (4) standards of care, (5) minimally safe nursing practice, and (6) differences between nursing and medical practice. In addition, state boards of nursing define specific nursing practices such as rules concerning the administration of intravenous therapy. Additionally, guidelines from professional nursing groups (American Nurses Association), nursing specialty groups, institutional policies and procedures, and state/federal hospital licensing laws all help to identify the legal boundaries of nursing practice. There is also case law or common law consisting of prior court rulings that affect professional nursing practice.

The American Nurses Association (ANA) has developed standards for nursing practice, policy statements, and similar resolutions. The standards describe the scope, function, and role of the nurse and establish clinical practice standards. The Joint Commission requires that accredited hospitals fulfill certain

---

### BOX 4-1 NURSE PRACTICE ACTS

Nurse Practice Acts (NPAs) are state laws that are instrumental in defining the scope of nursing practice and protect public health, safety, and welfare. In each state, the law directs entry into nursing practice, defines the scope of practices, and identifies disciplinary actions. State boards of nursing oversee this statutory law. NPAs are the most significant part of legislation as related to professional nursing practice. Together, it is NPAs and common law that define nursing practice. The National Council of State Boards of Nursing maintain an online database of each state's NPA, and each state has a website where the NPAs are defined and outlined. For example, if the nurse is practicing in Missouri, Virginia, or West Virginia, the websites are as follows: Missouri: http://pr.mo.gov/nursing-rules-statutes.asp; Virginia: www.dhp.virginia.gov/nursing/nursing_laws_regs.htm; West Virginia: http://www.wvrnboard.com/images/pdf/6707.pdf.

---

standards with regard to nursing practice. One such requirement is that these institutions must have written policies and procedures. These policies are usually quite specific and are contained in policy and procedures manuals found on most nursing units. For example, a policy and procedure will outline the steps to take when changing a dressing or administering a medication. The nurse must know the policies and procedures of the employing institution, because if the nurse is involved in a lawsuit, these are one of the standards by which the nurse will be measured. Nursing specialty organizations also define standards of care for nurses who are certified in specialty areas, such as oncology, surgical care, or critical care. Standards of care help to determine whether a nurse is acting appropriately when performing professional duties. It is critical to safe nursing practice to remain up to date on the ever-changing obligations and standards of practice and care. If standards of care are not met, the nurse becomes liable for negligence and malpractice (Box 4-2). Current nursing literature remains an authoritative resource for information on new standards of care. State governments and/or state boards of nursing have websites that include links to specific nurse practice acts and standards of care.

## TEAMWORK AND COLLABORATION: LEGAL AND ETHICAL PRINCIPLES

### Ethical Terms Related to Nursing Practice

**Autonomy:** Self-determination and the ability to act on one's own; related nursing actions include promoting a patient's decision making, supporting informed consent, and assisting in decisions or making a decision when a patient is posing harm to himself or herself.

**Beneficence:** The ethical principle of doing or actively promoting good; related nursing actions include determining how the patient is best served.

**Confidentiality:** The duty to respect privileged information about a patient; related nursing actions include not talking about a patient in public or outside the context of the health care setting.

**Justice:** The ethical principle of being fair or equal in one's actions; related nursing actions include ensuring fairness in distributing resources for the care of patients and determining when to treat.

**Nonmaleficence:** The duty to do no harm to a patient; related nursing actions include avoiding doing any deliberate harm while rendering nursing care.

**Veracity:** The duty to tell the truth; related nursing actions include telling the truth with regard to placebos, investigational new drugs, and informed consent.

---

### BOX 4-2 AREAS OF POTENTIAL LIABILITY FOR NURSES

| AREA | EXAMPLES RELATED TO DRUG THERAPY AND THE NURSING PROCESS |
|------|----------------------------------------------------------|
| Failure to assess/evaluate | Failure to see significant changes in patient's condition after taking a medication; Failure to report the changes in condition after medication; Failure to take a complete medication history and nursing assessment/history; Failure to monitor patient after medication administration |
| Failure to ensure safety | Lack of adequate monitoring; Failure to identify patient allergies and other risk factors related to medication therapy; Inappropriate drug adminstration technique; Failure to implement appropriate nursing actions based on a lack of proper assessment of patient's condition |
| Medication errors | Failure to clarify unclear medication order; Failure to identify and react to adverse drug reactions; Failure to be familiar with medication prior to its administration; Failure to maintain level of professional nursing skills for current practice; Failure to identify patient's identity prior to drug administration; Failure to document drug administration in medication profile |

---

The legal-ethical dimensions of professional nursing care are also addressed in the legislation passed to amplify the guidelines contained in the HIPAA (1996). Under these federal regulations (see p. 54), the privacy of patient information is protected, and standards are included for the handling of electronic data about patients. HIPAA also defines the rights and privileges of patients in order to protect privacy without diminishing access to quality health care. The assurance of privacy—even prior to establishment of the HIPAA guidelines—was based on the principle of respect of an individual's right to determine when, to what extent, and under what circumstances private information can be shared or withheld from others, including family members. In addition, confidentiality must be preserved; that is, the individual identities of patients or research study participants are not to be linked to information they provide and cannot be publicly divulged. HIPAA addresses the issues of confidentiality and privacy by prohibiting prescribers, nurses, and other health care providers from sharing with others any patient health care information, including laboratory results, diagnoses, and prognoses, without the patient's consent. Conflicting obligations arise when a patient wants to keep information away from insurance companies, and matters remain complicated and challenging in the era of improving technology and computerization of medical records. Health care facilities continue to work diligently, however, to adhere to HIPAA guidelines and use special access codes to limit who can access information in computerized documents and charts.

In summary, federal and state legislation, standards of care, and nurse practice acts provide the legal framework for safe nursing practice, including drug therapy and medication administration. Further, as discussed in Chapter 1, the standard "Six Rights" of medication administration are yet another measure for ensuring safety and adherence to laws necessary for protecting the patient. Chapter 1 also discusses other patient rights that are part of the standards of practice of every licensed registered nurse and every student studying the art and science of nursing.

## ETHICAL CONSIDERATIONS

Decisions in health care are seldom made independently of other people and are made with consideration of the patient, family, nurses, and other members of the health care team. All members of the health care team must make a concentrated effort to recognize and understand their own values and be considerate, nonjudgmental, and respectful of the values of others and ethics. The use of drug therapy has evolved from just administering whatever was prescribed to providing responsible drug therapy for the purpose of achieving defined outcomes that improve a patient's quality of life.

Ethical principles are useful strategies for members of the health care team (e.g., physician, pharmacist, nurse) and include standards or truths on which ethical actions are made. Some of the most useful principles in nursing and health care, specifically drug therapy, include autonomy, beneficence, nonmaleficence, and veracity (see the Teamwork and Collaboration: Legal and Ethical Principles box on p. 58). However, day-to-day practice in nursing and health care pose many potential ethical conflicts. Each situation is different and requires compassionate and humane solutions. When answers to ethical dilemmas remain unclear and ethical conflict occurs, then the appropriate action must be based on ethical principles.

for Nurses (available at www.nursingworld.org/codeofethics) and the International Council of Nurses (ICN) Code of Ethics for Nurses serve as frameworks of practice for all nurses and as ethical guidelines for nursing care (see the Teamwork and Collaboration: Legal and Ethical Principles box on the ICN Code of Ethics for Nurses below). Adherence to these ethical principles and codes of ethics ensures that the nurse is acting on behalf of the patient and with the patient's best interests at heart. As a professional, the nurse has the responsibility to provide safe nursing care to patients regardless of the setting, person, group, community, or family involved. Although it is not within the nurse's realm of ethical and professional responsibility to impose his or her own values or standards on the patient, it *is* within the nurse's realm to provide information and to assist the patient in making decisions regarding health care.

The nurse also has the right to refuse to participate in any treatment or aspect of a patient's care that violates the nurse's personal ethical principles. However, this must be done without deserting the patient, and in some facilities the nurse may be transferred to another patient care assignment only if the transfer is approved by the nurse manager or nurse supervisor. The nurse must always remember, however, that the ANA *Code of Ethics for Nurses* and professional responsibility and accountability require the nurse to provide nonjudgmental nursing care from the start of the patient's treatment until the time of the patient's discharge. If transferring to a different assignment is not an option because of institutional policy and because of the increase in the acuteness of patients' conditions and the high patient-to-nurse workload, the nurse must always act in the

### TEAMWORK AND COLLABORATION: LEGAL AND ETHICAL PRINCIPLES

#### *Elements of Liability for Nursing Malpractice*

| ELEMENT | EXAMPLE |
| --- | --- |
| Duty | Being responsible for accurate assessment of a patient's intravenous (IV) and site of IV during caustic drug infusion and the timely reporting of changes in the patient's condition. |
| Breach of duty | Nurse does not notice that the IV site is swollen, red, painful, and warm to touch nor that the IV has quit infusing properly. |
| Causation | Failure of the nurse to note the signs and symptoms of extravasation at IV site (with a chemotherapy drug or other caustic drug) that results in the need for skin grafting. |
| Damage | Extensive skin and nerve damage with several surgical skin grafts resulting in limited use of arm. |

## Ethical Nursing Considerations and Drug Therapy

Ethical nursing practice is based on fundamental principles such as beneficence, autonomy, justice, veracity, and confidentiality. The American Nurses Association (ANA) *Code of Ethics*

### TEAMWORK AND COLLABORATION: LEGAL AND ETHICAL PRINCIPLES

#### *International Council of Nurses* Code of Ethics for Nurses

The International Council of Nurses (ICN) first adopted the *ICN Code of Ethics for Nurses* in 1953; the *Code* has been revised several times since then, most recently in 2006. The 2006 revision is available in English, French, Spanish, and German. This Code is a guide for action based on social values and needs. The Preamble identifies the four fundamental responsibilities of nurses—promoting health, preventing illness, restoring health, and alleviating suffering—and points out that the need for nursing is universal. The Code makes it clear that inherent in professional nursing practice is respect for human rights including the right to life, dignity, and the right to be treated with respect. Nursing care is provided without regard to age, color, creed, culture, disability, illness, gender, nationality, politics, race, or social status. Nurses render services to the individual, family, and community. The *Code* describes four principal elements that provide a framework for the standards of ethical conduct it defines: nurses and people, nurses and practice, nurses and the profession, and nurses and co-workers. The *ICN Code of Ethics for Nurses* serves as a guide for action based on social values and needs and should be understood, internalized, and applied by nurses in all aspects of their work. Nurses can obtain assistance in translating these standards into conduct by discussing the *Code* with co-workers and collaborating with their national nurses' associations in the application of ethical standards in nursing practice, education, management, and research.

best interest of the patient while remaining an objective patient advocate. It is always the nurse's responsibility to provide the highest-quality nursing care and to practice within the professional standards of care. The ANA *Code of Ethics for Nurses*, the ICN *Code of Ethics for Nurses*, nurse practice acts, federal and state codes, ethical principles, and the previously mentioned legal principles and legislation are readily accessible and provide nurses with a sound, rational framework for professional nursing practice.

Another area of ethical consideration related to drug therapy and the nursing process is the use of placebos. A placebo is a drug dosage form (e.g., tablet or capsule) without any pharmacologic activity due to a lack of active ingredients. However, there may be reported therapeutic responses, and placebos have been found to be beneficial in certain patients, such as those being treated for anxiety. Placebos are also administered frequently in experimental studies of new drugs to evaluate and measure the pharmacologic effects of a new medicine compared with those of an inert placebo. Except in new drug studies, however, placebo use is often considered to be unethical and deceitful, possibly creating mistrust among the nurse, the prescriber, and the patient. In current clinical practice guidelines for pain management, the American Pain Society and the Agency for Health Care Policy and Research recommend the avoidance of placebos because their use is believed to be deceitful and to violate a patient's rights to the highest-quality care possible. Many health care agencies limit the use of placebos to research only to avoid the possible deceit and mistrust. If an order is received for a placebo for a patient, it is within the legal purview of a professional nurse to inquire about the order and to ask why a placebo is being prescribed; the order must never be taken lightly. If administration of the placebo is part of a research study or clinical trial, the informed consent process must be thorough and the patients must be informed of their right to (1) leave the study at any time without any pressure or coercion to stay, (2) leave the study without consequences to medical care, (3) receive full and complete information about the study, and (4) be aware of all alternative options and receive information on all treatments, including placebo therapy, being administered in the study.

## NURSING PROCESS

Only information on the cultural considerations related to drug therapy and the nursing process will be presented in the following sections. Legal issues and ethical principles are integrated into professional nursing practice, whereas there are specific racial-ethnic (cultural) factors that need to be addressed in each phase of the nursing process.

## ASSESSMENT

A thorough cultural assessment is needed for the provision of culturally competent nursing care. A variety of assessment tools and resources to incorporate into nursing care are provided in Box 4-3. However, various factors must be assessed and then applied to nursing care, specifically drug therapy and the nursing process. Some of the specific questions about

---

> **BOX 4-3**   **CULTURAL ASSESSMENT TOOLS AND RELATED WEB LINKS**
>
> • Several cultural assessment tools have been developed over the last decade. Madeline Leininger's Sunrise Model focuses on seven major areas of cultural assessment, including educational, economic, familial and social, political, technologic, religious and philosophic, and cultural values, beliefs, and practices.
>
> • Other comprehensive cultural assessment tools include those developed by Andrews and Bowls, 1999; Friedman, Bowden, and Jones, 2003; Giger and Davidhizar, 1999; and Purnell and Pcaulanka, 1998. Rani Srivastava's (2006), found in *The Healthcare Professional's Guide to Clinical Cultural Competence* (Healthcare Professional's Guides), contains further discussion on how populations are viewed by health care workers and not through the use of ethno-cultural/religious labels.

the patient's physical, mental, and spiritual health include the following:

### MAINTAINING HEALTH

• *For physical health:* Where are special foods and clothing items purchased? What types of health education are of the patient's culture? Where does the patient usually obtain information about health and illness? Folklore? Where are health services obtained? Who are health care providers (e.g., physicians, nurse practitioners, community services organizations, health departments, healers)?

• *For mental health:* What are examples of culturally specific activities for the mind and for maintaining mental health, as well as beliefs about stress reduction, rest, and relaxation?

• *For spiritual health:* What are resources for meeting spiritual needs?

### PROTECTING HEALTH

• *For physical health:* Where are special clothing and everyday essentials? What are examples of the patient's symbolic clothing, if any?

• *For mental health:* Who within the family and community teaches the roles in the patient's specific culture? Are there rules about avoiding certain persons or places? Are there special activities that must be performed?

• *For spiritual health:* Who teaches spiritual practices, and where can special protective symbolic objects such as crystals or amulets be purchased? Are they expensive, and how available are they for the patient when needed?

### RESTORING HEALTH

• *For physical health:* Where are special remedies purchased? Can individuals produce or grow their own remedies, herbs, and so on? How often are traditional and nontraditional services obtained?

• *For mental health:* Who are the traditional and nontraditional resources for mental health? Are there culture-specific activities for coping with stress and illness?

• *For spiritual health:* How often and where are traditional and nontraditional spiritual leaders or healers accessed?*

---

*Modified from Spector RE: *Cultural care: guides to heritage assessment and health traditions,* ed 2, Upper Saddle River, NJ, 2000, Pearson/Prentice Hall, pp 24-25.

## NURSING DIAGNOSES

1. Sleep deprivation related to a lack of adherence to cultural practices for encouraging stress release and sleep induction
2. Deficient knowledge (drug therapy) related to lack of experience and information about prescribed drug therapy
3. Risk for injury related to adverse and unpredictable reaction to drug therapy due to racial/ethnic or cultural factors

## PLANNING

### GOALS

1. Patient states the need for assistance with nonpharmacologic management of sleep deficit.
2. Patient requests written and verbal education about medication therapy.
3. Patient states need for information about the influence of racial/ethnic cultural factors upon specific drug therapy with emphasis on safety measures.

### OUTCOME CRITERIA

1. Patient describes specific measures to enhance sleep patterns such as regular sleep habits, decrease in caffeine, meditation, relaxation therapy, journaling sleep patterns, and noting those measures that enhance or take away sleep.
2. Patient lists the various medication(s) with their therapeutic and adverse effects, dosage routes, and specific methods of adequate self administration, drug interactions, and any other special considerations.
3. Patient describes the impact of his or her racial/ethnic influences (e.g., metabolic enzyme differences) on specific medications and the resulting potential for increase in adverse effects, toxicity, and/or increased or decreased effectiveness (medication therapy).

## IMPLEMENTATION

There are numerous interventions for implementation of culturally competent nursing care, but one very important requirement is that nurses maintain current knowledge about various cultures and related activities and practices of daily living, health beliefs, and emotional and spiritual health practices and beliefs. Specifically, knowledge about medications that may elicit varied responses due to racial/ethnic variations is most important with application of concepts of culturally competent care and ethnopharmacology to each patient care situation. Information of particular significance is the impact of cytochrome P-450 enzymes on certain phases of drug metabolism (see previous discussion on p. 27). Specific examples of differences in certain cytochrome P-450 enzymes can be found on p. 52. Consider additional factors, including the patient's verbal and nonverbal communication patterns; health belief systems; identification of health care provider and/or alternate healers; and interpretation of space, time, and touch. For example, with regard to adherence with the treatment regimen, Hispanics with hypertension have been found in some studies to be less likely than African Americans or whites to continue to take medication as prescribed, a finding that may reflect the patients' health belief systems. Other lifestyle decisions (e.g., use of tobacco or alcohol) may also affect responses to drugs and must be considered during drug administration. In addition, a patient's cultural background and associated socioeconomic status may create a situation that leads the patient to skip pills, split doses, and not obtain refills. This culture of poverty may be a causative factor in noncompliance and requires astute attention and individualized nursing actions.

## EVALUATION

Culturally competent nursing care related to drug therapy may be evaluated through the actual compliance (or lack thereof) to the medication regimen(s). Safe, effective, and therapeutic self-administration of drugs with minimal to no adverse/toxic effects will be present only when the patient is treated as an individual and has a thorough understanding of the medication regimen.

---

### CASE STUDY

#### Clinical Drug Trial

A patient on the cardiac telemetry unit has had a serious heart condition for years and has been through every known protocol for treatment. The cardiologist has admitted him to a telemetry unit for observation during a trial of a new investigational drug. The patient exclaims, "I have high hopes for this drug. I've read about it on the Internet and the reports are wonderful. I can't wait to get better!"

1. What is the best way for the nurse to answer this statement?

The physician meets with the patient and the nurse to explain the medication and how the double-blind experimental drug study will work. The purpose of the medication and potential hazards of the therapy are described, as well as the laboratory tests that will be performed to measure the drug's effectiveness. The physician then asks the nurse to have the patient sign the consent form. When the nurse goes to get the patient's signature, the patient says, "I'll sign it, but I really didn't understand what that doctor told me about the placebo."

2. Should the nurse continue with getting the consent form signed? Explain your answer.

3. The patient tells the nurse, "How can I make sure I have the real drug and not the fake drug? I really want to see if it will help my situation." What is the nurse's best response?

4. After a week, the patient tells the nurse, "I don't see that this drug is helping me. In fact, I feel worse. But I'm afraid to tell the doctor that I want to stop the medicine. What do I do?" What is the nurse's best response?

For answers, see http://evolve.elsevier.com/Lilley.

## KEY POINTS

- A variety of culturally based assessment tools are available for use in patient care and drug therapy.
- Drug therapy and subsequent patient responses may be affected by racial and ethnic variations in levels of specific enzymes and metabolic pathways of drugs.
- Various pieces of federal legislation, as well as state law, state practice acts, and institutional policies, have been established to help ensure the safety and efficacy of drug therapy and the nursing process.
- HIPAA guidelines have increased awareness concerning patient confidentiality and privacy. It is important to understand this federal legislation as it relates to drug therapy and the nursing process.
- The Controlled Substance Act of 1970 provides nurses and other health care providers with information on drugs that cause little to no dependence versus those associated with a high level of abuse and dependency.
- Always obtain informed consent as needed, with complete understanding of your role and responsibilities as patient advocate in obtaining such consent.
- In the IND research process, adhere to the study protocol while also acting as a patient advocate and honoring the patient's right to safe, quality nursing care.
- Adhere to legal guidelines, ethical principles, and the ANA *Code of Ethics for Nurses* so that your actions are based on a solid foundation.
- Placebo use remains controversial and if a placebo is ordered, question the prescriber about the specific cause for its use.

## NCLEX® EXAMINATION REVIEW QUESTIONS

1 A patient is undergoing major surgery and asks the nurse about a living will. He states, "I don't want anybody making decisions for me. And I don't want to prolong my life." The patient is demonstrating
   a  autonomy.
   b  beneficence.
   c  justice.
   d  veracity.

2 When caring for an elderly Chinese patient, the nurse recognizes that which of these cultural issues may influence the care of this patient?
   a  Radiographs are seen as a break in the soul's integrity.
   b  Hospital diets are interpreted as being healing and healthful.
   c  The use of heat may be an important practice for this patient.
   d  Being hospitalized is a source of peace and socialization for this culture.

3 A patient is being counseled for possible participation in a clinical trial for a new medication. After the patient meets with the physician, the nurse is asked to obtain the patient's signature on the consent forms. The nurse knows that this "informed consent" indicates which of the following?
   a  Once therapy has begun, the patient cannot withdraw from the clinical trial.
   b  The patient has been informed of all potential hazards and benefits of the therapy.
   c  The patient has received only the information that will help to make the clinical trial a success.
   d  No matter what happens, the patient will not be able to sue the researchers for damages.

4 A new drug has been approved for use, and the drug manufacturer has made it available for sale. During the first 6 months, the FDA receives reports of severe adverse effects that were not discovered during the testing and considers withdrawing the drug. This illustrates which phase of investigational drug studies?
   a  Phase I
   b  Phase II
   c  Phase III
   d  Phase IV

5 A patient of Japanese descent describes a family trait that manifests frequently: She says that members of her family often have "strong reactions" after taking certain medications, but her white friends have no problems with the same dosages of the same drugs. The nurse recognizes that, because of this trait, which statement applies?
   a  She may need lower dosages of the medications prescribed.
   b  She may need higher dosages of the medications prescribed.
   c  She should not receive these medications because of potential problems with metabolism.
   d  These situations vary greatly, and her accounts may not indicate a valid cause for concern.

6 When evaluating polymorphism and medication administration, the nurse considers which factors? (Select all that apply.)
   a  Nutritional status
   b  Drug route
   c  Patient's ethnicity
   d  Cultural beliefs
   e  Patient's age

## NCLEX® EXAMINATION REVIEW QUESTIONS — cont'd

7 The nurse is reviewing the four clinical phases of investigational drug studies. Place the four phases in the correct order of occurrence.

a Studies that are voluntarily conducted by pharmaceutical companies to obtain more information about the therapeutic and adverse effects of a drug.

b Studies that involve small numbers of volunteers who have the disease or ailment that the drug is designed to diagnose or treat.

c Studies that involve small numbers of healthy subjects who do not have the disease or ailment that the drug is intended to treat.

d Studies that involve large numbers of patients who have the disease that the drug is intended to treat; these studies establish the drug's clinical effectiveness, safety, and dosage range.

1. a, 2. c, 3. b, 4. d, 5. a, 6. a, c, d, e, 7. a = 4, b = 4, c = 2, c = 1, d = 3

For Critical Thinking and Prioritization Questions, see http://evolve.elsevier.com/Lilley.

# Medication Errors:
# Preventing and Responding

## OBJECTIVES

When you reach the end of this chapter, you will be able to do the following:

1  Compare the following terms related to drug therapy in the context of professional nursing practice: *adverse drug event, adverse drug reaction, allergic reaction, idiosyncratic reaction, medical error,* and *medication error.*
2  Describe the most commonly encountered medication errors.
3  Develop a framework for professional nursing practice for prevention of medication errors.
4  Identify potential physical and emotional consequences of a medication error.

5  Discuss the impact of culture and age on the occurrence of medication errors.
6  Analyze the various ethical dilemmas related to professional nursing practice associated with medication errors.
7  Identify agencies concerned with prevention of and response to medication errors.
8  Discuss the possible consequences of medication errors for professional nurses and other members of the health care team.

## KEY TERMS

**Adverse drug event** Any undesirable occurrence related to administration of or failure to administer a prescribed medication. (p. 65)

**Adverse drug reactions** Unexpected, unintended, or excessive responses to medications given at therapeutic dosages (as opposed to overdose); one type of adverse drug event. (p. 65)

**Allergic reaction** An immunologic reaction resulting from an unusual sensitivity of a patient to a particular medication; a type of adverse drug event and a subtype of adverse drug reactions. (p. 65)

**Idiosyncratic reaction** Any abnormal and unexpected response to a medication, other than an allergic reaction, that is peculiar to an individual patient. (p. 65)

**Medical errors** A broad term used to refer to any errors at any point in patient care that cause or have the potential to cause patient harm. (p. 65)

**Medication errors** Any preventable adverse drug events involving inappropriate medication use by a patient or health care professional; they may or may not cause the patient harm. (p. 65)

**Medication reconciliation** A procedure implemented by health care providers to maintain an accurate and up-to-date list of medications for all patients between all phases of health care delivery. (p. 70)

## GENERAL IMPACT OF ERRORS ON PATIENTS

Medical errors and medication errors in particular have received much national attention. The study that brought medical errors to the public was the landmark study done in 1999 by the Institute of Medicine (IOM). According to this study, the number of patient deaths from medical errors in U.S. hospitals ranged from 44,000 to 98,000 annually based on data from two large-scale studies. The IOM conducted a similar study in 2006 and found that medical errors harm at least 1.5 million people per year, including 117,000 hospitalizations at a cost of over $4 billion. A follow-up study in 2010 showed 25.1 "harms" per 100 admissions to the hospital. This study showed no significant change in rates of preventable errors since the IOM study. Numerous health institutions have made prevention of medical errors a top priority. The most important change is to recognize that reporting of errors should not be punitive toward the reporter. In fact, all health care professionals are encouraged to report errors. It has been shown that reporting of errors can prevent errors from occurring. This study also brought forth the notion that most errors occur as a breakdown in the medication use system, as opposed to being the fault of the individual. This concept has been taken a step further and has created "just culture." Just culture recognizes that systems are generally at fault when an error occurs, but that when professionals do not follow policies or have repeated errors, that professional needs remedial education and must be held accountable.

Medical errors can occur during all phases of health care delivery and involve all categories of health professionals. Some of the more common types of error include misdiagnosis, patient misidentification, lack of patient monitoring, wrong-site surgery, and medication errors. Most studies have looked at medical errors occurring in hospitals; however, many serious medication errors occur in the home. Errors occurring in homes can be quite harmful, as potent drugs once used only in hospitals are now being prescribed for outpatients. The majority of fatal errors at home involve the mixing of prescription drugs with alcohol or other drugs. Intangible losses resulting from such adverse outcomes include patient dissatisfaction with, and loss of trust in, the health care system. This, in turn, can lead to adverse health outcomes because patients are afraid to seek health services. This chapter focuses on the issues related to medication errors and ways to prevent and respond to these errors.

## MEDICATION ERRORS

An adverse drug event is a general term that encompasses all types of clinical problems related to medication use. These include medication errors and adverse drug reactions. The various subsets of adverse drug events and their interrelationships are illustrated in Figure 5-1. Adverse drug reactions are reactions that occur with the use of the particular drug. Two types of adverse drug reactions are allergic reaction (often predictable) and idiosyncratic reaction (usually unpredictable). Medication errors are a common cause of adverse health care outcomes and can range from having no significant effect to directly causing patient disability or death.

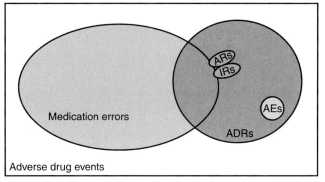

**FIGURE 5-1** Diagram illustrating the various classes and subclasses of adverse drug events. *ADRs,* Adverse drug reactions; *AEs,* adverse (drug) effects; *ARs,* allergic reactions; *IRs,* idiosyncratic reactions.

It is important to consider all of the steps involved in the medication use system when discussing medication errors. Identifying, responding to, and ultimately preventing medication errors require an examination of the entire medication use process. Attention must be focused on all persons and all steps involved in the medication use process, including the prescriber, the transcriber of the order, nurses, pharmacists, and any other ancillary staff involved. A systems approach takes the "Six Rights" one step further and examines the entire health care system, the health care professionals involved, and any other factor that has an impact on the error.

Drugs commonly involved in severe medication errors include central nervous system drugs, anticoagulants, and chemotherapeutic drugs. "High-alert" medications have been identified as those that, because of their potentially toxic nature, require special care when prescribing, dispensing, and/or administering. High-alert medications are not necessarily involved in more errors than other drugs; however, the potential for patient harm is higher. Some high-alert medications are listed in Box 5-1. Medication errors also result from the fact that there are large numbers of drugs that have similarities in spelling and/or pronunciation (i.e., look-alike or sound-alike names). Several acronyms have been created to refer to these drugs, including SALAD (sound-alike, look-alike drugs) and LASA (look-alike, sound-alike). Mix-ups between such drugs are most dangerous when two drugs from very different therapeutic classes have similar names. This can result in patient effects that are grossly different from those intended as part of the drug therapy. The Safety and Quality Improvement: Preventing Medication Errors box on p. 66 lists examples of commonly confused drug names. More information on high-alert medications and sound-alike, look-alike drugs can be found at the website of the Institute for Safe Medication Practices at http://www.ismp.org.

It is widely recognized that most medication errors result from weaknesses in the systems within health care organizations rather than from individual shortcomings. System weaknesses include failure to create a "just culture" or nonpunitive work atmosphere for reporting errors, excessive workload with

## BOX 5-1 EXAMPLES OF HIGH-ALERT MEDICATIONS

### Drug Classes/Categories

- Adrenergic agonists, IV (e.g., epinephrine, phenylephrine, norepinephrine)
- Adrenergic antagonists, IV (e.g., propranolol, metoprolol, labetalol)
- Anesthetic agents, general, inhaled and IV (e.g., propofol, ketamine)
- Antidysrhythmics, IV (e.g., lidocaine, amiodarone)
- Antithrombotic agents (anticoagulants), including warfarin, low–molecular-weight heparin, IV unfractionated heparin, factor Xa inhibitors (e.g., fondaparinux), direct thrombin inhibitors (e.g., argatroban, lepirudin, bivalirudin), thrombolytics (e.g., alteplase, reteplase, tenecteplase), and glycoprotein IIb/IIIa inhibitors (e.g., eptifibatide)
- Cardioplegic solutions
- Chemotherapeutic agents, parenteral and oral
- Epidural or intrathecal medications
- Hypoglycemics, oral
- Inotropic drugs, IV (e.g., digoxin, milrinone)
- Moderate sedation drugs, IV (e.g., midazolam)
- Narcotics/opiates, IV, transdermal, and oral (including liquid concentrates, immediate- and sustained-release formulations)
- Neuromuscular blocking agents (e.g., succinylcholine, rocuronium, vecuronium)
- Radiocontrast agents, IV
- Total parenteral nutrition solutions

### Specific Drugs

- Insulin, subcutaneous and IV
- Magnesium sulfate injection
- Methotrexate, oral, nononcologic use
- Oxytocin, IV
- Nitroprusside sodium for injection
- Potassium chloride for injection
- Potassium phosphates injection
- Promethazine, IV
- Sodium chloride for injection, hypertonic (greater than 0.9% concentration)
- Sterile water for injection, inhalation, and irrigation (excluding pour bottles) in containers of 100 mL or more

From Institute for Safe Medication Practices: ISMP's list of high-alert medications, available at http://www.ismp.org/Tools/highalertmedications.pdf.

## ⚡ SAFETY AND QUALITY IMPROVEMENT: PREVENTING MEDICATION ERRORS

### *Institute for Safe Medication Practices: Examples of Look-Alike, Sound-Alike (LASA) Commonly Confused Drug Names*

| NAMES OF MEDICATIONS | COMMENTS |
| --- | --- |
| carboplatin vs. cisplatin | Two different antineoplastic drugs |
| Celebrex vs. Celexa | Antiinflammatory drug vs. antidepressant drug |
| Depakote vs. Depakote ER | Same drug; immediate-release vs. extended-release dosage forms |
| dopamine vs. dobutamine | Vasopressor drugs of markedly different strengths; dobutamine is also a strong inotropic affecting the heart |
| fentanyl vs. sufentanil | Both are injectable anesthetics but with a significant difference in potency and duration of action |
| glipizide vs. glyburide | Two different antidiabetic drugs |
| Humulin vs. Humalog | Short-acting vs. rapid-acting insulin |
| Lamictal vs. Lamisil | Anticonvulsant/mood stabilizer vs. antifungal drug |
| metronidazole vs. metformin | Antibiotic vs. antidiabetic drug |
| MiraLax vs. Mirapex | Laxative vs. antiparkinson drug |
| morphine vs. hydromorphone | Two different potency opioids |
| oxycodone vs. OxyContin | Immediate-release vs. long-acting oxycodone |
| Paxil vs. Plavix | Antidepressant vs. antiplatelet drug |
| trazodone vs. tramadol | Antidepressant vs. analgesic |

Additional examples can be found at http://www.ismp.org/Tools/confuseddrugnames.pdf. Accessed February 23, 2011.

minimal time for preventive education, and lack of interdisciplinary communication and collaboration. All hospitals are required to analyze medication errors and implement ways to prevent them. Nurses must take the time to report errors, because without reporting, no changes can be made. When errors are reported, trends can be identified and processes can be changed to prevent the errors from occurring again.

## ISSUES CONTRIBUTING TO ERRORS

### Organizational Issues

Medication errors can occur at any step in the medication process: procuring, prescribing, transcribing, dispensing, administering, and monitoring. One study noted that half of all preventable adverse drug events begin with an error at the medication ordering (prescribing) stage. Most prescribing errors can be caught by the pharmacist before order entry and by nurses prior to administration. Administration is the next most common point in the process at which medication errors

occur, followed by dispensing errors and transcription errors. It is very important for nurses to have good relationships with pharmacists, because the two professions, working together, can have a major impact in preventing medication errors. Hospital pharmacists are usually available 24/7 and serve as great resources when the nurse has any question regarding drug therapy.

The Joint Commission, the major accreditation body for hospitals, began a patient public awareness campaign in 2006 called *Speak Up.* It encourages patients to take a more active role in their health care by "speaking up" and asking questions whenever they feel the need to do so. The value of this program is twofold: patients learn more about their illnesses and the care provided, and they can advocate for their own safety at each health care encounter. Specific topics on the campaign website (http://www.jointcommission.org/speakup.aspx) include asking questions about care in general, learning about living organ donation, preventing infections in the hospital, avoiding medication errors, participating in research studies, planning for follow-up care, avoiding errors in medical tests, and knowing about patients rights in general (see Box 5-2).

Effective use of technologies such as computerized prescriber order entry and bar coding of medication packages has been shown to reduce medication errors. In February 2004, the U.S. Food and Drug Administration (FDA) announced new regulations requiring bar codes for all prescription and over-the-counter medications. Unfortunately, only a small percentage of U.S. hospitals have implemented bar-code scanning technology, primarily due to prohibitive cost. Cost is a barrier to technologic improvements in general. The cost of implementing current technology, including automated drug dispensing cabinets with electronic charting and computerized order entry, may range from hundreds of thousands of dollars to over $20 million. Nonetheless, these various technologic advances have been shown to reduce medication errors. For example, computerized order entry (also known as computerized physician order entry [CPOE]) eliminates handwriting and standardizes many prescribing functions. Bar coding of medications allows the nurse to use electronic devices for verification of correct medication at the patient's bedside. Computer programs are used in the pharmacy to screen for potential drug interactions. Despite all the benefits technology has to offer, workload issues (i.e., nursing staff shortage), inadequate education in the use of the equipment, or difficulties in mastering the use of complex technology can prevent the technology from eliminating errors as it was designed to do. Self-medication by patients (e.g., patient-controlled analgesia) has been shown to reduce errors, provided patients have adequate cognitive ability and mental alertness.

## Educational System Issues and Their Potential Impact on Medication Errors

All health professionals have an obligation to double-check any necessary information before proceeding. This includes stopping and checking medication orders and being comfortable with one's knowledge of the drug *before* administering it. Numerous drug information guides are available to be utilized by the nurse. Even the most capable health care provider cannot know everything nor have immediate recall of every fact ever read. This is especially true given the increasing complexity of health care practice.

Patient safety begins in the educational process with nursing students and faculty members. Adopting the philosophy that "no question is a stupid question" allows students to begin their careers with greater confidence and with a healthy habit of self-monitoring. In contrast, berating or otherwise penalizing a student for not immediately recalling a given fact, or for simply asking questions, instills fear and shame. It also discourages dialogue that would otherwise promote and enhance student learning. Commonly reported student nurse errors involve the following situations: unusual dosing times, medication administration record issues (unavailability of the record, failure to document doses given resulting in administration of extra doses, failure to review the record before medicating patients), administration of discontinued or "held" medications, failure to monitor vital signs or laboratory results, administration of oral liquids as injections, preparation of medications for multiple patients at the same time, and dispensing of medications in different doses than those ordered (e.g., tablets that need to be broken in half). The World Health Organization has developed information about patient safety concerns, safety initiatives, and patient safety solutions (Box 5-2).

## Medication Errors and Related Sociologic Factors

Effective communication among all members of the health care team contributes to improved patient care. However, a 2008 study published in *American Nurse Today* identified disruptive physician behavior and lack of institutional response to it

---

### BOX 5-2   WORLD HEALTH ORGANIZATION COLLABORATING CENTRE FOR PATIENT SAFETY SOLUTIONS AND SPEAK UP INITIATIVES ABOUT MEDICATIONS AND HEALTH

The World Health Organization (WHO) posts information on its website regarding initiatives to promote patient safety in medication administration and other aspects of health care. As the WHO notes, no adverse event should ever occur anywhere in the world if the knowledge exists to prevent it from happening. Knowledge is of little use, however, if it is not applied in practice. The WHO Collaborating Centre for Patient Safety Solutions has developed patient safety initiatives that can serve as a guide in redesigning the patient care process to prevent the inevitable errors from ever reaching patients. Patient safety solutions are defined by the WHO as any system design feature or intervention that has demonstrated the ability to prevent or mitigate patient harm arising from the health care process. Information about the first group of patient safety solutions (2008/2009) approved by the WHO center is available at http://www.ccforpatient safety.org. These patient safety concerns include avoiding confusion of medications with look-alike, sound-alike names; ensuring correct patient identification; enhancing communication during patient "hand-overs" between care units or care teams; ensuring performance of the correct procedure at the correct body site; maintaining control of concentrated electrolyte solutions; ensuring medication accuracy at transition points in care; avoiding catheter and tubing misconnections; and promoting single use of injection devices and improved hand hygiene to prevent health care–associated infections.

More information about patient safety and safety initiatives is also provided in a national campaign supported by The Joint Commission and the Centers for Medicare and Medicaid. These initiatives encourage patients to take a role in preventing health care errors by becoming more active, involved, and informed regarding all aspects of their health care. The *Speak Up* campaign features various brochures, posters, and buttons addressing a variety of patient safety issues and encourages the public to do the following: **S**peak up if you have any questions. **P**ay attention to your health care, and make sure that any treatments or medications are appropriate and are ordered by the proper health care professionals. **E**ducate yourself about medical diagnoses and be informed. **A**sk a family member or friend you trust to be your advocate. **K**now the medications you take and the reason for taking them. **U**se a hospital, ambulatory, or urgent care center or other type of health care facility. **P**articipate in all decisions about your treatment because you are the very center and heart of the health care team. The success of the Speak Up initiatives is well documented in the results of a 2005 survey of more than 600 accredited health care organizations, of which approximately 81% reported that campaigns like Speak Up bring more value to the accreditation process and 82% would like to see The Joint Commission sponsor more patient education programs in the future. Some 91% of these 600 organizations viewed the initiatives and program as excellent, very good, or good. For more information on the use of Speak Up and to look at the materials available, visit http://www.jointcommission.org/speakup.aspx; or contact Joint Commission Resources at 877-223-6866 or visit http://www.jcrinc.com/. Other sources of information are listed at http://www.ccforpatientsafety.org.

*Use of Abbreviations*

Medication errors often occur as a result of misinterpretation of abbreviations. Therefore, the National Coordinating Council for Medication Error Reporting and Prevention recommends that the following abbreviations be written out in full and the abbreviations avoided. The U.S. Pharmacopeia and Institute of Safe Medication Practices endorse the avoidance of abbreviations whenever possible. Most hospitals and nursing care units are adopting this significant change in documentation. NOTE: It is the philosophy of the authors of this textbook to avoid abbreviations whenever possible.

| ABBREVIATION | INTENDED MEANING | COMMON ERROR |
| --- | --- | --- |
| U | Units | Mistaken for a zero (0), a four (4), or cc. |
| mcg (μg) | Micrograms | Mistaken for mg (milligrams). |
| Q.D. | Latin abbreviation for "every day" | The period after the "Q" can be mistaken for an "I" so that a medication is given "QID" (four times daily) instead of once daily. |
| Q.O.D. | Latin abbreviation for "every other day" | Misinterpreted as "QD" (daily) or QID. If "O" is poorly written it may look like a period or "I." |
| D/C | Discharge or discontinue | Medications have been prematurely discontinued when D/C (intended to mean "discharge") was misinterpreted as "discontinue" because it was followed by a list of drugs. Use the word "Stop." |
| HS | Half strength | Misinterpreted as the Latin abbreviation "HS" (hour of sleep). |
| cc | Cubic centimeters | Mistaken for "U" (units) when written poorly. |
| AU, AS, AD | Both ears, left ear, right ear | Misinterpreted as the Latin abbreviation "OU" (both eyes), "OS" (left eye), "OD" (right eye). Also, some people forget which is right or left, or both, and which is eye or ear. |

as significant factors affecting nurse job satisfaction and nursing staff retention. Ninety-six percent of the nurses surveyed said they had witnessed or experienced disruptive behavior by a physician. Other literature shows that nurses are the primary victims of disruptive behavior and that this behavior may not only undermine patient care but also lead to staff dissatisfaction and turnover. In response to this increasing problem, The Joint Commission requires hospitals to establish procedures for managing disruptive behavior by physicians and others who are granted clinical privileges. Disruptive behavior, as defined by the American Medical Association (AMA), is personal verbal or physical conduct that affects or potentially may affect patient care in a negative fashion. These behaviors are classified into four types by the AMA: (1) intimidation and violence, (2) inappropriate language or comments, (3) sexual harassment, and (4) inappropriate responses to patient needs or staff requests.

Fortunately, communication between prescribers and other members of the health care team has improved somewhat over the years with newer generations of prescribers. This is due in large part to more progressive approaches in medical education that emphasize a team orientation. Such approaches recognize the ever-increasing complexities of health care delivery and the reality that no one team member can know every fact and provide for all patient care needs.

## PREVENTING, RESPONDING TO, REPORTING, AND DOCUMENTING MEDICATION ERRORS: A NURSING PERSPECTIVE

### Preventing Medication Errors

Medication errors are considered to be any preventable event that could lead to inappropriate medication use or harm. The major categories of medication error are defined by the 2005 National Coordinating Council for Medication Error Reporting and Prevention as (1) no error, although circumstances or events occurred that could have led to an error, (2) medication error that causes no harm, (3) medication error that causes harm, and (4) medication error that results in death. Medication errors may be prevented through a variety of strategies, including: (1) Multiple systems of checks and balances should be implemented to prevent medication errors. (2) Prescribers should write legible orders that contain correct information, or orders should be written electronically if the technology is available. (3) Authoritative resources, such as pharmacists or current drug literature, should be consulted if there is any area of concern, beginning with the medication order and continuing throughout the entire medication administration process. (4) Nurses should always check the medication order three times before giving the drug and consult with authoritative resources (see earlier in the chapter) if any questions or concerns exist. Faculty members should not be the student's research source regarding medications, and the safe practice of using appropriate resources should begin early in the educational process. (5) The Six Rights of medication administration should be used consistently, which has been shown to substantially reduce the likelihood of a medication error. See the Safety and Quality Improvement: Preventing Medication Errors box on p. 69 for a more concise and detailed listing of ways to help prevent medication errors. See the Patient-Centered Care: Lifespan Considerations for the Pediatric Patient box on p. 69 for a discussion of medication errors in pediatric patients and special considerations for this age group.

### Responding to, Reporting, and Documenting Medication Errors

Responding to and reporting medication errors are part of the professional responsibilities for which the nurse is accountable. If a medication error does occur, it must be reported, regardless

## ⚡ SAFETY AND QUALITY IMPROVEMENT: PREVENTING MEDICATION ERRORS

### How to Prevent Medication Errors

- As the first step to defend against errors, assess information about drug allergies, vital signs, and laboratory test results.
- Use two patient identifiers before giving medications.
- Never give medications that you have not drawn up or prepared yourself.
- Minimize the use of verbal and telephone orders. If used, be sure to repeat the order to confirm with the prescriber. Speak slowly and clearly, and spell the drug name aloud.
- List the reason for use of each drug on the medication administration record and any educational materials.
- Avoid abbreviations, medical shorthand, and acronyms because they can lead to confusion, miscommunication, and risk of error (see the Teamwork and Collaboration: Legal and Ethical Principles box on p. 68.).
- Never assume anything about any drug order or prescription, including route. If a medication order is questioned for any reason (e.g., dose, drug, indication), never assume that the prescriber is correct. Always be the patient's advocate and investigate the matter until all ambiguities are resolved.
- Do not try to decipher illegibly written orders; instead, contact the prescriber for clarification. Illegible orders fall below applicable standards for quality medical care and endanger patient safety. If in doubt about any part of an order, always check with the prescriber. Compare the medication order against what is on hand by checking for the Right Drug, Right Dose, Right Time, Right Patient, and Right Route.
- Never use trailing zeros (e.g., 1.0 mg) in writing and/or transcribing medication orders. Use of trailing zeros is associated with increased occurrence of overdose. For example, "1.0 mg warfarin sodium" could be misread as "10 mg warfarin," a tenfold dose increase. Instead, use "1 mg" or even "one mg."
- Failure to use leading zeros can also lead to overdose. For example, .25 mg digoxin could be misread as 25 mg digoxin, a dose that is 100 times the dose ordered. Instead, write "0.25 mg."
- Carefully read all labels for accuracy, expiration dates, dilution requirements, and warnings (e.g., black box warnings).
- Remain current with new techniques of administration and new equipment.
- Encourage the use of generic names to avoid medication errors due to many sound-alike trade names.
- Listen to and honor any concerns expressed by patients. If the patient voices a concern about being allergic to a medication or states that a pill has already been taken or that the medication is not what he or she usually takes—then STOP, listen, and investigate.
- Strive to maintain your own health to remain alert, and never be too busy to stop, learn, and inquire. In addition, engage in ongoing continuing education.
- Become a member of professional nursing organizations to network with other nursing students or professional nurses to advocate for improved working conditions and to stand up for the rights of nurses and patients.
- Know where to find the latest information on which dosage forms can or should not be crushed or opened (e.g., capsules), and educate patients accordingly.
- Safeguard any medications that the patient had on admission or transfer so that additional doses are not given or taken by mistake. In such situations, safeguarding is accomplished by compiling a current medication history and resolving any discrepancies rather than ignoring them.
- Always verify new medication administration records if they have been rewritten or reentered for any reason, and follow policies and procedures about this action.
- Make sure the weight of the patient is always recorded before carrying out a medication order to help decrease dosage errors.
- Provide for mandatory recalculation of every drug dosage for high-risk drugs (e.g., highly toxic drugs) or high-risk patients (e.g., pediatric or elderly patients) because there is a narrow margin between therapeutic serum drug levels and toxic levels (e.g., for chemotherapeutic or digitalis drugs, or in the presence of altered liver or kidney function in a patient).
- Always suspect an error whenever an adult dosage form is dispensed for a pediatric patient.
- Seek translators when appropriate—never guess what patients are trying to say.
- Educate patients to take an active role in medication error prevention, both in the hospital setting and at home.
- Involve yourself politically in advocating for legislation that improves patient safety.

## PATIENT-CENTERED CARE: LIFESPAN CONSIDERATIONS FOR THE PEDIATRIC PATIENT

### Medication Errors

Of all the ways a pediatric patient may be harmed during medical treatment, medication errors are the most common. As with elderly patients, when medication errors occur, there is a higher risk of death. The findings of several studies indicate that medication errors involving inpatient pediatric patients occur at a rate of 4.5 to 5.7 errors per 100 drugs used. The most common medication errors in pediatrics are dosing errors. Research has begun to identify some of the groups of pediatric patients who are at highest risk of medication errors. These include the following patients: (1) those younger than 2 years of age, (2) those in intensive care units (ICUs), specifically the neonatal ICU, (3) those in the emergency department between the hours of 4 AM and 8 AM or on the weekend and who are seriously ill, (4) those receiving intravenous and/or chemotherapeutic drugs, and (5) those whose weight has not been determined or recorded. Mathematical dosage calculations for pediatric patients are also problematic. In determination of the correct dosage once the drug has been ordered, the problems of most concern include the following: (1) inability of the nurse to understand/perform the correct calculation or dilution, (2) infrequent use of calculations, and (3) decimal point misplacement, with potential overdosing or underdosing.

The following are some of the actions that can be taken to prevent pediatric medication errors:
- Report all medication errors, because this information is part of the practice of professional nursing and helps in identifying causes of medication error.

- Know the drug thoroughly, including its on- and off-label uses, action, adverse effects, dosage ranges, routes of administration, high-alert drug status cautions (see Box 5-1), and contraindications (e.g., Is it recommended for use in pediatric patients?).
- Confirm information about the patient each and every time a dose is given, and check three times before giving the drug by comparing the drug order with the patient's medication profile and verifying for the Right Drug, Right Dose, Right Time, Right Route, and Right Patient.
- Double-check and verify information in handwritten orders that may be incomplete, unclear, or illegible.
- Avoid verbal telephone orders in general. When they are unavoidable, always repeat them back to the prescriber over the telephone. Insist that the prescriber sign off any emergency in-person verbal orders before leaving the unit.
- Avoid distractions while giving medications.
- Communicate with everyone (e.g., parent, caregiver) involved in patient care.
- Make sure all orders are clear and understood with shift changes.
- Use authoritative resources such as drug handbooks, *Physicians' Desk Reference*, or information from the Food and Drug Administration website (http://www.fda.gov). For off-label use of drugs, see http://www.fda.gov/Drugs/ResourcesForYou/Consumers/ucm143565.htm.

of whether the error was made by a nursing student or a professional nurse. Follow facility policies and procedures for reporting and documenting the error closely and cautiously. Once the patient has been assessed and urgent safety issues have been addressed, report the error immediately to the appropriate prescriber and nursing management personnel, for example, the nurse manager or supervisor. If the patient cannot be left alone due to deterioration of the patient's condition or the need for close monitoring after the medication error, a fellow nurse or other qualified health care professional should remain with the patient and provide appropriate care while the prescriber is contacted. Follow-up procedures or tests may be ordered or an antidote prescribed. These orders should be implemented as indicated by the prescriber. Remember that the nurse's highest priority at all times during the medication administration process and during a medication error is the patient's physiologic status and safety.

When a medication error has occurred, complete all appropriate forms—including an incident report—as per the facility's policies and procedures, and provide appropriate documentation. Document the medication error, however, by providing only factual information about the error. Documentation should always be accurate, thorough, and objective. Avoid using judgmental words such as *error* in the documentation. Instead, chart factual information such as the medication that was administered, the actual dose given, and other details regarding the order (e.g., wrong patient, wrong route, and/or wrong time). Also note any observed changes in the patient's physical and mental status. In addition, document the fact that the prescriber was notified and any follow-up actions or orders that were implemented. Patient monitoring should be ongoing.

Most facilities require additional documentation when a medication error occurs consisting of an incident report or unusual occurrence report. Always follow facility policies and procedures or protocols in completing an incident report. Documentation should include only factual information about the error as well as all corrective actions taken. Complete any additional sections of the form to help with the investigation of the incident. Because these forms are forwarded to the facility's risk management department, this complete and factual information may help prevent errors in the future. Do not document on the patient's chart that an incident report was filled out, and a copy of the incident report should not be kept. Incident reports are not to be placed in the patient's chart. The reporting of actual and suspected medication errors should offer the option of anonymity. This may help to foster improved error reporting and safe medication practices. Internal, facility-based systems of error tracking may generate data to help customize policy and procedure development. All institutional pharmacy departments are required to have an adverse drug event monitoring program.

Nurses as well as health care facilities may also be involved in external reporting of medication errors. There are nationwide confidential reporting programs that collect and disseminate safety information on a larger scale. One such program is the U.S. Pharmacopeia Medication Errors Reporting Program (USPMERP). The U.S. Pharmacopeia (USP) has created a nationwide database of medication errors and their causes,

as well as potential errors. Any health care professional can report an error by contacting the USPMERP at 800-23-ERROR. Many important institutional changes have been made based on the data collected by this program. MedWatch is another useful error and adverse event reporting program provided by the FDA. Any member of the public can report problems with medications or medical devices via telephone or mail, or online at the FDA website. The Institute for Safe Medication Practices and the Joint Commission also provide useful information and reporting services to health care providers aimed at safety enhancement.

---

**CASE STUDY**

### *Preventing Medication Errors*

During your busy clinical day as a student nurse, the staff nurse assigned to your patient comes to you and says, "Would you like to give this injection? We have a 'now' order for Sandostatin (octreotide) 200 mcg subcutaneously. I've already drawn it up; 200 mcg equals 2 mL. It needs to be given as soon as possible, so I drew it up to save time." She hands you a syringe that has 2 mL of a clear fluid in it and the patient's medication administration record (MAR).

1. Should you give this medication "now," as ordered? Why or why not?

You decide to check the order that is handwritten on the MAR with the order written on the chart. The physician wrote, "Octreotide, 200 mcg now, subcutaneously, then 100 mcg every 8 hours as needed." Before you have a chance to find your instructor, the nurse returns and says, "Your instructor probably won't let you give the injection unless you can show the medication ampules. Here are the ampules I used to draw up the octreotide. Be quick—your patient needs it now!"

You take the order, the MAR, the two ampules, and the syringe to your instructor. Together you read the order and then check the ampules. Each ampule is marked "Sandostatin (octreotide) 500 mcg/mL."

2. If the nurse drew up 2 mL from these two ampules, how much octreotide is in the syringe? How does this amount compare with the amount on the order?

The nurse is astonished when you point out that the ampules read "500 mcg/mL." She goes into the automated medication dispenser and sees two identical boxes of Sandostatin next to each other in the refrigerated section. One box is labeled "100 mcg/mL," and the other box is labeled "500 mcg/mL." She then realizes that she chose ampules of the wrong strength of drug and drew up an incorrect dose.

3. What would have happened if you had given the injection?

4. What needs to be done at this point? What contributed to this potential medication error, and how can it be prevented in the future?

For answers, see http://evolve.elsevier.com/Lilley.

## Performing Medication Reconciliation

Medication reconciliation is a process in which medications are "reconciled" at all points of entry and exit to/from a health care entity. Medication reconciliation requires patients to provide a list of all the medications they are currently taking (including herbals and over-the-counter drugs). The prescriber is then to assess those medications and decide if they are to be continued upon hospitalization. Medication reconciliation was designed to ensure that there are no discrepancies between what the patient was taking at home and in the hospital. Medication reconciliation is to occur at entry into the facility, upon transfer from surgery, or into or out of the intensive care unit and at discharge.

Although this seems to be an easy process, numerous problems have been encountered since its inception in 2005. The first problem is that many times patients do not know exactly what medications they are taking and may report that they take a "blue pill for blood pressure." Sometimes the patient may have a list of medications but some of the medications were discontinued prior to admission, and they oftentimes fail to provide this vital piece of information. This can lead to the prescriber continuing a medicine based on faulty information. This particular problem has grown because many hospitals now use hospitalists (physicians that only take care of the patient in the hospital), and the primary care provider who has the most accurate list of medications is not involved. Hospitals throughout the country are working feverishly to figure out ways to avoid the problems described. This is an ongoing process. The Joint Commission has made medication reconciliation a National Patient Safety Goal since 2006; however, due to the problems encountered it has now scaled back its requirements (available at http://www.jointcommission.org/standards_infor mation/npsgs.aspx).

Medication reconciliation involves three steps (additional information can be found on either of the websites mentioned earlier in the chapter):

1. Verification—Collection of the patient's medication information with a focus on medications currently used (including prescription drugs as well as over-the-counter medications and supplements)
2. Clarification—Professional review of this information to ensure that medications and dosages are appropriate for the patient
3. Reconciliation—Further investigation of any discrepancies and documentation of relevant communications and changes in medication orders

To ensure ongoing accuracy of medication use, the steps listed need to be repeated at each stage of health care delivery:

a. Admission
b. Status change (e.g., from critical to stable). It is the role of the provider to evaluate current medications and specify in writing which medications are to be continued or discontinued with any status change, transfer, or discharge.
c. Patient transfer within or between facilities or provider teams
d. Discharge (the latest medication list should be provided to the patient to take to his or her next health care provider, or this information should be otherwise forwarded to the provider; applicable confidentiality guidelines should be followed)

Some applicable assessment and education tips regarding medication reconciliation are as follows:

1. Ask the patient open-ended questions, and gradually move to yes-no questions to help determine specific medication information. (Details are important, maybe even critical!)
2. Avoid the use of medical jargon unless it is clear that the patient understands and is comfortable with such language.
3. Prompt the patient to try to remember all applicable medications (e.g., patches, creams, eyedrops, inhalers, professional samples, injections, dietary supplements). If the patient provides a medication list, make a copy for the patient's chart.
4. Clarify unclear information to the extent possible (e.g., by talking with the home caregiver or the outpatient pharmacist who fills the patient's prescriptions, if needed).
5. Record the foregoing information in the patient's chart as the first step in the medication reconciliation process.
6. Emphasize to the patient the importance of always maintaining a current and complete medication list and bringing it to each health care encounter (e.g., as a wallet card or other list). Many patients use their own computers for this. Also encourage patients to learn the names and current dosages of their medications.

## OTHER ETHICAL ISSUES

### Notification of Patients Regarding Errors

A landmark article published in the *Journal of Clinical Outcomes Management* in 2001 recognized the obligation of institutions and health care providers to provide full disclosure to patients when errors have occurred in their care. The article not only emphasized the ethical basis for this practice but also addressed the legal implications and was a starting point for understanding the issue of notification of patients regarding medication errors. The point was made that patients who seek attorney services are often motivated primarily by a perceived imbalance in power between themselves and their health care providers and by fear of financial burden. Health care organizations can choose to proactively apologize and accept responsibility for obvious errors and even offer needed financial support (e.g., for travel expenses, temporary loss of wages). Research indicates that such actions help health care organizations to avoid litigation and potentially much larger financial settlements.

### Possible Consequences of Medication Errors for Nurses

The possible effects of medication errors on patients range from no significant effect to permanent disability and even death in the most extreme cases. However, medication errors may also affect health care professionals, including nurses and student nurses, in a number of ways. An error that involves significant patient harm or death may take an extreme emotional toll on the nurse involved in the error. Nurses may be named as defendants in malpractice litigation, with possibly serious financial consequences. Many nurses choose to carry personal malpractice insurance for this reason, although nurses working in institutional settings are usually covered by the institution's liability insurance policy. Nurses should obtain clear written documentation of any institutional coverage provided before deciding whether to carry individual malpractice insurance.

Administrative responses to medication errors vary from institution to institution and depend on the severity of the error. One possible response is a directive to the nurse involved to obtain continuing education or refresher training. Disciplinary action, including suspension or termination of employment, may also occur depending on the specific incident. However, many hospitals have implemented a nonpunitive approach to medication errors. Nurses who have violated regulations of their state's nurse practice act may also be counseled or disciplined by their state nursing board, which may suspend or permanently revoke their nursing license. Student nurses, given their lack of clinical experience, should be especially careful to avoid medication errors, as well as errors in general. When in doubt about the correct course of action, students should consult with clinical instructors or more experienced staff nurses. Nonetheless, if a student nurse realizes that he or she has committed an error, the student should notify the responsible clinical instructor immediately. The patient may require additional monitoring or medication, and the prescriber may also need to be notified. Although such events are preferably avoided, they can ultimately be useful, though stressful, learning experiences for the student nurse. However, student nurses who commit sufficiently serious errors or display a pattern of errors can expect more severe disciplinary action. This may range from a requirement for extra clinical time or repeating of a clinical course to suspension or expulsion from the nursing school program (see Educational System Issues and Their Potential Impact on Medication Errors earlier in the chapter).

## SUMMARY

The increasing complexity of nursing practice also increases the risk for medication errors. Widely recognized and common causes of error include misunderstanding of abbreviations, illegibility of prescriber handwriting, miscommunication during verbal or telephone orders, and confusing drug nomenclature. The structure of various organizational, educational, and sociologic systems involved in health care delivery may also contribute directly or indirectly to the occurrence of medication errors. Understanding these influences can help the nurse take proactive steps to improve these systems. Such actions can range from fostering improved communication with other health care team members, including students, to advocating politically for safer conditions for both patients and staff. The first priority when an error does occur is to protect the patient from further harm whenever possible. All errors should serve as red flags that warrant further reflection, detailed analysis, and future preventive actions on the part of nurses, other health care professionals, and possibly even patients themselves.

## ▌ KEY POINTS

- To prevent medication errors from misinterpretation of the prescriber's orders, avoid abbreviations. Medication errors include giving a drug to the wrong patient, confusing sound-alike and look-alike drugs, administering the wrong drug or wrong dose, giving the drug by the wrong route, and giving the drug at the wrong time.
- Measures to help prevent medication errors include being prepared and knowledgeable and taking time to always triple-check for the right patient, drug, dosage, time, and route. It is also important for nurses always to be aware of the entire medication administration process and to take a systems analysis approach to medication errors and their prevention.
- Encourage patients to ask questions about their medications and to question any concern about the drug or any component of the medication administration process.

- Encourage patients to always carry drug allergy information on their persons and to keep a current list of medications in their wallets or purses and on their refrigerators. This list should include the drug's name, reason the drug is being used, usual dosage range and dosage prescribed, expected adverse effects and possible toxicity of the drug, and the prescriber's name and contact information.
- Report medication errors. It is important to include in this documentation assessment of patient status before, during, and after the medication error, as well as specific orders carried out in response to the error.

## ▌ NCLEX® EXAMINATION REVIEW QUESTIONS

1 The nurse keeps in mind that which measure is used to reduce the risk of medication errors?
   a When questioning a drug order, keep in mind that the prescriber is correct.
   b Be careful about questioning the drug order a board-certified physician has written for a patient.
   c Always double-check the many drugs with sound-alike and look-alike names because of the high risk of error.
   d If the drug route has not been specified, use the oral route.
2 During the medication administration process, it is important that the nurse remembers which guideline?
   a When in doubt about a drug, ask a colleague about it before giving the drug.
   b Ask what the patient knows about the drug before giving it.

   c When giving a new drug, be sure to read about it after giving it.
   d If a patient expresses a concern about a drug, stop, listen, and investigate the concerns.
3 If a student nurse realizes that he or she has made a drug error, the instructor should remind the student of which concept?
   a The student bears no legal responsibility when giving medications.
   b The major legal responsibility lies with the health care institution at which the student is placed for clinical experience.
   c The major legal responsibility for drug errors lies with the faculty members.
   d Once the student has committed a medication error, his or her responsibility is to the patient and to being honest and accountable.

## NCLEX® EXAMINATION REVIEW QUESTIONS—cont'd

4 The nurse is giving medications to a newly admitted patient who is to receive nothing by mouth (NPO status) and finds an order written as follows: "Digoxin, 250 mcg stat." Which action is appropriate?
  a Give the medication immediately (stat) by mouth because the patient has no intravenous (IV) access at this time.
  b Clarify the order with the prescribing physician before giving the drug.
  c Ask the charge nurse what route the physician meant to use.
  d Start an IV line, then give the medication IV so that it will work faster, because the patient's status is NPO at this time.

5 The nurse is reviewing medication orders. Which digoxin dose is written correctly?
  a digoxin .25 mg
  b digoxin .250 mg
  c digoxin 0.250 mg
  d digoxin 0.25 mg

6 The nurse is administering medications. Examples of high-alert medications include: (Select all that apply.)
  a Insulins
  b Antibiotics
  c Opiates
  d Anticoagulants
  e Potassium chloride for injection

7 Convert 250 micrograms to milligrams. Be sure to depict the number correctly according to the guidelines for decimals and zeroes.

1. c, 2. d, 3. d, 4. b, 5. d, 6. a, c, d, e, 7. 0.25 mg

For Critical Thinking and Prioritization Questions, see http://evolve.elsevier.com/Lilley.

# 6

# Patient Education and Drug Therapy

## OBJECTIVES

When you reach the end of this chapter, you will be able to do the following:

1 Discuss the importance of patient education in the safe and efficient administration of drugs (e.g., prescription drugs, over-the-counter drugs, herbal preparations, dietary supplements).
2 Summarize the various teaching and learning principles appropriate to patient education and drug therapy across the lifespan as applicable to any health care setting.

3 Identify the impact of the various developmental phases (as described by Erikson) on patient education as it relates to drug therapy and the nursing process.
4 Develop a complete patient teaching plan as part of a comprehensive nursing care plan for drug therapy and the nursing process for the adult patient.

## KEY TERMS

**Affective domain** The most intangible domain of the learning process. It involves affective behavior, which is conduct that expresses feelings, needs, beliefs, values, and opinions; the feeling domain. (p. 75)

**Cognitive domain** The domain involved in the learning and storage of basic knowledge. It is the thinking portion of the learning process and incorporates a person's previous experiences and perceptions; the learning/thinking domain. (p. 75)

**Health literacy** The degree to which individuals have the capacity to obtain and then process and understand basic health information as well as basic health information

and services needed to make appropriate health decisions (p. 75)

**Learning** The acquisition of knowledge or skill. (p. 75)

**Psychomotor domain** The domain involved in the learning of a new procedure or skill; often called the *doing domain*. (p. 75)

**Teaching** A system of directed and deliberate actions intended to induce learning. (p. 75)

Given the constant change in today's health care climate and increased consumer awareness, the role of the nurse as an educator continues to increase and remains a significant part of patient care, both in and out of the hospital environment. Patient education is essential in any health care setting and is a critical component of quality and safe health care. Without patient education, the highest quality and safest of care cannot be provided. Patient education is also very crucial in assisting patients, family, significant others, and caregivers to adapt to illness, prevent illness, maintain health and wellness, and provide self-care. Patient education is a process, much like the nursing process; it provides patients with a framework of knowledge that assists in the learning of healthy behaviors and assimilation of these behaviors into a lifestyle.

Patient education may be one of the more satisfying aspects of nursing care because it is essential to improved health outcomes and can be easily measured. In fact, in the current era of increasing acuteness of patient conditions and the need to decrease length of stays in hospitals, patient education and family teaching become even more essential to effectively and efficiently meet outcome criteria. Patient education has also been identified as a valued and satisfying activity for the professional nurse. Additionally, patient education is a qualifier found in professional and accreditation standards. Health teaching is not only included in the American Nurses Association document *Nursing: Scope and Standards of Practice* (2004) but is also one of the grading criteria used by The Joint Commission (2011), which was formerly known as the Joint Commission on Accreditation of Healthcare Organizations (JCAHO). Visit http://www.thejointcommission.org for more information on accreditation, certification, standards, measurement, and related topics.

Contributing to the effectiveness of patient education is an understanding of and attention to the three domains of learning: the cognitive, affective, and psychomotor domains. It is recommended that one or a combination of these domains be addressed in any patient educational session. The cognitive domain refers to the level at which basic knowledge is learned and stored. It is the thinking portion of the learning process and incorporates a person's previous experiences and perceptions. Previous experiences with health and wellness influence the learning of new materials, and prior knowledge and experience can serve as the foundation for adding new concepts. Thus, the learning process begins with the identification of what experiences the person has had with the subject matter or content. However, it is important to remember that thinking involves more than the delivery of new information because a patient must build relationships between prior and new experiences to formulate new meanings. At a higher level in the thinking process, the new information is used to question something that is uncertain, to recognize when to seek additional information, and to make decisions during real-life situations.

The affective domain is the most intangible component of the learning process. Affective behavior is conduct that expresses feelings, needs, beliefs, values, and opinions. It is well known that individuals view events from different perspectives and often choose to internalize feelings rather than express them. You must be willing to approach patients in a nonjudgmental manner, listen to their concerns, recognize the nonverbal messages being given, and assess patient needs with an open mind. If you are successful in gaining the trust and confidence of patients and family members, it may have a powerful effect on their attitudes and thus on the learning process.

The psychomotor domain involves the learning of a new procedure or skill and is often called the *doing domain*. Learning is generally accomplished by demonstration of the procedure or task using a step-by-step approach with return demonstrations by the learner to verify whether the procedure or skill has been mastered. Using a teaching approach that engages these domains—whether one, two, or a combination of all three—will certainly add to the quality and effectiveness of patient education sessions and subsequent learning.

The result of effective patient education is learning. Learning is defined as a change in behavior, and teaching as a sharing of knowledge. Although you may never be certain that patients will take medications as prescribed, you may carefully assess, plan, implement, and evaluate the teaching you provide to help maximize outcome criteria. Just like the nursing process, the medication administration process and the teaching-learning process provide systematic frameworks for professional nursing practice. The remainder of this chapter provides a brief look at patient education as related to the nursing process and drug therapy.

## ASSESSMENT OF LEARNING NEEDS RELATED TO DRUG THERAPY

As previously mentioned, the patient education process is similar to the nursing process. A very important facet of the patient education process, like the nursing process, is a thorough assessment of learning needs. Complete this assessment before patients begin any form of drug therapy. As related to patient education and drug therapy, assessment includes gathering subjective and objective data about the following:

- Adaptation to any illnesses
- Age
- Barriers to learning (Box 6-1)
- Cognitive abilities
- Coping mechanisms
- Cultural background
- Developmental status for age group with attention to cognitive and mental processing abilities
- Education received including highest grade level completed and literacy level
- Emotional status
- Environment at home and at work
- Folk medicine, home remedies, or use of alternative/complementary therapies (e.g., physical therapy, chiropractic therapy, osteopathic medicine, meditation, yoga, aromatherapy)
- Family relationships
- Financial status
- Health literacy (Box 6-2)
- Psychosocial growth and development level according to Erikson's stages (Box 6-3)
- Health beliefs, including beliefs about health, wellness, and/or illness

## BOX 6-1   STRATEGIES TO ENHANCE PATIENT EDUCATION AND REDUCE BARRIERS TO LEARNING

- Work with available educational resources in nursing and pharmacy to collect or order and distribute materials about drug therapy. Make sure that written materials are available to all individuals and are prepared on a reading level that is most representative of the geographical area, such as an eighth-grade reading level. Most acute care and other health care facilities have electronic resources, so that printing educational materials is easy. Some examples of electronic or computerized programs are Micromedex and Lexi-PALS; these offer patient pamphlets that are in different languages and at appropriate reading levels.

- Be sure that written and verbal instructions are available in the language most commonly spoken, such as Spanish. Identify resources within the facility and in the community that can provide assistance with translation, such as nurses or other health care providers who are proficient in Spanish and other languages. Have the information available so that education is carried out in a timely and effective manner.

- Perform a cultural assessment that includes questions about level of education, learning experiences, past and present successes of therapies and medication regimens, language spoken, core beliefs, value system, meaning of health and illness, perceived cause of illness, family roles, social organization, and health practices or lack thereof.

- Make sure that written materials are available on the most commonly used medications and that all materials are updated annually to ensure that information is current.

- Have available information for patients on how they can prevent medication errors. The Institute for Safe Medication Practices offers informative

pamphlets on the patient's role in preventing medication errors as well as web-based resources such as alerts for consumers with the proper citation.

- Work collaboratively in the health care setting, inpatient and outpatient, to develop a listing of medications that may be considered error prone, such as cardiac drugs, chemotherapeutic drugs, low–molecular-weight heparin, digoxin, metered-dose inhaled drugs, and acetaminophen. Lack of time for patient education is often a concern for nurses, but efforts should be undertaken to make materials available and to review these with patients and those involved in their care. Use all available resources, such as videotapes, verbal instructions, pictures, and other health care providers.

- For the adolescent, be sure to provide clear and simple directions for each medication, including clarification of information that may well be misinterpreted. For example, teenage girls may have the false idea that oral contraceptives prevent them from contracting sexually transmitted diseases.

- Use readability tools in the development of patient education materials if you are involved in this process. Several tools are available, such as the SMOG (Simple Measure of Gobbledygook) readability measure and the Fry readability formula. It is important to know that evidenced-based measures such as these are available to help in the creation of written materials and verbal instructions for patients. Online resources include http://www.readabilityformulas.com/smog-readability-formula.php and http://www.readabilityformulas.com/fry-graph-readability-formula.php.

- Never wait until discharge to teach patients. Include family or caregivers whenever possible, so that they become contributors to patient education and not barriers!

## BOX 6-2   A BRIEF LOOK AT HEALTH LITERACY

- In 2004, the Institute of Medicine estimated that over 90 million Americans have difficulty in not only understanding information about their own health concerns but also have difficulty acting on the information.

- As related to patient education, assessing and addressing health literacy is only one aspect, but a very important aspect, of health communication and the cognitive domain of learning.

- If there is health illiteracy, studies have shown that issues of noncompliance to treatment regimens and disease complications as well as difficulty accessing health care are problematic, contributing to poor health as well as higher health care costs.

- Health illiteracy has been associated with less education, lower socioeconomic status, decrease in sensorial abilities, and multiple disease processes, so assessment of these factors is important to individualized patient education.

- Other areas to assess related to health literacy include reading level, ability to follow directions/instructions, as well as ability to manage everyday living activities such as self-care, grocery shopping, and meal preparation.

- Assessment of health literacy may be done with much sensitivity and does not only relate to education but also to levels of stress/inability to cope with a new diagnosis/process new and complex information (i.e., patients with higher level of education but are stressed and unable to process due to a disturbing diagnosis).

## BOX 6-3   ERIKSON'S STAGES OF DEVELOPMENT

**Infancy (birth to 1 year of age):** Trust versus mistrust. Infant learns to trust himself or herself, others, and the environment; learns to love and be loved.

**Toddlerhood (1 to 3 years of age):** Autonomy versus shame and doubt. Toddler learns independence; learns to master the physical environment and maintain self-esteem.

**Preschool age (3 to 6 years of age):** Initiative versus guilt. Preschooler learns basic problem solving; develops conscience and sexual identity; initiates activities as well as imitates.

**School age (6 to 12 years of age):** Industry versus inferiority. School-age child learns to do things well; develops a sense of self-worth.

**Adolescence (12 to 18 years of age):** Identity versus role confusion. Adolescent integrates many roles into self-identity through imitation of role models and peer pressure.

**Young adulthood (18 to 45 years of age):** Intimacy versus isolation. Young adult establishes deep and lasting relationships; learns to make commitment as a spouse, parent, and/or partner.

**Middle adulthood (45 to 65 years of age):** Generativity versus stagnation. Adult learns commitment to the community and world; is productive in career, family, and civic interests.

**Older adulthood (over 65 years of age):** Integrity versus despair. Older adult appreciates life role and status; deals with loss and prepares for death.

- Information the patient understands about past and present medical conditions, medical therapy, and medications
- Language(s) spoken
- Level of knowledge about any medication(s) being taken
- Limitations (physical, psychological, cognitive, and motor)
- Medications currently taken (including over-the-counter drugs, prescription drugs, and herbal products)
- Misinformation about drug therapy
- Mobility and motor skills
- Motivation
- Nutritional status
- Past and present health behaviors
- Past and present experience with drug regimens and other forms of therapy, including levels of compliance
- Race and/or ethnicity
- Readiness to learn
- Religion or religious beliefs
- Self-care ability
- Sensory status
- Social support

During the assessment of learning needs, be astutely aware of the patient's verbal and nonverbal communication. Often a patient will not tell you how he or she truly feels. A seeming discrepancy is an indication that the patient's emotional or physical state may need to be further assessed in relation to his or her actual readiness and motivation for learning. Use of open-ended questions is encouraged, because they stimulate more discussion and greater clarification from the patient than closed-ended questions that require only a "yes" or "no" answer. Assess level of anxiety, because mild levels of anxiety have been identified as being motivating, whereas moderate to severe levels may be obstacles. In addition, if there are physical needs that are not being met, such as relief from pain, vomiting, or other physical distress, these needs become obstacles to learning. These physical issues must be managed appropriately before any patient teaching occurs.

## NURSING DIAGNOSES RELATED TO LEARNING NEEDS AND DRUG THERAPY

Some of the most commonly used and currently approved NANDA-I (2012-2014) nursing diagnoses related to patient education and drug therapy are as follows (see Chapter 1 for a more complete listing):

- Deficient knowledge
- Falls, risk for
- Ineffective self-health management
- Readiness for enhanced self-health management
- Impaired memory
- Injury, risk for
- Noncompliance
- Sleep deprivation

As an example of how nursing diagnoses related to patient education are derived, the nursing diagnosis of *deficient knowledge* refers to a situation in which the patient, caregiver, or significant other has a limited knowledge base or skills with regard to the medication or medication regimen. A nursing diagnosis of *deficient knowledge* develops out of objective and/or subjective data showing that there is limited understanding, no understanding, or misunderstanding of the medication and its action, indications, adverse reactions, toxic effects, drug-drug and/or drug-food interactions, cautions, and contraindications. This diagnosis may also reflect decreased cognitive ability or impaired motor skill needed to perform self-medication. Deficient knowledge differs from noncompliance in that the latter occurs when the patient does not take the medication as prescribed or at all; in other words, the patient does not comply with or adhere to the instructions given about the medication. Noncompliance is usually a patient's choice. A nursing diagnosis of *noncompliance* is made when data collected from the patient show that the condition or symptoms for which the patient is taking the medication have recurred or were never resolved because the patient did not take the medication per the prescriber's orders or did not take the medication at all. Although noncompliance is usually a patient decision, other factors need to be assessed to determine the cause of the noncompliance (e.g., lack of ability of the parent, family, or caregiver to administer the medication; other physical, emotional, or socioeconomic factors). These factors are associated with the nursing diagnosis of ineffective health maintenance and provide a patient-centered approach to the plan of care.

## PLANNING RELATED TO LEARNING NEEDS AND DRUG THERAPY

The planning phase of the teaching-learning process occurs as soon as a learning need has been assessed and then identified in the patient, family, or caregiver. With mutual understanding, the nurse and patient identify goals and outcome criteria that are associated with the identified nursing diagnosis and are able to relate them to the specific medication the patient is taking. The following is an example of a measurable goal with outcome criterion related to a nursing diagnosis of *deficient knowledge* for a patient who is self-administering an oral antidiabetic drug and has many questions about the medication therapy. *Sample goal:* The patient safely self-administers the prescribed oral antidiabetic drug within a given time frame. *Sample outcome criterion:* The patient remains without signs and symptoms of overmedication while taking an oral antidiabetic drug, such as hypoglycemia with tachycardia, palpitations, diaphoresis, hunger, and fatigue. When drug therapy goals and outcome criteria are developed, appropriate time frames for meeting outcome criteria must be identified (see Chapter 1 for more information on the nursing process). In addition, goals and outcome criteria need to be realistic, based on patient needs, stated in patient terms, and include behaviors that are measurable, such as *list, identify, demonstrate, self-administer, state, describe,* and *discuss.*

## IMPLEMENTATION RELATED TO PATIENT EDUCATION AND DRUG THERAPY

After you have completed the assessment phase, identified nursing diagnoses, and created a plan of care, the implementation phase of the teaching-learning process begins. This phase includes conveying specific information about the medication

## EVIDENCE-BASED PRACTICE

### Building a Collaborative Nursing Practice to Promote Patient Education: An Inpatient and Outpatient Partnership

#### Review

This study took place in a large medical facility with an oncology nursing staff, located in the Midwestern region of the United States. The study looked at the communication among nurses as related to patient education to those with cancer. Specifically, the nurses were interested in looking at the lack of consistency in formal patient education between the inpatient and outpatient settings.

#### Type of Evidence

Initially a team was formed to help in identifying and then implementing potential solutions for improving communication about specialty-specific patient education. This team consisted of clinical nurse specialist in hematology/oncology/blood marrow transplantation (BMT), a nursing education specialist, and three nurse educators representing the facility's Cancer Education Center. The Cancer Education Center is responsible for an outpatient educational program with the mission of meeting educational needs of patients with cancer across the continuum of care. A thorough literature search was completed only to find out that there was minimal information written about nurse-to-nurse communication. The team then developed a pilot project to assist them in evaluating the effects of collaborative efforts in promoting patient education between inpatient and outpatient areas. Goals and objectives were identified and were twofold: (1) to build a collaborative nursing practice between their inpatient and outpatient practice settings, and (2) to provide an opportunity to increase the effectiveness of inpatient hematology/oncology and BMT nurses' professional development. A call for applications was sent out the staff of the hematology/oncology/BMT units with a total of 13 applicants. Five applicants were selected for formal interviews inclusive of the project team members and inpatient nurses. After orientation to the process and project, the participants began their work in the outpatient Cancer Education Center with an average patient population of about 140. A four-level evaluation model (see original journal article for more specific information) was used to help analyze the value of the pilot project.

#### Results of Study

Using an anonymous format, all of the information collected from interviews and surveys were analyzed for content themes. The five themes identified, after validation with nursing leadership and project participants, included increased awareness and application of knowledge, professional development, collaboration, the importance of continued collaboration, and the impact on nursing practice. The results showed a positive impact on all five themes despite the fact that each staff nurse worked only six times in the Cancer Education Center. Numerous patient responses reflected a feeling of increased comfort with the inpatient-to-outpatient transition process. For the nurse participants and other nurses in the setting, there was an increase in sharing of knowledge and experiences. Additionally, several barriers to collaboration occurred, which spurred the need for being prepared for such barriers. These potential barriers included barrier for project funding, level of participant motivation, length of time needed for acclimation to the project's setting (took longer!), and the need for more educational opportunities with specific strategies for how to best work with patients and families seeking out education in the outpatient versus inpatient setting.

#### Link of Evidence to Nursing Practice

There were several important findings from this study as discussed above; however, the need to foster and build strong networking and collaborative relationships among staff nurses in a continuum of settings is crucial to job satisfaction and more importantly, to the effectiveness of meeting patient education needs in cancer patients who are frequently moving from inpatient to outpatient settings. In addition, the educational needs of these patients continually change, requiring even more specific educational programs and nurses prepared for these programs. This study also found that as the nurse participant's knowledge increased, the patient benefited greatly, which is applicable to any type of patient care. It is well documented in the literature that as nurses expand their knowledge about the system and aspects of nursing care, the benefit to the patient is enhanced as noted in the depth of interactions and the level of care provided. The collaborative partnership between nurses and their patients regardless of setting is challenging, but nurses need to continue to discover opportunities to foster their education, experience, and collaborative relationships among the care continuum. In summary, this study had very positive results from the pilot evaluation and led to a shared communication and staffing model. The collaborative program in this study continues to be offered through a formal staff development program called Nursing Perspectives.

Reference: Negley DF, Ness S, Fee-Schroeder K, et al: Building a collaborative nursing practice to promote patient education: an inpatient and outpatient partnership, *Oncol Nurs Forum* 36(1):19-23, 2009.

to the patient, family, or caregiver. Teaching-learning sessions must incorporate clear, simple, concise written instructions (Box 6-4); oral instructions; and written pamphlets, pictures, videos, or any other learning aids that will help ensure patient learning. You may have to conduct several brief teaching-learning sessions with multiple strategies, depending on the needs of the patient. Several changes related to the growth and aging of patients affect teaching-learning, and Table 6-1 lists educational strategies for accommodating these changes in a plan of care. You may also need to identify aids to help the patient in the safe administration of medications at home, such as the use of medication day or time calendars, pill reminder stickers, daily medication containers with alarms, weekly pill containers with separate compartments for different dosing times for each day for the week, and/or a method of documenting doses taken to avoid overdosage or omission of doses.

Special issues arise when the patient speaks limited or no English. Communicate with the patient in the patient's native language, if at all possible. If you are not able to speak the patient's native language, a translator needs to be made available to prevent communication problems, minimize errors, and help boost the patient's level of trust and understanding. In practice, this translator may be another nurse or health care professional; a nonprofessional member of the health care team; or a layperson, family member, adult friend, or religious leader or associate. However, it is best to avoid using family members as translators if possible because of issues with bias and misinterpretation, as well as potential confidentiality issues. It is important to remember that some of these individuals may not be competent in or comfortable with communicating technical clinical information, and other resources must be used if this is the case. As the United States experiences

## BOX 6-4    GENERAL TEACHING AND LEARNING PRINCIPLES

- Make learning patient-centered and individualized to each patient's needs, including his or her learning needs. This includes assessment of the patient's cultural beliefs, educational level, previous experience with medications, level of growth and development (to best select a teaching-learning strategy), age, gender, family support system, resources, preferred learning style, and level of sophistication with health care and health care treatment.
- Assess the patient's motivation and readiness to learn.
- Assess the patient's ability to use and interpret label information on medication containers.
- Some studies have shown that as much as 20% of the U.S. population is functionally illiterate. Therefore, ensure that educational strategies and materials are at a level that the patient is able to understand, while taking care to not embarrass the patient.
- If a patient is illiterate, he or she still needs to be instructed on safe medication administration. Use pictures, demonstrations, and return demonstrations to emphasize instructions.
- Consider, assess, and appreciate language and ethnicity during patient teaching. Make every effort to educate non–English-speaking patients in their native language. Ideally the patient needs to be instructed by a health professional familiar with the patient's clinical situation who also speaks the patient's native language. At the very least, provide the patient detailed written instructions in his or her native language.
- Assess the family support system for adequate patient teaching. Family living arrangements, financial status, resources, communication patterns, the roles of family members, and the power and authority of different family members must always be considered.
- Make the teaching-learning session simple, easy, fun, thorough, effective, and not monotonous. Make it applicable to daily life, and schedule it at a time when the patient is ready to learn. Avoid providing extraneous information that may be confusing or overwhelming to the patient.
- Remember that learning occurs best with repetition and periods of demonstration and with the use of audiovisuals and other educational aids.
- Patient teaching must focus on the various processes in the cognitive, affective, and/or psychomotor domains (see earlier discussion).
- Consult online resources for help in obtaining the most up-to-date and accurate patient teaching materials and information.

## TABLE 6-1    EDUCATIONAL STRATEGIES TO ADDRESS COMMON CHANGES RELATED TO AGING THAT MAY INFLUENCE LEARNING

| CHANGE RELATED TO AGING | EDUCATIONAL STRATEGY |
| --- | --- |
| **Cognitive and Memory Impairment** | |
| Slowed cognitive functioning | Slow the pace of the presentation, and attend to verbal and nonverbal patient cues to verify understanding. |
| Decreased short-term memory | Provide smaller amounts of information at one time. Repeat information frequently. Provide written instructions for home use. |
| Decreased ability to think abstractly | Use examples to illustrate information. Use a variety of methods, such as audiovisuals, props, videotapes, large-print materials, materials with vivid color, return demonstrations, and practice sessions. |
| Decreased ability to concentrate | Decrease external stimuli as much as possible. |
| Increased reaction time (slower to respond) | Always allow sufficient time, and be patient. Allow more time for feedback. |
| **Disturbed Sensory Perception** | |
| **_Hearing Impairment_** | |
| Diminished hearing | Perform a baseline hearing assessment. Use tone- and volume-controlled teaching aids; use bright, large-print material to reinforce. |
| Decreased ability to distinguish sounds (e.g., differentiate words beginning with *S, Z, T, D, F,* and *G*) | Speak distinctly and slowly, and articulate carefully. |
| Decreased conduction of sound | Sit on the side of the patient's best ear. |
| Loss of ability to hear high-frequency sounds | Do not shout; speak in a normal voice but a lower voice pitch. |
| Partial to complete loss of hearing | Face the patient so that lip reading is possible. Use visual aids to reinforce verbal instruction. Reinforce teaching with easy-to-read materials. Decrease extraneous noise. Use community resources for the hearing impaired. |
| **_Visual Impairment_** | |
| Decreased visual acuity | Ensure that the patient's glasses are clean and in place and that the prescription is current. |
| Decreased ability to read fine detail | Use printed materials with large print that is brightly and clearly colored. |
| Decreased ability to discriminate among blue, violet, and green; tendency for all colors to fade, with red fading the least | Use high-contrast materials, such as black on white. Avoid the use of blue, violet, and green in type or graphics; use red instead. |
| Thickening and yellowing of the lenses of the eyes, with decreased accommodation | Use nonglare lighting, and avoid contrasts of light (e.g., a darkened room with a single light). |
| Decreased depth perception | Adjust teaching to allow for the use of touch to gauge depth. |
| Decreased peripheral vision | Keep all teaching materials within the patient's visual field. |
| **_Touch and Vibration Impairment_** | |
| Decreased sense of touch | Increase the time allowed for the teaching of psychomotor skills, the number of repetitions, and the number of return demonstrations. |
| Decreased sense of vibration | Teach the patient to palpate more prominent pulse sites (e.g., carotid and radial arteries). |

Modified from Weinrich SP, Boyd M, Nussbaum J: Continuing education: adapting strategies to teach the elderly, *J Gerontol Nurs* 15(11):17-21, 1989; McKenry LM, Salerno E: *Mosby's pharmacology in nursing*, ed 22, St Louis, 2006, Mosby.
NOTE: These strategies may also be appropriate for younger patients.

rapid growth in minority populations, our health care system will see a staggering increase in the percentage of non–English-speaking patients. According to the August 2008 projections of the U.S. Census Bureau, demographic changes will be significant, with minority groups—which currently compose one-third of the U.S. population—growing to become the majority by 2042 and projected to increase to 54% of the population by 2050. This growth in cultural diversity will continue to demand that nursing and related health care professions provide patient education materials in both English and Spanish. Publications provided for non–English-speaking patients may enable you to convey a sufficient amount of information in the patient's language to help effectively educate the patient and also allow you to share materials with family members and caregivers for their use. Companies now also publish a variety of patient education materials for the discharge process in both English and Spanish.

Non–English-speaking patients tend to notice and appreciate their health professionals' efforts to speak their own language and will often help teach them new words or phrases, if there is enthusiasm and interest. This experience may lead to significantly greater rapport, put the patient at ease, and show respect for his or her culture or race/ethnicity. Obtaining and keeping available a foreign language dictionary may be helpful. Keeping notes about newly learned words, phrases, or sentences may be helpful, too. Even if the professional does not use the correct verb tenses, he or she may often communicate sufficiently with the patient for the purpose at hand. As one begins to learn a foreign language, a major challenge may be to speak with a patient over the telephone. The important goal is to try to increase one's *listening* speed to match the *speaking* speed of the patient. With effort, this *can* be accomplished. If one can grasp even a few words of what the patient is saying, one may be able, with continued conversation with the patient, to determine and respond to the patient's needs. However, be aware that patients who are native English speakers may also have problems learning about their medications and treatment regimens because of learning deficits or difficulties, hearing and speech deficits, lack of education, or minimal previous exposure to treatment regimens and medication use.

The teaching of manual skills for specific medication administration is also part of the teaching-learning session. Sufficient time must be allowed for the patient to become familiar with any equipment and to perform several return demonstrations to you or another health care provider. Teaching-learning needs will vary from patient to patient. Make every effort to include family members, significant others, or caregivers in the teaching session(s) for reinforcement purposes. Audiovisual aids may be incorporated and based on findings from the learning needs and nursing assessment. Resources for information about medications include *USP Drug Information* volume II, *Advice for the Patient,* which is published annually (along with the *Health Care Professional* volume) by Thomson Micromedex; this information is appropriate to share with the patient. This type of resource may be helpful to the patient when he or she seeks information about a medication (e.g., purpose, adverse effects, method of administration, drug interactions) and helpful to you in developing a patient teaching plan. Create a safe, nonthreatening, nondistracting environment for learning needs, and be open and receptive to the patient's questions. The following strategies may help ensure an effective teaching-learning session:

- Begin the teaching-learning process upon the patient's admission to the health care setting (see the Teamwork and Collaboration: Legal and Ethical Principles box on p. 81).
- Individualize the teaching session to the patient.
- Provide positive rewards or reinforcement after accurate return demonstration of a procedure, technique, and/or skill during the teaching session.
- Complete a medication calendar that includes the names of the drugs to be taken along with the dosage and frequency. Allow the patient to see what the medications look like for future reference.
- Use audiovisual aids.
- Involve family members or significant others in the teaching session, as deemed appropriate.
- Keep the teaching on a level that is most meaningful to the given patient; general research on reading skills has shown that written materials must be written at an eighth-grade reading level.

---

### 🌐 PATIENT-CENTERED CARE: CULTURAL IMPLICATIONS

#### *Patient Education*

Research various cultures to enhance an individualized approach to nursing care. For example, with Mexican-American patients, aspects of nursing care must be approached in a sensitive manner with strong consideration for the family, communication needs, and religion. Approximately 90% of native Mexicans are Roman Catholic. To help meet the needs of these patients more effectively, consider speaking with them about their desire for clergy visits while in the hospital. Family members are generally involved, and Mexican Americans often have large extended families; therefore, take the time to include family members in the patient's care and when providing discharge instructions and medication instructions.

Health care professionals who work in a geographic area where a variety of non-English languages are widely spoken need to make an effort to learn one or more of these languages. Adult foreign language education is available in most U.S. cities, often at 2- and 4-year colleges or universities. Many classes are designed for working professionals and are scheduled at a variety of convenient times during the day and evening to accommodate demanding work schedules. Community colleges often offer quality courses that meet as little as 1 day or evening per week. Many employers will pay for job-related courses, and some courses may qualify for professional continuing education credits. Language courses provide a means of networking and developing quality friendships with other highly motivated, empathic individuals both within and outside of the health care profession. A variety of self-study materials are also available.

---

Modified from McKenry LM, Salerno E: *Mosby's pharmacology in nursing,* ed 22, St Louis, 2006, Mosby.

## TEAMWORK AND COLLABORATION: LEGAL AND ETHICAL PRINCIPLES

### Discharge Teaching

The safest practices for discharge teaching are as follows:

- Always follow the health care facility's policy on discharge teaching with regard to how much information to impart to the patient.
- Do not assume that any patient has received adequate teaching before interacting with you.
- Always begin discharge teaching as soon as possible when the patient is ready.
- Minimize any distractions during the teaching session.
- Evaluate any teaching of the patient and/or significant others by having the individuals repeat the instructions you have given them.
- Contact the institution's social services department or the discharge planner if there are any concerns regarding the learning capacity of the patient.
- Document what you taught, who was present with the patient during the teaching, what specific written instructions were given, what the responses of the patient and significant other or caregiver were, and what your own nursing actions were, such as specific demonstrations or referrals to community resources.
- Document teaching-learning strategies used, such as videotapes and pamphlets.

Modified from U.S. Pharmacopeia Safe Medication Use Expert Committee Meeting, Rockville, MD, May 2003, available at http://www.usp.org.

Box 6-4 lists some general teaching and learning principles to consider in providing patient education.

Upon completion of any teaching-learning process or patient education session, complete the documentation and include notes about the content provided, strategies used, and patient response to the teaching session, and an overall evaluation of learning. Because of the significance of patient education related to drug therapy and the nursing process, this textbook integrates patient education into each chapter in the implementation phase of the nursing process. In addition, a Patient Teaching Tips section is included at the end of most chapters.

## EVALUATION OF PATIENT LEARNING RELATED TO DRUG THERAPY

Evaluation of patient learning is a critical component of safe and effective drug administration. To verify the success—or lack of success—of patient education, ask specific questions related to patient outcomes and request that the patient repeat information or give a return demonstration of skills, if appropriate. The patient's behavior—such as adherence to the schedule for medication administration with few or no complications—is one key to determining whether or not teaching was successful and learning occurred. If a patient's behavior is characteristic of noncompliance or an inadequate level of learning, develop, implement, and evaluate a new plan of teaching.

## CASE STUDY

### Patient Education and Anticoagulant Therapy

M.S., an 82-year-old retired librarian, has developed atrial fibrillation. As part of his medical therapy, he is started on the oral anticoagulant warfarin (Coumadin). His wife reports that he has some trouble hearing yet refuses to consider getting hearing aids. In addition, this is his first illness and his wife states that he has "always hated taking medications. He's read about herbs and folk healing and would rather try natural therapy." The nurse is planning education about oral anticoagulant therapy, and M.S. says that he'll "give it a try" for now, but he "knows nothing about this drug."

1. What will the nurse assess, including possible barriers to learning, before teaching?
2. Formulate an education-related nursing diagnosis for this patient based on the information given above. In addition, provide a goal and one example of an outcome criterion for the nursing diagnosis.
3. What education strategies will the nurse plan to use, considering any age-related changes the patient may have?

For answers, see http://evolve.elsevier.com/Lilley.

## SUMMARY

Patient education is a critical part of patient care, and patient education about medication administration, therapies, or regimens is no exception. From the time of initial contact with the patient throughout the time you work with the patient, the patient is entitled to all information about medications prescribed as well as other aspects of his or her care. Evaluation of patient learning and compliance with the medication regimen remains a continuous process; be willing to listen to the patient about any aspect of the patient's drug therapy. Professional nurses are teachers and serve as patient advocates and thus have a responsibility to facilitate learning for patients, families, significant others, and caregivers. Accurate assessment of learning needs and readiness to learn always requires a look at the whole patient, including cultural values, health practices, and literacy issues. Every effort needs to be made to see that the patient receives effective learning to ensure successful outcomes with regard to drug therapy—and all parts of the patient's health care.

It is important to consult resources mentioned earlier, as well as the U.S. Pharmacopeia (at http://www.usp.org), which serves as an advocate for patient safety and establishes standards for medications. This organization is a tremendous resource for the health care professional in obtaining information for the patient so that quality patient education can be provided. The U.S. Pharmacopeia values patient education as a means of enhancing patient safety as well as a means of decreasing medication errors in the hospital setting or at home. In addition, the Institute for Safe Medication Practices (at http://www.ismp.org) provides nurses with a wealth of information related to patient education, safety, and prevention of medication errors. As a nonprofit organization, this institute works closely with nurses, prescribers, regulatory agencies, and professional organizations to provide education about medication errors and their prevention, and is a premier resource in all matters pertaining to safe medication practices in health care organizations.

Another resource is the National Council on Patient Information and Education (NCPIE), which may be accessed at www.talkaboutrx.org. This site was developed with the purpose of stimulating and improving communication of information on the appropriate use of medications to consumers and health care professionals (Box 6-5). In summary, it is professional nurses who usually have the most contact with patients and see patients in a variety of settings. Because of this, nurses need to continue to be patient advocates and take the initiative to plan, design, create, and present educational materials for teaching about drug therapy.

---

**BOX 6-5    NATIONAL COUNCIL ON PATIENT INFORMATION AND EDUCATION (NCPIE): A BRIEF REVIEW**

- NCPIE is composed of over 125 diverse organizations with the mission to stimulate and improve communication and information on appropriate medication use.
- It is the leading authority for informing the general public and health care professionals on safe medication use through use of more effective communication leading to better health outcomes and quality of life.
- NCPIE has been involved in promoting and sharing of information among consumers, prescribers, pharmacists, and other members of the health care team for approximately 25 years.

- With some 3.5 billion prescriptions being dispensed annually, taking the drugs properly and with full knowledge is a challenge; NCPIE attempts to make communication better about these issues.
- NCPIE's website, available at *www.talkaboutrx.org*, helps consumers make sound decisions about the use of medicines. Other resources available on the NCPIE's website are Educate Before You Medicate: Knowledge Is the Best Medicine; Communicate Before You Medicate, Team Up and Talk, Mustforseniors.org.
- Some of the programs that were launched in 2002 include the "Be MedWise" campaign at www.bemedwise.org, which targeted the use of over-the-counter medications.

Data from National Council on Patient Information and Education: National Council on Patient Information and Education website, 2011, available at http://www.talkaboutrx.org. Accessed February 4, 2011.

---

## PATIENT TEACHING TIPS

- Teaching needs to focus on either the cognitive, affective, or psychomotor domain or a combination of all three. The cognitive domain may involve recall for synthesis of facts, with the affective domain involving behaviors such as responding, valuing, and organizing. The psychomotor domain includes teaching someone how to perform a procedure.
- Realistic patient teaching goals and outcome criteria must be established with the involvement of the patient, caregiver, or significant other.
- Keep patient teaching on a level that is most meaningful to the individual. Most research indicates that reading materials need to be written at an eighth-grade reading level but adjusted accordingly to patient assessment.

- Follow teaching and learning principles when developing and implementing patient education.
- Be sure to control the environmental factors, such as lighting, noise, privacy, and odors. Provide dignified care while preparing the patient for teaching, and respect personal space. If there are distractions, such as television, radio, cell phone, or computer, work with the patient/family members to safely and appropriately quiet these items during teaching sessions.
- Make sure that all patient education materials are organized and at hand. If the patient wears eyeglasses or hearing aids, be sure they are made available prior to education.

## KEY POINTS

- The effectiveness of patient education relies on an understanding of and attention to the cognitive, affective, and psychomotor domains of learning. After you have completed the assessment phase, identified nursing diagnoses, and created a plan of care, the implementation phase of the teaching-learning process begins; reevaluation of the teaching plan must occur frequently and as needed. The growth in cultural diversity, in particular the increase in the Hispanic population, demands that nursing and related health care professions provide patient education materials in both English and Spanish.
- In educational sessions, patients need to receive information through as many senses as possible, such as verbally and visually (e.g., through pamphlets, videotapes, and diagrams), to maximize learning. Information must be presented at the patient's reading level (in the patient's native language, if possible) and suitable for the patient's level of cognitive development (see Erikson's stages in Box 6-3).
- Teaching and learning principles also must be integrated into patient education plans. Evaluation of patient learning is a critical component of safe and effective drug administration.
- To verify the success—or lack of success—of patient education, nurses need to be very specific in their questions related to patient outcomes and request that the patient repeat information or perform a return demonstration of skills, if appropriate.

## NCLEX® EXAMINATION REVIEW QUESTIONS

1  A 47-year-old patient with diabetes is being discharged to home and must take insulin injections twice a day. The nurse keeps in mind which concepts when considering patient teaching?
   a  Teaching needs to begin at the time of diagnosis or admission and is individualized to the patient's reading level.
   b  The nurse can assume that because the patient is in his forties he will be able to read any written or printed documents provided.
   c  The majority of teaching can be done with pamphlets that the patient can share with family members.
   d  A thorough and comprehensive teaching plan designed for an eleventh-grade reading level needs to be developed.

2  The nurse is developing a discharge plan regarding a patient's medication. Which of these statements about the discharge plan is true?
   a  It will be developed right before the patient leaves the hospital.
   b  It will be developed only after the patient is comfortable or after pain medications are administered.
   c  It will include videos, demonstrations, and instructions written at least at the fifth-grade level.
   d  It will be individualized and based on the patient's level of cognitive development.

3  The nurse is responsible for preoperative teaching for a patient who is mildly anxious about receiving pain medications postoperatively. The nurse recognizes that this level of anxiety may
   a  impede learning because anxiety is always a barrier to learning.
   b  lead to major emotional unsteadiness.
   c  result in learning by increasing the patient's motivation to learn.
   d  reorganize the patient's thoughts and lead to inadequate potential for learning.

4  What action by the nurse is the best way to assess a patient's learning needs?
   a  Quiz the patient daily on all medications.
   b  Begin with validation of the patient's present level of knowledge.

   c  Assess family members' knowledge of the prescribed medication even if they are not involved in the patient's care.
   d  Ask the caregivers what the patient knows about the medications.

5  Which technique would be most appropriate to use when the nurse is teaching a patient with a language barrier?
   a  Obtain an interpreter who can speak in the patient's native tongue for teaching sessions.
   b  Use detailed explanations, speaking slowly and clearly.
   c  Assume that the patient understands the information presented if the patient has no questions.
   d  Provide only written instructions.

6  A nursing student is identifying situations that involve the psychomotor domain of learning as part of a class project. Which are examples of learning activities that involve the psychomotor domain? (Select all that apply.)
   a  Teaching a patient how to self-administer eyedrops
   b  Having a patient list the adverse effects of an antihypertensive drug
   c  Discussing what foods to avoid while taking antilipemic drugs
   d  Teaching a patient how to measure the pulse before taking a beta blocker
   e  Teaching a family member how to give an injection
   f  Teaching a patient the rationale for checking a drug's blood level

7  The nurse is instructing an elderly patient on how to use his walker. Which education strategies are appropriate? (Select all that apply.)
   a  Speak slowly and loudly.
   b  Ensure a quiet environment for learning.
   c  Repeat information frequently.
   d  Allow for an increased number of return demonstrations.
   e  Provide all the information in one teaching session.

1. a, 2. d, 3. c, 4. b, 5. a, 6. a, d, e, 7. b, c, d

For Critical Thinking and Prioritization Questions, see http://evolve.elsevier.com/Lilley.

# 7

# Over-the-Counter Drugs and Herbal and Dietary Supplements

## OBJECTIVES

When you reach the end of this chapter, you will be able to do the following:

1 Discuss the differences between prescription drugs, over-the-counter (OTC) drugs, herbals, and dietary supplements.
2 Briefly discuss the differences between the federal legislation governing the promotion and sale of prescription drugs and the legislation governing OTC drugs, herbals, and dietary supplements.
3 Describe the advantages and disadvantages of the use of OTC drugs, herbals, and dietary supplements.

4 Discuss the role of nonprescription drugs, specifically herbals and dietary supplements, in the integrative (often called *alternative* or *complementary*) approach to nursing and health care.
5 Discuss the potential dangers associated with the use of OTC drugs, herbals, and dietary supplements.
6 Develop a nursing care plan related to OTC, herbal, and dietary supplement drug therapy and the nursing process.

## KEY TERMS

**Alternative medicine** Herbal medicine, chiropractic, acupuncture, massage, reflexology, and any other therapies traditionally not emphasized in Western medical schools but popular with many patients. (p. 88)

**Complementary medicine** Alternative medicine when used simultaneously with, rather than instead of, standard Western medicine. (p. 88)

**Conventional medicine** The practice of medicine as taught in Western medical schools. (p. 87)

**Dietary supplement** A product that contains an ingredient intended to supplement the diet, including vitamins, minerals, herbs, or other botanicals. (p. 87)

**Herbal medicine** The practice of using herbs to heal. (p. 87)

**Herbs** Plant components including bark, roots, leaves, seeds, flowers, fruit of trees, and extracts of these plants that are valued for their savory, aromatic, or medicinal qualities. (p. 87)

**Iatrogenic effects** Unintentional adverse effects that are caused by the actions of a prescriber, other health care professional, or by a specific treatment. (p. 87)

**Integrative medicine** Simultaneous use of both traditional and alternative medicine. (p. 88)

**Legend drugs** Medications that are not legally available without a prescription from a prescriber (e.g., physician, nurse practitioner, physician assistant; also called *prescription drugs*). (p. 88)

**Over-the-counter (OTC) drugs** Medications that are legally available without a prescription. (p. 85)

**Phytochemicals** The pharmacologically active ingredients in herbal remedies. (p. 89)

# OVER-THE-COUNTER DRUGS

Health care consumers are becoming increasingly involved in the diagnosis and treatment of common ailments. This has led to a great increase in the use of nonprescription or over-the-counter (OTC) drugs. More than 80 classes of OTC drugs are marketed to treat a variety of illnesses ranging from acne to cough and cold, pain relief, and weight control. There are currently more than 300,000 OTC products containing over 800 major active ingredients. OTC medications now account for about 60% of all medications used in the United States. Health care consumers use OTC drugs to treat or cure more than 400 different ailments. Over 40 medications that formerly required a prescription are now available OTC. Some 40% to 87% of people 65 years of age or older use one OTC product regularly, and 5.7% take five or more OTC or dietary supplements daily. Some of the most commonly used OTC products include acetaminophen (see Chapter 10), aspirin (see Chapter 44), ibuprofen (see Chapter 44), famotidine, omeprazole and antacids (see Chapter 50), loperamide (see Chapter 51), and cough and cold products (see Chapter 18).

For nurses to understand current OTC classification, it is helpful to have some knowledge of the U.S. Food and Drug Administration (FDA) approval process for these medications. In 1972, the FDA initiated an OTC Drug Review to ensure the safety and effectiveness of the OTC products available, as well as to establish appropriate labeling standards. As a result of this review, approximately one-third of the OTC products were determined to be safe and effective for their intended uses, and one-third were found to be ineffective. A small number were considered to be unsafe, and the remainder required submission of additional data before their safety and effectiveness could be established. Products determined to be unsafe were removed from the market. Some established products that were found to be ineffective but not unsafe were "grandfathered" in and allowed to remain on the market. Many of these have gradually slipped into obscurity and are no longer sold. The FDA now requires new stricter "drug facts" labeling for OTC products that includes information on the following: purpose and uses of the product; specific warnings, including when the product should not be used under any circumstances; and when it is appropriate to consult a doctor or pharmacist. This labeling also describes side effects that could occur; substances or activities to avoid; dosage instructions; and active ingredients, warnings, storage information, and inactive ingredients.

Another result of the OTC Drug Review was the reclassification from prescription to OTC status of more than 40 primary product ingredients. The FDA's Nonprescription Drugs Advisory Committee is responsible for the reclassification of prescription drug products to OTC status. A drug must meet the criteria listed in Box 7-1 to be considered for reclassification. The required information is obtained from clinical trials and postmarketing safety surveillance data, which are submitted to the FDA by the manufacturer. Although this reclassification procedure has been criticized as overly time consuming, it is structured to ensure that products reclassified to OTC status are safe and effective when used by the average consumer.

## BOX 7-1  CRITERIA FOR OVER-THE-COUNTER STATUS

**Indication for Use**

Consumer must be able to easily:
- Diagnose condition
- Monitor effectiveness

Benefits of correct usage must outweigh risks.

**Safety Profile**

Drugs must have:
- Favorable adverse event profile
- Limited interaction with other drugs
- Low potential for abuse
- High therapeutic index*

**Practicality for Over-the-Counter Use**

Drugs must be:
- Easy to use
- Easy to monitor

*Ratio of toxic to therapeutic dosage.

OTC status has many advantages over prescription status. Patients can conveniently and effectively self-treat many minor ailments. Some professionals argue that allowing patients to self-treat minor illnesses enables prescribers to spend more time caring for patients with serious health problems. Others argue that it delays patients from seeking medical care until they are very ill. The financial effect of this status change is enormous: by 2013, OTC sales in the United States will exceed $22 billion. Manufacturers often benefit by prolonging market exclusivity without competition from generic products.

Reclassification of a prescription drug as an OTC drug may increase out-of-pocket costs for many patients because third-party health insurance payers usually do not cover OTC products. However, overall health care costs tend to decrease when products are reclassified as OTC due to a direct reduction in drug costs, elimination of prescriber office visits, and avoidance of pharmacy dispensing fees. Some examples of drugs that have recently been reclassified as OTC products appear in Box 7-2.

The importance of patient education cannot be overstated. Many patients are inexperienced in the interpretation of medication labels (Figure 7-1), which results in misuse of the products. This lack of experience and possibly a lack of information or knowledge may lead to adverse events or drug interactions with prescription medications or other OTC medications. Small print on OTC package labels often complicates the situation, especially for elderly patients. According to a report of the Institute for Safe Medication Practices, one study found that parents gave children incorrect doses of OTC fever medications over 50% of the time. Use of OTC medications can be hazardous for patients with various chronic illnesses, including diabetes, enlarged prostate, hypertension, cardiovascular disease, and glaucoma. Patients are encouraged to read labels carefully and consult a qualified health professional when in doubt.

Another problem associated with OTC drugs is that their use may postpone effective management of chronic disease states and may delay treatment of serious and/or life-threatening

## BOX 7-2　RECLASSIFIED OVER-THE-COUNTER PRODUCTS

**Analgesics**

ibuprofen (Advil, Motrin)

naproxen sodium (Aleve, Naprosyn)

**Histamine Blockers**

*H₁ Receptors*

chlorpheniramine maleate (Chlor-Trimeton)

diphenhydramine hydrochloride (Benadryl)

fexofenadine (Allegra)

loratadine (Claritin)

cetirizine (Zyrtec)

*H₂ Receptors*

cimetidine (Tagamet HB)

famotidine (Pepcid AC)

nizatidine (Axid AR)

ranitidine (Zantac)

*Proton Pump Inhibitors*

lansoprazole (Prevacid-24)

omeprazole (Prilosec-OTC)

**Smoking Deterrents**

nicotine polacrilex gum (Nicorette)

nicotine transdermal patches (Nicoderm) (other dosage forms available)

**Topical Medications**

clotrimazole (Lotrimin)

butoconazole (Femstat)

miconazole (Monistat)

minoxidil solution and hydrocortisone acetate 1% cream (Rogaine)

terbinafine (Lamisil AT)

**Weight Loss Products**

orlistat (Allī)

FIGURE 7-1 Example of an over-the-counter drug label. (From U.S. Food and Drug Administration: The new over-the-counter medicine label: take a look, 2011, available at http://www.fda.gov/Drugs/EmergencyPreparedness/BioterrorismandDrugPreparedness/ucm133411.htm#.TnP-oVxzZyo.email. Accessed November 14, 2011.)

disorders. This is because the OTC medication may relieve symptoms without necessarily addressing the cause of the disorder. This situation is often complicated when patients are afraid to visit a provider, are uninsured/underinsured, have impaired health literacy (see Chapter 6), or simply want to avoid the inconvenience of visiting a provider and instead are hoping for a "quick fix" for themselves or their children.

OTC medications also have their own toxicity profiles. For example, cough and cold products usually include one or more of the following ingredients: nasal decongestants (for stuffy nose), expectorants (for loosening chest mucus), antihistamines (for sneezing and runny nose), and antitussives (for cough). In 2008, the FDA issued recommendations that OTC cough and cold products not be used in children younger than 2 years of age. This followed numerous case reports of symptoms such as oversedation, seizures, tachycardia, and even death in toddlers medicated with such products. There is also evidence that such medications are simply not efficacious in small children. A study in 2010 showed a dramatic decrease in young children emergency department visits since the FDA recommendation (Shehab et al., 2010). The FDA continues to evaluate the safety

and efficacy of cough and cold products for children 2 to 11 years of age but has issued no guidelines to date. Parents are advised to be mindful of how much medication they give to their children and to be careful not to give two products that contain the same active ingredient(s).

Two other examples of OTC drug hazards include products containing acetaminophen (e.g., Tylenol) and nonsteroidal antiinflammatory drugs (NSAIDs) such as ibuprofen (e.g., Advil, Motrin) and naproxen (e.g., Aleve). Hepatic toxicity is associated with excessive doses of acetaminophen and is a leading cause of liver failure. Acetaminophen doses are not to exceed a total of 3 to 4 g/day. The use of NSAIDs is associated with gastrointestinal ulceration, myocardial infarction, and stroke. Patients may sometimes choose excessive dosages of these and other OTC medications out of ignorance or simply in hopes of easing their symptoms. In 2009, the FDA finalized regulations requiring specific labeling for acetaminophen, aspirin, and NSAIDS to enhance consumer awareness of these risks.

Abuse can also be a potential hazard with the use of OTC drug products. Pseudoephedrine is found in a variety of cough and cold products (see Chapter 17); however, this drug is also used to manufacture the widely abused street drug methamphetamine. Because of the potential for abuse, products containing pseudoephedrine must be sold from behind the pharmacy counter, and patients must sign a log book held by the pharmacist. Many patients become addicted to OTC nasal sprays because they can cause rebound congestion and dependency. Dextromethorphan (used as a cough suppressant) is also

## TABLE 7-1  COMMON OVER-THE-COUNTER (OTC) DRUGS

| TYPE OF OTC DRUG | EXAMPLES | WHERE DISCUSSED IN THIS BOOK |
|---|---|---|
| Acid-controlling drugs (H₂ blockers), antacids, and proton pump inhibitors | cimetidine (Tagamet HB), famotidine (Pepcid AC), nizatidine (Axid AR), ranitidine (Zantac); aluminum- and magnesium-containing products (Maalox, Mylanta); calcium-containing products (Tums), lansoprazole (Prevacid-24), omeprazole (Prilosec-OTC) | Chapter 50: Acid-Controlling Drugs |
| Antifungal drugs (topical) | clotrimazole (Lotrimin), miconazole (Monistat), terbinafine (Lamisil AT) | Chapter 56: Dermatologic Drugs |
| Antihistamines and decongestants | brompheniramine (Dimetapp), cetirizine (Zyrtec), chlorpheniramine (Contac, Theraflu), diphenhydramine (Benadryl), fexofenadine (Allegra), guaifenesin (Robitussin), loratadine (Claritin), pseudoephedrine (Sudafed) | Chapter 36: Antihistamines, Decongestants, Antitussives, and Expectorants |
| Eyedrops | artificial tears (Moisture Eyes, Murine) | Chapter 57: Ophthalmic Drugs |
| Hair growth drugs (topical) | minoxidil (Rogaine) | Chapter 56: Dermatologic Drugs |
| Pain-relieving drugs | | |
|   Analgesics | acetaminophen (Tylenol) | Chapter 10: Analgesic Drugs |
|   Nonsteroidal antiinflammatory drugs | aspirin, ibuprofen (Advil, Motrin), naproxen sodium (Aleve) | Chapter 44: Antiinflammatory and Antigout Drugs |

commonly abused. It is known by the brand name of Robitussin, and abusing it is called *Robotripping*.

Several other OTC products can cause specific problems. The use of sympathomimetics (see Chapter 18) can cause problems in patients with type 1 diabetes and patients with hypertension or angina. Aspirin is not to be used in children as it can cause a rare condition called Reye's syndrome (see Chapter 44). Long-term use of antacids can result in constipation or impaction (see Chapter 50).

Normally, OTC medications are used only for short-term treatment of common minor illnesses. An appropriate medical evaluation is recommended for all chronic health conditions, even if the final decision is to prescribe OTC medications. Patient assessment includes questions regarding OTC drug use, including what conditions are being treated. Such questions may help uncover more serious ongoing medical problems. Inform patients that OTC drugs, including herbal products, are still medications. Their use may have associated risks depending on the specific OTC drugs used, concurrent prescription medications, and the patient's overall health status and disease states.

Health care professionals have an excellent opportunity to prevent common problems associated with the use of OTC drugs. Up to 60% of patients consult a health care professional when selecting an OTC product. Provide patients with information about choice of an appropriate product, correct dosing, common adverse effects, and drug interactions with other medications.

For specific information on various OTC drugs, see the appropriate drug chapters later in this text. (Table 7-1 provides cross-references to these chapters.)

## HERBALS AND DIETARY SUPPLEMENTS
### History

Dietary supplement is a broad term for orally administered alternative medicines and includes the category of herbal supplements. Dietary supplements are products that contain ingredients intended to augment the diet and include vitamins, minerals, herbs or other botanicals, amino acids, and

## TABLE 7-2  CONVENTIONAL MEDICINES DERIVED FROM PLANTS

| MEDICINE* | PLANT |
|---|---|
| atropine | *Atropa belladonna* |
| capsaicin | *Capsicum frutescens* |
| cocaine | *Erythroxylon coca* |
| codeine | *Papaver somniferum* |
| digoxin | *Digitalis lanata* |
| paclitaxel | *Taxis brevifolia* |
| quinine | *Cinchona officinalis* |
| scopolamine | *Datura fastuosa* |
| senna | *Cassia acutifolia* |
| vincristine | *Catharanthus roseus* |

*Includes both over-the-counter and prescription drugs.

substances such as enzymes, organ tissues, glandular products, metabolites, extracts, and concentrates. Dietary supplements may be produced in many forms, such as tablets, capsules, softgels, gelcaps, liquids, and powders. These supplements may also be found in nutritional, breakfast, snack, or health food bars; drinks; and shakes.

Herbs come from nature and include the leaves, bark, berries, roots, gums, seeds, stems, and flowers of plants. They have been used for thousands of years to help maintain good health. Herbs have been an integral part of society because of their culinary and medicinal properties. About 30% of all modern drugs are derived from plants (Table 7-2). In the early nineteenth century, scientific methods became more advanced and became the preferred means of healing. At this time, the practice of botanical healing was dismissed as quackery. Herbal medicine lost ground to new synthetic medicines during the early part of the twentieth century. These synthetically derived medicines were touted by scientists and physicians as more effective and reliable.

In the 1960s, concerns were expressed over the iatrogenic effects of conventional medicine. These concerns, along with a desire for more self-reliance, led to a renewed interest in "natural health," and, as a result, the use of herbal products increased. In 1974, the World Health Organization encouraged developing countries to use traditional plant medicines. In 1978, the German equivalent of the FDA published a series of herbal recommendations known as the *Commission E monographs*. These monographs focus on herbs whose effectiveness for specific indications is supported by the research literature. Recognition of the increasing use of herbal products and other nontraditional remedies, known as alternative medicine, led to the establishment of the Office of Alternative Medicine by the National Institutes of Health in 1992. This office was later renamed the National Center for Complementary and Alternative Medicine (NCCAM). Complementary medicine refers to the simultaneous use of both traditional and alternative medicine. This practice is also referred to as integrative medicine. NCCAM classifies complementary and alternative medicine into the following five categories: (1) alternative medical systems, (2) mind-body interventions, (3) biologically based therapies, (4) manipulative and body-based methods, and (5) energy therapies.

Many controversies remain about the safety and control of herbals and dietary supplements, although they continue to be used in the United States and abroad. Their uses and touted advantages are widely publicized. As a result, these products are sold in grocery stores, pharmacies, health food stores, and fitness gyms and can even be ordered through television, radio, and the Internet. Adverse effects are considered to be minimal by the public as well as by the companies that sell these supplements. However a false sense of security has been created because the view of the public tends to be that if a product is "natural," then it is safe. The information listed in this book regarding herbal products does not imply author or publisher endorsement of such products.

For many years, neither federal legislation nor the FDA provided any safeguards surrounding dietary supplements. Instead, manufacturers were responsible only for ensuring product safety and for not making unproven claims about their efficacy. In 1993, the FDA threatened to remove dietary supplements from the market. The American public reacted with a massive letter-writing campaign to Congress, and the 103rd Congress responded by passing the Dietary Supplement and Health Education Act (DSHEA) of 1994. The DSHEA defined dietary supplements and provided a regulatory framework. In 2002, the U.S. Pharmacopeia, an independent organization that is the government's official standard-setting authority for dietary supplements, began certifying products that it had independently tested as part of its Dietary Supplement Verification Program.

A major difference between legend drugs (prescription drugs) and OTC products and dietary supplements is that the DSHEA requires no proof of efficacy and sets no standards for quality control for supplements. In contrast, the FDA has specific and stringent requirements for manufacturers of legend drugs. However, in June 2007, the FDA announced that all manufacturers of dietary supplements would be required to comply with the same good manufacturing practices, as prescription manufacturers are required to do. Under these new requirements, manufacturers must provide data that demonstrate product identity, composition, quality, purity, and strength of active ingredients. They must also demonstrate that products are free from contaminants such as microbes, pesticides, and heavy metals (e.g., lead). Currently there is a bill in Congress, known as the Dietary Supplement Act of 2010, which would require more stringent control over dietary supplements. The fate of this bill is pending.

Manufacturers of supplements may currently claim an effect but cannot promise a specific cure on the product label. Dietary supplements do not need approval from the FDA before they are marketed. A manufacturer does not have to provide the FDA with the evidence to substantiate effectiveness before or after it markets the product, except in the case of a new dietary ingredient. The FDA posts warnings on herbal products on its website (http://www.fda.gov). In contrast, regulating agencies in Germany, France, the United Kingdom, and Canada require manufacturers to meet standards of herbal quality and safety.

## Consumer Use of Dietary Supplements

Consumer use of dietary supplements is growing, with an estimated 50% of U.S. adults using some form of alternative medicine, despite the fact that one-fourth of the 44 million people who use them experience adverse reactions. Consumers use dietary supplements for the treatment and prevention of diseases and proactively to preserve health and wellness and boost the immune system (e.g., reduce cardiovascular risk factors, increase liver and immune system functions, increase feelings of wellness). In addition, herbs may be used as adjunct therapy to support conventional pharmaceutical therapies.

Some herbal products may be used to treat minor conditions and illnesses (e.g., coughs, colds, stomach upset) in much the same way that conventional FDA-approved OTC nonprescription drugs are used. As the number of herbal products on the market increases, nurses will need to respond to patients' educational needs about these products.

## Safety

Dietary supplements, and especially herbal medicines, are often perceived as being natural and therefore harmless; however, this is not the case. Many examples exist of allergic reactions, toxic reactions, and adverse effects caused by herbs. Some herbs have been shown to have possible mutagenic effects and to interact with drugs (Table 7-3). It is estimated that 70% of patients using dietary supplements do not disclose this to their health care providers. In addition, one study identified a relatively low level of knowledge of these products and their risks, even among regular users. This demonstrates the need for health care providers to develop a clinical knowledge base regarding these products and know where to find key information as the need arises. Because of underreporting, present knowledge may represent but a small fraction of potential safety concerns. Also, the FDA has limited oversight of how dietary supplements are prepared, whether herbal or not.

There are few published scientific data regarding the safety of dietary supplements. Two recent examples indicating some of the growing concerns about herbal remedies include the FDA warnings about possible liver toxicity with the use of kava and

## TABLE 7-3   SELECTED HERBS AND DIETARY SUPPLEMENTS AND THEIR POSSIBLE DRUG INTERACTIONS

| HERB OR DIETARY SUPPLEMENT | POSSIBLE DRUG INTERACTION |
|---|---|
| Chamomile | Increased risk for bleeding with anticoagulants |
| Cranberry | Decreased elimination of many drugs that are renally excreted |
| Echinacea | Possible interference with or counteraction to immunosuppressant drugs and antivirals |
| Evening primrose | Possible interaction with antipsychotic drugs |
| Garlic | Possible interference with hypoglycemic therapy and the anticoagulant warfarin (Coumadin) |
| Gingko | May increase risk of bleeding with anticoagulants (warfarin, heparin) and antiplatelets (aspirin, clopidogrel) |
| Ginger root | At high dosages, possible interference with cardiac, antidiabetic, or anticoagulant drugs |
| Grapefruit | Decreases metabolism of drugs used for erectile dysfunction |
|  | Decreases metabolism of estrogens and some psychotherapeutic drugs (benzodiazepines, sertraline) |
|  | Increases risk of toxicity of immunosuppressants, HMG-CoA reductase inhibitors, and some psychotherapeutic drugs (pimozide, escitalopram) |
|  | Increases intensity and duration of effects of caffeine |
| Hawthorn | May lead to toxic levels of cardiac glycosides (e.g., digitalis) |
| Kava | May increase the effect of barbiturates and alcohol |
| Saw palmetto | May change the effects of hormones in oral contraceptive drugs, patches, or hormonal replacement therapies |
| St. John's wort | May lead to serotonin syndrome if used with other serotonergic drugs (e.g., selective serotonin reuptake inhibitors [see Chapter 16]) |
| Valerian | Increases central nervous system depression if used with sedatives |

possible cardiovascular and stroke risks with the use of ephedra. Sale of ephedra was officially banned by the FDA in April 2004. Kava remains on the market despite a 2002 FDA consumer warning letter regarding the risk of liver toxicity. Also, a state-of-the-art paper published in the *Journal of the American College of Cardiology* in 2010 suggests that many herbal products are best avoided in patients with cardiovascular diseases (Tachjian et al., 2010). Herbal products can increase bleeding risk with warfarin (see Chapter 26), potentiate digoxin toxicity (see Chapter 24), increase the effects of antihypertensive agents (see Chapter 22), and cause heart block or dysrhythmias (see Chapter 25).

The FDA has established MedWatch, which has a toll-free number (800-332-1088) consumers can call to report adverse effects of dietary supplements or of any drugs or medical devices. Other authoritative references that can be utilized for herbal information include Pharmacist's Letter/Prescriber's Letter Natural Medicines Comprehensive Database and Natural Standard, available at www.naturalstandard.com. Health care providers need to be on the alert for announcements about the safe and effective use of dietary supplements as well as reported adverse effects. The discriminating and proper use of some dietary supplements may provide some therapeutic benefits, but the indiscriminate or excessive use of dietary supplements can be dangerous.

## Level of Use

The FDA estimates that over 29,000 different dietary supplements are currently used in the United States, with approximately 1000 new products introduced annually. A great deal of public interest in the use of dietary supplements remains. Estimates of the prevalence of dietary supplement use differ greatly. The wide disparity in these estimates is most likely due to the use of varying terminology (e.g., "herbs" versus "dietary supplements") and differences in the wording of questions regarding

length of use (e.g., "have you ever used" versus "have you used in the last 12 months"). One recent estimate of the amount spent on dietary supplements was in excess of $20 billion annually in the United States. The use of botanical medicines is greater in other parts of the world than in the United States.

The many different herbs in these preparations contain a wide variety of active phytochemicals (plant compounds). Herbal medicine is based on the premise that plants contain natural substances that can promote health and alleviate illness. Some of the more common ailments and conditions treated with herbs are anxiety, arthritis, colds, constipation, cough, depression, fever, headache, infection, insomnia, intestinal disorders, premenstrual syndrome, menopausal symptoms, stress, ulcers, and weakness.

Herbal products constitute the largest growth area in retail pharmacy. Their use is increasing at a rate of 20% to 25% per year, which far exceeds the growth in the use of conventional drugs. Insurance plans and managed care organizations are beginning to offer reimbursement for alternative treatments. Some of the most commonly used herbal remedies are aloe, black cohosh, chamomile, echinacea, feverfew, garlic, ginger, ginkgo biloba, ginseng, goldenseal, hawthorn, St. John's wort, saw palmetto, and valerian. These products are covered in more detail in the Safety: Herbal Therapies and Dietary Supplements boxes that appear in the various drug chapters (see the inside back cover for a complete listing of these boxes with page numbers throughout the textbook).

## NURSING PROCESS

## ASSESSMENT

### OVER-THE-COUNTER DRUGS

Nursing assessments are always important to perform, but they are especially important in situations in which a patient

## PATIENT-CENTERED CARE: CULTURAL IMPLICATIONS

### Drug Responses and Cultural Factors

Responses to drugs—including over-the-counter (OTC) drugs, herbals, and dietary supplements—may be affected by beliefs, values, and genetics as well as by culture, race, and ethnicity (see Chapter 4 for more discussion of cultural considerations). As one example of the impact of culture on drug response and use, if patients who are Japanese experience nausea, vomiting, or bowel changes as adverse effects of OTC drugs, herbals, and/or dietary supplements, these often are not mentioned. The reason is that this culture finds it unacceptable to complain about gastrointestinal symptoms, and so they may go unreported to the point of causing risk to the patient.

Herbal and alternative therapies may also be used more extensively in some cultures than in others. Wide acceptance of herbal use without major concern for the effects on other therapies may be very problematic because of the many interactions of conventional drugs with herbals and dietary supplements. For example, the Chinese herb ginseng may inhibit or accelerate the metabolism of a specific medication and significantly affect the drug's absorption or elimination.

One genetic factor that has an influence on drug response is acetylation polymorphism; that is, prescription drugs, OTC drugs, herbals, and dietary supplements may be metabolized in different ways that are genetically determined and vary with race or ethnicity. For example, populations of European or African descent contain approximately equal numbers of individuals showing rapid and slow acetylation (which affects drug metabolism), whereas Japanese and Inuit populations may contain more rapid acetylators. See Chapter 4 for a more in-depth discussion of these specific genetic attributes.

Modified from Munoz C, Hilgenberg C: Ethnopharmacology, *Am J Nurs* 105(8):40-49, 2005.

is self-medicating. Reading level, cognitive level, motor abilities, previous use of *OTC drugs,* successes versus failures with drug therapies and self-medication, and caregiver support are just a few of the variables to be assessed, as deemed appropriate. Other assessment data include questioning about allergies to any of the ingredients of the drug. Include a list of *all* medications and substances used by the patient, including OTC drugs, prescription drugs, herbal products, vitamins, and minerals in the medication history. Also note use of alcohol, tobacco, and caffeine. Assess past and present medical history so that possible drug interactions, contraindications, and cautions are identified. Screen patients carefully before recommending an OTC drug because patients often assume that if a drug is sold OTC it is completely safe to take and without negative consequences. This is not true—OTC drugs can be just as lethal or problematic as prescription drugs if they are not taken properly or are taken in high dosages and without regard to directions (see discussion earlier in the chapter).

Assessment of the patient's knowledge about the components of self-medication, including the positive or negative consequences of the use of a given OTC drug, must be included. Assessment of the patient's (or caregiver's or family member's) level of knowledge and experience with OTC self-medication is critical to the patient's safety, as is assessment of attitudes toward and beliefs about their use, especially a too-casual attitude or a lack of respect for and concern about the use of OTC drugs. This is especially true if a casual attitude is combined with a lack of knowledge. Obviously this could result in overuse, overdosage, and potential complications. See Chapter 6 for more information on patient education.

Generally speaking, laboratory tests are not ordered before the use of OTC drugs, because they are self-administered and self-monitored. However, there are situations in which patients may be taking certain medications that react adversely with these drugs, and laboratory testing may be needed. Some patient groups are also at higher risk for adverse reactions to OTC drugs (as to most drugs in general), including pediatric and elderly patients; patients with single and/or multiple acute and chronic illnesses; those who are frail or in poor health, debilitated, or nutritionally deficient; and those with suppressed immune systems. OTC drugs must also be used with caution and may be contraindicated in patients with a history of renal, hepatic, cardiac, or vascular dysfunction. More assessment information for OTC drugs, herbals, and dietary supplements can be found in other chapters in this textbook when relevant (see Table 7-1). It is important to remember that consumer/patient safety and quality of care related to drug therapy of any kind begins with education. Thus, the best way for patients to help themselves is for them to learn how to assess each situation, weigh all the factors, and find out all they can about the OTC drug they wish to take *before* taking it!

## HERBAL PRODUCTS AND DIETARY SUPPLEMENTS

Many *herbal products* and *dietary supplements* are readily available in drug, health food, and grocery stores as well as in home gardens, kitchens, and medicine cabinets. As noted earlier in the chapter, among the more commonly used herbals are aloe, black cohosh, chamomile, echinacea, feverfew, garlic, ginger, ginkgo biloba, ginseng, goldenseal, hawthorn, St. John's wort, saw palmetto, and valerian. Although patients generally self-administer these products and do not perform an assessment, in various settings you may be able to assess the patient through a head-to-toe physical examination, medical and nursing history, and medication history. Share assessment data and factors and variables to consider with the patient for the patient's safety. This sharing of assessment information allows you to be sure that the patient is taking the herbal product in as safe a manner as possible.

Many herbals and dietary supplements may lead to a variety of adverse effects. For example, some may cause dermatitis when used topically, whereas some taken systemically may be associated with kidney disorders such as nephritis. Therefore, for example, patients with existing skin problems or kidney dysfunction must seek medical advice before using certain herbals. It is also crucial to patient safety to consider any other contraindications, cautions, and potential drug-drug and drug-food interactions. See Table 7-3 for more information on drug interactions.

## CASE STUDY

### Over-the-Counter Drugs and Herbal Products

J.V., a 28-year-old graduate student, is at the student health clinic for a physical examination that is required before he goes on a research trip out of the country. As he completes the paperwork, he asks the nurse, "The form is asking about my medications. I don't have any prescribed medicines, but I take several herbal products and over-the-counter medicines. Do you need to know about these?"

1. How should the nurse answer J.V.?

On the form, J.V. lists the following items:

  1 baby aspirin each day to prevent blood clots

  Sleep-Well herbal product with valerian at night if needed

  Benadryl as needed for allergies, especially at night

  Stress-Away herbal product with ginseng as needed

  Generic ibuprofen, 3 or 4 tablets three times a day for muscle aches from working out

  Memory Boost herbal product with ginkgo every morning

2. Examine the products on J.V.'s list, and state whether there are any concerns with interactions or adverse effects. You may need to refer to descriptions of the individual herbal products (see the inside back cover for a complete listing of Safety: Herbal Therapies and Dietary Supplements boxes located throughout the textbook) or to the appropriate drug chapters for more information.

3. Upon further questioning, J.V. remembers that he has had problems with "acid stomach" for about a year and takes Prilosec-OTC for that as needed. What concerns, if any, are there about this?

For answers, see http://evolve.elsevier.com/Lilley.

## NURSING DIAGNOSES

Nursing diagnoses appropriate for the patient who is taking *OTC drugs, herbals, and/or dietary supplements* include the following (without related causes, because these are too numerous to include):

1. Impaired physical mobility
2. Impaired memory
3. Impaired urinary elimination
4. Acute pain or Chronic pain
5. Fatigue
6. Activity intolerance
7. Insomnia
8. Ineffective health maintenance
9. Risk for injury

## PLANNING

### GOALS

1. Patient is able to increase mobility as tolerated and without distress.
2. Patient experiences increased alertness and improved short-term and long-term memory with continued use of the herbal product and/or dietary supplement.
3. Patient maintains normal elimination patterns during herbal drug use.
4. Patient experiences pain relief or relief of the symptoms of the disease process or injury.
5. Patient experiences increase in energy and/or function.
6. Patient's tolerance for activity remains within normal limits and/or improves during OTC drug or herbal therapy.
7. Patient experiences limited sleep pattern disturbance while on OTC drug or herbal therapy.
8. Patient seeks healthy maintenance behaviors with questions about the OTC drug, herbal, and/or dietary supplement, its action, therapeutic effects versus adverse effects, toxicity, cautions, contraindications, drug-drug or drug-food interactions, and appropriate dosage formulation administration.
9. Patient remains free from injury while taking OTC drug, herbal, and/or dietary supplement.

### OUTCOME CRITERIA

1. Patient states that the actions of the OTC drug, herbal, and/or dietary supplement have been beneficial with relief of symptoms and increased physical mobility.
   - Patient experiences improving overall well-being and health status with minimal adverse effects or complications.
2. Patient reports any change in orientation to person, place, time, or in short-term/long-term memory immediately and seeks appropriate directions regarding discontinuing therapy.
3. Patient identifies measures to increase urinary elimination and enhance urinary elimination patterns such as increasing fluid intake to 6 to 8 glasses of water per day, unless contraindicated, and taking time to void at regular intervals.
4. Patient describes nonpharmacologic approaches to the treatment of acute and chronic pain such as the use of hot or cold packs, physical therapy, massage, relaxation therapy, biofeedback, imagery, and hypnosis.
5. Patient takes measures to minimize fatigue through the use of herbal and dietary supplements, sleeping 6 to 8 hours per night, increasing fluid intake, and intake of recommended daily amounts of food/caloric/protein.
6. Patient states that the actions of the OTC drug, herbal, and/or dietary supplement have been beneficial with relief of symptoms and subsequent increased ability to participate in activities of daily living (ADLs) as well as increase in other physical activities.
7. Patient states increased hours of sleep (i.e., 6 to 8 hours of sleep) and less difficulty with onset of sleep while using OTC, herbal, and/or dietary supplement.
8. Patient experiences healthier behaviors as related to health maintenance by being more knowledgeable about self-medication administration with OTC drugs, herbals, and/or dietary supplements.
   - Patient inquires of pharmacist or health care provider about the safe daily healthy maintenance behavior of taking herbals and/or dietary supplements and deciphers information appropriately.
9. Patient states the importance of taking drugs as directed and of immediately reporting any severe adverse effects

or complications associated with the use of an OTC drug, herbal, and/or dietary supplement to the health care provider and pharmacist and to contact the poison control center, if needed.

- Patient is able to self-administer OTC drugs, herbals, and/or dietary supplements as directed and with proper administration technique (e.g., transdermal patch, suppository, liquid, quick-dissolve tablet) with experiencing of minimal adverse effects and decrease in risk for self-injury.

## IMPLEMENTATION

With *OTC drugs, herbals,* and *dietary supplements,* patient education is an important strategy to enhance patient safety. Patients need to receive as much information as possible about the safe use of these products and to be informed that, even though these are not prescription drugs, they are *not* completely safe and are not without toxicity. Include information about safe use, frequency of dosing and dose, specifics of how to take the medication (e.g., with food or at bedtime), as well as strategies to prevent adverse effects, drug interactions, and toxicity in the patient instructions. Another consideration is the dosage form, because a variety are available such as liquids, tablets, enteric-coated tablets, transdermal patches, gum, and quick-dissolve tablets or strips. For transdermal patches (e.g., for smoking cessation), it is important to emphasize proper use and application. Make sure the patient is aware that the FDA does not regulate these products unless there is sufficient data to support a recall of the product. The companies that manufacture OTC drugs, herbals, and/or dietary supplements are not

required to provide evidence of safety and effectiveness. As previously mentioned, many consumers believe that no risks exist if a medication is available OTC or is an herbal or a "natural" substance. See Box 7-1 for more information about the criteria for moving a drug from prescription to OTC status. The fact that a drug is an herbal or a dietary supplement does not mean that it can be safely administered to children, infants, pregnant or lactating women, or patients with certain health conditions that put them at risk.

## EVALUATION

Patients taking *OTC drugs, herbals,* and/or *dietary supplements* need to carefully monitor themselves for unusual or adverse reactions and therapeutic responses to the medication to prevent overuse and overdosing. The range of therapeutic responses will vary, depending on the specific drug and the indication for which it is used. Therapeutic responses also vary depending on the drug's action; a few examples are decreased pain; decreased stiffness and swelling in joints; decreased fever; increased activity or mobility, as in increased ease of carrying out ADLs; increased hair growth; increased ease in breathing; decrease in constipation, diarrhea, bowel irritability, or gastrointestinal reflux or hyperacidity; resolution of allergic symptoms; decreased vaginal itching and discharge; increased healing; increased sleep; and decreased fatigue or improved energy. For more specific information about nursing diagnoses, planning with goals and outcome criteria, implementation, and evaluation related to various OTC drugs, herbals, and/or dietary supplements, see the appropriate chapters later in the book. Table 7-1 provides cross-references to these chapters.

## ■ PATIENT TEACHING TIPS

- Provide verbal and written information about how to choose an appropriate OTC drug or herbal or dietary supplement as well as information about correct dosing, common adverse effects, and possible interactions with other medications.
- Many patients believe that no risks exist if a medication is herbal and "natural" or if it is sold OTC, so provide adequate education about the drug or product as well as all the advantages and disadvantages of its use, because this is crucial to patient safety.
- Provide instructions on how to read OTC drug, herbal, and dietary supplement labels and directions. Encourage the reading of ingredients if using more than one product, as the ingredient/chemical may occur in both products. For example, a multivitamin supplement may contain ginseng, and taking additional ginseng supplements may lead to toxicity. Another example is with products containing acetaminophen (Tylenol). If the patient is taking acetaminophen and then also takes a cold/flu product, there may also be acetaminophen in that product, and consequently the risk of adverse effects and toxicity increases.
- Emphasize the importance of taking all OTC drugs, herbals, and dietary supplements with extreme caution, and being aware of all the possible interactions and/or concerns associated with the use of these products.

- Instruct the patient that all health care providers (e.g., nurses, dentists, osteopathic and chiropractic physicians) need to be aware about the use of any OTC drugs, herbals, and dietary supplements (and, of course, any prescription drug use).
- Encourage journaling of any improvement of symptoms noted with the use of a specific OTC drug, herbal, and/or dietary supplement.
- Encourage the use of appropriate and authoritative resources for patient information, such as a registered pharmacist, literature provided from the drug company and pharmacist, and web-based information from reliable sites at an appropriate reading level for the patient (e.g., www.Webmd.com).
- Instruct the patient that all medications, whether an OTC drug, herbal, and/or dietary supplement, must be kept out of the reach of children and pets.
- Provide thorough instructions regarding the various dosage forms of OTC drugs, herbals, and dietary supplements. Provide specific instructions such as how to mix powders and how to properly use transdermal patches, inhalers, ointments, lotions, nose drops, ophthalmic drops, elixirs, suppositories, vaginal suppositories or creams, and all other dosage forms (see Chapter 9); also provide information about proper storage and cleansing of any equipment.

## KEY POINTS

- Consumers use herbal products therapeutically for the treatment of diseases and pathologic conditions, prophylactically for long-term prevention of disease, and proactively for the maintenance of health and wellness.
- The FDA has established the MedWatch program to track adverse events and/or problems related to drug therapy. The toll-free number for reporting adverse effects of prescription drugs, OTC drugs, herbals, and dietary supplements is 800-332-1088. Nurses may report adverse events anonymously and without consequence via telephone. Adverse

event reporting is also available inside of medical reference applications such as Epocrates or Medscape.
- Herbal products are not FDA-approved drugs, and therefore their labeling cannot be relied on to provide consumers and patients with adequate instructions for use or even information about warnings.
- The fact that a drug is an herbal product, dietary supplement, or OTC medication is no guarantee that it can be safely administered to children, infants, pregnant or lactating women, or patients with certain health conditions that may put them at risk.

## NCLEX® EXAMINATION REVIEW QUESTIONS

1 The nurse is reviewing dietary supplements and recalls that under the DSHEA, manufacturers of dietary supplements are required to
   a follow FDA standards for quality control.
   b prove efficacy and safety of dietary supplements.
   c identify the active ingredients on the label.
   d obtain FDA approval before the products are marketed.

2 When educating patients about the safe use of herbal products, the nurse remembers to include which concept?
   a Herbal and over-the-counter products are approved by the FDA and under strict regulation.
   b Herbal products are tested for safety by the FDA and the U.S. Pharmacopeia.
   c No adverse effects are associated with these products because they are natural and may be purchased without a prescription.
   d Take the product with caution because labels may not contain reliable information.

3 When taking a patient's drug history, the nurse asks about use of over-the-counter drugs. The patient responds by saying, "Oh, I frequently take aspirin for my headaches, but I didn't mention it because aspirin is nonprescription." What is the best response from the nurse?
   a "That's true, over-the-counter drugs are generally not harmful."
   b "Aspirin is one of the safest drugs out there."
   c "Although aspirin is over the counter, it's still important to know why you take it, how much you take, and how often."
   d "We need you to be honest about the drugs you are taking. Are there any others that you haven't told us about?"

4 When making a home visit to a patient who was recently discharged from the hospital, the nurse notes that she has a small pack over her chest and that the pack has a strong odor. She also is drinking herbal tea. When asked about the pack and the tea, the patient says, "Oh, my grandmother never used medicines from the doctor. She told me that this plaster and tea were all I would need to fix things." Which response by the nurse is most appropriate?

   a "You really should listen to what the doctor told you if you want to get better."
   b "What's in the plaster and the tea? When do you usually use them?"
   c "These herbal remedies rarely work, but if you want to use them, then it is your choice."
   d "It's fine if you want to use this home remedy, as long as you use it with your prescription medicines."

5 A patient tells the nurse that he has been using an herbal supplement that contains kava for several years to help him to relax in the evening. However, the nurse notes that he has a yellow tinge to his skin and sclera, and is concerned about liver toxicity. The nurse advises the patient to stop taking the kava and to see his health care provider for an examination. What else, if anything, should the nurse do at this time?
   a Report this incident to MedWatch.
   b Notify the state's pharmaceutical board.
   c Contact the supplement manufacturer.
   d No other action is needed.

6 The nurse is reviewing the drug history of a patient, and during the interview the patient asks, "Why are some drugs over-the-counter and others are not?" The nurse keeps in mind that criteria for over-the-counter status include: (Select all that apply.)
   a The condition must be diagnosed by a health care provider.
   b The benefits of correct usage of the drug outweigh the risks.
   c The drug has limited interaction with other drugs.
   d The drug is easy to use.
   e The drug company sells OTC drugs at lower prices.

7 A patient comes to the clinic complaining of elbow pain after an injury. He states that he has been taking two pain pills, eight times a day, for the past few days. The medication bottle contains acetaminophen, 325-mg tablets. Calculate how much medication he has been taking per day. Is this a safe dose of this medication?

1. c, 2. d, 3. c, 4. b, 5. a, 6. b, c, d, 7. 5200 mg/day, No

For Critical Thinking and Prioritization Questions, see http://evolve.elsevier.com/Lilley.

# 8

# Gene Therapy and Pharmacogenomics

## ⊝volve WEBSITE

*http://evolve.elsevier.com/Lilley*

- Animations
- Answer Key—Textbook Case Studies
- Critical Thinking and Prioritization Questions

- Key Points—Downloadable
- Review Questions for the NCLEX® Examination
- Unfolding Case Studies

## OBJECTIVES

When you reach the end of this chapter, you will be able to do the following:

1 Understand the basic terms related to genetics and drug therapy.
2 Briefly discuss the major concepts of genetics as an evolving segment of health care, such as principles of genetic inheritance; deoxyribonucleic acid (DNA), ribonucleic acid (RNA), and their functioning; the relationship of DNA to protein synthesis; and the importance of amino acids.
3 Describe the basis of the Human Genome Project and its impact on the role of genetics in health care.

4 Discuss the different gene therapies currently available.
5 Differentiate between direct and indirect forms of gene therapy.
6 Identify the regulatory and ethical issues related to gene therapy as related to nursing and health care professionals.
7 Briefly discuss pharmacogenomics and pharmacogenetics.
8 Discuss the evolving role of professional nurses as related to gene therapy.

## KEY TERMS

**Acquired disease** Any disease triggered by external factors and not *directly* caused by a person's genes (e.g., an infectious disease, noncongenital cardiovascular diseases). (p. 96)

**Alleles** The two or more alternative forms of a gene that can occupy a specific locus (location) on a chromosome (see *chromosomes*). (p. 95)

**Chromatin** A collective term for all of the chromosomal material within a given cell. (p. 96)

**Chromosomes** Structures in the nuclei of cells that contain threads of deoxyribonucleic acid (DNA), which transmit genetic information, and are associated with ribonucleic acid (RNA) molecules and synthesis of protein molecules. (p. 95)

**Gene** The biologic unit of heredity; a segment of a DNA molecule that contains all of the molecular information required for the synthesis of a biologic product such as an RNA molecule or an amino acid chain (protein molecule). (p. 95)

**Gene therapy** New therapeutic technologies that directly target human genes in the treatment or prevention of illness. (p. 97)

**Genetic disease** Any disorder caused directly by a genetic mechanism. (p. 96)

**Genetic material** DNA or RNA molecules or portions thereof. (p. 95)

**Genetic polymorphisms (PMs)** Variants that occur in the chromosomes of 1% or more of the general population (i.e., they occur too frequently to be caused by a random recurrent mutation). (p. 98)

**Genetic predisposition** The presence of certain factors in a person's genetic makeup, or *genome* (see next page), that increase the individual's likelihood of eventually developing one or more diseases. (p. 96)

## KEY TERMS—cont'd

**Genetics** The study of the structure, function, and inheritance of genes. (p. 96)

**Genome** The complete set of genetic material of any organism. It may be contained in multiple chromosomes (groups of DNA or RNA molecules) in higher organisms; in a single chromosome, as in bacteria; or in a single DNA or RNA molecule, as in viruses. (p. 96)

**Genomics** The study of the structure and function of the genome, including DNA *sequencing, mapping,* and *expression,* and the way genes and their products work in both health and disease. (p. 96)

**Genotype** The particular alleles present at a given site (locus) on the chromosomes of an organism that determine a specific genetic trait for that organism (compare *phenotype*). (p. 96)

**Heredity** The characteristics and qualities that are genetically passed from one generation to the next through reproduction. (p. 96)

**Human Genome Project (HGP)** A scientific project of the U.S. Department of Energy and National Institutes of Health to describe in detail the entire genome of a human being. (p. 97)

**Inherited disease** Genetic disease that results from defective alleles passed from parents to offspring. (p. 96)

**Nucleic acids** Molecules of DNA and RNA in the nucleus of every cell. DNA makes up the chromosomes and encodes the genes. (p. 95)

**Personalized medicine** The use of molecular and genetic characterizations of both the disease process and the patient for the customization of drug therapy. (p. 99)

**Pharmacogenetics** A general term for the study of the genetic basis for variations in the body's response to drugs, with a focus on variations related to a single gene. (p. 98)

**Pharmacogenomics** A branch of *pharmacogenetics* (see earlier) that involves the survey of the entire genome to detect multigenic (multiple-gene) determinants of drug response. (p. 98)

**Phenotype** The expression in the body of a genetic trait that results from a person's particular *genotype* (see earlier) for that trait. (p. 96)

**Proteome** The entire set of proteins produced from the information encoded in an organism's genome. (p. 97)

**Proteomics** The detailed study of the proteome, including all biologic actions of proteins. (p. 97)

**Recombinant DNA (rDNA)** DNA molecules that have been artificially synthesized or modified in a laboratory setting. (p. 97)

---

Genetic processes are a highly complex part of physiology and are far from completely understood. Genetic research is one of the most active branches of science today, involving many types of health care professionals, including nurses. Expected outcomes of this research include a deeper knowledge of the genetic influences on disease, along with the development of gene-based therapies. The practice of nursing requires an understanding of genetic concepts as well as genetically related health issues and therapeutic techniques. The goal of this chapter is to introduce some of the major concepts in this very complex and emerging branch of health science. In 1996, the National Coalition for Health Professional Education in Genetics (NCHPEG) was founded as a joint project of the American Medical Association, the American Nurses Association, and the National Human Genome Research Institute (http://www. nchpeg.org). The purpose of NCHPEG is to promote the education of health professionals and the public regarding advances in applied genetics.

Since the 1960s, published literature has described the role of nursing in genetics and genetic research. The Genetics Nursing Network was formed in 1984 and later became the International Society of Nurses in Genetics (ISONG). In 1997, the American Nurses Association designated genetics nursing as an official nursing specialty. In 2001, ISONG approved formation of the Genetic Nursing Credentialing Commission (GNCC). The growing understanding of genetics is quickly creating demand for clinicians in all fields who can educate patients and provide clinical care that tailors health care services to each patient's inherent genetic makeup. This reality also calls for increasing the level of genetics education in nursing school curricula as well as continuing nursing education. Interestingly, the study of genetics has become commonplace in secondary and even primary education.

## BASIC PRINCIPLES OF GENETIC INHERITANCE

Nucleic acids are biochemical compounds consisting of two types of molecules: deoxyribonucleic acid (DNA) and ribonucleic acid (RNA). DNA molecules make up the genetic material that is passed between all types of organisms during reproduction. In some viruses (e.g., human immunodeficiency virus), it is actually RNA molecules that pass the virus's genetic material between generations; however, this is an exception to the norm. A chromosome is a long strand of DNA that is contained in the nuclei of cells. DNA molecules, in turn, act as the template for the formation of RNA molecules, from which proteins are made. Humans normally have 23 pairs of chromosomes in each of their somatic cells. Somatic cells are the cells in the body other than the sex cells (sperm cells or egg cells), which have 23 single (unpaired) chromosomes. One pair of chromosomes in each cell is termed the sex chromosomes, which can be designated as either X or Y. The sex chromosomes are normally XX for females and XY for males. One member of each pair of chromosomes in somatic cells comes from the father's sperm and one from the mother's egg. Alleles are the alternative forms of a gene that can vary with regard to a specific genetic trait.

Genetic traits can be desirable (e.g., lack of allergies) or undesirable (e.g., predisposition toward a specific disease). Each person has two alleles for every gene-coded trait: one allele from the mother, the other from the father. An allele may be dominant or recessive for a given genetic trait. The particular combination of alleles, or genotype, for a given trait determines whether or not a person manifests that trait, or the person's phenotype. Genetic traits that are passed on differently to male and female offspring are said to be sex-linked traits because they are carried on either the X or Y chromosome. For example, hemophilia genes are carried by females but manifest as a bleeding disorder only in males. Hemophilia is an example of an inherited disease; that is, a disease caused by passage of a genetic defect from parents to offspring. A more general term is genetic disease, which is any disease caused by a genetic mechanism. Note, however, that not all genetic diseases are inherited. Chromosomal abnormalities (aberrations) can also occur spontaneously during embryonic development. In contrast, an acquired disease is any disease that develops in response to external factors and is not directly related to a person's genetic makeup. Genetics can play an indirect role in acquired disease, however. For example, atherosclerotic heart disease is often acquired in middle or later life. Many people have certain genes in their cells that increase the likelihood of this condition. This is known as a genetic predisposition. In some cases, a person may be able to offset his or her genetic predisposition by lifestyle choices, such as consuming a healthy diet and exercising to avoid developing heart disease.

Current literature differentiates "old genetics," which focused on single-gene inherited diseases such as hemophilia, from the "new genetics." The new genetic perspective recognizes that common diseases, including Alzheimer's disease, cancer, and heart disease, are the product of complex relationships between genetic and environmental factors. These environmental factors, such as diet or toxic exposures, can initiate or worsen disease processes. Research into disease treatment is beginning to look at genetically tailored therapy.

## DISCOVERY, STRUCTURE, AND FUNCTION OF DNA

Genetics is the study of the structure, function, and inheritance of genes. Heredity refers to the qualities that are genetically transferred from one generation to the next during reproduction. A major turning point in the understanding of genetics came in 1953, when Drs. James Watson and Francis Crick first reported the chemical structures of human genetic material and named the primary biochemical compound deoxyribonucleic acid (DNA). They later received a Nobel Prize for their discovery.

It is now recognized that DNA is the primary molecule in the body that serves to transfer genes from parents to offspring. It exists in the nucleus of all body cells as strands in chromosomes, collectively called chromatin. As described in Chapter 40, DNA molecules contain four different organic bases, each of which has its own alphabetical designation: adenine (A), guanine (G), thymine (T), and cytosine (C). These bases are linked to a type of sugar molecule known as deoxyribose. In turn, these sugar molecules are linked to a "backbone" chain of phosphate molecules, which results in the classic double-helix structure of two side-by-side spiral macromolecular chains. An important related biomolecule is ribonucleic acid (RNA). RNA has a chemical structure similar to that of DNA, except that its sugar molecule is the compound ribose instead of deoxyribose and it contains the base uracil (U) in place of thymine. RNA more commonly occurs as a single-stranded molecule, although in some genetic processes it can also be double-stranded. In double-stranded structures, the base of each strand binds (via hydrogen bonds) to that of the other strand in the space between the two strands. This binding is based on complementary base pairings determined by the chemistry of the base molecules themselves. Specifically, adenine can only bind with thymine or uracil, whereas cytosine can only bind with guanine.

A nucleotide is the structural unit of DNA and consists of a single base and its attached sugar and phosphate molecules. A nucleoside is the base and attached sugar without the phosphate molecule. A relatively small sequence of nucleotides is called an oligonucleotide (the prefix oligo- means "a small number"). Certain new drug therapies involve synthetic analogues of both nucleosides and nucleotides (see Chapters 40, 45, 46, and 47). A related field is targeted drug therapy. Targeted drug therapy focuses on modifying the function of immune system cells (T cells and B cells) and biochemical mediators of immune response (cytokines). However, it is expected to focus on modifying specific genes as well. Current examples of targeted drug therapy are presented in Chapters 45, 46, 48, and 49. One of these drugs, the ophthalmic antiviral drug fomivirsen, is an oligonucleotide with a chemical structure that is opposite (complementary) to that of a critical part of the messenger RNA (mRNA) of the cytomegalovirus. For this reason, it is called an antisense oligonucleotide, and it is the first of this new class of drugs.

An organism's entire DNA structure is its genome. This word is a combination of the terms gene and chromosome, and it refers to all the genes in an organism taken together. Genomics is the relatively new science of determining the location (mapping), structure (DNA base sequencing), identification (genotyping), and expression (phenotyping) of individual genes along the entire genome, and determining their function in both health and disease processes.

### Protein Synthesis

Protein molecules drive the functioning of all biochemical reactions. Protein synthesis is the primary function of DNA in human cells. There is a direct relationship between DNA nucleotide sequence and corresponding amino acid sequences. This allows for precision in protein synthesis. Interestingly, it is estimated that only 2% to 3% of the human genome is involved in protein synthesis. Amino acid sequences control the shape of protein molecules, which ultimately affects their ability to function in the body. Mutations, undesired changes in DNA sequence, can affect the shape of protein molecules and impair or destroy their functioning.

In the cell nuclei, the double strands of DNA uncoil and separate, and a strand of mRNA forms on each separate DNA strand through complementary base pairing as described earlier in the chapter. This process is called *transcription* of the DNA. These mRNA molecules then detach from their corresponding DNA strands, leave the cell nucleus, and enter the cytoplasm, where they are then "read," or translated, by the ribosomes. Ribosomes are composed of a second type of RNA known as *ribosomal* RNA (rRNA), as well as several accessory proteins. Individual sequences of three bases along the mRNA molecule serve to code for specific amino acid molecules. This translation process involves molecules of a third type of RNA, *transfer* RNA (tRNA). The tRNA molecules transport the corresponding amino acid molecules to the site of ribosomal translation along the mRNA strand in sequence according to the three-base codes along the mRNA strand. This in turn results in the creation of chains of multiple amino acids (polypeptide chains), which are known as protein molecules. The specificity of this genetic code is very important for proper protein synthesis, and the process is similar for all living organisms—plant and animal.

There are countless specific amino acid sequences (polypeptides) that result in the synthesis of many thousands of types of protein molecules. Proteins include hormones, enzymes, immunoglobulins, and numerous other biochemical molecules that regulate processes throughout the body. They are involved in both healthy physiologic processes and the pathophysiologic processes of many diseases. The biomedical literature continues to identify and describe many proteins that are part of disease processes. Manipulation of genetic material, as in gene therapy (see later in the chapter), can theoretically modify the synthesis of these proteins and therefore aid in the treatment of disease. This emerging science continues to give rise to novel terminology. The entire set of proteins produced by a genome is now known as the proteome. Proteomics is the study of the proteome, including protein expression, modification, localization, and function, as well as the protein-protein interactions that are part of biologic processes. This science is expected to provide new drug therapies in the future. Furthermore, most clinically approved drugs interact with body proteins such as cell membrane receptors, hormones, and enzymes.

## Human Genome Project

In 1990, an unprecedented genetic research project began in the United States, the Human Genome Project (HGP). It was coordinated by the U.S. Department of Energy and the National Institutes of Health (NIH). The project was completed in 2003, two years ahead of schedule. The goals of this project were to identify the estimated 30,000 genes and 3 billion base pairs in the DNA of an entire human genome. Additional goals included developing new tools for genetic data analysis and storage, transferring newly developed technologies to the private sector, and addressing the inherent ethical, legal, and social issues involved in genetic research and clinical practice. However, the ultimate goal was to develop improved prevention, treatment, and cures for disease. When the HGP began, there were 100 known human disease-related genes. By its completion, there were 1400.

## GENE THERAPY

### Background

Gene therapy is an experimental technique that uses genes to treat or prevent disease. It allows doctors to treat a disorder by inserting a gene into a patient's cells instead of using drugs or surgery. Researchers are testing several approaches to gene therapy, including:

- Replacing a mutated gene with a healthy copy of the gene
- Introducing a new gene into the body to help fight a disease
- Inactivating a mutated gene that is functioning improperly

Gene therapy research is based on the ongoing discovery of new details regarding cellular processes, including biochemical processes that occur at the molecular level. In addition, the increased understanding of allelic variation and its role in disease susceptibility can be used to guide attempts at preventive therapy based on a person's genotypic risk factors.

Although hundreds of gene therapy clinical trials have been approved by the U.S. Food and Drug Administration (FDA), no gene therapy to date has been approved for routine treatment of disease. The goal of gene therapy is to transfer exogenous genes that will either provide a temporary substitute for, or initiate permanent changes in, the patient's own genetic functioning to treat a given disease. Originally projected to provide treatment primarily for inherited genetic diseases, gene therapy techniques are now being researched for treatment of acquired illnesses such as cancer, cardiovascular diseases, diabetes, infectious diseases, and substance abuse. In the future, *in utero* gene therapy may be used to prevent the development of serious diseases as part of prenatal care for the unborn infant.

### Description

During gene therapy, segments of DNA are injected into the patient's body in a process called *gene transfer*. These artificially produced DNA splices are also known as recombinant DNA (rDNA) and must be inserted into some kind of carrier or vector for the gene transfer process. Vectors currently being evaluated include spherical lipid compounds known as *liposomes,* free DNA splices known as *plasmids,* DNA conjugates in which DNA splices are linked (conjugated) to either protein or gold particles, and various types of viruses. Viruses are the most widely studied rDNA vectors thus far. One commonly used group of viruses is the adenoviruses, which include the human influenza (flu) viruses.

### Limitations

Viruses used for gene transfer can also induce viral disease and can be immunogenic in the human host. The proteins produced by artificial methods can be immunogenic. Even in the absence of significant virus-induced disease, the positive effects (e.g., supplemented protein synthesis) may only be temporary, and further treatments may be required. As a result, viruses must be carefully chosen and modified in an effort to optimize therapeutic effects while minimizing undesirable adverse effects. The determination of an ideal gene transfer method remains a major challenge for gene therapy researchers. Figure 8-1 provides a clinical example of the potential use of gene therapy.

**In Vitro Manipulation**

Viral vector

Proliferation

Therapeutic ADA gene

Dysfunctional ADA gene

Self-replication

**Corrected Cell**

**FIGURE 8-1** Gene therapy for adenosine deaminase (ADA) deficiency attempts to correct this immunodeficiency state. The viral vector containing the therapeutic gene is inserted into the patient's lymphocytes. These cells can then make the ADA enzyme. (From Lewis SM et al: *Medical-surgical nursing: assessment and management of clinical problems,* ed 7, St Louis, 2007, Mosby.)

## Current Application

One indirect form of gene therapy is well established and is called *rDNA technology.* It involves the use of rDNA vectors in the laboratory to make recombinant forms of drugs, especially biologic drugs such as hormones, vaccines, antitoxins, and monoclonal antibodies. The most common example is the use of the *Escherichia coli* bacterial genome to manufacture a recombinant form of human insulin. When the human insulin gene is inserted into the genome of the bacterial cells, the resulting culture artificially generates human insulin on a large scale. Although this insulin must be isolated and purified from its bacterial culture source, the majority of the world's medical insulin supply has been produced by this method for well over a decade.

## Regulatory and Ethical Issues Regarding Gene Therapy

Gene therapy research is inherently complex and can also carry great risks for its recipients. Thus, the issue of patient safety becomes significant. Research subjects who receive gene therapy often have a life-threatening illness, such as cancer, which may justify the risks involved. However, case reports of patient deaths in gene therapy trials have underscored these risks and raised the awareness of patient safety. In the 1980s, the NIH Recombinant DNA Advisory Committee was assigned responsibility for oversight of gene therapy research in the United States. It reviews clinical trials involving human gene transfer. The FDA must also review and approve all human clinical gene therapy trials, as it does for any type of drug therapy.

Any institution that conducts any type of research involving human subjects must have an institutional review board,

whose purpose is to protect research subjects from unnecessary risks. Also required for institutions engaging in gene therapy research is an institutional biosafety committee. The role of this committee is to ensure compliance with the NIH *Guidelines for Research Involving Recombinant DNA Molecules.*

A major ethical issue related to gene therapy is that of eugenics. Eugenics is the intentional selection before birth of genotypes that are considered more desirable than others. For similar reasons, the prospect of being able to manipulate genes in human germ cells (sperm and eggs) is also a potential ethical hazard of gene therapy. Theoretically, even cosmetic modifications could be attempted by using such techniques as a part of routine family planning. Because of ethical concerns such as these, U.S. gene therapy research is limited to somatic cells only. Gene therapy in germ-line (reproductive) cells is currently not approved for funding by the National Institutes of Health. This limitation remains despite arguments from those who believe that human germ-cell research could potentially yield cures for many serious chronic illnesses and disabilities, such as Parkinson's disease and spinal paralysis.

## PHARMACOGENETICS AND PHARMACOGENOMICS

**Pharmacogenetics** is a general term for the study of genetic variations in drug response and focuses on single-gene variations. A related science that pertains more directly to the HGP is **pharmacogenomics.** Pharmacogenomics is the combination of two scientific disciplines: pharmacology and genomics. Pharmacogenomics involves how genetics (genome) affect the body's response to drugs. Pharmacogenomics offer physicians the opportunity to individualize drug therapy based on a patient's genetic makeup, rather than giving the "standard" dose to all patients. The ultimate goal is to predict patient drug response and proactively tailor drug selection and dosages for optimal treatment outcomes. Warfarin is an anticoagulant drug that is used to prevent blood clots (see Chapter 26). Research has shown that people with certain genetic variations (*CYP2C9\*2* or *CYP2C9\*3* alleles) are at increased risk of bleeding and require lower doses than those without the variation. In addition, variations in the gene that encodes *VKORC1* may make a patient more or less sensitive to warfarin. This genetic variation occurs most frequently in the Asian population.

Individual differences in alleles that occur in at least 1% of a population are known as **genetic polymorphisms (PMs).** The word *polymorphism* literally means "many forms." Polymorphisms are considered to be too frequent to result from random genetic mutations. Polymorphisms that alter the amount or actions of drug-metabolizing enzymes can alter the reactions to medications. Known examples include those PMs that affect the metabolism of certain antimalarial drugs, the antituberculosis drug isoniazid, and the variety of drugs that are metabolized by the subtypes of cytochrome (CYP) enzymes. They can also alter the functioning of drug receptor proteins, cell membrane ion channels and drug transport proteins, and intracellular second messenger proteins (which carry out drug actions after a drug molecule binds to a cell membrane receptor).

## TABLE 8-1   CLINICAL APPLICATIONS OF PHARMACOGENOMICS

| GENETIC TECHNIQUE | APPLICATION |
| --- | --- |
| Genotyping for the presence of the CYP2D6 isoenzyme and for *CYP2D6* alleles determining whether patients are poor, intermediate, extensive, or ultra- rapid metabolizers related to these enzymes (under study) | *Psychiatry* and *general medicine:* Helps guide the prescribing of selected medications such as anticoagulants, immunosuppressants, antidepressants, antipsychotics, mood stabilizers, anticonvulsants, beta blockers, and antidysrhythmics |
| Genotyping for the presence of the *p-glycoprotein* drug transport protein (under study) | *Cardiology, infectious diseases, oncology, and other practice areas:* Assists in drug selection and dosing for drugs such as digoxin, antiretrovirals, and antineoplastics |
| Genotyping for the presence of thiopurine methyltransferase enzyme | *Oncology:* Used to temper toxicity through more careful dosing of the cancer drug 6-mercaptopurine in pediatric leukemia patients |
| Genotyping for variations in beta-adrenergic receptors (under study) | *Pulmonology:* Determines which asthma patients are more or less responsive to beta-agonist therapy (e.g., albuterol) and which patients might benefit from other types of drug therapy |
| Genotyping for the presence of the Philadelphia chromosome | *Oncology:* Identifies those patients with chronic myelogenous leukemia who may be stronger candidates for therapy with the cancer drug imatinib (Gleevec) |
| Genotyping for the presence of the *HER2/neu* protooncogene | *Oncology:* Identifies a subset of breast cancer patients whose tumors express this gene, which indicates their suitability for treatment with the cancer drug trastuzumab (Herceptin) |
| Viral genotyping of hepatitis C viruses (under study) | *Infectious diseases:* Can determine whether a particular infection warrants 26 versus 48 weeks of drug therapy (thereby reducing both costs and adverse drug effects) |
| Genotyping for the presence of factor V gene mutation | *Women's health:* Identifies women with a 7 to 100 times greater risk of thrombosis with oral contraceptive use compared to women without the mutation |
| Muscle biopsy test for patients with a family history of malignant hyperthermia | *Surgery:* Assesses the patient's risk of this adverse effect known to occur with administration of various inhalation anesthetics and intraoperative paralyzing drugs |
| Genotyping for the presence of sodium channels associated with renin-angiotensin receptors and adrenal gland receptors | *Cardiology:* Allows refined antihypertensive drug selection |
| Race-based drug selection | *Cardiology:* Indicates use of the drug isosorbide dinitrate/hydralazine (BiDil) for treatment of hypertension in African-American patients due ultimately to genotypic variations in this patient population |

*CYP2D6,* Cytochrome P-450 enzyme subtype 2D6; *HER2/neu,* human epidermal growth factor receptor 2.

Differences in CYP enzymes (see Chapter 2) are the best studied PM effects thus far. Depending on their existing genes for these enzymes, patients can be genetically classified as "poor" or "rapid" metabolizers of CYP-metabolized drugs such as warfarin, phenytoin, codeine, and quinidine. With warfarin and phenytoin, a rapid metabolizer may need a higher dose of medication for the same effect, whereas a lower dose may be best for a poor metabolizer. With codeine, a poor metabolizer may actually need a higher dose to get the same analgesic effect that occurs when codeine is metabolized to morphine. In contrast, a rapid metabolizer may convert codeine to morphine too quickly, resulting in oversedation, and a lower dose may be sufficient. A similar situation is also likely to occur with quinidine. Because CYP enzymes are known to vary among racial and ethnic groups, the principle of "cultural safety" becomes one of the imperatives for routine gene-based drug dosing.

Studying both the genome of the patient and the genetic features of the pathology (e.g., tumor cells, infectious organisms) before treatment could allow for customized drug selection and dosing. Such analysis could permit the avoidance of drugs not likely to be effective as well as optimization of drug dosages to minimize the risk of adverse drug effects. These applications of pharmacogenomics are examples of personalized medicine.

## DNA Microarray Technology

Most drug dosage changes are still usually made on a trial-and-error basis by monitoring patient response. Researchers have developed an analytical tool known as a high-density microarray. This technology uses tiny microchip plates that contain thousands of microscopic DNA samples. A patient's blood can then be screened for thousands of corresponding DNA sequences that bind from the patient's blood sample to the sequences on the chip. This allows determination of the presence or absence of various genes, such as those related to drug metabolism. For example, the enzymes in the CYP system help metabolize from 25% to 30% of currently available drugs. Over 40 specific *CYP* genes have been identified thus far. In December 2004, the FDA approved the first DNA microchip for clinical use—the AmpliChip Microarray. It is used to screen blood samples for the individual's CYP enzyme profile. Although this type of genotypic profiling is not yet practical for widespread use, it will eventually become a standard in clinical practice.

Table 8-1 lists several other examples of current clinical applications of pharmacogenomics.

## APPLICATION OF GENETIC PRINCIPLES RELATED TO DRUG THERAPY AND THE NURSING PROCESS

As noted previously, the recognition that genetic factors contribute, at some level, to most diseases continues to grow. Thus, genetic influences on health, including the interaction of genetic and environmental (nongenetic) factors, will routinely affect nursing care delivery. In general, it is expected that in the next few years genetic research will move from the laboratory to more clinical practice settings.

Nurses in general practice settings will not be expected to perform in-depth genetic testing or counseling. Nurses—or other health care providers—with specialty certification in the field of genetics will conduct genetic testing and counseling. However, all nurses will need to have a working knowledge of relevant genetic principles. In this era of the "new genetics" paradigm, nurses are fully aware of the fact that nearly all diseases have a genetic component. Conditions such as myocardial infarction, cancer, mental illness, diabetes, and Alzheimer's disease are now viewed in a different light because of the known complex interactions between a number of factors, including the influence of one or more genes and a variety of environmental exposures for patients.

There are several other applicable skills regarding genetics for nurses in general practice settings. Assessment is the first step of the nursing process, and during the assessment the nurse may uncover factors that may point to a risk for genetic disorders. During the initial assessment, the nurse obtains a patient's personal and family history. The family history is most effective if it covers at least three generations and includes the current and past health status of each family member. Assessment of factors possibly indicating an increased risk for genetic disorders is also important. A few examples of such factors are a higher incidence of a particular disease or disorder in the patient's family than in the general population; diagnosis of a disease in family members at an unusually young age; or diagnosis of a family member with an unusual form of cancer or with more than one type of cancer.

It is also important to inquire about any unusual reactions to a drug—on the part of both the patient, family members, significant others, and/or caregivers. An unusual or other than expected reaction to a drug in family members may point to a difference in the patient's ability to metabolize certain drugs. As indicated earlier in the chapter (as well as in Chapter 2), genetic factors may alter a patient's metabolism of a particular drug, resulting in either increased or decreased drug action. Each and every time a medication is administered, the patient's response to that drug must be assessed. Any unusual medication responses in a patient may point to a need for further investigation. Once a genetic variation is known, drug therapy may be adjusted accordingly.

As DNA chip technology becomes more affordable and accessible, it will be possible for patients to know in advance their relative risks for different diseases in later life. Genotype testing to identify a patient's drug-metabolizing enzymes will help prescribers better predict a patient's response to drug therapy.

Teaching about genetic testing and counseling may be another responsibility of the nurse. Patients will have questions and concerns about genetic testing and other issues. Nurses in general practice are not experts in genetic issues. However, the nurse may help with suggestions about genetic counseling if appropriate. If genetic testing is ordered, the nurse may be a part of the testing process and will need to ensure that the informed decision-making and consent procedure has been carried out correctly.

Maintaining privacy and confidentiality is of utmost importance during genetic testing and counseling. The patient is the one who decides whether to include or exclude any family members from the discussion and from knowledge of the results of genetic testing. The patient needs to be reminded that he or she is not required to undergo the genetic test and that the patient has the right to disclose or withhold test results from anyone. Nurses must protect against improper disclosure of information to other family members, friends of the family, other health care providers, and insurance providers. Nurses share the responsibility with other health care providers to protect patients and their families against the misuse of the patients' genetic information.

Other responsibilities of the professional nurse may include development of clinical and social policy such as genetic nondiscrimination and prenatal testing policies, testing of genetic products for reliability, and tasks in genetic informatics to meet the challenge of sifting through a continually expanding body of knowledge.

## CASE STUDY

### Genetic Counseling

 During the nurse's assessment of a newly admitted 38-year-old patient, the patient tells the nurse, "I'm allergic to codeine. Whenever I take it, it just knocks me out!" The patient tells the nurse that codeine does the same thing to all of her sisters.

1. Does the patient have an actual allergy to codeine? What else could be happening?

The next day, the patient's oncologist comes in and explains the results of a genetic test that was performed on an outpatient basis. The patient agrees to allow the nurse to sit in on the conversation. The physician tells the patient that she has a type of gene which indicates that she has a strong chance of developing breast cancer within the next 5 years. The oncologist recommends that she undergo a bilateral mastectomy soon to avoid the possibility of developing breast cancer and suggests that she share this information with her sisters and her daughter, who is 18 years old. After the physician leaves, the patient tells the nurse, "I don't know what to do. I haven't talked to one of my sisters for years and I just know she won't believe me. I also don't want to worry my daughter. She is so young, and I'm sure she's too young to get cancer."

2. Should the nurse tell the patient's sister and daughter? Explain your answer.

3. What is the best way for the nurse to handle this situation?

For answers, see http://evolve.elsevier.com/Lilley.

## SUMMARY

Increasing scientific understanding of genetic processes is expected to revolutionize modern health care in many ways. The artificial manipulation and transfer of genetic material, although not yet a standard treatment for disease, is the focus of over 300 current human clinical gene therapy trials. The spectrum of diseases that may eventually be treatable by gene therapy includes inherited diseases that are present from birth, disabilities such as paralysis from spinal cord injuries, life-threatening illnesses such as cancer, and even chronic illnesses acquired later in life for which a person may have a genetic predisposition. The science of pharmacogenomics has already identified some of the genetic nuances in how different individuals' bodies metabolize drugs to their benefit or harm. Continued study in this area is expected to result in proactive customization of drug therapy to promote therapeutic benefits while minimizing or eliminating toxic effects. Genetic procedures and therapeutic techniques will likely become an increasing part of nursing practice as well as of health care delivery in general. As the role and impact of genetics and genetically based drug therapy increase, so will their role in the nursing process.

## KEY POINTS

- Genetic processes are a highly complex facet of human physiology, and genetics is becoming an integral part of health care that holds much promise in the form of new treatments for alterations in health.
- The Human Genome Project (HGP), spearheaded by the U.S. Department of Energy and the NIH, described in detail the entire genome of a human individual.
- Basic genetic inheritance is carried by 23 pairs of chromosomes in each of the somatic cells; one pair of chromosomes in each cell is the *sex chromosomes,* identified as XX for females and XY for males.
- Applicable skills for general nurses include taking thorough patient, family, and drug histories, recognizing situations that may warrant further investigation through genetic testing, identifying resources for patients, maintaining confidentiality and privacy, and ensuring that informed consent is obtained for genetic testing and counseling.

## NCLEX® EXAMINATION REVIEW QUESTIONS

1 Which is the most appropriate example of a product formed by an indirect form of gene therapy?
   a Stem cells
   b Insulin
   c Antigen substitution
   d Platelet inhibitors
2 The nurse is explaining the general goal of gene therapy to a patient. With gene therapy, the general goal is to transfer exogenous genes to a patient for which result?
   a To change the patient's own genetic functioning to treat a given disease
   b To improve drug metabolism
   c To prevent genetic disorders in the patient's future children
   d To stimulate the growth of stem cells
3 The NIH Recombinant DNA Advisory Committee has what responsibility?
   a Approving all forms of human clinical gene therapy
   b Identifying all major risks to the human subjects in a specific research protocol
   c Reviewing clinical trials involving human gene transfer
   d Analyzing genomes and determining whether they appear mutagenic
4 The presence of certain factors in a person's genetic makeup that increase the likelihood of eventually developing one or more diseases is known as a
   a genetic mutation.
   b genetic polymorphism.
   c genetic predisposition.
   d genotype.
5 The nurse is reviewing gene therapy. Which is a commonly studied adenovirus?
   a Hepatitis A and C virus
   b Genovirum
   c Human influenza virus
   d Pallodium
6 General responsibilities of the nurse regarding genetics may include which of these activities? (Select all that apply.)
   a Assessing the patient's personal and family history
   b Referring the patient to a genetic counselor or other genetics specialist
   c Communicating the results of genetic tests to the patient and patient's family
   d Maintaining privacy and confidentiality during the testing process
   e Answering questions about genetic test results
7 The nurse is assessing a patient for a possible increased risk for genetic disorders. Which of these, if present, may indicate an increased risk for a genetic disorder? (Select all that apply.)
   a Having a brother who died of a myocardial infarction at age 29
   b Having a family member who has been diagnosed with more than one type of cancer
   c Having an uncle who was diagnosed with prostate cancer at age 73
   d A history of allergy to shellfish and iodine
   e Having a maternal grandmother, two maternal aunts, and a sister who were diagnosed with colon cancer

1. b, 2. a, 3. b, 4. c, 5. c, 6. a, b, d, 7. a, b, e

For Critical Thinking and Prioritization Questions, see http://evolve.elsevier.com/Lilley.

# Photo Atlas of Drug Administration

## PREPARING FOR DRUG ADMINISTRATION

NOTE: This photo atlas is designed to illustrate general aspects of drug administration. For detailed instructions, please refer to a nursing fundamentals or nursing skills book.

When giving medications, remember safety measures and correct administration techniques to avoid errors and to ensure optimal drug actions. Keep in mind the basic "Six Rights":

1. Right drug
2. Right dose
3. Right time
4. Right route
5. Right patient (using two identifiers)
6. Right documentation

Refer to Chapter 1 for additional rights regarding drug administration. Other things to keep in mind when preparing to give medications are as follows:

- Remember to perform hand hygiene before preparing or giving medications (Box 9-1)
- If you are unsure about a drug or dosage calculation, do not hesitate to double-check with a drug reference or with a pharmacist. **DO NOT** administer a medication if you are unsure about it!
- Be punctual when giving drugs. Some medications must be given at regular intervals to maintain therapeutic blood levels.
- Figure 9-1 shows an example of a computer-controlled drug-dispensing system. To prevent errors, obtain the drugs for one patient at a time.
- Remember to check the drug at least three times before giving it. The nurse is responsible for checking original medication labels against the transcribed medication order. In Figure 9-2, the nurse is checking the drug against the medication administration record after taking it out of the dispenser drawer. The drug must then be checked before opening it and again after opening it but before giving it to the patient. Some drugs (i.e., heparin and insulin) must be checked by two licensed nurses.
- Health care facilities have various means of checking the medication record when a new one is printed, so be sure that

you are working from one that has been checked or verified before giving the medication. If the patient's medication record has a new drug order on it, the best rule of practice is to double-check that order against the original medication order on the patient's medical record.

- Check the expiration date of all medications. Medications used past the expiration date may be less potent or even harmful.
- Make sure that drugs that are given together are compatible. For example, bile acid sequestrants and antacids (see Chapters 27 and 50) must not be given with other drugs, because they will interfere with drug absorption and action. Check with a pharmacist if unsure. Before administering any medication, check the patient's identification bracelet (Figure 9-3). The Joint Commission's standards require two patient identifiers (name and birthday, or name and account number, according to the facility policy). In some facilities, patient information is in a barcode system that is scanned. In

FIGURE 9-1 Using a computer-controlled drug-dispensing system to remove medication.

addition, assess the patient's drug allergies before giving any medication.

- Be sure to take time to explain the purpose of each medication, its action, possible adverse effects, and any other pertinent information, especially drug-drug or drug-food interactions, to the patient and/or caregiver.
- Open the medication at the bedside into the patient's hand or into a medicine cup. Try not to touch the drugs with your hands. Leaving the drugs in their packaging until you get to the patient's room helps to avoid contamination and waste in case the patient refuses the drug.
- If the patient refuses a drug, the drug may be returned to the automated medication dispenser or to the pharmacy if the package is unopened. Check facility policy. Discard opened drugs per facility protocol. Scheduled drugs that are not given will need a witness if discarded. Note on the patient's record which drug was refused and the patient's reason for refusal.
- Discard any medications that fall to the floor or become contaminated by other means.

- Stay with the patient while the patient takes the drugs. Do not leave the drugs on the bedside table or the meal tray for the patient to take later.
- Document the medication given on the medication record (see Figure 9-9) as soon as it is given and before going to the next patient. Be sure also to document therapeutic responses, adverse effects (if any), and other concerns in the nurse's notes. Some facilities use manual documentation, and others use electronic documentation.
- Return to evaluate the patient's response to the drug. Remember that the expected response time will vary according to the drug route. For example, responses to sublingual nitroglycerin or intravenous (IV) push medications need to be evaluated within minutes, but it may take an hour or more for a response to be noted after an oral medication is given.
- See the Patient-Centered Care: Lifespan Considerations for the Pediatric Patient box on p. 41 (in Chapter 3) for age-related considerations for medication administration to infants and children.

---

### BOX 9-1    STANDARD PRECAUTIONS

Always adhere to Standard Precautions, including the following:

- Wear clean gloves when exposed to or when there is potential exposure to blood, body fluids, secretions, excretions, and any items that may contain these substances. Always wash hands immediately when there is direct contact with these substances or any item contaminated with blood, body fluids, secretions, or excretions. Gloves must always be worn when giving injections and may be necessary during medication preparation. Be sure to assess the patient for latex allergies and use nonlatex gloves if indicated.
- Perform hand hygiene after removing gloves and between patient contacts. According to the Centers for Disease Control and Prevention, the preferred method of hand decontamination is with an alcohol-based hand rub, but washing with an antimicrobial soap and water is an alternative to the alcohol rub. Use soap and water to wash hands when hands are visibly dirty.
- Perform hand hygiene:
  - Before direct contact with patients
  - After contact with blood, body fluids, excretions, mucous membranes, wound dressings, or nonintact skin

- After contact with a patient's skin (i.e., when taking a pulse or positioning a patient)
- After removing gloves
- Wear a mask, eye protective gear, and face shield during any procedure or patient care activity with the potential for splashing or spraying of blood, body fluids, secretions, or excretions. Use of a gown may also be indicated for these situations.
- When administering medications, once the exposure or procedure is completed and exposure is no longer a danger, remove soiled protective garments or gear and perform hand hygiene.
- Never remove, recap, cap, bend, or break any used needle or needle system. Be sure to discard any disposable syringes and needles in the appropriate puncture-resistant container.

For detailed information on Standard Precautions, see the guidelines posted on the Centers for Disease Control and Prevention website at http://www.cdc.gov/hicpac/pdf/isolation/Isolation2007.pdf. Accessed June 11, 2012.

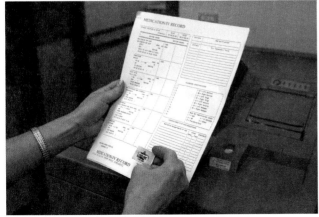

**FIGURE 9-2** Checking the medication against the order on the medication administration record.

**FIGURE 9-3** Always check the patient's identification, using two patient identifiers, and allergies before giving medications.

## ENTERAL DRUGS

### Administering Oral Drugs

Always begin by performing hand hygiene and maintain Standard Precautions (see Box 9-1). When administering oral drugs, keep in mind the following points:

#### Oral Medications

- Administration of some oral medications (and medications by other routes) requires special assessments. For example, it is recommended that the apical pulse be auscultated for 1 full minute before any digitalis preparation is given (Figure 9-4). Administration of other oral medications may require blood pressure monitoring. Be sure to document all parameters. In addition, do not forget to check the patient's identification and allergies before giving any oral medication (or medication by any other route).
- If the patient is experiencing difficulty swallowing (dysphagia), some types of tablets can be crushed with a pill-crushing device (Figure 9-5) for easier administration. Crush one type of pill at a time, because if you mix together all of the medications before crushing (instead of crushing them one at a time) and then spill some, there is no way to know which drug has been wasted. Also, if all are mixed together, you cannot check the Six Rights three times before giving the drug. Mix the crushed medication in a small amount of soft food, such as applesauce or pudding. Be sure that the pill-crushing device is clean before and after you use it. See Chapter 2 for more information on medications that are not to be crushed.
- **CAUTION:** Be sure to verify whether a medication can be crushed by consulting a drug reference book or a pharmacist. Some oral medications, such as capsules, enteric-coated tablets, and sustained-release or long-acting drugs, must *not* be crushed, broken, or chewed (Figure 9-6). These medications are formulated to protect the gastric lining from irritation or protect the drug from destruction by gastric acids, or are designed to break down gradually and slowly release the medication. If these drugs, designated with labels such as *sustained release* or *extended release,* are crushed or opened, then the intended action of the dosage form is destroyed. As a result, gastric irritation may occur, the drug may be inactivated by gastric acids, or the immediate availability of a drug that was supposed to be released slowly may cause *toxic* effects. Check with the prescriber to see if an alternate form of the drug is needed.
- Be sure to position the patient to a sitting or side-lying position to make it easier for the patient to swallow oral medications and to avoid the risk of aspiration (Figure 9-7). Always provide aspiration prevention measures as needed.
- Offer the patient a full glass of water; 4 to 6 oz of water or other fluid is recommended for the best dissolution and absorption of oral medications. *Age-related considerations:* Young patients and the elderly may not be able to drink a full glass of water but need to take enough fluid to ensure that the medication reaches the stomach. If the patient prefers another fluid, be sure to check for interactions between the medication and the fluid of choice. If fluid restriction is ordered, be sure to follow the guidelines.
- If the patient requests, you may place the pill or capsule in the patient's mouth with your gloved hand.
- Lozenges are not be chewed unless specifically instructed/ordered.
- Effervescent powders and tablets need to be mixed with water and then given immediately after they are dissolved.
- Remain with the patient until all medication has been swallowed. If you are unsure whether a pill has been swallowed, ask the patient to open his or her mouth so that you can inspect to see if it is gone. Assist the patient to a comfortable position after the medication has been taken.
- Document the medication given on the medication record (see Figure 9-9), and monitor the patient for a therapeutic response as well as for adverse reactions.

#### Sublingual and Buccal Medications

The sublingual and buccal routes prevent destruction of the drugs in the gastrointestinal tract and allow for rapid absorption into the bloodstream through the oral mucous membranes. These routes are not often used. Be sure to provide instruction to the patient before giving these medications.

- Sublingual tablets are placed under the tongue (Figure 9-8). Buccal tablets are placed between the upper or lower molar teeth and the cheek.
- Be sure to wear gloves if you are placing the tablet into the patient's mouth. Adhere to Standard Precautions (see Box 9-1).
- Instruct the patient to allow the drug to dissolve completely before swallowing.
- These drug forms are not taken with fluids. Instruct the patient not to drink anything until the tablet has dissolved completely.
- Be sure to instruct the patient not to swallow the tablet; saliva should not be swallowed until the drug is dissolved.
- When using the buccal route, alternate sides with each dose to reduce risk of oral mucosa irritation.
- Document the medication given on the medication record (Figure 9-9), and monitor the patient for a therapeutic response as well as for adverse reactions.

#### Orally Disintegrating Medications

Orally disintegrating medications, either in tablet or medicated strip form, dissolve in the mouth without water within 60 seconds. These medications are placed *on* the tongue, not under the tongue, as in the sublingual route. The absorption through the oral mucosa is rapid with a faster onset of action than for drugs that are swallowed. The patient must be instructed to allow the medication to dissolve on the tongue and not to chew or swallow the medication.

- Be sure to wear gloves if you are placing the medication on the patient's tongue. Adhere to Standard Precautions (see Box 9-1).
- Make sure the patient has not eaten or had anything to drink for 5 minutes before and after taking these medications.
- Orally disintegrating medications are often packed in foil blister packs. Do not open the package until just before giving the medication. Carefully open *one* dose at a time. These medications are fragile and may break if they are pushed through the blister pack. Once a blister or foil pack is

opened, the tablet must either be taken or discarded; it cannot be stored for another time.
- Orally disintegrating medications cannot be split, broken, or torn.
- Instruct the patient to hold the medication on the tongue to allow it to dissolve, instead of chewing or swallowing it. This

usually takes about a minute. Warn the patient that there may be a sweet or even slightly bitter taste. Remind the patient not to drink water or to eat for 5 minutes after taking the medication.
- Document the medication given on the medication record (see Figure 9-9), and monitor the patient for a therapeutic response as well as for adverse reactions.

FIGURE 9-4 Some medications require special assessment before administration, such as taking an apical pulse.

FIGURE 9-5 Using a pill-crushing device to crush a tablet.

FIGURE 9-6 Enteric-coated tablets and long-acting medications are not to be crushed, broken, or chewed.

FIGURE 9-7 Giving oral medications.

FIGURE 9-8 Proper placement of a sublingual tablet.

# MEDICATION ADMINISTRATION RECORD

| Effective: 11/04/12 at 0600 | 11/04/12 0600-2400 | 11/05/12 0001-0559 |
|---|---|---|
| *ROUTINE ORDERS* | *Time/Initials* | *Time/Initials* |
| lansoprazole (Prevacid) 15 mg<br>1 CAPSULE AC BREAKFAST PO<br>DOSE = 1 CAP = 15 mg<br><br>ORD#: 5 | 0730 *LLL* | |
| nitroglycerin 2% ointment 1 pkt<br>NITRO-BID 2% OINT(unit dose)<br>1 packet Q 6 H TP<br>1 inch = 1 packet<br><br>ORD#: 6 | 0900 *JSS*<br>1500 __<br>2100 __ | 0300 __ |
| enoxaparin (Lovenox) 30 mg<br>30 mg DAILY subcut<br>DOSE = 30 mg = 0.3 mL<br>(30 mg/0.3 mL premixed)<br>DOCUMENT SITE      ORD#: 7 | 0900 *JSS*<br>Site: *RA* | |
| digoxin (Lanoxin) 0.125 mg<br>ONE TABLET DAILY PO<br>DOSE = 1 TAB = 0.125 MG<br>CHECK & DOCUMENT<br>APICAL PULSE      ORD#: 8 | 0900 *JSS*<br>AP = *90* | |
| | | |
| *PRN ORDERS* | | |
| acetaminophen     650 mg<br>(Tylenol) 2 tablets Q 4 H prn PO<br>PRN pain or headache<br>DOSE = 650 mg = 2 TABLETS<br><br>ORD #: 10 | | |

**ALLERGIES** — INJECTION SITES

| **IVP DYE** | Abdomen |
|---|---|
| **PCN** | LA = Left abdomen |
| **SULFA** | RA = Right abdomen |
| | LT = Left thigh     RT = Right thigh |
| | LVG = Left ventrogluteal |
| | RVG = Right ventrogluteal |
| | LA = Left arm     RA = Right arm |
| | O = Other (specify) |

### STAT and SINGLE DOSE MEDS

| MED/DOSAGE/ROUTE | Date | Time | INITIALS |
|---|---|---|---|
| *Lasix, 40 mg IV STAT* | *11/04* | *1200* | *JSS* |
| | | | |
| | | | |
| | | | |
| | | | |
| | | | |
| | | | |
| | | | |
| | | | |
| | | | |

| INITIALS | MAR VERIFICATION/TIME |
|---|---|
| *CTR* | *Charles T. Ryan, RN/0500* |
| | |

***SIGNATURE LOG***

| INITIALS | FULL SIGNATURE / TITLE |
|---|---|
| *JSS* | *Julie S. Snyder, RN* |
| *LLL* | *Linda L. Lilley, RN* |
| | |
| | |
| | |
| | |

Patient Name:      *Rue, Jeannie*

MR#:  *06121958*      DOB:  *05/25/40*

Admitting Dr:  *Keadle, Ralph*      Room:  *6717*

**MAYFIELD GENERAL HOSPITAL**

**Virginia Shores, VA**

PAGE 1 of 1

**FIGURE 9-9** Example of a medication administration record.

## Liquid Medications

- Liquid medications may come in a single-dose (unit-dose) package, may be poured into a medicine cup from a multidose bottle, or may be drawn up in an oral-dosing syringe (Figure 9-10).
- When pouring a liquid medication from a container, first shake the bottle gently to mix the contents if indicated. Remove the cap and place it upside down on a paper towel on the counter. Hold the bottle with the label against the palm of your hand to keep any spilled medication from altering the label. Place the medicine cup at eye level, and fill to the proper level on the scale (Figure 9-11). Pour the liquid so that the base of the meniscus is even with the appropriate line measure on the medicine cup.
- If you overfill the medicine cup, discard the excess in the sink. Do not pour it back into the multidose bottle. Before replacing the cap, wipe the rim of the bottle with a paper towel.
- Doses of medications that are less than 5 mL cannot be measured accurately in a calibrated medicine cup. For small volumes, use a calibrated oral syringe. Do not use a hypodermic syringe or a syringe with a needle or syringe cap. If hypodermic syringes are used, the drug may be inadvertently given parenterally, or the syringe cap or needle, if not removed from the syringe, may become dislodged

and accidentally aspirated by the patient when the syringe plunger is pressed.
- Document the medication given on the medication record (see Figure 9-9), and monitor the patient for a therapeutic response as well as for adverse reactions.

## Oral Medications for Infants and Children

- Liquids are usually ordered for infants and young children because they cannot swallow pills or capsules.
- A plastic disposable oral-dosing syringe is recommended for measuring small doses of liquid medications. Use of an oral-dosing syringe prevents the inadvertent parenteral administration of a drug once it is drawn up into the syringe.
- Position the infant so that the head is slightly elevated to prevent aspiration. Not all infants will be cooperative, and many need to be partially restrained (Figure 9-12).
- Place the plastic dropper or syringe inside the infant's mouth, beside the tongue, and administer the liquid in small amounts while allowing the infant to swallow each time.
- A clean empty nipple may be used to administer the medication. Place the liquid inside the empty nipple and allow the infant to suck the nipple. Add a few milliliters of water to rinse any remaining medication into the infant's mouth, unless contraindicated.
- Take great care to prevent aspiration. A crying infant can easily aspirate medication. If the infant is crying, wait until the infant is calmer before trying again to give the medication.
- Do not add medication to a bottle of formula; the infant may refuse the feeding or may not drink all of it. Make sure that all of the oral medication has been taken, and then return the infant to a safe, comfortable position.
- A child will reject oral medications that taste bitter. The drug may be mixed with a teaspoon of a sweet-tasting food such as jelly, applesauce, ice cream, or sherbet. Using honey in infants is *not* recommended because of the risk of botulism. Do not mix the medication in an essential food item, such as formula, milk, or orange juice, because the child may reject that food later. After the medication is taken, offer the child juice, a flavored frozen ice pop, or water.

**FIGURE 9-10 A,** Liquid medication in a unit-dose package. **B,** Liquid measured into a medicine cup from a multidose container. **C,** Liquid medicine in an oral-dosing syringe.

**FIGURE 9-11** Measuring liquid medication.

**FIGURE 9-12** Administering oral liquid medication to an infant.

## Administering Drugs through a Nasogastric or Gastrostomy Tube

Always begin by performing hand hygiene and maintain Standard Precautions (see Box 9-1). Gloves must be worn. When administering drugs via these routes, keep in mind the following points:

- Before giving drugs via these routes, position the patient in a semi-Fowler's or Fowler's position and leave the head of the bed elevated for at least 30 minutes afterward to reduce the risk of aspiration (Figure 9-13).
- Assess whether fluid restriction or fluid overload is a concern. It will be necessary to give water along with the medications to flush the tubing.
- Check to see if it is recommended for the drug to be given on an empty or full stomach. In addition, some drugs are incompatible with enteral feedings. If the drug is to be given on an empty stomach, or if incompatibility exists, the feeding may need to be stopped before and/or after giving the medication. Follow the guidelines for the specific drug if this is necessary. Examples of drugs that are not compatible with enteral feedings are phenytoin and carbidopa-levodopa. Whenever possible, give liquid forms of drugs to prevent clogging the tube.
- If tablets must be given, crush the tablets individually into a fine powder. Administer the drugs separately (Figure 9-14). Keeping the drugs separate allows for accurate identification if a dose is spilled. Be sure to check whether the medication can be crushed; enteric-coated and sustained-release tablets or capsules are not to be crushed (see Chapter 2). Check with a pharmacist if you are unsure.

- Before administering the drugs, follow the institution's policy for verifying tube placement and checking gastric residual. Reinstill gastric residual per institutional policy, and then clamp the tube.
- Dilute a crushed tablet or liquid medication in 15 to 30 mL of warm water. Some capsules may be opened and dissolved in 30 mL of warm water; check with a pharmacist.
- Remove the piston from an adaptable-tip syringe and attach it to the end of the tube. Unclamp the tube and pinch the tubing to close it again. Add 30 mL of warm water and release the pinched tubing. Allow the water to flow in by gravity to flush the tube, and then pinch the tubing closed again before all the water is gone to prevent excessive air from entering the stomach. If a stopcock valve device is present on the enteral tube, then open and close the stopcock instead of pinching the tubing to clamp it.
- Pour the diluted medication into the syringe and release the tubing to allow it to flow in by gravity (Figure 9-15). Flush between each drug with 10 mL of warm water. Be careful not to spill the medication mixture. Adjust fluid amounts if fluid restrictions are ordered, but sufficient fluid must be used to dilute the medications and to flush the tubing.
- If water or medication does not flow freely, you may apply gentle pressure with the plunger or bulb of the syringe. Do not try to force the medicine through the tubing.
- After the last drug dose, flush the tubing with 30 mL of warm water, and then clamp the tube. Resume the tube feeding when appropriate.
- Have the patient remain in a high Fowler's or slightly elevated right-side-lying position to reduce the risk of aspiration.
- Document the medications given on the medication record (see Figure 9-9), the amount of fluid given on the patient's intake and output record, and the patient's response in the patient's record.

**FIGURE 9-14** Medications given through gastric tubes need to be administered separately. Dilute crushed pills in 15 to 30 mL of water before administration.

**FIGURE 9-13** Elevate the head of the bed before administering medications through a nasogastric or other enteric tube.

**FIGURE 9-15** Pour liquid medication into the syringe, then unclamp the tubing and allow it to flow in by gravity.

## Administering Rectal Drugs

Always begin by performing hand hygiene and maintain Standard Precautions (see Box 9-1). Gloves must be worn. When administering rectal drugs, keep in mind the following points:

- Assess the patient for the presence of active rectal bleeding or diarrhea, which generally are contraindications for the use of rectal suppositories.
- Suppositories should not be divided to provide a smaller dose. The active drug may not be evenly distributed within the suppository base.
- Position the patient on his or her left side, unless contraindicated. The uppermost leg needs to be flexed toward the waist (Sims' position). Provide privacy and drape.
- Do not insert the suppository into stool. Gently palpate the rectal wall for the presence of feces. If possible, have the patient defecate. DO NOT palpate the patient's rectum if the patient has had rectal surgery.
- Remove the wrapping from the suppository and lubricate the rounded tip with water-soluble gel (Figure 9-16).
- Insert the tip of the suppository into the rectum while having the patient take a deep breath and exhale through the mouth. With your gloved finger, quickly and gently insert the suppository into the rectum, alongside the rectal wall, at least 1 inch beyond the internal sphincter (Figure 9-17).
- Have the patient remain lying on his or her left side for 15 to 20 minutes to allow absorption of the medication.
- *Age-related considerations:* With children it may be necessary to gently but firmly hold the buttocks in place for 5 to 10 minutes until the urge to expel the suppository has passed. Older adults with loss of sphincter control may not be able to retain the suppository.
- If the patient prefers to self-administer the suppository, give specific instructions on the purpose and correct procedure. Be sure to tell the patient to remove the wrapper.
- Use the same procedure for medications administered by a retention enema, such as sodium polystyrene sulfonate (see Chapter 29). Drugs given by enemas are diluted in the smallest amount of solution possible. Retention enemas need to be held for 30 minutes to 1 hour before expulsion, if possible, for maximum absorption.
- Document the medication given on the medication record (see Figure 9-9), and monitor the patient for a therapeutic response as well as for adverse reactions.

FIGURE 9-16 Lubricate the suppository with a water-soluble lubricant.

FIGURE 9-17 Inserting a rectal suppository.

## PARENTERAL DRUGS

### Preparing for Parenteral Drug Administration

FIGURE 9-18 NEVER RECAP A USED NEEDLE! Always dispose of uncapped needles in the appropriate sharps container. See Box 9-1 for Standard Precautions.

FIGURE 9-19 An UNUSED needle may need to be recapped before the medication is given to the patient. The "scoop method" is one way to recap an unused needle safely. Be sure not to touch the needle to the countertop or to the outside of the needle cap.

FIGURES 9-20 and 9-21 There are several types of needlestick prevention syringes. This example (Figure 9-20) has a guard over the unused syringe. After the injection, the nurse pulls the guard up over the needle until it locks into place (Figure 9-21).

FIGURE 9-22 The parts of a syringe and hypodermic needle.

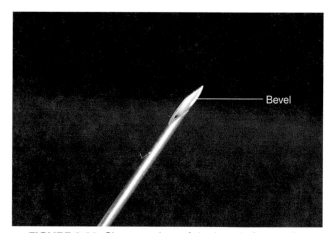

FIGURE 9-23 Close-up view of the bevel of a needle.

FIGURE 9-24 Be sure to choose the correct size and type of syringe for the drug ordered.

FIGURE 9-25 Needles come in various gauges and lengths. The larger the gauge number, the smaller the needle. Be sure to choose the correct needle—gauge and length—for the type of injection ordered.

FIGURES 9-26 and 9-27 Some medications come in prefilled sterile medication cartridges. Figures 9-26 and 9-27 show the Carpuject prefilled cartridge and syringe system. Follow the manufacturer's instructions for assembling prefilled syringes. After use, dispose of the syringe in a sharps container; the cartridge is reusable. Some prefilled syringes come with an air bubble in the syringe; do not expel the bubble before administration.

FIGURE 9-28 Ampules containing medications come in various sizes. The neck of the ampule must be broken carefully before the medication is withdrawn.

FIGURE 9-29 Use a filter needle when withdrawing medication from an ampule. Filter needles help to remove tiny glass particles that may result from the ampule breakage. DO NOT USE A FILTER NEEDLE FOR INJECTION INTO A PATIENT! Some facilities may also require the use of a filter needle to withdraw medications from a vial.

## Removing Medications from Ampules

Always begin by performing hand hygiene and maintain Standard Precautions (see Box 9-1). Gloves may be worn. When performing these procedures, keep in mind the following points:

- When removing medication from an ampule, use a sterile filter needle (Figure 9-29). These needles are designed to filter out glass particles that may be present inside the ampule after it is broken. The filter needle IS NOT intended for administration of the drug to the patient.
- Medication often rests in the top part of the ampule. Tap the top of the ampule lightly and quickly with your finger until all fluid moves to the bottom portion of the ampule (Figure 9-30).
- Place a small gauze pad or dry alcohol swab around the neck of the ampule to protect your hand. Snap the neck quickly and firmly, and break the ampule *away* from your body (Figures 9-31 and 9-32).
- To draw up the medication, either set the open ampule on a flat surface or hold the ampule upside down. Insert the filter needle (attached to a syringe) into the center of the ampule opening. Do not allow the needle tip or shaft to touch the rim of the ampule (Figure 9-33).

- Gently pull back on the plunger to draw up the medication. Keep the needle tip below the fluid within the vial; tip the ampule to bring all of the fluid within reach of the needle.
- If air bubbles are aspirated, do not expel them into the ampule. Remove the needle from the ampule, hold the syringe with the needle pointing up, and tap the side of the syringe with your finger to cause the bubbles to rise toward the needle. Draw back slightly on the plunger, and slowly push the plunger upward to eject the air. Do not eject fluid.
- Excess medication is disposed of into a sink. Hold the syringe vertically with the needle tip up and slanted toward the sink. Slowly eject the excess fluid into the sink, and then recheck the fluid level by holding the syringe vertically.
- Remove the filter needle and replace with the appropriate needle for administration. NEVER use a filter needle to administer medications to a patient!
- Be sure to ensure the sterility of the injection needle throughout the process. Do not touch the open end of the needle hub, or the tip of the syringe, when attaching a needle to a syringe.
- Dispose of the glass ampule pieces and the used filter needle in the appropriate sharps container.

## Removing Medications from Vials

Always begin by performing hand hygiene and maintain Standard Precautions (see Box 9-1). Gloves may be worn. When performing these procedures, keep in mind the following points:

- Vials can contain either a single dose or multiple doses of medication. Follow the institution's policy for using opened multidose vials, such as vials of insulin. Mark multidose vials with the date and time of opening and the discard date (per facility policy). If you are unsure about the age of an opened vial of medication, discard it and obtain a new one.
- Check institutional policies regarding which type of needle to use to withdraw fluid from a vial. With the exception of insulin, which must be withdrawn using an insulin syringe, fluid may be withdrawn from a vial using a blunt fill needle or a filter needle. Using a blunt fill needle reduces the chance of injury with a sharp needle (Figure 9-34).
- If the vial is unused, remove the cap from the top of the vial.

FIGURE 9-30 Tapping an ampule to move the fluid below the neck.

FIGURES 9-31 AND 9-32 Breaking an ampule. Carefully break the neck of the ampule in a direction *away* from you and away from others near you.

FIGURE 9-33 Using a filter needle to withdraw medication from an ampule.

- If the vial has been previously opened and used, wipe the top of the vial vigorously with an alcohol swab.
- Air must first be injected into a vial before fluid can be withdrawn. The amount of air injected into a vial needs to equal the amount of fluid that needs to be withdrawn.
- Determine the volume of fluid to be withdrawn from the vial. Pull back on the syringe's plunger to draw an amount of air into the syringe that is equivalent to the volume of medication to be removed from the vial. Insert the syringe into the vial, preferably using a needleless system. Figure 9-35 shows a needleless system for vial access. Inject the air into the vial.
- While holding onto the plunger, invert the vial and remove the desired amount of medication (Figure 9-36).
- Gently but firmly tap the syringe to remove air bubbles. Excess fluid, if present, must then be discarded into a sink.
- Some vials are not compatible with needleless systems and therefore require a needle for fluid withdrawals (Figure 9-37). Use a blunt fill needle if available (see Figure 9-34).
- When an injection requires two medications from two different vials, begin by injecting air into the first vial (without touching the fluid in the first vial), and then inject air into the second vial. Immediately remove the desired dose from the second vial. Change needles (if possible), and then remove the exact prescribed dose of drug from the first vial. Take great care not to contaminate the drug in one vial with the drug from the other vial. Check with a pharmacist to make sure the two drugs are compatible for mixing in the same syringe.
- For injections, if a needle has been used to remove medication from a vial, always change the needle before administering the dose. Changing needles ensures that a clean and sharp needle is used for the injection. Medication that remains on the outside of the needle may cause irritation to the patient's tissues. In addition, the needle may become dull if used to puncture a rubber stopper. However, some syringes, such as insulin syringes, have needles that are fixed onto the syringe and cannot be removed.
- Ensure the sterility of the injection needle throughout the process. Do not touch the open end of the needle hub, or the tip of the syringe, when attaching a needle to a syringe.

FIGURE 9-34 Comparison of the sharp tip of a needle for injection *(above)* with the blunt tip of a fill needle *(below)*, which is used to remove fluid from a vial.

FIGURE 9-35 Insert air into a vial before withdrawing medication (needleless system shown).

FIGURE 9-36 Withdrawing medication from a vial (needleless system shown).

FIGURE 9-37 Using a needle and syringe to remove medication from a vial.

# Injections Overview
## Needle Insertion Angles for Intramuscular, Subcutaneous, and Intradermal Injections

**FIGURE 9-38** Comparison of angles of needle insertion for injections.

- For any injection, if syringes are prepared at a medication cart or in a medication room, then each parenteral medication should be prepared separately and a label identifying the patient, the medication, the dose, and the route placed on the barrel of the syringe before the nurse leaves the preparation area.
- For intramuscular (IM) injections, insert the needle at a 90-degree angle (Figure 9-38). Intramuscular injections deposit the drug deep into muscle tissue, where the drug is absorbed through blood vessels within the muscle. The rate of absorption of medication given by the intramuscular route is slower than that of medications given by the intravenous route but faster than that of medications given by the subcutaneous route. Intramuscular injections generally require a longer needle to reach the muscle tissue, but shorter needles may be needed for older patients, children, and adults who are malnourished. The site chosen will also determine the length of the needle needed. In general, aqueous medications can be given with a 22- to 27-gauge needle, but oil-based or more viscous (thick) medications are given with an 18- to 25-gauge needle. Average needle lengths for children range from ⅝ to 1 inch, and needles for adults range from 1 to 1½ inches. The nurse must choose the needle length based on the size of the muscle at the injection site, the age of the patient, and the type of medication used. For a normal, well-developed adult, 3 mL is the maximum amount used in a single injection. Follow agency policy. If more than 3 mL is needed for the ordered dose, then the medication will need to be given in 2 separate injections. However, if the patient is an older adult, or thin, a smaller maximum volume, such as 2 mL, is recommended.
- For subcutaneous (subcut) injections, insert the needle at either a 45- or 90-degree angle. Subcutaneous injections deposit the drug into the loose connective tissue under the dermis. This tissue is not as well supplied with blood vessels as is the muscle tissue; as a result, drugs are absorbed more slowly than drugs given intramuscularly. Doses are usually 0.5 to 1 mL. In general, use a 25-gauge, ½- to ⅝-inch needle. A *90-degree angle* is used for an *average-sized* patient; a *45-degree angle* may be used for *thin, emaciated, and/or malnourished* adults and for children. To ensure correct needle

**FIGURE 9-39** Air-lock technique for intramuscular injections.

length, grasp the skinfold with thumb and forefinger, and choose a needle that is approximately half the length of the skinfold from top to bottom.
- Intradermal (ID) injections are given into the outer layers of the dermis in very small amounts, usually 0.01 to 0.1 mL. These injections are used mostly for diagnostic purposes, such as testing for allergies or tuberculosis, and for local anesthesia. Very little of the drug is absorbed systemically. In general, choose a tuberculin or 1-mL syringe with a 25- or 27-gauge needle that is ⅜ to ⅝ inch long. The angle of injection is 5 to 15 degrees.
- For specific information about giving injections to children, see Box 9-2.

## Air-Lock Technique

- Some facilities recommend administering intramuscular injections using the air-lock technique (Figure 9-39). Check institutional policies.
- After withdrawing the desired amount of medication into the syringe, withdraw an additional 0.2 mL of air. Be sure to inject using a 90-degree angle. The small air bubble that follows the medication during the injection may help prevent the medication from leaking through the needle track into the subcutaneous tissues.

## Intradermal Injections

**FIGURES 9-40 and 9-41** Intradermal injection.

Always begin by performing hand hygiene and maintain Standard Precautions (see Box 9-1). Gloves must be worn. When giving an intradermal injection, keep in mind the following points:

- Be sure to choose an appropriate site for the injection. Avoid areas of bruising, rashes, inflammation, edema, or skin discoloration.
- Help the patient to a comfortable position. Extend and support the elbow and forearm on a flat surface.
- In general, three to four finger widths below the antecubital space and one hand width above the wrist are the preferred locations on the forearm. Areas on the back that are also suitable for subcutaneous injection may be used if the forearm is not appropriate for the intradermal injection.
- Cleanse the site with an alcohol or antiseptic swab. Apply the swab at the center of the site, and cleanse outward in a circular direction for about 2 inches (5 cm) (see Figure 9-43); then let the skin dry.
- After cleansing the site, stretch the skin over the site with your nondominant hand.

- With the needle almost against the patient's skin, insert the needle, bevel UP, at a 5- to 15-degree angle until resistance is felt, and then advance the needle through the epidermis, approximately 3 mm (Figures 9-40 and 9-41). The needle tip should still be visible under the skin.
- Do not aspirate. This area under the skin contains very few blood vessels.
- Slowly inject the medication. It is normal to feel resistance, and a bleb that resembles a mosquito bite (about 6 mm in diameter) will form at the site if accurate technique is used.
- Withdraw the needle slowly while gently applying a gauze pad at the site, but do not massage the site.
- Dispose of the syringe and needle in the appropriate container. DO NOT RECAP the needle. Perform hand hygiene after removing gloves.
- Provide instructions to the patient as needed for a follow-up visit for reading the skin testing, if applicable.
- Document on the medication record the date of the skin testing and the date that results need to be read, if applicable.

## Subcutaneous Injections

Always begin by performing hand hygiene and maintain Standard Precautions (see Box 9-1). Gloves must be worn. When giving a subcutaneous injection, keep in mind the following points:

- Be sure to choose an appropriate site for the injection. Avoid areas of bruising, rashes, inflammation, edema, or skin discoloration (Figure 9-42).
- Ensure that the needle size is correct. Grasp the skinfold between your thumb and forefinger, and measure from top to bottom. The needle must be approximately one-half this length.
- Cleanse the site with an alcohol or antiseptic swab. Apply the swab at the center of the site, and cleanse outward in a circular direction for about 2 inches (5 cm) (Figure 9-43); then let the skin dry.
- Tell the patient that he or she will feel a "stick" as you insert the needle.
- For an average-sized patient, pinch the skin with your nondominant hand and inject the needle quickly at a 45- or 90-degree angle (Figure 9-44).
- For an obese patient, pinch the skin and inject the needle at a 90-degree angle. Be sure the needle is long enough to reach the base of the skinfold.
- *Age-related considerations:* For a child or a thin patient, pinch the skin gently and be sure to use a 45-degree angle when injecting the needle.
- Injections given in the abdomen must be given at least 2 inches away from the umbilicus because of the surrounding vascular structure (Figure 9-45). The injection site must also be 2 inches away from any incisions, stomas, or open wounds, if present.
- After the needle enters the skin, grasp the lower end of the syringe with your nondominant hand. Move your dominant hand to the end of the plunger—be careful not to move the syringe.
- Aspiration of medication to check for blood return is not necessary for subcutaneous injections, but some institutions may require it. Check institutional policy. Heparin injections and insulin injections are NOT aspirated before injection.
- With your dominant hand, slowly inject the medication.
- Withdraw the needle quickly, and place a swab or sterile gauze pad over the site.

- Apply gentle pressure but do not massage the site. If necessary, apply a bandage to the site.
- Dispose of the syringe and needle in the appropriate container. DO NOT RECAP the needle. Perform hand hygiene after removing gloves.
- Document the medication given on the medication record (see Figure 9-9), and monitor the patient for a therapeutic response as well as for adverse reactions.
- For injections of heparin or other subcutaneous anticoagulants, follow the manufacturer's instructions for injection technique as needed. Many manufacturers recommend the area of the abdomen known as the "love handles" for injection of anticoagulants. DO NOT ASPIRATE before injecting, and DO NOT massage the site after injection. These actions may cause a hematoma at the injection site.
- Heparin doses are ordered in units, but it is important to note that units of heparin are not the same as units of insulin. Heparin is *never* measured with insulin syringes.

### Insulin Syringes

- *Always use an insulin syringe to measure and administer insulin.* When giving small doses of insulin, use an insulin syringe that is calibrated for smaller doses. Figure 9-46 shows insulin syringes with two different calibrations. Notice that in the 100-unit syringe, each line represents 2 units; in the 50-unit syringe, each line represents 1 unit. NOTE: A unit of insulin is NOT equivalent to a milliliter of insulin!
- Figure 9-47 shows several examples of devices that can be used to help the patient self-administer insulin. These devices feature a multidose container of insulin and easy-to-read dials for choosing the correct dose. The needle is changed with each use. These devices are for single-patient use only and cannot be used by more than one patient due to the risk of blood contamination of the medication reservoir.
- When two different types of insulin are drawn up into the same syringe, always draw up the clear insulin into the syringe first (Figure 9-48). See p. 113 for information about mixing two types of insulin in one syringe.

**FIGURE 9-42** Potential sites for subcutaneous injections.

FIGURE 9-43 Before giving an injection, cleanse the skin with an alcohol or antiseptic swab using a circular motion.

FIGURE 9-44 Giving a subcutaneous injection at a 90-degree angle.

FIGURE 9-45 When giving a subcutaneous injection in the abdomen, be sure to choose a site at least 2 inches away from the umbilicus.

FIGURE 9-46 Insulin syringes are available in 100-unit and 50-unit calibrations.

FIGURE 9-47 A variety of devices are available for insulin injections.

FIGURE 9-48 Mixing two types of insulin in the same syringe. NOTE: The clear insulin is always drawn up into the syringe first.

## Intramuscular Injections

Always begin by performing hand hygiene and maintain Standard Precautions (see Box 9-1). Gloves must be worn. When giving an intramuscular (IM) injection, keep in mind the following points:

- Choose the appropriate site for the injection by assessing not only the size and integrity of the muscle but the amount and type of injection. Palpate potential sites for areas of hardness or tenderness, and note the presence of bruising or infection.
- The dorsogluteal injection site is no longer recommended for injections because of the close proximity to the sciatic nerve and major blood vessels. Injury to the sciatic nerve from an injection may cause partial paralysis of the leg. The dorsogluteal site is not to be used for intramuscular injections; instead, the ventrogluteal site is the preferred intramuscular injection site for adults and children.
- Assist the patient to the proper position, and ensure his or her comfort.
- Locate the proper site for the injection. Cleanse the site with an alcohol or antiseptic swab. Apply the swab at the center of the site, and cleanse outward in a circular direction for about 2 inches (5 cm) (see Figure 9-43); then let the skin dry. Keep a sterile gauze pad nearby for use after the injection.

- With your nondominant hand, pull the skin taut. Follow the instructions for the Z-track method (see later) if appropriate.
- Grasp the syringe with your dominant hand as if holding a dart and position the needle at a 90-degree angle to the skin. Tell the patient that he or she will feel a "stick" as you insert the needle.
- Insert the needle quickly and firmly into the muscle. Grasp the lower end of the syringe with the nondominant hand while still holding the skin back, to stabilize the syringe. With the dominant hand, pull back on the plunger for 5 to 10 seconds to check for blood return.
- If no blood appears in the syringe, inject the medication slowly, at the rate of 1 mL every 10 seconds. After injecting the drug, wait 10 seconds, and then withdraw the needle smoothly while releasing the skin.
- Apply gentle pressure at the site, and watch for bleeding. Apply a bandage if necessary.
- If blood does appear in the syringe, remove the needle, dispose of the medication and syringe, and prepare a new syringe with the medication.
- Dispose of the syringe and needle in the appropriate container. DO NOT RECAP the needle. Perform hand hygiene after removing gloves.
- Document the medication given on the medication record (see Figure 9-9), and monitor the patient for a therapeutic response as well as for adverse reactions.

### Z-Track Method

**FIGURES 9-49 and 9-50** Z-track method for intramuscular injections.

- The Z-track method is used for injections of irritating substances such as iron dextran and hydroxyzine. The technique reduces pain, irritation, and staining at the injection site. Some facilities recommend this method for *all* intramuscular injections (Figures 9-49 and 9-50).
- After choosing and preparing the site for injection, use your nondominant hand to pull the skin laterally and hold it in this position while giving the injection. Insert the needle at a 90-degree angle, aspirate for 5 to 10 seconds to check for blood return, and then inject the

medication slowly. After injecting the medication, wait 10 seconds before withdrawing the needle. Withdraw the needle slowly and smoothly, and maintain the 90-degree angle.
- Release the skin immediately after withdrawing the needle to seal off the injection site. This technique forms a Z-shaped track in the tissue that prevents the medication from leaking through the more sensitive subcutaneous tissue from the muscle site of injection. Apply gentle pressure to the site with a dry gauze pad.

## Ventrogluteal Site

- The ventrogluteal site is the *preferred* site for adults and children. It is considered the safest of all sites because the muscle is deep and away from major blood vessels and nerves (Figure 9-51).
- Position the patient on his or her side, with knees bent and upper leg slightly ahead of the bottom leg. If necessary, the patient may remain in a supine position.
- Palpate the greater trochanter at the head of the femur and the anterosuperior iliac spine. As illustrated in Figure 9-52, use the left hand to find landmarks when injecting into the patient's right ventrogluteal site, and use the right hand to find landmarks when injecting into the patient's

left ventrogluteal site. Place the palm of your hand over the greater trochanter and your index finger on the anterosuperior iliac spine. Point your thumb toward the patient's groin and fingers toward the patient's head. Spread the middle finger back along the iliac crest, toward the buttocks, as much as possible.

- The injection site is the center of the triangle formed by your middle and index fingers (see arrow in Figure 9-52).
- Before giving the injection, you may need to switch hands so that you can use your dominant hand to give the injection (Figure 9-53).
- Follow the general instructions for giving an intramuscular injection.

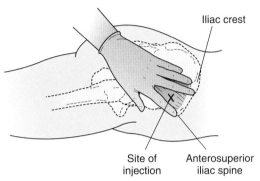

Iliac crest

Site of injection        Anterosuperior iliac spine

**FIGURE 9-51** Finding landmarks for a ventrogluteal injection.

**FIGURES 9-52 and 9-53** Ventrogluteal intramuscular injection.

## Vastus Lateralis Site

FIGURE 9-54 Vastus lateralis intramuscular injection in a small child. The nurse stabilizes the leg before giving the injection.

FIGURES 9-55, 9-56, and 9-57 Vastus lateralis intramuscular injection.

- Generally the vastus lateralis muscle is well developed and not located near major nerves or blood vessels. It is the preferred site of injection of drugs such as immunizations for infants (Figure 9-54). For specific information about giving injections to children, see Box 9-2.
- The patient may be sitting or lying supine; if supine, have the patient bend the knee of the leg in which the injection will be given.

- To find the correct site of injection, place one hand above the knee and one hand below the greater trochanter of the femur. Locate the midline of the anterior thigh and the midline of the lateral side of the thigh. The injection site is located within the rectangular area (Figures 9-55, 9-56, and 9-57).

---

### BOX 9-2 PEDIATRIC INJECTIONS

Site selection is crucial for pediatric injections. Factors to consider are the age of the child, the size of the muscle at the injection site, the type of injection, the thickness of the solution, and the ease with which the child can be positioned properly. There is no universal agreement in the literature on the "best" intramuscular injection site for children. For infants, the preferred site is the vastus lateralis muscle. The ventrogluteal site may also be used in children of all ages. For immunizations in toddlers and older children, the deltoid muscle may be used *if* the muscle mass is well developed. Intramuscular injections for older infants and small children should not exceed 1 mL in a single injection. Refer to facility policy.

Children are often extremely fearful of needles and injections. Even a child who appears calm may become upset and lose control during an injection procedure. For safety reasons, it is important to have another person available for positioning and holding the child.

Distraction techniques are helpful. Say to the child, "If you feel this you can ask me to take it out, please." Be quick and efficient when giving the injection.

Have a small, colorful bandage on hand to apply after the injection. If the child is old enough, have the child hold the bandage and apply it after the injection. If possible, offer a reward sticker after the injection.

After the injection, allow the child to express his or her feelings. For young children, encourage parents to offer comfort with holding and cuddling. Older children respond better if they receive praise.

EMLA (lidocaine/prilocaine) cream or a vapocoolant spray, if available, may be used before the injection to reduce the pain from the needle insertion. However, because these agents do not absorb down into the muscle, the child may still experience pain when the medication enters the muscle. Apply EMLA cream to the site at least 1 hour and up to 3 hours before the injection. Vapocoolant spray is applied to the site immediately before the injection. Another option is to apply a wrapped ice cube to the injection site for a minute before the injection.

From Hockenberry MJ, Wilson D: *Wong's nursing care of infants and children,* ed 9, St Louis, 2011, Mosby.

**Deltoid Site**

Deltoid muscle

Site of injection

**FIGURES 9-58, 9-59, and 9-60** Deltoid intramuscular injection. The deltoid site is not considered a primary site for intramuscular injections but is used for immunizations for toddlers, older children, and adults. This site is not used for infants.

- Even though the deltoid site (Figure 9-58) is easily accessible, it is *not* the first choice for intramuscular injections because the muscle may not be well developed in some adults, and the site carries a risk for injury because the axillary nerve lies beneath the deltoid muscle. In addition, the brachial artery and radial, brachial, and ulnar nerves are also located in the upper arm. Always check medication administration policies, because some facilities do not permit the use of the deltoid site for intramuscular injections. The deltoid site must only be used for administration of immunizations to toddlers, older children, and adults (not infants) and only for small volumes of medication (0.5 to 1 mL).
- The patient may be sitting or lying down. Remove clothing to expose the upper arm and shoulder; do not roll up tight-fitting sleeves. Have the patient relax his or her arm and slightly bend the elbow.
- Palpate the lower edge of the acromion process. This edge becomes the base of an imaginary triangle (Figure 9-59).
- Place three fingers below this edge of the acromion process. Find the point on the lateral arm in line with the axilla. The injection site will be in the center of this triangle, three finger widths (1 to 2 inches) below the acromion process.
- *Age-related considerations:* In children and smaller adults, it may be necessary to bunch the underlying tissue together before giving the injection and/or use a shorter (5/8-inch) needle (Figure 9-60).
- To reduce patient anxiety, have the patient look away before giving the injection.

## Preparing Intravenous Medications

Always begin by performing hand hygiene and maintain Standard Precautions (see Box 9-1). Gloves must be worn for most of these procedures. When administering intravenous (IV) drugs, keep in mind the following points:

- The intravenous route for medication administration provides for rapid onset and faster therapeutic drug levels in the blood than other routes. However, the intravenous route is also potentially more dangerous. Once an intravenous drug is given, it begins to act immediately and cannot be removed. The nurse must be aware of the drug's intended effects and possible adverse effects. In addition, hypersensitivity (allergic) reactions may occur quickly.
- Since the passage of the Needle Safety and Prevention Act of 2001, many institutions now use a needleless system for all infusion lines.
- Before giving an intravenous medication, assess the patient's drug allergies, assess the intravenous line for patency, and assess the site for signs of phlebitis or infiltration.
- When more than one intravenous medication is to be given, check with the pharmacy for compatibility if the medications are to be infused at the same time.
- Check the expiration date of both the medication and infusion bags.
- *Age-related considerations:* For children, infusion pumps *must* be used to prevent the risk of infusing the fluid and medication too fast.
- The Joint Commission requires that the pharmacy prepare intravenous solutions and intravenous piggyback (IVPB) admixtures under a special laminar airflow hood. Most IVPB medications come in vials that are added to the intravenous bag just before administration. On the rare occasion when you must dilute a drug for intravenous use, contact the pharmacist for instructions. Be sure to verify which type of fluid to use and the correct amount of solution for the dosage.
- It is important to choose the correct solution for diluting intravenous medications. For example, phenytoin must be infused with normal saline, not dextrose solutions (see Chapter 14). Check with the pharmacist if necessary.
- Most IVPB medications are provided as part of an "add-a-vial" system that allows the intravenous medication vial to be attached to a small-volume minibag for administration. Figure 9-61 shows two examples of IVPB medications attached to small-volume infusion bags.

- These IVPB medication setups allow for mixing of the drug and diluent immediately before the medication is given. Remember that if the seals are not broken and the medication is not mixed with the fluid in the infusion bag, then the medication stays in the vial! As a result, the patient does not receive the ordered drug dose; instead, the patient receives a small amount of plain intravenous fluid.
- One type of IVPB system that needs to be activated before administration is illustrated in Figure 9-62. To activate this type of IVPB system, snap the connection area between the intravenous infusion bag and the vial (Figure 9-63). Gently squeeze the fluid from the infusion bag into the vial and allow the medication to dissolve (Figure 9-64). After a few minutes, rotate the vial gently to ensure that all of the powder is dissolved. When the drug is fully dissolved, hold the IVPB apparatus by the vial and squeeze the bag; fluid will enter the bag from the vial. Make sure that all of the medication is returned to the IVPB bag.
- When hanging these IVPB medications, take care NOT to squeeze the bag. This may cause some of the fluid to leak back into the vial and alter the dose given.
- Always label the IVPB bag with the patient's name and room number, the name of the medication, the dose, the date and time mixed, your initials, and the date and time the medication was given.
- Some intravenous medications must be mixed using a needle and syringe. Again, in many facilities, this procedure will be performed in the pharmacy. Follow the facility policy. After checking the order and the compatibility of the drug and the intravenous fluid, wipe the port of the intravenous bag with an alcohol swab (Figure 9-65).
- Carefully insert the needle into the center of the port and inject the medication (Figures 9-66 and 9-67). Note how the medication remains in the lower part of the intravenous infusion bag. Turn the bag gently, end to end, to mix the fluid and added medication (Figure 9-68).
- Always add medication to a *new* bag of intravenous fluid, not to a bag that has partially infused. The concentration of the medication may be too strong if it is added to a partially full bag.
- Always label the intravenous infusion bag when a drug has been added (Figure 9-69). Label as per institution policy and include the patient's name and room number, the name of the medication, the date and time mixed, your initials, and the date and time the infusion was started. In addition, label all intravenous infusion tubing per institution policy.

**FIGURE 9-61** Two types of intravenous piggyback medication delivery systems. These intravenous systems must be activated before the drug is administered to the patient.

**FIGURE 9-62** Activating an intravenous piggyback infusion bag (step 1).

**FIGURE 9-63** Activating an intravenous piggyback infusion bag (step 2).

**FIGURE 9-64** Activating an intravenous piggyback infusion bag (step 3).

**FIGURES 9-65, 9-66, and 9-67** Adding a medication to an intravenous infusion bag with a needle and syringe.

**FIGURE 9-68** Mix the medication thoroughly before infusing by gently turning end to end. Do not shake the bag.

**FIGURE 9-69** Label the intravenous infusion bag when medication has been added.

## Infusions of Intravenous Piggyback Medications

Always begin by performing hand hygiene and maintain Standard Precautions (see Box 9-1). Gloves must be worn.

- Refrigerated medications may need to be left on the counter to warm to room temperature before administering. If you are infusing the IVPB medication for the first time, you will need to attach the medication bag to the appropriate tubing and "prime" the tubing by allowing just enough fluid through the tubing to flush out the air. Take care not to waste too much of the medication when flushing the tubing.
- If you are adding IVPB medication to an infusion that already has tubing, then use the technique of "backpriming" to flush the tubing (Figure 9-70). Backpriming allows for the administration of multiple intravenous medications without multiple disconnections, and thus reduces the risk of contamination of the intravenous tubing system.
- Backpriming allows the removal of the old medication fluid that has remained in the IVPB tubing from the previous dose of intravenous medication. After ensuring that the medication in the primary infusion (if any) is compatible with the medication in the IVPB bag, close the roller clamp on the primary infusion if the intravenous fluid is infusing by gravity flow (not necessary if an infusion pump is used). Remove the empty IVPB container from the intravenous pole, lower it to below the level of the primary infusion bag, and open the clamp on the IVPB tubing. This will allow fluid to flow from the primary intravenous bag into the empty IVPB bag. Then, close the clamp on the IVPB tubing and squeeze the fluid that is in the drip chamber into the old IVPB bag to remove the old medication fluid. At this point you may add the new dose of intravenous medication to the IVPB tubing.
- Backpriming will not be possible if the primary intravenous infusion contains heparin, aminophylline, a vasopressor, or multivitamins. Check with a pharmacist if unsure about compatibility.
- Stopping intravenous infusions of medications such as vasopressors for an IVPB medication may affect a patient's blood pressure; stopping intravenous heparin may affect the patient's coagulation levels. Be sure to assess carefully before adding an IVPB medication to an existing infusion. A separate intravenous line may be necessary.
- Figure 9-71 shows an IVPB medication infusion (also known as the *secondary infusion*) with a primary gravity infusion. When the IVPB bag is hung higher than the primary intravenous infusion bag, the IVPB medication will infuse until empty, then the primary infusion will take over again.
- When beginning the infusion, attach the IVPB tubing to the upper port on the primary intravenous tubing. A back-check valve above this port prevents the medication from infusing up into the primary intravenous infusion bag.
- Fully open the clamp of the IVPB tubing and regulate the infusion rate with the roller clamp of the primary infusion tubing. Be sure to note the drip factor of the tubing, and

calculate the drops per minute to set the correct infusion rate for the IVPB medication.

- Monitor the patient during the infusion. Observe for hypersensitivity and for adverse reactions. In addition, observe the intravenous infusion site for infiltration. Have the patient report if pain or burning occurs.
- Monitor the rate of infusion during the IVPB medication administration. Changes in arm position may alter the infusion rate.
- When the infusion is complete, clamp the IVPB tubing and check the primary intravenous infusion rate. If necessary, adjust the clamp to the correct infusion rate.
- Figure 9-72 shows an IVPB medication infusion with a primary infusion that is going through an electronic infusion pump.
- When giving IVPB drugs through an intravenous infusion controlled by a pump, attach the IVPB tubing to the port on the primary intravenous tubing above the pump. Open the roller clamp of the IVPB medication tubing. Make sure that the IVPB bag is higher than the primary intravenous infusion bag.
- Following the manufacturer's instructions, set the infusion pump to deliver the IVPB medication. Entering the volume of the IVPB bag and the desired time frame of the infusion (e.g., over a 60-minute period) will cause the pump to automatically calculate the flow rate for the IVPB medication. Start the IVPB infusion as instructed by the pump.
- Monitor the patient during the infusion, as described earlier.
- When the infusion is complete, the primary intravenous infusion will automatically resume.
- Document the medication given on the medication record (see Figure 9-9), and monitor the patient for a therapeutic response as well as for adverse reactions.
- When giving intravenous medications through a saline (heparin) lock, follow the facility's guidelines for the flushing protocol before and after the medication is administered.
- Figure 9-73 illustrates a volume-controlled administration set that can be used to administer intravenous medications. The chamber is attached to the infusion between the intravenous infusion bag and the intravenous tubing. Fill the chamber with the desired amount of fluid, and then add the medication via the port above the chamber, as shown in the photo. Be sure to cleanse the port with an alcohol swab before inserting the needle in the port. Label the chamber with the medication's name, dose, and time added and your initials. Infuse the drug at the prescribed rate.
- In patient-controlled analgesia (PCA), a specialized pump is used to allow patients to self-administer pain medications, usually opiates (Figure 9-74). These pumps allow the patient to self-administer only as much medication as needed to control the pain by pushing a button for intravenous bolus doses. Safety features of the pump prevent accidental overdoses. A patient receiving PCA pump infusions must be monitored closely for his or her response to the drug, excessive sedation, hypotension, and changes in mental and respiratory status. Follow the facility's guidelines for setup and use.

**FIGURE 9-70** Flush the intravenous piggyback (secondary) tubing by using the backpriming method. Fluid is drained through the tubing into the old intravenous piggyback bag, which is then discarded. The new dose of medication is then attached to the primed secondary tubing.

**FIGURE 9-71** Infusing an intravenous piggyback medication with a primary gravity infusion. Note how the primary bag is lower than the IVPB.

**FIGURE 9-72** Infusing an intravenous piggyback medication with the primary infusion on an electronic infusion pump.

**FIGURE 9-73** Adding a medication to a volume-controlled administration set.

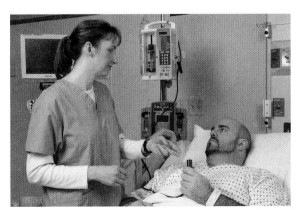

**FIGURE 9-74** Instructing the patient on the use of a patient-controlled analgesia pump.

- Figure 9-75 displays a smart pump, a new type of IV infusion safety system that has been designed to reduce IV medication errors. A smart pump contains built-in software that is programmed with facility-specific dosing profiles. The pump is able to "check" the dose-limits and other clinical guidelines, and when the pump is set up for patient use, it can warn the nurse if a potentially unsafe drug dose or therapy is entered.

## Intravenous Push Medications

Always begin by performing hand hygiene and maintain Standard Precautions (see Box 9-1).

When administering intravenous push (or bolus) medications, keep in mind the following points:

- Registered nurses are usually the only nursing staff members, besides a nurse anesthetist, allowed to give intravenous push medications. This may vary at different facilities.
- Intravenous push injections allow for rapid intravenous administration of a drug. The term *bolus* refers to a dose given all at once. Intravenous push injections may be given through an existing intravenous line, through an intravenous (saline or heparin) lock, or directly into a vein.
- Because the medication may have an immediate effect, monitor the patient closely for adverse reactions as well as for therapeutic effects.
- Follow the manufacturer's instructions carefully when preparing an intravenous push medication. Some drugs require careful dilution. Consult a pharmacist if you are unsure about the dilution procedure. Improper dilution may increase the risk of phlebitis and other complications.
- Some drugs are *never* given by intravenous push. Examples include dopamine, potassium chloride, and antibiotics such as vancomycin.
- Small amounts of medication, less than 1 mL, need to be diluted in 5 to 10 mL of normal saline or another compatible fluid to ensure that the medication does not collect in a "dead space" of the tubing (such as the Y-site port). Check the facility's policy.
- Most drugs given by intravenous push injection are to be given over a period of 1 to 5 minutes to reduce local or systemic adverse effects. Always time the administration with your watch, because it is difficult to estimate the time accurately. Adenosine, however, must be given very rapidly, within 2 to 3 seconds, for optimal action. ALWAYS check packaging information for guidelines, because many errors and adverse effects have been associated with too-rapid intravenous drug administration.

### Intravenous Push Medications through an Intravenous Lock

- Obtain two syringes of 0.9% normal saline (NS). Most facilities provide prefilled 10-mL syringes. Prepare medication for injection. (Facilities may differ in the protocol for intravenous lock flushes—follow institutional policies.) If ordered, prepare a syringe with heparin flush solution.
- Follow the guidelines for a needleless system, if used.
- Cleanse the injection port of the intravenous lock vigorously with an antiseptic swab for 15 seconds (Figure 9-76).

- Insert the syringe of NS into the injection port (Figure 9-77; a needleless system is shown). Open the clamp of the intravenous lock tubing, if present.
- Gently aspirate and observe for blood return. Absence of blood return does not mean that the intravenous line is occluded; further assessment may be required.
- Flush gently with saline while assessing for resistance. If resistance is felt, do not apply force. Stop and reassess the intravenous lock.
- Observe for signs of infiltration while injecting NS.
- Reclamp the tubing (if a clamp is present) and remove the NS syringe. Repeat cleansing of the port, and attach the medication syringe. Open the clamp again.
- Inject the medication over the prescribed length of time. Measure time with a watch or clock (Figure 9-78).
- When the medication is infused, clamp the intravenous lock tubing (if a clamp is present) and remove the syringe.
- Repeat cleansing of the port; attach an NS syringe and inject the contents into the intravenous lock slowly. If a heparin flush is ordered, attach the syringe containing heparin flush solution and inject slowly (per the institution's protocol).

### Intravenous Push Medications through an Existing Infusion

- Prepare the medication for injection. Follow the guidelines for a needleless system, if used.
- Check compatibility of the intravenous medication with the existing intravenous solution.
- Choose the injection port that is closest to the patient.
- Remove the cap, if present, and cleanse the injection port with an antiseptic swab.
- Occlude the intravenous line by pinching the tubing just above the injection port (Figure 9-79). Attach the syringe to the injection port.
- Gently aspirate for blood return.
- While keeping the intravenous tubing clamped, slowly inject the medication according to administration guidelines. Be sure to time the injection with a watch or clock.
- After the injection, release the intravenous tubing, remove the syringe, and check the infusion rate of the intravenous fluid.

### After Injection of Intravenous Push Medications

- Monitor the patient closely for adverse effects. Monitor the intravenous infusion site for signs of phlebitis and infiltration.
- Document medication given on the medication record (see Figure 9-9), and monitor the patient for a therapeutic response as well as for adverse reactions.

FIGURE 9-75 A smart pump.

**FIGURE 9-76** Cleanse the port vigorously for 15 seconds before attaching the syringe.

**FIGURE 9-77** Attaching the syringe to the intravenous lock, using a needleless system.

**FIGURE 9-78** Slowly inject the intravenous push medication through the intravenous lock; use a watch to time the injection.

**FIGURE 9-79** When giving an intravenous push medication through an intravenous line, pinch the tubing just above the injection port.

## TOPICAL DRUGS

### Administering Eye Medications

Always begin by performing hand hygiene and maintain Standard Precautions (see Box 9-1). Gloves must be worn. When administering eye preparations, keep in mind the following points:

- Assist the patient to a supine or sitting position. Tilt the patient's head back slightly. Make sure the patient is not wearing contact lenses.
- Remove any secretions with a sterile gauze pad; be sure to wipe from the inner to outer canthus (Figure 9-80).
- Have the patient tilt his or her head slightly back and look up. With your nondominant hand, gently pull the lower lid open to expose the conjunctival sac.

### Eyedrops

- With your dominant hand resting on the patient's forehead, hold the eye medication dropper 1 to 2 cm above the conjunctival sac. Do not touch the tip of the dropper to the eye or with your fingers (Figure 9-81).
- Drop the prescribed number of drops into the conjunctival sac. Never apply eyedrops to the cornea.
- If the drops land on the outer lid margins (if the patient moved or blinked), repeat the procedure.
- *Age-related considerations:* Infants often squeeze the eyes tightly shut to avoid eyedrops. To give drops to an uncooperative infant, restrain the head gently and place the drops at the corner near the nose where the eyelids meet. When the eye opens, the medication will flow into the eye.

### Eye Ointment

- Gently squeeze the tube of medication to apply an even strip of medication (about 1 to 2 cm) along the border of the conjunctival sac. Start at the inner canthus and move toward the outer canthus (Figure 9-82).

### After Instillation of Eye Medications

- Ask the patient to close the eye gently. Squeezing the eye shut may force the medication out of the conjunctival sac. A tissue may be used to blot liquid that runs out of the eye, but instruct the patient not to wipe the eye.
- You may apply gentle pressure to the patient's nasolacrimal duct for 30 to 60 seconds with a gloved finger wrapped in a tissue. This will help to reduce systemic absorption of the drug through the nasolacrimal duct and may also help to reduce the taste of the medication in the nasopharynx (Figure 9-83).
- If multiple eyedrops are due at the same time, then wait several minutes before administering the second medication. Check the instructions for the specific drug.
- Assist the patient to a comfortable position. Warn the patient that vision may be blurry for a few minutes.
- Document the medication given on the medication record (see Figure 9-9), and monitor the patient for a therapeutic response as well as for adverse reactions.

**FIGURE 9-80** Cleanse the eye, washing from the inner to outer canthus, before giving eye medications.

**FIGURE 9-81** Insert the eyedrop into the lower conjunctival sac.

FIGURE 9-82 Applying eye ointment. Move from the inner to outer canthus, along the border of the conjunctival sac.

FIGURE 9-83 Applying gentle pressure against the nasolacrimal duct after giving eye medication.

## Administering Eardrops

Always begin by performing hand hygiene and maintain Standard Precautions (see Box 9-1). Gloves may be worn. When administering ear preparations, keep in mind the following points:

- After explaining the procedure to the patient, assist the patient to a side-lying position with the affected ear facing up. If cerumen or drainage is noted in the outer ear canal, remove it carefully without pushing it back into the ear canal.
- Remove excessive amounts of cerumen before instillation of medication.
- If refrigerated, warm the ear medication by taking it out of refrigeration for at least 30 minutes before administration. Instillation of cold eardrops can cause nausea, dizziness, and pain.
- *Age-related considerations:* For an adult or a child older than 3 years of age, pull the pinna up and back (Figure 9-84). For an infant or a child younger than 3 years of age, pull the pinna down and back (Figure 9-85).

- Administer the prescribed number of drops. Direct the drops along the sides of the ear canal rather than directly onto the eardrum.
- Instruct the patient to lie on his or her side for 5 to 10 minutes. Gently massaging the tragus of the ear with a finger will help to distribute the medication down the ear canal.
- If ordered, a loose cotton pledget can be gently inserted into the ear canal to prevent the medication from flowing out. The cotton must remain somewhat loose to allow any discharge to drain out of the ear canal. To prevent the dry cotton from absorbing the eardrops that were instilled, moisten the cotton with a small amount of medication before inserting the pledget. Insertion of cotton too deeply may result in increased pressure within the ear canal and on the eardrum. Remove the cotton after about 15 minutes.
- If medication is needed in the other ear, wait 5 to 10 minutes after instillation of the first eardrops before administering.
- Document the medication given on the medication record (see Figure 9-9), and monitor the patient for a therapeutic response as well as for adverse reactions.

FIGURE 9-84 For adults, pull the pinna up and back.

FIGURE 9-85 For infants and children younger than 3 years of age, pull the pinna down and back.

## Administering Inhaled Drugs

Always begin by performing hand hygiene and maintain Standard Precautions (see Box 9-1). Gloves may be worn. Patients with asthma need to monitor their peak expiratory flow rates by using a peak flowmeter. A variety of inhalers are available (Figure 9-86). Be sure to check for specific instructions from the manufacturer as needed. Improper use will result in inadequate dosing. When administering inhaled preparations, keep in mind the following points.

### Metered-Dose Inhalers

- Shake the metered-dose inhaler (MDI) gently before using.
- Remove the cap; hold the inhaler upright and grasp with the thumb and first two fingers.
- Tilt the patient's head back slightly.
- If the inhaler is used without a spacer, do the following:
  1. Have the patient open his or her mouth; position the inhaler 1 to 2 inches away from the patient's mouth (Figure 9-87). For self-administration, some patients may measure this distance as 1 to 2 finger widths.
  2. Have the patient exhale, then press down once on the inhaler to release the medication; have the patient breathe in slowly and deeply for 5 seconds.
  3. Have the patient hold his or her breath for approximately 10 seconds, then exhale slowly through pursed lips.
- *Age-related considerations:* Spacers can be used with children and adults who have difficulty coordinating inhalations with activation of metered-dose inhalers (see Chapter 37). If the inhaler is used with a spacer, do the following:
  1. Attach the spacer to the mouthpiece of the inhaler after removing the inhaler cap.
  2. Place the mouthpiece of the spacer in the patient's mouth.
  3. Have the patient exhale.
  4. Press down on the inhaler to release the medication, and have the patient inhale deeply and slowly through the spacer. The patient then needs to breathe in and out slowly for 2 to 3 seconds, and then hold his or her breath for 10 seconds (Figure 9-88).

- If a second puff of the same medication is ordered, wait 1 to 2 minutes between puffs.
- If a second type of inhaled medication is ordered, wait 2 to 5 minutes between medication inhalations or as prescribed.
- If both a bronchodilator and a corticosteroid inhaled medication are ordered, the bronchodilator needs to be administered first so that the passages will be more open for the second medication.
- Instruct the patient to rinse his or her mouth after inhaling a corticosteroid medication to prevent the development of an oral fungal infection.
- Document the medication given on the medication record (see Figure 9-9), and monitor the patient for a therapeutic response as well as for adverse reactions.
- It is important to teach the patient how to calculate the number of doses in the inhaler and to keep track of uses. Simply shaking the inhaler to "estimate" whether it is empty is not accurate and may result in its being used when it is empty. Many MDIs now come with devices that help to count the remaining doses. If the inhaler does not have a dose-counting device, then the patient needs to be taught to count the number of puffs needed per day (doses) and divide this amount into the actual number of actuations (puffs) in the inhaler to estimate the number of days the inhaler will last. Then, a calendar can be marked a few days before this date with a note that it is time to obtain a refill. In addition, the date can be marked on the inhaler with a permanent marker. For example, an inhaler with 200 puffs, ordered to be used 4 times a day (2 puffs per dose, 8 puffs per day), would last for 25 days (200 divided by 8).
- Dry powder inhalers have varied instructions, so follow the manufacturer's instructions closely. Instruct patients to cover the mouthpiece completely with their mouths. Capsules that are intended for use with these inhalers must NEVER be taken orally. Some dry powder inhalers also have convenient built-in dose counters.

FIGURE 9-87 Using a metered-dose inhaler without a spacer.

FIGURE 9-88 Using a spacer device with a metered-dose inhaler.

FIGURE 9-86 **A,** Metered-dose inhaler (MDI). **B,** Automated, or breath-activated, MDI. **C,** Dry powder inhaler that delivers powdered medication.

## Small-Volume Nebulizers

- In some facilities, the air compressor is located in the wall unit of the room. In other facilities and at home, a small portable air compressor is used. Be sure to follow the manufacturer's instructions for use.
- In some facilities, nebulizer treatments may be performed by a respiratory therapist. However, closely monitor the patient before, during, and after the drug administration.
- Be sure to take the patient's baseline heart rate, especially if a beta-adrenergic drug is used. Some drugs may increase the heart rate.
- After gathering the equipment, add the prescribed medication to the nebulizer cup (Figure 9-89). Some medications will require a diluent; others are premixed with a diluent. Be sure to verify before adding a diluent.
- Have the patient hold the mouthpiece between his or her lips (Figure 9-90).
- *Age-related considerations:* Use a face mask for a child or an adult who is too fatigued to hold the mouthpiece. Special adaptors are available if the patient has a tracheostomy.
- Before starting the nebulizer treatment, have the patient take a slow, deep breath, hold it briefly, then exhale slowly. Patients who are short of breath should be instructed to hold their breath every fourth or fifth breath.
- Turn on the small-volume nebulizer machine (or turn on the wall unit) and make sure that a sufficient mist is forming.
- Instruct the patient to repeat the breathing pattern mentioned previously during the treatment.
- Occasionally tap the nebulizer cup during the treatment and toward the end to move the fluid droplets back to the bottom of the cup.
- Monitor the patient throughout treatment to ensure that the nebulizer medication is properly administered.
- Monitor the patient's heart rate during and after the treatment.
- If inhaled steroids are given, instruct the patient to rinse his or her mouth afterward.
- After the procedure, clean and store the tubing per institutional policy.
- Document the medication given on the medication record (see Figure 9-9), and monitor the patient for a therapeutic response as well as for adverse reactions.
- If the patient will be using a nebulizer at home, instruct the patient to rinse the nebulizer parts after each use with warm, clear water and to air-dry. Wash the parts daily with warm, soapy water and allowed to air-dry. Once a week, soak the nebulizer parts in a solution of vinegar and water (four parts water and one part white vinegar) for 30 minutes; rinse thoroughly with clear, warm water; and air-dry. Storing nebulizer parts that are still wet will encourage bacterial and mold growth.

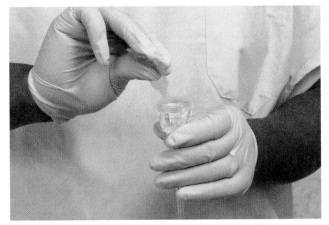

**FIGURE 9-89** Adding medication to the nebulizer cup.

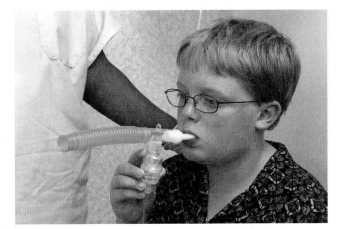

**FIGURE 9-90** Administering a small-volume nebulizer treatment.

## Administering Medications to the Skin

Always begin by performing hand hygiene and maintain Standard Precautions (see Box 9-1). Gloves must be worn. Avoid touching the preparations to your own skin. When administering skin preparations, keep in mind the following points.

### Lotions, Creams, Ointments, and Powders

- Apply powder to clean, dry skin. Have the patient turn his or her head to the other side during application to avoid inhalation of powder particles.
- Apply lotion to clean, dry skin. Remove residual from previous applications with soap and water.
- Before administering any dose of a topical skin medication, ensure that the site is dry and free of irritation. Thoroughly remove previous applications using soap and water, if appropriate for the patient's condition, and dry the area thoroughly. Be sure to remove any debris, drainage, or pus if present.
- *Age-related considerations:* The skin of an older patient may be more fragile and easily bruised. Be sure to handle the skin gently when cleansing to prepare the site for medication and when applying medications.
- With lotion, cream, or gel, obtain the correct amount with your gloved hand (Figure 9-91). If the medication is in a jar, remove the dose with a sterile tongue depressor and apply to your gloved hand. Do not contaminate the medication in the jar.
- Apply the preparation with long, smooth, gentle strokes that follow the direction of hair growth (Figure 9-92). Avoid excessive pressure. Be especially careful with the skin of elderly persons, because age-related changes may result in increased capillary fragility and tendency to bruise.
- Some ointments and creams may soil the patient's clothes and linens. If ordered, cover the affected area with gauze or a transparent dressing.
- Nitroglycerin ointment in a tube is measured carefully on clean ruled application paper before it is applied to the skin (Figure 9-93). Unit-dose packages are not to be measured. Do not massage nitroglycerin ointment into the skin. Apply the measured amount onto a clean, dry site, and then secure the application paper with a transparent dressing or a strip of tape. Always remove the old medication before applying a new dose. Rotate application sites.

### Transdermal Patches

- Be sure that the old patch is removed as ordered. Some patches may be removed before the next patch is due—check the order. Clear patches may be difficult to find, and patches may be overlooked in obese patients with skinfolds. Cleanse the site of the old patch thoroughly. Observe for signs of skin irritation at the old patch site. Rotate sites of application with each dose.
- Transdermal patches need to be applied at the same time each day if ordered daily.
- The old patch can be pressed together and then wrapped in a glove as you remove the glove from your hand. Dispose in the proper container according to the facility's policy.
- Select a new site for application and ensure that it is clean and without powder or lotion. For best absorption and fewest adverse effects, the site needs to be hairless and free from scratches or irritation. If it is necessary to remove hair, clip the hair instead of shaving to reduce irritation to the skin. Application sites may vary. Follow the drug manufacturer's specific instructions as to where to apply the patch.
- Remove the backing from the new patch (Figure 9-94). Take care not to touch the medication side of the patch with your fingers.
- Place the patch on the skin site and press firmly (Figure 9-95). Press around the edges of the patch with one or two fingers to ensure that the patch is adequately secured to the skin. If an overlay is provided by the drug manufacturer, apply it over the patch.
- Instruct the patient not to cut transdermal patches. Cutting transdermal patches releases all of the medication at once and may result in a dangerous overdose.

### After Administration of Topical Skin Preparations

- Document the medication given on the medication record (see Figure 9-9), and monitor the patient for a therapeutic response as well as for adverse reactions.
- Provide instruction on administration to the patient and/or caregiver.

**FIGURE 9-91** Use gloves to apply topical skin preparations.

**FIGURE 9-92** Spread the lotion on the skin with long, smooth, gentle strokes.

**FIGURE 9-93** Measure nitroglycerin ointment carefully before application.

**FIGURE 9-94** Opening a transdermal patch medication.

**FIGURE 9-95** Ensure that the edges of the transdermal patch are secure after applying.

## Administering Nasal Medications

Always begin by performing hand hygiene and maintain Standard Precautions (see Box 9-1). Patients may self-administer some of these drugs after proper instruction. Gloves must be worn. When administering nasal medications, keep in mind the following points:

- Before giving nasal medications, explain the procedure to the patient and tell him or her that temporary burning or stinging may occur. Instruct the patient that it is important to clear the nasal passages by blowing his or her nose, unless contraindicated (e.g., with increased intracranial pressure or nasal surgery), before administering the medication. Assess for deviated septum or a history of nasal fractures, because these may impede the patient's ability to inhale through the affected nostril.
- Figure 9-96 illustrates various delivery forms for nasal medications: sprays, drops, and metered-dose sprays.
- Assist the patient to a supine position. Support the patient's head as needed.
- If specific areas are targeted for the medication, position as follows:
  - For the posterior pharynx, position the head backward.
  - For the ethmoid or sphenoid sinuses, place the head gently over the top edge of the bed or place a pillow under the shoulders and tilt the head back.
  - For the frontal or maxillary sinuses, place the head back and turned toward the side that is to receive the medication.

### Nasal Drops

- Hold the nose dropper approximately ½ inch above the nostril. Administer the prescribed number of drops toward the midline of the ethmoid bone (Figure 9-97).

- Repeat the procedure as ordered, instilling the indicated number of drops per nostril.
- Keep the patient in a supine position for 5 minutes.
- *Age-related considerations:* Infants are nose breathers, and the potential congestion caused by nasal medications may make it difficult for them to suck. If nose drops are ordered, administer them 20 to 30 minutes before a feeding.

### Nasal Spray

- Have the patient sitting upright, and occlude one nostril by pressing a finger against the outer nare. After gently shaking the nasal spray container, insert the tip into the nostril. Squeeze the spray bottle into the nostril while the patient inhales through the open nostril (Figure 9-98).
- Repeat the procedure as ordered, instilling the indicated number of sprays per nostril.
- Keep the patient in a supine position for 5 minutes.

### After Administration of Nasal Medicines

- Offer the patient tissues for blotting any drainage, but instruct the patient to avoid blowing his or her nose for several minutes after instillation of the drops.
- Assist the patient to a comfortable position.
- Document the medication given on the medication record (see Figure 9-9), and document drainage, if any. Monitor the patient for a therapeutic response as well as for adverse reactions.

**FIGURE 9-96** Nasal medications may come in various delivery forms.

**FIGURE 9-97** Administering nose drops.

**FIGURE 9-98** Before self-administering the nasal spray, the patient needs to occlude the other nostril.

## Administering Vaginal Medications

Always begin by performing hand hygiene and maintain Standard Precautions (see Box 9-1). Gloves must be worn. When administering vaginal preparations, keep in mind the following points:

- Vaginal suppositories are larger and more oval than rectal suppositories (Figure 9-99).
- Figure 9-100 shows examples of a vaginal suppository in an applicator and vaginal cream in an applicator.
- Before giving these medications, explain the procedure to the patient and have her void the bladder.
- If possible, administer vaginal preparations at bedtime to allow the medications to remain in place as long as possible.
- Some patients may prefer to self-administer vaginal medications. Provide specific instructions if necessary.
- Position the patient in the lithotomy position and elevate the hips with a pillow, if tolerated. Be sure to drape the patient to provide privacy.

### Creams, Foams, or Gels Applied with an Applicator

- Fit the applicator to the tube of the medication, and then gently squeeze the tube to fill the applicator with the correct amount of medication.
- Lubricate the tip of the applicator with water-soluble lubricant.
- Use your nondominant hand to spread the labia and expose the vagina. Gently insert the applicator as far as possible into the vagina (Figure 9-101).
- Push the plunger to deposit the medication. Remove the applicator and wrap it in a paper towel for cleaning.

### Suppositories or Vaginal Tablets

- For suppositories or vaginal tablets, remove the wrapping and lubricate the suppository with a water-soluble lubricant. Be sure that the suppository is at room temperature.

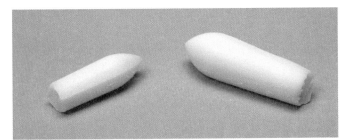

**FIGURE 9-99** Vaginal suppositories *(right)* are larger and more oval than rectal suppositories *(left)*.

**FIGURE 9-100** Vaginal cream and suppository, with applicators.

- Using the applicator provided, insert the suppository or tablet into the vagina, and then push the plunger to deposit the suppository. Remove the applicator.
- If no applicator is available, use your dominant index finger to insert the suppository about 2 inches into the vagina (Figure 9-102).
- Have the patient remain in a supine position with hips elevated for 5 to 10 minutes to allow the suppository to melt and the medication to be absorbed.
- If the patient desires, apply a perineal pad.
- If the applicator is to be reused, wash with soap and water and store in a clean container for the next use.
- Document the medication given on the medication record (see Figure 9-9), and monitor the patient for a therapeutic response as well as for adverse reactions.

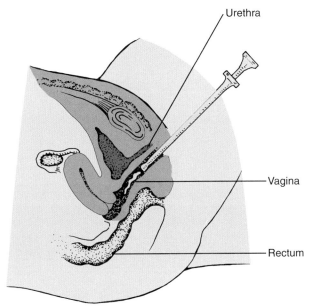

**FIGURE 9-101** Administering vaginal cream with an applicator.

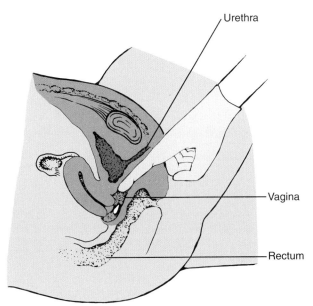

**FIGURE 9-102** Administering a vaginal suppository.

### PART 2

# Drugs Affecting the Central Nervous System

## VOCABULARY

In any subject matter, mastering the vocabulary is essential to mastering the content. However, in a complex, technical subject such as nursing pharmacology, if the vocabulary is not mastered, understanding the content will be almost impossible. Each chapter in this text contains a list of key terms at the beginning, and as an independent learner, you should spend some time and energy on the vocabulary contained in the key terms. Do not expect to completely understand and master the words from the key terms alone. The terms are further defined and explained in the body of the chapter, and it is when you  read the chapter that you should expect to fully master the vocabulary. However, the time you spend working on the key terms will pay off when you read the chapter.

Consider the terms *agonist* and *antagonist* in the Chapter 10 key terms. These terms share a common word part, which means the words are related in meaning. This is an important first step in mastering them. What does *agonist* mean? What is the similarity between *agonist* and *antagonist*? What is the essential difference between the two? Asking these questions as you start to work on Chapter 10 is a valuable technique for beginning to master the content. Do not simply memorize the terms. Learn what they mean and link relationships between words with common elements. As you practice this technique it will become easier to retain the meaning. The Chapter 10 key terms also contain other words that should be viewed as a group that shares an important relationship. The first of these words is *pain*. The definition provided is clear and relatively easy to understand, but your focus should be not just on that single word, because there are 13 other words that relate to pain: *acute, breakthrough, cancer, central, chronic, deep, neuropathic, phantom, referred, somatic, superficial, vascular,* and *visceral.* Each of these words defines and categorizes pain in a very specific way. As you go about setting up vocabulary cards, look at the opening pages in this chapter. You will find considerable discussion of these terms, which is useful in helping you obtain the fullest understanding of these terms. Do not simply focus on a meaning of each term, but also ask what the similarities and/or differences are and how these words relate to one another.

## TEXT NOTATION

The Study Skills Tips for Part 1 discussed a method for text underlining. If it is done carefully, this strategy is particularly useful for later review of text material. The object of text underlining is to pick out important terms, ideas, and key information so you can come back to it later for quick review. The three key elements in successful text notation are as follows:

1. Read the material once before attempting any underlining.
2. Be acutely aware of the author's language.
3. Be selective in underlining. The most common fault in underlining is to mark too much material.

The following are three paragraphs from Chapter 10 that have been underlined. The underlining should be viewed as an example of what can be done. Each reader will mark the text somewhat differently based on his or her background and  experience. As you study this example, think not only about what has been underlined but also about why that material was chosen.

    <u>Pain</u> is <u>most commonly defined</u> as an <u>unpleasant sensory and emotional experience</u> associated with either actual or potential tissue damage. It is a very personal and individual experience. Pain can be defined as whatever the patient says it is, and it exists whenever the patient says it does. Although the mechanisms of pain are becoming better understood, <u>a patient's perception of pain is a complex process. Pain involves physical, psychological, and even cultural factors.</u> Because pain intensity cannot be precisely quantified, health care providers must cultivate relationships of mutual trust with their patients to provide optimal care.

    There is <u>no single approach to effective pain management.</u> Instead, pain management is tailored to each patient's needs. The cause of the pain, the existence of concurrent medical conditions; the characteristics of the pain; and the psychological and cultural characteristics of the patient need to be considered. It also requires ongoing reassessment of the pain and the effectiveness of treatment. The patient's <u>emotional response to pain depends</u> on his or her <u>psychological experiences of pain.</u> Pain results from the <u>stimulation of sensory nerve fibers</u> known as <u>nociceptors.</u> These <u>receptors transmit pain signals</u> from various body regions to the <u>spinal cord and brain, which leads to the sensation of pain, or</u> <u>nociception.</u>

    The <u>physical impulses</u> that signal pain <u>activate various nerve pathways</u> from the <u>periphery to the spinal cord and to the brain.</u> The level of stimulus needed to produce a painful sensation is <u>referred to as the</u> <u>pain threshold.</u> Because this is a <u>measure of the physiologic response</u> of the nervous system, it is <u>similar for most persons.</u> However, <u>variations in pain sensitivity</u> may result from genetic factors.

## LANGUAGE CONVENTIONS

Certain words and phrases are like signal lights at an intersection. They serve to tell the reader that something special, important, or noteworthy is happening. To the attentive, active reader, these conventions contribute significantly to understanding what the author is trying to convey. Whether you are highlighting, underlining, writing margin notes, or studying the material using the PURR model, it is important that you become sensitive to these conventions.

The text following the topic heading *Anatomy, Physiology, and Pathophysiology Overview* in Chapter 10 contains several examples. The first sentence of the third paragraph contains the phrase *classified as.* Whenever an author says that something is being classified it means that there are at least two (and perhaps several more) elements of the term or idea that are being classified. This means that you should immediately ask a question about the reading, "What is being classified? How many classifications are there for this?" These questions will help you focus on what to learn and keep your attention firmly fixed on the process of learning.

As you read this chapter, or any other chapter, become aware of words and phrases like these that are intended to draw your attention to something the author wanted to emphasize. The more aware of language conventions you become, the easier it will be to become a selective reader. Selective readers do not try to remember everything they read, but they are able to select from the mass of information those concepts and/or terms that the writers tried to stress.

# Analgesic Drugs

## OBJECTIVES

When you reach the end of this chapter, you will be able to do the following:

1 Define *acute pain* and *chronic pain.*
2 Contrast the signs, symptoms, and management of acute and chronic pain.
3 Discuss the pathophysiology and characteristics associated with cancer pain and other special pain situations.
4 Describe pharmacologic and nonpharmacologic approaches for the management of acute and chronic pain.
5 Discuss the use of nonopioids, nonsteroidal antiinflammatory drugs, opioids (opioid agonists, opioids with mixed actions, opioid agonists-antagonists and antagonists), and miscellaneous drugs in the management of pain, including acute and chronic pain, cancer pain, and special pain situations.
6 Identify examples of drugs classified as nonopioids, nonsteroidal antiinflammatory drugs, opioids (opioid agonists, opioids with mixed actions, opioid agonists-antagonists and antagonists), and miscellaneous drugs.
7 Briefly describe the mechanism of action, indications, dosages, routes of administration, adverse effects, toxicity, cautions,

contraindications, and drug interactions of nonopioids, nonsteroidal antiinflammatory drugs (see Chapter 44), opioids (opioid agonists, opioids with mixed actions, opioid agonists-antagonists and antagonists), and miscellaneous drugs.
8 Contrast the pharmacologic and nonpharmacologic management of acute and chronic pain with the management of pain associated with cancer and pain experienced in terminal conditions.
9 Briefly describe the specific standards of pain management as defined by the World Health Organization and The Joint Commission.
10 Develop a nursing care plan based on the nursing process related to the use of nonopioid and opioid drug therapy for patients in pain.
11 Identify various resources, agencies, and professional groups that are involved in establishing standards for the management of all types of pain and for promotion of a holistic approach to the care of patients with acute or chronic pain and those in special pain situations.

## DRUG PROFILES

- ◆ **acetaminophen, p. 157**
  **codeine sulfate, p. 153**
  **fentanyl, p. 153**
  **lidocaine, transdermal, p. 157**
  **meperidine hydrochloride, p. 154**
  **methadone hydrochloride, p. 154**
- ◆ **morphine sulfate, p. 151**

- ◆ **naloxone hydrochloride, p. 155**
  **naltrexone hydrochloride, p. 155**
  **oxycodone hydrochloride, p. 154**
  **tramadol hydrochloride, p. 157**

  ---

- ◆ *Key drug*

## KEY TERMS

**Acute pain** Pain that is sudden in onset, usually subsides when treated, and typically occurs over less than a 6-week period. (p. 142)

**Addiction** A chronic, neurobiologic disease whose development is influenced by genetic, psychosocial, and environmental factors (same as *psychological dependence*). (p. 144)

**Adjuvant analgesic drugs** Drugs that are added for combined therapy with a primary drug and may have additive or independent analgesic properties, or both. (p. 141)

**Agonist** A substance that binds to a receptor and causes a response. (p. 147)

**Agonists-antagonists** Substances that bind to a receptor and cause a partial response that is not as strong as that caused by an agonist (also known as a *partial agonist*). (p. 147)

**Analgesic ceiling effect** What occurs when a given pain drug no longer effectively controls a patient's pain despite the administration of the highest safe dosages. (p. 147)

**Analgesics** Medications that relieve pain without causing loss of consciousness (sometimes referred to as *painkillers*). (p. 141)

**Antagonist** A drug that binds to a receptor and prevents (blocks) a response. (p. 147)

**Breakthrough pain** Pain that occurs between doses of pain medication. (p. 146)

**Cancer pain** Pain resulting from any of a variety of causes related to cancer and/or the metastasis of cancer. (p. 143)

**Central pain** Pain resulting from any disorder that causes central nervous system damage. (p. 143)

**Chronic pain** Persistent or recurring pain that is often difficult to treat. Includes any pain lasting longer than 3 to 6 months, pain lasting longer than 1 month after healing of an acute injury, or pain that accompanies a nonhealing tissue injury. (p. 142)

**Deep pain** Pain that occurs in tissues below skin level; opposite of *superficial pain*. (p. 143)

**Gate theory** The most well-described theory of pain transmission and pain relief. It uses a gate model to explain how impulses from damaged tissues are sensed in the brain. (p. 143)

**Narcotics** A legal term established under the Harrison Narcotic Act of 1914. It originally applied to drugs that produce insensibility or stupor, especially the opioids (e.g., morphine, heroin). Currently used to refer to any medically used controlled substances and in legal settings to refer to any illicit or "street" drug. (NOTE: This term is falling out of use in favor of *opioid* and will not be used further in this text.)

**Neuropathic pain** Pain that results from a disturbance of function or pathologic change in a nerve. (p. 143)

**Nociception** Processing of pain signals in the brain that gives rise to the feeling of pain. (p. 142)

**Nociceptors** A subclass of sensory nerves (A and C fibers) that transmit pain signals to the central nervous system from other body parts. (p. 142)

**Nonopioid analgesics** Analgesics that are not classified as opioids. (p. 143)

**Nonsteroidal antiinflammatory drugs (NSAIDs)** A large, chemically diverse group of drugs that are analgesics and also possess antiinflammatory and antipyretic activity but are not corticosteroids. (p. 143)

**Opioid analgesics** Synthetic drugs that bind to opiate receptors to relieve pain. (p. 141)

**Opioid naïve** Describes patients who are receiving opioid analgesics for the first time and who therefore are not accustomed to their effects. (p. 150)

**Opioid tolerance** A normal physiologic condition that results from long-term opioid use, in which larger doses of opioids are required to maintain the same level of analgesia and in which abrupt discontinuation of the drug results in withdrawal symptoms (same as *physical dependence*). (p. 144)

**Opioid tolerant** The opposite of opioid naïve; describes patients who have been receiving opioid analgesics (legally or otherwise) for a period of time (1 week or longer) and who are at greater risk of opioid withdrawal syndrome upon sudden discontinuation. (p. 145)

**Opioid withdrawal** The signs and symptoms associated with abstinence from or withdrawal of an opioid analgesic when the body has become physically dependent on the substance. (p. 150)

**Pain** An unpleasant sensory and emotional experience associated with actual or potential tissue damage. (p. 141)

**Pain threshold** The level of a stimulus that results in the sensation of pain. (p. 142)

**Pain tolerance** The amount of pain a patient can endure without its interfering with normal function. (p. 142)

**Partial agonist** A drug that binds to a receptor and causes a response that is less than that caused by a full agonist (same as *agonist-antagonist*). (p. 147)

**Phantom pain** Pain experienced in the area of a body part that has been surgically or traumatically removed. (p. 143)

**Physical dependence** A condition in which a patient takes a drug over a period of time and unpleasant physical symptoms (withdrawal symptoms) occur if the drug is stopped abruptly or smaller doses are given. The physical adaptation of the body to the presence of an opioid or other addictive substance. (p. 142)

**Psychologic dependence** A pattern of compulsive use of opioids or any other addictive substance characterized by a continuous craving for the substance and the need to use it for effects other than pain relief (also called *addiction*). (p. 144)

**Referred pain** Pain occurring in an area away from the organ of origin. (p. 143)

**Somatic pain** Pain that originates from skeletal muscles, ligaments, or joints. (p. 143)

**Special pain situations** The general term for pain control situations that are complex and whose treatment typically involves multiple medications, various health care personnel, and nonpharmacologic therapeutic modalities (e.g., massage, chiropractic care, surgery). (p. 164)

**Superficial pain** Pain that originates from the skin or mucous membranes; opposite of *deep pain*. (p. 143)

**Synergistic effects** Drug interactions in which the effect of a combination of two or more drugs with similar actions is greater than the sum of the individual effects of the same drugs given alone. For example, 1 + 1 is greater than 2. (p. 146)

**Tolerance** The general term for a state in which repetitive exposure to a given drug, over time, induces changes in drug receptors that reduce the drug's effects (same as *physical dependence*). (p. 142)

**Vascular pain** Pain that results from pathology of the vascular or perivascular tissues. (p. 143)

**Visceral pain** Pain that originates from organs or smooth muscles. (p. 143)

**World Health Organization (WHO)** An international body of health care professionals, including clinicians and epidemiologists among many others, that studies and responds to health needs and trends worldwide. (p. 146)

## ANATOMY, PHYSIOLOGY, AND PATHOPHYSIOLOGY OVERVIEW

The management of pain is a very important aspect of nursing care in a variety of settings and across the lifespan. Pain is the most common reason that patients seek health care, resulting in some 70 million office visits annually in the United States. Surgical and diagnostic procedures often require pain management, as do several diseases including arthritis, diabetes, multiple sclerosis, cancer, and acquired immunodeficiency syndrome (AIDS). Pain leads to much suffering and is a tremendous economic burden in terms of lost workplace productivity, workers' compensation payments, and other related health care costs.

To provide quality patient care, you must be well informed about both pharmacologic and nonpharmacologic methods of pain management. This chapter focuses on pharmacologic methods of pain management. Nonpharmacologic methods of pain management are listed in Box 10-1.

Medications that relieve pain without causing loss of consciousness are classified as analgesics. They are also commonly referred to as *painkillers*. There are various classes of analgesics, determined by their chemical structures and mechanisms of action. This chapter focuses primarily on the opioid analgesics, which are used to manage moderate to severe pain. Often drugs from other chemical categories are added to the opioid regimen as adjuvant analgesic drugs (or adjuvants) and are described later.

Pain is most commonly defined as an unpleasant sensory and emotional experience associated with either actual or potential tissue damage. It is a very personal and individual experience. Pain can be defined as whatever the patient says it is, and it exists whenever the patient says it does. Although the mechanisms of pain are becoming better understood, a patient's perception of pain is a complex process. Pain involves physical, psychological, and even cultural factors (see Patient-Centered Care: Cultural Implications box). Because pain intensity cannot be precisely quantified, health care providers must cultivate relationships of mutual trust with their patients to provide optimal care.

### 🌐 PATIENT-CENTERED CARE: CULTURAL IMPLICATIONS

#### *The Patient Experiencing Pain*

- Each culture has its own beliefs, thoughts, and ways of approaching, defining, and managing pain. Attitudes, meanings, and perceptions of pain vary with culture, race, and ethnicity.
- African Americans believe in the power of healers who rely strongly on the religious faith of people and often use prayer and the laying on of hands for relief of pain.
- Hispanic Americans believe in prayer, the wearing of amulets, and the use of herbs and spices to maintain health and wellness. Specific herbs are used in teas and therapies, often including religious practices, massage, and cleansings.
- Some traditional methods of healing for the Chinese include acupuncture, herbal remedies, yin and yang balancing, and cold treatment. *Moxibustion,* in which cones or cylinders of pulverized wormwood are burned on or near the skin over specific meridian points, is another form of healing.
- Asian and Pacific Islander patients are often reluctant to express their pain because they believe that the pain is God's will or is punishment for past sins.
- For many Native Americans, treatments for pain include massage, the application of heat, sweat baths, herbal remedies, and being in harmony with nature.
- In Arab culture, patients are expected to express their pain openly and anticipate immediate relief, preferably through injections or intravenous drugs.
- Remain aware of all cultural influences on health-related behaviors and on patients' attitudes toward medication therapy and thus, ultimately, on its effectiveness. A thorough assessment that includes questions about the patient's cultural background and practices is important to the effective and individualized delivery of nursing care.

### BOX 10-1  NONPHARMACOLOGIC TREATMENT OPTIONS FOR PAIN

- Acupressure
- Acupuncture
- Art therapy
- Behavioral therapy
- Biofeedback
- Comfort measures
- Counseling
- Distraction
- Hot or cold packs
- Hypnosis
- Imagery
- Massage
- Meditation
- Music therapy
- Pet therapy
- Physical therapy
- Reduction of fear
- Relaxation
- Surgery
- Therapeutic baths
- Therapeutic communication
- Therapeutic touch
- Transcutaneous electric nerve stimulation
- Yoga

There is no single approach to effective pain management. Instead, pain management is tailored to each patient's needs. The cause of the pain, the existence of concurrent medical conditions; the characteristics of the pain; and the psychological and cultural characteristics of the patient need to be considered. It also requires ongoing reassessment of the pain and the effectiveness of treatment. The patient's emotional response to pain depends on his or her psychological experiences of pain. Pain results from the stimulation of sensory nerve fibers known as nociceptors. These receptors transmit pain signals from various body regions to the spinal cord and brain, which leads to the sensation of pain, or nociception (Figure 10-1).

The physical impulses that signal pain activate various nerve pathways from the periphery to the spinal cord and to the brain. The level of stimulus needed to produce a painful sensation is referred to as the pain threshold. Because this is a measure of the physiologic response of the nervous system, it is similar for most persons. However, variations in pain sensitivity may result from genetic factors.

There are three main receptors believed to be involved in pain. The mu receptors in the dorsal horn of the spinal cord appear to play the most crucial role. Less important but still involved in pain sensations are the kappa and delta receptors. Pain receptors are located in both the central nervous system (CNS) and various body tissues. Pain perception—and, conversely, emotional well-being—is closely linked to the number of mu receptors. This number is controlled by a single gene, the mu opioid receptor gene. When the number of receptors is high, pain sensitivity is diminished. Conversely, when the receptors are reduced or missing altogether, relatively minor noxious stimuli may be perceived as painful.

The patient's emotional response to the pain is also molded by the patient's age, sex, culture, previous pain experience, and anxiety level. Whereas pain threshold is the physiologic element of pain, the psychological element of pain is called pain tolerance. This is the amount of pain a patient can endure without its interfering with normal function. Because it is a subjective response, pain tolerance can vary from patient to patient. Pain tolerance can be modulated by the patient's personality, attitude, environment, culture, and ethnic background. Pain tolerance can even vary within the same person depending on the circumstances involved. Table 10-1 lists the various conditions that can alter one's pain tolerance.

Pain can also be further classified in terms of its onset and duration as either acute or chronic. Acute pain is sudden and usually subsides when treated. One example of acute pain is postoperative pain. Chronic pain is persistent or recurring, lasting 3 to 6 months. It is often more difficult to treat, because changes occur in the nervous system that often require increasing drug dosages. This situation is known by the general term tolerance or physical dependence (see Chapter 17). Acute and chronic pain differ in their onset and duration, their associated diseases or conditions, and the way they are treated. Table 10-2 lists the different characteristics of acute and chronic pain and various diseases and conditions associated with each.

**FIGURE 10-1** Illustration of the four processes of nociception. (From Jarvis C: *Physical examination and health assessment,* ed 6, St Louis, 2012, Saunders.)

Pain can be further classified according to its source. The two most common sources of pain are somatic and visceral. Somatic pain originates from skeletal muscles, ligaments, and joints. Visceral pain originates from organs and smooth muscles. Sometimes pain is described as superficial. Superficial pain originates from the skin and mucous membranes. Deep pain occurs in tissues below skin level. Pain may be appropriately treated when the source of the pain is known. For example, visceral and superficial pain usually require opioids for relief, whereas somatic pain (including bone pain) usually responds better to nonopioid analgesics such as nonsteroidal antiinflammatory drugs (NSAIDs) (see Chapter 44).

Pain may be further subclassified according to the diseases or other conditions that cause it. Vascular pain is believed to originate from the vascular or perivascular tissues and is thought to account for a large percentage of migraine headaches. Referred pain occurs when visceral nerve fibers synapse at a level in the spinal cord close to fibers that supply specific subcutaneous tissues in the body. An example is the pain associated with cholecystitis, which is often referred to the back and scapular areas. Neuropathic pain usually results from damage to peripheral or CNS nerve fibers by disease or injury but may also be idiopathic (unexplained). Phantom pain occurs in the area of a body part that has been removed—surgically or traumatically—and is often described as burning, itching, tingling, or stabbing. It

can also occur in paralyzed limbs following spinal cord injury. Cancer pain can be acute or chronic or both. It most often results from pressure of the tumor mass against nerves, organs, or tissues. Other causes of cancer pain include hypoxia from blockage of blood supply to an organ, metastases, pathologic fractures, muscle spasms, and adverse effects of radiation, surgery, and chemotherapy. Central pain occurs with tumors, trauma, inflammation, or disease (e.g., cancer, diabetes, stroke, multiple sclerosis) affecting CNS tissues.

Several theories attempt to explain pain transmission and pain relief. The most common and well described is the gate theory. This theory, proposed by Melzack and Wall in 1965, uses the analogy of a gate to describe how impulses from damaged tissues are sensed in the brain. First, the tissue injury causes the release of several substances from injured cells, such as bradykinin, histamine, potassium, prostaglandins, and serotonin. Some current pain medications work by altering the actions and levels of these substances (e.g., NSAIDs → prostaglandins; antidepressants → serotonin). The release of these pain-mediating chemicals initiates action potentials (electrical nerve impulses) at the distal end of sensory nerve fibers through pain receptors known as *nociceptors*. These nerve impulses are conducted along sensory nerve fibers and activate pain receptors in the *dorsal horn* of the spinal cord. It is here that the so-called gates are located. These gates regulate the flow of sensory nerve impulses. If impulses are stopped by a gate at this junction, no impulses are transmitted to the higher centers of the brain. Conversely, if the gates permit a sufficient number and intensity of action potentials to be conducted from the spinal cord to the cerebral cortex, the sensation of pain is then felt. This is known as *nociception*. Figure 10-2 depicts the gate theory of pain transmission.

Both the opening and the closing of this gate are influenced by the relative activation of large-diameter A fibers and small-diameter C fibers (Table 10-3). Closing of the gate seems to be affected by the activation of A fibers. This causes the inhibition of impulse transmission to the brain and avoidance of pain sensation. Opening of the gate is affected by the stimulation of C fibers. This allows impulses to be transmitted to the brain and pain to be sensed. The gate is innervated by nerve fibers that originate in the brain and modulate the pain sensation by sending impulses to the gate in the spinal cord. These nerve fibers enable the brain to evaluate, identify, and localize the pain. Thus, the brain can control the gate, either keeping the gate closed or allowing it to open so that the brain is stimulated and pain is sensed. The cells that control the gate have a threshold. Impulses that reach these cells must rise above this threshold before an impulse is permitted to travel up to the brain.

The body is also equipped with certain endogenous neurotransmitters known as *enkephalins* and *endorphins*. These substances are produced within the body to fight pain and are considered the body's painkillers. Both are capable of bonding with opioid receptors and inhibiting the transmission of pain impulses by closing the spinal cord gates, in a manner similar to that of opioid analgesic drugs. The term *endorphin* is a condensed version of the term "endogenous morphine." These endogenous analgesic substances are released whenever the

| TABLE 10-1 | CONDITIONS THAT ALTER PAIN TOLERANCE | |
|---|---|---|
| **PAIN THRESHOLD** | **CONDITIONS** | |
| Lowered | Anger, anxiety, depression, discomfort, fear, isolation, chronic pain, sleeplessness, tiredness | |
| Raised | Diversion, empathy, rest, sympathy, medications (analgesics, antianxiety drugs, antidepressants) | |

| TABLE 10-2 | ACUTE VERSUS CHRONIC PAIN | | |
|---|---|---|---|
| **TYPE OF PAIN** | **ONSET** | **DURATION** | **EXAMPLES** |
| Acute | Sudden (minutes to hours); usually sharp, localized; physiologic response (SNS: tachycardia, sweating, pallor, increased blood pressure) | Limited (has an end) | Myocardial infarction, appendicitis, dental procedures, kidney stones, surgical procedures |
| Chronic | Slow (days to months); long duration; dull, persistent aching | Persistent or recurring (endless) | Arthritis, cancer, lower back pain, peripheral neuropathy |

*SNS*, Sympathetic nervous system.

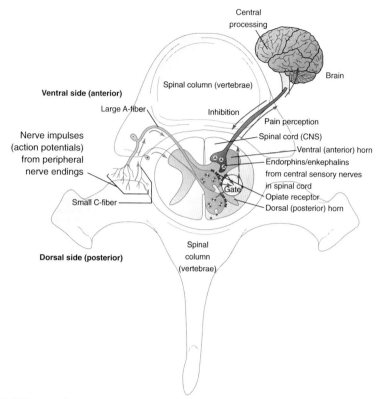

**FIGURE 10-2** Gate theory of pain transmission. *CNS*, Central nervous system.

| TABLE 10-3 | | **A AND C NERVE FIBERS** | | |
|---|---|---|---|---|
| TYPE OF FIBER | MYELIN SHEATH | FIBER SIZE | CONDUCTION SPEED | TYPE OF PAIN |
| A | Yes | Large | Fast | Sharp and well localized |
| C | No | Small | Slow | Dull and nonlocalized |

body experiences pain or prolonged exertion. For example, they are responsible for the phenomenon of "runner's high." Figure 10-1 depicts this entire process.

Another phenomenon of pain relief that may be explained by the gate theory is the fact that massaging a painful area often reduces the pain. When an area is rubbed or liniment is applied, large sensory A nerve fibers from peripheral receptors carry pain-modulating impulses to the spinal cord. Remember, the A fibers tend to close the gate, which reduces pain sensation in the brain.

## TREATMENT OF PAIN IN SPECIAL SITUATIONS

It is estimated that one of every three Americans experiences ongoing pain. Pain is poorly understood and often undertreated. In addition to enduring their baseline chronic pain, patients with illnesses such as cancer, AIDS, and sickle cell anemia may also experience crisis periods of acute pain. Effective management of acute pain is often different from management of chronic pain in terms of medications and dosages used.

Routes of drug administration may include oral, intravenous (IV), intramuscular (IM), subcutaneous (subcut), transdermal, and rectal. One intravenous route commonly used in the hospital setting is patient-controlled analgesia (PCA). In this situation, patients are able to self-medicate by pressing a button on a PCA infusion pump. This has been shown to be very effective and reduces the total opioid dose used. Morphine and hydromorphone are commonly given by PCA. Potential hazards of PCA include well-meaning family members' pressing the dosing button rather than letting able patients do so on their own. For patients truly not able to self-medicate using the PCA pump, a different method of pain control needs to be used. Numerous deaths have occurred when well-meaning family members have administered too much of the opioid drug. This is called *PCA by proxy*. The Institute for Safe Medication Practices (www.ismp.org) advises against PCA by proxy.

Patients with complex pain syndromes often benefit from a holistic or multimodal clinical approach that involves pharmacologic and/or nonpharmacologic treatment. Effective drug therapy may include use of opioid and/or nonopioid drugs. The goals of pain management include reducing and controlling pain, and improving body function and quality of life.

In situations such as pain associated with cancer, the main consideration in pain management is patient comfort and not trying to prevent drug addiction (or psychologic dependence; see Chapter 17). Opioid tolerance is a state of adaptation in which exposure to a drug causes changes in drug receptors that result in reduced drug effects over time. This can occur in as little as 1 week. Because of increasing pathology (e.g., tumor burden), cancer patients usually require increasingly higher opioid doses and thus do become physically dependent on the drugs. Cancer patients are likely to experience withdrawal symptoms (see Chapter 17) if opioid doses are abruptly reduced or discontinued; however, actual psychological dependence or addiction in such patients is unusual. For long-term pain control, oral, intravenous, subcutaneous, transdermal, and sometimes even rectal dosing routes are favored over multiple intramuscular injections due to associated puncture trauma (bruising) and erratic drug absorption.

One controversial issue in pain management is the use of placebos, inert dosage forms that actually lack medication. Some prescribers feel that this practice may be helpful by taking advantage of the well-documented placebo effect. The placebo effect is a psychological therapeutic effect that occurs even in the absence of actual medication. It is believed to arise from activation of the patient's own endorphins. It is also attributed to the patient's belief that any "treatment" is effective, as well as the patient's high level of trust in the health care provider. Critics argue that the use of placebos is unethical, because it requires that the patient be deceived in the process. The use of placebos for pain management has fallen out of favor, and they are rarely used today (see Chapter 4 for further discussion).

The treatment of acute pain in patients who are addicted to opioids is of great concern to clinicians, who may be reluctant to prescribe opioid therapy. However, habitual street opioid users are opioid tolerant and generally require high dosages. Longer-acting opioids such as methadone or extended-release oxycodone are usually better choices than shorter-acting immediate-release drug products for these patients. This is because the shorter-acting drugs are more likely to produce a psychological "high" or euphoria, which only reinforces addictive tendencies. Genetic differences in cytochrome P-450 enzymes (see Chapters 2 and 8) can cause different patients, whether addicted or not, to respond more or less effectively to a given drug. For this reason, patients must not automatically be viewed with suspicion if they complain that a given drug does not work for them.

The label of "addict" can be used unfairly to justify refusal to prescribe pain medications, resulting in undertreatment of pain, even in patients who do not use street drugs. This is now regarded as an inappropriate and inhumane clinical practice. In these situations, control of the patient's pain takes ethical and clinical priority over concerns regarding drug addiction. Nonetheless, prescribers must contend with the reality of abuse of street and/or prescription drugs by patients without genuine pain conditions (see Chapter 17). Such patients often request excessive numbers of prescriptions and may use multiple prescribers and/or pharmacies. At times, they may also forge prescriptions and/or use a telephone to call in prescriptions for non–Schedule II opioids such as hydrocodone/acetaminophen (Vicodin). Community pharmacists work collaboratively to detect such abuses and notify law enforcement authorities. Creating a phony prescription for a controlled substance is a felony under federal and state laws.

---

## EVIDENCE-BASED PRACTICE

### Student Nurses' Misconceptions of Adults with Chronic Nonmalignant Pain

#### Review

The purpose of this study was to identify some of the misconceptions that student nurses have, across 3 years of undergraduate education, about adults who are experiencing chronic nonmalignant pain. Previously identified misconceptions about patients with chronic nonmalignant pain reported in an extensive literature search served as the basis of the study. The rationale for this study was to identify potential gaps in attitudes and knowledge of student nurses. The results were then used to discuss educational approaches focused on improving care of the patient experiencing chronic nonmalignant pain. The two major questions that this study sought to explore included the following: (1) Do student nurses hold misconceptions about adults with chronic nonmalignant pain, and (2) If so, to what extent do they develop during their undergraduate education?

#### Type of Evidence

The researchers developed, tested, and validated a survey tool specifically for this cross-sectional study to evoke responses from students at three points during their undergraduate nursing education in New Zealand. The survey began with a vignette of a 22-year-old client who was experiencing back pain for 6 months. The injury that caused the pain resulted when the woman suffered a fall while lifting a patient. It was thought that the vignette represented demographics that would be most familiar to the participants. Part of the vignette also purposely alluded to some of the basic details of misconceptions of pain (McCaffery and Pasero, 1999) but without giving many specific details. The patient in the vignette was also someone who was a healthy, fit young adult prior to the injury. There were two slight variations in the vignettes with the hopes of eliciting possible differences in responses toward patients, depending on whether a specific pathology had been identified. A series of eight items, the misconception items, were directly linked to each of the misconceptions identified by McCaffery and Pasero (1990), and the responses were gathered using a seven-point Likert scale seeking differing levels of agreement in relation to the items. A tool was designed and used with another group of students from a different discipline but within the same facility. This was done to get feedback from a group of students similar to the participants but prior to the final study. Some minor changes were made in the tool before moving forward with the study.

#### Results of Study

Some 435 students were approached to participate in the research study, and 430 completed and returned the surveys for a total response rate of 99%. A convenience sampling was used because the students were easily accessible; they represented about 75% of students enrolled in the facility in semesters one, four, and six of the undergraduate nursing degree program in the city of Auckland and around 13% of those enrolled in New Zealand. These participants were distributed over a 3-year period of undergraduate studies during six semesters of full-time studies. The majority were female students, although there was no further specific demographic data collected about the participants. A cross-sectional design meant that data gathered came from each participant only once during the study. A research assistant, and one who had not taught the students, met with the students and invited them to participate in the study. Sessions were held in the middle of the semester to increase the response rate as well as diminish anxiety during final exam time. More than 38% of the participants demonstrated a misconception about people with chronic pain and that they were tolerant to some degree of pain. More than 60% did not hold this misconception about tolerance to pain. More than one-half of the students' (59%) responses indicated that they held the misconception that psychological impairment is related to chronic pain.

*Continued*

**EVIDENCE-BASED PRACTICE—cont'd**

## *Student Nurses' Misconceptions of Adults with Chronic Nonmalignant Pain*

Approximately 79% of the students suggested that they believed stress was a contributory cause of chronic pain, whereas less than one-fourth indicated that they accurately understood that this was not the case. The misconception of compensation and exaggeration in chronic pain was held by 47.9% of the participants, and 51.7% did not hold this same misconception. About one-third of the students indicated that they held the misconception that patients with chronic pain were manipulative, and the majority indicated that they did not.

Approximately 64% of the participants held the misconception that depression plays a role in the chronic pain experience. Opioid addiction was a misconception held by about one-half of the participants, such that 54.8% believed that patients taking opioids were likely to be addicted. Some 58% of the students indicated that they did hold the misconception that patients with chronic pain were non-compliant and dependent, whereas 41.4% indicated that they did not hold this misconception. Another question that was posed to the students was the extent to which they had developed their misconceptions of patients with chronic pain during their undergraduate education. There were significantly positive trends across the semesters, suggesting that students held their misconceptions to a lesser degree as they progressed through their course of study. In summary, analysis of the results indicate that a substantial proportion of students who participated in the study hold misconceptions about patients with chronic pain to some extent.

The analysis of the misconception scores across the semesters indicates that the knowledge and attitudes of students toward adults experiencing chronic nonmalignant pain developed to some degree because their misconceptions were held to a lesser degree by the end of the program of study.

### Link of Evidence to Nursing Practice

It is a known phenomenon that a gap exists between theory and practice across many areas of professional nursing practice. Therefore, it would be ideal for nursing educators and the nursing educational experience to equip students with the knowledge, skills, and attitudes to participate in the discussion, planning, and implementing of care for patients suffering from chronic nonmalignant pain. Nursing faculty and schools of nursing need to make available experiential learning situations that will enhance the blending of knowledge, skills, and attitudes into professional nursing practice so that these gaps in care are closed. The findings of this study show that students, like many practicing nurses, hold misconceptions about adults with chronic nonmalignant pain, representing a lack of knowledge and inappropriate attitudes. An integrated approach to teaching chronicity and disability needs to be included in the nursing curriculum; however, critical thinking, linking theory to practice, and developing compassion also need to be part of the educational process.

References: Shaw S, Lee A: Student nurses' misconceptions of adults with chronic nonmalignant pain, *Pain Manag Nurs* 11(1):2-14, 2010; McCaffery M, Pasero C: *Pain: clinical manual*, St Louis, 1990, Mosby; McCaffery M, Pasero C: *Pain: clinical manual*, ed 2, St Louis, 1999, Mosby.

For patients receiving long-acting opioids, breakthrough pain often occurs between doses of pain medications. This is because the analgesic effects wear off as the drug is metabolized and eliminated from the body. Treatment with prn (as needed) doses of immediate-release dosage forms (e.g., oxycodone IR) given between scheduled doses of extended-release dosage forms (e.g., oxycodone ER) is often helpful in these cases. Chewing or crushing of any extended-release opioid drug can cause oversedation, respiratory depression, and even death due to rapid drug absorption. If the patient is requiring larger doses for breakthrough pain, the dose of the scheduled extended-release opioid may need to be shortened or a more potent drug started.

Drugs from other chemical categories are often added to the opioid regimen as adjuvant drugs. These assist the primary drugs in relieving pain. Such adjuvant drug therapy may include NSAIDs (see Chapter 44), antidepressants (see Chapter 16), antiepileptic drugs (see Chapter 14), and corticosteroids (see Chapter 33), all of which are discussed further in their corresponding chapters. This approach allows the use of smaller dosages of opioids and reduces some of the adverse effects that are seen with higher dosages of opioids, such as respiratory depression, constipation, and urinary retention. It permits drugs with different mechanisms of action to produce synergistic effects. Antiemetics (see Chapter 52) and laxatives (see Chapter 51) may also be needed to prevent or relieve associated constipation, nausea, and vomiting (Box 10-2).

One common use of adjuvant drugs is in the treatment of neuropathic pain. Opioids are not completely effective in such cases. Neuropathic pain usually results from some kind of nerve damage secondary to disease (e.g., diabetic neuropathy, postherpetic neuralgia secondary to shingles, trigeminal neuralgia, AIDS or injury, including nerve damage secondary to surgical procedures [e.g., post-thoracotomy pain syndrome occurring after cardiothoracic surgery]). Common symptoms include hypersensitivity or hyperalgesia to mild stimuli such as light touch or a pinprick, or the bed sheets on a person's feet. This is also known as *allodynia*. It can also manifest as hyperalgesia to uncomfortable stimuli, such as pressure from an inflated blood pressure cuff on a patient's limb. It may be described as heat, cold, numbness and tingling, burning, or electrical sensations. Examples of adjuvants commonly used in these cases are the antidepressant amitriptyline and the anticonvulsants gabapentin and pregabalin.

The three-step analgesic ladder defined by the World Health Organization (WHO) is often applied as the pain management standard for cancer pain. Examples of nonopioid analgesic drugs include NSAIDs (see Chapter 44) as well as acetaminophen and tramadol (see Drug Profiles). Step 1 is the use of nonopioids (with or without adjuvant medications) once the pain has been identified and assessed. If pain persists and/or increases, treatment moves to step 2, which is defined as the use of opioids with or without nonopioids and with or without adjuvants. If pain persists or increases, management then rises to step 3, which is the use of opioids indicated for moderate to severe pain, administered with or without nonopioids or adjuvant medications. Many experts now question the effectiveness of Step 2, and the WHO is considering adjusting the ladder. Not all patients will be treated effectively using the ladder method and may need to seek an experienced pain management physician.

---

### BOX 10-2 POTENTIAL OPIOID ADVERSE EFFECTS AND THEIR MANAGEMENT

**Constipation**

Opioids decrease gastrointestinal (GI) tract peristalsis because of their central nervous system (CNS) depression, with subsequent constipation as an adverse effect. Stool becomes excessively dehydrated because it remains in the GI tract longer. **Preventative measures:** Constipation may be managed with increased intake of fluids, stool softeners such as docusate sodium, or the use of stimulants such as bisacodyl or senna. Agents such as lactulose, sorbitol, and polyethylene glycol (Miralax) have been proven effective. Less commonly used are bulk-forming laxatives such as psyllium, for which increased fluid intake is especially important to avoid fecal impactions or bowel obstructions.

**Nausea and Vomiting**

Opioids decrease GI tract peristalsis, and some also stimulate the vomiting center in the CNS, so nausea and vomiting are often experienced. **Preventative measures:** Nausea and vomiting may be managed with the use of antiemetics such as phenothiazines.

**Sedation and Mental Clouding**

Any change in mental status should always be evaluated to ensure that causes other than drug-related CNS depression are ruled out. **Preventative measures:** Persistent drug-related sedation may be managed with a decrease in the dosage of opioid or change in drug used. The prescriber may also order various CNS stimulants (see Chapter 13).

**Respiratory Depression**

Long-term opioid use is generally associated with tolerance to respiratory depression. **Preventative measures:** For severe respiratory depression, opioid antagonists (naloxone) may be used to improve respiratory status and, if they are titrated in small amounts, the respiratory depression may be reversed without analgesia reversal.

**Subacute Overdose**

Subacute overdose may be more common than acute respiratory depression and may progress slowly (over hours to days), with somnolence and respiratory depression. Before analgesic dosages are changed or reduced, advancing disease must be considered, especially in the dying patient. **Preventative measures:** Often, holding one or two doses of an opioid analgesic is enough to judge if the mental and respiratory depression is associated with the opioid. If there is improvement with this measure, the opioid dosage is often decreased by 25%.

**Other Opioid Adverse Effects**

Dry mouth, urinary retention, pruritus, myoclonus, dysphoria, euphoria, sleep disturbances, sexual dysfunction, and inappropriate secretion of antidiuretic hormone may occur but are less common than the aforementioned adverse effects. **Preventative measures:** Ongoing assessment is needed for each of the adverse effects so that appropriate measures may be implemented (e.g., sucking of sugar-free hard candy or use of artificial saliva drops or gum for dry mouth; use of diphenhydramine for pruritus).

---

## PHARMACOLOGY OVERVIEW

Opioids are classified as both mild agonists (codeine, hydrocodone) and strong agonists (morphine, hydromorphone, levorphanol, oxycodone, oxymorphone, meperidine, fentanyl, and methadone). Meperidine is not recommended for long-term use because of the accumulation of a neurotoxic metabolite, *normeperidine*. In fact, many hospitals have tried to prohibit the use of meperidine due to its adverse CNS effects, including seizures. In 2010, the mild agonist, propoxyphene (Darvocet) was withdrawn from the market due to adverse effects. The opiate agonists-antagonists such as pentazocine and nalbuphine are associated with an analgesic ceiling effect. This means that the drug reaches a maximum analgesic effect, so that analgesia does not improve even with higher dosages (see Drug Profiles). Such drugs are useful only in patients who have not been previously exposed to opioids and can be used for nonescalating moderate to severe pain. Finally, because of associated bruising and bleeding risks, as well as injection discomfort, there is now a strong trend away from intramuscular injections in favor of intravenous, oral, and transdermal routes of drug administration.

## OPIOID DRUGS

The pain-relieving drugs currently known as *opioid analgesics* originated from the opium poppy plant. The word *opium* is a Greek word that means "juice." More than 20 different alkaloids are obtained from the unripe seed of the poppy. The properties of opium and its many alkaloids have been known for centuries. Opium-smoking immigrants brought opium to the United States, where unrestricted availability of opium prevailed until the early twentieth century.

## Chemical Structure

Opioid analgesics are very strong pain relievers. They can be classified according to their chemical structure or their action at specific receptors. Of the 20 different natural alkaloids available from the opium poppy plant, only three are clinically useful: morphine, codeine, and papaverine. Of these, only morphine and codeine are pain relievers; papaverine is a smooth muscle relaxant. Relatively simple synthetic chemical modifications of these opium alkaloids have produced the three different chemical classes of opioids: morphine-like drugs, meperidine-like drugs, and methadone-like drugs (Table 10-4).

## Mechanism of Action and Drug Effects

Opioid analgesics can also be characterized according to their mechanism of action. They are agonists, agonists-antagonists, or antagonists (nonanalgesic). An *agonist* binds to an opioid pain receptor in the brain and causes an analgesic response—the reduction of pain sensation. An *agonist-antagonist*, also called a partial agonist or a *mixed agonist*, binds to a pain receptor and causes a weaker pain response than does a full agonist. Different drugs in this class exert their agonist and/or antagonist effects by binding in different degrees to kappa and mu opioid receptors. Although not normally used as first-line analgesics, they are sometimes useful in pain management in opioid-addicted patients as well as obstetrical patients (because they avoid oversedation of the mother and/or fetus). An antagonist binds to a pain receptor but does not reduce pain signals. It functions as a *competitive antagonist* because it competes with

## TABLE 10-4　CHEMICAL CLASSIFICATION OF OPIOIDS

| CHEMICAL CATEGORY | OPIOID DRUGS |
| --- | --- |
| Meperidine-like drugs | Meperidine, fentanyl, remifentanil, sufentanil, alfentanil |
| Methadone-like drugs | Methadone |
| Morphine-like drugs | Morphine, heroin, hydromorphone, oxymorphone, levorphanol, codeine, hydrocodone, oxycodone |
| Other | Tramadol, tapentadol |

## TABLE 10-5　OPIOID RECEPTORS AND THEIR CHARACTERISTICS

| RECEPTOR TYPE | PROTOTYPICAL AGONIST | EFFECTS OF OPIOID STIMULATION |
| --- | --- | --- |
| mu | morphine | Supraspinal analgesia, respiratory depression, euphoria, sedation* |
| kappa | ketocyclazocine | Spinal analgesia, sedation,† miosis |
| delta | Enkephalins | Analgesia |

*Moderate level of sedation.
†Twice as much sedation compared to mu receptors.

and reverses the effects of agonist and agonist-antagonist drugs at the receptor sites.

The receptors to which opioids bind to relieve pain are listed in Table 10-5. The mu, kappa, and delta receptors are most responsive to drug activity, with the mu being the most important. Many of the characteristics of a particular opioid, such as its ability to sedate, its potency, and its ability to cause hallucinations, can be attributed to relative affinity for these various receptors.

Understanding the relative potencies of various drugs becomes important in clinical settings. *Equianalgesia* refers to the ability to provide equivalent pain relief by calculating dosages of different drugs and/or routes of administration that provide comparable analgesia. Box 10-3 lists equianalgesic doses for several common opioids and shows how to calculate dosage conversions for patients. Because fentanyl is most commonly used transdermally, it is discussed separately in its drug profile.

## Indications

The main use of opioids is to alleviate moderate to severe pain. The amount of pain control or unwanted adverse effects depends on the specific drug, the receptors to which it binds, and its chemical structure.

Strong opioid analgesics such as fentanyl, sufentanil, and alfentanil are commonly used in combination with anesthetics during surgery. These drugs are used not only to relieve pain but also to maintain a balanced state of anesthesia. The practice of using combinations of drugs to produce anesthesia is referred to as *balanced anesthesia* (see Chapter 11). Use of fentanyl injection for management of postoperative and procedural pain has become popular due to its rapid onset and short duration.

Transdermal fentanyl comes in a patch formulation for use in long-term pain management and is not to be used for postoperative or any other short-term pain control (see the Safety and Quality Improvement: Preventing Medication Errors box).

## ⚡ SAFETY AND QUALITY IMPROVEMENT: PREVENTING MEDICATION ERRORS

### Fentanyl Transdermal Patches

When giving fentanyl transdermal patches, keep in mind several important points to avoid improper administration:

- These patches are recommended to be used only by patients who are considered opioid tolerant. To be considered opioid tolerant, a patient needs to have been taking, for a week or longer, morphine 60 mg daily, oral oxycodone 30 mg daily, or oral hydromorphone 8 mg daily (or an equianalgesic dose of another opioid). Giving fentanyl transdermal patches to non–opioid-tolerant patients may result in severe respiratory depression. Thorough assessment is important.
- Inform patients that heat, such as in the form of a heating pad/pack, must never be applied over a fentanyl transdermal patch. The increased circulation that results from the application of heat may result in increased absorption of medication, causing an overdose.
- Teach about the proper disposal of transdermal patches. Children have pulled used patches from the trash, which has resulted in death due to exposure to the drug. For disposal at home, the product insert recommends that the patch be disposed of by flushing down the toilet. However, disposal practices may vary by area because of concerns for the water systems. Disposal policies in facilities also vary, but some require that used patches be placed in a sharps container rather than be flushed.
- Keep patches, as well as all medications, away from children and pets. Do not store medications in warm, moist places such as medicine cabinets in the bathroom.

The Institute for Safe Medication Practices has described examples of fatal patient incidents resulting from failure to follow the above points. It is essential for the patient's safety to read the product labeling and follow instructions precisely. For more information, go to www.ismp.org.

Strong opioids such as morphine, meperidine, hydromorphone, and oxycodone are often used to control postoperative and other types of pain. Because morphine and hydromorphone are available in injectable forms, they are often first-line analgesics in the immediate postoperative setting. There is a trend away from using meperidine due to its greater risk for toxicity (see Drug Profile). All available oxycodone dosage forms are orally administered. The product OxyContin is a sustained-release form of oxycodone that is designed to last up to 12 hours. The "Contin" in the product name is a trademark of the original drug manufacturer, and refers to the "continuous-release" nature of the drug formulation. Recall that a continuous- or extended-release dosage form of a drug means that it has a prolonged duration of action, most often 8 to 24 hours (see Chapter 2). Similarly, the drug product MS Contin is a long-acting or sustained-release form of morphine that is also designed to provide 8 to 12 hours of pain relief. The "MS" stands for morphine sulfate. Both drugs are also available generically.

There are also immediate-release dosage forms of oxycodone and morphine in tablet, capsule, and liquid form. Meperidine is available only in immediate-release dosage forms, both oral

## BOX 10-3 CALCULATING DOSAGE CONVERSIONS BETWEEN COMMONLY USED OPIOIDS

### EQUIANALGESIC DOSES

| | ORAL DOSE (mg) | PARENTERAL DOSE (mg) | ORAL-TO-PARENTERAL DOSE RATIO | DOSING INTERVAL (hr) |
|---|---|---|---|---|
| morphine | 30 | 10 | 3:1 | 12 (continuous release) 4 (immediate release) |
| hydromorphone | 7.5 | 1.5 | 5:1 | 4 (immediate release) |
| oxycodone | 15 | N/A | N/A | 4 (immediate release) |
| hydrocodone | 30 | N/A | N/A | N/A |
| fentanyl | See fentanyl Drug Profile | | | |

**Basic Conversion Equation**

$$\frac{\text{24-hour amount of current drug}}{x} = \frac{\text{EA dose of current drug}}{\text{EA dose of desired drug}}$$

*Where x = amount of desired opioid in 24 hours and EA = equianalgesic dose obtained from the table above*

For example: A patient with colon cancer is currently taking oral oxycodone 80 mg every 12 hours and needs to be converted to intravenous morphine due to a bowel obstruction. What is the equivalent IV morphine dose?

Step 1: **Determine the 24-hour amount of oxycodone taken by this patient:**

80 mg × 2 doses per 24 hours = 160 mg per 24 hours

Step 2: **Using the conversion table above, find the equianalgesic (EA) doses of oxycodone and parenteral morphine:**

15 mg oxycodone = 10 mg parenteral morphine

Step 3: **Use the above equation and solve for *x* by cross-multiplying:**

$$\frac{\text{24-hour amount of oxycodone (160 mg)}}{x} = \frac{\text{EA of current oxycodone (15 mg)}}{\text{EA dose of parenteral morphine (10 mg)}}$$

*Where x = amount of parenteral morphine in 24 hours (solve by cross-multiplying)*

$$160 \text{ mg} \times 10 \text{ mg} = 15 \text{ mg } x \quad x = \frac{1600 \text{ mg}}{15 \text{ mg}}$$

x = 107 mg (approximately 100 mg of injectable morphine per 24 hours)

*N/A*, Not applicable.

and injectable. The analgesic effects of immediate-release oral dosage forms of all three drugs typically last for about 4 hours.

Opioids also suppress the medullary cough center, which results in cough suppression. The most commonly used opioid for this purpose is codeine (see Chapter 36). Hydrocodone is also used in many cough suppressants, either alone or in combination with other drugs. Sometimes they have a depressant effect on the CNS and cause sedation. To avoid this problem, dextromethorphan, a nonopioid cough suppressant, is often given instead (see Chapters 17 and 36).

Constipation is often an unwanted side effect of opioids due to decreased gastrointestinal (GI) tract motility. It occurs because opioid drugs bind to intestinal opioid receptors. However, this effect is sometimes helpful in treating diarrhea. Some of the opioid-containing antidiarrheal preparations are camphorated opium tincture (paregoric) and diphenoxylate/atropine (Lomotil) tablets.

## Contraindications

Contraindications to the use of opioid analgesics include known drug allergy and severe asthma. It is not uncommon for patients to state they are allergic to codeine, when in the overwhelming majority of these patients nausea was the "allergic" reaction.

Many patients will claim to be allergic to morphine because it causes itching. Itching is a pharmacologic effect due to histamine release and not an allergic reaction. Thus, it is important to determine the exact nature of a patient's stated allergy. Although not absolute contraindications, extreme caution is to be used in cases of respiratory insufficiency, especially when resuscitative equipment is not available; conditions involving elevated intracranial pressure (e.g., severe head injury); morbid obesity and/or sleep apnea; myasthenia gravis; paralytic ileus (bowel paralysis); and pregnancy, especially with long-term use or high dosages.

## Adverse Effects

Many of the unwanted effects of opioid analgesics are related to their pharmacologic effects in areas other than the CNS. Some of these unwanted effects can be explained by the drug's selectivity for the receptors listed in Table 10-5. The various body systems that the opioids affect and their specific adverse effects are summarized in Table 10-6.

Opioids that have an affinity for mu receptors and have rapid onset of action produce marked euphoria. These are the opioids that are most likely to be abused. All opioid drugs have a strong abuse potential. They are common recreational drugs of abuse among the lay public and also among health care professionals,

## TABLE 10-6 OPIOID-INDUCED ADVERSE EFFECTS BY BODY SYSTEM

| BODY SYSTEM | ADVERSE EFFECTS |
| --- | --- |
| Cardiovascular | Hypotension, flushing, bradycardia |
| Central nervous | Sedation, disorientation, euphoria, lightheadedness, dysphoria |
| Gastrointestinal | Nausea, vomiting, constipation, biliary tract spasm |
| Genitourinary | Urinary retention |
| Integumentary | Itching, rash, wheal formation |
| Respiratory | Respiratory depression and possible aggravation of asthma |

For further information on transdermal fentanyl, visit http://www.ismp.org/Newsletters/acutecare/articles/20050811.asp.

## TABLE 10-7 OPIOID ANTAGONISTS (REVERSAL DRUGS)

| GENERIC NAME | TRADE NAME | ADVERSE EFFECTS |
| --- | --- | --- |
| naloxone (IV) | Narcan | Raised or lowered blood pressure, dysrhythmias, pulmonary edema, withdrawal |
| naltrexone (PO) | ReVia | Nervousness, headache, nausea, vomiting, pulmonary edema, withdrawal |

*IV,* Intravenous; *PO,* oral.

who often have relatively easy access. The person taking them to alter his or her mental status will soon become psychologically dependent (addicted; see Chapter 17).

In addition, opioids cause histamine release. It is thought that this histamine release is responsible for many of the drugs' unwanted adverse effects, such as itching or pruritus, rash, and hemodynamic changes. Histamine release causes peripheral arteries and veins to dilate, which leads to flushing and orthostatic hypotension. The amount of histamine release that an opioid analgesic causes is related to its chemical class. The naturally occurring opiates (e.g., morphine) elicit the most histamine release; the synthetic opioids (e.g., meperidine) elicit the least histamine release. (See Table 10-4 on p. 148 for a list of the various opioids and their respective chemical classes.)

The most serious adverse effect of opioid use is CNS depression, which may lead to respiratory depression. When death occurs from opioid overdose, it is almost always due to respiratory depression. When opioids are given, care must be taken to titrate the dose so that the patient's pain is controlled without affecting respiratory function. Individual responses to opioids vary, and patients may occasionally experience respiratory compromise despite careful dose titration. Respiratory depression can be prevented in part by using drugs with very short duration of action and no active metabolites. Respiratory depression seems to be more common in patients with a preexisting condition causing respiratory compromise, such as asthma, chronic obstructive pulmonary disease, or sleep apnea. Respiratory depression is strongly related to the degree of sedation (see Toxicity and Management of Overdose later).

GI tract adverse effects are common in patients receiving opioids due to stimulation of GI opioid receptors. Nausea, vomiting, and constipation are the most common adverse effects. Opioids can irritate the GI tract, stimulating the chemoreceptor trigger zone in the CNS, which in turn may cause nausea and vomiting. Opioids slow peristalsis and increase absorption of water from intestinal contents. These two actions combine to produce constipation. This is more pronounced in hospitalized patients who are nonambulatory. Patients may require laxatives (see Chapter 51) to help maintain normal bowel movements.

Urinary retention, or the inability to void, is another unwanted adverse effect of opioid analgesics, caused by increasing bladder tone. This is sometimes prevented by giving low

dosages of an opioid agonist-antagonist or an opioid antagonist or a cholinergic agonist (see Chapter 20), such as bethanechol.

Severe hypersensitivity or anaphylactic reaction to opioid analgesics is rare. Many patients will experience GI discomforts or histamine-mediated reactions to opioids and call these "allergic reactions." However, true anaphylaxis is rare, even with intravenously administered opioids. Some patients may complain of flushing, itching, or wheal formation at the injection site, but this is usually local and histamine mediated, and not a true allergy. Box 10-2 (p. 147) provides additional information on opioid adverse effects and their management.

### Toxicity and Management of Overdose

Naloxone and naltrexone are opioid antagonists, and they bind to and occupy all of the receptor sites (mu, kappa, delta). They are competitive antagonists with a strong affinity for these binding sites. Through such binding they can reverse the adverse effects induced by the opioid drug, such as respiratory depression. These drugs are used in the management of both opioid overdose and opioid addiction. The commonly used opioid antagonists (reversal drugs) are listed in Table 10-7.

When treating an opioid overdose or toxicity, the symptoms of withdrawal need to be considered. However, regardless of potential withdrawal symptoms, when a patient experiences severe respiratory depression, naloxone must be given. Some degree of physical dependence is expected in opioid-tolerant patients. The extent of opioid tolerance is most visible when an opioid drug is discontinued abruptly or when an opioid antagonist is administered. This usually leads to symptoms of opioid withdrawal, also known as *abstinence syndrome* (see Chapter 17). This can occur after as little as 2 weeks of opioid therapy in opioid-naïve patients. Gradual dosage reduction after chronic opioid use, when possible, helps to minimize the risk and severity of withdrawal symptoms.

Respiratory depression is the most serious adverse effect associated with opioids. Stimulating the patient may be adequate to reverse mild hypoventilation. If this is unsuccessful, ventilatory assistance using a bag and mask or endotracheal intubation may be needed to support respiration. Administration of opioid antagonists (e.g., naloxone) may also be necessary to reverse severe respiratory depression. Careful titration of dose until the patient begins to breathe independently will prevent overreversal. The effects of naloxone are short lived and usually last about 1 hour. With long-acting opioids, respiratory depressant effects may reappear, and naloxone may need to be redosed.

The onset of withdrawal symptoms is directly related to the half-life of the opioid analgesic being used. Withdrawal symptoms resulting from the discontinuance or reversal of therapy with short-acting opioids (codeine, hydrocodone, morphine, and hydromorphone) will appear within 6 to 12 hours and peak at 24 to 72 hours. Withdrawal symptoms associated with the long half-life drugs (methadone, levorphanol, and transdermal fentanyl) may not appear for 24 hours or longer after drug discontinuation and may be milder.

## Interactions

Potential drug interactions with opioids are significant. Coadministration of opioids with alcohol, antihistamines, barbiturates, benzodiazepines, phenothiazine, and other CNS depressants can result in additive respiratory depressant effects. The combined use of opioids (such as meperidine) with monoamine oxidase inhibitors, such as selegiline, can result in respiratory depression, seizures, and hypotension.

### Laboratory Test Interactions

Opioids can cause an abnormal increase in the serum levels of amylase, alanine aminotransferase, alkaline phosphatase, bilirubin, lipase, creatinine kinase, and lactate dehydrogenase (see the Safety: Laboratory Values Related to Drug Therapy box). Other abnormal results include a decrease in urinary 17-ketosteroid levels and an increase in the urinary alkaloid and glucose concentrations.

## Dosages

For the recommended initial dosages of selected analgesic drugs in opioid-naïve patients, see the Dosages table on p. 152.

## DRUG PROFILES

### OPIOID AGONISTS

#### ◆ morphine sulfate

Morphine, a naturally occurring alkaloid derived from the opium poppy, is the drug prototype for all opioid drugs. It is classified as a Schedule II controlled substance. Morphine is indicated for severe pain and has a high abuse potential. It is available in oral, injectable, and rectal dosage forms. Extended-release forms include MS Contin, Kadian, and Avinza. Morphine also has a potentially toxic metabolite known as *morphine-6-glucuronide*. Accumulation of this metabolite is more likely to occur in patients with renal impairment. For this reason, other Schedule II opioids such as hydromorphone (Dilaudid), fentanyl (see fentanyl drug profile), and oxymorphone (Opana) may be safer analgesic choices for patients with renal insufficiency. Drug profile information for hydromorphone is similar to that for morphine and meperidine. However, it is essential that all health care professionals realize that hydromorphone is about eight times more potent than morphine. One milligram of IV, IM, or subcut hydromorphone is equivalent to 7 mg of IV, IM, or subcut morphine. This difference in potency often is not taken into account when prescribing, and deaths have been reported

## SAFETY: LABORATORY VALUES RELATED TO DRUG THERAPY

### *Analgesics*

| LABORATORY TEST | NORMAL RANGES | RATIONALE FOR ASSESSMENT |
|---|---|---|
| Alkaline phosphatase (ALP) | 30-120 units/L | ALP is found in many tissues but in highest concentrations in the liver, biliary tract, and bone. Detection of this enzyme is important for determining liver and bone disorders. Enzyme levels of ALP are increased in both extrahepatic and intrahepatic obstructive biliary disease and cirrhosis and/or other liver abnormalities. |
| Alanine aminotransferase (ALT); formerly serum glutamic-pyruvic transaminase (SGPT) | 4-36 units/L Elderly may have slightly higher levels than the adult | ALT is found mainly in the liver and lesser amounts in the kidneys, heart, and skeletal muscle. If there is injury or disease to the liver parenchyma (cells), it will cause a release of this liver cellular enzyme into the bloodstream and thus elevate serum ALT levels. Most ALT elevations are from liver disease. Therefore, if medications are then metabolized by the liver, this metabolic process will be altered and possibly lead to toxic levels of drugs. |
| Gama-glutamyl transferase (GGT) | Male/female 45 years of age and older: 8-38 units/L | GGT is an enzyme that is present in liver tissue; when there is damage to the liver cells (hepatocytes) that manufacture bile, the enzyme will be released throughout the cell membranes and released into the blood. Individuals of African ancestry have normal values that are double the values of those who are white. |
| Aspartate aminotransferase (AST); formerly called serum glutamic-oxalocetic transaminase (SGOT) | 0-35 units/L | AST is elevated with hepatocellular diseases. With disease or injury of liver cells, the cells lyse and the AST is released and picked up by the blood; the elevation of AST is directly related to the number of cells affected by disease or injury. |
| Lactic dehydrogenase (LDH) | 100-190 units/L | LDH is found in cells of many body tissues including the heart, liver, red blood cells, kidneys, skeletal muscles, brain, and lungs. Because it is in so many tissues, the total LDH level is not a specific indicator of one disease. If there is disease or injury affecting cells containing LDH, the cells lyse and LDH is released from the cells into the bloodstream, thus increasing LDH levels. This enzyme is just part of the total picture of altered liver function which, if present, will then decrease the breakdown/metabolism of drugs and other chemical compounds, resulting in elevated blood levels of drugs. |

## DOSAGES

### Selected Analgesic Drugs and Related Drugs

| DRUG (PREGNANCY CATEGORY) | PHARMACOLOGIC CLASS | USUAL DOSAGE RANGE | INDICATIONS/USES |
|---|---|---|---|
| **Opioids** | | | |
| codeine sulfate (D) | Opiate analgesic; opium alkaloid | **Adult**<br>15-60 mg tid-qid | Opioid analgesia |
| | | **Pediatric 2-5 yr**<br>PO/subcut/IM: 2.5-5 mg q4-6h—do not exceed 30 mg/day | Relief of cough |
| | | **Pediatric 6-11 yr**<br>5-10 mg q4-6h | Relief of cough |
| | | **Adult and pediatric older than 12 yr**<br>10-20 mg q4-6h—do not exceed 120 mg/day | Relief of cough |
| | | **Adult**<br>15-60 mg tid-qid | Opioid analgesia |
| fentanyl (Duragesic, Oralet, Actiq*) (D) | Opioid analgesic | All doses titrated to response, starting with lowest effective dose | Procedural sedation or adjunct to general anesthesia |
| | | **Pediatric**<br>IV/IM: 0.5-2 mcg/kg/dose | |
| | | **Adult**<br>IV/IM: 50-100 mcg/dose titrated to response via continuous infusion | Relief of moderate to severe acute pain |
| | | Duragesic (transdermal patch): 12.5-200 mcg/hr q72h; Oralet, Actiq (buccal lozenges): begin with lowest dose (200 mcg) and titrate as needed<br>NOTE: The FDA has placed restrictions on transmucosal fentanyl (only allowed for chronic pain) | Relief of chronic pain, including cancer pain |
| meperidine HCl (Demerol) (D) | Opioid analgesic | **Pediatric**<br>PO/IM/IV/subcut: 1-1.8 mg/kg q3-4h prn (max 100 mg/dose) | Meperidine use not recommended because of the unpredictable effects of neurometabolites at analgesic doses and risk for seizures |
| | | **Adult**<br>PO/IV/IM/subcut: 50-150 mg q3-4h prn | Obstetric analgesia, preoperative sedation |
| methadone HCl (Dolophine) (D) | Opioid analgesic | **Adult**<br>PO/IM/IV/subcut: 2.5-10 mg q8-12h; | Opioid analgesia, relief of chronic pain, opioid detoxification |
| | | 40 mg or more once daily | Opioid addiction maintenance |
| morphine sulfate (MSIR, Roxanol, others) (D) | Opiate analgesic; opium alkaloid | **Pediatric younger than 6 mo**<br>PO: less than 6 months: 0.1 mg/kg/dose q3-4h prn<br>IV/IM/subcut: 0.03-0.05 mg/kg q3-8h prn | Opioid analgesia |
| | | **Older than 6 mo**<br>PO: 0.2-0.5 mg/kg/dose q4h prn<br>IV/IM/subcut: 0.05-0.2 mg/kg q2-4h prn | |
| | | **Adult**<br>PO: 10-30 mg q4h prn<br>IV/IM /subcut: 2.5-15 mg q2-6h prn | Opioid analgesia |
| ◆ morphine sulfate, continuous-release (MS Contin, Oramorph, Kadian, Avinza) (D) | Opiate analgesic; opium alkaloid | **Adult only**<br>PO: 15 mg q8h to 200 mg q8-12h | Relief of moderate to severe pain |
| oxycodone, immediate-release (OxyIR) (D) | Opioid, synthetic | **Pediatric**<br>PO: 0.1-0.3 mg/kg q3h prn | Relief of moderate to severe pain |
| | | **Adult**<br>PO: 5-20 mg q4-6h prn | Relief of moderate to severe pain |
| oxycodone, continuous-release (OxyContin) (D) | Opioid, synthetic | **Adult only**<br>PO: 10-160 mg q8-12h | Relief of moderate to severe pain |

## DOSAGES—cont'd

### Selected Analgesic Drugs and Related Drugs

| DRUG (PREGNANCY CATEGORY) | PHARMACOLOGIC CLASS | USUAL DOSAGE RANGE | INDICATIONS/USES |
|---|---|---|---|
| **Opioid Antagonists** | | | |
| ◆ naloxone HCl (Narcan) | Opioid antagonist | **Pediatric** | Treatment of opioid overdose |
| | | IV: 0.01 mg/kg IV followed by 0.1 mg/kg if needed (Note: PALS doses vary) | |
| | | IV: 0.0005-0.01 mg/kg IV—repeat at 2-3 min intervals | Postoperative anesthesia reversal |
| | | **Adult** | Treatment of opioid overdose |
| | | IV: 0.4-2 mg IV—repeat in 2-8 min if needed | |
| | | IV: 0.1-0.2 mg IV—repeat at 2-3 min intervals | Postoperative anesthesia reversal |
| naltrexone HCl | Opioid antagonist | **Adult** | Maintenance of opioid-free state |
| | | PO: 50 mg q24h or 100 mg every other day | |
| **Nonopioids** | | | |
| ◆ acetaminophen (Tylenol, others) (B) | Nonopioid analgesic, antipyretic | **Pediatric** | Relief of mild to moderate pain |
| | | PO/PR: Variable doses by age from 40 to 480 mg q4-6h | |
| | | **Adult** | Relief of mild to moderate pain |
| | | PO/PR: 325-650 mg q4-6h; not to exceed 3 g/day | |
| | | In alcoholics, not to exceed 2 g/day | |
| tramadol (Ultram) | Nonopioid analgesic (with opioid-like activity) | **Adult** PO: 50-100 mg q4-6h; not to exceed 400 mg/day | Relief of moderate to moderately severe pain |

*FDA*, U.S. Food and Drug Administration; *HCl*, hydrochloride; *IM*, intramuscular; *IV*, intravenous; *IR*, immediate release; *MS*, morphine sulfate; *MSIR*, morphine sulfate immediate-release; *PCA*, patient-controlled analgesia; *PO*, oral; *PR*, rectal; *subcut*, subcutaneous.
*Actiq is not approved for use in patients younger than 16 years of age.
The maximum recommended daily dose of acetaminophen for a typical adult patient with normal liver function is 3000 mg/24 hr. For hepatically compromised patients, this dosage may be 2000 mg or even lower. If in doubt, check with a pharmacist or prescriber regarding a particular patient.

when larger doses of hydromorphone are given. Morphine is available in oral, rectal, epidural, and injectable dosage forms, including PCA cartridges. Epidural dosage forms are injected onto the dura mater of the spinal cord. DepoDur is a liposomal epidural morphine product. Liposomes are a lipid-based drug vehicle that facilitates drug absorption through the lipid layer of cell membranes. Epidural analgesics have the potential for causing increased intracranial pressure, especially with multiple injections, and increased CNS depression when given with other CNS depressant drugs. Other CNS depressant drugs are not to be given without orders from an anesthesiologist. For dosage information, see the table on p. 152.

### Pharmacokinetics

| Route | Onset of Action | Peak Plasma Concentration | Elimination Half-life | Duration of Action |
|---|---|---|---|---|
| IM | Rapid | 30-60 min | 1.7-4.5 hr | 6-7 hr |

### codeine sulfate

Codeine sulfate is a natural opiate alkaloid (Schedule II) obtained from opium. It is similar to morphine in terms of its pharmacokinetic and pharmacodynamic properties. In fact, about 10% of a codeine dose is metabolized to morphine in the body. However, codeine is less effective as an analgesic and is the only agonist to possess a ceiling effect (meaning increasing the dose will not increase response). Therefore it is more commonly used as an antitussive drug in an array of cough preparations (see Chapter 36). Codeine combined with acetaminophen (tablets or elixir) is classified as a Schedule III controlled substance and is commonly used for control of mild to moderate pain as well as cough. When codeine is not combined with other drugs, it is classified as a Schedule II controlled substance, which implies a high abuse potential. Codeine causes GI tract upset, and many patients will say they are allergic to codeine, when in fact it just upsets their stomach. For dosage information, see the table on p. 152.

### Pharmacokinetics

| Route | Onset of Action | Peak Plasma Concentration | Elimination Half-life | Duration of Action |
|---|---|---|---|---|
| PO | 15-30 min | 34-45 min | 2.5-4 hr | 4-6 hr |

### fentanyl

Fentanyl is a synthetic opioid (Schedule II) used to treat moderate to severe pain. Like other opioids, it also has a high abuse potential. It is available in several dosage forms: parenteral injections, transdermal patches (Duragesic), buccal lozenges (Fentora), and buccal lozenges on a stick (Actiq). The buccal dosage forms are absorbed through the oral mucosa.

They may be especially helpful in managing breakthrough and procedural pain. The injectable form is used most commonly in perioperative settings and in intensive care unit settings for sedation during mechanical ventilation. The oral and transdermal forms are used primarily for long-term control of both malignant and nonmalignant chronic pain. Fentanyl is a very potent analgesic. Fentanyl in a dose of 0.1 mg intravenously is roughly equivalent to 10 mg of morphine intravenously.

The transdermal delivery system (patch) has been shown to be highly effective in the treatment of various chronic pain syndromes such as cancer-induced pain, especially in patients who cannot take oral medications. This route is not to be used in opioid-naïve patients or for acute pain relief. Fentanyl patches are difficult to titrate and are best used for nonescalating pain. To perform a conversion using the table in Box 10-3, first determine the daily (24-hour) opioid requirement of the patient. Second, if the opioid is not morphine, convert its dose to the equianalgesic dose of morphine using Box 10-3. Finally, calculate the equipotent transdermal fentanyl dosage. These tables are conservative in their dosages for achieving pain relief, and supplemental short-acting opioid analgesics are be added as needed.

Fentanyl patches take 6 to 12 hours to reach steady-state pain control after the first patch is applied, and supplemental short-acting therapy may be required. Most patients will experience adequate pain control for 72 hours with this method of fentanyl delivery. A new patch is to be applied every 72 hours. It is important to remove the old patch when applying a new one. It takes about 17 hours for the amount of fentanyl to reduce by 50% once the patch is removed.

The U.S. Food and Drug Administration (FDA) has issued many safety warnings about the use of fentanyl patches. Fentanyl patches are intended for management of chronic or cancer pain in opioid-tolerant patients whose pain is not adequately controlled by other types of medications. These patches are not recommended for acute pain situations such as postoperative pain. Deaths have occurred from drug-induced respiratory arrest when these conditions have not been met. According to the FDA, patients who are considered opioid tolerant are those who have been taking at least 60 mg of oral morphine daily or at least 30 mg of oral oxycodone daily or at least 8 mg of oral hydromorphone daily or an equianalgesic dose of another opioid. Other hazards associated with the use of fentanyl patches are cutting the patch and exposing the patch to heat (e.g., via a heating pad or sauna), both of which accelerate the diffusion of the drug into the patient's body.

For dosage information, see the table on p. 152.

## Pharmacokinetics

| Route | Onset of Action | Peak Plasma Concentration | Elimination Half-life | Duration of Action |
|-------|-----------------|---------------------------|----------------------|--------------------|
| IV | Rapid | Minutes | 1.5-6 hr | 30-60 min |
| Transdermal | 12-24 hr | 48-72 hr | Delayed | 13-40 hr |
| PO | 5-15 min | 20-30 min | 5-15 hr | Unknown |

### meperidine hydrochloride

Meperidine hydrochloride (Demerol) is a synthetic opioid analgesic (Schedule II). Meperidine must be used with caution, if at all, in elderly patients and in patients who require long-term analgesia or who have kidney dysfunction. An active metabolite, normeperidine, can accumulate to toxic levels and lead to seizures. For this reason, meperidine is now used less commonly than before and is definitely not recommended for long-term pain treatment. However, it is still used for acute pain during postoperative periods, as well as in emergency department settings for acute migraine headaches. Meperidine is available in oral and injectable forms. For dosage information, see the table on p. 152.

## Pharmacokinetics

| Route | Onset of Action | Peak Plasma Concentration | Elimination Half-life | Duration of Action |
|-------|-----------------|---------------------------|----------------------|--------------------|
| IM | Rapid | 30-60 min | 3-5 hr | 2-4 hr |

### methadone hydrochloride

Methadone hydrochloride (Dolophine) is a synthetic opioid analgesic (Schedule II). It is the opioid of choice for the detoxification treatment of opioid addicts in methadone maintenance programs. Use of agonist-antagonist opioids (e.g., pentazocine) in heroin-addicted patients or those in methadone maintenance programs can induce significant withdrawal symptoms. There has been renewed interest in the use of methadone for chronic (e.g., neuropathic) and cancer-related pain. The drug is readily absorbed through the GI tract with peak plasma concentrations at 4 hours for single dosing. Methadone is unique in that its half-life is longer than its duration of activity because it is bound into the tissues of the liver, kidneys, and brain. With repeated doses, the drug accumulates in these tissues and is slowly released, thus allowing for 24-hour dosing. Methadone is eliminated through the liver, which makes it a safer choice than some other opioids for patients with renal impairment. Recent FDA reports have cited the prolonged half-life of the drug as a cause of unintentional overdoses and deaths. There is also concern that methadone may cause cardiac dysrhythmias. Methadone is available in oral and injectable forms. For dosage information, see the table on p. 152.

## Pharmacokinetics

| Route | Onset of Action | Peak Plasma Concentration | Elimination Half-life | Duration of Action |
|-------|-----------------|---------------------------|----------------------|--------------------|
| PO | 30-60 min | 1.5-2 hr | 25 hr | 22-48 hr |

### oxycodone hydrochloride

Oxycodone hydrochloride is an analgesic drug that is structurally related to morphine and has comparable analgesic activity (Schedule II). It is also commonly combined in tablets with acetaminophen (Percocet) and with aspirin (Percodan). Oxycodone is also available in immediate-release formulations (Oxy IR) and sustained-released formulations (OxyContin).

A somewhat weaker but commonly used opioid is hydrocodone (Schedule III), which is available only in tablet form, most commonly in combination with acetaminophen (Vicodin) but also with aspirin and ibuprofen. It is available only for oral use. For dosage information, see the table on p. 152.

### Pharmacokinetics (Immediate Release)

| Route | Onset of Action | Peak Plasma Concentration | Elimination Half-life | Duration of Action |
|-------|----------------|---------------------------|----------------------|--------------------|
| PO | 10-15 min | 1 hr | 2-3 hr | 3-6 hr |

### OPIOID AGONISTS-ANTAGONISTS

Opioids with mixed actions are often called *agonists-antagonists* (Schedule IV). They bind to the mu receptor and can therefore compete with other substances for these sites. They either exert no action (i.e., they are competitive antagonists) or have only limited action (i.e., they are partial agonists). They are similar to the opioid agonists in terms of their therapeutic indications; however, they have a lower risk of misuse and addiction. The antagonistic activity of this group can produce withdrawal symptoms in opioid-dependent patients. Their use is contraindicated in patients who have shown hypersensitivity reactions to the drugs.

These drugs have varying degrees of agonist and antagonist effects on the different opioid receptor subtypes. They are used in situations requiring short-term pain control, such as after obstetric procedures. They are sometimes chosen for patients who have a history of opioid addiction. These medications can both help prevent overmedication and reduce posttreatment addictive cravings in these patients. Combination products of buprenorphine and naloxone offer physicians an in-office treatment of addiction (see Chapter 17). These drugs are normally not strong enough for management of longer-term chronic pain (e.g., cancer pain, chronic lower back pain). They are *not* to be given concurrently with full opioid agonists, because they may both reduce analgesic effects and cause withdrawal symptoms in opioid-tolerant patients. Adverse reactions are similar to opioids but with a lower incidence of respiratory depression. Four opioid agonists-antagonists are currently available: buprenorphine (Buprenex), butorphanol (Stadol), nalbuphine (Nubain), and pentazocine (Talwin). They are available in various oral, injectable, and intranasal dosage forms as indicated in the dosage table. All except butorphanol are also available in combination with the opioid antagonist naloxone to enhance their opioid antagonistic effects, which are usually weaker than the agonistic effects of these drugs.

### OPIOID ANTAGONISTS

Opioid antagonists produce their antagonistic activity by competing with opioids for CNS receptor sites.

#### ♦ naloxone hydrochloride

Naloxone hydrochloride (Narcan) is a pure opioid antagonist. It has no agonistic morphine-like properties and works as a blocking drug for the opioid drugs. Accordingly, the drug does not produce analgesia or respiratory depression. Naloxone is the drug of choice for the complete or partial reversal of opioid-induced respiratory depression. It is also indicated in cases of suspected acute opioid overdose. Failure of the drug to significantly reverse the effects of the presumed opioid overdose indicates that the condition may not be related to opioid overdose. The primary adverse effect is opioid withdrawal syndrome, which can occur with abrupt overreversal in opioid-tolerant patients. Naloxone is available only in injectable dosage forms. Use of the drug is contraindicated in patients with a history of hypersensitivity to it. For dosage information, see the table on p. 152.

### Pharmacokinetics

| Route | Onset of Action | Peak Plasma Concentration | Elimination Half-life | Duration of Action |
|-------|----------------|---------------------------|----------------------|--------------------|
| IV | Less than 2 min | Rapid | 64 min | 0.5-2 hr |

#### naltrexone hydrochloride

Naltrexone hydrochloride (ReVia) is an opioid antagonist used as an adjunct for the maintenance of an opioid-free state in former opioid addicts. The FDA has identified it as a safe and effective adjunct to psychosocial treatments of alcoholism. It is also indicated for reversal of postoperative opioid-induced respiratory depression. Nausea and tachycardia are the most common adverse effects and are related to reversal of the opioid effect. Use of naltrexone hydrochloride is contraindicated in cases of known drug allergy and in patients with hepatitis or other severe liver dysfunction. It is available only for oral use. For dosage information, see the table on p. 152.

### Pharmacokinetics

| Route | Onset of Action | Peak Plasma Concentration | Elimination Half-life | Duration of Action |
|-------|----------------|---------------------------|----------------------|--------------------|
| PO | Rapid | 1 hr | 4-13 hr | 24-72 hr |

## NONOPIOID AND MISCELLANEOUS ANALGESICS

Acetaminophen (Tylenol) is the most widely used nonopioid analgesic. Acetaminophen is commonly abbreviated APAP in the U.S.; however, this abbreviation is not recognized in Canada. There is a current movement to stop using APAP as an abbreviation, because of the potential that patients will not realize they are receiving a prescription with acetaminophen and may take additional over-the-counter acetaminophen.

All of the drugs in the NSAID class (which includes aspirin, ibuprofen, naproxen, the cyclooxygenase-2 [COX-2] inhibitor celecoxib [Celebrex], and others) are nonopioid analgesics. These drugs are discussed in greater detail in Chapter 44. They are used for management of pain, especially pain associated with inflammatory conditions such as arthritis, because they have significant antiinflammatory effects in addition to their analgesic effects.

Miscellaneous analgesics include tramadol and transdermal lidocaine and are discussed in depth in their respective drug profiles in this chapter. Capsaicin is a topical product made from several different types of peppers. It works by decreasing or interfering with substance P, a pain signal in the brain. Capsaicin is available over the counter. It can be used for muscle pain, joint pain, and nerve pain. Milnacipran (Savella) is a selective serotonin and norepinephrine dual-uptake inhibitor. It is indicated for the treatment of fibromyalgia. It is thought that patients with fibromyalgia have reduced levels of norepinephrine in their brains, and milnacipran increases norepinephrine levels, which helps reduce pain associated with the disease.

## Mechanism of Action and Drug Effects

The mechanism of action of acetaminophen is similar to that of the salicylates. It blocks peripheral pain impulses by inhibition of prostaglandin synthesis. Acetaminophen also lowers febrile body temperatures by acting on the hypothalamus, the structure in the brain that regulates body temperature. Heat is dissipated through vasodilation and increased peripheral blood flow. In contrast to NSAIDs, acetaminophen lacks antiinflammatory effects. Although acetaminophen shares the analgesic and antipyretic effects of the salicylates and other NSAIDs, it does not have many of the unwanted effects of these drugs. For example, acetaminophen products are not usually associated with cardiovascular effects (e.g., edema) or platelet effects (e.g., bleeding), as are aspirin and other NSAIDs. They also do not cause the aspirin-related GI tract irritation or bleeding nor any of the aspirin-related acid-base changes.

## Indications

Acetaminophen is indicated for the treatment of mild to moderate pain and fever. It is an appropriate substitute for aspirin because of its analgesic and antipyretic properties. Acetaminophen is a valuable alternative for those patients who cannot tolerate aspirin or for whom aspirin may be contraindicated.

Acetaminophen is also the antipyretic (antifever) drug of choice in children and adolescents with flu syndromes, because the use of aspirin in these populations is associated with a condition known as *Reye's syndrome.*

## Contraindications

Contraindications to acetaminophen use include known drug allergy, severe liver disease, and the genetic disease known as *glucose-6-phosphate dehydrogenase (G6PD) deficiency.*

## Adverse Effects

Acetaminophen is generally well tolerated and is therefore available over the counter and in many combination prescription drugs. Possible adverse effects include rash, nausea, and vomiting. Much less common but more severe are the adverse effects of blood disorders or dyscrasias (e.g., anemias) and nephrotoxicities, and, of most concern, hepatotoxicity.

### Toxicity and Management of Overdose

Many people do not realize that acetaminophen, despite its over-the-counter status, is a potentially lethal drug when taken in overdose. Depressed patients (especially adolescents) may intentionally overdose on the drug as an attention-seeking gesture without realizing the grave danger involved.

The ingestion of large amounts of acetaminophen, as in acute overdose, or chronic unintentional misuse can cause hepatic necrosis. Acute ingestion of acetaminophen doses of 150 mg/kg (approximately 7 to 10 grams) or more may result in hepatic toxicity. Acute hepatotoxicity can usually be reversed with acetylcysteine, whereas long-term toxicity is more likely to be permanent.

The standard maximum daily dose of acetaminophen for healthy adults is 4000 mg. However, limitation to 2000 mg or less may be necessary for patients with risk factors such as advanced age (elderly) or liver dysfunction. Excessive dosing may occur inadvertently with the use of combination products that include a fixed ratio of an opioid drug plus acetaminophen (e.g., hydrocodone plus acetaminophen). Prescribers must be mindful of recommended daily dose limits when prescribing these medications. In 2011, the FDA announced that combination products are to be limited to 325 mg of acetaminophen, and a maximum daily dose of 3000 mg/day is being considered.

The long-term ingestion of large doses of acetaminophen is more likely to result in severe hepatotoxicity, which may be irreversible. Because the reported or estimated quantity of drug ingested is often inaccurate and not a reliable guide to the therapeutic management of the overdose, serum acetaminophen concentration is determined no sooner than 4 hours after the ingestion. If a serum acetaminophen level cannot be determined, it is assumed that the overdose is potentially toxic and treatment with acetylcysteine needs to be started. Acetylcysteine is the recommended antidote for acetaminophen toxicity and works by preventing the hepatotoxic metabolites of acetaminophen from forming. It is most effective when given within 10 hours of an overdose. Historically, the usual dosage regimen is a 140 mg/kg oral loading dose, followed by 70 mg/kg every 4 hours for 17 additional doses. This drug is notoriously bad tasting with an odor of rotten eggs, and vomiting of an oral dose is common. It is recommended that the dose be repeated if vomiting occurs within 1 hour of dosing. An intravenous dosage formulation of acetylcysteine (Acetadote) is also available.

## Interactions

A few drugs can interact with acetaminophen. Alcohol is potentially the most dangerous. Chronic heavy alcohol abusers may be at increased risk of liver toxicity from excessive acetaminophen use. For this reason, a maximum daily dose of 2000 mg is generally recommended. Health care professionals need to warn patients with regular intake of alcohol not to exceed recommended dosages of acetaminophen because of the risk of liver dysfunction and possible liver failure. Ideally, alcohol consumption is not to exceed three drinks daily. Other hepatotoxic drugs need to be avoided. Other drugs that potentially can interact with acetaminophen include phenytoin, barbiturates, warfarin, isoniazid, rifampin, beta blockers, and anticholinergic drugs, all of which are discussed in greater detail in later chapters.

# DRUG PROFILES

## ◆ acetaminophen

Acetaminophen (Tylenol) is an effective and relatively safe nonopioid analgesic used for mild to moderate pain relief. It is best avoided in patients who are alcoholic or who have hepatic disease. Acetaminophen is available in oral, rectal, and most recently, IV form. Acetaminophen is also a component of several prescription combination drug products, including hydrocodone/acetaminophen (Vicodin) and oxycodone/acetaminophen (Percocet).

### Pharmacokinetics

| Route | Onset of Action | Peak Plasma Concentration | Elimination Half-life | Duration of Action |
|-------|-----------------|---------------------------|-----------------------|--------------------|
| PO | 10-30 min | 0.5-2 hr | 1-4 hr | 3-4 hr |

## tramadol hydrochloride

Tramadol hydrochloride (Ultram) is categorized as a miscellaneous analgesic due to its unique properties. It is a centrally acting analgesic with a dual mechanism of action. It creates a weak bond to the mu opioid receptors and inhibits the reuptake of both norepinephrine and serotonin. Although it does have weak opioid receptor activity, tramadol is not currently classified as a controlled substance. Tramadol is indicated for the treatment of moderate to moderately severe pain. Tramadol is rapidly absorbed, and its absorption is unaffected by food. It is metabolized in the liver to an active metabolite and eliminated via renal excretion. Adverse effects are similar to those of opioids and include drowsiness, dizziness, headache, nausea, constipation, and respiratory depression. Seizures have been reported in patients taking tramadol and occur in patients taking both normal and excessive dosages. Patients who may be at risk are those receiving tricyclic antidepressants, selective serotonin reuptake inhibitors (SSRIs), monoamine oxidase inhibitors, neuroleptics, or other drugs that reduce the seizure threshold. There is also an increased risk of developing serotonin syndrome when tramadol is taken concurrently with SSRIs (see Chapter 16).

Use of tramadol is contraindicated in cases of known drug allergy, which may include allergy to opioids due to potential cross-reactivity. It is also contraindicated in cases of acute intoxication with alcohol, hypnotics, centrally acting analgesics, opioids, or psychotropic drugs. The drug is only available in oral dosage forms, including a combination with acetaminophen (Ultracet), as well as extended-release formulation (ConZip, Ryzolt, Ultram ER) and as an orally disintegrating tablet called Rybix. A new drug, tapentadol (Nucynta), is structurally related to tramadol with a duel mechanism of action. It is a mu agonist and a norepinephrine reuptake inhibitor. It is a Schedule II narcotic.

### Pharmacokinetics

| Route | Onset of Action | Peak Plasma Concentration | Elimination Half-life | Duration of Action |
|-------|-----------------|---------------------------|-----------------------|--------------------|
| PO | 30 min | 2 hr | 5-8 hr | 6 hr |

## lidocaine, transdermal

Transdermal lidocaine is a topical anesthetic (see Chapter 11) and cardiac antidysrhythmic (see Chapter 23) that is formulated into a patch (Lidoderm), which is placed onto painful areas of the skin. It is indicated for the treatment of postherpetic neuralgia, a painful skin condition that remains after a skin outbreak of shingles. Shingles is caused by the herpes zoster virus, also known as the varicella-zoster virus, which causes chickenpox in children. Lidocaine patches provide local pain relief, and up to three patches may be placed on a large painful area. However, the patches are not to be worn for longer than 12 hours a day to avoid potential systemic drug toxicity (e.g., cardiac dysrhythmias). Because they act topically, there are minimal systemic adverse effects. However, the skin at the site of treatment may develop redness or edema, and unusual skin sensations may occur. These reactions are usually mild and transient and resolve within a few minutes to hours. Patches are applied only to intact skin with no blisters. They can be used either alone or as part of adjunctive treatment with systemic therapies such as antidepressants (see Chapter 16), opioids, or anticonvulsants (see Chapter 14). Used patches must be disposed of securely because they may be dangerous to children or pets. Specific pharmacokinetic data are not listed due to the continuous nature of dosing. Studies have demonstrated that a patch can provide varying degrees of pain relief for 4 to 12 hours.

# NURSING PROCESS

Pain may be acute or chronic and occurs in patients in all settings and across the lifespan, thus leading to much suffering and distress. Patients experiencing pain pose many challenges to the nurse, prescribers, and other health care providers involved in their care. The challenge is that pain is a complex and multifaceted problem that requires astute assessment skills with appropriate interventions based on the individual, the specific type of pain, related diseases, and/or health status.

Medical associations, health care organizations, governing bodies, and professional nursing organizations have been involved in defining standards and outcomes of care related to assessment and management of pain. For example, The Joint Commission (www.jointcommission.org) and the Agency for Healthcare Research and Quality (www.ahrq.gov/whatsnew.asp#qt) have developed such standards. In addition, the WHO (www.who.int/en) has developed standards related specifically to cancer pain. Professional nursing organizations, such as the Oncology Nursing Society and the American Nurses Association, have also created standards of care related to pain assessment and management. In 2009, the American Pain Society also published opioid guidelines available at http://www.ampainsoc.org/.

# ASSESSMENT

Adequate analgesia requires a holistic, comprehensive, and individualized patient assessment with specific attention to the type, intensity, and characteristics of the pain and the levels of comfort. Comfort, in this situation, is defined as the extent of physical and psychological ease that an individual experiences. Perform a thorough health history, nursing assessment, and medication history as soon as possible or upon the first encounter with the patient, including questions about the following: (1) allergies to nonopioids, opioids, partial or mixed agonists, and/or opioid antagonists (see previous pharmacologic discussion for examples of specific drugs); (2) potential drug-drug and/or drug-food interactions; (3) presence of diseases or CNS depression; (4) history of the use of alcohol, street drugs, or any illegal drug or substance and/or history of substance abuse, with information about the substance, dose, and frequency of use; (5) results of laboratory tests ordered, such as levels of serum ALT, ALP, GGT, 5′-nucleotidase, and bilirubin (indicative of liver function), and/or levels of BUN and creatinine (reflective of renal function); abnormal liver or renal function may require that lower doses of analgesic be used to prevent toxicity or overdosage (see the Safety: Laboratory Values related to Drug Therapy box on p. 151); (6) character and intensity of the pain, including onset, location, and quality (e.g., stabbing/knifelike, throbbing, dull ache, sharp, diffuse, localized, or referred); actual rating of the pain using a pain assessment scale (see later); and any precipitating, aggravating, and/or relieving factors; (7) duration of the pain (acute versus chronic); and (8) types of pharmacologic, nonpharmacologic, and/or adjunctive measures that have been implemented, with further explanation of the treatment's duration of use and overall effectiveness.

To be thorough and effective, include in your assessment the factors or variables that may impact an individual's pain experience, such as physical factors (e.g., age, gender, pain threshold, overall state of health, disease processes or pathologies) and emotional, spiritual, and cultural variables (e.g., reaction to pain, pain tolerance, fear, anxiety, stressors, sleep patterns, societal influences, family roles, phase of growth and development, and religious, racial, and/or ethnic beliefs or practices). Age-appropriate assessment tools are recommended in assessing pain across the lifespan (see later discussion). For pediatric and elderly patients, nonverbal behavior or cues and information from family members or caregivers may be helpful in identifying pain levels. In an elderly individual, physical and cognitive impairments may affect reporting of pain; however, this does not mean that the elderly patient is not experiencing pain—the patient's reporting may just be altered. Chronic pain and pain associated with cancer are both complex and multifactorial problems requiring a holistic approach with attention to other patient complaints, such as a decrease in activities of daily living, insomnia, depression, social withdrawal, anxiety, personality changes, and quality of life issues.

Perform a system-focused nursing assessment with collection of both subjective and objective data as follows: neurologic status (e.g., level of orientation and alertness, level of sedation, sensory and motor abilities, reflexes); respiratory status (e.g., respiratory rate, rhythm, and depth; breath sounds); GI status (e.g., presence of bowel sounds; bowel patterns; complaints of constipation, diarrhea, nausea, vomiting, or abdominal discomfort); genitourinary status (e.g., urinary output; any burning or discomfort on urination; urinary retention); and cardiac status (e.g., pulse rate and rhythm, blood pressure, any problems with

---

## PATIENT-CENTERED CARE: LIFESPAN CONSIDERATIONS FOR THE PEDIATRIC PATIENT

### *Opioid Use*

- Assessment of the pediatric patient is challenging, and all types of behavior that may indicate pain, such as muscular rigidity, restlessness, screaming, fear of moving, and withdrawn behavior, must be carefully considered.
- Adequacy of pain management is more difficult to determine in children because of their inability to express themselves. Frequently the reason older pediatric patients do not verbalize their pain is their fear of treatment, such as injections. Compassionate and therapeutic communication skills, as well as the use of alternate routes of administration, as ordered, will help in these situations.
- The "ouch scale" is often used to determine the level of pain in children. This scale is used to obtain the child's rating of the intensity of pain from 0 to 5 by means of simple face diagrams, from a very happy face for level 0 (no pain) to a sad, tearful face for level 5 (severe pain). Pain assessment is very important in pediatric patients because they are often undermedicated. Always thoroughly assess the pediatric patient's verbal and nonverbal behavior, and never underestimate the patient's complaints! Remember that parents and caregivers can play a very important role in this assessment.
- The patient's baseline age, weight, and height are important to document, because drug calculations are often based on these variables. With the pediatric patient, check and double-check *all* mathematical calculations for accuracy to avoid excessive dosages; this is especially true for opioids.
- Analgesics must be given, as ordered, before pain becomes severe, with oral dosage forms used first, if appropriate.
- If suppositories are used, be careful to administer the exact dose and not to split, halve, or divide an adult dose into a child's dose. This may result in the administration of an unknown amount of medication and possible overdose.

- When subcutaneous, intramuscular, and intravenous medications are used, the principle of atraumatic care in the delivery of nursing care must be followed. One technique used to help ensure atraumatic care is the application of a mixture of local anesthetics or other prescribed substances to the injection site before the injection is given. EMLA (lidocaine/prilocaine) is a topical cream that anesthetizes the site of the injection; if ordered, apply 1 to 2½ hours before the injection. Consult institutional policies and procedures for further instructions regarding its use.
- Distraction and creative imagery may be used for older children such as toddlers or preschool-age children.
- Always monitor pediatric patients very closely for any unusual behavior while receiving opioids.
- Report the following signs and symptoms of central nervous system changes to the prescriber immediately if they occur: dizziness, lightheadedness, drowsiness, hallucinations, changes in the level of consciousness, and sluggish pupil reaction. Do not administer further medication until the nurse receives further orders from the prescriber.
- Always monitor and document vital signs before, during, and after the administration of opioid analgesics. An opioid medication is usually withheld if a patient's respirations are less than 12 breaths/min or if there are any changes in the level of consciousness. Always follow protocol, and never ignore a patient's status!
- Generally speaking, smaller doses of opioids, with very close and frequent monitoring, are indicated for the pediatric patient. Giving oral medications with meals or snacks may help to decrease GI upset.

dizziness or syncope). Assess and document vital signs, including blood pressure, pulse rate, respirations, temperature, and level of pain (now considered as the fifth vital sign). It is important to pull from one's knowledge base and remember that during the acute pain response, stimulation of the sympathetic nervous system may result in elevated values for vital signs, with an increase in blood pressure (120/80 mm Hg or higher), pulse rate (100 beats/min or higher), and respiratory rate and depth (20 breaths/min or higher and shallow breathing).

A variety of pain assessment tools are available that may be used to gather information about the fifth vital sign. One very basic assessment tool is the Numeric Pain Intensity Scale (0 to 10 pain rating scale); patients are asked to rate their pain intensity by picking the number that most closely represents their level of pain. The Verbal Rating Scale, another pain assessment tool, uses verbal descriptors for pain, including words such as *mild, moderate, severe, aching, agonizing,* or *discomfort.* The FACES Pain Rating Scale is helpful in assessing pain in patients of all ages and educational levels because it relies on a series of faces ranging from happy to sad to sad with tears. The patient is asked to identify the face that best represents the pain he or she is experiencing at that moment. When the patient is in acute pain, when pain intensity is a primary focus for assessment, and/or when the need is to determine the efficacy of pain management intervention, the simple, one-dimensional scales (e.g., the Numeric Pain Intensity Scale) work best. The elderly, especially those with cognitive impairment, may need more time to respond to the assessment tool and may also require large-print versions of written tools. There are other assessment tools that are multidimensional scales and are more beneficial in assessing patients who experience chronic rather than acute pain. One example is the Brief Pain Inventory assessment tool, which includes a body map so that the patient can identify on the figure the exact area where pain is felt. This tool also helps in obtaining information about the impact of pain on functioning. Assess pain before, during, and after the pain intervention, as well as the level of pain during activity and at rest. The following sections provide assessment information for specific drug classes.

### NONOPIOIDS

For patients receiving *nonopioid analgesics,* focus the assessment not only on general data as described earlier but also on the specific drug being given. For example, in those patients taking acetaminophen, begin the assessment by determining whether the patient has allergies, is pregnant, and/or is breastfeeding. As mentioned in the pharmacology section, acetaminophen is contraindicated in those with severe liver disease and in patients with G6PD deficiency. Additionally, due to possible adverse effects of blood disorders (anemias), renal/liver toxicity, cautious use is necessary. See pharmacology discussion for more information about acute overdose and chronic unintentional misuse. Also assess for any other medications the patient is taking, because of the risk of excessive doses when taking combination products consisting of acetaminophen. Inadvertent overdosing is a possible consequence of this situation. Other drug interactions and concerns are addressed in the pharmacology discussion.

Once therapy has been initiated, closely monitor for chronic acetaminophen poisoning, looking for symptoms such as rapid, weak pulse, dyspnea, and cold and clammy extremities. Long-term daily use of acetaminophen may lead to increased risk of permanent liver damage, and therefore you must frequently monitor the results of liver function studies. Adults who ingest higher than recommended dosages may be at higher risk of liver dysfunction as well as other adverse effects such as loss of appetite, jaundice, nausea, and vomiting. Children are also at high risk of liver dysfunction if the recommended dosage ranges are exceeded. With the use of NSAIDs (e.g., ibuprofen, aspirin, and COX-2 inhibitors), assess renal and liver functioning and gather information about GI disorders such as ulcers (see Chapter 44 for more information on antiinflammatory drugs). With aspirin, age is important; this drug is not to be given to children and adolescent patients because of the risk of Reye's syndrome. Aspirin may also lead to bleeding and ulcers, so ruling out conditions that represent contraindications and cautions to its use before therapy begins is important to patient safety. With tramadol hydrochloride, assessment of age is important because this drug is not recommended for use in individuals 75 years of age or older.

A miscellaneous nonopioid analgesic, lidocaine transdermal, is another option for managing different types of pain. For lidocaine transdermal patches, understand that this transdermal drug is indicated in those with postherpetic neuralgia, and thus assess the herpetic lesion(s) and surrounding skin. When these patches are used, they must be kept away from children and are not to be prescribed for very young, small, or debilitated patients because these patients are at higher risk for toxicity. Liver function also needs to be assessed and monitored.

### OPIOIDS

When *opioid analgesics,* or any other CNS depressants, are prescribed, focus assessment on vital signs; allergies; respiratory disorders; respiratory function (rate, rhythm, depth, and breath sounds); presence of head injury (which will mask signs and symptoms of increasing intracranial pressure); neurologic status, with attention to level of consciousness or alertness and the level of sedation; sensory and motor functioning; GI tract functioning (bowel sounds and bowel patterns); and genitourinary functioning (intake and output). In addition, all opioids may cause spasms of the sphincter of Oddi. If renal and liver function studies are ordered, monitor results, because the risk of toxicity increases with diminished function of these organs. An additional concern is any past or present history of neurologic disorders such as Alzheimer's disease, dementia, multiple sclerosis, muscular dystrophy, myasthenia gravis, or cerebrovascular accident or stroke, because the use of opioids may alter symptoms of the disease process, possibly masking symptoms or worsening the clinical presentation when no actual pathologic changes have occurred. In these situations, use of another analgesic or pain protocol may be indicated. Attention to age is also important, because both elderly and very young patients are more sensitive to opioids—as to many other medications. In fact, old or young age may be a contraindication to opioid use, depending on the specific drug. See the earlier pharmacology discussion regarding cautions, contraindications, and drug interactions.

### OPIOID AGONISTS-ANTAGONISTS

In patients taking *opioid agonists-antagonists,* such as buprenorphine hydrochloride, assess vital signs with attention to respiratory rate and breath sounds. The opioid agonists-antagonists still possess opioid agonist effects, and therefore the assessment information related to opioids is applicable to these drugs as well. It is also very important to remember during assessment that these drugs are still effective analgesics and still have CNS depressant effects but are subject to a ceiling effect (see earlier definition). Given the action of these drugs, the assessment may help determine whether the patient is an abuser of opioids. This is important because the simultaneous administration of agonists-antagonists with another opioid will lead to reversal of analgesia and possible opioid withdrawal. Age is another factor to assess, because these drugs are not recommended for use in patients 18 years of age or younger. See previous discussion for a listing of contraindications, cautions, and drug interactions.

### OPIOID ANTAGONISTS

Remember that the *opioid antagonists* are used mainly in reversing respiratory depression secondary to opioid overdosage. Naloxone may be used in patients of all ages, including neonates and children. Assess and document vital signs before, during, and after the use of the antagonist so that the therapeutic effects can be further assessed and documented and the need for further doses determined. In addition, remember that the antagonist drug may not work with just one dosing and that repeated doses are generally needed to reverse the effects of the opioid. See the pharmacology section for information about contraindications, cautions, and drug interactions.

## NURSING DIAGNOSES

1. Impaired gas exchange related to opioid-induced CNS effects and respiratory depression
2. Acute pain related to specific disease processes or conditions and other pathologies leading to various levels and types of pain
3. Chronic pain related to various disease processes, conditions, or syndromes causing pain
4. Constipation related to the CNS depressant effects on the GI system
5. Deficient knowledge related to lack of familiarity with opioids, their use, and their adverse effects

## PLANNING

### GOALS

1. Patient regains/maintains a respiratory rate between 10 and 20 breaths per minute without respiratory depression.
2. Patient states adequate acute pain relief associated with appropriate analgesic drug therapy regimen.
3. Patient experiences relief from chronic pain associated with appropriate pharmacologic therapy regimen.

4. Patient identifies measures to help maintain normal bowel elimination patterns and avoids/minimizes opioid-induced constipation.
5. Patient demonstrates adequate knowledge about the analgesic and/or other drug therapy and nondrug regimen.

### OUTCOME CRITERIA

1. Patient states correct technique for coughing and deep breathing and adequate fluid intake while taking opioids and/or other analgesics for pain.
   - Patient's respiratory rate is within normal depth, rate, and patterns with clearing breath sounds.
2. Patient relates increased comfort levels as seen by decreased use of analgesics, increased activity and performance of activities of daily living, decreased complaints of acute pain, as well as decreased levels of pain as rated on a scale of 1 to 10.
3. Patient relates increased comfort levels as seen by decreased use of analgesics, increased activity and performance of activities of daily living, decreased complaints of chronic pain, as well as decreased levels of pain as rated on a scale of 1 to 10.
   - Patient uses nonpharmacologic measures such as relaxation therapy, distraction, and music therapy to help improve comfort and enhance any drug therapy regimens for chronic pain.
4. Patient states various measures to help minimize or avoid the occurrence of constipation with forcing of fluids, increasing fiber in the diet, and improving mobility.
5. Patient reports appropriate use of analgesics with minimal complications/adverse effects.
   - Patient states rationale for the use, action, and therapeutic effects associated with analgesic drugs for management of acute and/or chronic pain.
   - Patient states rationale for the use of nondrug approaches to pain management.
   - Patient states importance of taking medication as prescribed.

## IMPLEMENTATION

Once the cause of pain has been diagnosed or other assessment and data gathering have been completed, begin pain management immediately and aggressively in conformity with the needs of each individual patient and situation. Pain management is varied and multifaceted and needs to incorporate pharmacologic as well as nonpharmacologic approaches (see Box 10-1 on p. 141 and the Safety: Herbal Therapies and Dietary Supplements box on p. 161). Pain management strategies must also include consideration of the type of pain and pain rating as well as pain quality, duration, and precipitating factors, and interventions that help the pain. Some general principles of pain management are as follows: (1) Individualize a plan of care based on the patient as a holistic and cultural being (see the Patient-Centered Care: Cultural Implications box on p. 141). (2) Manage mild pain with the use of nonopioid drugs such as acetaminophen, tramadol, and NSAIDs (see Chapter 44).

(3) Manage moderate to severe pain with a stepped approach using opioids. Other analgesics or types of analgesics may be used in addition to other categories of medication (see pharmacology discussion). (4) Administer analgesics as ordered but before the pain gets out of control. (5) Always consider the use of nonpharmacologic comfort measures (see Box 10-1) such as homeopathic and folk remedies, exercise, distraction, music or pet therapy, massage, and transcutaneous electrical stimulation. Although not always effective, these measures may prove beneficial for some patients. See Patient Teaching Tips for more information related to analgesics.

## SAFETY: HERBAL THERAPIES AND DIETARY SUPPLEMENTS

### *Feverfew* (Chrysanthemum parthenium)

**Overview**
A member of the marigold family known for its antiinflammatory properties

**Common Uses**
Treatment of migraine headaches, menstrual cramps, inflammation, and fever

**Adverse Effects**
Nausea, vomiting, constipation, diarrhea, altered taste sensations, muscle stiffness, and joint pain

**Potential Drug Interactions**
Possible increase in bleeding with the use of aspirin and other nonsteroidal antiinflammatory drugs, dipyridamole, and warfarin

**Contraindications**
Contraindicated in those allergic to ragweed, chrysanthemums, and marigolds, as well as those about to undergo surgery

### NONOPIOIDS

Give *nonopioid analgesics* as ordered or as indicated for fever or pain. Acetaminophen is to be taken as prescribed and within the recommended dosage range over a 24-hour period because of the risk of liver damage and acute toxicity. If a patient is taking other over-the-counter medications with acetaminophen, he or she needs to understand the importance of reading the labels very carefully (of other medications) to identify the total amount of acetaminophen taken and any other drug-drug interactions. In educating the patient, emphasize the signs and symptoms of acetaminophen overdose: bleeding, loss of energy, fever, sore throat, and easy bruising (due to hepatotoxicity). These must be reported immediately by the patient, family member, or caregiver to the nurse and/or prescriber. Any worsening or changing in the nature and/or characteristic of pain must also be reported. Suppository dosage forms of acetaminophen—like suppository forms of other drugs—are recommended to be placed into a medicine cup of ice. Once the suppository is unwrapped, cold water may be run over it to moisten the suppository for easier insertion. The suppository is inserted into the rectum using a gloved finger and water-soluble lubricating gel, if necessary. Acetaminophen tablets may be crushed if needed. Adult patients who take 3000 mg/day or greater of acetaminophen are at increased risk for acute

hepatotoxicity. Death may occur after ingestion of more than 15 g. Liver damage from acetaminophen may be minimized by timely dosing with acetylcysteine (see previous discussion). If acetylcysteine is indicated, warn the patient about the drug's foul taste and odor. Many patients report that the drug smells and tastes like rotten eggs. Acetylcysteine is better tolerated if it is disguised by mixing with a drink such as cola or flavored water to increase its palatability. Use of a straw may help minimize contact with the mucous membranes of the mouth and is recommended. This antidote may be given through a nasogastric or orogastric tube or intravenously, if necessary.

Tramadol may cause drowsiness, dizziness, headache, nausea, constipation, and respiratory depression. If dizziness, blurred vision, or drowsiness occur, be sure to assist the patient with ambulation (as with the use of any analgesic that may lead to dizziness or lightheadedness) to minimize the risk of fall and injury. Educate the patient about injury prevention, including the need to dangle the feet over the edge of the bed before full ambulation, changing positions slowly, and asking for assistance when ambulating. In addition, while the patient is taking tramadol—as well as any other analgesics, and especially opioids—the patient needs to avoid any tasks that require mental clarity and alertness. Increasing fluids and fiber in the diet may help with constipation. Use of flat cola, ginger ale, or dry crackers may help to minimize nausea.

### OPIOIDS

When *opioids* (and other analgesics) are prescribed, administer the drug as ordered after checking for the "Six Rights" of medication administration (see Chapter 1). After the prescriber's order has been double-checked, closely examine the medication profile and documentation to determine the last time the medication was given before another dose is administered. Monitor the patient's vital signs at frequent intervals with special attention to respiratory changes. A respiratory rate of 10 breaths/min (some protocols still adhere to the parameter of 12 breaths/min) may indicate respiratory depression and must be reported to the prescriber. The drug dosage, frequency, and/or route may need to be changed or an antidote (opioid antagonist) given if respiratory depression occurs. Naloxone must always be available, especially with the use of intravenous and/or other parenteral dosage forms of opioids, such as PCA (see Chapter 9 and the discussion to follow), and/or epidural infusions. Naloxone is indicated to reverse CNS depression, specifically respiratory depression, but remember that this antidote also reverses analgesia. Monitor the patient's urinary output as well; it should be at least 600 mL/24 hr. Monitor bowel sounds during therapy; decreased peristalsis may indicate the need for a dietary change, such as increased fiber, or use of a stool softener or mild laxative (see Box 10-2). Assess the patient's pupillary reaction to light. Pinpoint pupils indicate a possible overdose.

Opioids or any analgesic must be given before the pain reaches its peak to help maximize the effectiveness of the opioid or other analgesic. Once the drug is administered, return at the appropriate time (taking into consideration the times of onset and peak effect of the drug and the route) to assess the effectiveness of the drug and/or other interventions as well as observe for the presence of adverse effects (see previous discussion of pain assessment tools). With regard to the route of administration, the recommendation is that oral dosage forms be used first, but only if ordered and if there is no nausea or vomiting. Taking the dose with food may help minimize GI upset. Should nausea or vomiting be problematic, an antiemetic may be ordered for administration before or with the dosing of medication. Crucial safety measures include keeping bed side rails up, turning bed alarms on (depending on the policies and procedures of the specific facility), and making sure the call bell/alarm is within the patient's reach. These measures will help to prevent falls or injury related to opioid use. Opioids

and similar drugs lead to CNS depression with possible confusion, altered sensorium or alertness, hypotension, and altered motor functioning. Because of these drug effects, all patients are at risk for falls or injury, and the elderly are at higher risk (see Box 10-2 on p. 147 and the Patient-Centered Care: Lifespan Considerations for the Elderly Patient box below). See Box 10-4 below for more specific information concerning the handling of controlled substances and opioid counts.

When managing pain with morphine and similar drugs, withhold the dose and contact the prescriber if there is any decline in the patient's condition or if the vital signs are abnormal (see parameters mentioned earlier), especially if the respiratory rate

---

## PATIENT-CENTERED CARE: LIFESPAN CONSIDERATIONS FOR THE ELDERLY PATIENT

### Opioid Use

- Record the patient's weight and height before opioid therapy is begun, if appropriate. Monitor the patient carefully for any changes in vital signs, level of consciousness, or respiratory rate, as well as any changes indicative of central nervous system depression, and report and document any such changes.
- Many institutionalized or hospitalized elderly patients are very stoic about pain; elderly patients may also have altered presentations of common illnesses so that the pain experience manifests in a different way or may simply be unable to state how they feel in a clear manner. Each and every patient—regardless of age—has the right to a thorough pain assessment and adequate and appropriate pain management. It is a myth that aging increases one's pain threshold. The problem is that cognitive impairment and dementia are often major barriers to pain assessment. Nevertheless, many elderly patients are still reliable in their reporting of pain, even with moderate to severe cognitive impairment.
- Over time, the elderly may lose reliability in recalling and accurately reporting chronic pain. The elderly, especially those 75 years of age or older, are at higher risk for too much or too little pain management, so you must remember that drugs have a higher peak and longer duration of action in these patients than in their younger counterparts.
- Smaller dosages of opioids are generally indicated for elderly patients because of their increased sensitivity to the central nervous system depressants and diminished renal and hepatic function. Paradoxical (opposite) reactions and/or unexpected reactions may also be more likely to occur in patients of this age group.

- In elderly male patients, benign prostatic hyperplasia or obstructive urinary diseases must be considered because of the urinary retention associated with the use of opioids. Urinary outflow can become further diminished in these patients and result in adverse reactions or complications. Dosage adjustments may need to be made by the prescriber.
- Polypharmacy is often a problem in older adults; therefore, have a complete list of all medications the patient is currently taking, and assess for drug interactions and treatment (drug) duplication.
- Frequent assessments of elderly patients are needed. Pay attention to level of consciousness, alertness, and cognitive ability while ensuring that the environment is safe by keeping a call bell or light at the bedside. Using bed alarms and/or raising side rails are indicated when appropriate.
- Decreased circulation causes variation in the absorption of intramuscular or intravenous dosage forms and often results in the slower absorption of parenteral forms of opioids.
- As stated by the American Geriatric Society on the Management of Pain, nonsteroidal antiinflammatory drugs must be used with caution because of their potential for renal and gastrointestinal toxicity. Acetaminophen is the drug of choice for relieving mild to moderate pain, but with cautious dosing because of hepatic and renal concerns. The oral route of administration is preferred for analgesia. The regimen needs to be as simple as possible to enhance compliance. Be sure to note, report, and document any unusual reactions to the opioid drugs. Hypotension and respiratory depression may occur more frequently in elderly patients taking opioids; thus very careful vital sign monitoring is needed.

---

## BOX 10-4   CONTROLLED SUBSTANCE/OPIOID COUNTS—A MUST-DO!

Any medication that has the potential for abuse or is a controlled substance—often opioids—is handled differently from other medications. Opioids are delivered to a nursing unit by the pharmacy, and these and other controlled substances (see Chapter 4) are kept in a locked cabinet or in an automated dispensing system (see Chapter 9). At the beginning of each shift, two registered nurses must count all of the opioids and/or other controlled substances located in the locked cabinet and record the count on a controlled substance and/or opioid administration record. When opioids and other controlled substances are dispensed through an automated medication-dispensing system, the drug is counted before the nurse removes the dose from the system. Any discrepancies found in the count of opioids or other controlled substances are investigated by registered nurses. If any opioids are unaccounted for, the nurse manager or supervisor needs to be contacted immediately. The following guidelines must be adhered to when giving opioids and other controlled substances: (1) Check

the opioid administration record for the number left in stock. (2) Compare this number with the actual supply available. (3) If the count is accurate, obtain the desired dose of drug. (4) If the count is incorrect, notify the nurse manager or supervisor and follow any institutional policy. (5) Record the count of the remaining supply. Once the dose is removed, the nurse may be required to record the patient's name, prescriber's name, patient's medical record number, dose of medication ordered, and the nurse's signature. (6) Administer the drug according to policy and procedures. If the controlled substance cannot be given to the patient because of patient refusal, medication contamination, changes in vital signs or status, or some other reason, the medication will need to be "wasted." However, wasting of controlled substances requires the signature of another nurse who witnesses the discarding or wasting of the medication and documentation on the appropriate form. Automated systems record this information within the computer system.

is less than 10 breaths/min. Intramuscular injections are rarely used because of the availability of other effective and convenient dosage forms, such as PCA pumps, transdermal patches, continuous subcutaneous infusions, and epidural infusions.

For transdermal patches (e.g., transdermal fentanyl), two systems are used. The oldest type of patch contains a reservoir system consisting of four layers beginning with the adhesive layer and ending with the protective backing. Between these two layers are the permeable rate-controlling membrane and the reservoir layer, which holds the drug in a gel or liquid form. The newer type of patch has a matrix system consisting of two layers: one layer containing the active drug with the releasing and adhesive mechanisms, and the protective impermeable backing layer. The advantages of the matrix system over the reservoir system are that the patch is slimmer and smaller, it is more comfortable, it is worn for up to 7 days (the older reservoir system patch is worn for up to 3 to 4 days), and it appears to result in more constant serum drug levels. In addition, the matrix system is alcohol-free; the alcohol in the reservoir system often irritates the patient's skin. It is important to know what type of delivery system is being used so that proper guidelines are followed to enhance the system's and drug's effectiveness.

Apply transdermal patches to only a clean, nonhairy area. When the patch is changed, place the new patch on a new site, but only after the old patch has been removed and the old site cleansed of any residual medication. Rotation of sites helps to decrease irritation and enhance drug effects. Transdermal patches require special discarding of old/used patches (see the Safety and Quality Improvement: Preventing Medication Errors box on p. 148). Transdermal systems are beneficial for the delivery of many types of medications, especially analgesics, and have the benefits of allowing multiday therapy with a single application, avoiding first-pass metabolism, improving patient compliance, and minimizing frequent dosing. However, the patient must be watched carefully for the development of any type of contact dermatitis caused by the patch (the prescriber is to be contacted immediately if this occurs) and maintain his or her own pain journal when at home. Journal entries are a valid source of information for the nurse, other health care professionals, the patient, and family members to assess the patient's pain control and to monitor the effectiveness not only of transdermal analgesia but also any medication regimen.

With the intravenous administration of *opioid agonists,* follow manufacturer guidelines and institutional policies regarding specific dilutional amounts and solutions as well as the time period for infusion. When PCA is used, the amounts and times of dosing must be noted in the appropriate records and tracked by appropriate personnel. The fact that a pump is being used, however, does not mean that it is 100% reliable or safe. Closely monitor and frequently check all equipment. Additionally, frequently monitor pain levels, response to medication, and vital signs with the use of other parenteral opioid administration. Always follow dosage ranges for all opioid agonists and agonists-antagonists, and pay special attention to the dosages of morphine and morphine-like drugs. For intravenous infusions, you are responsible for monitoring the intravenous needle site and infusion rates and documenting any adverse effects or complications. Another point to remember when administering opioids—as well as any other analgesics—is that each medication has a different onset of action, peak, and duration of action, with the intravenous route producing the most rapid onset (e.g., within minutes) (Table 10-8).

To reverse an opioid overdose or opioid-induced respiratory depression, an *opioid antagonist,* such as naloxone, must be

## TABLE 10-8 OPIOID ADMINISTRATION GUIDELINES

| OPIOID | NURSING ADMINISTRATION |
| --- | --- |
| buprenorphine and butorphanol | When giving IV, infuse over the recommended time (usually 3-5 min). Always assess respirations before, during, and after use. Give IM as ordered. |
| codeine | Give PO doses with food to minimize GI tract upset; ceiling effects occur with oral codeine resulting in no increase in analgesia with increased dosage. |
| fentanyl | Administer parenteral doses as ordered and as per manufacturer guidelines in regard to mg/min to prevent CNS depression and possible cardiac or respiratory arrest. Transdermal patches come in a variety of dosages. Fentanyl lozenges on a stick are also available. Be sure to remove residual amounts of the old patch before application of a new patch. Dispose of patches properly to avoid inadvertent contact with children or pets. |
| hydromorphone | May be given subcut, rectally, IV, PO, or IM. |
| levorphanol | May be given PO, subcut, or IV; give IV forms over 5 min or as indicated by manufacturer guidelines; longer acting, lasting up to 6-8 hr. |
| meperidine | Given by a variety of routes: IV, IM, or PO; highly protein bound, so watch for interactions and toxicity. Monitor elderly patients for increased sensitivity. |
| morphine | Available in a variety of forms: subcut, IM, PO, IV, extended- and immediate-release; morphine sulfate (Duramorph) for epidural infusion. Always monitor respiratory rate. |
| nalbuphine | IV doses of 10 mg given undiluted over 5 min. |
| naloxone | Antagonist given for opioid overdose; 0.4 mg usually given IV over 15 sec or less. Reverses analgesia as well. |
| oxycodone | Often mixed with acetaminophen or aspirin; PO and suppository dosage forms. Now available in both immediate and sustained-release tabs. |
| oxymorphone | Available in PO, IM, IV, subcut, and rectal suppository dosage forms. Extended-release oral form (Opana) is the only form commonly used. |
| pentazocine | Subcut, IV, and IM forms; mixed agonist-antagonist; IV dose of 5 mg to be given over 1 min. |

*CNS,* Central nervous system; *GI,* gastrointestinal; *IM,* intramuscular(ly); *IV,* intravenous(ly); *PO,* oral(ly); *subcut,* subcutaneous(ly).

administered. Naloxone is given intravenously in diluted form and administered slowly (such as over 15 seconds, or as ordered; see Table 10-7). However, consider the packaging and manufacturer guidelines. Emergency resuscitative equipment must always be available in the event of respiratory or cardiac arrest.

## OPIOID AGONISTS-ANTAGONISTS

Remember when giving *agonists-antagonists* that they react very differently depending on whether they are given by themselves or with other drugs. When administered alone, they are effective analgesics because they bind with opiate receptors and produce an agonist effect (see discussion in pharmacology section). If given at the same time as other opioids, however, they lead to reversal of analgesia and acute withdrawal because of the blocking of opiate receptors. Be very careful to check dosages and routes as well as to perform the interventions mentioned for opioid agonist drugs, including closely assessing vital signs, especially respiratory rate. Emphasize the importance of reporting any dizziness, unresolved constipation, urinary retention, and sedation. See Table 10-6 for additional adverse effects of opioid agonists as they are similar to the opioid agonist-antagonist drugs. Other points to emphasize with the patient include that the drug also has the ability to reverse analgesia as well as precipitate withdrawal (if taken with other opioid agonists). A list of other opioid agonists must be shared with the patient, as well.

## OPIOID ANTAGONISTS

*Opioid antagonists* must be given as ordered and be readily available, especially when the patient is receiving PCA with an opioid, is opioid naïve, or is receiving continuous doses of opioids. Several doses of these drugs are often required to ensure adequate opioid agonist reversal (see earlier discussion). Encourage patients to report any nausea or tachycardia.

## GENERAL CONSIDERATIONS

You are always responsible and accountable to maintain a current, updated knowledge base on all forms of analgesics as well as protocols for pain management with focus on the specific drug(s) as well as differences in the treatment of mild to moderate pain, severe pain, and pain in special situations (e.g., cancer pain). The WHO's three-step analgesic ladder provides a standard for pain management in cancer patients and must be reviewed and considered, as needed.

Dosing of medications for pain management is very important to the treatment regimen. As noted earlier, once a thorough assessment has been performed, it is best to treat the patient's pain before it becomes severe, which is the rationale for considering pain to be the fifth vital sign. When pain is present for more than 12 hours a day, analgesic doses are individualized and are best administered around the clock rather than on an as-needed basis, while always staying within safe practice guidelines for each drug used. Around-the-clock (or scheduled) dosing maintains steady-state levels of the medication and prevents drug troughs and pain escalation. No given dosage of an analgesic will provide the same level of pain relief for every patient; thus there is a need for a process of titration—upward or even downward—to be carried out based on the individual's needs.

Aggressive titration may be necessary in difficult pain control cases and in cancer pain situations. Patients with severe pain, metastatic pain, or bone metastasis pain may need increasingly higher dosages of analgesic. These special pain situations may require an opiate such as morphine that needs to be titrated until the desired response is achieved or until adverse effects occur. A patient-rated pain level of less than 4 on a scale of 1 to 10 is considered to indicate effective pain relief.

If pain is not managed adequately by monotherapy, other drugs or adjuvants may need to be added to enhance analgesic efficacy. This includes the use of NSAIDs (for analgesic, antiinflammatory effects), acetaminophen (for analgesic effects), corticosteroids (for mood elevation and antiinflammatory, antiemetic, and appetite stimulation effects), anticonvulsants (for treatment of neuropathic pain), tricyclic antidepressants (for treatment of neuropathic pain and for their innate analgesic properties and opioid-potentiating effects), neuroleptics (for treatment of chronic pain syndromes), local anesthetics (for treatment of neuropathic pain), hydroxyzine (for mild antianxiety properties as well as sedating effects and antihistamine and mild antiemetic actions), or psychostimulants (for reduction of opioid-induced sedation when opioid dosage adjustment is not effective). Table 10-9 provides a listing of drugs that are *not* to be used in patients experiencing cancer pain.

Dosage forms are also important, especially with chronic pain and cancer pain. Oral administration is always preferred but is not always tolerated by the patient and may not even be a viable option for pain control. If oral dosing is not appropriate, less invasive routes of administration include rectal and transdermal routes. Rectal dosage forms are safe, inexpensive, effective, and helpful if the patient is experiencing nausea or vomiting or altered mental status; however, this route is not suitable for those with diarrhea, stomatitis, and/or low blood cell counts. Transdermal patches may provide up to 7 days of pain control but are not for rapid dose titration and are used only when stable analgesia has been previously achieved. Long-acting forms of morphine and fentanyl may be delivered via transdermal patches when a longer duration of action is needed. Intermittent injections or continuous infusions via the intravenous or subcutaneous route are often used for opioid delivery and may be administered at home in special pain situations, such as in hospice care or management of chronic cancer pain. Subcutaneous infusions are often used when there is no intravenous access. PCA pumps may be used to help deliver opioids intravenously, subcutaneously, or even intraspinally and can be managed in home health care or hospice care for the patient at home. Use of the intrathecal or epidural route requires special skill and expertise, and delivery of pain medications using these routes is available only from certain home health care agencies for at-home care. The main reason for long-term intraspinal opioid administration is intractable pain. Transnasal dosage forms are approved only for butorphanol, an agonist-antagonist drug, and this dosage form is generally not used or recommended. Regardless of the specific drug or dosage form used, a fast-acting rescue drug needs to be ordered and available for patients with cancer pain and patients presenting other special challenges in pain management.

## TABLE 10-9   DRUGS NOT RECOMMENDED FOR TREATMENT OF CANCER PAIN

| CLASS | DRUG | REASON FOR NOT RECOMMENDING |
|---|---|---|
| Opioids with dosing around the clock | meperidine | Short (2-3 hr) duration of analgesia; administration may lead to CNS toxicity (tremor, confusion, or seizures) |
| Miscellaneous | Cannabinoids | Adverse effects of dysphoria, drowsiness, hypotension, and bradycardia, which preclude their routine use as analgesics; may be indicated for use in treating severe chemotherapy-induced nausea and vomiting |
| Opioid agonists-antagonists | pentazocine butorphanol nalbuphine | May precipitate withdrawal in opioid-dependent patients; analgesic ceiling effect; possible production of unpleasant psychological adverse effects, including dysphoria, delusions, and hallucinations |
| | buprenorphine | Analgesic ceiling effect; can precipitate withdrawal if given with an opioid |
| Opioid antagonists | naloxone naltrexone | Reverses analgesia as well as CNS depressant effects, such as respiratory depression |
| Combination preparations | Brompton cocktails | No evidence of analgesic benefit over use of single opioid analgesic |
| | DPT* (meperidine, promethazine, and chlorpromazine) | Efficacy poor compared with that of other analgesics; associated with a higher incidence of adverse effects |
| Anxiolytics (as monotherapy) or sedatives-hypnotics (as monotherapy) | Benzodiazepines (e.g., alprazolam) | Analgesic properties not associated with these drugs except in some situations of neuropathic pain; common risk of sedation, which may put some patients at higher risk for neurologic complications |
| | Barbiturates | Analgesic properties not demonstrated; sedation is problematic and limits use |

*CNS,* Central nervous system.
*DPT is the abbreviation for the trade names Demerol, Phenergan, and Thorazine.

## CASE STUDY

### *Opioid Administration*

You are assigned to care for a patient who is in the terminal phases of breast cancer. As a home health care nurse, you have many responsibilities; however, you have not cared for many patients who are in the terminal phase of their illness. In fact, most of your patients are postoperative and have only required assessments, dressing changes, and wound care.

Mrs. D. is 48 years of age and underwent bilateral mastectomy 4 years ago. She had lymph node involvement at the time of surgery, and recently has been diagnosed with metastasis to the bone. She has been taking oxycodone (one 5-mg tab every 6 hours) at home but is not sleeping through the night and is now complaining of increasing pain to the point that her quality of life has decreased significantly. She wants to stay at home

during the terminal phases of her illness but needs to have adequate and safe pain control. Her husband of 18 years is very supportive. They have no children. They are both college graduates and have medical insurance.

1. Mrs. D.'s recent increase in pain has been attributed to bone metastasis in the area of the lumbar spine. At this time, the oxycodone is not beneficial, and you as the home health care nurse need to advocate for Mrs. D. to receive adequate pain relief. When discussing her pain medications with her physician, what type of medication would you expect to be ordered to relieve the bone pain, and what is the rationale for this medication? (Provide references from within this chapter to support the selection of the specific opioid drug.)
2. Mrs. D.'s husband confides in you that he is worried that she will become addicted to the new medication. He is not sure he agrees with around-the-clock dosing. How do you address his concerns?
3. What should Mr. D. do if he feels that Mrs. D. has had an overdose?

For answers, see http://evolve.elsevier.com/Lilley.

Regardless of the drug(s) used for the pain management regimen, always remember that individualization of treatment is one of the most important considerations for effective and quality pain control. Also consider implementing the following:

- At the initiation of pain therapy, conduct a review of all relevant histories, laboratory test values, nurse-related charting entries, and diagnostic study results in the patient's medical record. If there are underlying problems, consider these variables while never forgetting to treat the patient with dignity and empathy. Never let compounding variables and any other problems overshadow the fact that there is a patient

who is in pain and deserving of safe, quality care. Always look and listen!
- Develop goals for pain management in conjunction with the patient, family members, significant others, and/or caregiver. These goals include improving the level of comfort with increased levels of activities of daily living and ambulation.
- Collaborate with other members of the health care team to select a regimen that will be easy for the patient to follow while in the hospital and, if necessary, at home (e.g., for cancer patients and other patients with chronic pain).

- Be aware that most regimens for acute pain management include treatment with short-acting opioids plus the addition of other medications such as NSAIDs.
- Be familiar with equianalgesic doses of opioids, because lack of knowledge may lead to inadequate analgesia or overdose.
- Use an analgesic appropriate for the situation (e.g., short-acting opioids for severe pain secondary to a myocardial infarction, surgery, or kidney stones). For cancer pain, the regimen usually begins with short-acting opioids with eventual conversion to sustained-release formulations.
- Use preventative measures to manage adverse effects. In addition, a switch is made to another opioid as soon as possible if the patient finds that the medication is not controlling the pain adequately.
- Consider the option of analgesic adjuvants, especially in cases of chronic pain or cancer pain; these might include other prescribed drugs such as NSAIDs, acetaminophen, corticosteroids, anticonvulsants, tricyclic antidepressants, neuroleptics, local anesthetics, hydroxyzine, and/or psychostimulants. Over-the-counter drugs and herbals may be helpful.
- Be alert to patients with special needs, such as patients with breakthrough pain. Generally, the drug used to manage such pain is a short-acting form of the longer-acting opioid being given (e.g., immediate-release morphine for breakthrough pain while sustained-release morphine is also used).
- Identify community resources that can assist the patient, family members, and/or significant others. These resources may include various websites for patient education such as http://www.theacpa.org; www.painconnection.org; and www.painaction.com. Many other pain management sites may be found on the Internet by using the search terms *pain, pain clinic,* or *pain education* and looking for patient-focused materials/sites.
- Conduct frequent online searches to remain current on the topic of pain management, pain education, drug and non-drug therapeutic regimens for pain, and special pain situations. The following professional nurse and/or prescriber-focused websites are listed at www.painedu.org/resources.asp as resources for the topic of general pain management: www.aapainmanage.org, www.painmed.org; www.painfoun dation.org; www.ampainsoc.org; www.aspmn.org; www. asam.org; www.paineducators.org; www.asra.com; www. iasp-pain.org; www.painpolicy.wisc.edu; www.painmedic inenews.com; www.pain-topics.org; www.pain.com; and www.painandhealth.org. On the topic of chronic pain, websites are as follows: www.theacpa.org and www.arthritis.org.

On the topic of cancer pain, websites are as follows: www. cancer.org; www.apos-society.org; www.asco.org; www.cancer care.org; www.cancer.gov; and www.ons.org.

- Because fall prevention is of utmost importance in patient care (after the ABCs [airway, breathing, circulation] of care are addressed), monitor the patient frequently after an analgesic is given. Frequent measurement of vital signs, inclusion of the patient in a frequent watch program, and/or use of bed alarms is encouraged.
- Restraints may cause many injuries; therefore, if restraints are necessary, follow the appropriate procedures, including specific institutional policies and rules. Assess, monitor, evaluate, and document the reason for the restraint; also document the patient's behavior, the type of restraint used, and the assessment of the patient after the placement of restraints. Use of restraints has been largely replaced with a bed watch system and the use of bed and/or wheelchair alarms. Give instructions to the patient, family members, and/or caregivers about the risk for falls and the need for safety measures. Restraints are not used in long-term care facilities.

## EVALUATION

Positive therapeutic outcomes of acetaminophen use are decreased symptoms, fever, and pain. Monitor for the adverse reactions of anemias and liver problems due to hepatotoxicity and report patient complaints of abdominal pain and/or vomiting to the prescriber. During and after the administration of other *nonopioid analgesics* such as tramadol, *opioids,* and *mixed opioid agonists,* monitor the patient for both therapeutic effects and adverse effects frequently and as needed. Therapeutic effects of analgesics include increased comfort levels as well as decreased complaints of pain and longer periods of comfort, with improvements in performance of activities of daily living, appetite, and sense of well-being. Monitoring for adverse effects will vary with each drug (see earlier discussions), but effects may consist of nausea, vomiting, constipation, dizziness, headache, blurred vision, decreased urinary output, drowsiness, lethargy, sedation, palpitations, bradycardia, bradypnea, dyspnea, and hypotension. If the patient's vital signs change, the patient's condition declines, or pain continues, contact the prescriber immediately and continue to closely monitor. Respiratory depression may be manifested by a respiratory rate of less than 10 breaths/min, dyspnea, diminished breath sounds, and/or shallow breathing. Include review of the effectiveness of multimodal and nonpharmacologic approaches to pain management in your evaluation.

## PATIENT TEACHING TIPS

- Capsaicin is a topical product made from different types of peppers that may help with muscle pain and joint/nerve pain. It may cause local, topical reactions, so be sure to share information with the patient about its safe use.
- Opioids are not to be used with alcohol or with other CNS depressants, unless ordered, because of worsening of the depressant effects.
- A holistic approach to pain management may be appropriate, with the use of complementary modalities including the following: biofeedback, imagery, relaxation, deep breathing, humor, pet therapy, music therapy, massage, use of hot or cold compresses, and use of herbal products.
- Dizziness, difficulty breathing, low blood pressure, excessive sleepiness (sedation), confusion, or loss of memory must be promptly reported to the nurse, prescriber, or other health care providers.
- Opioids may result in constipation, so forcing fluids (up to 3 L/day unless contraindicated), increasing fiber consumption, and exercising as tolerated is recommended. Stool softeners may also be necessary.
- Report any nausea or vomiting. Antiemetic drugs may be prescribed.
- Any activities requiring mental clarity or alertness may need to be avoided if experiencing drowsiness or sedation. Ambulate with caution and/or assistance as needed.
- It is important for the patient to share any history of addiction with health care providers, but when such a patient experiences pain and is in need of opioid analgesia, understand that the patient has a right to comfort. Any further issues with addiction may be managed during and after the use of opioids. Keeping an open mind regarding the use of resources, counseling, and other treatment options is important in dealing with addictive behaviors.
- If pain is problematic and not managed by monotherapy, a combination of a variety of medications may be needed. Other drugs that may be used include antianxiety drugs, sedatives, hypnotics, or anticonvulsants.
- For the cancer patient or patient with special needs, the prescriber will monitor pain control and the need for other options for therapy or for dosing of drugs. For example, the use of transdermal patches, buccal tablets, and continuous infusions while the patient remains mobile or at home is often helpful in pain management. It is also important to understand that if morphine or morphine-like drugs are being used, the potential for addiction exists; however, in specific situations, the concern for quality of life and pain management is more important than the concern for addiction.
- Most hospitals have inpatient and outpatient resources such as pain clinics. Patients need to constantly be informed and aware of all treatment options and remain active participants in their care for as long as possible.
- Tolerance does occur with opioid use, so if the level of pain increases while the patient remains on the prescribed dosage, the prescriber or health care provider must be contacted. Dosages must not be changed, increased, or doubled unless prescribed.

## KEY POINTS

- Pain is individual and involves sensations and emotions that are unpleasant. It is influenced by age, culture, race, spirituality, and all other aspects of the person.
- Pain is associated with actual or potential tissue damage and may be exacerbated or alleviated depending on the treatment and type of pain.
- Types of analgesics include the following:
  - Nonopioids, including acetaminophen, aspirin, and NSAIDs
  - Opioids, which are natural or synthetic drugs that either contain or are derived from morphine (opiates) or have opiate-like effects or activities (opioids), and opioid agonist-antagonist drugs
- Pediatric dosages of morphine must be calculated very cautiously with close attention to the dose and kilograms of body weight. Cautious titration of dosage upward is usually the standard.
- Elderly patients may react differently than expected to analgesics, especially opioids and opioid agonists-antagonists.
- In treating the elderly, remember that these patients experience pain the same as does the general population, but they may be reluctant to report pain and may metabolize opiates at a slower rate and thus are at increased risk for adverse effects such as sedation and respiratory depression. The best rule is to start with low dosages, reevaluate often, and go slowly during upward titration.

## ▌NCLEX® EXAMINATION REVIEW QUESTIONS

1 For best results when treating severe pain associated with pathologic spinal fractures related to metastatic bone cancer, the nurse should remember that the best type of dosage schedule is to administer the pain medication
  a as needed.
  b around the clock.
  c on schedule during waking hours only.
  d around the clock, with additional doses as needed for breakthrough pain.

2 A patient is receiving an opioid via a PCA pump as part of his postoperative pain management program. During rounds, the nurse finds him unresponsive, with respirations of 8 breaths/min and blood pressure of 102/58 mm Hg. After stopping the opioid infusion, what should the nurse do next?
  a Notify the charge nurse
  b Draw arterial blood gases
  c Administer an opiate antagonist per standing orders
  d Perform a thorough assessment, including mental status examination

3 A patient with bone pain caused by metastatic cancer will be receiving transdermal fentanyl patches. The patient asks the nurse what benefits these patches have. The nurse's best response includes which of these features?
  a More constant drug levels for analgesia
  b Less constipation and minimal dry mouth
  c Less drowsiness than with oral opioids
  d Lower dependency potential and no major adverse effects

4 Intravenous morphine is prescribed for a patient who has had surgery. The nurse informs the patient that which common adverse effects can occur with this medication? (Select all that apply.)
  a Diarrhea
  b Constipation
  c Pruritus
  d Urinary frequency
  e Nausea

5 Several patients have standard orders for acetaminophen as needed for pain. When the nurse reviews their histories and assessments, the nurse discovers that one of the patients has a contraindication to acetaminophen therapy. Which patient should receive an alternate medication?
  a A patient with a fever of 103.4° F (39.7° C)
  b A patient admitted with deep vein thrombosis
  c A patient admitted with severe hepatitis
  d A patient who had abdominal surgery 1 week earlier

6 The nurse is administering an intravenous dose of morphine sulfate to a 48-year-old postoperative patient. The dose ordered is 3 mg every 3 hours as needed for pain. The medication is supplied in vials of 4 mg/mL. How much will be drawn into the syringe for this dose?

7 An opioid analgesic is prescribed for a patient. The nurse checks the patient's medical history knowing this medication is contraindicated in which disorder?
  a Renal insufficiency
  b Severe asthma
  c Liver disease
  d Diabetes mellitus

1. d, 2. c, 3. a, 4. b, c, e 5. c, 6. 0.75 mL, 7. b

For Critical Thinking and Prioritization Questions, see http://evolve.elsevier.com/Lilley.

# General and Local Anesthetics

## evolve WEBSITE

*http://evolve.elsevier.com/Lilley*

- Animations
- Answer Key—Textbook Case Studies
- Critical Thinking and Prioritization Questions

- Key Points—Downloadable
- Review Questions for the NCLEX® Examination
- Unfolding Case Studies

## OBJECTIVES

When you reach the end of this chapter, you will be able to do the following:

1 Define *anesthesia*.
2 Describe the basic differences between general and local anesthesia.
3 List the most commonly used general and local anesthetics and associated risks.
4 Discuss the differences between depolarizing neuromuscular blocking drugs and nondepolarizing blocking drugs and their impact on the patient.

5 Compare the mechanisms of action, indications, adverse effects, routes of administration, cautions, contraindications, and drug interactions for general and local anesthesia as well as drugs used for moderate or conscious sedation.
6 Develop a nursing care plan for patients before anesthesia (preanesthesia), during anesthesia, and after anesthesia (postanesthesia) related to general anesthesia.
7 Develop a nursing care plan for patients undergoing local anesthesia and/or moderate or conscious sedation.

## DRUG PROFILES

dexmedetomidine, p. 173
isoflurane, p. 173
ketamine, p. 173
♦ lidocaine, p. 176
nitrous oxide, p. 173
pancuronium, p. 180

♦ propofol, p. 173
sevoflurane, p. 173
♦ succinylcholine, p. 179
♦ vecuronium, p. 180

_____

♦ *Key drug*

## KEY TERMS

Adjunct anesthetics Drugs used in combination with anesthetic drugs to control the adverse effects of anesthetics or to help maintain the anesthetic state in the patient. (See *balanced anesthesia*.) (p. 170)

Anesthesia The loss of the ability to feel pain resulting from the administration of an anesthetic drug. (p. 170)

Anesthetics Drugs that depress the central nervous system (CNS) or peripheral nerves to produce decreased or loss of consciousness, or muscle relaxation. (p. 170)

Balanced anesthesia The practice of using combinations of different drug classes rather than a single drug to produce anesthesia. (p. 171)

**General anesthesia** A drug-induced state in which the CNS nerve impulses are altered to reduce pain and other sensations throughout the entire body. It normally involves complete loss of consciousness and depression of normal respiratory drive. (p. 170)

**Local anesthesia** A drug-induced state in which peripheral or spinal nerve impulses are altered to reduce or eliminate pain and other sensations in tissues innervated by these nerves. (p. 170)

**Malignant hyperthermia** A genetically linked major adverse reaction to general anesthesia characterized by a rapid rise in body temperature, as well as tachycardia, tachypnea, and sweating. (p. 172)

**Moderate sedation** A milder form of general anesthesia that causes partial or complete loss of consciousness but does not generally reduce normal respiratory drive (also referred to as *conscious sedation*). (p. 173)

**Overton-Meyer theory** A theory that describes the relationship between the lipid solubility of anesthetic drugs and their potency. (p. 171)

**Spinal anesthesia** Local anesthesia induced by injection of an anesthetic drug near the spinal cord to anesthetize nerves that are distal to the site of injection (also called *intraspinal anesthesia*). (p. 174)

## ANATOMY, PHYSIOLOGY, AND PATHOPHYSIOLOGY OVERVIEW

**Anesthetics** are drugs that reduce or eliminate pain by depressing nerve function in the central nervous system (CNS) and/or the peripheral nervous system (PNS). This state of reduced neurologic function is called *anesthesia*. Anesthesia is further classified as *general* or *local*. General anesthesia involves complete loss of consciousness, loss of body reflexes, elimination of pain and other sensations throughout the entire body, and skeletal and smooth muscle paralysis, including paralysis of respiratory muscles. This loss of normal respiratory function requires mechanical or manual ventilatory support to avoid brain damage and suffocation (death from respiratory arrest). Local anesthesia does not involve paralysis of respiratory function but does involve elimination of pain sensation in the tissues innervated by *anesthetized* nerves. Functions of the *autonomic nervous system,* which is a branch of the parasympathetic nervous system, may also be affected.

## PHARMACOLOGY OVERVIEW

### GENERAL ANESTHETICS

General anesthetics are drugs that induce general anesthesia and are most commonly used to induce anesthesia during surgical procedures. General anesthetics are given only under controlled situations by anesthesiologists or nurse anesthetists. General anesthesia is achieved by the use of one or more drugs. Often a synergistic combination of drugs is used, which allows for smaller doses of each drug and better control of the patient's anesthetized state. Inhalational anesthetics are volatile liquids or gases that are vaporized or mixed with oxygen to induce anesthesia. For a historical perspective on general anesthesia, see Box 11-1.

Parenteral anesthetics (Table 11-1) are given intravenously and are used for induction and/or maintenance of general anesthesia, induction of amnesia, and as adjuncts to inhalation-type anesthetics (Table 11-2). The specific goal varies with the drug. Common intravenous anesthetic drugs include drugs classified solely as general anesthetics, such as etomidate and propofol.

**Adjunct anesthetics** or simply adjuncts are also used. *Adjunct* is a general term for any drug that enhances clinical therapy when used simultaneously with another drug. Adjunct drugs can be thought of as "helper drugs" when their use complements the use of any other drug(s). They are used simultaneously with general anesthetics for anesthesia initiation (induction), sedation, reduction of anxiety, and amnesia. Adjuncts include neuromuscular blocking drugs (NMBDs; see Neuromuscular Blocking Drugs later in the chapter), sedative-hypnotics or anxiolytics (see Chapter 12) such as propofol (this chapter), benzodiazepines (e.g., diazepam, midazolam),

---

**BOX 11-1    GENERAL ANESTHESIA: A HISTORICAL PERSPECTIVE**

Until recently, general anesthesia was described as having several definitive stages. This was especially true with the use of many of the ether-based inhaled anesthetic drugs. Features of these distinctive stages were easily observable to the trained eye. They included specific physical and physiologic changes that progressed gradually and predictably with the depth of the patient's anesthetized state. Gradual changes in pupil size, progression from thoracic to diaphragmatic breathing, vital sign changes, and several other changes all characterized the various stages. Newer inhalational and intravenous general anesthetic drugs, however, often have a much more rapid onset of action and body distribution. As a result, the specific stages of anesthesia once observed with older drugs are no longer sufficiently well defined to be observable. Thus, the concept of stages of anesthesia is an outdated one in most modern surgical facilities. Registered nurses who pursue advanced training to become certified registered nurse anesthetists often find this to be a rewarding and interesting area of nursing practice. Some nurses also find that this type of work offers greater flexibility in their work schedule than do other practice areas.

---

**TABLE 11-1    PARENTERAL GENERAL ANESTHETICS**

| GENERIC NAME | TRADE NAME |
| --- | --- |
| etomidate | Amidate |
| ketamine | Ketalar |
| methohexital | Brevital |
| propofol | Diprivan |
| thiopental | Pentothal |

barbiturates (e.g., thiopental, methohexital; see Chapter 12), opioid analgesics (e.g., morphine, fentanyl, sufentanil; see Chapter 10), anticholinergics (e.g., atropine; see Chapter 21), and antiemetics (e.g., ondansetron; see Chapter 52). Note that propofol can be used as a general anesthetic and/or sedative-hypnotic, depending on the dose. The simultaneous use of both general anesthetics and adjuncts is called balanced anesthesia. Common adjunctive anesthetic drugs are listed in Table 11-3.

## Mechanism of Action and Drug Effects

Many theories have been proposed to explain the actual mechanism of action of general anesthetics. The drugs vary widely in their chemical structures, and their mechanism of action is not easily explained by a structure-receptor relationship. The concentrations of various anesthetics required to produce a given state of anesthesia also differ greatly. The Overton-Meyer theory has been used to explain some of the properties of anesthetic drugs since the early days of anesthesiology. In general terms, it proposes that, for all anesthetics, potency varies directly with lipid solubility. In other words, across a continuum of drug potency, fat-soluble drugs are stronger anesthetics than water-soluble drugs. Nerve cell membranes have high lipid content, as does the blood-brain barrier (see Chapter 2). Lipid-soluble anesthetic drugs can therefore easily cross the blood-brain barrier to concentrate in nerve cell membranes.

The overall effect of general anesthetics is a progressive reduction of sensory and motor CNS functions. The degree and speed of this process varies with the anesthetics and adjuncts used along with their dosages and routes of administration. General anesthesia initially produces a loss of the senses of sight, touch, taste, smell, and hearing, along with loss of consciousness. Cardiac and pulmonary functions are usually the last to be interrupted, because they are controlled by the *medulla* of the *brainstem*. These are the classical "stages" of anesthesia. Mechanical ventilatory support is absolutely necessary. In more extensive surgical procedures, especially those involving the heart, pharmacologic cardiac support involving adrenergic drugs (see Chapter 18) and inotropic drugs (see Chapter 24) may also be required.

The reactions of various body systems to general anesthetics are further described in Table 11-4.

## Indications

General anesthetics are used to produce unconsciousness as well as relaxation of skeletal and visceral smooth muscles for surgical procedures as well as in electroconvulsive therapy for severe depression (see Chapter 16).

## Contraindications

Contraindications to the use of anesthetic drugs include known drug allergy. Depending on the drug type, contraindications may also include pregnancy, narrow-angle glaucoma, and known susceptibility to malignant hyperthermia (see Adverse Effects) from prior experience with anesthetics.

### TABLE 11-2  INHALATIONAL GENERAL ANESTHETICS

| GENERIC NAME | TRADE NAME |
| --- | --- |
| **Inhaled Gas** | |
| nitrous oxide (laughing gas) | |
| | |
| **Inhaled Volatile Liquid** | |
| desflurane | Suprane |
| enflurane | Ethrane |
| halothane | Fluothane |
| isoflurane | Forane |
| methoxyflurane | Penthrane |
| sevoflurane | Ultane |

### TABLE 11-3  ADJUNCTIVE ANESTHETIC DRUGS (ADULT DOSES)

| DRUG | PHARMACOLOGIC CLASS | USUAL DOSAGE RANGE | INDICATIONS/USES |
| --- | --- | --- | --- |
| alfentanil (Alfenta) | Opioid analgesic | 130-245 mcg/kg IV | Anesthesia induction |
| fentanyl (Sublimaze) | | 50-100 mcg/kg IV | |
| sufentanil (Sufenta) | | 8-30 mcg/kg IV | |
| diazepam (Valium) | Benzodiazepine | 5-15 mg PO/IV/IM | Amnesia and anxiety reduction |
| midazolam (Versed) | | 1-5 mg IV | |
| atropine | Anticholinergic | 0.2-1 mg IV/IM/subcut | Drying up of excessive secretions |
| glycopyrrolate (Robinul) | | 4 mcg/kg IM | |
| scopolamine | | 0.3-0.6 mg subcut/IM/IV | |
| meperidine (Demerol) | Opioid analgesic | 50-100 mg IV/IM | Pain prevention and pain relief |
| morphine | | 5-20 mg IV/IM | |
| hydroxyzine (Atarax, Vistaril) | Antihistamine | 25-100 mg IM | Sedation, prevention of nausea and vomiting, anxiety reduction |
| promethazine (Phenergan) | | 25-50 mg IM | |
| pentobarbital (Nembutal) | Sedative-hypnotic | 150-200 mg IM | Amnesia and sedation |
| secobarbital (Seconal) | | 100 mg PO | |
| dexmedetomidine (Precedex) | Alpha$_2$ agonist | 0.2-0.7 mcg/kg/hr IV (doses up to 1.4 mcg/kg/hr have been shown to be effective) | Sedation |

*IM*, Intramuscularly; *IV*, intravenously; *PO,* orally; *subcut,* subcutaneously

## TABLE 11-4   EFFECTS OF INHALED AND INTRAVENOUS GENERAL ANESTHETICS

| ORGAN/SYSTEM | REACTION |
| --- | --- |
| Respiratory system | Depressed muscles and patterns of respiration; altered gas exchange and impaired oxygenation; depressed airway-protective mechanisms; airway irritation and possible laryngospasm |
| Cardiovascular system | Depressed myocardium; hypotension and tachycardia; bradycardia in response to vagal stimulation |
| Cerebrovascular system | Increased intracranial blood volume and increased intracranial pressure |
| Gastrointestinal system | Reduced hepatic blood flow and thus reduced hepatic clearance |
| Renal system | Decreased glomerular filtration |
| Skeletal muscles | Skeletal muscle relaxation |
| Cutaneous circulation | Vasodilation |
| Central nervous system (CNS) | CNS depression; blurred vision; nystagmus; progression of CNS depression to decreased alertness, sensorium, and decreased level of consciousness |

## PATIENT-CENTERED CARE: LIFESPAN CONSIDERATIONS FOR THE ELDERLY PATIENT

### Anesthesia

- The elderly patient is affected more adversely by anesthesia than the young or middle-aged adult. With aging comes organ system deterioration. Declining liver function results in decreased metabolism of drugs, and a decline in renal functioning leads to decreased drug excretion. Either of these can lead to drug toxicity, unsafe levels, and/or overdose. If both of these organs are not functioning properly, the risk of drug toxicity or overdose is even greater. In addition, the elderly are more sensitive to the effects of drugs affecting the central nervous system.
- Presence of cardiac and respiratory diseases places the elderly patient at higher risk for cardiac dysrhythmias, hypotension, respiratory depression, atelectasis, and/or pneumonia during the postanesthesia and postoperative phases.
- The practice of polypharmacy is yet another concern in the elderly with regard to administration of any type of anesthetic. Because of the presence of various age-related diseases, the older patient is generally taking more than one medication. The more drugs a patient is taking, the higher the risk of adverse reactions and drug-drug interactions, including interactions with anesthetics.

## Adverse Effects

Adverse effects of general anesthetics are dose dependent and vary with the individual drug. The heart, peripheral circulation, liver, kidneys, and respiratory tract are the sites primarily affected. Myocardial depression is a common adverse effect. All of the halogenated anesthetics are capable of causing hepatotoxicity, and methoxyflurane can cause significant respiratory depression.

With the development of newer drugs, many of the unwanted adverse effects characteristic of the older drugs (such as hepatotoxicity and myocardial depression) are now a thing of the past. In addition, many of the bothersome adverse effects such as nausea, vomiting, and confusion are less common since balanced anesthesia is widely used. Substance abuse (e.g., alcohol abuse; see Chapter 17) can predispose a patient to anesthetic-induced complications (e.g., liver toxicity). A positive history of substance abuse may lead to dosage adjustments in one or more of the drugs used. A drug-abusing patient with a high tolerance for street drugs may require larger doses of anesthesia-related drugs (e.g., benzodiazepines, opioids) to achieve the desired sedative effects.

Malignant hyperthermia is an uncommon, but potentially fatal, genetically linked adverse metabolic reaction to general anesthesia. It is classically associated with the use of volatile inhalational anesthetics as well as the depolarizing NMBD succinylcholine (see Neuromuscular Blocking Drugs later in this chapter). Signs include rapid rise in body temperature, tachycardia, tachypnea, and muscular rigidity. Patients known to be at greater risk for malignant hyperthermia include children, adolescents, and individuals with muscular and/or skeletal abnormalities such as hernias, strabismus, ptosis, scoliosis, and muscular dystrophy. Malignant hyperthermia is treated with cardiorespiratory supportive care as needed to stabilize heart and lung function along with the skeletal muscle relaxant dantrolene (see Chapter 12). In fact, by law, all facilities that provide general anesthesia must maintain a certain amount of dantrolene on hand in case of malignant hyperthermia.

## PATIENT-CENTERED CARE: LIFESPAN CONSIDERATIONS FOR THE PEDIATRIC PATIENT

### Anesthesia

- Premature infants, neonates, and pediatric patients are more adversely affected by anesthesia than the young or middle-aged adult patient. The reason for this difference in response is the increased sensitivity of the pediatric patient to anesthetics and related drugs because of immature functioning of the liver and kidneys, which leads to possible drug accumulation, toxicity, and subsequent complications. The central nervous system of pediatric patients is also more sensitive to the effects of anesthetics. Because of these risks of toxicity and complications with all forms of anesthesia, take every precaution to ensure that the patient remains safe and free from harm.
- Cardiac and respiratory systems are not fully developed in the neonate, premature infant, and newborn, which makes this age group more susceptible to problems with the metabolism and excretion of drugs. Some of the more common problems include central nervous system depression with subsequent respiratory and cardiac depression, development of atelectasis, pneumonia, and cardiac abnormalities.
- Neonates in particular (see age group definitions and further discussion in Chapter 3) are at higher risk of upper airway obstruction during general anesthesia. During the anesthetic process, the risk of laryngospasm related to the intubation process may be increased for neonates because of the specific physical characteristics of the larynx and respiratory structures in this age group. Their higher metabolic rate and small airway diameter also put neonates at greater risk of experiencing complications during general anesthesia.
- Before any medications are given to the pediatric patient, perform a careful check and double-check of mathematical drug calculations. In addition to weight, body surface area and laboratory test results that may indicate organ dysfunction should always be taken into consideration in the actual drug calculation.
- Resuscitative equipment should be readily available on any neonatal or pediatric nursing care unit.

## Toxicity and Management of Overdose

In large doses, anesthetics are potentially life threatening, with cardiac and respiratory arrest as the ultimate causes of death. However, these drugs are almost exclusively administered in a very controlled environment by personnel trained in advanced cardiac life support. These drugs are also very quickly metabolized. In addition, the medullary center, which governs the vital functions, is the last area of the brain to be affected by anesthetics and the first to regain function. These factors combined make an anesthetic overdose rare and easily reversible.

## Interactions

Some of the common drugs that interact with general anesthetics are antihypertensives and beta blockers, which have additive effects when combined with general anesthetics (i.e., increased hypotensive effects from antihypertensives, and increased myocardial depression with beta blockers). No significant laboratory test interactions have been reported.

## DRUG PROFILES

The dose of any anesthetic depends on the complexity of the surgical procedure to be performed and the physical characteristics of the patient. All of the general anesthetics have a rapid onset of action along with rapid elimination upon discontinuation. Anesthesia is maintained intraoperatively by continuous administration of the drug.

### isoflurane

Isoflurane (Forane) is a fluorinated ether that is a chemical isomer of the older fluorinated ether enflurane. It has a more rapid onset of action, causes less cardiovascular depression, and has little or no associated toxicity. This is in contrast to enflurane, which can cause seizures, and halothane, which is associated with liver toxicity.

### sevoflurane

Sevoflurane (Ultane) is a fluorinated ether and is now widely used. Its pharmacokinetics, with rapid onset and rapid elimination, make it especially useful in outpatient surgery settings. It is also nonirritating to the airway, which greatly facilitates induction of an unconscious state, especially in pediatric patients.

### ketamine

Ketamine is a unique drug with multiple properties. Given intravenously, it can be used for both general anesthesia and moderate sedation. It is commonly used in the emergency department for setting broken bones. It can also provide moderate sedation when given intravenously and by other routes, including subcutaneous, intramuscular, epidural, oral, intranasal, rectal, transdermal, and topical. It binds to receptors in both central and peripheral nervous systems, including opioid receptors. The most important receptors for the therapeutic activity of this drug, however, are the N-methyl-D-aspartate (NMDA) receptors located in the dorsal horn of the spinal cord. The drug is highly lipid soluble and penetrates the blood-brain barrier rapidly, which results in a rapid onset of action. It has a low incidence of reduction of cardiovascular, respiratory, and bowel function.

Adverse effects can include disturbing psychomimetic effects, including hallucinations. However, these are less likely to occur when benzodiazepines (see Chapter 12) are coadministered with the drug. Interacting drugs include NMBDs (prolonged paralysis) and halothane (reduced cardiac output and blood pressure). The drug is contraindicated in cases of known drug allergy.

### nitrous oxide

Nitrous oxide, also known as *laughing gas,* is the only inhaled gas currently used as a general anesthetic. It is the weakest of the general anesthetic drugs and is used primarily for dental procedures or as a supplement to other, more potent anesthetics.

### ◆ propofol

Propofol (Diprivan) is a parenteral general anesthetic used for the induction and maintenance of general anesthesia and also for sedation for mechanical ventilation in intensive care unit (ICU) settings. In lower doses, it can also be used as a sedative-hypnotic for moderate sedation. Some states allow nurses to administer propofol as part of a moderate sedation protocol. However, many state boards of nursing prohibit administration by nurses. Propofol also is typically well tolerated, producing few undesirable effects. Propofol is a lipid-based emulsion, and prolonged use, or if given in conjunction with total parenteral nutrition, requires serum lipids to be monitored.

### dexmedetomidine

Dexmedetomidine (Precedex) is an alpha-2 adrenergic receptor agonist (see Chapter 13). It produces dose-dependent sedation, decreased anxiety, and analgesia without respiratory depression. It is used for procedural sedation and for surgeries of short duration. It has a short half-life, and the patient awakens quickly upon withdrawal of the drug. Dexmedetomidine is also used in the intensive care setting for sedation of mechanically ventilated patients. Lower doses may be needed with concurrent anesthetics, sedatives, or opioids. Side effects include hypotension, bradycardia, transient hypertension, and nausea. Doses are listed in Table 11-3. Although the prescribing information states that dexmedetomidine is to be used for only 24 hours, multiple studies have shown it to be safe and effective at longer durations.

## DRUGS FOR MODERATE SEDATION

Moderate sedation, *conscious sedation,* and *procedural sedation* are synonymous terms for anesthesia that does not cause complete loss of consciousness and does not normally cause respiratory arrest. As more minor surgical procedures move from traditional operating room settings to outpatient surgery centers or office-based practices, the use of moderate sedation will continue to increase. Moderate sedation allows the patient to relax and have markedly reduced or no anxiety, yet still maintain his or her own open airway, and response to verbal commands. Standards must be followed when providing moderate sedation. Health care personnel who administer moderate sedation are required to have advanced cardiac life support training; one professional must have no duties other than to monitor the patient, and someone with the ability to intubate the patient must be present in case the patient slips into a deeper state of sedation and is unable to maintain an open airway. The American Society of Anesthesiologists has published guidelines on moderate sedation, which can be found at www.asahq.org.

The most commonly used drugs for moderate sedation include a benzodiazepine, usually midazolam (see Chapter 12), with an opioid, usually fentanyl or morphine. Propofol is also a common agent used. Propofol is usually given by an anesthesiologist, although there is some debate among physician specialties as who should be allowed to administer propofol. The doses of midazolam used in moderate sedation are 0.02 to 0.1 mg over a 2-minute period, not to exceed 2.5 mg. If needed, a repeat dose of 25% of the initial dose may be used. If midazolam is combined with an opioid such as fentanyl or morphine, the dose should be reduced by 30% to 50%. The most common dose of fentanyl is 1 to 2 mcg/kg, which may be repeated every 30 minutes. The dose of morphine for moderate sedation is 2 mg IV. When these drugs are combined with a benzodiazepine, smaller doses should be used. The dose of propofol for moderate sedation is 0.5 to 1 mg/kg followed by 0.5 mg/kg every 3 to 5 minutes. Mild amnesia is also a common effect, due to the midazolam. This is often desirable for helping patients not to remember painful medical procedures. Moderate sedation is associated with a more rapid recovery time than general anesthesia as well as a better safety profile because of lower cardiopulmonary risks.

The oral route of drug administration is commonly used in pediatric patients. This often involves administering an oral syrup form of midazolam with or without concurrent use of injected medications such as opiates. This is especially helpful for pediatric patients who must undergo uncomfortable procedures such as wound suturing or diagnostic procedures requiring reduced movement such as computed tomography and magnetic resonance imaging. See the Patient-Centered Care: Lifespan Considerations for the Pediatric Patient box below for other considerations.

## LOCAL ANESTHETICS

Local anesthetics are the second major class of anesthetics. They reduce pain sensations at the level of peripheral nerves, although this can involve *intraspinal anesthesia* (see later). They are also called *regional anesthetics* because they render a specific portion of the body insensitive to pain. They work by interfering with nerve transmission in specific areas of the body, blocking nerve conduction only in the area in which they are applied without causing loss of consciousness. They are most commonly used in clinical settings in which loss of consciousness is undesirable or unnecessary. These include childbirth and other situations in which spinal anesthesia is desired, dental procedures, suturing of skin lacerations, and diagnostic procedures (e.g., lumbar puncture, thoracentesis, biopsy).

Most local anesthetics belong to one of two major groups of organic compounds: esters and amides. They are classified as either *parenteral* (injectable) or *topical* anesthetics. Parenteral anesthetics are most commonly given intravenously but may also be administered by various spinal injection techniques (Box 11-2). Topical anesthetics are applied directly to the skin and mucous membranes. They are available in the form of solutions, ointments, gels, creams, powders, suppositories, and ophthalmic drops. Their dosage strengths are listed in Table 11-5.

The injection of parenteral anesthetic drugs into the area near the spinal cord is known as *spinal* or *intraspinal* anesthesia. This type of anesthesia is generally used to block all peripheral nerves that branch out distal to the injection site. The result is elimination of pain and paralysis of the skeletal and smooth muscles of the corresponding innervated tissues. Some of the medications used for spinal anesthesia include the opioids morphine, hydromorphone, fentanyl, and meperidine (see Chapter 10), and the local anesthetics lidocaine and bupivacaine. Because spinal anesthesia does not depress the CNS at a level that causes loss of consciousness, it can be thought of as

---

### PATIENT-CENTERED CARE: LIFESPAN CONSIDERATIONS FOR THE PEDIATRIC PATIENT

#### *Moderate or Conscious Anesthesia*

- The American Academy of Pediatrics recommends that moderate or conscious sedation (anesthesia) be used to reduce anxiety, pain, and fear in the pediatric patient. The use of moderate anesthesia in the pediatric patient allows a procedure to be performed restraint free in most situations while keeping the patient responsive.
- Pediatric dosing often conforms to the following guidelines:
  - Morphine—pediatric dosing may be at 0.05 to 0.1 mg/kg intravenously (IV) over a 2-minute period and is ideal for long procedures or cases in which pain is anticipated after the procedure.
  - Fentanyl—pediatric dosing may be at 0.5 to 1 mcg/kg with increments over 3 minutes to a maximum of three doses. Too rapid an IV injection may result in chest rigidity, which may need to be treated with muscle relaxants and possibly mechanical ventilation. Fentanyl is used often for short procedures.
  - Hydromorphone—pediatric dosing is at 0.015 to 0.02 mg/kg.
  - Meperidine—pediatric dosing is at 0.5 to 1 mg/kg over 2 minutes.

- Discharge status of the pediatric patient depends on the type of drugs and drug combinations used. Discharge after conscious or moderate sedation is based mainly on whether the following criteria are met:
  - Patient is alert and oriented compared with the baseline neurologic assessment.
  - Protective swallowing and gag reflexes are intact.
  - Vital signs are stable and consistent with baseline values for at least 30 minutes after the last dosing. Different health care facilities set different criteria that must be met and documented (blood pressure and pulse rate within normal limits or within 20 points of baseline, temperature lower than 101° F [38.3° C]).
  - Oxygen saturation is at least 95% on room air 30 minutes after the last dose.
  - Pain rating is at baseline levels or less.
  - Ambulation is at baseline level.
  - An adult is present to get the patient home and remain with the patient for at least two half-lives of the various drugs used for the anesthesia.
  - If a reversal drug was administered, there has been time for the drug to be excreted.

NOTE: Drugs given as anesthesia for moderate sedation procedures are given only under controlled situations by anesthesiologists or nurse anesthetists.

## BOX 11-2 TYPES OF LOCAL ANESTHESIA

**Central**

- **Spinal or intraspinal anesthesia:** Anesthetic drugs are injected into the area near the spinal cord within the vertebral column. Intraspinal anesthesia is commonly accomplished by one of two injection techniques: intrathecal and epidural.
  - **Intrathecal anesthesia** involves injection of anesthetic into the subarachnoid space. Intrathecal anesthesia is commonly used for patients undergoing major abdominal or limb surgery for whom the risks of general anesthesia are too high or for patients who prefer this technique instead of complete loss of consciousness during their surgical procedure. More recently, intrathecal injection of anesthetics through implantable drug pumps is even being used on an outpatient basis in patients with severe chronic pain syndromes, such as those resulting from occupational injuries.
  - **Epidural anesthesia** involves injection of anesthetic via a small catheter into the epidural space without puncturing the dura. Epidural anesthesia is commonly used to reduce maternal discomfort during labor and delivery and to manage postoperative acute pain after major abdominal or pelvic surgery. This route is becoming more popular for the administration of opioids for pain management.

**Peripheral**

- **Infiltration:** Small amounts of anesthetic solution are injected into the tissue that surrounds the operative site. This approach to anesthesia is commonly used for such procedures as wound suturing and dental surgery. Often drugs that cause constriction of local blood vessels (e.g., epinephrine, cocaine) are also administered to limit the site of action to the local area.
- **Nerve block:** Anesthetic solution is injected at the site where a nerve innervates a specific area such as a tissue. This allows large amounts of anesthetic drug to be delivered to a very specific area without affecting the whole body. This method is often reserved for more difficult-to-treat pain syndromes such as cancer pain and chronic orthopedic pain.
- **Topical anesthesia:** The anesthetic drug is applied directly onto the surface of the skin, eye, or any mucous membrane to relieve pain or prevent it from being sensed. It is commonly used for diagnostic eye examinations and skin suturing.

## TABLE 11-5 SELECTED TOPICAL ANESTHETICS

| DRUG | ROUTE | DOSE STRENGTH |
|---|---|---|
| benzocaine (Dermoplast, Lanacane, Solarcaine) | Topical, aerosol, and spray | 0.5%-20% ointment or cream |
| cocaine | Topical | 4%-10% solution, jelly |
| dibucaine (Nupercainal) | Injection and topical | 0.5%-1% solution, ointment, or cream |
| dibucaine | Topical | 1% ointment |
| dyclonine (Dyclone, Sucrets) | Topical | 0.5%-1% solution |
| ethyl chloride (Chloroethane) | Topical | Spray |
| lidocaine (Lidoderm) | Topical | 5% patch |
| proparacaine (Alcaine, Ophthetic) | Ophthalmic | 0.5% solution |
| prilocaine/lidocaine (EMLA) | Topical | 2.5% prilocaine and 2.5% lidocaine cream |
| tetracaine (Pontocaine) | Injection, topical, and ophthalmic | 0.5%-2% solution, ointment, or cream |

## TABLE 11-6 SELECTED PARENTERAL LOCAL ANESTHETIC DRUGS*

| GENERIC NAME | TRADE NAME | POTENCY | ONSET | DURATION |
|---|---|---|---|---|
| lidocaine | Xylocaine | Moderate | Immediate | 60-90 min |
| mepivacaine | Carbocaine | Moderate | Immediate | 120-150 min |
| procaine | Novocain | Lowest | 2-5 min | 30-60 min |
| tetracaine | Pontocaine | Highest | 5-10 min | 90-120 min |

*Other common parenteral anesthetic drugs include bupivacaine (Marcaine, Sensorcaine), chloroprocaine (Nesacaine), etidocaine (Duranest), propoxycaine (Ravocaine), and ropivacaine (Naropin).

a large-scale type of *local* rather than general anesthesia. Common types of local anesthesia are described in Box 11-2. The parenteral local anesthetic drugs and their pharmacokinetics are summarized in Table 11-6.

Local anesthesia of specific peripheral nerves is accomplished by *nerve block anesthesia* or *infiltration anesthesia*. Nerve block anesthesia involves relatively deep injections of drugs into locations adjacent to major nerve trunks or ganglia. It focuses on a relatively large body region but not necessarily as extensive as that affected by spinal anesthesia. In contrast, infiltration anesthesia involves multiple small injections (intradermal, subcutaneous, submucosal, or intramuscular) to produce a more limited or "local" anesthetic field. Another subtype of local anesthesia involves *topical* application of a drug (e.g., lidocaine) onto the surface of the skin, mucous membranes, or eye. A new method of administering local anesthetics is

via a peripheral nerve catheter attached to a pump containing the local anesthetic. These pumps are designed to infuse local anesthetic around the nerves that innervate the surgical site for several days postoperatively. The catheter is implanted during surgery and is normally taken out by the patient at home once the anesthetic has been infused. Common trade names include Pain Buster and On-Q pump.

## Mechanism of Action and Drug Effects

Local anesthetics work by rendering a specific portion of the body insensitive to pain by interfering with nerve transmission. Nerve conduction is blocked only in the area in which the anesthetic is applied, and there is no loss of consciousness. Local anesthetics block both the generation and conduction of impulses through all types of nerve fibers (sensory, motor, and autonomic) by blocking the movement of certain ions (sodium, potassium, and calcium) important to this process. They do this by making it more difficult for these ions to move in and out of the nerve fiber. For this reason, some of these drugs are also described as *membrane-stabilizing* because they alter the cell membrane of the nerve so that the free movement of ions is inhibited. The membrane-stabilizing effects occur first in the small fibers, then in the large fibers. In terms of paralysis, usually autonomic activity is affected first, and then pain and other sensory functions are lost. Motor activity is the last to be lost. When the effects of the local anesthetic wear off, recovery occurs in reverse order: motor activity returns first, then sensory functions, and finally autonomic activity.

Possible systemic effects of local anesthetics include effects on circulatory and respiratory function. The systemic adverse effects depend on where and how the drug is administered (e.g., injection at a certain level in the spinal cord or topical application of a drug that gains access to the circulation). Such adverse effects are unlikely unless large quantities of a drug are injected. Local anesthetics also produce *sympathetic blockade;* that is, they block the action of the two *neurotransmitters* of the sympathetic nervous system: *norepinephrine* and *epinephrine* (see Chapter 18). The cardiac effects include a decrease in stroke volume, cardiac output, and peripheral resistance. The respiratory effects include reduced respiratory function and altered breathing patterns, but complete paralysis of respiratory function is unlikely.

## Indications

Local anesthetics are used for surgical, dental, or diagnostic procedures, as well as for the treatment of various types of chronic pain. Spinal anesthesia is used to control pain during surgical procedures and childbirth. Nerve block anesthesia is used for surgical, dental, and diagnostic procedures and for the therapeutic management of chronic pain. Infiltration anesthesia is used for relatively minor surgical and dental procedures.

## Contraindications

Contraindications for local anesthetics include known drug allergy. Only specially formulated dosage forms are intended for ophthalmic use (see Chapter 57).

## Adverse Effects

The adverse effects of the local anesthetics are limited and of little clinical importance in most circumstances. The undesirable effects usually occur with high plasma concentrations of the drug, which result from inadvertent intravascular injection, an excessive dose or rate of injection, slow metabolic breakdown, or injection into a highly vascular tissue. One notable complication of spinal anesthesia is *spinal headache.* Spinal headache occurs in up to 70% of patients who either experience inadvertent dural puncture during epidural anesthesia or undergo intrathecal anesthesia. Spinal headache is most often self-limiting and is treated with bed rest and conventional analgesic medications. Oral or intravenous forms of the CNS stimulant caffeine (see Chapter 13) are also sometimes used. Severe cases of spinal headache may be treated by the anesthetist by injection of a small volume (roughly 15 mL) of venous sample of the patient's own blood into the patient's epidural space. The exact mechanism by which this *blood patch* provides relief is unknown, but it is effective in treating spinal headache in over 90% of cases. See Box 11-9 for more information on spinal headaches.

True allergic reactions to local anesthetics are rare. However, allergic reactions can occur, ranging from skin rash, urticaria, and edema to anaphylactic shock. Such allergic reactions are generally limited to a particular chemical class of anesthetics called the *ester type.* Box 11-3 categorizes the local anesthetic drugs into the

| BOX 11-3 | CHEMICAL GROUPS OF LOCAL ANESTHETICS | |
| --- | --- | --- |
| **Ester Type** | | **Amide Type** |
| benzocaine | | bupivacaine |
| chloroprocaine | | dibucaine |
| cocaine | | etidocaine |
| procaine | | lidocaine |
| proparacaine | | mepivacaine |
| propoxycaine | | prilocaine |
| tetracaine | | |

ester and amide chemical families. Different enzymes are responsible for the breakdown of these two groups of anesthetics in the body. Anesthetics belonging to the ester family are metabolized by cholinesterase in the plasma and liver. They are converted into a para-aminobenzoic acid (PABA) compound. This compound is responsible for the allergic reactions. In contrast, the *amide type* of anesthetics is metabolized uneventfully to active and inactive metabolites in the liver by other enzymes. Often when an individual has an adverse reaction to one of the local anesthetics, using a drug from the alternate chemical class avoids this problem.

### Toxicity and Management of Overdose

Local anesthetics have little opportunity to cause toxicity under most circumstances. However, systemic reactions are possible if sufficiently large quantities are absorbed into the systemic circulation. To prevent this from occurring, a *vasoconstrictor* such as epinephrine is often coadministered with the local anesthetic to maintain localized drug activity (e.g., lidocaine/epinephrine or bupivacaine/epinephrine). This property of epinephrine also serves to reduce local blood loss during minor surgical procedures. If significant amounts of the locally administered anesthetic are absorbed systemically, cardiovascular and respiratory function may be compromised. In extreme cases, such as inadvertent injection of drug into a major blood vessel, symptomatic and supportive cardiovascular and/or respiratory therapy may be required until the drug is metabolized and eliminated.

### Interactions

Few clinically significant drug interactions occur with the local anesthetics. When given with enflurane, halothane, or epinephrine, these drugs can lead to dysrhythmias.

## DRUG PROFILES

Besides lidocaine, profiled here, local anesthetics include bupivacaine, chloroprocaine, etidocaine, mepivacaine, prilocaine, procaine, propoxycaine, ropivacaine, and tetracaine. There are two major types of local anesthetics as determined by chemical structure: amides and esters. These designations refer to the type of linkage between the aromatic ring and the amino group of the chemical structures of the drug molecules. These structural components give these drugs their anesthetic properties.

◆ **lidocaine**

Lidocaine belongs to the amide class of local anesthetics. Some patients may report that they have allergic or anaphylactic reactions to the "caines," as they may refer to lidocaine and the other amide drugs. In these situations, it may be wise to try a local anesthetic of the ester type.

Lidocaine (Xylocaine) is one of the most commonly used local anesthetics. It is available in several strengths, both alone and in different concentrations with epinephrine, and is used for both infiltration and nerve block anesthesia. Lidocaine is also available in topical forms, including the unique product EMLA. This is a cream mixture of lidocaine and prilocaine that is applied to skin to ease the pain of needle punctures (e.g., starting an intravenous line). There is also a transdermal lidocaine patch for relief of *postherpetic neuralgia* (see Chapter 10). Parenteral lidocaine is also used to treat certain cardiac dysrhythmias (see Chapter 23). Contraindications include known drug allergy. Lidocaine is a pregnancy category B drug.

## NEUROMUSCULAR BLOCKING DRUGS

*Neuromuscular blocking drugs (NMBDs)* prevent nerve transmission in skeletal and smooth muscles, leading to paralysis. They are often used as adjuncts with general anesthetics for surgical procedures. Neuromuscular blocking drugs also paralyze the skeletal muscles required for breathing: the *intercostal* muscles and the *diaphragm*. The patient is rendered unable to breathe on his or her own, and mechanical ventilation is required to prevent brain damage or death by suffocation. Deaths have been reported when an NMBD is accidentally mistaken for a different drug and given to a patient who is not mechanically ventilated. Most hospitals have taken extra precautions to keep NMBDs separated from other drugs, or at least marked with warning stickers. It is essential that the nurse ensure that the patient is ventilated before giving an NMBD and double-check that an NMBD is not inadvertently given. In the event of an error, the patient would experience a horrendous death, because the mind is alert but the patient cannot speak or move (see the Safety and Quality Improvement: Preventing Medication Errors box).

---

### ⚡ SAFETY AND QUALITY IMPROVEMENT: PREVENTING MEDICATION ERRORS

#### *Neuromuscular Blocking Drugs*

Neuromuscular blocking drugs are considered high-alert drugs, because improper use may lead to severe injury or death. The Institute for Safe Medication Practices has reported several cases of patient death or injury as a result of medication errors involving neuromuscular blocking drugs. Because these drugs paralyze the respiratory muscles, incorrect administration without sufficient ventilator support has resulted in patient deaths. There have been medication errors due to "sound-alike" drug names as well (e.g., vancomycin and vecuronium). Most facilities have followed recommendations to restrict access to these drugs, provide warning labels and reminders, and increase staff awareness of the dangers of these drugs.

For more information, visit www.ismp.org/Newsletters/acutecare/articles/20050922.asp.

---

Historically, snakes and plants have played a role in the identification of substances that cause paralysis and to the discovery of related receptor proteins in animals and humans. The beginning steps involved study of the irreversible nerve transmission inhibition caused by toxins in the venoms of krait snake species and the venoms of certain varieties of cobra. *Curare,* a general term for various South American arrow poisons, has a long and intriguing history. It has been used for centuries by natives of the Amazon River region and other parts of South America to kill wild animals for food. Animals shot with arrows soaked in this plant substance normally die from paralysis of respiratory muscles. Once the receptor sites of action of these venoms and toxins were identified, pharmacologic drugs were developed that mimic these substances. Curare can be considered the grandfather of modern NMBDs. Several curare-like drugs are now used in clinical practice. The first drug derived from curare to be used medicinally was d-tubocurarine, which was introduced into anesthesia practice in 1940; it has now been replaced by newer drugs such as pancuronium. Pancuronium has a pharmacodynamic profile similar to that of curare but produces fewer adverse effects.

## Mechanism of Action and Drug Effects

NMBDs are classified into two groups based on mechanism of action: depolarizing and nondepolarizing. Depolarizing NMBDs work similarly to the neurotransmitter acetylcholine (ACh). They bind in place of ACh to cholinergic receptors at the motor endplates of muscle nerves or neuromuscular junctions. Thus they are competitive agonists (see Chapter 2). There are two phases of depolarizing block. During phase I (depolarizing phase), the muscles fasciculate (twitch). Eventually, after continued depolarization has occurred, muscles are no longer responsive to the ACh released; thus muscle tone cannot be maintained and the muscle becomes paralyzed. This is phase II, or the desensitizing phase. Depolarizing NMBDs include d-tubocurarine and succinylcholine (see later). The duration of action of succinylcholine after a single dose to facilitate intubation is only about 5 to 9 minutes because of the rapid breakdown of the drug by cholinesterase, the enzyme responsible for metabolizing succinylcholine.

Nondepolarizing NMBDs also bind to ACh receptors at the neuromuscular junction, but instead of mimicking ACh, they block its actions. Therefore, these drugs are *competitive antagonists* (see Chapter 2) of ACh. Consequently, the nerve cell membrane is not depolarized, the muscle fibers are not stimulated, and skeletal muscle contraction does not occur. Nondepolarizing NMBDs include vecuronium and pancuronium and are typically classified into three groups based on their duration of action: short-acting, intermediate-acting, and long-acting drugs.

The typical time course of NMBD-induced paralysis during a surgical procedure is as follows: The first sensation that is typically felt is muscle weakness. This is usually followed by a total flaccid paralysis. Small, rapidly moving muscles such as those of the fingers and eyes are generally the first to be paralyzed. The next are those of the limbs, neck, and trunk. Finally, the intercostal muscles and the diaphragm are paralyzed, which causes respiratory arrest. The patient can no longer breathe on his or her own. It must be noted that NMBDs, when used alone, do *not* cause sedation or relieve pain or anxiety. Therefore, the patient needs to also receive appropriate medications

## TABLE 11-7   EFFECTS OF GANGLIONIC BLOCKADE BY NEUROMUSCULAR BLOCKING DRUGS

| SITE | PART OF NERVOUS SYSTEM BLOCKED | PHYSIOLOGIC EFFECT |
|------|-------------------------------|--------------------|
| Arterioles | Sympathetic | Vasodilation and hypotension |
| Veins | Sympathetic | Dilation |
| Heart | Parasympathetic | Tachycardia |
| Gastrointestinal tract | Parasympathetic | Reduced tone and tract motility; constipation |
| Urinary bladder | Parasympathetic | Urinary retention |
| Salivary glands | Parasympathetic | Dry mouth |

## BOX 11-4   CONDITIONS THAT PREDISPOSE PATIENTS TO TOXIC EFFECTS FROM NEUROMUSCULAR BLOCKING DRUGS

Acidosis
Amyotrophic lateral sclerosis
Hypermagnesemia
Hypocalcemia
Hypokalemia
Hypothermia
Myasthenia gravis
Myasthenic syndrome
Neonatal status
Neurofibromatosis
Paraplegia
Poliomyelitis

## BOX 11-5   CONDITIONS THAT OPPOSE THE EFFECTS OF NEUROMUSCULAR BLOCKING DRUGS

Cirrhosis with ascites
Clostridial infections
Hemiplegia
Hypercalcemia
Hyperkalemia
Peripheral nerve transection
Peripheral neuropathies
Thermal burns

to manage pain and/or anxiety. Neuromuscular blocking drugs temporarily inactivate the body's natural drive to control respirations. Recovery of muscular activity after discontinuation of anesthesia usually occurs in the reverse order of the paralysis, and thus the diaphragm is ordinarily the first to regain function.

## Indications

The main therapeutic use of NMBDs is for maintaining skeletal muscle paralysis to facilitate controlled ventilation during surgical procedures. Shorter-acting NMBDs are often used to facilitate intubation with an endotracheal tube. This is commonly done for a variety of diagnostic procedures such as laryngoscopy, bronchoscopy, and esophagoscopy. When used for this purpose, NMBDs are frequently combined with anxiolytics, analgesics, and anesthetics. Additional nonsurgical applications include reduction of laryngeal or general muscle spasms, reduction of spasticity from tetanus and neurologic diseases such as multiple sclerosis, and prevention of bone fractures during electroconvulsive therapy (see Chapter 16). These drugs are also used for the diagnosis of *myasthenia gravis*, a disease characterized by chronic muscular weakness.

## Contraindications

Contraindications to NMBDs include known drug allergy and also may include previous history of malignant hyperthermia, penetrating eye injuries, and narrow-angle glaucoma.

## Adverse Effects

The muscle paralysis induced by depolarizing NMBDs (e.g., succinylcholine) is sometimes preceded by muscle spasms, which may damage muscles. These muscle spasms are termed *muscle fasciculations* and are most pronounced in the muscle groups of the hands, feet, and face. Injury to muscle cells may cause postoperative muscle pain and release potassium into the circulation, resulting in hyperkalemia, which is usually self-limiting and reversible. Small doses of nondepolarizing NMBDs are sometimes administered with succinylcholine to minimize these muscle fasciculations. In spite of these disadvantages, succinylcholine is still popular due to its rapid onset of action, its depth of neuromuscular blockade, and its short duration of action. For these reasons, it is often preferred to nondepolarizing NMBDs for *rapid-sequence induction* of anesthesia (e.g., for emergency intubation).

The effects on the cardiovascular system vary depending on the NMBD used and the individual patient. Increases and decreases in blood pressure and heart rate have been seen. Some NMBDs cause a release of histamine, which can result in bronchospasm, hypotension, and excessive bronchial and salivary secretion. The gastrointestinal tract is seldom affected by NMBDs. When it is affected, decreased tone and motility typically result, which can lead to constipation or even ileus. Use of succinylcholine has been associated with hyperkalemia; dysrhythmias; fasciculations; muscle pain; myoglobinuria; increased intraocular, intragastric, and intracranial pressure; and malignant hyperthermia.

The key to limiting adverse effects with most NMBDs is to use only enough of the drug to block the neuromuscular receptors. If too much is used, the risk is increased that other ganglionic receptors will be affected. Blockade of these other ganglionic receptors leads to most of the undesirable effects of NMBDs. The effects of ganglionic blockade in various areas of the body are listed in Table 11-7.

## Toxicity and Management of Overdose

The primary concern when NMBDs are overdosed is prolonged paralysis requiring prolonged mechanical ventilation (see the Safety and Quality Improvement: Preventing Medication Errors box on p. 177). Cardiovascular collapse may be seen and is thought to be the result of histamine release. Multiple medical conditions can predispose an individual to toxicity. These conditions increase the sensitivity of the individual to NMBDs and prolong their effects. These predisposing conditions are listed in Box 11-4. Some conditions make it more difficult for NMBDs to work, and therefore higher doses of NMBDs are required in these cases. Although these conditions do not necessarily lead to toxicity or overdose, they are worthy of mention and are listed in Box 11-5.

Anticholinesterase drugs such as neostigmine, pyridostigmine, and edrophonium are antidotes and are used to reverse muscle paralysis. They work by preventing the enzyme cholinesterase from breaking down ACh. This causes ACh to build up at the motor endplate, and it eventually displaces the nondepolarizing NMBD molecule, returning the nerve to its original

---

**BOX 11-6 DRUGS THAT INTERACT WITH NEUROMUSCULAR BLOCKING DRUGS**

| Additive Effects | Opposing Effects |
|---|---|
| Aminoglycosides | carbamazepine |
| Calcium channel blockers | Corticosteroids |
| clindamycin | phenytoin |
| cyclophosphamide | |
| cyclosporine | |
| dantrolene | |
| furosemide | |
| Inhalation anesthetics | |
| Local anesthetics | |
| magnesium | |
| quinidine | |

---

**BOX 11-7 CLASSIFICATION OF NONDEPOLARIZING NEUROMUSCULAR BLOCKING DRUGS**

| Short-Acting Drug | Long-Acting Drugs |
|---|---|
| mivacurium (Mivacron) | doxacurium (Nuromax) |
| | pancuronium (Pavulon) |
| **Intermediate-Acting Drugs** | tubocurarine (dTC) |
| atracurium (Tracrium) | |
| rocuronium (Zemuron) | |
| vecuronium (Norcuron) | |

---

## DOSAGES

### *Selected Neuromuscular Blocking Drugs*

| DRUG | PHARMACOLOGIC CLASS | USUAL DOSAGE RANGE | INDICATIONS/USES |
|---|---|---|---|
| pancuronium (Pavulon) | Nondepolarizing NMBD (long-acting) | **Adults, children older than 1 month**<br>IV: 60-100 mcg/kg<br>**Neonates up to 1 month**<br>Because neonates are very sensitive to nondepolarizing NMBDs, give a test dose of 20 mcg/kg IV | Intubation |
| ♦ succinylcholine (Anectine, Quelicin) | Depolarizing NMBD (short-acting) | **Adult**<br>IV: 0.04-0.1 mg/kg<br>Continuous infusion: 0.1 mg/kg/hr<br>**Pediatric**<br>IV: 1-2 mg/kg<br>IM: 3-4 mg/kg<br>**Adult**<br>IV: 0.3-1.1 mg/kg<br>IM: 3-4 mg/kg | Intubation<br>Mechanical ventilation<br>Intubation<br><br>Intubation |
| ♦ vecuronium (Norcuron) | Nondepolarizing NMBD (intermediate-acting) | **Pediatric**<br>IV: 0.08-0.1 mg/kg<br>**Adult**<br>IV: 0.08-0.1 mg/kg<br>Continuous infusion: 0.1 mg/kg/hr | Intubation<br><br>Intubation<br>Mechanical ventilation |

*IM,* Intramuscular; *IV,* intravenous; *NMBD,* neuromuscular blocking drug.

---

state. Dysmetabolic syndrome known as malignant hyperthermia (see General Anesthetics earlier in the chapter) can also occur with NMBDs, especially succinylcholine.

## Interactions

Many drugs interact with NMBDs, which may lead to either synergistic or opposing effects. Aminoglycoside antibiotics, when given with an NMBD, can have additive effects. The tetracycline antibiotics can also produce neuromuscular blockade, possibly by chelation of calcium, and calcium channel blockers have also been shown to enhance neuromuscular blockade. Other notable drugs that interact with NMBDs are listed in Box 11-6.

## Dosages

For dosage information of selected NMBDs, see the table on this page.

## DRUG PROFILES

Neuromuscular blocking drugs are one of the most commonly used classes of drugs in the operating room. They are given primarily with general anesthetics to facilitate endotracheal intubation and to relax skeletal muscles during surgery. In addition to their use in the operating room, they are given in the ICU to paralyze mechanically ventilated patients. There are two basic types of NMBDs: depolarizing and nondepolarizing drugs. Nondepolarizing NMBDs are generally classified by their duration of action. Box 11-7 lists examples of currently used nondepolarizing drugs.

### DEPOLARIZING NEUROMUSCULAR BLOCKING DRUGS
#### ♦ succinylcholine

Succinylcholine is the only currently available drug in the *depolarizing* subclass of NMBDs. Succinylcholine (Anectine) has a structure similar to that of the parasympathetic neurotransmitter ACh. It stimulates the same neurons as ACh and produces the same physiologic responses initially. Compared to ACh, however, succinylcholine is metabolized more slowly. Because of this slower metabolism, succinylcholine subjects the motor endplate to ongoing depolarizing stimulation. Repolarization cannot occur. As long as sufficient succinylcholine concentrations are present, the muscle loses its ability to contract, and flaccid muscle paralysis results. Because of its quick onset of action, succinylcholine is most commonly used to facilitate endotracheal intubation. It is seldom used over long periods because of its tendency to cause muscular fasciculations. It is contraindicated in patients with personal or familial history of malignant hyperthermia, skeletal muscle myopathies, and known hypersensitivity to the drug. It is available only in injectable form. For dosage information, see the table on p. 179.

### Pharmacokinetics

| Route | Onset of Action | Peak Plasma Concentration | Elimination Half-life | Duration of Action |
|---|---|---|---|---|
| IV | Rapid, less than 1 min | 60 sec | Less than 1 min | 4-6 min |

### NONDEPOLARIZING NEUROMUSCULAR BLOCKING DRUGS

Nondepolarizing NMBDs are commonly used to facilitate endotracheal intubation, reduce muscle contraction, and facilitate a variety of diagnostic procedures. They are often combined with anxiolytics or anesthetics. They may also be used to induce respiratory arrest in patients on mechanical ventilation.

### pancuronium

Pancuronium (Pavulon) is a long-acting nondepolarizing NMBD. It is used as an adjunct to general anesthesia to facilitate endotracheal intubation and to provide skeletal muscle relaxation during surgery or mechanical ventilation. It is most commonly employed for long surgical procedures that require prolonged muscle paralysis. Use of pancuronium is contraindicated in cases of known drug allergy. It is available only in injectable form. For dosage information, see the table on p. 179.

### Pharmacokinetics

| Route | Onset of Action | Peak Plasma Concentration | Elimination Half-life | Duration of Action |
|---|---|---|---|---|
| IV | 3-5 min | 5 min | 100 min | 45-60 min |

### ◆ vecuronium

Vecuronium (Norcuron) is an intermediate-acting nondepolarizing NMBD. It is used as an adjunct to general anesthesia to facilitate tracheal intubation and to provide skeletal muscle relaxation during surgery or mechanical ventilation, and it is one of the most commonly used NMBDs. Long-term use in the ICU setting has resulted in prolonged paralysis and subsequent difficulty weaning from mechanical ventilation. This is believed to be due to an active metabolite, 3-desacetyl vecuronium, which tends to accumulate with prolonged use. Use of vecuronium is

contraindicated in cases of known drug allergy. It is available only in injectable form. For dosage information, see the table on p. 179.

### Pharmacokinetics

| Route | Onset of Action | Peak Plasma Concentration | Elimination Half-life | Duration of Action |
|---|---|---|---|---|
| IV | 2.5-3 min | 3-5 min | 65-76 min | 25-40 min |

### TEAMWORK AND COLLABORATION: PHARMACOKINETIC BRIDGE TO NURSING PRACTICE

With moderate (conscious or procedural) sedation or anesthesia, it is always important to understand the pharmacokinetic properties of the drug(s) used. For example, the intravenous form of midazolam has an onset of action of 1 to 5 minutes, a peak plasma effect of 20 to 60 minutes, an elimination half-life of 1 to 4 hours (time it takes for 50% of the drug to be excreted), and a duration of action of 2 to 6 hours. Therefore, if midazolam is used for moderate sedation, you will begin to see the sedating properties within 1 to 5 minutes and peak effects on the patient between 20 to 60 minutes. Since the drug's action only lasts for 2 to 6 hours, midazolam is an attractive option for use in outpatient procedures because of fast onset and short duration of action. Therefore, as noted with this drug's pharmacokinetic properties, you may then be able to predict the drug's onset of action, peak effect, and duration of action.

## NURSING PROCESS

## ASSESSMENT

It is important to note that anesthetics are not drugs that are typically given by the registered nurse unless the nurse is a licensed nurse anesthetist. Exceptions to this statement are orders for topical forms, such as oral swish-and-swallow solutions that may be used during chemotherapy and lidocaine patches for pain relief. Associated with each drug used for general and local anesthesia are some very broad as well as specific assessment parameters. First, for any form of anesthesia and during any of the phases of anesthesia, the major parameters to assess are airway, breathing, and circulation (ABCs). Include in your assessment questions regarding allergies and use of prescription as well as over-the-counter drugs, herbals, supplements, and social and/or illegal drugs.

Another important area to assess is the patient's use of alcohol and nicotine. Excessive use of alcohol may alter the patient's response to general anesthesia, especially if there is liver impairment. Also, if the patient has a history of alcohol abuse, withdrawal symptoms may occur during the recovery from anesthesia and/or surgery. Perform a respiratory assessment (e.g., respiratory rate, rhythm, and depth; breath sounds; oxygen saturation level), especially if the patient has a history of smoking or is currently a smoker. The patient's history of smoking is important because nicotine has a paralyzing effect on the cilia within the respiratory tract. Once they are malfunctioning, these cilia cannot perform their main function of keeping foreign bodies out of the lungs and allowing mucus and secretions to be coughed up with ease. Malfunctioning of the cilia can potentially lead to atelectasis or pneumonia. Other objective data include weight and height, because these parameters are often used in the dosing of anesthesia. Other studies that may be ordered by the anesthesiologist and/or surgeon include an electrocardiogram, chest radiograph, and tests of renal function (e.g., BUN level, creatinine level, urinalysis with specific gravity) and hepatic function (e.g., total protein and albumin levels; bilirubin level; ALP, AST, and ALT levels). Additional laboratory tests may include Hgb, Hct, WBC with differential, and tests that indicate clotting abilities, such as PT-INR, aPTT, and platelet count. Also assess results for serum electrolytes, specifically potassium, sodium, chloride, phosphorus, magnesium, and calcium, because abnormalities may lead to further complications from the anesthesia. You must assess the results of a pregnancy test in females of childbearing age, if ordered, because of the possibility of teratogenic effects (adverse effects on the fetus) related to the anesthetic drug.

## CASE STUDY

### Moderate (Conscious) Sedation

A 53-year-old woman is scheduled to have a colonoscopy this morning, and she is very anxious. The nurse anesthetist has explained the moderate (conscious) sedation that is planned, but the patient says after the anesthetist leaves the room, "I'm so afraid of feeling it during the test. Why don't they just put me to sleep?"

1. How does moderate sedation differ from general anesthesia?
2. What is the nurse's best answer to the patient's question?
3. What is important for the nurse to assess before this procedure is performed?

The certified registered nurse anesthetist prepares to administer morphine and midazolam (Versed) before the procedure.

4. Explain the purpose of these two medications during moderate sedation. How are the dosages adjusted when these are given together?

For answers, see http://evolve.elsevier.Lilley.

Neurologic assessment includes a thorough survey of the patient's mental status. Determine and document level of consciousness, alertness, and orientation to person, place, and time prior to the anesthesia. Additional neurologic assessment includes motor assessments, with left-right and upper extremity versus lower extremity comparisons of strength, reflexes, grasp, and ability to move on command. Sensory assessment focuses on the same anatomic areas, with comparisons of the response to various types of stimuli such as sharp, dull, soft, and cold versus warm. Swallowing ability and gag reflexes are also important to assess and document for baseline status and comparisons. When these motor, sensory, and cognitive parameters are within normal limits, there is proof of an intact neurologic system.

One very significant reaction to assess for in patients receiving *general anesthesia* is that of malignant hyperthermia. This is a rapid progression of hyperthermia that may be fatal if not promptly recognized and aggressively treated. The tendency is inherited, so

questions about related signs and symptoms in the family's and patient's medical histories are important to document and report. A familial history of malignant hyperthermia would put the patient at risk. Signs and symptoms of malignant hyperthermia include a rapid rise in body temperature, tachycardia, tachypnea, muscle rigidity, cyanosis, irregular heartbeat, mottling of the skin, diaphoresis (profuse sweating), and an unstable blood pressure. If there is no documented problem with general anesthesia or if the patient is undergoing general anesthesia for the first time, perform an astute and careful examination of all medical and medication histories. With any type of anesthesia, it is often very slight changes in vital signs, other vital parameters, and laboratory test results that may provide nursing and other health care providers with a possible clue to the patient's reaction to anesthesia. Note that malignant hyperthermia occurs during the anesthesia process and in the surgical suite; nevertheless, close observation after anesthesia is still important and much needed. Intravenously administered anesthetic drugs are usually combined with adjuvant drugs (given at the same time) such as sedative-hypnotics, antianxiety drugs, opioid and nonopioid analgesics, antiemetics, and anticholinergics. These drugs are used to decrease some of the undesirable aftereffects of inhaled anesthetics. If they are used, perform a complete assessment for each of the drugs, including obtaining a medical history and medication profile. Liver and kidney function studies are important in these patients as well, so that any risks of toxicity and complications can be anticipated.

For patients about to undergo anesthesia with *neuromuscular blocking drugs (NMBDs)*, perform a complete head-to-toe assessment with a thorough medical and medication history. Which specific drug is being used and whether it is depolarizing or nondepolarizing will guide your assessment, because of the action of NMBDs on the patient's neuromuscular functioning (see pharmacology discussion). Assess all cautions, contraindications, and drug interactions. Another concern with the use of these drugs is that they are associated with an increase in intraocular pressure and intracranial pressure. Therefore, these anesthetic drugs should not be used or used with extreme caution (close monitoring of these pressures) in patients with glaucoma or closed head injuries.

Complete a thorough respiratory assessment in patients receiving NMBDs because of the effect of these drugs on the respiratory system. In particular, these drugs have a paralyzing effect on the muscles used for breathing and—for this very reason—are used to facilitate intubation for mechanical ventilation. Paralysis of respiratory muscles allows patient relaxation to the point where the patient will not fight against the breaths delivered by the ventilator. Also indicated with the use of NMBDs is careful assessment of serum electrolyte levels, specifically potassium and magnesium levels. Imbalances in these electrolytes may lead to increased action of the NMBD with exacerbation of the drug's actions and toxic effects. Allergic reactions to these drugs are most commonly characterized by rash, fever, respiratory distress, and pruritus. Drug interactions with herbal products are outlined in the Safety: Herbal Therapies and Dietary Supplements box on p. 182. For more specific information on the differences between depolarizing and nondepolarizing NMBDs, see the pharmacology section of this chapter.

## SAFETY: HERBAL THERAPIES AND DIETARY SUPPLEMENTS

### Possible Effects of Popular Herbal Products When Combined with Anesthetics

**Feverfew:** Migraine headaches, insomnia, anxiety, joint stiffness, risk of increased bleeding times with increased risk of bleeding

**Garlic:** Changes in blood pressure, risk of increased bleeding

**Ginger:** Sedating effects; risk of bleeding, especially if taken with either aspirin or ginkgo

**Ginseng:** Irritability and insomnia, risk of cardiac adverse effects

**Kava:** Sedating effects, potential liver toxicity, risk of additive effects with medications

**St. John's Wort:** Sedation, blood pressure changes, risk of interaction with other medications that prolong the effects of anesthesia

For more information, see www.aana.com, www.anesthesiapatient safety.com, www.herbalgram.com, and http://nccam.NIH.gov.

With the use of *conscious or moderate sedation,* as with any anesthesia technique, assessment for allergies, cautions, contraindications, and drug interactions is important. Because moderate sedation is commonly used across the lifespan, closely assess organ function and note diseases or conditions that could lead to excessive levels of the drug in the body, such as liver or kidney impairment. See Chapters 10 and 12 for more information about the assessment associated with the use of opioids and sedative-hypnotics/CNS depressants.

Use of *spinal anesthesia* requires thorough assessment with an emphasis on the ABCs, respiratory function, and vital signs, specifically blood pressure. Baseline respirations with attention to rate, rhythm, depth, and breath sounds are important to note, as are oxygen saturation levels obtained via pulse oximetry. Because of possible problems with vasodilatation from the spinal anesthetic, document baseline blood pressure levels and pulse rate. Record history of previous reactions to this form of anesthesia, allergies, and a listing of all medications, and report any abnormal reactions to the anesthesiologist and surgeon. Neurologic assessment with notation of sensory and motor intactness in the lower extremities, as well as documentation of any abnormalities, is important. The use of epidural anesthesia requires special attention to overall hemostasis through monitoring of vital signs and oxygen saturation levels. Assess baseline sensory and motor function in the extremities, and document an intact neurologic system (see Implementation for more detailed discussion). Spinal headaches may occur with either spinal anesthesia or epidural injections, and thus baseline assessment for the presence of headaches is important.

*Local-topical anesthetics,* such as lidocaine, used for either infiltration or nerve block anesthesia may be administered with or without a vasoconstrictor (e.g., epinephrine). The vasoconstrictors are used to help confine the local anesthetic to the injected area, prevent systemic absorption of the anesthetic, and reduce bleeding. If there is systemic absorption of the vasoconstrictor into the bloodstream, the patient's blood pressure could elevate to life-threatening levels, especially in patients who are at high risk (e.g., those with underlying arterial disease). Therefore, review the patient's medical history to assess for any preexisting illnesses, such as vascular disease, aneurysms, or hypertension, because these may be contraindications to the use of the vasoconstrictor with the anesthetic. In addition, with these local anesthetics, assess for allergies to the drug as well as baseline vital signs. Also assess for possible drug interactions, and note prescription medications, herbal products, supplements, and over-the-counter medications. In summary, it is important with any type of anesthesia to assess the patient's level of homeostasis prior to actual administration of the drug. This assessment may include taking vital signs as well as checking the ABCs. Other parameters of interest may be oxygen saturation levels measured by pulse oximetry, cardiovascular and respiratory function, and neurologic function.

## NURSING DIAGNOSES

1. Impaired gas exchange related to the general anesthetic's CNS depressant effect with altered respiratory rate and effort (decreased rate, decreased depth)
2. Decreased cardiac output related to the systemic effects of anesthesia
3. Acute pain related to the adverse effect of spinal headache from epidural anesthesia
4. Deficient knowledge related to lack of information about anesthesia
5. Risk for injury related to the impact of any form of anesthesia on the CNS (e.g., CNS depression and decreased sensorium)

## PLANNING

### GOALS

1. Patient maintains normal and effective respiratory patterns and status.
   - Patient demonstrates an understanding about the potential complications of anesthesia related to the respiratory system.
2. Patient maintains blood pressure and pulse rate within normal limits.
   - Patient demonstrates an understanding about the potential complications of anesthesia related to cardiac functioning.
3. Patient fully understands the potential for the adverse effect of spinal headache associated with epidural anesthesia.
4. Patient demonstrates sound knowledge base about the action and adverse effects of anesthesia.
5. Patient states the potential complications of anesthesia and possible risks related to CNS depression, specifically decreased sensorium.

### OUTCOME CRITERIA

1. Patient states measures to increase respiratory expansion through coughing, deep breathing, turning, and ambulating (when allowed).
2. Patient remains well hydrated with increase in fluids and remains ambulating to help increase circulation and minimize complications, unless contraindicated.

3. Patient states measures to help minimize and/or prevent acute pain from possible complication of spinal headache with bed rest, hydration, and following postanesthesia/postepidural orders for up to 24 to 48 hours after procedure.

4. Patient experiences maximal effects of anesthesia as noted by following preanesthesia orders, such as remaining NPO, taking medications only as prescribed, as well as experiencing minimal adverse effects from an adequate knowledge about the postanesthesia period and ways to minimize problems (see all measures listed in outcome criteria 1 to 3 and 5).

5. Patient remains free of injury and/or falls by asking for assistance while ambulating or having assistance if at home and recovering alone as well as taking medications only as prescribed, sitting up for brief periods prior to ambulating, forcing fluids, and resuming adequate nutritional intake during the postanesthesia period.

## IMPLEMENTATION

Regardless of the type of anesthesia used, one of the most important nursing considerations during the preanesthesia, intraanesthesia, and postanesthesia periods is close and frequent observation of all body systems. Begin with a focus on the ABCs of nursing care, vital signs, and oxygen saturation levels as measured by pulse oximetry as well as by the clinical presentation of the patient. Remember that the way a patient looks is very important at any point in time! Document the observations from these interventions, and repeat the interventions as needed, depending on the patient's status and in keeping with the standard of care for the type of anesthesia. Monitor vital signs frequently and as needed, and based on the patient's condition, including assessing the fifth vital sign of pain (see discussion later in this section and in Chapter 10).

For patients undergoing *general anesthesia,* assessing the patient's temperature is especially important because of the risk of malignant hyperthermia, and close monitoring is required if malignant hyperthermia occurred during the anesthesia process. This sudden elevation in the patient's body temperature (e.g., higher than 104° F [40° C]) not only requires critical care during and immediately after anesthesia but also calls for close monitoring even during regular postoperative care (see earlier discussion). When intravenous, inhaled, or other forms of anesthesia are used, resuscitative equipment and medications, including opioid antidotes, are readily available in the surgical and postsurgical areas in case of cardiorespiratory distress or arrest. The anesthesiologist keeps control of the anesthetic drug, and he or she is well prepared for any emergency—as is the entire group of individuals in the surgical suite and postanesthesia recovery area. Continual monitoring of the status of breath sounds is an important intervention, because hypoventilation may be a complication of general and other forms of anesthesia. Oxygen is administered after a patient has received general and/or other forms of anesthesia to compensate for the respiratory depression that may have occurred during the anesthesia and surgical process. Because oxygen is a drug, a doctor's order is needed for its administration. Continuous monitoring of oxygen saturation levels is therefore an important intervention. In addition, hypotension and orthostatic hypotension are possible problems after anesthesia, so postural blood pressure measurements (supine and standing), in addition to regular blood pressure monitoring, may be needed. Additional nursing interventions include monitoring of neurologic parameters such as reflexes, response to commands, level of consciousness or sedation, and pupil reaction to light. Monitor for changes in sensation and movement in the extremities, distal pulses, temperature, and color when nerve blocks and spinal anesthesia are used, because it is important to confirm that areas distal to the anesthetic site have remained intact.

Should the patient require pain management once the anesthesia has been terminated, remember that the anesthetic and any adjuvant drugs used continue to have an effect on the patient until the period of the drugs' action has passed. Therefore, administer sedative-hypnotics, opioids, nonopioids, and other CNS depressants for pain relief cautiously and *only* with close monitoring of vital signs. If the patient has received some of these medications during postanesthesia, document dosages of drugs used, and then pass them on during a report when the patient is transferred to another unit. Additional orders are usually provided by the physician/surgeon or anesthesiologist regarding doses of analgesics to administer once the patient has been transferred or if discharged to home. If such orders have not been provided, however, and the patient is experiencing pain, contact the appropriate prescriber. The concern here is that the patient may receive either too much or not enough analgesic.

Patients who receive *NMBDs* as part of an induction process for mechanical ventilation need to be monitored closely during and after initiation of mechanical ventilation. Patients receiving NMBDs and who are awake may need to receive other medications for sedation and/or pain. These patients are in intensive care or critical care units, and many protocols are provided regarding interventions after the intubation. These include measurement of vital signs and determination of neurologic status, including sensation and hand grasp strength. When mechanical ventilation is used, educate patients and family members about the purpose of the drug-induced paralysis while receiving mechanical ventilation (e.g., to prevent the patient from fighting against the ventilation provided by the machine, resisting the effects of the mechanical ventilatory assistance and possibly leading to hypoventilation). Inform the family and remember in the nursing care of these patients that they can still hear the spoken word. Knowing what to expect is key to helping decrease fears and anxiety—for both the patient and those visiting the patient.

Patients undergoing *moderate sedation* as the method of anesthesia should receive patient education before the procedure. As noted earlier in the chapter, recovery from this type of anesthesia is more rapid, and the safety profile is better than that of general anesthesia with its inherent cardiorespiratory risks. As with general anesthesia, however, monitor the ABCs of care, vital signs, pulse oximetry oxygen saturation levels, and level of consciousness or sedation. See Box 11-8 for more information on moderate sedation.

With *spinal anesthesia,* nursing interventions need to include constant monitoring for a return of sensation and motor

---

### BOX 11-8 MODERATE OR CONSCIOUS SEDATION: WHAT TO EXPECT AND QUESTIONS TO ASK

1. What questions do the patient or caregiver need to ask about the technique of moderate or conscious sedation?
   - Who will be providing this type of anesthesia?
   - Who will be monitoring me or my loved one?
   - Will there be constant monitoring of blood pressure, pulse rate, respiratory rate, and temperature?
   - Will there be emergency equipment in the room, in case of need?
   - Are the personnel qualified to administer these drugs? To administer advanced cardiac life support?
   - What do I need to know about care at home? Will I need help? Can I drive after having the procedure?
2. What are the adverse effects of moderate or conscious sedation?
   - Brief periods of amnesia (loss of memory)
   - Headache
   - Hangover feeling
   - Nausea and vomiting
3. What is to be expected immediately following the procedure?
   - Frequent monitoring
   - Written postoperative instructions and care
   - If the patient is of driving age, no driving for at least 24 hours after undergoing moderate sedation
   - A follow-up contact by phone to check on the patient
4. Who administers the conscious sedation?
   - Moderate or conscious sedation is safe when administered by qualified providers. Certified registered nurse anesthetists, anesthesiologists, other physicians, dentists, and oral surgeons are qualified to administer conscious sedation.

5. Which procedures generally require moderate sedation?
   - Breast biopsy
   - Vasectomy
   - Minor foot surgery
   - Minor bone fracture repair
   - Plastic or reconstructive surgery
   - Dental prosthetic or reconstructive surgery
   - Endoscopy (such as diagnostic studies and treatment of stomach, colon, and bladder cancer)
6. What are the overall benefits of this type of anesthesia?
   - It is a safe and effective option for patients undergoing minor surgeries or diagnostic procedures.
   - It allows patients to recover quickly and resume normal activities in a relatively short period of time.
7. Are there any concerns about daily medications or herbals if undergoing conscious sedation?
   - As with any form of anesthesia, being open and honest with the nurse anesthetist or anesthesiologist is of significant importance to patient safety.
   - Be sure to follow instructions closely regarding the intake of all medications including herbals, food, or liquids before anesthesia as such substances may react negatively with the drugs being administered.
   - Inquire about any brochures or written pamphlets such as the AANA brochure titled "Before anesthesia: Your active role makes a difference."

Data from Brenman EK (editor): Pain management: spinal headaches, 2007, available at http://www.WebMD.com; American Association of Nurse Anesthetists (AANA), available at www.aana.com. Accessed February 25, 2011.

---

activity below the anesthetic insertion site. Because of the risk that the anesthetic drug may move upward in the spinal cord and breathing may be affected, continually monitor respiratory and breathing status. In addition, because positioning is important to the movement of the anesthetic drug, keep the head of the bed elevated. Remember, though, that this complication is usually identified and treated by the anesthesiologist, and patients will not return to their rooms on a nursing unit until all respiratory risks are identified and managed appropriately. Another major area of concern with spinal anesthesia is the risk for a sudden decrease in blood pressure. This drop in blood pressure is secondary to vasodilation caused by the anesthetic block to the sympathetic vasomotor nerves. Vital signs and oxygen saturation levels should return to normal before the patient is transferred out of postanesthesia care; however, continue to monitor these vital signs frequently after transfer.

Another adverse reaction to intraspinal anesthesia is the occurrence of spinal headaches. These may occur with both intrathecal and epidural injections but are actually more frequent with the latter. Because intrathecal spinal needle designs have been technologically improved, the occurrence of spinal headaches is rare. Larger-bore needles are used to deliver epidural anesthetics, however, and these are more likely to give rise to spinal headache if they are inadvertently passed through the dura mater (the covering of the spinal cord). Keep the patient hydrated and on bedrest as recommended by the anesthesiologist. See Box 11-9 for more information about these headaches and their treatment.

---

### BOX 11-9 SPINAL HEADACHES: A BRIEF LOOK AT A TERRIBLE PAIN!

*Why do spinal headaches occur?* As a result of penetration into and through the dura mater of the spinal cord (the covering of the spinal cord), a leakage of cerebrospinal fluid occurs from the insertion site. If enough of the spinal fluid leaks out, a spinal headache results. These headaches are more likely to be associated with epidural anesthesia than with intrathecal anesthesia because of the larger needles used with epidurals.

*What are the symptoms of a spinal headache?* Patients say that these headaches are worse than any other type! They are more severe when the patient is in an upright position and improve upon lying down. They may occur up to 5 days after the procedure and may be prevented with bed rest after the epidural procedure.

*How are spinal headaches treated?* Adequate hydration using intravenous fluids is often tried to help increase cerebral spinal fluid pressure. Other recommendations include the drinking of a beverage high in caffeine and strict bed rest for 24 to 48 hours. If the headaches are intolerable, however, the anesthesiologist may create a "blood patch" to help close up or seal the leak. This requires insertion of a needle into the same space or right next to the area that was injected with the anesthesia. A small amount of blood is then taken from the patient and injected into the epidural space. The blood clots and forms a seal over the hole that caused the leak, and the headache is relieved.

Data from American Association of Nurse Anesthetists: Conscious sedation: what patients should expect, 2005, available at http://www.aana.com; Bezov D, Ashina S, Lipton R: Post-dural puncture headache: part II—prevention, management, and prognosis, *Headache* 50(9):1482-1498, 2010.

The use of epidural anesthesia (also called *regional anesthesia* in some textbooks) does not pose the same risk of respiratory complications as general anesthesia; however, monitoring is still needed to confirm overall homeostasis. You must measure vital signs and pulse oximetry to determine oxygen saturation levels. In addition, patients undergoing this form of anesthesia require monitoring for the return of motor function and tactile sensation. Check the patient frequently for the return of sensation bilaterally along the dermatome (area of the skin innervated by specific segments of the spinal cord); such monitoring is important to ensure patient safety as well as to maximize comfort. Assess touch sensation through hand pressure or a gentle pinch of the skin. You need to know the level at which the epidural anesthesia was given to monitor properly for return of sensation. This monitoring process generally occurs in a post-anesthesia care unit, and the patient is not returned to a regular nursing unit until all sensation and/or voluntary movement of the lower extremities is regained.

With regard to the use of *topical or local anesthetics* (e.g., lidocaine with or without epinephrine), solutions that are not clear and appear cloudy or discolored are not to be used. Some anesthesiologists mix the solution with sodium bicarbonate to minimize local pain during infiltration, but this also causes a more rapid onset of action and a longer duration of sensory analgesia. If an anesthetic ointment or cream is used, the nurse will thoroughly cleanse and dry the area to be anesthetized before applying the drug. If a topical or local anesthetic is being used in the nose or throat, remember that it may cause paralysis and/or numbness of the structures of the upper respiratory tract, which can lead to aspiration. If the patient receives a solution form of anesthetic, exact amounts of the drug are used and at the exact dosing times or intervals. Local anesthetics are not to be swallowed unless the prescriber has so instructed. Should this occur, closely observe the patient, check for the gag reflex, and expect to withhold food or drink until the patient's sensation and/or gag reflex has returned.

Once the patient has recovered from the anesthesia and procedure and is ready for discharge, complete your patient teaching. Focus the patient education on the patient's needs and how these needs can be met at home. Home health care and/or rehabilitation services may be indicated, and arrangements should be made before the patient is discharged. If additional care or resources are needed at home (e.g., for a patient who lives alone), these arrangements should be completed in a timely fashion. Some examples of procedures for which help might be needed are wound care, dressing changes, surgical site care, drawing of blood for laboratory studies, and administration of various medications through the intravenous, intramuscular, or subcutaneous route. Some patients may also need assistance with taking oral medications at home. Pain management requires thorough and individualized patient teaching and also includes any necessary education for patients who will require home health care. See Chapter 10 for more information on analgesics. Provide simple instructions using age-appropriate teaching strategies (see Chapter 6). Sharing of information about community resources is also important, especially for patients who need transportation, assistance with meals, housekeeping during recovery, and/or the services of additional health care providers (e.g., physical therapists, occupational therapists) in the home setting. Some of these community resources may be agencies that are supported by city or state social service programs. Meals on Wheels, senior citizen support groups, and church-sponsored groups are just a few examples of important resource groups. Many of these resources are free or have income-based fees. Additional suggestions regarding patient education are provided in the Patient Teaching Tips.

## EVALUATION

The therapeutic effects of any *general or local anesthesia* include the following: loss of consciousness and reflexes during general anesthesia and loss of sensation to a particular area during local anesthesia (e.g., loss of sensation to the eye during corneal transplantation). Constantly monitor the patient who has undergone general anesthesia for the occurrence of adverse effects of the anesthesia. These may include myocardial depression, convulsions, respiratory depression, allergic rhinitis, and decreased renal or liver function. Constantly monitor patients who have received a local anesthetic for the occurrence of adverse effects, including bradycardia, myocardial depression, hypotension, and dysrhythmias. In addition, as mentioned earlier in this chapter, significant overdoses of local anesthetic drugs or direct injection into a blood vessel may result in cardiovascular collapse or cardiac or respiratory depression. For those receiving spinal anesthesia, therapeutic effects include loss of sensation below the area of administration, and adverse effects include hypotension, hypoventilation, urinary retention, the possibility of a prolonged period of decreased sensation or motor ability, and infection at the site. With *epidural anesthesia,* therapeutic effects are similar to those seen with intrathecal anesthesia; however, adverse effects include possible spinal headache (often severe) and/or loss of motor function or sensation below the area of administration. *Moderate sedation* provides the therapeutic effect of a decreased sensorium but without the complications of general anesthesia; however, there are CNS depressant effects associated with the drugs used.

## KEY POINTS

- Anesthesia is the loss of the ability to feel pain resulting from the administration of an anesthetic drug. General anesthesia is a drug-induced state in which the nerve impulses of the CNS are altered to reduce pain and other sensations throughout the entire body and normally involves complete loss of consciousness and respiratory drive depression.
- General anesthetics are drugs that induce general anesthesia, including the administration of specific parenteral anesthetics. Inhalational anesthetic drugs are also general anesthetics and include volatile liquids or gases.
- Local anesthetics are used to induce a state in which peripheral or spinal nerve impulses are altered to reduce or eliminate pain and other sensations. Spinal anesthesia, or regional anesthesia, is a form of local anesthesia.
- Conscious or moderate sedation is a form of general anesthesia resulting in partial or complete loss of consciousness but without reducing normal respiratory drive.

- Adjunct anesthetics are drugs that assist with the induction of general anesthesia and include neuromuscular blocking drugs (NMBDs), sedative-hypnotics, and/or anxiolytics and antiemetics.
- Nondepolarizing NMBDs are used as an adjunct to general anesthesia to provide skeletal muscle relaxation during surgery and/or mechanical ventilation.
- Nursing assessment is very important to patient safety during and after all forms of anesthesia. With general anesthesia, however, one major problem to be concerned with is that of malignant hyperthermia, which may be fatal if not promptly recognized and aggressively treated. Signs and symptoms include rapid rise in body temperature, increased pulse rate (tachycardia)/respiratory rate (tachypnea), muscle rigidity, and unstable blood pressure.

## PATIENT TEACHING TIPS

- Whenever general anesthesia is used, emphasize the prescriber's recommendations/orders about whether any medications should be discontinued or tapered before anesthetic administration.
- Make sure information about the anesthetic, route of administration, adverse effects, and special precautions is included in preprocedure and surgical education.
- Openly discuss with the patient all fears and anxieties about anesthesia and related procedures/surgery.
- Share with the patient and family instructions about the postanesthesia process and the need for close monitoring of vital signs, breath sounds, and neurologic intactness. Patients should expect frequent turning, coughing, and deep breathing to prevent atelectasis or pneumonia.
- Encourage patients to ambulate with assistance as needed and as ordered. Mobility helps increase circulation and improve ventilation to the alveoli of the lungs; consequently, circulation to the legs will be improved (which helps to prevent stasis of blood and possible blood clot formation in the leg veins). Assistance is needed to prevent falls or injury until recovery from the anesthetic.
- Encourage the patient to request pain medication, if needed, before pain becomes moderate to severe. Inform the patient that,

even though anesthesia has been administered, there may still be discomfort or pain from the procedure or surgery. The anesthesia will wear off, and adequate analgesia will be needed. Ask the patient to rate his or her pain on a scale of 0 to 10, with 0 being no pain and 10 being the worst possible pain. See Chapter 10 for more information on pain assessment and its management.

- Explain the rationale for any other treatments or procedures related to the anesthesia (e.g., epidural catheter placement; delivery of oxygen; administration of a gas; use of various tubes, catheters, or intravenous lines). Adequate patient education will help ease fears and anxieties and help in preventing adverse effects or complications.
- For a patient with diminished sensorium, the bed side rails should be up and a call button at the bedside. These actions are critical to patient safety. Note that bed alarms may be used instead of side rails. Everyone involved in the postanesthesia and postsurgical care (e.g., family members) should be educated about these safety measures.
- With local anesthesia, the patient should understand the purpose and action of the local anesthetic as well as adverse effects.
- Inform a patient receiving spinal anesthesia about the need for frequent assessments, measurement of vital signs, and system assessments during and after the procedure.

## NCLEX® EXAMINATION REVIEW QUESTIONS

1 The physician has requested "lidocaine *with* epinephrine." The nurse recognizes that the most important reason for adding epinephrine is that it
   a helps to calm the patient before the procedure.
   b minimizes the risk of an allergic reaction.
   c enhances the effect of the local lidocaine.
   d reduces bleeding in the surgical area.
2 The surgical nurse is reviewing operative cases scheduled for the day. Which of these patients is more prone to complications from general anesthesia?

   a A 79-year-old woman who is about to have her gallbladder removed
   b A 49-year-old male athlete who quit heavy smoking 12 years ago
   c A 30-year-old woman who is in perfect health but has never had anesthesia
   d A 50-year-old woman scheduled for outpatient laser surgery for vision correction

3 Which nursing diagnosis is possible for a patient who is now recovering after having been under general anesthesia for 3 to 4 hours during surgery?
   a Impaired urinary elimination related to the use of vasopressors as anesthetics
   b Increased cardiac output related to the effects of general anesthesia
   c Risk for falls related to decreased sensorium for 2 to 4 days postoperatively
   d Impaired gas exchange due to the CNS depressant effect of general anesthesia

4 A patient is recovering from general anesthesia. What is the nurse's main concern during the immediate postoperative period?
   a Airway
   b Pupillary reflexes
   c Return of sensations
   d Level of consciousness

5 A patient is about to undergo cardioversion, and the nurse is reviewing the procedure and explaining moderate sedation. The patient asks, "I am afraid of feeling it when they shock me?" What is the nurse's best response?
   a "You won't receive enough of a shock to feel anything."
   b "You will feel the shock but you won't remember any of the pain."
   c "The medications you receive will reduce any pain and help you not to remember the procedure."
   d "They will give you enough pain medication to prevent you from feeling it."

6 The nurse is administering an NMBD to a patient during a surgical procedure. Number the following phases of muscle paralysis in the order in which the patient will experience them. (Number 1 is the first step.)
   a Paralysis of intercostals and diaphragm muscles
   b Muscle weakness
   c Paralysis of muscles of the limbs, neck, and trunk
   d Paralysis of small rapidly moving muscles (fingers, eye)

7 During a patient's recovery from a lengthy surgery, the nurse monitors for signs of malignant hyperthermia. In addition to a rapid rise in body temperature, which assessment findings would indicate the possible presence of this condition? (Select all that apply.)
   a Respiratory depression
   b Tachypnea
   c Tachycardia
   d Seizure activity
   e Muscle rigidity

1. d, 2. a, 3. d, 4. a, 5. c, 6. a = 4, b = 2, c = 3, d = 1, 7. b, c, e

For Critical Thinking and Prioritization Questions, see http://evolve.elsevier.com/Lilley.

# Central Nervous System Depressants and Muscle Relaxants

## OBJECTIVES

When you reach the end of this chapter, you will be able to do the following:

1. Briefly describe the functions of the central nervous system.
2. Contrast the effects of central nervous system depressant drugs and central nervous system stimulant drugs (see Chapter 13) as relates to their basic actions.
3. Define the terms *hypnotic, rapid eye movement, rapid eye movement sleep interference, rapid eye movement rebound, sedative, sedative-hypnotic, sleep,* and *therapeutic index.*
4. Briefly discuss the problem of sleep disorders.
5. Identify the specific drugs within each of the following categories of central nervous system depressant drugs: benzodiazepines, nonbenzodiazepines, muscle relaxants, and miscellaneous drugs.

6. Contrast the mechanism of action, indications, adverse effects, toxic effects, cautions, contraindications, dosage forms, routes of administration, and drug interactions of the following medications: benzodiazepines, nonbenzodiazepines, muscle relaxants, and miscellaneous drugs.
7. Discuss the nursing process as it relates to the nursing care of a patient receiving any central nervous system depressants and/or muscle relaxant.
8. Develop a thorough nursing care plan related to the use of pharmacologic and nonpharmacologic approaches to the treatment of sleep disorders.

## DRUG PROFILES

- **baclofen, p. 197**
- **cyclobenzaprine, p. 197**
- **diazepam, p. 192**
- **eszopiclone, p. 193**
- **midazolam, p. 192**
- **pentobarbital, p. 195**
- **phenobarbital, p. 195**

- **ramelteon, p. 193**
- **temazepam, p. 193**
- **zaleplon, p. 193**
- **zolpidem, p. 193**

———————

- *Key drug*

## KEY TERMS

**Barbiturates** A class of drugs that are chemical derivatives of barbituric acid. They are used to induce sedation. (p. 193)

**Benzodiazepines** A chemical category of drugs most frequently prescribed as anxiolytic drugs and less frequently as sedative-hypnotic agents. (p. 190)

**Gamma-aminobutyric acid (GABA)** The primary inhibitory neurotransmitter found in the brain. A key compound affected by sedative, anxiolytic, psychotropic, and muscle-relaxing medications. (p. 190)

## KEY TERMS—cont'd

**Hypnotics** Drugs that, when given at low to moderate dosages, calm or soothe the central nervous system (CNS) without inducing sleep but when given at high dosages cause sleep. (p. 189)

**Non–rapid eye movement (non-REM) sleep** The largest portion of the sleep cycle. It has four stages and precedes REM sleep. Most of a normal sleep cycle consists of non-REM sleep. (p. 189)

**Rapid eye movement (REM) sleep** One of the stages of the sleep cycle. Some of the characteristics of REM sleep are rapid movement of the eyes, vivid dreams, and irregular breathing. (p. 189)

**REM interference** A drug-induced reduction of REM sleep time. (p. 189)

**REM rebound** Excessive REM sleep following discontinuation of a sleep-altering drug. (p. 189)

**Sedatives** Drugs that have an inhibitory effect on the CNS to the degree that they reduce nervousness, excitability, and irritability without causing sleep. (p. 189)

**Sedative-hypnotics** Drugs that can act in the body either as sedatives or as hypnotics. (p. 189)

**Sleep** A transient, reversible, and periodic state of rest in which there is a decrease in physical activity and consciousness. (p. 189)

**Sleep architecture** The structure of the various elements involved in the sleep cycle, including normal and abnormal patterns of sleep. (p. 189)

**Therapeutic index** The ratio between the toxic and therapeutic concentrations of a drug. If the index is low, the difference between the therapeutic and toxic drug concentrations is small, and use of the drug is more hazardous. (p. 193)

## ANATOMY, PHYSIOLOGY, AND PATHOPHYSIOLOGY OVERVIEW

*Sedatives* and *hypnotics* are drugs that have a calming effect or that depress the central nervous system (CNS). A drug is classified as either a sedative or a hypnotic drug depending on the degree to which it inhibits the transmission of nerve impulses to the CNS. Sedatives reduce nervousness, excitability, and irritability without causing sleep, but a sedative can become a hypnotic if it is given in large enough doses. Hypnotics cause sleep and have a much more potent effect on the CNS than do sedatives. Many drugs can act as either a sedative or a hypnotic, depending on dose and patient responsiveness, and for this reason are called sedative-hypnotics. Sedative-hypnotics can be classified chemically into three main groups: barbiturates, benzodiazepines, and miscellaneous drugs.

## PHYSIOLOGY OF SLEEP

Sleep is defined as a transient, reversible, and periodic state of rest in which there is a decrease in physical activity and consciousness. Normal sleep is cyclic and repetitive, and a person's responses to sensory stimuli are markedly reduced during sleep. During waking hours, the body is bombarded with stimuli that provoke the senses of sight, hearing, touch, smell, and taste. These stimuli elicit voluntary and involuntary movements or functions. During sleep, a person is no longer aware of the sensory stimuli within his or her immediate environment.

Sleep research involves study of the patterns of sleep, or what is sometimes referred to as sleep architecture. The architecture of sleep consists of two basic elements that occur cyclically: rapid eye movement (REM) sleep and non–rapid eye movement (non-REM) sleep. The normal cyclic progression of the stages of sleep is summarized in Table 12-1. Various sedative-hypnotic drugs affect different stages of the normal sleep pattern. Prolonged sedative-hypnotic use may reduce the cumulative amount of REM sleep; this is known as REM interference. This can result in daytime fatigue, because REM sleep provides a certain component

| TABLE 12-1 | STAGES OF SLEEP | |
|---|---|---|
| **STAGE** | **CHARACTERISTICS** | **AVERAGE PERCENTAGE OF SLEEP TIME IN STAGES (FOR YOUNG ADULT)** |
| **Non-REM Sleep** | | |
| 1 | Dozing or feelings of drifting off to sleep; person can be easily awakened; insomniacs have longer stage 1 periods than normal. | 2%-5% |
| 2 | Relaxation, but person can easily be awakened; person has occasional REMs and also slight eye movements. | 50% |
| 3 | Deep sleep; difficult to wake person; respiratory rates, pulse, and blood pressure may decrease. | 5% |
| 4 | Very difficult to wake person; person may be very groggy if awakened; dreaming occurs, especially about daily events; sleepwalking or bedwetting may occur. | 10%-15% |
| **REM Sleep** | | |
| | REMs occur; vivid dreams occur; breathing may be irregular. | 25%-33% |

Modified from McKenry LM, Tessier E, Hogan MA: *Mosby's pharmacology in nursing*, ed 22, St Louis, 2006, Mosby. *REM*, Rapid eye movement.

of the "restfulness" of sleep. Upon discontinuance of a sedative-hypnotic drug, REM rebound can occur in which the patient has an abnormally large amount of REM sleep, often leading to frequent and vivid dreams. Abuse and misuse of sedative-hypnotic drugs is common and is discussed in Chapter 17.

**PATIENT-CENTERED CARE: CULTURAL IMPLICATIONS**

### Understanding Your Patient's Sleep Needs

- Question the patient of another culture about his or her usual sleep patterns and habits and what is practiced to promote sleep.
- Collect a thorough health, medication, and diet history to identify food and herbal practices used to manage common everyday problems, such as insomnia.
- Asians, Pacific Islanders, Hispanics, and African Americans have a high incidence of lactose intolerance, so use of warm milk at bedtime to help with sleep may lead to GI distress, abdominal cramping, and bloating. Lactose-free milk may be used.
- Some Asian Americans believe in the yin and the yang and may practice meditation, herbology, nutritional interventions, and acupuncture for sleep.
- Chinese patients have been found to require lower doses of benzodiazepines (diazepam [Valium] and alprazolam [Xanax]).
- Some Hispanics believe that maintaining a balance in diet and physical activity are methods for preventing evil or poor health. Nondrug therapies and/or home remedies of vegetables and herbs may be used for sleep and other health issues.
- Jewish Americans may tend to be less accepting of therapeutic touch as compared to some cultures. Nurses must be sensitive to this and find alternatives to massage.

**TABLE 12-2   SEDATIVE-HYPNOTIC BENZODIAZEPINES AND MISCELLANEOUS DRUGS**

| GENERIC NAME | TRADE NAME |
| --- | --- |
| **Long Acting** | |
| clonazepam | Klonopin |
| diazepam | Valium |
| flurazepam | Dalmane |
| **Intermediate Acting** | |
| alprazolam | Xanax |
| lorazepam | Ativan |
| temazepam | Restoril |
| **Short Acting** | |
| eszopiclone* | Lunesta |
| midazolam | Versed |
| ramelteon* | Rozerem |
| triazolam | Halcion |
| zaleplon* | Sonata |
| zolpidem* | Ambien |

*These drugs share many characteristics with the benzodiazepines but are classified as miscellaneous hypnotic drugs.

## PHARMACOLOGY OVERVIEW

### BENZODIAZEPINES AND MISCELLANEOUS HYPNOTIC DRUGS

Historically, benzodiazepines were the most commonly prescribed sedative-hypnotic drugs; however, the nonbenzodiazepine drugs are now more frequently prescribed. Other drugs commonly used for sleep include the antihistamine diphenhydramine (see Chapter 36), trazodone, and amitriptyline (see Chapter 16). The benzodiazepines show favorable adverse effect profiles, efficacy, and safety when used appropriately. Benzodiazepines are classified as either sedative-hypnotics or anxiolytics depending on their primary usage. Anxiolytic drugs are used to reduce the intensity of feelings of anxiety. However, any of these drugs can function along a continuum as a sedative and/or hypnotic and/or anxiolytic depending on the dosage and patient sensitivity. See Chapter 16 for a further discussion of the anxiolytic use of benzodiazepines. There are five benzodiazepines commonly used as sedative-hypnotic drugs. In addition, there are several miscellaneous drugs that are used as hypnotics. They function much like benzodiazepines but are chemically distinct from them. All are listed in Table 12-2. Ramelteon is a hypnotic drug not related to any other hypnotics. It has a new mechanism of action and is profiled separately later in the chapter.

### Mechanism of Action and Drug Effects

The sedative and hypnotic action of benzodiazepines is related to their ability to depress activity in the CNS. The specific areas that are affected include the hypothalamic, thalamic, and limbic systems of the brain. Although the mechanism of action is not certain, research suggests that there are specific receptors in the brain for benzodiazepines. These receptors are thought to be either gamma-aminobutyric acid (GABA) receptors or other adjacent receptors. GABA is the primary inhibitory neurotransmitter of the brain, and it serves to modulate CNS activity by inhibiting overstimulation. Like GABA itself, benzodiazepine activity appears to be related to their ability to inhibit stimulation of the brain. They have many favorable characteristics compared with the older drug class *barbiturates* (see the next section of this chapter). They do not suppress REM sleep to the same extent, nor do they induce hepatic microsomal enzyme activity as do the barbiturates. They are safe to administer to patients who are taking medications metabolized by this enzyme system.

### Indications

Benzodiazepines have a variety of therapeutic applications. They are commonly used for sedation, relief of agitation or anxiety, treatment of anxiety-related depression, sleep induction, skeletal muscle relaxation, and treatment of acute seizure disorders. Benzodiazepines are often combined with anesthetics, analgesics, and neuromuscular blocking drugs in balanced anesthesia and also moderate sedation (see Chapter 11) for their amnesic properties to reduce memory of painful procedures. Finally, benzodiazepine receptors in the CNS are in the same area as those that play a role in alcohol addiction. Therefore, some benzodiazepines (e.g., diazepam, chlordiazepoxide) are used in the treatment and prevention of the symptoms of alcohol withdrawal (see Chapter 17). When benzodiazepines are used to treat insomnia, it is recommended that they be used short term if clinically feasible to avoid dependency. Two newer products that have been approved by the U.S. Food and Drug Administration (FDA) for long-term use for insomnia include eszopiclone (Lunesta) and an extended-release form of zolpidem (Ambien CR). These two drugs are classified as nonbenzodiazepines.

## Contraindications

Contraindications to the use of benzodiazepines include known drug allergy, narrow-angle glaucoma, and pregnancy.

## Adverse Effects

As a class, benzodiazepines have a relatively favorable adverse effect profile; however, they can be harmful if given in excessive doses or when mixed with alcohol. Adverse effects associated with their use usually involve the CNS. Commonly reported undesirable effects are headache, drowsiness, paradoxical excitement or nervousness, dizziness or vertigo, cognitive impairment, and lethargy. Benzodiazepines can create a significant fall hazard in elderly patients, and the lowest effective dose must be used in this patient population. Although these drugs have comparatively less intense effects on the normal sleep cycle, a "hangover" effect is sometimes reported (e.g., daytime sleepiness). Withdrawal symptoms such as rebound insomnia (i.e., greater insomnia than pretreatment) may occur with abrupt discontinuation.

### Toxicity and Management of Overdose

An overdose of benzodiazepines may result in one or all of the following symptoms: somnolence, confusion, coma, and diminished reflexes. Overdose of benzodiazepines alone rarely results in hypotension and respiratory depression. These effects are more commonly seen when benzodiazepines are taken with other CNS depressants such as alcohol or barbiturates. The same holds true for their lethal effects. In the absence of the concurrent ingestion of alcohol or other CNS depressants, benzodiazepine overdose rarely results in death.

Treatment of benzodiazepine intoxication is generally symptomatic and supportive. Flumazenil, a benzodiazepine antidote, can be used to acutely reverse the sedative effects of benzodiazepines. It antagonizes the action of benzodiazepines on the CNS by directly competing with the benzodiazepine for binding at the receptors. Flumazenil is used in cases of oral overdose or excessive intravenous sedation. The dosage regimens to be followed for the reversal of conscious sedation or general anesthesia induced by benzodiazepines and the management of suspected overdose are summarized in Table 12-3.

## Interactions

Potential drug interactions with the benzodiazepines are significant because of their intensity, particularly when they involve other CNS depressants (e.g., alcohol, opioids, muscle relaxants). These drugs result in further CNS depressant effects, including reduced blood pressure, reduced respiratory rate, sedation, confusion, and diminished reflexes. This and other major drug interactions are listed in Table 12-4. Herbal remedies that interact with the benzodiazepines include kava and valerian, which

| TABLE 12-3 | **FLUMAZENIL TREATMENT REGIMEN** | |
|---|---|---|
| **INDICATION** | **RECOMMENDED REGIMEN** | **DURATION** |
| Reversal of moderate sedation or general anesthesia | 0.2 mg (2 mL) IV over 15 sec, then 0.2 mg if consciousness does not occur; may be repeated at 60-sec intervals prn up to 4 additional times (maximum total dose, 1 mg) | 1-4 hr |
| Management of suspected benzodiazepine overdose | 0.2 mg (2 mL) IV over 30 sec; wait 30 sec, then give 0.3 mg (3 mL) over 30 sec if consciousness does not occur; further doses of 0.5 mg (5 mL) can be given over 30 sec at intervals of 1 min up to a cumulative dose of 3 mg | 1-4 hr |

NOTE: Flumazenil has a relatively short half-life and a duration of effect of 1 to 4 hr; therefore, if flumazenil is used to reverse the effects of a long-acting benzodiazepine, the dose of the reversal drug may wear off and the patient may become sedated again, requiring more flumazenil. *IV,* Intravenously.

| TABLE 12-4 | **BENZODIAZEPINES: DRUG/ FOOD INTERACTIONS** | |
|---|---|---|
| **DRUG** | **MECHANISM** | **RESULT** |
| Azole antifungals, verapamil, diltiazem, protease inhibitors, macrolide antibiotics, grapefruit juice | Decreased benzodiazepine metabolism | Prolonged benzodiazepine action |
| CNS depressants | Additive effects | Increased CNS depression |
| olanzapine | Unknown | Increased benzodiazepine effects |
| rifampin | Increased metabolism | Decreased benzodiazepine effects |

*CNS,* Central nervous system; *MAOIs,* monoamine oxidase inhibitors.

may also lead to further CNS depression. Food-drug interactions include interactions with grapefruit and grapefruit juice, which alter drug metabolism via inhibition of the cytochrome P-450 system and can result in prolonged effect, increased effect, and toxicity.

## Dosages

For dosage information, see the table on p. 192.

## DRUG PROFILES

Benzodiazepines and miscellaneous sedative-hypnotic drugs are prescription-only drugs, and they are designated as Schedule IV controlled substances. Uses for benzodiazepines can vary,

**SAFETY: HERBAL THERAPIES AND DIETARY SUPPLEMENTS**

### Kava (Piper methysticum)

**Overview**

Kava consists of the dried rhizomes of *Piper methysticum*. The drug contains kava pyrones (kawain). Extended continuous intake can cause a temporary yellow discoloration of the skin, hair, and nails.

**Common Uses**

Relief of anxiety, stress, restlessness; promotion of sleep

**Adverse Effects**

Skin discoloration, possible accommodative disturbances and pupillary enlargement, scaly skin (with long-term use)

**Potential Drug Interactions**

Alcohol, barbiturates, psychoactive drugs

**Contraindications**

Contraindicated in patients with Parkinson's disease, liver disease, depression, or alcoholism; in those operating heavy machinery; and in pregnant and breastfeeding women

 **SAFETY: HERBAL THERAPIES AND DIETARY SUPPLEMENTS**

### Valerian (Valeriana officinalis)

**Overview**

Valerian root, consisting of fresh underground plant parts, contains essential oil with monoterpenes and sesquiterpenes (valerianic acids).

**Common Uses**

Relief of anxiety, restlessness, sleep disorders

**Adverse Effects**

Central nervous system depression, hepatotoxicity, nausea, vomiting, anorexia, headache, restlessness, insomnia

**Potential Drug Interactions**

Central nervous system depressants, monamine oxidase inhibitors, phenytoin, warfarin; may have enhanced relative and adverse effects when taken with other drugs (including other herbal products) that have known sedative properties (including alcohol)

**Contraindications**

Contraindicated in patients with cardiac disease, liver disease, or those operating heavy machinery

including treatment of insomnia, moderate sedation (see Chapter 11), muscle relaxation, anticonvulsant therapy (see Chapter 14), and anxiety relief (see Chapter 16). The miscellaneous drugs are normally used only for their hypnotic purposes to treat insomnia. Dosage information appears in the Dosages table on this page.

## BENZODIAZEPINES

### diazepam

Diazepam (Valium) was the first clinically available benzodiazepine drug. It has varied uses, including treatment of anxiety,

---

**DOSAGES**

### Selected Benzodiazepine and Other Sedative-Hypnotic Drugs

| DRUG (PREGNANCY CATEGORY) | ONSET AND DURATION | USUAL DOSAGE RANGE | INDICATIONS/ USES |
|---|---|---|---|
| diazepam (Valium) (D) | Long acting | **Adult** PO: 2-10 mg 3-4 times daily IV: 2-10 mg IV (supplied 5 mg/mL) IM: infrequent use | Muscle relaxation, preprocedure sedation, status epilepticus, acute anxiety/ agitation |
| ◆ temazepam (Restoril) (D) | Intermediate acting | **Adult** PO: 7.5-30 mg at bedtime | Sleep induction |
| ◆ zaleplon (Sonata) (C) | Short acting | **Adult** PO: 5-10 mg at bedtime | Sleep induction |
| ◆ zolpidem* (Ambien) (C) | Short acting | **Adult** PO: 5-10 mg at bedtime | Sleep induction |
| eszopiclone* (Lunesta) (C) | Short acting | **Adult** PO: 1-3 mg at bedtime | Sleep induction |
| ramelteon* (Rozerem) (C) | Short acting | **Adult** PO: 8 mg at bedtime | Sleep induction |

*IM*, Intramuscular; *IV*, intravenous; *N/A*, not applicable; *PO*, oral.
*Nonbenzodiazepine drugs.

procedural sedation and anesthesia adjunct, anticonvulsant therapy, and skeletal muscle relaxation following orthopedic injury or surgery. It is available in oral, rectal, and injectable forms.

### Pharmacokinetics

| Route | Onset of Action | Peak Plasma Concentration | Elimination Half-life | Duration of Action |
|---|---|---|---|---|
| IV | Immediate | 8 min | 20-50 hr | 15-60 min |
| PO | 30 min | 1-2 hr | 20-60 hr | 12-24 hr |

### midazolam

Midazolam (Versed) is most commonly used preoperatively and for moderate sedation (see Chapter 11). It is useful for this indication due to its ability to cause amnesia and anxiolysis (reduced anxiety) as well as sedation. This helps patients to feel less anxious about, and avoid remembering, uncomfortable medical procedures. The drug is normally given by injection in adults. However, a liquid oral dosage form is also available for children. See Chapter 11 for dosage information.

### Pharmacokinetics

| Route | Onset of Action | Peak Plasma Concentration | Elimination Half-life | Duration of Action |
|---|---|---|---|---|
| IV | 1-5 minutes | 20-60 minutes | 1-4 hours | 2-6 hours |

#### ◆ temazepam

Temazepam (Restoril), an intermediate-acting benzodiazepine, is actually one of the metabolites of diazepam and normally induces sleep within 20 to 40 minutes. Temazepam has a long onset of action, so it is recommended that patients take it about 1 hour prior to going to bed. Although it is still an effective hypnotic, it has been replaced by the newer drugs.

#### Pharmacokinetics

| Route | Onset of Action | Peak Plasma Concentration | Elimination Half-life | Duration of Action |
|-------|-----------------|---------------------------|-----------------------|--------------------|
| PO | 30-60 min | 2-3 hr | 9.5-12 hr | 7-8 hr |

### NONBENZODIAZEPINES

#### ◆ zaleplon

Zaleplon (Sonata) is a short-acting nonbenzodiazepine hypnotic. A unique advantage of this drug stems from its very short half-life. Patients whose sleep difficulties include early awakenings can take a dose in the middle of the night as long as it is at least 4 hours before they must arise.

#### Pharmacokinetics

| Route | Onset of Action | Peak Plasma Concentration | Elimination Half-life | Duration of Action |
|-------|-----------------|---------------------------|-----------------------|--------------------|
| PO | Rapid | 1 hr | 1 hr | 6-8 hr |

#### ◆ zolpidem

Zolpidem (Ambien) is also a short-acting nonbenzodiazepine hypnotic. Its relatively short half-life and its lack of active metabolites contribute to a lower incidence of daytime sleepiness compared with benzodiazepine hypnotics. A unique dosage form, Ambien CR, is a longer-acting form with two separate drug reservoirs. One releases zolpidem faster than the other to induce hypnosis (sleep) more rapidly. The second reservoir also releases zolpidem but does so more slowly throughout the night to help maintain sleep. One special concern with this particular dosage form is the possibility of *somnambulation* or sleepwalking, which has been reported with its use. Nevertheless, Ambien CR is currently one of only two hypnotics to be FDA-approved for long-term use; the other is eszopiclone (Lunesta; see next profile).

#### Pharmacokinetics

| Route | Onset of Action | Peak Plasma Concentration | Elimination Half-life | Duration of Action |
|-------|-----------------|---------------------------|-----------------------|--------------------|
| PO | 30 min | 1.6 hr | 1.4-4.5 hr | 6-8 hr |

#### eszopiclone

Eszopiclone (Lunesta) is the first hypnotic to be FDA-approved for long-term use. It is designed to provide a full 8 hours of sleep. It is considered a short- to intermediate-acting agent. As with other hypnotics, patients should allot 8 hours of sleep time and should avoid taking hypnotics when they must awaken in less than 6 to 8 hours.

#### Pharmacokinetics

| Route | Onset of Action | Peak Plasma Concentration | Elimination Half-life | Duration of Action |
|-------|-----------------|---------------------------|-----------------------|--------------------|
| PO | 30-60 min | 1 hr | 6 hr | 8 hr |

#### ramelteon

Ramelteon (Rozerem) is the first prescription hypnotic in 35 years with a new mechanism of action. This drug is structurally similar to the hormone melatonin, which is believed to regulate circadian rhythms (day-night sleep cycles) in the body. Over-the-counter dietary supplements containing melatonin have been available for several years. Ramelteon works as an agonist at melatonin receptors in the CNS. Technically it is not a CNS depressant, but it is included here because of its use as a hypnotic. It is also not classified as a controlled substance because of its lack of observed dependency risk. It has a shorter duration of action than other hypnotics and is therefore indicated primarily for patients who have difficulty with sleep *onset* rather than sleep maintenance. Its use is contraindicated in cases of severe liver dysfunction. It is best avoided in patients receiving fluvoxamine (see Chapter 16), fluconazole, or ketoconazole (see Chapter 42), all of which can impede its metabolism. Rifampin (see Chapter 41) can reduce the efficacy of ramelteon by speeding its metabolism via the induction of hepatic enzymes.

#### Pharmacokinetics

| Route | Onset of Action | Peak Plasma Concentration | Elimination Half-life | Duration of Action |
|-------|-----------------|---------------------------|-----------------------|--------------------|
| PO | 30-60 min | 45 min | 1-2.5 hr | 6-8 hr |

## BARBITURATES

Barbiturates were first introduced into clinical use in 1903 and were the standard drugs for treating insomnia and producing sedation. Chemically they are derivatives of barbituric acid. Although 50 different barbiturates are approved for clinical use in the United States, only a few are in clinical use today. This is due to the favorable safety profile and proven efficacy of the benzodiazepines. Barbiturates can produce many unwanted adverse effects. They are physiologically habit forming and have a low therapeutic index (i.e., there is only a narrow dosage range within which the drug is effective, and above that range it is rapidly toxic). Barbiturates can be classified into four groups based on their onset and duration of action. Table 12-5 lists the barbiturates in each category and summarizes their pharmacokinetic characteristics.

### Mechanism of Action and Drug Effects

Barbiturates are CNS depressants that act primarily on the brainstem in an area called the *reticular formation*. Their sedative and hypnotic effects are dose related, and they act by reducing the nerve impulses traveling to the area of the brain called the *cerebral cortex*. Their ability to inhibit nerve impulse transmission is due in part to their ability to potentiate the action of the inhibitory neurotransmitter GABA, which is found in high

| TABLE 12-5 | SEDATIVE-HYPNOTIC BARBITURATES |
| --- | --- |
| **GENERIC NAME** | **TRADE NAME** |
| **Ultrashort Acting** | |
| methohexital | Brevital |
| thiopental | Pentothal |
| **Short Acting** | |
| pentobarbital | Nembutal |
| secobarbital | Seconal |
| **Intermediate Acting** | |
| butabarbital | Butisol |
| **Long Acting** | |
| phenobarbital | Generic |
| mephobarbital | Mebaral |

| TABLE 12-6 | BARBITURATES: ADVERSE EFFECTS |
| --- | --- |
| **BODY SYSTEM** | **ADVERSE EFFECTS** |
| Cardiovascular | Vasodilation and hypotension, especially if given too rapidly |
| Gastrointestinal | Nausea, vomiting, diarrhea, constipation |
| Hematologic | Agranulocytosis, thrombocytopenia |
| Nervous | Drowsiness; lethargy; vertigo |
| Respiratory | Respiratory depression, cough |
| Other | Hypersensitivity reactions: urticaria, angioedema, rash, fever, Stevens-Johnson syndrome |

concentrations in the CNS. Barbiturates also raise the seizure threshold and can be used to treat seizures (see Chapter 14).

## Indications

All barbiturates have the same sedative-hypnotic effects but differ in their potency, time to onset of action, and duration of action. They can be used as hypnotics, sedatives, and anticonvulsants and also for anesthesia during surgical procedures. It is important to note that the use of barbiturates is no longer recommended for sleep induction. The various categories of barbiturates can be used for the following therapeutic purposes: (1) ultrashort acting: anesthesia for short surgical procedures, anesthesia induction, control of convulsions, and reduction of intracranial pressure in neurosurgical patients; (2) short acting: sedation and control of convulsive conditions; (3) intermediate acting: sedation and control of convulsive conditions; and (4) long acting: epileptic seizure prophylaxis.

## Contraindications

Contraindications to barbiturate use include known drug allergy, pregnancy, significant respiratory difficulties, and severe kidney or liver disease. These drugs must be used with caution in elderly patients due to their sedative properties and increased fall risk.

## Adverse Effects

Adverse effects of barbiturates relate to the CNS and include drowsiness, lethargy, dizziness, hangover (prolongation of drowsiness, lethargy, and dizziness), and paradoxical restlessness or excitement. Their long-term effects on normal sleep architecture can be detrimental. Sleep research has shown that adequate rest is obtained from the sleep process only when there are proper amounts of REM sleep, which is sometimes referred to as *dreaming sleep*. Barbiturates deprive people of REM sleep, which can result in agitation and an inability to deal with normal daily stress. When the barbiturate is stopped and REM sleep once again takes place, a rebound phenomenon can occur. During this rebound, the proportion of REM sleep is increased,

dream time constitutes a larger percentage of total sleep, and nightmares often ensue. Common adverse effects of barbiturates are listed in Table 12-6. As is the case with most sedative drugs, barbiturates are also associated with an increased incidence of falls when used in the elderly. If they are recommended for older adults at all, the usual dose is reduced by half whenever possible.

### Toxicity and Management of Overdose

Phenobarbital is also used to treat status epilepticus (prolonged uncontrolled seizures). In extreme cases, patients may be intentionally overdosed to the extent of causing therapeutic phenobarbital or pentobarbital coma. Because of the inhibitory effects on nerve transmission in the brain (possibly GABA mediated), the uncontrollable seizures can be stopped until sufficient serum levels of anticonvulsant drugs are achieved. An overdose of barbiturates produces CNS depression ranging from sleep to profound coma and death. Respiratory depression progresses to Cheyne-Stokes respirations, hypoventilation, and cyanosis. Patients often have cold, clammy skin or are hypothermic, and later they can exhibit fever, areflexia, tachycardia, and hypotension.

Treatment of an overdose is mainly symptomatic and supportive. The mainstays of therapy are maintenance of an adequate airway, assisted ventilation, and oxygen administration if needed, along with fluid and pressor support as indicated. Barbiturates are highly metabolized by the liver, where they also induce enzyme activity. In an overdose, however, the amount of barbiturate may overwhelm the liver's ability to metabolize it. This is a situation in which administration of activated charcoal may be helpful. Activated charcoal adsorbs (binds to) drug molecules in the stomach. It also has the effect of drawing the drug from the circulation into the GI tract for elimination. Multiple-dose (every 4 hours) nasogastric administration of activated charcoal is a common regimen. Phenobarbital and mephobarbital are relatively acidic and can be eliminated more quickly by the kidneys when the urine is alkalized (pH is raised). This keeps the drug in the urine and prevents it from being resorbed back into the circulation. Alkalization, along with forced diuresis using diuretics (e.g., furosemide [see Chapter 28]), can hasten elimination of the barbiturate.

### Interactions

Barbiturates as a class are notorious enzyme inducers. They stimulate the action of enzymes in the liver that are responsible for the metabolism or breakdown of many drugs. By stimulating the action of these enzymes, they cause many drugs to be metabolized more quickly, which usually shortens their duration of action. Other drugs that are enzyme inducers are warfarin, rifampin, and phenytoin.

Additive CNS depression occurs with the coadministration of barbiturates with alcohol, antihistamines, benzodiazepines, opioids, and tranquilizers. Most of the drug-drug interactions are secondary to the effects of barbiturates on the hepatic enzyme system. Barbiturates increase the activity of hepatic microsomal or cytochrome P-450 enzymes (see Chapter 2). This process is called *enzyme induction*. Induction of this enzyme system results in increased drug metabolism and breakdown. However, if two drugs are competing for the same enzyme system, the result can be inhibited drug metabolism and possibly increased toxicity for the wide variety of drugs that are metabolized by these enzymes. Drugs most likely to have marked interactions with the barbiturates include monoamine oxidase inhibitors (MAOIs), tricyclic antidepressants (see Chapter 16), anticoagulants (see Chapter 26), glucocorticoids (see Chapter 30), and oral contraceptives (see Chapter 34) with barbiturates. Coadministration of MAOIs and barbiturates can result in prolonged barbiturate effects. Coadministration of anticoagulants with barbiturates can result in decreased anticoagulation response and possible clot formation. Coadministration of barbiturates with oral contraceptives can result in accelerated metabolism of the contraceptive drug and possible unintended pregnancy. Women taking both types of medication concurrently need to be advised to consider an additional method of contraception as a backup.

## Dosages

Barbiturates can act as either sedatives or hypnotics depending on the dosage. For information on selected barbiturates and their recommended sedative and hypnotic dosages, see the table on this page.

### DOSAGES

#### *Selected Barbiturates*

| DRUG | ONSET AND DURATION | USUAL DOSAGE RANGE | INDICATIONS/USES |
|------|--------------------|--------------------|--------------------|
| pentobarbital (Nembutal) | Short acting | **Pediatric** IM/IV/PO/PR: 2-6 mg/kg/day (max 100 mg) | Anticonvulsant, preoperative sedative, sedative |
|  |  | **Adult** IM: 150-200 mg IV: 100 mg | Preoperative sedative |
| phenobarbital | Long acting | **Pediatric** PO: 6 mg/kg in 3 divided doses | Sedative |
|  |  | IM/IV: 1-3 mg/kg | Preoperative sedative |
|  |  | **Adult** PO: 30-120 mg/day divided | Sedative |
|  |  | IM/IV: 100-200 mg 60-90 min before surgery | Preoperative sedative |

*IM*, Intramuscularly; *IV*, intravenously; *PO*, orally; *PR*, rectally.

### TABLE 12-7 BARBITURATES: CONTROLLED SUBSTANCE SCHEDULE

| SCHEDULE | BARBITURATES |
|----------|--------------|
| C-II | pentobarbital, secobarbital |
| C-III | butabarbital, thiopental |
| C-IV | mephobarbital, methohexital, phenobarbital |

## DRUG PROFILES

Like benzodiazepines, barbiturates can also have varied uses, including preoperative sedation, anesthesia adjunct, and anticonvulsant therapy. All barbiturates are controlled substances, but not all are on the same schedule, as illustrated in Table 12-7. Dosage information appears in the Dosages table for barbiturates.

### pentobarbital

Pentobarbital (Nembutal) is a short-acting barbiturate. Formerly prescribed as a sedative-hypnotic for insomnia, pentobarbital is now principally used preoperatively to relieve anxiety and provide sedation. In addition, it is used occasionally to control status epilepticus or acute seizure episodes resulting from meningitis, poisons, eclampsia, alcohol withdrawal, tetanus, and chorea. Pentobarbital may also be used to treat withdrawal symptoms in patients who are physically dependent on barbiturates or nonbarbiturate hypnotics. It is available in oral, injectable, and rectal dosage forms.

#### Pharmacokinetics

| Route | Onset of Action | Peak Plasma Concentration | Elimination Half-life | Duration of Action |
|-------|-----------------|---------------------------|-----------------------|--------------------|
| PO | 30-60 min | 1-2 hr | 20-45 min | 3-4 hr |

### phenobarbital

Phenobarbital is the most commonly prescribed barbiturate, either alone or in combination with other drugs. It is considered the prototypical barbiturate and is classified as a long-acting drug. Phenobarbital is used for the prevention of generalized tonic-clonic seizures and fever-induced convulsions. In addition, it has been useful in the treatment of hyperbilirubinemia in neonates. It is only rarely used today as a sedative and is no longer recommended to be used as a hypnotic drug. It is available in oral and injectable forms.

#### Pharmacokinetics

| Route | Onset of Action | Peak Plasma Concentration | Elimination Half-life | Duration of Action |
|-------|-----------------|---------------------------|-----------------------|--------------------|
| IV | 5 min | 30 min | 50-120 hr | 6-12 hr |
| PO | 30 min | 1-6 hr | 50-120 hr | 6-12 hr |

### OVER-THE-COUNTER HYPNOTICS

Nonprescription sleeping aids often contain antihistamines (see Chapter 36). These drugs have a CNS depressant effect. The most common antihistamines contained in over-the-counter sleeping aids are doxylamine (Unisom) and diphenhydramine (Sominex). Analgesics (e.g., acetaminophen [see Chapter 10]) are sometimes added to offer some pain relief if pain is a component of the sleep disturbance (e.g., acetaminophen/diphenhydramine [Extra Strength Tylenol PM]). As with other CNS depressants, concurrent use of alcohol can cause respiratory depression or arrest.

## MUSCLE RELAXANTS

A variety of conditions such as trauma, inflammation, anxiety, and pain can be associated with acute muscle spasms. Although there is no perfect therapy available for relief of skeletal muscle spasticity, muscle relaxant drugs are capable of providing some relief. The muscle relaxants are a group of compounds that act predominantly within the CNS to relieve pain associated with skeletal muscle spasms. Most muscle relaxants are known as *centrally acting* skeletal muscle relaxants because their site of action is the CNS. Centrally acting skeletal muscle relaxants are similar in structure and action to other CNS depressants such as diazepam. It is believed that the muscle relaxant effects are related to this CNS depressant activity. Only one of these compounds, dantrolene, acts directly on skeletal muscle. It belongs to a group of relaxants known as direct-acting skeletal muscle relaxants. It closely resembles GABA.

Muscle relaxants are most effective when they are used in conjunction with rest and physical therapy. When taken with alcohol, other CNS depressants, or opioid analgesics, enhanced CNS depressant effects are seen. In such cases, close monitoring and dosage reduction of one or both drugs need to be considered.

### Mechanism of Action and Drug Effects

The majority of the muscle relaxants work within the CNS. Their beneficial effects are believed to come from their sedative effects rather than from direct muscle relaxation. Dantrolene acts directly on the excitation-contraction coupling of muscle fibers and not at the level of the CNS. It directly affects skeletal muscles by decreasing the response of the muscle to stimuli. It appears to exert its action by decreasing the amount of calcium released from storage sites in the sarcoplasmic reticula of muscle fibers. All other muscle relaxants have no direct effects on muscles, nerve conduction, or muscle-nerve junctions and have a depressant effect on the CNS. Their effects are the result of CNS depression in the brain primarily at the level of the brainstem, thalamus, and basal ganglia and also at the spinal cord. The effects of muscle relaxants are relaxation of striated muscles, mild weakness of skeletal muscles, decreased force of muscle contraction, and muscle stiffness. Other effects include generalized CNS depression manifested as sedation, somnolence, ataxia, and respiratory and cardiovascular depression. Baclofen is one of the more effective drugs in this class and is a derivative of GABA. It is believed to work by depressing nerve transmission in the spinal cord. The other drugs in this class are not derivatives of GABA but act by enhancing GABA's central inhibitory effects at the level of the spinal cord.

### Indications

Muscle relaxants are primarily used for the relief of painful musculoskeletal conditions such as muscle spasms, often following injuries such as low back strain. They are most effective when used in conjunction with physical therapy. They may also be used in the management of spasticity associated with severe chronic disorders such as multiple sclerosis and other types of cerebral lesions, cerebral palsy, and rheumatic disorders. Some relaxants are used to reduce choreiform movement in patients with Huntington's chorea, to reduce rigidity in patients with parkinsonian syndrome, or to relieve the pain associated with trigeminal neuralgia. Intravenous dantrolene is used for the management of the hypermetabolic skeletal muscle spasms that accompany the crisis condition known as malignant hyperthermia (see Chapter 11). Baclofen has been shown to be effective in relieving hiccups.

### Contraindications

The only usual contraindication to the use of muscle relaxants is known drug allergy, but contraindications for some drugs may include severe renal impairment.

### Adverse Effects

The primary adverse effects of muscle relaxants are an extension of their effects on the CNS and skeletal muscles. Euphoria, lightheadedness, dizziness, drowsiness, fatigue, confusion, and muscle weakness are often experienced early in treatment. These adverse effects are generally short-lived, as patients grow tolerant to them over time. Less common adverse effects seen with muscle relaxants include diarrhea, GI upset, headache, slurred speech, muscle stiffness, constipation, sexual difficulties in males, hypotension, tachycardia, and weight gain.

### Toxicity and Management of Overdose

The toxicities and consequences of an overdose of muscle relaxants primarily involve the CNS. There is no specific antidote (or reversal drug) for muscle relaxant overdoses. They are best treated with conservative supportive measures. More aggressive therapies are generally needed when muscle relaxants are taken along with other CNS depressant drugs in an overdose. An adequate airway must be maintained, and means of artificial respiration must be readily available. Electrocardiographic monitoring needs to be instituted, and large quantities of intravenous fluids are administered to avoid crystalluria.

### Interactions

When muscle relaxants are administered along with other depressant drugs such as alcohol and benzodiazepines, caution needs to be used to avoid overdosage. Mental confusion, anxiety, tremors, and additive hypoglycemic activity have been reported with this combination as well. A dosage reduction and/or discontinuance of one or both drugs is recommended.

### Dosages

For dosage information for commonly used muscle relaxants, see the table on p. 197.

## DOSAGES

### Selected Muscle Relaxants

| DRUG (PREGNANCY CATEGORY) | PHARMACOLOGIC CLASS | USUAL DOSAGE RANGE | INDICATIONS/USES |
|---|---|---|---|
| ◆ baclofen (Lioresal) (C) | Centrally acting | **Adult**<br>PO: 5 mg three times daily (tid) for 3 days, then 10 mg tid for 3 days, then 20 mg tid, then titrated to response (max: 20 mg po qid) | Spasticity |
| ◆ cyclobenzaprine (Flexeril) (B) | Centrally acting | **Adult**<br>PO: 5-10 mg tid<br>**Adults and adolescents 15 yrs and younger**<br>5 mg PO tid<br>Dosage may be increased to 10 mg po tid if needed | Spasticity |

*PO, Orally.*

## DRUG PROFILES

With the exception of dantrolene (Dantrium), which acts directly on skeletal muscle tissues, muscle relaxants are classified as centrally acting drugs because of their site of action in the CNS. These include baclofen (Lioresal), carisoprodol (Soma), chlorzoxazone (Paraflex), cyclobenzaprine (Flexeril), metaxalone (Skelaxin), methocarbamol (Robaxin), and tizanidine (Zanaflex). Some evidence suggests that carisoprodol has abuse potential; however, it and other muscle relaxants are not controlled substances. Use of all muscle relaxants is contraindicated in patients who have shown a hypersensitivity reaction to them or have compromised pulmonary function, active hepatic disease, or impaired myocardial function. Dosage information appears in the Dosages table for muscle relaxants.

### ◆ baclofen

Baclofen (Lioresal) is available in both oral and injectable dosage forms. The injectable form is for use with an implantable baclofen pump device. This method is sometimes used to treat chronic spastic muscular conditions. With this route, a test dose needs to be administered initially to test for a positive response. The injection is diluted before infusion. Both oral and injectable doses are titrated to desired response.

### Pharmacokinetics

| Route | Onset of Action | Peak Plasma Concentration | Elimination Half-life | Duration of Action |
|---|---|---|---|---|
| PO | 0.5-1 hr | 2-3 hr | 2.5-4 hr | 8 hr or longer |

### ◆ cyclobenzaprine

Cyclobenzaprine (Flexeril) is available in a 5-mg and 10-mg dose and an extended-release formulation (Amrix). Cyclobenzaprine is a centrally acting muscle relaxant that is structurally and pharmacologically related to the tricyclic antidepressants. It is the most commonly used drug in this class to reduce spasms following musculoskeletal injuries. It is very common for patients to exhibit marked sedation from its use.

### Pharmacokinetics

| Route | Onset of Action | Peak Plasma Concentration | Elimination Half-life | Duration of Action |
|---|---|---|---|---|
| PO | 1 hr | 3-8 hr | 8-37 hr | 12-24 hr |

## NURSING PROCESS

## ASSESSMENT

Before administering any *CNS depressant drug,* such as a benzodiazepine, nonbenzodiazepine, miscellaneous drug, muscle relaxant, or barbiturate, perform an assessment focusing on some of the more common parameters and data, including the following: (1) complaints of any insomnia with attention to onset, duration, frequency, and pharmacologic as well as nonpharmacologic measures used; (2) any concerns by the patient or family of sleep disorders, sleep patterns, difficulty in sleeping, or frequent awakenings; (3) the time it takes to fall asleep and the energy level upon awakening; (4) vital signs with attention to blood pressure (both supine and standing measurements); pulse rate and rhythm; respiratory rate, rhythm, and depth; body temperature; and presence of pain; (5) thorough physical assessment/examination for baseline comparisons; (6) neurologic findings with a focus on any changes in mental status, memory, cognitive abilities, alertness, level of orientation (to person, place, and time) or level of sedation, mood changes, depression or other mental disorder, changes in sensations, anxiety, and panic attacks; and (7) miscellaneous information about medical history; allergies; use of alcohol; smoking history; caffeine intake; past and current medication profile, with notation of use of any prescription drugs, over-the-counter drugs, and herbals; alternative or folk practices; and any changes in health status, weight, nutrition, exercise, life stressors (including loss and grief), or lifestyle.

For patients taking *benzodiazepines* or *benzodiazepine-like drugs,* assessment needs to also the identification of disorders or conditions that represent cautions or contraindications to use of these drugs as well as drugs the patient is taking that might interact with benzodiazepines or benzodiazepine-like drugs (see pharmacology discussion). Closely monitor those who are anemic, are suicidal, or have a history of abusing drugs, alcohol, or other substances. Other significant cautions pertain to use of these drugs in the elderly and the very young because of their increased sensitivity to these drugs, as well as in pregnant or lactating women. The elderly and very young may require lower dosages due to potential ataxia and excessive sedation. In addition, before initiating drug therapy with the benzodiazepines and other sedative-hypnotic drugs, including barbiturates, the prescriber may order blood studies such as CBC. Renal function studies (BUN or creatinine levels) and/or hepatic function studies (ALP level) may be ordered to rule out organ impairment and prevent potential toxicity or complications resulting from decreased excretion and/or metabolism. Potential drug interactions for benzodiazepines are presented in Table 12-4. Pay particular attention to the concurrent use of other CNS depressants (e.g., opioids), because this may lead to severe decreases in blood pressure, respiratory rate, reflexes, and level of consciousness.

With the *nonbenzodiazepines* such as zaleplon and zolpidem tartrate, include a head-to-toe physical assessment and a thorough medication history with measurement of vital signs and other parameters previously mentioned. Assess and document for allergies to these drugs and to aspirin. If the patient is allergic to aspirin, there is an associated risk of allergies to nonbenzodiazepines. Other considerations include the need for assessment of any confusion and lightheadedness, especially in the elderly because of their increased sensitivity. Do not use zaleplon and eszopiclone in those younger than 18 years of age, and use extreme caution if there is a history of compromised respiratory status or drug, alcohol, or other substance abuse. Drug interactions include other CNS depressants.

For *muscle relaxants,* always note drug allergies before use, and perform a complete head-to-toe assessment with focus on the neurologic system. In the elderly, there is increased risk of CNS toxicity with possible hallucinations, confusion, and excessive sedation. Assessment includes taking a thorough health/medication history and examining the complete patient profile with results of associated laboratory studies. See pharmacology discussion about cautions, contraindications, and drug interactions.

The *miscellaneous* drug ramelteon is a newer medication that is used for insomnia but is not associated with CNS depression, does not carry the potential for abuse or dependence, and does not lead to withdrawal symptoms when treatment stops. Therefore, this drug can be used for patients who are likely to be abusers of CNS depressants. Include inquiry into sleep patterns and habits in your assessment. Because this drug is not to be used in patients with liver impairment, liver function studies are needed prior to beginning the medication. Perform respiratory assessment and assessment of other vital signs as well. If the patient has a history of respiratory disorders such as chronic obstructive pulmonary disease or sleep apnea, or if the patient is a child, this medication would not be indicated.

*Barbiturates* are discussed further in Chapter 14 along with other antiepileptic drugs. However, a brief description is needed to emphasize the importance of conducting a thorough patient assessment as well as evaluating for cautions, contraindications, and drug interactions. Barbiturates are not to be used by pregnant or lactating women. These drugs cross the placenta and breast-blood barriers, posing the risk of respiratory depression in the fetus and neonate. Withdrawal symptoms may appear in neonates born to women who have taken barbiturates during their last trimester of pregnancy. Barbiturates may also produce paradoxical excitement in children and confusion and mental depression in the elderly, so baseline neurologic assessment is needed. Assessment of renal and liver function is also important in those with compromised organ function and in the elderly to help avoid toxicity.

## NURSING DIAGNOSES

1. Impaired gas exchange related to the respiratory depression associated with CNS depressants
2. Deficient knowledge related to inadequate information about the various CNS drugs and their first-time use
3. Disturbed sleep patterns related to the drug's interference with REM sleep
4. Risk for injury and falls related to adverse effect of decreased sensorium
5. Risk for injury related to possible drug overdose or adverse reactions related to drug-drug interactions (e.g., combined use of the drug with alcohol, tranquilizers, and/or analgesics) and decreased level of alertness and an unsteady gait
6. Risk for injury and addiction related to physical or psychological dependence on CNS drugs

## PLANNING

### GOALS

1. Patient maintains normal gas exchange and is free of respiratory depression.
2. Patient demonstrates adequate knowledge about the drugs, how they work, and their adverse effects and interactions.
3. Patient remains free of further disturbed sleep patterns.
4. Patient remains free of self-injury and falls due to safety measures for decreased sensorium.
5. Patient remains free of injury due to adequate information about drug interactions that lead to further CNS depression.
6. Patient remains free of injury to self with no drug dependence.

### OUTCOME CRITERIA

1. Patient states measures to maintain normal gas exchange such as coughing, deep breathing, taking only the prescribed amount of medication, and reporting any difficulty breathing to prescriber.
2. Patient demonstrates adequate knowledge about the medication(s) used including sedating/hypnotic properties, CNS depressant effects, and side effects of altered respirations, decreased depth/rate of respirations, altered cough, confusion, drowsiness, and interactions with other CNS depressants.

3. Patient states risk for REM interference from sedative-hypnotic drugs with associated sleep interference with most of these drugs as well as known hangover effects.
   - Patient states importance of trying nonpharmacologic measures for enhancing sleep as appropriate prior to drug therapy, such as massage, relaxation therapy, music, biofeedback.
4. Patient demonstrates understanding of safety measures to decrease risk of injury/falls while taking sedative/hypnotics, such as taking medication only as prescribed, removing all throw rugs from walking areas (especially at night), moving and changing positions slowly, ambulating with caution, and reporting any excessive drowsiness or sedation to prescriber.
5. Patient ably states common drug interactions associated with and to avoid with sedative/hypnotics, (i.e., other CNS depressants, opioids, herbals [kava, valerian], alcohol, and sedating products found over the counter [diphenhydramine]).
6. Patient remains free of risk of drug dependence issues through appropriate use of sedative/hypnotics, taking medication only as prescribed, reporting any problems with increased resistance to drug's effects, as well as excessive sedation and the feeling that more medication is needed to get the same drug effect.
   - Patient tries nonpharmacologic measures to promote sleep, as needed.

## IMPLEMENTATION

Patients taking *benzodiazepines* and other CNS depressants experience sedation and possible ataxia, thus the need for patient safety measures. Hospital or facility policies mandate the type of safety precautions to be taken, such as the use of side rails or bed alarms. Ambulation needs to occur safely and with assistance when patients are sedated or are experiencing the adverse effects of these drugs. In addition, dependence may be a problem with the benzodiazepines, but not to the same degree as with the barbiturates. While taking these drugs, patients need to avoid driving or participating in any activities that require mental alertness. It is recommended that these drugs be taken on an empty stomach for faster onset of action; however, this often results in GI upset so, practically speaking, they need to be taken with food, a light snack, or meals. Orally administered benzodiazepines have an onset of action of 30 minutes to 6 hours depending on the drug (see the Pharmacokinetics tables in the Drug Profiles section), and the appropriate timing and intervals of dosing will be determined by these characteristics. For example, if a patient takes a benzodiazepine or other CNS drug to induce sleep and the drug's onset of action is 30 to 60 minutes, then the drug needs to be dosed 60 minutes prior to bedtime. In addition, it is crucial to patient compliance and safety to understand that drug tolerance may develop to many of these drugs, and so the patient may require larger dosages to produce the same therapeutic effect at some point. Interrupting therapy helps to decrease drug tolerance.

Among the benzodiazepines, REM interference is less problematic with flurazepam, quazepam, and estazolam, primarily because they produce fewer active metabolites. Educate patients about the REM interference and rebound insomnia that may occur with just a 3- to 4-week regimen of drug therapy. To minimize REM interference, benzodiazepines and other drugs are only used when nonpharmacologic methods fail and must be used with caution in all patients with sleep disorders and for short periods of time. Zolpidem is also available in a sustained-release product used for long-term management of sleep disorders. Gradual weaning-off periods are recommended for benzodiazepines and all CNS depressants. Hangover effects are also associated with many of the CNS depressants but occur less frequently with benzodiazepines and nonbenzodiazepines than with barbiturates.

It is recommended that *nonbenzodiazepines* (e.g., zaleplon) be taken for the prescribed time. Take zaleplon as directed and immediately before bedtime due to its quick onset of action. Avoid consumption of very heavy and/or high-fat meals within 2 hours of taking this drug because of interference with the drug's action. Zolpidem has optimal absorption if taken at bedtime on an empty stomach with no crushing, chewing, or breaking of the oral dosage form. This drug may infrequently lead to temporary memory loss. To help avoid this adverse effect, it is important to encourage the patient to not take a dose of the drug without a full night's sleep (e.g., at least 7 to 8 hours) the previous night. As with any CNS depressant drug, avoid tasks requiring mental alertness until response to the drug is known. Tolerance and dependence are possible with prolonged use, and this drug is to be gradually weaned before discontinuation.

*Muscle relaxants* have different indications than the barbiturates and benzodiazepines and are not used to treat insomnia. They are generally indicated for some forms of spasticity (see Pharmacology Overview). However, when used they may lead to adverse effects and toxicities, so frequently monitor airway, breathing, and circulation. Early identification of toxicity is critical to provide prompt treatment and to prevent respiratory and other CNS depressant effects. Closely monitor all vital parameters, level of consciousness, and presence of sedation when these muscle relaxants are used. Encourage cautious ambulation. Recommend that the patient change positions purposefully and slowly to prevent syncope or dizziness. The greatest risk for hypotension associated with these drugs is usually within 1 hour of dosing, so the patient must be more cautious about activity during this time.

The *miscellaneous* drug ramelteon must be used with caution, with emphasis on the fact that the drug is not to be mixed with alcohol. In the patient education, include that the drug is to be taken 30 minutes before bedtime and is *not* to be taken along with or immediately following a high-fat meal.

*Barbiturates* are to be used with very close monitoring and extreme caution. Observe and document the patient's level of consciousness or sedation; orientation to person, place, and time; respiratory rate; oxygen saturation; and other vital signs. Advise the patient to take oral doses with food or a light snack, and not to alter dosage forms. Use a bed alarm system or side rails and provide assistance with ambulation, as needed or indicated, to help prevent injury. Barbiturates also produce a hangover effect, and this residual drowsiness occurs upon awakening and results in impaired reaction times. The intermediate- and long-acting hypnotics are often the culprits for this adverse effect. Abrupt withdrawal of barbiturates after prolonged therapy may produce adverse effects ranging from nightmares, hallucinations, and delirium to seizures. In addition, while the patient is taking barbiturates, monitor the patient's red blood cell count and hemoglobin and hematocrit levels because of the possible adverse effect of anemia. Long-term use of barbiturates also requires monitoring of therapeutic blood levels of the drug. For example, the therapeutic level of phenobarbital must range between 10 and 40 mcg/mL. Patients with serum levels above 40 mcg/mL may experience toxicity manifested by cold and clammy skin, respiratory rate of less than 10 breaths/min, and other signs of severe CNS depression.

Intravenous use of barbiturates, as with some benzodiazepines (e.g., diazepam), requires dilution of the drug with normal saline or other recommended solutions. Recommendations regarding diluents and rates of intravenous administration must be strictly followed for safe use. Most of the drugs are not to be given any faster than 1 mg/kg per minute, and a maximum amount per minute may be specified. Consult authoritative drug sources (e.g., a current drug handbook/reference or the manufacturer's insert) for the recommended rate of infusion before giving any of these drugs. Too rapid an infusion of a barbiturate may produce profound hypotension and marked respiratory depression. If intravenous infiltration is present, the site may become swollen, erythematous, and tender. Tissue necrosis may occur with this infiltration, depending on the irritating qualities of the particular drug. There are antidote protocols for some of the intravenous barbiturates. For example, with phenobarbital intravenous infiltration, the solution must be discontinued, a 0.5% procaine solution injected into the affected area, and moist heat applied, as per institutional policy or procedure. Always check protocol for management of infiltration of an intravenous drug before intervening because, in certain situations, the intravenous catheter may be left in place until antidotes are administered. Another area of concern with intravenous drugs is incompatibilities with other intravenously administered medications, and barbiturates have several. Some intravenous drugs that are incompatible with barbiturates include amphotericin B, hydrocortisone, and hydromorphone. Only give these particular drugs after the intravenous line has been adequately flushed with normal saline. With intramuscular injection, give the solution deep into a large muscle mass to prevent tissue sloughing; however, avoid this route and use only when absolutely necessary.

In summary, before giving any CNS depressant, it is always important to try nonpharmacologic measures to induce sleep.

However, if medication therapy is indicated, preventing respiratory depression and other problems associated with CNS depression is of prime importance, as is maintaining patient safety and preventing injury. Documentation must be timely, clear, and concise and reflect follow-up of the patient's response to the drug. It is also important to document the dose, route, time of administration, and safety measures taken after each dose is given.

## CASE STUDY

### *Drugs for Sleep*

 P.S., a 68-year-old retired secretary, comes to the office complaining of feeling "so tired" during the day. She has had trouble sleeping off and on for years, and a few weeks ago received a prescription for the benzodiazepine alprazolam (Xanax) to take "as needed for nerves." Upon closer questioning, the nurse discovers that P.S. has been using alprazolam almost every night for 3 weeks to help her get to sleep. She says, "I just could not fall asleep before! I am sleeping very well, but I'm so tired during the day. I don't understand how I can get such good sleep and still feel tired!"

1. Can you explain the reason for her tiredness?
2. P.S.'s nurse practitioner prescribes a period of decreasing doses of the alprazolam each evening, then every other evening, until the medication is stopped. Explain the rationale behind the tapering dosage schedule.
3. P.S. receives a prescription for ramelteon (Rozerem). How is this drug different from alprazolam?
4. What nonpharmacologic measures can P.S. try to improve her sleep?

For answers, see http://evolve.elsevier.com/Lilley.

## EVALUATION

Some of the criteria by which to confirm a patient's therapeutic response to a *CNS depressant* include the following: an increased ability to sleep at night, fewer awakenings, shorter sleep induction time, few adverse effects such as hangover effects, and an improved sense of well-being because of improved sleep. Therapeutic effects related to *muscle relaxants* include decreased spasticity, reduction of choreiform movements in Huntington's chorea, decreased rigidity in parkinsonian syndrome, and relief of pain from trigeminal neuralgia. Constantly watch for and document the occurrence of any of the adverse effects of benzodiazepines, barbiturates, and muscle relaxants. See the previous discussions of adverse effects for each type of drug. Evaluation for CNS depressant toxic effects includes monitoring for severe CNS depression of all body systems, especially respiratory and circulatory collapse, with decrease in respiratory rate/depth and decrease in blood pressure.

## PATIENT TEACHING TIPS

- Encourage individuals to keep a journal recording sleep habits, sleep patterns, and response to both drug and nondrug therapy (Box 12-1).
- Implement nonpharmacologic measures first to enhance sleep. This is important because the use of CNS depressants for treatment of sleep deficit or insomnia often leads to interference with the REM stage of sleep, hangover effects, and/or tolerance, as well as other adverse effects.
- Always check with the prescriber or pharmacist before taking any over-the-counter medications because of the many drug interactions with CNS depressants.
- Keep these drugs and all medications out of the reach of children.
- Emphasize that medications are to be taken only as prescribed. The patient is usually told that if one dose does not work, not to double up on the dosage unless otherwise prescribed or directed.
- Educate about any time constraints related to driving, operation of heavy machinery or equipment, and participation in activities requiring mental alertness while the patient is taking these medications.

- Do not abruptly discontinue or withdraw these medications, if possible, to avoid rebound insomnia.
- Sedative-hypnotic drugs (for sleep promotion) are not intended for long-term use because of their adverse effects, interference with REM sleep, and addictive properties.
- Advise the patient that hangover effects may occur with most of these drugs and that this is more problematic in the elderly or in patients with altered renal and hepatic function.
- Provide the patient with thorough instructions about safety with these drugs, such as avoiding smoking in bed or when lounging.
- Teach the patient about significant drug/drug and drug/food interactions with all these medications.
- Educate patients about the effect of grapefruit and grapefruit juice on benzodiazepines. The grapefruit results in decreased drug metabolism via inhibition of the cytochrome P-450 system and may lead to a prolonged effect and possible toxicity (of the benzodiazepine).

## BOX 12-1   SLEEP DIARIES AND NONPHARMACOLOGIC TREATMENT OF SLEEP DISORDERS

### Information for a Sleep Diary

- What time do you usually go to bed and wake up?
- How long and how well do you sleep?
- When were you awake during the night, and for how long?
- How easy was it to go to sleep?
- How easy was it to wake up in the morning?
- How much caffeine or alcohol do you consume?
- What time did you last eat or drink (if after dinner)?
- Did you have any bedtime snacks?
- What emotions or stressors are present?
- What medications do you take daily?
- Do you smoke? If so, how much and for how long?
- Do you consume alcohol? If so, how much and for how long?
- Do you take any over-the-counter drugs? If so, what drug and for what reason? How much and for how long?
- Do you take any herbals? If so, which ones? For what and for how long?

### Nonpharmacologic Sleep Interventions

- Establish a set sleep pattern with a time to go to bed at night and a regular time to get up in the morning, and stick to it. This will help to reset your internal clock.
- Sleep only as much as you need to feel refreshed and renewed. Too much sleep may lead to fragmented sleep patterns and shallow sleep.

- Keep bedroom temperatures moderate, if possible.
- Avoid caffeine-containing beverages and food within 6 hours of bedtime.
- Decrease exposure to loud noises.
- Avoid daytime napping.
- Avoid exercise late in the evening (i.e., not past 7 PM).
- Avoid alcohol in the evening. Rather than putting you to sleep, it actually results in fragmented sleep.
- Avoid tobacco at bedtime, because it disturbs sleep.
- Try to relax before bedtime with soft music, yoga, relaxation therapy, deep breathing, or light reading on a topic that is not intense or anxiety provoking.
- Drink a warm decaffeinated beverage, such as warm milk or chamomile tea, 30 minutes to 1 hour before bedtime.
- If you are still awake 20 minutes after going to bed, get up and engage in a relaxing activity (as noted previously) and go back to bed once you feel drowsy. Repeat as necessary.

## KEY POINTS

- Nonpharmacologic measures to improve sleep need to be tried before resorting to treatment with medications.
- Recognize and understand the classification and pharmacokinetic properties of barbiturates. Short-acting barbiturates include pentobarbital and secobarbital. Intermediate-acting barbiturates include butabarbital. Long-acting barbiturates include phenobarbital and mephobarbital.
- The pharmacokinetics of each group of barbiturates lends specific characteristics to the drugs in that group. You need to understand how these drugs are absorbed orally and used parenterally, as well as their onset time, time until peak effect, and duration of action. You must understand the life-threatening potential of these drugs because too rapid an infusion may precipitate respiratory and/or cardiac arrest.

- Benzodiazepines are commonly used for sedation, relief of anxiety, skeletal muscle relaxation, and treatment of acute seizure disorders.
- Most sedative-hypnotic drugs suppress REM sleep and should be used only for the recommended period of time. This time frame varies, depending on the specific drug used.
- Long-acting benzodiazepines include clonazepam, diazepam, and flurazepam. Intermediate-acting benzodiazepines include alprazolam, lorazepam, and temazepam. Short-acting benzodiazepines include eszopiclone, midazolam, ramelteon, triazolam, zaleplon, and zolpidem.

## NCLEX® EXAMINATION REVIEW QUESTIONS

1 A patient has been admitted to the emergency department because of an overdose of an oral benzodiazepine. He is very drowsy but still responsive. The nurse will prepare for which immediate intervention?
   a Hemodialysis to remove the medication
   b Administration of flumazenil
   c Administration of naloxone
   d Intubation and mechanical ventilation

2 An older adult has been given a benzodiazepine for sleep induction, but the night nurse noted that the patient was awake most of the night, watching television and reading in bed. The nurse documents that the patient has had which type of reaction to the medication?
   a Allergic
   b Teratogenic
   c Paradoxical
   d Idiopathic

3 The nurse is preparing to administer a medication for sleep. Which intervention applies to the administration of a non-benzodiazepine, such as zaleplon (Sonata)?
   a These drugs need to be taken about 1 hour before bedtime.
   b Because of their rapid onset, these drugs need to be taken just before bedtime.
   c The patient needs to be cautioned about the high incidence of morning drowsiness that may occur after taking these drugs.
   d These drugs are less likely to interact with alcohol.

4 The nurse will monitor the patient who is taking a muscle relaxant for which adverse effect?
   a CNS depression
   b Hypertension
   c Peripheral edema
   d Blurred vision

5 A hospitalized patient is complaining of having difficulty sleeping. Which action will the nurse take first to address this problem?
   a Administer a sedative-hypnotic drug if ordered.
   b Offer tea made with the herbal preparation valerian.
   c Encourage the patient to exercise by walking up and down the halls a few times if tolerated.
   d Provide an environment that is restful, and reduce loud noises.

6 Which considerations are important for the nurse to remember when administering a benzodiazepine as a sedative-hypnotic drug? (Select all that apply.)
   a These drugs are intended for long-term management of insomnia.
   b The drugs can be administered safely with other CNS depressants for insomnia.
   c The dose needs to be given about 1 hour before the patient's bedtime.
   d The drug is used as a first choice for treatment of sleeplessness.
   e The patient needs to be evaluated for the drowsiness that may occur the morning after a benzodiazepine is taken.

7 A child is to receive phenobarbital 2 mg/kg IV on call as a preoperative sedative. The child weighs 64 pounds. How many milligrams will the child receive for this dose?

1. b, 2. c, 3. b, 4. a, 5. d, 6. c, e, 7. 58.2 mg

For Critical Thinking and Prioritization Questions, see http://evolve.elsevier.com/Lilley.

# Central Nervous System Stimulants and Related Drugs

## evolve WEBSITE

*http://evolve.elsevier.com/Lilley*

- Animations
- Answer Key—Textbook Case Studies
- Critical Thinking and Prioritization Questions

- Key Points—Downloadable
- Review Questions for the NCLEX® Examination
- Unfolding Case Studies

## OBJECTIVES

When you reach the end of this chapter, you will be able to do the following:

1 Briefly review the anatomy, physiology, and functions of the central nervous system with attention to the stimulant effects on its function.
2 Review the key terms as they relate to the central nervous system and stimulant drugs.
3 Identify the various central nervous system stimulant drugs.

4 Discuss the mechanisms of action, indications, dosages, routes of administration, contraindications, cautions, drug interactions, adverse effects, and any related toxicity for the various central nervous system stimulants and related drugs.
5 Develop a nursing care plan based on the nursing process for patients using central nervous system stimulants and related drugs.

## DRUG PROFILES

♦ **amphetamines, p. 207**
  **atomoxetine, p. 208**
♦ **caffeine, p. 212**
  **doxapram, p. 213**
♦ **methylphenidate, p. 207**

  **modafinil, p. 208**
  **orlistat, p. 209**
♦ **phentermine, p. 209**
♦ **sumatriptan, p. 211**

_____

♦ *Key drug*

## KEY TERMS

**Amphetamines** A class of stimulant drugs that includes amphetamine sulfate and all of its drug derivatives. (p. 206)

**Analeptics** Central nervous system (CNS) stimulants that have generalized effects on the brainstem and spinal cord, which produce an increase in responsiveness to external stimuli and stimulate respiration. (p. 212)

**Anorexiants** Drugs used to control or suppress appetite. (p. 208)

**Attention deficit hyperactivity disorder (ADHD)** A syndrome characterized by difficulty in maintaining concentration on a given task and/or hyperactive behavior; may affect children,

adolescents, and adults. The term *attention deficit disorder (ADD)* has been absorbed under this broader term. (p. 205)

**Cataplexy** A condition characterized by abrupt attacks of muscular weakness and hypotonia triggered by an emotional stimulus such as joy, laughter, anger, fear, or surprise. It is often associated with narcolepsy. (p. 205)

**Central nervous system (CNS) stimulants** Drugs that stimulate specific areas of the brain or spinal cord. (p. 204)

**Ergot alkaloids** Drugs that narrow or constrict blood vessels in the brain and provide relief of pain for certain migraine headaches. (p. 209)

**Migraine** A common type of recurring painful headache characterized by a pulsatile or throbbing quality, incapacitating pain, and photophobia. (p. 205)

**Narcolepsy** A syndrome characterized by sudden sleep attacks, *cataplexy*, sleep paralysis, and visual or auditory hallucinations at the onset of sleep. (p. 205)

**Serotonin receptor agonists** A class of CNS stimulants used to treat migraine headaches; they work by stimulating 5-hydroxytryptamine 1 receptors in the brain and are sometimes referred to as *selective serotonin receptor agonists* or *triptans.* (p. 209)

**Sympathomimetic drugs** CNS stimulants such as noradrenergic drugs (and, to a lesser degree, dopaminergic drugs) whose actions resemble or mimic those of the sympathetic nervous system. (p. 204)

## ANATOMY, PHYSIOLOGY, AND PATHOPHYSIOLOGY OVERVIEW

The central nervous system (CNS) is a very complex system in the human body. Many therapeutic drugs either work in the CNS or cause adverse effects in the CNS. Activity of the CNS is regulated by a checks-and-balances system that consists of excitatory and inhibitory neurotransmitters and their corresponding receptors in the brain and spinal cord tissues. CNS stimulation results from either excessive stimulation of excitatory neurons or blockade of inhibitory neurons. Central nervous system (CNS) stimulants are a broad class of drugs that stimulate specific areas of the brain or spinal cord. Most CNS stimulant drugs act by stimulating the excitatory neurons in the brain. These neurons contain receptors for excitatory neurotransmitters, including dopamine (dopaminergic drugs), norepinephrine (adrenergic drugs), and serotonin (serotonergic drugs). Dopamine is a metabolic precursor of norepinephrine, which is also a neurotransmitter in the sympathetic nervous system. Actions of adrenergic drugs often resemble or mimic the actions of the sympathetic nervous system. For this reason, adrenergic drugs (and, to a lesser degree, dopaminergic drugs as well) are also called sympathomimetic drugs. Other sympathomimetic drugs are discussed further in Chapter 18.

CNS stimulant drugs are classified in three ways. The first is on the basis of chemical structural similarities. Major chemical classes of CNS stimulants include amphetamines, serotonin agonists, sympathomimetics, and xanthines (Table 13-1). Second, these drugs can be classified according to their site of therapeutic action in the CNS (Table 13-2). Finally, they can be categorized according to five major therapeutic usage categories for CNS stimulant drugs (Table 13-3). These include anti–attention deficit, antinarcoleptic, anorexiant, antimigraine, and analeptic drugs. Anorexiants are drugs used to control obesity by suppression of appetite. Analeptics are drugs used for specific CNS stimulation in certain clinical situations. Some therapeutic overlap exists among these drug categories.

| TABLE 13-2 | CNS STIMULANTS: SITE OF ACTION |
| --- | --- |
| **PRIMARY SITE OF ACTION** | **CNS STIMULANTS** |
| Cerebrovascular system, 5-HT$_{1D/1B}$ receptors | Serotonin agonists |
| Cerebral cortex | Amphetamines, phenidates, modafinil, armodafinil |
| Hypothalamic and limbic regions | Anorexiants |
| Medulla and brainstem | Analeptics |

*CNS,* Central nervous system.

| TABLE 13-1 | STRUCTURALLY RELATED CNS STIMULANTS |
| --- | --- |
| **CHEMICAL CATEGORY** | **CNS STIMULANTS AND RELATED DRUGS** |
| Amphetamines and related stimulants | dextroamphetamine, methamphetamine, benzphetamine, methylphenidate, dexmethylphenidate, |
| Serotonin agonists | almotriptan, eletriptan, frovatriptan, naratriptan, rizatriptan, sumatriptan, zolmitriptan |
| Sympathomimetics | phentermine, phendimetrazine |
| Xanthines | caffeine, theophylline, aminophylline |
| Miscellaneous | modafinil, armodafinil, orlistat (lipase inhibitor), doxapram (analeptic) |

*CNS,* Central nervous system.

| TABLE 13-3 | CNS STIMULANTS AND RELATED DRUGS: THERAPEUTIC CATEGORIES |
| --- | --- |
| **CATEGORY** | **DRUGS** |
| Anti-ADHD | dextroamphetamine, lisdexamfetamine, methamphetamine, methylphenidate, atomoxetine (norepinephrine reuptake inhibitor) |
| Antinarcoleptic | dextroamphetamine, methamphetamine, methylphenidate, modafinil, armodafinil |
| Anorexiant | methamphetamine, phentermine, phendimetrazine, diethylpropion, benzphetamine, orlistat (lipase inhibitor) |
| Antimigraine | almotriptan, eletriptan, frovatriptan, naratriptan, rizatriptan, sumatriptan, zolmitriptan (serotonin agonists); dihydroergotamine mesylate, ergot-amine tartrate with caffeine (ergot alkaloids) |
| Analeptic | caffeine, doxapram, aminophylline, theophylline, modafinil, armodanafil (antinarcoleptic) |

*ADHD,* Attention deficit hyperactivity disorder; *CNS,* central nervous system.

# ATTENTION DEFICIT HYPERACTIVITY DISORDER

Attention deficit hyperactivity disorder (ADHD), formerly known as *attention deficit disorder (ADD)*, is the most common psychiatric disorder in children, affecting 3% to 10% of school-age children. Boys are affected from two to nine times more often than girls, although the disorder may be underdiagnosed in girls. Primary symptoms of ADHD are a developmentally inappropriate ability to maintain attention span and/or the presence of hyperactivity and impulsivity. The disorder may involve predominantly attention deficit, predominantly hyperactivity or impulsivity, or a combination of both. It usually begins before 7 years of age, sometimes earlier than 4 years of age. It can officially be diagnosed when symptoms last at least 6 months and occur in at least two different settings (e.g., home and school), according to the *Diagnostic and Statistical Manual of Mental Disorders.* Many children outgrow ADHD, but adult ADHD is also common. Drug therapy for both childhood and adult ADHD is essentially the same. There is some social controversy regarding possible overdiagnosis of, and overmedication for this disorder. Studies in twins indicate a degree of genetic predisposition and familial heritability. The disorder is commonly associated with other forms of mental illness, including depression, bipolar disorder, anxiety, and learning difficulties.

# NARCOLEPSY

Narcolepsy is an incurable neurologic condition in which patients unexpectedly fall asleep in the middle of normal daily activities. These "sleep attacks" are reported to cause car accidents or near-misses in 70% or more of patients. Another major symptom of the disease is dysfunctional *rapid eye movement sleep* (see Chapter 12). Cataplexy is an associated symptom in at least 70% of narcolepsy cases. It involves sudden acute skeletal muscle weakness. The condition is often associated with strong emotions (e.g., joy, anger), and commonly the knees buckle and the individual falls to the floor while still awake. Men and women are equally affected, with approximately 100,000 cases in the United States. Some genetic markers have been identified. Roughly half of patients with narcolepsy experience migraine headaches as well.

# OBESITY

According to the National Institutes of Health and the Centers for Disease Control and Prevention, approximately 30% of Americans are obese and nearly two thirds (64.5%) are overweight. This translates into more than 72 million obese adults, with a higher incidence of obesity among women and minorities. Obesity was formerly defined as being 20% or more above one's ideal body weight based on population statistics for height, body frame, and gender. More recent data are based on a measurement known as the body mass index (BMI), defined as weight in kilograms divided by height in meters squared (i.e., $BMI = weight [kg] \div [height (m)]^2$). *Overweight* is now defined as a BMI of 25 to 29.9, whereas *obesity* is now defined as a BMI

of 30 or higher. At any given time, one third of women and one quarter of men are trying to lose weight. Moreover, the incidence of obesity in young people 6 to 19 years of age has more than tripled since 1980. The pathophysiology of obesity is not fully understood, but calorie excess, disordered metabolism, and other factors are hypothesized. Obesity increases the risk for hypertension, dyslipidemia, coronary artery disease, stroke, type 2 diabetes mellitus, gallbladder disease, gout, osteoarthritis, sleep apnea, and certain types of cancer, including breast and colon cancer. An estimated 80% of diabetes risk in the United States can be attributed to excess weight. Some 112,000 deaths each year are linked to obesity. The related health care costs alone are currently estimated at more than $140 billion. Yet many people who attempt weight loss do so for cosmetic reasons rather than health reasons. Obese people are often stigmatized, at times even by the health care professionals treating them.

# MIGRAINE

A migraine is a common type of recurring headache, usually lasting from 4 to 72 hours. Typical features include a pulsatile quality with pain that worsens with each pulse. The pain is most commonly unilateral but may occur on both sides of the head. Associated symptoms include nausea, vomiting, *photophobia* (avoidance of light), and *phonophobia* (avoidance of sounds). In addition, some migraines are accompanied by an *aura,* which is a predictive set of altered visual or other senses (formerly termed *classic migraine*). However, the majority of migraines are without an aura (formerly termed *common migraine*). Migraines affect about 30 million people in the United States, with a reported incidence in females roughly three times that in males. Migraine headaches have been classified by the World Health Organization as one of the 19 most disabling diseases worldwide, with approximately 64 to 150 million workdays lost annually. Migraines commonly begin after 10 years of age and peak between the mid-twenties and early forties. They often fade after 50 years of age. Familial inheritance of migraine is well recognized. Precipitating factors include stress, hypoglycemia, menses, endogenous estrogen (including oral contraceptives), exercise, and intake of alcohol, caffeine, cocaine, nitroglycerin, aspartame, and the food additive monosodium glutamate (MSG). Over 50% of patients with narcolepsy report nocturnal migraines. Historically, there have been several theories regarding the cause of migraines, including the "vascular hypothesis" and the "neurovascular hypothesis." Most recent evidence points to decreased serotonin levels. Thus, the majority of current investigations involve drugs that can increase the serotonin levels.

# ANALEPTIC-RESPONSIVE RESPIRATORY DEPRESSION SYNDROMES

*Neonatal apnea,* or periodic cessation of breathing in newborn babies, is a common condition seen in neonatal intensive care units. It occurs in about 25% of premature infants whose pulmonary and CNS structures, including the medullary centers that control breathing, have not completed their gestational development because of preterm birth. Infants undergoing prolonged mechanical ventilation, especially at high pressures, often develop a chronic lung disease known as *bronchopulmonary dysplasia,* for which caffeine can be helpful. *Postanesthetic respiratory depression* occurs when a patient's spontaneous respiratory drive does not resume adequately and in a timely manner after general anesthesia. Respiratory depression may also be secondary to abuse of some drugs. Hypercapnia, or elevated blood levels of carbon dioxide, is often associated with later stages of chronic obstructive pulmonary disease (COPD). Analeptic drugs such as theophylline, aminophylline, caffeine, and doxapram may be used to treat one or more of these conditions. Analeptic drugs are now used much less frequently than they were in the earlier days of general anesthesia. This is because of advances in intensive respiratory care, including mechanical ventilation and improved anesthetic techniques, as well as the availability of newer medications with less toxicity.

## PHARMACOLOGY OVERVIEW

## DRUGS FOR ATTENTION DEFICIT HYPERACTIVITY DISORDER AND NARCOLEPSY

CNS stimulants are the first-line drugs of choice for both ADHD and narcolepsy. They are potent drugs with a strong potential for tolerance and psychological dependence (addiction; see Chapter 17). They are classified as Schedule II drugs under the Controlled Substance Act. Although there has been some public controversy regarding their use in ADHD, these drugs have led to a 65% to 75% improvement in symptoms in treated patients compared with a placebo. In general, CNS stimulants elevate mood, produce a sense of increased energy and alertness, decrease appetite, and enhance task performance impaired by fatigue or boredom. Two of the oldest known stimulants are cocaine and amphetamine, which are prototypical drugs for this class. Caffeine, contained in coffee and tea, is another plant-derived CNS stimulant.

Amphetamine sulfate was first synthesized in the late 1800s. It was subsequently used to treat narcolepsy and then to prolong the alertness of soldiers during World War II. Later derivatives of this drug, which are still used clinically, include its d-isomer dextroamphetamine sulfate, methamphetamine hydrochloride, benzphetamine, and mixed amphetamine salts—salts of both amphetamine and dextroamphetamine. They are often collectively referred to simply as amphetamines. Methylphenidate, a synthetic amphetamine derivative, was first introduced for the treatment of hyperactivity in children in 1958. Its d-isomer is the drug dexmethylphenidate. The phenidates are also Schedule II drugs. All of these amphetamine-related drugs are used to treat ADHD and/or narcolepsy. Nonamphetamine stimulants include pemoline and modafinil. In 2005, pemoline was taken off the market because of reports of liver failure associated with its use.

Atomoxetine is a nonstimulant drug that is also used to treat ADHD. Atomoxetine is a norepinephrine reuptake inhibitor. Because it is not an amphetamine, it is associated with a low incidence of insomnia and has low abuse potential. Another advantage is that phone-in refills are allowed for this drug (as opposed to Schedule CII drugs, which require a written prescription). One of the newest drugs in the ADHD arsenal is lisdexamfetamine (Vyvanse). It is a prodrug for dextroamphetamine, meaning it is converted in the body to dextroamphetamine.

## Mechanism of Action and Drug Effects

Amphetamines stimulate areas of the brain associated with mental alertness, such as the cerebral cortex and the thalamus. Pharmacologic actions of CNS stimulants are similar to the actions of the sympathetic nervous system in that the CNS and respiratory systems are the primary systems affected. CNS effects include mood elevation or euphoria, increased mental alertness and capacity for work, decreased fatigue and drowsiness, and prolonged wakefulness. The respiratory effects most commonly seen are relaxation of bronchial smooth muscle, increased respiration, and dilation of pulmonary arteries.

The amphetamines and phenidates increase the effects of norepinephrine and dopamine in CNS synapses by increasing their release and blocking their reuptake. As a result, both neurotransmitters are in contact with their receptors longer, which lengthens their duration of action. Modafinil is also classified as an analeptic. It promotes wakefulness like the amphetamines and phenidates. It lacks sympathomimetic properties, however, and appears to work primarily by reducing gamma-aminobutyric acid (GABA)–mediated neurotransmission in the brain. GABA is the principal inhibitory neurotransmitter in the brain. The nonstimulant drug atomoxetine is also being used to treat ADHD. It works in the CNS by selective inhibition of norepinephrine reuptake.

## Indications

Various amphetamine derivatives, including methylphenidate, are currently used to treat both ADHD and narcolepsy. Dexmethylphenidate is currently indicated for ADHD alone. Amphetamine sulfate was also used to treat obesity in the early to mid twentieth century. However, the only amphetamines currently approved for this indication are benzphetamine and methamphetamine (see Anorexiants). The nonamphetamine stimulant modafinil is indicated for narcolepsy.

Specialists sometimes recommend periodic "drug holidays" (e.g., 1 day per week) without medication to diminish the addictive tendencies of the stimulant drugs. School-age children often do not take these drugs on weekends and school vacations.

## Contraindications

Contraindications to the use of amphetamine and nonamphetamine stimulants include known drug allergy or cardiac structural abnormalities. These drugs can also exacerbate the following conditions: marked anxiety or agitation, Tourette's syndrome and other tic disorders (hyperstimulation), hypertension, and glaucoma (can increase intraocular pressure; see Chapter 57). The drugs must not be used in patients who have received therapy with any monoamine oxidase inhibitor (MAOI) in the preceding 14 days (see Chapter 16). Contraindications specific to atomoxetine include drug allergy, glaucoma, and recent MAOI use.

## TABLE 13-4 CNS STIMULANTS: COMMON DRUG INTERACTIONS

| DRUG | INTERACTING DRUGS | MECHANISM | RESULT |
|---|---|---|---|
| **Amphetamine and Nonamphetamine Stimulants** | | | |
| Amphetamines (various salts) methylphenidate | CNS stimulants | Additive toxicities | Cardiovascular adverse effects, nervousness, insomnia |
| | MAOIs | Increased release of catecholamines | Headaches, dysrhythmias, severe hypertension |
| **Atomoxetine** | Sympathomimetic drugs | Enhanced SNS effects | Cardiovascular adverse effects (dysrhythmias, tachycardia, hypertension) |
| | CYP2D6 inhibitors (MAOIs, paroxetine) | Reduced metabolism of atomoxetine | Enhanced atomoxetine toxicity |
| **Anorexiants and Analeptics** | | | |
| phentermine | CNS stimulants | Additive toxicities | Nervousness, insomnia, dysrhythmias, seizures |
| | MAOIs | Increased release of catecholamines | Headaches, dysrhythmias, severe hypertension |
| | Serotonergic drugs | Additive toxicity | Cardiovascular adverse effects, nervousness, insomnia, convulsions |
| **Serotonin Agonists** | | | |
| sumatriptan and others | Ergot alkaloids, SSRIs, MAOIs | Additive toxicity | Cardiovascular adverse effects, nervousness, insomnia, convulsions |
| **Ergot Alkaloids** | | | |
| D.H.E.45, Caffergot | Protease inhibitors, azole antifungals, macrolide antibiotics | Increased ergot levels | Acute ergot toxicity; nausea, vomiting, hypotension or hypertension, seizures, coma, death; use with ergot alkaloids is contraindicated |

*CNS,* Central nervous system; *CYP2D6,* cytochrome P-450 enzyme 2D6; *MAOIs,* monoamine oxidase inhibitors; *SNS,* sympathetic nervous system; *SSRIs,* selective serotonin reuptake inhibitors.

## Adverse Effects

Both amphetamine and nonamphetamine stimulants have a wide range of adverse effects that most often arise when these drugs are administered at high doses. These drugs tend to "speed up" body systems. For example, effects on the cardiovascular system include increased heart rate and blood pressure. Other adverse effects include angina, anxiety, insomnia, headache, tremor, blurred vision, increased metabolic rate (beneficial in treatment of obesity), gastrointestinal (GI) distress, dry mouth, and worsening of or new onset of psychiatric disorders, including mania, psychoses, or aggression. Common adverse effects associated with atomoxetine include headache, abdominal pain, vomiting, anorexia, and cough.

## Interactions

Drug interactions associated with these drugs vary greatly from class to class. Table 13-4 summarizes some of the more common interactions for all drug classes in this chapter.

## Dosages

For dosage information, see the table on p. 211.

## DRUG PROFILES

### AMPHETAMINES AND RELATED STIMULANTS

The principal drugs used to treat ADHD and narcolepsy are amphetamines and nonamphetamine stimulants. Atomoxetine, a nonstimulant drug, is also used for ADHD.

### ◆ amphetamines

The various amphetamine salts are the prototypical CNS stimulants used to treat ADHD and narcolepsy. Amphetamine is available in prescription form only for oral use, both as single-component dextroamphetamine sulfate (Dexedrine) and as a mixture of dextroamphetamine sulfate, dextroamphetamine saccharate, amphetamine sulfate, and amphetamine aspartate (Adderall).

### Pharmacokinetics (dextroamphetamine)

| Route | Onset of Action | Peak Plasma Concentration | Elimination Half-life | Duration of Action |
|---|---|---|---|---|
| PO | 30-60 min | 90-120 min | 7-14 hr | 10 hr |

### ◆ methylphenidate

Methylphenidate (Ritalin) was the first prescription drug indicated for ADHD and continues to be the most widely prescribed drug for the treatment of ADHD and is also used for narcolepsy. Extended-release dosage forms include Ritalin SR, Concerta, and Metadate CD. There is some controversy regarding drug therapy for ADHD. Some parents may be understandably apprehensive regarding this type of drug therapy. However, with proper diagnosis of the disorder, proper dosing of the drug, and regular medical monitoring, many children can achieve significant improvement in school performance and social skills. Psychosocial problems within a child's family need to be ruled out or addressed if they are contributing to the child's problems, regardless of whether the medication is prescribed.

### Pharmacokinetics (immediate release)

| Route | Onset of Action | Peak Plasma Concentration | Elimination Half-life | Duration of Action |
|---|---|---|---|---|
| PO | 30-60 min | 6-8 hr | 1-3 hr | 4-6 hr |

### atomoxetine

Atomoxetine (Strattera) is approved for treating ADHD in children older than 6 years of age and in adults. This medication is not a controlled substance because it lacks addictive properties, unlike amphetamines and phenidates. For this reason, it has rapidly gained popularity as a therapeutic option for treating ADHD. In September 2005, however, the FDA issued a warning describing cases of suicidal thinking and behavior in small numbers of adolescent patients receiving this medication, similar to its previous warnings regarding adolescent use of antidepressant medications (see Chapter 16). Prescribers are advised to work with parents in providing prudent monitoring of any young patients taking this medication and to promptly reevaluate patients showing any behavioral symptoms of concern.

### Pharmacokinetics

| Route | Onset of Action | Peak Plasma Concentration | Elimination Half-life | Duration of Action |
|---|---|---|---|---|
| PO | 60 min | 1-2 hr | 5-24 hr | 24-120 hr |

### modafinil

Modafinil (Provigil) is indicated for improvement of wakefulness in patients with excessive daytime sleepiness associated with narcolepsy and also with *shift work sleep disorder.* It has less abuse potential than amphetamines and methylphenidate and is a Schedule IV drug. A related drug is armodafinil (Nuvigil), which is similar to modafinil.

### Pharmacokinetics

| Route | Onset of Action | Peak Plasma Concentration | Elimination Half-life | Duration of Action |
|---|---|---|---|---|
| PO | 1-2 months* | 2-4 hr | 8-15 hr | Unknown |

*Therapeutic effects.

## ANOREXIANTS

By definition, an *anorexiant* is any substance that suppresses appetite. Anorexiants are CNS stimulant drugs used to promote weight loss in obesity; however, their effectiveness has not been proved. These drugs include phentermine (Ionamin), benzphetamine (Didrex), methamphetamine (Desoxyn), and diethylpropion (Tenuate). In 2010, sibutramine (Meridia) was withdrawn from the market due to safety concerns. Benzphetamine and methamphetamine are the

only amphetamines currently approved for treating obesity. Orlistat (Xenical) is a related nonstimulant drug used to treat obesity. It works locally in the small and large intestines where it inhibits absorption of caloric intake from fatty foods.

## Mechanism of Action and Drug Effects

Anorexiants are CNS stimulants that are believed to work by suppressing appetite control centers in the brain. Some evidence suggests that they also increase the body's basal metabolic rate, including mobilization of adipose tissue stores and enhanced cellular glucose uptake, as well as reduce dietary fat absorption.

There are some minor differences between these drugs in terms of their individual actions. Phentermine, diethylpropion, methamphetamine, and benzphetamine resemble amphetamine sulfate in their chemical structures and CNS effects. These drugs are classified as both anorexiants and adrenergic (sympathomimetic) drugs. However, all appear to suppress appetite centers in the CNS through dopamine- and norepinephrine-mediated pathways.

Orlistat differs from other antiobesity drugs in that it is not a CNS stimulant. It works by inhibiting the enzyme lipase. This results in reduced absorption of dietary fat from the intestinal tract and increased fat elimination in the feces.

## Indications

Anorexiants are used for the treatment of obesity. However, their effects are often minimal without accompanying behavioral modifications involving diet and exercise. Current evidence-based guidelines for the treatment of obesity do not support the use of anorexiants as monotherapy. They are most commonly used in higher-risk patients. These include obese patients with a BMI of 30 or higher, or patients with a BMI of 27 who are also hypertensive or have high cholesterol or diabetes.

## Contraindications

Contraindications to anorexiants include drug allergy, any severe cardiovascular disease, uncontrolled hypertension, hyperthyroidism, glaucoma, mental agitation, history of drug abuse, eating disorders (e.g., anorexia, bulimia), and use of MAOIs (see Chapter 16) within the previous 14 days. Orlistat is contraindicated in cases of chronic malabsorption syndrome (e.g. Crohn's disease, colitis, short bowel syndrome) or cholestasis.

## Adverse Effects

With the exception of diethylpropion, anorexiants may raise blood pressure and cause heart palpitations and even dysrhythmias at higher dosages. Ironically, at therapeutic dosages, they may actually reflexively slow the heart rate. Diethylpropion, however, has little cardiovascular activity. These drugs may also cause anxiety, agitation, dizziness, and headache. The most common adverse effects of orlistat include headache, upper respiratory tract infection (mechanism uncertain), and GI distress, including fecal incontinence and oily stools.

## Interactions

See Table 13-4.

## Dosages

For dosage information, see the table on p. 211.

## DRUG PROFILES

Amphetamine salts are no longer used for treatment of obesity because of their high abuse potential. The nonstimulant drug orlistat, a lipase inhibitor, is available over the counter.

### ◆ phentermine

Phentermine (Ionamin) is a sympathomimetic anorexiant that is structurally related to amphetamines but with much lower abuse potential. It is classified as a Schedule IV drug. This drug is not to be confused with several other drugs that were recalled by the FDA in the late 1990s (fenfluramine/dexfenfluramine [Phen-Fen]) and in 2000 (phenylpropanolamine) because of case reports of various adverse cardiovascular and/or pulmonary effects.

### orlistat

Orlistat (Xenical) is unrelated to other drugs in its category. Alli is an over-the-counter (OTC) version released in 2007. It works by binding to gastric and pancreatic enzymes called *lipases*. Blocking these enzymes reduces fat absorption by roughly 30%. Restricting dietary intake of fat to less than 30% of total calories

can help reduce some of the GI adverse effects, which include oily spotting, flatulence, and fecal incontinence in 20% to 40% of patients. Decreases in serum concentrations of vitamins A, D, and E and beta carotene are seen as a result of the blocking of fat absorption. Supplementation with fat-soluble vitamins corrects this deficiency.

### Pharmacokinetics

| Route | Onset of Action | Peak Plasma Concentration | Elimination Half-life | Duration of Action |
|-------|-----------------|---------------------------|-----------------------|---------------------|
| PO | 3 mo* | 6-8 hr | 1-2 hr | Unknown |

*Therapeutic effects.

## ANTIMIGRAINE DRUGS

Serotonin receptor agonists, first introduced in the 1990s, have revolutionized the treatment of migraine headache. They work by stimulating serotonin receptors in the brain. They include sumatriptan (Imitrex), almotriptan (Axert), eletriptan (Relpax), naratriptan (Amerge), rizatriptan (Maxalt), zolmitriptan (Zomig), and frovatriptan (Frova). Collectively, these drugs are referred to as *triptans*. They are to be used cautiously in patients with severe cardiovascular disease (especially angina pectoris). Historically, ergot alkaloids were the mainstay of treatment of migraine headaches but have been replaced by the triptans for first-line therapy. The ergot alkaloids are obtained from a fungus and cause vasoconstriction of dilated blood vessels in the brain and of the carotid arteries. They are contraindicated in patients with peripheral vascular disease, coronary artery disease, sepsis, impaired renal or hepatic function, and severe hypertension.

## Mechanism of Action and Drug Effects

The chemical name for serotonin is 5-hydroxytryptamine, or 5-HT. Physiologists have further identified two 5-HT receptor subtypes on which these drugs have their greatest effect: $5\text{-HT}_{1B}$ and $5\text{-HT}_{1D}$. Triptans stimulate these receptors in cerebral arteries, causing vasoconstriction and normally reducing or eliminating headache symptoms. They also reduce the production of inflammatory neuropeptides. This is known as *abortive* drug therapy because it treats a headache that has already started. Ergot alkaloids also narrow or constrict blood vessels in the brain. Although the cause of migraines is not fully understood, they are thought to be related to abnormal dilation of the blood vessels within the brain.

## Indications

The triptan antimigraine drugs, also referred to as *selective serotonin receptor agonists (SSRAs)*, are indicated for abortive therapy of an acute migraine headache. Although they may be taken during aura symptoms in patients who have auras with their headaches, these drugs are not indicated for *preventive* migraine therapy. Preventive therapy is indicated if migraine attacks occur one or more days per week. A variety of drugs are used for preventive therapy; most of them are discussed in more detail in other chapters. First-line drugs for preventive therapy include propranolol (see Chapter 19), amitriptyline (see Chapter 16), valproic acid, and topiramate (see Chapter 15). Second-line therapies include the ergot alkaloid dihydroergotamine mesylate (D.H.E. 45); nonsteroidal antiinflammatory drugs, including naproxen (see Chapter 44), calcium channel blockers, and angiotensin receptor blockers (see Chapter 22). In many cases, preventive drug therapy is sufficient to prevent a full-blown migraine. However, when prevention fails, treatment is needed and the triptans are the most commonly prescribed drug class. Another frequently used product as abortive therapy is a combination of acetaminophen or aspirin plus the barbiturate butalbital plus the analeptic caffeine, with or without codeine (Fioricet). In addition to potentiating the effects of the analgesics, caffeine can also enhance intestinal absorption of the ergot alkaloids and has a vasoconstricting effect, which can reduce cerebral blood flow to ease headache pain. Caffeine also has a diuretic effect, which may ultimately also reduce cerebral blood flow owing to reduced vascular volume secondary to enhanced urinary output.

## Contraindications

Contraindications to triptans include drug allergy and the presence of serious cardiovascular disease, because of the vasoconstrictive potential of these medications. Contraindications to the use of ergot alkaloids include uncontrolled hypertension; cerebral, cardiac, or peripheral vascular disease; dysrhythmias; glaucoma; and coronary or ischemic heart disease.

## Adverse Effects

Triptans have potential vasoconstrictor effects, including effects on the coronary circulation. Injectable dosage forms may cause local irritation at the site of injection. Other adverse effects include feelings of tingling, flushing (skin warmth and redness), and a congested feeling in the head or chest. Ergot alkaloids are associated with the adverse effects of nausea, vomiting, cold or clammy hands and feet, muscle pain, dizziness, numbness, a vague feeling of anxiety, a bitter or foul taste in the mouth or throat, and irritation of the nose (with the nasal spray dosage form). Overuse of abortive therapy may result in rebound headaches.

---

## EVIDENCE-BASED PRACTICE

### Ibuprofen May Help Relieve Acute Migraine Headaches

**Review**

Migraine headache is a common, disabling condition that has a major impact on the individual, health care services, and society. Many migraine sufferers do not seek proper medical attention and often rely on the use of over-the-counter (OTC) analgesics/medications. The goal of this review of literature was to assess the effectiveness and tolerability of ibuprofen on migraine headaches in adults. Additionally, this review is to assess ibuprofen when given as monotherapy or together with an antiemetic as compared to placebo treatment or other drug treatment for the relief of acute migraines in adults.

**Type of Evidence**

The investigators searched the databases of Cochrane CENTRAL, MEDLINE, EMBASE and the Oxford Pain Relief Database. These sources were used to identify studies published through April 2010 about ibuprofen and migraines. Criteria used to determine inclusion included randomized, double-blind trials of self-given ibuprofen versus active comparators to treat a migraine episode with outcome data for at least 10 participants per treatment group. Once data were collected, two independent investigators performed a methodological trial from which nine studies comparing ibuprofen and placebo or other active drugs were identified. Over 4300 participants were studied for a total of over 5220 migraine attacks. Of these studies, none were representative of the protocol of using ibuprofen and an antiemetic. Single doses of medications were used to treat all the attacks. Relative risk and number needed to treat (NNT) or harm versus placebo or other active drug were calculated from the participants.

**Results of Study**

When comparing ibuprofen 400 mg with use of the placebo, the numbers needed to treat (NNTs) were 7.2 for 2 hours pain-free (26% versus 12%), 3.2 for 2 hours of headache relief (57% versus 25%), and 4.0 for 24-hour sustained headache relief (45% versus 19%). Ibuprofen 200 mg versus the placebo showed that the NNTs were 9.7 for 2 hours pain-free (20% versus 10%) and 6.3 for 2 hours of

headache relief (52% versus 37%). The ibuprofen dose of 400 mg offered significantly better 2-hour headache relief than the 200-mg dose, and the soluble dosage forms of ibuprofen offered better 1 hour relief but not the 2-hour headache relief as compared to standard tablet dosage forms. Another set of symptoms that were looked at were those of nausea, vomiting, photophobia, phonophobia, and functional disability. These symptoms were reduced within 2 hours with the ibuprofen versus placebo. Additionally, fewer participants used rescue medication. Side effects were mostly mild and temporary and occurred similarly in participants across treatment groups. The major limitation of this review includes weaknesses inherent in the reviewed studies as well as the fact that a small number of events were used to calculate some of the results.

**Link of Evidence to Nursing Practice**

Over 30 million people in the United States suffer from migraines with significant impacts on quality of life. Migraine management remains a huge challenge for health care professionals and has a subsequent negative impact on health care costs. Migraines have been classified as one of the 19 most disabling diseases worldwide. Therefore, adequate management or treatment is crucial to patient quality of life and to helping trim the costs of health care. Ibuprofen has been identified as an effective treatment for acute migraine headaches leading to pain relief in about 50% of sufferers but only complete relief from pain (and other symptoms) in a minority of participants. This review is just one example of the need for more effective, larger sample-sized studies. Additionally, there is the need for further studies on migraines and looking at a variety of outcomes for pain relief, types of management, and multisymptom management. Dosage formulations and their advantages and effectiveness also need to be studied. Nurse researchers need to continue to take the lead in identifying patient problems as well as helping to identify a variety of medical, holistic and alternative approaches to their short and long-term treatment.

Reference: Rabbie R, Derry S, Moore RA, et al: Ibuprofen with or without an antiemetic for acute migraine headaches in adults, *Cochrane Database Syst Rev* 10:CD008039, 2010.

## Interactions

See Table 13-4.

## Dosages

For dosage information, see the table on this page.

## DRUG PROFILES

### SEROTONIN RECEPTOR AGONISTS

Serotonin receptor agonists are used to treat migraine headache. They can produce relief from moderate to severe migraines within 2 hours in 70% to 80% of patients. They work by stimulating 5-HT$_1$ receptors in the brain and are sometimes referred to as *SSRAs* or *triptans*. They are available in a variety of formulations, including oral tablets, sublingual tablets, subcutaneous self-injections, and nasal sprays. A common effect of migraines is nausea and vomiting. Orally administered medications are therefore not tolerated by some patients. Non-oral (including sublingual) forms are advantageous for this reason. They also often have a more rapid onset of action, producing relief in some patients in 10 to 15 minutes, compared with 1 to 2 hours for tablets taken orally. For dosage information, see the table on this page.

### ◆ sumatriptan

Sumatriptan (Imitrex) was the original prototype drug for this class. As noted earlier, there are now seven triptans. Slight pharmacokinetic differences exist between some of these products, but their effects are comparable overall.

#### Pharmacokinetics

| Route | Onset of Action | Peak Plasma Concentration | Elimination Half-life | Duration of Action |
|---|---|---|---|---|
| PO | 0.5-1 hr | 2.5 hr | 2.5 hr | 4 hr |

## DOSAGES

### *Selected CNS Stimulants and Related Drugs*

| DRUG (PREGNANCY CATEGORY) | PHARMACOLOGIC CLASS | USUAL DOSAGE RANGE | INDICATIONS/USES |
|---|---|---|---|
| ◆ amphetamine/dextroamphetamine (Adderall) (C) | CNS stimulant | **Pediatric 3-5 yr**<br>PO: 2.5 mg/day, increased weekly until desired effect<br>**Pediatric 6 yr and older and Adult**<br>PO: 5 mg once or twice daily, increased weekly until desired effect to a daily max of 40 mg | ADHD, narcolepsy |
| atomoxetine (Strattera) (C) | Selective norepinephrine reuptake inhibitor | **Pediatric (less than 70 kg)**<br>PO: 0.5-1.2 mg/kg/day divided once or twice daily<br>**Adult** (70 kg or more)<br>PO: 40-100 mg/day divided once or twice daily | ADHD |
| ◆ caffeine (B) | Xanthine cerebral stimulant | **Adult**<br>PO: 300-400 mg<br>IV: 500 mg<br>**Premature infants**<br>IV (caffeine citrate only): 20 mg/kg load followed by 5 mg/kg once daily | Treatment of spinal headache<br><br>Neonatal apnea, bronchopulmonary dysplasia |
| doxapram (Dopram) (B) | Respiratory stimulant (analeptic) | **Adult, pediatric older than 12 yr**<br>IV: 0.5-1 mg/kg, may repeat up to 2 mg/kg<br>Infusion of 1-2 mg/min for up to 2 hr | Drug-induced respiratory depression<br>COPD-associated hypercapnia |
| ◆ methylphenidate, extended release (Concerta) (C) | CNS stimulant | **Pediatric and adult**<br>18-72 mg/day in a single dose | ADHD, narcolepsy |
| ◆ methylphenidate (Ritalin) (C) | CNS stimulant | **Pediatric 6 yr and older**<br>PO: 5 mg bid before breakfast and lunch and increased weekly until desired effect to max of 60 mg/day<br>**Adult**<br>PO: 20-60 mg/day divided bid-tid | ADHD, narcolepsy |
| ◆ methylphenidate, extended release (Ritalin-SR) (C) | CNS stimulant | **Pediatric and adult**<br>20-60 mg/day in a single dose | ADHD, narcolepsy |
| modafinil (Provigil) (C) | CNS stimulant | **Adult**<br>PO: 200 mg q AM; if second dose needed, give at noon | Narcolepsy |
| orlistat (Xenical, Alli) (B) | Lipase inhibitor | **Adult**<br>PO: 120 mg tid with each meal containing fat | Obesity |
| ◆ sumatriptan (Imitrex) (C) | Serotonin receptor agonist | **Adult**<br>PO: 25, 50, or 100 mg, can repeat after 2 hr (max 200 mg/day)<br>Subcut: 4-6 mg, can repeat in 1 hr (max 2 injections/day)<br>Nasal spray: 5, 10, or 20 mg, can repeat after 2 hr (max 40 mg/day) | Acute migraine with or without aura |

*ADHD*, Attention deficit hyperactivity disorder; *CNS*, central nervous system; *COPD*, chronic obstructive pulmonary disease; *IM*, intramuscular; *IV*, intravenous; *PO*, oral; *subcut*, subcutaneous.

## ERGOT ALKALOIDS

Ergot alkaloids, such as ergotamine, are still used in treatment and prevention of migraines but are rapidly being replaced by the triptans. Dihydroergotamine mesylate (D.H.E. 45) is available in injectable form and as a nasal spray (Migranal). Ergotamine tartrate with caffeine (Cafergot) is available in tablet form.

## DRUGS FOR SPECIFIC RESPIRATORY DEPRESSION SYNDROMES: ANALEPTICS

Analeptics include doxapram (Dopram) and the methylxanthines aminophylline, theophylline, and caffeine. These drugs are sometimes used to treat neonatal and postoperative respiratory depression. Neonatal uses are more common. Postoperative respiratory depression is a less common problem today due to the design of newer anesthetic drugs with shorter durations of action.

## Mechanism of Action and Drug Effects

Analeptics work by stimulating areas of the CNS that control respiration, mainly the medulla and spinal cord. Methylxanthine analeptics (caffeine, aminophylline, and theophylline) also inhibit the enzyme *phosphodiesterase*. This enzyme breaks down a substance called *cyclic adenosine monophosphate (cAMP)*. When analeptics block this enzyme, cAMP accumulates. This results in relaxation of smooth muscle in the respiratory tract, dilation of pulmonary arterioles, and stimulation of the CNS in general. Aminophylline is a *prodrug* (a drug that is formulated for greater solubility to facilitate administration but must be metabolized to an active form); it is *hydrolyzed* to theophylline in the body. Theophylline, in turn, is metabolized to caffeine. Caffeine is inherently a stronger CNS stimulant, hence its popularity in coffee, tea, and soft drinks. It also helps to potentiate the effects of analgesics used for migraine therapy and has a diuretic effect. The stimulant effects of caffeine are attributed to its antagonism (blocking) of adenosine receptors in the brain. Adenosine is associated with sleep promotion. The mechanism of action of doxapram is similar to that of the methylxanthines, but it has a greater stimulant effect in the area of the brain that senses carbon dioxide content. When the carbon dioxide content of the blood is high, the respiratory center in the brain is stimulated to induce deeper and faster breathing in an attempt to exchange more carbon dioxide for inhaled oxygen.

## Indications

Currently listed indications for analeptics include neonatal apnea, bronchopulmonary dysplasia, hypercapnia associated with COPD, postanesthetic respiratory depression, and respiratory depression secondary to drugs of abuse (e.g., opioids, alcohol, or barbiturates). In newborns, administration of caffeine is associated with less tachycardia, CNS stimulation, and feeding intolerance than administration of theophylline or aminophylline. The latter are also used to treat neonatal bradycardia and are infrequently used to treat asthma in older children and adults.

## Contraindications

Contraindications to the use of analeptics include drug allergy, peptic ulcer disease (especially for caffeine), and serious cardiovascular conditions. Concurrent use of other phosphodiesterase-inhibiting drugs such as sildenafil and similar drugs is also not recommended.

Doxapram use is contraindicated in newborns because of the benzyl alcohol contained in the injectable formulation of the drug. Benzyl alcohol is associated with *gasping syndrome* in infants and may also displace bilirubin into the blood from albumin binding sites in the circulation. This, in turn, could cause or worsen hyperbilirubinemia, a common condition in high-risk infants.

Its use is also contraindicated in patients with epilepsy or other convulsive disorders, those who have shown a hypersensitivity reaction to it, those showing evidence of head injury, those suffering from cardiovascular impairment or severe hypertension, and patients who have experienced a stroke.

## Adverse Effects

At higher dosages, analeptics stimulate the vagal, vasomotor, and respiratory centers of the medulla in the brainstem, as well as increasing blood flow to skeletal muscles. Vagal effects include stimulation of gastric secretions, diarrhea, and reflex tachycardia. Vasomotor effects include flushing (warmth, redness) and sweating of the skin. Respiratory effects include elevated respiratory rate (which is normally desired). Skeletal muscle effects include muscular tension and tremors. Neurologic effects include reduced deep tendon reflexes.

## Interactions

See Table 13-4.

## Dosages

For dosage information, see the table on p. 211.

## DRUG PROFILES

Analeptic drugs include doxapram (Dopram), aminophylline, theophylline, and caffeine. The profiles for aminophylline and theophylline can be found in Chapter 37. The antinarcoleptic analeptic drug modafinil was discussed earlier in the narcolepsy section of this chapter. For dosage information, see the table on p. 211.

◆ **caffeine**

Caffeine is a CNS stimulant that can be found in OTC drugs (e.g., NoDoz) and combination prescription drugs (e.g., Fioricet, Fiorinal). It is also contained in many beverages and foods. A few of the many foods and drugs that contain caffeine are listed in Table 13-5. Caffeine is contraindicated in patients with a known hypersensitivity to it and is used with caution in patients who have a history of peptic ulcers or cardiac dysrhythmias or who have recently experienced a myocardial infarction. Caffeine is available in oral and injectable dosage forms.

### Pharmacokinetics

| Route | Onset of Action | Peak Plasma Concentration | Elimination Half-life | Duration of Action |
|---|---|---|---|---|
| PO | 15-45 min | 1 hr | 3-4 hr | 6 hr |

There are two forms of intravenous caffeine: caffeine citrate and caffeine sodium benzoate. Caffeine citrate is recommended for neonatal apnea, including cases not responsive to other methylxanthines such as theophylline. Caffeine sodium benzoate is used for respiratory depression in adults only, because it contains the preservative benzyl alcohol.

### doxapram

Doxapram (Dopram) is an analeptic that is commonly used in conjunction with supportive measures in cases of respiratory depression that involve anesthetics or drugs of abuse and in COPD-associated hypercapnia. Deep tendon reflexes, in addition to vital signs and heart rhythm, are monitored to prevent overdosage of this drug.

### Pharmacokinetics

| Route | Onset of Action | Peak Plasma Concentration | Elimination Half-life | Duration of Action |
|-------|-----------------|---------------------------|----------------------|--------------------|
| IV | Less than 30 sec | Less than 2 min | 2-4 hr | 5-12 min |

## NURSING PROCESS

## ASSESSMENT

*CNS stimulants* are used for a variety of conditions and disorders. They have addictive potential, and so the following assessment data need to be collected before their use, regardless of indication: (1) a thorough medical history with attention to preexisting diseases or conditions, especially those of the cardiovascular, cerebrovascular, neurologic, renal, and liver systems; (2) past and current history of addictive or substance abuse behaviors; (3) complete medication profile with a listing of prescription, OTC, and herbal drugs and any use

### TABLE 13-5 CAFFEINE-CONTAINING BEVERAGES AND DRUGS

| MEDICATION OR BEVERAGE | AMOUNT OF CAFFEINE |
|------------------------|--------------------|
| **Nonprescription Medications** | |
| *Analgesics* | |
| Anacin | 32 mg/tab |
| Excedrin, Excedrin Aspirin-Free, Excedrin Migraine | 65 mg/tab |
| | |
| **Stimulants** | |
| NoDoz Maximum Strength | 100 mg/tab |
| Vivarin | 200 mg/tab |
| Zantrex-3 (marketed as anorexiant) | 200 mg/tab |
| | |
| **Prescription Medications (for Migraines)** | |
| Fioricet, Fiorinal | 40 mg/tab |
| Esgic | 40 mg/tab |
| Cafergot | 10 mg/suppository |
| | |
| **Beverages** | |
| Coffee (brewed, instant) | 80-150 mg/5-oz cup |
| Coffee (decaffeinated) | 2-20 mg/5-oz cup |
| Tea (brewed) | 30-75 mg/5-oz cup |
| Soft drinks | 35-60 mg/12-oz cup |
| Cocoa | 5-40 mg/5-oz cup |
| Supplemented water (Red Bull, Propel, Vitamin Water) | ~50 mg/12-oz cup |
| Coffee-flavored or chocolate ice cream | 30-45 mg/0.5-oz cup |

of alcohol, nicotine, and/or social or illegal drugs; and (4) a complete nutritional and dietary history. Assess all of these areas because of the mechanism of action of CNS stimulants, which increases pulse rate and blood pressure, and can lead to seizures, intracerebral bleeding, and toxicity (due to decreased drug metabolism and excretion). Stimulation of the respiratory system is actually desirable, and this action is beneficial in those patients suffering from CNS depression, such as postoperatively. Improvement of attention span is beneficial for those in need of the medication, but the possibility of adverse effects requires a thorough assessment to obtain baseline information. The anorexiant action may cause complications if the drugs are used or ordered inappropriately. When these drugs are taken for appetite suppression, assess and document baseline height, weight, and dietary intake. Measure vital signs with specific attention to blood pressure and pulse rate whenever these drugs are used.

To add to the thoroughness of the assessment, include in your nursing history the following information: inquiry about lifestyle, exercise, nutritional habits and patterns (e.g., a reduction in fat-soluble vitamins, history of any type of eating disorder), educational level, previous teaching and learning successes and failures, available support structures (e.g., family and friends), self-esteem, stress levels, mental status and mental health problems (drugs may exacerbate psychosis), presence of diabetes (diabetic patients need closer monitoring and tighter glucose control when taking stimulant medications due to increased glucogenolysis), and information related to contraindications, cautions, and drug interactions (see Table 13-4).

With *drugs used for the management of attention deficit hyperactivity disorder,* very cautiously and continuously assess the patient. For the pediatric patient, gather the following information during assessment: baseline weight, height, growth and development patterns, and vital signs. Complete blood counts may be ordered. Thoroughly document any changes in emotional status as well. Adults also require thorough assessment of baseline weight, height, and vital signs. Assess and document usual sleep habits and patterns so that sleep disturbances may be anticipated and managed appropriately. Atypical behavior, loss in attention span, and history of social problems or problems in school are also important to assess and document before and during therapy for baseline comparison. For children with ADHD, parental support is important to the success of treatment, and so a home assessment may be needed. Attention to and documentation of daily dietary intake before drug therapy is important because of the risk of drug-related weight loss. It is also important that the pediatric patient not experience too rapid or too much weight loss; a thorough nutritional and dietary assessment is needed. Cardiac assessment is important because of the CNS stimulation. Blood pressure, pulse rate, heart sounds, and any history of chest pain or palpitations must be noted. Other data to gather during assessment include possible contraindications, cautions, and drug interactions (see previous discussion). Document findings and note the patient's use of any prescription drugs, OTC drugs (e.g., nasal decongestants, which are also stimulants), and herbal preparations, specifically ginseng and caffeine (see the Safety: Herbal Therapies and Dietary Supplements box on p. 214).

## SAFETY: HERBAL THERAPIES AND DIETARY SUPPLEMENTS

### Selected Herbal Compounds Used for Nervous System Stimulation

| COMMON NAME(S) | USES | POSSIBLE DRUG INTERACTIONS (AVOID CONCURRENT USE) |
|---|---|---|
| *Ginkgo biloba,* ginkgo | To enhance mental alertness; to improve memory or dementia | Warfarin, aspirin |
| Ginseng | To enhance impaired mental function and concentration | Drugs for diabetes that lower blood sugar (e.g., insulin, oral hypoglycemic drugs), monoamine oxidase inhibitors |
| Guarana | To stimulate nervous system, suppress appetite | Adenosine, disulfiram, quinolones, oral contraceptives, beta blockers, iron, lithium, phenylephrine (e.g., nasal spray), cimetidine, theophylline, tobacco |

The *serotonin agonists* commonly used in the treatment of migraines are not without adverse reactions, contraindications, cautions, and drug interactions (see previous discussion). Include in your assessment a thorough cardiac history as well as measurement of blood pressure and pulse rate and rhythm. If a patient has a history of hypertension, there is risk of further increases in blood pressure to dangerous levels with use of these drugs, and thus the need for careful assessment and documentation. In fact, generally these drugs are not prescribed for patients with migraines who also have coronary artery disease unless a thorough cardiac evaluation has been performed. Conduct a careful assessment to identify other drugs the patient is taking that might lead to significant drug interactions, such as ergot alkaloids, selective serotonin receptor inhibitors, and MAOIs. If serotonin agonists are taken within 2 weeks of the use of these drugs, there is high risk for an additive toxicity. Such toxicity would be manifested by nervousness, insomnia, cardiovascular complications, and convulsions (serotonin syndrome).

*Ergot alkaloids* also have cautions, contraindications, and drug interactions (see previous discussion), which you need to assess for and document. Obtain a history of the migraines and their pattern, exacerbating factors, measures that provide relief, and previous treatments.

An *analeptic* such as doxapram is used as a central respiratory stimulant; therefore, it is most likely to be used in a hospital setting, specifically in intensive care units or postanesthesia units. The same concerns regarding contraindications, cautions, and drug interactions exist for this drug as for all CNS stimulants, and even closer attention must be paid to vital signs, especially heart rate and rhythm, and blood pressure. Any elevations in blood pressure and pulse rate may put the patient at a higher risk of complications. Perform a thorough neurologic assessment with specific attention to any possibility of seizures. Assess

baseline deep tendon reflexes, and document for comparative purposes.

## NURSING DIAGNOSES

1. Decreased cardiac output related to the adverse effects of CNS stimulants (e.g., palpitations and tachycardia)
2. Imbalanced nutrition, less than body requirements, related to adverse effects of CNS stimulants (e.g., amphetamines and anorexiants)
3. Chronic pain related to the experience of or a history of migraine headaches
4. Disturbed sleep patterns related to the action and adverse effects of CNS stimulants

## PLANNING

### GOALS

1. Patient remains free of cardiac symptoms and adverse effects.
2. Patient's nutritional status remains intact and without excess weight loss.
3. Patient regains adequate comfort level with adequate and efficient management of migraines.
4. Patient experiences minimal disturbed sleep patterns.

### OUTCOME CRITERIA

1. Patient vital signs, especially blood pressure (120/80) and pulse rate (60 to 100) remain within normal limits and without major fluctuations or changes.
   - Patient states symptoms (e.g., palpitations, chest pain) that need to be reported to the prescriber immediately.
2. Patient maintains appropriate weight without too rapid losses during drug therapy regimen.
   - Patient regains or maintains near normal body weight and BMI during therapy.
   - Patient continues to undergo close to normal growth and development while taking medications.
3. Patient reports a decrease in headaches and improved activities of daily living and well being while taking medications as prescribed.
   - Patient reports minimal adverse effects from antimigraine medications.
   - Patient states improved quality of life with efficient and adequate self-administration of medication.
4. Patient experiences more restful sleep while experiencing efficient drug therapy.
   - Patient uses nonpharmacologic measures to enhance sleep such as massage, biofeedback, music therapy, relaxation breathing, and keeping the room quiet and at a comfortable temperature.

## IMPLEMENTATION

With *drugs used for the treatment of attention deficit hyperactivity disorder,* some pediatric patients may respond better to certain dosage forms such as immediate release. However, dosing needs to be individualized and based on the patient's needs at different times during the school day (e.g., a noon dose to help with music lessons later in the afternoon). Well-planned scheduling of these medications and close communication among the school, teachers, school nurse, and the family and patient is very important to successful treatment. It is also important to time the dosing of medications—but as ordered—for periods in which symptom control is most needed but without causing alterations in sleep patterns. Generally speaking, once-a-day dosing is used with extended-release or long-acting preparations. Adequate and proper dosing will be manifested by good control of inattentive/impulsive behavior during school time. If extended-release dosage forms lead to acceptable outcomes for the pediatric patient, taking medications at school may not be necessary. Many times a stigma is associated with taking medications at school. This may be preventable with use of long-acting preparations or other scheduling. To help decrease the occurrence of insomnia, it is recommended that the last daily dose be taken 4 to 6 hours before bedtime, as ordered. During therapy, monitor the patient for continued physical growth, with specific attention to weight and height. The prescriber may order medication-free times on weekends, holidays, and/or vacations; that is, the drug may be discontinued periodically so that the need for the medication can be reassessed and sensitivity increased.

Because *anorexiants* are generally used for a short period of time, emphasize to the patient and all members of the patient's support system that a suitable diet, appropriate independent and/or supervised exercise program, and behavioral modifications are necessary to support a favorable result and to help the patient cease overeating and experience healthy weight loss. With a drug regimen, medications are usually taken first thing in the morning, as ordered, to minimize interference with sleep. Therefore, it is recommended that these drugs not be taken within 4 to 6 hours of sleep. If the patient has been taking these drugs for a prolonged period, an interval period of weaning before discontinuation is needed to avoid withdrawal symptoms and to avoid any chance of a rebound increase in appetite. Weights must be assessed weekly or as ordered. Encourage journal keeping so that the patient can keep record of food intake as well as responses to the drug regimen, any adverse effects, socialization, exercise, and notes about how they are feeling day to day. Dry mouth may be managed with frequent mouth care and the use of sugar-free gum or hard candy. Sucking ice chips, as well as keeping a bottle of fresh water on hand at all times, may also be helpful. If headaches occur, acetaminophen will most likely be suggested. Caffeine in any form needs to be avoided including coffee, tea, sodas, and chocolate. Other products that may contain caffeine include some OTC analgesics; OTC compounds to treat menstrual symptoms; OTC products for cough, cold, flu, or congestion; and prescription drugs such as analgesics with ergotamine and caffeine, and butalbital with aspirin and caffeine. Supplementation with fat-soluble vitamins may be indicated with use of these drugs. It is also important to watch for tolerance to the anorexiant during the course of treatment. Other nursing considerations include emphasis on a holistic approach to treatment of obesity, including the possible use of hypnosis, biofeedback, and guided imagery, as ordered. Encourage patients to keep follow-up visits with their prescribers and others involved in their care.

*SSRAs* come in a variety of dosage forms. Rizatriptan is available in oral tablets as well as in a disintegrating tablet or wafer that dissolves on the tongue. The latter dosage form leads to a more rapid absorption. Use of the nasal spray or self-injectable forms of the serotonin agonists is especially desirable in patients experiencing the nausea and vomiting that may occur with migraine headaches. Self-injectable forms and nasal sprays also have the benefit of an onset of action of 10 to 15 minutes compared with 1 to 2 hours for tablet forms. Administration of a test dose of the injectable and all other dosage forms is usually recommended. If the injectable form is prescribed, provide instructions and demonstrations of the technique. See the Patient Teaching Tips for more information.

*Ergot alkaloids* are taken exactly as prescribed; for example, tablets need to be taken with 6 to 8 ounces of water or other fluid and work best when taken at the first sign of the migraine. This allows more successful treatment. With ergotamine tartrate and related drugs, the maximum dose is usually 6 tablets for a single headache and 10 tablets in any 7-day period. Dependence may occur with the ergots, and if they are withdrawn suddenly, rebound headaches may occur. Encourage the patient to report to the prescriber any headaches that are uncharacteristic or unusual, as well as any persistent headache, worsening of headaches, severe nausea, vomiting, dizziness, or restlessness. Any of the following also need to be reported immediately to the prescriber: slow, fast, or irregular heartbeat; tingling, pain, or coldness in the fingers or toes; loss of feeling in the fingers or toes; muscle pain or weakness; chest pain; severe stomach or abdominal pain; lower back pain; little or no urine. Emphasize that the patient must seek immediate medical attention if there is any chest pain, vision changes, confusion, or slurred speech. As mentioned previously, these medications are not to be taken with triptans.

The *analeptic* doxapram may be administered intravenously, but at different dosages depending on the purpose. (For dosage information, see the table on p. 211.) Give doxapram infusions using an intravenous pump, and closely monitor the patient. Because the patient's sensorium is generally diminished in this situation, place the patient in the Sims' or semi-Fowler's position to prevent aspiration. The patient's airway, breathing, and circulation (ABCs of care) are of highest priority. If adverse effects occur (see the pharmacology discussion), notify the prescriber.

## EVALUATION

Therapeutic responses to *drugs for attention deficit hyperactivity disorder* include decreased hyperactivity, increased attention span and concentration, improved behavior, and, for adults, increased effectiveness at work. Adverse effects range from loss of appetite to increased irritability, insomnia, palpitations, nausea, and headaches. Therapeutic effects of *anorexiants* include appetite control and weight loss for the treatment of obesity. Adverse effects of these drugs include dry mouth, headache, insomnia, constipation, tachycardia, cardiac irregularities, hypertension, changes in mental status or sensorium, changes in mood or affect, alteration of sleep patterns, and seizures (all due to excess CNS stimulation). Evaluating for any increased irritability and withdrawal symptoms

## TEAMWORK AND COLLABORATION: LEGAL AND ETHICAL PRINCIPLES

### Handling of Prescription Drugs

It is important for the nurse to understand the following amendments to the federal laws that apply to the handling of all prescription drugs by the registered nurse. (NOTE: This is a summary and does not reflect the laws in their entirety.) The registered nurse is prohibited from doing the following:

- Compounding or dispensing the designated drugs for legal distribution and administration.
- Distributing the drugs to any individuals who are not licensed or authorized by federal or state law to receive the drugs (e.g., those outside the health care provider–patient relationship); the penalties for such actions are generally severe.
- Making, selling, keeping, or concealing any counterfeit drug equipment.
- Possessing any type of stimulant or depressant drug unless authorized to do so by a legal prescription (as a patient); any unauthorized possession is illegal.

It is important to adhere to these legal guidelines in the practice of drug administration to avoid legal penalties, including possible loss of license or other severe penalties.

(e.g., headache, nausea and vomiting) is also important. If the anorexiant affects fat metabolism, then there may be adverse effects such as flatulence with an oily discharge, spotting, and fecal urgency. The patient also needs to be closely evaluated for decreased levels of fat-soluble vitamins (A, D, E, and K), because their levels may be affected by the decreased absorption of fats. For *drugs used to treat narcolepsy*, therapeutic responses include a decrease in daytime sleepiness. Adverse effects for which to monitor include headache, nausea, nervousness, insomnia, and anxiety. Therapeutic responses to the *serotonin agonists* include aborting of migraine headache with improved daily functioning and performance because of the reduction in headaches. Adverse effects for which to monitor include pain at the injection site (if a self-injectable form is used; such pain is temporary), flushing, chest tightness or pressure, weakness, sedation, dizziness, sweating, increase in blood pressure and pulse rate, and bad taste with the nasal spray formulation, which may precipitate nausea.

## PATIENT TEACHING TIPS

### General Information

- Serotonin agonists are to be taken as prescribed on a prn (as needed) basis at the onset of the migraine but within the frequency and dosage amount prescribed.
- Medications need to be taken exactly as prescribed without skipping, omitting, or adding doses.
- Alcohol, OTC cold products, cough syrups that contain alcohol, nicotine, and caffeine-containing food items and/or beverages must be avoided.
- Keeping a journal of daily activities and response to drug therapy and any adverse effects is encouraged. Medications or foods/beverages identified as triggers to a migraine may vary from person to person. Encourage the patient to track food/beverage intake as well as sleep habits and other practices/factors that may be identified as precipitators of migraines.
- Avoid any abrupt or sudden withdrawal of medications.

### Drugs Used to Treat Attention Deficit Hyperactivity Disorder

- For maximal drug effects, medications are to be taken on an empty stomach 30 to 45 minutes before eating.
- Keeping all follow-up appointments is important to monitoring drug therapy.
- If the prescriber decides to discontinue the medication, a weaning process with careful supervision is recommended.
- Extended-release or long-acting preparations are to be taken in their original dosage form and only as directed. They are not to be crushed, chewed, broken, or altered in any way.
- Dosage amounts are not to be increased or decreased by the patient or family, because this may lead to drug-related complications. If there is any concern about the drug and its dosage amount or adverse effects, encourage parents or caregivers to contact the prescriber.

### Anorexiants

- The patient must follow all prescriber instructions regarding medications, diet, and exercise.
- Some of these medications may impair alertness and the ability to think, so patients need to remain very cautious if engaging in activities that may be adversely affected until these impairments are resolved.
- An unpleasant taste of the medicine and/or dry mouth may be minimized by the use of mouth rinses, ice chips, sugarless chewing gum, and/or hard candies.

### Antimigraine Drugs

- Encourage patients who experience migraines to avoid foods/beverages that are known triggers to severe or other forms of migraine headaches.
- Other triggers for some individuals may include food additives, preservatives (including MSG, nitrates, and nitrites), artificial sweeteners (especially aspartame when used for extended periods of time), and chocolate.
- Before using a nasal spray dosage form of an antimigraine drug, instruct the patient to first gently blow the nose to clear the nasal passages. With the head upright, the patient then closes one nostril and inserts the nozzle into the open nostril. While a breath is taken through the nose, the spray is released. The nozzle is removed, and then the patient gently breathes in through the nose and out through the mouth for 10 to 20 seconds. Some bad taste may be experienced.
- Until migraine is resolved, the patient may find comfort by avoiding doing things that require alertness and rapid skilled movements. It may be helpful to keep the room darkened and noise to a minimum. If the headache is not resolved and/or vomiting occurs, the patient may need further

## PATIENT TEACHING TIPS—cont'd

medical attention to help avoid additional problems, such as dehydration.

- Encourage keeping a journal about the experience of all headaches, precipitators/relievers, and the rating of each headache on a scale of 0 to 10 (where 0 is no pain and 10 is the worst pain ever). Recording of other symptoms (e.g., photophobia, nausea, and vomiting) as well as their frequency and duration is recommended.
- When taking SSRAs, the patient must understand the importance of contacting the prescriber immediately if there are any problems with palpitations, chest pain, and/or pain or weakness in the extremities.
- Injectable forms of sumatriptan are to be given subcutaneously and as ordered. Have the patient practice administering injections (without the medication) with you at the prescriber's office so that proper technique is used and a moderate comfort level is achieved.
- Autoinjectors with prefilled syringes may be used. The syringe needs to be discarded in an appropriate container or receptacle after use and kept out of the reach of children.

- Administer no more than two injections of sumatriptan during a 24-hour period, and allow at least 1 hour between injections.
- When using injectable sumatriptan, contact the prescriber or emergency services immediately if there is swelling around the eyes, pain or tightness in the chest or throat, wheezing, and/or heart throbbing.
- Treatment for migraine headaches may relieve the pain and symptoms of a migraine attack as well as prevent further migraine attacks. Some abortive therapies, such as sumatriptan, may offer rapid relief if drugs are given as ordered and before the headache worsens. Drugs may be given orally, sublingually, or by subcutaneous injection in the thigh. When a triptan does not work, an ergot alkaloid (e.g., dihydroergotamine or ergotamine tartrate) may be ordered but is not to be used concurrently. Other drugs that may also be used to try to prevent migraine headache include antidepressants, antiseizure medications, and beta blockers.

## KEY POINTS

- CNS stimulants are drugs that stimulate the brain or spinal cord.
- The actions of these stimulants mimic those of the neurotransmitters of the sympathetic nervous system (e.g., norepinephrine, dopamine, and serotonin).
- Included in the family of CNS stimulants are amphetamines, analeptics, and anorexiants with therapeutic uses for attention deficit hyperactivity disorder, narcolepsy, and appetite control. Adverse effects associated with CNS stimulants include changes in mental status or sensorium, changes in mood or affect, tachycardia, loss of appetite, nausea, altered sleep patterns (e.g., insomnia), physical dependency, irritability, and seizures.
- Serotonin agonists may be administered as a subcutaneous injection, as a nasal spray, and as oral tablets. Any chest pain or tightness, tremors, vomiting, or worsening symptoms needs to be reported to the prescriber immediately.

- Anorexiants control or suppress appetite. They are used to stimulate the CNS and result in suppression of appetite control centers in the brain.
- Contraindications to the use of anorexiants, as well as other CNS stimulants, include hypersensitivity, seizure activity, convulsive disorders, and liver dysfunction.
- The SSRAs are a newer class of CNS stimulants and are used to treat migraine headaches. They are not to be given to patients with coronary heart disease.
- Amphetamines elevate mood or produce euphoria, increase mental alertness and capacity for work, decrease fatigue and drowsiness, and prolong wakefulness.
- Journaling is helpful in evaluating the effects of all drugs used to treat attention deficit hyperactivity disorder, obesity, migraines, and narcolepsy.

## NCLEX® EXAMINATION REVIEW QUESTIONS

1 A patient with narcolepsy will begin treatment with a CNS stimulant. The nurse expects to see which adverse effect?
   a Bradycardia
   b Nervousness
   c Mental clouding
   d Drowsiness at night

2 A patient at a weight management clinic who was given a prescription for orlistat (Xenical) calls the clinic hotline complaining of a "terrible side effect." The nurse suspects that the patient is referring to which problem?
   a Nausea
   b Sexual dysfunction
   c Urinary incontinence
   d Fecal incontinence

3 The nurse is developing a plan of care for a patient receiving an anorexiant. Which nursing diagnosis is most appropriate?
   a Deficient fluid volume
   b Sleep deprivation
   c Impaired memory
   d Imbalanced nutrition, less than body requirements

4 A patient has a new prescription for sumatriptan (Imitrex). The nurse providing patient teaching on self-administration will include which information?
   a Correct technique for intramuscular injections
   b Take the medication before the headache worsens.
   c Allow at least 30 minutes between injections.
   d Take no more than 4 doses in a 24-hour period.

5  The nurse is reviewing the history of a patient who will be starting the triptan sumatriptan (Imitrex) as part of treatment for migraine headaches. Which condition, if present, may be a contraindication to triptan therapy?
   a  Cardiovascular disease
   b  Chronic bronchitis
   c  History of renal calculi
   d  Diabetes mellitus type 2

6  The nurse is reviewing medication therapy with the parents of an adolescent with ADHD. Which statement is correct? (Select all that apply.)
   a  "Be sure to have your child blow his nose before administering the nasal spray."
   b  "This medication is used only when symptoms of ADHD are severe."
   c  "The last dose should be taken 4 to 6 hours before bedtime to avoid interference with sleep."
   d  "Be sure to contact the physician right away if you notice expression of suicidal thoughts."
   e  "We will need to check your child's height and weight periodically to monitor physical growth."
   f  "If adverse effects become severe, stop the medication for 3 to 4 days."

7  The medication order reads: "Atomoxetine (Strattera) 1.2 mg/kg/day in 2 divided doses." The child weighs 66 lbs. How much will be given with each dose?

1. b, 2. d, 3. d, 4. b, 5. a, 6. c, d, e, 7. 18 mg per dose

For Critical Thinking and Prioritization Questions, see http://evolve.elsevier.com/Lilley.

# Antiepileptic Drugs

## OBJECTIVES

When you reach the end of this chapter, you will be able to do the following:

1  Briefly describe the pathophysiology of epilepsy.
2  Discuss the rationale for the use of the various classes of antiepileptic drugs (AEDs) in the management of the different forms of epilepsy.
3  Identify the various drugs in each of the following drug classes: iminostilbenes, benzodiazepines, barbiturates, hydantoins, and miscellaneous drugs.

4  Identify the mechanisms of action, indications, cautions, contraindications, dosages, routes of administration, adverse effects, toxic effects, therapeutic blood levels, and drug interactions for each antiepileptic drug.
5  Develop a nursing care plan, including patient education, based on the nursing process for patients receiving AEDs.

## DRUG PROFILES

♦ **carbamazepine, p. 229**
  ethosuximide, p. 229
♦ **gabapentin, p. 229**
  lamotrigine, p. 230
  levetiracetam, p. 230
  oxcarbazepine, p. 229
♦ **phenobarbital and primidone, p. 226**

♦ **phenytoin and fosphenytoin, p. 228**
  pregabalin, p. 230
  tiagabine, p. 230
  topiramate, p. 230
♦ **valproic acid, p. 231**
  zonisamide, p. 231

───────────

♦ *Key drug*

## KEY TERMS

**Anticonvulsants** Substances or procedures that prevent or reduce the severity of *epileptic* or other *convulsive* seizures. (p. 221)

**Antiepileptic drugs** Prescription drugs that prevent or reduce the severity of epilepsy and different types of epileptic seizures, not just convulsive seizures. (p. 221)

**Autoinduction** A metabolic process in which a drug stimulates the production of enzymes that enhance its own metabolism

over time, which leads to a reduction in therapeutic drug concentrations. (p. 229)

**Convulsion** A type of seizure involving excessive stimulation of neurons in the brain and characterized by the spasmodic contraction of voluntary muscles. (See also *seizure.*) (p. 220)

**Electroencephalogram (EEG)** A recording of the electrical activity that arises from spontaneous currents in nerve cells in the brain, derived from electrodes placed on the outer skull. (p. 220)

Epilepsy A general term for any of a group of neurologic disorders characterized by *recurrent* episodes of *convulsive seizures,* sensory disturbances, abnormal behavior, loss of consciousness, or any combination of these. (p. 220)

Generalized onset seizures Seizures originating simultaneously in both cerebral hemispheres. (p. 220)

Gingival hyperplasia Overgrowth of gum tissue and often a side effect of phenytoin. (p. 228)

Partial onset seizures Seizures originating in a more localized region of the brain (also called *focal* seizures). (p. 221)

Primary epilepsy Epilepsy in which there is no identifiable cause. Also known as *idiopathic.* (p. 220)

Seizure Excessive stimulation of neurons in the brain leading to a sudden burst of abnormal neuron activity that results in temporary changes in brain function, primarily affecting sensory and motor activity. (p. 220)

Status epilepticus A seizure disorder characterized by generalized tonic-clonic convulsions that occur repeatedly; considered a medical emergency. (p. 221)

Tonic-clonic seizures Seizures involving initial muscular contraction throughout the body (tonic phase), progressing to alternating contraction and relaxation (clonic phase). (p. 220)

## ANATOMY, PHYSIOLOGY, AND PATHOPHYSIOLOGY OVERVIEW

### EPILEPSY

Epilepsy is a syndrome of central nervous system (CNS) dysfunction that can cause symptoms ranging from momentary sensory disturbances to convulsive seizures. It is the most common chronic neurologic illness, affecting 3 million people in the United States and 50 million people worldwide. It results from excessive electrical activity of neurons (nerve cells) located in the superficial area of the brain known as the *cerebral cortex* or *gray matter.* The terms *seizure, convulsion,* and *epilepsy* are often used interchangeably, but they do not have the same meaning. A seizure is a brief episode of abnormal electrical activity in the nerve cells of the brain, which may or may not lead to a convulsion. A convulsion is a more severe seizure characterized by involuntary spasmodic contractions of any or all voluntary muscles throughout the body, including skeletal, facial, and ocular muscles. Commonly reported symptoms include abnormal motor function, loss of consciousness, altered sensory awareness, and psychic changes. In contrast, epilepsy is a chronic, recurrent pattern of seizures. Excessive electrical discharges can often be detected by an electroencephalogram (EEG), which is obtained to help diagnose epilepsy. Fluctuations in the brain's electrical potential are seen in the form of waves. These waves correlate well with different neurologic conditions and are used as diagnostic indicators. In the case of epilepsy, they are used to identify specific seizure subtypes.

Up to 50% of patients with epilepsy have normal EEGs; therefore a careful history is very important for accurate diagnosis. Other applicable diagnostic tests include skull radiography, *computed tomography,* and *magnetic resonance imaging.* These procedures help to rule out structural causes of epilepsy, such as brain tumors. In particularly severe cases, patients may be observed in a hospital setting or sleep study laboratory. This allows for continuous EEG and video monitoring to identify detailed patterns of seizure activity and to allow tailoring of an effective treatment.

Epilepsy occurs most commonly in children and the elderly. Epilepsy without an identifiable cause is known as primary epilepsy or *idiopathic* epilepsy. Primary epilepsy accounts for roughly 50% of cases. Evidence indicates genetic predispositions,

but these have yet to be clearly defined. Studies in the field of *pharmacogenomics* (see Chapter 8) are beginning to clarify genetic factors that can help optimize antiepileptic drug therapy. In other cases, epilepsy has a distinct cause, such as trauma, infection, cerebrovascular disorder, or other illness. This is known as *secondary* or *symptomatic* epilepsy. The chief causes of secondary epilepsy in children and infants are developmental defects, metabolic disease, and injury at birth. *Febrile seizures* occur in children 6 months to 5 years of age, and by definition are caused by fever. Children usually outgrow the tendency to have such seizures, and thus these seizures do not constitute a chronic illness. Antipyretic drugs (e.g., acetaminophen [see Chapter 10]) are normally adequate for acute treatment.

In adults, acquired brain disorder is the major cause of secondary epilepsy. Examples include head injury, disease or infection of the brain and spinal cord, stroke, metabolic disorders, adverse drug reactions (e.g., meperidine [see Chapter 10], theophylline [see Chapter 37]), primary or metastatic brain tumor, or other nonspecific neurologic diseases. The elderly have the highest incidence of new-onset epilepsy. Fortunately, seizures in the elderly are often well controlled with drug therapy.

Seizures are classified into different categories based on their presenting features. There are three major categories: *partial onset, generalized onset,* and *unclassified* seizures (Box 14-1). Evidence provided by EEG and other diagnostic techniques indicates that different types of seizures originate from disruptions of normal brain electrical activity in different regions or *lobes* of the brain.

Generalized onset seizures, formerly called *grand mal* seizures, are characterized by neuronal activity that originates simultaneously in the gray matter of both hemispheres. There are several subtypes of generalized seizures. Tonic-clonic seizures begin with muscular contraction throughout the body (tonic phase) and progress to alternating contraction and relaxation (clonic phase). *Tonic* seizures involve spasms of the upper trunk with flexion of the arms. *Clonic* seizures are the same as tonic-clonic seizures but without the tonic phase. *Atonic* seizures, also known as *drop attacks,* involve sudden global muscle weakness and syncope. *Myoclonic seizures* are characterized by brief muscular jerks, but not as extreme as in other subtypes. Finally, *absence* seizures involve a brief loss of awareness that commonly occurs

## BOX 14-1 CLASSIFICATION OF SEIZURES

**Partial Seizures**
*Description*
Short alterations in consciousness, repetitive unusual movements (chewing or swallowing movements), psychologic changes, and confusion

*Simple Seizures*
- No impaired consciousness
- Motor symptoms (most commonly related to the face, arm, or leg)
- Hallucinations of sight, hearing, or taste along with somatosensory changes (tingling)
- Autonomic nervous system responses
- Personality changes

*Complex Seizures*
- Impaired consciousness
- Memory impairment
- Behavioral effects
- Purposeless behaviors
- Aura, chewing and swallowing movements, unreal feelings, and bizarre behavior
- Tonic, clonic, or tonic-clonic seizures

**Generalized Seizures**
*Description*
Most often seen in children and commonly characterized by temporary lapses in consciousness lasting a few seconds. Staring off into space, daydreaming, and inattentive look are common symptoms. Patients may exhibit rhythmic movements of their eyes, head, or hands but do not experience convulsions. Patients may have several attacks per day.
- Both cerebral hemispheres involved
- Tonic, clonic, myoclonic, atonic, or tonic-clonic seizures and infantile spasms possible
- Brief loss of consciousness for a few seconds with no confusion
- Head drop or falling-down symptoms

**Unclassified Seizures**
*Description*
Seizures that are not officially classified due to inadequate data, as well as seizures that do not fit into the above categories. These include neonatal seizures such as those manifested by rhythmic eye movements, chewing, and swimming movements.

with repetitive spasmodic eye blinking for up to 30 seconds. This type occurs primarily in childhood and rarely after 14 years of age.

Partial onset seizures originate in a localized or *focal* region (e.g., one lobe) of the brain. There are three types of partial onset seizures. *Simple partial onset seizure,* formerly called *petit mal* seizure, is characterized by brief loss of awareness (e.g., blank stare) but without loss of consciousness or spasmodic eye blinking as in absence seizures. In *complex partial onset seizure,* the level of consciousness is reduced but is not completely lost. Partial onset seizures can progress to generalized tonic-clonic seizures in up to 40% of patients. This third type is known as a *secondary generalized tonic-clonic seizure.* The latter two types are also associated with *postictal confusion,* a term for the confused mental state that follows seizure activity. *Unclassified seizures* are those that do not clearly fit into any of the other categories.

Seizure episodes can sometimes start off as partial and then become generalized. If the partial component is not noticed, the patient may be misdiagnosed and receive suboptimal drug therapy. Another important seizure condition is status epilepticus. In status epilepticus, multiple seizures occur with no recovery between them. If appropriate therapy is not started promptly, hypotension, hypoxia, brain damage, and death can quickly ensue. Thus, status epilepticus is considered a true medical emergency (see Table 14-3 for drugs used to treat status epilepticus). Febrile seizures can also sometimes progress to status epilepticus. In addition to the website of the International League Against Epilepsy, other helpful websites include www.epilepsyfoundation.org and www.epilepsy.com.

## PHARMACOLOGY OVERVIEW

### ANTIEPILEPTIC DRUGS

Antiepileptic drugs are also called *anticonvulsants.* Antiepileptic drugs is a more appropriate term, because many of these medications are indicated for the management of all types of epilepsy, and not necessarily just convulsions. Anticonvulsants, on the other hand, are medications that are used to prevent the *convulsive* seizures typically associated with epilepsy.

The goal of antiepileptic drug therapy is to control or prevent seizures while maintaining a reasonable quality of life. Approximately 70% of patients can expect to become seizure free while taking only one drug. The remaining 30% of cases are more complicated, and often require multiple medications. Antiepileptic drugs have many adverse effects, and it is often difficult to achieve seizure control while avoiding adverse effects. In most cases, the therapeutic goal is not to eliminate seizure activity but rather to maximally reduce the incidence of seizures while minimizing drug-induced toxicity. Many patients must take these drugs for their entire lives. Treatment may eventually be stopped in some, but others will experience repeated seizures if constant levels of antiepileptic drugs are not maintained in the blood. Abrupt discontinuation of these drugs can result in withdrawal seizures. In both children and adults, there is only a 40% chance of recurrence after the first partial or generalized seizure. Therefore, antiepileptic drug therapy is *not* recommended after a single isolated seizure event.

There are numerous antiepileptic drugs available. To optimize drug selection, neurologists must consider the known efficacy of a drug for a certain type of seizure, the adverse effects and drug interaction profile, the cost, ease of use, and the availability of pediatric dosage forms. Many antiepileptic drugs are also used to treat other types of illnesses, including psychiatric disorders (see Chapter 16), migraine headaches (see Chapter 13), and neuropathic pain syndromes (see Chapter 10).

It is sometimes difficult to control a patient's seizures using a single drug. Single-drug therapy must fail before multidrug therapy is attempted. Patients are normally started on a single antiepileptic drug, and the dosage is slowly increased until the seizures are controlled or until clinical toxicity occurs. If the first antiepileptic drug is not effective, the drug is tapered slowly while a second drug is introduced. Antiepileptic drugs are never to be stopped abruptly unless a severe adverse effect occurs.

Therapeutic drug monitoring (see Chapter 2) of serum drug concentrations provides a useful guideline in assessing the effectiveness of and adherence to therapy. For example, if a patient has a very low serum level, it may mean the patient is not taking the medication as prescribed. This gives the nurse an opportunity to ask about why the patient may not be taking the medication. If the level is above normal, the nurse needs to contact the physician before giving the next dose. Maintaining serum drug levels within therapeutic ranges helps not only to control seizures but also to reduce adverse effects. Drugs that are routinely monitored in this way have a low *therapeutic index* (see Chapter 2). There are established normal therapeutic ranges for many antiepileptic drugs, but these are only guidelines (see Table 14-6). The serum concentrations of phenytoin, phenobarbital, carbamazepine, and primidone correlate better with seizure control and toxicity than do those of valproic acid, ethosuximide, and clonazepam. Each patient must be monitored and dosed based on the individual case. In many patients, maintenance is successful at levels below or above the usual therapeutic range. The goal is to slowly titrate to the lowest effective serum drug level that controls the seizure disorder. This reduces the risk for adverse drug effects and drug interactions. Successful control of a seizure disorder hinges on selection of the appropriate drug class and drug dosage, avoidance of drug toxicity, and patient compliance with the treatment regimen.

The antiepileptic drugs traditionally used to manage seizure disorders include barbiturates, hydantoins, and iminostilbenes, plus valproic acid. Second- and third-generation antiepileptics are also available (Table 14-1). The latter drugs may have fewer adverse effects and drug interactions than the more traditional drugs. This may benefit elderly patients, who are more likely to be taking multiple medications and, therefore, are more prone to drug interactions. However, there is currently debate in the neurologic literature as to whether patients actually benefit more from newer than from older drugs. It is now believed that the majority of pediatric and adult epilepsy patients who have been seizure free for 1 to 2 years while taking antiepileptic drugs can eventually stop taking them with medical supervision.

For many years, only the name-brand form of phenytoin, Dilantin, was available. However, generic dosage forms are also available now. Both name-brand and generic phenytoin are commonly prescribed. Phenobarbital and valproic acid are used almost exclusively in the generic forms. The remainder of the newer antiepileptic drugs is still available in brand-name forms only, with the exception of gabapentin and levetiracetam. All generic drug manufacturers are required to provide research data that demonstrate *bioequivalency* of their generic drugs to the corresponding original brand-name drugs. This means that the generic drug product must meet federal standards that include equality of absorption and distribution *(bioavailability)*, as well as equal clinical efficacy compared with the brand-name drug. In spite of the existence of these standards, both the American Academy of Neurology and the American Epilepsy

### TABLE 14-1 CURRENTLY AVAILABLE ANTIEPILEPTIC DRUGS

| GENERIC NAME | TRADE NAME | ROUTE |
|---|---|---|
| **Traditional Antiepileptic Drugs** | | |
| *Barbiturates* | | |
| phenobarbital | Generic | PO |
| | Generic | IV |
| primidone | Mysoline | PO |
| | | |
| *Hydantoins* | | |
| phenytoin | Dilantin | PO, IV |
| fosphenytoin | Cerebyx | IV, IM |
| | | |
| *Iminostilbenes* | | |
| carbamazepine | Tegretol, Carbatrol | PO |
| oxcarbazepine | Trileptal | PO |
| | | |
| **Miscellaneous Antiepileptic Drugs** | | |
| gabapentin | Neurontin | PO |
| lacosamide | Vimpat | PO, IV |
| lamotrigine | Lamictal | PO |
| levetiracetam | Keppra | PO |
| pregabalin | Lyrica | PO |
| tiagabine | Gabitril | PO |
| topiramate | Topamax | PO |
| valproic acid | Depakene, Depakote | PO |
| | Depacon | IV |
| zonisamide | Zonegran | PO |

*IM*, Intramuscular; *IV*, intravenous; *PO*, oral.

Society are concerned that generic drug products may be less clinically efficacious than brand-name drug products. Of particular concern is the common requirement of health insurance companies that patients receive generic drugs when available. Increased monitoring of patients is necessary when switching from brand-name products to generics.

## Mechanism of Action and Drug Effects

As with many classes of drugs, the exact mechanism of action of the antiepileptic drugs is not known with certainty. However, evidence indicates that they alter the movement of sodium, potassium, calcium, and magnesium ions. The changes in the movement of these ions result in more stabilized and less excitable cell membranes.

The major pharmacologic effects of antiepileptics are threefold. First, they *increase the threshold* of activity in the area of the brain called the *motor cortex*. In other words, they make it more difficult for a nerve to be excited, or they reduce the nerve's response to incoming electrical or chemical stimulation. Second, they act to *limit the spread* of a seizure discharge from its origin. They do this by suppressing the transmission of impulses from one nerve to the next. Third, they can *decrease the speed* of nerve impulse conduction within a given neuron. Less well understood are mechanisms that involve drug effects outside the neuron. For example, some drugs may indirectly affect seizure *foci* (locations) in the brain by altering the blood supply to these areas. Some drugs

## PATIENT-CENTERED CARE: LIFESPAN CONSIDERATIONS FOR THE PEDIATRIC PATIENT

### Antiepileptic Drugs

- If a skin rash develops in a child or infant taking phenytoin, discontinue the drug immediately and notify the prescriber.
- Chewable dosage forms of antiepileptic drugs are not recommended for once-a-day administration. Intramuscular injections of barbiturates or phenytoin must never be used.
- Encourage family members, parents, significant others, or caregivers to keep a journal with a record of the signs and symptoms before, during, and after a seizure and before, during, and after treatment with an antiepileptic drug.
- Encourage the wearing of a medical alert bracelet or necklace at all times with information about the diagnosis, drug therapy, and any drug allergies.
- Shake suspension dosage forms thoroughly before use. A graduated device or oral syringe may be used for more accurate dosing of this liquid.

- Pediatric patients are more sensitive to barbiturates and may respond to lower than expected dosages. They may also experience more profound central nervous system depressive effects related to the antiepileptic drug or show depression, confusion, or excitement (a paradoxical reaction).
- Any excessive sedation, confusion, lethargy, hypotension, bradypnea, tachycardia, and/or decreased movement in pediatric patients taking any antiepileptic drug must be reported to the prescriber immediately.
- Carbamazepine may be given with meals to reduce risk of gastrointestinal distress. All suspension forms are to be shaken and mixed thoroughly before use.
- Oral forms of valproic acid are not to be given with milk, because this may cause the drug to dissolve early and irritate the mucosa. Carbonated beverages must also be avoided.

## TABLE 14-2   COMMON SEIZURE INDICATIONS FOR ANTIEPILEPTIC DRUGS

|  | PARTIAL | SECONDARY GENERAL | GENERALIZED TONIC CLONIC | ABSENCE | MYOCLONIC |
|---|---|---|---|---|---|
| **First Line** | carbamazepine<br>phenobarbital<br>primidone<br>phenytoin<br>fosphenytoin | carbamazepine<br>phenobarbital<br>primidone<br>phenytoin<br>fosphenytoin | carbamazepine<br>phenobarbital<br>primidone<br>phenytoin<br>fosphenytoin<br>valproic acid | valproic acid | valproic acid |
| **Adjunct Drugs** | clonazepam<br>clorazepate<br>oxcarbazepine<br>gabapentin<br>pregabalin<br>lamotrigine<br>levetiracetam<br>tiagabine<br>topiramate<br>zonisamide | clonazepam<br>oxcarbazepine<br>gabapentin<br>lamotrigine<br>levetiracetam<br>tiagabine<br>topiramate<br>zonisamide | clonazepam<br>lamotrigine<br>topiramate<br>zonisamide | acetazolamide<br>ethosuximide<br>zonisamide | clonazepam<br>zonisamide |

work by enhancing the effects of the inhibitory neurotransmitter gamma-aminobutyric acid (GABA). GABA plays a role in regulating neuron excitability in the brain. Low levels of GABA are associated with seizures. Many antiepileptic drugs increase GABA levels to the normal range, and thus reduce the potential for seizures. Regardless of the mechanism, the overall effect is that antiepileptics stabilize neurons and keep them from becoming hyperexcited and generating excessive nerve impulses to adjacent neurons.

## Indications

Antiepileptic drugs are used to prevent or control seizure activity. As evidenced by the wide range of seizure disorders listed in Box 14-1, epilepsy is a very diverse disorder. As a result, specific indications vary among drugs. The most recent indications are noted, drug by drug, in Table 14-2, the Dosages table on p. 227, and specific drug profiles. It is important to have an accurate diagnosis of the seizure type, because some drugs may not be ideal for specific seizures. For example, it is known that carbamazepine may worsen myoclonic or absence seizures. Other

evidence supports the following generalizations: Phenobarbital, phenytoin, primidone, carbamazepine, and valproic acid are equally effective for partial onset seizures. Lamotrigine, topiramate, gabapentin, oxcarbazepine, zonisamide, levetiracetam, and tiagabine are all effective as adjunctive therapy for refractory (not responsive to other therapy) partial onset seizures. Specific antiepileptic drugs and the seizure disorders they are used to treat are listed in Table 14-2.

Antiepileptics are used for the long-term maintenance treatment of epilepsy. However, they are also useful for the acute treatment of status epilepticus. In this case, diazepam or lorazepam are considered to be the drugs of choice. Other commonly used drugs in status epilepticus are listed in Table 14-3. Once status epilepticus is controlled, long-term drug therapy is begun with other drugs for the prevention of future seizures. Patients who undergo brain surgery or who have experienced severe head injuries may receive prophylactic antiepileptic therapy. These patients are at high risk for acquiring a seizure disorder, and often severe complications will arise if seizures are not controlled.

**TABLE 14-3 ANTIEPILEPTIC DRUGS USED TO TREAT STATUS EPILEPTICUS**

| DRUG | IV DOSE | ONSET | DURATION | HALF-LIFE | ADVERSE EFFECTS |
|---|---|---|---|---|---|
| diazepam | **Pediatric:** 0.15-0.25 mg/kg* **Adult:** 5-30 mg | Immediate | 15-60 min | 20-50 hr | Apnea, hypotension, somnolence |
| fosphenytoin | 15-20 phenytoin equivalents/kg | 15-30 min | 12-24 hr | 10-60 hr | Comparable to those for phenytoin (see below) |
| lorazepam[†] | **Pediatric:** 0.05-0.1 mg/kg **Adult:** 4 mg | 1-20 min | Hours | 15 hr | Apnea, hypotension, somnolence |
| phenobarbital | 15-20 mg/kg | 5 min | 6-12 hr | 50-120 hr | Apnea, hypotension, somnolence |
| phenytoin | 15-20 mg/kg | 1-2 hr | 12-24 hr | 7-42 hr | Cardiac dysrhythmias, hypotension |

*IV,* Intravenous.
*Rectal products are also available for emergency use for both adults and children of all ages.
[†]Off-label use (not a Food and Drug Administration–approved indication), but still sometimes used for this purpose.

## Contraindications

The only usual contraindication to antiepileptics is known drug allergy. Pregnancy is also a common contraindication; however, the prescriber must consider the risks to mother and infant of untreated maternal epilepsy and the increased risk for seizure activity. Many women take antiepileptics throughout their pregnancy. The newer generation antiepileptic drugs appear to be safer in pregnancy than the traditional drugs.

## Adverse Effects

Antiepileptic drugs are plagued by many adverse effects, which often limit their usefulness. Many patients cannot tolerate the adverse effects, and therapy must be withdrawn. Birth defects in infants of epileptic mothers are higher than normal, regardless of whether the mother was receiving drug therapy. Epileptic women need to be monitored closely during pregnancy by both an obstetrician and a neurologist. Each antiepileptic drug is associated with its own diverse set of adverse effects. The various antiepileptic drugs and their most common adverse effects are listed in Table 14-4.

In December 2008, the U.S. Food and Drug Administration (FDA) required black box warnings on all antiepileptic drugs regarding the risk of suicidal thoughts and behavior. Patients being treated with antiepileptic drugs for any indication need to be monitored for the emergence or worsening of depression, suicidal thoughts or behavior, or any unusual changes in mood or behavior. The FDA's action was based on a review of 199 clinical trials of 11 antiepileptic drugs, which showed that patients receiving antiepileptic drugs had almost twice the risk of suicidal behavior compared with those receiving a placebo.

## Interactions

Drug interactions that can occur with antiepileptic drugs are numerous and are summarized in Table 14-5. Many of the antiepileptic drugs can interact with each other, requiring close monitoring of the patient. Since many of these drugs induce hepatic metabolism, the effects of other drugs may be reduced, including oral contraceptives. There is a prime opportunity to counsel the patient about need for alternative birth control methods due to reduced efficacy. Carbamazepine is not to be given with grapefruit because this leads to increased toxicity of the antiepileptic drug.

**TABLE 14-4 ADVERSE EFFECTS OF SELECTED ANTIEPILEPTIC DRUGS**

| DRUG OR DRUG CLASS | ADVERSE EFFECTS |
|---|---|
| **First-Line Drugs** | |
| Barbiturates: phenobarbital, primidone | Dizziness, drowsiness, lethargy, paradoxical restlessness |
| Hydantoins: phenytoin, fosphenytoin | Nystagmus, ataxia, drowsiness, rash, gingival hyperplasia, thrombocytopenia, agranulocytosis, hepatitis |
| Iminostilbenes: carbamazepine, oxcarbazepine | Nausea, headache, dizziness, unusual eye movements, visual change, behavioral changes, rash, abdominal pain, abnormal gait |
| valproic acid and derivatives, including valproate sodium and divalproex sodium | Dizziness, drowsiness, GI upset, weight gain, hepatotoxicity, pancreatitis |
| **Adjunct Drugs** | |
| gabapentin | Dizziness, drowsiness, nausea, visual and speech changes, edema |
| pregabalin | Dizziness, drowsiness, peripheral edema, blurred vision |
| lamotrigine | Drowsiness, ataxia, headache, nausea, blurred or double vision |
| levetiracetam | Dizziness, drowsiness, hyperactivity, behavior changes such as anxiety, hostility, agitation, or suicidal ideation, uncoordination |
| Succinimides: ethosuximide | Nausea, abdominal pain, dizziness, drowsiness |
| tiagabine | Dizziness, drowsiness, agitation, asthenia, GI upset, abdominal pain, rash, tremor |
| topiramate | Dizziness, drowsiness, GI upset, ataxia |
| zonisamide | Drowsiness, anorexia, ataxia, confusion, agitation, cognitive impairment |

*GI,* Gastrointestinal.

## Dosages

For certain antiepileptic drugs, the safe and toxic levels are very close together; that is, they have a narrow therapeutic range. Table 14-6 lists the various drugs for which monitoring of therapeutic plasma levels is required and their corresponding therapeutic values. For dosage information see the table on p. 227.

| TABLE 14-5 | SIGNIFICANT DRUG INTERACTIONS OF ANTIEPILEPTIC DRUGS | | |
|---|---|---|---|
| **AED DRUG OR DRUG CLASS** | **INTERACTING DRUG** | **MECHANISM** | **RESULTS** |
| **Barbiturates** | | | |
| | Beta blockers, corticosteroids (e.g., prednisone), oral contraceptives, dihydropyridine, calcium channel blockers, metronidazole, quinidine, theophylline | Altered CYP450 enzyme metabolism | Reduced effects of listed drugs |
| | ethanol (alcohol) | Enhanced CNS depression | Can be fatal |
| **Hydantoins** | | | |
| phenytoin | amiodarone, benzodiazepines, azole antifungals, isoniazid, proton pump inhibitors, sulfonamide antibiotics, SSRIs | Altered CYP450 enzyme metabolism | Reduced hydantoin clearance and increased effects |
| | carbamazepine | Altered CYP450 enzyme metabolism | Increased hydantoin clearance and reduced effects |
| | cyclosporine, loop diuretics, meperidine, methadone, rifampin, quinidine, quetiapine, theophylline, zonisamide | Increased metabolism | Reduced effects of listed drugs |
| | warfarin | Displacement of warfarin from plasma protein binding sites | Increased free warfarin levels and bleeding risk |
| **Iminostilbenes** | | | |
| carbamazepine | Azole antifungals, diltiazem, isoniazid, macrolides, protease inhibitor antiretrovirals, SSRIs, valproic acid, verapamil | Altered CYP450 enzyme metabolism | Increased carbamazepine levels and toxicity risk |
| | Barbiturates, hydantoins, rifampin, succinimides, theophylline | Altered CYP450 enzyme metabolism | Reduced carbamazepine levels and efficacy |
| | acetaminophen | Altered CYP450 enzyme metabolism | Increased hepatic metabolism of acetaminophen and toxicity risk, and reduced efficacy |
| | Antipsychotics, antidepressants, benzodiazepines, cyclosporine, oral contraceptives | Altered CYP450 enzyme metabolism | Reduced efficacy; patient response must be monitored |
| | Monoamine oxidase inhibitors (MAOIs) | Altered CYP450 metabolism | Increased MAOI toxicity risk |
| oxcarbazepine | Barbiturates, hydantoins | Altered CYP450 enzyme metabolism | Increased barbiturate and hydantoin levels and reduced oxcarbazepine levels |
| | valproic acid, verapamil | Altered CYP450 enzyme metabolism | Reduced oxcarbazepine levels |
| | lamotrigine | Altered CYP450 enzyme metabolism | Reduced lamotrigine levels |
| | Oral contraceptives | Altered CYP450 enzyme metabolism | Reduced oral contraceptive levels and increased likelihood of pregnancy |
| **Valproic Acid and Derivatives** | | | |
| valproic acid valproate sodium and divalproex sodium | aspirin | Displacement of valproic acid from plasma protein binding sites | Increased free valproic acid levels and toxicity risk |
| | carbamazepine, oxcarbazepine, lamotrigine | Altered CYP450 enzyme metabolism | Reduced valproic acid efficacy; increased lamotrigine levels; increased or decreased carbamazepine levels |
| | lorazepam | Altered hepatic metabolism | Increased lorazepam toxicity risk |
| | rifampin | Altered CYP450 enzyme metabolism | Reduced valproic acid efficacy |
| | Tricyclic antidepressants | Altered CYP450 enzyme metabolism | Increased tricyclic antidepressant toxicity risk |
| **Succinimides** | | | |
| ethosuximide | Hydantoins, barbiturates, valproic acid | Altered CYP450 enzyme metabolism | Increased or reduced involved drug clearance |
| **Miscellaneous AEDs** | | | |
| gabapentin | Alcohol | Additive CNS depression | Increased CNS depression |
| pregabalin | None listed | | |
| lamotrigine | Hydantoins, oral contraceptives, oxcarbazepine, rifampin | Altered CYP450 enzyme metabolism | Reduced lamotrigine levels and efficacy; may need dosage increase |
| lamotrigine | CNS depressants | Additive effects | Increased CNS depression |

*Continued*

**TABLE 14-5**   **SIGNIFICANT DRUG INTERACTIONS OF ANTIEPILEPTIC DRUGS—cont'd**

| AED DRUG OR DRUG CLASS | INTERACTING DRUG | MECHANISM | RESULTS |
|---|---|---|---|
| lamotrigine | valproic acid | Altered CYP450 enzyme metabolism | Increased lamotrigine levels and toxicity risk; may need dosage reduction |
| levetiracetam | None listed | | |
| tiagabine | CNS depressants | Additive effects | Increased CNS depression |
| topiramate | carbamazepine, hydantoins, valproic acid, oral contraceptives | Altered CYP450 enzyme metabolism | Reduced object drug activity |
| zonisamide | CYP450 enzyme inducers or inhibitors | Altered CYP450 enzyme metabolism | Increased or reduced clearance and effects |

*AED,* Antiepileptic drug; *CNS,* central nervous system; *CYP450,* cytochrome P-450; *GI,* gastrointestinal; *SSRIs,* selective serotonin reuptake inhibitors.

**TABLE 14-6**   **THERAPEUTIC PLASMA LEVELS OF ANTIEPILEPTIC DRUGS WITH A NARROW THERAPEUTIC RANGE**

| ANTIEPILEPTIC DRUG | THERAPEUTIC PLASMA LEVEL (mcg/mL) |
|---|---|
| carbamazepine | 4-12 |
| phenobarbital | 10-40 |
| phenytoin | 10-20 |
| primidone | 5-12 |
| valproic acid | 50-100 |

## DRUG PROFILES

In most children and adults, epilepsy can be controlled with a first-line antiepileptic drug such as carbamazepine (Tegretol), phenobarbital, phenytoin (Dilantin), or valproic acid (Depakene). For patients who do not respond to these first-line drugs, there are a number of second-line or *adjunct* antiepileptic drugs that are used occasionally, such as ethosuximide (Zarontin), primidone (Mysoline), the benzodiazepines (see Chapter 16), diazepam (Valium), clonazepam (Klonopin), clorazepate (Tranxene), and the diuretic acetazolamide (Diamox [see Chapter 28]).

After valproic acid was introduced in 1978, no major new drugs for the treatment of epilepsy were introduced in the United States until the 1990s. Gabapentin (Neurontin), lamotrigine (Lamictal), and felbamate (Felbatol) all were approved during this decade. Although felbamate initially appeared to be a promising antiepileptic drug, there were several case reports of aplastic anemia and acute liver failure associated with its use. As a result, the FDA recommends that felbamate be given only to patients with seizures who do not respond to treatment with all other medications. Because of its rare clinical use, this drug is not discussed further in this book.

Antiepileptic drugs most recently approved include levetiracetam (Keppra), topiramate (Topamax), zonisamide (Zonegran), tiagabine (Gabitril), and pregabalin (Lyrica). These drugs fall into the miscellaneous category of antiepileptics and have greatly expanded the options currently available to treat patients with seizure disorders. Common adverse effects and drug interactions are listed in the individual drug profiles and/or in Tables 14-3 and 14-4. For dosage information, see the table on p. 227.

### BARBITURATES

#### ♦ phenobarbital and primidone

Historically, two of the most commonly used antiepileptic drugs were the barbiturates phenobarbital and primidone (Mysoline). Primidone is metabolized in the liver to phenobarbital and phenylethylmalonamide, both of which have anticonvulsant properties. Use of primidone can provide anticonvulsant activity with a lower serum level of phenobarbital than that attained with phenobarbital itself. This can reduce the likelihood of sedation and fatigue associated with phenobarbital. Phenobarbital is a Schedule IV controlled substance, whereas primidone is not controlled. Phenobarbital has been used since 1912, principally for controlling tonic-clonic and partial seizures. Phenobarbital is used for the management of status epilepticus and is an effective prophylactic drug for the control of febrile seizures. Although phenobarbital is still used to treat seizure emergencies, the use of oral phenobarbital for seizure prevention is much less common. In third-world countries, oral phenobarbital is often the drug of choice for routine seizure prophylaxis because of its low cost. The most common adverse effect of phenobarbital is sedation, although tolerance to this effect usually develops with continued therapy. Therapeutic effects are generally seen at serum drug levels of 10 to 40 mcg/mL. A major advantage of this drug is its long half-life, which allows once-a-day dosing. This can be a substantial advantage for patients who have a difficult time remembering to take their medication or for those who have erratic schedules. Even if a patient takes his or her dose 12 or even 24 hours late, therapeutic blood levels may still be maintained. Contraindications include known drug allergy, porphyria (a disorder of the synthesis of *heme,* a component of hemoglobin), liver or kidney impairment, and respiratory illness. Adverse effects include cardiovascular, CNS, gastrointestinal (GI), and dermatologic reactions (see Table 14-4). Phenobarbital interacts with many drugs because it is a major inducer of hepatic microsomal enzymes, including the cytochrome P-450 system enzymes (see Chapter 2), which causes more rapid clearance of some drugs (see Table 14-5). Phenobarbital is available in oral and injectable forms, whereas primidone is available only for oral use.

## DOSAGES

### Selected Antiepileptic Drugs*

| DRUG (PREGNANCY CATEGORY) | PHARMACOLOGIC CLASS | USUAL DOSAGE RANGE | SEIZURE INDICATIONS |
|---|---|---|---|
| ◆ carbamazepine (Tegretol, Tegretol XR) (D) | Iminostilbene | **Pediatric**<br>PO: younger than 6 yr, 10-20 mg/kg/day<br>PO: 6-12 yr, 200-1000 mg/day<br>**Adult and pediatric older than 12 yr**<br>PO: 400-1200 mg/day | Partial, secondary generalized, generalized tonic-clonic seizures |
| ethosuximide (Zarontin) (C) | Succinimide | **Pediatric**<br>PO: 3-6 yr, 250 mg/day then adjust;<br>older than 6 yr, 500 mg/day then adjust<br>**Adult**<br>PO: 500 mg/day then adjust | Absence seizures |
| ◆ fosphenytoin (Cerebyx) (D) | Hydantoin | **Pediatric**<br>IV: 10-20 PE†/kg loading dose; may begin maintenance dosing 8-12 hr later using pediatric phenytoin dosing guidelines (see below)<br>**Adult**<br>IV: 10-20 PE†/kg loading dose; maintenance dose 4-6 mg/kg/day | Partial, secondary generalized, generalized tonic-clonic seizures |
| ◆ gabapentin (Neurontin) (C) | Miscellaneous | **Pediatric**<br>PO: 10-15 mg/kg/day divided tid, then adjust<br>**Adult**<br>PO: Older than 18 yr, 900-1800 mg/day | Partial, secondary generalized seizures |
| lamotrigine (Lamictal) (C) | Miscellaneous | **Pediatric**<br>PO: 2-12 yr, 5-15 mg/kg/day depending on other AEDs used<br>**Adult**<br>PO: 50-200 mg once daily or divided bid | Partial, secondary generalized, generalized tonic-clonic seizures; seizures associated with Lennox-Gastaut syndrome |
| levetiracetam (Keppra) (C) | Miscellaneous | **Pediatric**<br>20 mg/kg/day in two divided doses<br>**Adult**<br>PO: 500 mg bid to 3000 mg/day | Partial, secondary generalized seizures |
| oxcarbazepine (Trileptal) (C) | Iminostilbene | **Pediatric**<br>PO: 8-10 mg/kg/day divided bid; max 600 mg/day<br>**Adult**<br>300-600 mg bid | Partial, secondary generalized seizures |
| ◆ phenobarbital (oral, injectable) (D) | Barbiturate | **Pediatric**<br>PO: 3-6 mg/kg/day<br><br>**Adult**<br>PO: 1-3 mg/kg/day | Partial, secondary generalized, generalized tonic-clonic seizures, prophylaxis for febrile seizures, psychomotor seizures<br>Partial, secondary generalized, generalized tonic-clonic seizures |
| ◆ phenytoin (Dilantin) (D) | Hydantoin | **Pediatric**<br>PO: 5-10 mg/kg/day, depending on age<br>**Adult**<br>PO: 300-600 mg/day | Partial, secondary generalized, generalized tonic-clonic seizures<br>Generalized tonic-clonic seizures |
| pregabalin (Lyrica) (C) | Miscellaneous | **Adult**<br>PO: 150-600 mg/day divided into 2 or 3 doses | Partial seizures |
| ◆ primidone (Mysoline) (D) | Barbiturate | **Pediatric**<br>PO: younger than 8 yr, 125-250 mg/tid; doses vary based on age<br>**Adult and pediatric older than 8 yr**<br>250 mg orally 4-6 times/day; max 2 g/day | Partial, secondary generalized, generalized tonic-clonic seizures<br><br>Partial, secondary generalized, generalized tonic-clonic seizures |
| tiagabine (Gabitril) (C) | Miscellaneous | **Pediatric**<br>PO: 12-18 yr, 4-32 mg divided bid-qid<br>**Adult**<br>4 mg daily to 56 mg divided bid-qid | Partial, secondary generalized seizures |

*Continued*

## DOSAGES—cont'd

### Selected Antiepileptic Drugs*

| DRUG (PREGNANCY CATEGORY) | PHARMACOLOGIC CLASS | USUAL DOSAGE RANGE | SEIZURE INDICATIONS |
|---|---|---|---|
| topiramate (Topamax) (C) | Miscellaneous | **Pediatric**<br>PO: Doses vary by type of seizure<br>**Adult**<br>PO: 25-1600 mg/day | Partial, secondary generalized, generalized tonic-clonic seizures |
| ◆ valproic acid (Depacon, IV Depakote, Depakene oral) (D) | Miscellaneous | **Adult and pediatric**<br>PO: 15-60 mg/kg/day divided bid-tid<br>IV: 10-15 mg/kg/day as a 60-min infusion | Generalized tonic-clonic, absence, myoclonic seizures |
| zonisamide (Zonegran) (C) | Miscellaneous | **Pediatric**<br>Older than 16 yr, 100-400 mg/day<br>**Adult**<br>100-400 mg/day | Partial, secondary generalized, generalized tonic-clonic, absence, myoclonic seizures |

*AED,* Antiepileptic drug; *IM,* intramuscular; *IV,* intravenous; *PE,* phenytoin equivalent; *PO,* oral.
†One PE = 1.5 mg fosphenytoin = 1 mg phenytoin. Therefore, 1.5 mg fosphenytoin is given for each milligram of phenytoin desired.
*See Table 14-3 for doses of drugs used for status epilepticus.

### Pharmacokinetics (phenobarbital)

| Route | Onset of Action | Peak Plasma Concentration | Elimination Half-life | Duration of Action |
|---|---|---|---|---|
| PO | 20-60 min | 8-12 hr | 50-120 hr | 6-12 hr |
| IV | 5 min | 30 min | 50-120 hr | 6-12 hr |

### Pharmacokinetics (primidone)

| Route | Onset of Action | Peak Plasma Concentration | Elimination Half-life | Duration of Action |
|---|---|---|---|---|
| PO | Unknown | 3-4 hr | 10-12 hr* | Unknown |

*Longer for active metabolites, including phenobarbital.

## HYDANTOINS

### ◆ phenytoin and fosphenytoin

Phenytoin (Dilantin) has been used as a first-line drug for many years and is the prototypical drug. It is indicated for the management of tonic-clonic and partial seizures. Contraindications include known drug allergy and heart conditions that involve bradycardia or blockage of electrocardiac function. Adverse effects and drug interactions both are numerous and are listed in Table 14-4 and 14-5, respectively. The most common adverse effects are lethargy, abnormal movements, mental confusion, and cognitive changes. Gingival hyperplasia is a well-known adverse effect of long-term oral phenytoin therapy. Scrupulous dental care can help prevent gingival hypertrophy. Long-term phenytoin therapy can cause gingival hyperplasia, acne, hirsutism, and hypertrophy of subcutaneous facial tissue resulting in an appearance known as *Dilantin facies.* Another long-term consequence of phenytoin therapy is osteoporosis. Vitamin D therapy may help to prevent this, particularly in women. Therapeutic drug levels are usually 10 to 20 mcg/mL. At toxic levels, phenytoin can cause nystagmus, ataxia, dysarthria, and encephalopathy. Phenytoin can interact with other medications for two main reasons. First, it is highly bound to plasma proteins and competes with other highly protein-bound medications for

binding sites. Second, it induces hepatic microsomal enzymes, mainly cytochrome P-450 enzymes (see Chapter 2). This increases the metabolism of other drugs that are metabolized by these enzymes and reduces their blood levels.

Exaggerated phenytoin effects can be seen in patients with very low serum albumin concentrations. This most commonly occurs in patients who are malnourished or have chronic renal failure. In these patients, it may be necessary to maintain phenytoin levels well below 20 mcg/mL. With lower levels of albumin, more of the free, unbound, pharmacologically active phenytoin molecules will be present in the blood.

Phenytoin has many advantages for long-term therapy. It is usually well tolerated, highly effective, and relatively inexpensive. It can also be given intravenously if needed. Most often, however, phenytoin is taken orally. The long half-life of the drug allows for twice- or even once-daily dosing. This encourages patient adherence to drug therapy, which helps reduce seizure frequency.

Parenteral phenytoin is adjusted chemically to a pH of 12 for reasons of drug stability. It is very irritating to veins when injected and must be given by slow intravenous (IV) push (not exceeding 50 mg/min in adults) directly into a large vein through a large-gauge (20-gauge or larger) venous catheter. Phenytoin is only to be diluted in normal saline (NS) for IV infusion, and a filter must be used. Follow each dose by an injection of a saline flush to avoid local venous irritation. Soft-tissue irritation and inflammation can occur at the site of injection with or without extravasation. This can vary from slight tenderness to extensive necrosis and sloughing, and in rare instances can require amputation. Avoid improper administration, including subcutaneous or perivascular injection, to help prevent the possibility of such occurrences.

Fosphenytoin (Cerebyx) is an injectable prodrug of phenytoin that was developed in an attempt to overcome some of the chemical disadvantages of phenytoin injection. Fosphenytoin is a water-soluble phenytoin derivative that can be given intramuscularly or intravenously—by IV push or continuous

## TABLE 14-7  COMPARISON OF PHENYTOIN SODIUM AND FOSPHENYTOIN SODIUM

| | PHENYTOIN SODIUM (DILANTIN IV) | FOSPHENYTOIN SODIUM (CEREBYX IM/IV) |
|---|---|---|
| pH | 12 | 8.6-9 |
| Maximum infusion rate | 50 mg/min | 150 mg PE*/min |
| Admixtures | 0.9% saline | 0.9% saline or 5% dextrose |

*IM*, Intramuscular; *IV*, intravenous; *PE*, phenytoin sodium equivalents.
*150 mg fosphenytoin sodium = 100 mg phenytoin sodium.

infusion—without causing burning on injection associated with phenytoin. Fosphenytoin is dosed in *phenytoin equivalents (PE)* as indicated in Table 14-7. Fosphenytoin is given at a rate of 150 mg PE/min or less to avoid hypotension or cardiorespiratory depression. If dysrhythmias or hypotension occur, discontinue the infusion. Implement fall prevention measures after infusion of either phenytoin or fosphenytoin because of possible ataxia and dizziness. Take vital signs up to 2 hours after infusion. Check available references and/or consult with a pharmacist before administering because there are numerous IV incompatibilities with both drugs.

### Pharmacokinetics (phenytoin)

| Route | Onset of Action | Peak Plasma Concentration | Elimination Half-life | Duration of Action |
|---|---|---|---|---|
| PO | Unknown | 12 hr | 7-42 hr | 12-36 hr |
| IV | 1-2 hr | 2-3 hr | 7-42 hr | 12-24 hr |

## IMINOSTILBENES
### ♦ carbamazepine

Carbamazepine (Tegretol) is the second most commonly prescribed antiepileptic drug in the United States, after phenytoin. It was marketed in the late 1960s for the treatment of epilepsy after its efficacy and safety were proven for the treatment of *trigeminal neuralgia* (a painful facial nerve condition). It is chemically related to the *tricyclic* antidepressants (see Chapter 16) and is considered a first-line treatment for partial seizures and generalized tonic-clonic seizures. It may actually worsen myoclonic or absence seizures. Therefore its use is contraindicated in both of these conditions as well as in cases of known drug allergy and bone marrow depression. Carbamazepine is associated with autoinduction of hepatic enzymes. Autoinduction is a process in which, over time, a drug stimulates the production of enzymes that enhance its own metabolism, which leads to lower than expected drug concentrations. With carbamazepine, this process usually occurs within the first 2 months after starting the drug. Carbamazepine has numerous adverse reactions and drug interactions; examples are given in Tables 14-4 and 14-5. It is available for oral use only.

### Pharmacokinetics

| Route | Onset of Action | Peak Plasma Concentration | Elimination Half-life | Duration of Action |
|---|---|---|---|---|
| PO | Slow | 4-8 hr | 25-65 hr | 12-24 hr |

### oxcarbazepine

Oxcarbazepine (Trileptal) is a chemical analogue of carbamazepine. Its precise mechanism of action has not been identified, although it is known to block voltage-sensitive sodium channels, which aids in stabilizing excited neuronal membranes. It is indicated for partial seizures and secondarily generalized seizures. Contraindications include known drug allergy. Common adverse reactions include headache, dizziness, and nausea (see also Table 14-4). Unlike carbamazepine, this drug is not a hepatic enzyme inducer. As a result, it is associated with far fewer common drug interactions than is carbamazepine (see Table 14-5). Oxcarbazepine is available for oral use only.

### Pharmacokinetics

| Route | Onset of Action | Peak Plasma Concentration | Elimination Half-life | Duration of Action |
|---|---|---|---|---|
| PO | 2-4 hr | 2-3 days | 2-9 hr | Unknown |

## SUCCINIMIDE
### ethosuximide

Ethosuximide (Zarontin) is used in the treatment of uncomplicated absence seizures. It is not effective for secondary generalized tonic-clonic seizures. The only listed contraindication for either use is known allergy to succinimides. Adverse effects include GI and CNS effects (see Table 14-4). Drug interactions most commonly involve hepatic enzyme–inducing drugs (see Table 14-5). Succinimides are available for oral use only.

### Pharmacokinetics

| Route | Onset of Action | Peak Plasma Concentration | Elimination Half-life | Duration of Action |
|---|---|---|---|---|
| PO | Unknown | 4 hr | 60 hr | Unknown |

## MISCELLANEOUS DRUGS
### ♦ gabapentin

Gabapentin (Neurontin) is a chemical analogue of *GABA*, a neurotransmitter that inhibits brain activity. The exact mechanism of action of gabapentin is unknown. Many believe that it works by increasing the synthesis and synaptic accumulation of GABA between neurons, hence, the drug name. It is indicated as an adjunct drug for the treatment of partial seizures and for prophylaxis of partial seizures. Evidence also shows gabapentin to be effective as single-drug therapy for new-onset epilepsy. It is most commonly used to treat neuropathic pain (see Chapter 10). Contraindications include known drug allergy. Adverse effects include CNS and GI symptoms (see Table 14-4). Drug interactions are listed in Table 14-5. Gabapentin is available for oral use only.

**Pharmacokinetics**

| Route | Onset of Action | Peak Plasma Concentration | Elimination Half-life | Duration of Action |
|---|---|---|---|---|
| PO | Unknown | Unknown | 5-7 hr | Unknown |

### pregabalin

Pregabalin (Lyrica), like gabapentin, is structurally related to the inhibitory neurotransmitter GABA. However, it does not bind to GABA receptors but rather to the alpha$_2$-delta receptor sites, which affect calcium channels in CNS tissues. Its mechanism of action is still not fully understood. Pregabalin is a Schedule V controlled substance. The drug is indicated as adjunct therapy for partial seizures, although it is most commonly used for *neuropathic pain* (see Chapter 10), and *postherpetic neuralgia* (see Chapter 40). Contraindications include known drug allergy. Adverse drug reactions are primarily CNS related (see Table 14-4). No clinically significant drug interactions are listed to date; however, as with all antiepileptic drugs, the potential for additive CNS depression exists when other sedating drugs are used. Pregabalin is available for oral use only.

**Pharmacokinetics**

| Route | Onset of Action | Peak Plasma Concentration | Elimination Half-life | Duration of Action |
|---|---|---|---|---|
| PO | Unknown | 1.5 hr | 6 hr | Unknown |

### lamotrigine

Lamotrigine (Lamictal) is indicated for simple or complex partial seizures, for generalized seizures related to *Lennox-Gastaut syndrome* (an atypical form of absence epilepsy that may persist into adulthood), and, most recently, for primary generalized tonic-clonic seizures. It is also used for the treatment of bipolar disorder. It has no known contraindications other than drug allergy. Common adverse effects include relatively minor CNS and GI symptoms (see Table 14-4). One potentially serious adverse effect is a rash that can progress to the major dermatologic reaction known as *Stevens-Johnson syndrome.* This condition involves inflammation and sloughing of skin, potentially over the entire body, in a manner that resembles a third-degree burn. It is often reversible but can also be fatal. To avoid this condition, patients' doses are very slowly titrated over several weeks. Drug interactions chiefly involve other antiepileptic drugs as well as other CNS depressants and oral contraceptives (see Table 14-5). Lamotrigine is available for oral use only.

**Pharmacokinetics**

| Route | Onset of Action | Peak Plasma Concentration | Elimination Half-life | Duration of Action |
|---|---|---|---|---|
| PO | Unknown | 1.4-2.3 hr | 24 hr | Unknown |

### levetiracetam

Levetiracetam (Keppra) is indicated as adjunct therapy for partial seizures with and without secondary generalization. It is contraindicated in cases of known drug allergy. Its mechanism of action is unknown. It is generally well tolerated, with the most common adverse effects being CNS related (see Table 14-4). No drug interactions are currently listed; however, like all antiepileptic drugs, the potential for excessive CNS depression exists when it is used in combination with other sedating drugs. Levetiracetam is available in both oral and injectable forms.

**Pharmacokinetics**

| Route | Onset of Action | Peak Plasma Concentration | Elimination Half-life | Duration of Action |
|---|---|---|---|---|
| PO | Rapid | 1 hr | 6-8 hr | Unknown |

### tiagabine

Tiagabine (Gabitril) is indicated as adjunct therapy for partial seizures. Contraindications include known drug allergy. Its exact mechanism of action has not been identified, but is known to have beneficial effects by inhibiting the reuptake of GABA from the neuronal synapses (spaces between neurons) in the brain. In February 2005, the FDA issued a special warning regarding the use of tiagabine for "off-label" (non–FDA-approved) indications. Although tiagabine is effective in controlling epileptic seizures, there have been several case reports of *paradoxical* seizures (opposite of what would intuitively be expected) in nonepileptic patients who are treated with the drug for other indications. Most of these cases involved patients being treated for psychiatric disorders such as bipolar disorder. Of even greater concern is that in some of these cases the seizure episodes progressed to status epilepticus. For these reasons, prescribers are currently advised to avoid off-label use of tiagabine. Common adverse effects are CNS and GI symptoms (see Table 14-4). Drug interactions chiefly involve other CNS depressant drugs (see Table 14-5). Tiagabine is available for oral use only.

**Pharmacokinetics**

| Route | Onset of Action | Peak Plasma Concentration | Elimination Half-life | Duration of Action |
|---|---|---|---|---|
| PO | Rapid | 45 min | 7-9 hr | Unknown |

### topiramate

Topiramate (Topamax) is a structurally unique drug chemically related to fructose. It is indicated as adjunct therapy for partial and secondarily generalized seizures, for generalized tonic-clonic seizures, and for drop attacks in Lennox-Gastaut syndrome. Contraindications include known drug allergy. Its exact mechanism of action is unknown. Common adverse effects are primarily CNS related (see Table 14-4). Angle-closure glaucoma can also occur, and the patient must immediately report any visual changes. Common drug interactions involve chiefly other antiepileptic drugs and oral contraceptives (see Table 14-5). Topiramate is available for oral use only. In 2011, the FDA notified health care professionals about an increased risk of cleft palate in children born to mothers who were taking topiramate during pregnancy.

## Pharmacokinetics

| Route | Onset of Action | Peak Plasma Concentration | Elimination Half-life | Duration of Action |
|---|---|---|---|---|
| PO | Unknown | 2-4 hr | 21 hr | Unknown |

### ◆ valproic acid

Valproic acid is used primarily in the treatment of generalized seizures (absence, myoclonic, and tonic-clonic). It is also used for bipolar disorder (see Chapter 16) and has been shown to be effective in controlling partial seizures. Contraindications include known drug allergy, liver impairment, and *urea cycle* disorders (genetic disorders of urea metabolism). Common adverse effects include drowsiness; nausea, vomiting, and other GI disturbances; tremor; weight gain; and transient hair loss (see Table 14-4). The most serious adverse effects are hepatotoxicity and pancreatitis. Valproic acid can interact with many medications (see Table 14-5). The main reasons for these interactions are protein binding and liver metabolism. It is highly bound to plasma proteins and competes with other highly protein-bound medications for binding sites. It also is metabolized by hepatic microsomal enzymes and competes for metabolism with other drugs. In contrast to phenobarbital and phenytoin, it is not a hepatic enzyme inducer. It is available in both oral and injectable forms. Valproic acid itself is chemically the simplest dosage form and is available as an oral liquid. Long-acting oral dosage forms are also available as divalproex sodium (Depakote), which comes in delayed- and extended-release tablets as well as capsules with long-acting granules (Depakote Sprinkles) that can be opened and sprinkled into food. The injectable form is the salt valproate sodium (Depacon).

## Pharmacokinetics

| Route | Onset of Action | Peak Plasma Concentration | Elimination Half-life | Duration of Action |
|---|---|---|---|---|
| PO, IV | 15-30 min | 1-4 hr | 6-16 hr | 4-6 hr |

### zonisamide

Zonisamide (Zonegran) is a sulfonamide derivative (see Chapter 38) indicated for a variety of seizure types, including partial and secondary generalized, primary generalized, absence, and myoclonic. It is contraindicated in patients with known drug allergy to the drug itself or to sulfa drugs (see Chapter 38). Common adverse effects include CNS and GI symptoms (see Table 14-4). Zonisamide interacts with a number of drugs metabolized by cytochrome P-450 enzymes, which increase or decrease clearance of zonisamide (see Table 14-5). Zonisamide is available for oral use only.

## Pharmacokinetics

| Route | Onset of Action | Peak Plasma Concentration | Elimination Half-life | Duration of Action |
|---|---|---|---|---|
| PO | Rapid | 2-6 hr | 63 hr | Unknown |

## ⚡ SAFETY AND QUALITY IMPROVEMENT: PREVENTING MEDICATION ERRORS

### Sound-Alike/Look-Alike Drugs: Cerebryx and Celebrex

Be careful with drug names! When using their trade names, Cerebryx and Celebrex sound and look very much alike. However, they are quite different. Cerebryx is a trade name for fosphenytoin, a hydantoin class antiepeliptic drug. It is used to treat a variety of seizure disorders. Celebrex is the trade name for celecoxib, a COX-2 inhibitor antiinflammatory drug used for pain and various disorders such as osteoarthritis and rheumatoid arthritis (see Chapter 44). Although the trade names are very similar, the indications are very different! These two drugs illustrate the importance of using both the trade name and generic name when ordering medications.

## NURSING PROCESS

## ASSESSMENT

With use of any of the *antiepileptic drugs,* perform a thorough physical assessment and obtain a comprehensive health and medication history, so that any possible allergies, drug interactions, adverse reactions, cautions, and contraindications can be identified. Thoroughly review the patient's medical history, and note any type of seizure disorder, precipitating events, and the duration, frequency, and intensity of the seizure activity. Other information to assess for includes the occurrence of any other problems or signs and symptoms occurring before, during, or after the seizure. Question the patient about the occurrence of panic attacks because of the possible association between high levels of anxiety or stress and the precipitation of seizures in those at risk. Assess the patient for signs and symptoms of autonomic nervous system responses associated with anxiety or stress such as cold, clammy hands, excessive sweating (diaphoresis), agitation, and trembling of the extremities. Additional assessment about other problems or symptoms is important because some antiepileptic medications may be indicated for other medical diagnoses, such as prevention of migraines or treatment of postherpetic neuralgia and neuropathic pain. A complete neurologic assessment with documentation of baseline CNS functioning is also important before administering antiepileptic drugs. This may include testing and grading the response of deep tendon reflexes, bilateral and upper and lower extremity sensory and motor testing, and questioning about the presence of any headaches, photosensitivity, occurrence of auras, or visual changes.

Before giving these drugs, review the laboratory test results, which may include the results of red blood cell and white blood cell counts, clotting studies, and renal and/or liver function studies. Knowing baseline levels of these laboratory values is important to help identify any initial abnormalities as well as to provide a comparison value when assessing for possible adverse effects, cautions, contraindications, and interactions. Assess urinary output (at least 30 mL/hr) and urine specific gravity. Conditions other than epilepsy or seizure disorders may also cause loss of or alterations in consciousness and are worthy of consideration during assessment. These conditions include syncope, breath-holding practices, transient ischemic attacks, drug use, metabolic disorders, infections, head trauma, tumors, and psychogenic problems. Therefore, an attempt will most likely be made to rule out or eliminate many of these disorders or conditions during the diagnosing of epilepsy, and therein lies the importance of analyzing all available points of data. An EEG may also be ordered to provide more information related to the diagnosis of epilepsy. Another diagnostic procedure, magnetic resonance imaging, may be performed for neuroimaging and further data gathering.

The use of a *succinimide,* such as ethosuximide, requires assessment for the specific indication for this medication, that is, generalized absence seizures. In addition to performing a baseline neurologic assessment, other questions to pose to the patient include inquiring about any problems with nausea, abdominal pain, or dizziness. Always assess for any allergies to this drug.

*Miscellaneous* drugs such as tiagabine, topiramate, and zonisamide are some of the more recently available antiepileptic drugs and have significant contraindications, cautions, and drug interactions, which have been discussed previously in the Pharmacology Overview in this chapter and are summarized in Tables 14-4 and 14-5. Assess vital signs and mental status with attention to the patient's sensorium, level of alertness or consciousness, and any mental depression before, during, and after drug therapy and/or seizure activity. Document any of the following baseline problems if administering tiagabine or topiramate: dizziness, drowsiness, GI upset, ataxia, and/or agitation.

If *barbiturates* have been ordered, carefully assess not only the neurologic system but also vital signs because of the CNS depression associated with this class of drugs. Obtain and document all of the aforementioned general assessment data when barbiturates are prescribed. In addition, identify patients at high risk for excessive sedation for safety purposes. If the patient is in an acute care facility, assess the room and environment to ensure that safety measures are in place (e.g., side rails up or a bed alarm system in use depending on facility policy), noise level is controlled, and seizure precautions are available (oxygen, suctioning equipment, and airway devices nearby; padded side rails being used; and IV access obtained per facility policy). Note the patient's age, because the very young and the elderly react with more sensitivity to these drugs with paradoxical reactions, irritability, and hyperactivity (as compared to CNS depressant effects). Cautions, contraindications, and drug interactions have been previously discussed in the Pharmacology Overview.

With *hydantoins* like phenytoin, the previously mentioned assessment data are also appropriate. Perform a skin assessment and document intactness and the presence or absence of any rashes, because of the possibility of a measles-like rash. In addition, baseline dental hygiene habits and an oral assessment, such as the status of the patient's gums and teeth, are important because of the adverse effects of gingival hyperplasia. Assessment of baseline neurologic functioning is crucial with the use of these CNS-altering medications and needs to include the following: (1) a focus on vision with attention to any abnormalities, especially those related to eye movement; (2) baseline neuromuscular stability with attention to coordinated movements, gait, and reflexes; and (3) assessment of speech for clarity and ability to form and express words appropriately. In addition, when the phenytoins are taken, baseline liver function studies and complete blood counts are needed. Attention must also be given to specific drug-related cautions, contraindications, and drug interactions.

Before administering carbamazepine, an *iminostilbene,* a complete blood count is often ordered. Document these laboratory findings for baseline comparisons because of the possible adverse effect of drug-related anemias (e.g., aplastic anemia). Measure baseline vision and any abnormalities because of the potential visual changes. Significant contraindications include conditions involving bone marrow suppression because it is an adverse effect (though rare).

*Gabapentin* requires a thorough neurologic assessment with attention to baseline energy levels, visual intactness, sensory and motor functioning, and any changes in speech. It is also important to understand the rationale for gabapentin's use so that appropriate education and instructions can be shared with the patient and family. For example, gabapentin may be used for seizure therapy, but it is also used to treat postherpetic neuralgia and neuropathic pain and to prevent migraines. Thus, an individualized plan of care with proper education needs to be developed from the appropriate assessment data. Pregabalin is similar to gabapentin and requires the same assessment.

*Valproic acid* requires a careful assessment, as well. Gather and document information about the patient's medical history, medication profile, and neurologic system with information about seizure activity (see previous discussion). Assessment for drug allergies, cautions, contraindications, and drug interactions has been previously discussed. Other assessment areas include baseline weight, liver function studies, and notation of a history of pancreatitis.

*Lamotrigine* use requires a thorough neurologic assessment and documentation of baseline energy levels, vision acuity, and history of headaches for comparative purposes due to common adverse effects of headaches, vision changes, and drowsiness. Several newer *miscellaneous antiepileptic drugs* are available, such as levetiracetam, topiramate, zonisamide, tiagabine, and pregabalin. These miscellaneous drugs require the same thorough, general assessment as with other antiepileptic drugs. A few additional points must be kept in mind. For example, in patients taking levetiracetam, you must document the presence of any neuropsychiatric symptoms because of the potential for drug-related agitation, depression, anxiety, and other mood or behavioral changes. Although these adverse effects are rare, the assessment data must still be thorough. One interesting fact, as noted in the pharmacology section, is the lack of drug interactions with levetiracetam; however, because all antiepileptic drugs depress the CNS in some manner, assessment for the use of other CNS depressant drugs is important to note. In addition, assess liver and renal functioning before therapy is initiated. Topiramate is used not only for management of seizures but also for other indications such as cluster headaches and neuropathic pain. Therefore, include a thorough review of the medical and medication history in the assessment to understand the reason for the drug's use. Document energy levels as well.

## Medications for Seizures

Devin, a 21-year-old patient, has been brought to the emergency department in status epilepticus. Measures are taken to ensure her safety and prevent injury, and an intravenous (IV) line is started. The emergency department physician has ordered diazepam (Valium) 8 mg IV push, STAT.

1. The diazepam is supplied in a vial of 5 mg/mL. How much medication will the nurse draw up into the syringe?

The IV diazepam is given at a rate of 2 mg/min. Soon after the IV diazepam is given, Devin's seizures stop, and she regains consciousness. She is admitted to a medical-surgical unit, and her mother goes to the room with her. The admitting orders call for an initial IV dose of phenytoin, followed by oral doses twice a day.

2. Why was the loading dose given intravenously?

After 2 days of observation, Devin is ready for discharge to her mother's home. Her phenytoin level is 16 mcg/mL. She is very concerned about how the phenytoin will affect her.

3. Evaluate the phenytoin level of 16 mcg/mL.

4. What teaching should the patient receive regarding self-care and the adverse effects of phenytoin?

5. After 4 months, the patient's mother calls to report that Devin has seemed "very sad lately" and has not wanted to join her friends for evenings out. "Devin just goes to work, then comes home and stays in her room." What is the priority in this situation?

For answers, see http:/evolve.elsevier.com/Lilley.

## NURSING DIAGNOSES

1. Deficient knowledge related to lack of familiarity and minimal experience with and lack of information concerning the use of antiepileptic drugs

2. Noncompliance with the therapeutic regimen related to the patient's misuse of drugs or lack of understanding about the seizure disorder and its treatment

3. Chronic low self-esteem related to diagnosis of a lifelong disease and the adverse effects associated with antiepileptic drugs

4. Risk for injury related to decreased sensorium and CNS depression associated with the actions and adverse effects of antiepileptic drugs

## PLANNING

### GOALS

1. Patient demonstrates adequate knowledge about diagnosis and associated drug therapy.

2. Patient remains compliant with the therapy regimen, avoids adverse effects as much as possible, and experiences minimal problems with either overtreatment or undertreatment.

3. Patient maintains positive self-esteem and body image.

4. Patient remains free from injury during drug therapy.

### OUTCOME CRITERIA

1. Patient states the therapeutic drug effects (e.g., minimal to no seizure activity) as well as adverse effects of antiepileptic drugs and measures to decrease drug-related sedation, confusion, ataxia, and drowsiness.

2. Patient and/or family states the importance of taking the medication exactly as prescribed, such as at the same time every day, to help maximize therapeutic effectiveness and minimize adverse effects.
   • Patient states the dangers associated with sudden withdrawal of the medication, such as rebound seizure activity.

3. Patient communicates openly and frequently about diagnosis-related and drug-related changes in self-esteem as well as increase in feelings of anxiety, stress, and/or altered body image.

4. Patient experiences a safe and protective environment while at home/work while implementing safety measures to minimize injury to self such as changing positions slowly and purposely, keeping throw rugs off the floor.
   • Patient reports symptoms of excessive sedation, confusion, lethargy, and dizziness to prescriber.

## IMPLEMENTATION

For patients taking *antiepileptic* drugs, interventions are aimed at monitoring the patient while providing safety measures (see previous discussion) and securing the airway, breathing, and circulation. Airway maintenance is of critical importance for epileptic patients because the tongue relaxes during seizure activity, falling backward and subsequently blocking the airway. Maintain the patient's airway in the same way as during cardiopulmonary resuscitation, using the chin lift or jaw thrust method. Provide rescue breathing, if the patient is not breathing on his or her own, at a rate of 1 breath every 5 seconds. If the patient is breathing, keep the airway open through proper positioning (as just described). In addition to performing these critical components of care, maintain seizure precautions according to hospital policy. This may include making sure the patient is gently kept in bed or kept from falling, putting the side rails up, placing the patient in a side-lying position if needed. Avoid use of a tongue blade or other instrument to pry open the patient's mouth or clenched teeth, and ensure quick access to oxygen and suctioning equipment at all times.

With antiepileptic drug administration, adhere closely to the drug dose and frequency of dosing, as ordered. Close monitoring of dosing is important to attain therapeutic blood levels. For example, if an antiepileptic drug is ordered to be administered every 6 hours, it is crucial to dose the drug so that it is given around the clock to maintain blood levels. Administering the antiepileptic drug at the same time every day is also important to maintain blood levels. Educate patients on the importance of adhering to the medication regimen due to the impact one dose may have on maintaining steady states and therapeutic blood levels (see Chapter 2). If one or more doses of the antiepileptic drug is missed, the prescriber needs to be contacted immediately due to the increased risk of seizure activity. See Patient Teaching Tips for more information.

With oral dosing, it is recommended that these drugs be taken with at least 6 to 8 oz of fluid, preferably water, and with food, meals, or a snack to help decrease the risk of GI upset, a frequently encountered adverse effect. Juices, milk, and carbonated beverages are best avoided as the fluids of choice because of possible interactions with the drug. Oral suspensions are to be shaken and the solution mixed thoroughly. Capsules are *not* to be crushed, opened, or chewed—especially if extended- or long-release forms. Chewing or altering these long-release type formulations would allow for the entire dosage to be released at once versus over a period of time. Extended-release dosage forms are usually ordered once a day, and so checking and double-checking the dosage and frequency is critical to patient safety. These actions will help to prevent the patient from experiencing either too high or too low drug serum levels.

If there are any questions regarding the type of capsule, pill, or tablet or questions about other dosage forms and recommended administration guidelines, use appropriate authoritative sources. These sources would include a licensed pharmacist, manufacturer-package insert, and/or a current (within last 3 years) nursing drug handbook or pharmacology book. If there are any questions about the medication order or the medication prescribed, contact the prescriber immediately for clarification. *Topiramate* and *valproic acid* tablets and delayed- or extended-release dosage forms are not to be altered in any way and must be given as prescribed.

The following interventions are specific to drugs and/or drug classes:

- *Carbamazepine:* This drug is *not* to be given with grapefruit/grapefruit juice because this leads to increased toxicity of the antiepileptic drug. If the drug is to be replaced with another antiepileptic drug, a plan needs to be in place to decrease the dosages of the older drug before beginning low doses (at first) of the newer drug. Serum therapeutic levels are given in Table 14-6.
- *Hydantoins:* As a point of reference, 150 mg of fosphenytoin is the equivalent of 100 mg of phenytoin, and the dose, concentration solution, and infusion rate of fosphenytoin is expressed as a phenytoin equivalent (PE). With parenteral forms, the only dilutional fluid to use with these drugs is normal saline (NS). A filter must also be used. Rates of infusion must follow manufacturer's guidelines and are usually 150 mg PE/min or less to avoid hypotension and cardiorespiratory depression. If dysrhythmias or hypotension occur, discontinue the infusion immediately, monitor patient vital signs, and contact the prescriber immediately. Implement safety measures, such as assisting the patient with ambulation and having the patient move slowly and purposefully, when this drug (or any other antiepileptic drug) is given because of the adverse effects of ataxia and dizziness. IV dose administration requires even more cautious use because of the rapid onset of action. CNS depression is always a concern; thus, there is a need to frequently monitor the patient's vital signs. If existing IV lines contain D$_5$W or other solutions, the line must be flushed with normal saline before and after dosing to avoid precipitate

formation. If infiltration of the IV site leads to subcutaneous tissue access, ischemia and sloughing may occur because of the high alkalinity of the drug. Review hospital or facility policy as well as manufacturer's guidelines regarding the use of possible antidotes. If infiltration occurs, discontinue infusion of the solution immediately, but leave the IV catheter/needle in place until all orders from the prescriber have been received. This practice allows any antidote medication to be administered through the IV catheter, if ordered. Sustained- or extended-release oral dosage forms are never to be opened, punctured, chewed, or broken in pieces. Other regular forms of the drug may be crushed, as needed. Gingival hyperplasia is an adverse effect and requires that the patient receive daily oral care as well as frequent dental visits. Complete blood counts are often monitored very closely within the first year of therapy (e.g., measured monthly for 1 year, then every 3 months).

- *Barbiturates* (e.g., phenobarbital): Abrupt withdrawal of these drugs, as well as of any antiepileptic drugs, must be avoided due to possible rebound seizure activity. Most of the oral dosage forms of this class of drugs are to be taken with water. Elixir dosage forms may be safely mixed with fruit juice, milk, or water. If IV infusions are indicated, calculate the dose carefully and use an IV infusion pump to administer the drug. Too rapid an infusion of IV dosage forms may lead to cardiovascular collapse and respiratory depression. In addition, frequently monitor vital signs and IV infusion rates and document in the patient's chart. If any signs or symptoms of cardiovascular or respiratory depression are noted, withhold the drug and contact the prescriber immediately while providing supportive care through maintenance of the airway, breathing, and circulation.
- *Gabapentin:* This is one of the antiepileptic drugs that can be taken without regard to meals. If discontinuation of the drug is indicated, taper the dosage, as ordered, over at least 1 week to avoid rebound seizures.
- *Lamotrigine:* The dosing regimen must be followed, as ordered. Checking for possible drug interactions is important to patient safety. If the patient shares any suicidal thoughts or actions, contact the prescriber immediately.
- *Levetiracetam:* The most common adverse effect is sleepiness. Contact the prescriber if any extreme adverse effects or any problems with moving, walking, or changes in mood/behavior occur. Any suicidal thoughts or psychotic symptoms must also be reported immediately. With the beginning of antiepileptic therapy, encourage the patient not to drive, operate heavy machinery, or make major decisions due to the sedation and CNS depression.
- *Oxcarbazepine:* This drug is to be taken as prescribed and is usually given in two divided doses. Always check for any potential drug interactions before administering (see previous discussion). The drug must be taken with food or snacks. Rash, abnormal walking or moving, or abdominal pain must also be reported, if present.
- *Pregabalin:* The daily dosage is usually given in two or three divided doses. Sudden or abrupt withdrawal is to be avoided.

Monitor the patient for any excessive dizziness, ocular or visual changes, or edema. If these are present, report immediately.

- *Tiagabine:* This drug is to be taken with food. Report any problems with tremors, rash, or abdominal pain.
- *Valproic acid:* Oral dosage forms are not to be taken with carbonated beverages. It is recommended that this drug be taken with at least 4 to 6 oz of water, food, or a snack to minimize GI upset.

## EVALUATION

The occurrence of a therapeutic response to *antiepileptic drugs* does not mean that the patient has been cured of the seizures but only that seizure activity is decreased or absent. Thoroughly document any response to the medication in the nurse's notes. These classes of medications have other indications, such as management of chronic pain and migraines, so the existing problem or disorder would show improvement with minimal adverse effects. In addition, when monitoring and evaluating the effects of antiepileptic drugs, constantly assess the patient for changes in mental status/level of consciousness, affect, eye problems, or visual disorders. Monitoring CBC is also important because of the occurrence of blood dyscrasias. Measurements of serum levels of the specific antiepileptic drug are ordered at baseline or at the start of therapy and frequently thereafter to determine if subsequent serum levels are subtherapeutic, therapeutic, or toxic. Subtherapeutic levels indicate that the dosage may need to be increased (by the prescriber), and toxic levels require withholding or decreasing the dose—but only if prescribed! Serum therapeutic levels are found in Table 14-6.

## PATIENT TEACHING TIPS

- Educate the patient about the sedating effects of drug therapy so that appropriate steps can be taken to ensure patient safety until a steady state is achieved (usually after four or five drug half-lives). The patient is not to drive, operate heavy machinery, or make major decisions until steady state is achieved.
- The patient needs to understand the importance of reporting any suicidal thoughts or ideas immediately. Alcohol, caffeine intake, and smoking are to be avoided.
- Antiepileptic drugs must never be abruptly discontinued as it may precipitate rebound seizure activity.
- The adverse effects most commonly associated with these drugs are drowsiness, GI upset, and CNS-depressing effects. Remind the patient that these adverse effects often decrease after the drug has been taken for several weeks. Taking the antiepileptic drug with food and/or 6 to 8 oz of fluids will help to minimize GI upset, unless otherwise noted.
- Advise the female patient contemplating pregnancy to seek education and medical advice from the prescriber due to the teratogenic effects of some of the medications.
- Educate the patient about drug interactions between antiepileptic drugs and beta blockers, corticosteroids, calcium channel blockers, ethanol (alcohol), and other CNS depressants.
- Inform the patient that a recurrence of seizure activity is usually due to a lack of compliance with the drug regimen. If a dose or doses of medication are missed, the prescriber needs to be contacted for further instructions. Adherence to medication regimen is critical to the prevention of seizure activity.
- Emphasize to the patient that treatment of epilepsy is lifelong and that compliance with the treatment regimen is important for effective therapy. Share information with the patient and family about community and other appropriate resources (e.g., national and local support groups).

- Discuss with the patient important ways to improve *safety* in day-to-day activities while taking antiepileptic drugs: *In the kitchen:* Use an electric stove with no open flame, wear oven mitts, and cook only on rear burners. Cook in the microwave—it is the safest option. Have a plumber install a heat-control device on faucets to avoid burns. Carpet floors to help cushion falls, and use plastic dishes and containers instead of glass when possible. *In the bathroom:* Use heat-control devices on faucets. Carpet floors instead of using tile. Do not put a lock on the bathroom door so that help can be obtained if needed. Bathe with only a few inches of water in the tub, and if seizure activity has not been fully controlled, bathe while someone else is present in the home. *During activities:* Always have someone along when engaging in sports, and make sure the person is knowledgeable about the management of airway and seizures. Bike riding with a helmet, swimming, and water sports are okay if an accompanying adult is present who knows how to manage seizure activity and its consequences.
- Each state has different driving regulations for individuals with epilepsy, and the Waiting Period for Drivers License Following Seizures provides specific requirements/guidelines. Contact each state's Division of Motor Vehicles for current and relevant information.
- Many people with epilepsy work at steady jobs and have successful careers. Some are unable to work, but epilepsy should not prevent the individual from getting a job; such discrimination has been outlawed by the Americans with Disabilities Act of 1990 (Public Law 101-336).
- Encourage the patient to wear a medical alert bracelet or necklace and to keep a medical alert card on his or her person at all times.
- Keeping a daily diary or journal is important and is a helpful tool for the patient, prescriber, and/or caregivers. Entries need to include the date and time of any seizure as well as any details such as omitted drug doses, illnesses, and so on.

## KEY POINTS

- *Epilepsy* is a disorder of the brain manifested as a chronic, recurrent pattern of seizures. A *seizure* is abnormal electrical activity in the brain.
- Seizures are classified as follows: partial-onset seizures or those originating in a more localized region of the brain; status epilepticus, characterized by generalized tonic-clonic convulsions that occur repeatedly in succession; and tonic-clonic seizures involving initial muscular contraction throughout the body (tonic) and progressing to alternating contraction and relaxation (clonic phase).
- You must be able to distinguish between the different types of seizure, and assess/document all symptoms, events, and problems that occur before, during, and after any seizure activity. This information may aid in the diagnosis of the type of seizure the patient is experiencing.

- Noncompliance with the drug regimen is the most important factor leading to treatment failure.
- Monitor therapeutic blood levels at all times. Avoid abrupt withdrawal of the antiepileptic drug to prevent rebound seizure activity.
- IV infusions of antiepileptic drugs are very dangerous and must be managed cautiously, with adherence to hospital or facility policy and manufacturer's guidelines. Avoid rapid infusions because of the risk for cardiac and/or respiratory arrest.
- Elderly patients may experience paradoxical reactions to antiepileptic drugs, resulting in hyperactivity and irritability versus sedation.

## NCLEX® EXAMINATION REVIEW QUESTIONS

1 The nurse is preparing to give medications. Which is the most appropriate nursing action for intravenous (IV) phenytoin (Dilantin)?
   a Give IV doses via rapid IV push.
   b Administer in normal saline solutions.
   c Administer in dextrose solutions.
   d Ensure continuous infusion of the drug.
2 The nurse is reviewing the drugs currently taken by a patient who will be starting drug therapy with carbamazepine (Tegretol). Which drug may raise a concern for interactions?
   a digoxin (Lanoxin)
   b acetaminophen (Tylenol)
   c diazepam (Valium)
   d warfarin (Coumadin)
3 Which response would the nurse expect to find in a patient with a phenytoin (Dilantin) level of 35 mcg/mL?
   a Ataxia
   b Hypertension
   c Seizures
   d No unusual response; this level is therapeutic.
4 A patient is taking pregabalin (Lyrica) but does not have a history of seizures. The nurse recognizes that this drug is also indicated for
   a postherpetic neuralgia.
   b viral infections.
   c Parkinson's disease.
   d depression.

5 The nurse is assessing a newly admitted patient who has a history of seizures. During the assessment, the patient has a generalized seizure that does not stop for several minutes. The nurse expects that which drug will be ordered for this condition?
   a valproic acid (Depakote)
   b neurontin (Gabapentin)
   c carbamazepine (Tegretol)
   d diazepam (Valium)
6 The nurse is administering an antiepileptic drug and will follow which guidelines? (Select all that apply.)
   a Monitor the patient for drowsiness.
   b Medications may be stopped if seizure activity disappears.
   c Give the medication at the same time every day.
   d Give the medication on an empty stomach.
   e Notify the prescriber if the patient is unable to take the medication.
7 The nurse is preparing to administer valproic acid to a child. The order reads: "Give valproic acid, 15 mg/kg/day PO in three divided doses." The child weighs 33 pounds. How many milligrams will the child receive with each dose?

1. b, 2. b, 3. a, 4. a, 5. d, 6. a, c, e, 7. 75 mg per dose

For Critical Thinking and Prioritization Questions, see http://evolve.elsevier.com/Lilley.

# Antiparkinson Drugs

## ℮volve WEBSITE

*http://evolve.elsevier.com/Lilley*

- Animations
- Answer Key—Textbook Case Studies
- Critical Thinking and Prioritization Questions

- Key Points—Downloadable
- Review Questions for the NCLEX® Examination
- Unfolding Case Studies

## OBJECTIVES

When you reach the end of this chapter, you will be able to do the following:

1 Briefly discuss the impact of acetylcholine and dopamine on the brain.
2 Describe the pathophysiology of Parkinson's disease.
3 Identify the different classes of medications used to manage Parkinson's disease, and list the drugs in each class.

4 Discuss the mechanisms of action, dosages, indications, routes of administration, contraindications, cautions, drug interactions, adverse effects, and toxic effects of antiparkinson drugs.
5 Develop a nursing care plan that includes all phases of the nursing process for patients taking antiparkinson drugs.

## DRUG PROFILES

amantadine, p. 243
♦ benztropine mesylate, p. 246
bromocriptine, p. 244
♦ carbidopa-levodopa, p. 246
entacapone, p. 244

♦ ropinirole, p. 245
selegiline and rasagiline, p. 242

_____

♦ *Key drug*

## KEY TERMS

**Adjunctive drugs** Drugs that are added as a second drug for combined therapy with a primary drug and may have additive or independent properties. (p. 241)

**Akinesia** Classically defined as "without movement." Absence or poverty of movement that results in a masklike facial expression and impaired postural reflexes. (p. 239)

**Bradykinesia** Slowness of movement; a classic symptom of Parkinson's disease. (p. 239)

**Chorea** A condition characterized by involuntary, purposeless, rapid motions such as flexing and extending the fingers, raising and lowering the shoulders, or grimacing. (p. 239)

**Dyskinesia** Term for abnormal and distressing involuntary movements; inability to control movements, which often occurs as a side effect of levodopa therapy. (p. 239)

**Dystonia** Impaired or distorted voluntary movement, often involving the head, neck, or feet. (p. 239)

**Exogenous** A term describing any substance produced outside of the body that may be taken into the body (e.g., a medication, food, or environmental toxin). (p. 245)

**On-off phenomenon** A common experience of patients taking medication for Parkinson's disease in which they experience periods of greater symptomatic control ("on" time) alternating with periods of lesser symptomatic control ("off" time). (p. 239)

**237**

## KEY TERMS—cont'd

**Parkinson's disease** A slowly progressive, degenerative neurologic disorder characterized by resting tremor, pill-rolling of the fingers, masklike facies, shuffling gait, forward flexion of the trunk, loss of postural reflexes, and muscle rigidity and weakness. (p. 238)

**Postural instability** A decrease or change in motor and muscle movements that leads to unsteadiness and hesitation in movement and gait when the individual starts or stops walking, or causes leaning to the left or right when sitting; occurs in Parkinson's disease. (p. 239)

**Presynaptic** Drugs that exert their antiparkinson effects before the nerve synapse. (p. 243)

**Rigidity** Resistance of the muscles to passive movement; leads to the "cogwheel" rigidity seen in Parkinson's disease. (p. 239)

**TRAP** (*Tremor, rigidity, akinesia, postural instability); an acronym for symptoms of Parkinson's disease. (p. 239)

**Tremor** In Parkinson's disease, shakiness of the extremities seen mostly at rest. (p. 239)

**Wearing-off phenomenon** A gradual worsening of parkinsonian symptoms as a patient's medications begin to lose their effectiveness, despite maximal dosing with a variety of medications. (p. 239)

---

# ANATOMY, PHYSIOLOGY, AND PATHOPHYSIOLOGY OVERVIEW

## PATHOPHYSIOLOGY OF PARKINSON'S DISEASE

**Parkinson's disease** is a chronic, progressive, neurodegenerative disorder affecting the dopamine-producing neurons in the brain. Other chronic central nervous system (CNS) neuromuscular disorders are myasthenia gravis and Alzheimer's disease. Parkinson's disease was initially recognized in 1817, at which time it was called *shaking palsy.* James Parkinson later described in more detail the symptoms of both the early and advanced stages of the disease. The underlying pathologic defect was not discovered until the1960s. It was then recognized that Parkinson's disease involves a dopamine deficit in the area of the cerebral cortex called the *substantia nigra,* which is contained within another brain structure known as the *basal ganglia.* Also relevant is the adjacent structure called the *globus pallidus.* All three structures are parts of the brain that make up the *extrapyramidal system,* which is involved in motor function, including posture, muscle tone, and smooth muscle activity. In addition, the *thalamus* serves as a relay station for brain impulses, whereas the *cerebellum* regulates muscle coordination (Figure 15-1).

*Dopamine* is an inhibitory neurotransmitter and *acetylcholine* is an excitatory neurotransmitter in this area of the brain. A correct balance between these two neurotransmitters is needed for the proper regulation of posture, muscle tone, and voluntary movement. Parkinson's disease results from an imbalance in these two neurotransmitters in the basal ganglia. This imbalance is caused by failure of the nerve terminals in the substantia nigra to produce dopamine. Dopamine acts in the basal ganglia to control movements. Destruction of the substantia nigra by Parkinson's disease leads to dopamine depletion. This often results in excessive, unopposed acetylcholine (cholinergic) activity due to the lack of a normal dopaminergic balancing effect. Figure 15-2 illustrates the difference in neurotransmitter concentrations in persons with normal balance and in patients with Parkinson's disease.

Some theorize that Parkinson's disease is the result of an earlier head injury or of excess iron in the substantia nigra, which undergoes oxidation and causes the generation of toxic free radicals. Another theory postulates that, because dopamine levels naturally decrease with age, Parkinson's disease represents a premature aging of the *nigrostriatal cells* of the substantia nigra resulting from environmental or intrinsic biochemical factors, or both. Evidence from animal studies suggests that environmental toxins, such as pesticides and metals, also may contribute to the development of Parkinson's disease.

Parkinson's disease affects at least 1 million Americans and 4 million people worldwide. It is the second most common neurodegenerative disease after Alzheimer's disease. Some patients may have symptoms of both conditions. In most patients, the disease becomes apparent between 45 and 65 years of age, with

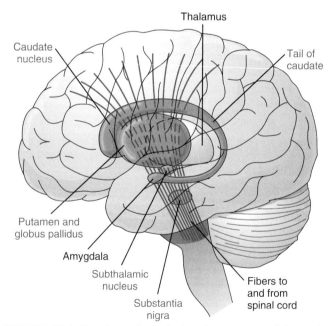

**FIGURE 15-1** Basal ganglia and related structures of the brain. (From Copstead-Kirkhorn LC, Banasik JL: *Pathophysiology,* ed 4, St Louis, 2010, Saunders.)

a mean age of onset of 56 years. The number of patients with Parkinson's disease is expected to continue to increase as our elderly population grows. The disease occasionally occurs in younger people, especially after acute encephalitis, or carbon monoxide or metallic poisoning. However, it is usually idiopathic (of no known cause). Overall, there is a 2% chance of developing the disease in one's lifetime. Men are affected more often than women in a ratio of up to 3:2. Evidence now suggests a possible genetic link, with up to 20% of patients having a family history of the disease.

There are no readily available laboratory tests that can detect or confirm Parkinson's disease. The diagnosis is usually made on the basis of the classic symptoms and physical findings. The classic symptoms of Parkinson's disease include bradykinesia, postural instability, rigidity, and tremors (TRAP [Tremor, rigidity, akinesia, postural instability] with akinesia really manifesting as bradykinesia) (see Table 15-1). Computed tomography (CT), magnetic resonance imaging (MRI), cerebrospinal fluid analysis, and electroencephalography (EEG) are usually normal and of little diagnostic value. Positron emission tomography (PET) may offer some additional information. CT, MRI, and PET may be useful tools for ruling out other possible

diseases as causes of the symptoms, as well as for follow-up imaging after drug and surgical treatments.

Unfortunately, Parkinson's disease is a progressive condition. Over time, there is substantial reduction in the number of surviving dopaminergic terminals that can take up pharmacologically administered levodopa and convert it into dopamine. Rapid swings in the response to levodopa, called the on-off phenomenon, also occur. The result is worsening of the disease when too little dopamine is present, or dyskinesias when too much is present. In contrast, the wearing-off phenomenon occurs when anti–Parkinson's disease medications begin to lose their effectiveness, despite maximal dosing, as the disease progresses. Dyskinesia is the difficulty in performing voluntary movements and is commonly seen in the disease. The two dyskinesias most frequently associated with antiparkinson therapy are chorea (irregular, spasmodic, involuntary movements of the limbs or facial muscles) and dystonia (abnormal muscle tone leading to impaired or abnormal movements). Dystonia commonly involves the head, neck, or feet and is a symptom common to patients with Parkinson's disease. These motor complications make Parkinson's disease a prominent cause of disability. Dementia may also be a result of the disease and is referred to as *Parkinson's disease–associated dementia*.

Symptoms of Parkinson's disease do not appear until approximately 80% of the dopamine store in the substantia nigra has been depleted. This means that by the time the disease is diagnosed, only approximately 20% of the patient's original dopaminergic terminals are functioning normally.

## TREATMENT OF PARKINSON'S DISEASE

The first step in the treatment of Parkinson's disease is to provide a full explanation of the disease to the patient and his or her family members or significant others. Physical therapy, speech therapy, and occupational therapy are almost always needed when the patient is in the later stages of the disease.

Treatment of the disease centers around drug therapy. However, physical activity is a must for these patients. Many experts believe that physical activity is as important as any drug

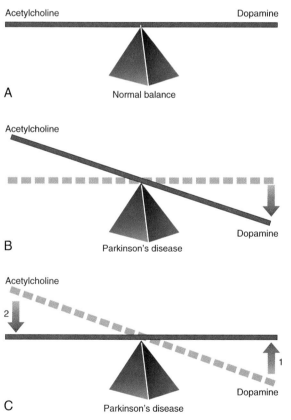

A, Normal balance of acetylcholine and dopamine in the CNS.
B, In Parkinson's disease, a decrease in dopamine results in an imbalance.
C, Drug therapy in Parkinson's disease is aimed at correcting the imbalance between acetylcholine and dopamine. This can be accomplished by:
1. increasing the supply of dopamine
2. blocking or lowering acetylcholine levels

**FIGURE 15-2** The neurotransmitter abnormality in Parkinson's disease.

| TABLE 15-1 | CLASSIC PARKINSONIAN SYMPTOMS |
|---|---|
| **SYMPTOM** | **DESCRIPTION** |
| Akinesia | Absence of psychomotor activity resulting in mask-like facial expression |
| Bradykinesia | Slowness of movement |
| Rigidity | "Cogwheel" rigidity, resistance to passive movement |
| Tremor | Pill rolling: tremor of the thumb against the forefinger, seen mostly at rest and less severe during voluntary activity; usually starts on one side then progresses to the other; is the presenting sign in 70% of cases; also seen as tremor of the hand and extremities. |
| Postural instability | Unsteadiness (associated with bradykinesia and rigidity) that leads to danger of falling; leaning to one side, even when sitting |

therapy, and together they greatly improve mobility. For severe cases, the surgical technique of *deep brain stimulation* may be used. This involves electrical stimulation of dopamine-deficient brain tissues in a way that helps to reduce Parkinson-associated dyskinesias. Surgical treatments are for the more severe cases, and the patient must still respond well to drug therapy.

## PHARMACOLOGY OVERVIEW

Because Parkinson's disease is thought to be due to an imbalance of dopamine and acetylcholine, drug therapy is aimed at increasing the levels of dopamine and/or antagonizing the effects of acetylcholine. Unfortunately, current drug therapy does not slow the progression of the disease, but rather is used to slow the progression of symptoms. The drugs available for the treatment of Parkinson's disease are listed in Table 15-2.

Antiparkinson drug therapy is based upon the fact that nerve terminals can take up substances, store them, and release them for use when needed. As long as there are functioning nerve terminals that can take up dopamine, the symptoms of

Parkinson's disease can be at least partially controlled. Since Parkinson's disease is essentially a deficiency of dopamine in certain areas of the brain, it seems logical that drug therapies focus primarily on restoring and enhancing dopaminergic activity in these neurons. A variety of both indirect- and direct-acting drugs are available for this purpose. The indirect-acting drugs are often administered first in the disease process.

## INDIRECT-ACTING DOPAMINERGIC DRUGS
### MONOAMINE OXIDASE INHIBITORS

The enzyme *monoamine oxidase (MAO)* causes the breakdown of *catecholamines* in the body, which include dopamine, norepinephrine, and epinephrine. There are two subclasses of MAO in the body: MAO-A and MAO-B. As early as 1965, nonselective monoamine oxidase inhibitors (MAOIs), which inhibit both MAO-A and MAO-B, were being used to improve the therapeutic effect of levodopa by preventing its metabolic breakdown. They were also among the first medications used to treat depression but have been replaced by newer drug

---

| TABLE 15-2 | **REVIEW OF PHARMACOLOGIC THERAPY FOR PARKINSON'S DISEASE** | | |
|---|---|---|---|
| **GENERIC NAME** | **TRADE NAME** | **ROUTE** | **INDICATIONS** |
| **Indirect-Acting Dopamine Receptor Agonists (MAO-B Inhibitors)** | | | |
| selegiline | Eldepryl, Zelapar* | PO | Used in conjunction with carbidopa-levodopa in early stages of disease; help- |
| rasagiline | Azilect | PO | ful with symptom fluctuations |
| **Dopamine Modulator** | | | |
| amantadine | Symmetrel | PO | Used in early stages; can be effective in moderate or advanced stages; reduces tremor or muscle rigidity |
| **COMT Inhibitors** | | | |
| tolcapone | Tasmar | PO | Usually added to carbidopa-levodopa to treat symptom fluctuations; delays "off" periods; has levodopa dose-sparing effect |
| entacapone | Comtan | PO | |
| **Direct-Acting Dopamine Receptor Agonists** | | | |
| *Ergot* | | | |
| bromocriptine | Parlodel | PO | Usually used as drug of choice for young patients; first- or second-line therapy of choice for elderly; can be used as adjunct to levodopa for "off" periods; can be used to reduce dyskinesia associated with later stages |
| *Nonergot* | | | |
| pramipexole | Mirapex | PO | |
| ropinirole | Requip | PO | |
| **Dopamine Replacement Drugs** | | | |
| carbidopa-levodopa | Sinemet, Parcopa* | PO | Usually started as soon as patient becomes functionally impaired; drug of choice for most elderly patients |
| **Anticholinergic Drugs**† | | | |
| benztropine | Cogentin | PO, IV | Used as secondary drug for tremor/muscle rigidity |
| trihexyphenidyl | Generic only (formerly Artane) | PO | |
| **Antihistamines**‡ | | | |
| diphenhydramine | Benadryl | PO, IV | Used as secondary drug for tremor/muscle rigidity |

*COMT,* Catechol ortho-methyltransferase; *IV,* intravenous; *MAO-B,* monoamine oxidase type B; *PO,* oral.
*Orally disintegrating tablet (see Chapter 2).
†See Chapter 21.
‡See Chapter 36.

categories (see Chapter 16). A major adverse effect of the non-selective MAOIs is that they interact with tyramine-containing foods (cheese, red wine, beer, and yogurt) because of their inhibitory activity against MAO-A. This has been called the *cheese effect,* and can result in severe hypertension. Selegiline is a selective MAO-B inhibitor and is much less likely to elicit the classic cheese effect. It is approved for use in conjunction with levodopa therapy in the treatment of Parkinson's disease. There was earlier speculation that selegiline, as well as possibly vitamins E and C, might have antiparkinson effects due to "neuroprotective" activity at the neuronal (nerve cell) level. However, no studies to date have demonstrated this to be true. Nonetheless, this theoretical neuroprotective effect is still debated in the literature.

Rasagiline is the newest antiparkinson drug and received FDA approval in 2008. Like selegiline, rasagiline is a selective MAO-B inhibitor. It is approved to be given once a day as monotherapy in the early stages of the disease, as well as in combination with other drugs in advanced cases. Drug interactions and adverse effects are similar to those of selegiline.

## Mechanism of Action and Drug Effects

The MAO enzymes are widely distributed throughout the body, with the highest concentrations found in the liver, kidney, stomach, intestinal wall, and brain. Most MAO-B occurs in the CNS, primarily in the brain. The primary role of MAO enzymes is the breakdown of catecholamines, such as dopamine, norepinephrine, and epinephrine, as well as serotonin. Giving an MAO-B inhibitor such as selegiline or rasagiline causes an increase in the levels of dopaminergic stimulation in the CNS. This helps to counter the dopaminergic deficiency seen in Parkinson's disease. Administration of selegiline can also allow the dose of levodopa (discussed later in this chapter) to be reduced. Improvement in functional ability and decreased severity of symptoms can occur; however, only approximately 50% to 60% of patients show a positive response.

## Indications

Selegiline and rasagiline are currently approved for use in combination with carbidopa-levodopa. They are adjunctive drugs used when a patient's response to levodopa is fluctuating. They may also be somewhat beneficial as a prophylactic drug to delay reduction in a patient's response to levodopa. Studies have shown that selegiline-treated patients required levodopa therapy approximately 1.8 times later than control patients. As Parkinson's disease progresses, it becomes more difficult to manage it with levodopa. Ultimately, levodopa no longer controls the disease, and the patient is seriously debilitated. This generally occurs between 5 and 10 years after the start of levodopa therapy.

## Contraindications

Selegiline and rasagiline are contraindicated in cases of known drug allergy. Concurrent use with the opioid analgesic meperidine (see Chapter 10) is also contraindicated due to well-documented drug interactions between MAOIs and meperidine.

## Adverse Effects

The most common adverse effects associated with selegiline use are mild and are listed in Table 15-3. At recommended dosages of 10 mg/day, the drug maintains its selective MAO-B inhibition. However, at dosages that exceed 10 mg/day, selegiline becomes a nonselective MAOI, which contributes to the development of the cheese effect described earlier.

## Interactions

Selegiline interacts with meperidine and has been associated with delirium, muscle rigidity, hyperpyrexia (high fever), and hyperirritability. Other reported reactions are listed in Table 15-4. Selegiline may safely be taken concurrently with catechol ortho-methyltransferase (COMT) inhibitors (see later drug section). Patients taking higher doses of selegiline need to avoid tyramine-containing foods such as aged cheese, sausages, and draft beer.

## Dosages

For dosage information, see the table on p. 242. Also see the Safety and Quality Improvement: Preventing Medication Errors box on p. 243.

| TABLE 15-3 | ADVERSE EFFECTS OF SELECTED ANTIPARKINSON DRUGS |
| --- | --- |
| **DRUG OR DRUG CLASS** | **ADVERSE EFFECTS** |
| **MAO-B inhibitor:** selegiline | Dizziness, insomnia, hallucinations, ataxia, agitation, depression, paresthesia, somnolence, headache, dyskinesia, nausea, diarrhea, hypotension or hypertension, chest pain, weight loss, dermatologic reactions, rhinitis, pharyngitis |
| **Dopamine modulator:** amantadine | Dizziness, insomnia, agitation, anxiety, headache, hallucinations, nausea, orthostatic hypotension, peripheral edema, dry mouth |
| **COMT inhibitors:** entacapone, tolcapone | GI upset, dyskinesia, urine discoloration, orthostatic hypotension, syncope, dizziness, fatigue, hallucinations, anxiety, somnolence, rash, dyspnea, worsening of dyskinesia *tolcapone:* liver failure |
| **Anticholinergic agent:** benztropine | Tachycardia; confusion; memory impairment; rash; hyperthermia; constipation; dry throat, nose, or mouth; nausea; vomiting; urinary retention; blurred vision; fever |
| **Ergot derivative:** bromocriptine | Ataxia, dizziness, headache, depression, drowsiness, GI upset, visual changes |
| **Nonergot derivatives:** pramipexole, ropinirole | Edema, fatigue, syncope, dizziness, drowsiness, GI upset |
| **Dopamine replacement drugs:** levodopa, carbidopa-levodopa combination | Palpitations, hypotension, urinary retention, depression, dyskinesia |

*COMT,* Catechol ortho-methyltransferase; *GI,* gastrointestinal; *MAO-B,* monoamine oxidase type B.

## TABLE 15-4    SELECTED DRUG INTERACTIONS OF ANTIPARKINSON DRUGS

| DRUG OR DRUG CLASS | INTERACTING DRUG | MECHANISM | RESULT |
|---|---|---|---|
| **MAO-B inhibitor:** selegiline | meperidine and other opioids, tramadol, cyclobenzaprine, dextromethorphan, other MAOIs, serotonergic antidepressants, oxcarbazepine | Additive CNS stimulation | Serotonin syndrome |
| | carbamazepine, oral contraceptives | Reduced selegiline clearance | Potential selegiline toxicity |
| | buspirone | Uncertain | Hypertension |
| **Dopamine modulator:** amantadine | Anticholinergics | Additive effects | Increased anticholinergic adverse effects |
| **COMT inhibitor:** entacapone | MAOIs, catecholamines | Reduced catecholamine metabolism | Tachycardia, cardiac dysrhythmias, hypertension |
| **Ergot derivative:** bromocriptine | erythromycin | Cytochrome P-450 interactions | Increased bromocriptine effects with risk of toxicity |
| | Sympathomimetics | Additive effects | Hypertension, cardiac dysrhythmias |
| | Antihypertensives | Additive effects | Hypotension |
| **Nonergot:** ropinirole | warfarin, ciprofloxacin | Cytochrome P-450 interactions | Reduced ropinirole clearance with risk of toxicity |
| | Antipsychotics | Antidopaminergic activity | Reduced efficacy of ropinirole |
| **Dopamine replacement:** levodopa, carbidopa | Nonselective MAOIs | Additive toxicity | Hypertensive reactions |
| | Benzodiazepines, antipsychotics | Reduced levodopa effects | Reduced therapeutic effects |

*CNS,* Central nervous system; *COMT,* catechol ortho-methyltransferase; *ECG,* electrocardiogram; *MAO-B,* monoamine oxidase type B; *MAOI,* monoamine oxidase inhibitor.

## DOSAGES

### Selected Antiparkinson Drugs

| DRUG (PREGNANCY CATEGORY) | PHARMACOLOGIC CLASS | USUAL ADULT DOSAGE RANGE | INDICATIONS |
|---|---|---|---|
| amantadine (Symmetrel) (C) | Dopamine modulator | PO: 100-400 mg/day divided q12h | |
| ◆ benztropine (Cogentin) (C) | Anticholinergic | PO: 0.5-6 mg/day | |
| bromocriptine (Parlodel) (D) | Direct-acting dopamine agonist; ergot derivative | PO: 2.5-90 mg/day | |
| carbidopa-levodopa (Sinemet, Sinemet CR, Parcopa) (C) | Antiparkinson agent | PO: 10/100, 1 tab 3-8 times/day; 25/100, 1 tab 3-6 times/day; 25/250, 1 tab tid-qid<br>CR: 1 tab bid; up to 2-8 tabs at 4- to 8-hr intervals<br>PO (orally disintegrating tablet [Parcopa]): same as above | Parkinson's disease |
| entacapone (Comtan) (C) | COMT inhibitor | PO: 200 mg with each dosage of levodopa, up to 8 times/day | |
| ◆ ropinirole (Requip) (C) | Direct-acting dopamine agonist; nonergot derivative | PO: 0.25 mg tid, slowly titrating to max dose of 24 mg/day | |
| selegiline (Eldepryl, Zelapar) (C) | Selective MAO-B inhibitor | PO: 5 mg bid with breakfast and lunch in combination with carbidopa-levodopa, or 10 mg q AM<br>PO (orally disintegrating tablet [Zelapar]): 1.25-2.5 mg once daily | |

*CR,* Controlled release; *MAOI,* monoamine oxidase inhibitor; *PO,* oral; *subcut,* subcutaneous.

## DRUG PROFILES

### selegiline and rasagiline

Selegiline (Eldepryl) is a selective MAO-B inhibitor which is indicated for Parkinson's disease. It is used as an adjunctive drug along with levodopa to reduce the dosage of levodopa needed for symptom control. Adverse effects increased with doses greater than 10 mg when it loses its selectivity for MAO-B are listed in Table 15-3. Drug interactions are listed in Table 15-4. Selegiline is available as an oral tablet and an orally disintegrating tablet for buccal use known as Zelapar, which can provide improved drug absorption. In addition, a transdermal form of the drug known as Emsam is available. Emsam is currently indicated only for major depressive disorder (see Chapter 16). Rasagiline (Azilect) is a newer selective MAO-B inhibitor comparable to selegiline. Its advantage is that it is approved as monotherapy for Parkinson's disease, whereas selegiline is normally used adjunctively with the dopamine replacement drug levodopa.

### Pharmacokinetics

| Route | Onset of Action | Peak Plasma Concentration | Elimination Half-life | Duration of Action |
|---|---|---|---|---|
| PO | 1 hr | 0.5-2 hr | 2 hr | 1-3 days |

## ⚡ SAFETY AND QUALITY IMPROVEMENT: PREVENTING MEDICATION ERRORS

### *Look-Alike/Sound-Alike Drugs: Selegiline and Salagen*

Be careful with look-alike/sound-alike drugs! Medication errors often occur when drug names are similar.

Selegiline is a monoamine oxidase inhibitor that is used to treat Parkinson's disease. Salagen, an oral form of pilocarpine hydrochloride, is prescribed for relief of dry mouth symptoms, also known as *xerostomia*, in patients who have Sjögren's syndrome or who have received radiation therapy. To make it more confusing, both drugs are available in 5-mg dosage forms. Be sure to double-check the name and use of these drugs when receiving orders, and instruct patients to check the drug names when getting these drugs filled at pharmacies.

For more information, visit www.ismp.org/Newsletters/acutecare/articles/20050922_1.asp.

## DOPAMINE MODULATOR

Only one drug is currently known to function as a dopamine modulator. Amantadine (Symmetrel) was first recognized as an antiviral drug and was used for treating influenza virus infections. It is still used for this purpose (see Chapter 40) as well as for management of Parkinson's disease.

## Mechanism of Action and Drug Effects

Amantadine appears to work by causing the release of dopamine and other catecholamines from their storage sites, or vesicles, in the presynaptic fibers of nerve cells within the basal ganglia that have not yet been destroyed by the disease process. Amantadine also blocks the reuptake of dopamine into the nerve fibers. This results in higher levels of dopamine in the synapses between nerves and improved dopamine neurotransmission between neurons. Because amantadine does not directly stimulate dopaminergic receptors, it is considered to be indirect acting. Amantadine also has some anticholinergic properties (see Chapter 21). This may further help by controlling symptoms of dyskinesia.

## Indications

Amantadine is generally indicated in the early stages of Parkinson's disease while there are still some intact neurons in the basal ganglia. However, it can be used in the moderate to advanced stages. It is usually effective for only 6 to 12 months, after which it often fails to relieve hypokinesia and rigidity. Once it becomes ineffective, a dopamine agonist such as bromocriptine is usually tried next (see later drug section). It is often used to treat dyskinesia associated with carbidopa-levodopa. It is also indicated for influenza virus infection (see Chapter 40).

## Contraindications

Amantadine is contraindicated in cases of known drug allergy.

## Adverse Drug Effects

Common adverse effects associated with amantadine are relatively mild and include dizziness, insomnia, and nausea.

## Drug Interactions

Amantadine causes increased anticholinergic adverse effects when given with anticholinergic drugs.

## Dosage

For dosage information, see the table on p. 242.

## DRUG PROFILE

### amantadine

Amantadine (Symmetrel) is actually an antiviral drug that is used most often for influenza virus infection (see Chapter 40). It is also indicated for treatment of moderate Parkinson's disease, for which it helps to control symptoms of tremor, including motor rigidity, by virtue of both its dopaminergic and anticholinergic effects. Common adverse reactions include dizziness, insomnia, and nausea. Interacting drugs include anticholinergics (additive effects) (see Table 15-4). Amantadine is available only for oral use.

### Pharmacokinetics

| Route | Onset of Action | Peak Plasma Concentration | Elimination Half-life | Duration of Action |
|-------|-----------------|---------------------------|-----------------------|--------------------|
| PO | 48 hr | 2-4 hr | 11-15 hr | 6-12 wk |

## CATECHOL ORTHO-METHYLTRANSFERASE INHIBITORS

The third category of indirect-acting dopaminergic drugs is the *catechol ortho-methyltransferase (COMT)* inhibitors. There are currently two drugs in this category: tolcapone (Tasmar) and entacapone (Comtan).

## Mechanism of Action and Drug Effects

Tolcapone and entacapone, like amantadine, work presynaptically. Both drugs block COMT. COMT is the enzyme that catalyzes the breakdown of the body's catecholamines. Tolcapone acts both centrally and peripherally, whereas entacapone cannot cross the blood-brain barrier and therefore can act only peripherally. The positive effect of these drugs is that they prolong the duration of action of levodopa. This is especially true when levodopa is given with carbidopa (see section on dopamine replacement drugs later in the chapter). This results in reduction of the wearing-off phenomenon.

## Indications

COMT inhibitors are indicated for the treatment of Parkinson's disease.

## Contraindications

Both COMT inhibitors (tolcapone and entacapone) are contraindicated in cases of known drug allergy. Tolcapone is also contraindicated in cases of liver failure.

## Adverse Effects

Commonly reported adverse effects with both COMT inhibitors include gastrointestinal (GI) upset and urine discoloration. In addition, they also can worsen dyskinesia that may already be present (see Table 15-3). Tolcapone has been associated with cases of severe liver failure. For this reason, the FDA announced in 1998 that this drug is to be considered only in patients who do not respond to other Parkinson's disease drug therapy.

## Interactions

Neither tolcapone nor entacapone are to be taken with non-selective MAOIs because of cardiovascular risk due to reduced catecholamine metabolism. However, the selective MAO-B inhibitor selegiline may be safely taken concurrently with COMT inhibitors.

## Dosages

For dosage information, see the table on p. 242.

## DRUG PROFILE

Inhibition of the enzyme in the body known as COMT is a strategy for prolonging the duration of action of levodopa. Two compounds were developed for this purpose: tolcapone (Tasmar) and entacapone (Comtan). Both drugs are reversible inhibitors of COMT. Tolcapone has been associated with severe liver failure and is rarely used. To date, no similar pattern of adverse outcomes has been shown with entacapone.

### entacapone

Entacapone (Comtan) is a COMT inhibitor indicated for the adjunctive treatment of Parkinson's disease. Entacapone is taken with levodopa and is effective from the first dose. A patient can feel the benefit of entacapone within a few days. Entacapone benefits patients who are experiencing wearing-off effects. When used with levodopa, it can also reduce on-off effects. The levodopa dosage can often be reduced. Adverse reactions include GI upset, dyskinesias, and urine discoloration (see Table 15-3). Entacapone is contraindicated in patients who have shown a hypersensitivity reaction to it and used with caution in patients with preexisting liver disease. Entacapone is available only for oral use. It is also available in combination tablets that contain various doses of entacapone, carbidopa, and levodopa (Stalevo).

### Pharmacokinetics

| Route | Onset of Action | Peak Plasma Concentration | Elimination Half-life | Duration of Action |
|---|---|---|---|---|
| PO | 1 hr | 0.5-1.5 hr | 1-5.3.5 hr | 6 hr |

## DIRECT-ACTING DOPAMINE RECEPTOR AGONISTS

Direct-acting dopamine receptor agonists are drugs used to treat Parkinson's disease, often as first-line agents used upon diagnosis. These drugs include two subclasses: *nondopamine dopamine receptor agonists (NDDRAs)* and *dopamine replacement drugs*. NDDRAs are further subdivided into the ergot derivatives bromocriptine (Parlodel) and the nonergot drugs pramipexole (Mirapex) and ropinirole (Requip). Pergolide was taken off the U.S. market after severe adverse effects were reported.

## NONDOPAMINE DOPAMINE RECEPTOR AGONISTS

### Mechanism of Action and Drug Effects

All of the NDDRAs work by direct stimulation of presynaptic and/or postsynaptic dopamine receptors in the brain. They may be used in early or late stages of the disease.

Chemically, bromocriptine is an ergot alkaloid similar to ergotamine (see Chapter 13). (*Ergot* is the name of a pathologic fungal growth on plants.) Bromocriptine works by activating presynaptic dopamine receptors to stimulate the production of more dopamine. It chief site of activity is the $D_2$ subclass of dopamine receptors. Pramipexole and ropinirole are two newer *nonergot* NDDRAs. Both are effective in early and late stages of Parkinson's disease.

### Indications

Both ergot and nonergot NDDRAs are used to treat various stages of Parkinson's disease, either alone or in combination with other drugs. Bromocriptine also inhibits the production of the hormone *prolactin*, which stimulates normal lactation. For this reason, it is used to treat women with excessive or undesired breast milk production (*galactorrhea*) and is also used for treatment of prolactin-secreting tumors. Ropinirole is also used to treat a disorder known as *restless legs syndrome*, a nocturnal movement of the legs that disrupts sleep.

### Contraindications

Known allergy is a contraindication to dopaminergic drug therapy. These drugs are not to be used concurrently with adrenergic drugs (see Chapter 18) due to the cardiovascular risks of excessive catecholamine activity.

### Adverse Effects

Many potential adverse effects are associated with the dopaminergic drugs. They are listed in Table 15-3.

### Interactions

Interactions vary among drugs and are listed in Table 15-4.

### Dosages

For dosage information, see the table on p. 242.

## DRUG PROFILES

The traditional role of the NDDRAs bromocriptine, pramipexole, and ropinirole has been as adjuncts to levodopa for management of motor fluctuations; however, they are now often used as first-line therapy. These drugs differ from levodopa in that they do not replace dopamine itself but act by stimulation of dopaminergic receptors in the brain. They have been used as initial monotherapy and as combination therapy with low-dose levodopa in an attempt to either delay levodopa therapy or reduce the dosage of levodopa and its associated motor complications (see drug profile for levodopa).

### bromocriptine

Bromocriptine stimulates only the $D_2$ receptors and antagonizes the $D_1$ receptors. Eventually, carbidopa-levodopa is needed to control the patient's symptoms. Using amantadine or a nondopamine agonist until it fails may postpone the need for levodopa therapy for up to 3 years. Bromocriptine may also be given with carbidopa-levodopa so that lower dosages of the levodopa are needed. This often results in prolonging the "on" periods and minimizing the "off" periods of the disease. Bromocriptine is indicated for Parkinson's disease as well as hyperprolactinemia. Bromocriptine is contraindicated in cases of known drug allergy to any ergot alkaloids. It is also contraindicated in patients with severe ischemic disease of any kind (e.g., peripheral vascular disease) due to the ability of bromocriptine to stimulate dopamine receptors in the peripheral tissues outside of the brain. This can result in vasoconstriction, which can worsen peripheral vascular disease. Adverse reactions include GI upset, dyskinesias, sleep disturbances, and others as listed in Table 15-3. Drug interactions occur with erythromycin (see Chapter 38) and adrenergic drugs (see Chapter 18). Drug interactions are listed in Table 15-4. Bromocriptine is available only for oral use.

### Pharmacokinetics

| Route | Onset of Action | Peak Plasma Concentration | Elimination Half-life | Duration of Action |
|-------|-----------------|---------------------------|-----------------------|---------------------|
| PO | 0.5-1.5 hr | 1-3 hr | 3-5 hr | 4-8 hr |

### ♦ ropinirole

Ropinirole (Requip) is a nonergot NDDRA. A similar drug is pramipexole (Mirapex). These nonergot drugs have a better adverse effects profile (e.g., fewer dyskinesias) than bromocriptine. Ropinirole is more specific than bromocriptine for the $D_2$ subfamily of dopamine receptors ($D_2$, $D_3$, and $D_4$). This in turn results in more specific antiparkinson effects with fewer of the adverse effects associated with more generalized dopaminergic stimulation. Ropinirole can be effective in both early- and late-stage Parkinson's disease and appears to delay the need for levodopa therapy. Ropinirole is indicated for both monotherapy and adjunctive therapy with levodopa. It is also approved by the FDA for moderate to severe primary restless legs syndrome. The drug is contraindicated in patients with known drug allergy. Adverse effects include dizziness, GI upset, and somnolence (see Table 15-3). Drug interactions occur with any drug metabolized by cytochrome P-450 enzyme 1A2 (e.g., warfarin, ciprofloxacin) (see Table 15-4). Ropinirole is available only for oral use.

### Pharmacokinetics

| Route | Onset of Action | Peak Plasma Concentration | Elimination Half-life | Duration of Action |
|-------|-----------------|---------------------------|-----------------------|---------------------|
| PO | 30 min | 1-2 hr | 3-5 hr | 6-10 hr |

## DOPAMINE REPLACEMENT DRUGS

The traditional cornerstone of therapy for Parkinson's disease has been with the drug levodopa. It is a biologic precursor of dopamine required by the brain for dopamine synthesis. However, levodopa cannot be used by itself in the brain and must be combined with another substance, carbidopa. The combination product carbidopa-levodopa provides exogenous sources of dopamine that directly replace dopamine in the substantia nigra. These drugs are thus classified as *dopamine replacement* drugs and are drugs of choice in the later stages of Parkinson's disease.

## Mechanism of Action and Drug Effects

Dopamine replacement drugs stimulate presynaptic dopamine receptors to increase brain levels of dopamine. Dopamine must be administered orally as levodopa, because exogenously administered dopamine cannot pass through the blood-brain barrier. Levodopa is the biologic precursor of dopamine and can penetrate into the CNS.

Levodopa is given in combination with carbidopa. Very large oral doses of levodopa are required to obtain adequate dopamine replacement, because much of the levodopa administered is broken down outside the CNS by the enzyme dopa decarboxylase. Large doses result in high peripheral levels of dopamine and lead to many unwanted adverse effects (see Table 15-3). These adverse effects include confusion, involuntary movements, GI distress, hypotension, and even cardiac dysrhythmias. These problems may be avoided when levodopa is given with carbidopa. Carbidopa is a peripheral decarboxylase inhibitor with little or no pharmacologic activity when given alone. When given in combination with levodopa, carbidopa inhibits the breakdown of levodopa in the periphery and thus allows smaller doses of levodopa to be used. Lesser amounts of levodopa result in fewer unwanted adverse effects.

## Indications

Dopamine replacement drugs are used to directly restore dopaminergic activity in Parkinson's disease. Dopamine itself is also given by injection in critical care settings (see Chapter 18) as a pressor drug to raise blood pressure and enhance renal perfusion.

## Contraindications

Levodopa and carbidopa are both contraindicated in cases of angle-closure glaucoma, because they can raise intraocular pressure. However, they may be used cautiously in patients with open-angle glaucoma (see Chapter 57). Neither drug is to be used in patients with any undiagnosed skin condition, because both drugs can activate malignant melanoma.

## Adverse Effects

Adverse effects of dopamine replacement drugs include cardiac dysrhythmias, hypotension, chorea, muscle cramps, and GI distress (see Table 15-3).

## Interactions

A possible drug interaction can occur with pyridoxine (vitamin $B_6$). Other interactions are listed in Table 15-4.

## DRUG PROFILE

### ♦ carbidopa-levodopa

Carbidopa-levodopa (Sinemet), available orally, is one of the most commonly used drugs for Parkinson's disease. Carbidopa (Lodosyn) alone is not used as therapy, rather as an adjunct to treat nausea associated with Sinemet. A variety of studies have shown that the controlled-release product Sinemet CR (or generic) increases "on" time and decreases "off" time. As with all sustained-release products, Sinemet CR must not be crushed; however, it can be split one time, unlike most other CR or XR drugs on the market. Drug interactions occur with tricyclic antidepressants and other drugs (see Table 15-4). A possible drug interaction may occur with pyridoxine (vitamin $B_6$). Pyridoxine reduces the effectiveness of carbidopa-levodopa; however, the dose can usually be adjusted to overcome this interaction. See the nursing implementation section for discussion of the possible interaction of carbidopa-levodopa with dietary protein. Carbidopa-levodopa is best taken on an empty stomach; however, to minimize GI side effects, it can be taken with food.

### Pharmacokinetics

| Route | Onset of Action | Peak Plasma Concentration | Elimination Half-life | Duration of Action |
|---|---|---|---|---|
| PO | 2-3 wk* | 0.5-2 hr | 1.5 hr | 5 hr |

*Therapeutic effect.

## ANTICHOLINERGIC DRUGS

Anticholinergic drugs block the effects of the neurotransmitter acetylcholine at cholinergic receptors in the brain as well as in the rest of the body. They are discussed in greater detail in Chapter 21. Anticholinergics are used as adjunct drug therapy in Parkinson's disease due to their anti-tremor properties. The purpose of their use is to reduce excessive cholinergic activity in the brain. Accumulation of acetylcholine in Parkinson's disease causes an overstimulation of the cholinergic excitatory pathways, which results in tremors and muscle rigidity. Cogwheel rigidity is an example and is defined as resistance to passive movement. It can be observed when an arm that is flexed toward the body is then extended at the elbow. Muscle tremors are usually worse when the patient is at rest and consist of a pill-rolling movement and bobbing of the head. Anticholinergic drugs help to alleviate these bothersome and often disabling symptoms. However, anticholinergics do little to relieve the *bradykinesia* (extremely slow movements) that is also associated with Parkinson's disease.

Acetylcholine is responsible for causing increased *s*alivation, *l*acrimation (tearing of the eyes), *u*rination, *d*iarrhea, increased *G*I motility, and possibly *e*mesis (vomiting). The acronym *SLUDGE* is often used to describe these cholinergic effects. Anticholinergics have the opposite effects. They can cause dry mouth or decreased salivation, urinary retention, decreased GI motility (constipation), dilated pupils (mydriasis), and smooth muscle relaxation. Anticholinergic drugs readily cross the blood-brain barrier and therefore can get to the site of Parkinson's disease pathology in the brain, the substantia nigra.

Historically, the anticholinergic drugs atropine and scopolamine were used. However, the anticholinergic adverse effects of dry mouth, urinary retention, and blurred vision associated with these original anticholinergics can be excessive. Therefore, synthetic anticholinergics were developed that have better adverse effect profiles. The anticholinergics most commonly used include benztropine (Cogentin) and trihexyphenidyl (generic only; formerly Artane). Antihistamines (see Chapter 36) also have significant anticholinergic properties; they can also be used to manage cholinergic symptoms in Parkinson's disease. The most common choice is the drug diphenhydramine (Benadryl). Anticholinergics must be used cautiously in older adults because of significant potential adverse effects such as confusion, urinary retention, visual blurring, palpitations, and increased intraocular pressure.

## DRUG PROFILE

### ♦ benztropine mesylate

Benztropine (Cogentin) is an anticholinergic drug used for Parkinson's disease and also for extrapyramidal symptoms from antipsychotic drugs (see Chapter 16). Benztropine is to be used with caution in hot weather or during exercise because it may cause hyperthermia. Other adverse effects include tachycardia, confusion, disorientation, toxic psychosis, urinary retention, dry throat, constipation, nausea, and vomiting. Anticholinergic syndrome can occur when it is given with other drugs such as amantadine, phenothiazine, or tricyclic antidepressants that are associated with a high incidence of anticholinergic effects. Alcohol is to be avoided. Benztropine is available as tablets and in injectable form. The normal dosage is 0.5 to 6 mg/day in one or two divided doses.

### Pharmacokinetics

| Route | Onset of Action | Peak Plasma Concentration | Elimination Half-life | Duration of Action |
|---|---|---|---|---|
| PO | 1 hr | 2-4 hr | 4-8 hr | 6-10 hr |

## NURSING PROCESS

### ASSESSMENT

After patients are confronted with the diagnosis of Parkinson's disease, they soon experience the impact of the disease with every movement and activity of daily living. Not only will their lives never be the same, they will soon learn that their quality of life depends on drug therapy and nondrug measures. Before medications for Parkinson's disease are given, assess and document vital signs (e.g., blood pressure, pulse, respirations, temperature, pain) and ABCs (airway, breathing, and circulation). In addition, obtain a complete nursing history with a thorough physical assessment, including compiling a comprehensive medication profile. Because it may take several weeks to see a therapeutic response to medication regimens, a keen assessment and careful patient monitoring are even more critical to quality nursing care. A thorough assessment includes a health history, review of systems, and determination of sensory and motor abilities. Also gather the following information: complaint(s) upon admission or the symptom(s)/event that led the patient to obtain medical treatment; past and current medical history with a focus on the presence or absence of head injury, seizures, diabetes, hypertension, heart disease, and/or cancer; family history of any neuromuscular or neurologic disorders, heart disease, diabetes, cancer, seizures, cerebrovascular accident (stroke), and/or Parkinson's disease. Additionally, complete a thorough systems assessment with gathering of subjective and objective information in the following areas as related to the possible impact of Parkinson's disease:

- *Central nervous system*—Inquire about any headaches, fatigue, weakness, paralysis, dizziness, and/or syncope. Note any changes in walking or mobility, increase in rigidity or muscle movements, and/or changes in the ability to carry out activities of daily living. Also important are any changes in sensation in the extremities, changes in vision or hearing, loss of or changes in coordination, changes in gait and balance, and/or any changes in energy level. Also include questions about any changes in baseline levels of alertness; changes in memory (short-term or long-term); blackouts or seizures; numbness, tingling, or abnormal sensations in the extremities; changes in mood; changes in muscle movement or strength (e.g., paralysis) or voluntary versus involuntary motor control; and any muscle rigidity or tremors. Assess response to stimuli, and assess pupils with attention to size, shape, response to light, and symmetry (in reactions). Assess deep tendon reflexes with attention to strength bilaterally. Observe and document the patient's ability to walk, his or her gait, and upper/lower, left/right extremity strength. Also assess and document ability to feed self and carry out activities of daily living.
- *Genitourinary and gastrointestinal systems*—Perform a general survey of the abdominal area with inspection, auscultation of bowel sounds, and palpation for any distention or tenderness. Determine daily baseline urinary and bowel patterns with attention to any changes in or loss of control of bladder or bowel functioning as well as the patient's ability to engage in toileting activities. Inquire about the need for assistance with these daily functions. Ask the patient about any difficulty in swallowing (dysphagia) and any problems in feeding self or preparing meals. If such difficulties are identified, assess further for any subsequent nutritional excesses or deficits.
- *Skin and oral mucus membranes*—Assess the skin's color, texture, turgor, and fragility, and note any breaks in the skin, bruises, lesions, masses, and/or swelling. Also document color and moisture of the oral cavity and mucus membranes.
- *Respiratory system*—Focus attention on respiratory rate, rhythm, depth, effort, and breath sounds.
- *Psychological and emotional status*—Assess the patient for any recent or past changes in mood, affect, or personality. Also note any other disease-related concerns such as depression, emotional ups and downs, increase in irritability, social withdrawal, or changes in sexual functioning or intimacy.
- *Functional abilities*—Inquire about any changes in everyday function in the patient's personal and/or professional life. Assess and note any changes in daily task performance at the place of employment or need to take sick leave or sick days,

as well as the patient's ability to exercise, drive, and/or shop for groceries and other necessities.

With *indirect-acting dopamine receptor agonists,* such as amantadine, and *direct-acting dopamine receptor agonists,* such as carbidopa-levodopa, and ropinirole, include in your assessment vital signs with supine and standing blood pressures (because of drug-related postural hypotension), height, weight, medication and medical history, and nursing history. Include family, significant others, and/or caregiver in the assessment and data collection process. Note contraindications, cautions, and drug interactions prior to administering these drugs (see previous pharmacology discussion). Assess motor skills, including abilities and deficiencies, and for the presence of akinesia, bradykinesia, postural instability, rigidity, tremors, staggering gait, or drooling (see Key Terms and Table 15-1). Assessment of urinary patterns is also important because of the possibility of drug-induced urinary retention. If BUN and creatinine measurements are ordered, the results need to be routinely examined because these values are indicators of renal function. Alkaline phosphatase levels are indicators of liver function and also need to be assessed, if ordered. These laboratory values are important to determine in patients with decreased renal or liver function so that dosage amounts of antiparkinson drugs may be altered by the prescriber.

As related to lifespan considerations, it is important to understand the gynecologic history of the patient and to know if the patient is pregnant and/or lactating. Some of the *dopamine replacement drugs* cross into the placenta and into breast milk and have unknown actions in the pediatric patient. Drug interactions related to these drugs are presented in Table 15-4. See Table 15-3 for a listing of selected antiparkinson drugs and their related classifications and subclassifications.

When *anticholinergic drugs* are prescribed, assess the patient carefully to determine gross level of organ functioning—especially in those systems most affected by Parkinson's disease, including the GI, genitourinary, visual, cardiac, and neurologic systems. Assess mental status, and pay close attention to any present or past changes as well as the presence of confusion, disorientation, or psychotic-like behavior. This is important to consider in elderly patients because of decline in liver function and a subsequent higher risk for adverse effects and possible toxicity (with antiparkinson drugs and drugs in general) and an overall increased sensitivity to the effects of drugs (see Chapter 3). Cautions, contraindications, and drug interactions have been previously discussed.

For the *indirect-acting dopamine receptor agonist drugs (subclass of presynaptic dopamine release enhancers)* that are also antiviral (e.g., amantadine), the previously discussed baseline and general assessment information is also applicable. The patient's knowledge of the drug's use for Parkinson's disease (versus its use as an antiviral) and awareness that its onset of action will be delayed for several days or longer needs to be confirmed. Continual assessment of the patient's status and improvement of disease-related symptoms is important, because a decline in this drug's effectiveness (specifically a failure in the ability to control hypokinesia and rigidity of Parkinson's) may occur within

## PATIENT-CENTERED CARE: LIFESPAN CONSIDERATIONS FOR THE ELDERLY PATIENT

### *Antiparkinson Drugs*

- Carbidopa-levodopa must be used cautiously and with close monitoring in elderly patients, especially those with a history of cardiac, renal, hepatic, endocrine, pulmonary, ulcer, or psychiatric disease.
- Elderly patients taking carbidopa-levodopa are at an increased risk for experiencing adverse effects, especially confusion, loss of appetite, and orthostatic hypotension.
- Carbidopa-levodopa is often started at a low dose because of the increased sensitivity of older patients to these medications and the need to save higher dosages for a later time during treatment.
- Overheating is a problem in patients taking anticholinergics, and so elderly patients taking these drugs must avoid excessive exercise during warm weather and excessive heat exposure.
- One of the main problems with the long-term use of carbidopa-levodopa is that its duration of effectiveness decreases over time; this is even more problematic in elderly patients. Catechol ortho-methyltransferase (COMT) inhibitors hold much promise for elderly patients who are experiencing the wearing-off phenomenon; they help turn "off" times into "on" times so that the drug begins to work throughout the day.

6 to 12 months after initiation of therapy. If amantadine (also a prolactin inhibitor) is prescribed, the nurse must understand that this drug is also used for suppression of lactation and must assess for the appropriateness of its use. Patients taking these drugs also require additional CNS assessment because of the possible adverse effects of dizziness, headache, insomnia, and anxiety. Also, if the patient is taking this medication long term, assessment for orthostatic hypotension and dizziness is crucial to patient safety.

The antiparkinson drugs classified as *indirect-acting dopamine receptor agonists (subclass of MAO-B inhibitors),* such as selegiline, require assessment of many of the same parameters discussed earlier. In addition, however, cardiac status is important to assess and document because of the possible adverse effects of hypotension/hypertension and chest pain. Assessment of dosing is also important because, as with other antiparkinson drugs, a low dose is used initially with gradual increases over approximately a 3- to 4-week period. The lowest possible dose is recommended for initiation of therapy so that plenty of room exists for further increases in dosing as the disease progresses. These drugs also require careful neurologic assessment due to drug-adverse effects of depression, hallucinations, ataxia, and agitation (see Table 15-3).

For the *indirect-acting dopamine receptor agonist-COMT inhibitors* (e.g., entacapone and tolcapone), assessment of baseline vital signs is also required, with a focus on standing and supine blood pressure because of the adverse effects of orthostatic hypotension and syncope. In fact, these adverse effects occur more frequently with the COMT inhibitors than with the other antiparkinson drugs, and thus increased caution and concern is needed. Assessment of dosing time is also important because if these drugs are not given 1 hour before or 2 hours after meals, the bioavailability of the drug may be

adversely affected. Assess serum transaminase levels before and during drug therapy with tolcapone due to the adverse effect of liver failure. If the patient's ALT level is elevated to the upper range of normal or higher, the prescriber will most likely discontinue the drug because of the increased risk of hepatic failure.

## NURSING DIAGNOSES

1. Urinary retention related to the pathophysiologic effects of the disease process on the bladder with incomplete emptying
2. Constipation related to decreased GI peristalsis associated with the disease process
3. Imbalanced nutrition, less than body requirements, related to the disease process as well as adverse effects of drug therapy
4. Impaired physical mobility related to the disease process and adverse effects of the various antiparkinson medications
5. Disturbed body image related to changes in appearance and mobility due to the disease process
6. Deficient knowledge related to lack of exposure to and experience with a complex and long-term treatment regimen
7. Risk for injury related to the physical limitations and changes in mobility, gait, balance, and coordination produced by the disease process

## PLANNING

### GOALS

1. Patient regains as normal as possible bladder elimination patterns.
2. Patient maintains as normal as possible bowel elimination patterns.
3. Patient maintains adequate and balanced nutritional status.
4. Patient is able to maintain safe mobility and activities of daily living.
5. Patient maintains a positive self-image and body image.
6. Patient demonstrates adequate knowledge and comprehension about the illness, medication therapy, and drug-related adverse and toxic effects.
7. Patient remains free from injury and self harm.

### OUTCOME CRITERIA

1. Patient discusses ways to minimize problems associated with drug-induced alterations in bladder elimination patterns (retention) such as forcing fluids, taking medications as prescribed, attempting to empty the bladder at regular intervals, and reporting any unresolved urinary problems.
2. Patient implements various measures to decrease constipation such as increasing bulk and fiber in the diet with fruits and vegetables, forcing fluids, and remaining as active as possible.
3. Patient states the importance and gives examples of daily menus for increased dietary protein, increased intake from the major food groups divided in six small frequent meals, and use of nutritional supplements and vitamins.

4. Patient participates in daily care with use of assistive devices, as appropriate, as well as walking/ambulating.
   - Patient removes any barriers to safe mobility in the home environment and uses handrails throughout the home
   - Patient maintains mobility with the use of active/passive range-of-motion exercises or through use of physical and/or occupational therapy resources at home.
5. Patient openly verbalizes fears, anxieties, and changes in self-image with members of the health care team, supportive staff, family, and support groups.
6. Patient (and family, significant others, and/or caregiver) openly discusses impact of the disease process on relationships, daily activities, future activities; the lifelong need for daily medication; and monitoring for adverse and toxic effects (e.g., dizziness, nausea, vomiting, GI upset, and palpitations).
   - Patient states purposes of medication therapy such as decrease in symptoms of Parkinson's, improved comfort, improved activities of daily living, increase in nutritional status.
   - Patient states information for point of contact with prescriber and symptoms to report such as dry mouth, unresolved nausea/vomiting, fainting, loss of appetite.
7. Patient (and family, significant others, and/or caregiver) describes ways of preventing self-injury, such as the use of assistive devices, removing throw rugs, use of night lights, and handrail placement throughout the home.

## CASE STUDY

### *Drugs for Parkinson's Disease*

Ben, a 62-year-old retired contractor, is undergoing surgery to repair an umbilical hernia. He has had Parkinson's disease for 5 years and is currently taking carbidopa-levodopa (Sinemet CR) and selegiline (Eldepryl). Other than the Parkinson's disease, he has no health problems. He has enjoyed fairly good control up until this week but is now experiencing more "bad times," as he calls them.

1. Patients who are taking long-term levodopa treatment often experience an "on-off" phenomenon in symptoms. Explain the physiology behind this phenomenon.
2. Explain the reason for giving selegiline along with the carbidopa-levodopa. Ben undergoes the surgery without any difficulties, and the following medication orders are noted on the chart:
   Continue previous orders for carbidopa-levodopa (Sinemet CR) 1 tablet bid and selegiline (Eldepryl) 5 mg bid (taken with the Sinemet CR)
   Meperidine (Demerol) 10 mg IV every 4 hours as needed for pain
   Ondansetron (Zofran) 4 mg IV one time if needed for nausea
   Begin entacapone (Comtan) 200 mg bid with each dose of Sinemet
3. Are there any concerns regarding drug interactions? Explain your answer.
4. What is the purpose of the entacapone?
5. Before administering the entacapone, the nurse reviews Ben's history for any potential contraindications. What condition(s) would be a potential contraindication to entacapone?

*IV,* Intravenous.
For answers, see http://evolve.elsevier.com/Lilley.

## IMPLEMENTATION

Nursing interventions associated with the various antiparkinson drugs will vary somewhat depending on the drug class, but close monitoring and comprehensive patient education are required for all of these drugs. With the onset of drug therapy, encourage patients, family, or caregivers to begin keeping a daily drug calendar or journal with entries including the drugs prescribed, dosage, frequency/timing, therapeutic changes, and adverse effects. During the start of *dopaminergic replacement drug* therapy, the patient will most likely need assistance when walking because of the dizziness and possible syncope caused by these drugs. Doses are given several hours before bedtime to decrease the incidence of insomnia, a known adverse effect of these drugs. Oral doses are given with food to help minimize GI upset. Interaction of vitamin $B_6$ (pyridoxine) with levodopa was once a major concern because this vitamin was found to block the uptake of plain levodopa. However, a majority of patients taking a carbidopa-levodopa combination drug were found to have no problems with vitamin $B_6$. The National Parkinson's Disease Foundation (available at www.pdf.org) reports that only patients who are very sensitive to the effects of any of these drugs will have problems with vitamin $B_6$. If it is a problem, the prescriber needs to be consulted for further instructions (see p. 246). In addition, amino acids from dietary protein may interfere with the uptake of levodopa in the brain. While taking carbidopa-levodopa, the patient may continue to eat high-protein foods (e.g., meat, fish, poultry, and dairy products) but use portion control (meat portion about the size of a deck of cards) and take the drug dose one-half hour before a protein-containing meal. Timing is the issue, not the quantity of protein consumed over the course of the day. A nutritional consult may be beneficial to assist the patient in menu planning. A nutritionist may also be helpful in teaching the patient about how to divide the total quantity of protein among small frequent meals so that minimal amounts of protein are ingested throughout the day and are consumed at the proper time. Consumption of well-balanced meals is important, as is increasing fluids. Patients need to aim at drinking at least 3000 mL/day unless contraindicated. Drinking water is important, even if the patient is not thirsty or in need of hydration, to prevent and manage the adverse effect of constipation. Encourage the intake of foods that are natural laxatives, such as prunes, vegetables, and other foods high in fiber. If the adverse effect of dry mouth is problematic, taking fluids and sucking on hard candy or lozenges may be helpful. If nausea or vomiting occurs or problems with edema are persistent (the patient gains 2 pounds or more in 24 hours or 5 pounds or more in 1 week), the prescriber needs to be contacted immediately.

With *anticholinergic drugs,* patients need to take the medication as prescribed, after meals or at bedtime and not at the same time as with other medications. Patients also need to know that it may take a few days to several weeks for the drugs to show their therapeutic effectiveness (e.g., improvement in tremors). Because of the risk of stomach upset (i.e., nausea, vomiting), it is recommended that these drugs be taken with a snack, such as ginger ale and crackers. These medications are generally taken at night because of their sedating properties. Measures to help prevent and treat dry mouth are encouraged, such as increasing fluids and sucking on sugar-free hard candies. See Chapter 21 for further information about the use of these drugs, interventions, and adverse effects to report. *Bromocriptine* is to be taken as prescribed and not abruptly stopped. Because this drug may cause GI upset, it is best taken with a snack. Any severe dizziness, GI upset, ataxia, excess drowsiness, or visual changes must be reported immediately.

*MAO-B inhibitors,* such as selegiline, are to be given exactly as ordered. Selegiline is often given in upwardly titrated dosages while carbidopa-levodopa dose amounts are decreased. Place oral disintegrating dosage forms on the tongue, and do not swallow dosage form until it is completely melted. This dosage form is to be taken without liquids and given in the morning before breakfast. Foods and fluids are not to be consumed for 5 minutes before or after the drug is taken. Postural hypotension may be a transient problem, and so the patient needs to move and change positions slowly and purposely. If dizziness is severe or if the patient experiences hallucinations, the prescriber needs to be contacted for further instructions.

The newer *COMT inhibitors* have been shown to have greater efficacy in patients with advanced forms of Parkinson's disease. After treatment using the various dosage forms of levodopa or carbidopa-levodopa, a COMT inhibitor may then be added to the therapeutic regimen. Onset of therapeutic effects is rapid. These drugs are to be administered as prescribed and may be taken without regard to meals or food. These and other antiparkinson drugs are never to be discontinued abruptly and require a gradual weaning period to avoid worsening of Parkinson's disease or other dangerous effects. Emphasize to patients and caregivers that all appointments with the prescriber must be kept and all laboratory testing performed, as ordered. Patients need to also understand the importance of changing positions slowly and with purpose to avoid syncope due to drug-related orthostatic hypotension. Inform patients that entacapone may turn their urine brownish orange but that this is not harmful. As with all medications, patients must keep on their person a written list of prescription drugs, over-the-counter drugs, vitamins, minerals, and herbal therapies they are taking at all times. This list of medications needs updating frequently and should be taken each time the prescriber is visited and/or the patient is hospitalized. This allows continuity of information with health care providers and helps to prevent errors or omission of medications. Encourage patients to report to the prescriber any back

and/or abdominal pain (especially in the right upper quadrant), bruising, or jaundice as these may be indicative of liver dysfunction associated with tolcapone (see Table 15-3).

It is most important in the care of patients with Parkinson's disease to be aware of all other forms of therapies that may be beneficial, such as support groups, water aerobics, and occupational and physical therapy. Some community resources that are available are community-wide recreation facilities, transportation services, and Meals on Wheels. Educational materials and emotional support resources need to be made available and shared with family members, caregivers, and significant others because of the long-term and progressive nature of the disease. Contacting research institutes about new treatment protocols may be a viable option for patients and family members during the course of the disease. See Patient Teaching Tips for more specific information.

## EVALUATION

Monitoring the patient's response to any of the *antiparkinson drugs* is crucial to documenting treatment success or failure. Therapeutic responses to the antiparkinson drugs include an improved sense of well-being, improved mental status, increased appetite, ability to perform activities of daily living, improved concentration and ability to think more clearly, and a decrease in the intensity of parkinsonian symptoms (e.g., less tremor, shuffling of gait, and muscle rigidity, and fewer involuntary movements). In addition to monitoring for therapeutic responses, also monitor for adverse effects such as dizziness, hallucinations, nausea, insomnia (associated with *indirect-acting dopamine receptor agoninsts* such as selegiline, amantadine, entacapone, and tolcapone), ataxia, depression (associated with *direct-acting dopamine receptor agonists* such as bromocriptine and *dopamine replacement drugs* such as levodopa and carbidopa), palpitations, hypotension, and urinary retention. Patients need to understand the importance of immediately reporting to their prescriber any of the following signs and symptoms indicating possible overdose: excessive twitching, drooling, or eye spasms. Therapeutic effects of *COMT inhibitors* (e.g., entacapone) may be noticed within a few days, whereas therapeutic effects of other antiparkinson drugs may take weeks to manifest. Adverse effects for which to monitor with COMT inhibitors include those mentioned previously, but fewer dyskinesias are seen than with dopamine agonists.

## ▮ PATIENT TEACHING TIPS

- All medications must be taken exactly as ordered. Around-the-clock dosing is usually prescribed to achieve steady blood levels, especially with dopamine agonists.
- Some patients will be allowed a certain amount of freedom in the dosing of their medications depending on their individual needs. An example is when a patient is traveling or attending a function where an extra dose of medication may be indicated/needed to help with movement disorder.

- Alcohol, over-the-counter drugs, and herbals are to be avoided unless approved by the prescriber.
- Emphasize the importance of taking the medication as prescribed and not quitting the medication. It is important for the patient/family/caregiver to understand that medication(s) must be taken at the dosage and time prescribed. Inability to adhere to or remain compliant may lead to exacerbation of symptoms and development of complications. Missing a dose by even 30 minutes may lead to an "off" period and last hours.

- If the patient misses a dose of medication, the prescriber must be notified for further instructions. Some prescribers tell patients initially that if they miss a dose to take it as soon as they remember, and if it is close to the next dose time, then to skip the missed dose and take the next dose.
- If experiencing postural hypotension, the patient needs to understand the rationale for changing positions slowly and the need to increase fluids and wear compression stockings, unless contraindicated. If the patient has a history of congestive heart failure, fluid intake must be done very cautiously.
- Sustained-released drug forms are not to be crushed, chewed, or altered in any way. The drug is to be taken in its whole form. The exception to this standard of care is with Sinemet CR, which may be split only once and is available in scored dosage form for this reason (see pharmacology discussion).
- With anticholinergics, warn the patient about the adverse effect of dry mouth. Use of artificial saliva drops/gum, frequent mouth care, fluids, and sucking on sugarless gum or hard candy may be helpful.
- Inform the patient that urine color may darken if taking entacapone and that this adverse effect is harmless.
- Encourage the patient to report any change in vision (e.g., blurring), decline in mental alertness, confusion, or lethargy experienced while taking any of the antiparkinson drugs. Any difficulty with urination, irregular pulse rate, or severe, uncontrolled movements of the arms or legs must also be reported.
- The patient and family must understand that some antiparkinson drugs are often titrated to the patient's response and that it may take 3 to 4 weeks for a therapeutic response to become evident.
- The nonergot drug ropinirole may result in drowsiness, fatigue, and syncope. Emphasis on safety and how to handle these adverse effects is important.
- Fluids and dietary fiber must be increased to help prevent constipation associated with the disease process. Constipation is also an adverse effect of drug therapy.
- Inform the patient that the COMT inhibitors entacapone and tolcapone need to be taken with food, meals, or a snack to minimize GI upset. Other instructions with the use of entacapone include reporting any signs and symptoms of possible liver dysfunction such as jaundice and back or abdominal pain.
- Any abnormal contractions of the head, neck, or trunk, as well as any syncope, falls, itching, and/or jaundice must be reported immediately to the prescriber.
- Educate the patient about the goal of therapy, especially if entacapone is being used to help manage the wearing-off phenomenon. The wearing-off phenomenon is a waning of the effects of a dose of levodopa before the scheduled time of the next dose, resulting in diminished motor ability and the experience of more disease symptoms. If a COMT inhibitor is added to carbidopa-levodopa, the wearing-off phenomenon is minimized, and the therapeutic effects of the regimen are maximized. The patient can then expect that the "off" time will be minimized and that the drugs will work throughout the day, which is the goal in the treatment of Parkinson's disease.

## ■ KEY POINTS

- The neurotransmission-related abnormalities in Parkinson's disease include the chronic, progressive degeneration of dopamine-producing neurons in the brain. Patients with this disease also have elevated acetylcholine levels and lowered dopamine levels.
- Signs and symptoms of this disease process include bradykinesia (slow movements), muscle rigidity (cogwheel rigidity), tremor (pill rolling), postural instability, and dystonias (abnormal muscle tone in any tissue).
- Dyskinesias occur as adverse effects of some of the antiparkinson drugs. Dyskinesias include motor difficulties while performing voluntary movements.
- Drugs used in the treatment of Parkinson's disease include amantadine, benztropine, bromocriptine, carbidopa-levodopa, entacapone, ropinirole, and selegiline.
- Patient considerations include providing individual and family support along with options for care of the family member with Parkinson's disease. The disease is long-term and lifelong, as well as debilitating. A holistic approach in which all aspects of the patient and family are considered and respected is the key to quality nursing care.

# NCLEX® EXAMINATION REVIEW QUESTIONS

1 Which condition will alert the nurse to a potential caution or contraindication regarding the use of a dopaminergic drug for treatment of mild Parkinson's disease?
   a Diarrhea
   b Tremors
   c Angle-closure glaucoma
   d Unstable gait

2 A patient is taking entacapone (Comtan) as part of the therapy for Parkinson's disease. Which intervention by the nurse is appropriate at this time?
   a Notify the patient that this drug causes discoloration of the urine.
   b Limit the patient's intake of tyramine-containing foods.
   c Monitor results of renal studies because this drug can seriously affect renal function.
   d Force fluids to prevent dehydration.

3 During a patient teaching session about antiparkinson drugs, the nurse will include which statement?
   a "The drug will be stopped when tremors and weakness are relieved."
   b "If a dose is missed, take two doses to avoid significant decreases in blood levels."
   c "Be sure to notify your physician if your urine turns brownish-orange in color."
   d "Take care to change positions slowly to prevent falling due to a drop in blood pressure."

4 A patient will be taking selegiline (Eldepryl), 10 mg daily, in addition to dopamine replacement therapy for Parkinson's disease. The nurse will implement which precautions regarding selegiline?
   a Teach the patient to avoid foods containing tyramine.
   b Monitor for dizziness.
   c Inform the patient that this drug may cause urine discoloration.
   d Monitor for tachycardia and palpitations.

5 A patient with Parkinson's disease will start taking entacapone (Comtan) along with the carbidopa-levodopa (Sinemet) he has been taking for a few years. The nurse recognizes that the advantage of taking entacapone is that
   a the entacapone can reduce on-off effects.
   b the levodopa may be stopped in a few days.
   c there is less GI upset with entacapone.
   d it does not cause the cheese effect.

6 The nurse is assessing a patient who has begun therapy with amantadine (Symmetrel) for Parkinson's disease. The nurse will look for which possible adverse effects? (Select all that apply.)
   a Nausea
   b Palpitations
   c Dizziness
   d Insomnia
   e Edema

7 The order reads: bromocriptine (Parlodel) 10 mg per day PO. The medication is available in 2.5-mg tablets. How many tablets will the nurse give per dose?

1. c, 2. a, 3. d, 4. b, 5. a, 6. a, c, d, 7. 4 tablets

For Critical Thinking and Prioritization Questions, see http://evolve.elsevier.com/Lilley.

# Psychotherapeutic Drugs

## evolve WEBSITE

*http://evolve.elsevier.com/Lilley*

- Animations
- Answer Key—Textbook Case Studies
- Critical Thinking and Prioritization Questions

- Key Points—Downloadable
- Review Questions for the NCLEX® Examination
- Unfolding Case Studies

## OBJECTIVES

When you reach the end of this chapter, you will be able to do the following:

1 Briefly discuss the various mental illnesses.
2 Identify the various psychotherapeutic drug classes, such as anxiolytic drugs, antidepressants, mood-stabilizing drugs, and antipsychotics.
3 Discuss the mechanisms of action, indications, therapeutic effects, adverse effects, toxic effects, drug interactions,

contraindications, and cautions associated with the various psychotherapeutic drugs.
4 Develop a nursing care plan that includes all phases of the nursing process for patients taking psychotherapeutic drugs.
5 Develop patient education guidelines for patients taking psychotherapeutic drugs.

## DRUG PROFILES

- **alprazolam, p. 257**
- **amitriptyline, p. 262**
- **bupropion, p. 266**
  buspirone, p. 258
  clozapine, p. 271
- **diazepam, p. 258**
  duloxetine, p. 267
- **fluoxetine, p. 266**
  haloperidol, p. 269

- **lithium, p. 259**
- **lorazepam, p. 258**
- **mirtazapine, p. 266**
- **risperidone, p. 271**
  selegiline transdermal patch, p. 264
  trazodone, p. 266

---

- *Key drug*

## KEY TERMS

**Affective disorders** Emotional disorders that are characterized by changes in mood. (p. 255)

**Agoraphobia** An anxiety disorder that involves an intense fear of being in unfamiliar situations or places that may be difficult to leave or in which help may not be available in the event of having an unexpected panic attack or panic-like symptoms. (p. 255)

**Akathisia** A movement disorder in which there is an inability to sit still; motor restlessness. It can occur as an adverse effect of psychotropic medications. (p. 268)

**Anxiety** The unpleasant state of mind in which real or imagined dangers are anticipated and/or exaggerated. (p. 255)

**Biogenic amine hypothesis** A theory suggesting that depression and mania are caused by alterations in the concentrations of dopamine and norepinephrine, and serotonin and histamine in the brain. (p. 260)

**Bipolar disorder** A major psychological disorder characterized by episodes of *mania* or *hypomania*, cycling with depression; formerly called *manic-depressive illness*. (p. 255)

**Depression** An abnormal emotional state characterized by exaggerated feelings of sadness, melancholy, dejection, worthlessness, emptiness, and hopelessness that impact the patient's life and may be out of proportion to reality. Signs include withdrawal from social contact, loss of appetite, and insomnia. (p. 255)

**Dopamine hypothesis** A theory suggesting that dopamine dysregulation in certain parts of the brain is one of the primary contributing factors to the development of psychotic disorders (psychoses). (p. 256)

**Dyskinesia** Term for abnormal and distressing involuntary movements; inability to control movements. (p. 268)

**Dysregulation hypothesis** A theory that views depression and affective disorders as caused not simply by decreased or increased catecholamine and serotonin activity but by failure of the brain to *regulate* the levels of these neurotransmitters. (p. 260)

**Dystonia** A syndrome of abnormal muscle contraction that produces repetitive involuntary twisting movements and abnormal posturing of the neck, face, trunk, and extremities; often caused as an adverse reaction to psychotropic medications. (p. 268)

**Extrapyramidal symptoms** The term for signs and symptoms that resemble pathologic changes to the *pyramidal* portions of the brain. Such symptoms include various motion disorders similar to those seen in Parkinson's disease, and are an adverse effect associated with use of various antipsychotic drugs. (p. 268)

**Gamma-aminobutyric acid** An amino acid in the brain that functions to inhibit nerve transmission in the central nervous system. (p. 255)

**Hypomania** A less severe and less potentially hazardous form of mania. (p. 255)

**Mania** An acute illness characterized by an expansive emotional state, including extreme excitement, elation, hyperactivity, agitation, talkativeness, flight of ideas, reduced attention span, increased psychomotor activity, impulsivity, insomnia, anorexia, and sometimes violent, destructive, and self-destructive behavior. (p. 255)

**Metabolic syndrome** A cluster of conditions (increased glucose level, increased blood pressure, abnormal cholesterol levels, excess body fat around the waist) occurring together that increases the risk of heart disease, stroke, and diabetes. (p. 269)

**Neuroleptic malignant syndrome** An uncommon but serious adverse effect associated with the use of antipsychotic drugs and characterized by symptoms such as fever, cardiovascular instability, and myoglobinemia (presence in the blood of muscle breakdown proteins). (p. 268)

**Neurotransmitters** Endogenous chemicals in the body that serve to conduct nerve impulses between nerve cells (neurons). (p. 254)

**Permissive hypothesis** A theory postulating that reduced concentrations of serotonin (5-hydroxytryptamine) is the predisposing factor in individuals with affective disorders. (p. 260)

**Psychosis** (Plural: *psychoses*) A type of serious mental illness that can take several different forms and is associated with being out of touch with reality; that is, the individual is unable to distinguish imaginary from real circumstances and events. (p. 255)

**Psychotherapeutics** The treatment of emotional and mental disorders. (p. 255)

**Psychotropic** Capable of affecting mental processes; usually said of a medication. (p. 256)

**Serotonin syndrome** A rare collection of symptoms resulting from elevated levels of the neurotransmitter *serotonin;* may occur with the use of any psychotropic drug (e.g., antidepressants, buspirone, tramadol) that enhances brain serotonin activity (see Box 16-1). (p. 265)

**Stigma** Widespread negative perceptions of and prejudice toward a specific group of people such as those with mental illness. (p. 255)

**Tardive dyskinesia** A serious drug adverse effect characterized by abnormal and distressing involuntary body movements and muscle tension that is associated with the use of antipsychotic medications. (p. 268)

## ANATOMY, PHYSIOLOGY, AND PATHOPHYSIOLOGY OVERVIEW

From time to time, most people experience the normal emotions of anxiety, depression, excitement, and grief. Many times such emotions are simply situational. They arise because of a specific event and subside with time. Treatment, if any, is often limited to psychotherapy, and possibly short-term drug therapy. However, longer-term pharmacotherapy in conjunction with psychotherapy is usually recommended when a person's emotions or behaviors compromise his or her quality of life, ability to carry out normal activities of daily living, social functioning (interactions and relationships with others), or occupational

functioning (e.g., employment, school) over a prolonged period (at least several months).

The exact causes of mental disorders are not fully understood. There are many theories that attempt to explain the etiology and pathophysiology of mental dysfunction. In the biochemical imbalance theory, mental disorders are thought to arise as the result of abnormal levels of endogenous chemicals in the brain known as **neurotransmitters.** The conduction of messages between neurons (nerve cells) by neurotransmitters is called *neurotransmission.* This occurs in both the central nervous system (CNS) and the peripheral nervous system. The proposed mechanisms of both the pathology of and drug therapy for mental illness center around neurotransmission within the brain. There is evidence indicating that the brain levels of catecholamines (especially dopamine and norepinephrine; see Chapter 18) and indolamines (serotonin and histamine) play an important role in maintaining mental health. Other biochemical substances necessary for the maintenance of normal mental function are the inhibitory neurotransmitter gamma-aminobutyric acid, the cholinergic neurotransmitter acetylcholine (see Chapter 20), and some inorganic ions such as sodium, potassium, and magnesium. Drugs used to treat mental illnesses, including anxiety, affective disorders, and psychoses, work by blocking or stimulating the release of various endogenous neurotransmitters.

The symptoms of the different psychiatric disorders often overlap, which can make them difficult to accurately diagnose. Complicating this issue further is the subjectivity of patients' experience of their symptoms. The *Diagnostic and Statistical Manual of Mental Disorders*, 4th edition, Text Revision *(DSM-IV-TR)* is a widely used reference published by the American Psychiatric Association. It presents demographic information and diagnostic criteria for recognized psychiatric disorders. Often a patient has ongoing symptoms that meet the criteria for several mental disorders. Such patients may be said to have a spectrum disorder. For example, research shows that more than half of chronically depressed adults also have a comorbid personality disorder, and one third have a comorbid anxiety disorder and/or a substance abuse disorder. The problem of comorbid substance abuse is especially troublesome. Usually, a patient must discontinue use of the abused substance(s) to have a chance at significant success in treating the concurrent psychiatric disorder. Unfortunately, this does not happen in the majority of patients.

Patients with mental illness may be more susceptible to various physical health problems than the general population. Obesity and tobacco use is significantly more common in patients with certain mental disorders. These patients are at greater risk for physical illnesses associated with obesity, including diabetes, hypertension, and heart disease. Economic, educational, and psychosocial issues may preclude a mentally ill person from seeking psychiatric health care. Thus, many patients self-medicate with substances of abuse, including alcohol, tobacco, and illegal or unauthorized prescription drugs. This compounds the problem of their baseline psychiatric illness.

Despite the development of newer, more effective treatments for mental illness, a longstanding societal stigma continues to be an obstacle for diagnosed patients. The National Alliance on Mental Illness (NAMI) is an organization that works to reduce this stigma. NAMI seeks to promote consumer well-being and autonomy through public education, research funding, and legislative advocacy.

The treatment of mental disorders is called psychotherapeutics. Ideal mental health care involves many components, including a carefully detailed patient interview (to help ensure accurate and complete diagnosis) and carefully chosen and regularly monitored drug therapy. Nonpharmacologic treatments include psychotherapy, support groups, social and family support systems, and often spiritual support systems. Other practices that promote mental health include physical exercise, good nutrition, and mental exercises such as meditation and visualization. In extreme cases, such as refractory depression, electroconvulsive therapy may be used.

This chapter focuses on three common types of mental illness: anxiety, affective, and psychotic disorders. The drugs used to treat anxiety are anxiolytics. Mood stabilizers and antidepressants are used to treat affective disorders, while antipsychotics are used to treat psychotic disorders.

Anxiety is the unpleasant state of mind characterized by a sense of dread and fear. It may be based on anticipated or past experiences. It may also stem from exaggerated responses to imaginary negative situations or to common everyday experiences. Persistent anxiety is divided clinically into several distinct disorders, including the following:
- Obsessive-compulsive disorder
- Posttraumatic stress disorder
- Generalized anxiety disorder
- Panic disorder with or without agoraphobia
- Social phobia (also called social anxiety disorder)
- Simple phobia

Anxiety is a normal reaction to stress; however, results of epidemiologic studies show that 5% to 8% of adults suffer from generalized anxiety disorder, 2.7% from panic disorder, 6.8% to 12% from posttraumatic stress disorder, and 3.8% from agoraphobia (the fear of being in unfamiliar situations or places). Obsessive-compulsive disorder is twice as common as schizophrenia or panic disorder in the general population. Anxiety may occur as a result of medical illnesses (e.g., cardiovascular or pulmonary disease, hypothyroidism, hyperthyroidism, pheochromocytoma, Cushing syndrome, and hypoglycemia).

Affective disorders, also called *mood disorders,* are characterized by changes in mood and range from mania (exaggerated emotions) to depression (fewer emotions or emotional range). Some patients may exhibit both mania and depression, experiencing periodic swings in emotions between these two extremes. This is referred to as bipolar disorder. Hypomania is a form of mania that is less severe and less potentially dangerous (to patient and others).

Bipolar disorder occurs in an estimated 2% of the population. Depression is currently reported to have prevalence rates ranging from 8% to 12%. Major depressive disorders are expected to become the second leading cause of disability by the year 2020. Common depressive symptoms include feelings of worthlessness, loss of interest in normally pleasurable activities, reduced energy level, reduced motivation and ability to meet routine responsibilities, drastic increase or decrease in appetite, insomnia or hypersomnia, and recurrent thoughts of death or suicide. In addition to being associated with reductions in quality of life and occupational and social functioning, depression is also accompanied by the occurrence of major sleep disturbances in up to 80% of patients. Despite recent advances in pharmacotherapy for depression, it remains undertreated in many cases.

Psychosis is a severe mental disorder that often impairs mental function to the point of causing significant disability in performing the activities of daily living. A hallmark of psychosis is a loss of contact with reality. The primary psychotic disorders are schizophrenia and depressive and drug-induced psychoses. Schizophrenia may trigger hallucinations, paranoia, and delusions (false beliefs), and it is estimated to affect 1% of the population. The dopamine hypothesis of psychotic illness grows out of the observation that psychotic patients often have excessive dopaminergic activity in the brain. Drug therapy is therefore aimed at reducing this activity. Note that this is in direct contrast to the treatment of Parkinson's disease (see Chapter 15), in which the therapeutic goal is to enhance brain dopaminergic activity.

## PHARMACOLOGY OVERVIEW

Psychotropic drugs are among the most commonly prescribed drugs in the United States. Because of the inherent variability in the description of symptoms and the diagnoses, the effects of these drugs are less easily quantified than many other types of medications. For example, it is usually not known how long a given psychotropic drug works in the body (duration of action). Thus, the effectiveness of psychotropic drug therapy is often measured by verbal reports from patients regarding the level of improvement (if any) in their social and occupational functioning. Drug selection is often a trial-and-error process, which can be long and frustrating for both prescribers and patients.

It is hoped that the emerging field of pharmacogenomics (see Chapter 8) will eventually allow more proactive and improved customization of psychotropic drug therapy. Also, as more information is learned about a drug after initial marketing, it is common for the approved indications for a given drug to expand over time. For example, a drug initially approved to treat depression may later be approved to treat social anxiety disorder or additional conditions.

A common problem with psychotropic drug therapy, as with other types of drug therapy, is nonadherence to the prescribed regimen. Many people do not want to accept a psychiatric diagnosis because of the associated stigma. As a result, they may remain in denial about the reality of their mental illness, including the need to take psychotropic medications. They may also have legitimate fears about adverse effects, as well as fear of the unknown regarding their illness. For example, the weight gain that is associated with antipsychotics can be a reason for patient noncompliance. Finally, they may dread the prospect of having to remain on medication to control their symptoms. Such patients can often be helped by support groups and other social supports. As they adjust to their diagnosis, it is hoped they will see enough benefits of treatment to strengthen their own role in maintaining their mental health.

## ANXIETY DISORDERS
### ANXIOLYTIC DRUGS

Primary anxiolytic drugs include the benzodiazepine drug class and the miscellaneous drug buspirone (Table 16-1). The benzodiazepines are commonly used as first-line drug therapy for both acute and chronic anxiety disorders; they are the focus of this section. In addition, other drugs that

are effective as anxiolytics include selective serotonin reuptake inhibitors (SSRIs), tricyclic antidepressants (TCAs), and monoamine oxidase inhibitors (MAOIs) (all discussed in the section on antidepressants), antipsychotics (see later section on antipsychotic drugs), and the antihistamine hydroxyzine (see Chapter 36).

## Mechanism of Action and Drug Effects

All anxiolytic drugs decrease anxiety by reducing overactivity in the CNS. Benzodiazepines exert their effects by depressing activity in the areas of the brain called the *brainstem* and the *limbic system*. Benzodiazepines are believed to increase the action of gamma-aminobutyric acid (GABA), which is an inhibitory neurotransmitter in the brain that blocks nerve transmission in the CNS.

The drug buspirone is a miscellaneous anxiolytic in its own class and is described in further detail in its drug profile.

## Indications

Benzodiazepines are the largest and most commonly prescribed anxiolytic drug class because they offer several advantages over the other drugs used to treat anxiety. Because of their wide range of therapeutic effects, they are sometimes used for other indications such as ethanol withdrawal (see Chapter 17), insomnia and muscle spasms (see Chapter 12), seizure disorders (see Chapter 14), and as adjuncts in anesthesia (see Chapter 11). They are also commonly used as adjunct therapy for depression because depressive and anxious symptoms often occur together.

## Contraindications

Contraindications to benzodiazepines include known drug allergy; narrow-angle glaucoma, due to their ability to cause mydriasis; and pregnancy, due to their sedative properties and risk for teratogenic effects.

## Adverse Effects

The most common undesirable effect of these drugs is an overexpression of their therapeutic effects, in particular CNS depression. Benzodiazepines can also cause hypotension. Of

| TABLE 16-1 | CURRENTLY AVAILABLE ANXIOLYTIC DRUGS | |
|---|---|---|
| **GENERIC NAME** | **TRADE NAME** | **ROUTE** |
| **Benzodiazepines** | | |
| alprazolam | Xanax | PO |
| clorazepate | Tranxene T-Tab | PO |
| chlordiazepoxide | Librium | PO, IM, IV |
| clonazepam | Klonopin | PO |
| diazepam | Valium | PO, PR, IM, IV |
| lorazepam | Ativan | PO, IM, IV |
| oxazepam | Serax | PO |
| **Miscellaneous** | | |
| buspirone | BuSpar | PO |
| meprobamate | Miltown | PO |
| hydroxyzine | Vistaril | PO, IM |

particular note are paradoxical reactions (opposite of those that would normally be expected) to the benzodiazepines and antihistamines, including hyperactivity and aggressive behavior. Such reactions are relatively uncommon. They are more likely to occur in children, in adolescents, and in the elderly with dementia. Rebound disinhibition can occur in elderly patients upon tapering of doses or discontinuation of the benzodiazepines. In rebound disinhibition, an elderly patient experiences marked sedation for 1 to 2 hours, followed by marked agitation and confusion for several hours afterward. All benzodiazepines are potentially habit-forming and addictive (Schedule IV). Although they can provide significant symptom relief, they must be used judiciously and at the lowest effective doses needed for symptom control. See Table 16-2 for more information on adverse effects. Elderly patients tend to be more sensitive to the sedating effects of benzodiazepines, which can increase their risk for falls; thus lower doses are usually needed.

## Toxicity and Management of Overdose

When benzodiazepines are taken alone, an overdose is generally not life threatening. When they are combined with alcohol or other CNS depressants, the outcome is much more severe. An overdose of benzodiazepines may result in any of the following symptoms: somnolence, confusion, coma, and respiratory depression. The treatment of benzodiazepine intoxication is generally symptomatic and supportive. Flumazenil (Romazicon) is a benzodiazepine receptor blocker (antagonist) that is used to reverse the effects of benzodiazepines. It is sometimes given to reverse benzodiazepine effects after procedures involving moderate sedation (see Chapter 11). The treatment regimen for the acute reversal of benzodiazepine effects is summarized in Chapter 12. Flumazenil may cause acute withdrawal syndrome, including seizures in patients taking long-term benzodiazepines or those with a history of substance abuse.

## Interactions

Several notable drug interactions occur with the use of benzodiazepines. Alcohol and CNS depressants, when coadministered with benzodiazepines, can result in additive CNS depression and even death. This serious consequence is more likely to occur in patients with renal and/or hepatic compromise (e.g., the elderly). Other drug interactions are listed in Table 16-3.

## Dosages

Recommended dosages of selected anxiolytic drugs are given in the table on this page.

## DRUG PROFILES

### BENZODIAZEPINES

Benzodiazepines are widely used anxiolytic drugs. Benzodiazepines are all classified as Schedule IV controlled substances. For dosage and indication information, see the table on this page.

♦ **alprazolam**

Alprazolam (Xanax) is most commonly used as an anxiolytic. It is also indicated for the specific anxiety disorder known as *panic disorder*. Adverse effects include confusion, ataxia, headache, and others listed in Table 16-2. Interacting drugs include alcohol, antacids, oral contraceptives, and others listed in Table 16-3. Alprazolam is available only for oral use, in both tablet and orally dissolving tablet forms. The orally dissolving tablet is indicated for the treatment of anxiety disorder, short-term relief of anxiety symptoms, treatment of anxiety associated with

| TABLE 16-2 | ADVERSE EFFECTS OF SELECTED ANXIOLYTIC DRUGS* |
|---|---|
| **DRUG OR DRUG CLASS** | **ADVERSE EFFECTS** |
| **Benzodiazepines** | Amnesia, anorexia, sedation, lethargy, fatigue, confusion, drowsiness, dizziness, ataxia, headache, visual changes, hypotension, weight gain or loss, nausea, weakness |
| **Miscellaneous** buspirone | Paradoxical anxiety, dizziness, blurred vision, headache, nausea |

*See also drug profiles for drug-specific information.

## DOSAGES

### Selected Anxiolytic Drugs

| DRUG (PREGNANCY CATEGORY) | PHARMACOLOGIC CLASS | USUAL DOSAGE RANGE* | CURRENT FDA-APPROVED INDICATIONS/USES |
|---|---|---|---|
| ♦ alprazolam (Xanax) (D) | Benzodiazepine | **Adult** PO: 0.25-2 mg tid; do not exceed 4 mg/day | Anxiety |
| ♦ diazepam (Valium) (D) | Benzodiazepine | **Adult** PO: 2-10 mg 2-3 times/day **Pediatric** PO: 1-2.5 mg 3-4 times/day | Anxiety |
| ♦ lorazepam (Ativan) (D) | Benzodiazepine | **Adult** PO: 0.5-6 mg/day in 2-3 divided doses | Anxiety, alcohol withdrawal, agitation |

*All dosages reflect usual adult dosage ranges. Pediatric dosages may be more variable and are best prescribed by a pediatric practitioner.

depression, and treatment of panic disorder with or without agoraphobia.

### Pharmacokinetics

| Route | Onset of Action | Peak Plasma Concentration | Elimination Half-life | Duration of Action |
|---|---|---|---|---|
| PO | 30-60 min | 1-2 hr | 10-15 hr | 6 hr |

#### ◆ diazepam

Diazepam (Valium) used to be the most commonly prescribed benzodiazepine; however, for treatment of anxiety, it has generally been replaced by the shorter-acting benzodiazepines alprazolam and lorazepam. Diazepam is indicated for the relief of anxiety, management of alcohol withdrawal, reversal of status epilepticus, preoperative sedation, and less frequently as an adjunct for the relief of skeletal muscle spasms. Diazepam has active metabolites that can accumulate in patients with hepatic dysfunction, because it is metabolized primarily in the liver. This can result in additive, cumulative effects that may be manifested as prolonged sedation, respiratory depression, or coma. For this reason, it is probably best avoided in patients with major hepatic compromise. Adverse drug effects include headache, confusion, slurred speech, and others listed in Table 16-2. Diazepam interacts with alcohol, oral contraceptives, and others as shown in Table 16-3. Diazepam is available in oral, rectal, and injectable dosage forms.

### Pharmacokinetics

| Route | Onset of Action | Peak Plasma Concentration | Elimination Half-life | Duration of Action |
|---|---|---|---|---|
| PO | 30-60 min | 1-2 hr | 20-80 hr | 12-24 hr |

#### ◆ lorazepam

Lorazepam (Ativan) is an intermediate-acting benzodiazepine. Of those mentioned here, alprazolam is the shortest acting, whereas diazepam is the longest acting. Lorazepam is available in oral and injectable forms. It may be given intravenously or intramuscularly. It has excellent absorption and bioavailability when given intramuscularly, but it is irritating to the muscle and must be diluted. The conversion between injectable and oral dosage forms is 1:1. Lorazepam can be given by intravenous push, which is useful in the treatment of an acutely agitated patient. It is often administered as a continuous infusion to agitated patients who are undergoing mechanical ventilation. It is also used to treat or prevent alcohol withdrawal (see Chapter 17). Indications, contraindications, and adverse effects are similar to those of alprazolam.

### Pharmacokinetics

| Route | Onset of Action | Peak Plasma Concentration | Elimination Half-life | Duration of Action |
|---|---|---|---|---|
| PO | 30-60 min | 2 hr | 11-16 hr | 8 hr |

### MISCELLANEOUS DRUG

#### buspirone

Buspirone (BuSpar) is an anxiolytic drug that is different both chemically and pharmacologically from the benzodiazepines. Its precise mechanism of action is unknown, but it appears to have agonist activity at both serotonin and dopamine receptors. It is indicated for the treatment of anxiety and is always administered on a scheduled (not "as-needed") basis, as opposed to the benzodiazepines that may be administered as needed or on a schedule. The only reported contraindication is drug allergy. Buspirone lacks the sedative properties and dependency potential of the benzodiazepines. Adverse effects include paradoxical anxiety, dizziness, blurred vision, headache, and nausea. Potential drug interactions include a risk for serotonin syndrome (see section on antidepressants). Patients receiving buspirone and antidepressants together need to be monitored carefully. It is recommended that monoamine oxidase inhibitors (MAOIs) not be used concurrently with buspirone due to

| TABLE 16-3 | DRUG INTERACTIONS OF SELECTED ANXIOLYTIC DRUGS* | | |
|---|---|---|---|
| **DRUG CLASS** | **INTERACTING DRUG(S)** | **MECHANISM** | **RESULT** |
| **Benzodiazepines** | CNS depressants (e.g., alcohol, opioids) | Additive effects | Enhanced CNS depression (e.g., sedation, confusion, ataxia) |
| | Oral contraceptives, azole antifungals, SSRIs, verapamil, diltiazem, opioids, valproic acid | Impaired hepatic elimination of benzodiazepine | Enhanced benzodiazepine effects (e.g., CNS depression) |
| | rifampin | Enhanced benzodiazepine clearance | Reduced therapeutic effects |
| | theophylline | Antagonistic effects | Reduced sedative effects |
| | phenytoin | Reduced clearance | Potential for digoxin toxicity and phenytoin toxicity |
| **Miscellaneous** buspirone | CYP3A4 inhibitors, azole antifungals, verapamil, diltiazem | Impaired hepatic metabolism of buspirone | Enhanced buspirone effects |
| | rifampin | Enhanced buspirone clearance | Reduced therapeutic effects |
| | MAOIs | Unknown | Increased blood pressure |

*CNS*, Central nervous system; *CYP3A4*, cytochrome P-450 enzyme 3A4; *MAOIs*, monoamine oxidase inhibitors; *NSAIDs*, nonsteroidal antiinflammatory drugs; *SSRIs*, selective serotonin reuptake inhibitors.
*See also drug profiles for drug-specific information.

the risk of hypertension. A washout period of at least 14 days after discontinuation of MAOI therapy must be allowed before buspirone is started. Other drugs that interact with buspirone include *inhibitors* of the cytochrome P-450 enzyme system (see Chapter 2)—specifically with CYP3A4 (e.g., ketoconazole [see Chapter 42], clarithromycin [see Chapter 38])—which can reduce buspirone clearance; and *inducers* of these same enzymes, which can enhance buspirone clearance and decrease its therapeutic effect. In either case, the buspirone dosage may need to be adjusted. Other interactions are listed in Table 16-3. Buspirone is available only for oral use.

## Pharmacokinetics

| Route | Onset of Action | Peak Plasma Concentration | Elimination Half-life | Duration of Action |
|-------|-----------------|---------------------------|-----------------------|--------------------|
| PO | 2-3 wk | 40-60 min | 2-3 hr | Unknown |

## AFFECTIVE DISORDERS

Several classes of drugs are used in the treatment of the affective (emotional) disorders. The two main drug categories are mood-stabilizing drugs and antidepressant drugs.

## MOOD-STABILIZING DRUGS

Mood stabilizers are drugs used to treat bipolar illness (cycles of mania, hypomania, and depression). Clinical evidence indicates that the catecholamines (dopamine and norepinephrine) play an important pathophysiologic role in the development of mania. Serotonin also appears to be involved. Lithium has been in use for many years and is still used to effectively alleviate the symptoms of acute mania. Lithium is available in two salt forms: lithium carbonate and lithium citrate. Lithium is also effective for the maintenance treatment of bipolar disorder. Lithium is thought to potentiate serotonergic neurotransmission. A variety of medications may be used in conjunction with lithium to regulate mood or achieve stability; they include benzodiazepines (described earlier), antipsychotic drugs (see later in the chapter), antiepileptic drugs (see Chapter 14), and dopamine receptor agonists (see Chapter 15). The antiepileptics valproic acid, lamotrigine, oxcarbazepine, and topiramate are preferred to lithium because lithium has a narrow therapeutic range and requires blood level monitoring. These drugs are often effective in treating mania, hypomania, and, to a lesser degree, depressive symptoms. Other evidence has shown that the atypical antipsychotic drugs risperidone, olanzapine, quetiapine, and ziprasidone (see later) can also be effective in treating mania and hypomania. Available mood-stabilizing drugs are listed in Table 16-4.

## DRUG PROFILE

### lithium

The antimanic effect of lithium is not fully understood. Research indicates that lithium ions alter sodium ion transport in nerve cells, which results in a shift in catecholamine metabolism. The levels of lithium required to produce a therapeutic effect are close to the toxic levels. For the management of acute mania, a lithium serum level of 1 to 1.5 mEq/L is usually required. Desirable long-term maintenance levels range between 0.6 and 1.2 mEq/L. Blood levels are best measured 8 to 12 hours after the last dose (roughly the midpoint of the drug half-life), because the half-life is usually between 18 and 24 hours. Both sodium and lithium are monovalent positive ions, and one can affect the other. Therefore, the patient's serum sodium levels require monitoring. Keeping the sodium level in the normal range (135 to 145 mEq/L) helps to maintain therapeutic lithium levels. Patients should be advised not to drastically change their sodium intake while taking lithium and to avoid overhydration as well as dehydration.

Lithium is indicated for the treatment of manic episodes in bipolar disorder as well as for maintenance therapy to prevent such episodes. Contraindications to lithium therapy are relative and include dehydration, known sodium imbalance, and major renal or cardiovascular disease, because all of these conditions increase the risk of lithium toxicity. Renal dysfunction of any degree can increase lithium levels. Elderly patients are particularly prone to this effect, because renal function normally declines with advancing age. Adverse effects tend to correlate with serum levels. Levels exceeding 1.5 to 2.5 mEq/L begin to produce toxicity, including gastrointestinal discomfort, tremor, confusion, somnolence, seizures, and possibly death. The most serious adverse effect is cardiac dysrhythmia. Other effects include drowsiness, slurred speech, epilepsy-type seizures, choreoathetotic movements (involuntary wavelike movements of the extremities), ataxia (generalized disturbance of muscular coordination), and hypotension. Long-term treatment may cause hypothyroidism. Potentially interacting drugs include the thiazide diuretics (see Chapter 28), angiotensin-converting enzyme inhibitors (see Chapter 22), and nonsteroidal antiinflammatory drugs (see Chapter 44), all of which can increase lithium toxicity. Lithium carbonate is available only for oral use.

## Pharmacokinetics*

| Route | Onset of Action | Peak Plasma Concentration | Elimination Half-life | Duration of Action |
|-------|-----------------|---------------------------|-----------------------|--------------------|
| PO | 7-14 days† | 0.5-2 hr | 18-24 hr | 2-24 hr |

*Information provided is for immediate-release lithium.
†Therapeutic benefit for maintenance control of mania.

## ANTIDEPRESSANT DRUGS

Antidepressants are the pharmacologic treatment of choice for major depressive disorders. Not only are they very effective in treating depression, they are also useful in treating other disorders, such as dysthymia (chronic low-grade depression), schizophrenia (as an adjunctive drug), eating disorders, and personality disorders. Some of the antidepressants are also used in the treatment of various medical conditions, including migraine headaches, chronic pain syndromes, sleep disorders, premenstrual syndrome, and hot flashes associated with menopause. Available antidepressants are listed in Table 16-4.

| TABLE 16-4 | CURRENTLY AVAILABLE MOOD STABILIZERS AND ANTIDEPRESSANTS | |
|---|---|---|
| **GENERIC NAME** | **TRADE NAME** | **ROUTE** |
| **Mood Stabilizers** | | |
| lithium carbonate* | Lithobid | PO |
| lithium citrate* | Generic | PO |
| Antiepileptics (valproic acid, lamotrigine, topiramate. oxcarbazepine) | Depakote, Depakene, Lamictal, Topamax, Trileptal | PO |
| **Antidepressants** | | |
| *First Generation* | | |
| *Tricyclics* | | |
| amitriptyline | Elavil | PO |
| amoxapine | Generic | PO |
| clomipramine | Anafranil | PO |
| desipramine | Norpramin | PO |
| doxepin | Sinequan | PO |
| imipramine | Tofranil | PO |
| nortriptyline | Pamelor | PO |
| protriptyline | Vivactil | PO |
| trimipramine | Surmontil | PO |
| *Tetracyclics* | | |
| maprotiline (first generation) | Generic | PO |
| mirtazapine (second generation) | Remeron | PO |
| *MAOIs* | | |
| isocarboxazid | Marplan | PO |
| phenelzine | Nardil | PO |
| tranylcypromine | Parnate | PO |
| *Second Generation* | | |
| *SSRIs* | | |
| citalopram | Celexa | PO |
| escitalopram | Lexapro | PO |
| fluoxetine | Prozac | PO |
| fluvoxamine | Generic | PO |
| paroxetine | Paxil | PO |
| sertraline | Zoloft | PO |
| *SNRIs* | | |
| duloxetine | Cymbalta | PO |
| venlafaxine | Effexor | PO |
| desvenlafazine | Pristiq | PO |
| *Miscellaneous* | | |
| bupropion | Wellbutrin | PO |
| nefazodone | Generic | PO |
| trazodone | Generic, Oleptro | PO |
| vilazodone | Viibrya | PO |

*Also classified as an antipsychotic.

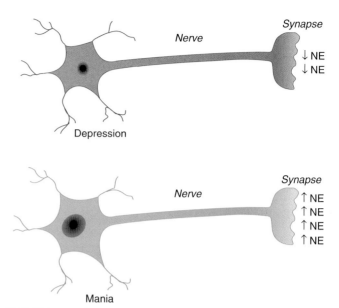

**FIGURE 16-1** Biologic amine hypothesis. *NE,* Norepinephrine.

Many of the drugs used to treat affective disorders increase the levels of neurotransmitter concentrations in the CNS; these neurotransmitters include serotonin (also known as 5-hydroxytryptamine, or 5-HT), dopamine, and norepinephrine. This treatment is based on the belief that alterations in the levels of these neurotransmitters are responsible for causing depression. A widely held hypothesis advanced to explain depression in these terms is the biogenic amine hypothesis. It postulates that depression results from a deficiency of neuronal and synaptic catecholamines (primarily norepinephrine) and mania from an excess of amines at the adrenergic receptor sites in the brain. This hypothesis is illustrated in Figure 16-1.

Another hypothesis regarding the cause of depression is the permissive hypothesis, which led to the creation of the selective serotonin reuptake inhibitor (SSRI) drug class. The permissive theory postulates that reduced concentrations of serotonin are the predisposing factor in patients with affective disorders. Depression results from decreases in both the serotonin and catecholamine levels, whereas mania results from increased dopamine and norepinephrine levels but decreased serotonin levels. The permissive hypothesis is illustrated in Figure 16-2. The dysregulation hypothesis is essentially a reformulation of the biogenic amine hypothesis. This theory views depression and other affective disorders not simply in terms of decreased or increased catecholamine activity but as a failure of the regulation of these systems.

Research indicates that early and aggressive antidepressant treatment increases the chances for full remission. The first 6 to 8 weeks of therapy constitute the acute phase. The primary goals during this time are to obtain a response to drug therapy and to improve the patient's symptoms. It is currently recommended that antidepressant drug therapy be maintained at the effective dose for an additional 8 to 14 months after remission of depressive symptoms. In choosing an antidepressant, the patient's previous psychotropic drug response history (if any) needs to be considered. Family history of depression with known drug responses are also helpful. Therapeutic response is measured primarily by subjective patient feedback. In addition, a few measurement tools are available that attempt to quantify the patient's response to drug therapy, such as the Hamilton Rating Scale for Depression and the Symptom Checklist-90 anxiety factor scale.

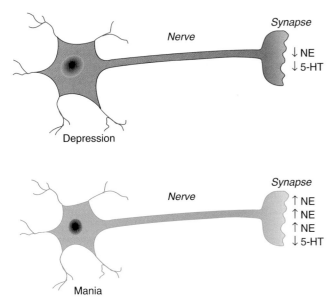

**FIGURE 16-2** Permissive hypothesis. *NE,* Norepinephrine; *5-HT,* serotonin.

Anxiety and depression commonly occur together and reinforce each other. Similarly, there is much crossover in terms of symptom control between antidepressant and anxiolytic drugs. A nonresponse to antidepressant drug therapy is defined as failure to respond to at least 6 weeks of therapy with adequate drug dosages. Twenty percent to 30% of patients who do not respond to the usual dosage of an antidepressant will respond to higher dosages. Therefore, dosage optimization, which involves careful upward titration of dose for several weeks, is recommended before concluding that a given drug is ineffective. Often times a switch to a different pharmacologic class of antidepressant is necessary. Forty percent to 60% of patients will respond to the second drug class tried. Anxiolytic and antipsychotic drugs may also be used, either alone or as adjunct therapy. Evidence suggests that psychotherapy given with antidepressant medication is more effective than medication alone.

The most severe cases of refractory depression may warrant an attempt at treatment with electroconvulsive therapy. Electroconvulsive therapy treatment is generally carried out in a postanesthesia care unit setting under brief general anesthesia. Seizure activity is induced in the anesthetized patient via externally applied electric shocks to the brain.

Treatment failure in cases of depression may be due to a misdiagnosis or failure to treat comorbid mental illness (e.g., anxiety disorder, substance abuse) and/or comorbid nonpsychiatric illness (e.g., hypothyroidism). It may also be due to nonadherence to drug therapy. Careful choice of drug therapy to minimize adverse effects may improve patient compliance with treatment and therapeutic outcome. Another reason for treatment failure may be the discouragement associated with depression itself. This alone may cause patients to give up prematurely on their drug therapy, especially because antidepressants often take several weeks to reach their full effect. Effective psychotherapy and support groups can help encourage patients to be consistent with prescribed psychotropic drug therapy.

In 2005, the U.S. Food and Drug Administration (FDA) issued special black box warnings regarding the use of all classes of antidepressants in both adult and pediatric patient populations. Data from the FDA indicated a higher risk for suicide in patients receiving these medications (up to 4% of patients taking the drugs showed suicidal thoughts or behaviors compared with 2% receiving a placebo). As a result, current recommendations for all patients receiving antidepressants include regular monitoring for signs of worsening depressive symptoms, especially when the medication is started or the dosage is changed. Patients need immediate evaluation if they report, or others observe, signs of worsening depression or other emotional instability. Most patients do not experience severe adverse effects from these medications, and many patients obtain significant relief.

## TRICYCLIC ANTIDEPRESSANTS

Tricyclic antidepressants (TCAs) were the original first-generation antidepressants. Their use has largely been replaced with the SSRIs and serotonin-norepinephrine reuptake inhibitors (SNRIs). The TCAs are considered second-line drug therapy in patients for whom the SSRIs are ineffective or as adjunct therapy with newer drugs. The TCAs are so named because of their characteristic three-ring chemical structure.

### Mechanism of Action and Drug Effects

TCAs are believed to work by correcting imbalance in the neurotransmitter concentrations of serotonin and norepinephrine at the nerve endings in the CNS (the biogenic amine hypothesis). This is accomplished by blocking the presynaptic reuptake of the neurotransmitters, which makes them available for transmission of nerve impulses to adjacent neurons in the brain. Some also believe that these drugs may help regulate malfunctioning neurons (the dysregulation hypothesis).

### Indications

Originally used to treat depression, currently TCAs are most commonly used to treat neuropathic pain syndromes and insomnia. With the advent of the newer-generation antidepressant classes, their use as antidepressants is rare. Some of the TCAs have additional specific indications. For example, imipramine is used as an adjunct in the treatment of childhood enuresis (bedwetting), and clomipramine is useful in the treatment of obsessive-compulsive disorder. Because TCAs tend to increase appetite leading to weight gain, they are sometimes used to treat anorexia nervosa.

### Contraindications

Contraindications for TCAs include known drug allergy, use of MAOIs within the previous 14 days, and pregnancy. TCAs are also not recommended in patients with any acute or chronic cardiac problems or history of seizures, because both conditions are associated with a greater likelihood of death upon TCA overdose.

### Adverse Effects

Undesirable effects of TCAs are a result of their effects on various receptors, especially the muscarinic receptors (a type of

## TABLE 16-5 ADVERSE EFFECTS OF SELECTED MOOD STABILIZERS AND ANTIDEPRESSANTS*

| DRUG OR DRUG CLASS | ADVERSE EFFECTS |
| --- | --- |
| **Mood Stabilizers** | |
| lithium salts | GI discomfort, tremor, confusion, sedation, seizures, cardiac dysrhythmia, drowsiness, slurred speech, slowed motor abilities, weight gain, ataxia, hypotension |
| Antiepileptic drugs | Dizziness, drowsiness, GI upset, weight gain, hepatotoxicity, pancreatitis, unusual eye movements, visual changes, behavioral changes, ataxia |
| **Antidepressants** | |
| **First Generation** | |
| Tricyclics | Anorexia, dry mouth, blurred vision, constipation, gynecomastia, sexual dysfunction, altered blood glucose level, urinary retention, agitation, anxiety, ataxia, cognitive impairment, sedation, headache, insomnia, skin rash, photosensitivity, weight changes, orthostatic hypotension, blood dyscrasias |
| MAOIs | Dizziness, dyskinesias, nausea, syncope, hypotension |
| **Second Generation** | |
| **Tetracyclics** | |
| mirtazapine, maprotiline | Drowsiness, abnormal dreams, dry mouth, constipation, increased appetite, asthenia (muscle weakness) |
| SSRIs | Anxiety, dizziness, drowsiness, headache, mild GI disturbance, sexual dysfunction, asthenia, tremor |
| SNRIs | Dizziness, drowsiness, headache, GI upset, anorexia, hepatotoxicity |
| **Miscellaneous** | |
| trazodone, bupropion | Dizziness, headache, sedation, nausea, blurred vision, tachycardia |

*See also drug profiles for drug-specific information.

cholinergic receptor) and, to a lesser degree, adrenergic, histaminergic, dopaminergic, and serotonergic receptors. Blockade of cholinergic receptors results in undesirable anticholinergic adverse effects, the most common being constipation and urinary retention. Nortriptyline and desipramine have less anticholinergic activity, and they are preferred for use in the elderly. Adrenergic and dopaminergic receptor blockade can lead to disturbances in cardiac conduction and hypotension. Histaminergic blockade can cause sedation, and serotonergic blockade can alter the seizure threshold, and cause sexual dysfunction (see Table 16-5).

### Toxicity and Management of Overdose

Tricyclic antidepressant overdoses are notoriously lethal. It is estimated that 70% to 80% of patients who die of TCA overdose do so before reaching the hospital, especially if the drugs are taken with alcohol. The primary organ systems affected are the CNS and cardiovascular system. Death usually results from either seizures or dysrhythmias. Historically it was taught that

patients should not receive more than a 1-month supply of antidepressants because of the risk of suicide attempts. However, with the cost of drugs today, it is not uncommon to see a 3-month supply given with only one copay. This is a double-edged sword: the patient saves money, but now the depressed patient has more than enough drugs to cause death by overdose.

There is no specific antidote for TCA poisoning. Management efforts are aimed at reducing drug absorption by administering multiple doses of activated charcoal. Administration of sodium bicarbonate speeds up elimination of the TCA by alkalinizing the urine. CNS damage may be minimized by the administration of diazepam, and cardiovascular events may be minimized by giving antidysrhythmics. Other care includes basic life support in an intensive care setting to maintain vital organ functions. These interventions must continue until enough of the TCA is eliminated to permit restoration of normal organ function.

### Interactions

Increased anticholinergic effects are seen when TCAs are taken with anticholinergics and phenothiazines. When MAOIs are taken with TCAs, the result may be increased therapeutic and toxic effects, including hyperpyretic crisis (excessive fever). Other drug interactions are listed in Table 16-6.

### Dosages

Recommended dosages of selected TCA drugs are given in the table on p. 263.

### DRUG PROFILE

TCAs are effective drugs in the treatment of various affective disorders, but they are associated with serious adverse effects. Therefore, patients taking them need to be monitored closely. For this reason, all antidepressants are available only with a prescription. Some herbal products used to treat depression, such as St. John's wort (see the Safety: Herbal Therapies and Dietary Supplements box on p. 264), are available over the counter but should not be taken with prescription antidepressants. Many drugs in this class are rated as pregnancy category D drugs, which makes their use by pregnant women relatively more hazardous than that of most of the newer drugs.

#### ♦ amitriptyline

Amitriptyline (Elavil) is the oldest and most widely used of all the TCAs. Its original indication was depression, but it is now more commonly used to treat insomnia and neuropathic pain. Contraindications include known drug allergy, pregnancy, and recent myocardial infarction. It has very potent anticholinergic properties, which can lead to many adverse effects such as dry mouth, constipation, blurred vision, urinary retention, and dysrhythmias (see Table 16-5). Drug interactions are listed in Table 16-6. Amitriptyline is available only for oral use.

#### Pharmacokinetics

| Route | Onset of Action | Peak Plasma Concentration | Elimination Half-life | Duration of Action |
| --- | --- | --- | --- | --- |
| PO | 7-21 days | 2-12 hr | 10-50 hr | 6-12 hr |

CHAPTER 16   Psychotherapeutic Drugs   **263**

## DOSAGES

### Selected Mood-Stabilizing and Antidepressant Drugs

| DRUG (PREGNANCY CATEGORY) | PHARMACOLOGIC CLASS | USUAL DOSAGE RANGE* | CURRENT FDA-APPROVED INDICATIONS/USES |
|---|---|---|---|
| **Mood Stabilizers** | | | |
| ◆ lithium carbonate (D) | Inorganic salt | 600-1800 mg/day divided bid-tid | Acute mania, prevention of mania |
| **Antidepressants** *First Generation* | | | |
| ◆ amitriptyline (generic only; formerly Elavil) (C) | Tricyclic | Adult PO: 10-300 mg/day | Depression (more commonly used for insomnia and neuropathic pain) |
| *Second Generation* | | | |
| ◆ bupropion (Wellbutrin, Zyban) (C) | Miscellaneous | PO: 200-300 mg/day, divided bid PO, SR: 150-300 mg/day | Depression (Wellbutrin), smoking cessation (Zyban) |
| duloxetine (Cymbalta) (C) | SNRI | PO: 20-40 mg/day; or 60 mg/day divided bid | Depression, GAD, diabetic peripheral neuropathy |
| ◆ fluoxetine (Prozac) (C) | SSRI | PO: 10-20 mg/day; higher doses up to 80 mg/day divided bid | Depression, OCD, bulimia nervosa, panic disorder, premenstrual dysphoric disorder |
| ◆ mirtazapine (Remeron) (C) | Tetracyclic | PO: 15-45 mg at bedtime | Depression, bipolar disorder |
| trazodone (Desyrel) (C) | Triazolopyridine | PO: 25-600 mg/day, with larger doses divided | Depression (more commonly used for insomnia) |

*GAD,* Generalized anxiety disorder; *OCD,* obsessive-compulsive disorder; *PO,* oral; *SNRI,* serotonin norepinephrine reuptake inhibitor; *SSRI,* selective serotonin reuptake inhibitor.

*All dosages reflect usual adult dosage ranges. Pediatric dosages may be more variable and are best prescribed by a pediatric practitioner.

### TABLE 16-6   DRUG INTERACTIONS OF SELECTED MOOD-STABILIZING AND ANTIDEPRESSANT DRUGS*

| DRUG CLASS | INTERACTING DRUG(S) | MECHANISM | RESULT |
|---|---|---|---|
| **Mood Stabilizers** | | | |
| lithium salts | Thiazide diuretics, angiotensin converting enzyme inhibitors, verapamil, diltiazem, NSAIDs | Decreased lithium excretion | Increased lithium toxicity |
| Antiepileptic drugs | See Table 14-5. | | |
| **Antidepressants** *First Generation* | | | |
| Tricyclics (TCAs) | carbamazepine, rifamycins | Enhanced TCA clearance | Reduced therapeutic effects |
| | carbamazepine | Reduced carbamazepine clearance | Potential for carbamazepine toxicity |
| | MAOIs | Enhance serotonergic effects | Potential for serotonin syndrome |
| | valproic acid | Reduced TCA clearance | Potential for TCA toxicity |
| | Anticholinergics | Additive anticholinergic effects | Potential for paralytic ileus |
| | Sympathomimetics | Enhanced sympathomimetic effects | Potential for cardiac dysrhythmias |
| *Second Generation* **Tetracyclics** | | | |
| mirtazapine, maprotiline | Alcohol, CYP inhibitors | Additive effects | Increased toxicity |
| **SSRIs** | MAOIs, linezolid, lithium, metoclopramide, buspirone, sympathomimetics, tramadol | Additive effects | Potential for serotonin syndrome |
| | Benzodiazepines | Reduced metabolism | Potential benzodiazepine toxicity |
| | warfarin, phenytoin | Protein binding displacement | Potential for warfarin or phenytoin toxicity |
| | propafenone | Increased propafenone levels | Potential for propafenone toxicity |
| **SNRIs** | | | |
| duloxetine | SSRIs, triptans | Additive effects | Risk of serotonin syndrome |
| | NSAIDs, warfarin | Additive effects | Risk of bleeding |
| | Alcohol | Additive liver toxicity | Increased risk of hepatotoxicity |
| **Miscellaneous** | | | |
| trazodone, bupropion | Azole antifungals, phenothiazines, protease inhibitors | Impaired hepatic metabolism | Increased effects |
| | Carbamazepine | Increased metabolism | Decreased therapeutic effects |
| | Alcohol, CNS depressants | Additive effects | Increased CNS depression |

*CNS,* Central nervous system; *CYP,* cytochrome P-450; *MAOIs,* monoamine oxidase inhibitors; *NSAIDs,* nonsteroidal antiinflammatory drugs; *SNRIs,* serotonin-norepinephrine reuptake inhibitors; *SSRIs,* selective serotonin reuptake inhibitors.

*See also drug profiles for drug-specific information.

**SAFETY: HERBAL THERAPIES AND DIETARY SUPPLEMENTS**

### St. John's Wort (Hypericum perforatum)

**Overview**

St. John's wort herbal preparations consist of the dried above-ground parts of the plant species *Hypericum perforatum* gathered during flowering season. The herb is available over the counter in numerous oral dosage forms. St. John's wort is sometimes referred to as the *herbal Prozac*.

**Common Uses**

Depression, anxiety, sleep disorders, nervousness

**Adverse Effects**

Gastrointestinal upset, allergic reactions, fatigue, dizziness, confusion, dry mouth, possible photosensitization (especially in fair-skinned individuals)

**Potential Drug Interactions**

Monoamine oxidase inhibitors, selective serotonin reuptake inhibitors, cyclosporine, sympathomimetic amines, piroxicam, tetracycline, tyramine-containing foods, opioids, digoxin, estrogens, theophylline, warfarin

**Contraindications**

Contraindicated in patients with bipolar depression, schizophrenia, Alzheimer's disease, and dementia

## MONOAMINE OXIDASE INHIBITORS

Monoamine oxidase inhibitors (MAOIs), along with TCAs, represent the first generation of antidepressant drug therapy; they are rarely used as antidepressants, but are used to treat Parkinson's disease. A serious disadvantage to MAOI use is their potential to cause a hypertensive crisis when taken with stimulant medications or with a substance containing tyramine, which is found in many common foods and beverages (Table 16-7).

Currently four MAOI antidepressants are available. Isocarboxazid, phenelzine, and tranylcypromine are nonselective inhibitors of both MAO type A and MAO type B. Selegiline is a selective MAO-B inhibitor that comes in a transdermal dosage form. An oral form of this drug is also used to treat Parkinson's disease (see Chapter 15). Because these drugs inhibit the MAO enzyme system in the CNS, amines such as dopamine, serotonin, and norepinephrine are not broken down, and therefore higher levels of these substances occur. This, in turn, alleviates the symptoms of depression.

Most adverse effects of MAOIs stem from their interactions with food and other medications. A variety of over-the-counter drugs (especially for cough and cold) also can interact with MAOIs to cause adverse cardiovascular effects. For example, MAOIs may increase the CNS depressant effects of diphenhydramine and cetirizine. Patients taking MAOIs need to read labels and/or consult the pharmacist when using any such products. Dosage information for selected MAOIs is given in the table on p. 263.

Sympathomimetic drugs can also interact with MAOIs, and together these drugs can cause a hypertensive crisis. MAOIs can markedly potentiate the effects of meperidine, and therefore their concurrent use is contraindicated. In addition, concurrent use of MAOIs with SSRIs carries the risk for serotonin

| TABLE 16-7 | FOOD AND DRINK TO AVOID WHEN TAKING MONOAMINE OXIDASE INHIBITORS | |
|---|---|
| **FOOD/DRINK** | **EXAMPLES** |
| **High Tyramine Content (Not Permitted)** | |
| Aged mature cheeses | Cheddar, blue, Swiss |
| Smoked or pickled meats | Herring, sausage, corned beef, smoked fish or poultry, salami, pepperoni |
| Aged or fermented meats | Chicken or beef liver pâté, game fish or poultry |
| Yeast extracts | Brewer's yeast |
| Red wines | Chianti, burgundy, sherry, vermouth |
| Italian broad beans | Fava beans |
| **Moderate Tyramine Content (Limited Amounts Allowed)** | |
| Meat extracts | Bouillon, consommé |
| Pasteurized light and pale beer | |
| Ripe avocado | |
| **Low Tyramine Content (Permissible)** | |
| Distilled spirits | Vodka, gin, rye, scotch (in moderation) |
| Non-aged cheeses | American cheese, mozzarella, cottage cheese, cream cheese |
| Chocolate and caffeinated beverages | |
| Fruit | Figs, bananas, raisins, grapes, pineapple, oranges |
| Soy sauce | |
| Yogurt, sour cream | |

syndrome. A washout period of 2 to 5 weeks between drugs is recommended.

### Toxicity and Management of Overdose

Clinical symptoms of MAOI overdose generally do not appear until about 12 hours after ingestion. The primary signs and symptoms are cardiovascular and neurologic. The most serious cardiovascular effects are tachycardia and circulatory collapse, and the neurologic symptoms of major concern are seizures and coma. Hyperthermia and miosis are also generally present in overdose. Treatment is aimed at eliminating the ingested toxin and protecting the organs at greatest risk for damage—the brain and the heart. Recommended treatments are urine acidification to a pH of 5 and hemodialysis. Treatment of hypertensive crisis resulting from consumption of tyramine-containing foods or beverages may require intravenous administration of hypotensive drugs along with careful monitoring in an intensive care setting.

### DRUG PROFILE

**selegiline transdermal patch**

The selegiline transdermal patch (Emsam) is a selective MAO-B inhibitor. It is currently indicated for major depression. The lowest strength of the selegiline transdermal patch (6 mg/24 hr) can be used without dietary restrictions. However, to date there are insufficient data to permit the same dietary freedom with the 9- and 12-mg patch strengths. Contraindications include known drug allergy. Adverse drug effects and drug interactions are the same as for the oral dosage form and can be found earlier in the discussion of MAOIs in general and in Chapter 15 for selegiline in particular. Patients need to avoid exposing the patch to external sources of heat, such as a heating pad, electric blanket, sauna, or even prolonged direct sunlight, as these heat sources speed absorption. Standard pharmacokinetic parameters for the transdermal dosage form are not known at this time.

## SECOND-GENERATION ANTIDEPRESSANTS

The period from the 1980s to the present was one of much development in psychotropic pharmacotherapy. Several new antidepressants alone were introduced, including trazodone (Desyrel, Oleptro) and bupropion (Wellbutrin). Both are still commonly used. The selective serotonin reuptake inhibitors (SSRIs) were also introduced. These include fluoxetine (Prozac), sertraline (Zoloft), paroxetine (Paxil), fluvoxamine (generic only; formerly Luvox), citalopram (Celexa), and escitalopram (Lexapro). The 1990s saw the introduction of still more antidepressants, including the serotonin-norepinephrine reuptake inhibitors (SNRIs) venlafaxine (Effexor) and miscellaneous drugs nefazodone (Serzone) and mirtazapine (Remeron). Two new SNRIs were introduced in the 2000s, including duloxetine (Cymbalta) and desvenlafaxine (Pristiq). Desvenlafaxine is the major active metabolite of venlafaxine. Currently available second-generation drugs are listed in Table 16-4. The second-generation antidepressants are generally considered superior to TCAs and MAOIs in terms of their adverse effect profiles. They are associated with significantly fewer and less severe systemic adverse effects, especially anticholinergic and cardiovascular adverse effects. It takes approximately the same amount of time to reach maximum clinical effectiveness with the second-generation antidepressants as it does with the TCAs and MAOIs, typically 4 to 6 weeks.

### Mechanism of Action and Drug Effects

The inhibition of serotonin reuptake is the primary mechanism of action of the SSRIs, although SSRIs may also have weak effects on norepinephrine and dopamine reuptake (see individual drug profiles). SNRIs inhibit the reuptake of both serotonin and norepinephrine. Educate patients that antidepressant drugs commonly must be taken for several weeks before full therapeutic effects are realized. This requires some patience and faithful dosing on the part of patients.

### Indications

Although depression is their primary indication, they have shown benefit in treating a variety of other mental and physical disorders. Examples include bipolar disorder, obesity, eating disorders, obsessive-compulsive disorder, panic attacks or disorders, social anxiety disorder, posttraumatic stress disorder, premenstrual dysphoric disorder, the neurologic disorder myoclonus, and various substance abuse problems such as alcoholism. This list is expanding with continued research on these drugs.

---

### BOX 16-1  COMMON SYMPTOMS OF SEROTONIN SYNDROME

Common symptoms include:
- Delirium
- Agitation
- Tachycardia
- Sweating
- Myoclonus (muscle spasms)
- Hyperreflexia
- Shivering
- Coarse tremors
- Extensor plantar muscle (sole of foot) responses

In more severe cases, the following may occur:
- Hyperthermia
- Seizures
- Rhabdomyolysis
- Renal failure
- Cardiac dysrhythmias
- Disseminated intravascular coagulation

---

### Contraindications

Contraindications include known drug allergy, use of MAOIs in the previous 14 days, and therapy with certain antipsychotic drugs such as thioridazine or mesoridazine. In addition, a significant history of cardiac disease or seizure may be a contraindication due to the relatively uncommon, but reported, cardiac effects and alterations in seizure threshold (see later discussion). Bupropion is also contraindicated in cases of eating disorders and seizure disorders because it can lower the seizure threshold.

### Adverse Effects

The second-generation antidepressants offer advantages over TCAs and MAOIs due to their improved adverse effect profiles. However, up to two thirds of all depressed patients may still discontinue therapy due to drug adverse effects. Some of the most common adverse effects are insomnia (partly due to reduced rapid eye movement sleep), weight gain, and sexual dysfunction. Sexual dysfunction caused by the SSRIs is primarily related to inability to achieve orgasm. One potentially hazardous adverse effect of any drug or combination of drugs that have serotoninergic activity is known as serotonin syndrome. The symptoms of this condition are listed in Box 16-1. Fortunately, it is usually self-limiting on discontinuation of the causative drugs. (See also Table 16-5.)

### Interactions

The second-generation antidepressants are highly bound to albumin. When given with other drugs that are also highly protein bound (e.g., warfarin and phenytoin), they compete for binding sites on the surface of albumin. This results in more free, unbound drug and therefore a more pronounced drug effect.

Some of the drugs may also inhibit cytochrome P-450 enzymes, although there is debate about this in the literature. The cytochrome P-450 system is an enzyme system in the liver that is responsible for the metabolism of several drugs (see Chapter 2). Inhibition of this enzyme system results in higher levels of these drugs with the potential for toxicity.

To prevent the potentially fatal pharmacodynamic interactions that can occur between these drugs and the MAOIs, a 2- to 5-week washout period is recommended between uses of these two classes of medications. Other drug interactions are listed in Table 16-6.

## Dosages

Recommended dosages of selected newer-generation antidepressants are given in the table on p. 263.

## DRUG PROFILES

The second-generation drugs have proved to be effective antidepressants. They also have generally better adverse effect profiles than first-generation antidepressants. They are now considered first-line drugs in the treatment of patients with depression, including patients with concurrent symptoms of anxiety and patients with depression with suicidal ideations.

### trazodone

Trazodone (Desyrel, Oleptro) is in the triazolopyridine drug class. It was the first of the second-generation antidepressants that could selectively inhibit serotonin reuptake but minimally affect norepinephrine reuptake. Trazodone has minimal adverse effects on the cardiovascular system, which is an advantage over the TCAs. It is indicated for the treatment of depression, and it is also commonly used as a nonaddictive drug treatment for insomnia. Contraindications include known drug allergy. Adverse effects include strongly sedative qualities. These can be severe and can impair cognitive function in older adults. However, the sedating effect of trazodone is often advantageous in helping depressed patients, who commonly have comorbid anxiety and/or insomnia, obtain effective sleep. Trazodone also has been associated in rare cases with transient nonsexual *priapism*. This is a dangerously sustained penile erection that is reportedly the result of alpha-adrenergic blockade. Trazodone interacts with azole antifungals (see Chapter 42), phenothiazines (see later in the chapter), and protease inhibitors (see Chapter 40), all of which can increase the risk of trazodone toxicity; carbamazepine (see Chapter 14), which can reduce trazodone levels, while carbamazepine levels are increased; and CNS depressants (e.g., alcohol), whose effects can be potentiated by trazodone. It is also recommended that trazodone be started gradually after a patient has recently stopped MAOI therapy. Trazodone is available only for oral use. Vilazodone (Viibryd), marketed in 2011, is similar to trazodone in both structure and action. Vilazodone is a SSRI and a 5-HT$_{1A}$ receptor agonist.

### Pharmacokinetics

| Route | Onset of Action | Peak Plasma Concentration | Elimination Half-life | Duration of Action |
|---|---|---|---|---|
| PO | 1-2 wk | 2-4 wk | 6-9 hr | Several weeks |

### ◆ fluoxetine

Fluoxetine (Prozac) was the first SSRI marketed for the treatment of depression and is considered the prototypical SSRI. Since that time, it has become the top-prescribed antidepressant in the United States and one of the most commonly prescribed of all drugs. Although it was initially indicated for the treatment of depression, the indications for fluoxetine have since expanded to include bulimia, obsessive-compulsive disorder, panic disorder, and premenstrual dysphoric disorder. Contraindications include known drug allergy and concurrent MAOI therapy. Adverse effects include anxiety, dizziness, drowsiness, insomnia,

and others listed in Table 16-5. Interacting drugs include benzodiazepines (reduced benzodiazepine clearance) (see Chapter 12); buspirone (reduced buspirone effects) (see earlier in the chapter); antipsychotics (elevated antipsychotic levels); and propafenone (see Chapter 24). Other drug interactions are listed in Table 16-6. Fluoxetine is available only for oral use.

### Pharmacokinetics

| Route | Onset of Action | Peak Plasma Concentration | Elimination Half-life | Duration of Action |
|---|---|---|---|---|
| PO | 1-4 wk | 6-8 hr | 1-3 days* | 2-4 wk |

*Active metabolite has a half-life of 7 to 10 days.

### ◆ bupropion

Bupropion is a unique antidepressant in terms of both its structure and mechanism of action. It has relatively weak, but measurable, effects on brain serotonin activity, but little to no effect on monoamine oxidase. Its strongest therapeutic activity appears to be primarily dopaminergic and noradrenergic.

Bupropion was originally indicated for treatment of depression but is now also indicated as an aid in smoking cessation. It is sometimes added as an adjunct antidepressant for patients experiencing sexual adverse effects secondary to SSRI therapy. Although the mechanism is unclear, the drug is often effective in this situation. A sustained-release form of bupropion, Zyban, was approved for smoking cessation treatment. Sustained-release bupropion was an innovative new treatment because it was the first nicotine-free prescription medicine used to treat nicotine dependence. Its exact mechanism of action in treating nicotine dependence is unknown, but it is believed to be related to the drug's ability to modulate dopamine and norepinephrine levels in the brain. Both of these neurotransmitters are believed to play an important role in maintaining nicotine addiction. However, the newer smoking cessation drug varenicline (Chantix; see Chapter 17) is becoming popular for this purpose.

Bupropion is contraindicated in patients who have a known drug allergy, those with a seizure disorder (bupropion can lower the seizure threshold), those who currently have anorexia nervosa or bulimia or have had one of these disorders in the past, and those currently taking an MAOI. Common adverse effects include dizziness, confusion, tachycardia, agitation, tremor, and dry mouth. Drugs that interact with bupropion include the azole antifungals (see Chapter 42) as well as other drugs metabolized by the cytochrome P-450 enzyme system (see Chapter 2) and CNS depressants. Other drug interactions are listed in Table 16-6. Bupropion is available only for oral use.

### Pharmacokinetics

| Route | Onset of Action | Peak Plasma Concentration | Elimination Half-life | Duration of Action |
|---|---|---|---|---|
| PO | Up to 4 wk | 3 hr | 10-14 hr | Weeks to months |

### ◆ mirtazapine

Mirtazapine (Remeron) is unique in that it promotes the presynaptic release of both serotonin and norepinephrine in the brain.

This is due to its antagonist activity in the presynaptic alpha$_2$-adrenergic receptors. It does not inhibit the reuptake of either of these neurotransmitters. It is strongly associated with sedation in more than 50% of patients due to its histamine 1 (H$_1$) receptor activity and therefore is usually dosed once daily at bedtime. Furthermore, although clearance of the drug may be somewhat reduced in elderly patients, no dosage adjustment is currently recommended. Mirtazapine is indicated for treatment of depression, including that associated with bipolar disorder. It is also sometimes helpful (mechanism unknown) in reducing the sexual adverse effects in male patients receiving SSRI therapy. Mirtazapine is known to be an appetite stimulant and thus can be helpful in underweight depressed patients or harmful in those who are already overweight. Mirtazapine is contraindicated in cases of drug allergy and concurrent use of MAOIs. Adverse effects include drowsiness, abnormal dreams, dry mouth, constipation, increased appetite, and asthenia. Drug interactions include additive CNS depressant effects with alcohol and CYP inhibitors (see Chapter 2). Mirtazapine is available only for oral use.

### Pharmacokinetics

| Route | Onset of Action | Peak Plasma Concentration | Elimination Half-life | Duration of Action |
|---|---|---|---|---|
| PO | 1-3 wk | 2 hr | 20-40 hr | Unknown |

### duloxetine

Duloxetine (Cymbalta), like venlafaxine, is a serotonin-norepinephrine reuptake inhibitor (SSNRI). It is indicated for depression and generalized anxiety disorder. It is also indicated for pain resulting from diabetic peripheral neuropathy or fibromyalgia. It is contraindicated in cases of known drug allergy and concurrent MAOI use, and it can worsen uncontrolled angle-closure glaucoma. Adverse effects include dizziness, drowsiness, headache, gastrointestinal upset, anorexia, and hepatotoxicity. Drugs with which duloxetine interacts include SSRIs and triptans (increased risk of serotonin syndrome) and alcohol (increased risk of liver injury). Duloxetine is available only for oral use.

### Pharmacokinetics

| Route | Onset of Action | Peak Plasma Concentration | Elimination Half-life | Duration of Action |
|---|---|---|---|---|
| PO | 2-6 weeks | 6 hr | 12 hr | Unknown |

## PSYCHOTIC DISORDERS
### ANTIPSYCHOTIC DRUGS

Antipsychotic drugs are used to treat serious mental illnesses such as drug-induced psychoses, schizophrenia, and autism. Antipsychotics are also used to treat extreme mania (as an adjunct to lithium), bipolar disorder, depression that is resistant to other therapy, certain movement disorders (e.g., Tourette's syndrome), and certain other medical conditions (e.g., nausea, intractable hiccups). Antipsychotics have also been referred to as *tranquilizers* or *neuroleptics* because they produce a state of tranquility and act on abnormally

### TABLE 16-8 CURRENTLY AVAILABLE ANTIPSYCHOTIC DRUGS

| GENERIC NAME | TRADE NAME | ROUTE |
|---|---|---|
| **Conventional** | | |
| ***Phenothiazines*** | | |
| chlorpromazine | Thorazine | PO, PR, IM, IV |
| fluphenazine | generic | PO, IM |
| perphenazine | generic | PO |
| prochlorperazine | Compazine | PO, PR, IM, IV |
| trifluoperazine | generic | PO |
| thioridazine | generic | PO |
| ***Thioxanthene*** | | |
| thiothixene | Navane | PO |
| ***Phenylbutylpiperidines*** | | |
| haloperidol | Haldol | PO, IM |
| pimozide | Orap | PO |
| ***Dihydroindolone*** | | |
| molindone | Moban | PO |
| **Atypical** | | |
| ***Dibenzodiazepines*** | | |
| clozapine | Clozaril | PO |
| loxapine | Loxitane | PO |
| olanzapine | Zyprexa | PO, IM |
| quetiapine | Seroquel | PO |
| asenapine | Saphris | sublingual |
| ***Benzisoxazoles*** | | |
| lurasidone | Latuda | PO |
| paliperidone | Invega | PO |
| risperidone | Risperdal | PO, IM |
| ziprasidone | Geodon | PO, IM |
| iloperidone | Fanapt | PO |
| ***Quinolinone*** | | |
| aripiprazole | Abilify | PO, IM |

*IM,* Intramuscular; *IV,* intravenous; *MAOIs,* monoamine oxidase inhibitors; *PO,* oral; *PR,* per rectum; *SNRIs,* serotonin-norepinephrine reuptake inhibitors; *SSRIs,* selective serotonin reuptake inhibitors.

functioning nerves. However, these are both older terms that are now less commonly used.

Antipsychotic drugs represent a significant advance in the treatment of mental illnesses, as borne out by the fact that the early treatment of mental illnesses (before the 1950s) consisted of such extreme measures as isolation, physical restraint, shock therapy, and even lobotomy.

The phenothiazines are the largest chemical class of antipsychotic drugs, constituting about two thirds of all antipsychotics. They were also the original drugs in this category. Like many other drugs, phenothiazines were discovered by chance, in this case during research for new antihistamines. Chlorpromazine, isolated in 1951, was the first phenothiazine to be discovered in this way. The currently available antipsychotics are listed in Table 16-8.

Overall, there are few differences between conventional, or first-generation, antipsychotics in terms of mechanism of action. Therefore, selection of an antipsychotic is based primarily on the patient's tolerance and the need to minimize adverse effects. Of the currently available antipsychotic drugs, no single drug stands out for all patients as either more or less effective in the treatment of psychotic symptoms. Antipsychotic drug therapy does not normally provide a cure for psychoses but is a way of chemically controlling the symptoms of the illness.

More recently, a new generation of antipsychotic medications has evolved. These are referred to as *atypical antipsychotics,* as opposed to the conventional drugs, which can also be thought of as older-generation antipsychotics. Atypical antipsychotics differ from conventional drugs in that they tend to have better adverse effect profiles. The atypical antipsychotics still have adverse effects, but they are usually not as severe as the conventional antipsychotic drugs.

## Mechanism of Action and Drug Effects

All antipsychotics block dopamine receptors in the brain, which decreases the dopamine concentration in the CNS. Specifically, the conventional phenothiazines block the dopamine receptors postsynaptically in certain areas of the CNS, such as the limbic system and the basal ganglia. These are the areas associated with emotions, cognitive function, and motor function. This receptor blocking produces a tranquilizing effect in psychotic patients. Both the therapeutic and toxic effects of these drugs are the direct result of the dopamine blockade in these areas. The atypical antipsychotic drugs block specific dopamine receptors called dopamine 2 ($D_2$) receptors, as well as specific serotonin receptors in the brain known as serotonin 2 (5-$HT_2$) receptors. These more refined mechanisms of action of the atypicals are responsible for their improved efficacy and safety profiles, compared with older drugs (see Adverse Effects).

All antipsychotics show efficacy in improving the positive symptoms of schizophrenia, and these beneficial effects may even increase over time. So-called *positive symptoms* include hallucinations, delusions, and conceptual disorganization. Unfortunately, conventional drugs are less effective in managing negative symptoms. Negative symptoms are apathy, social withdrawal, blunted affect, poverty of speech, and catatonia. It is these negative symptoms that account for most of the social and vocational disability caused by schizophrenia. Fortunately, atypical antipsychotics have improved efficacy in treating both positive and negative symptoms.

## Indications

Antipsychotic drugs are indicated for psychotic illness, most commonly schizophrenia. As more has been learned about these drugs, especially the atypical antipsychotic drugs, their indications have expanded to include anxiety and mood disorders as well. Certain antipsychotics (e.g., prochlorperazine) are used as antiemetics (see Chapter 52). They block serotonin receptors and dopamine receptors in the chemoreceptor trigger zone in the brain and inhibit neurotransmission in the vagus nerve in the gastrointestinal tract. Additional blocking of dopamine receptors in the brainstem reticular system also allows atypical drugs to have anxiolytic or antianxiety effects.

## Contraindications

Contraindications to the use of antipsychotic drugs include known drug allergy, comatose state, and, possibly, significant CNS depression, brain damage, liver or kidney disease, blood dyscrasias, or uncontrolled epilepsy.

## Adverse Effects

Common adverse effects caused by blockade of the alpha-adrenergic, dopamine, endocrine, histamine, and muscarinic (cholinergic) receptors are listed in Table 16-9. Possible severe hematologic effects include agranulocytosis (lack of granulocytes in the blood) and hemolytic anemia. CNS effects include drowsiness, neuroleptic malignant syndrome, extrapyramidal symptoms, and tardive dyskinesia. Neuroleptic malignant syndrome is a potentially life-threatening adverse effect that may include high fever, unstable blood pressure, and myoglobinemia. Extrapyramidal symptoms are involuntary motor symptoms similar to those associated with Parkinson's disease (see Chapter 15). This drug-induced state is known as *pseudoparkinsonism* and is characterized by symptoms such as akathisia (distressing motor restlessness) and acute dystonia (painful muscle spasms). Two anticholinergic medications, benztropine (Cogentin) and trihexyphenidyl (Artane), are commonly used to treat these symptoms (see Chapter 15). *Tardive* is a word that means "late appearing." Tardive dyskinesia is characterized by involuntary contractions of oral and facial muscles (e.g., involuntary tongue thrusting) and choreoathetosis (wavelike movements of the extremities) and usually appears only after continuous long-term antipsychotic therapy. Theoretically these effects are possible with atypical antipsychotics as well; however, evidence suggests that the incidence is lower.

Cardiovascular effects, caused by alpha receptor blockade, include postural hypotension. In addition, electrocardiogram (ECG) changes, notably prolonged QT interval, are associated with all classes of antipsychotic drugs. Baseline and periodic ECGs, as well as measurement of serum potassium and magnesium levels, can help to determine if a patient is at risk for such

| TABLE 16-9 | ANTIPSYCHOTICS: RECEPTOR-RELATED ADVERSE EFFECTS | |
|---|---|---|
| **RECEPTOR** | **ADVERSE EFFECTS** | **DRUG CATEGORY** |
| Alpha-adrenergic | Postural hypotension, lightheadedness, reflex tachycardia | Conventional drugs |
| Dopamine | Extrapyramidal movement disorders, dystonia, parkinsonism, akathisia, tardive dyskinesia | Atypical drugs |
| Endocrine | Prolactin secretion (galactorrhea, gynecomastia), menstrual changes, sexual dysfunction | Conventional drugs |
| Histamine | Sedation, drowsiness, hypotension, weight gain | Conventional drugs |
| Muscarinic (cholinergic) | Blurred vision, worsening of angle-closure glaucoma, dry mouth, tachycardia, constipation, urinary retention, decreased sweating | Conventional drugs |

effects or to diagnose newly acquired cardiac dysrhythmias. The conventional drugs such as the phenothiazines and haloperidol can also augment prolactin release, which can result in swelling of the breasts and milk secretion in women taking these drugs. Gynecomastia (breast tissue enlargement) can also be a distressing adverse effect in male patients (Table 16-10).

Adverse effects on the endocrine system associated with antipsychotics include insulin resistance, weight gain, and changes in serum lipid levels. Antipsychotics are associated with development of metabolic syndrome, which can cause serious long-term health problems.

In 2011, the FDA required manufacturers to change a product's labeling to include stronger wording regarding the use of antipsychotics in pregnant women. The new labeling includes more consistent information about the potential risk for abnormal muscle movements (extrapyramidal symptoms) and withdrawal symptoms in newborns whose mothers were treated with these drugs during the third trimester of pregnancy.

## Interactions

Major drug interactions are listed in Table 16-11. Antihypertensives may have additive hypotensive effects and CNS depressants may have additive CNS depressant effects when taken with antipsychotics. Grapefruit juice can enhance the effects of clozapine (by reducing its metabolism via the cytochrome P-450 enzyme system). Because grapefruit juice affects many enzymes in the P-450 system, it is wise to avoid this food for patients taking multiple medications.

## Dosages

Recommended dosages of selected antipsychotic drugs are given in the table on this page.

## DRUG PROFILES

The conventional antipsychotic drugs are currently still available on the U.S. market (see Table 16-8). However, much of their use in clinical practice has been replaced by the atypical antipsychotic drugs, which have better adverse effects profiles. All antipsychotics are prescription-only medications that are indicated for the treatment of various psychotic disorders. No single drug stands out as being either more or less effective in the treatment of the symptoms of psychosis. Some of the factors to be considered before selecting an antipsychotic are the patient's history of response to a drug and the possible adverse effects profile. Starting at a low dose with titration to the lowest effective dose helps achieve a balance between symptom relief and adverse effects. For dosage information on profiled drugs, see the table on this page.

### BUTYROPHENONE
**haloperidol**

Haloperidol (Haldol) is structurally different from the thioxanthenes and the phenothiazines but has similar antipsychotic

| TABLE 16-10 | ADVERSE EFFECTS OF SELECTED PSYCHOTROPIC DRUGS* | |
|---|---|---|
| **DRUG OR DRUG CLASS** | **ADVERSE EFFECTS** | |
| Conventional (e.g., haloperidol) | Akathisia, extrapyramidal symptoms, hypertension, neuroleptic malignant syndrome, confusion, headache, mild GI disturbance, dry mouth, amenorrhea, gynecomastia, visual disturbances, hyperpyrexia, edema, tardive dyskinesia, skin rash, photosensitivity, weight gain, urinary retention | |
| Atypical (e.g., clozapine, risperidone) | Tachycardia, akathisia, agitation, asthenia, ataxia, seizures, dyskinesia, dizziness, drowsiness, headache, insomnia, dry mouth, dyspepsia, anxiety, increased appetite, weight gain | |

GI, Gastrointestinal; MAOIs, monoamine oxidase inhibitors; SNRIs, serotonin-norepinephrine reuptake inhibitors; SSRIs, selective serotonin reuptake inhibitors.
*See also drug profiles for drug-specific information.

## DOSAGES

### Selected Antipsychotic Drugs

| DRUG (PREGNANCY CATEGORY) | PHARMACOLOGIC CLASS | USUAL DOSAGE RANGE* | CURRENT FDA-APPROVED INDICATIONS/USES |
|---|---|---|---|
| **First Generation (Conventional)** | | | |
| haloperidol (Haldol) (C) | Butyrophenone, phenylbutylpiperidine | **Adult** PO, IM/IV: 0.5-5 mg bid-tid **Pediatric** PO: 0.05-0.15 mg/kg/day IM/IV (acute care only): 1-3 mg q4-8h | Schizophrenia, Tourette's syndrome, severe refractory behavioral problems or hyperactivity |
| **Second Generation (Atypical)** | | | |
| clozapine (Clozaril) (B) | Dibenzodiazepine | PO: 12.5 mg bid, titrate up to maximum of 900 mg/day. Larger doses divided tid | Schizophrenia; recurrent suicidal behavior in patients with schizophrenia or schizoaffective disorder |
| ◆ risperidone (Risperdal) (C) | Benzisoxazole | PO: 2-8 mg/day in either one or two doses IM depot form (Risperdal Consta): 25-50 mg every 2 wk | Schizophrenia, mania, irritability associated with autism |

IM, intramuscular; IV, intravenous; PO, oral.
*All dosages reflect usual adult dosage ranges. Pediatric dosages may be more variable and are best prescribed by a pediatric practitioner.

properties. It is indicated primarily for the long-term treatment of psychosis. However, it has been largely replaced by the atypical antipsychotics because of its adverse effects (see later). Haloperidol is contraindicated in patients who have shown a hypersensitivity reaction to it, those in a comatose state, those taking large amounts of CNS depressants, and those with Parkinson's disease (due to its antidopaminergic effects). It is a high-potency neuroleptic drug that has a favorable cardiovascular, anticholinergic, and sedative adverse effect profile, but it can cause extrapyramidal symptoms as well as tardive dyskinesia. Haloperidol is available in three salt forms: base (for oral use), decanoate injection (for IM only), and lactate injection (IM or IV). Haloperidol decanoate has an extremely long duration of action, which has historically made it useful in treating patients with schizophrenia who were nonadherent with their drug regimen. The lactate formulation is commonly given intravenously in acute situations. It is important to note that, although the manufacturer states that it is not to be given intravenously, clinical experience and case reports have shown the intravenous route to be safe and effective. Other adverse effects are listed in Table 16-10. Drugs with which haloperidol interacts are listed in Table 16-11.

### Pharmacokinetics

| Route | Onset of Action | Peak Plasma Concentration | Elimination Half-life | Duration of Action |
|---|---|---|---|---|
| PO | 2 hr | 2-6 hr | 13-35 hr | 8-12 hr |
| IM | Lactate: 20-30 min | Lactate: 30-45 min | 13-35 hr | Lactate: 4-8 hr |
| | Decanoate: 3-9 days | Decanoate: unknown | | Decanoate: 1 mo |

## ATYPICAL ANTIPSYCHOTICS

Between 1975 and 1990, not a single new antipsychotic drug was approved in the United States. In 1990, clozapine (Clozaril), the first of the atypical antipsychotics, was approved. Clozapine was followed by risperidone (Risperdal), olanzapine (Zyprexa), quetiapine (Seroquel), ziprasidone (Geodon), aripiprazole (Abilify), paliperidone (Invega), iloperidone (Fanapt), asenapine (Saphris), and lurasidone (Latuda).

The term *atypical antipsychotics* refers to the following advantageous properties of these drugs: reduced effect on prolactin levels compared with conventional drugs and improvement in the negative symptoms associated with schizophrenia. They also seem to show a lower risk for neuromuscular malignant syndrome, extrapyramidal adverse effects, and tardive dyskinesia. All ten of the currently available atypical drugs have several pharmacologic properties in common. Antagonist activity at the $D_2$ receptor is believed to be the mechanism of their antimanic activity. Serotonergic (serotonin agonist) activity at various 5-HT receptor subtypes and alpha$_2$-adrenergic (agonist) activity are associated with antidepressant activity. Alpha$_1$-adrenergic receptor antagonist activity is associated with orthostatic hypotension, and $H_1$ receptor antagonist activity is associated with both sedative and appetite-stimulating effects. This latter activity accounts for the common adverse effect of weight gain that is associated to various degrees with antipsychotic drugs. This can cause or worsen obesity and even lead to diabetes. Clozapine and olanzapine are associated with the most weight gain, risperidone and quetiapine with less, and ziprasidone is considered weight-neutral. Other atypical antipsychotics fall between the aforementioned drugs. Sedative effects may diminish over time and can actually be helpful for patients with insomnia. Although these drugs all have similar pharmacologic properties, they vary in the degree of affinity for the various types of receptors. These subtle pharmacologic differences, along with often unknown and unpredictable patient physiologic variation, help to explain why some patients respond better (or do not respond) to one medication versus another.

In April 2005, the FDA issued a special public health advisory concerning the use of atypical antipsychotic drugs in elderly patients for off-label (non–FDA-approved) uses. These medications are currently approved for the treatment of schizophrenia and mania. In practice, however, they are also commonly used to control behavioral symptoms of agitation in elderly patients with dementia, including dementia related to Alzheimer's disease. The FDA data found that elderly patients given atypical antipsychotics for this reason were up to 1.7 times more likely to die during treatment. The FDA recommends that patients so treated have their treatment plans reevaluated by their prescribers.

| TABLE 16-11 | DRUG INTERACTIONS OF SELECTED ANTIPSYCHOTICS* | | |
|---|---|---|---|
| **DRUG CLASS** | **INTERACTING DRUG(S)** | **MECHANISM** | **RESULT** |
| **Conventional and Atypical** | Alcohol, other CNS depressants | Additive drug effects | Enhanced CNS depression; dystonia with alcohol |
| | Antihypertensives | Enhanced antihypertensive effects | Potential for hypotension |
| **Conventional: Phenothiazines** | Anticholinergics | Additive and antagonistic drug effects | Reduced phenothiazine efficacy; enhanced anticholinergic effects |
| | Beta blockers | Additive drug effects | Potential toxicity of either drug |
| | Opioids | Additive drug effects | Excessive sedation, hypotension |
| | levodopa/carbidopa | Uncertain | Diminished antiparkinson effects |
| | phenytoin | Uncertain | Can increase or reduce phenytoin levels |
| | Thiazide diuretics | Reduced diuretic clearance | Potential for hypotension |
| **Atypicals*** | CYP3A4 inhibitors (e.g., ketoconazole) | Reduced antipsychotic clearance | Potential for antipsychotic toxicity |
| | carbamazepine | Enhanced antipsychotic clearance | Reduced therapeutic effects |

*CNS,* Central nervous system; *CYP3A4,* cytochrome P-450 enzyme 3A4.
*See also drug profiles for drug-specific information.

Dosage information for atypical antipsychotics is given in the table on p. 269.

### clozapine

Clozapine (Clozaril) was the first of the *atypical* antipsychotics. Compared to conventional antipsychotic drugs, it more selectively blocks the dopaminergic receptors in the *mesolimbic* region of the brain. Conventional antipsychotic drugs block dopamine receptors in an area of the brain called the *neostriatum*, but blockade in this area is believed to give rise to extrapyramidal adverse effects. Because clozapine has very weak dopamine-blocking abilities in this area of the brain, it is associated with minor or no extrapyramidal symptoms. This often makes clozapine the drug of choice for treatment of psychotic disorders in patients who also have Parkinson's disease, because it will not worsen motor symptoms.

Clozapine has been extremely useful for the treatment of patients for whom therapy with other antipsychotic drugs has failed, especially those with schizophrenia. In particular, it is indicated for schizophrenic patients who have shown high risk for suicidal behavior. Adverse effects include the potential for agranulocytosis, a dangerous disorder of white blood cell (WBC) underproduction that is drug induced. For this reason, patients beginning clozapine therapy require weekly monitoring of WBC counts for the first 6 months of therapy. The drug needs to be discontinued if the count falls below 3000/mm³ and withheld until it rises above this value. It is also recommended that WBC counts be evaluated weekly for 4 weeks after discontinuation of the drug. Clozaril is available only through the Clozapine National Registry, with which the patient and prescriber must be registered. Other adverse effects are listed in Table 16-10. Clozapine is contraindicated in patients with known drug allergy; in those with myeloproliferative disorders, severe granulocytopenia, CNS depression, or angle-closure glaucoma; and in comatose patients. Interacting drugs include alcohol and other CNS depressants (increased CNS depression), levodopa (diminished therapeutic effects), antihypertensives (risk of hypotension), and others listed in Table 16-11. Clozapine is available only for oral use.

Other atypical antipsychotics have features comparable to those of clozapine but do not require extensive WBC monitoring. Risperidone is described in the following profile as an example of these drugs. Orally disintegrating tablets are available for clozapine and risperidone, and asenapine is available as a sublingual tablet. These dosage forms may improve compliance. The dosage is the same as that for regular tablets (see the Dosages table on p. 269).

### Pharmacokinetics

| Route | Onset of Action | Peak Plasma Concentration | Elimination Half-life | Duration of Action |
|---|---|---|---|---|
| PO | 1-6 hr | Weeks | 6 hr | 4-12 hr |

### ◆ risperidone

Risperidone (Risperdal) is an atypical antipsychotic that was introduced a few years after clozapine. It is even more active than clozapine at the serotonin (5-HT$_{2A}$ and 5-HT$_{2C}$) receptors. It also has a high affinity for alpha$_1$- and alpha$_2$-adrenergic receptors and histamine H$_1$ receptors. This drug is indicated for schizophrenia, including negative symptoms, and causes minimal extrapyramidal adverse effects at therapeutic dosages of 1 to 6 mg/day.

Risperidone is contraindicated in cases of known drug allergy. Adverse effects include elevated prolactin levels, abnormal dreams, insomnia, dizziness, headache, and others listed in Table 16-10. Drugs interacting with risperidone include CNS depressants, antihypertensives, and others listed in Table 16-11. Risperidone is available for oral and injectable use. The long-acting injectable form is called Risperdal Consta, and one intramuscular injection lasts approximately 2 weeks. This is at least one option for helping patients maintain adherence with the prescribed drug regimen. Patients must continue to take oral risperidone for 3 weeks after the first injection of the Consta dosage form to ensure adequate blood levels from the injection. Paliperidone also comes as a long-acting injection (Invega Sustenna), which lasts 1 month.

### Pharmacokinetics

| Route | Onset of Action | Peak Plasma Concentration | Elimination Half-life | Duration of Action |
|---|---|---|---|---|
| PO | 1-2 wk | 1-2 hr | 20-30 hr | 7 days |
| IM | 3 wk | Unknown | 20-30 hr | 2 wk |

## NURSING PROCESS

## ASSESSMENT

Before administering any of the psychotherapeutic drugs, perform a complete head-to-toe physical assessment and mental status examination. Document your findings. This data will serve as a comparative baseline for the patient during and after initiation of therapy.

Thoroughly assess the patient's neurologic functioning, including level of consciousness, mental alertness, and level of motor and cognitive functioning. The Mini-Mental State Examination (MMSE) is one tool that you may use to assess cognitive status and help identify impairments often found in mental illnesses. The MMSE is simple to use, is cost-effective, and may be completed in about 20 minutes. The MMSE is available in most nursing assessments, nursing fundamentals, and/or psychiatric or mental health nursing textbooks. Points are scored in the areas of level of orientation, attention and calculation ability, recall, and language skills. Other mental health assessment tools include the six-item Blessed Orientation-Memory-Concentration Test, clock-drawing tasks, and Functional Activities Questionnaire (for those with dementia), Alzheimer's Disease Assessment Scale, Mattis Dementia Rating Scale, Severe Impairment Battery, and the Hamilton Rating Scale for Depression. In addition to performing examinations such as these, note baseline levels of motor responses and reflexes as well as the presence of any tremors and/or personality changes. Assess for the presence of cold clammy hands, sweating, and/or pallor. These particular findings may be indicative of an altered autonomic nervous system response.

Constantly assess the patient for any suicidal ideations or tendencies, with attention not only to overt cues and behaviors but also to covert thoughts and ideation. This is important because of the potential for suicide with the use of psychotherapeutic drugs, with or without the concurrent use of other medications or alcohol. Suicide assessment tools are available and may help you identify an individual's risk for suicidal behaviors. One such tool, the Suicide Assessment Scale, has been found to be valid, reliable, and easy to use. The following are some questions that may be helpful: "What brings you to the doctor's office today?" "How has life been treating you?" "What are some of your worries or concerns?" "How would you describe your mood?" "Tell me about your thoughts." If an assessment reveals any concerns and/or the patient acknowledges suicidal thoughts, make an appropriate referral for immediate assessment and/or treatment.

Remember that many of the patients who require psychotherapeutic drugs are depressed and, as such, suffer from insomnia and possibly from self-neglect. Deterioration in health status and weight loss or gain may also occur. Therefore, it is important to assess sleep habits and nutritional intake and to perform a head-to-toe physical examination for baseline and comparative purposes. Note any drug allergies as well as any contraindications, cautions, and potential drug interactions (see pharmacology discussion and Tables 16-3, 16-6, and 16-11). Assess and document blood pressure and pulse rate before, during, and after drug therapy. Postural blood pressures (i.e., blood pressure taken supine then standing) are particularly important to note because of the possible drug-related adverse effects of postural hypotension and dizziness. The more potent older drugs (e.g., MAOIs or TCAs) may lead to a significant drop in blood pressure and possible syncope, warranting even more skillful assessment and close monitoring (of blood pressure readings).

Review the results of any laboratory studies performed before and during the drug therapy. This is especially important for patients who are receiving long-term drug therapy to prevent or identify any early complications or other possible adverse effects or toxicity. Laboratory studies may include, but are not limited to, tests to confirm therapeutic serum levels of the specific drug and, if appropriate, a complete blood count, erythrocyte sedimentation rate, serum electrolyte and glucose levels, BUN, liver function studies, serum level of vitamin $B_{12}$, and thyroid studies. If the patient is experiencing forms of dementia, other types of testing may be needed, such as genetic studies, computed tomography, or magnetic resonance imaging.

With psychotherapeutic drug therapy, assess the patient's mouth and oral cavity to make sure the patient has swallowed the entire oral dosage. This helps to prevent hoarding or "cheeking" of medications, a form of noncompliance that may lead to drug toxicity or overdose. If the assessment shows that this is a potential risk, using liquid dosage forms, when available, may minimize such problems. Other areas to assess include the patient's appetite, sleeping patterns, addictive behaviors, elimination difficulties, and allergic reactions. Note any new symptoms or problems.

## ANXIOLYTIC DRUGS

Anxiety disorders are treated with the anxiolytic drugs. *Anxiolytic drugs*, specifically the benzodiazepines, are associated with many contraindications, cautions, and drug interactions (see pharmacology discussion). When these drugs are used, the prescriber may order laboratory studies, such as complete blood counts,

---

### PATIENT-CENTERED CARE: LIFESPAN CONSIDERATIONS FOR THE ELDERLY PATIENT

#### Psychotherapeutic Drugs

- Elderly patients show higher serum levels of psychotherapeutic drugs because they have age-related changes in drug distribution and metabolism, less serum albumin, decreased lean body mass, less water in tissues, and increased body fat. They also have decreased renal function. Because of these changes, elderly patients generally require lower dosages of antipsychotic and antidepressant drugs and are at greater risk for toxicity.
- Orthostatic hypotension, anticholinergic adverse effects, sedation, and extrapyramidal symptoms are more common in elderly patients taking psychotherapeutic drugs.
- Careful evaluation and documentation of baseline parameters, including neurologic findings, are important to the safe use of these drugs.
- Increased anxiety is often associated with the use of tricyclic antidepressants.
- Patients with a history of cardiac disease may be at a greater risk for experiencing dysrhythmias, tachycardia, stroke, myocardial infarction, or heart failure.
- Lithium toxicity is more common in elderly patients, and lower dosages are often necessary to achieve therapeutic levels. Close monitoring is important to its safe use in this age group. Central nervous system toxicity, lithium-induced goiter, and hypothyroidism are more common in elderly patients.

---

### PATIENT-CENTERED CARE: LIFESPAN CONSIDERATIONS FOR THE PEDIATRIC PATIENT

#### Psychotherapeutic Drugs

- Pediatric patients are more likely to experience adverse effects from psychotropic drugs, especially extrapyramidal effects.
- The incidence of Reye's syndrome and other adverse reactions is greater in pediatric patients who have had chickenpox, central nervous system infections, measles, acute illnesses, or dehydration and are taking psychotropic drugs.
- Lithium may lead to decreased bone density or bone formation in children; therefore, children receiving it need to be closely monitored for signs and symptoms of lithium toxicity and bone disorders. The safety and efficacy of lithium dosing for those younger than 6 years of age is not established.
- Tricyclic antidepressants generally are not prescribed for patients younger than 12 years of age. However, some antidepressants are used in children with enuresis, attention deficit disorders, and major depressive disorders, and may be associated with adverse reactions such as electrocardiographic changes, nervousness, sleep disorder, fatigue, elevated blood pressure, and gastrointestinal upset.
- Pediatric patients are generally more sensitive to the effects of most drugs, and psychotherapeutic drugs are no exception. Be aware of the risk of toxicity, which can be fatal. If confusion, lethargy, visual disturbances, insomnia, tremors, palpitations, constipation, or eye pain occur, contact the prescriber immediately.

---

serum electrolyte levels, and hepatic/renal function studies (see earlier discussion). Blood pressure readings are also very important to assess because of drug-related postural hypotension. The baseline neurologic examination needs to include assessment of alertness, orientation, and sensory/motor functioning as well as any complaints of ataxia, headache, or other neurologic abnormalities. To complete a thorough medication profile, create a list of all medications taken along with any other psychotherapeutic drugs, all prescription drugs, over-the-counter drugs, vitamins, minerals, and herbal products. Diazepam, although one of the more commonly prescribed benzodiazepines, is generally used for seizure disorders and preoperative sedation and requires assessment related to these uses (see Chapters 11 and 14). Specific concerns for pediatric and elderly patients are presented in the boxes on p. 272. Closely observe and assess elderly patients for oversedation and/or profound CNS depression during drug therapy. The elderly are often more sensitive to drugs and therefore more likely to experience adverse effects; their safety needs to be a constant concern.

Since eye problems may occur with use of *benzodiazepines,* baseline visual testing using a Snellen chart or an eye examination conducted by the appropriate health care provider (e.g., an ophthalmologist or optometrist) is recommended. Allergic reactions to some of these medications (e.g., clonazepam) are characterized by a red raised rash. In addition, obese patients may experience toxicity in a shorter period of time than those who are not obese. This occurs because several anxiolytic drugs are lipid soluble and have greater affinity for fatty tissues; therefore, their half-life is increased in patients who are obese. Give lorazepam cautiously (under very close supervision) if the patient is suicidal, because its use may be associated with suicide attempts. Administer alprazolam only after very careful assessment of mental status, mood, sensorium, and sleep patterns.

Some benzodiazepines are also associated with medication errors because of the existence of sound-alike or look-alike drugs. Assessing the drug order for the right drug is important because of the possibility of such an error and the negative consequences to the patient. Benzodiazepine drugs and the sound-alike medications with which they could be confused include the following: Klonopin (clonazepam) and clonidine; diazepam and Ditropan (oxybutynin); lorazepam and alprazolam; and Versed (midazolam) and VePesid (etoposide) and Vistaril (hydroxyzine).

*Buspirone* is another anxiolytic drug that is not a benzodiazepine. It is used because it has fewer adverse effects, such as decreased sedation and lack of dependency potential. However, it is associated with many drug interactions, cautions, and contraindications (see pharmacology discussion). General assessment of the neurologic system and a mental health assessment are also important to complete.

---

### ⚡ SAFETY AND QUALITY IMPROVEMENT: PREVENTING MEDICATION ERRORS

#### *Sound-Alike Drugs: Bupropion and Buspirone*

Is it bupropion or buspirone? Be careful—these two central nervous system drugs have sound-alike names but very different uses.

Bupropion (Wellbutrin) is an antidepressant that is used to relieve depression. The Zyban formulation of bupropion is given to treat nicotine withdrawal symptoms. Bupropion is available in various formulations ranging from 75- to 100-mg tablets to extended- or sustained-release formulations of 100-mg, 150-mg, 200-mg, and 300-mg tablets.

Buspirone hydrochloride (BuSpar) is an anxiolytic drug that is used for short-term treatment of anxiety symptoms or long-term management of anxiety disorders. It is available in tablets ranging from 5 mg to 30 mg.

---

### MOOD-STABILIZING DRUGS

As previously discussed in the pharmacology section, affective disorders are treated with *mood-stabilizing drugs* and antidepressant drugs. Before antimanic drugs such as lithium are administered, perform a thorough neurologic examination. Also assess vital signs, especially blood pressure, hydration status, dietary intake, skin tone, and presence of edema. Baseline levels of consciousness and alertness, gait and mobility levels, and overall motor functioning are also important to assess. These are particularly important to assess because poor coordination, tremors, and weakness may be symptoms of toxic blood levels of antimanic drugs. Laboratory studies often ordered before and during drug therapy include serum sodium, albumin, and uric acid levels. Serum levels of sodium are important to know because lithium toxicity is potentiated by the presence of hyponatremia and hypovolemia. During the initial phase of therapy, serum lithium levels must be assessed every 3 to 4 days (therapeutic levels are 0.6 mEq/L to 1.2 mEq/L; toxic levels are above 1.5 mEq/L). A urinalysis with specific gravity may also be ordered to assess volume status.

### ANTIDEPRESSANTS

You must assess for many cautions, contraindications, and drug interactions before giving *antidepressants* (see pharmacology discussion). Continuous assessment for any suicidal ideations or tendencies is important because indicators of suicide risk may be covert as well as overt. Suicide must always be considered a potential risk when any psychotherapeutic medication, whether an antidepressant or other CNS-altering drug, is taken alone or in combination with other drugs or alcohol.

The *second-generation antidepressants* are associated with fewer and less severe adverse effects as compared to the older TCA and MAOI antidepressants. These second-generation drugs include *SSRIs* (fluoxetine [Prozac]) and *SNRIs* (duloxetine [Cymbalta]). However, with SSRIs it is still important to assess and document neuromuscular and gastrointestinal systems. Cautious use in the elderly is recommended due to their increased risk for toxicity. Additionally, there is concern for the occurrence of serotonin syndrome. Serotonin syndrome (see Box 16-1) includes symptoms such as agitation, tachycardia, sweating, and muscle tremors. Contraindications include the use of these drugs within 14 days of use of MAOIs and with some antipsychotic drugs. Assess for significant drug interactions, such as warfarin and phenytoin, due to their increased protein binding. Do not give *SNRIs*, such as duloxetine (Cymbalta), to patients with closed-angle glaucoma or those taking MAOIs. Liver function studies may be ordered prior to use of this drug because of the risk of liver toxicity. The *miscellaneous antidepressant,* bupropion, may be preferred over some of the other antidepressants because of fewer anticholinergic, antiadrenergic, and cardiotoxic effects (see pharmacology discussion). Assess the patient's baseline neurologic, mental, and cardiac status before the drug is used. Because of delayed therapeutic effects, closely assess the patient for any suicidal tendencies or ideas. Assess the availability of family support systems as well as the need for any supportive resources.

*TCAs*, as an older class of antidepressants, are effective drugs but are associated with serious adverse effects. However, some patients do tolerate the TCAs. When patients are taking TCAs, monitor closely for potential adverse effects. Use with the herbal product, St. John's wort, is not recommended. Amitriptyline is not to be used in patients with recent myocardial infarction and is associated with potent anticholinergic properties leading to dry mouth, constipation, blurred vision, urinary retention, and alterations in cardiac rhythm.

Closely monitor patients receiving *MAOIs* who have a history of suicide attempts or suicidal ideations. Suicidal thoughts and suicide attempts are important to consider, because these drugs may be hoarded by the patient and then used to carry out suicide. These patients must be under the care of a health care professional (e.g., psychiatrist, physician, or nurse practitioner) so that they may be closely monitored for destructive behaviors. MAOIs are also known for their significant drug interactions (see Table 15-4) such as with meperidine, other opioids, other MAOIs, SSRIs, oral contraceptives, and buspirone. MAOIs, if taken with foods high in tyramine (see Table 16-7), are associated with a hypertensive crisis; therefore, closely monitor blood pressure readings, including postural blood pressure measurements. Postural hypotension, an adverse effect of MAOIs, may lead to a high risk of dizziness, fainting, and possible falls or injury. If the patient is hospitalized, monitor supine/standing or sitting blood pressures at least every 8 hours or more frequently, if needed. A period of 1 to 2 minutes needs to elapse after taking the supine blood pressure before measuring standing or sitting pressures and pulse rate. Laboratory tests that are often ordered for patients taking these drugs include complete blood counts and renal and liver function studies. In addition, it is crucial to understand that elderly patients be given these drugs only if it is deemed absolutely necessary by the prescriber and only with

### SAFETY: HERBAL THERAPIES AND DIETARY SUPPLEMENTS

#### *Ginseng*

**Overview**
Comes from the *Panax quinquefolius* plant in North America (American ginseng), the *Panax ginseng* plant in Asia (Panax ginseng), and the *Acanthopanax senticosus* plant in Russia (Siberian ginseng). All three are different herbs, with Siberian ginseng being markedly different from the other two but often less expensive. Used for more than 5000 years.

**Common Uses**
Improvement of physical endurance and concentration, stress reduction (NOTE: This is a very abbreviated list of uses for these products.)

**Adverse Effects**
Elevated blood pressure, chest pain or palpitations, anxiety, insomnia, headache, nausea, vomiting, diarrhea

**Potential Drug Interactions**
May reduce the effectiveness of anticoagulants and immunosuppressants, but enhance the effectiveness of anticonvulsants and antidiabetic drugs

**Contraindications**
Contraindicated in children and pregnant women

careful monitoring. The extrapyramidal adverse effects (e.g., tremors) are often worse in the elderly and may result in inability to perform activities of daily living. This extrapyramidal reaction may lead to progressive deterioration of motor activities; thus, there is a need for a thorough motor and neurologic assessment.

### ANTIPSYCHOTICS

The use of *antipsychotics* requires careful assessment of all body systems. Assessment of cardiovascular, cerebrovascular, neurologic, gastrointestinal, genitourinary, renal, hepatic, and hematologic functioning is important to safe and efficacious drug therapy. The presence of significant disease in one or several organ systems may lead to a more adverse response to a drug and may even be dose limiting; therefore, perform a careful and skillful assessment of the patient before and during drug therapy. Weight gain may occur, and if the patient is experiencing deleterious health effects because of this, another drug may be ordered. Suicidal ideations, orthostatic changes in blood pressure, extrapyramidal symptoms, confusion, headache, gastrointestinal upset, abnormal muscle movements, rashes, and dry mouth may be associated with many of these drugs; therefore, perform and document a thorough nursing history and mental status examination prior to the initiation of drug therapy. Identify possible drug interactions with any prescription drugs, over-the-counter medications, and/or herbals the patient is taking, as well as any conditions that represent cautions or contraindications to use of the antipsychotic drug (see pharmacology discussion). The phenothiazine antipsychotics may still be prescribed in some situations but are mentioned here mainly for historical purposes. These antipsychotics are associated with significant extrapyramidal adverse effects (see earlier discussion) as well as anticholinergic adverse effects such as dry mouth, urinary hesitancy, and constipation.

Haloperidol is similar to other high-potency antipsychotics because its sedating effects are low but the incidence of extrapyramidal symptoms is high. Assessment of baseline motor, sensory, and neurologic functioning is therefore very important to patient safety. With some of the antipsychotic drugs, patients may experience adverse effects of tremors and muscle twitching from the drug's blockade of dopamine receptors (dopamine generally has an inhibitory effect on specific motor activity in the musculoskeletal system). These extrapyramidal movements are like those in parkinsonism (see Chapter 15) and may be very bothersome and uncomfortable.

Atypical antipsychotics such as clozapine and risperidone have many contraindications, cautions, and drug interactions. Perform a thorough mental status examination, and document the findings prior to initiation of treatment with these and other antipsychotic drugs. An assessment of musculoskeletal functioning and monitoring for any extrapyramidal reaction is also important to patient safety. Monitor liver and renal function studies, complete blood count, and urinalysis before and during therapy. Make sure to document blood pressure readings with close attention to postural readings because of the potential for the adverse effect of postural hypotension. A drop of 20 mm Hg or more in the systolic blood pressure requires immediate attention and implementation of safety precautions. In addition, for the elderly patient, the prescriber may order reduced dosages to help prevent toxicity. These drugs are also associated with a high degree of sedation and must be used only when absolutely necessary and with extreme caution (close monitoring) in the elderly and other patients who are at risk for falls or have limited motor and sensory capabilities. Carefully monitor heart sounds, and observe for any abnormal heart rhythms in patients taking these drugs.

## NURSING DIAGNOSES

1. Imbalanced nutrition, less than body requirements, related to the consequences of the mental health disorder and/or the use of psychotherapeutic drugs
2. Urinary retention related to the adverse effects of psychotherapeutic drugs
3. Constipation related to the adverse effects of psychotherapeutic drugs
4. Sexual dysfunction related to the adverse effects associated with psychotherapeutic drugs
5. Sleep deprivation related to the mental health disorder and/or related drug therapy
6. Deficient knowledge related to lack of information about the specific psychotherapeutic drugs and their adverse effects
7. Impaired social interaction related to various inadequacies felt by the patient due to illness or isolation from others
8. Situational low self-esteem related to the mental health disorder and from the adverse effects of psychotherapeutic drugs, including sexual dysfunction
9. Risk for injury to self related to the mental health disorder and/or possible adverse effects of psychotherapeutic drugs

## PLANNING

### GOALS

1. Patient exhibits improved nutritional status and without weight loss.
2. Patient remains free from any alterations in urinary elimination patterns.
3. Patient regains/maintains normal bowel elimination patterns.
4. Patient remains free from or experiences minimal alterations in sexual function.
5. Patient implements measures to minimize sleep deprivation.
6. Patient is compliant to medication therapy, takes medication(s) as ordered, and is free from complications associated with drug therapy.
7. Patient regains/maintains social interaction and open communication with family, friends, significant others, and members of the health care team.
8. Patient exhibits more positive self-image, healthier thought processes, and interactive processes.
9. Patient maintains safety with drug therapeutic regimen and without injury to self.

### OUTCOME CRITERIA

1. Patient shows healthy nutritional habits with appropriate weight gain and a diet that includes foods from the U.S. Department of Agriculture MyPlate (www.choosemyplate.gov/).
2. Patient reports any problems with urinary hesitancy, urgency, retention, or discomfort over the lower abdominal area.
3. Patient states measures to increase bowel elimination, such as increasing dietary bulk/fiber with fruits and vegetables, while also increasing fluid intake.
   - Patient reports any problems with bowel elimination, such as constipation or passing of hard stool.
4. Patient openly communicates with the prescriber and his or her partner about difficulty with sexual functioning as related to drug therapy.
   - Patient openly identifies/discusses with the prescriber options for improving sexual functioning to assist with any altered patterns of sexual behavior.
5. Patient reports measures to increase healthier sleeping habits through journaling, use of nondrug sleep enhancement measures such as going to bed at a regular time nightly, decreasing room noise/light, calming music, aromatherapy, and avoiding caffeine in the late afternoon/evening (see Chapter 12 for sleep hygiene nursing interventions).
6. Patient states reasoning for compliance to medication regimen, as well as the need to take the medication exactly as prescribed, and related drug safety measures.
   - Patient has assistance at home in the daily monitoring of self-administration of medication(s).
   - Patient states common adverse effects of psychotherapeutic drug therapy, such as confusion, sedation, constipation, nausea, dizziness, unsteady gait, dry mouth, changes in sexual performance, weight gain/loss, and loss or increase in appetite.
   - Patient states adverse effects that need reporting to the prescriber, such as unresolved constipation, urinary retention, increasing levels of sedation, and dizziness/fainting upon standing or changing of positions.
7. Patient demonstrates improved or no further deterioration in social integration with healthier patterns of communication and participation in activities.
   - Patient interacts openly and frequently with family, friends, significant others, and members of the health care team without suspicion or paranoia.
   - Patient participates daily or more frequently in social interactions/activities and plans to engage in more social activities, as appropriate.
8. Patient demonstrates improved self-concept/self-esteem in daily interactions with family/friends/significant others while experiencing fewer episodes of self-destructive and negative behaviors.
   - Patient feels more positive about self as seen with increased participation in activities of daily living, social activities, and family functions.
9. Patient demonstrates safety with activities of daily living and self-care measures by moving slowly, changing positions slowly, and reporting excess dizziness as well as fainting episodes.

# IMPLEMENTATION

Regardless of the psychotherapeutic drug prescribed, several general nursing actions are important for safe administration. First and foremost, demonstrate a firm but patient attitude and use therapeutic communication if appropriate. Once the patient's reading level and effective means of teaching and learning are identified, provide the patient with simple explanations about the drug, its action, and the length of time before therapeutic effects can be expected. Always use a thorough psychosocial and holistic approach when caring for any patient with any illness. Monitor vital signs and document findings, especially during the initiation of therapy. Of great concern is administration of these medications to those who are elderly and to patients with a history of hypertension and cardiac disease. All of the psychotherapeutic drugs are to be taken exactly as prescribed and at the same time every day and without failure. If omission occurs, contact the prescriber immediately. Abrupt withdrawal may have negative effects on the patient's physical and mental status. Solicit help from family members or others providing support in the care of the patient so that there are options for assistance with drug administration. Adherence to the medication regimen is crucial to effective management; identify and utilize all support systems and resources to accomplish this.

## ANXIOLYTIC DRUGS

Specific nursing interventions related to the use of *anxiolytic drugs* include frequent monitoring of vital signs with special attention to blood pressure and postural blood pressures. Encourage the use of elastic compression stockings and changing positions slowly to minimize dizziness and falls from orthostatic hypotension. Create a therapeutic environment for open communication—especially of all disturbing thoughts, including those of suicide. Check the patient's oral cavities for hoarding or cheeking of drugs. Dispense medications only as ordered to help minimize the risk for suicide attempts. Use intravenous routes of administration only as prescribed and give the drug over the recommended time with the proper diluent and at a rate indicated by the manufacturer and prescriber. Always administer intramuscular dosage forms in a large muscle mass and only as ordered or indicated (see Chapter 9 for more information on parenteral administration). See Patient Teaching Tips for more information.

## MOOD-STABILIZING DRUGS

Safe use of the *mood-stabilizing drug lithium* depends on adequate hydration and electrolyte status, because lithium levels may become toxic with dehydration and hyponatremia. See Patient Teaching Tips for more information.

## ANTIDEPRESSANTS

Administer all antidepressants carefully and exactly as ordered. With *second-generation antidepressants,* emphasize that it may take up to 4 to 6 weeks before therapeutic effects are evident. This 4- to 6-week time frame is also associated with the TCAs and MAOIs. Make sure the patient understands this and continues to take the medication as prescribed—even if the patient feels his

or her condition is not improving. Carefully monitor the patient, be readily available, and provide supportive care during this time. The period before therapeutic effects are seen may be the time the patient is at highest risk for self-harm and/or suicide. Advise the patient to take the drug(s) with food and at least 4 to 6 oz of fluid. Assist with ambulation and other activities if the patient is weak, elderly, or dizzy (from postural hypotension). Counsel patients about potential sexual dysfunction (if appropriate) and if an adverse effect of the drug. If sexual dysfunction occurs, provide information to the patient about various options (e.g., waiting to see if the adverse effect resolves, reducing the current dosage of the drug as ordered, taking a "drug holiday" if ordered by the prescriber). A drug holiday, if indicated, generally occurs in a hospital setting, and the drug is removed but only under very close monitoring. See Patient Teaching Tips for more specific information regarding *SSRIs* and *SNRIs.*

With the use of *TCAs* and *MAOIs,* educate the patient on adverse effects and drug/food interactions. Emphasize the importance of keeping a list of all medications on their person at all times. Advise to change positions purposely and slowly. All health care providers need to be informed that the patient is taking these drugs and that weaning must occur when these drugs are to be discontinued. With TCAs, advise the patient to report any of the following to the prescriber if they occur: blurred vision, excessive drowsiness, sleepiness, urinary retention, constipation, and cognitive impairment. It is also important to inform patients that tolerance to sedation will occur with some second-generation antidepressants.

## PATIENT-CENTERED CARE: CULTURAL IMPLICATIONS

### Psychotherapeutic Drugs

Many racial and ethnic groups respond to drugs differently. For example, Asians have lower drug metabolism activity than whites related to lower levels of various enzymes. Asians often require lower dosages of benzodiazepines and tricyclic antidepressants because they have lower levels of the enzymes metabolizing these drugs (e.g., CYO2D6) and are therefore more sensitive to the drugs.

Diazepam follows a different metabolic pathway in the Chinese and Japanese populations. These two groups are found to be poor metabolizers of this drug and its metabolite. Approximately 20% of Chinese and Japanese individuals metabolize diazepam poorly, which results in rapid drug accumulation. To prevent possible toxicity, lower dosages are generally required. Nurses need to be aware of this cultural variable and assess these patients for sedation, overdosage, and other adverse reactions.

Researchers have also identified genetic factors that help predict a response to antidepressants. A study of some 80 Mexican Americans with depression found that depressed and highly anxious patients with certain variant genes had a 70% higher reduction in anxiety and a 30% higher reduction in depression in response to treatment with fluoxetine than did other racial and ethnic groups without the specific gene variation.

## ANTIPSYCHOTICS

Patients need to be aware that *antipsychotic drugs* are to be taken exactly as prescribed to be effective. Different levels of paranoia or delusions may lead the patient to mistrust you and other members of the health care team, so maintain a sufficient level of trust through consistency, empathy, and the establishment of therapeutic communication to help ensure compliance. Adherence/compliance is always a critical issue for patients with psychotic illnesses, because these patients are at higher risk for not taking medications and not keeping follow-up appointments. Nonadherence to the medical and treatment regimen is of major concern because the serum levels of drugs such as haloperidol must be within a specified therapeutic range for the patient to feel better and be functional. If serum levels of haloperidol are less than 4 ng/mL, the patient may show symptoms of the mental disorder, whereas levels higher than 22 ng/mL may result in toxicity. Therefore, selection of an antipsychotic drug and its dosage, route of administration, risk for toxicity, and/or suicidal potential, as well as therapeutic communication and patient education, are all important factors for successful therapy. Because most antipsychotic drugs are quite potent, be sure that oral dosage forms have actually been swallowed and have not been intentionally hidden in the side of the mouth (see previous discussion on cheeking of medications). Oral forms of the antipsychotics are generally well absorbed and will cause less gastrointestinal upset if taken with food or a full glass of water. Sucking on hard candy or gum may help to relieve dry mouth. With any of the dosage forms, perspiration may be increased; therefore, encourage the patient to avoid engaging in excessive activity or being exposed to heat or humidity. Excessive sweating can lead to dehydration and subsequent drug toxicity.

Haloperidol may not necessarily be the best drug to use because of the risk for undermedication or overmedication and troubling adverse effects (see Table 16-10). Therefore, other antipsychotics (e.g., clozapine and risperidone) may be preferred, as previously discussed. Clozapine and risperidone are therapeutically effective and carry a minimal risk of tardive dyskinesia and extrapyramidal symptoms. In addition, they usually lead to improvement in cognitive behavior. Clozapine is to be taken as ordered and usually given in divided doses; proper dosing is very important to therapeutic effectiveness. If any changes in blood counts (e.g., leukopenia) are noted or if abnormal cardiac functioning (e.g., tachycardia) is identified, contact the prescriber immediately. In such a case, the medication may need to be discontinued, but only as ordered, and the patient monitored closely. Titration of doses of clozapine, either upward or downward, needs to be done very carefully with close monitoring of the patient for any exacerbation of the mental illness or suicidal tendencies.

Risperidone is to be given as ordered and administered by injection into a deep muscle mass. Always check hospital or facility policy and/or drug insert guidelines regarding the administration of this drug. Intramuscular injection dosage forms may be ordered along with oral doses of risperidone or possibly of another antipsychotic drug for several weeks, with maintenance doses of an intramuscular injection given every 2 to 4 weeks, as ordered. Always alternate intramuscular injection sites to maintain tissue integrity and muscle mass, and be sure that the site is not red, swollen, or irritated. Document and report any changes. Oral solution, tablets, and orally disintegrating tabs are other available dosage forms. Do not give oral solutions with cola or tea. Disintegrating tabs need to be dissolved under the tongue before swallowing with or without liquid. Always follow the prescriber's orders for administering this and all other drugs. The daily amount is usually given in two divided doses, with dosage decreased in the elderly and in those with impaired renal or hepatic function. Make sure you report any excess sedation, anxiety, extrapyramidal symptoms, tardive dyskinesia, seizures, or strokelike symptoms immediately. Measuring vital signs and monitoring for any postural hypotension is also important during treatment.

Once therapy with any of the antipsychotic drugs has been initiated, it is important for you and other health care providers involved in the patient's care to monitor drug therapy closely, including measuring serum drug levels during follow-up visits. If the patient is suspected of being nonadherent and serum drug levels are subtherapeutic, the patient needs to be reevaluated by the prescriber for a possible change of drug or dosage form. The parenteral dosage forms usually come in a depot (longer-releasing) dosage formulation that releases the drug over 2 to 4 weeks, leading to increased compliance and often a better therapeutic outcome.

Patient education (see Patient Teaching Tips) and patient adherence with the drug regimen are keys to successful treatment, regardless of the mental illness. Often it is the mental disorder itself that causes patient nonadherence. Keeping communication open with the patient, family, and/or caregiver is important to develop trust and a sense of empathy. Although patient education may have been thorough, emphasize that the patient may call the prescriber, clinic, or hotline 24 hours a day. Keep phone numbers continually updated. Make constant and ongoing professional counseling available with a mental health care provider (psychiatrist, nurse practitioner, or other licensed mental health professional) so that the patient's progress is consistently monitored. Group therapy and support groups are also available for the patient and significant others.

## EVALUATION

Monitor the therapeutic effects of psychotherapeutic medications and the patient's progress before and during drug therapy. Mental alertness, cognition, affect, mood, ability to carry out activities of daily living, appetite, and sleep patterns are all areas that need to be closely monitored and documented. The patient must continue with other forms of therapy, in addition to drug therapy, with the goal of acquiring more effective coping skills. Other forms of treatment may include intense psychotherapy, relaxation therapy, stress reduction, and lifestyle changes. It is important to mention that blood levels of these drugs will be measured during follow-up visits to ensure that therapeutic levels are maintained. Such monitoring of serum drug levels helps identify both subtherapeutic and toxic levels.

The therapeutic effects of *anxiolytic drugs* are evidenced by improved mental alertness, cognition, and mood; fewer anxiety and panic attacks; improved sleep patterns and appetite; more interest in self and others; less tension and irritability; and fewer feelings of fear, impending doom, and stress. Watch for

## CASE STUDY
### Antidepressants

A 49-year-old patient comes to the clinic with a history of depression. He tells you that he was treated for it by a doctor in another country, but he "ran out of pills" a week ago and did not know how to get a refill. He could not remember the name of the medication but said it was for "depression." He has also been having trouble sleeping. After a psychiatric evaluation, he is given a 2-week prescription for fluoxetine (Prozac).

1. A few days later, his wife calls to describe "a terrible reaction" that he is having. She says that he is shaking and shivering, has a fever, and is somewhat confused and upset. She thinks he has a bad infection. What do you think has happened, and why?
2. What could have been done to prevent this problem?
3. After 2 weeks, the patient is given a prescription for trazodone (Desyrel) and is instructed to return to the office in 2 weeks. What advantage does this medication have for this patient?

For answers, see http://evolve.elsevier.com/Lilley.

the adverse effects of hypotension, lethargy, fatigue, drowsiness, and confusion in patients taking anxiolytic drugs. In general, adverse reactions to *antidepressants* consist of drowsiness, dry mouth, constipation, dizziness, postural hypotension, sedation, blood dyscrasias, sexual dysfunction, and dyskinesias. Overdose is evidenced by seizures or dysrhythmias.

Therapeutic effects of the *mood stabilizer lithium* are decreased mania and stabilization of the patient's mood. Lithium is usually better tolerated by the patient during the manic phase. Adverse reactions to lithium include dysrhythmias, hypotension, sedation, slurred speech, slowed motor abilities, and weight gain. Gastrointestinal adverse effects include GI discomfort.

When used as antidepressants, *SSRIs* and *SNRIs* may take up to 6 weeks to reach full therapeutic effect. A therapeutic response to these drugs includes improved depression or mental status, improved ability to carry out activities of daily living, less insomnia, and improved mood disorder with minimal adverse effects of weight gain, headache, gastrointestinal upset, insomnia, dizziness, drowsiness, and sexual dysfunction. Monitor the patient for symptoms of serotonin syndrome such as agitation, tachycardia, hyperreflexia, and tremors.

The therapeutic effects of the *antipsychotic drugs* include improvement in mood and affect, and alleviation or decrease in psychotic symptoms (decrease in hallucinations, paranoia, delusions, garbled speech) once the patient has been taking the medication for several weeks. Careful monitoring of the patient's potential to injure self or others during the delay between the start of therapy and symptomatic improvement is critical. Evaluation for adverse effects includes monitoring blood counts (clozapine) as well as tic-like trembling movements of the hands, face, neck, and head; hypotension; and dry mouth (haloperidol).

## PATIENT TEACHING TIPS

### Anxiolytic Drugs
- Encourage patients to avoid operating heavy machinery and driving until the adverse effects of sedation or drowsiness have resolved.
- Educate about the development of tolerance to the sedating properties of benzodiazepines with chronic use (see Chapter 12).
- Instruct patients not to take over-the-counter drugs or herbals without seeking advice from the prescriber.
- Keep these and all psychotherapeutic drugs out of the reach of children.
- Alcohol and other CNS depressants must be avoided.
- Advise patients to carry a medical alert or other identification bracelet/necklace with their diagnoses and a list of their drugs and allergies at all times. The drug list needs to be updated at least every 3 months.
- Medications must always be taken exactly as ordered. Avoid sudden withdrawal. If withdrawal of a drug is necessary, tapering/weaning of doses is needed.

### Mood-Stabilizing Drugs
- Instruct the patient that lithium must be taken at the same time each day, and give specific instructions on how to handle missed doses. Make sure the patient understands the importance of adequate hydration.

- Inform the patient that the adverse effects of lithium are usually transient; however, excessive tremors, seizures, confusion, ataxia, and excessive sedation must be reported to the prescriber immediately.

### Monoamine Oxidase Inhibitors and Tricyclic Antidepressants
- Advise the patient taking MAOIs to contact the prescriber immediately if any of the following signs and symptoms of overdosage or toxicity occur: tachycardia, hyperthermia, or seizures.
- If the patient is taking an MAOI, caution him or her about avoiding over-the-counter cold and flu products. Foods or beverages high in tyramine are to be avoided (see Table 16-7).
- When the patient is taking a TCA, any blurred vision, agitation, urinary retention, or ataxia needs to be reported to the prescriber immediately.
- Encourage wearing of a medical alert necklace or bracelet showing the diagnosis and a list of current drugs.

### Selective Serotonin Reuptake Inhibitors and Serotonin-Norepinephrine Reuptake Inhibitors
- Consumption of fiber supplements must occur at least 2 hours before or after the dosing of medication to avoid interference with drug absorption; however, dietary fiber intake is appropriate.

## PATIENT TEACHING TIPS—cont'd

- Encourage the patient to openly discuss any concerns about the medication and adverse effects such as gastrointestinal upset, sexual dysfunction, or tremors.
- Provide a listing of drug-drug interactions, such as the strong interaction between SSRIs and MAOIs, St. John's wort (an herbal product), and tryptophan (a serotonin precursor found in foods). Such interactions may pose a risk for serotonin syndrome (see earlier discussion). Cold products and over-the-counter medications must be approved by the prescriber.
- SSRIs must be taken carefully and as prescribed. Any increase in suicidal thoughts or extreme changes in mood needs to be reported immediately to the prescriber.
- Emphasize that all follow-up visits must be kept and prescriber contacted if there are any concerns. Educate that discontinuation of SSRIs and SNRIs requires a tapering period of up to 1 to 2 months, as ordered. Discontinuation syndrome may occur with or without a tapering period; this includes symptoms of dizziness, diarrhea, movement disorders, insomnia, irritability, visual disturbance, lethargy, anorexia, and lowered mood.

- If there is ever doubt that too much of an antidepressant has been taken, contact the prescriber and/or seek emergency medical treatment immediately.
- If transdermal patches are the dosage form used, emphasize the importance of rotating the patch site with each application and to place patch on a nonhairy, healthy, intact area. Any residue from the previous patch is to be gently cleansed off prior to application of a new patch.

### Antipsychotics

- Advise patients to avoid hot baths, saunas, and hot climates with antipsychotics because of the risk of further drop in blood pressure, especially upon standing (postural hypotension). Injury to self may occur due to dizziness or fainting.
- Haloperidol and other antipsychotics must never be stopped abruptly because of the high risk of inducing a withdrawal psychosis.
- Drug interactions with clozapine include alcohol, CNS depressants, levodopa, and antihypertensives.
- Any sore throat, malaise, fever, or bleeding must be reported to the prescriber immediately because of the drop in WBC counts with clozapine.

## KEY POINTS

- Psychosis is a major emotional disorder that impairs mental function. A person experiencing psychosis cannot participate in everyday life and shows the hallmark sign of loss of contact with reality.
- Affective disorders are emotional disorders characterized by changes in mood. They range from mania (abnormally elevated emotions) to depression (abnormally reduced emotions) and include anxiety, a normal emotion that may be a healthy reaction but becomes pathologic when it is life-altering.

- Situational anxiety arises in response to specific life events, and nursing assessment is key to identifying patients at risk.
- SSRIs and SNRIs are often prescribed because of their superiority to older antidepressants.
- Nursing considerations related to psychotherapeutic drugs include the need for skillful patient assessment with an emphasis on past and present medical history, physical examination, and a thorough medication history and profile.

## NCLEX® EXAMINATION REVIEW QUESTIONS

1 In caring for a patient experiencing ethanol withdrawal, the nurse expects to administer which medication or medication class as treatment for this condition?
   a lithium (Eskalith)
   b Benzodiazepines
   c buspirone (BuSpar)
   d Antidepressants

2 Patient teaching for a patient receiving an MAOI would include instructions to the patient to avoid which food product?
   a Orange juice
   b Milk
   c Shrimp
   d Swiss cheese

3 After a patient has been treated for depression for 4 weeks, the nurse calls the patient to schedule a follow-up visit. What concern will the nurse assess for during the conversation with the patient?

   a Weakness
   b Hallucinations
   c Suicidal ideations
   d Difficulty with urination

4 The nurse is caring for a patient who has been taking clozapine (Clozaril) for 2 months. Which laboratory test(s) should be performed regularly while the patient is taking this medication?
   a Platelet count
   b WBC count
   c Liver function studies
   d Renal function studies

5 The nurse is giving medications to a patient. Which drug or drug class, when administered with lithium, increases the risk for lithium toxicity?
   a Thiazides
   b levofloxacin
   c calcium citrate
   d Beta blockers

6  The nurse is teaching a patient about treatment with an SSRI antidepressant. Which teaching considerations are appropriate? (Select all that apply.)

a  The patient should be told which foods contain tyramine and instructed to avoid these foods.

b  The patient should be instructed to use caution when standing up from a sitting position.

c  The patient should not take any products that contain the herbal product St. John's wort.

d  This medication should not be stopped abruptly.

e  Drug levels may become toxic if dehydration occurs.

f  The patient should be told to check with the prescriber before taking any over-the-counter medications.

7  A patient with a feeding tube will be receiving risperidone (Risperdal) 8 mg in 2 divided doses via the feeding tube. The medication is available in a 1 mg/mL solution. How many milliliters will the nurse administer for each dose?

1. b, 2. d, 3. c, 4. b, 5. a, 6. b, c, d, f, 7. 4 mL per dose

For Critical Thinking and Prioritization Questions, see http://evolve.elsevier.com/Lilley.

# Substance Abuse

## OBJECTIVES

When you reach the end of this chapter, you will be able to do the following:

1. Discuss substance abuse and the significance of the problem in the United States.
2. Identify the drugs or chemicals that are most frequently abused.
3. Contrast the signs and symptoms of the most commonly abused drugs/chemicals.
4. Compare the treatments for drug withdrawal for the most commonly abused opioids (narcotics), central nervous system (CNS) depressants, amphetamines and other CNS stimulants, nicotine, and alcohol.
5. Describe alcohol abuse syndrome with a focus on signs and symptoms, mild to severe alcohol withdrawal symptoms, and associated treatment.
6. Describe other drug abuse syndromes, signs and symptoms, withdrawal symptoms, and treatment regimens.
7. Identify various assessment tools used in the nursing assessment of substance abuse.
8. Develop a nursing care plan encompassing all phases of the nursing process for a patient undergoing treatment for substance abuse and dependency.

## KEY TERMS

**Addiction** Strong psychological or physical dependence on a drug or other psychoactive substance. (p. 282)

**Amphetamine** A drug that stimulates the central nervous system. (p. 284)

**Detoxification** A process of eliminating a toxic substance from the body; a medically supervised program for alcohol or opioid addiction (p. 284)

**Enuresis** Urinary incontinence. (p. 285)

**Habituation** Development of tolerance to a substance following prolonged medical use but without psychological or physical dependence (addiction). (p. 282)

**Illicit drug use** The use of a drug or substance in a way that it is not intended to be used or the use of a drug that is not legally approved for human administration. (p. 284)

**Intoxication** Stimulation, excitement, or stupefaction produced by a chemical substance. (p. 282)

**Korsakoff's psychosis** A syndrome of amnesia with confabulation (making up of stories) associated with chronic alcohol abuse; it often occurs together with *Wernicke's encephalopathy.* (p. 287)

**Micturition** Urination, the desire to urinate, or the frequency of urination. (p. 285)

**Narcolepsy** A sleep disorder characterized by sleeping during the day, disrupted nighttime sleep, cataplexy, sleep paralysis, and hallucinations. (p. 285)

**Opioid analgesics** Synthetic pain-relieving substances that were originally derived from the opium poppy. Naturally occurring opium derivatives are called *opiates.* (p. 283)

**Physical dependence** A condition characterized by physiologic reliance on a substance, usually indicated by tolerance to the effects of the substance and development of withdrawal symptoms when use of the substance is terminated. (p. 282)

**Psychoactive properties** Drug properties that affect mood, behavior, cognitive processes, and mental status. (p. 284)

**Psychological dependence** A condition characterized by strong desires to obtain and use a substance. (p. 282)

**Raves** Increasingly popular all-night parties that typically involve dancing, drinking, and the use of various illicit drugs. (p. 285)

**Roofies** Pills that are classified as benzodiazepines. They have recently gained popularity as a recreational drug; chemically known as *flunitrazepam*. (p. 286)

**Substance abuse** The use of a mood- or behavior-altering substance in a maladaptive manner that often compromises health, safety, and social and occupational functioning, and causes legal problems. (p. 282)

**Wernicke's encephalopathy** A neurologic disorder characterized by apathy, drowsiness, ataxia, nystagmus, and ophthalmoplegia; it is caused by thiamine (vitamin $B_1$) deficiency secondary to chronic alcohol abuse. (p. 287)

**Withdrawal** A substance-specific mental disorder that follows the cessation or reduction in use of a psychoactive substance that has been taken regularly to induce a state of intoxication. (p. 282)

## ANATOMY, PHYSIOLOGY, AND PATHOPHYSIOLOGY OVERVIEW

**Substance abuse** affects people of all ages, sexes, and ethnic and socioeconomic groups. **Physical dependence** and **psychological dependence** on a substance are chronic disorders with remissions and relapses, such as occur with any other chronic illness. Relapses are not to be seen as failures but as indications to intensify treatment. Recognizing physical or psychological dependence and understanding the various treatment guidelines are important skills for those caring for these patients. **Habituation** refers to situations in which a patient becomes accustomed to a certain drug (develops tolerance) and may have mild psychological dependence on it but does not show compulsive dose escalation, drug-seeking behavior, or major withdrawal symptoms on drug discontinuation. This might occur, for example, in a postsurgical patient who receives opioid pain therapy regularly for only a few weeks.

In 2010, the Office of Applied Studies of the U.S. Substance Abuse and Mental Health Services Administration conducted a survey indicating that some 22.6 million Americans 12 years of age or older were current illicit drug users; that is, they reported using an illicit drug during the month prior to the survey interview. This number represents 8.9% of the population 12 years of age and older. Marijuana was identified as the most commonly used illicit drug, followed by psychotherapeutic drugs, pain relievers, tranquilizers, stimulants, and sedatives used for nonmedical purposes.

Nearly 50% of the adult patients seen in many family practice clinics have an alcohol or drug disorder. Some 25% to 40% of hospital admissions are related to substance abuse and its sequelae. Of patients seen in a general medicine practice, 10% to 16% are seeking treatment for problems related to substance abuse. Substance abuse is strongly associated with many types of mental illness. Treatment of both disorders is often very difficult, in part because of the high risk of drug interactions with the abused substances. Assessment, intervention, use of certain medications, specific **addiction** treatment strategies, and monitoring of recovery are essential to the care of this patient population.

This chapter focuses on three major classes of commonly abused substances and two commonly abused individual drugs. A description of the category or the individual drug, possible effects, signs and symptoms of **intoxication** and **withdrawal**, peak period and duration of withdrawal symptoms, and drugs used to treat withdrawal are discussed. The list of substances of abuse in Box 17-1 is not all-inclusive, but it contains some of the substances most commonly abused at this time. Not all of these substances are discussed in this chapter. Refer to The National Institute on Drug Abuse, available at www.nida.nih.gov/nidahome.html for further information.

Specific drugs used to treat withdrawal symptoms are discussed in the sections covering the drug whose withdrawal symptoms they are intended to treat. Pharmacologic therapies are indicated for patients with addictive disorders to prevent life-threatening withdrawal complications, such as seizures and delirium tremens, and to increase compliance with psychosocial forms of addiction treatment.

---

**BOX 17-1   COMMONLY ABUSED SUBSTANCES**

**Major Categories**
Opioids
Stimulants
Depressants

**Individual Drugs**
Alcohol
Anabolic steroids (see Chapter 35)
Dextromethorphan
Lysergic acid diethylamide (LSD)
Marijuana
Methamphetamine
Methylenedioxymethamphetamine (MDMA, ecstasy)
Nicotine
Phencyclidine (PCP)

## PHARMACOLOGY OVERVIEW

### OPIOIDS

Opioid analgesics are synthetic versions of pain-relieving substances that were originally derived from the opium poppy plant (see Chapter 10). More than 20 different alkaloids are obtained from the unripe seed of the opium poppy plant, only a few of which are clinically useful, including morphine and codeine. The other opioid analgesics that are currently used in medical practice are synthetic or semisynthetic derivatives of these two drugs.

Diacetylmorphine (better known as *heroin*) and opium are classified as Schedule I drugs and are not available in the United States for therapeutic use. Heroin was banned in the United States in 1924 because of its high potential for abuse and the increasing number of heroin addicts. In Europe, heroin is available for medical treatment of pain, and governmental programs also exist to provide heroin to addicts with the goal of reducing crime.

Heroin is one of the most commonly abused opioids. Some of the other commonly abused substances in the opioid category are codeine, hydrocodone, hydromorphone, meperidine, morphine, and oxycodone. Currently heroin remains one of the top 10 most abused drugs in the United States and often is used in combination with the stimulant drug cocaine (discussed later in Stimulants). When heroin is injected (called *mainlining* or *skin popping*), sniffed (known as *snorting*), or smoked, it binds with opiate receptors found in many regions of the brain. The result is intense euphoria, often referred to as a *rush*. This rush lasts only briefly and is followed by a relaxed, contented state that persists for a couple of hours. In large doses, heroin, like other opioids, can reduce or stop respiration.

### Mechanism of Action and Drug Effects

Opioids work by blocking receptors in the central nervous system (CNS). When these receptors are blocked, the perception of pain is blocked. There are three main receptor types to which opioids bind. These receptors and their physiologic effects when stimulated are discussed in Chapter 10. One of the reasons that opioids are abused is their ability to produce euphoria.

The drug effects of opioids are primarily centered in the CNS. However, these drugs also act outside the CNS, and many of their unwanted effects stem from these actions. In addition to analgesia, opioids produce drowsiness, euphoria, tranquility, and other alterations of mood. The mechanism by which opioids produce the latter effects is not entirely clear. The effects of opioids can be collectively referred to as *narcosis* or *stupor,* which involves reduced sensory response, especially to painful stimuli. For this reason, opioid analgesics are also referred to as *narcotics* (see Chapter 4), especially by law enforcement authorities.

### Indications

The intended drug effects of opioids are to relieve pain, reduce cough, relieve diarrhea, and induce anesthesia. Many have a high potential for abuse and are therefore classified as Schedule II controlled substances. Relaxation and euphoria are the most common drug effects that lead to abuse and psychological dependence. Sustained-release oxycodone (e.g., OxyContin) is

an example of an opioid narcotic that is controversial because it is often overprescribed, misused, and grossly abused. Numerous deaths have been reported when sustained-release oxycodone was crushed and the entire 12-hour supply was released at one time.

Certain opioid drugs are themselves used to treat opioid dependence. Historically, methadone has been used most commonly for this purpose. Its long half-life of up to 12 to 24 hours allows patients to be dosed once daily at federally approved methadone maintenance clinics. In theory, the goal of such programs is to reduce the patient's dosage gradually so that eventually the patient can live permanently drug free. Unfortunately, relapse rates are often high in these programs. However, patients who remain on long-term opioid maintenance therapy still benefit by avoiding the hazards associated with obtaining and using illegal "street" drugs.

### Contraindications

Contraindications to the therapeutic use of opioid medications include known drug allergy, pregnancy (high dosage or prolonged use is contraindicated), respiratory depression or severe asthma when resuscitative equipment is not available, and *paralytic ileus* (bowel paralysis).

### Adverse Effects

Adverse effects of opioids can be broken down into two groups: CNS and non-CNS. The primary adverse effects of opioids are related to their actions in the CNS. The major CNS-related adverse effects include diuresis, miosis, convulsions, nausea, vomiting, and respiratory depression. Many of the non-CNS adverse effects are secondary to the release of histamine. Histamine release can cause vasodilation leading to hypotension, spasms of the colon leading to constipation, increased spasms of the ureter resulting in urinary retention, and dilation of cutaneous blood vessels leading to flushing of the skin of the face, neck, and upper thorax. The release of histamine is also thought to cause sweating, urticaria, and pruritus.

#### Management of Withdrawal, Toxicity, and Overdose

Box 17-2 lists the signs and symptoms of opioid withdrawal. The box also indicates the time when these symptoms are most likely to occur and their duration. Many patients require a

---

**BOX 17-2 SIGNS AND SYMPTOMS OF OPIOID WITHDRAWAL**

**Peak Period**
1 to 3 days

**Duration**
5 to 7 days

**Signs**
Drug seeking, mydriasis, piloerection, diaphoresis, rhinorrhea, lacrimation, vomiting, diarrhea, insomnia, elevated blood pressure and pulse rate

**Symptoms**
Intense desire for drugs, muscle cramps, arthralgia, anxiety, nausea, malaise

formal detoxification program while withdrawal symptoms are occurring. See Chapter 10 for a detailed discussion of physical dependence and the management of acute intoxication, toxicity, and overdose. Withdrawal symptoms include nausea, dysphoria, muscle aches, lacrimation, rhinorrhea, pupillary dilation, piloerection (hair standing on end) or sweating, diarrhea, yawning, fever, and insomnia. Medications listed in Box 17-3 are intended to help decrease the desire for the abused opioid and reduce the severity of these withdrawal symptoms. The most serious adverse effect and the most common cause of death with opioids is respiratory depression.

Certain medications are used to prevent relapse use once an initial remission is achieved. They are useful only when concurrent counseling is provided and offer additional insurance against return to illicit drug use. For opioid abuse or dependence, naltrexone, an opioid antagonist, is administered. Naltrexone, which is also available as an injection called Vivitrol, works by blocking the opioid receptors so that use of opioid drugs does not produce euphoria. When euphoria is eliminated, the reinforcing effect of the drug is lost. The patient needs to be free from opioids for at least 1 week before beginning this medication, because naltrexone can produce withdrawal symptoms if given too soon. Naltrexone is also approved for use by alcohol-dependent patients to reduce cravings for alcohol and the likelihood of a full relapse if a slip occurs. Another opioid antagonist, naloxone, is used for opioid dependence. It is combined with buprenorphine (Subutrex) or used alone (Suboxone) (see Chapter 10).

## STIMULANTS

The abuse of stimulants is related to their ability to cause elevation of mood, reduction of fatigue, a sense of increased alertness, and invigorating aggressiveness. Amphetamine is a stimulant drug that is commonly abused. Chemically, three classes of amphetamine exist: salts of racemic amphetamine, dextroamphetamine, and methamphetamine. These classes vary with respect to their potency and peripheral effects. Another stimulant drug of abuse is cocaine, which also produces strong CNS stimulation. Cocaine was originally classified as a narcotic. It is considered a narcotic by the penal system and has been treated as a narcotic in terms of secured storage in health care facilities. However, unlike the opioid analgesics, cocaine does not normally induce a state of narcosis or stupor and is therefore more correctly categorized as a stimulant drug. Other commonly abused substances in this category include methylphenidate, dextroamphetamine, phenmetrazine, and methamphetamine. Multiple slight chemical variants of amphetamine exist. They are commonly referred to as "designer drugs," which have psychoactive properties along with their stimulant properties, which further enhances their abuse potential. Table 17-1 lists commonly abused forms of amphetamine and cocaine with their street names.

Methamphetamine is a chemical class of amphetamine, but it has a much stronger effect on the CNS than the other two classes of amphetamine. Methamphetamine is generally used in pill form orally or in powder form by snorting or injecting. It has 15 to 20 times the potency of amphetamine sulfate, the original drug in this class. Crystallized methamphetamine, known as *ice, crystal,* or *crystal meth,* is a smokable and more powerful form of the drug. Methamphetamine users who inject the drug and share needles are at risk for acquiring human immunodeficiency virus (HIV) infection and acquired immunodeficiency syndrome (AIDS), as well as hepatitis B and C. Marijuana and alcohol are commonly listed as additional drugs of abuse in those admitted for treatment of methamphetamine abuse. Most of the recorded methamphetamine-related deaths involved the use of methamphetamine in combination with at least one other drug, such as alcohol, heroin, or cocaine. The over-the-counter (OTC) decongestant pseudoephedrine is commonly used to synthesize methamphetamine in secret drug laboratories, often in private homes. This practice has lead to dramatic increases in the abuse of this drug. In 2005, the Combat Methamphetamine Epidemic Act required restricted retail sales of all nonprescription drug products containing pseudoephedrine. Specific restrictions include allowing sales only from *behind* the pharmacy counter, requiring photo identification and electronic or paper record keeping of purchasers (which must remain on file for 2 years), and setting maximum allowable amount (in grams) of pseudoephedrine that can be sold per consumer per month.

---

### BOX 17-3    MEDICATIONS FOR TREATMENT OF OPIOID WITHDRAWAL

**Clonidine (Catapres) Substitution**

Clonidine, 0.1 or 0.2 mg orally, is given every 4 to 6 hours as needed for signs and symptoms of withdrawal for 5 to 7 days. Days 2 to 4 are typically the most difficult days for the patient in detoxification. Check blood pressure before each dose, and do not give medication if patient is hypotensive.

**Methadone Substitution**

Methadone test dose of 10 mg is given orally in liquid form or as a crushed tablet. Additional 10- to 20-mg doses are given for signs and symptoms of withdrawal every 4 to 6 hours for 24 hours after initial dose. Range for total daily dose is 15 to 30 mg. Repeat total first-day dose in two divided doses (stabilization dose) for 2 to 3 days, then reduce dosage by 5 to 10 mg/day until medication is completely withdrawn.

---

### TABLE 17-1    VARIOUS FORMS OF AMPHETAMINE AND COCAINE WITH STREET NAMES

| CHEMICAL NAME | STREET NAMES |
| --- | --- |
| dimethoxymethylamphetamine | DOM, STP |
| methamphetamine (crystallized form) | Ice, crystal, glass |
| methamphetamine (powdered form) | Speed, meth, crank |
| methylenedioxyamphetamine | MDA, love drug |
| methylenedioxymethamphetamine | MDMA, ecstasy |
| cocaine (powdered form) | Coke, dust, snow, flake, blow, girl |
| cocaine (crystallized form) | Crack, crack cocaine, freebase rocks, rock |

Another synthetic amphetamine derivative is methylene-dioxymethamphetamine (MDMA, "ecstasy," or "E"), which is also usually prepared in secret home laboratories. This drug tends to have more calming effects than other amphetamine drugs. It is usually taken in pill form but can also be snorted or injected. Users often feel a strong sense of social bonding with and acceptance of other people, hence the nickname "love drug." The drug can also be very energizing, which makes it popular at raves (all-night dance parties). Originally synthesized by Merck Pharmaceuticals in 1914, it was studied by the U.S. Army as a "brainwashing" drug in the 1950s. Its popularity has grown widely since the Drug Enforcement Administration classified it as a Schedule I controlled substance in 1985.

Another illicit drug use problem is cocaine use. Cocaine is a white powder that is derived from the leaves of the South American coca plant. Cocaine is either snorted or injected intravenously. Cocaine tends to give a temporary illusion of limitless power and energy but afterward leaves the user feeling depressed, edgy, and craving more. Crack is a smokable form of cocaine that has been chemically altered. Cocaine and crack are highly addictive. The psychological and physical dependence can erode physical and mental health and can become so strong that these drugs dominate all aspects of the addict's life.

## Mechanism of Action and Drug Effects

Stimulants work by releasing *biogenic amines* from their storage sites in the nerve terminals. The primary biogenic amine released is norepinephrine. Its release results in stimulation of the CNS, as well as cardiovascular stimulation, which results in increased blood pressure and heart rate and possibly cardiac dysrhythmias. The effect on smooth muscle is seen primarily in the urinary bladder and results in contraction of the sphincter. This is helpful in treating enuresis (urinary incontinence) but results in painful and difficult micturition (voiding or urination) otherwise.

Stimulants, particularly amphetamines, are very potent CNS stimulants. This CNS stimulation commonly results in wakefulness, alertness, and a decreased sense of fatigue; elevation of mood, with increased initiative, self-confidence, and ability to concentrate; often elation and euphoria; and an increase in motor and speech activity.

## Indications

Many therapeutic uses for stimulants exist. Currently their most common use is in the treatment of attention deficit disorder or attention deficit hyperactivity disorder (see Chapter 13). Stimulants may be used to prevent or reverse fatigue and sleep, such as when they are used to treat narcolepsy (episodes of acute sleepiness). Another therapeutic effect of amphetamines is their ability to stimulate the respiratory center. Occasionally they are used after anesthesia to stimulate the respiration. Stimulants are also used to reduce food intake and treat obesity; however, this therapeutic effect is limited because of rapid development of tolerance.

## Contraindications

Contraindications to the therapeutic use of stimulant medications include drug allergy, diabetes, cardiovascular disorders, states of agitation, hypertension, known history of drug abuse, and Tourette's syndrome.

## Adverse Effects

Adverse effects of stimulants are commonly an extension of their therapeutic effects. The CNS-related adverse effects are restlessness, syncope (fainting), dizziness, tremor, hyperactive reflexes, talkativeness, tenseness, irritability, weakness, insomnia, fever, and sometimes euphoria. Confusion, aggression, increased libido, anxiety, delirium, paranoid hallucinations, panic states, and suicidal or homicidal tendencies occur, especially in mentally ill patients. Fatigue and depression usually follow the CNS stimulation. Cardiovascular effects are common and include headache, chilliness, pallor or flushing, palpitations, tachycardia, cardiac dysrhythmias, anginal pain, hypertension or hypotension, and circulatory collapse. Excessive sweating can also occur. Gastrointestinal (GI) effects include dry mouth, metallic taste, anorexia, nausea, vomiting, diarrhea, and abdominal cramps. A sometimes fatal hyperthermia can also occur, driven partly by excessive drug-induced muscular contractions.

## Management of Withdrawal, Toxicity, and Overdose

Box 17-4 lists the signs and symptoms of withdrawal from stimulants, and also indicates the peak period when these symptoms are most likely to occur and their duration. Death due to poisoning or toxic levels is usually a result of convulsions, coma, or cerebral hemorrhage and may occur during periods of intoxication or withdrawal. Treatment of overdose is supportive and generally requires sedation of the patient.

## DEPRESSANTS

Depressants are drugs that relieve anxiety, irritability, and tension when used as intended. They are also used to treat seizure disorders and induce anesthesia. The two main pharmacologic classes of depressant are benzodiazepines and barbiturates. Both of these drug classes are discussed further in Chapter 12.

Benzodiazepines are relatively safe. They offer many advantages over older drugs used to relieve anxiety and insomnia.

---

### BOX 17-4   SIGNS AND SYMPTOMS OF STIMULANT WITHDRAWAL

**Peak Period**
1 to 3 days

**Duration**
5 to 7 days

**Signs**
Social withdrawal, psychomotor retardation, hypersomnia, hyperphagia

**Symptoms**
Depression, suicidal thoughts and behavior, paranoid delusions

**Treatment**
No specific pharmacologic treatments to reduce cravings or reverse acute toxicity and no known antidotes.

However, they are often intentionally and unintentionally misused. Ingestion of benzodiazepines together with alcohol can be lethal. Another depressant that is neither a benzodiazepine nor a barbiturate is marijuana. Derived from the cannabis plant, marijuana ("pot," "grass," "weed") is the most commonly abused drug worldwide. Marijuana is generally smoked as a cigarette ("joint") or in a pipe ("bong") but can be mixed in food or tea.

A benzodiazepine that has gained popularity as a recreational drug is flunitrazepam. Flunitrazepam is not legally available for prescription in the United States, but it is legally sold in over 60 countries for treatment of insomnia. The drug, known as roofies among young people, creates a sleepy, relaxed, drunken feeling that lasts 2 to 8 hours. Roofies are commonly used in combination with alcohol and other drugs. They are sometimes taken to enhance a heroin high or to mellow or ease the experience of coming down from a cocaine or crack high. Used with alcohol, roofies produce disinhibition and amnesia.

Roofies have recently gained a reputation as a "date rape" drug. Girls and women around the country have reported being raped after being involuntarily sedated with roofies, which were often slipped into their drinks by their attackers. The drug has no taste or odor, so the victims do not realize what is happening. About 10 minutes after ingesting the drug, the woman may feel dizzy and disoriented, simultaneously too hot and too cold, and nauseous. She may experience difficulty speaking and moving and then pass out. Such a victim will have no memories of what happened while under the influence of the drug. Another popular date rape drug used in similar fashion is gamma-hydroxybutyric acid (GHB). GHB works by mimicking the natural inhibitory brain neurotransmitter gamma-aminobutyric acid (GABA). It is also known as "liquid ecstasy." These drugs are also used simply for their depressant and hallucinogenic effects.

## Mechanism of Action and Drug Effects

Benzodiazepines and barbiturates work by increasing the action of GABA. GABA is an amino acid in the brain that inhibits nerve transmission in the CNS. The alteration of GABA action in the CNS results in relief of anxiety, sedation, and muscle relaxation. The effects of depressants are primarily limited to the CNS. They can also cause amnesia and unconsciousness. They have moderate effects outside the CNS, causing slight blood pressure decreases.

The active ingredients of the marijuana plant are known as cannabinoids, the most active of which is delta-9-trans-tetrahydrocannabinol, abbreviated *THC*. THC exerts its effects on the body by chemically binding to and stimulating two cannabinoid receptors in the CNS (CB1 and CB2). Smoking the drug leads to acute sensorial changes that start within 3 minutes, peak in 20 to 30 minutes, and last for 2 to 3 hours. Effects are longer when the drug is taken via the oral route. Specific effects include mild euphoria, memory lapses, dry mouth, enhanced appetite, motor awkwardness, and distorted sense of time and space. THC also stimulates sympathetic receptors and inhibits parasympathetic receptors in cardiac tissue, which leads to tachycardia. Other effects include hallucinations, anxiety, paranoia, and unsteady gait.

## Indications

Many therapeutic uses of depressants exist. Benzodiazepines are used primarily to relieve anxiety, to induce sleep, to sedate, and to prevent seizures. Barbiturates are used as sedatives and anticonvulsants and to induce anesthesia. Controversial medical uses for marijuana include treatment of chronic pain, reduction of nausea and vomiting associated with cancer treatment, and appetite stimulation in those with wasting syndromes, such as patients with cancer or AIDS. In 1996, California became the first state to legalize the medical use of marijuana. Since that time, 14 other states have legalized the use of marijuana for medical purposes, and others have legislation pending. Dronabinol is a synthetic THC prescription capsule approved by the Food and Drug Administration (FDA) for the previously mentioned indications (see Chapter 52 for further discussion of this drug). However, it is often not popular with those who claim that it is not as effective as inhaled marijuana.

## Contraindications

Contraindications to the therapeutic use of depressant medications include known drug allergy, dyspnea or airway obstruction, narrow-angle glaucoma, and porphyria (a metabolic disorder).

## Adverse Effects

The most common undesirable effect of benzodiazepines and barbiturates is an overexpression of their therapeutic effects. The CNS is the primary area of the body adversely affected by these drugs. Drowsiness, sedation, loss of coordination, dizziness, blurred vision, headaches, and paradoxical reactions (insomnia, increased excitability, hallucinations) are the primary CNS adverse effects. Occasional GI effects include nausea, vomiting, constipation, dry mouth, and abdominal cramping. Other possible adverse effects are pruritus and skin rash. Long-term use of marijuana may result in chronic respiratory symptoms (similar to those of tobacco abuse) and memory and attention deficit problems. A chronic depressive "amotivational" syndrome has also been observed, especially among younger users.

### Management of Withdrawal, Toxicity, and Overdose

Box 17-5 lists the signs, symptoms, and treatment of withdrawal from depressants, and also indicates the peak periods when these symptoms are most likely to occur and their duration. Fatal poisoning is unusual with benzodiazepines when they are taken alone. When benzodiazepines are ingested with alcohol or barbiturates, however, the combination can be lethal. Death is typically due to respiratory arrest. Abrupt withdrawal of benzodiazepines when they have been taken for prolonged periods has resulted in autonomic withdrawal symptoms, seizures, delirium, rebound anxiety, myoclonus (involuntary muscle contractions), myalgia, and sleep disturbances.

Flumazenil is a benzodiazepine reversal agent. Flumazenil antagonizes the action of benzodiazepines on the CNS by directly competing with them for binding at the benzodiazepine receptor in the CNS and thus reversing sedation. The dosage regimen to be followed for the reversal of conscious sedation or general anesthesia induced by a benzodiazepine and the management of suspected benzodiazepine overdoses are summarized in Chapter 12 (Table 12-3).

Barbiturates and benzodiazepines are commonly implicated in suicides, especially in combination with alcohol. Generally speaking, depressants are not regularly prescribed over a long period. Relatively safe hypnotic drugs such as the benzodiazepines are preferred whenever possible, especially in emotionally disturbed patients. Combinations of sedative-hypnotic drugs or in combination with alcohol need to be avoided. Long-term use of hypnotic drugs leads to ineffective control of insomnia, decrease in rapid eye movement sleep, dependence, and drug withdrawal symptoms.

Effects of marijuana use are usually self-limiting and resolve within a few hours.

## ALCOHOL

Alcoholic beverages have been used since the beginning of human civilization. Individuals of Arab descent introduced the technique of distillation to Europe in the Middle Ages. Alcohol has been called the "elixir of life" and has been touted as a remedy for practically all diseases, which led to the use of the term *whisky,* Gaelic for "water of life." Over time, it has been determined that the therapeutic value of alcohol is extremely limited, and long-term ingestion of excessive amounts is a major social and medical problem.

## Mechanism of Action and Drug Effects

Alcohol, which is more accurately known as *ethanol* and abbreviated as *ETOH,* is a CNS depressant. It results in CNS depression by dissolving in the lipid membranes within the CNS. The latest hypothesis is that ethanol causes a local disordering in the lipid matrix of the brain. This has been termed *membrane fluidization.* Some also believe that ethanol may augment GABA-mediated synaptic inhibition and fluxes of chloride. This enhancement of the action of GABA, an inhibitory neurotransmitter in the brain, causes CNS depression. The CNS is continuously depressed in the presence of ethanol. Moderate amounts of ethanol may stimulate or depress respirations. Effects of ethanol on the circulation are relatively minor. In moderate doses, ethanol causes vasodilation, especially of the cutaneous vessels, and produces warm, flushed skin. Ingestion of ethanol causes a feeling of warmth because it enhances cutaneous and gastric blood flow. Increased sweating may also occur. Heat is therefore lost more rapidly, and the internal body temperature consequently falls. The short-term (versus long-term) ingestion of ethanol, even in intoxicating doses, produces little lasting change in hepatic function. Long-term ingestion of ethanol is one of the primary causes of liver failure. Ethanol exerts a diuretic effect by virtue of its inhibition of antidiuretic hormone secretion and the resultant decrease in renal tubular reabsorption of water.

## Indications

Few legitimate uses of ethanol and alcoholic beverages exist. Ethanol is an excellent solvent for many drugs and is commonly employed as a vehicle for medicinal mixtures. When applied topically to the skin, ethanol acts as a coolant. Ethanol sponges are therefore used to treat fever. Ethanol may also be used in liniments (oily medications used on the skin). Applied topically, ethanol is the most popular skin disinfectant. More commonly, however, the type of alcohol used on the skin is isopropyl alcohol, which is similar in structure to ethanol but is more toxic and is not drinkable.

Systemic uses of ethanol are limited to the treatment of methyl alcohol and ethylene glycol intoxication (e.g., from drinking automotive antifreeze solution). However, small amounts of ethanol preparations (such as red wine) have been shown to have cardiovascular benefits.

## Adverse Effects

Long-term excessive ingestion of ethanol is directly associated with serious neurologic and mental disorders. These neurologic disorders can result in seizures. Nutritional and vitamin deficiencies, especially of the B vitamins, can occur and can lead to Wernicke's encephalopathy, Korsakoff's psychosis, polyneuritis, and nicotinic acid deficiency encephalopathy.

Moderate amounts of ethanol may stimulate or depress respirations. Large amounts produce dangerous or lethal depression of respiration. Although circulatory effects of ethanol are relatively minor, acute severe alcoholic intoxication may cause cardiovascular depression. Long-term excessive use of ethanol has largely irreversible effects on the heart, such as cardiomyopathy.

When consumed on a regular basis in large quantities, ethanol produces a constellation of dose-related negative effects such as alcoholic hepatitis or its progression to cirrhosis. Teratogenic effects can be devastating and are caused by the direct action of ethanol, which inhibits embryonic cellular proliferation early in gestation. This often results in a condition known as *fetal alcohol syndrome,* which is characterized by craniofacial abnormalities, CNS dysfunction, and both prenatal and postnatal growth retardation in the infant. Pregnant women need to be strongly advised not to consume alcohol during pregnancy, and appropriate treatment and counseling need to be arranged for pregnant women addicted to alcohol or any other drug of abuse.

## Interactions

Alcohol can intensify the sedative effects of any medications that work in the CNS (e.g., sedative-hypnotics, benzodiazepines, antidepressants, antipsychotics, opioids). It can interact with the antibiotic metronidazole, causing a disulfiram reaction. Alcohol can also cause severe hepatotoxicity when taken with acetaminophen. Acute ingestion of alcohol can increase the bioavailability of the blood thinner warfarin, which increases the chances of bleeding. Chronic ingestion can cause warfarin to be less effective, leading to increased risks of clots.

### Management of Withdrawal, Toxicity, and Overdose

Box 17-6 lists the common signs and symptoms of ethanol withdrawal. Signs and symptoms may vary depending on the individual's usage pattern, the preferred type of ethanol, and the presence of comorbidities. Treatment of ethanol toxicity is supportive and strives to stabilize the patient and maintain the airway. Ethanol withdrawal can be life threatening.

One pharmacologic option for the treatment of alcoholism is disulfiram (Antabuse). Disulfiram works by altering the metabolism of alcohol. It is not a cure for alcoholism, but it helps patients who have a sincere desire to stop drinking. The rationale for its use is that patients know that if they are to avoid the devastating experience of *acetaldehyde syndrome,* they cannot drink for at least 3 or 4 days after taking disulfiram. Table 17-2 outlines acetaldehyde syndrome. These adverse effects are obviously very uncomfortable and potentially dangerous for someone with any other major illnesses. For this reason, disulfiram is usually reserved as the treatment of last resort for "hard core" alcoholic patients for whom other treatment options (e.g., Alcoholics Anonymous, psychotherapy) have failed but who still hope to avoid continued alcohol abuse. When ethanol is ingested by an individual previously treated with disulfiram, the blood acetaldehyde concentration rises 5 to 10 times higher than in an untreated individual. Within about 5 to 10 minutes of alcohol ingestion, the individual's face feels hot, and soon afterward it is flushed and scarlet. After this, throbbing in the head and neck, nausea, copious vomiting, diaphoresis, dyspnea, hyperventilation, vertigo, blurred vision, and confusion occur. As little as 7 mL of alcohol will cause mild symptoms in a sensitive person. The effects last from 30 minutes to several hours. After the symptoms wear off, the patient is exhausted and may sleep for several hours. Most of the signs and symptoms observed after the ingestion of disulfiram plus alcohol are attributable to the

---

### BOX 17-6  SIGNS, SYMPTOMS, AND TREATMENT OF ETHANOL WITHDRAWAL

**Mild Withdrawal**
*Signs and Symptoms*
Systolic blood pressure higher than 150 mm Hg, diastolic blood pressure higher than 90 mm Hg, pulse rate higher than 110 beats/min, temperature above 100° F (37.7° C), tremors, insomnia, agitation

**Moderate Withdrawal**
*Signs and Symptoms*
Systolic blood pressure 150 to 200 mm Hg, diastolic blood pressure 90 to 140 mm Hg, pulse rate 110 to 140 beats/min, temperature 100° to 101° F (37.7° to 38.3° C), tremors, insomnia, agitation

**Severe Withdrawal (Delirium Tremens)**
*Signs and Symptoms*
Systolic blood pressure higher than 200 mm Hg, diastolic blood pressure higher than 140 mm Hg, pulse rate higher than 140 beats/min, temperature above 101° F (38.3° C), tremors, insomnia, agitation

**Treatment**
Benzodiazepines are the treatment of choice for ethanol withdrawal. The dosages are variable and differ from institution to institution. Lower dosages are used for mild symptoms, and higher dosages are needed for severe withdrawal. The oral route is preferred; however, it is often necessary to use the intravenous route for patients experiencing severe withdrawal. Patients who are experiencing severe withdrawal often require monitoring in an intensive care unit for cardiac and respiratory function, fluid and nutrition replacement, vital signs, and mental status. Restraints are indicated for a patient who is confused or agitated to protect the patient from self and to protect others (delirium tremens can be a terrifying and life-threatening state). Thiamine administration, hydration, and magnesium replacement may be indicated depending on the severity of the withdrawal state.

---

### TABLE 17-2  DISULFIRAM ADVERSE EFFECTS: ACETALDEHYDE SYNDROME

| BODY SYSTEM AFFECTED | RESULT |
|---|---|
| Cardiovascular | Vasodilation over the entire body, hypotension, orthostatic syncope, chest pain |
| Central nervous | Intense throbbing of the head and neck leading to a pulsating headache, sweating, marked uneasiness, weakness, vertigo, blurred vision, confusion |
| Gastrointestinal | Nausea, copious vomiting, thirst |
| Respiratory | Difficulty breathing |

---

resulting increase in the concentration of acetaldehyde in the body. There have even been a few published reports of localized disulfiram-alcohol skin reactions when alcohol preparations—even beer-containing shampoo—were placed on the skin. The usual dosage of disulfiram is 250 mg/day, or 125 mg/day in patients who experience adverse effects such as sedation, sexual dysfunction, and elevated liver enzyme levels.

A less noxious drug therapy option is the use of naltrexone, as mentioned previously in the section on opioids earlier in the chapter. The newest drug treatment indicated for alcoholism is acamprosate. Approved in 2004, it is used to maintain abstinence from alcohol in patients who are abstinent when starting the drug and who have additional psychosocial support. Its mechanism of action is not completely understood, but it may interact with *glutamate* and *GABA* receptors in the brain. The usual dosage is two 333-mg tablets taken three times daily.

## NICOTINE

Nicotine was first isolated from the leaves of tobacco in 1828. The medical significance of nicotine grows out of its toxicity, presence in tobacco, and propensity for eliciting dependence in its users. The long-term effects of nicotine and the untoward effects of the long-term use of tobacco are considerable. Although many people smoke because they believe cigarettes calm their nerves, smoking releases epinephrine, a hormone that creates physiologic stress in the smoker rather than relaxation. The apparent calming effects may be related to the increased deep breathing associated with smoking. The use of tobacco is addictive. Most users develop tolerance for nicotine and need greater amounts to produce the desired effect. Smokers become physically and psychologically dependent and will suffer withdrawal symptoms. Smoking is particularly dangerous in adolescents because their bodies are still developing and changing. The chemicals, including 200 known poisons, present in cigarette smoke can adversely affect this maturation. One third of young people who are "just experimenting" end up becoming addicted by the time they are 20 years of age.

### Mechanism of Action and Drug Effects

Nicotine works by directly stimulating the autonomic ganglia of the nicotinic receptors (see Chapter 20). Its site of action is the ganglion itself rather than the preganglionic or postganglionic nerve fiber. The organs throughout the body that are innervated by nerves stimulated by nicotine actually contain nicotinic receptors. These receptors are so named because they were originally tested with nicotine to measure their responses. Nicotine can have multiple unpredictable and dramatic effects on the body because nicotinic receptors are found in several systems, including the adrenal glands, skeletal muscles, and CNS.

The major action of nicotine is transient stimulation, followed by more persistent depression of all autonomic ganglia. Small doses of nicotine stimulate the ganglion cells directly and facilitate the transmission of impulses. When larger doses of the drug are applied, the initial stimulation is followed quickly by a blockade of transmission.

Nicotine markedly stimulates the CNS, including respiratory stimulation. This stimulation of the CNS is followed by depression. Nicotine can have dramatic effects on the cardiovascular system as well, resulting in increases in heart rate and blood pressure. The GI system is generally stimulated by nicotine, which produces increased tone and activity in the bowel. This often leads to nausea and vomiting and occasionally to diarrhea.

## Indications

The nicotine found in nature (i.e., tobacco plants) has no known therapeutic uses. It is medically significant because of its addictive and toxic properties. However, nicotine that is formulated into various drug products to reduce cravings and promote smoking cessation can be considered a therapeutic drug. It is available for this purpose as chewing gum, transdermal patches, and nasal spray.

## Adverse Effects

Nicotine primarily affects the CNS. Large doses can produce tremors and even convulsions. Respiratory stimulation also commonly occurs. The initial stimulation of the CNS induced by nicotine is quickly followed by depression. Death can even result from respiratory failure, which is thought to be due to both central paralysis and peripheral blockade of respiratory muscles. The cardiovascular effects of nicotine are an increase in heart rate and blood pressure. The effects of nicotine on the GI system are largely due to parasympathetic stimulation, which results in increased tone and motor activity of the bowel. Nicotine induces vomiting by both central and peripheral actions. Centrally, nicotine's emetic effects are due to stimulation of the *chemoreceptor trigger zone* in the brain.

### Management of Withdrawal, Toxicity, and Overdose

Acute nicotine toxicity generally occurs in children who accidentally ingest cigarettes. Treatment is supportive and may include treatment with activated charcoal. Smoking cessation is the primary cause of nicotine withdrawal, although discontinuation of any tobacco product can lead to this syndrome. An important and often overlooked problem in hospitalized patients is nicotine withdrawal, which manifests largely as cigarette craving. Irritability, restlessness, and a decrease in heart rate and blood pressure occur. Cardiac symptoms resolve over 3 to 4 weeks, but cigarette craving may persist for months or even years.

The nicotine transdermal system (patch), nicotine polacrilex (gum), and inhalers or nasal spray can be used to provide nicotine without the carcinogens in tobacco and are now available OTC. The patch system uses a stepwise reduction in subcutaneous delivery to gradually decrease the nicotine dose, and patient treatment compliance seems higher than with the gum. Acute relief from withdrawal symptoms is most easily achieved with the use of the gum, because rapid chewing releases an immediate dose of nicotine. The dose is approximately half the dose the average smoker receives in one cigarette, however, and the onset of action is 30 minutes versus 10 minutes or less from smoking. These pharmacologic changes in delivery minimize the immediate reinforcement and self-reward effects that are prominent with the rapid nicotine delivery of cigarette smoking.

A sustained-release form of the antidepressant bupropion (see Chapter 16) called *Zyban* has been approved as first-line therapy to aid in smoking cessation treatment. Sustained-release bupropion is an innovative treatment because it is the first nicotine-free prescription medicine to treat nicotine dependence. Table 17-3 lists the currently available drugs for nicotine withdrawal therapy.

Varenicline (Chantix) both activates and antagonizes the *alpha-4-beta-2* nicotinic receptors in the brain. This effect

### TABLE 17-3 NICOTINE WITHDRAWAL THERAPIES

| DRUG | DOSAGE | RECOMMENDED DURATION OF USE |
|---|---|---|
| **Transdermal Nicotine Systems** | | |
| Habitrol, Nicoderm | 7 mg/24 hr | 2-4 wk |
| | 14 mg/24 hr | 2-4 wk |
| | 21 mg/24 hr | 4-8 wk |
| Nicotrol | 5 mg/16 hr | 2-4 wk |
| | 10 mg/16 hr | 2-4 wk |
| | 15 mg/16 hr | 4-12 wk |
| ProStep | 11 mg/24 hr | 2-4 wk |
| | 22 mg/24 hr | 4-8 wk |
| Nicotrol inhaler | 10 mg/inhalation | 6-12 wk |
| Nicotrol NS nasal spray | 10 mg/spray | |
| nicotine gum (Resin) | When the patient has a strong urge to smoke, a stick of gum is chewed; use gradually reduced over a 2-3 mo period. | |
| **Antidepressant** | | |
| bupropion (Zyban) | 15-mg sustained-release tabs | 15 mg on days 1-3, then 150 mg bid for 7-12 wk |
| **Partial Nicotine Agonist** | | |
| varenicline (Chantix) | 0.5 or 1 mg tabs | 12-wk regimen, beginning with 0.5 mg orally bid, titrated to 1 mg daily by day 8. |

provides some stimulation to nicotine receptors, while also reducing the pleasurable effects of nicotine from smoking. This drug has demonstrated greater efficacy than bupropion. The recommended 12-week treatment regimen begins with 0.5 mg orally twice daily, titrating up to 1 mg twice daily by day 8. An optional second 12-week regimen may be prescribed to help the patient maintain tobacco abstinence. The most common adverse effects are nausea, vomiting, headache, flatulence, insomnia, and taste disturbances. Drowsiness has also been reported, which prompted the FDA to recommend caution in driving and engaging in other potentially hazardous activities until the patient can determine how the drug affects his or her mental status. Although many highly addicted smokers are reporting significant success with varenicline, the FDA issued warnings in January 2008 regarding its use. Specifically, case reports of psychiatric symptoms including agitation, depression, and suicidality, as well as worsening of preexisting psychiatric illness while using the drug have emerged. The FDA recommends appropriate patient education and follow-up regarding these adverse effects. Varenicline is a pregnancy category C drug.

## NURSING PROCESS

## ASSESSMENT

The purpose of a substance abuse assessment is to determine whether substance abuse exists, to evaluate the relationship between the abuse and other health concerns, and to begin the implementation of an effective health promotion and health restoration plan. Because of the prevalence of substance abuse and the role played by the professional nurse in a variety of settings, the nurse may be the first one to identify the risky behavior in a patient. Indications of abuse problems in patients may also present themselves during an abuser's hospitalization for an injury, illness, or surgery. However, even when substance abuse is not suspected, include questions about use of alcohol, nicotine, opioids, and so on in the general nursing assessment and medication history (see Pharmacology Overview). Question all patients about the use and misuse of substances, because addiction is found across the lifespan, in all cultures and in all types of individuals, and may therefore be encountered in all clinical specialties. Additionally, abuse/misuse of substances/prescription medications may need to be assessed in family members because adolescents and other individuals in the home may be stealing their parents' prescription drugs.

The nurse's responsibilities relative to drug abuse and the nursing process must begin with the cultivation of excellent interpersonal communication skills. It is important for you to acknowledge and address your own individual beliefs about drug and alcohol use as well as any personal history of coping with addiction or dealing with addicted family members. This process will allow you to anticipate potential responses and behaviors toward this patient population and seek out resolution about these feelings. Acknowledging feelings and beliefs about this group of patients within a proper perspective and ethical framework will allow you to resolve any personal animosity, judgmental attitudes, rejection, and/or enabling behaviors. Once detrimental behaviors and possible barriers to responsible and nonjudgmental care have been dealt with, focus on the patient and avoid being drawn into the manipulative and other negative behaviors of the abuser.

A thorough patient assessment and history must include specific questions about the substance(s) being used, the duration of abuse, related physical and mental health concerns, and withdrawal potential. In patients with suspected or confirmed substance abuse, honesty—on the part of the patient as well as the family or significant other—may be problematic when it comes to answering questions about drug use. Therefore, establishing a more communicative environment is needed and may be possible through the use of open-ended questions during assessment. Additionally, be sure to maintain a nonjudgmental approach during the assessment phase as well as other phases of the nursing process. A medication history needs to include information about all drugs being used, including prescription drugs, OTC drugs, herbals, dietary supplements, and illegal or street drugs. Include the names of these drugs, doses, frequency, and duration of use. Be attentive to any clues the patient, family, or significant other may reveal, including behavioral and mood changes. A patient's reported use of multiple prescribed drugs as well as contact with multiple prescribers raises a red flag as a possible sign of drug abuse. In addition, laboratory findings are important to assess, including results of renal and liver function studies and any drug screening studies. Assess

## BOX 17-7   DIAGNOSIS OF DEPENDENCE

The *Diagnostic and Statistical Manual of Mental Disorders IV, Text Revision* (American Psychiatric Association, 2000) identified criteria for the diagnosis of a dependence. The occurrence of at least *three* of the following symptoms within a 12-month period helps confirm a diagnosis of dependence:

- Tolerance or a marked need for increased amounts of the substance to achieve the desired effect
- Withdrawal symptoms
- Unsuccessful attempts to cut down or control use of the substance
- Abandonment or reduction of important social, occupational, or recreational activities due to substance use. The use continues regardless of recurrent physical/psychological problems.

Modified from Maurer FA, Smith CM: *Community/public health nursing practice: health for families and populations,* ed 4, Philadelphia, 2009, Saunders.

and monitor results of HIV and hepatitis laboratory tests, once ordered. Measure and document baseline vital signs.

A number of assessment tools with established validity and reliability are available to nurses and health care professionals for use with patients suspected of drug or substance. The goal of adequate screening for alcohol and other drug abuse or addiction is to identify patients who have or are at risk for developing alcohol or drug-related problems and to further engage them in discussion. This may help in further diagnosing and more accurately treating the patient's abuse problem. Laboratory tests are available to detect alcohol and other drugs in the blood and/or urine. These are used to identify more recent drug abuse rather than long-term use or dependence. However, there are other tests that are best used when assessing someone for confirmation of a diagnosis rather than screening (Box 17-7). The CAGE Questionnaire is available as a screening tool for alcohol use in adults and is used by many health care professionals in the field of alcohol addiction. Even though it is simple and brief (consisting of only four questions), it has a noted accuracy rate of 93%. The CAGE Questionnaire has also been adapted to include drug use in adults (CAGE-AID). Other available screening tools include the Substance Abuse Subtle Screening Inventory (SASSI), the Michigan Alcoholism Screening Test (MAST-G) for use in geriatric patients, and the Problem Oriented Screening Instrument for Teenagers (POSIT). If the findings of an assessment questionnaire are positive, the next step would be to explore the history of the patient's alcohol or drug use and problems. Further observation is needed to identify any physical, psychological, and social signs of dependence and dysfunction. Maintaining communication with family members may also provide useful information. If abuse is identified by a history-taking process, physical assessment, drug history profile, screening tests, or patient's confession of abuse, then confidentiality, privacy, and nonjudgmental behavior are keys to ethical nursing practice. Although the substance abuse must be reported to the necessary health care professionals, adhere to the American Nurses Association *Code of Ethics for Nurses* in making this report (see Chapter 4).

Assessment of *opioid* abuse includes, in addition to the assessment information above, determination of the route being used for drug delivery (e.g., oral versus intravenous use). The use of intravenous drugs may give rise to health concerns such as HIV/AIDS or hepatitis. Respiratory assessment with attention to rate and rhythm are important because of the risk for respiratory depression with opioid overdose or overuse. Other more specific signs and symptoms have been described earlier in the chapter.

Assessment of *CNS stimulant* abuse requires careful questioning about and observation for adverse effects, toxicity, and withdrawal signs and symptoms. Some of the more commonly abused CNS stimulants are dextroamphetamine, methamphetamine (crystallized and powdered forms), and cocaine (see Table 17-1). Signs and symptoms of CNS stimulant abuse have been previously discussed, such as changes in blood pressure and an increased heart rate. However, the following information needs to be assessed and documented: (1) frequent vital signs; (2) thorough head-to-toe physical examination; (3) assessment of neurologic functioning with attention to mydriasis (pupil dilation), hyperactive reflexes, headache, increased motor/speech activity, agitation, syncope, tremors, altered level of consciousness, and seizure activity; and (4) cardiac assessment with attention to increased heart rate (tachycardia), irregular heart rhythm (dysrhythmia), and hypertension or hypotension. Document and immediately report any abnormal assessment findings and/or the presence of an elevated temperature (hyperthermia which may be fatal), complaints of vomiting, headache or flushing of the face, and elevated temperature.

The most dangerous substances in terms of withdrawal are *CNS depressants* such as barbiturates, benzodiazepines, and cannabinoids. Abuse of CNS depressants is manifested by a decrease in vital signs and mental functioning (see previous discussion); therefore, frequent monitoring of vital signs and neurologic status is needed for safe and prudent care. As with any drug, obtain a comprehensive, thorough nursing history and medication profile. Additional signs and symptoms of abuse are tremors and agitation with possible progression to hallucinations and sometimes death with continued abuse. Early withdrawal (see Table 17-5) may be manifested by increased blood pressure and pulse rate and altered mental status. Because of the risk of respiratory and circulatory depression, always perform an assessment of the patient's ABCs (*a*irway, *b*reathing, and *c*irculation). See Pharmacology Overview for more specific information. Marijuana, as a depressant, may cause dizziness, disorientation, euphoria, and difficulty with speech and motor activities. Long-term use of marijuana may lead to a chronic, depressive, a motivational behavior. Be sure you always assess for any different or unusual behavioral changes. Assessment of marijuana use includes appraisal of cognitive and motor function and assessment for the inability to carry out minor tasks.

The signs and symptoms of ethanol (alcohol) withdrawal and toxicity are presented in Box 17-6. Include gathering data about possible drug interactions, especially the use of other CNS depressants such as opioids, sedatives, and hypnotics in the assessment. Blood alcohol levels are important to monitor, because the health issues and signs and symptoms that appear are directly related to the blood alcohol level.

Abuse of *nicotine* (a CNS stimulant) is associated with adverse effects such as increase in heart rate and blood pressure. It can also result in vomiting and increased bowel tone and motor activity. If the patient has a history of malnutrition, chronic lung disease, stroke, cancer, cardiac disease, or renal or liver dysfunction, relevant laboratory tests are generally ordered, and their results need to be examined by the nurse and those involved in the patient's care. Assessment needs to include vital signs, breath sounds, oxygen saturation levels, and monitoring for changes in neurologic functioning (e.g., level of consciousness, sensory/motor problems). Remember that smoking cessation and signs and symptoms of nicotine withdrawal may happen abruptly in hospitalized patients. Signs and symptoms of a craving for nicotine include irritability, restlessness, and decrease in pulse rate and blood pressure, which will help in early identification of more serious problems.

## CASE STUDY

### Substance Abuse and Adolescents

You are having a discussion with a neighbor who has a 14-year-old son. The neighbor expresses concern about his son and substance abuse problems he has heard about.

1. The neighbor describes his son's friend, who was a bright and motivated student but has become sullen and withdrawn, and lacks the motivation he once had. In addition, he has a chronic cough but denies that he smokes cigarettes. This behavior change may indicate abuse of what substance? Are there any long-term effects?

2. The neighbor mentions "huffing," which his son told him has happened at several parties this year. The neighbor says, "Huffing is not harmful, right?" What will you tell him?

   A few weeks later, the neighbor calls you because his son is extremely drowsy and unable to speak. The neighbor notes that his bottle of alprazolam (Xanax) is almost empty and worries that his son has taken an overdose.

3. What will you do first? What treatment would you expect his son to receive?

For answers, see http://evolve.elsevier.com/Lilley.

## NURSING DIAGNOSES

1. Ineffective health management of self related to perceived barriers of care due to substance abuse
2. Deficient knowledge related to lack of information about addictive behaviors and drugs being abused
3. Chronic low self-esteem related to the influence of substance abuse
4. Risk for injury and falls related to substance abuse and/or abrupt withdrawal

## PLANNING

### GOALS

1. Patient demonstrates patterns of more effective health maintenance.
2. Patient openly discusses his or her substance abuse and the benefits of a treatment regimen.

3. Patient gains improved self-esteem during treatment for substance abuse.
4. Patient remains free from injury during treatment for substance abuse and addictive disorder.

### OUTCOME CRITERIA

1. Patient openly discusses individual, family, and other perceived barriers to his or her own effective health maintenance.
   - Patient exhibits a healthy participation and cooperation with therapeutic regimen for addictive and abusive disorders.
2. Patient demonstrates knowledge base about addictive and abusive behaviors through discussion of expectations of recovery, benefits, and short-/long-term effects of treatment as well as signs and symptoms of withdrawal regimen.
3. Patient verbalizes feelings of improved self-esteem as well as healthy adaptation and coping skills in an open and secure treatment environment.
4. Patient undergoes safe withdrawal from the abused substance with stabilization of the aggravated and dysfunctional physical and emotional state without injury to self or others.

## IMPLEMENTATION

The nurse plays a vital role in the care of patients manifesting abuse behaviors, intoxication, and withdrawal. It is also the nurse who, through the nursing process, helps to meet the patient's basic needs after developing a therapeutic relationship and teaches the patient, family, and/or significant others about addiction and its effect on the entire family. Nursing strategies for meeting actual or potential health problems are implemented for nursing diagnoses generated from assessment data. Nurses working with substance abuse patients need their own sound knowledge base as well as special understanding and empathy. Participation in training, seminars, and education about the process of substance abuse and related lifestyles is encouraged to assist in understanding the patient and developing a comprehensive plan of care. In general, nursing interventions involve maximizing all of the therapeutic plans and minimizing those factors contributing to the abusive behaviors. Once a therapeutic rapport has been established and a patient-nurse-health care provider contract has been agreed upon, maximizing recovery is the plan. Interventions are based on the patient's specific physical and emotional problems and are carried out accordingly and in order of priority of basic needs. For example, if a patient is experiencing hallucinations (from either use of a substance or from its withdrawal), manage the ABCs of care and monitor vital signs and neurologic and mental status while providing a calm, quiet, nonjudgmental, and nonthreatening environment. Seizures may occur, so safety precautions are needed, including the use of protective measures such as attention to the airway, padding of side rails, and implementation of other seizure precautions (consult facility policies and procedures). For more information related to lifespan considerations (for adolescent and elderly patients), see the boxes on p. 293.

## PATIENT-CENTERED CARE: LIFESPAN CONSIDERATIONS FOR THE ELDERLY PATIENT

### Alcohol and Substance Abuse

Alcohol and substance abuse among the elderly is a hidden national epidemic. A substantial number of older adults are drinking at higher than recommended levels; thus, alcohol abuse is becoming a growing problem in this population and is one that is often ignored and/or missed by many health care providers.

Alcohol abuse and alcoholism cut across gender, race, and nationality with some statistics showing 10% of the country's population identified as abusing alcohol. Additionally, in adults 18 years of age or older, individuals identified as current drinkers were at 52%. However, in a study of some 12,000 Medicare beneficiaries 65 years of age or older, 9% consumed more alcohol than recommended in health guidelines. Conversely, a study conducted at Brandeis University identified the fact that about two-thirds of Medicare beneficiaries did not drink at all, and some 25% drank within recommended guidelines; however, the remaining 9% were found to drink more than 30 drinks a month or more than four drinks in any one session during a month. Obviously, alcohol abuse is of major concern for the older population and renders the necessity of thorough assessment for drug/chemical abuse in this group of patients.

Abuse of other substances by older adults is also an overlooked and often ignored problem. Older drug abusers are often poor, frail, and hidden from health professionals and service providers. The stigma associated with these problems keeps them, as well as family members, from coming forward to report problems. Although the overall rate of substance abuse is lower in older adults than in younger people, substance abuse in the elderly is a significant and growing problem. Alcohol abuse in the elderly is complicated by the fact that many abusers in this age group also use prescription and OTC medications. OTC drugs may cause adverse effects even when taken alone, and serious consequences may result when they are taken with alcohol. The main problems are seen when the combining of alcohol with a drug results in intensification of the drug's action (e.g., heightened hypotensive effects when an antihypertensive drug is taken with alcohol); this can lead to increased adverse effects with significant negative consequences (such as dizziness and possible syncope due to the greater drop in blood pressure, which can result in falls and injury). Some of the signals indicating an alcohol- or alcohol and medication–related problem in the elderly include trouble with memory after having a drink or taking a medication; loss of coordination, unsteadiness in walking or frequent falls; changes in sleeping habits; unexplained bruises; and irritability, sadness, depression, and being unsure of oneself.

Data from Buddy T: Unhealthy drinking increasing among older adults, 2009, available at www.alcoholism.about.com/b/2009/03/19/unhealthy-drinking-increasing-among-older-adults.htm. Accessed March 26, 2011; New York Office of Alcoholism and Substance Abuse Services: Elderly alcohol and substance abuse, 2005, available at http://www.oasas.ny.gov/AdMed/FYI/FYIInDepth-Elderly.cfm. National Institute on Alcohol Abuse and Alcoholism: Summary Health Statistics, available at www.niaaa.nih.gov/FAQs/General-English/Pages/default.aspx#olderpeople. Accessed March 26, 2011.

## PATIENT-CENTERED CARE: LIFESPAN CONSIDERATIONS FOR THE PEDIATRIC PATIENT

### Abuse of Over-the-Counter Drugs and Huffing Practices in Adolescents

Adolescent patients are exposed to very real drug hazards connected with some everyday products within the home. Two major problems involving hazardous drug use are seen in this population. The first is the abuse of OTC cold products, specifically *dextromethorphan*-containing products. Dextromethorphan is the most commonly used and most effective nonprescription cough suppressant and is an ingredient in several OTC products, including Robitussin DM cough syrup and Mucinex DM tablets. Some adolescents have discovered that taking dextromethorphan in large amounts leads to a "high" that is accompanied by hallucinations. The hallucinations have been documented to be similar to those associated with the street drug phencyclidine (PCP) and the anesthetic ketamine (see Chapter 11). The incidence of abuse varies and has rapidly increased. In April 2005, the *Medical News Today* reported that 1 in 11 teens has abused dextromethorphan-containing medications (17th annual study; Partnership for a Drug-Free America). However, a 2008 study found that 1 in 10 American teenagers had abused products with dextromethorphan to get high, making this OTC cough medicine more popular in this age group than cocaine, ecstasy, LSD, and meth. DXM is found in almost half of all of the OTC drugs sold in the United States, and for teens experimenting with drugs, DXM is cheap, easily obtained, and legal!

Additionally, it has been found that teens who abuse dextromethorphan may also abuse other drugs such as lysergic acid diethylamide (LSD), PCP, ecstasy, and inhalants. The hazardous short- or long-term effects that may occur with these drugs include nausea, hot flashes, reduced mental status, dizziness, seizures, loss of coordination and balance, brain damage, and death. The second problem is that of "huffing" or the abuse of inhalants, including the following substances: (1) *volatile solvents*—nail polish and paint thinner, (2) *aerosols*—deodorants and cooking sprays, (3) *gases*—butane cigarette lighter fluid and nitrous oxide (laughing gas), and (4) *nitrites*—cyclohexyl nitrite (found in room deodorizers) and amyl nitrite and butyl nitrite (sold on the street in small sealed containers). While some studies reported an increase in inhalant abuse by teens in the past 10 years, a new report based upon the National Survey on Drug Use and Health found that fewer adolescents are using inhalants such as glue and lighter fluid, but that the number of inhalant abusers in U.S. teens has not declined. The Associated Press (2009) reported that the number of adolescents actually abusing inhalants, as compared to those just trying them, remained at a stable rate between 2002 and 2007. Inhalant use often results in a euphoric feeling, but brain damage and even death can occur with just one huff. While the rate may be "stable," there is still a tremendous need for continued prevention and treatment efforts. Education needs to begin early on in elementary school, so that children learn of the problem and the related damaging effects to the brain before actual exposure to the practice. Education and awareness are important to prevent abuse and abuse behaviors, and a child is never too young to learn about these types of dysfunctional and life-threatening behaviors. Parents, other family members and relatives, and caregivers need to be actively involved in any educational sessions about this specific practice, as well as about other drugs that are abused, and related signs and symptoms.

Data from Griffin MR: Teen drug abuse of cough and cold medicine, WebMD Feature in collaboration with Consumer Healthcare Products Association (CHPA), available at www.webmd.com/parenting/teen-abuse-cough-medicine-9/teens-and-dxm-drug-abuse. Accessed March 25, 2011; Werner, E: Fewer teens sniffing inhalants to get high, Associated Press, Washington, DC, March 16, 2009; Join Together: Inhalant use declines among U.S. teens, March 19, 2009, available at http://www.drugfree.org/join-together/drugs/inhalant-use-declines-among. Prescription for danger: A report on the troubling trend of prescription and over-the-counter drug abuse among the nation's teens, January 2008, available at http:// www.promoteprevent.org/resources/prescription-danger-report-prescription-and-over-counter-drug-abuse-among-nations-teens.; The Partnership for a Drug-Free America: Generation RX: National study reveals new category of substance abuse emerging: Teens abusing RX and OTC medications intentionally to get high, Robert Wood Johnson Foundation, April 21, 2005, Washington, D.C.

Substance withdrawal is treated with a multimodal approach that includes pharmacologic and nonpharmacologic interventions. You have the responsibility to remain nonjudgmental while assisting in the patient's recovery and rehabilitation. You need to remain current in your knowledge about the different substances being abused as well as the various treatment and rehabilitation protocols. Of all interventions, ensuring patient safety is of utmost importance. The patient's movement through the plan of care for withdrawal, recovery, and rehabilitation must be individualized and in a safe, secure, and nonthreatening environment. Patient education remains an essential part of patient care to help the patient, family, and/or significant others understand the need for long-term lifestyle changes. Whether it is disulfiram treatment for alcohol abuse or bupropion therapy for nicotine withdrawal, patients need careful instructions and information about their treatment regimen.

Substance abuse has a major impact on family members and significant others. The family will also be in need of treatment and therapeutic support. But it is the caring, empathic, supportive, and educative responses by the nurse that will convey acceptance to the patient and family and help in the overall process of recovery and rehabilitation. A nonjudgmental attitude, caring, empathy, and quality care must always be the center of Patient Rights as well as the American Nurses Association *Code of Ethics for Nurses* (see Chapter 4) regardless of the admitting diagnosis and/or the type of substance being abused. Lifelong treatment is often indicated; the need for support during the long-term process of recovery must be emphasized and support recommended from within the family unit and extending outward to the community. (See Box 17-8 for a listing of various organizations and resources.) Methods to encourage recovery and minimize relapse need to be individualized for each patient and draw on all available resources, whether private or public. Communication techniques must be reinforcing and firm, yet sensitive to the patient's values and beliefs. Family members must be an integral part of all treatment and must participate in all educational sessions.

**BOX 17-8   ORGANIZATIONS AND AGENCIES CONCERNED WITH SUBSTANCE ABUSE**

Alcoholics Anonymous
American Council for Drug Education
American Society of Addiction Medicine
International Nurses Society on Addictions
National Center on Addiction and Substance Abuse at Columbia University
National Clearinghouse for Alcohol and Drug Information
National Council on Alcoholism and Drug Dependence
National Inhalant Prevention Coalition
National Institute on Alcohol Abuse and Alcoholism
National Institute on Drug Abuse
Partnership for a Drug-Free America
Substance Abuse and Mental Health Services Administration
U.S. Drug Enforcement Administration

## EVALUATION

Patient safety is of utmost importance at all times during patient care but especially when the patient is experiencing the signs and symptoms of withdrawal. Patients may go from mild withdrawal to severe withdrawal and enter into life-threatening situations within a period of a day or two, and therefore complete evaluation of the patient and environment must be ongoing. Evaluation of the recovery and rehabilitation process is important as well, with monitoring of the therapeutic effects of the treatment regimen and monitoring for any ill effects from the physiologic and/or psychological withdrawal of the substance. Part of this evaluation process also is appraisal of the support provided by others such as family members, as well as review of the availability of needed resources during and after hospitalization. In addition, report any abnormality in vital signs, laboratory test results, mental status, or other parameters immediately. An ongoing evaluation needs to also examine the availability of emotional, social, cultural, spiritual, and financial support, and revise the nursing care plan as needed.

## PATIENT TEACHING TIPS

- Ensure that relevant, nondiscriminatory, current, and accurate information—at various reading levels—is available to the patient, family, or significant others regarding the specific abuse disorder, signs and symptoms, withdrawal, and treatment regimens. Making an informed decision is best for everyone involved in the process of recovery and rehabilitation.
- Educate the patient, family, and/or significant other about available support groups and community resources.
- Be sure that the patient understands the importance of having—on his or her person at all times—a current list of all

medications, including treatment regimens for the abuse disorder. Include information about the drug, its action, why it is used and how, adverse effects, cautions, drug-drug and drug-food interactions, cautions, contraindications, dosing, and consequences of any missed doses.
- Patients must be educated about their rights to ethical and empathic treatment, regardless of the reason for treatment. One online resource available is at www.healthline.com/ga lecontent/center-for-substance-abuse-prevention. This site provides written information, resources, and video clips about drug/chemical abuse.

## KEY POINTS

- Physical dependence is a condition characterized by physiologic reliance on a substance, usually indicated by tolerance to the effects of the substance and development of withdrawal symptoms when use of the substance is terminated.
- Psychological dependence is a condition characterized by strong desires to obtain and use a substance.
- Habituation refers to situations in which a patient becomes accustomed to a certain drug (develops tolerance) and may have mild psychological dependence on it but does not show compulsive dose escalation, drug-seeking behavior, or major withdrawal symptoms upon drug discontinuation.
- Acamprosate is used to maintain abstinence from alcohol in patients who are abstinent when starting the drug and who have additional psychosocial support. Its mechanism of action is not completely understood.
- A new medication for smoking cessation is varenicline, which has shown better efficacy than bupropion.
- Drug withdrawal symptoms vary with the class of drug and may even be the opposite of the drug's action. Signs and symptoms of *opioid withdrawal* include seeking the drug from more than one prescriber, mydriasis (pupil dilatation), rhinorrhea, diaphoresis, piloerection (goose bumps), lacrimation, diarrhea, insomnia, and elevated blood pressure and pulse rate. Signs and symptoms of *CNS stimulant withdrawal* include social isolation or withdrawal, psychomotor retardation, and hypersomnia. Signs and symptoms of *CNS depressant withdrawal* include increased psychomotor activity; agitation; muscular weakness; hyperthermia; diaphoresis; delirium; convulsions; elevated blood pressure, pulse rate, and temperature; and eyelid tremors. *Ethanol withdrawal* produces varying degrees of signs and symptoms depending on the specific blood alcohol level. Delirium tremens are characterized by hypertensive crisis, tachycardia, and hyperthermia and may be life threatening.
- Evaluation of the recovery and rehabilitation process is important, including monitoring of the therapeutic effects of the treatment regimen and monitoring for any physiologic and/or psychological ill effects from the withdrawal of the abused substance.

## NCLEX® EXAMINATION REVIEW QUESTIONS

1 A patient is experiencing withdrawal from opioids. The nurse expects to see which assessment finding most commonly associated with acute opioid withdrawal?
   a Elevated blood pressure
   b Decreased pulse
   c Lethargy
   d Constipation

2 During treatment for withdrawal from opioids, the nurse expects which medication to be ordered?
   a amphetamine (Dexedrine)
   b clonidine (Catapres)
   c diazepam (Valium)
   d disulfiram (Antabuse)

3 The nurse is presenting a seminar on substance abuse. Which drug is the most commonly used illicit drug in the United States?
   a Crack cocaine
   b Heroin
   c Marijuana
   d Methamphetamine

4 A patient who is taking disulfiram as part of an alcohol treatment program accidentally takes a dose of cough syrup that contains a small percentage of alcohol. The nurse expects to see which symptom as a result of acetaldehyde syndrome?
   a Lethargy
   b Copious vomiting
   c Hypertension
   d No ill effect because of the small amount of alcohol in the cough syrup

5 The nurse is assessing a patient for possible substance abuse. Which assessment finding indicates possible use of amphetamines?
   a Lethargy and fatigue
   b Cardiovascular depression
   c Talkativeness and euphoria
   d Difficulty swallowing and constipation

6 A patient experiencing ethanol withdrawal is beginning to show severe manifestations of delirium tremens. The nurse will plan to implement which interventions for this patient? (Select all that apply.)
   a Doses of an oral benzodiazepine
   b Doses of an intravenous benzodiazepine
   c Restraints if the patient becomes confused, agitated, or a threat to himself or others
   d Thiamine supplementation
   e Oral disulfiram (Antabuse) treatment
   f Monitoring in the intensive care unit

7 A patient has been admitted to the emergency department after a suspected overdose of benzodiazepines mixed with alcohol. The patient is lethargic and cannot speak. The nurse expects which immediate measures to be implemented? (Select all that apply.)
   a Prepare to administer naloxone (Narcan).
   b Prepare to administer flumazenil.
   c Monitor the patient for convulsions.
   d Prepare for potential respiratory arrest.
   e Apply restraints.

1. a, 2. b, 3. c, 4. b, 5. c, 6. b, c, d, f, 7. b, c, d

For Critical Thinking and Prioritization Questions, see http://evolve.elsevier.com/Lilley.

# Drugs Affecting the Autonomic Nervous System

## PURR APPLICATION

### Planning for the Part

The basic explanation provided for the PURR model in the Study Skills Tips for Part 1 demonstrates the application process as it relates to individual chapters. There is another application for the PURR model that can be very useful. This application encourages the learner to take a broader view of the assignment. In the case of this text, you have noticed that the chapters are grouped together into multiple chapter blocks called *parts*. Part organization is not some random process applied by the author to further complicate the subject. Part organization is a carefully considered process to put content together in a fashion that is logical and meaningful. Since the authors have spent considerable time trying to link the chapters together in the most logical pattern, it is to your benefit as a student to learn to take advantage of the work already done for you.

### Part Title

Begin the process of part planning by looking at the Part 3 title, "Drugs Affecting the Autonomic Nervous System." Then look at the part structure. There are four chapters contained in Part 3. All of these chapters must be concerned with the autonomic nervous system. Even before you have read any chapter, you are beginning to look for the links that will establish a relationship—not only the links among the ideas in individual chapters but also the broader links that connect the four chapters in this part with each other and with the ideas that have come in earlier parts and will follow in later parts.

There is a clear example here of the way in which parts relate to one another. Look back at Part 2, "Drugs Affecting the Central Nervous System." Clearly that part deals with some aspect of the nervous system, as does this part. One learning objective you should establish for yourself is determining the relationship between these two parts. You must be able to define and explain *central nervous system* and *autonomic nervous system*. However, just defining these terms and moving on limits the learning you can achieve. Ask yourself some additional questions that will help you establish a connection between these parts. What are the differences in function of the central and the autonomic nervous systems? Are there pharmacologic drugs that have application in both the central and autonomic nervous systems? The principle is to keep stressing the links that must exist throughout all the parts and chapters you are studying. The normal study pattern that most students apply is one that focuses on the individual chapters, but it is essential to remain aware of the broader scope of chapter and part.

## Part Chapters

After considering the part title and looking for relationships between the new part and the previous parts, the next step in applying the *Plan* step of PURR is to spend a few minutes studying the chapter titles and looking for the relationships that must exist. Part 3 has four chapters, and there is a clear pattern in these chapters. Chapters 18 and 19 both contain the term *adrenergic*. Clearly the two chapters are dealing with the same broad topic. However, Chapter 18 covers adrenergic drugs and Chapter 19 covers adrenergic-blocking drugs. Apply questioning strategies at this point. What does *adrenergic* mean? What is an *adrenergic drug?* These two questions are essential in mastering the content of Chapter 18 and should be questions that you ask yourself almost without thinking.

The next step is one that can greatly enhance your understanding when you start to read the material. This is a step that is easily overlooked. Notice that Chapter 18 deals with drugs and Chapter 19 deals with blocking drugs. There must be a difference between a *drug* and a *blocking drug*. Focus now with a few questions that will keep you aware that the content in Chapter 18 has a direct relationship to the content in Chapter 19. What is the difference between a drug and a blocking drug? When is the pharmacologic application of a drug appropriate? Under what conditions should a blocking drug be chosen? Then ask a question to help maintain the focus on the concept of the entire part: What aspects of the autonomic nervous system are related to the adrenergic drugs and blocking drugs?

Once you begin to focus on the relationship of chapters within a part, certain things will begin to become apparent. Chapters 20 and 21 also cover drugs and blocking drugs. These two chapters develop the concept in relation to cholinergics rather than adrenergics. However, the same questions you used as a focus for Chapters 18 and 19 can be recycled in setting up the study of Chapters 20 and 21. Simply replace the term *adrenergic* with *cholinergic* and you are ready to begin reading these two chapters with a clear personal learning objective.

## Active Questioning

Active questioning is the key concept to master in working through the process of planning your learning for an entire part rather than for single chapters. The idea is to view the part as a whole rather than seeing only the content of individual chapters. The preceding discussion has provided a number of sample questions to help you begin the process. These questions should not be seen as the only questions you should ask, but rather as examples to help you develop a questioning process.

Keep in mind that you may or may not ask questions that are useful and appropriate when you are using only the chapter titles as the question stimulus. Some of the questions you devise will prove to be very useful when reading the chapter. On the other hand, some of the initial questions you generate may have little or no application as you read and understand the content of an individual chapter. Do not worry about the quality of your questions when planning at the part level. Questions can (and sometimes should) be revised or discarded when the details of the chapter become clearer. The important point is that you begin the part with some questions to help you focus your own reading and learning. Also, you will find that the more you apply active questioning as a part of your learning strategy, the better your questions will become.

## STUDY GROUPS

A significant part of the PURR approach to learning is active questioning and rehearsing. When we engage others in this process, we have access to their ideas and understanding. We must also think through our own thoughts and make them clear to others. The best way to learn is to teach others.

Study groups are particularly helpful when anticipating test questions. With several minds working, you increase your odds of being correct. In nursing, your textbook learning is of no value until you are able to apply the knowledge and skills you are learning. Study groups provide a discussion venue to stimulate thinking about the nursing process. Study group members can share lecture notes, which is of value if you need to be absent or if you have an instructor who talks too fast. Relating with a study group keeps you alert while you are studying. It is hard to fall asleep or daydream when you are in the middle of a discussion. There are many advantages to working with a study group; however, you must be careful when selecting the people to be in your group. Consider these four guidelines when establishing your study group:

1. Choose students who have **similar abilities and motivation** to yours. Socializing and gossiping can eat up valuable study time. Noncommitted and underprepared classmates can be a drain.
2. Look for students who have a **common time to meet.**
3. Select classmates who have learning styles **different** from yours. They might understand the reading material or lecture material better than you. They may be able to draw a diagram that will help your learning.
4. Find students that have **good communication skills;** that is, people who know how to listen, ask good questions, and explain concepts.

Study groups are not for everyone; however, they may be an alternative for you if you are having difficulty staying focused during your personal study time.

# Adrenergic Drugs

## OBJECTIVES

When you reach the end of this chapter, you will be able to do the following:

1 Briefly describe the functions of the sympathetic nervous system and the specific effects of adrenergic stimulation.
2 List the various drugs classified as adrenergic agonists or sympathomimetics.
3 Discuss the mechanisms of action, therapeutic effects, indications, adverse and toxic effects, cautions, contraindications, drug interactions, and available antidotes to overdosage for the various adrenergic agonists or sympathomimetic drugs.
4 Develop a nursing care plan that includes all phases of the nursing process for patients taking adrenergic agonists.

## DRUG PROFILES

- ◆ **dobutamine, p. 305**
- ◆ **dopamine, p. 305**
- ◆ **epinephrine, p. 305**
  **fenoldopam, p. 305**
  **midodrine, p. 305**

- ◆ **norepinephrine, p. 306**
  **phenylephrine, p. 306**

  _____

- ◆ *Key drug*

## KEY TERMS

**Adrenergic agonists** Drugs that stimulate and mimic the actions of the sympathetic nervous system. Also called *sympathomimetics*. (p. 299)

**Adrenergic receptors** Receptor sites for the sympathetic neurotransmitters norepinephrine and epinephrine. (p. 299)

**Alpha-adrenergic receptors** A class of adrenergic receptors that are further subdivided into alpha$_1$- and alpha$_2$-adrenergic receptors. (p. 299)

**Autonomic functions** Bodily functions that are involuntary and result from the physiologic activity of the autonomic nervous system. The functions often occur in pairs of opposing actions between the sympathetic and parasympathetic divisions of the autonomic nervous system. (p. 299)

**Autonomic nervous system** A branch of the peripheral nervous system that controls autonomic bodily functions. It consists of the sympathetic nervous system and the parasympathetic nervous system. (p. 299)

**Beta-adrenergic receptors** Receptors located on postsynaptic cells that are stimulated by specific autonomic nerve fibers. Beta$_1$-adrenergic receptors are located primarily in the heart, whereas beta$_2$-adrenergic receptors are located in the smooth muscle fibers of the bronchioles, arterioles, and visceral organs. (p. 299)

**Catecholamines** Substances that can produce a sympathomimetic response. They are either endogenous catecholamines (such as epinephrine, norepinephrine, and dopamine) or synthetic catecholamine drugs (such as dobutamine). (p. 299)

**Dopaminergic receptor** A third type of adrenergic receptor (in addition to alpha-adrenergic and beta-adrenergic receptors) located in various tissues and organs and activated by the binding of the neurotransmitter dopamine, which can be either endogenous or a synthetic drug form. (p. 300)

**Mydriasis** Pupillary dilation, whether natural (physiologic) or drug induced. (p. 303)

**Ophthalmics** Drugs that are used in the eye. (p. 302)

**Positive chronotropic effect** An increase in heart rate. (p. 302)

**Positive dromotropic effect** An increase in the conduction of cardiac electrical impulses through the atrioventricular node, which results in the transfer of nerve action potentials

from the atria to the ventricles. This ultimately leads to a systolic heartbeat (ventricular contractions). (p. 302)

**Positive inotropic effect** An increase in the force of contraction of the heart muscle (myocardium). (p. 302)

**Sympathomimetics** Drugs used therapeutically that mimic the catecholamines epinephrine, norepinephrine, and dopamine. Also called *adrenergic agonists*. (p. 299)

**Synaptic cleft** The space either between two adjacent nerve cell membranes or between a nerve cell membrane and an effector organ cell membrane (also called *synapse*). (p. 300)

## ANATOMY, PHYSIOLOGY, AND PATHOPHYSIOLOGY OVERVIEW

The body's nervous system is divided into two major branches: the central nervous system and the peripheral nervous system (Figure 18-1). The central nervous system contains the brain and the spinal cord. The peripheral nervous system is further subdivided into somatic and autonomic. The autonomic nervous system is yet further subdivided into the parasympathetic (cholinergic) and the sympathetic (adrenergic). Understanding the autonomic nervous system and its subclasses is critical in the study of pharmacology, as numerous drugs act in these systems. This chapter will focus on the adrenergic nervous system and related compounds.

Adrenergic compounds include several exogenous (synthetic) and endogenous (produced in the body naturally) substances. They have a wide variety of therapeutic uses depending on their site of action and their effect on different types of adrenergic receptors. Adrenergics stimulate the sympathetic nervous system (SNS) and are also called adrenergic agonists. They are also known as sympathomimetics, because they mimic the effects of the SNS neurotransmitters norepinephrine, epinephrine, and dopamine. These three neurotransmitters are chemically classified as catecholamines. In considering the adrenergic class of medications, it is helpful to understand how the SNS operates in relation to the rest of the nervous system.

## SYMPATHETIC NERVOUS SYSTEM

Figure 18-1 depicts the divisions of the nervous system and shows the relationship of the SNS to the entire nervous system. The SNS is the counterpart of the parasympathetic nervous system; together they make up the autonomic nervous system. They provide a checks-and-balances system for maintaining the normal homeostasis of the autonomic functions of the human body.

There are receptor sites for the catecholamines norepinephrine and epinephrine throughout the body. These are referred to as adrenergic receptors. It is at these receptor sites that adrenergic drugs bind and produce their effects. Many physiologic

responses are produced when they are stimulated or blocked. Adrenergic receptors are further divided into alpha-adrenergic receptors and beta-adrenergic receptors, depending on the specific physiologic responses caused by their stimulation. Both types of adrenergic receptors have subtypes (designated 1 and 2), which provide a further means of checks and balances that control stimulation and blockade, vasoconstriction and vasodilation of blood vessels, and the increased and decreased production of various substances. The alpha$_1$- and alpha$_2$-adrenergic receptors are differentiated by their location relative to nerves. The alpha$_1$-adrenergic receptors are located on postsynaptic effector cells (the tissue, muscle, or organ that the nerve stimulates). The alpha$_2$-adrenergic receptors are located on the presynaptic nerve terminals. They control the release of neurotransmitters. The predominant alpha-adrenergic agonist response is vasoconstriction and central nervous system (CNS) stimulation.

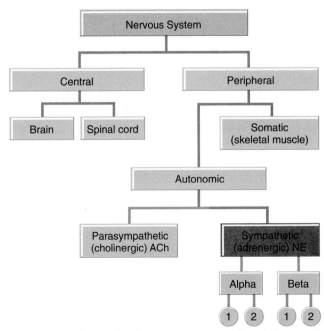

**FIGURE 18-1** Sympathetic nervous system in relation to the entire nervous system. *ACh,* Acetylcholine; *NE,* norepinephrine.

**TABLE 18-1** **ADRENERGIC RECEPTOR RESPONSES TO STIMULATION**

| LOCATION | RECEPTOR | RESPONSE |
|---|---|---|
| **Cardiovascular** | | |
| Blood vessels | Alpha$_1$ | Vasoconstriction |
| | Beta$_2$ | Vasodilation |
| Cardiac muscle | Beta$_1$ | Increased contractility |
| Atrioventricular node | Beta$_1$ | Increased heart rate |
| Sinoatrial node | Beta$_1$ | Increased heart rate |
| **Endocrine** | | |
| Liver | Alpha$_1$, beta$_2$ | Glycogenolysis |
| Kidney | Beta$_1$ | Increased renin secretion |
| **Gastrointestinal** | | |
| Muscle | Alpha$_1$, beta$_2$ | Decreased motility (relaxation of gastrointestinal smooth muscle) |
| **Genitourinary** | | |
| Bladder sphincter | Alpha$_1$ | Constriction |
| Penis | Alpha$_1$ | Ejaculation |
| Uterus | Alpha$_1$ | Contraction |
| | Beta$_2$ | Relaxation |
| **Respiratory** | | |
| Bronchial muscles | Beta$_2$ | Dilation (relaxation of bronchial smooth muscles) |
| **Ocular** | | |
| Pupillary muscles of the iris | Alpha$_1$ | Mydriasis (dilated pupils) |

The beta-adrenergic receptors are all located on postsynaptic effector cells. The beta$_1$-adrenergic receptors are primarily located in the heart, whereas the beta$_2$-adrenergic receptors are located in the smooth muscle fibers of the bronchioles, arterioles, and visceral organs. A beta-adrenergic agonist response results in bronchial, gastrointestinal (GI), and uterine smooth muscle relaxation; glycogenolysis; and cardiac stimulation. Table 18-1 provides a more detailed listing of the adrenergic receptors and the responses elicited when they are stimulated by a neurotransmitter or a drug that acts like a neurotransmitter (Figure 18-2).

Another type of adrenergic receptor is the dopaminergic receptor. When stimulated by dopamine, these receptors cause the vessels of the renal, mesenteric, coronary, and cerebral arteries to dilate, which increases blood flow to these tissues. Dopamine is the only substance that can stimulate these receptors.

Catecholamine neurotransmitters are produced by the SNS and are stored in vesicles or granules located in the ends of nerves. Here the transmitter waits until the nerve is stimulated, then the vesicles move to the walls of nerve endings and release their contents into the space between the nerve ending and the effector organ, known as the synaptic cleft or *synapse.* The released contents of the vesicles (catecholamines) then have the opportunity to bind to the receptor sites located all along

the effector organ (see Figure 18-2). Once the neurotransmitter binds to the receptors, the effector organ responds. Depending on the function of the particular organ, this response may involve smooth muscle contraction (e.g., skeletal muscles) or relaxation (e.g., GI and airway smooth muscles), an increased heart rate, the increased production of one or more substances (e.g., stress hormones), or constriction of a blood vessel.

This process is halted by the action of specific enzymes and by reuptake of the neurotransmitter molecules back into the nerve cell (neuron). Catecholamines are metabolized by two enzymes, monoamine oxidase (MAO) and catechol ortho-methyltransferase (COMT). Each enzyme breaks down catecholamines but is responsible for doing it in different areas. MAO breaks down the catecholamines that are in the nerve ending, whereas COMT breaks down the catecholamines that are outside the nerve ending at the synaptic cleft (see Figure 18-2). Neurotransmitter molecules may also be taken back up into the presynaptic nerve fiber by various protein pumps within the cell membrane. This phenomenon is known as *active transport.* This restores the catecholamine to the vesicle and provides another means of maintaining an adequate supply of the substance for future sympathetic nerve impulses. This process is illustrated in Figure 18-2. The sympathetic branch of the autonomic nervous system is often described as having a "fight-or-flight" function, because it allows the body to respond in a self-protective manner to dangerous situations.

## PHARMACOLOGY OVERVIEW

### ADRENERGIC DRUGS

Adrenergics are drugs with effects that are similar to or mimic the effects of the SNS neurotransmitters norepinephrine, epinephrine, and dopamine. These neurotransmitters are known as *catecholamines.* Catecholamines produce a sympathomimetic response. They are either endogenous substances such as epinephrine, norepinephrine, and dopamine or synthetic substances such as dobutamine and phenylephrine. The three endogenous catecholamines, (epinephrine, norepinephrine, and dopamine) are also available in synthetic drug form.

Catecholamine drugs that are used therapeutically produce the same result as endogenous catecholamines. When any of the adrenergic drugs is given, it bathes the area between the nerve and the effector cell (i.e., the synaptic cleft). Once there, the drug has the opportunity to induce a response. This can be accomplished in one of three ways: by direct stimulation, by indirect stimulation, or by a combination of the two (mixed-acting).

A direct-acting sympathomimetic binds directly to the receptor and causes a physiologic response (Figure 18-3). Epinephrine is an example of such a drug. An indirect-acting sympathomimetic causes the release of the catecholamine from the storage sites (vesicles) in the nerve endings; it then binds to the receptors and causes a physiologic response (Figure 18-4). Amphetamine and other related anorexiants (see Chapter 13) are examples of such drugs. A mixed-acting sympathomimetic both directly stimulates the receptor by binding to it and indirectly stimulates

**FIGURE 18-2** Mechanism by which stimulation of a nerve fiber results in a physiologic process; adrenergic drugs mimic this same process. *COMT,* Catechol ortho-methyltransferase; *MAO,* monoamine oxidase; *NE,* norepinephrine.

**FIGURE 18-3** Mechanism of physiologic response to direct-acting sympathomimetics. *D,* Drug; *NE,* norepinephrine.

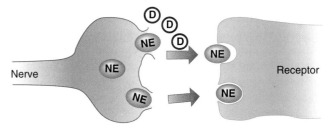

**FIGURE 18-4** Mechanism of physiologic response to indirect-acting sympathomimetics. *D,* Drug; *NE,* norepinephrine.

the receptor by causing the release of the neurotransmitter stored in vesicles at the nerve endings (Figure 18-5). Ephedrine is an example of a mixed-acting adrenergic drug.

There are also noncatecholamine adrenergic drugs such as phenylephrine, metaproterenol, and albuterol. These are structurally dissimilar to the endogenous catecholamines and have a longer duration of action than either the endogenous or synthetic catecholamines. The noncatecholamine drugs show similar patterns of activity.

Adrenergic agents can also be classified as either selective or nonselective in their actions. For example, phenylephrine and

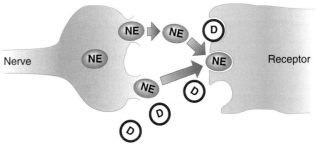

**FIGURE 18-5** Mechanism of physiologic response to mixed-acting sympathomimetics. *D,* Drug; *NE,* norepinephrine.

## TABLE 18-2 CATECHOLAMINES AND THEIR DOSE-RESPONSE RELATIONSHIP

| DRUG | DOSAGE | RECEPTOR |
|------|--------|----------|
| dobutamine (Dobutrex) | Maintenance: 2-15 mcg/kg/min | Beta$_1$ more than beta$_2$ |
| | High: 40 mcg/kg/min | Beta$_2$ more than alpha$_1$ |
| dopamine (Intropin) | Low: 0.5-2 mcg/kg/min | Dopaminergic |
| | Moderate: 2-4 or less than 10 mcg/kg/min | Beta$_1$ |
| | High: 20-30 mcg/kg/min | Alpha$_1$ |
| epinephrine (Adrenalin) | Low: 1-4 mcg/min | Beta$_1$ more than beta$_2$ more than alpha$_1$ |
| | High: 4-40 mcg/min | Alpha$_1$ more than/equal to beta$_1$ |

clonidine are considered selective agonists, meaning they only affect one receptor subtype. Epinephrine and norepinephrine are considered nonselective agonists, because they have action at both alpha and beta receptors. Adrenergic drugs can also act at different types of adrenergic receptors depending on the amount of drug administered. For example, dopamine may produce dopaminergic, beta$_1$, or alpha$_1$ effects, depending on the dose given. See Table 18-2 for other examples of catecholamines and the dose-specific selectivity.

Although adrenergics work primarily at postganglionic receptors (the receptors that immediately innervate the effector organ, gland, or muscle) peripherally, they may also work more centrally in the nervous system at the preganglionic sympathetic nerve trunks. The ability to do so depends on the potency of the specific drug and the dose used.

Adrenergic drugs are classified most technically by their specific receptor activities; they may also be categorized in terms of their clinical effects. For example, phenylephrine is both an alpha$_1$ agonist and a vasopressive drug (pressor), whereas albuterol is both an alpha$_2$ agonist and a bronchodilator. Both classifications are suitable for most clinical purposes. Clinically, it may be necessary to carefully choose an adrenergic drug with greater selectivity for a particular receptor type to avoid undesired clinical effects. In such a situation, detailed knowledge of the type and degree of receptor selectivity of different drugs becomes important.

## Mechanism of Action and Drug Effects

To fully understand the mechanism of action of adrenergics, one must have a working knowledge of normal adrenergic transmission. This transmission takes place at the junction between the nerve (postganglionic sympathetic neuron) and the receptor site of the innervated organ or tissue (effector). The process of SNS stimulation is illustrated in Figure 18-2 and was discussed earlier in this chapter. When adrenergic drugs stimulate alpha$_1$-adrenergic receptor sites located on smooth muscles, vasoconstriction usually occurs. Binding to these alpha$_1$ receptors can also cause the relaxation of GI smooth muscle, contraction of the uterus and bladder, male ejaculation, and contraction of

the pupillary muscles of the eye, which causes the pupils to dilate (see Table 18-1). Stimulation of alpha$_2$-adrenergic receptors, on the other hand, actually tends to reverse sympathetic activity but is not of great significance either physiologically or pharmacologically.

There are beta$_1$-adrenergic receptors on the myocardium and in the conduction system of the heart, including the sinoatrial node and the atrioventricular node. When these beta$_1$-adrenergic receptors are stimulated by an adrenergic drug, three things result: (1) an increase in the force of contraction (positive inotropic effect), (2) an increase in heart rate (positive chronotropic effect), and (3) an increase in the conduction of cardiac electrical nerve impulses through the atrioventricular node (positive dromotropic effect). In addition, stimulation of beta$_1$ receptors in the kidney causes an increase in renin secretion. Activation of beta$_2$-adrenergic receptors produces relaxation of the bronchi (bronchodilation) and uterus, and also causes increased glycogenolysis (glucose release) from the liver (see Table 18-1).

## Indications

Adrenergics, or sympathomimetics, are used in the treatment of a wide variety of illnesses and conditions. Their selectivity for either alpha- or beta-adrenergic receptors and their affinity for certain tissues or organs determine the settings in which they are most commonly used. Some adrenergics are used as adjuncts to dietary changes in the short-term treatment of obesity. These drugs are discussed in more detail in Chapter 13.

### Respiratory Indications

Bronchodilators are adrenergic drugs that have an affinity for the adrenergic receptors located in the respiratory system. They tend to preferentially stimulate the beta$_2$-adrenergic receptors and cause bronchodilation. Of the two subtypes of beta-adrenergic receptors, these drugs are attracted more to the beta$_2$-adrenergic receptors located on the bronchial, uterine, and vascular smooth muscles as opposed to the beta$_1$-adrenergic receptors located on the heart. The beta$_2$ agonists are helpful in treating conditions such as asthma and bronchitis. Common bronchodilators that are classified as predominantly beta$_2$-selective adrenergic drugs include albuterol, ephedrine, formoterol, levalbuterol, metaproterenol, pirbuterol, salmeterol, and terbutaline. These drugs are discussed in more detail in Chapter 37.

### Indications for Topical Nasal Decongestants

The intranasal application of certain adrenergics can cause the constriction of dilated arterioles and a reduction in nasal blood flow, which thus decreases congestion. These adrenergic drugs work by stimulating alpha$_1$-adrenergic receptors and have little or no effect on beta-adrenergic receptors. The nasal decongestants include ephedrine, naphazoline, oxymetazoline, phenylephrine, and tetrahydrozoline. They are discussed in more detail in Chapter 36.

### Ophthalmic Indications

Some adrenergics are applied to the surface of the eye. These drugs are called ophthalmics. They work in much the same way as nasal decongestants except that they affect the vasculature of the eye. They stimulate alpha-adrenergic receptors located on small arterioles in the eye and temporarily relieve conjunctival congestion by causing arteriolar vasoconstriction. The ophthalmic adrenergics include epinephrine, naphazoline, phenylephrine, and tetrahydrozoline.

Adrenergics can also be used to reduce intraocular pressure, which makes them useful in the treatment of open-angle glaucoma. They can also dilate the pupils (mydriasis), which makes them useful for diagnostic eye examinations. They produce these effects by stimulating alpha- or beta$_2$-adrenergic receptors, or both. The two adrenergics used for this purpose are epinephrine and dipivefrin. Ocular adrenergic drugs are discussed in more detail in Chapter 57.

## Cardiovascular Indications

The final group of adrenergic agents is used to support the cardiovascular system during cardiac failure or shock. These drugs are referred to as *vasoactive sympathomimetics, vasoconstrictive drugs* (also known as *vasopressive drugs, pressor drugs,* or *pressors), inotropes,* or *cardioselective sympathomimetics.* They have a variety of effects on the various alpha- and beta-adrenergic receptors, and the effects can be related to the specific dose of the adrenergic drug. Common vasoactive adrenergic drugs include dobutamine, dopamine, ephedrine, epinephrine, fenoldopam, midodrine, norepinephrine, and phenylephrine.

It is important to note that a common medication error is confusion between norepinephrine and the brand name for phenylephrine, which is Neo-Synephrine. These drugs are often both ordered for a patient at the same time, and, because the names sound alike, the wrong drug may be given. To avoid this confusion, many pharmacies list these drugs by their trade names as well: norepinephrine is called *Levophed,* and phenylephrine is called *Neo-Synephrine.*

## Contraindications

The only usual contraindications to the use of adrenergic drugs are known drug allergy and severe hypertension.

## Adverse Effects

Unwanted CNS effects of the alpha-adrenergic drugs include headache, restlessness, excitement, insomnia, and euphoria. Possible cardiovascular adverse effects of the alpha-adrenergic drugs include chest pain, vasoconstriction, hypertension, tachycardia, and palpitations or dysrhythmias. Effects on other body systems include anorexia (loss of appetite), dry mouth, nausea, vomiting, and, rarely, taste changes.

The beta-adrenergic drugs can adversely stimulate the CNS, causing mild tremors, headache, nervousness, and dizziness. These drugs can also have unwanted effects on the cardiovascular system, including increased heart rate (positive chronotropy), palpitations (dysrhythmias), and fluctuations in blood pressure. Other significant effects include sweating, nausea, vomiting, and muscle cramps. See the Patient-Centered Care: Lifespan Considerations for the Elderly Patient box on this page for additional information.

## Toxicity and Management of Overdose

The toxic effects of adrenergic drugs are an extension of their common adverse effects (e.g., seizures from excessive CNS stimulation, hypotension or hypertension, dysrhythmias, palpitations, nervousness, dizziness, fatigue, malaise, insomnia, headache, tremor, dry mouth, and nausea). The two most life-threatening effects involve the CNS and cardiovascular system. In the acute setting, seizures can be effectively managed with diazepam. Intracranial bleeding can also occur, often as the result of an extreme elevation in blood pressure. Such elevated blood pressure poses the risk of hemorrhage not only in the brain but elsewhere in the body as well. The best and most effective treatment in this situation is to lower the blood pressure using a rapid-acting sympatholytic drug (e.g., esmolol; see Chapter 19). This can directly reverse the adrenergic-induced state.

The majority of the adrenergic compounds have very short half-lives, and thus their effects are short-lived. Therefore, when these drugs are taken in overdose or toxicity develops, stopping the drug causes the toxic symptoms to subside in a relatively short period of time. The recommended treatment for overdose is often to manage the symptoms and support the patient. If

## DOSAGES

### *Selected Vasoactive Adrenergics*

| DRUG | PHARMACOLOGIC CLASS | USUAL DOSAGE RANGE | INDICATIONS |
|---|---|---|---|
| ◆ dobutamine (Dobutrex) (D) | Beta$_1$-adrenergic | **Pediatric**<br>IV infusion: 2.5-20 mcg/kg/min<br>**Adult**<br>IV infusion: 2.5-40 mcg/kg/min | Cardiac decompensation |
| ◆ dopamine (Intropin) (C) | Beta$_1$-adrenergic | **Adult and pediatric**<br>IV infusion: 1-50 mcg/kg/min | Shock syndrome, cardiopulmonary arrest |
| ◆ epinephrine (Adrenalin) (C) | Alpha- and beta-adrenergic | **Pediatric**<br>Subcut: 10 mcg/kg repeated q15min ×2 then q4h prn<br>**Adult**<br>Subcut: 0.3-0.5 mg repeated q10-15min if required<br>**Neonatal**<br>IV: 10-30 mcg/kg q3-5min if required<br>**Pediatric**<br>IV: 10 mcg/kg q3-5min if required<br>**Adult**<br>IV: 1 mg q3-5min if required | Anaphylaxis<br><br><br><br>Cardiopulmonary arrest |
| fenoldopam (Corlopam) (C) | Dopamine 1 agonist | **Adult only**<br>IV: 0.1-1.6 mcg/kg/min for up to 48 hr | Hypertensive emergency in hospital setting |
| midodrine (ProAmatine) (C) | Alpha$_1$-adrenergic | **Adult only**<br>PO: 10 mg tid, max 40 mg/day | Orthostatic hypotension |
| ◆ norepinephrine (Levophed) (C) | Alpha- and beta-adrenergic | **Pediatric**<br>IV infusion: 0.1-0.2 mcg/kg/min<br>**Adult**<br>IV infusion: 2-30 mcg/min | Hypotensive states |
| phenylephrine (Neo-Synephrine) (C) | Alpha-adrenergic | **Pediatric (for hypotension during spinal anesthesia)**<br>Subcut/IM: 0.1 mg/kg/dose<br>**Adult**<br>IV infusion: 10 mg/250 or 500 mL IV solution, start at 100-180 mcg/min and titrate down to 40-60 mcg/min<br>IM/subcut: 2-5 mg<br>IV: 0.1-0.5 mg | Hypotension or shock |

*IM*, Intramuscular; *IV*, intravenous; *PO*, oral; *subcut*, subcutaneous.

death occurs, it is usually the result of either respiratory failure or cardiac arrest. The treatment of overdose is therefore aimed at supporting the respiratory and cardiac systems.

## Interactions

Numerous drug interactions can occur with adrenergic drugs. Although many of the interactions result only in a diminished effect because of direct antagonism at and competition for receptor sites, some reactions can be life-threatening. The following are some of the more serious drug-drug interactions involving adrenergic drugs: When alpha- and beta-adrenergic drugs are given with adrenergic antagonists (e.g., some classes of antihypertensive drugs), the drugs directly antagonize each other, which results in reduced therapeutic effects. Administration of adrenergics with anesthetic drugs (see Chapter 11) can increase the risk of cardiac dysrhythmias. Tricyclic antidepressants (see Chapter 16), when given with adrenergics, can cause increased vasopressor effects, acute hypertensive crisis. Administration of adrenergic drugs with monoamine oxidase inhibitors (MAOIs) may cause a possibly life-threatening hypertensive crisis

(see Chapter 16). Antihistamines (see Chapter 36) and thyroid preparations (see Chapter 31) can also increase the effects of adrenergic drugs.

### Laboratory Test Interactions

Alpha-adrenergic drugs can cause an increase in serum levels of endogenous corticotropin (i.e., adrenocorticotropic hormone), corticosteroids, and glucose. Therefore, the results of laboratory tests for these substances need to be interpreted with caution in patients receiving any of these medications.

### Dosages

For dosage information on various adrenergic drugs, see the table on this page.

## DRUG PROFILES

The four frequently used classes of adrenergic drugs are bronchodilators (see Chapter 37), ophthalmic drugs (see Chapter 57), nasal decongestants (see Chapter 36), and vasoactive drugs, which are emphasized in this chapter (see

Drug Profiles) and in Chapter 24. The receptor selectivity for the alpha$_1$, beta$_1$, and beta$_2$ receptor subtypes is *relative* (as opposed to *absolute*). Thus, there may be some overlap of drug effects between the different adrenergic classes of drugs, especially at higher dosages. In contrast, dopamine receptors are more specific for dopamine itself and/or specific dopaminergic drugs.

## VASOACTIVE ADRENERGICS

Adrenergics that have primarily cardioselective effects are referred to as *vasoactive adrenergics.* They are used to support a failing heart or to treat shock. They may also be used to treat orthostatic hypotension. These drugs have a wide range of effects on alpha- and beta-adrenergic receptors, depending on the dosage. The vasoactive adrenergics are very potent, quick-acting, injectable drugs. Although dosage recommendations are given in the table on p. 304, all of these drugs are titrated to the desired physiologic response. All of the vasoactive adrenergics (with the exception of midodrine) are rapid in onset, and their effects very quickly cease when administration is stopped. Therefore, careful titration and monitoring of vital signs and electrocardiogram (ECG) are required.

#### ◆ dobutamine

Dobutamine (Dobutrex) is a beta$_1$-selective vasoactive adrenergic drug that is structurally similar to the naturally occurring catecholamine dopamine. Through stimulation of the beta$_1$ receptors on heart muscle (myocardium), it increases cardiac output by increasing contractility (positive inotropy), which increases the stroke volume, especially in patients with heart failure. Dobutamine is available only as an intravenous drug and is given by continuous infusion. (See Dosages table on p. 304.)

**Pharmacokinetics**

| Route | Onset of Action | Peak Plasma Concentration | Elimination Half-life | Duration of Action |
|---|---|---|---|---|
| IV | Less than 2 min | Less than 10 min | 2-5 min | Less than 10 min |

#### ◆ dopamine

Dopamine (Intropin) is a naturally occurring catecholamine neurotransmitter. It has potent dopaminergic as well as beta$_1$- and alpha$_1$-adrenergic receptor activity, depending on the dosage. Dopamine, when used at low dosages, can dilate blood vessels in the brain, heart, kidneys, and mesentery, which increases blood flow to these areas (dopaminergic receptor activity). At higher infusion rates, dopamine can improve cardiac contractility and output (beta$_1$-adrenergic receptor activity). At highest doses, dopamine causes vasoconstriction (alpha$_1$-adrenergic receptor activity). Use of dopamine is contraindicated in patients who have a catecholamine-secreting tumor of the adrenal gland known as a *pheochromocytoma.* The drug is available only as an intravenous injectable drug and is given by continuous infusion. (See Dosages table on p. 304.)

**Pharmacokinetics**

| Route | Onset of Action | Peak Plasma Concentration | Elimination Half-life | Duration of Action |
|---|---|---|---|---|
| IV | 2-5 min | Rapid | Less than 2 min | 10 min |

#### ◆ epinephrine

Epinephrine (Adrenalin) is an endogenous vasoactive catecholamine. It acts directly on both the alpha- and beta-adrenergic receptors of tissues innervated by the SNS. It is considered the prototypical nonselective adrenergic agonist. Epinephrine is administered in emergency situations and is one of the primary vasoactive drugs used in many advanced cardiac life support protocols. The physiologic response it elicits is dose related. At low dosages, it stimulates mostly beta$_1$-adrenergic receptors, increasing the force of contraction and heart rate. It is also used to treat acute asthma (see Chapter 37) and anaphylactic shock at these dosages because it has significant bronchodilatory effects via the beta$_2$-adrenergic receptors in the lungs. At high dosages (e.g., intravenous drip), it stimulates mostly alpha-adrenergic receptors, causing vasoconstriction, which elevates the blood pressure. (See Dosages table on p. 304.) Epinephrine is available in two strengths for IV use, which has led to many medication errors. It is available as 1:1000 (1 mg/mL) and also as 1:10,000 (0.1 mg/mL). Be aware of these differences in strength and associated indications. Reading the label carefully before administering the drug is critical to patient safety.

**Pharmacokinetics**

| Route | Onset of Action | Peak Plasma Concentration | Elimination Half-life | Duration of Action |
|---|---|---|---|---|
| Subcut | 5-10 min | 20 min | Variable | Unknown |
| IV | Less than 2 min | Rapid | Less than 5 min | 5-30 min |

#### ◆ fenoldopam

Fenoldopam (Corlopam) is a peripheral dopamine 1 (D$_1$) agonist indicated for parenteral use in lowering blood pressure. Fenoldopam produces its blood pressure–lowering effects by inducing arteriolar vasodilation mainly through stimulation of D$_1$ receptors. It appears to be as effective as sodium nitroprusside for short-term treatment of severe hypertension and may have beneficial effects on renal function because it increases renal blood flow. It is available as a 10-mg/mL injection. (See Dosages table on p. 304.)

**Pharmacokinetics**

| Route | Onset of Action | Peak Plasma Concentration | Elimination Half-life | Duration of Action |
|---|---|---|---|---|
| IV | 5 min | 20 min | More than 5 min | 10 min |

#### ◆ midodrine

Midodrine (ProAmatine) is a prodrug that is converted in the liver to its active form, desglymidodrine. This active metabolite is responsible for the primary pharmacologic action of midodrine, which is alpha$_1$-adrenergic receptor stimulation. This alpha$_1$ stimulation causes constriction of both arterioles and veins, resulting in peripheral vasoconstriction. Midodrine is primarily indicated for the treatment of symptomatic orthostatic hypotension. Midodrine is available as 2.5- and 5-mg tablets (see Dosages table on p. 304.) Midodrine is usually given two to three times per day. The last dose of the day should not be given after 6 PM.

### Pharmacokinetics

| Route | Onset of Action | Peak Plasma Concentration | Elimination Half-life | Duration of Action |
|---|---|---|---|---|
| PO | 45-90 min | 1 hr | More than 3-4 hr | 6-8 hr |

#### ◆ norepinephrine

Norepinephrine (Levophed) acts predominantly by directly stimulating alpha-adrenergic receptors, which leads to vasoconstriction. It also has some direct-stimulating beta-adrenergic effects on the heart (beta$_1$-adrenergic receptors) but none on the lung (beta$_2$-adrenergic receptors). Norepinephrine is directly metabolized to dopamine and is used primarily in the treatment of hypotension and shock. It is given only by continuous infusion. (See Dosages table on p. 304.)

### Pharmacokinetics

| Route | Onset of Action | Peak Plasma Concentration | Elimination Half-life | Duration of Action |
|---|---|---|---|---|
| PO | Rapid | 1-2 min | Less than 5 min | 1-2 min |

#### ◆ phenylephrine

Phenylephrine (Neo-Synephrine) works almost exclusively on the alpha-adrenergic receptors. It is used primarily for short-term treatment to raise blood pressure in patients in shock, to control some dysrhythmias (supraventricular tachycardias), and to produce vasoconstriction in regional anesthesia. It is also administered topically as an ophthalmic drug (see Chapter 57) and as a nasal decongestant (see Chapter 36). (See Dosages table on p. 304.)

### Pharmacokinetics

| Route | Onset of Action | Peak Plasma Concentration | Elimination Half-life | Duration of Action |
|---|---|---|---|---|
| IV | Rapid | Rapid | Less than 5 min | 15-20 min |

# NURSING PROCESS

# ASSESSMENT

*Adrenergic agonist drugs* have a variety of effects depending on the receptors they stimulate. Stimulation of the alpha-adrenergic receptors results in vasoconstriction of blood vessels. Stimulation of beta$_1$-adrenergic receptors produces cardiac stimulation, and beta$_2$-adrenergic receptor stimulation results in bronchodilation. Because of these sympathomimetic properties, use of adrenergic agonists requires careful patient assessment and monitoring to maximize therapeutic effects and minimize possible adverse effects. Focus assessment on

## ⚡ SAFETY AND QUALITY IMPROVEMENT: PREVENTING MEDICATION ERRORS

### *Ratio Solutions: Which Strength Is Stronger?*

- When giving epinephrine, it is important to choose the correct dosage form. Ratio solutions indicate the number of grams of the medication per total milliliters of solution. Be sure you know what the numbers mean!
- A medication that is designated 1:1000 has 1 gram of medication per 1000 mL of solution.
- A medication that is designated 1:10,000 has 1 gram of medication per 10,000 mL of solution.
- Which is the more potent dose? 1:1000 or 1:10,000? 1:10,000 strength contains 0.1 mg/mL of medication; 1:1000 strength contains 1 mg/mL of medication, which is *ten times* stronger than the 1:10,000 strength. Therefore, the solution with the smaller number of milliliters is actually the more potent dose!

a comprehensive health history with past and present medical history, and obtain a past/present medication history. Also include specific system-based questions, and identify cautions, contraindications, and drug interactions. Include the following health history questions in your assessment: (1) Medication history and allergies: What prescription medications are taken regularly? What about the self-administration of over-the-counter medications and herbals? Are there allergies to any medications, over-the-counter drugs, herbals, foods, topical products, and/or environmental pollutants/products? (2) Respiratory: Is there a history of asthma, and, if present, how frequent and severe are the acute episodes? What factors exacerbate or help to alleviate asthma? Any other asthma-related symptoms such as dyspnea, chest pain? Treatments used for asthma and associated successes or failures? (3) Cardiovascular: Is there a history of transient ischemic attacks or any history of cerebrovascular accident or stroke? Is there a history of hypertension, hypotension, cardiac irregularities, or other cardiovascular disease? (4) Renal/liver: Is there a history of kidney problems? Has anyone ever reported that kidney/liver function studies are abnormal? History of chronic kidney infections? Any jaundice? With altered renal/liver function, there is the risk for altered excretion/metabolism of drugs thus leading to possible toxicity.

Performing a thorough head-to-toe physical assessment is also a very important part of data collection with these drugs. Thorough assessment of the cardiac system is important because the adrenergic agonist drugs may exacerbate preexisting cardiac disorders. Other parameters that need to be thoroughly assessed with the adrenergic drugs include baseline vital signs. Assess and document breath sounds, heart sounds, peripheral pulses, skin color, and capillary refill. Specifically with the use of midodrine, assess postural blood pressures and pulse rates in supine, sitting, and standing positions before and during drug administration. In addition to measurement of postural blood pressures and pulse rates, inquire about other significant symptoms such as dizziness, lightheadedness, and syncope. Assessment of the patient's symptoms and the patient's perception of either disease progression or a decrease in symptoms is very important for effective and successful treatment.

With other adrenergic drugs, such as those used for bronchodilating effects, perform a thorough respiratory assessment and document the patient's respiratory rate, rhythm, and depth as well as the presence of normal and/or adventitious (abnormal) breath sounds. Asking questions about any complaints of difficulty in breathing and activity/exercise intolerance is also important. Assess and document pulse oximetry readings for oxygen saturation levels. Include in the assessment measurement of respiratory peak flow using a flow meter as well as measurement of the anterior-posterior diameter of the chest wall. A decrease in peak flow readings may indicate bronchospasms, whereas an increased anterior-posterior chest wall diameter is seen in chronic lung disorders such as emphysema. Prescribers may also order additional respiratory function studies such as measurement of arterial blood gas levels.

Elderly and very young patients may react with increased sensitivity to these drugs. In addition, some of these drugs are used only for acute episodes of asthma, whereas other drugs are used year-round as preventative drugs. For example, the drugs salmeterol (see Chapter 37) and formoterol are *not* used to treat acute asthmatic episodes, whereas albuterol is indicated for treatment of acute episodes.

Epinephrine and similar drugs are used for their cardiac, bronchial, antiallergic, ophthalmic, and vasopressor effects. Focus assessment on vital signs, breath sounds, arterial blood gas levels, and ECG findings, if ordered. Assess and document liver and renal function test results. In addition, assess each system related to the specific action of the drug.

Overall, adrenergic drugs work in similar ways, but individual drugs may have some differences with regard to action, indications, and overall considerations. If the general class of drugs and the way in which they work is known, then the relevant assessment parameters, cautions, contraindications, drug interactions, and lifespan considerations are easy to determine. If the drug is a pure adrenergic agonist, the net effect is stimulation of alpha-adrenergic receptors with vasoconstriction of blood vessels and subsequent elevation of blood pressure and heart rate. You would then know to expect specific actions from the drug as well as to anticipate certain adverse effects. The drug may be used for the therapeutic effect of increased blood pressure, but an unwanted adverse effect could then be a hypertensive crisis. If the drug is a beta-adrenergic agonist, it will stimulate both beta$_1$ and beta$_2$ receptors, which will lead to cardiac stimulation and bronchodilation. This beta$_1$ action can also result in too much stimulation with severe tachycardia and possibly chest pain, if coronary artery disease is present. Thus, by knowing the actions of a given drug, you may draw conclusions about, anticipate, and be very alert to the drug's therapeutic action, adverse effects, cautions, contraindications, drug interactions, and toxicity.

# NURSING DIAGNOSES

1. Impaired gas exchange related to asthma-induced bronchospasms
2. Decreased cardiac output related to cardiovascular adverse effects of adrenergic agonist drugs
3. Ineffective peripheral tissue perfusion related to intense vasoconstrictive actions of medications
4. Acute pain related to adverse effects of tachycardia and palpitations
5. Disturbed sleep patterns related to CNS stimulation caused by adrenergic drugs
6. Deficient knowledge of the therapeutic regimen, adverse effects, drug interactions, and precautions related to the use of adrenergic drugs
7. Noncompliance with drug therapy related to lack of information about the importance of taking the medication as ordered
8. Risk for injury related to possible adverse effects (nervousness, vertigo, hypertension, or tremors) or to potential drug interactions

# PLANNING

## GOALS

1. Patient experiences normal patterns of gas exchange and open airways.
2. Patient maintains normal cardiac output status.
3. Patient displays adequate peripheral vascular/tissue perfusion.
4. Patient experiences relief of pain and increased levels of comfort.
5. Patient experiences improved sleep patterns.
6. Patient demonstrates adequate knowledge about the use of specific medication.
7. Patient remains adherent to the drug therapy regimen and without drug-related complications.
8. Patient remains free from injury related to drug therapy.

## OUTCOME CRITERIA

1. Patient shows improvement in gas exchange and respiratory status with normal respiratory rate (12 to 20 breaths/minute), regular rhythm and depth, clearing breath sounds, and pulse oximetry reading above 90%.
2. Patient's blood pressure and pulse rate remain within normal limits (BP 120/80; pulse 60 to 100 beats/min).
   - Patient's capillary refill is less than 5 seconds in fingers and toes.
3. Patient's circulation in extremities remains intact.
   - Patient's capillary refill is intact, with skin color pink and extremities warm to touch.
   - Patient's pedal pulses intact and strong to palpation.
4. Patient remains comfortable during drug therapy and takes medications exactly as prescribed.
   - Patient remains free of increased heart rate and irregular heart rhythm.
5. Patient uses relaxation therapy, massage, and maintains healthy sleep patterns in a quiet, temperate room environment.
   - Patient demonstrates proper use of drug therapy regimen and avoids overuse of medication to decrease adverse effects.
6. Patient states rationale for use of medications as well as timing/dosing and scheduling of drug therapy.

- Patient states most common adverse effects of drug therapy.
- Patient states adverse effects to report if they occur, such as increased occurrence of palpitations, chest pain, irregular heart rhythm, dizziness, and overall feeling of discomfort, anxiety, and restlessness.

7. Patient reports taking medication exactly as prescribed for maintenance and/or acute use and without adverse and/or toxic reactions.

8. Patient remains free from self-injury as related to safe and as-prescribed self-administration of drug therapy.

---

## CASE STUDY

### Dopamine Infusion

 Mr. P., age 82 years, is receiving dopamine at a dose of 5 mcg/kg/min for heart failure. He has a history of hypothyroidism and takes a daily dose of thyroid replacement hormone. Yesterday, Mr. P's vital signs were as follows:

Blood pressure: 150/88 mm Hg

Pulse rate: 92 beats/min

Respiration rate: 16 breaths/min

His heart rhythm showed sinus rhythm with rare ectopic beats. While at rest, he had no shortness of breath but did experience some dyspnea when getting up to the bedside commode. He has edema in his lower legs rated as 2+ edema.

1. Explain how this dose of dopamine works to help treat Mr. P's heart failure.
2. What would you expect to happen if the dose were set to 1 mcg/kg/min? 20 mcg/kg/min?

This morning, you make rounds and find that Mr. P's vital signs are as follows:

Blood pressure: 170/94 mm Hg

Pulse rate: 120 beats/min

Respiration rate: 22 breaths/min

The heart monitor shows sinus tachycardia with two to three ectopic beats per minute. Mr. P. is complaining of palpitations and some shortness of breath at rest but says, "I've felt this before when I've had bad spells with my heart. I'm sure it will pass."

3. Do you think there is a concern at this time? Explain your reasoning and what should be done.

The physician decides to titrate the dopamine infusion to 3 mcg/kg/min, which you do immediately.

4. How quickly should you see a response from the patient to this decrease in dosage?

For answers, see http://evolve.elsevier.com/Lilley.

---

## ▌IMPLEMENTATION

There are several nursing interventions that may maximize the therapeutic effects of *adrenergic drugs* and minimize their adverse effects. These interventions include checking package inserts for the types and amounts of dilutional solutions to use with parenteral dosage forms (and for all dosage forms). For example, subcutaneous administration of the adrenergic agonist epinephrine to patients with asthma requires safe calculations and accurate dosing. A tuberculin syringe may be used for subcutaneous administration of epinephrine to help in accurate dosing for both adult and pediatric patients.

Use of epinephrine and some of the other pure *alpha-adrenergics* may not be indicated for shock-related symptoms because these drugs lead to vasoconstriction of the renal vessels and subsequent renal damage or shutdown. Therefore, when a patient is in shock and requires medications, dopamine is generally the drug of choice (rather than epinephrine). Dopamine is used because in specific dosage ranges it helps treat a shock-related syndrome through its ability to produce vasoconstriction of peripheral blood vessels and increase blood pressure, but without vasoconstriction of the renal vasculature. This lack of renal vasculature vasoconstriction helps improve perfusion through the kidneys and thus salvages the kidneys (while increasing blood pressure). With administration of dopamine and similar drugs, check the intravenous site frequently for infiltration (e.g., every hour, as needed) to be sure that the site remains intact and that the drug is being infused at the proper rate. Infiltration of an intravenous solution containing an adrenergic drug may lead to tissue necrosis from excessive vasoconstriction around the intravenous site. Phentolamine is often used for the treatment of infiltration (see Chapter 19). Also, with intravenous infusions, use only clear solutions and a proper dilutional fluid, always administer the drug with an intravenous infusion pump, and closely monitor the cardiac system (e.g., vital signs, heart sounds, and/or ECG monitoring). Give all of these drugs per the manufacturer's instructions and suggested infusion rates to avoid precipitating dangerously high blood pressure and pulse rate and subsequent complications.

When these drugs are given via an inhaler or nebulizer, provide the patient with complete, thorough, and age-appropriate instructions about correct use, storage, and care of equipment. Instruct the patient on how to use a spacer correctly, because use of this device with the inhaler is often ordered. A spacer provides more effective delivery of inhaled doses of drug (see Patient Teaching Tips, as well as Chapter 9). When the adrenergics are dosed for bronchodilating effects, often two adrenergics are prescribed. This is because different medications are associated with different pharmacokinetics and actions. One inhaler may be for use in *acute* situations, and the other may be for *long-term* and/or *preventative* use. With this type of treatment regimen, the patient needs to receive thorough, simple, and complete instructions and explanations about the method of delivery as well as the drugs used. This will help to minimize overdosage and reduce the risk of severe adverse effects such as hypertension, severe tachycardia, tremors, and CNS overstimulation.

Emphasize in patient teaching that these medications are to be used only as prescribed with regard to amount, timing, and spacing of doses. Because of their synergistic effects, when these medications (especially asthmatics) are used in combination with other types of bronchodilators, the patient must be very clear about what to do before, during, and after the dose is delivered. If the patient is taking an inhaled dosage form, he or she may also be taking an oral or parenteral form of the same or a similar drug. The reason for the use of more than one drug of the same drug class and the use of more than one route of administration is to achieve combined therapeutic effects. In educating the patient, pay extremely close attention to these regimens because of the need to prevent exacerbation of adverse effects, minimize drug interactions, and prevent severe vascular and cardiovascular adverse effects. Advise the patient to immediately report any complaints of chest pain, palpitations, headache, or seizures.

Patients with chronic lung disease who are receiving adrenergic drugs also need to avoid anything that may exacerbate their respiratory condition (e.g., food or other allergens, cigarette smoking) and implement measures that may help diminish the risk of respiratory infection. These measures may include avoiding those who are ill with colds or flu, avoiding crowded areas, remaining well nourished and rested, and maintaining fluid intake of up to 3000 mL/day to ensure adequate hydration (unless contraindicated). Keeping a journal of symptoms and noting any improvement or worsening in the treated condition while taking the medications may also be very helpful.

Salmeterol is not to be used for relief of acute symptoms, and education about its dosing is important. The dosage of salmeterol is usually 1 puff twice daily, 12 hours apart. Always recheck these orders and directions. If another type of inhalant is used, such as a corticosteroid, instruct the patient to use the bronchodilator first, with a 5-minute waiting period prior to taking the second drug. All equipment must be rinsed after use. Provide patients with instructions about the importance of rinsing their mouth thoroughly after the use of any inhalant form of medication. Oral rinsing and mouth care after use of the inhaled drug is needed to prevent irritation and infection. See Chapter 37 for further discussion of salmeterol.

If ophthalmic forms of these drugs are used, make sure that the medication has not expired and is a clear solution. Do not allow the eyedropper to touch the eye when the drug is applied to help prevent contamination of the remaining solution. With ophthalmic administration, apply drops and ointments into the conjunctival sac—not directly onto the eye (cornea) itself.

Oral midodrine is to be taken exactly as prescribed. This medication is usually ordered to be given with forcing of fluids before the patient gets out of bed in the morning. Doses of the drug are often front-loaded in their dosing schedule so that most of the doses occur in the morning when patients with orthostatic intolerance are usually more symptomatic. Patients need to avoid taking this medication after 6 PM *if at all possible* to prevent insomnia and possible supine hypertension.

## TEAMWORK AND COLLABORATION: LEGAL AND ETHICAL PRINCIPLES

### *Infiltrating Intravenous Infusions*

Nurses often encounter infiltrating intravenous (IV) infusions in the routine care of many of their patients. Every action taken is very important in meeting the standard of care for the patient and in ensuring that the nurse has acted as any prudent nurse would. The assessment and action of the nurse can be important for the patient, as in the case of *Macon-Bibb County Hospital Authority v. Ross* (335 SE2d 633-GA).

#### Situation and Outcome

At approximately 2:52 PM, Ms. Ross arrived at the emergency department with dyspnea, bradycardia, and a blood pressure (BP) of 250/150 mm Hg. She became unresponsive, and at 2:55 PM went into respiratory arrest. She was intubated by a respiratory therapist. At approximately 2:58 PM, she received intravenous (IV) Nipride in an IV site in her right wrist. Nipride was used to decrease the severely elevated blood pressure. By 3:13 PM, the patient's blood pressure was 120/90 and the Nipride was discontinued as prescribed by the physician. Actual events are documented as follows: At 3:28 PM, the patient had no blood pressure at all and the physician had prescribed IV administration of dopamine to elevate her blood pressure; dopamine was actually administered at 3:31 PM to increase the then nonexistent blood pressure. She was then transferred to the cardiac care unit at approximately 4:30 PM after her blood pressure had stabilized. At midnight, a nurse noted that the IV catheter site had a "bruise bluish in color." The next notation was at 11:00 AM that morning. The patient's right arm was noted to be swollen, sore, and with a large blistered area located around the IV catheter site. The same description was noted again at 4:00 PM. There was no evidence that a physician was consulted or informed until 6:50 PM. At this time, the blistered area was shown to a physician but it wasn't until later in the evening that another physician cleansed the blistered area and treated it as a burn. The patient's lower right arm was permanently scarred and, it was undisputed, that the injury was a result of the infiltration of the dopamine. A nurse expert testified that she believed that the hospital personnel had been negligent in inserting the IV in the smaller vein at the patient's wrist or at least in the failure to document why it was not placed in the recommended vein initially or subsequently. However, most significant was the fact that there was a failure to notify the physician of the swollen and blistered arm. On a jury verdict, the court entered judgment for the patient. The hospital appealed.

The court of appeals affirmed the judgment of the lower court. It was noted that, although an infiltration may result from an improper technique, it may also be due to the size of the needle, the status of the patient's veins, or specific intolerance to an IV catheter. However, according to the expert nurse's testimony, supported by suitable references, dopamine must be infused into a large vein such as a vein in the antecubital fossa, to minimize the risk for extravasation. In addition, a dopamine infusion needs to be monitored continuously and the infusion very closely regulated. The antidote to counter the effects of dopamine extravasation is phentolamine (Regitine), and damage may be decreased or reversed if given within a specified time period. The nurses were criticized for not being sufficiently knowledgeable regarding dopamine, which resulted in their failure to notify a physician of the patient's impaired tissue integrity.

Data from *Macon-Bibb County Hospital Authority v Ross,* 70785 (176 Ga. App. 221) (335 SE2d 633), 1985, available at www.lawskills.com/case/ga/id/427/29/index.html. Accessed November 2, 2011.

## EVALUATION

Therapeutic effects of *adrenergic drugs* include the following: For vasoactive drugs, therapeutic effects include improved cardiac output (with increased urinary output), return to normal vital signs (e.g., blood pressure of 120/80 mm Hg or higher or gradual increases in blood pressure as indicated, pulse rate greater than 60 but less than 100 beats/min), improved skin color (pallor to pink) and temperature (cool to warm) in the extremities, improved peripheral pulses, and increased level of consciousness. Therapeutic effects of drugs given for bronchial indications include a return to normal respiratory rate (more than 12 but fewer than 20 breaths/min), improved breath sounds throughout the lung field with fewer adventitious (abnormal) sounds, increased air exchange in all areas of the lungs, decreased to no coughing, less dyspnea, improved partial pressure of oxygen and pulse oximeter readings, and tolerance of slowly increasing levels of activity. Therapeutic effects of midodrine include improved level of functioning and improved performance of the activities of daily living, fewer episodes of postural intolerance (dizziness, lightheadedness, and syncopal episodes), and more energy.

To evaluate for the occurrence of adverse effects with *adrenergic drugs,* monitor for stimulation of the systems that are affected, such as the cardiac system and the CNS. Adverse effects such as cardiac irregularities, hypertension, and tachycardia may occur. Be sure to monitor for chest pain.

## PATIENT TEACHING TIPS

- Medications must always be taken as prescribed. Excessive dosing may cause CNS and cardiovascular stimulation with tremors, nervousness, tachycardia, and palpitations.
- Instructions must be clear and concise for use of inhaled forms of medication, including nebulizers, inhalers, and metered-dose inhalers (see Chapter 9).
- Instruct the patient to report to the prescriber immediately any worsening of respiratory symptoms, dyspnea, distress, chest pain, and/or cardiac palpitations.
- Over-the-counter medications and herbal supplements are to be avoided unless the prescriber's approval is obtained.
- Midodrine requires careful dosing, as ordered. Encourage the patient to keep a journal to record adverse effects, improvements in symptoms, and any worsening of symptoms.

## KEY POINTS

- Catecholamines are substances that produce a sympathomimetic response (stimulate the SNS). The naturally occurring or endogenous catecholamines include epinephrine, norepinephrine, and dopamine. An example of an exogenous catecholamine is dobutamine.
- If the patient has a chronic respiratory disease, such as emphysema or chronic asthma or bronchitis, it is important for the patient to avoid contact with individuals who may have infections to help minimize situations that would exacerbate the original problem. Respiratory irritants must be avoided.
- Midodrine use requires careful blood pressure monitoring, so patient education about supine blood pressure measurement and journaling of measured blood pressure values is very important to the effective use of the drug.
- Inhaled forms of beta$_2$ agonists are used for their bronchodilating action and must be taken only as prescribed, with caution to avoid any overuse of the drug. Overdosage of these drugs may lead to severe cardiovascular, CNS, and cerebrovascular adverse effects and stimulation.

## NCLEX® EXAMINATION REVIEW QUESTIONS

1 The nurse caring for a patient who is receiving beta$_1$ agonist drug therapy needs to be aware that these drugs cause which effect?
   a Increased cardiac contractility
   b Decreased heart rate
   c Bronchoconstriction
   d Increased GI tract motility
2 During a teaching session for a patient who is receiving inhaled salmeterol, the nurse emphasizes that the drug is indicated for which condition?
   a Rescue treatment of acute bronchospasms
   b Prevention of bronchospasms
   c Reduction of airway inflammation
   d Long-term treatment of sinus congestion
3 For a patient receiving a vasoactive drug such as intravenous dopamine, which action by the nurse is most appropriate?
   a Monitor the gravity drip infusion closely, and adjust as needed.
   b Assess the patient's cardiac function by checking the radial pulse.
   c Assess the intravenous site hourly for possible infiltration.
   d Administer the drug by intravenous boluses according to the patient's blood pressure.

4  A patient is receiving dobutamine for shock and is complaining of feeling more "skipping beats" than yesterday. What will the nurse do next?
   a  Monitor for other signs of a therapeutic response to the drug.
   b  Titrate the drug to a higher dose to reduce the palpitations.
   c  Discontinue the dobutamine immediately.
   d  Assess the patient's vital signs and cardiac rhythm.

5  When a drug is characterized as having a negative chronotropic effect, the nurse knows to expect which effect?
   a  Reduced blood pressure
   b  Decreased heart rate
   c  Decreased ectopic beats
   d  Increased force of cardiac contractions

6  The nurse is monitoring a patient who is receiving an infusion of a beta-adrenergic agonist. Which adverse effects may occur with this infusion? (Select all that apply.)
   a  Mild tremors
   b  Bradycardia
   c  Tachycardia
   d  Palpitations
   e  Drowsiness
   f  Nervousness

7  The order reads: "Dopamine 3 mcg/kg/min IV." The solution available is 400 mg in 250 mL D$_5$W, and the patient weighs 176 pounds. The nurse will set the IV infusion pump to run at how many mL/hour?

1. a, 2. b, 3. c, 4. d, 5. b, 6. a, c, d, f, 7. 9 mL/hr

For Critical Thinking and Prioritization Questions, see http://evolve.elsevier.com/Lilley.

# CHAPTER

# 19

# Adrenergic-Blocking Drugs

## ⊖volve WEBSITE

*http://evolve.elsevier.com/Lilley*
- Animations
- Answer Key—Textbook Case Studies
- Critical Thinking and Prioritization Questions
- Key Points—Downloadable
- Review Questions for the NCLEX® Examination
- Unfolding Case Studies

## OBJECTIVES

When you reach the end of this chapter, you will be able to do the following:

1   Briefly review the functions of the sympathetic nervous system and the specific effects of adrenergic-blocking drugs.
2   List the various drugs classified as adrenergic antagonists (blockers) or sympatholytics.
3   Discuss the mechanisms of action, therapeutic effects, indications, adverse and toxic effects, cautions, contraindications, drug interactions, dosages, routes of administration, and any antidotal management for the various alpha antagonists (blockers), beta nonselective blockers, and the beta$_1$- and beta$_2$-blockers.
4   Develop a nursing care plan that includes all phases of the nursing process for patients taking adrenergic antagonists.

## DRUG PROFILES

- ♦ **atenolol, p. 318**
  **carvedilol, p. 318**
- ♦ **esmolol, p. 319**
  **labetalol, p. 319**
- ♦ **metoprolol, p. 319**
- ♦ **phentolamine, p. 316**

- ♦ **propranolol, p. 319**
  **sotalol, p. 319**
  **tamsulosin, p. 316**

  _____

- ♦ *Key drug*

## KEY TERMS

**Acrocyanosis** Decreased amount of oxygen delivered to the extremities, causing the feet or hands to turn blue. (p. 313)

**Adrenergic receptors** Specific receptor sites located throughout the body for the endogenous sympathetic neurotransmitters norepinephrine and epinephrine. (p. 313)

**Agonists** Drugs with a specific receptor affinity that mimic the body's natural chemicals (e.g., hormones, neurotransmitters). (p. 313)

**Angina** Paroxysmal (sudden) chest pain caused by myocardial ischemia. (p. 317)

**Antagonists** Drugs that bind to specific receptors and inhibit or block the response of the receptors. (p. 313)

**Dysrhythmias** Irregular heart rhythms; almost always called *arrhythmias* in clinical practice. (p. 317)

**Extravasation** The leaking of fluid from a blood vessel into the surrounding tissues, as in the case of an infiltrated intravenous infusion. (p. 314)

**First-dose phenomenon** Severe and sudden drop in blood pressure after the administration of the first dose of an alpha-adrenergic blocker. (p. 314)

**Intrinsic sympathomimetic activity** The paradoxical action of some beta-blocking drugs (e.g., acebutolol) that mimics the action of the sympathetic nervous system. (p. 316)

**Lipophilicity** The chemical attraction of a substance (e.g., drug molecule) to lipid or fat molecules. (p. 317)

**Orthostatic hypotension** A sudden drop in blood pressure when a person stands up. Also referred to as *postural hypotension* or *orthostasis*. (p. 314)

**Pheochromocytoma** A vascular adrenal gland tumor that is usually benign but secretes epinephrine and norepinephrine and thus often causes central nervous system stimulation and substantial blood pressure elevation. (p. 313)

**Raynaud's disease** A narrowing of small arteries that limits the amount of blood circulation to the extremities, causing numbness of the nose, fingers, toes, and ears in response to cold temperatures or stress. (p. 313)

**Sympatholytics** Drugs that inhibit the postganglionic functioning of the sympathetic nervous system. (p. 313)

## ANATOMY, PHYSIOLOGY, AND PATHOPHYSIOLOGY OVERVIEW

The autonomic nervous system consists of the parasympathetic and sympathetic nervous systems. The class of drugs discussed in this chapter works primarily on the sympathetic nervous system (SNS). As discussed in Chapter 18, the adrenergic agonist drugs stimulate the SNS. Those drugs are called agonists because they bind to receptors and cause a response. Adrenergic blockers have the opposite effect and are therefore referred to as antagonists. They bind to adrenergic receptors, but in doing so inhibit or block stimulation by the SNS. They are also referred to as sympatholytics because they "lyse," or inhibit, SNS stimulation.

Throughout the body, there are receptor sites for the endogenous sympathetic neurotransmitters norepinephrine and epinephrine. Such receptors are known as adrenergic receptors, and two basic types are found: alpha and beta. There are subtypes of the alpha- and beta-adrenergic receptors, designated 1 and 2. The $alpha_1$- and $alpha_2$-adrenergic receptors are differentiated by their location on nerves. The $alpha_1$-adrenergic receptors are located on the tissue, muscle, or organ that the nerve is stimulating (postsynaptic effector cells). The $alpha_2$-adrenergic receptors are located on the actual nerves that stimulate the presynaptic effector cells. The $alpha_2$ receptors are inhibitory in nature. Thus, it is actually the stimulation of $alpha_2$ receptors that causes the inhibitory effects of the SNS. $Alpha_2$–active drugs (e.g., clonidine) are discussed in Chapter 22. The $beta_1$-adrenergic receptors are located primarily in the heart. The $beta_2$-adrenergic receptors are located primarily on the smooth muscles of the bronchioles and blood vessels. It is at these various receptors that adrenergic blockers act. They are classified by the type of adrenergic receptor they block—alpha or beta or, in a few cases, both. Hence, they are called *alpha blockers, beta blockers,* or *alpha/beta blockers.*

## PHARMACOLOGY OVERVIEW

### ALPHA BLOCKERS

#### Mechanism of Action and Drug Effects

The alpha-adrenergic–blocking drugs, or alpha blockers, interrupt stimulation of the SNS at the $alpha_1$-adrenergic receptors. More specifically, alpha blockers work either by direct competition with norepinephrine or by a noncompetitive process.

Figure 19-1 illustrates these two mechanisms. Alpha blockers have a greater affinity for the alpha-adrenergic receptor than norepinephrine does and therefore can chemically displace norepinephrine molecules from the receptor. Adrenergic blockade at these receptors leads to effects such as vasodilation, reduced blood pressure, miosis (pupillary constriction), and reduced smooth muscle tone in organs such as the bladder and prostate. Currently available alpha blockers are listed in Table 19-1.

### Indications

The alpha blockers such as doxazosin, prazosin, and terazosin cause both arterial and venous dilation, which reduces peripheral vascular resistance and blood pressure. These drugs are used to treat hypertension (see Chapter 22). There are also alpha-adrenergic receptors in the prostate and bladder. By blocking stimulation of $alpha_1$ receptors, these drugs reduce smooth muscle contraction of the bladder neck and the prostatic portion of the urethra. For this reason, alpha blockers are given to patients with benign prostatic hyperplasia (BPH) to decrease resistance to urinary outflow. This reduces urinary obstruction and relieves some of the effects of BPH. Tamsulosin and alfuzosin are used exclusively for treating BPH, whereas terazosin and doxazosin can be used for both hypertension and BPH.

Other alpha blockers can inhibit responses to adrenergic stimulation. These drugs noncompetitively block alpha-adrenergic receptors on smooth muscle and various exocrine glands. Because of this action, they are very useful in controlling or preventing hypertension in patients who have a pheochromocytoma, a tumor that forms on the adrenal gland on top of the kidney and secretes norepinephrine, thus causing SNS stimulation. The alpha blockers are also useful in the treatment of patients who have increased endogenous alpha-adrenergic agonist activity, which results in vasoconstriction. Three conditions in which this occurs are Raynaud's disease, acrocyanosis, and frostbite. Phenoxybenzamine, in particular, is an alpha blocker that is beneficial in the treatment of these syndromes, although its use is uncommon.

Still other alpha blockers (e.g., phentolamine) are effective at counteracting the effects of injected epinephrine and norepinephrine. They do this by causing peripheral vasodilation and reducing peripheral resistance by blocking catecholamine-stimulated vasoconstriction. Because of their potent vasodilating properties and their fast onset of action, they are used to prevent skin necrosis and sloughing after the

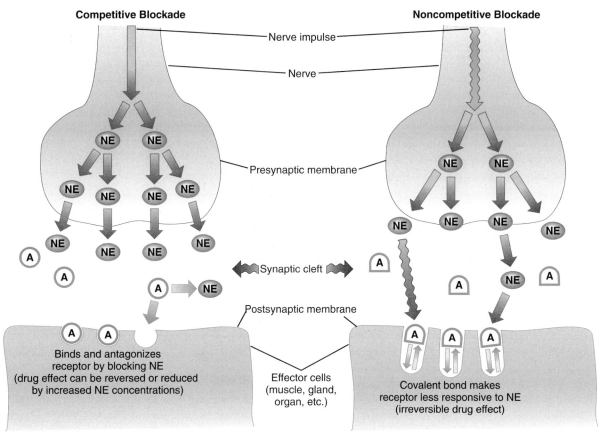

**FIGURE 19-1** Mechanisms for alpha-adrenergic competitive and noncompetitive blockade by alpha blocker drugs. *A,* Alpha blocker; *NE,* norepinephrine.

extravasation of vasopressors such as norepinephrine or epinephrine. When these drugs extravasate (leak out of the blood vessel into the surrounding tissue), they cause vasoconstriction and ultimately tissue death, or necrosis. If the vasoconstriction is not reversed quickly, the entire limb can be lost. Phentolamine, in particular, can reverse this potent vasoconstriction and restore blood flow to the ischemic tissue.

## Contraindications

Contraindications to the use of alpha-blocking drugs include known drug allergy and peripheral vascular disease and may include hepatic and renal disease, coronary artery disease, peptic ulcer, and sepsis.

## Adverse Effects

The primary adverse effects of alpha blockers are those related to their effects on the vasculature. First-dose phenomenon, which is a severe and sudden drop in blood pressure after the administration of the first dose of an alpha-adrenergic blocker, can cause patients to fall or pass out. All patients must be warned about this adverse effect before they take their first dose of an alpha blocker. Orthostatic hypotension can occur with any dose of an alpha blocker, and patients must be warned to get up slowly from a supine position. The primary adverse effects of the alpha blockers are listed by body system in Table 19-2.

## Toxicity and Management of Overdose

In an acute oral overdose, activated charcoal is administered to bind the drug and remove it from the stomach and the circulation. With overdoses of both oral and injectable forms, symptomatic and supportive measures are to be instituted as needed. Blood pressure support with the administration of fluids, volume expanders, and vasopressor drugs and the administration of anticonvulsants such as diazepam for the control of seizures are examples of such measures.

## Interactions

The most severe drug interactions with alpha blockers are the ones that potentiate the effects of the alpha blockers. The alpha blockers are very highly protein bound and compete for binding sites with other drugs that are highly protein bound (see Chapter 2). Because of the limited sites for binding on proteins and the increased competition for these sites, more free alpha blocker molecules circulate in the bloodstream. More active drug results in a more pronounced drug effect. Some of the common drugs that interact with alpha blockers and the results of these interactions are listed in Table 19-3.

## Dosages

For dosage information on alpha blockers, see the table on p. 315.

| TABLE 19-1 | CURRENTLY AVAILABLE ADRENERGIC-BLOCKING DRUGS | |
| --- | --- | --- |
| **GENERIC NAME** | **TRADE NAME** | **ROUTE** |
| **Alpha₁ Blockers** | | |
| alfuzosin | Uroxatral | PO |
| doxazosin | Cardura | PO |
| phenoxybenzamine | Dibenzyline | PO |
| phentolamine | Generic | IV, IM, IM/subcut/ intradermal (for ex- travasation wounds) |
| prazosin | Minipress | PO |
| terazosin | Hytrin | PO |
| tamsulosin | Flomax | PO |
| **Beta Blockers** | | |
| *Nonselective* | | |
| carvedilol* | Coreg, Coreg CR | PO |
| labetalol* | Normodyne, Trandate | PO, IV |
| nadolol | Corgard | PO |
| penbutolol | Levatol | PO |
| pindolol | Visken | PO |
| propranolol* | Inderal | PO, IV |
| sotalol | Betapace | PO |
| timolol | Blocadren, Timoptic | PO, IV, ophthalmic |
| *Cardioselective* | | |
| acebutolol | Sectral | PO |
| atenolol | Tenormin | PO |
| betaxolol | Kerlone | PO |
| bisoprolol | Zebeta | PO |
| esmolol | Brevibloc | IV |
| nebivolol | Bystolic | PO |
| metoprolol | Lopressor, Toprol-XL | PO, IV |

*IM,* Intramuscular; *IV,* intravenous; *PO,* oral; *subcut,* subcutaneous.
*Has antagonist activity at alpha₁, beta₁, and beta₂ receptors.

| TABLE 19-2 | ALPHA BLOCKERS: ADVERSE EFFECTS |
| --- | --- |
| **BODY SYSTEM** | **ADVERSE EFFECTS** |
| Cardiovascular | Palpitations, orthostatic hypotension, tachycardia, edema, chest pain |
| Central nervous | Dizziness, headache, anxiety, depression, weakness, numbness, fatigue |
| Gastrointestinal | Nausea, vomiting, diarrhea, constipation, abdominal pain |
| Other | Incontinence, dry mouth, pharyngitis |

| TABLE 19-3 | ALPHA BLOCKERS: COMMON DRUG INTERACTIONS | | |
| --- | --- | --- | --- |
| **DRUG** | **INTERACTING DRUG** | **MECHANISM** | **RESULT** |
| phentolamine | Beta blockers, alcohol Erectile dysfunction drugs | Additive effects | Profound hypotension |
| | Epinephrine | Antagonism | Reduced phentolamine effects |
| tamsulosin | Warfarin | Competition for plasma protein-binding sites | Risk of bleeding |
| | Antihypertensives Erectile dysfunction drugs, alcohol | Additive effects | Risk of hypotension |

## DOSAGES

### Selected Alpha-Adrenergic–Blocking Drugs

| DRUG (PREGNANCY CATEGORY) | PHARMACOLOGIC CLASS | USUAL DOSAGE RANGE | INDICATIONS |
| --- | --- | --- | --- |
| ◆ phentolamine (Regitine) (C) | Alpha blocker | **Adult** IM/IV: 5 mg; repeat if necessary | Hypertensive episodes with pheochromocytoma |
| | | **Adult** 5-10 mg diluted in 10 mL NS injected into extravasation site | Alpha-adrenergic drug extravasation |
| | | **Pediatric** 0.1-0.2 mg/kg into extravasation site | |
| tamsulosin (Flomax) (B)* | Alpha₁ blocker | **Adult** PO: 0.4 mg once daily; max dose 0.8 mg | Benign prostatic hyperplasia |

*IM,* Intramuscular; *IV,* intravenous; *NS,* normal saline; *PO,* oral.
*Not indicated for use in women; however, it is sometimes used for kidney stones.

## DRUG PROFILES

The alpha blockers are commonly used to treat hypertension and/or benign prostatic hyperplasia. They include phentolamine, phenoxybenzamine, terazosin, alfuzosin, tamsulosin, silodosin, and prazosin. Prazosin is discussed in Chapter 22.

### ♦ phentolamine

Phentolamine (Regitine) is an alpha blocker that reduces peripheral vascular resistance and is also used to treat hypertension. Like phenoxybenzamine, it is used to treat the high blood pressure caused by pheochromocytoma, but phentolamine can also be used in the diagnosis of this catecholamine-secreting tumor. To help establish a diagnosis of pheochromocytoma, a single intravenous dose of phentolamine is given to the hypertensive patient. If the blood pressure declines rapidly, it is highly likely that the patient has a pheochromocytoma. Phentolamine is available only as an injectable preparation. It is most commonly used to treat the extravasation of vasoconstricting drugs such as norepinephrine, epinephrine, and dopamine, which when given intravenously can leak out of the vein, especially if the intravenous tube is not correctly positioned. If such a drug is allowed to extravasate into the surrounding tissue, the result is intense vasoconstriction, decreased blood flow, necrosis, and potential loss of the limb. When phentolamine is injected subcutaneously in a circular fashion around the extravasation site, it causes alpha-adrenergic receptor blockade and vasodilation, which in turn increases blood flow to the ischemic tissue and thus prevents permanent damage. Its use is contraindicated in patients who have shown a hypersensitivity to it, those who have experienced a myocardial infarction (MI), and those with coronary artery disease. Adverse effects include tachycardia, dizziness, gastrointestinal upset, and others listed in Table 19-2. Drugs with which phentolamine interacts include alcohol (a disulfiram-like reaction; see Chapter 17) and erectile dysfunction medications such as sildenafil (additive hypotensive effects; see Chapter 35). Epinephrine and ephedrine can counteract the desired effects of phentolamine. The recommended dosages are given in the table on p. 315.

### Pharmacokinetics

| Route | Onset of Action | Peak Plasma Concentration | Elimination Half-life | Duration of Action |
|-------|-----------------|----------------------------|------------------------|---------------------|
| IV | 1 hr | 4-6 hr | 24 hr | 3-4 days |

### tamsulosin

Tamsulosin (Flomax) is an alpha blocker used primarily to treat BPH and is exclusively indicated for male patients. Similar drugs with the same indication are alfuzosin and silodosin. These drugs block alpha-adrenergic receptors on smooth muscle within the prostate and bladder. This results in relaxation of these smooth muscle fibers and improved urinary flow. Other similar drugs include terazosin and doxazosin, which can be used to treat both BPH and hypertension. Contraindications to tamsulosin include known drug allergy and concurrent use of erectile dysfunction drugs such as sildenafil. Adverse effects include headache, abnormal ejaculation, rhinitis, and others listed in Table 19-2. Interacting drugs include other alpha blockers, calcium channel blockers, and erectile dysfunction drugs (additive hypotensive effects); drugs that induce or inhibit hepatic enzymes may reduce or enhance the effects of tamsulosin. It is available only for oral use.

### Pharmacokinetics

| Route | Onset of Action | Peak Plasma Concentration | Elimination Half-life | Duration of Action |
|-------|-----------------|----------------------------|------------------------|---------------------|
| PO | Unknown | 4-7 hr | 15 hr | Unknown |

## BETA BLOCKERS

### Mechanism of Action and Drug Effects

The beta-adrenergic–blocking drugs (beta blockers) block SNS stimulation of the beta-adrenergic receptors by competing with norepinephrine and epinephrine. The beta blockers can be either selective or nonselective, depending on the type of beta-adrenergic receptors they antagonize. Beta$_1$-adrenergic receptors are located primarily in the heart. Beta blockers that are selective for these receptors are called *cardioselective beta blockers* or *beta$_1$-blocking drugs*. Other beta blockers block both beta$_1$- and beta$_2$-adrenergic receptors and are referred to as *nonselective beta blockers*. Beta$_2$ receptors are located primarily on the smooth muscles of the bronchioles and blood vessels. In addition, beta blockers can be further categorized according to whether or not they have intrinsic sympathomimetic activity. Drugs with intrinsic sympathomimetic activity (acebutolol, penbutolol, pindolol) not only block beta-adrenergic receptors but also partially stimulate them. This was initially believed to be an advantageous characteristic, but clinical experience has not borne this out. Two beta blockers, carvedilol and labetalol, also have an alpha-receptor–blocking activity, especially at higher dosages. Table 19-1 lists the currently available beta blockers.

Cardioselective beta$_1$-blockers block the beta$_1$ receptors on the surface of the heart. This reduces myocardial stimulation, which in turn reduces heart rate, slows conduction through the atrioventricular (AV) node, prolongs sinoatrial (SA) node recovery, and decreases myocardial oxygen demand by decreasing myocardial contractile force (contractility). Nonselective beta blockers not only have these cardiac effects, but they block beta$_2$ receptors on the smooth muscle of the bronchioles and blood vessels as well.

Smooth muscle that surrounds the airways in the lungs is called the *bronchioles*. When the beta$_2$ receptors in the bronchioles are blocked, the end result is bronchial smooth muscle contraction and narrowing of the airways. This may lead to shortness of breath. In addition, the smooth muscle that surrounds blood vessels can cause dilation or constriction, depending on whether the beta$_1$ or beta$_2$ receptors are stimulated. When this beta$_2$ stimulation is blocked, the muscles are then stimulated by unopposed sympathetic activity at the beta$_1$ receptors, which causes them to contract. This causes increased peripheral vascular resistance. Furthermore, catecholamines promote *glycogenolysis* (the production of glucose from glycogen) and mobilize glucose in response to hypoglycemia. Nonselective beta blockers impair this process and also impede the secretion of insulin from the pancreas, which causes elevation of blood glucose level.

Finally, beta blockers can cause the release of free fatty acids from adipose tissue. This may result in moderately elevated blood levels of triglycerides and reduced levels of the "good cholesterol" known as *high-density lipoprotein (HDL).*

## Indications

Indications for beta blockers include angina, MI, cardiac dysrhythmias, hypertension, and heart failure.

Beta blockers are commonly used in the treatment of angina, or chest pain (see Chapter 23). These drugs work by decreasing the demand for myocardial energy and oxygen consumption, which helps shift the supply/demand ratio to the supply side and allows more oxygen to get to the heart muscle. This in turn helps to relieve the pain in the heart muscle caused by the lack of oxygen.

Beta blockers are also considered to be *cardioprotective* because they inhibit stimulation of the myocardium by circulating catecholamines. Myocardial infarction causes catecholamines to be released. Unopposed stimulation by catecholamines would further increase the heart rate and the contractile force and thereby increase myocardial oxygen demand. When a beta blocker occupies myocardial $beta_1$ receptors, circulating catecholamine molecules are prevented from binding to the receptors. Thus, the beta blockers protect the heart from being stimulated by these catecholamines. Because of this characteristic, beta blockers are commonly given to patients after they have experienced an MI to protect the heart.

Beta blockers also have a profound effect on the conduction system of the heart. The AV node normally receives impulse stimulation from the SA node and slows it down so that the ventricles have time to fill before they are stimulated to contract. Conduction in the SA node is slowed by beta blockers, which results in a decreased heart rate. These drugs also slow conduction through the AV node. These effects of the beta blockers on the conduction system of the heart make them useful in the treatment of various types of irregular heart rhythms called dysrhythmias (see Chapter 25).

Beta blockers are useful in treating hypertension because of their ability to reduce SNS stimulation of the heart, including reducing heart rate and the force of myocardial contraction (systole). Traditionally beta blockers were thought to worsen heart failure. However, recent studies have shown benefit to the use of beta blockers. Certain beta blockers such as carvedilol and metoprolol have produced the best results to date. The form of heart failure that includes a component of diastolic dysfunction responds especially favorably to beta blockers.

Because of their lipophilicity (attraction to lipid or fat), some beta blockers (e.g., propranolol) can easily gain entry into the central nervous system and are used to treat migraine headaches. In addition, the topical application of timolol to the eye has been very effective in treating ocular disorders such as glaucoma (see Chapter 57).

| TABLE 19-4 | BETA BLOCKERS: COMMON ADVERSE EFFECTS |
| --- | --- |
| **BODY SYSTEM** | **ADVERSE EFFECTS** |
| Cardiovascular | Atrioventricular block, bradycardia, heart failure |
| Central nervous | Dizziness, fatigue, depression, drowsiness, unusual dreams |
| Gastrointestinal | Nausea, vomiting, constipation, diarrhea |
| Hematologic | Agranulocytosis, thrombocytopenia |
| Metabolic | Hyperglycemia and/or hypoglycemia, hyperlipidemia |
| Other | Impotence, alopecia, bronchospasm, wheezing, dry mouth |

## Contraindications

Contraindications to the use of beta blockers include known drug allergies and may include uncompensated heart failure, cardiogenic shock, heart block or bradycardia, pregnancy, severe pulmonary disease, and Raynaud's disease.

## Adverse Effects

The adverse effects of beta blockers are primarily extensions of their pharmacologic activity. Most such effects are mild and diminish with time. Some of the most serious undesirable effects can be caused by acute withdrawal of the drug. For example, such sudden withdrawal may exacerbate underlying angina, precipitate an MI, or cause rebound hypertension. Beta blockers also delay the recovery from hypoglycemia in patients with type 1 diabetes (rarely in those with type 2). In addition, the nonselective beta blockers can interfere with the normal responses to hypoglycemia, such as tremor, tachycardia, and nervousness, in essence masking the signs and symptoms of hypoglycemia. Adverse effects induced by beta blockers are listed by body system in Table 19-4.

### Toxicity and Management of Overdose

For overdoses of both oral and injectable dosage forms, treatment consists primarily of symptomatic and supportive care. Atropine may be given intravenously for the management of bradycardia. If the bradycardia still persists, placement of a transvenous cardiac pacemaker may be considered. For the treatment of severe hypotension, vasopressors are titrated until the desired blood pressure and heart rate are achieved. Intravenously administered diazepam may be useful for the treatment of seizures. Most beta blockers are dialyzable; therefore, hemodialysis may be useful in enhancing elimination in the event of severe overdose.

## Interactions

Most of the drug interactions with beta blockers result from either the additive effects of coadministered medications with similar mechanisms of action or the antagonistic effects of various drugs. Nonselective beta blockers may mask the tachycardia from hypoglycemia caused by insulin and sulfonylureas, and the hypoglycemic effect of insulin and sulfonylureas may be enhanced (see Chapter 32). Some of the common drugs that

## DOSAGES

### Selected Beta-Adrenergic–Blocking Drugs

| DRUG (PREGNANCY CATEGORY) | PHARMACOLOGIC CLASS | USUAL DOSAGE RANGE | INDICATIONS |
|---|---|---|---|
| ◆ atenolol (Tenormin) (C) | Beta₁ blocker | **Adult**<br>PO: 50-200 mg/day daily or divided bid, (max 200 mg/day) | Hypertension, angina |
| carvedilol (Coreg) (C) | Alpha and beta blocker | **Adult**<br>PO: 3.125 mg bid; may double dose every 2 wk to highest tolerated dose, max 50 mg/day (100 mg/day for patients with heart failure who weigh over 85 kg) | Heart failure, angina, hypertension |
| ◆ esmolol (Brevibloc) (C) | Beta₁ blocker | **Adult**<br>IV: Bolus of 500 mcg/kg over 1 min, followed by 50 mcg/kg/min for 4 minutes and evaluate | Supraventricular tachydysrhythmias |
| labetalol (Normodyne, Trandate) (C) | Alpha₁ and beta blocker | **Adult**<br>PO: 200-800 mg/day divided bid<br>IV: 20 mg with additional doses of 40-80 mg at 10-min intervals until desired effect or a total dose of 300 mg is injected; maintenance infusion of 2 mg/min initially and titrated to response | Hypertension<br>Severe hypertension |
| ◆ metoprolol (Lopressor, Toprol XL) (C) | Beta₁ blocker | **Adult**<br>PO: 100-400 mg/day divided bid-tid<br>IV/PO: 3 bolus injections of 5 mg at 2-min intervals followed in 15 min by 50 mg PO q6h for 48 hr; thereafter 100 mg PO bid | Hypertension, late MI<br>Early MI |
| ◆ propranolol (Inderal) (C) | Beta blocker | **Adult**<br>PO: 80-320 mg/day divided bid-qid<br>120-640 mg/day divided bid-tid<br>10-30 mg tid-qid<br>180-240 mg divided tid-qid<br>160-240 mg/day divided | Angina<br>Hypertension<br>Dysrhythmias<br>Post-MI<br>Migraine |
| sotalol (Betapace) (B) | Beta blocker | **Adult**<br>PO: 160-320 mg/day divided | Life-threatening ventricular dysrhythmias |

*IV,* Intravenous; *MI,* myocardial infarction; *PO,* oral.

| TABLE 19-5 | BETA BLOCKERS: DRUG INTERACTIONS | |
|---|---|---|
| **INTERACTING DRUG** | **MECHANISM** | **RESULT** |
| Antacids (aluminum hydroxide type) | Decrease absorption | Decreased beta blocker activity |
| Antimuscarinics, anticholinergics | Antagonism | Reduced beta blocker effects |
| digoxin | Additive effect | Enhanced bradycardic effects of digoxin |
| Diuretics, cardiovascular drugs, alcohol | Additive effect | Additive hypotensive effects |
| Neuromuscular blocking drugs | Additive effect | Prolonged neuromuscular blockade |
| Oral hypoglycemic drugs, insulin | Mask signs of hypoglycemia | Delayed recovery from hypoglycemia |

interact with beta blockers and the resulting effects are given in Table 19-5.

## Dosages

For dosage information on selected beta blockers, see the table on this page.

## DRUG PROFILES

Numerous beta blockers currently available are listed in Table 19-1. Several beta blockers are profiled in the following sections. Contraindications, adverse reactions, and drug interactions are comparable for these drugs and are listed in the previous text, Table 19-4, and Table 19-5, respectively.

### ◆ atenolol

Atenolol (Tenormin) is a cardioselective beta blocker that is commonly used to prevent future heart attacks in patients who have had one. It is also used in the treatment of hypertension and angina and in the management of thyrotoxicosis to help block the symptoms of excessive thyroid activity. Atenolol is available for oral use. Recommended dosages are given in the table on this page.

### Pharmacokinetics

| Route | Onset of Action | Peak Plasma Concentration | Elimination Half-life | Duration of Action |
|---|---|---|---|---|
| PO | 1 hr | 2-4 hr | 6-7 hr | 24 hr |

### carvedilol

Carvedilol (Coreg) has many effects, including acting as a nonselective beta blocker, an alpha₁-blocker, a calcium channel blocker, and possibly an antioxidant. It is used primarily in the treatment of heart failure but is also beneficial for hypertension and angina. It has been shown to slow the progression of heart failure and to decrease the frequency of hospitalization in patients with mild to moderate (class II or III) heart failure. Carvedilol is most commonly added to digoxin, furosemide, and angiotensin-converting enzyme inhibitors when used to treat heart failure. Carvedilol is available only for oral use. A controlled-release formulation, Coreg CR, was recently approved. The dosages are different from those for immediate-release Coreg, and the two cannot be interchanged. Recommended dosages are given in the table on p. 318.

### Pharmacokinetics

| Route | Onset of Action | Peak Plasma Concentration | Elimination Half-life | Duration of Action |
|-------|-----------------|---------------------------|----------------------|-------------------|
| PO | 20-120 min | 1-4 hr | 6-8 hr | 8-24 hr |

#### ♦ esmolol

Esmolol (Brevibloc) is a very strong short-acting $beta_1$-blocker. It is primarily used in acute situations to provide rapid temporary control of the ventricular rate in patients with supraventricular tachydysrhythmias. Because of its very short half-life, it is given only as an intravenous infusion and is titrated to achieve the serum levels that control the patient's symptoms. Recommended dosages are given in the table on p. 318.

### Pharmacokinetics

| Route | Onset of Action | Peak Plasma Concentration | Elimination Half-life | Duration of Action |
|-------|-----------------|---------------------------|----------------------|-------------------|
| IV | Immediate | 6 min | 9 min | 15-20 min |

#### labetalol

Labetalol (Normodyne) is unusual in that it can block both alpha- and beta-adrenergic receptors. It is used in the treatment of severe hypertension and hypertensive emergencies to quickly lower the blood pressure before permanent damage is done. Labetalol is available for oral and injectable use. Recommended dosages are given in the table on p. 318.

### Pharmacokinetics

| Route | Onset of Action | Peak Plasma Concentration | Elimination Half-life | Duration of Action |
|-------|-----------------|---------------------------|----------------------|-------------------|
| IV | 2-5 min | 5-15 min | 2.5-8 hr | 2-4 hr |
| PO | 20-120 min | 1-4 hr | 2.5-8 hr | 8-24 hr |

#### ♦ metoprolol

Metoprolol (Lopressor) is a $beta_1$-blocker that has become a favorite of cardiologists for use in patients after MI. Recent studies of metoprolol have shown increased survival in patients given the drug after they have experienced an MI. Metoprolol is available for oral and injectable use. Recommended dosages are given in the table on p. 318.

### Pharmacokinetics

| Route | Onset of Action | Peak Plasma Concentration | Elimination Half-life | Duration of Action |
|-------|-----------------|---------------------------|----------------------|-------------------|
| IV | 1 min | 20 min | 3-8 hr | 5-8 hr |
| PO | 1 hr | 2-4 hr | 3-8 hr | 10-20 hr |

#### ♦ propranolol

Propranolol (Inderal) is the prototypical nonselective $beta_1$- and $beta_2$-blocking drug. It was one of the very first beta blockers to be used. Lengthy experience with it has revealed many uses for it. In addition to the indications mentioned for metoprolol, propranolol has been used for the treatment of tachydysrhythmias associated with cardiac glycoside intoxication and for the treatment of hypertrophic subaortic stenosis, pheochromocytoma, thyrotoxicosis, migraine headache, essential tremor, and many other conditions. The same contraindications that apply to the cardioselective beta blockers discussed earlier hold for propranolol as well. In addition, its use is contraindicated in patients with bronchial asthma. Propranolol is available for oral and injectable use. Recommended dosages are given in the table on p. 318.

### Pharmacokinetics

| Route | Onset of Action | Peak Plasma Concentration | Elimination Half-life | Duration of Action |
|-------|-----------------|---------------------------|----------------------|-------------------|
| IV | 2 min | 1-4 hr | 3-5 hr | 3-6 hr |
| PO | 1-2 hr | 1-4 hr | 3-5 hr | 6-12 hr |

#### sotalol

Sotalol (Betapace) is a nonselective beta blocker that has very potent antidysrhythmic properties. It is commonly used for the management of difficult-to-treat dysrhythmias. Often these dysrhythmias are life-threatening ventricular dysrhythmias such as sustained ventricular tachycardia. It has properties characteristic of both a class II and class III antidysrhythmic drug (see Chapter 25). Because it is a nonselective beta blocker, it causes some of the unwanted adverse effects typical of these drugs (e.g., hypotension). Sotalol is available only for oral use. Recommended dosages are given in the table on p. 318.

### Pharmacokinetics

| Route | Onset of Action | Peak Plasma Concentration | Elimination Half-life | Duration of Action |
|-------|-----------------|---------------------------|----------------------|-------------------|
| PO | 1-2 hr | 2.5-4 hr | 12 hr | 8-16 hr |

## NURSING PROCESS

## ASSESSMENT

*Adrenergic-blocking drugs,* or sympatholytics, produce a variety of effects on the patient, depending on the type of receptor(s) blocked. Because of the impact of these drugs, primarily on the cardiac and respiratory systems, their use requires careful assessment to help minimize the adverse effects and maximize the therapeutic effects. Understanding the basic anatomy and

## ⚡ SAFETY AND QUALITY IMPROVEMENT: PREVENTING MEDICATION ERRORS

### *Look-Alike Drugs: Toprol-XL, Topamax, and Tegretol*

Be careful about look-alike drugs! Medication errors often occur when drug names are similar. The Food and Drug Administration has reported errors in prescribing and dispensing involving a mix-up between Topamax (topiramate), which is indicated for the treatment of epilepsy and prophylaxis of migraines, and Toprol-XL (metoprolol succinate), which is used for the treatment of hypertension and heart failure as well as the long-term treatment of angina pectoris. Other errors have occurred when Toprol-XL and Tegretol (carbamazepine), a drug used for various types of seizures and trigeminal neuralgia, have been confused. Consider what would happen if a patient with a history of seizures receives a beta blocker instead of the prescribed antiepileptic drug! These cases reinforce the importance of checking the drug name carefully (using both trade and generic names).

For more information, go to http://www.fda.gov/Safety/MedWatch/Safety Information/SafetyAlertsforHumanMedicalProducts/default.htm.

physiology of adrenergic receptors and their subsequent actions if stimulated or blocked is also critical in carrying out assessment and other aspects of the nursing process and drug therapy. If an adrenergic-blocking drug is nonselective, it blocks both alpha and beta (beta$_1$ and beta$_2$) receptors. Alpha receptor blocking affects blood vessels, whereas beta$_1$ receptor blocking affects heart rate and beta$_2$ blocking affects bronchial smooth muscle. Therefore, a nonselective adrenergic blocker will have the following actions: (1) alpha blocking leading to blockade of the sympathetic stimulation of blood vessels (i.e., vasoconstriction) and resulting in vasodilation and a subsequent decrease in blood pressure; (2) beta$_1$ blocking leading to blockade of the sympathetic effects on heart rate, contractility, and conduction with resulting bradycardia, negative inotropic effects (i.e., decrease in contractility), and a decrease in conduction; and (3) beta$_2$ blocking leading to blockade of the sympathetic effects on bronchial smooth muscle with the net effect of bronchoconstriction. However, if the drug is only an alpha-, beta$_1$-, or beta$_2$-blocker, the resulting effect will be related to the specific receptor being blocked (or combination of receptors, depending on the drug). An understanding of these basic physiologic concepts is necessary to critical thinking and decision making in the administration of these drugs.

Begin a thorough assessment by gathering information about the patient's allergies and past and present medical conditions. Conducting a system overview and taking a thorough medication history is also a part of this process. Pose the following questions and document the findings: Are there any allergies to medications and/or foods? Is there a history of chronic obstructive pulmonary disease (e.g., emphysema, asthma, chronic bronchitis), other respiratory diseases, hypertension or hypotension, cardiac disease, bradycardia, congestive heart failure, and/or cardiac dysrhythmias? This information is crucial because the action and adverse effects of alpha and beta blockers may pose additional health risks to individuals with these problems. For example, alpha blockers may precipitate hypotension, thus patients with baseline low blood pressure readings need more frequent blood pressure monitoring, or they may not tolerate the drug at all.

Beta-blocking drugs may precipitate bradycardia, hypotension, heart block, heart failure, bronchoconstriction, and/or increased airway resistance. Therefore, any preexisting condition that might be worsened by the concurrent use of any of these medications may then represent a contraindication or caution. More specifically, with beta$_1$-blocking drugs, patients with preexisting bradycardia, decreased cardiac contractility, heart failure, and/or decreased conduction with heart block cannot take these drugs without exacerbation of these conditions. As another example, patients with a history of asthma, emphysema, bronchitis, or any condition with increased airway resistance or bronchoconstriction cannot take beta$_2$-blocking drugs without experiencing further bronchoconstriction and negative effects on their underlying disease condition. Given the actions and adverse effects of the drug, it is also important, to assess intake and output, daily weights, breath sounds, and blood glucose levels, especially if the patient has diabetes. For a complete listing of drug interactions, see Tables 19-3 and 19-5.

## ▌NURSING DIAGNOSES

1. Ineffective airway clearance related to the adverse effect of bronchoconstriction caused by beta-adrenergic drugs as well as any underlying restrictive airway conditions
2. Ineffective peripheral tissue perfusion related to the adverse effects of the disease of hypertension and the adverse effects of the adrenergic-blocking drugs (hypotension)
3. Imbalanced nutrition, less than body requirements, due to nausea and vomiting related to the adverse effects of the adrenergic blockers
4. Deficient knowledge related to lack of information about the therapeutic regimen, drug adverse effects, drug interactions, and precautions to be taken during drug treatment
5. Risk for injury related to possible adverse effects of the adrenergic-blocking drugs (e.g., postural hypotension, dizziness, syncope, numbness and tingling of the fingers and toes)

## ▌PLANNING

### ▌GOALS

1. Patient maintains/regains effective airway clearance and airway exchange.
2. Patient maintains/regains adequate peripheral tissue perfusion.
3. Patient experiences improved nutritional status.
4. Patient demonstrates adequate knowledge about use of the specific medications, their adverse effects, and the appropriate dosing routine to be followed at home.
5. Patient remains free from injury related to minimal problems with adverse effects of the medications.

### ▌OUTCOME CRITERIA

1. Patient states that respirations are performed with ease and in a regular rhythm, and without any bronchospasm, wheezing, or difficulty.
2. Patient states that blood pressure readings are within normal ranges.

- Patient experiences minimal adverse effects of drug therapy, specifically hypotension.
3. Patient states adequate dietary intake of the following: grains, vegetables, fruits, dairy, and protein foods (see www.choose myplate.gov/).
4. Patient states the rationale for both pharmacologic and non-pharmacologic treatment of hypertension or other indications for drug therapy.
   - Patient states importance of adhering with the medication therapy regimen and taking medication as prescribed.
   - Patient reports effective blood pressure lowering or other treatment with an adrenergic blocker without risks and complications such as syncope, dizziness, and hypotension.
   - Patient demonstrates the correct method of self-measurement of blood pressure using a digital cuff device.
   - Patient states the conditions that may occur of which the prescriber must be informed immediately, such as palpitations, chest pain, insomnia, and excessive agitation.
5. Patient remains free from injury due to taking medication as prescribed and preventing/managing adverse reactions.
   - Patient keeps all follow-up appointments with the prescriber to maintain safe therapy.
   - Patient follows instructions to avoid sudden withdrawal of hypertensive drugs to prevent rebound hypertensive crises and experiences minimal complications/injury to self.

## IMPLEMENTATION

Several nursing interventions may help maximize therapeutic effects of *adrenergic-blocking drugs* and minimize their adverse effects. To help minimize dry mouth, encourage intake of water within any restrictions and frequent rinsing/spraying of mouth with over-the-counter dental products indicated for dry mouth. Sugarless gum/candy may also be helpful with dry mouth. If any of the medications are given intravenously, an ECG monitor/cardiac monitoring is usually recommended. Encourage patients taking alpha blockers to change positions slowly and with purpose to prevent or minimize postural hypotension with subsequent dizziness and/or syncope. Alpha blockers and their indications in treatment of hypertensive disease and/or hypertensive crises are discussed further in Chapter 22. Use of the newer alpha blocker tamsulosin in patients with BPH is quite common, and patients taking this drug need to inform all health care providers—including dentists—that this is part of their medical regimen, especially before any type of surgery. In addition, anything leading to vasodilation needs to be avoided to prevent postural hypotension with resultant dizziness, light-headedness, and syncope. This includes alcohol intake, excessive exercise, exposure to hot climates, and use of saunas, hot tubs, and heated showers or baths. See Patient Teaching Tips for more information.

When either an alpha blocker or beta blocker is used, count the apical pulse for 1 full minute. Measure and document both supine and standing blood pressures. Contact the prescriber immediately if the patient has any problems with dizziness,

fainting, or lightheadedness, or if the systolic blood pressure is lower than 100 mm Hg or the pulse rate is lower than 60 beats/min. Daily weight measurement is important to monitor the progress of therapy and check for the adverse effect of edema. A good rule of thumb is to contact the prescriber if the patient shows an increase of 2 pounds or more over a 24-hour period or 5 pounds or more within 1 week. Keeping a daily journal documenting daily weights, blood pressure readings, pulse rates, adverse effects, and overall feelings of wellness or lack thereof will be important to the monitoring of the therapeutic regimen. Other symptoms to report to the prescriber include muscle weakness, shortness of breath, and collection of fluid in the lower extremities as manifested by difficulty in putting on shoes or socks and weight gain. Patients taking any of these medications must be weaned off the drug slowly because an abrupt discontinuation could lead to rebound hypertension or chest pain. The prescriber will designate a period of time for weaning; however, it is generally over a period of 1 to 2 weeks. Understanding basic anatomy and physiology and how receptors work will help guide nursing actions related to these drugs. See Patient Teaching Tips for more specific information.

# EVALUATION

Therapeutic effects for which to monitor in patients receiving *adrenergic-blocking drugs* include, but are not limited to, a decrease in blood pressure, pulse rate, and palpitations (in patients with these specific problems before drug therapy); alleviation of the symptoms of the disorder for which the drug was indicated; a return to normal blood pressure and pulse with lowering of the blood pressure toward 120/80 mm Hg and the pulse toward 60 beats/min in patients with diagnosed hypertension; and a decrease in chest pain in patients with angina. Also monitor patients for adverse effects associated with these medications, including bradycardia, depression, fatigue, and hypotension. See Tables 19-2 and 19-4 for other potential adverse effects.

## PATIENT TEACHING TIPS

- Give patients written and verbal information about drug indications, actions, adverse effects, cautions, contraindications, and drug interactions. This information needs to be age-specific and tailored to the specific learning needs of the patient.
- Emphasize the need to wear a medical alert bracelet or necklace identifying the specific medical diagnoses and provide a list of all medications. The patient needs to understand the importance of carrying this information in written form on his or her person at all times and update the information at least every few months or whenever there are major changes in the diagnosis and treatment regimen. Recommend to the patient that he or she also keep a card in his or her wallet or purse to record blood pressure readings by date and time. This information may then be shared with other health care professionals.
- Caution the patient to take medications exactly as prescribed and to never abruptly discontinue them due to the risk of rebound hypertension. If there is concern about omitted or skipped doses, the patient needs to contact the prescriber immediately.
- Caffeine and other central nervous system stimulants must be avoided while taking adrenergic-blocking drugs to prevent further irritability of the cardiac and central nervous systems and subsequent negative effects on health status.

- Alcohol ingestion is to be avoided because it causes vasodilation, which increases the risk of hypotension and postural blood pressure changes.
- Encourage the patient to contact the prescriber if he or she experiences palpitations, chest pain, confusion, weight gain (2 pounds or more in 24 hours or 5 pounds or more in 1 week), dyspnea, nausea, or vomiting. Other problems to report include swelling in the feet and ankles, shortness of breath, excessive fatigue, dizziness, and syncope.
- The alpha blocker tamsulosin must be taken as directed and with caution in patients with blood pressure problems (e.g., hypotension). The drug must also be used with caution by the elderly and while driving or engaging in other activities requiring alertness, because the adverse effects of this drug include blurred vision, dizziness, and drowsiness.
- Caution patients to change positions slowly to avoid dizziness and/or syncope. Excessive exercise, exposure to hot climates, use of a sauna or tanning bed, and alcohol consumption exacerbate vasodilation from the adrenergic-blocking drugs and lead to a greater drop in blood pressure with even more risk of dizziness and syncope.
- Constipation may develop as an adverse effect. Increasing fluids as well as fiber may help to prevent constipation.

## KEY POINTS

- Adrenergic-blocking drugs block the stimulation of the alpha-, $beta_1$-, and/or $beta_2$-adrenergic receptors, with the net result of blocking the effects of either norepinephrine or epinephrine on the receptors. This blocking action leads to a variety of physiologic responses depending on which receptors are blocked. Knowing how these receptors work allows the nurse to understand and predict the expected therapeutic effects of the drugs as well as the expected adverse effects.
- With alpha blockers, the predominant response is vasodilation. This is due to blocking of the alpha-adrenergic effect of vasoconstriction, which results in blood vessel relaxation.
- Vasodilation of blood vessels with the alpha blockers results in a drop in blood pressure and a reduction in urinary obstruction, which may lead to increased urinary flow rates. Monitor for these effects in patients taking alpha blockers.

- Beta blockers inhibit the stimulation of beta-adrenergic receptors by blocking the effects of the SNS neurotransmitters norepinephrine, epinephrine, and dopamine. Stimulation of $beta_1$ receptors leads to an increase in heart rate, conduction, and contractility. Stimulation of $beta_2$ receptors results in bronchial smooth muscle relaxation or bronchodilation. Blocking of $beta_1$ receptors results in a *decrease* in heart rate, conduction, and contractility. Blocking of $beta_2$ receptors leads to a *decrease* in bronchial smooth muscle relaxation, or bronchoconstriction.
- Beta blockers are classified as either selective or nonselective. Selective beta blockers are also called *cardioselective beta blockers* and block only the beta-adrenergic receptors in the heart that are located on the postsynaptic effector cells (i.e., the cells that nerves stimulate). The beneficial effects of the cardioselective beta blockers include decreased heart rate, reduced cardiac conduction, and

## KEY POINTS—cont'd

decreased myocardial contractility with no bronchoconstriction. These drugs are a good choice for patients with hypertension who also have bronchospastic airway disease or other pulmonary disease.

- Nonselective beta blockers block both beta$_1$- and beta$_2$-adrenergic receptors and affect the heart and bronchial smooth muscle. These drugs are used to treat patients with hypertension who do not have a problem with bronchospasm or pulmonary airway disease.

- Nursing considerations for patients taking alpha and beta blockers include teaching patients that they must weigh themselves daily, avoid sudden changes in position, and increase intake of fluids and fiber. Weight gain, dizziness, fainting, and/or a decrease in heart rate below 60 beats/min or a blood pressure of less than 100 mm Hg systolic or less than 80 mm Hg diastolic need to be reported immediately.

## NCLEX® EXAMINATION REVIEW QUESTIONS

1  When a patient has experienced extravasation of a peripheral infusion of dopamine, the nurse will inject the alpha blocker phentolamine (Regitine) into the area of extravasation and expect which effect?
   a  Vasoconstriction
   b  Vasodilation
   c  Analgesia
   d  Hypotension

2  When administering beta blockers, the nurse will follow which guideline for administration and monitoring?
   a  The drug may be discontinued at any time.
   b  Postural hypotension rarely occurs with this drug.
   c  Tapering off the medication is necessary to prevent rebound hypertension.
   d  The patient needs to stop taking the medication at once if he or she gains 3 to 4 pounds in a week.

3  The nurse providing teaching for a patient who has a new prescription for beta$_1$ blockers will keep in mind that these drugs may result in which effect?
   a  Tachycardia
   b  Tachypnea
   c  Bradycardia
   d  Bradypnea

4  A patient who has recently had a myocardial infarction (MI) has started therapy with a beta blocker. The nurse explains that the main purpose of the beta blocker for this patient is to
   a  cause vasodilation of the coronary arteries.
   b  prevent hypertension.
   c  increase conduction through the SA node.
   d  protect the heart from circulating catecholamines.

5  Before initiating therapy with a nonselective beta blocker, the nurse will assess the patient for a history of which condition?
   a  Hypertension
   b  Liver disease
   c  Pancreatitis
   d  Asthma

6  A patient is taking an alpha blocker as treatment for benign prostatic hyperplasia. The nurse will monitor for which potential drug effects? (Select all that apply.)
   a  Orthostatic hypotension
   b  Increased blood pressure
   c  Increased urine flow
   d  Headaches
   e  Bradycardia

7  A child in the pediatric ICU has been receiving a dopamine infusion. This morning while on rounds, the nurse noted that the IV has infiltrated. After stopping the infusion, the nurse prepares to administer phentolamine (Regitine). The ordered dose is 0.2 mg/kg, to be injected into the area of extravasation. The child weighs 39 lb. How many milligrams will the nurse administer? (Round to tenths.)

1. b, 2. c, 3. c, 4. d, 5. d, 6. a, c, d, 7. 3.5 mg

For Critical Thinking and Prioritization Questions, see http://evolve.elsevier.com/Lilley.

# CHAPTER
# 20

# Cholinergic Drugs

## OBJECTIVES

When you reach the end of this chapter, you will be able to do the following:

1. Briefly review the functions of the autonomic nervous system and the impact of the parasympathetic division.
2. List the various drugs classified as cholinergic agonists (also called *parasympathomimetics*).
3. Discuss the mechanisms of action, therapeutic effects, indications, adverse and toxic effects, drug interactions,

cautions, contraindications, dosages, routes of administration, and any antidotal management for the various cholinergic agonists (or parasympathomimetics).

4. Develop a nursing care plan that includes all phases of the nursing process for patients taking cholinergic agonists.

## DRUG PROFILES

- ♦ **bethanechol, p. 327**
- ♦ **donepezil, p. 328**
- ♦ **memantine, p. 328**

- ♦ **pyridostigmine, p. 329**

- ♦ *Key drug*

## KEY TERMS

**Acetylcholine** The neurotransmitter responsible for transmission of nerve impulses to effector cells in the parasympathetic nervous system. (p. 325)

**Acetylcholinesterase** The enzyme responsible for the breakdown of acetylcholine (also referred to simply as *cholinesterase*). (p. 325)

**Alzheimer's disease** A disease of the brain that is characterized by progressive mental deterioration manifested by confusion, disorientation, and loss of memory, ability to calculate, and visual-spatial orientation. (p. 327)

**Atony** A lack of normal muscle tone (p. 326)

**Cholinergic crisis** Severe muscle weakness and respiratory paralysis due to excessive acetylcholine; often seen in patients with myasthenia gravis as an adverse effect of drugs used to treat the disorder (p. 327)

**Cholinergic receptor** A nerve receptor that is stimulated by acetylcholine. (p. 325)

**Miosis** The contraction of the pupil. (p. 326)

**Muscarinic receptors** Cholinergic receptors that are located postsynaptically in the *effector organs* such as smooth muscle, cardiac muscle, and glands supplied by parasympathetic fibers. (p. 325)

**Nicotinic receptors** Cholinergic receptors located in the *ganglia* (where presynaptic and postsynaptic nerve fibers meet) of both the parasympathetic nervous system and the sympathetic nervous system; so named because they can be stimulated by the alkaloid nicotine. (p. 325)

**Parasympathomimetics** Drugs that mimic the parasympathetic nervous system; also referred to as *cholinergic agonist drugs*. (p. 325)

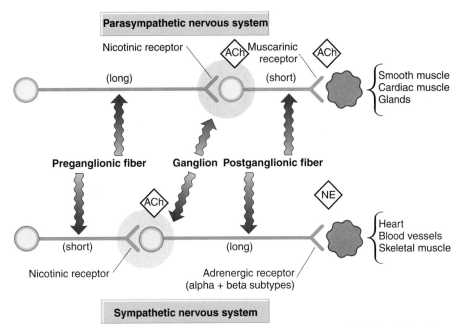

**FIGURE 20-1** Parasympathetic and sympathetic nervous systems and their relationship to one another. *ACh,* Acetylcholine; *NE,* norepinephrine.

## ANATOMY, PHYSIOLOGY, AND PATHOPHYSIOLOGY OVERVIEW

*Cholinergic drugs, cholinergic agonists,* and *parasympathomimetics* are all terms that refer to the class of drugs that stimulate the parasympathetic nervous system.

## PARASYMPATHETIC NERVOUS SYSTEM

The parasympathetic nervous system (PNS) is the branch of the autonomic nervous system with functions opposite those of the sympathetic nervous system (Figure 20-1). Acetylcholine is the neurotransmitter responsible for the transmission of nerve impulses to effector cells in the parasympathetic nervous system. A cholinergic receptor is a receptor that binds acetylcholine and mediates its actions. There are two types of cholinergic receptors, as determined by their location and their action. Nicotinic receptors are located in the ganglia of both the parasympathetic nervous system and sympathetic nervous system. They are called *nicotinic* because they can also be stimulated by nicotine. The other type of cholinergic receptor is the muscarinic receptor. Muscarinic receptors are located postsynaptically in the effector organs (i.e., smooth muscle, cardiac muscle, and glands) supplied by the parasympathetic fibers. They are called *muscarinic* because they are stimulated by the alkaloid muscarine, a substance isolated from mushrooms. Figure 20-2 shows how the nicotinic and muscarinic receptors are arranged in the parasympathetic nervous system.

## PHARMACOLOGY OVERVIEW
## CHOLINERGIC DRUGS

Cholinergic drugs, also known as cholinergic *agonists* or parasympathomimetics, mimic the effects of acetylcholine. These

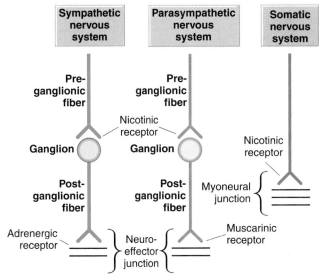

**FIGURE 20-2** Sympathetic, parasympathetic, and somatic nervous systems. Note the location of the nicotinic and muscarinic receptors in the parasympathetic nervous system.

drugs can stimulate cholinergic receptors either directly or indirectly. *Direct-acting* cholinergic agonists bind directly to cholinergic receptors and activate them. *Indirect-acting* cholinergic agonists stimulate the postsynaptic release of acetylcholine at the receptor site. This then allows acetylcholine to bind to and stimulate the receptor. Indirect-acting cholinergic drugs (also known as *cholinesterase inhibitors*) work by inhibiting the action of acetylcholinesterase, the enzyme responsible for breaking down acetylcholine. Acetylcholinesterase is also referred to as *cholinesterase.* There are two categories of cholinesterase inhibitors: reversible inhibitors and irreversible inhibitors. *Reversible* cholinesterase inhibitors bind to cholinesterase for a short period of time, whereas *irreversible* cholinesterase inhibitors

## BOX 20-1   CHOLINERGIC DRUGS

**Direct-Acting Drugs**
bethanechol (Urecholine)
carbachol (Carboptic, others)
pilocarpine (Salagen, Pilocar [see Chapter 57], others)
succinylcholine (Anectine, Quelicin; see Chapter 11)

**Indirect-Acting Drugs**
donepezil (Aricept)
echothiophate (Phospholine Iodide; see Chapter 57)
edrophonium (Tensilon, others)
galantamine (Razadyne)
neostigmine (Prostigmin)
physostigmine (Antilirium)
pyridostigmine (Mestinon)
rivastigmine (Exelon)
tacrine (Cognex)

## TABLE 20-1   CHOLINERGIC AGONISTS: DRUG EFFECTS

| BODY TISSUE/ ORGAN | RESPONSE TO STIMULATION | |
| --- | --- | --- |
| | MUSCARINIC | NICOTINIC |
| Bronchi (lung) | Increased secretions, constriction | None |
| Cardiovascular | | |
| Blood vessels | Dilation | Constriction |
| Heart rate | Slowed | Increased |
| Blood pressure | Decreased | Increased |
| Eye | Miosis (pupil constriction), decreased accommodation | Miosis (pupil constriction), decreased accommodation |
| Gastrointestinal | | |
| Tone | Increased | Increased |
| Motility | Increased | Increased |
| Sphincters | Relaxed | None |
| Genitourinary | | |
| Tone | Increased | Increased |
| Motility | Increased | Increased |
| Sphincter | Relaxed | Relaxed |
| Glandular secretions | Increased intestinal, lacrimal, salivary, and sweat gland secretion | — |
| Skeletal muscle | — | Increased contraction |

have a long duration of activity, and the body must generate new cholinesterase enzymes to override the effects of the irreversible drugs. Box 20-1 lists the direct- and indirect-acting cholinergics.

## Mechanism of Action and Drug Effects

When acetylcholine directly binds to its receptor, stimulation occurs. Once binding takes place on the membranes of an effector cell (cell of the target tissue or organ), the permeability of the cell changes, and calcium and sodium are permitted to flow into the cell. This then depolarizes the cell membrane and stimulates the effector organ.

The effects of direct- and indirect-acting cholinergic drugs are seen when the parasympathetic nervous system is stimulated. There are many mnemonics to aid in remembering these effects. One is to think of the parasympathetic nervous system as the "rest and digest" system, in contrast to the "flight or fight" sympathetic nervous system.

Cholinergic drugs are used primarily for their effects on the gastrointestinal tract, bladder, and eye. These drugs stimulate the intestine and bladder, which results in increased gastric secretions, gastrointestinal (GI) motility, and urinary frequency. They also stimulate constriction of the pupil, termed miosis. This helps decrease intraocular pressure. In addition, cholinergic drugs cause increased salivation and sweating. Cardiovascular effects include reduced heart rate and vasodilation. Pulmonary effects include causing the bronchi of the lungs to constrict and the airways to narrow.

At recommended dosages, cholinergic drugs primarily affect the muscarinic receptors, but at high dosages the nicotinic receptors can also be stimulated. The desired effects come from muscarinic receptor stimulation; many of the undesirable adverse effects are due to nicotinic receptor stimulation. The various effects of the cholinergic drugs are listed in Table 20-1 according to the receptors stimulated.

## Indications
### Direct-Acting Drugs
Direct-acting drugs, such as carbachol, pilocarpine, and echothiophate, are used topically to reduce intraocular pressure in

patients with glaucoma or in those undergoing ocular surgery (see Chapter 57). They are poorly absorbed orally, which limits their use mostly to topical application. One exception is the direct-acting cholinergic drug bethanechol, which is administered orally. Bethanechol affects the detrusor muscle of the urinary bladder and also the smooth muscle of the GI tract. It causes increased bladder and GI tract tone and motility, which increases the movement of contents through these areas. It also causes the sphincters in the bladder and the GI tract to relax, allowing them to empty. Bethanechol is also used to treat atony of the bladder and GI tract. Atony can occur after a surgical procedure. The direct-acting drug, cevimeline, is used to treat excessively dry mouth (xerostomia) resulting from a disorder known as *Sjögren's syndrome.* Oral pilocarpine can also be used for this purpose. Another direct-acting cholinergic is succinylcholine, which is used as a neuromuscular blocker in general anesthesia (see Chapter 11).

### Indirect-Acting Drugs
Indirect-acting drugs work by increasing acetylcholine concentrations at the receptor sites, which leads to stimulation of the effector cells. Indirect-acting drugs cause skeletal muscle contraction and are used for the diagnosis and treatment of myasthenia gravis. Their ability to inhibit acetylcholinesterase also makes them useful for the reversal of neuromuscular blockade produced either by neuromuscular blocking drugs or by anticholinergic poisoning. For this reason, the indirect-acting drug physostigmine is considered the antidote for anticholinergic poisoning as well as poisoning by irreversible cholinesterase

inhibitors such as the organophosphates and carbonates, common classes of insecticides.

Indirect-acting drugs are also used to treat Alzheimer's disease, which is a neurologic disorder in which patients have decreased levels of acetylcholine. In the treatment of Alzheimer's disease, cholinergic drugs increase concentrations of acetylcholine in the brain by inhibiting cholinesterase. This increase in acetylcholine levels helps to enhance and maintain memory and learning capabilities. There are three cholinesterase inhibitors used to treat Alzheimer's disease, including donepezil (Aricept), galantamine (Razadyne), and rivastigmine (Exelon); all are indirect-acting cholinergic drugs. Although their therapeutic efficacy is often limited (it has been reported that only 15% to 30% of patients treated actually see benefits), these drugs may enhance a patient's mental status enough to cause a noticeable, if temporary, improvement in the quality of life for patients as well as caregivers and family members. The most commonly used of these medications at this time is donepezil. Patient response to these drugs is highly variable. For this reason, failure to respond to maximally titrated dosages of one of these drugs does not necessarily rule out an attempt at therapy with another drug in this same class. Memantine (Namenda) is also used to treat Alzheimer's disease, but it is not a cholinesterase inhibitor. For dosage information on all of these drugs, see the table on p. 328.

## Contraindications

Contraindications to the use of cholinergic drugs include known drug allergy, GI or genitourinary (GU) tract obstruction, bradycardia, defects in cardiac impulse conduction, hyperthyroidism, epilepsy, hypotension, or chronic obstructive pulmonary disease. Parkinson's disease (see Chapter 15) is listed as a precaution to these drugs; however, rivastigmine (Exelon) is used in patients with Parkinson's disease who also have dementia.

## Adverse Effects

The primary adverse effects of cholinergic drugs are the consequence of overstimulation of the parasympathetic nervous system. They are extensions of the cholinergic reactions that affect many body functions. The major effects are listed by body system in Table 20-2. The effects on the cardiovascular system are complex and may include syncope, hypotension with reflex tachycardia, hypertension, or bradycardia, depending on if the muscarinic or nicotinic receptors are stimulated.

### Toxicity and Management of Overdose

There is little systemic absorption of the topically administered drugs and therefore little systemic toxicity. When administered locally in the eye, they can cause temporary ocular changes such as transient blurring and dimming of vision. Systemic toxicity with topically applied cholinergics is seen most commonly when longer-acting drugs are given repeatedly over a long period. This can result in overstimulation of the parasympathetic nervous system and all the attendant responses. Treatment is generally symptomatic and supportive, and the administration of a reversal drug (e.g., atropine) is rarely required.

| TABLE 20-2 | CHOLINERGIC AGONISTS: ADVERSE EFFECTS |
|---|---|
| **BODY SYSTEM** | **ADVERSE EFFECTS** |
| Cardiovascular | Bradycardia or tachycardia, hypotension or hypertension, syncope, conduction abnormalities (atrioventricular block and cardiac arrest) |
| Central nervous | Headache, dizziness, convulsions, ataxia |
| Gastrointestinal | Abdominal cramps, increased secretions, nausea, vomiting, diarrhea |
| Respiratory | Increased bronchial secretions, bronchospasm |
| Other | Lacrimation, sweating, salivation, miosis |

The likelihood of toxicity is greater for cholinergics that are given orally or intravenously. The most severe consequence of an overdose of a cholinergic drug is a cholinergic crisis. Symptoms include circulatory collapse, hypotension, bloody diarrhea, shock, and cardiac arrest. Early signs include abdominal cramps, salivation, flushing of the skin, nausea, and vomiting. Transient syncope, transient complete heart block, dyspnea, and orthostatic hypotension may also occur. These can be reversed promptly by the administration of atropine, a cholinergic antagonist. Severe cardiovascular reactions or bronchoconstriction may be alleviated by epinephrine, an adrenergic agonist. One way of remembering the effects of cholinergic poisoning is to use the acronym *SLUDGE*, which stands for salivation, lacrimation, urinary incontinence, diarrhea, GI cramps, and emesis.

## Interactions

Anticholinergics (such as atropine), antihistamines, and sympathomimetics may antagonize cholinergic drugs and lead to a reduced response to them. Other cholinergic drugs may have additive effects.

## Dosages

For the recommended dosages of the cholinergic drugs, see the Dosages table on p. 328.

## DRUG PROFILES

### ♦ bethanechol

Bethanechol (Urecholine) is a direct-acting cholinergic agonist. It is used in the treatment of acute postoperative and postpartum nonobstructive urinary retention and for the management of urinary retention associated with neurogenic atony of the bladder. It has also been used to prevent and treat bladder dysfunction induced by phenothiazine and tricyclic antidepressants (see Chapter 16). In addition, it is used in the treatment of postoperative GI atony and gastric retention, chronic refractory heartburn, as well as in diagnostic testing for infantile cystic fibrosis. Bethanechol is available orally and subcutaneously. Contraindications include known drug allergy, hyperthyroidism, peptic ulcer, active bronchial asthma, cardiac disease or coronary artery disease, epilepsy, and Parkinsonism. The drug is to be avoided in patients in whom the strength or integrity of the GI tract or bladder wall is questionable or with conditions

## DOSAGES

### Selected Cholinergic Agonist Drugs

| DRUG (PREGNANCY CATEGORY) | PHARMACOLOGIC CLASS | USUAL DOSAGE RANGE | INDICATIONS/USES |
|---|---|---|---|
| ◆ bethanechol (Urecholine) (C) | Muscarinic (direct-acting) | **Adult**<br>PO: 10-50 mg tid-qid (usually start with 5-10 mg, repeating hourly until urination, max 50 mg/cycle) | Postoperative and postpartum functional urinary retention |
| ◆ donepezil (Aricept) (C) | Anticholinesterase (indirect-acting) | **Adult**<br>PO: 5-10 mg/day as a single dose | Alzheimer's dementia |
| ◆ memantine (Namenda) (B) | NMDA-receptor antagonist | **Adult only**<br>PO: Initial dose is 5 mg/day; titrate by 5 mg/wk up to a target dose of 10 mg/bid (20 mg/day). Maximum dose in renal impairment is 10 mg/day. | Alzheimer's dementia |
| physostigmine (Antilirium) (C) | Anticholinesterase (indirect-acting) | **Pediatric**<br>IM/IV: 0.01-0.03 mg/kg repeated at 5-10 min intervals until desired effect or 2 mg is reached<br>**Adult**<br>IM/IV; 0.5-2 mg repeated q20 min if needed | Reversal of anticholinergic drug effects and tricyclic antidepressant overdose |
| ◆ pyridostigmine (Mestinon) (C) | Anticholinesterase (indirect-acting) | **Adult**<br>PO: 600 mg/day in divided doses<br>IV: 0.1-0.25 mg/kg | Myasthenia gravis<br>Antidote for neuromuscular blocker toxicity |

*IM,* Intramuscular; *IV,* intravenous; *NMDA,* N-methyl-D-aspartate; *PO,* oral.

in which increased muscular activity could prove harmful, such as known or suspected mechanical obstruction.

Adverse effects include syncope, hypotension with reflex tachycardia, headache, seizure, GI upset, and asthmatic attacks. Drugs that interact with bethanechol include acetylcholinesterase inhibitors (i.e., indirect-acting cholinergics), which can enhance the adverse effects of bethanechol. Recommended dosages are given in the table on this page.

### Pharmacokinetics

| Route | Onset of Action | Peak Plasma Concentration | Elimination Half-life | Duration of Action |
|---|---|---|---|---|
| PO/injection | 30-90 min | Less than 30 min | Unknown | 1-6 hr |

### ◆ donepezil

Donepezil (Aricept) is a cholinesterase inhibitor drug that works centrally in the brain to increase levels of acetylcholine by inhibiting acetylcholinesterase. It is used in the treatment of mild to moderate Alzheimer's disease. Similar cholinesterase inhibitors include tacrine, galantamine, and rivastigmine. Rivastigmine is also approved for treating dementia associated with Parkinson's disease. Contraindications for donepezil include known drug allergy. Adverse effects are normally mild and resolve on their own. They can often be avoided by careful dose titration. They include GI upset (including ulcer risk due to increased gastric secretions), drowsiness, dizziness, insomnia, and muscle cramps. The effects on the cardiovascular system are complex and may include bradycardia, syncope, hypotension with reflex tachycardia, or hypertension. Interacting drugs include anticholinergics (counteract donepezil effects) and nonsteroidal antiinflammatory drugs (see Chapter 44). Donepezil is available only for oral use as both a tablet and a rapid-acting, orally

disintegrating tablet. Recommended dosages are given in the table on this page.

### Pharmacokinetics

| Route | Onset of Action | Peak Plasma Concentration | Elimination Half-life | Duration of Action |
|---|---|---|---|---|
| PO | 3 wk | 3-4 hr | 70 hr | 2 wk |

### ◆ memantine

Memantine (Namenda) is not a cholinergic drug, but is being included here in the discussion of drugs for Alzheimer's dementia. It is classified as an N-methyl-D-aspartate (NMDA) receptor antagonist owing to its inhibitory activity at the NMDA receptors in the central nervous system. Stimulation of these receptors is believed to be part of the Alzheimer's disease process. Memantine blocks this stimulation and thereby helps to reduce or arrest the patient's degenerative cognitive symptoms. As with all other currently available medications for this debilitating illness, the effects of this drug are likely to be temporary but may still afford some improvement in quality of life and general functioning for some patients. Its only current contraindication is known drug allergy. Reported adverse effects are relatively uncommon but include hypotension, headache, GI upset, musculoskeletal pain, dyspnea, ataxia, and fatigue. No clearly defined drug interactions are listed. Memantine is available only for oral use. The recommended dosage is given in the table on this page.

### Pharmacokinetics

| Route | Onset of Action | Peak Plasma Concentration | Elimination Half-life | Duration of Action |
|---|---|---|---|---|
| PO | Unknown | 5 hr | 70 hr | Unknown |

### ◆ pyridostigmine

Pyridostigmine (Mestinon) is a synthetic quaternary ammonium compound that is similar in structure to other drugs in this class, including edrophonium, physostigmine, and neostigmine. All are indirect-acting cholinergic drugs that work to increase acetylcholine by inhibiting acetylcholinesterase. Pyridostigmine has been shown to improve muscle strength and is used to relieve the symptoms of myasthenia gravis, and it is the most commonly used drug for symptomatic treatment of myasthenia gravis. Edrophonium (Tensilon) is an indirect-acting cholinergic drug that is commonly used to diagnose myasthenia gravis. It can also be used to differentiate between myasthenia gravis and cholinergic crisis. Neostigmine, pyridostigmine, and physostigmine are also useful for reversing the effects of nondepolarizing neuromuscular blocking drugs (see Chapter 11) after surgery. They are also used in the treatment of severe overdoses of tricyclic antidepressants because of the significant anticholinergic effects associated with the tricyclic antidepressants. Physostigmine, neostigmine, and pyridostigmine are also used as an antidote after toxic exposure to nondrug anticholinergic agents, including those used in chemical warfare. Contraindications to these drugs include known drug allergy, prior severe cholinergic reactions, asthma, gangrene, hyperthyroidism, cardiovascular disease, and mechanical obstruction of the GI or GU tracts. Adverse effects include GI upset and excessive salivation. Interacting drugs include the anticholinergic drugs, which counteract the therapeutic effects of indirect-acting cholinergic drugs. Pyridostigmine is available in oral and injectable forms. Recommended dosages are given in the table on p. 328.

### Pharmacokinetics

| Route | Onset of Action | Peak Plasma Concentration | Elimination Half-life | Duration of Action |
|---|---|---|---|---|
| Oral/IM | 15-45 min | 1-2 hours | 3-4 hr | Up to 6 hr |
| IV | 2-5 min | Immediate | 1-2 hr | 2-3 hr |

## █ NURSING PROCESS

## █ ASSESSMENT

*Cholinergic drugs,* or parasympathomimetics, produce a variety of effects stemming from their ability to stimulate the parasympathetic nervous system and mimic the action of acetylcholine. These effects include a decrease in heart rate, increase in GI and GU tone through increased contractility of the smooth muscle of the bowel and bladder, increase in the contractility and tone of bronchial smooth muscle, increased respiratory secretions, and miosis or pupillary constriction. Therefore, if the patient has any preexisting conditions, such as heart block, or the patient is taking other drugs that mimic the actions of the parasympathetic nervous system, adverse effects or toxicity may be increased. Before cholinergic drugs are given, perform a thorough head-to-toe physical examination, and obtain a nursing history and medication history (including prescription drugs, over-the-counter drugs, and herbals). Document drug allergies and past and present medical conditions as well. Identify cautions, contraindications, and drug interactions. Assess vital signs and document with special attention to baseline blood pressure readings because of the potential for orthostatic hypotension.

Before a drug for Alzheimer's disease, such as donepezil or memantine, is used, assess the patient for allergies, cautions, contraindications, and drug interactions. Perform a close assessment and documentation of the patient's neurologic status with attention to short- and long-term memory; level of alertness; motor, cognitive, and sensory functioning; any suicidal tendencies or thoughts; musculoskeletal intactness; and GI, GU, and cardiovascular functioning. Assess urinary patterns so that any problems with urinary retention may be identified. Report any abnormalities and/or complaints to the prescriber immediately. Presence or absence of family support systems is important to note because of the chronic nature of this illness. Once the patient has begun taking medication, it is critical for you to continue to assess the patient's response to the drug. Especially note any changes in symptoms within the first 6 weeks of therapy. Journaling may be helpful to the prescriber to assess any positive changes and any adverse effects and/or lack of improvement. Ginkgo may be used by some health care providers for organic brain syndrome (see the Safety: Herbal Therapies and Dietary Supplements box on p. 328).

### CASE STUDY

#### *Donepezil (Aricept) for Alzheimer's Disease*

 E. is a 72-year-old woman married to F., age 73 years. F. has noticed that E. is becoming more forgetful but did not worry about it until she got lost while driving home from the grocery store. F. makes an appointment for E. to see their primary care physician, Dr. S. After the examination, Dr. S. tells F., in private, that she thinks that E. is in the early stages of Alzheimer's disease but will order some tests to rule out other problems. F. then accompanies Dr. S. while she tells E. of the tentative diagnosis. Understandably, E. is upset to hear this news.

1. In her discussion with E. and her husband, Dr. S. mentioned a drug called donepezil (Aricept) that can be used in the early stages of Alzheimer's disease. It may be started after a few diagnostic tests are performed. After Dr. S. leaves the room, E. asks the nurse, "What will this drug do for me? Will it stop the Alzheimer's disease?" How will the nurse reply?

   Several diagnostic tests are performed, including a complete blood count, serum electrolyte levels, vitamin $B_{12}$ levels, liver and thyroid function tests, and a magnetic resonance imaging scan to rule out other neurologic disease. Results of all tests are within normal limits. Dr. S. decides to prescribe donepezil, 5 mg, daily, for E.

2. After a week, F. calls the nurse to ask about giving E. an over-the-counter antihistamine for her allergies. "She always needs an allergy pill this time of year." He also says that she needs to take a pain pill for her mild arthritis but is not sure whether to use acetaminophen or ibuprofen. What will the nurse tell F.?

3. After 6 weeks, F. brings E. back to the doctor's office for a follow-up appointment. F. privately tells Dr. S. that he is "upset" because he has noticed very little improvement. E. tells Dr. S. that she feels "fine" and has not noticed any problems. What do you think will be Dr. S.'s next order at this time? Is E.'s response to the donepezil typical? Explain your answer.

For answers, see http://evolve.elsevier.com/Lilley.

**SAFETY: HERBAL THERAPIES AND DIETARY SUPPLEMENTS**

### *Ginkgo* (Ginkgo biloba)

**Overview**
The dried leaf of the ginkgo plant contains flavonoids, terpenoids, and organic acids that help ginkgo preparations exert their positive effects as an antioxidant and inhibitor of platelet aggregation.

**Common Uses**
To prevent memory loss, peripheral arterial occlusive disease, vertigo, tinnitus

**Adverse Effects**
Stomach or intestinal upset, headache, bleeding, allergic skin reaction

**Potential Drug Interactions**
Aspirin, nonsteroidal antiinflammatory drugs, warfarin, heparin, anticonvulsants, ticlopidine, clopidogrel, dipyridamole, tricyclic antidepressants

**Contraindications**
None

## NURSING DIAGNOSES

1. Decreased cardiac output related to adverse cardiovascular effects of hypotension and bradycardia
2. Deficient knowledge of the therapeutic regimen, adverse effects, drug interactions, and precautions for cholinergic drugs related to lack of experience with drug therapies
3. Risk for injury related to the possible adverse effects of cholinergic drugs, such as bradycardia and hypotension, with subsequent risk for falls or syncope

## PLANNING

### GOALS

1. Patient maintains normal cardiac output/status due to proper taking of medication as prescribed.
2. Patient demonstrates adequate knowledge about the safe use of prescribed medication, its adverse effects, and the appropriate dosing at home.
3. Patient remains free from injury resulting from the adverse effects of the medication.

### OUTCOME CRITERIA

1. Patient, caregiver, or family member states symptoms to report to the prescriber immediately such as the occurrence of dizziness, syncope, excess fatigue, and lightheadedness with heart rate changes.
   - Patient has blood pressure and pulse rate monitored and recorded daily.
   - Patient's blood pressure and pulse rate stay within normal ranges or without significant drops while on medication.
2. Patient, caregiver, or family member states the importance of scheduling and keeping follow-up appointments with the prescriber related to the management of the disorder for

which medication has been prescribed and the monitoring for therapeutic or adverse effects.
   - Patient, caregiver, or family member demonstrates understanding that medications are not curative but are for symptomatic control.
   - Patient, caregiver, or family member demonstrates understanding that it may take several weeks for medications (i.e., medications for Alzheimer's disease) to have therapeutic effects.
3. Patient, caregiver, or family member demonstrates an understanding about the need to implement safety measures to avoid falls such as taking time to move slowly from lying/sitting to standing, taking purposeful movements, and using compression stockings.

## IMPLEMENTATION

Several nursing interventions may help to maximize the therapeutic effects of cholinergic drugs and minimize their adverse effects. If the patient has undergone surgery and cholinergic drugs are indicated, encourage ambulation and increased intake of fluids and fiber, unless contraindicated. Early ambulation helps to increase GI peristalsis and possibly prevent the need for drugs such as bethanechol, which is used to treat decreased or absent peristalsis related to the surgery and/or anesthesia. However, do not administer these drugs if a mechanical obstruction is suspected. Use of these drugs in such a situation may possibly result in bowel perforation. Subcutaneous injections of bethanechol need to be administered as ordered (see Chapter 9 for information on injection techniques) and sites rotated if injections are frequent. It is always preferable to use nonpharmacologic measures rather than pharmacologic regimens to treat the anticipated postoperative problems of decreased peristalsis and/or urinary retention. For drugs used to treat myasthenia gravis, give the oral medication about 30 minutes before meals to allow for onset of action and therapeutic effects (e.g., decreased dysphagia or decreased difficulty swallowing). Atropine is the antidote to a cholinergic overdose; therefore, this medication needs to be readily available and given per the prescriber's order.

None of the drugs used for treatment of Alzheimer's disease provide a cure, but these drugs do improve function and cognition to some degree. It is crucial to discuss, with empathy and compassion, the fact that the disease has no cure. The diagnosis of Alzheimer's disease and/or dementia is shocking, at best. Those involved in the care of the patient need to be honest in sharing information with the patient, family, significant others, and caregivers. Always follow ethical standards of practice when working with patients, and adhere to the American Nurses Association *Code of Ethics for Nurses*. This code outlines behaviors required to maintain a high level of professionalism and specific actions that demonstrate respect for patient rights in any patient care situation. However, any sharing of information with the patient, family, significant others, and caregivers must be done with the approval of the prescriber, with good intent, in compliance with any research protocol, and/or with the goal of being a patient advocate. When beginning any of these medications, the patient will most likely need continued assistance and help with activities of daily living (ADLs) and ambulation (because the medication may increase dizziness and subsequent gait imbalances at the initiation of treatment). The patient, family members, and caregivers also need to understand the importance of taking the medication exactly as ordered. Dosages and exact scheduling of medications is critical for the patient and family/caregiver to understand in order to achieve the drug's maximum therapeutic effects. In addition, instruct the patient and anyone involved in the patient's daily care about how to take the medication (e.g., taking the drug with food to decrease GI upset). Encourage the patient and family/caregiver to educate themselves about the use of the drug, its adverse effects, possible interactions, and potential for harm, and emphasize the importance of *not* withdrawing the medication abruptly. The patient must be weaned off all drugs over a period of time designated by the prescriber, because of the potential for a rapid decline in cognitive functioning.

Most of the cholinergic agonists have dose-limiting adverse effects that include severe GI disturbances such as nausea and vomiting. Blood pressure readings and pulse rates need to be taken and recorded before, during, and after initiation of drug therapy. Dizziness may occur with therapy, resulting in the need for assistance with ambulation and other ADLs. Maintenance of a journal that records daily doses of drugs, ability of the patient to participate in ADLs, motor ability, gait, mental status, cognition, and any adverse effects will provide valuable information to any health care provider or caregiver involved in the patient's day-to-day care.

Dosages of these medications may be changed by the prescriber after about 6 weeks if no therapeutic response occurs. For patient safety, blood pressure, pulse rate, and electrocardiogram need to be carefully monitored throughout therapy. Instruct the patient, family, or caregiver to report any cardiac problems such as decrease in pulse rate (less than 60 beats/min) and/or drop in blood pressure. A cholinergic crisis, resulting from overdosage of medication, may be manifested by abdominal cramps, flushing of the skin, nausea and vomiting (early signs and symptoms) progressing to circulatory collapse, hypotension, and cardiac arrest. Dissolving forms of the medication donepezil are to be placed on the tongue and allowed to dissolve before the patient drinks fluids or swallows.

In summary, because most of the cholinergic drugs are used to treat patients diagnosed with Alzheimer's disease, monitor the patient's family and other support personnel closely, and be sure that their questions are answered fully and completely and their needs met. Often family members, significant others, and caregivers have many questions as well as short- and long-term concerns. Preplanning education addressing these concerns is an important part of a holistic approach to patient care and to the meeting of patient needs. Often the best place to begin in terms of education is to prepare answers to the following questions that are often posed: What should we expect for our loved one? What will happen to the person emotionally and physically? What treatments are available, and what drugs are deemed safe? What are the common adverse effects of drug therapy, and how can they be minimized? What about diet, fluids, and exercise for our loved one? Are there herbals or any supplements or over-the-counter drugs that would help with the disease, or should they be avoided? What will we need to do for long-term care or other living situations for our loved one? What are the expected costs of our lived one's care now and in the future? What are the costs of drug therapy? Other costs? What kind of help can we all receive emotionally? What about emotional support for our loved one? How can this disease affect intimate relationships? What type of attorney should we seek out? What about durable power of attorney and living wills? Other types of wills? Are these needed right away if we don't have these legal documents already? How do we all go on with our lives when our loved one is changing so drastically? Will life ever be normal again? What about research and clinical trials for treatment regimens? Should we pursue other treatments or do nothing new? What about drugs that are not yet FDA-approved? How long will this process take? Just what can we expect over time?

## EVALUATION

Monitor patients for the following therapeutic effects: (1) in patients with myasthenia gravis, a decrease in the signs and symptoms of the disease; (2) in patients experiencing a decrease in GI peristalsis postoperatively, an increase in bowel sounds, the passage of flatus, and the occurrence of bowel movements (all indicating an increase in peristalsis); and (3) in patients who have a hypotonic bladder with urinary retention, micturition (voiding) within about 60 minutes of the administration of bethanechol. Also monitor for adverse effects of these medications, including increased respiratory secretions, bronchospasm, nausea, vomiting, diarrhea, hypotension, bradycardia, and conduction abnormalities. For other adverse effects, see Table 20-2.

Therapeutic effects of the drugs used to manage Alzheimer's disease–related dementia or cognitive impairment include an improvement of the symptoms of the disease, but in most cases it takes up to 6 weeks for these effects to become apparent. Varying degrees of improvement in mood and a decrease in confusion usually occur. Adverse effects include nausea, vomiting, dizziness, and others (see individual drug profiles for specific information).

## EVIDENCE-BASED PRACTICE

### Exercise and Improved Cognition

#### Review

As the average age of the population in the United States and elsewhere continues to increase, the number of people living with Alzheimer's disease is expected to rise from the current 26.6 million to more than 106 million by 2050. It has been estimated that if the onset of dementia could be delayed by about 12 months, there would be approximately 9.2 million fewer cases worldwide. Several clinical trials have examined the ability of pharmacologic therapies such as cholinesterase inhibitors (e.g., donepezil), vitamin E, and rofecoxib to prevent progression to dementia in those at risk for Alzheimer's disease, but outcomes have been largely negative. However, many observational studies have suggested that physical activity may reduce the risk for cognitive decline. Because the evidence supporting a preventative effect of exercise is sparse, a randomized trial was designed to determine whether a program of regular exercise could slow the rate of cognitive decline in older adults at risk. This study is one of the first to demonstrate that exercise improves cognitive functioning in older adults experiencing subjective and objective mild cognitive impairment.

#### Type of Evidence

This study was a randomized, controlled trial in which one group of patients participated in a 24-week home-based program of physical activity consisting mainly of walking, whereas a second control group received only education and the usual care. Study participants were individuals who reported memory problems but did not meet the criteria for dementia. A total of 170 participants were randomly assigned to the two study groups, but only 138 actually completed the 18-month assessment. Those participating in the exercise program increased their physical activity by the relatively modest amount of about 20 minutes per day. Cognitive function was measured over a period of 18 months using the Alzheimer's Disease Assessment Scale—Cognitive Subscale (ADAS-Cog).

#### Results of Study

In an intent-to-treat analysis, participants in the physical activity group showed an average improvement of 0.26 points in their ADAS-Cog scores at the end of the 6-month intervention, while those in the usual care group showed deterioration by an average of 1.04 points; thus, the absolute improvement of the

physical activity group over the usual care group was 1.3 points. The researchers noted that this result compares favorably with the reported improvement of 0.5 points associated with the use of donepezil. After the 6-month intervention period, patients in the physical activity group were encouraged to remain active, and a newsletter was sent out periodically to reinforce the goals of the program. No further intervention was offered. By 18 months, those in the physical activity group had improved by an average of 0.73 points in ADAS-Cog score, compared with an improvement of 0.04 points for those in the usual care group. Modest improvements were also seen in scores on some other tests, including word list delayed recall and Clinical Dementia Rating sum of boxes, but no significant changes were seen in scores on tests of word list total immediate recall, digit symbol coding, or verbal fluency. Beck Depression Inventory scores and scores on the Medical Outcomes 36-Item Short Form Health Survey physical and mental component summaries also improved in the physical activity group.

#### Link of Evidence to Nursing Practice

A very important achievement of this study is its demonstration of the potential benefit of the simple, nonpharmacologic intervention of exercise, which is almost universally available, in the prevention of cognitive decline. For these participants as well as many other patients with physical and/or mental disease, the benefits of exercise go beyond improvement in cognition and include a positive impact on depression, quality of life, and cardiovascular function, as well as a decrease in falls and disability. Although advances are being made in health and technology and people are living longer, there is a need to find alternative therapies as well as therapies that are nonpharmacologic and simple to implement to prevent and treat diseases such as Alzheimer's dementia and other catastrophic brain disorders. Nurses can educate patients and family members on the importance of habitual exercise as well as encourage the provision of consistent medical care, a suitable environment, adequate nutritional intake, and social interaction to help prevent mental and physical deterioration associated with certain disease states. These simple measures are easy to implement and may contribute significantly to the improvement of the individual's well-being in later life.

Reference: Jeffery S: Exercise may improve cognition in adults with memory impairment, *JAMA* 300:1027-1037, 1077-1079, 2008.

## ▌ PATIENT TEACHING TIPS

- Medications must be taken exactly as ordered and with meals to minimize GI upset. Medications are never to be increased except on the advice of the prescriber. Give specific instructions on what to do if a medication dose has been omitted.
- Intervals between doses of medication need to be timed consistently to optimize therapeutic effects and minimize adverse effects and toxicity.
- Encourage patients, family, significant others, and/or caregivers to call the prescriber or other health care provider if there is any increased muscle weakness, abdominal cramps, diarrhea, dizziness, ataxia, and/or difficulty breathing.
- Share information about community resources with patients, caregiver(s), family, and significant others. Such resources may include, but are not be limited to, Meals on Wheels; local, state, and national chapters of the Alzheimer's Association; adult day care and/or alternate care resources; special prescription services (e.g., Nationwide Prescription Assistance at the toll-free number 888-812-5152 or online at

www.freemedicinefoundation.com); and respite care and/or home health care services.
- Signs and symptoms of improvement of myasthenia gravis include a decrease in or absence of ptosis (eyelid drooping) and diplopia (double vision), less difficulty swallowing and chewing, and an improvement in muscle weakness. If the medication is being taken for myasthenia gravis, the patient needs to take it 30 minutes before meals so that the drug begins to work before the patient chews and swallows. This will help strengthen the muscles for chewing and eating.
- Sustained-released or extended-release dosage forms must be taken in their entirety and should not be crushed, chewed, or broken in any way.
- The patient needs to wear a medical alert bracelet or necklace or carry a medical alert card on his or her person at all times that gives the medical diagnoses and provides access to a list of medications and allergies, and any special requirements regarding emergency treatment.

## KEY POINTS

- *Cholinergics, cholinergic agonists,* and *parasympathomimetics* are all appropriate terms for the class of drugs that stimulate the parasympathetic nervous system, which is the branch of the autonomic nervous system that opposes the sympathetic nervous system.
- The primary neurotransmitter of the parasympathetic nervous system is acetylcholine, and there are two types of cholinergic receptors: nicotinic and muscarinic.
- Nursing considerations for the administration of cholinergic drugs include giving the drug as directed and monitoring the patient carefully for the occurrence of bradycardia, hypotension, headache, dizziness, respiratory depression, and bronchospasms. If these occur in a patient taking cholinergics, the prescriber must be contacted immediately.
- It may take up to 6 weeks for a therapeutic response to occur with some of the medications used with Alzheimer's disease.
- Patients taking cholinergics need to change positions slowly to avoid dizziness and fainting that may result from the adverse effect of postural hypotension.

## NCLEX® EXAMINATION REVIEW QUESTIONS

1 The nurse is reviewing the use of bethanechol (Urecholine) in a patient who is experiencing postoperative urinary retention. Which statement best describes the mechanism of action of bethanechol?
   a It causes decreased bladder tone and motility.
   b It causes increased bladder tone and motility.
   c It increases the sensation of a full bladder.
   d It causes the sphincters in the bladder to become tighter.

2 The family of a patient who has recently been diagnosed with Alzheimer's disease is asking about the new drug prescribed to treat this disease. The patient's wife says, "I'm so excited that there are drugs that can cure this disease! I can't wait for him to start treatment." Which reply from the nurse is appropriate?
   a "The sooner he starts the medicine, the sooner it can have this effect."
   b "These effects won't be seen for a few months."
   c "These drugs do not cure Alzheimer's disease. Let's talk about what the physician said to expect with this drug therapy."
   d "His response to this drug therapy will depend on how far along he is in the disease process."

3 The nurse is giving a dose of bethanechol (Urecholine) to a postoperative patient. The nurse is aware that contraindications to bethanechol include:
   a bladder atony.
   b peptic ulcer.
   c urinary retention.
   d hypothyroidism.

4 A patient took an accidental overdose of a cholinergic drug while at home. He comes to the emergency department with severe abdominal cramping and bloody diarrhea. The nurse expects that which drug will be used to treat this patient?

   a atropine (generic)
   b physostigmine (Antilirium)
   c bethanechol (Urecholine)
   d phentolamine (Regitine)

5 The nurse is reviewing the orders for a newly admitted patient and sees an order for edrophonium (Tensilon). The nurse expects that this drug is ordered for which reason?
   a To reduce symptoms and delay the onset of Alzheimer's disease
   b To treat the symptoms of myasthenia gravis
   c To aid in the diagnosis of myasthenia gravis
   d To reverse the effects of nondepolarizing neuromuscular blocking drugs after surgery

6 When giving intravenous cholinergic drugs, the nurse must watch for symptoms of a cholinergic crisis, such as: (Select all that apply.)
   a peripheral tingling.
   b hypotension.
   c dry mouth.
   d syncope.
   e dyspnea.
   f tinnitus.

7. A patient who has had an accidental overdose of tricyclic antidepressants is to receive physostigmine (Antilirium), 1.5 mg IM stat. The medication is available in a vial that contains 2 mL, with a concentration of 1 mg/mL. How much medication will the nurse draw up into the syringe for this dose?

1. b, 2. c, 3. b, 4. a, 5. c, 6. b, d, e, 7. 1.5 mL.

For Critical Thinking and Prioritization Questions, see http://evolve.elsevier.com/Lilley.

# Cholinergic-Blocking Drugs

## OBJECTIVES

When you reach the end of this chapter, you will be able to do the following:

1. Briefly review the functions of the sympathetic nervous system and the specific effects of blocking cholinergic receptors (parasympatholytic effects).
2. List the various drugs classified as cholinergic antagonists (blocking) or sympatholytics.
3. Discuss the mechanisms of action, therapeutic effects, indications, adverse and toxic effects, drug interactions, cautions, contraindications, dosages, routes of administration, and any antidotal management for the various cholinergic antagonists (blockers).
4. Develop a nursing care plan that includes all phases of the nursing process for patients taking cholinergic antagonists.

## DRUG PROFILES

- ◆ **atropine, p. 337**
- ◆ **dicyclomine, p. 337**
- **glycopyrrolate, p. 338**
- **oxybutynin, p. 339**

- **scopolamine, p. 339**
- ◆ **tolterodine, p. 339**

- ◆ *Key drug*

## KEY TERMS

**Cholinergic-blocking drugs** Drugs that block the action of acetylcholine and substances similar to acetylcholine at receptor sites in the synapse. (p. 335)

**Mydriasis** Dilation of the pupil of the eye caused by contraction of the dilator muscle of the iris. (p. 336)

**Parasympatholytics** Drugs that reduce the activity of the parasympathetic nervous system; also called *anticholinergics*. (p. 335)

## ANATOMY, PHYSIOLOGY, AND PATHOPHYSIOLOGY OVERVIEW

### PARASYMPATHETIC NERVOUS SYSTEM

The parasympathetic nervous system is the branch of the autonomic nervous system with nerve functions generally opposite those of the sympathetic nervous system (see Chapters 18 and 19 for a discussion of the sympathetic nervous system). Acetylcholine is the neurotransmitter responsible for the transmission of nerve impulses to effector cells in the parasympathetic nervous system. A cholinergic receptor is one that binds acetylcholine and mediates its actions. This chapter focuses on cholinergic-blocking drugs, which inhibit the effects of the parasympathetic nervous system.

## PHARMACOLOGY OVERVIEW

### CHOLINERGIC-BLOCKING DRUGS

*Cholinergic blockers, anticholinergics,* parasympatholytics, and *antimuscarinic drugs* are all terms that refer to the class of drugs that block or inhibit the actions of acetylcholine in the parasympathetic nervous system. These drugs were first discussed in Chapter 15 in relation to treatment of Parkinson's disease.

Cholinergic blockers have many therapeutic uses and are one of the oldest groups of therapeutic drugs. Originally they were derived from various plant sources, but today they are only part of a larger group of cholinergic blockers that also include synthetic and semisynthetic drugs. Box 21-1 lists the currently available cholinergic blockers.

### Mechanism of Action and Drug Effects

Cholinergic-blocking drugs block the action of the neurotransmitter acetylcholine at the muscarinic receptors in the parasympathetic nervous system (PNS). Acetylcholine that is released from a stimulated nerve fiber is then unable to bind to the receptor site and fails to produce a cholinergic effect. This is why the cholinergic blockers are also referred to as *anticholinergics.* Blocking the parasympathetic nerves allows the sympathetic (adrenergic) nervous system to dominate. Because of this, cholinergic blockers have many of the same effects as the adrenergics (see Chapter 18). Figure 21-1 illustrates the site of

action of the cholinergic blockers in the parasympathetic nervous system.

Cholinergic blockers are *competitive antagonists.* They compete with acetylcholine for binding at the muscarinic receptors of the parasympathetic nervous system. Once they have bound to the receptor, they inhibit cholinergic nerve transmission. This generally occurs at the neuroeffector junction, or the point where the nerve ending reaches the effector organs such as smooth muscle, cardiac muscle, and glands. Cholinergic blockers have little effect at the nicotinic receptors, although at high doses they can have partial blocking effects.

The major sites of action of the anticholinergics are the heart, respiratory tract, gastrointestinal (GI) tract, urinary bladder, eye, and exocrine glands (sweat gland, salivary gland). Anticholinergics have the opposite effects of the cholinergics

---

**BOX 21-1   CHOLINERGIC BLOCKERS GROUPED ACCORDING TO CHEMICAL CLASS**

**Natural Plant Alkaloids**
atropine (generic)
belladonna (Belladonna tincture)
hyoscyamine (Levsin)
scopolamine (Transderm-Scōp)

**Synthetic and Semisynthetic Drugs**
benztropine (Cogentin; see Chapter 16)
biperiden (Akineton)
darifenacin (Enablex)
dicyclomine (Bentyl)
fesoterodine (Toviaz)
glycopyrrolate (Robinul)
homatropine (Isopto Homatropine; see Chapter 57)
ipratropium (Atrovent; see Chapter 37)
mepenzolate (Cantil)
methscopolamine (Pamine)
oxybutynin (Ditropan)
procyclidine (Kemadrin)
propantheline (Pro-Banthine)
solifenacin (Vesicare)
tolterodine (Detrol)
trihexyphenidyl (generic; see Chapter 15)
trospium (Sanctura)

---

**FIGURE 21-1** Site of action of cholinergic blockers in the parasympathetic nervous system. *ACh,* Acetylcholine.

| TABLE 21-1 | CHOLINERGIC BLOCKERS: DRUG EFFECTS |
|---|---|
| **BODY SYSTEM** | **CHOLINERGIC-BLOCKING EFFECTS** |
| Cardiovascular | Small doses: decrease heart rate |
| | Large doses: increase heart rate |
| Central nervous | Small doses: decrease muscle rigidity and tremors |
| | Large doses: cause drowsiness, disorientation, hallucinations |
| Eye | Dilate pupils (mydriasis), decrease accommodation by paralyzing ciliary muscles (cycloplegia) |
| Gastrointestinal | Relax smooth muscle tone of gastrointestinal tract, decrease intestinal and gastric secretions, decrease motility and peristalsis |
| Genitourinary | Relax detrusor muscle of bladder, increase constriction of internal sphincter; these two effects may result in urinary retention |
| Glandular | Decrease bronchial secretions, salivation, and sweating |
| Respiratory | Decrease bronchial secretions, dilate bronchial airways |

(see Chapter 20) at these sites of action. Anticholinergic effects on the cardiovascular system are seen as an increase in heart rate. Respiratory system effects are dry mucous membranes and bronchial dilation. In the GI tract, cholinergic blockers cause a decrease in GI motility, GI secretions, and salivation. In the genitourinary (GU) system, they lead to decreased bladder contraction, which can result in urinary retention. In the skin they reduce sweating, and finally, anticholinergics cause the pupils to dilate and increase intraocular pressure. This occurs because the ciliary muscles and the sphincter muscle of the iris are innervated by cholinergic nerve fibers. Cholinergic blockers keep the sphincter muscle of the iris from contracting. The result is dilation of the pupil (mydriasis) and paralysis of the ocular lens (cycloplegia). This can be detrimental to patients with glaucoma because it results in increased intraocular pressure (see Chapter 57). These and other effects are listed by body system in Table 21-1. Many of the cholinergic-blocking drugs are available in a variety of forms, including intravenous, intramuscular, oral, and subcutaneous preparations.

## Indications

In the central nervous system, cholinergic blockers have the therapeutic effect of decreasing muscle rigidity and diminishing tremors. This is of benefit in the treatment of both Parkinson's disease (see Chapter 15) and drug-induced extrapyramidal reactions such as those associated with antipsychotic drugs (see Chapter 16). These conditions involve dysfunction of the extrapyramidal parts of the brain and include motor dysfunctions such as chorea, dystonia, and dyskinesia.

Cardiovascular effects of anticholinergics are related to their cholinergic-blocking actions on the heart's conduction system. At low dosages, the anticholinergics may actually slow the heart rate through their effects on the cardiac center in the portion of the brain called the *medulla.* At high dosages, cholinergic blockers block the inhibitory vagal (i.e.,

parasympathetic or cholinergic) effects on the pacemaker cells of the sinoatrial and atrioventricular nodes, which leads to acceleration of the heart rate due to unopposed sympathetic activity. Atropine is used primarily in the management of cardiovascular disorders, such as in the diagnosis of sinus node dysfunction, the treatment of patients with symptomatic second-degree atrioventricular block, and provision of advanced life support in the treatment of sinus bradycardia that is accompanied by hemodynamic compromise. It also has ophthalmic uses (see Chapter 57).

When the cholinergic stimulation of the parasympathetic nervous system is blocked by cholinergic blockers, the sympathetic nervous system effects go unopposed. In the respiratory tract, this results in decreased secretions from the nose, mouth, pharynx, and bronchi. It also causes relaxation of the smooth muscles in the bronchi and bronchioles, which results in decreased airway resistance and bronchodilation. Because of this, the cholinergic blockers have proved beneficial in treating exercise-induced bronchospasm, chronic bronchitis, asthma, and chronic obstructive pulmonary disease. They are also used preoperatively to reduce salivary secretions, which aids in intubation and other procedures (e.g., endoscopy) involving the oral cavity.

Gastric secretions and the smooth muscles responsible for producing gastric motility are both controlled by the parasympathetic nervous system, which is primarily under the control of muscarinic receptors. Cholinergic blockers antagonize these receptors, causing reduced secretions, relaxation of smooth muscle, and reduced GI motility and peristalsis. For these reasons, cholinergic blockers are commonly used in the treatment of irritable bowel disease and GI hypersecretory states.

Anticholinergics are useful in the treatment of such GU tract disorders as reflex neurogenic bladder and incontinence. They relax the detrusor muscles of the bladder and increase constriction of the internal sphincter. The ability of cholinergic blockers to decrease glandular secretions also makes them potentially useful drugs for reducing gastric and pancreatic secretions in patients with acute pancreatitis.

## Contraindications

Contraindications to the use of anticholinergic drugs include known drug allergy, angle-closure glaucoma, acute asthma or other respiratory distress, myasthenia gravis, acute cardiovascular instability (some exceptions were listed previously), and GI or GU tract obstruction (e.g., benign prostatic hyperplasia) or other acute GI or GU illness.

## Adverse Effects

Anticholinergic drugs cause widely varied adverse effects, with many body systems affected. The various adverse effects of cholinergic blockers are listed by body system in Table 21-2. Certain patient populations are more susceptible to the effects of the anticholinergics. These populations include infants, children with Down syndrome, those with spastic paralysis or brain damage, and the elderly. The elderly are extremely sensitive to the CNS effects of anticholinergics, and it is not uncommon for elderly patients to develop delirium due to anticholinergic effects.

## TABLE 21-2   CHOLINERGIC BLOCKERS: ADVERSE EFFECTS

| BODY SYSTEM | ADVERSE EFFECTS |
| --- | --- |
| Cardiovascular | Increased heart rate, dysrhythmias (tachycardia, palpitations) |
| Central nervous | Excitation, restlessness, irritability, disorientation, hallucinations, delirium, ataxia, drowsiness, sedation, confusion |
| Eye | Dilated pupils (causing blurred vision), increased intraocular pressure |
| Gastrointestinal | Decreased salivation, gastric secretions, and motility (causing constipation) |
| Genitourinary | Urinary retention |
| Glandular | Decreased sweating |
| Respiratory | Decreased bronchial secretions |

## Toxicity and Management of Overdose

The dosage of cholinergic blockers is particularly important, because there is a very small difference between therapeutic and toxic dosages. Drugs with this characteristic are commonly referred to as having a *low therapeutic index* (see Chapter 2). The treatment of cholinergic blocker overdose consists of symptomatic and supportive therapy. The patient should be hospitalized, with continuous monitoring, including continuous electrocardiographic monitoring. Activated charcoal has proven very effective in removing from the GI tract any drug that has not yet been absorbed.

Fluid therapy and other standard measures used for the treatment of shock are instituted as needed. Delirium, hallucinations, coma, and cardiac dysrhythmias respond favorably to treatment with the cholinergic drug physostigmine. Its routine use as an antidote for cholinergic blocker overdose is controversial because it has the potential to produce severe adverse effects (e.g., seizures and cardiac asystole) and is usually reserved for the treatment of patients who show extreme delirium or agitation or who could inflict injury upon themselves.

## Interactions

Drug interactions most commonly reported for the anticholinergics are additive anticholinergic effects when taken with other drugs that possess anticholinergic side effects such as amantadine (see Chapter 15), antihistamines (see Chapter 36), and tricyclic antidepressants (see Chapter 16). Reduced antipsychotic effects of phenothiazines (see Chapter 16) are seen when taken with anticholinergic drugs, and increased effects of digoxin (see Chapter 24) are seen when combined with anticholinergics.

## Dosages

For dosage information on selected cholinergic blockers, see the table on p. 338.

## DRUG PROFILES

Among the oldest and best known naturally occurring cholinergic blockers are the belladonna alkaloids. Of these, atropine is the prototypical drug. It has been in use for hundreds of years and continues to be widely administered because of its effectiveness. Besides atropine, scopolamine and hyoscyamine are the other major naturally occurring drugs. These drugs come from a variety of plants in the potato family.

Cholinergic blockers are used in the treatment of a variety of illnesses and conditions ranging from irritable bowel syndrome to the symptoms of the common cold and are also administered preoperatively to dry up secretions. They are the synthetic counterparts of the plant-derived belladonna alkaloids and are more specific in binding predominantly with muscarinic receptors. They are also associated with fewer adverse effects. Adverse effects and drug interactions are comparable for the different anticholinergic drugs and are detailed in Table 21-2 and previous text, respectively, unless otherwise noted.

### ♦ atropine

Atropine is a naturally occurring antimuscarinic. Atropine is more potent than scopolamine in its cholinergic-blocking effects on the heart and in its effects on the smooth muscles of the bronchi and intestines. Atropine is effective in the treatment of many of the conditions that are previously listed in the Indications section. Because atropine causes increased heart rate, it is used to treat bradycardia and ventricular asystole. Atropine is also used as an antidote for anticholinesterase inhibitor toxicity or poisoning. It is also used preoperatively to reduce salivation and GI secretions, as is glycopyrrolate. Atropine is contraindicated in patients with angle-closure glaucoma, adhesions between the iris and lens, certain types of asthma (not cholinergic associated), advanced hepatic and renal dysfunction, hiatal hernia associated with reflux esophagitis, intestinal atony, obstructive GI or GU conditions, and severe ulcerative colitis. Use with caution in patients with dysrhythmias (see Chapter 25). It is available in injectable, oral, and ophthalmic forms (see Chapter 57). It is also combined with the opiate diphenoxylate to make Lomotil tablets, a common antidiarrheal preparation. Overdose of atropine (usually from taking excessive Lomotil) is associated with flushing, dry skin and mucous membranes, mydriasis, altered mental status, and fever. Other serious effects include sinus tachycardia, urinary retention, hypertension, hallucinations, respiratory depression, and cardiovascular collapse. Activated charcoal is usually given along with supportive care. The reversible anticholinesterase inhibitor, physostigmine (see Chapter 20) is the antidote for atropine overdose. Recommended dosages are given in the table on p. xxx.

### Pharmacokinetics

| Route | Onset of Action | Peak Plasma Concentration | Elimination Half-life | Duration of Action |
| --- | --- | --- | --- | --- |
| IV | Immediate | 2-4 min | 2.5 hr | 4-6 hr |

### ♦ dicyclomine

Dicyclomine (Bentyl) is a synthetic antispasmodic cholinergic blocker used primarily in the treatment of functional disturbances of GI motility such as irritable bowel syndrome. It has

## DOSAGES

### Selected Cholinergic Antagonist (Anticholinergic) Drugs

| DRUG (PREGNANCY CATEGORY) | USUAL DOSAGE RANGE | INDICATIONS/USES |
|---|---|---|
| ◆ atropine (generic) (C) | **Pediatric**<br>0.02 mg/kg, max 0.5 mg<br>0.05 mg/kg initial dose, repeat q10-30min prn<br><br>**Adult**<br>IV: 0.5-1 mg (max 3 mg)<br>IV: 1-3 mg/dose, repeat prn until signs of atropine intoxication appear (e.g., tachycardia) | Treatment of bradycardia<br>Anticholinesterase effect for organophosphate or carbamate poisoning (e.g., insecticides)<br><br>Treatment of bradycardia, cardiopulmonary resuscitation<br>Anticholinesterase effect for organophosphate or carbamate poisoning (e.g., insecticides) |
| ◆ dicyclomine (Bentyl) (B) | **Pediatric**<br>PO: 5-10 mg tid-qid<br>**Adult**<br>PO: 80-160 mg/day divided qid | Treatment of irritable bowel syndrome |
| glycopyrrolate (Robinul) (B) | **Pediatric**<br>IM/IV: 4-9 mcg/kg/dose<br>**Adult and pediatric 12 yr and older**<br>IM: 4 mcg/kg 30-60 min preoperative<br>**Adult and pediatric**<br>0.2 mg for each 1 mg of neostigmine or 5 mg of pyridostigmine | Preoperative control of secretions<br><br>Preoperative control of secretions<br><br>Reversal of neuromuscular blockade |
| oxybutynin (Ditropan, Ditropan XL, Oxytrol [transdermal patch]) | **Pediatric 1-5 yr**<br>PO: 0.2 mg/kg/dose bid-qid<br>**Adult and pediatric older than 5 yr**<br>PO: 5 mg bid-qid<br>**Adult only**<br>PO ER tab: 5-30 mg/day in single or divided doses<br>**Adult**<br>Transdermal patch: 1 patch (3.9 mg/day) applied twice weekly (every 3-4 days) (for overactive bladder) | Antispasmodic for neurogenic bladder (e.g., following spinal cord injury), overactive bladder |
| scopolamine (generic injection; Transderm-Scōp patch) (C) | **Pediatric**<br>6 mcg/kg/dose, max 0.3 mg/dose; may repeat q6-8h<br>**Adult**<br>IM/IV/subcut: 0.3-0.65 mg<br>Transdermal patch: 1.5 mg patch behind ear every 3 days (delivers approx 1 mg scopolamine over 3 days); apply at least 4 hr before transportation | Preoperative control of secretions<br><br>Preoperative control of secretions<br>Motion sickness prevention |
| ◆ tolterodine (Detrol, Detrol XL) (C) | **Adult only**<br>PO: 1-2 mg bid<br>PO ER cap: 2-4 mg daily | Treatment of overactive bladder |

*ER,* Extended release; *IM,* intramuscular; *IV,* intravenous; *PO,* oral; *subcut,* subcutaneous.

also been used alone and in combination with phenobarbital for the treatment of colic and enterocolitis in infants. It is contraindicated in patients who have a known hypersensitivity to anticholinergics and in those with angle-closure glaucoma, GI tract obstruction, myasthenia gravis, paralytic ileus, GI atony, or toxic megacolon. It is available in injectable and oral form. Recommended dosages are given in the table on this page.

### Pharmacokinetics

| Route | Onset of Action | Peak Plasma Concentration | Elimination Half-life | Duration of Action |
|---|---|---|---|---|
| PO | 1-2 hr | 60-90 min | 9-10 hr | 3-4 hr |

### glycopyrrolate

Glycopyrrolate (Robinul) is a synthetic antimuscarinic drug that blocks receptor sites in the autonomic nervous system that control the production of secretions and the concentration of free acids in the stomach. It is most commonly used preoperatively to reduce salivation and excessive secretions in the respiratory and GI tracts. It is contraindicated in patients who are hypersensitive to it and in those with angle-closure glaucoma, myasthenia gravis, GI or GU tract obstruction, tachycardia, myocardial ischemia, hepatic disease, ulcerative colitis, or toxic megacolon. Glycopyrrolate is available in injectable and oral form. Recommended dosages are given in the table on this page.

## Pharmacokinetics

| Route | Onset of Action | Peak Plasma Concentration | Elimination Half-life | Duration of Action |
|---|---|---|---|---|
| IV | 1 min | 10-15 min | Variable | 4 hr |
| PO | Up to 45 min | 1 hr | Variable | 6 hr |

### oxybutynin

Oxybutynin (Ditropan) is a synthetic antimuscarinic drug used for the treatment of overactive bladder. It is also used as an antispasmodic for neurogenic bladder associated with spinal cord injuries and congenital conditions such as spina bifida. Contraindications include drug allergy, urinary or gastric retention, and uncontrolled angle-closure glaucoma. Oxybutynin is available for oral use. A transdermal patch (Oxytrol) is also available and approved for treatment of overactive bladder. Recommended dosages are given in the table on p. 338.

## Pharmacokinetics

| Route | Onset of Action | Peak Plasma Concentration | Elimination Half-life | Duration of Action |
|---|---|---|---|---|
| PO | Unknown | 1 hr | 2-3 hr | Unknown |

### scopolamine

Scopolamine is a naturally occurring cholinergic blocker and one of the principal belladonna alkaloids. It is the most potent antimuscarinic for the prevention of motion sickness. It works by correcting the imbalance between acetylcholine and norepinephrine in the higher centers in the brain, particularly in the vomiting center. Ipratropium, a derivative of scopolamine, has potent therapeutic effects on the lungs and is discussed in Chapter 37. Scopolamine is available in several different delivery systems. For the prevention of motion sickness, it is available in a transdermal delivery system (Transderm-Scōp), a patch that can be applied just behind the ear 4 to 5 hours before travel (see Chapter 52). Transdermal scopolamine may cause drowsiness, dry mouth, and blurred vision. Using scopolamine with central nervous system depressants or alcohol may increase sedation. Scopolamine is also available in parenteral formulations for injection by various routes: intravenous, intramuscular, and subcutaneous. Scopolamine is available for ocular indications and in oral form. The contraindications that apply to atropine apply to scopolamine as well. Recommended dosages are given in the table on p. 338.

## Pharmacokinetics

| Route | Onset of Action | Peak Plasma Concentration | Elimination Half-life | Duration of Action |
|---|---|---|---|---|
| IV | 30-60 min | 30-45 min | Variable | 4 hr |
| Transdermal | 4-5 hr | 6 hr | Variable | 72 hr |

### ◆ tolterodine

Tolterodine (Detrol) is a muscarinic receptor blocker used for the treatment of urinary frequency, urgency, and urge incontinence caused by bladder (detrusor) overactivity. Another drug that is commonly used to treat these conditions is oxybutynin (profiled previously). Other older-generation drugs include propantheline, hyoscyamine, and the tricyclic antidepressant imipramine. These drugs are less commonly used today because of their antimuscarinic adverse effects, particularly dry mouth. Newer drugs for this purpose include solifenacin (Vesicare), darifenacin (Enablex), trospium (Sanctura), and fesoterodine (Toviaz). The newer drugs are associated with a much lower incidence of dry mouth, in part because of their pharmacologic specificity for the bladder as opposed to the salivary glands.

Tolterodine is to be avoided in patients with angle-closure glaucoma or urinary retention. In patients with markedly decreased hepatic function or poor metabolizers taking drugs that inhibit cytochrome P-450 enzyme 3A4 (e.g., erythromycin or ketoconazole), the dose is reduced to 1 mg twice a day instead of the normal recommended dose of 2 mg twice a day. Tolterodine is available only for oral use. Recommended dosages are given in the table on p. 338.

## Pharmacokinetics

| Route | Onset of Action | Peak Plasma Concentration | Elimination Half-life | Duration of Action |
|---|---|---|---|---|
| PO | 1 hr | 1-2 hr | 2-4 hr | 5 hr |

# NURSING PROCESS

# ASSESSMENT

The drugs known as *parasympatholytics, cholinergic blockers, cholinergic antagonists,* or *anticholinergics* (an older term) produce a number of physiologic effects that result from the blocking of cholinergic receptors. These effects include smooth muscle relaxation, decreased glandular secretion, and mydriasis (pupil dilation). Knowing the way these drugs work and the related physiology will assist you in the safe assessment and nursing care of patients taking these drugs. A thorough medical history; complete medication history with a listing of prescription drugs, over-the-counter drugs, and herbals; as well as a thorough head-to-toe examination will help you identify the presence of any contraindications, cautions, and/or potential drug interactions associated with the cholinergic blocking drugs (see Pharmacology Overview). The assessment data will help you document baseline findings and provide information for evaluating drug effectiveness. Lifespan considerations for the very young and/or elderly patient include the need for close assessment and monitoring because of the increased susceptibility of these groups to the adverse effects of restlessness, irritability, disorientation, constipation, urinary retention, blurred vision (from pupil dilation), and tachycardia.

In your assessment associated with atropine and other cholinergic blockers, check for allergies, glaucoma, certain eye conditions (e.g., adhesions in the iris and lens of the eye), gastroesophageal reflux disease, poor intestinal motility, obstructions of the GI and GU systems, and severe ulcerative colitis. These conditions and others may be exacerbated

## PATIENT-CENTERED CARE: LIFESPAN CONSIDERATIONS FOR THE ELDERLY PATIENT

### Overactive Bladder

- Overactive bladder affects more than 12 million American adults, and the incidence of this disorder increases with age.
- Some questions to pose to the elderly patient regarding this condition are as follows:
  - Do you ever have a sudden and strong urge to urinate?
  - Do you urinate more than eight times in a 24-hour period?
  - Do you have to get up more than two times during the night to urinate?
  - Do you have "wetting" accidents?
  - Are these "wetting" accidents related to the uncontrollable urge to urinate?

  NOTE: If the patient answers yes to some of these questions, the patient needs to be encouraged to contact his or her primary health care provider. Referral to a urologist may or may not be necessary.

- Various treatments for overactive bladder are available nationwide in the United States including the use of solifenacin succinate (Vesicare), which is to be taken once daily and treats all of the major symptoms of overactive bladder, including urgency, frequency, and urge-related incontinence.
- Solifenacin succinate was found to reduce the number of incontinence episodes over 12 weeks in studies of the drug involving more than 3000 patients with overactive bladder symptoms. Five- to 10-mg dosing of the drug produced improvement in all of the major symptoms. Use of this drug is contraindicated in patients with glaucoma, certain gastrointestinal or genitourinary tract problems, severe constipation, and/or urinary retention. Adverse effects include dry mouth, constipation, and blurred vision. If a patient experiences severe abdominal pain or is constipated for 3 or more days, the patient needs to contact the prescriber immediately.

Data from WebMD: Overactive bladder health check, 2011, available at www.webmd.com/urinary-incontinence-oab/overactive-bladder-health-check/default.htm. Accessed November 16, 2011; Vesicare (solifenacin succinate) website, 2011, available at www.vesicare.com.

by the cholinergic blockers (see Pharmacology Overview in this chapter and in Chapters 18 to 20) and would be considered contraindications. Address the associated cautions, contraindications, and drug interactions with dicyclomine, glycopyrrolate, and oxybutynin. Also, note any disorders of the bladder or GI tract. Apply the transdermal dosage form of scopolamine only after the order has been reviewed and the skin assessed.

## NURSING DIAGNOSES

1. Constipation related to adverse effects of cholinergic-blocking drugs
2. Deficient knowledge related to lack of information about the therapeutic regimen, adverse effects, drug interactions, and precautions related to the use of cholinergic-blocking drugs
3. Risk for injury related to decreased sweating and loss of normal heat-regulating mechanisms due to the impact of the drug on the temperature-regulating mechanisms

## PLANNING

### GOALS

1. Patient experiences minimal adverse effects such as constipation.
2. Patient demonstrates adequate knowledge about the use of the specific medication, adverse effects, and appropriate dosing at home.
3. Patient is free from injury resulting from the adverse effect of inability to regulate sweating.

### OUTCOME CRITERIA

1. Patient states various measures to regain normal bowel patterns and avoids constipation by forcing fluids and increasing fiber in daily dietary intake.
   - Patient increases fluids up to 8 glasses (preferably of water) per day.

- Patient starts foods high in fiber, such as generous amounts of vegetables, fruits and legumes, to help take in approximately 40 g/day.
- Patient uses a natural fiber supplement, if not contraindicated, such as a psyllium-based fiber product.
2. Patient states the rationale for the use of cholinergic blockers, such as preoperative preparation, decreasing side effects associated with drugs used for Alzheimer's disease, and irritable bowel syndrome.
   - Patient states the more common adverse effects associated with cholinergic blockers, such as dry mouth, constipation, and urinary retention.
   - Patient states those adverse effects that need to be reported immediately to the prescriber if they occur, such as unresolved constipation, pain over the bladder region and inability to urinate, and/or chest pain.
3. Patient states measures to help decrease impact of decreased ability to sweat such as avoiding hot climates, vigorous exercising (especially in heated or hot environments), saunas, and hot tubs.
   - Patients who are elderly identify their increased risk to being overwhelmed by the decreased ability to sweat and the need for adherence to the above situations.

## IMPLEMENTATION

A preventative focus for nursing care is important to the effective use of *cholinergic-blocking drugs*, especially with regard to patient teaching about how to decrease the need for these medications. There are several nursing interventions that may maximize the therapeutic effects of these drugs and minimize the adverse effects. Some important nursing interventions include giving the drug at the same time each day and per the prescriber's orders, and giving the medication with adequate fluid intake (6 to 8 glasses of water daily).

Because drugs such as atropine and glycopyrrolate are compatible with some of the commonly used opioids (e.g., meperidine and morphine), they may be used in combination with these drugs and mixed in the same syringe for parenteral dosing. Checking for the compatibility of drugs combined in the same syringe is important with any medication. Always double-check compatibility for patient safety. If a cholinergic-blocking drug is given via the ophthalmic route, always check the concentration of the drug and, once it is given, apply light pressure with a tissue to the inner canthus of the eye for approximately 30 to 60 seconds. This helps to minimize the possibility of systemic absorption of the drug.

Atropine may be combined with other cholinergic-blocking drugs (e.g., hyoscyamine) for treatment of lower urinary tract discomfort or to help decrease GI and GU hypermotility, but give the drug via the correct route and with proper dosing as prescribed. The anticholinergic adverse effect of dry mouth may be managed with frequent mouth care, oral rinses, increase in fluids, and use of sugar-free gum or hard candy. Oxybutynin needs to be taken as directed either 1 hour before or 2 hours after meals, if tolerated. Tolterodine must be taken as directed and with food. Transdermal forms of these medications (e.g., scopolamine, oxybutynin) are to be applied to the skin only after the previous dosage form has been removed and the area gently cleansed of residual medication. Transdermal patches may be applied to any dry, nonhairy, nonirritated area. Rotation of transdermal sites is recommended to decrease skin irritation. Also associated with the cholinergic-blocking drugs are the adverse effects of constipation and inability to sweat or perspire. Because these may be significant to patients, include education on how to minimize these adverse effects. See the Patient Teaching Tips below for more information on these specific drugs.

## EVALUATION

Monitoring of goals and outcome criteria is a starting place for effective evaluation of therapy with these medications. In particular, therapeutic effects of cholinergic-blocking drugs include the following: (1) improved ability to carry out activities of daily living and fewer problems with tremors, salivation, and drooling in patients with Parkinson's disease; (2) decreased GI symptoms, such as hyperacidity, abdominal pain, and

nausea and vomiting, with improved comfort; (3) decreased GU hypermotility, with increased comfort and improved patterns of voiding with an increase in time between voidings; and (4) fewer bronchospasms with induction of anesthesia and fewer problems with thickened, viscous secretions in patients before, during, and after surgery. Monitor the patient for the occurrence of adverse effects such as constipation, tachycardia, palpitations, confusion, sedation, drowsiness, hallucinations, urinary retention, and decreased sweating leading to hot, dry skin. Toxic effects of anticholinergics include delirium, hallucinations, and cardiac dysrhythmias.

---

## CASE STUDY

### Transdermal Scopolamine

Jan, a 53-year-old schoolteacher, is going on a cruise to Alaska with her husband, Jake, for their thirtieth anniversary. She is very excited about the trip but is also worried because she gets "very seasick" whenever she is on a boat. She calls her doctor's office for a prescription for a medicine for motion sickness. Her physician prescribes transdermal scopolamine (Transderm-Scōp).

1. Before Jan picks up the prescription, the nurse assesses for contraindications to scopolamine. What are the contraindications to the use of the scopolamine patch?

The nurse provides patient education, and Jan indicates that she understands how to use the patch. On the first day of the cruise, she applies the patch 4 hours before they board the ship.

2. That evening, Jan and Jake go to dinner. Jan is feeling somewhat drowsy, but thirsty. The waiter asks if they would like to have champagne as part of the first-night-of-the-cruise celebration. How should Jan respond?

3. The next morning, while out on the deck, Jake and Jan are taking pictures of the bright, snow-covered shoreline views. Jake looks at Jan and exclaims, "Look at your eyes! Is that a side effect of that patch?" What has Jake noticed about Jan's blue eyes? What would you suggest for Jan because of what Jake has noticed?

4. Later that day, Jan tells Jake, "I'm feeling great! I don't think I need this patch. I'm going to take it off, but I'll save it for later in case I get nauseated." Is this a good idea? Explain your answer.

For answers, see http://evolve.elsevier.com/Lilley.

---

## PATIENT TEACHING TIPS

- Medications need to be taken exactly as prescribed. Overdosage of anticholinergics may cause life-threatening problems, especially in the cardiovascular and central nervous systems.
- Anticholinergics may lead to dry mouth. Regular and thorough oral hygiene is required with brushing of teeth twice daily and dental flossing. Dry mouth may be minimized by forcing fluids, if not contraindicated, use of artificial saliva drops/gum, or sucking on sugar-free hard candy, as needed. Encourage regularly scheduled dental visits because of the risk of dental caries and gum disease with dry mouth. The use of water pick devices may stimulate gums and help prevent gum disease.

- Exercise must be done with caution and excessive sweating avoided because of drug-induced altered sweating. This may cause hyperthermia in the elderly or those with already altered sweating mechanisms.
- If there is sedation and/or blurred vision, the patient needs to avoid driving or engaging in activities that require quick decision making, alertness, or clear vision, such as operating heavy machinery, taking tests, and making important decisions. The adverse effects of sedation will decrease over time.
- Encourage the patient to wear dark or tinted glasses or sunglasses because of the increased sensitivity to light associated with these medications.

## PATIENT TEACHING TIPS—cont'd

- The patient must understand the importance of always consulting the prescriber or other health care provider before taking any other medications, including prescription drugs, over-the-counter medications, herbals, and supplements.
- The elderly patient has existing age-related changes in body temperature–regulating mechanisms. With these medications, especially at high dosages, there is an increased risk of heat stroke or hyperthermia because of the drug's interference with the body's heat-regulating mechanisms. To prevent hyperthermia in the elderly, they need to stay in shaded areas or inside in an air-conditioned or cooled environment when external temperatures are warm; remain well hydrated with cool fluids; wear protective clothing and hats; avoid saunas, hot tubs, excessive heat, and strenuous exercise in warm environments; and keep portable fans on hand and maintain adequate ventilation in heated environments.
- All health care providers need to be informed about the treatment regimen, and a list of the patient's drugs must be given to all involved in the care of a patient taking anticholinergics or cholinergic blockers. The prescriber needs to be contacted if there is any unresolved constipation, palpitations, alterations in gait or balance, excessive dizziness, or inability to void.
- Constipation may be managed by the increased dietary intake of fluids and fiber and/or the use of over-the-counter fiber-containing supplements, such as psyllium products.

## KEY POINTS

- *Cholinergic blockers, parasympatholytics, anticholinergics,* and *antimuscarinics* are all terms that refer to the drugs that block or inhibit the actions of acetylcholine in the parasympathetic nervous system.
- The use of these cholinergic blockers allows the sympathetic nervous system to dominate. These drugs are classified chemically as natural, semisynthetic, and synthetic cholinergic blockers. These drugs may be competitive antagonists (blockers) and compete with acetylcholine at the muscarinic receptors. In high dosages, they result in partial blocking actions at the nicotinic receptors.

## NCLEX® EXAMINATION REVIEW QUESTIONS

1. The nurse is providing education about cholinergic-blocking drug therapy to an elderly patient. Which is an important point to emphasize for this patient?
   a Avoid exposure to high temperatures.
   b Limit liquid intake to avoid fluid overload.
   c Begin an exercise program to avoid adverse effects.
   d Stop the medication if excessive mouth dryness occurs.
2. The nurse is giving a cholinergic-blocking drug and will assess the patient for which contraindications to these drugs?
   a Chronic bronchitis
   b Peptic ulcer disease
   c Irritable bowel syndrome
   d Benign prostatic hyperplasia
3. When assessing for adverse effects of cholinergic-blocking drug therapy, the nurse would expect to find that the patient complains of which drug effect?
   a Diaphoresis
   b Dry mouth
   c Diarrhea
   d Urinary frequency
4. The nurse administering a cholinergic-blocking drug to a patient who is experiencing drug-induced extrapyramidal effects would assess for which therapeutic effect?
   a Decreased muscle rigidity and tremors
   b Increased heart rate
   c Decreased bronchial secretions
   d Decreased GI motility and peristalsis
5. During the assessment of a patient about to receive a cholinergic-blocking drug, the nurse will determine whether the patient is taking any drugs that may potentially interact with the anticholinergic, including:
   a opioids, such as morphine sulfate.
   b antibiotics, such as penicillin.
   c tricyclic antidepressants, such as amitriptyline.
   d anticonvulsants, such as phenobarbital.
6. A patient has been given a prescription for transdermal scopolamine patches (Transderm-Scōp) for motion sickness for use during a vacation cruise. The nurse will include which instructions? (Select all that apply.)
   a "Apply the patch as soon as you board the ship."
   b "Apply the patch 3 to 4 hours before boarding the ship."
   c "The patch needs to be placed on a nonhairy area on your upper chest or upper arm."
   d "The patch needs to be placed on a nonhairy area just behind your ear."
   e "Change the patch every 3 days."
   f "Rotate the application sites."
7. The preoperative order for an adult patient reads: "Give scopolamine, 0.7 mg IM on call for surgery." The medication is available in vials of 0.4 mg/mL. How many milliliters will the nurse administer for this dose? (Round to tenths.)

*For answers see back of book.*

1. a, 2. d, 3. b, 4. a, 5. c, 6. b, d, e, f, 7. 1.8 mL.

For Critical Thinking and Prioritization Questions, see http://evolve.elsevier.com/Lilley.

# Drugs Affecting the Cardiovascular and Renal Systems

Linking Learning • Text Notation

## LINKING LEARNING

The Part 3 Study Skills Tips stressed the importance of planning for the part as a whole. With that in mind, what is the focus of Part 4? The part title is Drugs Affecting the Cardiovascular and Renal Systems. What is the first question you think you should ask about this part? I would begin by asking, "What are the cardiovascular and renal systems?" This is a very obvious question and might seem to be so basic that it need not be asked, but the next eight chapters will all develop around this part title. Asking the obvious question is sometimes exactly the thing that should be done to get started.

### Chapter Structure

Just as there is a structure to each part in the text, which is constant from one part to the next, there is also a structure in the chapters. This structure is a repeating model that was created by the authors in an attempt to organize the material and present it in the clearest way possible. The chapter structure is a valuable learning asset for those who make use of it .

### Chapter Objectives

Each chapter begins with a set of objectives. These are established by the authors and serve to tell you what they expect you will know and be able to do when you have completed the chapter. It is sometimes tempting to ignore the objectives and get right on with the task of reading the chapter. Do not give in to that temptation. Read the objectives and spend some time thinking about what they reveal about the content of the chapter.

#### Example Based on Chapter 24 Objectives

*Objective 1:* Differentiate between the terms *inotropic*, *chronotropic*, and *dromotropic*.

What can you learn from this objective? First, there is the vocabulary. This objective makes it clear that you have some terms to learn. This means that you may want to have some blank note cards available to start setting up vocabulary cards for this chapter. In fact, you should write each of the terms in Objective 1 on a separate card and be ready to complete the card as the terms are introduced and explained in the chapter.

The next thing that stands out in this first objective is that the three terms contain a common element: -*tropic*. This should bring active questioning into play. What does the suffix -*tropic* mean? Asking this question now is a way of noting that these three terms do have some common meaning. Also it serves to provide an immediate focus for personal learning when you begin to read the chapter.

*Objective 2:* Briefly discuss the pathophysiology of heart failure.

From this comes the potential for a new question relating to the first objective. What do *inotropic, chronotropic,* and *dromotropic* have to do with the heart? Just as it is essential to see the relationship between parts and chapters, it is also essential to see relationships within the chapters. These first two objectives should cause you to consider those relationships and make your own learning much more active.

## Chapter Headings

The next chapter structure to consider in this process is the chapter headings. Chapter 24 has the major sections Anatomy, Physiology, and Pathophysiology Overview; Pharmacology Overview; and Nursing Process. What is the importance of this heading structure? It tells you that the authors will focus on the pharmacologic aspects first and then explain how this relates to nursing. This does not tell the learner a great deal about what to anticipate in terms of chapter content, but it does make clear a structure that is consistent in most of the chapters in this text.

Heart failure drugs are broken down into subsections in this chapter. Spend several minutes considering the organization of these subsections. The first subtopic to consider is Mechanism of Action and Drug Effects. What is meant by mechanism of action? How do heart failure drugs act? On what do they act? It does not matter that you cannot answer these questions at this point. What is important is that you ask them as a means of fostering an active and participatory learning attitude when you begin to read the chapter. Think, question, anticipate, and then read. This sequence will enhance your learning.

Continue this process of looking at the subtopics and thinking ahead to what will be explained in the chapter. These subsections are the same in every chapter, and this thinking process should become automatic very quickly.

## Key Terms

The next chapter structure is one that has already been stressed in previous Study Skills Tips, and it is one that is essential to learning. The list of key terms is a mini-dictionary for each chapter. Words that have not been introduced earlier in the text and that are central to the content of this chapter are presented here. The listing is in alphabetical order, which means that the key terms will not necessarily occur in the same order in the body of the chapter.

Hypercholesterolemia, a condition in which greater-than-normal amounts of cholesterol...

As you read the key terms, be aware of the nature of the definition. A key term definition is specific and brief. It is a very useful place to begin to learn the new terms in the chapter, but the definition presented may not be enough for full understanding. You will find that full understanding will come after reading the chapter and encountering the term within the fuller context of sentences and paragraphs of text that explain not only the term but how it applies in the particular situation.

### Key Terms and Text Relationship

The term *inotropic drugs* is defined in the Chapter 24 key terms list. As I read it, I understand that inotropic has to do with force or energy of muscle contractions. Some of this information is clear, and some of it is still somewhat hazy. It should become clearer when connected with the chapter text. The first paragraph of the *Pharmacology Overview* section introduces inotropic drugs: "Drugs that increase the force of myocardial contraction are called positive inotropic drugs, and they have a role in the treatment of failing heart muscle."

With this sentence, I find I have a much clearer understanding of what is meant by *inotropic drugs,* and I have the added benefit of knowing that there are positive inotropic drugs. This is what must happen to fully master the content-specific vocabulary. You must see the core definition as presented in the list of key terms, but you must also read to determine how that core definition is expanded and exemplified in the body of the text.

When preparing vocabulary cards, it is not a good idea simply to copy the definition from the key terms list and assume that this definition will serve your purpose. Wait to fill out the card until after you encounter the same term in the body of the chapter, and then pick and choose the information from the key terms list and the chapter body that will provide you with the clearest understanding of the term. Also, when placing information on vocabulary cards, it is always useful to include a chapter number and page numbers so that you can locate the source of your definition quickly should you find it necessary later.

These chapter structures can provide you with a clear picture of what you are expected to learn and the organizational pattern in which the material will be presented. Being aware of the structures and making use of them in this way will improve your concentration when you begin  to read the chapter for understanding and memory. The time spent working with chapter structure is not wasted and does not significantly increase the study time for the chapter. In fact, the time you spend working with the objectives, headings, and key terms will generally save time when you are doing intensive reading and study.

## TEXT NOTATION

Highlighting or underlining text material is a tool that can be very helpful when rehearsing and reviewing materials after the study reading. The problem, as discussed in the *Study Guide,* is that it is often difficult to limit the quantity of material that is marked. Although a good general guideline is to try to limit yourself to marking no more than 20% to 25% of the total material, this guideline applies to large blocks of material. Some paragraphs contain essential information and must be marked extensively, whereas in other paragraphs only one or two sentences may need to be marked. In this Study Skills Tips section, the object is to look at how the author's structure and language can help you to select what should be marked.

## Text Notation Application

Reproduced here are two paragraphs from Chapter 29 with my model underlining completed, followed by a discussion of the reasons for which I made the choices. You should not view the model underlining as a "perfect" example. The decision as to what to mark is very much an individual choice based on a number of factors, including prior experience with the subject matter and awareness of personal learning objectives and needs. These model paragraphs with accompanying discussion are intended to provide you with a basic model to adapt to your own learning style and needs.

### Chapter 29, Paragraphs 1 and 2

*<u>Fluid and electrolyte management</u> is one of the <u>cornerstones of patient care</u>. Most disease processes, tissue injuries, and surgical procedures greatly influence the physiologic status of fluids and electrolytes in the body. <u>Understanding fluid and electrolyte management requires knowledge of the extent and composition of the various body fluid compartments.</u>*

*Approximately 60% of the adult human body is water. This is referred to as the <u>total body water (TBW),</u> and it is distributed in the <u>three main compartments</u> in the following proportions: <u>intracellular fluid (ICF), 67%; interstitial fluid (ISF), 25%; and plasma volume, 8%.</u> This distribution is illustrated in Figure 29-1. The actual volume of fluid that would normally be in each compartment in an average 70-kg man with a TBW content of 60% is shown in Table 29-1.*

### Discussion

The first thing you should notice is that the underlining I have done exceeds the 20% to 25% guideline. These are the first paragraphs in the chapter. First paragraphs are usually introductions to the topic and may vary a great deal in the quantity of important information. This chapter, in my view, contains a number of key points that must be considered. Because the content seems important, I have chosen to underline more text.

The first sentence was chosen because of the word *cornerstones*. This word suggests that fluid management is extremely important in patient care and that I must be sure to keep that focus throughout the chapter. Paying careful attention to the author's word choices plays a major role in selecting materials for text notation.

Paying attention to language led me to the third sentence, which begins, "Understanding fluid and electrolyte management requires…" That phrase should immediately capture your attention. The phrase says that there is something that is required before anything else that follows will make complete sense. The phrase should also serve as an instant cue to generate a question for reading. "What is required for the understanding fluid and electrolyte management?" This question is answered directly by the sentence containing the phrase. The question helps you select what you may possibly want to underline or highlight. Everything you do at this point serves as a guide to help you establish clear learning objectives and makes the process of selecting the best information for marking easier to accomplish.

The next segment was chosen because it stands out from the body of the paragraph. *Total body water* is italicized in Chapter 29. This is a print convention used as a means of putting emphasis on something that the author believes to be of special importance. The decision to underline words and phrases that are already emphasized is a personal one. You may feel that, since the author has already marked it, you have no need to add your own marks. I find that my own marking, even of italicized or bold print material, serves as a double reminder of the importance of the information. This is an excellent example of what I mean when I say that text notation is highly personal. Whether you choose to add your own marking or not, there is one aspect of this phrase that is essential. *Total body water* is part of the vocabulary of fluids and electrolytes. That means it is time to add to your vocabulary cards.

This term served as a lead-in to the next key point that I have marked. The next part of the sentence is, "…it is distributed in the three main compartments…" Whenever you see a phrase with a number and a word such as *main,* you should be aware that this is potentially important material. This phrase should generate a new question that will aid in your selection of material to mark: "What are the three main compartments?" You can see immediately that the rest of this sentence answers that question and therefore identifies what needs to be marked. This marking also identifies three additional vocabulary items to be added to your cards for this chapter. As you set up your cards, be careful. One fluid is *intra-* and the second is *inter-*. It would be easy to confuse the two, but they have very different meanings.

### Chapter 29, Paragraph 3

*The terms used to identify the various spaces within which the TBW is distributed can be quite confusing, and there are two basic approaches to distinguishing among the locations of the fluid. <u>The TBW can be described as being in or out of the <u>blood</u> vessels (vasculature).</u> If this point of reference is used, then the term <u>intravascular fluid (IVF)</u> is used to describe the fluid inside the blood vessels and the term <u>extravascular fluid (EVF)</u> is used to refer to the fluid outside the blood vessels. Examples of EVF include lymph and cerebrospinal fluid. As these concepts are learned, it is important to remember the difference between the <u>prefixes intra- (inside), inter- (between), and extra- (outside).</u> The term <u>plasma</u> is used to describe the <u>fluid that flows through the blood vessels (intravascular fluid).</u> <u>Serum</u> is a closely related term (see Key Terms). The interstitial fluid (ISF) is the <u>fluid that is in the space between cells, tissues,</u>*

*and organs.* When discussing blood vessels, the term *extravascular volume is used; extravascular volume is made up of plasma and ISF.* When discussing cells, the term *extracellular volume is used; extracellular volume is composed of ISF and intracellular fluid (ICF). These terms are often confused and misused. Table 29-1 lists these definitions for further clarity and understanding.*

## Discussion

The language conventions and the print conventions are the same that were used to help in the previous paragraph. This paragraph also makes a point about the possibility of confusing and/or misusing the terms introduced. Being told that there is confusing material suggests that it is crucial that you be able to identify, define, and explain each of the terms used, and that it will take some careful thought to do so. There is one additional point in this paragraph that is important. The last sentence points you to a table, Table 29-1. There are many tables in this text. Always remember that tables are often used in an effort to simplify complex material and to clarify the relationships between the items presented in the table. In these opening paragraphs, with the repeated reference to the confusing nature of the descriptions, Table 29-1 will almost certainly be important to your learning.

# Antihypertensive Drugs

## OBJECTIVES

When you reach the end of this chapter, you will be able to do the following:

1  Briefly discuss the normal anatomy and physiology of the autonomic nervous system, including the events that take place within the sympathetic and parasympathetic divisions as related to long-term and short-term control of blood pressure.
2  Define *hypertension*.
3  Compare primary and secondary hypertension and their related manifestations.
4  Describe the protocol for treating hypertension as detailed in the *Seventh Report of the Joint National Committee on Prevention, Detection, Evaluation, and Treatment of High Blood Pressure (JNC 7)*, including the rationale for its use.

5  List the criterion pressure values (in millimeters of mercury) for the hypertension categories of normal blood pressure, prehypertension, hypertension stage 1, and hypertension stage 2 as defined in *JNC 7*.
6  Using the most recent guidelines, compare the various drugs used in the pharmacologic management of hypertension with regard to mechanism of action, specific indications, adverse effects, toxic effects, cautions, drug interactions, contraindications, dosages, and routes of administration.
7  Discuss the rationale for the nonpharmacologic management of hypertension.
8  Develop a nursing care plan that includes all phases of the nursing process for patients receiving antihypertensive drugs.

## DRUG PROFILES

bosentan, p. 359
♦ captopril, p. 356
carvedilol, p. 353
♦ clonidine, p. 353
doxazosin, p. 353
enalapril, p. 356
eplerenone, p. 359

♦ hydralazine, p. 359
♦ losartan, p. 357
nebivolol, p. 353
sodium nitroprusside, p. 359
treprostinil, p. 360

♦ *Key drug*

## KEY TERMS

**Alpha₁ blockers** Drugs that primarily cause arterial and venous dilation through their action on peripheral sympathetic neurons. (p. 351)

**Antihypertensive drugs** Medications used to treat hypertension. (p. 349)

**Cardiac output** The amount of blood ejected from the left ventricle, measured in liters per minute. (p. 348)

**Centrally acting adrenergic drugs** Drugs that modify the function of the sympathetic nervous system in the brain by stimulating alpha₂ receptors. Alpha₂ receptors are inhibitory in nature and thus have a reverse sympathetic effect and cause decreased blood pressure. (p. 351)

**Essential hypertension** Elevated systemic arterial pressure for which no cause can be found; also called *primary* or *idiopathic hypertension*. (p. 349)

**Hypertension** A common, often asymptomatic disorder in which systolic blood pressure persistently exceeds 140 mm Hg and/or diastolic pressure exceeds 90 mm Hg. (p. 348)

**Orthostatic hypotension** A common adverse effect of adrenergic blocking drugs involving a sudden drop in blood pressure when a person changes position, especially when rising from a seated or horizontal position. (p. 352)

**Prodrug** A drug that is inactive in its given form, and which must be metabolized to its active form in the body, generally by the liver, to be effective. (p. 354)

**Secondary hypertension** High blood pressure caused by another disease such as renal, pulmonary, endocrine, or vascular disease. (p. 349)

## ANATOMY, PHYSIOLOGY, AND PATHOPHYSIOLOGY OVERVIEW

Hypertension, defined as a persistent systolic pressure of greater than 140 mm Hg and/or a diastolic pressure greater than 90 mm Hg, affects approximately 50 million people in the United States and approximately 1 billion people worldwide, designating it as the most common disease state. As the population ages, the incidence of hypertension will continue to increase.

Hypertension is a major risk factor for coronary artery disease, cardiovascular disease (CVD), and death resulting from cardiovascular causes. It is the most important risk factor for stroke and heart failure, and it is also a major risk factor for renal failure and peripheral vascular disease. There is indisputable evidence regarding the relationship between blood pressure and risk of CVD; the higher the blood pressure, the greater the chance of developing CVD. For people 40 to 70 years of age, the risk of developing CVD doubles with each 20 mm Hg increase in systolic blood pressure or 10 mm Hg increase in diastolic pressure.

To gain insight into the treatment of hypertension, it is necessary to have a basic understanding of blood pressure. Blood pressure is determined by the product of cardiac output (4 to 8 L/min) and systemic vascular resistance (SVR). Cardiac output is the amount of blood that is ejected from the left ventricle and is measured in liters per minute. SVR is the resistance to blood flow that is determined by the diameter of the blood vessel and the vascular musculature. It is calculated by the blood pressure divided by the cardiac output. Numerous factors interact to regulate these two major variables and keep the blood pressure within normal limits. These are illustrated in Figure 22-1. These are the same factors that can cause high blood pressure, or hypertension, and are the targets of action of many of the antihypertensive drugs.

The diagnosis and treatment of hypertension have varied considerably over the years. The *Seventh Report of the Joint National Committee on Prevention, Detection, Evaluation, and Treatment of High Blood Pressure (JNC 7)* was released in May 2003. This report provides treatment guidelines for hypertension assembled by two large expert panels based on a review of the latest clinical research publications on the disease. As with previous such reports, the development of *JNC 7* was sponsored by the National Heart, Lung, and Blood Institute of the National Institutes of Health, the major governmental health research entity of the United States. The efforts of the Joint National Committee are intended to educate both health care professionals and the general public about the dangers of the disease and the importance of its treatment. The *Eighth Report of the Joint National Committee on Prevention, Detection, Evaluation, and Treatment of High Blood Pressure (JNC 8)* is scheduled to be published in 2012, and more information is available at www.nhlbi.nih.gov/guidelines/hypertension/jnc8/index.htm.

A new classification system for blood pressure was identified in the *Sixth Report of the Joint National Committee on Prevention, Detection, Evaluation, and Treatment of High Blood Pressure (JNC 6)* in 1997. The previously applied term *mild hypertension* did not adequately reflect the serious nature of the condition. This became evident when it was found that most of the morbidity and mortality actually occur in this group. In addition, whereas pre-*JNC 6* reports had recommended a stepped-care pharmacologic approach to treating the illness, many practitioners believed that this approach no longer adequately reflected the current range of pharmacologic alternatives. In the *JNC 6*, individualized therapy was proposed as a more appropriate treatment strategy. This individualized approach continues to be emphasized in the *JNC 7* and will most likely be continued in the *JNC-8*. Many patients will require two or more medications, even as initial therapy, depending on their individual cardiovascular risk factors such as obesity, diabetes, and family history.

The classification scheme used to categorize individual cases of hypertension has been simplified to the following four stages based on blood pressure measurements: normal, prehypertension, stage 1 hypertension, and stage 2 hypertension. (Refer to the *JNC 7* at www.nhlbi.nih.gov/guidelines/hypertension.)

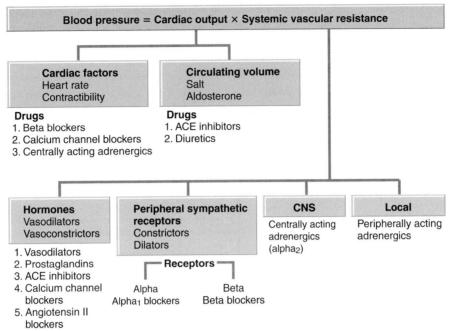

**FIGURE 22-1** Normal regulation of blood pressure and corresponding medications. *ACE,* Angiotensin-converting enzyme; *CNS,* central nervous system.

Hypertension can also be defined by its cause. When the specific cause of hypertension is unknown, it may be called essential hypertension (or idiopathic or primary hypertension). About 90% of cases of hypertension are of this type. Secondary hypertension accounts for the other 10%. Secondary hypertension is most commonly the result of another disease such as pheochromocytoma (adrenal tumor), preeclampsia of pregnancy (a pregnancy complication involving acute hypertension, among other symptoms), renal artery disease, sleep apnea, thyroid disease, or parathyroid disease. It may also result from the use of certain medications. If the cause of secondary hypertension can be eliminated, blood pressure usually returns to normal. If untreated, hypertension can cause damage to end organs such as the heart, brain, kidneys, and eyes.

The goal of antihypertensive therapy is the reduction of cardiovascular and renal morbidity and mortality. According to the *JNC 7,* the goal is to achieve a pressure of less than 140/90, which is associated with a decrease in CVD complications. In patients with hypertension and diabetes or renal disease, the goal is less than 130/80 mm Hg.

Fortunately, many significant advances have been made in both the ways to treat hypertension and in the understanding of the disease process. Large numbers of clinical trials have shown that adequately treating hypertension can prevent or delay CVD. Over the past 40 years, the development of new antihypertensive medications has had an enormous impact on the quality of life of people with hypertension. Drug therapy for hypertension first became available in the early 1950s with the introduction of ganglionic blocking drugs. However, unpleasant adverse effects and inconsistent therapeutic effects were common problems with these antihypertensive drugs. In 1953, the vasodilator hydralazine was introduced, and in 1958 the thiazide diuretics became available. Since that time, several additional drug categories have been developed, including loop diuretics (also called

*potassium-wasting diuretics*), potassium-sparing diuretics, beta blockers (beta receptor antagonists), angiotensin-converting enzyme (ACE) inhibitors, alpha$_1$ antagonists, alpha$_2$ agonists, angiotensin II receptor blockers (ARBs), calcium channel blockers (CCBs), vasodilators, and the newest class, the direct renin inhibitors. Although some of the medications mentioned in this chapter represent older classes of drugs, all are current therapeutic options listed in the treatment guidelines for hypertension published by the National Heart, Lung, and Blood Institute.

## PHARMACOLOGY OVERVIEW

Drug therapy for hypertension needs to be individualized. Important considerations in planning drug therapy are whether the patient has multiple medical problems and what impact drug therapy will have on the patient's quality of life. For example, sexual dysfunction in males is a common adverse effect of almost any antihypertensive drug and is the most common reason for nonadherence to drug therapy. Demographic factors, cultural implications, the ease of medication administration (e.g., a once-a-day dosing schedule or transdermal administration), and cost are other important considerations.

There are essentially seven main categories of pharmacologic drugs used to treat hypertension: diuretics, adrenergic drugs, vasodilators, angiotensin converting enzyme (ACE) inhibitors, angiotensin receptor blockers (ARBs), calcium channel blockers (CCBs), and direct renin inhibitors. All of these antihypertensive drugs (with the exception of diuretics) have some vasodilatory action. Those drugs in the vasodilator category are also called *direct vasodilators.* Drugs in any of these classes may be used either alone or in combination. The various categories and subcategories of antihypertensive drugs are listed in Box 22-1. The diuretics are discussed in detail in Chapter 28 and therefore are not covered in this chapter.

## REVIEW OF AUTONOMIC NEUROTRANSMISSION

There are two divisions of the autonomic nervous system (ANS): the parasympathetic nervous system (PSNS) and sympathetic nervous system (SNS). Stimulation of the ANS is controlled by the neurotransmitters acetylcholine and norepinephrine. Receptors for both divisions of the ANS are located throughout the body in a variety of tissues. ANS physiology is reviewed in greater detail in the introductory sections of Chapters 18 to 21. Receptors located between the postganglionic fiber and the effector cells (i.e., the postganglionic receptor) are called the *muscarinic* or *cholinergic* receptors in the PSNS. Receptors in the SNS are called *adrenergic* or *noradrenergic* receptors (i.e., alpha or beta receptors). Physiologic activity at muscarinic receptors is stimulated by acetylcholine and cholinergic agonist drugs (see Chapter 20) and is inhibited by cholinergic antagonists (anticholinergic drugs; see Chapter 21). Similarly, physiologic activity at adrenergic receptors is stimulated by norepinephrine and epinephrine and adrenergic agonists (see Chapter 18) and inhibited by antiadrenergics (adrenergic blockers; i.e., alpha or beta receptor blockers) (see Chapter 19). Figure 22-2 shows how these various receptors are arranged in both the PSNS and SNS and indicates their corresponding neurotransmitters.

---

**BOX 22-1  CATEGORIES AND SUBCATEGORIES OF ANTIHYPERTENSIVE DRUGS**

**Adrenergic Drugs**
- Centrally and peripherally acting adrenergic neuron blockers
- Centrally acting alpha$_2$ receptor agonists
- Peripherally acting alpha$_1$ receptor blockers
- Peripherally acting beta receptor blockers (beta blockers)
  - Cardioselective (beta$_1$ receptor blockers)
  - Nonselective (beta$_1$ and beta$_2$ receptor blockers)
- Peripherally acting dual alpha$_1$ and beta receptor blockers

**Angiotensin-Converting Enzyme Inhibitors**
**Angiotensin II Receptor Blockers**
**Calcium Channel Blockers**
- Benzothiazepines
- Dihydropyridines
- Phenylalkylamines

**Diuretics**
- Loop diuretics
- Potassium-sparing diuretics
- Thiazides and thiazide-like diuretics

**Vasodilators**
Act directly on vascular smooth muscle cells, *not* through alpha or beta receptors.

**Direct Renin Inhibitors**

---

## ADRENERGIC DRUGS

Adrenergic drugs are a large group of antihypertensive drugs, as shown in Box 22-1. The alpha blockers and combined alpha/beta blockers were described in detail in Chapter 19. The adrenergic drugs discussed here exert their antihypertensive action at different sites.

### Mechanism of Action and Drug Effects

Five specific drug subcategories are included in the adrenergic antihypertensive drugs as indicated in Box 22-1. Each of these subcategories of drugs can be described as having central action (in the brain) or peripheral action (at the heart and blood vessels). These drugs include the adrenergic neuron blockers (central and peripheral), the alpha$_2$ receptor agonists (central), the alpha$_1$ receptor

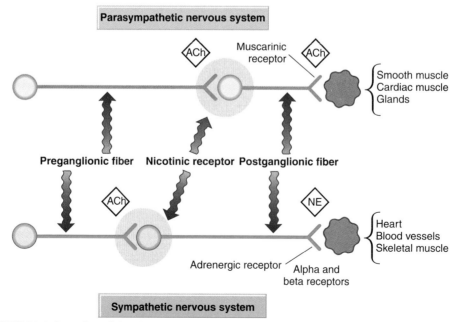

**FIGURE 22-2** Location of the nicotinic receptors in the parasympathetic and sympathetic nervous systems. *ACh,* Acetylcholine; *NE,* norepinephrine.

blockers (peripheral), the beta receptor blockers (peripheral), and the combination alpha$_1$ and beta receptor blockers (peripheral).

The centrally acting alpha$_2$-adrenergic receptor agonists clonidine and methyldopa act by modifying the function of the SNS. Stimulation of the SNS leads to an increase in heart rate and force of contraction, the constriction of blood vessels, and the release of renin from the kidney, resulting in hypertension. The centrally acting adrenergic drugs work by stimulating the alpha$_2$-adrenergic receptors in the brain. The alpha$_2$-adrenergic receptors are unique in that receptor stimulation actually reduces sympathetic outflow, in this case from the central nervous system (CNS). This results in a lack of norepinephrine production, which reduces blood pressure. Stimulation of the alpha$_2$-adrenergic receptors also affects the kidneys, reducing the activity of renin. Renin is the hormone and enzyme that converts the protein precursor angiotensinogen to the protein angiotensin I, the precursor of angiotensin II (AII), a potent vasoconstrictor that raises blood pressure.

In the periphery, the alpha$_1$ blockers doxazosin, prazosin, and terazosin also modify the function of the SNS. They do so by blocking the alpha$_1$-adrenergic receptors. When alpha$_1$-adrenergic receptors are stimulated by circulating norepinephrine, they produce increased blood pressure. Thus, when these receptors are blocked, blood pressure is decreased. The drug effects of the alpha$_1$ blockers are primarily related to their ability to dilate arteries and veins, which reduces peripheral vascular resistance and subsequently decreases blood pressure. This produces a marked decrease in the systemic and pulmonary venous pressures and an increase in cardiac output. The alpha$_1$ blockers also increase urinary flow rates and decrease outflow obstruction by preventing smooth muscle contractions in the bladder neck and urethra. This can be beneficial in cases of benign prostatic hyperplasia (BPH).

The beta blockers also act in the periphery and include propranolol, metoprolol, and atenolol as well as several other drugs. These drugs are discussed in more detail in Chapters 23 and 25 because they are also used for angina and conduction problems. Their antihypertensive effects are related to their reduction of the heart rate through beta$_1$ receptor blockade. Furthermore, beta blockers also cause a reduction in the secretion of the hormone renin (see section on ACE inhibitors), which in turn reduces both AII-mediated vasoconstriction and aldosterone-mediated volume expansion. Long-term use of beta blockers also reduces peripheral vascular resistance.

Two dual-action alpha$_1$ and beta receptor blockers, labetalol and carvedilol, also act in the periphery at the heart and blood vessels. They have the dual antihypertensive effects of reduction in heart rate (beta$_1$ receptor blockade) and vasodilation (alpha$_1$

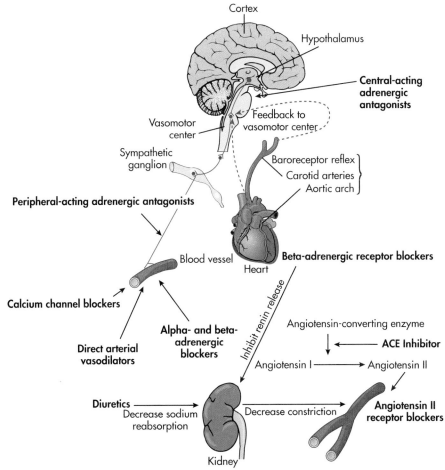

**FIGURE 22-3** Site and mechanism of action of the various antihypertensive drugs. (Modified from Lewis SM et al: *Medical-surgical nursing: assessment and management of clinical problems,* ed 8, St Louis, 2011, Mosby.)

**TABLE 22-1    ADRENERGIC DRUGS: DRUG INTERACTIONS**

| DRUG | INTERACTS WITH | MECHANISM | RESULT |
|------|----------------|-----------|--------|
| clonidine | TCAs, MAOIs, appetite suppressants, amphetamines | Opposing actions | Decreased hypotensive effects |
| | Diuretics, nitrates, other antihypertensive drugs | Additive | Increased hypotensive effects |
| | Beta blockers | Additive | May potentiate bradycardia and increase the rebound hypertension in clonidine withdrawal |
| doxazosin | CNS depressants, alcohol | Additive | Increased CNS depression |
| | Beta blockers and other hypotensive drugs | Additive | Increased hypotension |
| | verapamil | Increased serum prazosin levels | Increased hypotension |

*CNS,* Central nervous system; *MAOIs,* monoamine oxidase inhibitors; *TCAs,* tricyclic antidepressants.

receptor blockade). Figure 22-3 illustrates the site and mechanism of action of the various antihypertensive drugs.

## Indications

All of the drugs mentioned in this section are used primarily for the treatment of hypertension, either alone or in combination with other antihypertensive drugs. Various forms of glaucoma may also respond to treatment with some of these drugs. Clonidine also has several off-label uses (not approved by the U.S. Food and Drug Administration but still common in practice), including prophylaxis against migraine headaches and treatment of severe dysmenorrhea or menopausal flushing. It is also useful in the management of withdrawal symptoms in persons with opioid, nicotine, or alcohol dependency (see Chapter 17). The alpha$_1$ blockers doxazosin, prazosin, and terazosin have been used to relieve the symptoms associated with BPH (see Chapter 19). They have also proved effective in the management of severe heart failure when used with cardiac glycosides (see Chapter 24) and diuretics (see Chapter 28).

## Contraindications

Contraindications to the use of the adrenergic antihypertensive drugs include known drug allergy and may also include acute heart failure, concurrent use of monoamine oxidase inhibitors (see Chapter 16), severe mental depression, peptic ulcer, and severe liver or kidney disease. Asthma may also be a contraindication to the use of any noncardioselective beta blocker (e.g., carvedilol). The use of vasodilating drugs may also be contraindicated in cases of heart failure that is secondary to diastolic dysfunction.

## Adverse Effects

The most common adverse effects of adrenergic drugs are bradycardia with reflex tachycardia, postural and postexercise hypotension, dry mouth, drowsiness, dizziness, depression, edema, constipation, and sexual dysfunction (e.g., impotence). Other effects include headaches, sleep disturbances, nausea, rash, and palpitations. There is a high incidence of orthostatic hypotension (a sudden drop in blood pressure during changes in position) in patients taking alpha blockers. Orthostatic hypotension is commonly referred to as *postural hypotension.* When the patient changes positions, a situation known as *first-dose syncope,* in which the hypotensive effect is severe enough to cause the patient to lose consciousness with even the first dose of medication, can occur. Educate the patient to change positions slowly.

In addition, the abrupt discontinuation of the centrally acting alpha$_2$ receptor agonists can result in rebound hypertension, characterized by a sudden and very high elevation of blood pressure. This may also be true for other antihypertensive drug classes, especially beta blockers. Nonselective blocking drugs are also commonly associated with bronchoconstriction (due to unrestrained parasympathetic tone) as well as metabolic inhibition of glycogenolysis in the liver, which can lead to hypoglycemia. However, hyperglycemic episodes are also among the adverse effects reported for this drug class.

Any change in the dosing regimen for cardiovascular medications should be undertaken gradually and with appropriate patient monitoring and follow-up. Although the same is also true for most other classes of medications, abrupt dosage changes of cardiovascular medications, either up or down, can be especially hazardous for the patient. Some of these drugs can also cause disruptions in blood count as well as in serum electrolyte levels and renal function. Periodic monitoring of white blood cell count, serum potassium and sodium levels, and urinary protein levels is recommended.

## Interactions

Adrenergic drugs can cause additive CNS depression when taken with alcohol, benzodiazepines, and opioids. Other drug interactions that can occur with selected adrenergic drugs are summarized in Table 22-1. This list is merely representative and is not exhaustive. Always keep a drug information handbook available to check in cases in which a specific drug interaction is suspected. Hospital pharmacists are also excellent resources.

## Dosages

For dosage information on selected adrenergic antihypertensive drugs, see the table on p. 353.

## DRUG PROFILES

### ALPHA$_2$-ADRENERGIC RECEPTOR STIMULATORS (AGONISTS)

Of the two alpha$_2$ receptor agonists—clonidine and methyldopa—clonidine is by far the most commonly used and is the prototypical drug for this class. Methyldopa is commonly used to treat hypertension in pregnancy. However, these drugs are not typically prescribed as first-line antihypertensive drugs, because their use is associated with a high incidence of unwanted adverse effects such as orthostatic hypotension, fatigue, and dizziness. They may be used as adjunct drugs in the treatment of hypertension after other drugs have failed or may be used in conjunction with other antihypertensives such as diuretics.

## DOSAGES

### Selected Antihypertensive Drugs: Adrenergic Agonists and Antagonists

| DRUG (PREGNANCY CATEGORY) | PHARMACOLOGIC CLASS | USUAL DOSAGE RANGE | INDICATIONS/USES |
|---|---|---|---|
| carvedilol (Coreg) (C) | Peripherally acting alpha$_1$, beta$_1$, and beta$_2$ receptor antagonist (blocker) | PO: 3.125-25 mg bid | Hypertension (also used in heart failure) |
| ♦ clonidine (Catapres, Catapres-TTS) (C) | Centrally acting alpha$_2$ receptor agonist | PO: 0.2-0.6 mg/day Transdermal patch: 0.1, 0.2, or 0.3 mg/24 hr, applied weekly | Hypertension (may have other unlabeled uses including treatment of psychiatric, cardiovascular, and gastrointestinal problems) |
| doxazosin (Cardura) (C) | Peripherally acting alpha$_1$ receptor antagonist | PO: Initial dose 1 mg/day; may titrate up to maximum of 16 mg/day | Hypertension |

*PO*, Oral.

### ♦ clonidine

Clonidine (Catapres) is used primarily for its ability to decrease blood pressure. It is also useful in the management of opioid withdrawal. It has a better safety profile than the other centrally acting adrenergics and has the advantage of being available in several dosage formulations, including both topical and oral preparations. When the patch dosage form is used, it is important to remove the old patch before applying a new one. Clonidine must not be discontinued abruptly, as this will lead to severe rebound hypertension. Its use is contraindicated in patients who have shown hypersensitivity reactions to it. Recommended dosages are given in the table on this page.

### Pharmacokinetics

| Route | Onset of Action | Peak Plasma Concentration | Elimination Half-life | Duration of Action |
|---|---|---|---|---|
| PO | 30-60 min | 3-5 hr | 6-20 hr | 8 hr |

### ALPHA$_1$ BLOCKERS

The alpha$_1$ blockers are doxazosin (Cardura), prazosin (Minipress), tamsulosin (Flomax), and terazosin (Hytrin). Their use is contraindicated in patients who have shown a hypersensitivity to them. They are classified as pregnancy category C drugs. They are available only as oral preparations. Tamsulosin is not used to control blood pressure but is indicated solely for symptomatic control of benign prostatic hyperplasia (BPH). This use is described further in Chapters 19 and 35.

### doxazosin

Doxazosin (Cardura) is a commonly used alpha$_1$ blocker. It reduces peripheral vascular resistance and blood pressure by dilating both arterial and venous blood vessels. It has been shown to be beneficial in the treatment of hypertension and the relief of the symptoms of obstructive BPH. It is available in immediate- and extended-release formulations. When the drug is released from the extended-release form, the matrix of the capsule is expelled in the stool. Educate patients that this will happen, and reassure that the active drug has been absorbed. Confusion over the presence of the capsule matrix could cause patients to take more than the prescribed dosage. Recommended dosages are given in the table on this page.

### Pharmacokinetics

| Route | Onset of Action | Peak Plasma Concentration | Elimination Half-life | Duration of Action |
|---|---|---|---|---|
| PO | 1-2 hr | 2-3 hr | 15-22 hr | Less than 24 hr |

### DUAL-ACTION ALPHA$_1$ AND BETA RECEPTOR BLOCKERS
#### carvedilol

Carvedilol (Coreg) is a widely used drug and is well tolerated by most patients. In addition to treatment of hypertension, it is also indicated for treatment of mild to moderate heart failure in conjunction with digoxin, diuretics, and ACE inhibitors. Its contraindications include known drug allergy, cardiogenic shock, severe bradycardia or heart failure, bronchospastic conditions such as asthma, and various cardiac problems involving the conduction system. For dosage information, see the table on this page.

### Pharmacokinetics

| Route | Onset of Action | Peak Plasma Concentration | Elimination Half-life | Duration of Action |
|---|---|---|---|---|
| PO | 20-120 min | 1-4 hr | 6-8 hr | 8-24 hr |

### BETA RECEPTOR BLOCKER
#### nebivolol

Nebivolol (Bystolic) is the newest beta blocker, released in 2008. It is a beta$_1$-selective beta blocker approved for use in hypertension. It is also used for the treatment of heart failure. Nebivolol is similar to other beta$_1$-selective blockers; however, in addition to blocking beta$_1$ receptors, it also produces an endothelium-derived nitric oxide–dependent vasodilatation, which results in a decrease in SVR. It is promoted as causing less sexual dysfunction. Like other beta blockers, it should not be stopped abruptly but must be tapered over 1 to 2 weeks. Dosing starts at 5 mg/day and may be increased at 2-week intervals to a maximum of 40 mg/day.

## ANGIOTENSIN-CONVERTING ENZYME (ACE) INHIBITORS

The ACE inhibitors are a large group of antihypertensive drugs. Currently, there are ten ACE inhibitors available for clinical use. In addition, various combination drug products

| TABLE 22-2 | ACE INHIBITORS | |
|---|---|---|
| **DRUG (TRADE NAME)** | **COMBINATION WITH HYDROCHLOROTHIAZIDE** | **DOSING SCHEDULE** |
| benazepril (Lotensin) | Lotensin HCT | Once a day |
| captopril (Capoten) | Capozide | Multiple |
| enalapril (Vasotec) | Vaseretic | Multiple |
| fosinopril (Monopril) | None | Once a day |
| lisinopril (Prinivil) | Prinzide | Once a day |
| lisinopril (Zestril) | Zestoretic | Once a day |
| moexipril (Univasc) | None | Once a day |
| perindopril (Aceon) | None | Once to twice daily |
| quinapril (Accupril) | None | Once a day |
| ramipril (Altace) | None | Once a day |
| trandolapril (Mavik) | None | Once a day |

*ACE,* Angiotensin-converting enzyme.

are available in which a thiazide diuretic or a calcium channel blocker (CCB) is combined with an ACE inhibitor. Combination products tend to increase adherence since the patient is taking fewer drugs. The available ACE inhibitors are captopril (Capoten), benazepril (Lotensin), enalapril (Vasotec), fosinopril (Monopril), lisinopril (Prinivil), moexipril (Univasc), perindopril (Aceon), quinapril (Accupril), ramipril (Altace), and trandolapril (Mavik). These drugs are very safe and efficacious and are often used as first-line drugs in the treatment of both heart failure and hypertension. Some of the available drug combinations and dosing schedules for the various drugs that make up this large class of antihypertensives are summarized in Table 22-2. The ACE inhibitors as a class are very similar to one another and differ in only a few of their chemical properties; however, there are some differences among them in their clinical properties.

Captopril has the shortest half-life and therefore must be dosed more frequently than any of the other ACE inhibitors. This may be an important drawback for patients with a history of nonadherence to their medication regimen. On the other hand, it may be best to start with a drug that has a short half-life in a patient who is critically ill, so that if problems arise they will be short-lived. Both captopril and enalapril can be dosed multiple times a day.

Captopril and lisinopril are the only two ACE inhibitors that are not prodrugs. A prodrug is a drug that is inactive in its administered form and must be metabolized to its active form in the body, generally by the liver, to be effective. This characteristic of captopril and lisinopril is an important advantage in treating a patient with liver dysfunction; all of the other ACE inhibitors are prodrugs, and their transformation to active form is dependent upon liver function to reveal the active drug.

Enalapril is the only ACE inhibitor that is available in a parenteral preparation. All of the newer ACE inhibitors, such as benazepril, fosinopril, lisinopril, quinapril, and ramipril, have long half-lives and long durations of action, which allows them to be given orally only once a day. A once-a-day medication regimen promotes better patient adherence.

All ACE inhibitors have detrimental effects on the unborn fetus and neonate. They are classified as pregnancy category C drugs for women in their first trimester and as pregnancy category D drugs for women in their second or third trimester. ACE inhibitors are to be used by pregnant women only if there are no safer alternatives. Fetal and neonatal morbidity and mortality have been reported to have occurred in at least 50 cases in which women received ACE inhibitors during their pregnancies.

## Mechanism of Action and Drug Effects

The development of the ACE inhibitors was spurred by the discovery of an animal substance found to have beneficial effects in humans. This particular substance was the venom of a South American viper, which was found to inhibit kininase activity. Kininase is an enzyme that normally breaks down bradykinin, a potent vasodilator in the human body.

As their name implies, these drugs inhibit angiotensin-converting enzyme, which is responsible for converting AI (formed through the action of renin) to AII. AII is a potent vasoconstrictor and induces aldosterone secretion by the adrenal glands. Aldosterone stimulates sodium and water resorption, which can raise blood pressure. Together, these processes are referred to as the renin-angiotensin-aldosterone system. By inhibiting this process, blood pressure is lowered.

The primary effects of the ACE inhibitors are cardiovascular and renal. Their cardiovascular effects are due to their ability to reduce blood pressure by decreasing systemic vascular resistance (SVR). They do this by preventing the breakdown of the vasodilating substance bradykinin and also of substance P (another potent vasodilator), and preventing the formation of AII. These combined effects decrease afterload, or the resistance against which the left ventricle must pump to eject its volume of blood during contraction. The ACE inhibitors are beneficial in the treatment of heart failure because they prevent sodium and water resorption by inhibiting aldosterone secretion. This causes diuresis, which decreases blood volume and return to the heart. This in turn decreases preload, or the left ventricular end-diastolic volume, and the work required of the heart.

## Indications

The therapeutic effects of the ACE inhibitors are related to their potent cardiovascular effects. They are excellent antihypertensives and adjunctive drugs for the treatment of heart failure. They may be used alone or in combination with other drugs such as diuretics in the treatment of hypertension or heart failure.

The beneficial hemodynamic effects of the ACE inhibitors have been studied extensively. Because of their ability to decrease SVR (a measure of afterload) and preload, ACE inhibitors can stop the progression of left ventricular hypertrophy, which is sometimes seen after a myocardial infarction (MI). This pathologic process is known as *ventricular remodeling.* The ability of ACE inhibitors to prevent this is termed a *cardioprotective effect.* ACE inhibitors have been shown to decrease morbidity and mortality in patients with heart failure. They are considered the drugs of choice for hypertensive patients with heart failure. ACE inhibitors also have been shown to have a protective effect on the kidneys, because they

## TABLE 22-3 ACE INHIBITORS: THERAPEUTIC EFFECTS

| BODY SUBSTANCE | EFFECT IN BODY | ACE INHIBITOR ACTION | RESULTING HEMODYNAMIC EFFECT |
|---|---|---|---|
| aldosterone | Causes sodium and water retention | Prevents its secretion | Diuresis = ↓ plasma volume = ↓ filling pressures or ↓ preload |
| angiotensin II | Potent vaso-constrictor | Prevents its formation | ↓SVR = ↓ afterload |
| bradykinin | Potent vasodilator | Prevents its breakdown | ↓ SVR = ↓ afterload |

↓, Decreased; *ACE,* angiotensin-converting enzyme; *SVR,* systemic vascular resistance.

reduce glomerular filtration pressure. This is one reason that they are among the cardiovascular drugs of choice for diabetic patients. Numerous studies have shown that the ACE inhibitors reduce proteinuria, and they are considered by many to be standard therapy for diabetic patients to prevent the progression of diabetic nephropathy. The various therapeutic effects of the ACE inhibitors are listed in Table 22-3, which lists the biochemicals on which ACE inhibitors act and the resulting beneficial hemodynamic effects.

## Contraindications

Contraindications to the use of ACE inhibitors include known drug allergy, especially a previous reaction of angioedema (e.g., laryngeal swelling) to an ACE inhibitor. Patients with a baseline potassium level of 5 mEq/L or higher may not be suitable candidates for ACE inhibitor therapy, because these drugs can promote hyperkalemia (see later discussion). All ACE inhibitors are contraindicated in lactating women, children, and in patients with bilateral renal artery stenosis.

## Adverse Effects

Major CNS effects of the ACE inhibitors include fatigue, dizziness, mood changes, and headaches. A characteristic dry, nonproductive cough may occur that is reversible with discontinuation of the therapy. A first-dose hypotensive effect can

cause a significant decline in blood pressure. Other adverse effects include loss of taste, hyperkalemia, rash, anemia, neutropenia, thrombocytosis, and agranulocytosis. In patients with severe heart failure whose renal function may depend on the activity of the renin-angiotensin-aldosterone system, treatment with ACE inhibitors may cause acute renal failure. ACE inhibitors promote potassium resorption in the kidney, although they promote sodium excretion due to their reduction of aldosterone secretion. For this reason, serum potassium levels must be monitored regularly. This is especially true when there is concurrent therapy with potassium-sparing diuretics, although many patients tolerate both types of drug therapy with no major problems. One rare, but potentially fatal, adverse effect is angioedema. Angioedema is a strong vascular reaction involving inflammation of submucosal tissues, which can progress to anaphylaxis.

### Toxicity and Management of Overdose

The most pronounced symptom of an overdose of an ACE inhibitor is hypotension. Treatment is symptomatic and supportive and includes the administration of intravenous fluids to expand the blood volume. Hemodialysis is effective for the removal of captopril and lisinopril.

### Interactions

Nonsteroidal antiinflammatory drugs (NSAIDs), such as ibuprofen, can reduce the antihypertensive effect of ACE inhibitors (see Chapter 44). The use of NSAIDs and ACE inhibitors may also predispose patients to the development of acute renal failure. Concurrent use of ACE inhibitors and other antihypertensives or diuretics can have hypotensive effects. Giving lithium and ACE inhibitors together can result in lithium toxicity. Potassium supplements and potassium-sparing diuretics, when administered with ACE inhibitors, may result in hyperkalemia. The monitoring of serum potassium levels becomes important in these cases. False-positive results on tests for acetone in the urine may occur in patients taking captopril.

### Dosages

For dosage information on selected ACE inhibitors, see the table on this page.

## DOSAGES

### Selected Antihypertensive Drugs: ACE Inhibitors and Angiotensin II Receptor Blockers

| DRUG (PREGNANCY CATEGORY) | PHARMACOLOGIC CLASS | USUAL DOSAGE RANGE | INDICATIONS |
|---|---|---|---|
| ◆ captopril (Capoten) (C, first trimester; D, second and third trimesters) | ACE inhibitor | **Adult** PO: 25-150 mg bid-tid | Hypertension, heart failure |
| enalapril (Vasotec) (C, first trimester; D, second and third trimesters) | ACE inhibitor | **Adult** PO: 10-40 mg/day as a single dose or in 2 equal doses | Hypertension |
| | | PO: 2.5-20 mg bid | Heart failure |
| | | IV: 1.25-5 mg q6h over a 5-min period | Hypertension |
| ◆ losartan (Cozaar) (C, first trimester; D, second and third trimesters) | Angiotensin II receptor blocker | **Adult** PO: 25-100 mg as a single dose or divided bid | Hypertension, heart failure |

*ACE,* Angiotensin-converting enzyme; *IV,* intravenous; *PO,* oral.

## DRUG PROFILES

### ◆ captopril

Captopril (Capoten) was the first available ACE inhibitor and is considered the prototypical drug for the class. Several large multicenter studies have shown its clinical efficacy in minimizing or preventing the left ventricular dilatation and dysfunction (also called *ventricular remodeling*) that can arise in the acute period after an MI and thereby improving the patient's chances of survival. It can also reduce the risk of heart failure in these patients. It has the shortest half-life of all of the currently available ACE inhibitors, and it must be given three or four times a day. Recommended dosages are given in the table on p. 355.

Pharmacokinetics

| Route | Onset of Action | Peak Plasma Concentration | Elimination Half-life | Duration of Action |
|-------|-----------------|---------------------------|-----------------------|--------------------|
| PO | 15 min | 1-2 hr | 2 hr | 2-6 hr |

### enalapril

Enalapril (Vasotec) is the only ACE inhibitor currently marketed that is available in both oral and parenteral preparations. The parenteral formulation (enalaprilat) is an active drug. It offers the hemodynamic benefit of inhibiting ACE activity in an acutely ill patient who cannot tolerate oral medications. The other benefit to intravenous enalapril is that it does not require cardiac monitoring as do the intravenous beta blockers and calcium channel blockers. Although its half-life is slightly longer than that of captopril, it may still have to be given twice a day. The oral form of enalapril differs from captopril in that it is a prodrug, and the patient must have a functioning liver for the drug to be converted into its active form. As with captopril, it has been shown in many large studies to improve a patient's chances of survival after an MI and to reduce the incidence of heart failure. Recommended dosages are given in the table on p. 355.

Pharmacokinetics

| Route | Onset of Action | Peak Plasma Concentration | Elimination Half-life | Duration of Action |
|-------|-----------------|---------------------------|-----------------------|--------------------|
| PO | 1 hr | 4-6 hr | 2 hr | 12-24 hr |
| IV | 15 min | 1-4 hr | 2 hr | 4-6 hr |

## ANGIOTENSIN II RECEPTOR BLOCKERS

Angiotensin II receptor blockers (ARBs) are similar to the ACE inhibitors. The class includes losartan (Cozaar), eprosartan (Teveten), valsartan (Diovan), irbesartan (Avapro), candesartan (Atacand), olmesartan (Benicar), telmisartan (Micardis), and azilsartan (Edarbi).

### Mechanism of Action and Drug Effects

The ARBs block the binding of AII to type 1 AII receptors. The ACE inhibitors such as enalapril block conversion of AI to AII, but AII also may be formed by other enzymes that are not blocked by ACE inhibitors. For comparison, recall that ACE inhibitors block the breakdown of bradykinins and substance P, which accumulate and may cause adverse effects such as cough but might also contribute to the drugs' antihypertensive and cardiac and nephroprotective effects. Bradykinins are potent vasodilators and help to reduce blood pressure by dilating arteries and decreasing SVR.

In contrast to ACE inhibitors, the ARBs affect primarily vascular smooth muscle and the adrenal gland. By selectively blocking the binding of AII to the type 1 AII receptors in these tissues, ARBs block vasoconstriction and the secretion of aldosterone. AII receptors have been found in other tissues throughout the body, but the effects of ARB blocking of these receptors is unknown.

Clinically, ACE inhibitors and ARBs appear to be equally effective for the treatment of hypertension. Both are well tolerated, but ARBs do not cause cough. There is evidence that ARBs are better tolerated and are associated with lower mortality after MI than ACE inhibitors. It is not yet clear whether ARBs are as effective as ACE inhibitors in treating heart failure (cardioprotective effects) or in protecting the kidneys, as in diabetes. Both types of drugs are contraindicated for use in the second or third trimester of pregnancy. Whether one or more of these drugs could prove to have unique adverse effects with long-term use is unknown at this time.

### Indications

The therapeutic effects of ARBs are related to their potent vasodilating properties. They are excellent antihypertensives and adjunctive drugs for the treatment of heart failure. They may be used alone or in combination with other drugs such as diuretics in the treatment of hypertension or heart failure. The beneficial hemodynamic effect of ARBs is their ability to decrease SVR (a measure of afterload). Their use is rapidly growing, and multiple studies have verified their beneficial effects.

### Contraindications

Contraindications to the use of ARBs are known drug allergy, pregnancy, and lactation. They need to be used cautiously in elderly patients and in patients with renal dysfunction because of increased sensitivity to its effects and risk for adverse effects in these patients. As with other antihypertensives, blood pressure and apical pulse rate need to be assessed before and during drug therapy.

### Adverse Effects

The most common adverse effects of ARBs are upper respiratory infections and headache. Occasionally dizziness, inability to sleep, diarrhea, dyspnea, heartburn, nasal congestion, back pain, and fatigue can occur. Hyperkalemia is much less likely to occur than with the ACE inhibitors.

### Toxicity and Management of Overdose

Overdose may manifest as hypotension and tachycardia; bradycardia occurs less often. Treatment is symptomatic and supportive, and includes the administration of intravenous fluids to expand the blood volume.

| TABLE 22-4 | ANGIOTENSIN II RECEPTOR BLOCKERS: DRUG INTERACTIONS | |
|---|---|---|
| DRUG | MECHANISM | RESULT |
| NSAIDs | Decreased anti-hypertensive | Decreased effect of ARB and potential to renal failure |
| lithium | Inhibits lithium elimination | Increased lithium concentrations |
| rifampin | Increased metabolism | Decreased ARB effectiveness |
| Potassium supplements and potassium-sparing diuretics | Additive potassium-increasing effects | Possible hyperkalemia |

*ARB,* Angiotensin II receptor blocker.

## Interactions

The drugs that interact with ARBs, the mechanism responsible, and the result of the interaction are summarized in Table 22-4. In addition, as is the case with ACE inhibitors, ARBs can promote hyperkalemia, especially when taken concurrently with potassium supplements (although this occurs much less frequently than with ACE inhibitors). Patients' individual chemistries vary widely, however, so monitoring of the serum potassium level is necessary for all patients. Potassium supplements may still be indicated for patients with a tendency toward hypokalemia (whether acute or chronic).

## Dosages

For dosage information on selected ARBs, see the table on p. 355.

## DRUG PROFILE

### ♦ losartan

Losartan (Cozaar) has been shown to be beneficial in patients with hypertension and heart failure. Studies indicate that ARBs are better tolerated and produce a marginally lower mortality rate after MI than treatment with ACE inhibitors.

The use of losartan is contraindicated in patients who are hypersensitive to any component of this product. It is to be used with caution in patients with renal or hepatic dysfunction and in patients with renal artery stenosis. Breastfeeding women must not take losartan, because it can cause serious adverse effects on the nursing infant. Recommended dosages are given in the table on p. 355.

### Pharmacokinetics

| Route | Onset of Action | Peak Plasma Concentration | Elimination Half-life | Duration of Action |
|---|---|---|---|---|
| PO | 1 hr | 6 hr | 6-9 hr | 24 hr |

## CALCIUM CHANNEL BLOCKERS

Calcium channel blockers (CCBs) are also discussed in detail in the chapters on antidysrhythmic drugs (see Chapter 25) and antianginal drugs (see Chapter 23). As a class, they are used for several indications and have many beneficial effects and relatively few adverse effects. Their primary use is for the treatment of hypertension and angina. Their effectiveness in treating hypertension is related to their ability to cause smooth muscle relaxation by blocking the binding of calcium to its receptors, which thereby prevents contraction. Because of their effectiveness and safety, they have been added to the list of first-line drugs for the treatment of hypertension. Amlodipine (Norvasc) is the CCB most commonly used for hypertension. Calcium channel blockers are also effective antidysrhythmics (see Chapter 25). One specific CCB, nimodipine, can prevent the cerebral artery spasms that can occur after a subarachnoid hemorrhage. CCBs are also sometimes used in the treatment of Raynaud's disease and migraine headache. They are also used in combination with other drugs. Some examples are amlodipine/atorvastatin (Caduet), which is both an antihypertensive and a cholesterol-lowering drug (see Chapter 27); amlodipine/benazepril (Lotrel); amlodipine/olmesartan (Azar); and amlodipine/valsartan (Exforge).

## DIURETICS

The diuretics are a highly effective class of antihypertensive drugs. They are listed as the current first-line antihypertensives in the *JNC 7* guidelines for the treatment of hypertension. They may be used as monotherapy (single-drug therapy) or in combination with drugs of other antihypertensive classes. Their primary therapeutic effect is decreasing the plasma and extracellular fluid volumes, which results in decreased preload. This leads to a decrease in cardiac output and total peripheral resistance, all of which decrease the workload of the heart. This large group of antihypertensives is discussed in detail in Chapter 28. The thiazide diuretics (e.g., hydrochlorothiazide) are the most commonly used diuretics for treatment of hypertension.

## VASODILATORS

Vasodilators act directly on arteriolar and/or venous smooth muscle to cause relaxation. They do not work through adrenergic receptors. Vasodilator drugs include minoxidil, hydralazine (Apresoline), diazoxide (Hyperstat), and nitroprusside (Nitropress).

### Mechanism of Action and Drug Effects

Direct-acting vasodilators are useful as antihypertensive drugs because of their ability to directly cause peripheral vasodilation. This results in a reduction in systemic vascular resistance (SVR). In general, the most notable effect of the vasodilators is their hypotensive effect. However, minoxidil (Rogaine) (in its topical form) has also received attention because of its effectiveness in restoring hair growth. This application is described further in Chapter 56. Diazoxide, hydralazine, and minoxidil work primarily through arteriolar vasodilation, whereas nitroprusside has both arteriolar and venous effects.

### Indications

All of the vasodilators can be used to treat hypertension, either alone or in combination with other antihypertensives. Sodium nitroprusside and intravenous diazoxide are reserved for the management of hypertensive emergencies, in which blood pressure is severely elevated.

## Contraindications

Contraindications include known drug allergy and may also include hypotension, cerebral edema, head injury, acute MI, and coronary artery disease. They may also be contraindicated in cases of heart failure that is secondary to diastolic dysfunction.

## Adverse Effects

Diazoxide has many undesirable adverse effects including dizziness, headache, orthostatic hypotension, dysrhythmias, sodium and water retention, nausea, vomiting, and hyperglycemia in diabetic patients. These adverse effects have dramatically reduced the use of diazoxide. Adverse effects of hydralazine include dizziness, headache, anxiety, tachycardia, edema, dyspnea, nausea, vomiting, diarrhea, hepatitis, systemic lupus erythematosus (SLE), vitamin $B_6$ deficiency, and rash. Minoxidil adverse effects include T-wave electrocardiographic changes, pericardial effusion or tamponade, angina, breast tenderness, rash, and thrombocytopenia. Adverse effects of sodium nitroprusside include bradycardia, decreased platelet aggregation, rash, hypothyroidism, hypotension, methemoglobinemia, and, rarely, cyanide toxicity. Cyanide ions are a by-product of nitroprusside metabolism. Cyanide and thiocyanate toxicity are seen clinically when nitroprusside is used at high dosages for long periods of time and/or in patients with renal insufficiency. When nitroprusside is combined with sodium thiosulfate, the potential for cyanide toxicity is greatly reduced.

## Toxicity and Management of Overdose

Hydralazine toxicity or overdose produces hypotension, tachycardia, headache, and generalized skin flushing. Treatment is supportive and symptomatic and includes the administration of intravenous fluids, digitalization if needed, and the administration of beta blockers for the control of tachycardia.

Minoxidil overdose or toxicity can precipitate excessive hypotension. Treatment is supportive and symptomatic and includes the administration of intravenous fluids. Norepinephrine and epinephrine should not be used to reverse the hypotension because of the possibility of causing excessive cardiac stimulation.

The main symptom of sodium nitroprusside overdose or toxicity is severe hypotension. This drug is normally administered only to patients receiving intensive care. Under these conditions, the infusion rate is usually carefully titrated, yielding immediately visible results on a cardiovascular monitor that provides constant measurements of blood pressure from centrally placed venous or arterial catheters. For this reason, excessive hypotension is usually avoidable. When it does occur, discontinuation of the infusion has an immediate effect because the drug is metabolized very rapidly (half-life of 10 minutes). Treatment for the hypotension is supportive and symptomatic; if necessary, pressor drugs can be infused to quickly raise blood pressure. The chemical structure of nitroprusside does contain cyanide groups, which are released upon its metabolism in the body and can result in cyanide or thiocyanate toxicity. This usually occurs clinically when the drug is used at high dosages for prolonged periods and/or in patients with renal failure. If cyanide or thiocyanate toxicity occurs, treatment can be administered using a standard cyanide antidote kit that includes sodium nitrite and sodium thiosulfate for injection and amyl nitrite for inhalation.

## Interactions

The incidence of drug interactions is low for the direct-acting vasodilators as a class. Hydralazine can produce additive hypotensive effects when given with adrenergic or other antihypertensive drugs.

## Dosages

For dosage information for selected vasodilator drugs, see the table on this page.

## DOSAGES

### Selected Antihypertensive Drugs: Vasodilators

| DRUG (PREGNANCY CATEGORY) | PHARMACOLOGIC CLASS | USUAL DOSAGE RANGE | INDICATIONS |
|---|---|---|---|
| ◆ hydralazine (Apresoline) (C) | Direct-acting peripheral vasodilators | **Pediatric**<br>PO: 0.75-7.5 mg/kg/day to a max of 200 mg/day<br>**Adult**<br>PO: 10-25 mg 2-4 times/day × 7 days, then increase to 50 mg bid-qid. Titrate to effect to max dose of 300 mg/day<br>IV: 20-40 mg prn | Hypertension |
| sodium nitroprusside (Nipride, Nitropress) (C) | | **Pediatric and adult**<br>IV: 0.3-0.5 mcg/kg/min, titrate to desired effect. Max of 10 mcg/kg/min | |

*IV,* Intravenous; *PO,* oral.

## DOSAGES

### Miscellaneous Antihypertensive Drugs

| DRUG (PREGNANCY CATEGORY) | PHARMACOLOGIC CLASS | USUAL DOSAGE RANGE | INDICATIONS |
|---|---|---|---|
| bosentan (Tracleer) (X) | Endothelin receptor antagonist | **Adult only** PO: 62.5 mg bid | Pulmonary artery hypertension in patients with moderate to severe heart failure |
| eplerenone (Inspra) (B) | Aldosterone receptor antagonist | **Adult only** PO: Initial dose of 50 mg once/day ×4 wk, then increase as tolerated to max dose of 50 mg bid | Hypertension and post-MI status (to improve post-MI survival in patients with stable heart failure) |
| treprostinol (Remodulin) (B) | Vasodilator and platelet aggregation inhibitor | **Adult only** Continuous subcutaneous infusion: 1.25-2.5 ng/kg/min | Pulmonary artery hypertension in patients with severe heart failure |

*MI*, Myocardial infarction; *PO*, oral.

## DRUG PROFILES

### ♦ hydralazine

Hydralazine (Apresoline) is less commonly used now than when it first became available, but it is still effective for selected patients. It can be taken orally to treat routine cases of essential hypertension. It is also available in injectable form for hypertensive emergencies and is useful for patients who cannot tolerate oral therapy in the hospital. Hydralazine may be given intravenously. Some hospitals do not require cardiac monitoring when it is given intravenously. Contraindications include drug allergy, coronary artery disease, and mitral valve dysfunction, such as that related to childhood rheumatic fever. A new combination drug product is a tablet that contains both 37.5 mg of hydralazine and 20 mg of the antianginal drug isosorbide dinitrate (see Chapter 23). This drug combination is known as BiDil, and it is specifically indicated as an adjunct for treatment of heart failure in African-American patients. This drug combination has been shown to improve patient survival and prolong time to hospitalization for heart failure in African-American patient populations.

#### Pharmacokinetics

| Route | Onset of Action | Peak Plasma Concentration | Elimination Half-life | Duration of Action |
|---|---|---|---|---|
| IV | 5-20 min | 30-45 min | 2-8 hr | 1-4 hr |
| PO | 20-30 min | 1-2 hr | 2-8 hr | 8 hr |

### sodium nitroprusside

Sodium nitroprusside (Nitropress), like diazoxide, is normally used in the intensive care setting for severe hypertensive emergencies and is titrated to effect by intravenous infusion. Its use is contraindicated in patients with a known hypersensitivity to the drug, severe heart failure, and known inadequate cerebral perfusion (especially during neurosurgical procedures). Recommended dosages are given in the table on p. 358.

#### Pharmacokinetics

| Route | Onset of Action | Peak Plasma Concentration | Elimination Half-life | Duration of Action |
|---|---|---|---|---|
| IV | Less than 2 min | 2-5 min | 2 min | 1-10 min |

## MISCELLANEOUS ANTIHYPERTENSIVE DRUGS

Four newer medications exemplify some of the antihypertensive drugs most recently made available in the United States. These include eplerenone, bosentan, and treprostinil. All of these drugs are currently indicated for adult use only.

## DRUG PROFILES

### eplerenone

Eplerenone (Inspra) is currently the only drug in a new class of antihypertensive drugs called *selective aldosterone blockers*. It reduces blood pressure by blocking the actions of the hormone aldosterone at its corresponding receptors in the kidney, heart, blood vessels, and brain. Eplerenone is indicated for both routine treatment of hypertension and for post-MI heart failure. Its use is contraindicated in patients with known drug allergy, elevated serum potassium levels (higher than 5.5 mEq/L), or severe renal impairment and in those using a medication that inhibits the action of cytochrome P-450 enzyme 3A4. Many commonly used medications inhibit the action of this enzyme, including several antibiotic, antifungal, and antiviral drugs. Recommended dosages are given in the table on this page.

### bosentan

Bosentan (Tracleer) works by blocking the receptors of the hormone endothelin. Normally this hormone acts to stimulate the narrowing of blood vessels by binding to endothelin receptors ($ET_A$ and $ET_B$) in the endothelial (innermost) lining of blood vessels and in vascular smooth muscle. Bosentan reduces blood pressure by blocking this action. However, currently it is specifically indicated only for the treatment of pulmonary artery hypertension in patients with moderate to severe heart failure. It is available only through a limited distribution program directly from the manufacturer. Its use is contraindicated in patients with known drug allergy, pregnancy, or significant liver impairment, and in patients receiving concurrent drug therapy with cyclosporine or glyburide. Recommended dosages are given in the table on this page.

Ambrisentan (Letairis) is a new drug similar to bosentan. Other drugs used to treat pulmonary hypertension include epoprostenol, treprostinil, and iloprost. The erectile dysfunction drugs sildenafil and tadalafil are also used (see Chapter 35). Both of these drugs go by different trade names when used for pulmonary hypertension. Sildenafil, which is commonly known as Viagra, also has the trade name Revatio; and tadalafil, which is commonly known as Cialis, is called Adcirca when used for pulmonary hypertension.

### treprostinil

Treprostinil (Remodulin) lowers blood pressure through a combined mechanism of action by dilating both pulmonary and systemic blood vessels and by inhibiting platelet aggregation. Like bosentan, it is indicated specifically for treatment of pulmonary artery hypertension in patients with moderate to severe heart failure. Its only current contraindication is known drug allergy. It is also unique to date in being the only drug diluted to the nanogram level for administration. Recommended dosages are given in the table on p. 359.

## NURSING PROCESS

Over the last several decades, the diagnosis and treatment of hypertension has changed greatly from a stepped approach to a medical regimen that is now based on guidelines from the National Institutes of Health (issued in May 2003). These guidelines apply to adults 18 years of age and older and describe evaluation, classification, diagnosis, risk factors, identifiable causes, and blood pressure measurement techniques. One of the major differences in these guidelines, contained in *JNC 7*, is the creation of a "prehypertension" category, defined as a systolic blood pressure of 120 to 139 mm Hg and/or a diastolic blood pressure of 80 to 89 mm Hg. This is a change from previous guidelines and provides a more aggressive approach to the identification and subsequent management of the disease process, instead of a later diagnosis and treatment when multiple organ damage may be present. The nursing process discussion that follows provides both general and specific information related to the pharmacologic and nonpharmacologic treatment of all stages of hypertension.

## ASSESSMENT

Before any antihypertensive drug is given to a patient, obtain a thorough health history and perform a head-to-toe physical assessment. Measure and document blood pressure, pulse rate, respirations, and pulse oximetry readings. Monitor laboratory tests, including: (1) serum sodium, potassium, chloride, magnesium, and calcium levels; (2) serum level of troponin, which is usually elevated within 4 to 6 hours after a heart attack begins and may be a reliable indicator up to 14 days after a heart attack; (3) renal function studies, including BUN, serum, and urinary creatinine levels; and (4) hepatic function studies, including serum levels of ALT and AST.

Laboratory tests will most likely be complemented by more sophisticated scans and imaging studies. Noninvasive ophthalmoscopic examination of the eye structures (e.g., optic nerve, optic disk, vessels) by a professionally trained health care practitioner (e.g., nurse practitioner, physician assistant, physician, ophthalmologist, optometrist) allows easy visualization of the structures impacted by hypertension. If hypertensive retinopathy is present, the examination will reveal narrowing of blood vessels in the eye, oozing of fluid from these blood vessels, spots on the retina, swelling of the macula and optic nerve, and/or bleeding in the back of the eye. These problems may be prevented by controlling the blood pressure or treating hypertension with appropriate follow-up once it is diagnosed.

Assess also for conditions, factors, or variables that may be underlying causes of a patient's hypertension, such as:

- Addison's disease
- Coarctation of the aorta
- Coronary heart disease
- Culture and race or ethnicity
- Cushing's disease
- Family history of hypertension
- Nicotine use
- Obesity
- Peripheral vascular disease
- Pheochromocytoma
- Preeclampsia of pregnancy
- Renal artery stenosis
- Renal or liver insufficiency
- Stressful lifestyle

Many of these factors demand very cautious use of antihypertensive drugs. Other cautions and contraindications include the use of these drugs in the elderly and those with chronic illnesses because of further compromise of the physical condition these patients due to uncontrolled or untreated hypertension or the adverse effects of antihypertensives (e.g., fluid loss, dehydration, electrolyte imbalances, hypotension). For a complete listing of adverse effects as well as drug interactions associated with antihypertensives, see the pharmacology section of this chapter.

Use of *alpha-adrenergic agonists* demands close assessment of the patient's blood pressure, pulse rate, and weight before and during treatment because of their strong vasodilating properties and subsequent hypotensive adverse effects. These drugs may also be associated with fluid retention and edema, so assess heart and breath sounds and intake and output, as well as dependent edema. The *alpha-adrenergic antagonists* need to be used cautiously because of the potential for hypotension-induced dizziness and syncope. The use of either of these groups of drugs requires close assessment of all parameters, especially in the elderly or other patients with preexisting dizziness or syncope, or a debilitated state. With doxazosin, first-dose orthostatic hypotension may occur within 2 to 6 hours; therefore, carefully assess blood pressures (supine and standing) and measure corresponding pulse rates before the first dose and 2 to 6 hours afterward, as well as with any subsequent increase in the dosage. When any antihypertensive drug is used, measure blood pressures and pulse rates (supine and standing), and assess for cautions, contraindications, and drug interactions. With *centrally acting alpha blockers,* also assess white blood cell counts, serum potassium and sodium levels and level of protein in the urine (to identify proteinuria). Note the route of administration specified in the drug order because of concerns associated with different routes. For example, with clonidine transdermal patches, assess the skin for rash, redness, drainage, or broken integrity prior to application.

Review the *beta blockers* and their mechanisms of action before administering these drugs to a patient because of the risk for complications in certain patient populations. If the drug is a nonselective beta blocker, it blocks both beta$_1$ and beta$_2$ receptors and will have both cardiac and respiratory effects, whereas if a drug is only a beta$_1$-blocking drug, the cardiac system will be affected (pulse rate and blood pressure will decrease) but there will be no beta$_2$ effects. This limits any concern regarding respiratory problems (e.g., bronchoconstriction). Therefore, if a patient needs a beta blocker but has restrictive airway problems, a beta$_1$ blocker is recommended (to avoid bronchoconstriction). If there is no history of respiratory illness or concerns, however, the nonselective beta blockers may be very effective as antihypertensives. In addition, for patients with heart failure, understand that beta blockers also have a negative inotropic effect on the heart (decreased contractility); their use would lead to worsening of heart failure, which calls for a completely different class of antihypertensive.

With the use of beta blockers, assess blood pressure and apical pulse rate immediately before each dose. If the systolic blood pressure is less than 90 mm Hg or the pulse rate is less than 60 beats/min, notify the prescriber because of the risk of adverse effects (e.g., hypotension, bradycardia). In such cases, the drug would usually be withheld, as ordered or per protocol. These blood pressure and pulse rate parameters are also applicable with use of other antihypertensives. Also assess breath sounds and heart sounds before and during drug therapy.

With the use of *ACE inhibitors*, assess blood pressure, apical pulse rate, and respiratory status (because of the adverse effect of a dry, hacking, chronic cough). Take blood pressure readings immediately before initial and subsequent doses of the drug so that extreme fluctuations may be identified early. Also assess serum potassium, sodium, and chloride levels as ordered. Tests of baseline cardiac functioning will most likely be ordered prior to initiation of therapy. Because of the potential adverse effects of neutropenia and other blood disorders, assess complete blood count before and during therapy, as ordered. *Angiotensin receptor blockers (ARBs)* are to be used very cautiously in elderly patients and in patients with renal dysfunction because of their increased sensitivity to the drug's effects and increased risk for adverse effects.

Perform a baseline neurologic assessment with the use of *vasodilators*, with attention to level of consciousness and cognitive ability. Use these drugs with extreme caution with the elderly, because they are more sensitive to the drugs' blood pressure–lowering effects and may experience more problems with hypotension, dizziness, and syncope.

In summary, many assessment parameters are similar for the various groups of antihypertensives. The difference in the level of assessment depends on the drug's impact on blood pressure as well as the individual's response to the medication and any preexisting illnesses or conditions. Other factors to be assessed in any patient receiving these drugs, as well as most other drugs, include the patient's cultural background, racial or ethnic group, reading level, learning needs, developmental and cognitive status, financial status, mental health status, available support systems, and overall physical health. Encourage patients to learn how to assess and monitor themselves and their individual responses to drug therapy.

## ⊕ PATIENT-CENTERED CARE: CULTURAL IMPLICATIONS

### *Antihypertensive Drug Therapy*

The following are some important generalizations about demographics and the drugs used to treat hypertension:

- Beta blockers and angiotensin-converting enzyme (ACE) inhibitors have been found to be more effective in lowering blood pressure in whites than in African Americans.
- Calcium channel blockers and diuretics have been shown to be more effective in African-American patients than in white patients.
- Captopril, used as monotherapy to treat hypertension, has been found to elicit a lesser response in African-American patients, who are considered to be low-renin hypertensives, than in the general treatment population.
- Losartan, used as monotherapy for hypertension, has been found to be less effective in African-American patients than in other racial groups because African-American patients are low-renin hypertensives.

These findings are important to remember in the care of patients, whether they are in an inpatient setting; are being seen by a physician, physician's assistant, or nurse practitioner; or are being screened by a nurse in the community. The significance of these cultural-ethnic factors is that they allow a better understanding of the dynamics of pharmacologic treatment in hypertensive patients of different ethnic groups and also underscore the importance of a thorough nursing assessment that includes attention to cultural influences. These factors also allow an appreciation of individual responses to drug therapy and aid in achieving more successful treatment of the disease. These responses are often considered by health care providers in selecting first-line therapy.

Modified from Kelerman RD, Rakel RE: *Conn's current therapy 2010,* Philadelphia, 2010, St Louis: Elsevier.

## ▌NURSING DIAGNOSES

1. Ineffective peripheral tissue perfusion related to the impact of the hypertensive disease process and/or possible severe hypotensive adverse effects associated with antihypertensive drug therapy
2. Sexual dysfunction related to adverse effects of some antihypertensive drugs
3. Constipation related to the adverse effects of antihypertensive drugs
4. Noncompliance with drug therapy related to lack of familiarity with or acceptance of the disease process
5. Risk for injury (e.g., possible falls) related to possible antihypertensive drug–induced orthostatic hypotension with dizziness and syncope

## ▌PLANNING

Focus nursing goals for antihypertensive therapy on educating the patient, family, and/or caregiver about the critical importance of adequate management to prevent end-organ damage. Goals must include making sure the patient understands the nature of the disease, its symptoms and treatment, and the importance of adhering to the treatment regimen. The patient must also come to terms with the diagnosis as well as with the fact that there is no cure for the disease and treatment will be lifelong. Emphasize the influence of chronic illness and the importance of nonpharmacologic therapy, stress reduction, and follow-up care. Plan for ongoing assessment of blood pressure, weight, diet, exercise, smoking habits, alcohol intake, compliance with therapy, and sexual function in the patient receiving therapy for hypertension.

## GOALS

1. Patient regains control of hypertension with return of adequate tissue perfusion.
2. Patient experiences minimal changes in sexual functioning while managing adverse drug effects.
3. Patient experiences minimal changes in bowel elimination patterns.
4. Patient remains compliant with antihypertensive drug therapy.
5. Patient remains free from injury during drug therapy.

## OUTCOME CRITERIA

1. Patient states the importance of taking antihypertensive drug therapy as prescribed to maintain normal to near-normal blood pressure control.
   - Patient regains control of hypertension with a return of blood pressure to below the ranges set by the Joint National Committee, such as a systolic blood pressure of 120 to 139 mm Hg and/or a diastolic blood pressure of 80 to 89 mm Hg.
   - Patient states the importance of keeping follow-up appointments with prescriber as well as monitoring blood pressure.
2. Patient openly discusses any difficulty in sexual functioning during antihypertensive therapy.
   - Patient implements suggestions/interventions as shared by the prescriber to assist in decreasing any problems with sexual function.
   - Patient states the importance of avoiding abrupt discontinuation of drug therapy with antihypertensives while experiencing changes in sexual functioning to avoid rebound hypertension and risk for complications.
3. Patient manages constipation with healthy lifestyle/dietary changes.
   - Patient implements forcing fluids (unless contraindicated), increasing dietary fiber with increase in fruits and vegetables, and/or taking prescriber-suggested psyllium-based product for improving constipation.
4. Patient demonstrates an understanding of the importance of taking antihypertensive medication(s) exactly as prescribed.
   - Patient reports to prescriber any adverse effects such as dizziness, syncope, excessive fatigue, constipation, and/or changes in sexual functioning while continuing medication regimen unless prescribed by health care provider.
   - Patient's blood pressure begins to return to a range as defined by the prescriber and the Joint National Committee.
5. Patient follows instructions to maintain safety and minimize dizziness and syncope while on medication regimen.
   - Patient changes position slowly, carefully, and purposefully.
   - Patient keeps daily journal with entries about diet, exercise, adverse effects, blood pressure readings, and daily weights.

## IMPLEMENTATION

Nursing interventions may help patients achieve stable blood pressure while minimizing adverse effects during treatment with antihypertensives. Many patients have problems complying with treatment because the disease itself is silent or without symptoms. Because of this, some patients are unaware of their increased blood pressure or think that if they do not feel bad there is nothing wrong with them, which poses many problems for treatment. Also, the antihypertensives are often associated with multiple adverse effects that may impact patients' self-concept and/or sexual integrity. These adverse effects may lead patients to abruptly stop taking the medication. Inform patients that any abrupt withdrawal is a serious concern because of the risk of developing rebound hypertension, which is a sudden and very high elevation of blood pressure. This places the patient at risk for a cerebrovascular accident or other cerebral or cardiac adverse events. It is important to understand that with *all* antihypertensives there is a risk of rebound hypertension (with abrupt withdrawal), and prevention of this through patient education is critical to patient safety. Other interventions related to each major group of drugs are discussed in the following paragraphs. See the Patient Teaching Tips for more information.

Because of the potential for drug-related orthostatic hypotensive effects, patients taking *alpha-adrenergic agonists* will need to monitor their blood pressure and pulse rate at home or have these parameters measured by a family member who has received instructions or by local fire department, rescue, or emergency medical personnel or health care provider. The blood pressure machines found in grocery stores do not provide as accurate readings as measurement in the aforementioned ways. *Alpha-adrenergic antagonist drugs* are associated with first-dose syncope, so, to avoid injury, advise patients to remain supine for the first dose of the drug. More than likely, these drugs will be prescribed to be given at bedtime to allow the patient to sleep through the drug's first-dose syncope. It may take 4 to 6 weeks for the drug to achieve its full therapeutic effects. Educate the patient about this delayed onset of action and bedtime dosing to avoid injury. The patient needs continued monitoring for dizziness, syncope, edema, and other adverse effects (e.g., shortness of breath, exacerbation of pre-existing cardiac disorders). Diuretics may be ordered as adjunctive therapy to minimize the adverse effects of edema, but they may lead to more dizziness and electrolyte problems. *Centrally acting alpha blockers* require the same type of nursing interventions as other alpha blockers; however, as their name indicates, the mechanism of action of these drugs is central, so adverse effects are often more pronounced (e.g., hypotension, sedation, bradycardia, edema). See the Patient Teaching Tips for more information.

The *beta blockers* are either nonselective (block both beta$_1$ and beta$_2$ receptors; e.g., propranolol) or cardioselective (block mainly beta$_1$ receptors; e.g., atenolol). With any beta blocker, careful adherence to the drug regimen is critical to patient safety. Patients taking beta blockers may experience an exacerbation of respiratory diseases such as asthma, bronchospasm, and chronic obstructive pulmonary disease (because of increased bronchoconstriction due to beta$_2$ blocking) or an exacerbation of heart failure (because of the drug's negative inotropic effects, i.e., decreased contractility due to beta₁ blocking). Provide clear and concise instructions about reporting adverse effects and instructions for taking blood pressure and pulse rates. If a beta₁ blocker causes shortness of breath, it is most likely due to edema and/or exacerbation of heart failure. Any dizziness, postural hypotension, edema, constipation, or sexual dysfunction needs to be reported to the prescriber immediately. See Patient Teaching Tips for more information.

*ACE inhibitors* must also be taken exactly as prescribed. If angioedema occurs, contact the prescriber immediately. If the drug must be discontinued, weaning is recommended (as with all antihypertensives) to avoid rebound hypertension. Monitor serum sodium and potassium levels during therapy. Serum potassium levels increase as an adverse effect of these drugs, resulting in hyperkalemia and possible complications. Impaired taste may occur as an adverse effect and last up to 2 to 3 months after the drug has been discontinued. It is also important to educate the patient that it takes several weeks to see the full therapeutic effects and that potassium supplements are not needed with the ACE inhibitors because of the adverse effect of hyperkalemia.

*Angiotensin receptor blockers (ARBs)* must also be taken exactly as prescribed. They are often tolerated best with meals, as with many antihypertensives. The dosage must not be changed nor the medication discontinued except on the order of the prescriber. With ARBs, if the patient has hypovolemia or hepatic dysfunction, the dosage may need to be reduced. A diuretic such as hydrochlorothiazide may be ordered in combination with an ARB for patients who have hypertension with left ventricular hypertrophy. Losartan is also an option for patients at risk for stroke and for those who are hypertensive and have left ventricular hypertrophy. Most importantly, with ARBs, report any unusual dyspnea, dizziness, or excessive fatigue to the prescriber immediately.

Nursing considerations for *vasodilators* are similar to those for other antihypertensives; however, the impact of the vasodilators on blood pressure may be more drastic, depending on the specific drug and dosage. Hydralazine given by injection may result in reduced blood pressure within 10 to 80 minutes after administration and requires that you closely monitor the patient. With hydralazine, systemic lupus erythematosus (SLE) may be an adverse effect if the patient is taking more than 200 mg/day orally. If signs and symptoms of SLE occur, such as photosensitivity, characteristic skin rashes, CNS changes, or various blood dyscrasias (hemolytic anemia, leukopenia, thrombocytopenia), discontinue the drug, contact the prescriber immediately, and continue to closely monitor the patient. Electrocardiographic changes, cardiovascular inadequacies, and hypotension may have pronounced effects on the patient's cardiac status, so *never* give the drug without adequate monitoring and frequent assessment. Always dilute sodium nitroprusside per manufacturer's guidelines. Because this drug is a potent vasodilator, it may lead to extreme decreases in the patient's blood pressure. Severe drops in blood pressure may lead to irreversible ischemic injury and even death, so close monitoring is needed during drug administration. Remember that sodium nitroprusside should never be infused at the maximum dose rate for more than 10 minutes. If this drug does not control a patient's blood pressure after 10 minutes, it will most likely be discontinued by the prescriber.

Cyanide ions are a by-product of nitroprusside metabolism. Cyanide and thiocyanate toxicity are seen clinically when nitroprusside is used at high dosages for long periods of time and/or in patients with renal insufficiency. When nitroprusside is combined with sodium thiosulfate, the potential for cyanide toxicity is greatly reduced. To help prevent complications of cyanide and thiocyanate toxicity, (1) dilute the medication properly and avoid use of any solution that has turned blue, green, or red; (2) infuse only with use of a volumetric infusion pump, not through ordinary intravenous sets; (3) continuously monitor blood pressure during the infusion (often by invasive measures); and (4) when more than 500 mcg/kg of sodium nitroprusside is administered at a rate faster than 2 mcg/kg/min, be aware that this may result in production of cyanide at a faster rate than it can be eliminated by the patient unaided (see the Safety: Laboratory Values Related to Drug Therapy box below).

## SAFETY: LABORATORY VALUES RELATED TO DRUG THERAPY

### *Sodium Nitroprusside*

| LABORATORY TEST | NORMAL RANGES | RATIONALE FOR ASSESSMENT |
|---|---|---|
| Serum methemoglobin and serum cyanide levels | Normally there are no detectable amounts with appropriate drug levels of sodium nitroprusside. | Use of sodium nitroprusside may be associated with sequestration of hemoglobin as methemoglobin. The appearance of this clinically significant adverse effect of methemoglobinemia is rare (less than 10% of cases). Serum laboratory testing is used to measure the amount of methemoglobin. One significant clinical sign of this adverse effect is impaired oxygen delivery despite adequate cardiac output. When the sequestration is diagnosed, the treatment of choice is 1 to 2 mg/kg of methylene blue given intravenously over several minutes to allow binding of the metabolic by-product of cyanide to methemoglobin as cyanmethemoglobin, but this must be given only as ordered and with extreme caution. In addition, sodium nitroprusside may lead to toxic reactions, even at dosages that are within the recommended ranges. Toxic reactions are manifested by extreme hypotension, cyanide toxicity, or thiocyanate toxicity. Cyanide toxicity is manifested by severe hypotension. Cyanide assays are performed to detect cyanide in body fluids, but the results of this test are difficult to interpret and so it is not the most reliable method of monitoring. Other laboratory tests that may be helpful in diagnosing cyanide toxicity are alterations of acid-base balance and venous oxygen concentrations. Actual cyanide levels in the blood may lag behind peak cyanide levels by 1 hour or longer. |

*Calcium channel blockers* (CCBs) and related nursing interventions are discussed only briefly here, because these drugs are covered in other chapters. Drugs like enalapril are to be taken exactly as prescribed with a warning to the patient not to puncture, open, or crush the extended-release or sustained-release tablets and capsules. Be aware that CCBs are negative inotropic drugs (decrease cardiac contractility), because this action may induce more signs of heart failure if these drugs are given with drugs that are used to increase cardiac contractility, such as digitalis glycosides. Monitoring of blood pressure and pulse rate before and during therapy will aid in prevention or early detection of any problems related to the negative inotropic effects, negative chronotropic effects (decreased heart rate), and negative dromotropic effects (decreased conduction).

Remember always to base nursing interventions on a thorough assessment and plan of care that also includes consideration of the patient's cultural and ethnic group. This is particularly important with antihypertensives, because research studies have documented differences in responses to antihypertensives among different racial and ethnic groups. Some ethnic groups respond less favorably to certain drugs than to others. As for patients with any disease, patients with hypertension must be treated with respect and with an appreciation for a holistic approach to health care in which all physical, psychosocial, and spiritual needs are taken into consideration (see the Patient-Centered Care: Cultural Implications box on p. 361). Remember also that patient education is of critical importance and plays an important role in ensuring adherence to the drug regimen and in decreasing the incidence of problems related to these medications.

# EVALUATION

Because patients with hypertension are at high risk for cardiovascular injury, it is critical for them to adhere to both their pharmacologic and nonpharmacologic treatment regimens. Monitoring patients for the adverse effects (e.g., orthostatic hypotension, dizziness, fatigue) and toxic effects of the various types of antihypertensive drugs helps to identify potentially life-threatening complications. The most important aspect of the evaluation process is collecting data and monitoring patients for evidence of controlled blood pressure. Blood pressure must be maintained at values lower than the parameters established by the Joint National Committee or below the levels set by the Joint National Committee for "prehypertension," namely, a systolic blood pressure of 120 to 139 mm Hg and/or a diastolic blood pressure of 80 to 89 mm Hg. If compelling indications are present, such as diabetes mellitus or kidney disease, the blood pressure goal is often lower. Blood pressure needs to be monitored at periodic intervals. Patient education about self-monitoring is very important to the safe use of these drugs. Updated information on hypertension and its diagnosis, treatment, and evaluation is available at the National Heart, Lung, and Blood Institute website at www.nhlbi.nih.gov/guidelines/hypertension.

In addition to measuring blood pressure, the prescriber will examine the fundus of the patient's eye. Changes in the fundus have been found to be a more reliable indicator of the long-term effectiveness of treatment than blood pressure readings because of the changes in the vasculature of the eye caused by high blood pressure. Continually monitor the patient for the development of end-organ damage and for the presence of the specific problems that the medication can cause. Counsel and constantly

## EVIDENCE-BASED PRACTICE

### *Storytelling to Improve Blood Pressure*

**Review**

Is it possible that patient-to-patient storytelling, such as the use of narrative communication, has the benefit of lowering blood pressure? In this study of hypertensive black patients in Alabama, researchers identified a focus group of patients who were able to clearly and persuasively describe their experiences with hypertension. There were patients who were selected to serve as storytellers on DVDs and offer lessons about how to interact with physicians as well as discuss ways to better achieve medication adherence, diet, and exercise. The benefits of this intervention will be compared to that of the use of some antihypertensive medications.

**Type of Evidence**

There were 231 participants in the study. Participants were randomly selected to receive either the storytellers' DVDs or DVDs about general health issues that were totally unrelated to hypertension. The intervention patients spent an average of about 88 minutes watching the storytellers' DVDs.

**Results of Study**

Patients in both groups who had controlled hypertension at baseline were found to exhibit no significant changes in blood pressure 6 to 9 months after the intervention. However, in comparison, patients with uncontrolled hypertension at baseline were found to have significant reductions in mean blood pressure, a 15 mm Hg drop in systolic pressure (versus 3 mm Hg in the control group), and a 3 mm Hg drop in diastolic pressure (versus no change in the control group). In this randomized study, storytelling by black patients for use in black hypertensive patients achieved dramatic reductions in blood pressure (as stated above) as compared to the control groups.

**Link of Evidence to Nursing Practice**

For black patients with hypertension, it is important to note that the authors state "listeners may be influenced if they actively engage in a story, identify themselves with the storyteller and picture themselves taking part in the action." The authors go on to discuss the fact that the magnitude of the effect in this study with these participants was similar to the use of antihypertensive medications for lowering blood pressure. The important connection to nursing practice is that this study can be replicated in a larger sample size of black patients, and, if the benefits are sustained over time, the intervention of storytelling would be a substantial achievement.

Reference: Houston TK, Allison JJ, Sussman M, et al: Culturally appropriate storytelling to improve blood pressure: a randomized trial, *Ann Intern Med* 154(2):77, 2011.

## CASE STUDY

### Drugs for Hypertension

Hypertension was diagnosed in G.S., who is 30 years old. Both her mother and sister have hypertension, and both were also in their thirties when it was diagnosed. G.'s most current blood pressure reading is 150/96 mm Hg, and for this reason the nurse practitioner has recommended therapy with captopril (Capoten), light exercise in the form of walking, and relaxation therapy. After 1 month of therapy, G.'s blood pressure is 145/86 mm Hg. Stress reduction has been the biggest obstacle in her treatment, because she is a lawyer with a prominent law firm and has found that her blood pressure is consistently elevated (160/100 mm Hg) whenever she measures it at work. At this follow-up visit, she is also given a prescription for a diuretic to help with her blood pressure control.

1. What type of diuretic was probably prescribed for G.S. at this time? Explain your answer.
2. What possible adverse effects does G. need to be aware of while taking captopril?
3. G. tells you that she uses an over-the-counter pain reliever for occasional headaches. What potential interaction is of concern?
4. G.S. states that she and her husband are planning to start a family in 1 year. What will you, as her nurse, tell her about pregnancy and therapy with these drugs?
5. What lifestyle changes would you, as her nurse, recommend that she make, and, even more important, what information would you give her to help her change her lifestyle and more effectively reduce the stress in her life?

For answers, see http://evolve.elsevier.com/Lilley.

monitor male patients receiving antihypertensives for complaints of sexual dysfunction. This is important because the patient may experience sexual dysfunction and, if the patient is not expecting it, may not report the problem and decide to stop taking the medication abruptly. Once an antihypertensive drug is stopped abruptly, the patient is then placed at high risk for rebound hypertension and possible stroke or other complications. Communication is critical in these situations. Follow-up visits to the prescriber are important for monitoring these and other adverse effects and checking patient adherence to the drug regimen.

Therapeutic effects of antihypertensives in general include an improvement in blood pressure and in the disease process. Other therapeutic effects include a return to a normal baseline level of blood pressure with improved energy levels and decreased signs and symptoms of hypertension, such as less edema, improved breath sounds, no abnormal heart sounds, capillary refill in less than 5 seconds, and less shortness of breath. Monitor for the adverse effects discussed in the pharmacology section of the chapter as well as those described for each group of drugs earlier in the Nursing Process section.

## PATIENT TEACHING TIPS

### Antihypertensives in General

- Medications are to be taken exactly as ordered with avoidance of doubling up or omitting doses.
- Successful therapy requires adherence to the medication regimen as well as to any dietary restrictions (e.g., decreasing consumption of fatty or high-cholesterol foods).
- The patient needs to monitor stress levels and use biofeedback, imagery, and/or relaxation techniques or massage, as needed. Exercise, if approved by the prescriber, may also help in the management of hypertension and serves to relieve stress; supervised, prescribed exercise is usually ordered.
- Emphasize the importance of safety and the need to avoid smoking and excessive alcohol intake as well as excessive exercise, hot climates, saunas, hot tubs, and hot environments. Heat may precipitate vasodilation and lead to worsening of hypotension with the risk of fainting and injury to self.
- Frequent laboratory tests may be needed for the duration of therapy; emphasize the importance of keeping follow-up appointments to the patient.
- All medications must be kept out of the reach of children because of the potential for extreme toxicity. If a transdermal patch is used, instruct the patient on how to periodically check on its placement. There have been cases in which a patch that was placed on an adult later fell off and was accidentally picked up on the skin of a crawling infant, with severe consequences.

- Encourage the patient to wear a medical alert bracelet or necklace and to carry a medical identification card specifying his or her diagnosis, noting allergies, and listing all medications taken (e.g., prescribed drugs, over-the-counter medications, herbals, vitamins, and supplements). The same information must be kept in a visible location in the patient's car as well as in the patient's home (i.e., on the refrigerator) for emergency medical personnel.
- Emphasize the importance of recording blood pressure readings (and orthostatic blood pressure readings) and daily weights in a journal. Daily weights are to be done each morning, before breakfast, at the same time, and with the same amount of clothing. The patient must report to the prescriber an increase in weight by 2 pounds or more over a 24-hour period or 5 pounds or more in 1 week.
- Assess the patient's ability and comfort level in taking his or her own blood pressure and pulse rate. Monitor the patient's progress in the proper technique.
- Encourage patient to inform all health care providers (e.g., dentist, surgeon) about his or her antihypertensive medication regimen.
- Careful, purposeful, and cautious changing of positions is encouraged because of the possible adverse effect of postural hypotension and associated risk for dizziness, lightheadedness, and possible fainting and falls.

- Instruct the patient to always keep an adequate supply of antihypertensive medications on hand, especially while traveling.
- Scheduling of periodic eye examinations is recommended every 6 months due to the need to evaluate treatment effectiveness because of the impact of hypertension on the vasculature of the eyes.
- With successful therapy, the patient's condition will improve; however, the patient must understand to never abruptly stop taking the medication just because he or she is feeling better. Lifelong therapy is usually required.
- Saliva substitutes, use of sugar-free hard candy/gum, and forcing fluids (unless contraindicated) may help with dry mouth. Forcing fluids and increasing dietary fiber may help with preventing constipation. Instruct the patient to contact the prescriber if constipation remains a problem.
- Sexual dysfunction may occur with antihypertensives, and so encourage the patient to be open in reporting and discussing any problems or concerns. Inform the patient that, if this adverse effect occurs, options are available to help alleviate the problem, such as combination therapy that allows lower dosages of drugs to be used, as well as a change to other types of antihypertensives. Always reinforce the fact that these medications are to never be abruptly stopped because of the risk of severe hypertensive rebound.
- Inform the patient that antihypertensives may lead to depression and to report any change in emotional status to the prescriber.

### Alpha-Adrenergic Agonists
- First-dose syncope is associated with alpha adrenergic agonists, so patients need to avoid conditions/situations/drugs that would exacerbate this.

- Caution the patient to be careful at first with driving and other activities requiring alertness. The patient may have to postpone driving and other activities until the drug-related drowsiness subsides.
- Instruct the patient to report any dizziness, palpitations, and orthostatic hypotension to the prescriber immediately.
- Because centrally acting alpha blockers may also affect the patient's sexual functioning (e.g., causing impotence or decreased libido), inform the patient of these possible adverse effects and advise the patient to contact the prescriber if these effects are problematic. Other treatment options may be indicated.
- Transdermal patches of clonidine are to be applied to nonhairy areas of the skin as ordered, and application sites rotated. All residual drug on the skin must be cleansed with a washcloth soaked in lukewarm water and the area thoroughly dried (avoid excess rubbing of site) before applying a new patch.

### Beta Blockers
- Encourage the patient to move and change positions slowly to avoid possible dizziness, fainting, and falls. Instruct the patient to report a pulse rate lower than 60 beats/min, dizziness, or a systolic blood pressure of 90 mm Hg or lower to the prescriber.
- Prolonged sitting or standing and excessive physical exercise may also lead to exacerbation of hypotensive effects, so counsel the patient to avoid these activities or counteract them with healthy practices such as pumping the feet up and down while sitting.
- Heat may also exacerbate hypotensive effects of the beta blocker. Educate patient to avoid saunas, hot tubs and excessive heat or syncope (fainting) may result.

■ KEY POINTS

- All antihypertensives in some way affect cardiac output. Cardiac output is the amount of blood ejected from the left ventricle and is measured in liters per minute.
- The major groups of antihypertensives are diuretics (see Chapter 28), alpha blockers, centrally acting alpha blockers, beta blockers, ACE inhibitors, vasodilators, CCBs, and ARBs.
- ACE inhibitors work by blocking a critical enzyme system responsible for the production of AII (angiotensin II; a potent vasoconstrictor). They (1) prevent vasoconstriction caused by AII, (2) prevent aldosterone secretion and therefore sodium and water resorption, and (3) prevent the breakdown of bradykinin (a potent vasodilator) by AII.
- ARBs work by blocking the binding of angiotensin at the receptors; the end result is a decrease in blood pressure.
- Calcium channel blockers may be used to treat angina, dysrhythmias, and hypertension and help to reduce blood pressure by causing smooth muscle relaxation and dilatation of blood vessels. If calcium is not present, then the smooth muscle of the blood vessels cannot contract.

- A thorough nursing assessment includes determining whether the patient has any underlying causes of hypertension, such as renal or liver dysfunction, a stressful lifestyle, Cushing's disease, Addison's disease, renal artery stenosis, peripheral vascular disease, or pheochromocytoma.
- Always assess for the presence of contraindications, cautions, and potential drug interactions before administering any of the antihypertensive drugs. Contraindications include a history of MI or chronic renal disease. Cautious use is recommended in patients with renal insufficiency or glaucoma. Drugs that interact with antihypertensive drugs include other antihypertensive drugs, anesthetics, and diuretics.
- Hypertension is managed by both pharmacologic and nonpharmacologic measures. Patients need to consume a diet low in fat, make any other necessary modifications in their diet (such as possibly decrease the intake of sodium and increase fiber intake), engage in regular supervised exercise, and reduce the amount of stress in their lives.

## NCLEX® EXAMINATION REVIEW QUESTIONS

1 The nurse is administering antihypertensive drugs to older adult patients. The nurse knows that which adverse effect is of most concern for these patients?
a Dry mouth
b Hypotension
c Restlessness
d Constipation

2 When giving antihypertensive drugs, the nurse will consider giving the first dose at bedtime for which class of drugs?
a Alpha blockers such as doxazosin (Cardura)
b Diuretics such as furosemide (Lasix)
c ACE inhibitors such as captopril (Capoten)
d Vasodilators such as hydralazine (Apresoline)

3 A 56-year-old man started antihypertensive drug therapy 3 months earlier and is in the office for a follow-up visit. While the nurse is taking his blood pressure, he informs the nurse that he has had some problems with sexual intercourse. Which would be the most appropriate response by the nurse?
a "Not to worry. Eventually, tolerance will develop."
b "The physician can work with you on changing the dose and/or drugs."
c "Sexual dysfunction happens with this therapy, and you will learn to accept it."
d "This is an unusual occurrence, but it is important to stay on your medications."

4 When a patient is being taught about the potential adverse effects of an ACE inhibitor, which of these effects should the nurse mention as possibly occurring when this drug is taken to treat hypertension?
a Diarrhea
b Nausea
c Dry, nonproductive cough
d Sedation

5 A patient has a new prescription for an ACE inhibitor. During a review of the patient's list of current medications, which would cause concern for a possible interaction with this new prescription? (Select all that apply.)
a A benzodiazepine taken as needed for allergies
b A potassium supplement taken daily
c An oral anticoagulant taken daily
d An opioid used for occasional severe pain
e An NSAID taken as needed for headaches

6 The order reads: Give hydralazine (Apresoline) 0.75 mg/kg/day. The child weighs 16 pounds. How much hydralazine will be given? Round to hundredths.

1. b, 2. a, 3. b, 4. c, 5. b, e, 6. 5.45 mg/kg/day

For Critical Thinking and Prioritization Questions, see http://evolve.elsevier.com/Lilley.

# CHAPTER

# 23

# Antianginal Drugs

## ℮volve WEBSITE

*http://evolve.elsevier.com/Lilley*

- Animations
- Answer Key—Textbook Case Studies
- Critical Thinking and Prioritization Questions

- Key Points—Downloadable
- Review Questions for the NCLEX® Examination
- Unfolding Case Studies

## OBJECTIVES

When you reach the end of this chapter, you will be able to do the following:

1 Briefly describe the pathophysiology of myocardial ischemia and the subsequent occurrence of angina.
2 Describe the various factors that may precipitate angina as well as measures that decrease its occurrence.
3 Contrast the major classes of antianginal drugs (nitrates, calcium channel blockers, and beta blockers) with regard to their mechanisms of action, dosage forms, routes of

administration, cautions, contraindications, drug interactions, adverse effects, patient tolerance, and toxicity.
4 Develop a nursing care plan incorporating all phases of the nursing process related to the administration of antianginal drugs.

## DRUG PROFILES

amlodipine, p. 376
♦ atenolol, p. 374
♦ diltiazem, p. 376
♦ isosorbide dinitrate, p. 371
♦ isosorbide mononitrate, p. 371

♦ metoprolol, p. 374
♦ nitroglycerin, p. 372
ranolazine, p. 376

_____

♦ *Key drug*

## KEY TERMS

Angina pectoris Chest pain that occurs when the heart's supply of blood carrying oxygen is insufficient to meet the demands of the heart. (p. 369)

Atherosclerosis A common form of arteriosclerosis involving deposits of fatty, cholesterol-containing material (plaques) within arterial walls. (p. 369)

Chronic stable angina Chest pain that is primarily caused by atherosclerosis, which results in a long-term but relatively stable level of obstruction in one or more coronary arteries. (p. 369)

Coronary arteries Arteries that deliver oxygen to the heart muscle. (p. 369)

Coronary artery disease (CAD) Any one of the abnormal conditions that can affect the arteries of the heart and produce various pathologic effects, especially a reduced supply of oxygen and nutrients to the myocardium. (p. 369)

Ischemia Poor blood supply to an organ. (p. 369)

Ischemic heart disease Poor blood supply to the heart via the coronary arteries. (p. 369)

Myocardial infarction (MI) Necrosis of the myocardium following interruption of blood supply; it is almost always caused by atherosclerosis of the coronary arteries and is commonly called a *heart attack.* (p. 369)

Reflex tachycardia A rapid heartbeat caused by a variety of autonomic nervous system effects, such as blood pressure changes, fever, or emotional stress. (p. 371)

Unstable angina Early stage of progressive coronary artery disease. (p. 369)

Vasospastic angina Ischemia-induced myocardial chest pain caused by spasms of the coronary arteries; also referred to as *Prinzmetal* or *variant angina*. (p. 369)

## ANATOMY, PHYSIOLOGY, AND PATHOPHYSIOLOGY OVERVIEW

The heart is a very efficient organ that pumps blood to all the tissues and organs of the body. It is very demanding in an aerobic sense because it requires a large supply of oxygen to meet the incredible demands placed on it. The heart's much-needed oxygen supply is delivered to the heart muscle by means of the coronary arteries. When the heart's supply of blood carrying oxygen and energy-rich nutrients is insufficient to meet the demands of the heart, the heart muscle (or myocardium) aches. This is called angina pectoris, or chest pain. Poor blood supply to an organ is referred to as ischemia. When the heart is involved, the condition is called ischemic heart disease.

Ischemic heart disease is the number-one killer in the United States today. The primary cause is a disease of the coronary arteries known as atherosclerosis (fatty plaque deposits in the arterial walls). When atherosclerotic plaques project from the walls into the lumens of these vessels, the vessels become narrow. The supply of oxygen and energy-rich nutrients needed for the heart to meet its demand is then decreased. This disorder is called coronary artery disease (CAD). An acute result of CAD and of ischemic heart disease is myocardial infarction (MI), or heart attack. An MI occurs when blood flow through the coronary arteries to the myocardium is completely blocked so that part of the heart muscle cannot receive any of the blood-borne nutrients (especially oxygen). If this process is not reversed immediately, that area of the heart will die and become necrotic (dead or nonfunctioning). Damage to a large enough area of the myocardium can be disabling or fatal.

The rate at which the heart pumps and the strength of each heartbeat (contractility) influence oxygen demands on the heart. There are many substances and situations that can increase heart rate and contractility and thus increase oxygen demand. These include caffeine, exercise, and stress, among others, and result in stimulation of the sympathetic nervous system, which leads to increased heart rate and contractility. In a patient with CAD who has an already overburdened heart, this stimulation can worsen the balance between myocardial oxygen supply and demand and result in angina. Some of the drugs used to treat angina are aimed at correcting the imbalance between myocardial oxygen supply and demand by decreasing heart rate and contractility.

The pain of angina is a result of the following process: Under ischemic conditions when the myocardium is deprived of oxygen, the heart shifts to anaerobic metabolism to meet its energy needs. One of the byproducts of anaerobic metabolism is lactic acid. Accumulation of lactic acid and other metabolic byproducts causes the pain receptors surrounding the heart to be stimulated, which produces the heart pain known as *angina*. This is the same pathophysiologic mechanism responsible for causing the soreness in skeletal muscles after vigorous exercise.

There are three classic types of chest pain, or angina pectoris. Chronic stable angina has atherosclerosis as its primary cause. *Classic angina* and *effort angina* are other names for it. Chronic stable angina can be triggered by exertion or other stress (e.g., cold, emotions). The nicotine in tobacco as well as alcohol, coffee, and other drugs that stimulate the sympathetic nervous system can also exacerbate it. The pain of chronic stable angina is commonly intense but subsides within 15 minutes of either rest or appropriate antianginal drug therapy. Unstable angina is usually the early stage of progressive coronary artery disease (CAD). It often ends in an MI in subsequent years. For this reason, unstable angina is also called *preinfarction angina*. Another term for this type of angina is *crescendo angina*, because the pain increases in severity, as does the frequency of attacks. In later stages, pain may even occur while the patient is at rest. Vasospastic angina results from spasms in the layer of smooth muscle that surrounds atherosclerotic coronary arteries. In contrast to chronic stable angina, this type of pain often occurs at rest and without any precipitating cause. It does seem to follow a regular pattern, however, usually occurring at the same time of day. This type of angina is also called *Prinzmetal angina* or *variant angina*. Dysrhythmias and electrocardiogram (ECG) changes often accompany these different types of anginal attacks.

## PHARMACOLOGY OVERVIEW

The three main classes of drugs used to treat angina pectoris are the nitrates and nitrites, the beta blockers, and the calcium channel blockers (CCBs). Their various therapeutic effects are summarized and compared in Table 23-1. There are three main therapeutic objectives of antianginal drug therapy: (1) minimize the frequency of attacks and decrease the duration and intensity of the anginal pain; (2) improve the patient's functional capacity with as few adverse effects as possible; and (3) prevent or delay the worst possible outcome, myocardial infarction. The overall goal of antianginal drug therapy is to increase blood flow to ischemic myocardium, decrease myocardial oxygen demand, or both. Figure 23-1 illustrates how drug therapy works to alleviate angina. Evidence exists to suggest that drug therapy may be at least as effective as angioplasty in treating angina.

## TABLE 23-1 ANTIANGINAL DRUGS: THERAPEUTIC EFFECTS

| THERAPEUTIC EFFECT | NITRATES | BETA BLOCKERS* | AMLODIPINE | VERAPAMIL | DILTIAZEM |
|---|---|---|---|---|---|
| **Supply** | | | | | |
| Blood flow | ↑↑ | ↑ | ↑↑↑ | ↑↑↑ | ↑↑↑ |
| Duration of diastole | 0 | ↑↑↑ | 0/↑ | ↑↑↑ | ↑↑ |
| | | | | | |
| **Demand** | | | | | |
| Preload† | ↓↓ | ↑ | ↓/0 | 0 | 0/↓ |
| Afterload | ↓ | 0/↓ | ↓↓↓ | ↓↓ | ↓↓ |
| Contractility | 0 | ↓↓↓ | ↓ | ↓↓↓ | ↓↓ |
| Heart rate | 0/↑ | ↓↓↓ | 0/↓ | ↓↓ | ↓↓ |

↑, Increase; ↓, decrease; 0, little or no effect.
*In particular, those that are cardioselective and do not have intrinsic sympathomimetic activity.
†Preload is pressure in the heart caused by blood volume. The nitrates effectively move part of this blood out of the heart and into blood vessels, thereby decreasing preload or filling pressure.

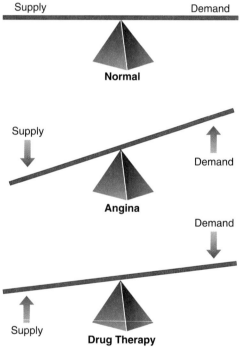

**FIGURE 23-1** Benefit of drug therapy for angina through increasing oxygen supply and decreasing oxygen demands.

## NITRATES AND NITRITES

Nitrates have long been the mainstay for both the prophylaxis and treatment for angina and other cardiac problems. Today there are several chemical derivatives of the early precursors, all of which are organic nitrate esters. They are available in a wide variety of preparations, including sublingual and oral tablets; capsules; ointments; patches; a translingual spray; and intravenous solutions. The following are the rapid- and long-acting nitrates available for clinical use:

- Amyl nitrite (rapid acting)
- Nitroglycerin (both rapid and long acting)
- Isosorbide dinitrate (both rapid and long acting)
- Isosorbide mononitrate (primarily long acting)

## Mechanism of Action and Drug Effects

Medicinal nitrates and nitrites, more commonly referred to simply as *nitrates,* dilate all blood vessels. They predominantly affect venous vascular beds; however, they also have a dose-dependent arterial vasodilator effect. These vasodilatory effects are the result of relaxation of the smooth muscle cells that are part of the wall structure of veins and arteries. The nitrates have a potent dilating effect on the large and small coronary arteries. This causes redistribution of blood and oxygen to previously ischemic myocardial tissue and reduction of anginal symptoms. By causing venous dilation, the nitrates reduce venous return and, in turn, reduce the left ventricular end-diastolic volume (or preload), which results in a lower left ventricular pressure. Left ventricular systolic wall tension is thus reduced, as is myocardial oxygen demand. These and other drug effects are summarized in Table 23-1.

Coronary arteries that have been narrowed by atherosclerosis can still be dilated as long as smooth muscle surrounding the coronary artery and the atherosclerotic plaque does not completely obstruct the arterial lumen. Exercise-induced spasms in atherosclerotic coronary arteries can also be reversed or prevented by administration of nitrates, which encourages healthy physical activity in patients.

## Indications

The nitrates are used to treat stable, unstable, and vasospastic (Prinzmetal) angina. Long-acting dosage forms are used more for prevention of anginal episodes. Rapid-acting dosage forms, most often sublingual nitroglycerin tablets, or an intravenous drip in the hospital setting, are used to treat acute anginal attacks.

## Contraindications

Contraindications to the use of nitrates include known drug allergy, as well as severe anemia, closed-angle glaucoma, hypotension, and severe head injury. This is because the vasodilatory effects of nitrates can worsen these latter conditions. In anemia, a drug-induced hypotensive episode can further compromise already reduced tissue oxygenation. Nitrates are also contraindicated with the use of the erectile dysfunction drugs sildenafil (Viagra), tadalafil (Cialis), and vardenafil (Levitra) (see Chapter 35).

## Adverse Effects

Nitrates are well tolerated, and most adverse effects are usually transient and involve the cardiovascular system. The most common undesirable effect is headache, which generally diminishes soon after the start of therapy. Other cardiovascular effects include tachycardia and postural hypotension. If nitrate-induced vasodilation occurs too rapidly, the cardiovascular system overcompensates and increases the heart rate, a condition referred to as reflex tachycardia. This may occur with significant vasodilation that involves the systemic veins. There is a large shift in blood volume toward the systemic venous circulation and away from the heart. Baroreceptors (blood pressure receptors) in the heart then falsely sense that there has been a dramatic loss of blood volume. At this point, the heart begins beating more rapidly to move the apparently smaller volume of blood more quickly throughout the body, especially toward the vital organs (including the heart itself). However, the same baroreceptors soon sense that there has not been a loss of blood volume but that the volume of blood missing in the heart is now in the periphery (e.g., venous system), and the heart rate slows back to normal.

Topical nitrate dosage forms can produce various types of contact dermatitis (skin inflammation), but these are actually reactions to the dosage delivery system and not to the nitroglycerin itself; thus, it is not a true drug allergy. It is important for the nurse to document the type of allergic reaction, so that clinicians do not avoid this important drug class if the reaction is only a contact dermatitis.

Tolerance to the antianginal effects of nitrates can occur surprisingly quickly in some patients, especially those taking long-acting formulations or taking nitrates around the clock. In addition, cross-tolerance can arise when a patient receives more than one nitrate dosage form. To prevent this, a regular nitrate-free period is arranged to allow certain enzymatic pathways to replenish themselves. A common regimen with transdermal patches is to remove them at night for 8 hours and apply a new patch in the morning. This has been shown to prevent tolerance to the beneficial effects of nitrates. However, some studies have questioned the advisability of this practice.

## Interactions

Nitrate antianginal drugs can produce additive hypotensive effects when taken in combination with alcohol, beta blockers, calcium channel blockers, phenothiazines, and erectile-dysfunction drugs such as sildenafil, tadalafil, and vardenafil. In fact, numerous deaths have been reported due to interactions with erectile-dysfunction drugs.

## Dosages

The organic nitrates are available in an array of forms and doses. For dosage information, see the table on this page.

## DOSAGES

### Selected Antianginal Nitrate Coronary Vasodilators

| DRUG (PREGNANCY CATEGORY) | USUAL DOSAGE RANGE | INDICATIONS |
|---|---|---|
| ◆ isosorbide dinitrate (Isordil, Dilatrate-SR) (C) | **Adult** PO: 5-20 mg bid-tid and 40-80 mg at 8 AM and 2 PM for SR formulations | |
| ◆ isosorbide mononitrate (Imdur, Monoket) (C) | **Adult** PO: 20 mg bid given 7 hr apart and 30-120 mg/day for SR formulations (Imdur) | Angina |
| ◆ nitroglycerin (Nitro-Bid, Nitrostat, Nitrol, others) (C) | **Adult** IV (continuous infusion): 5-20 mcg/min Ointment, 2%: 1-2 inch ribbon q8h Spray: 1-2 sprays onto or under the tongue at onset of attack; repeat as needed to max of 3 sprays in 15 min Sublingual: 1 tab under the tongue at first sign of chest pain; if pain not relieved after 1 dose, call 911; may repeat up to 3 tablets Patch: 0.1 to 0.8 mg/hr applied once daily | |

*IV,* Intravenous; *PO,* oral; *SL,* sublingual; *SR,* sustained release.

## DRUG PROFILES

### ◆ isosorbide dinitrate

Isosorbide dinitrate (Isordil) is an organic nitrate. It exerts the same effects as the other nitrates. When isosorbide dinitrate is metabolized in the liver, it is broken down into two active metabolites, both of which have the same therapeutic actions as isosorbide dinitrate itself. This drug is available in rapid-acting sublingual tablets, immediate-release tablets, and long-acting oral dosage forms.

#### Pharmacokinetics

| Route | Onset of Action | Peak Plasma Concentration | Elimination Half-life | Duration of Action |
|---|---|---|---|---|
| PO | 1 hr | Unknown | 3-5 hr | 4-6 hr |

### ◆ isosorbide mononitrate

Isosorbide mononitrate (Imdur) is one of the two active metabolites of isosorbide dinitrate, but it has no active metabolites itself. Because of these qualities, it produces a more consistent, steady therapeutic response, with less variation in response within the same patient and between patients. It is available in both immediate- and sustained-release oral dosage forms but is most commonly used in the sustained-release form.

### Pharmacokinetics (isosorbide mononitrate)

| Route | Onset of Action | Peak Plasma Concentration | Elimination Half-life | Duration of Action |
|-------|------|------|------|------|
| PO | 15-30 min | 0.5-1 hr | 5 hr | 5-12 hr |

#### ◆ nitroglycerin

Nitroglycerin is the prototypical nitrate and is manufactured by many pharmaceutical companies; therefore, it goes by many different trade names (e.g., Nitro-Bid, Nitrostat). It is often abbreviated as NTG or TNG. It has traditionally been the most important drug used in the symptomatic treatment of ischemic heart conditions such as angina. When given orally, nitroglycerin goes to the liver to be metabolized before it can become active in the body. During this process, a very large amount of the nitroglycerin is removed from the circulation. This is called a *large first-pass effect* (see Chapter 2). For this reason, nitroglycerin is administered by other routes to avoid the first-pass effect. Tablets administered by the sublingual route are used for the treatment of chest pain or angina of acute onset. They are also used for the prevention of angina when patients find themselves in situations likely to provoke an attack. Use of these routes is advantageous for relieving these acute conditions because the area under the tongue and inside the cheek is highly vascular. This means that the nitroglycerin is absorbed quickly and directly into the bloodstream, and hence its therapeutic effects occur rapidly. Sublingual nitroglycerin tablets must be stored in their original container, because exposure to air and moisture can inactivate the drug. Nitroglycerin also comes as a metered-dose aerosol that is sprayed under the tongue. Nitroglycerin is available in an intravenous form that is used for blood pressure control in hypertensive patients perioperatively; for the treatment of ischemic pain, heart failure, and pulmonary edema associated with acute MI; and in hypertensive emergency situations. Oral and topical dosage formulations are used for the long-term prophylactic management of angina pectoris. The topical formulation offers the same advantages as the sublingual formulation in that it also bypasses the liver and the first-pass effect. This formulation allows for the continuous slow delivery of nitroglycerin, so that a steady dose of nitroglycerin is supplied to the patient. See the Safety: Preventing Medication Errors box on p. 372.

### Pharmacokinetics

| Route | Onset of Action | Peak Plasma Concentration | Elimination Half-life | Duration of Action |
|-------|------|------|------|------|
| Sublingual | 2-3 min | Unknown | 1-4 min | 0.5-1 hr |

## BETA BLOCKERS

The beta-adrenergic blockers, more commonly referred to as *beta blockers,* have become the mainstay in the treatment of several cardiovascular diseases. These include angina, MI, hypertension (see Chapter 22), and dysrhythmias (see Chapter 25). Most available beta blockers demonstrate antianginal efficacy, although not all have been approved for this use. Those beta

### ⚡ SAFETY AND QUALITY IMPROVEMENT: PREVENTING MEDICATION ERRORS

#### *Understanding Rate Versus Dose*

The Institute for Safe Medication Practices (ISMP) reported an incident in which a nitroglycerin intravenous drip was set to infuse at 60 mL/hr rather than 60 mcg/min. With the medication concentration used (50 mg/250 mL) the patient actually received 200 mcg/min instead of the ordered 60 mcg/min. Investigation of this incident revealed that the nurses were using a handwritten, nonstandard dosing table rather than one that corresponded to the available concentrations of premixed solutions in the hospital. According to the report, the patient became hypotensive but recovered.

It is crucial to understand the difference between "mL/hr" and "mcg/min" when programming infusion pumps; rates are not interchangeable with ordered doses! In addition, using standardized dosing charts that correspond to available concentrations of solutions is important. Some facilities also require double-checking of infusion pump settings before medication therapy is begun.

For more information, see Improvised dosing charts can cause errors, *Nurse Advise-ERR* 3(6):3, 2005, available at http://www.ismp.org/Newsletters/nursing/Issues/NurseAdviseERR200506.pdf.

blockers approved as antianginal drugs are atenolol, metoprolol, nadolol, and propranolol.

## Mechanism of Action and Drug Effects

The primary effects of the beta blockers are related to the cardiovascular system. As discussed in Chapters 19 and 22, the predominant beta-adrenergic receptors in the heart are the $beta_1$ receptors. $Beta_1$ receptors are located in the heart's conduction system and throughout the myocardium. The beta receptors are normally stimulated by the binding of the neurotransmitters epinephrine and norepinephrine. These catecholamines are released in greater quantities during times of exercise or other stress to stimulate the heart muscle to contract more strongly. At the normal heart rate of 60 to 80 beats/min, the heart spends 60% to 70% of its time in diastole. As the heart rate increases during stress or exercise, the heart spends more time in systole and less time in diastole. The physiologic consequence is that the coronary arteries receive increasingly less blood, and eventually the myocardium becomes ischemic.

In an ischemic heart, the increased oxygen demand from increasing contractility (systole) also leads to increasing degrees of ischemia and chest pain. The physiologic act of systole requires energy in the form of adenosine triphosphate (ATP) and oxygen. Therefore, any decrease in the energy demands on the heart is beneficial for alleviating conditions such as angina. When beta receptors are blocked by beta blockers, the rate at which the pacemaker (sinoatrial [SA] node) fires decreases, and the time it takes for the node to recover increases. The beta blockers also slow conduction through the atrioventricular (AV) node and reduce myocardial contractility (negative inotropic effect). Both of these effects serve to slow the heart rate (negative chronotropic effect). These effects reduce myocardial oxygen demand, which aids in the treatment of angina by reducing the workload of the heart. Slowing the heart rate is also beneficial in patients with ischemic heart disease, because the coronary arteries have more diastolic time to fill with oxygen- and nutrient-rich blood and deliver these substances to the myocardial tissues.

The beta blockers also have many therapeutic effects after an MI. Following an MI, there is a high level of circulating catecholamines (norepinephrine and epinephrine). These catecholamines will produce harmful consequences if their actions go unopposed. They cause the heart rate to increase, which leads to a further imbalance in the supply-and-demand ratio, and they irritate the conduction system of the heart, which can result in potentially fatal dysrhythmias. The beta blockers block all of these harmful effects, and their use has been shown to improve the chances for survival in patients after MI. Unless strongly contraindicated, beta blockers are given to all patients in the acute stages after an MI.

The beta blockers also suppress the activity of the hormone renin, which is the first step in the renin-aldosterone-angiotensin system. Renin is a potent vasoconstrictor released by the kidneys when they sense that they are not being adequately perfused. When beta blockers inhibit the release of renin, blood vessels to and in the kidney dilate, causing reduced blood pressure (see Chapter 22).

## Indications

The beta blockers are most effective in the treatment of exertional angina (i.e., that caused by exercise). This is because the usual physiologic effects of an increase in the heart rate and systolic blood pressure that occurs during exercise or stress are blunted by the beta blockers, thereby decreasing the myocardial oxygen demand. For an individual (often elderly) with significant angina, "exercise" may simply be carrying out the activities of daily living, such as bathing, dressing, cooking, or housekeeping. Performing such activities with significant angina can become a major stressor for these patients. The beta blockers are also approved for the treatment of MI, hypertension (see Chapter 22), cardiac dysrhythmias (see Chapter 25), and essential tremor. Some uses that are common but are not U.S. Food and Drug Administration (FDA) approved are treatment of migraine headache and, in low dosages, even treatment of the tachycardia associated with stage fright.

## Contraindications

There are a number of contraindications to the use of beta blockers, including systolic heart failure and serious conduction disturbances, because of the effects of beta blockade on heart rate and myocardial contractility. These drugs should be used with caution in patients with bronchial asthma, because any level of blockade of beta$_2$ receptors can promote bronchoconstriction. These contraindications are relative rather than absolute and depend on patient-specific risks and expected benefits of this drug therapy. Other relative contraindications include diabetes mellitus (due to masking of hypoglycemia-induced tachycardia) and peripheral vascular disease (the drug may further compromise cerebral or peripheral blood flow).

## Adverse Effects

The adverse effects of the beta blockers result from their ability to block beta-adrenergic receptors (beta$_1$ and beta$_2$

**TABLE 23-2  BETA BLOCKERS: ADVERSE EFFECTS**

| BODY SYSTEM | ADVERSE EFFECTS |
|---|---|
| Cardiovascular | Bradycardia, hypotension, atrioventricular block |
| Central nervous | Dizziness, fatigue, depression, lethargy |
| Metabolic | Hyperglycemia and/or hypoglycemia, hyperlipidemia |
| Other | Wheezing, dyspnea, impotence |

**TABLE 23-3  BETA BLOCKERS: COMMON DRUG INTERACTIONS**

| INTERACTING DRUG | MECHANISM | RESULT |
|---|---|---|
| Diuretics and antihypertensives | Additive effects | Hypotension |
| Calcium channel blockers (diltiazem, verapamil) | Additive atrioventricular node suppression | Hypotension, bradycardia, heart block |
| Insulin and oral antidiabetic drugs | Masking of hypoglycemic effects | Unrecognized hypoglycemia |

receptors) in various areas of the body. Blocking of beta$_1$ receptors may lead to a decrease in heart rate, cardiac output, and cardiac contractility. Blocking of beta$_2$ receptors may result in bronchoconstriction and increased airway resistance in patients with asthma or chronic obstructive pulmonary disease. Beta blockers may lead to cardiac rhythm problems, decreased SA and AV nodal conduction, a decrease in systolic and diastolic blood pressures, and possible peripheral receptor blockade and/or decreased renin release from the kidneys. Beta blockers can mask the tachycardia associated with hypoglycemia, and diabetic patients may not be able to tell when their blood sugar falls too low. Fatigue, insomnia, and weakness may occur because of the negative effects on the cardiac and central nervous systems. The beta blockers can also cause both hypoglycemia and hyperglycemia, which is of particular concern in diabetic patients. Other common beta blocker–related adverse effects are listed in Table 23-2.

## Interactions

There are many important drug interactions that involve the beta blockers. The more common and important of these are listed in Table 23-3.

## Dosages

For dosage information on selected beta blockers, see the table on p. 374.

## DRUG PROFILES

Beta blockers are the mainstay in the treatment of a wide range of cardiovascular diseases, mainly hypertension, angina, and the acute stages of MI. The three most commonly used beta blockers are carvedilol, metoprolol, and atenolol. Carvedilol (Coreg) is not indicated for angina per se, but it is instead indicated for

## DOSAGES

### Selected Beta₁-Adrenergic–Blocking Drugs

| DRUG (PREGNANCY CATEGORY) | PHARMACOLOGIC CLASS | USUAL DOSAGE RANGE | INDICATIONS |
|---|---|---|---|
| ◆ atenolol (Tenormin) (C) | Beta₁ blocker | **Adult** PO: 50-200 mg/day as a single dose | Angina |
| ◆ metoprolol (Lopressor, Toprol-XL) (C) | | **Adult** PO: 100-400 mg/day in 2 divided doses IV: 5 mg every 2 min × 3 doses, then PO therapy as indicated | |

*IV,* Intravenous; *PO,* oral.

heart failure, essential hypertension, and left ventricular dysfunction. The newest beta blocker, nebivolol (Bystolic), is used to treat hypertension. Atenolol, metoprolol, nadolol, and propranolol all are indicated for angina. The drug profile for carvedilol appears in Chapter 19 on p. 318.

### ◆ atenolol

Atenolol (Tenormin) is a cardioselective beta₁-adrenergic receptor blocker and is indicated for the prophylactic treatment of angina pectoris. Use of atenolol after MI has been shown to decrease mortality. It was formerly available in an injectable form, but it is now only available in oral form.

#### Pharmacokinetics

| Route | Onset of Action | Peak Plasma Concentration | Elimination Half-life | Duration of Action |
|---|---|---|---|---|
| PO | 1 hr | 2-4 hr | 6-7 hr | 24 hr |

### ◆ metoprolol

Metoprolol (Lopressor, Toprol-XL) is also a cardioselective beta₁-adrenergic receptor blocker that is used for the prophylactic treatment of angina and has many of the same characteristics as atenolol. It has shown similar efficacy in reducing mortality in patients after MI and in treating angina. It is available in both oral (immediate-release and long-acting) and parenteral (injectable) forms. Intravenous metoprolol is commonly administered to hospitalized patients after an MI and is used for treatment of hypertension in patients unable to take oral medicine.

#### Pharmacokinetics

| Route | Onset of Action | Peak Plasma Concentration | Elimination Half-life | Duration of Action |
|---|---|---|---|---|
| IV | 1 min | 20 min | 3-8 hr | 5-8 hr |
| PO | 1 hr | 2-4 hr | 3-8 hr | 10-20 hr |

## CALCIUM CHANNEL BLOCKERS

There are three chemical classes of calcium channel blockers (CCBs): phenylalkylamines, benzothiazepines, and dihydropyridines, commonly represented by verapamil, diltiazem, and

| TABLE 23-4 | CLASSIFICATION OF CALCIUM CHANNEL BLOCKERS | |
|---|---|---|
| **GENERIC NAME** | **TRADE NAME** | **AVAILABLE ROUTES** |
| **Benzothiazepines** | | |
| diltiazem | Cardizem, Dilacor, Tiazac, Dilacor XR, Cartia XT, Matzim LA, Taztia XT, Diltia XT | PO/IV |
| **Dihydropyridines** | | |
| amlodipine | Norvasc | PO |
| felodipine | Plendil | PO |
| isradipine | DynaCirc | PO |
| nicardipine | Cardene | PO/IV |
| nifedipine | Adalat, Procardia | PO |
| nimodipine | Nimotop | PO |
| **Phenylalkylamines** | | |
| verapamil | Calan, Isoptin, Verelan | PO/IV |

*IV,* Intravenous; *PO,* oral.

amlodipine, respectively (Table 23-4). Although they all block calcium channels, their chemical structures and therefore their mechanisms of action differ slightly. More than nine CCBs are available today. Those that are used for the treatment of chronic stable angina are amlodipine, diltiazem, nicardipine, nifedipine, and verapamil.

### Mechanism of Action and Drug Effects

Calcium plays an important role in the excitation-contraction coupling process that occurs in the heart and vascular smooth muscle cells, as well as in skeletal muscle. Preventing calcium from entering into this process prevents muscle contraction and promotes muscle relaxation. Relaxation of the smooth muscles that surround the coronary arteries causes them to dilate. This dilation increases blood flow to the ischemic heart, which in turn increases the oxygen supply and helps shift the supply/demand ratio back to normal. Dilation also occurs in the arteries throughout the body, which results in a decrease in the force (systemic vascular resistance) against which the heart must exert itself when delivering blood to the body

| TABLE 23-5 | CALCIUM CHANNEL BLOCKERS: ADVERSE EFFECTS |
|---|---|

| BODY SYSTEM | ADVERSE EFFECTS |
|---|---|
| Cardiovascular | Hypotension, palpitations, tachycardia or bradycardia |
| Gastrointestinal | Constipation, nausea |
| Other | Dyspnea, rash, flushing, peripheral edema |

(afterload). Decreasing the afterload reduces the workload of the heart and therefore reduces myocardial oxygen demand. This is the primary beneficial antianginal effect of the dihydropyridine CCBs such as amlodipine and nifedipine. These drugs have a less negative inotropic effect than do verapamil and diltiazem.

Another cardiovascular effect of the CCBs is depression of the automaticity of and conduction through the SA and AV nodes. For this reason, they are useful in treating cardiac dysrhythmias (see Chapter 25). Finally, the CCBs reduce myocardial contractility and peripheral and coronary artery tone. Verapamil and diltiazem also decrease heart rate. Their strongest antianginal properties are secondary to their effects on myocardial contractility and the smooth muscle tone of peripheral and coronary arteries.

## Indications

The therapeutic benefits of the CCBs are numerous. Because of their very acceptable adverse effect and safety profiles, they are considered first-line drugs for the treatment of such conditions as angina, hypertension, and supraventricular tachycardia. They are often effective for the treatment of coronary artery spasms (vasospastic or Prinzmetal angina). However, they may not be as effective as the beta blockers in blunting exercise-induced elevations in heart rate and blood pressure. CCBs are also used for the short-term management of atrial fibrillation and flutter (see Chapter 25), migraine headaches (see Chapter 13), and Raynaud's disease (a type of peripheral vascular disease). The dihydropyridine CCB nimodipine is indicated solely for cerebral artery spasms associated with aneurysm rupture.

## Contraindications

Contraindications include known drug allergy, acute MI, second- or third-degree AV block (unless the patient has a pacemaker), and hypotension.

## Adverse Effects

The adverse effects of the CCBs are limited and primarily relate to overexpression of their therapeutic effects. The most common adverse effects are listed in Table 23-5. Historically, immediate-release nifedipine was used to lower blood pressure in acute hypertensive emergencies (the capsule was punctured and given sublingually). However, negative outcomes were reported with the rapid, dramatic reduction in blood pressure. For this reason, only the extended-release form of nifedipine is used today. (The exception is the use of immediate-release

| TABLE 23-6 | CALCIUM CHANNEL BLOCKERS: COMMON DRUG INTERACTIONS |
|---|---|

| INTERACTING DRUG | MECHANISM | RESULT |
|---|---|---|
| Beta blockers | Additive effects | Bradycardia and atrioventricular block |
| digoxin | Interference with drug elimination | Possible increased digoxin levels |
| amiodarone | Decreased metabolism | Bradycardia and decreased cardiac output |
| Azole antifungals, clarithromycin, erythromycin, HIV drugs | Decreased metabolism | Elevated levels and effects of calcium channel blockers |
| Statins | Inhibited statin metabolism | Increased risk of statin toxicity |
| cyclosporine | Decreased metabolism of either drug | Possible toxicity of either drug |

nifedipine for the treatment of premature labor.) Medication errors have occurred when a nurse drew up the contents of the capsule to be given sublingually, but inadvertently gave it intravenously. For this reason, the Institute for Safe Medication Practice recommends that the contents be drawn up into an oral syringe by the pharmacy.

## Interactions

Important drug interactions are listed in Table 23-6. A particular food interaction of note is the interaction with grapefruit juice, which can reduce the metabolism of the CCBs, especially nifedipine.

## Dosages

For dosage information on selected CCBs, see the table below.

### DOSAGES

**Selected Calcium Channel–Blocking Drugs**

| DRUG (PREGNANCY CATEGORY) | USUAL DOSAGE RANGE | INDICATIONS |
|---|---|---|
| amlodipine (Norvasc) (C) | **Adult** PO: 5-10 mg/day | ⎫ |
| ◆ diltiazem (Cardizem, Dilacor XR, Tiazac, Cartia XT, Diltia XT, Matzim LA, Taztia XT) (C) | **Adult** PO: Initial dose 30 mg qid before meals and at bedtime; range of 180-360 mg divided in 3-4 doses, or 1 daily for extended-release capsule; dosages of 480 mg/day may be needed | ⎬ Angina ⎭ |

*PO,* Oral.

# DRUG PROFILES

## ◆ diltiazem

Diltiazem (Cardizem, Dilacor, Tiazac) is the only benzothiazepine CCB. It has a particular affinity for the cardiac conduction system and is very effective for the treatment of angina pectoris resulting from coronary insufficiency and hypertension. It is one of the few CCBs that are also available in parenteral form, for which it is used in the treatment of atrial fibrillation and flutter along with paroxysmal supraventricular tachycardia (see Chapter 25). Verapamil is another CCB with similar indications. Several sustained-delivery formulations of diltiazem are available, which can be confused with each other. For example, there is Cardizem SR, which is taken twice a day, and Cardizem CD, which is taken once a day. In addition to other brands of these two dosage forms, the drug is also available in several strengths of immediate-release capsule as well as in intravenous form.

### Pharmacokinetics

| Route | Onset of Action | Peak Plasma Concentration | Elimination Half-life | Duration of Action |
|---|---|---|---|---|
| PO | 0.5-1 hr | 2-3 hr | 3.5-9 hr | 4-12 hr |

## amlodipine

Amlodipine (Norvasc) is currently the most popular CCB of the dihydropyridine subclass. It is indicated for both angina and hypertension and is available only for oral use.

### Pharmacokinetics

| Route | Onset of Action | Peak Plasma Concentration | Elimination Half-life | Duration of Action |
|---|---|---|---|---|
| PO | 30-50 min | 6-12 hr | 30-50 hr | 24 hr |

# MISCELLANEOUS ANTIANGINAL DRUG

# DRUG PROFILE

## ranolazine

Ranolazine (Ranexa) is the newest antianginal drug, approved by the FDA in 2006 for chronic angina. Its mechanism of action is unknown. Unlike other antianginal drugs, its antianginal and antiischemic effects do not involve reductions in heart rate or blood pressure. Ranolazine is known to prolong the QT interval on the ECG. For this reason, this drug is reserved for patients who have failed to benefit from other antianginal drug therapy. In fact, ranolazine is contraindicated in patients with preexisting QT prolongation or hepatic impairment, in those taking other QT-prolonging drugs (see Chapter 25), and in patients taking moderately potent cytochrome P-450 enzyme 3A4 inhibitors such as diltiazem. Other significant drug interactions include interactions with ketoconazole and verapamil, both of which can raise ranolazine levels. Ranolazine can also raise digoxin levels. The usual dose of ranolazine is 500 mg orally twice daily, which may be advanced to 1000 mg orally twice daily based on clinical symptoms. The drug is available only for oral use.

# SUMMARY OF ANTIANGINAL PHARMACOLOGY

In patients with coronary artery disease, clinical symptoms result from a lack of or inadequate delivery of blood carrying oxygen and nutrients to the heart, which results in ischemic heart disease. Antianginal drugs such as nitrates, nitrites, beta blockers, and calcium channel blockers are used to reduce ischemia by increasing the delivery of oxygen-rich blood to cardiac tissues or by reducing oxygen consumption by the coronary vessels. Either of these mechanisms can reduce ischemia and lead to a decrease in anginal pain. Nitrates and nitrites work mainly by decreasing venous return to the heart (preload) and decreasing systemic vascular resistance (afterload). Calcium channel blockers decrease calcium influx into the smooth muscle, causing vascular relaxation. This either reverses or prevents the spasms of coronary vessels that cause the anginal pain associated with Prinzmetal or chronic angina. Beta blockers help by slowing the heart rate and decreasing contractility, thereby decreasing oxygen demands. Although these groups of drugs have similar clinical effects, the nursing process required for each is somewhat specific because of the characteristics and effects of the drugs and the indications for and contraindications to their use.

---

## TEAMWORK AND COLLABORATION: PHARMACOKINETIC BRIDGE TO NURSING PRACTICE

Not only are the pharmacokinetic properties of the nitrates very interesting, but knowledge of these specific properties is critical to safe and accurate nursing care. Moreover, the patient's understanding of nitrate pharmacokinetics is important because the level of the patient's knowledge may strongly influence adherence to the drug regimen and the effectiveness of treatment for angina. The pharmacokinetics differ for the various dosage forms of nitroglycerin and include the following:

*Intravenous infusion:* Onset of action 1 to 2 minutes (fastest of all dosage forms), peak action not applicable, duration of action 3 to 5 minutes

*Sublingual tablet:* Onset of action 2 to 3 minutes, peak action unknown, duration of action 0.5 to 1 hour

*Immediate-release tablet:* Onset of action 1 hour, peak action unknown, duration of action 4 to 6 hours

*Transdermal patch:* Onset 30 to 60 minutes, peak action 1 to 3 hours, duration of action 8 to 12 hours

If the goal of treatment is to abort or treat a sudden attack of angina, then *rapid* onset of action is needed, so the clinical decision (by the prescriber) would be to order either intravenous infusion, sublingual tablet, and/or translingual spray, which has a similar onset time. These dosage forms have pharmacokinetics that allow quick entry of the drug into the bloodstream and lead to more rapid vasodilation. This provides more oxygenated blood to the myocardium and aborts acute attacks. If symptoms persist, more drastic medical management would be indicated. The quick-onset nitroglycerin dosage forms may also be used by the patient before engaging in activities known to provoke angina, such as increased physical activity, sexual intercourse, or other forms of physical exertion. If the purpose of treatment is maintenance therapy, the nitrate form must have other pharmacokinetic properties, such as a longer duration of action to provide protection against angina; a longer onset of action is acceptable because stopping an attack is not needed in this situation. Use of ointments, transdermal patches, or extended-release preparations would be appropriate in such cases. If an acute episode of angina occurs while the patient is taking maintenance therapy, a dosage form with a rapid onset of action is indicated (as ordered). It is easy to see that thorough knowledge of a drug and its pharmacokinetics allows for safe and sound decisions about drug therapy for patients with angina.

# NURSING PROCESS

## ASSESSMENT

Before *antianginal* drugs are administered, obtain a thorough past and present medical-health history and medication history (e.g., listing of all prescription drugs, over-the-counter products, herbals, vitamins, and supplements being taken) and document the findings. Also measure weight, height, and vital signs, with attention to supine, sitting, and standing blood pressures. Report a systolic blood pressure reading of less than 90 mm Hg to the prescriber before administering a dose of any of these drugs. With use of any drugs affecting blood pressure or pulse rate, such as antianginals, take the apical pulse rate for 1 full minute. If the pulse rate is 60 beats/min or less or 100 beats/min or greater (reflex tachycardia is an adverse effect), contact the prescriber for further instructions. In addition to rate, assess the quality and rhythm of the heartbeat and document prior to the administration of antianginal drugs. If the patient is experiencing any chest pain, include in your assessment description of onset, character (e.g., sharp, dull, piercing, squeezing, radiating), intensity, location, duration, precipitating factors (e.g., physical exertion, exercise, eating, stress, sexual intercourse), alleviating factors, and presence of nausea or vomiting. The prescriber may order an ECG, and you must review these results as well. Thoroughly assess for any contraindications, cautions, and drug interactions prior to giving these drugs. Significant interactions include alcohol, beta blockers, calcium channel blockers, phenothiazines, and erectile-dysfunction drugs such as sildenafil, tadalafil, and vardenafil. Taking these drugs with nitrates will result in worsening of hypotensive responses, paradoxical bradycardia, and a resultant increase in angina with subsequent significant risk of cardiac or cerebrovascular complications due to the decreased perfusion. Elderly patients often have difficulty with blood pressure control because of the occurrence of normal age-related periods of hypotension, and the use of antianginals may lead to worsening of hypotensive responses. If patients are taking nitrates on a long-term basis, it is important to assess continued therapeutic responses because of the development of tolerance to the drug's effects. During assessment and initiation of drug therapy, it is critical to patient safety to notify the prescriber of any increased angina, because another antianginal or vasodilating drug may be needed.

Concerns arise with the use of *nonselective beta blockers* and *beta₂ blockers* (as vasodilators) in patients with bronchospastic disease because of the drug-related effects of bronchoconstriction and increased airway resistance, which results in wheezing and dyspnea as adverse effects. Therefore, if asthma or other respiratory problems are present, beta blockers would not be indicated because bronchoconstriction could be exacerbated. In addition, there are also concerns about the use of beta blockers in patients with peripheral vascular disease, hypotension, hyperglycemia or hypoglycemia (see pharmacology discussion), and bradycardia. Nonselective beta blockers may also exacerbate preexisting heart failure. Assessment for edema is important in patients with cardiac risk factors and a weight gain of 2 pounds or more in 24 hours or 5 pounds or more in 1 week. This weight gain is to be reported to the prescriber immediately. Assess for significant drug interactions, including the concurrent use of other antihypertensives, calcium channel blockers, and oral antidiabetic drugs (see Table 23-3 for more information).

In patients taking *calcium channel blockers* (CCBs), assess for possible drug-food interactions, including grapefruit. Grapefruit juice reduces the metabolism of nifedipine, leading to possible toxicity; grapefruit must be avoided. Another area to be thoroughly assessed is that of the dosage form of nifedipine, which is available in extended and immediate-release forms. Therefore, follow the orders for administration of nifedipine carefully, and closely monitor the patient (e.g., vital signs). Diltiazem (Cardizem) is available in several sustained-delivery forms; closely assess the order to avoid medication error. Cautious use is important in patients with a history of hypotension, palpitations, tachycardia/bradycardia, constipation, dyspnea, and edema. Significant drug interactions are included in Table 23-6.

Assess patients taking *ranolazine (Ranexa)*, one of the newest antianginal drugs, for liver dysfunction through specific liver function testing prior to taking the medication. Additionally, assess for other medications the patient is taking, with an emphasis on medications that prolong the QT interval for which an EKG may also be ordered. Other medications to be concerned about include those that inhibit cytochrome P450, such as diltiazem.

## NURSING DIAGNOSES

1. Decreased cardiac output related to the pathology of coronary artery disease
2. Deficient knowledge related to first-time use of antianginal drugs and a new diagnosis of coronary artery disease
3. Risk for injury to self related to possible adverse drug effect of hypotension with subsequent dizziness and/or syncope/falls

## PLANNING

### GOALS

1. Patient exhibits therapeutic effects of antianginal drug therapy, such as improved cardiac output, with fewer episodes of chest pain.
2. Patient demonstrates increased knowledge about disease process and drug therapy.
3. Patient remains free from injury while receiving antianginal drug therapy.

### OUTCOME CRITERIA

1. Patient states that there are more frequent periods of comfort while carrying out activities of daily living, engaging in supervised exercise, and performing moderate activity, without recurring angina and without major adverse effects on follow-up with the prescriber.
   - Patient experiences fewer episodes to no episodes of chest pain (angina).

### Nitroglycerin for Angina

M.S., a 68-year-old accountant, has been diagnosed with coronary artery disease (CAD) after experiencing chest pain at times when he jogs. After undergoing a thorough physical examination, including cardiac catheterization, he is given a prescription for extended-release nitroglycerin capsules, 6.5 mg, three times a day. He also has a prescription for 0.4-mg sublingual nitroglycerin tablets to take as needed for chest pain.

1. What type of angina is M.S. experiencing, and what are the therapeutic goals of the drug therapy he has received?

M.S. asks you, "Why do I have two prescriptions for the same drug? It doesn't make sense to me!"

2. What is the best answer to his question?
3. Two days after he begins the nitroglycerin, M.S. calls the office and says, "I'm having awful headaches. What is wrong?" What is the best explanation, and what can he do about the headaches?

After 1 month, M.S. is switched from the extended-release capsules to a transdermal nitroglycerin patch. He says that he is glad he does not have to remember to "take those pills" three times a day. However, 2 months later, he calls and says, "I don't think this patch is working. I'm having more episodes of chest pain now when I jog."

4. What could be the explanation for this, and what can be done?

For answers, see http://evolve.elsevier.com/Lilley

2. Patient states rationale for antianginal drug therapy and importance of taking medication exactly as prescribed.
   - Patient states adverse effects of antianginal drug therapy, such as postural hypotension, dizziness, and severe headache, as well as measures to decrease their occurrence.
   - Patient states appropriate time frame of when to seek out emergency care (i.e., no relief after 1 dose of sublingual nitrates) and call 911.
3. Patient states measures to decrease risk for injury, such as changing positions slowly, keeping legs moving when in a still position, increasing fluid intake with medication regimen, and removing rugs or carpets that can cause tripping or slipping.

## IMPLEMENTATION

Always review and/or record the patient's vital signs and description of chest pain for the duration of therapy. Take into account the following considerations associated with the use of the various dosage forms and routes of administration: (1) *For any dosage form:* Administer the drug while the patient is seated to avoid falls or injury from drug-induced hypotension. This hypotension may last for up to 30 minutes after dosing of the drug. When administering nitrates, monitor the patient's chest pain, and have the patient rate the pain on a scale of 1 to 10 before, during, and after therapy. Monitor the patient's response to drug therapy by measuring the patient's blood pressure and pulse rate and assessing for the presence of headache, dizziness, and/or lightheadedness. When the patient is in a supine position, an appropriate dose of a nitrate will produce a clinical response of a fall in blood pressure of about 10 mm Hg and/or a rise in heart rate of 10 beats/min. However, the following parameters are alerts that there may be a problem with the patient and to contact the prescriber: a systolic blood pressure of 90 mm Hg or less and/or a pulse rate of 60 beats/min or less or a pulse rate greater than 100 beats/min. (2) *For oral dosage forms:* Counsel the patient that these forms are to be taken as ordered before meals and with 6 oz of water. Extended-release preparations must not be crushed, chewed, or altered in any way. Acetaminophen may be given if there is a drug-related headache and if not contraindicated. (3) *For sublingual forms:* Advise the patient to place the tablet under the tongue as directed and *not* to swallow until the drug is completely dissolved. Metered-dose aerosol sprays are applied onto or under the tongue (see Dosages table). Instruct the patient to keep nitrates in their original packaging or container (e.g., sublingual tablets come in a small amber-colored glass container with a metal lid). Exposure to light, plastic, cotton filler, and moisture must be avoided. (4) *For ointment:* Use the proper dosing paper supplied by the drug company to apply a thin layer on clean, dry, hairless skin of the upper arms or body. Avoid areas below the knees and elbows. Do not apply the ointment with the fingers unless a glove is worn to avoid contact with the skin and subsequent absorption. A tongue depressor may also be used, but in most situations the ointment may be squeezed directly from the tube onto the proper dosing paper. Once the ointment is in place, do *not* rub it into the skin; cover the area with an occlusive dressing if not provided (e.g., plastic wrap). Rotate application sites, and remove all residual from the previous dose of ointment gently with soap and water and pat the area dry. (5) *For transdermal forms:* Apply patches to a clean, residue-free, hairless area, and rotate sites. If cardioversion or use of an automated electrical defibrillator is required, remove the transdermal patch to avoid burning of the skin and damage to the defibrillator paddles. Before a new patch is applied, locate and remove the old patch and clean the skin of any residual drug. Carefully dispose of used, unneeded, or defective transdermal patches of any medication as indicated by hospital policy or per discharge instructions. It is important to follow any packaging insert instructions and/or facility policy because transdermal patches delivering potent medications need to be flushed down the toilet to avoid possible contact of residual drug by babies, children, pets and even adults (see Chapter 2). For more information visit www.fda.gov/downloads/Drugs/ResourcesForYou/Consumers/BuyingUsingMedicineSafely/UnderstandingOver-the-CounterMedicines/ucm107163 or www.ismp.org. (6) *For intravenous forms:* Intravenous dosing is for use in emergency situations only and in settings that provide close automatic monitoring of the blood pressure and pulse as well as constant ECG monitoring. Intravenous administration of nitrates may lead to sudden and severe hypotension, cardiovascular collapse, and shock. Always check for incompatibilities and the proper diluent. Only give intravenous solutions through an infusion pump and as ordered. Intravenous dosage forms are available as ready-to-use injectable doses and are administered using *specific nonpolyvinylchloride* (non-PVC) plastic intravenous bags and tubing. The non-PVC infusion kits are used to avoid absorption or uptake of the nitrate by the intravenous tubing and bag. This prevents decomposition of the nitrate with breakdown into cyanide when the drug is exposed to light. Intravenous forms of nitroglycerin are stable for about 96 hours after preparation. If parenteral solutions are not clear and are discolored, discard the solution.

With *isosorbide,* tablets are best taken on an empty stomach; however, if the patient complains of headache or gastrointestinal upset, the medicine needs to be taken with meals. Oral tablets of isosorbide can be crushed; however, the sublingual and extended-release forms are *not* to be crushed or chewed. As with sublingual nitroglycerin, instruct the patient not to swallow the medication until it is completely dissolved. If dizziness or lightheadedness occurs, assist the patient and encourage him or her to change positions slowly. Closely monitor the patient's blood pressure, including orthostatic blood pressures. Document the occurrence of anginal episodes, their character, precipitating factors, severity, and frequency noted.

*Beta blockers* need to be given as ordered and may be taken with or without food. Abrupt withdrawal must be avoided. Daily weights need to be measured every day at the same time and with the patient wearing the same amount of clothing. If there is a weight gain of 2 pounds or more in 24 hours or 5 pounds or more in 1 week, contact the prescriber immediately. When these drugs are used, take measures to reduce the incidence of orthostatic hypotension, such as advising the patient to dangle the legs on the side of the bed before standing and to move slowly and purposefully. Instruct the patient to contact the prescriber immediately if any excessive or intolerable dizziness, fatigue/lethargy, wheezing, or dyspnea occurs (see Chapter 19 for further discussion).

*Calcium channel blockers (CCBs)* are to be taken as ordered and without sudden withdrawal. Abrupt withdrawal can precipitate rebound hypertension and worsening of tissue ischemia.

Weight needs to be measured daily (see later discussion). Constantly monitor the patient for edema and shortness of breath. Instruct the patient to move and change positions slowly and cautiously to prevent syncope. Constipation may be prevented by increasing fluids and fiber in the diet. If the patient experiences palpitations, pronounced dizziness, nausea, or dyspnea, contact the prescriber immediately. Intravenous administration of any CCB requires the use of an infusion pump and careful monitoring (see Chapter 25).

Patients taking any of the vasodilators must avoid alcohol, saunas, hot tubs, hot showers, and hot weather or a hot environment. These conditions will exacerbate vasodilation and increase the occurrence of orthostatic hypotension, increasing the risk for dizziness, syncope, and falls. Caution the patient that with certain sustained-release forms of medication, the wax matrix may appear in the stool. Advise patients that the passing of the wax matrix occurs after the drug has been absorbed and that, even though the matrix is visible, it is of no concern. Instruct the patient on how to self-monitor blood pressure and pulse rate, as well as how to document the findings in a journal so that the information can be shared with health care providers. The journal can also list daily weights, response to the medication regimen, and any adverse effects. See the Patient Teaching Tips for more information.

## EVALUATION

Carefully monitor patients taking antianginals for the occurrence of an allergic reaction, which may be manifested by dyspnea, swelling of the face, or hives. Include in your evaluation a review for accomplishment of goals and outcomes, such as appropriate decrease in blood pressure, increase in cardiac output and tissue perfusion with decrease in angina, and a gradual increase in activity and performance of activities of daily living without exacerbation of anginal episodes. In addition, monitor the patient for adverse reactions such as headache, lightheadedness, dizziness, and decreased blood pressure, which may indicate the need to decrease the dosage. If the patient is receiving intravenous nitroglycerin, evaluate for excessive drops in blood pressure, worsening of angina, and significant changes in pulse rate (less than 60 beats/min or greater than100 beats/min), and contact the prescriber immediately.

## PATIENT TEACHING TIPS

### Nitroglycerin
- Emphasize to the patient the importance of keeping a daily journal with documentation of how he or she feels and number of anginal episodes, noting their intensity, frequency, duration, and character, as well as precipitating and/or relieving factors. Any evidence of possible tolerance to the medication is important to note and report to the prescriber.
- *Capsules* or *extended-release* dosage forms are never to be chewed, crushed, or altered in any way.

- Instruct the patient taking *aerosol* (spray) dosage forms not to shake the canister before lingual spraying and to avoid inhaling or swallowing the lingual aerosol until the drug is dispersed. With *sublingual* forms, the medication must be taken at the first sign of chest pain and not delayed until the pain is severe. The patient needs to sit or lie down and take one sublingual tablet. According to current guidelines, if the chest pain or discomfort is not relieved in 5 minutes, after *one* dose, the patient (or family member) must call 911 immediately. The patient can take one more tablet while awaiting emergency care and a third tablet 5 minutes later, but no more than three tablets total. These guidelines reflect the fact that angina pain that does not respond to nitroglycerin may indicate a myocardial infarction. The sublingual dose is to be placed under the tongue and the patient must avoid swallowing until the tablet is dissolved. Instruct the patient not to eat or drink until the drug has completely dissolved.

• Educate the patient about the best place to store the medication, such as keeping medicine away from moisture, light, heat, and cotton filler material. The *sublingual* dosage form of nitroglycerin needs to be kept in its original amber-colored glass container with metal lid to avoid loss of potency from exposure to heat, light, moisture, and cotton filler.

• Potency of the sublingual nitroglycerin is noted if there is burning or stinging once the medication is placed under the tongue; if the medication does not burn, then the drug has lost its potency, and a new prescription must be obtained.

• It is important to emphasize that the medication is potent only for 3 to 6 months. Remind the patient to always have a fresh supply of the drug on hand, to plan ahead if traveling, and (no matter the dosage form) to sit or lie down when taking the medication to avoid falls secondary to a drop in blood pressure.

• With *all forms of nitrates,* educate the patient about adverse effects such as flushing of the face, dizziness, fainting, brief throbbing headache, increase in heart rate, and lightheadedness. Headaches associated with nitrates last approximately 20 minutes (with sublingual forms) and may be managed with acetaminophen. If headaches are bothersome when an oral dosage form is used, the drug may be taken with meals, and the patient must contact the prescriber if adverse effects continue. Blurred vision, dry mouth, or severe headaches may indicate drug overdose and require immediate medical attention. While taking an antianginal, the patient must avoid alcohol, hot environmental temperatures, saunas, hot tubs, and excessive exertion. These increase vasodilation with subsequent worsening of hypotension, which possibly can lead to syncope (fainting) and/or other cardiac events.

• In many situations, the prescriber specifies that nitroglycerin be taken *before* stressful activities or events such as emotional situations, consumption of large meals, smoking, or sudden increase in activity (e.g., sexual intercourse). The patient needs to follow the prescriber's directions regarding prophylactic dosing very closely.

• With *ointment* forms, remind the patient to use the appropriate dosage paper for application of the ointment and not to use the fingers to apply the medicine. The medication can be pressed evenly and directly from the tube onto the printed dosing line on the paper. Instruct the patient to squeeze a thin line of ointment onto the paper and follow instructions regarding its application, such as measuring and applying ½ inch of ointment. An occlusive covering must be used, such as applying a piece of plastic wrap taped around the edges to adhere the dose to the skin. Only clean, nonirritated, and nonhairy areas free of residual medication are to be used for these ointments.

• With *transdermal nitrate* use, the patient must apply the patch at the same time each day and be sure to have only one patch in place at a time, cleansing all residue off the skin before applying a new patch. Advise the patient to avoid skinfolds, hairy areas, and any area distal to the knees or elbows as application sites. A transdermal patch must never be applied to irritated or open skin, and if the patch becomes loose, the patient needs to remove it and gently wash off the residue with lukewarm soap and water, *pat* the area dry, and place another patch in another area. Encourage rotation of sites to prevent irritation (with ointments, too). The prescriber may order the removal of the patch for an 8-hour period on specific days to help decrease or prevent drug tolerance, which may develop over time. Emphasize all instructions with both written and verbal instructions.

**Isosorbide Dinitrate or Isosorbide Mononitrate**

• Educate the patient about the basic differences in oral nitrates (e.g., the mononitrate form is well absorbed after oral dosing; the dinitrate form is poorly absorbed, but its metabolite, isosorbide mononitrate, is active and well absorbed). It is important that the patient know that these drugs are *not interchangeable.*

• Inform the patient to take the medication exactly as ordered with emphasis on the need to lie down when doses are taken to avoid injury from the sudden drop in blood pressure. The sudden drop in blood pressure may lead to dizziness, lightheadedness, and fainting.

• Isosorbide dinitrate is generally given three times a day with a 12-hour drug-free interval, such as dosing at 0700, 1300, and 1900. The 12-hour drug-free interval helps prevent the development of tolerance.

• Oral dosage forms are not to be altered in any way and must be taken with 6 to 8 oz of water.

• The patient must be cautious while taking these drugs and encouraged to rise slowly and move the legs about before standing up from a lying or sitting position to help prevent dizziness, possible fainting, and falls. The avoidance of alcohol, heat, and saunas must be emphasized because these factors exacerbate the hypotensive effects of the drug and may result in bodily harm/injury.

• Advise the patient that these and other antianginals are not to be stopped abruptly.

## KEY POINTS

- Angina pectoris (chest pain) occurs because of a mismatch between the oxygen supply and oxygen demand, with either too high a demand for oxygen or too little oxygen delivery.
- The heart is a very aerobic (oxygen-requiring) muscle, and when it does not receive enough oxygen, pain (angina) occurs. When the coronary arteries that deliver oxygen to the heart muscle become blocked, a heart attack or MI occurs.
- Coronary artery disease is an abnormal condition of the arteries (blood vessels) that deliver oxygen to the heart muscle. These arteries may become narrowed, which results in reduced flow of oxygen and nutrients to the myocardium.
- Nitrates, CCBs, and beta blockers may be used to treat the symptoms of angina.
- Nitroglycerin is the prototypical nitrate. Nitrates dilate constricted coronary arteries, helping to increase the supply of oxygen and nutrients to the heart muscle. Nitrates also dilate all other blood vessels. The venous dilation results in a decrease in blood return to the heart (decreased preload), whereas the arterial dilation results in a decrease of peripheral resistance (decreased afterload—that is, the pressure or force against which the left ventricle must pump). Isosorbide

dinitrates were the first group of oral drugs used to treat angina; isosorbide mononitrates are new and improved nitrates used for angina therapy. Beta blockers are also used to relieve angina and do so by decreasing the heart rate, reducing workload on the heart, and decreasing oxygen demands.
- Dosage forms for nitrates include conventional tablets, translingual spray, controlled-release and sustained-release capsules, transdermal patch, topical ointment, and intravenous injection.
- Quick-onset nitrates are used to treat acute anginal attacks, while longer-onset nitrates are used for prophylaxis.
- Instruct patients to always keep a fresh supply of sublingual nitroglycerin on their person and in their home, because the drug is only stable for 3 to 6 months.
- CCBs and beta blockers may be associated with the adverse effects of postural hypotension, dizziness, headache, and edema. The nonselective beta blockers may exacerbate congestive heart failure, problems related to respiratory bronchospasm, and hypoglycemia. Check the patient's pulse rate before drug administration, and if it is 60 beats/min or lower, contact the prescriber for further instructions.

## NCLEX® EXAMINATION REVIEW QUESTIONS

1 A patient has a new prescription for transdermal nitroglycerin patches. The nurse teaches the patient that these patches are most appropriately used for which reason?
   a  To relieve exertional angina
   b  To prevent palpitations
   c  To prevent the occurrence of angina
   d  To stop an episode of angina

2 A nurse with adequate knowledge about the administration of intravenous nitroglycerin will recognize that which statement is correct?
   a  The intravenous form is given by IV push injection.
   b  Because the intravenous forms are short-lived, the dosing must be every 2 hours.
   c  Intravenous nitroglycerin must be protected from exposure to light through use of special tubing.
   d  Intravenous nitroglycerin can be given via gravity drip infusions.

3 Which statement by the patient reflects the need for additional patient education about the calcium channel blocker diltiazem (Cardizem)?
   a  "I can take this drug to stop an attack of angina."
   b  "I understand that food and antacids alter the absorption of this oral drug."
   c  "When the long-acting forms are taken, the drug cannot be crushed."
   d  "This drug may cause my blood pressure to drop, so I need to be careful when getting up."

4 While assessing a patient with angina who is to start beta blocker therapy, the nurse is aware that the presence of which condition may be a problem if these drugs are used?
   a  Hypertension
   b  Essential tremors

   c  Exertional angina
   d  Asthma

5 A 68-year-old man has been taking the nitrate isosorbide dinitrate (Isordil) for 2 years for angina. He recently has been experiencing erectile dysfunction and wants a prescription for sildenafil (Viagra). Which response would the nurse most likely hear from the prescriber?
   a  "He will have to be switched to isosorbide mononitrate if he wants to take sildenafil."
   b  "Taking sildenafil with the nitrate may result in severe hypotension, so a contraindication exists."
   c  "I'll write a prescription, but if he uses it, he needs to stop taking the isosorbide for one dose."
   d  "These drugs are compatible with each other, and so I'll write a prescription."

6 The nurse is reviewing drug interactions with a male patient who has a prescription for isosorbide dinitrate (Isordil) as treatment for angina symptoms. Which substances listed below could potentially result in a drug interaction? (Select all that apply.)
   a  A glass of wine
   b  Thyroid replacement hormone
   c  tadalafil (Cialis), an erectile dysfunction drug
   d  metformin (Glucophage), an antidiabetic drug
   e  carvedilol (Coreg), a beta blocker

7. The order reads, "Give metoprolol (Lopressor) 300 mg/day PO in 2 divided doses." The tablets are available in 50-mg strength. How many tablets will the patient receive per dose?

For answers see http://evolve.elsevier.com/Lilley.

1. c, 2. c, 3. a, 4. d, 5. b, 6. a, c, e, 7. 3 tablets per dose (150 mg per dose)

For Critical Thinking and Prioritization Questions, see http://evolve.elsevier.com/Lilley.

## OBJECTIVES

When you reach the end of this chapter, you will be able to do the following:

1  Differentiate between the terms *inotropic, chronotropic,* and *dromotropic.*
2  Briefly discuss the pathophysiology of heart failure.
3  Identify the approach to treatment of heart failure as outlined by the American Heart Association and American College of Cardiology Guidelines for the Diagnosis and Management of Heart Failure in Adults (last updated in 2009).
4  Compare the mechanisms of action, pharmacokinetics, indications, dosages, dosage forms, routes of administration, cautions, contraindications, adverse effects, and toxicity of the following drugs used in treatment of heart failure: lisinopril, valsartan, carvedilol, metoprolol, dobutamine, nesiritide, hydralazine/isosorbide dinitrate, milrinone, and digoxin.

5  Briefly discuss the process of rapid versus slow digitalization as well as the use of the antidote digoxin immune Fab.
6  Identify significant drug-drug, drug–laboratory test, and drug-food interactions associated with digoxin and other heart failure drugs.
7  Develop a nursing care plan that includes all phases of the nursing process for patients undergoing treatment for heart failure and that reflects the American Heart Association and American College of Cardiology Guidelines for the Diagnosis and Management of Heart Failure in Adults.

## DRUG PROFILES

- **digoxin, p. 389**
  **digoxin immune Fab, p. 390**
- **dobutamine, p. 385**
  **hydralazine/isosorbide dinitrate, p. 385**
- **lisinopril, p. 385**

- **milrinone, p. 387**
- **nesiritide, p. 386**
- **valsartan, p. 385**

  ⧫ *Key drug*

## KEY TERMS

**Atrial fibrillation** A common cardiac dysrhythmia with atrial contractions that are so rapid that they prevent full repolarization of myocardial fibers between heartbeats. (p. 387)

**Automaticity** A property of specialized excitable tissue in the heart that allows self-activation through the spontaneous development of an action potential, such as in the pacemaker cells of the heart. (p. 385)

**Chronotropic drugs**  Drugs that influence the rate of the heart-beat. (p. 384)

**Dromotropic drugs**  Drugs that influence the conduction of electrical impulses within tissues. (p. 384)

**Ejection fraction**  The proportion of blood that is ejected during each ventricular contraction compared with the total ventricular filling volume. (p. 383)

**Heart failure**  An abnormal condition in which the heart cannot pump enough blood to keep up with the body's demand. It is often the result of myocardial infarction, ischemic heart disease, or cardiomyopathy. (p. 383)

**Inotropic drugs**  Drugs that influence the force of muscular contractions, particularly contraction of the heart muscle. (p. 384)

**Left ventricular end-diastolic volume**  The total amount of blood in the ventricle immediately before it contracts, or the preload. (p. 383)

**Refractory period**  The period during which a *pulse generator* (e.g., the *sinoatrial node* of the heart) is unresponsive to an electrical input signal, and during which it is impossible for the myocardium to respond. This is the period during which the cardiac cell is readjusting its sodium and potassium levels and cannot be depolarized again. (p. 388)

## ANATOMY, PHYSIOLOGY, AND PATHOPHYSIOLOGY OVERVIEW

Heart failure is a not a specific disease per se but rather a clinical syndrome caused by numerous different cardiac disorders. More than 5.7 million people in the United States have heart failure. It is one of the most common causes for hospitalization in the United States, estimated to result in more than 3.5 million hospitalizations annually. This is especially true for elderly patients. Heart failure also causes more than 300,000 deaths annually. The findings of one of the largest and most frequently cited studies involving patients with heart failure, the Framingham study, show that the 5-year survival rate in patients with heart failure is approximately 50%. The best way to prevent heart failure is to control risk factors associated with heart failure including hypertension, coronary artery disease, obesity, and diabetes.

*Heart failure* is a pathologic state in which the heart is unable to pump blood in sufficient amounts from the ventricles (i.e., cardiac output is insufficient) to meet the body's metabolic needs, or can do so only at elevated filling pressures. The signs and symptoms typically associated with this insufficiency make up the syndrome of heart failure. Initially, the patient is asymptomatic. As the disease progresses, so do the symptoms. Failure of the ventricle(s) to eject blood efficiently results in fluid volume overload, chamber dilation, and elevated intracardiac pressure. This syndrome can affect the left ventricle, the right ventricle, or both ventricles simultaneously. Left ventricular or "left-sided" heart failure often leads to pulmonary edema, coughing, shortness of breath, and dyspnea. Right ventricular heart failure typically involves systemic venous congestion, pedal edema, jugular venous distension, ascites, and hepatic congestion. Both syndromes occur due to increased hydrostatic pressure from the ventricles into the pulmonary and/or systemic circulation.

More specifically, heart failure occurs due to a reduced ratio of ejection fraction to left ventricular end-diastolic volume. The ejection fraction is the amount of blood ejected with each contraction, whereas the left ventricular end-diastolic volume is the total amount of blood in the ventricle just before contraction. The ejection fraction is an index of left ventricular function, and the normal value is approximately 65% (0.65) of the total volume in the ventricle.

When a person has heart failure, the heart cannot then meet the increased demands, and the blood supply to certain organs is reduced. The organs that are most dependent on blood supply, the brain and heart, are the last to be deprived of blood. The kidney is relatively less dependent on blood supply and has its blood supply shunted away from it. Therefore, the filtration of fluids and removal of waste products is impaired. This can lead to acute or chronic renal failure. It also contributes to conditions such as pulmonary edema, shortness of breath, and peripheral edema.

The physical defects causing heart failure are of two types: (1) a myocardial defect such as myocardial infarction or valve insufficiency, which leads to inadequate cardiac contractility and ventricular filling; and (2) a defect outside the myocardium (e.g., coronary artery disease, pulmonary hypertension, or diabetes), which results in an overload on an otherwise normal heart. Either or both of these defects may be present in a given patient. These and other common causes of myocardial deficiency and systemic defects are listed in Box 24-1.

The emphasis of this chapter is on systolic dysfunction or inadequate ventricular contractions (systole) during the pumping of the heart. Less common, but still important, is diastolic dysfunction or inadequate ventricular filling during ventricular relaxation (diastole). This condition is most commonly associated with left ventricular hypertrophy secondary to chronic hypertension. However, it may also result from cardiomyopathy (e.g., virus induced), pericardial disease, and diabetes.

Heart failure is stratified into classes using The New York Heart Association's functional classification. Class I describes a patient who is not limited with normal physical activity by symptoms. Class II occurs when ordinary physical activity results in fatigue, dyspnea, or other symptoms. Class III is characterized by a marked limitation in normal physical activity.

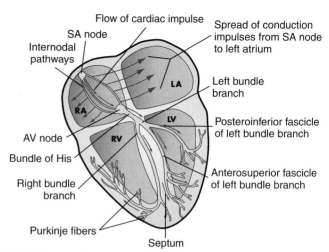

FIGURE 24-1 Conduction system of the heart. *AV,* Atrioventricular; *LA,* left atrium; *LV,* left ventricle; *RA,* right atrium; *RV,* right ventricle; *SA,* sinoatrial. (Modified from Kinney MR, Packa DR: *Andreoli's Comprehensive cardiac care,* ed 8, St Louis, 1996, Mosby; Lewis SM, Dirksen SR, Heitkemper MM, et al: *Medical-surgical nursing: assessment and management of clinical problems,* ed 7, St Louis, 2007, Mosby.)

Class IV is defined by symptoms at rest or with any physical activity. Drug therapy is individualized based on the patient's class of heart failure.

## PHARMACOLOGY OVERVIEW

Drugs that increase the force of myocardial contraction are called positive inotropic drugs, and they have a role in the treatment of failing heart muscle. Negative inotropic drugs reduce the force of contraction. Drugs that increase the rate at which the heart beats are called positive chronotropic drugs. Negative chronotropic drugs do the opposite. Drugs may also affect how quickly electrical impulses travel through the conduction system of the heart (the sinoatrial [SA] node, atrioventricular [AV] node, bundle of His, and Purkinje fibers) (Figure 24-1). Drugs that accelerate conduction are referred to as positive dromotropic drugs. Negative dromotropic drugs do the opposite. This chapter focuses on the positive inotropic drugs, phosphodiesterase inhibitors and cardiac glycosides, as well as the newest class of medications for heart failure, B-type natriuretic peptides. Although several other drugs are used in the treatment of heart failure, they are discussed in detail in other chapters; for example, angiotensin-converting enzyme (ACE) inhibitors and angiotensin receptor blockers (ARBs) are covered in Chapter 22; beta blockers are discussed in Chapters 19, 22 and 23; and diuretics are discussed in Chapter 28. These drugs are mentioned in this chapter as well, but for specifics, refer to the indicated chapters.

The treatment of heart failure has changed dramatically over the past decade. Digoxin used to be the mainstay in heart failure treatment, but because of adverse effects and drug interactions, it has been replaced by other drugs. According to the latest American Heart Association and American College of Cardiology Guidelines for the Diagnosis and Management of Heart Failure in Adults (2005, updated in 2009), the approach to the treatment of chronic heart failure revolves around reducing the effects of the renin-angiotensin-aldosterone system and the sympathetic nervous system. Therefore, the drugs of choice at the start of therapy are the ACE inhibitors (lisinopril, enalapril, captopril, and others) or the angiotensin II receptor blockers (valsartan, candesartan, losartan, and others) and certain beta blockers (metoprolol, a cardioselective beta blocker; carvedilol, a nonspecific beta blocker). Loop diuretics (furosemide) are used to reduce the symptoms of heart failure secondary to fluid overload, and the aldosterone inhibitors (spironolactone, eplerenone) are added as the heart failure progresses. Only after these drugs are used is digoxin added. Dobutamine, a positive inotropic drug, has also been used to treat heart failure. In 2005, a combination drug containing hydralazine and isosorbide dinitrate became the first drug approved for a specific ethnic group. Hydralazine/isosorbide dinitrate (BiDil) was approved specifically for use in the African-American population.

## ANGIOTENSIN-CONVERTING ENZYME INHIBITORS

The angiotensin-converting enzyme (ACE) inhibitors are a class of drugs that, as their name implies, inhibit angiotensin-converting enzyme, which is responsible for converting angiotensin I (formed through the action of renin) to angiotensin II. Angiotensin II is a potent vasoconstrictor and induces aldosterone secretion by the adrenal glands. Aldosterone stimulates sodium and water resorption, which can raise blood pressure. Together, these processes are referred to as the renin-angiotensin-aldosterone system. The ACE inhibitors are beneficial in the treatment of heart failure because they prevent sodium and water resorption by inhibiting aldosterone secretion. This causes diuresis, which decreases blood volume and blood return to the heart. This in turn decreases preload, or the left ventricular end-diastolic volume, and the work required of the heart.

Numerous ACE inhibitors are available, including lisinopril, enalapril, fosinopril, quinapril, captopril, ramipril, trandolapril, and perindopril. These drugs are all very similar, and lisinopril will be used as the class representative.

## DRUG PROFILE

**♦ lisinopril**

Lisinopril (Prinivil, Zestril) is a commonly used ACE inhibitor and is available in a generic form. It is used for hypertension, heart failure, and acute myocardial infarction. Like all ACE inhibitors, it is classified as a category C drug for women in the first trimester of pregnancy and a category D drug for women in the second and third trimesters; it can cause fetal death when used in the last two trimesters. Hyperkalemia may occur with any ACE inhibitor, and potassium supplementation or potassium-sparing diuretics need to be used with caution. Like all ACE inhibitors, lisinopril can cause a dry cough, which will not harm the patient but is annoying. Lisinopril (and all ACE inhibitors) may be associated with a decrease in renal function and hyperkalemia. For drug interactions, see Chapter 22.

### Pharmacokinetics

| Route | Onset of Action | Peak Plasma Concentration | Elimination Half-life | Duration of Action |
|---|---|---|---|---|
| PO | 1 hr | 6 hr | 11-12 hr | 24 hr |

## ANGIOTENSIN II RECEPTOR BLOCKERS

The therapeutic effects of angiotensin II receptor blockers (ARBs) in heart failure are related to their potent vasodilating properties. They may be used alone or in combination with other drugs such as diuretics in the treatment of hypertension or heart failure. The beneficial hemodynamic effect of ARBs is their ability to decrease systemic vascular resistance (a measure of afterload). Seven ARBs are currently available: valsartan (Diovan), candesartan (Atacand), eprosartan (Teveten), irbesartan (Avapro), telmisartan (Micardis), olmesartan (Benicar), and losartan (Cozaar). All of the ARBs are similar in action. Valsartan will be used as the class representative.

## DRUG PROFILE

**♦ valsartan**

Valsartan (Diovan) is a commonly used ARB. Like all ARBs, it is a pregnancy category D drug. Valsartan shares many of the same adverse effects as lisinopril, profiled earlier. The ARBs are not as likely to cause the cough associated with the ACE inhibitors, nor are they as likely to cause hyperkalemia. For drug interactions, see Chapter 22.

### Pharmacokinetics

| Route | Onset of Action | Peak Plasma Concentration | Elimination Half-life | Duration of Action |
|---|---|---|---|---|
| PO | 2 hr | Unknown | 6 hr | 12 hr |

## BETA BLOCKERS

Beta blockers (also discussed in Chapters 19, 22, and 23) work by reducing or blocking sympathetic nervous system stimulation to the heart and the heart's conduction system. By doing

this, beta blockers prevent catecholamine-mediated actions on the heart. This is known as a cardioprotective quality of beta blockers. The resulting cardiovascular effects include reduced heart rate, delayed AV node conduction, reduced myocardial contractility, and decreased myocardial automaticity. Metoprolol is the beta blocker most commonly used to treat heart failure. Metoprolol is available as an immediate-release and a sustained-release product, as well as an intravenous formulation.

Carvedilol (Coreg) has many effects, including acting as a nonselective beta blocker, an alpha$_1$ blocker, and possibly a calcium channel blocker and antioxidant. It is used primarily in the treatment of heart failure but is also beneficial for hypertension and angina. It has been shown to slow the progression of heart failure and to decrease the frequency of hospitalization in patients with mild to moderate (class II or III) heart failure. Carvedilol is most commonly added to digoxin, furosemide, and ACE inhibitors when used to treat heart failure. Carvedilol is available only for oral use. A controlled-release formulation, called Coreg CR, was recently approved. The dosages are different from those for immediate-release Coreg, and the two dosage forms cannot be interchanged.

## ALDOSTERONE ANTAGONISTS

Aldosterone antagonists spironolactone and eplerenone are useful in severe stages of heart failure. Activation of the renin-angiotensin-aldosterone system causes increased levels of aldosterone, which causes retention of sodium and water, leading to edema that can worsen heart failure. Spironolactone (Aldactone) is a potassium-sparing diuretic and is discussed in detail in Chapter 28. It also acts as an aldosterone antagonist, which has been shown to reduce the symptoms of heart failure. Eplerenone (Inspra) is a *selective aldosterone blocker*, blocking aldosterone at its receptors in the kidney, heart, blood vessels, and brain. It is discussed in detail in Chapter 22.

## MISCELLANEOUS HEART FAILURE DRUGS

### DRUG PROFILES

**hydralazine/isosorbide dinitrate**

Hydralazine/isosorbide dinitrate (BiDil) was the first drug approved for a specific ethnic group, namely African Americans. This combination of two older drugs contains 37.5 mg of hydralazine and 20 mg of isosorbide dinitrate. The individual drugs are discussed in detail in Chapter 22 (hydralazine) and Chapter 23 (isosorbide). Peak plasma levels of hydralazine/isosorbide dinitrate are achieved in 1 hour. The dose is 1 tablet three times a day, titrated up to a maximum of 2 tablets three times a day.

**♦ dobutamine**

Dobutamine (generic, formerly Dobutrex) is a beta$_1$-selective vasoactive adrenergic drug that is structurally similar to the naturally occurring catecholamine dopamine. Through stimulation of the beta$_1$ receptors on heart muscle (myocardium), it increases cardiac output by increasing contractility (positive inotropy), which increases the stroke volume, especially in patients with heart failure. Dobutamine is available only as an intravenous drug and is given by continuous infusion. See Chapter 18 for further discussion on this drug.

## B-TYPE NATRIURETIC PEPTIDE

The newest class of medications for heart failure, the B-type natriuretic peptides, currently includes only one drug, nesiritide.

## DRUG PROFILE

### ◆ nesiritide

Nesiritide (Natrecor) is classified as a synthetic version of *human B-type natriuretic peptide.* B-type natriuretic peptide (BNP) is a substance secreted from the ventricles of the heart in response to changes in pressure that occur when heart failure develops. The level of BNP in the blood increases when heart failure symptoms worsen. A related hormone that occurs naturally in the body is *atrial natriuretic peptide,* which affects vascular permeability. *Vascular permeability* refers to the ability of plasma to flow between blood vessels and their surrounding tissues, and it serves as one way for the body to regulate blood pressure.

Nesiritide is a synthetic b-type natriuretic hormone that has vasodilating effects on both arteries and veins. This vasodilation takes place in the heart itself and throughout the body. The effects of nesiritide have been shown to include diuresis (urinary fluid loss), *natriuresis* (urinary sodium loss), and vasodilation. These properties lead to an indirect increase in cardiac output and suppression of neurohormonal systems such as the renin-angiotensin system.

Nesiritide is used in the intensive care setting as a final effort to treat severe, life-threatening heart failure, often in combination with several other cardiostimulatory medications. It is no longer recommended to be used as a first-line drug for heart failure. In 2005, an expert panel reviewed nesiritide at the request of the U.S. Food and Drug Administration in response to reports of worsened renal function and mortality. The expert panel stated that the use of nesiritide be strictly limited to treatment of patients with acutely decompensated heart failure who have dyspnea at rest. It is not to be used to replace diuretics and is not to be used repetitively or to improve renal function. Its only current contraindication is drug allergy, although it is not recommended for use in patients with low cardiac filling pressures, as typically measured in the intensive care unit. Adverse effects include hypotension, cardiac dysrhythmias, insomnia, headache, and abdominal pain. Currently identified drug interactions include additive hypotensive effects with coadministration of ACE inhibitors and diuretics. This drug is available only in injectable form. Recommended dosages are given in the table below.

### Pharmacokinetics

| Route | Onset of Action | Peak Plasma Concentration | Elimination Half-life | Duration of Action |
|---|---|---|---|---|
| IV | 15 min | 1 hr | 18 min | 1 to several hr |

## DOSAGES

### *Selected Drugs for Heart Failure*

| DRUG (PREGNANCY CATEGORY) | PHARMACOLOGIC CLASS | USUAL DOSAGE RANGE | INDICATIONS |
|---|---|---|---|
| ◆ digoxin (Lanoxin) (C) | Digitalis cardiac glycoside | **Pediatric** <br> Digitalizing dose: <br> IV: 8-35 mcg/kg, divided into 3 doses, depending on age from premature infant to child older than 10 yr <br> PO: 20-40 mcg/kg, divided into 3 doses, depending on age from premature infant to child older than 10 yr <br> Usual maintenance dose: 20%-35% of digitalizing dose <br> **Adult** <br> PO/IV: Usual digitalizing dose: 1-1.5 mg divided into 3 doses; usual oral maintenance dose: 0.125-0.25 mg/day | Heart failure, supraventricular dysrhythmias |
| ◆ milrinone (Primacor) (C) | Phosphodiesterase inhibitor | **Adult** <br> IV loading dose: 50 mcg/kg <br> IV continuous infusion dose: 0.375-0.75 mcg/kg/min | Heart failure |
| ◆ nesiritide (Natrecor) (C) | Recombinant human B-type natriuretic peptide | **Adult only (pediatric use not yet established)** <br> IV: Initial bolus of 2 mcg/kg, followed by continuous infusion of 0.01 mcg/kg/min | Acutely decompensated heart failure in patients with dyspnea at rest or with minimal activity |

*IV,* Intravenous; *PO,* oral.

## PHOSPHODIESTERASE INHIBITORS

As the name implies, phosphodiesterase inhibitors (PDIs) are a group of inotropic drugs that work by inhibiting the action of an enzyme called phosphodiesterase. These drugs were discovered in the search for positive inotropic drugs with a wider therapeutic window than digoxin. Presently only one drug in this category is available in the United States: milrinone (Primacor).

### Mechanism of Action and Drug Effects

The mechanism of action of PDIs differs from other inotropic drugs such as digoxin and the catecholamines. PDIs share a similar pharmacologic action with methylxanthines such as theophylline (see Chapter 37). Both types of drug inhibit the action of phosphodiesterase, which results in an increase in intracellular cyclic adenosine monophosphate (cAMP). However, milrinone is more specific for phosphodiesterase type III, which is common in the heart and vascular smooth muscles.

The beneficial effects of milrinone come from the intracellular increase in cAMP, which results in two beneficial effects in a patient with heart failure: a positive inotropic response and vasodilation. For this reason, this class of drugs may also be referred to as *inodilators* (inotropics and dilators). Milrinone has a 10 to 100 times greater affinity for smooth muscle fibers surrounding pulmonary and systemic blood vessels than they do for cardiac muscle. This suggests that the primary beneficial effects of inodilators come from their vasodilating effects, which cause a reduction in the force against which the heart must pump to eject its volume of blood.

Finally, inhibition of phosphodiesterase results in the availability of more calcium for myocardial muscle contraction. This leads to an increase in the force of contraction (i.e., positive inotropic action). The increased calcium present in heart muscle is taken back up into its storage sites in the sarcoplasmic reticulum at a much faster rate than normal. As a result, the heart muscle relaxes more than normal and is also more compliant. In summary, PDIs have positive inotropic and vasodilatory effects. They may also increase heart rate in some instances and therefore may also have positive chronotropic effects as well.

### Indications

Phosphodiesterase inhibitors (PDIs) are primarily used in the intensive care unit setting for the short-term management of acute heart failure. The American Heart Association and American College of Cardiology guidelines, last updated in 2009, do not recommend long-term infusion of the PDIs.

### Contraindications

Contraindications to the use of PDIs include known drug allergy and may include the presence of severe aortic or pulmonary valvular disease and heart failure resulting from diastolic dysfunction.

### Adverse Effects

The primary adverse effect seen with milrinone therapy is dysrhythmia. Milrinone-induced dysrhythmias are mainly ventricular. Ventricular dysrhythmias occur in approximately 12% of patients treated with this drug. Some other adverse effects associated with milrinone therapy are hypotension, angina (chest pain), hypokalemia, tremor, and thrombocytopenia.

### Toxicity and Management of Overdose

No specific antidote exists for an overdose of milrinone. Hypotension secondary to vasodilation is the primary effect seen with excessive dosages. The recommendation is to reduce the dosage or temporarily discontinue the drug if excessive hypotension occurs. This is to be done until the patient's condition has stabilized. Initiation of general measures for circulatory support is also recommended.

### Interactions

Concurrent administration of diuretics may cause significant hypovolemia and reduced cardiac filling pressure. Appropriately monitor the patient in an intensive care setting to detect and respond to these problems. Additive inotropic effects may be seen with coadministration of digoxin. Furosemide must not be injected into intravenous lines with milrinone because it will precipitate immediately.

### Dosages

For dosage information, see the table on p. 386.

## DRUG PROFILE

#### ◆ milrinone

Milrinone (Primacor) is the only presently available PDI after the discontinuation of inamrinone (Inocor) in May 2011. Milrinone is also referred to as an *inodilator* because it exerts both a positive inotropic effect and a vasodilatory effect. Milrinone is contraindicated in cases of known drug allergy. Adverse effects include cardiac dysrhythmias, headache, hypokalemia, tremor, thrombocytopenia, and elevated liver enzyme levels. Interacting drugs include diuretics (additive hypotensive effects) and digoxin (additive inotropic effects). Milrinone is available only in injectable form. Recommended dosages are given in the table on p. 386.

#### Pharmacokinetics

| Route | Onset of Action | Peak Plasma Concentration | Elimination Half-life | Duration of Action |
|---|---|---|---|---|
| IV | 5-15 min | Immediate | 2-3 hr | 8-10 hr |

## CARDIAC GLYCOSIDES

Cardiac glycosides are one of the oldest groups of cardiac drugs. Not only do they have beneficial effects on the failing heart, but they also help control the ventricular response to atrial fibrillation. They were originally obtained from either the *Digitalis purpurea* or *Digitalis lanata* plant, both commonly known as foxglove. For this reason, cardiac glycosides are sometimes referred to as *digitalis glycosides*. Cardiac glycosides were the mainstay of therapy for heart failure for more than 200 years; however, they are no longer used as first-line drugs. Digoxin is the only cardiac glycoside currently available in the United States. Although digoxin is a powerful positive inotropic drug, it has not been shown to reduce mortality.

## Mechanism of Action and Drug Effects

The beneficial effect of digoxin is thought to be an increase in myocardial contractility—known as a *positive inotropic effect.* This occurs secondarily to the inhibition of the sodium-potassium adenosine triphosphatase pump. When the action of this enzyme-complex is inhibited, the cellular sodium and calcium concentrations increase. The overall result is enhanced myocardial contractility. Digoxin also augments cholinergic (or parasympathetic) stimulation via the vagus nerve of the parasympathetic nervous system. This is more commonly referred to as *vagal tone* and results in increased diastolic filling between heartbeats secondary to reduced heart rate. Vagal tone is also believed to sensitize cardiac barorecep-tors, which reduces sympathetic stimulation from the central nervous system. All of these processes further enhance cardiac efficiency and output.

Digoxin changes the electrical conduction properties of the heart, and this markedly affects the conduction system and cardiac automaticity. Digoxin decreases the velocity (rate) of electrical conduction and prolongs the refractory period in the conduction system. The particular site in the conduction system where this occurs is the area between the atria and the ventricles (SA node to AV node). The cardiac cells remain in a state of depolarization longer and are unable to start another electrical impulse, which also reduces heart rate and improves cardiac efficiency.

The following is a summary of the inotropic, chronotropic, dromotropic, and other effects produced by digoxin:
- A positive inotropic effect—an increase in the force and velocity of myocardial contraction without a corresponding increase in oxygen consumption
- A negative chronotropic effect—reduced heart rate
- A negative dromotropic effect—decreased automaticity at the SA node, decreased AV nodal conduction, reduced conductivity at the bundle of His, and prolongation of the atrial and ventricular refractory periods
- An increase in stroke volume
- A reduction in heart size during diastole
- A decrease in venous blood pressure and vein engorgement
- An increase in coronary circulation
- Promotion of tissue perfusion and diuresis as a result of improved blood circulation
- Decrease in exertional and paroxysmal nocturnal dyspnea, cough, and cyanosis
- Improved symptom control, quality of life, and exercise tolerance, but no apparent reduction in mortality

## Indications

Digoxin is primarily used in the treatment of systolic heart failure and atrial fibrillation. However, the latest heart failure treatment guidelines recommend that it be used as an adjunct to drugs of other classes, including beta blockers, diuretics, ACE inhibitors, and ARBs.

| TABLE 24-1 | DIGOXIN: COMMON ADVERSE EFFECTS |
|---|---|
| **BODY SYSTEM** | **ADVERSE EFFECTS** |
| Cardiovascular | Bradycardia or tachycardia; hypotension |
| Central nervous | Headache, fatigue, confusion, convulsions |
| Eye | Colored vision (i.e., green, yellow, or purple), halo vision |
| Gastrointestinal | Anorexia, nausea, vomiting, diarrhea |

Normal therapeutic level = 0.5 to 2 ng/mL.

## Contraindications

Contraindications to the use of digoxin include known drug allergy and may include second- or third-degree heart block, atrial fibrillation, ventricular tachycardia or fibrillation, heart failure resulting from diastolic dysfunction, and subaortic stenosis (obstruction in the left ventricle below the aortic valve). However, digoxin may be used to treat some of these conditions, if recommended by a competent cardiologist, depending on the given clinical situation.

## Adverse Effects

The common undesirable effects associated with digoxin use are cardiovascular, central nervous system, ocular, and gastrointestinal effects. These are outlined in Table 24-1.

### Toxicity and Management of Overdose

Digoxin has a low therapeutic index (see Chapter 2). Digoxin levels are monitored when the patient first starts taking the drug. However, monitoring of digoxin levels after the drug reaches steady state is usually necessary only if there is suspicion of toxicity, noncompliance, or deteriorating renal function. Normal therapeutic levels for digoxin are 0.5 to 2 ng/mL. Low potassium or magnesium levels may increase the potential for digoxin toxicity. Therefore, frequent monitoring of serum electrolytes is also important. Estimates are that as many as 20% of patients taking digoxin exhibit symptoms of toxicity. A decrease in renal function is also a common cause of digoxin toxicity, because digoxin is excreted almost exclusively via the kidneys. Signs and symptoms of digoxin toxicity include bradycardia, headache, dizziness, confusion, nausea, and visual disturbances (blurred vision or yellow vision). With toxicity, ECG findings may include heart block, atrial tachycardia with block, or ventricular dysrhythmias. Predisposing factors to digoxin toxicity are listed in Table 24-2.

The treatment strategies for digoxin toxicity depend on the severity of the symptoms. These strategies can range from simply withholding the next dose to instituting more aggressive therapies. The steps usually taken in the management of digoxin toxicity are listed in Table 24-3.

When significant toxicity develops as a result of digoxin therapy, the administration of digoxin immune Fab may be indicated. Digoxin immune Fab is an antibody that recognizes digoxin as an antigen and forms an antigen-antibody complex with the drug, thus inactivating the free digoxin. Digoxin immune Fab therapy is not indicated for every patient who is

## TABLE 24-2  CONDITIONS PREDISPOSING TO DIGITALIS TOXICITY

| CONDITION/DISEASE | SIGNIFICANCE |
|---|---|
| Use of cardiac pacemaker | A patient with this device may exhibit digitalis toxicity at lower dosages than usual. |
| Hypokalemia | The patient's risk of serious dysrhythmias is increased, and the patient is more susceptible to digitalis toxicity. |
| Hypercalcemia | The patient is at higher risk of experiencing sinus bradycardia, dysrhythmias, and heart block. |
| Atrioventricular block | Heart block may worsen with increasing levels or digitalis. |
| Dysrhythmias | Dysrhythmias may occur that did not exist before digitalis use and thus could be related to digitalis toxicity. |
| Hypothyroidism, respiratory or renal disease | Patients with these disorders require lower dosages because they cause delayed renal drug excretion. |
| Advanced age | Because of decreased renal function and the resultant diminished drug excretion along with decreased body mass in this patient population, a lower dosage than usual is needed to prevent toxicity. The practice of polypharmacy may also lead to toxicity. |
| Ventricular fibrillation | Ventricular rate may actually increase with digitalis use. |

## TABLE 24-3  DIGOXIN TOXICITY: STEP-BY-STEP MANAGEMENT

| STEP | ACTIONS |
|---|---|
| 1 | Discontinue administration of drug. |
| 2 | Begin continuous electrocardiographic monitoring for cardiac dysrhythmias; administer any appropriate antidysrhythmic drugs as ordered. |
| 3 | Determine serum digoxin and electrolyte levels. |
| 4 | Administer potassium supplements for hypokalemia if indicated, as ordered. |
| 5 | Institute supportive therapy for gastrointestinal symptoms (nausea, vomiting, or diarrhea). |
| 6 | Administer digoxin antidote (i.e., digoxin immune Fab) if indicated, as ordered. |

## TABLE 24-4  DIGOXIN: DRUG INTERACTIONS

| INTERACTING DRUG | MECHANISM | RESULT |
|---|---|---|
| Antidysrhythmics calcium (parenteral) | Increase cardiac irritability | Increased digoxin toxicity |
| cholestyramine colestipol sucralfate | Decrease oral absorption | Reduced therapeutic effect |
| Beta blockers | Block beta₁ receptors in the heart | Enhanced bradycardic effect of digoxin |
| Calcium channel blockers | Block beta₁ receptors in the heart | Enhanced bradycardic effect of digoxin |
| quinidine | Block calcium channels in the myocardium | Enhanced bradycardic and negative inotropic effects of digoxin |
| verapamil amiodarone dronedarone cyclosporine Azole antifungals | Decrease clearance | Digoxin levels increased by 50%; digoxin dose should be reduced by 50% |

showing signs of digoxin toxicity. The following are the clinical settings in which its use may be indicated:

- Hyperkalemia (serum potassium level higher than 5 mEq/L) in a patient with digoxin toxicity
- Life-threatening cardiac dysrhythmias, sustained ventricular tachycardia or fibrillation, and severe sinus bradycardia or heart block unresponsive to atropine treatment or cardiac pacing
- Life-threatening digoxin overdose: more than 10 mg digoxin in adults; more than 4 mg digoxin in children

## Interactions

A wide variety of significant drug interactions are possible with digoxin. Common examples are given in Table 24-4. The most important drug-drug interactions occurring with digoxin are interactions with amiodarone, quinidine, and verapamil. These three drugs can increase digoxin levels by 50%. When large amounts of bran are ingested, the absorption of oral digoxin may be decreased. Certain herbal supplements may interact with digoxin; for example, ginseng may increase digoxin levels, hawthorn may potentiate the effects of digoxin, licorice may increase the risk of cardiac toxicity due to potassium loss, and St. John's wort may reduce digoxin levels. Drugs that lower serum potassium or magnesium levels can predispose patients to digoxin toxicity.

## Dosages

For dosage information, see the table on p. 386. Also see the Safety and Quality Improvement: Preventing Medication Errors box on p. 390.

## DRUG PROFILES

### ◆ digoxin

Digoxin (Lanoxin) is indicated for the treatment of heart failure and atrial fibrillation and flutter. Digoxin use is contraindicated in patients who have shown a hypersensitivity to it and in those with ventricular tachycardia and fibrillation. Normal therapeutic drug levels of digoxin are between 0.5 and 2 ng/mL. However, levels higher than 2 ng/mL are used for the treatment of atrial fibrillation. Digoxin is available in oral and injectable forms. Because of digoxin's fairly long duration of action and half-life, a loading, or "digitalizing," dose is often given to bring serum levels of the drug up to a desirable therapeutic level more quickly. Recommended digitalizing doses and the daily oral and intravenous adult and pediatric dosages are given in the table on p. 386.

Pharmacokinetics

| Route | Onset of Action | Peak Plasma Concentration | Elimination Half-life | Duration of Action |
|---|---|---|---|---|
| PO | 1-2 hr | 2-8 hr | 35-48 hr | 3-4 days |
| IV | 5-30 min | 1-4 hr | 35-48 hr | 3-4 days |

### digoxin immune Fab

Digoxin immune Fab (Digifab) is the antidote for severe digoxin overdose and is indicated for the reversal of such life-threatening cardiotoxic effects as severe bradycardia, advanced heart block, ventricular tachycardia or fibrillation, and severe hyperkalemia. Use of digoxin immune Fab is contraindicated in patients who have shown a hypersensitivity to it. It is available only in parenteral form as a 40-mg vial. It is dosed based on the patient's serum digoxin level in conjunction with his or her weight. The recommended dosages vary according to the amount of cardiac glycoside ingested. One vial binds 0.5 mg of digoxin. It is important to bear in mind that after digoxin immune Fab is given, all subsequent measurements of serum digoxin level will be elevated for days to weeks. Therefore, after its administration, the clinical signs and symptoms of digoxin toxicity, rather than the digoxin serum levels, are the primary focus in monitoring for the effectiveness of reversal therapy.

Pharmacokinetics

| Route | Onset of Action | Peak Plasma Concentration | Elimination Half-life | Duration of Action |
|---|---|---|---|---|
| IV | Immediate | Immediate | 14-20 hr | Days to weeks |

### ⚡ SAFETY AND QUALITY IMPROVEMENT: PREVENTING MEDICATION ERRORS

#### The Importance of Decimal Points

Incorrect decimal placement can be lethal when calculating digoxin dosages! According to the Institute for Safe Medication Practices (ISMP), trailing zeros are *not* to be used after decimal points. In the case of digoxin, if a "1 mg" dose is ordered and is written as "1.0 mg," the order could be misread as "10 mg," and the patient would receive 10 times the ordered dose.

The ISMP also recommends that leading zeroes be used if a dose is less than a whole number. For example, ".25 mg" can look like "25 mg," which is a dose that is 100 times the ordered dose. Instead, the order must be written as "0.25 mg" to avoid any errors.

Of course, such an error hopefully would be caught when the nurse realizes how many 250-mcg digoxin tablets it would take to give a "25 mg" dose, or how many milliliters would be needed for an intravenous dose. However, such errors have occurred. Consider what would happen if a digoxin overdose leads to digoxin toxicity and the serious effects this would have on the patient!

Data from Institute for Safe Medication Practices: ISMP's list of error-prone abbreviations, symbols, and dose designations, Huntington Valley, PA, 2007, available at www.ismp.org/Tools/errorproneabbreviations.pdf. Accessed February 1, 2012.

## NURSING PROCESS

## ASSESSMENT

Before a drug used to treat heart failure is given, perform a thorough assessment, including assessment of the patient's past and present medical history, drug allergies, and family medical history with emphasis on any history of cardiac, hypertensive, or renal diseases. Your review may yield findings that either dictate very cautious use of the drug or even represent contraindications to its use. Assess the following clinical parameters and other data:

- Blood pressure
- Pulse rate—both apical and radial, measured for 1 full minute
- Peripheral pulse location and grading of strength
- Capillary refill
- Presence or absence of edema
- Heart sounds
- Breath sounds
- Weight
- Intake and output amounts
- Serum laboratory values such as potassium, sodium, magnesium, and calcium levels
- Electrocardiogram
- Results of renal function tests, including BUN and creatinine levels
- Results of liver function tests such as levels of AST, ALT, CPK, LDH, and ALP
- Medication history and profile, including all prescription drugs, over-the-counter drugs, herbals, and nutritional supplements taken; for example, herbal products (e.g., Siberian ginseng) may increase digitalis drug levels; consumption of large amounts of bran with digoxin will decrease the drug's absorption
- Dietary habits and all meals and snacks consumed over the previous 24 hours
- Smoking history
- Alcohol intake

*ACE inhibitors,* such as lisinopril, require thorough assessment of cautions, contraindications, and drug interactions (see Chapter 22). Hyperkalemia is an adverse effect; therefore, perform an assessment of serum potassium before giving these drugs and administer potassium supplementation and/or potassium-sparing diuretics with caution. Assess respiratory history, specifically any previous problems of cough. ACE inhibitors may cause a dry cough, which is not harmful but may be annoying. Patients may be switched to an *ARB,* such as valsartan (see Chapter 22), if the cough becomes problematic for the patient.

As mentioned earlier, metoprolol is the *beta blocker* most commonly used to treat heart failure. Carvedilol also has many therapeutic effects (see Chapters 19, 22, and 23 for a detailed discussion) and is commonly added to existing regimens of digoxin, furosemide (loop diuretic), and ACE inhibitors in the management of heart failure. Related assessment information for alpha- and beta-blocking drugs may be found in Chapter 19.

Dobutamine, a beta$_1$-selective adrenergic, is also used to treat heart failure and is discussed further in Chapter 18. The status of the patient's veins is important to assess when this drug is indicated because it is only given intravenously.

*Aldosterone antagonists,* such as spironolactone and eplerenone, require close assessment of heart and breath sounds as well as for the occurrence of edema, which is a known adverse effect (see Chapter 22 for more information). *Hydralazine/isosorbide dinitrate* is used mainly in African-American patients and is discussed further in Chapter 22.

The newest class of medications for heart failure, the *B-type natriuretic peptides,* includes the drug nesiritide. Carefully assess all body functions, especially cardiac function, with attention to heart sounds, blood pressure, pulse rate, and the presence of any cardiac dysrhythmias, hypotension, insomnia, and headache. These may be exacerbated with the use of this drug. See previous discussion for other cautions, contraindications, and drug interactions.

With any medication regimen, it is always important to assess support systems at home, because safe and effective therapy depends on close observation, monitoring of appropriate parameters (e.g., daily weight), attention to patient complaints, and evaluation of how the patient is feeling and functioning. With milrinone, a *phosphodiesterase inhibitor,* closely monitor cardiac status, which is critical to patient safety. These patients are usually in an ICU setting and require frequent assessment of heart sounds, vital signs, and any evidence of ventricular dysrhythmias on ECG readings. Assess also for any history of angina, hypotension, and hypokalemia, which may all be exacerbated with this drug. Significant drug interactions to assess for include parenteral furosemide that will precipitate immediately if milrinone is present in the IV lines.

Before giving *digoxin,* closely monitor serum electrolytes. Specifically, assess potassium levels because low levels or hypokalemia may precipitate digoxin toxicity. Hypokalemia is manifested by muscle weakness, confusion, lethargy, anorexia, nausea, and changes in the ECG. Low levels of magnesium or hypomagnesemia may also precipitate digoxin toxicity. Hypomagnesemia is manifested by agitation, twitching, hyperactive reflexes, nausea, vomiting, and ECG changes. You also need to closely assess digoxin levels once it has been administered because of the narrow range between the therapeutic and toxic levels of digoxin (also called a low therapeutic index; see Chapter 2). Measure and document baseline weight as well. Perform a careful assessment of the following systems: (1) Neurologic system: Note any history of headaches, fatigue, confusion, and/or convulsions; assess level of alertness and orientation; (2) Gastrointestinal system: Document any changes in appetite (decreased) and/or complaints of diarrhea, nausea, or vomiting; (3) Cardiac system: Note the history of any irregularities, pulse rate of lower than 60 beats/min or higher than 100 beats/min, hypotension, abnormal heart sounds, and abnormal ECG findings (if this test is ordered); and (4) Visual and sensory system: Document baseline vision as well as any changes in vision, such as green, yellow, or purple halo surrounding the peripheral field of vision. See Table 24-1 for more information on adverse effects of digoxin. Also assess for any cautions, contraindications, and drug interactions (see Table 24-2).

## PATIENT-CENTERED CARE: LIFESPAN CONSIDERATIONS FOR THE PEDIATRIC PATIENT

### Heart Failure

The cause, symptoms, treatment, and prognosis of heart failure in children vary depending on age. In infants, the cause of heart failure is generally due to holes in the heart or other structural problems. In older children, the structure of the heart may be normal but the heart muscle may be weakened. Symptoms of heart failure differ depending on age and become worse with age because the heart must keep up with increased oxygen demands and energy demands (with increased growth).

- Symptoms may include poor growth, difficulty in feeding, and tachypnea; in older children, inability to tolerate exercise and other activities, the need to rest more often, and dyspnea with minimal exertion occur more frequently.
- Treatment is generally age- and cause-specific. For septal defects, surgery or medication may be indicated. For more complex problems, surgery may be needed within the first few weeks of life.
- Drug therapy may include furosemide (a loop diuretic), angiotensin-converting enzyme inhibitors, beta blockers, and sometimes digoxin to help improve heart pumping efficiency.
- Correct calculation of dosages for any of the medications used is very important to safe and cautious nursing care. A one-decimal-point placement error will result in a tenfold dosage error, which could be fatal.
- Digoxin toxicity is manifested in children by nausea, vomiting, bradycardia, anorexia, and dysrhythmias.
- The prescriber needs to be notified immediately if any of the following develop or worsen: fatigue, sudden weight gain (2 pounds or more in 24 hours), palpitations, tachycardia or bradycardia, and/or respiratory distress.

Modified from Cincinnati Children's Hospital Medical Center: Signs and symptoms: congestive heart failure, 2006, available at http://www.cincinnatichildrens.org/health/c/chf. Accessed February 1, 2012.

## NURSING DIAGNOSES

1. Ineffective peripheral tissue perfusion related to the pathophysiologic influence of heart failure
2. Deficient knowledge related to lack of information and experience with heart failure as well as the first-time use of drugs indicated for heart failure
3. Noncompliance with therapy regimen related to lack of information about the disease process as well as the drug(s) and adverse effects

## PLANNING

### GOALS

1. Patient exhibits improved cardiac output with improved tissue perfusion once drug therapy is initiated.
2. Patient states use, action, adverse effects, and toxic effects of therapy.
3. Patient remains compliant with drug therapy regimen.

### OUTCOME CRITERIA

1. Patient experiences improved to strong peripheral pulses; pink, warm extremities and improved ability to carry out activities of daily living (ADLs).

2. Patient demonstrates sufficient knowledge about disease process related to heart failure, stating the importance of the need for life-long therapy, constant monitoring by physicians/health care provider, conserving of energy, and other measures to minimize oxygen demands.
   - Patient demonstrates proper technique for measuring radial pulse for 1 full minute before taking medication.
   - Patient states the most common adverse effects to expect with digoxin therapy, such as bradycardia or tachycardia (pulse rate less than 60 beats/min or greater than 100 beats/min as indicated by prescriber), headache, fatigue, confusion, halo vision, anorexia, nausea, and vomiting.
   - Patient states the importance of reporting to the prescriber symptoms that are indicative of digoxin toxicity, specifically anorexia, nausea, vomiting, and loss of appetite.
3. Patient's compliance with therapy results in improved heart function with subsequent heart rate above 60 beats/min and below 100 beats/min with regular rhythm.
   - Patient reports improved ability to perform simple ADLs with minimal dyspnea and increased energy levels.
   - Patient reports the consistent taking of medication at the same time every day along with performing daily weights.
   - Patient remains free from exacerbations of heart failure and states no severe adverse effects while taking medication exactly as ordered.

## ▌IMPLEMENTATION

Nursing interventions associated with the use of *ACE inhibitors, ARBs, beta blockers,* and *adrenergic drugs* are discussed further in Chapters 18, 19, and 22. When administering the *b-type natriuretic peptide* nesiritide, give the drug as ordered and with extreme caution. Nesiritide is strictly used in an intensive care setting in very ill patients who are experiencing acute decompensated heart failure and receiving continuous cardiac monitoring. While the drug is being administered intravenously, monitor the patient for all of its severe adverse effects, such as hypotension, dysrhythmias, headache, and abdominal pain. Avoid co-administration of drugs that decrease the patient's blood pressure, such as ACE inhibitors and diuretics, if at all possible. Hydralazine/isosorbide dinitrate must also be used with extreme caution because of the associated syncope. If this occurs, the drug will most likely be discontinued. Monitor blood pressure and other vital signs, especially with the first few doses of hydralazine/isosorbide dinitrate (because of the syncope). Drug interactions, cautions, and contraindications have been previously discussed.

Always check for compatibility of solutions when giving the *phosphodiesterase inhibitor* milrinone. Record intake and output, heart rate, blood pressure, daily weight, and respiration rate as well as heart and breath sounds. Report any evidence of hypokalemia to the prescriber immediately, and monitor the patient closely (vital signs). When heart failure drugs such as digoxin, milrinone, and digoxin immune Fab are administered parenterally, use an infusion pump unless the order is to administer them as an intravenous push.

Before administering any dose of the *cardiac glycoside* digoxin, check the serum potassium and magnesium levels to be sure they are within normal limits and to prevent toxicity. *Always* measure the patient's apical pulse rate (auscultate the apical heart rate, found at the apical impulse located at the fifth left midclavicular intercostal space) for 1 full minute. If the pulse rate is 60 beats/min or lower, or if it is higher than 100 beats/min, you will generally withhold the dose and notify the prescriber of the problem immediately. Although withholding of the dose is usually indicated, health care facilities and prescribers often have their own protocols that apply to individual patients. In addition, contact the prescriber if the patient experiences any of the following signs and symptoms of digoxin toxicity: headache, dizziness, confusion, nausea, and visual disturbances (yellow-green halo or blurred vision). ECG findings in a patient with digoxin toxicity would show heart block, atrial tachycardia with block, or ventricular dysrhythmias. Remember that most institutions and/or nursing units follow protocol or policy with regard to digitalis and its administration.

Other nursing interventions include checking the dosage form and prescribed amounts and the prescriber's order carefully to make sure that the correct drug dosage has been dispensed (e.g., 0.125 or 0.25 mg). Oral digoxin may be administered with meals but not with foods high in fiber (bran), because the fiber will bind to the digitalis and lead to altered absorption/bioavailability of the drug. If the medication is to be given intravenously, the following interventions are critical to patient safety: infuse undiluted intravenous forms at around 0.25 mg/min or over longer than a 5-minute period, or as per hospital protocol. The administration of intramuscular forms of cardiac glycosides is extremely painful and is not indicated or recommended, because tissue necrosis and erratic absorption are often the outcome. Digoxin is incompatible with many other medications in solution or syringe; therefore, double-check compatibility before parenteral administration.

Consider the interventions for patients undergoing digitalization separately from other drugs. Again, although digitalization is not commonly used in contemporary practice, it may still be performed in some areas of practice for the management of heart failure. Rapid digitalization (to achieve faster onset of action) is generally reserved for patients who have heart failure and are in acute distress. Such patients are hospitalized because digitalis toxicities can appear quickly (in this setting) and are directly correlated with the high drug concentrations used. If the patient undergoing rapid digitalization exhibits any of the manifestations of toxicity, contact the prescriber immediately. Continuously observe these patients, with frequent measurement of vital signs and serum drug and potassium levels. Slow digitalization (rarely used) is generally performed on an outpatient basis in patients with heart failure who are not in acute distress. In this situation, it takes longer for toxic effects to appear (depending on the drug's half-life) than with rapid digitalization. The main advantages of slow digitalization are that it can be performed on an outpatient basis, oral dosage forms can be used, and it is safer than rapid digitalization. The disadvantages are that it takes longer for the therapeutic effects to occur and the symptoms of toxicity are more gradual in onset and therefore more insidious.

If toxicity occurs and digoxin rises to a life-threatening level, administer the antidote, *digoxin immune Fab*, as ordered. It is given parenterally over 30 minutes, and in some scenarios it is given as an intravenous bolus (e.g., if cardiac arrest is imminent). All vials of the drug need to be refrigerated. The drug is stable for 4 hours after being mixed; use it immediately, and if not used within 4 hours, discard the drug. One vial of digoxin immune Fab binds 0.5 mg of digoxin. Check compatible solutions for dilution prior to infusion of the antidote. Closely monitor blood pressure, apical pulse rate and rhythm, electrocardiogram, and serum potassium levels, and record the findings. Document baseline data, and begin to observe closely for changes in assessment findings such as changes in muscle strength, occurrence of tremors and muscle cramping, changes in mental status, irregular cardiac rhythms (from hypokalemia), and confusion, thirst, and cold clammy skin (from hyponatremia). If the treatment does reduce the toxicity, these problems will improve considerably compared with the patient's baseline.

## ▌EVALUATION

Monitoring patients after the administration of drugs to improve heart contractility, or *positive inotropic drugs*, is critical for identifying therapeutic effects and adverse effects. Because *positive inotropic drugs* increase the force of myocardial contractility; alter electrophysiologic properties, leading to a decrease in heart rate (negative chronotropic effect); and decrease AV node conduction properties (negative dromotropic effect), the therapeutic effects of these drugs include the following:

- Increased urinary output
- Decreased edema
- Decreased dyspnea and crackles
- Decreased fatigue
- Resolution of paroxysmal nocturnal dyspnea
- Improved peripheral pulses, skin color, and temperature

For patients taking *lisinopril, valsartan, metoprolol, dobutamine, nesiritide,* and *hydralazine/isosorbide dinitrate*, therapeutic effects include improvement in symptoms of heart failure and improved cardiac function. During therapy, the evaluation must also monitor for the adverse effects of these medications, which have been discussed previously in the pharmacology section.

Therapeutic effects of *milrinone* include an improvement in cardiac function with a corresponding improvement in the patient's heart failure. Monitor for the adverse effects of hypotension, dysrhythmias, headache, ventricular fibrillation, chest pain, and hypokalemia. Evaluate patients taking milrinone for significant hypotension. If hypotension occurs, contact the prescriber, and discontinue the infusion or decrease the rate while waiting to hear from the prescriber.

While monitoring for the therapeutic effects of *digoxin*, assess the patient for the development of toxicity because of the drug's low therapeutic index. Toxic effects associated with digoxin may include nausea, vomiting, and anorexia. Monitoring laboratory values such as serum creatinine, potassium, calcium, sodium, and chloride levels—as well as watching the serum levels of digoxin (normal levels between 0.5 and 2 ng/mL)—is important to ensure safe and efficacious treatment.

## CASE STUDY

### *Phosphodiesterase Inhibitor for Heart Failure*

Jim, a 58-year-old retired bus driver, has been in the hospital for a week for treatment of heart failure. He had a myocardial infarction a year earlier and tells the nurse that he "hasn't felt well for weeks." He is currently receiving carvedilol, lisinopril, furosemide, and potassium supplements (all orally), but he has had little improvement.

Today during morning rounds, the nurse notes that Jim is having increased difficulty with breathing, and his heart rate is up to 120 beats/min. His weight has increased from 72 to 76 kg overnight, and his lower legs and ankles show edema rated as 3+. Crackles are heard over both lungs, and his pulse oximetry reading is 91% (down from 98% earlier). In addition, Jim is very restless. Oxygen is started, a Foley catheter is inserted, and Jim is transferred to the intensive care unit.

After examining Jim, Dr. Horne writes new medication orders as follows:

Change furosemide to 60 mg intravenously twice a day

Continue carvedilol and lisinopril

Start an infusion of milrinone as follows:

Loading dose: 50 mcg/kg over 10 minutes, followed by an infusion of 0.5 mcg/kg/min

1. Describe the drug effects of the medications Jim is receiving for the heart failure.
2. What laboratory values will you need to monitor while Jim is receiving the milrinone?

The charge nurse is in Jim's room when another nurse comes in to give Jim the intravenous dose of furosemide. As the nurse reaches for the tubing of the milrinone infusion to administer the diuretic, the charge nurse gently stops the nurse from giving the medication. Out in the hallway, the charge nurse speaks to the nurse.

3. What was the potential problem?

The next morning, Jim's breathing is better, his lungs are clearer, and his peripheral edema is now evaluated as trace edema. However, he complains of feeling his heart "skip" more than usual.

4. Is there a concern? What will the nurse need to do at this point?

After a week, Jim's condition has improved greatly. The milrinone was stopped, he was transferred to a regular room, and today he is ready to go home.

5. In addition to receiving education regarding his medications, what should Jim be taught to monitor while recovering at home?

For answers, see http://evolve.elsevier.com/Lilley.

## PATIENT TEACHING TIPS

- Hydralazine/isosorbide dinitrate may cause syncope, and this needs to be explained to the patient, with instructions to change positions carefully.
- Instruct the patient on how to take the radial pulse before each dose of digoxin or as indicated. Daily weights are important and need to be done the same time every morning and with the exact amount of clothing. For elderly or physically or mentally challenged patients, it is important that home health care personnel or a heart failure/hospital-based clinic supervise the medication regimen. This is important because these individuals are at risk for adverse effects, toxicity, and drug interactions. If the pulse rate is below 60 beats/min or is erratic, if the pulse rate is 100 beats/min or higher, or if there is anorexia, nausea, or vomiting, the health care provider must be contacted. Emphasize the importance of the patient reporting any palpitations or a feeling that the heart is racing, change in heart rate and/or irregular heart rate, the occurrence of dizziness or fainting, any changes in vision, and weight gain (2 pounds or more in 24 hours or 5 pounds or more in 1 week).
- Advise the patient to keep a daily journal with notation of medications, daily weights, dietary intake and appetite, any adverse effects or changes in condition, and a rating of how the he or she is feeling day to day.
- Instruct the patient to wear a medical alert bracelet or necklace and to keep a current medication and medical history card on his or her person at all times that lists allergies, medical diagnosis, and medications. Medical information and lists of medications need to be updated frequently or with each visit to the prescriber.
- Digoxin is usually taken once a day. Encourage the patient to take it at the same time every day. If a dose is missed, the patient may take the omitted dose if no more than 12 hours have passed from the time the drug was to have been taken. Instruct the patient that if more than 12 hours have passed since the missed dose, the patient should *not* skip that dose, *not* double up on the next digoxin dose, and contact the prescriber immediately for further instructions.
- Instruct the patient to *never* abruptly stop any of the medications being taken for heart failure. If problems occur, advise the patient to always contact the prescriber.
- If potassium-depleting diuretics are being taken as part of the therapy, encourage the patient to consume foods high in potassium and to report any weakness, fatigue, or lethargy. In addition, any worsening of dizziness or dyspnea or the occurrence of any unusual problems should be reported immediately.
- With medication regimens for heart failure, most patients are encouraged to avoid using antacids or eating ice cream, milk products, yogurt, cheese (dairy products), or bran for 2 hours before or 2 hours after taking medication to avoid interference with the absorption of the oral dosage forms of these medications.

## KEY POINTS

- Inotropic drugs affect the force of myocardial contraction; positive inotropics (e.g., digoxin) increase the force of contractions, and negative inotropics (e.g., beta blockers, calcium channel blockers) decrease myocardial contractility. Chronotropics affect heart rate per minute, with positive chronotropics increasing heart rate and negative chronotropics decreasing the heart rate. Dromotropic drugs affect the conduction of electrical impulses through the heart; positive dromotropic drugs increase the speed of electrical impulses through the heart, whereas negative drugs have the opposite effect.
- Know the protocol for heart failure management, because digoxin, once the cornerstone of treatment for heart failure, is now used only after all other recommended drugs have been tried. The American Heart Association and American College of Cardiology treatment guidelines (last updated in 2009) provide the protocol guidelines of treatment for heart failure, including the following: Drugs of choice to initiate treatment are the ACE inhibitors (lisinopril, enalapril, captopril, and others) or the ARBs (valsartan, candesartan, losartan) and beta blockers (metoprolol, a cardioselective beta blocker; carvedilol, a nonspecific beta blocker). The loop diuretics (furosemide) are used to reduce the symptoms of heart failure secondary to fluid overload, and the aldosterone inhibitors (spironolactone, eplerenone) are added as the heart failure progresses. Only after these drugs are used is digoxin added. Hydralazine/isosorbide dinitrate became the first drug approved for use in the African-American population. Nesiritide is used in special situations in intensive care.
- Be aware of the important physiologic concepts such as ejection fraction. A patient's ejection fraction reflects the contractility of the heart and is about 65% (0.65) in a normal heart. This value decreases as heart failure progresses; therefore, patients with heart failure have low ejection fractions because their hearts are failing to pump effectively.
- Recognize that hypotension, dysrhythmias, and thrombocytopenia are major adverse effects of milrinone.
- Keep informed of the contraindications to the use of digoxin, which include a history of allergy to the digitalis medications, ventricular tachycardia and fibrillations, and AV block.

## NCLEX® EXAMINATION REVIEW QUESTIONS

1  When teaching the patient about the signs and symptoms of cardiac glycoside toxicity, the nurse should alert the patient to watch for
   a  visual changes such as photophobia.
   b  flickering lights or halos around lights.
   c  dizziness when standing up.
   d  increased urine output.

2  During assessment of a patient who is receiving digoxin, the nurse monitors for findings that would indicate an increased possibility of toxicity, such as:
   a  apical pulse rate of 62 beats/min.
   b  digoxin level of 1.5 ng/mL.
   c  serum potassium level of 2.0 mEq/L.
   d  serum calcium level of 9.9 mEq/L.

3  When monitoring a patient who is receiving an intravenous infusion of nesiritide (Natrecor), the nurse will look for which adverse effect?
   a  Dysrhythmia
   b  Proteinuria
   c  Hyperglycemia
   d  Hypertension

4  A patient is taking a beta blocker as part of the treatment plan for heart failure. The nurse knows that the purpose of the beta blocker for this patient is to
   a  increase urine output.
   b  prevent stimulation of the heart by catecholamines.
   c  increase the contractility of the heart muscle.
   d  cause peripheral vasodilation.

5  The nurse is assessing a patient who is receiving a milrinone infusion and checks the patient's cardiac rhythm on the heart monitor. What adverse cardiac effect is most likely to occur in a patient who is receiving intravenous milrinone?
   a  Tachycardia
   b  Bradycardia
   c  Atrial fibrillation
   d  Ventricular dysrhythmia

6  The nurse is administering an intravenous infusion of a phosphodiesterase inhibitor to a patient who has heart failure. The nurse will evaluate the patient for which therapeutic effects? (Select all that apply.)
   a  Positive inotropic effects
   b  Vasodilation
   c  Decreased heart rate
   d  Increased blood pressure
   e  Positive chronotropic effects

7  The medication order for a 5-year-old child reads: "Give digoxin elixir, 15 mcg/kg, PO now." The child weighs 20 kg. How many milligrams will this child receive?

1. b, 2. c, 3. a, 4. b, 5. d, 6. a, b, e, 7. 0.3 mg

For Critical Thinking and Prioritization Questions, see http://evolve.elsevier.com/Lilley.

# Antidysrhythmic Drugs

## evolve WEBSITE

*http://evolve.elsevier.com/Lilley*

- Animations
- Answer Key—Textbook Case Studies
- Critical Thinking and Prioritization Questions

- Key Points—Downloadable
- Review Questions for the NCLEX® Examination
- Unfolding Case Studies

## OBJECTIVES

When you reach the end of this chapter, you will be able to do the following:

1 Describe the anatomy and physiology of the heart as well as cardiac electrophysiology, including normal conduction patterns, rate, and rhythm.
2 Briefly discuss the various disorders of cardiac electrophysiology and consequences to the patient.
3 Define the terms *dysrhythmia* and *arrhythmia*.
4 Identify the various causes of abnormal heart rhythms and their impact on the patient's health and activities of daily living.
5 Identify the most commonly encountered dysrhythmias.
6 Compare the various dysrhythmias with regard to their basic characteristics, impact on the structures of the heart, and related symptoms.

7 Contrast the various classes of antidysrhythmic drugs, citing prototypes in each class and describing their mechanisms of action, indications, routes of administration, dosing, any related drug protocols, adverse effects, cautions, contraindications, drug interactions, and any toxic reactions.
8 Develop a nursing care plan that includes all phases of the nursing process for patients receiving each class of antidysrhythmic drug.

## DRUG PROFILES

adenosine, p. 413
◆ amiodarone, p. 411
◆ atenolol, p. 410
◆ diltiazem, p. 412
◆ dofetilide, p. 412
esmolol, p. 410
flecainide, p. 409
ibutilide, p. 411
◆ lidocaine, p. 409

◆ metoprolol, p. 410
procainamide, p. 406
propafenone, p. 409
◆ quinidine, p. 408
◆ sotalol, p. 412
◆ verapamil, p. 413

———————

◆ *Key drug*

## KEY TERMS

**Action potential** Electrical activity that consists of a series of polarizations and depolarizations that travel across the cell membrane of a nerve fiber during transmission of a nerve impulse and across the cell membranes of a muscle cell during contraction. (p. 398)

**Action potential duration** The interval beginning with baseline (resting) membrane potential followed by depolarization and ending with repolarization to baseline membrane potential. (p. 399)

**Arrhythmia** Technically "no rhythm," meaning absence of heart rhythm (i.e., no heartbeat at all). More commonly used in clinical practice to refer to any variation from the normal rhythm of the heart. A synonymous term is *dysrhythmia*, which is the primary term used in this chapter and book. (p. 397)

**Cardiac Arrhythmia Suppression Trial (CAST)** The name of the major research study conducted by the National Heart, Lung, and Blood Institute to investigate the possibility of eliminating sudden cardiac death in patients with asymptomatic ectopy after a myocardial infarction. (p. 409)

**Depolarization** The movement of positive and negative ions on either side of a cell membrane across the membrane in a direction that brings the net charge to zero. (p. 398)

**Dysrhythmia** Any disturbance or abnormality in heart rhythm. (p. 397)

**Effective refractory period** The period after the firing of an impulse during which a cell may respond to a stimulus but the response will not be passed along or continued as another impulse. (p. 399)

**Internodal pathways (Bachmann bundle)** Special pathways in the atria that carry electrical impulses generated by the sinoatrial node. These impulses cause the heart to beat. (p. 400)

**Relative refractory period** The time after generation of an action potential during which a nerve fiber will show a (reduced) response only to a strong stimulus. (p. 399)

**Resting membrane potential (RMP)** The voltage that exists when the cell membranes of heart muscle (or other muscle or nerve cells) are at rest. (p. 397)

**Sodium-potassium adenosine triphosphatase (ATPase) pump** A mechanism for transporting sodium and potassium ions across the cell membrane against an opposing concentration gradient. Energy for this transport is obtained from the hydrolysis of adenosine triphosphate (ATP) by means of the enzyme ATPase. (p. 397)

**Sudden cardiac death** Unexpected, fatal cardiac arrest. (p. 410)

**Threshold potential** The critical state of electrical tension required for spontaneous depolarization of a cell membrane. (p. 400)

**Torsades de pointes** A rare ventricular arrhythmia that is associated with long QT interval and can degenerate into ventricular fibrillation and sudden death without medical intervention; often simply referred to as *torsades*. (p. 403)

**Vaughan Williams classification** The system most commonly used to classify antidysrhythmic drugs. (p. 403)

## ANATOMY, PHYSIOLOGY, AND PATHOPHYSIOLOGY OVERVIEW

### DYSRHYTHMIAS AND NORMAL CARDIAC ELECTROPHYSIOLOGY

A dysrhythmia is any deviation from the normal rhythm of the heart. The term arrhythmia (literally "no rhythm") implies asystole, or no heartbeat at all. Thus, the more accurate term for an irregular heart rhythm is *dysrhythmia*. However, *arrhythmia* is commonly used in clinical practice. Dysrhythmias can develop in association with many conditions, such as after a myocardial infarction (MI), cardiac surgery, or as the result of coronary artery disease. Dysrhythmias are usually serious and may require treatment with an antidysrhythmic drug or nonpharmacologic therapies; however, not all dysrhythmias require medical treatment. A cardiologist is usually consulted to make the judgment.

Disturbances in cardiac rhythm are the result of abnormally functioning cardiac cells. Thus, an understanding of the mechanism responsible for dysrhythmias first requires review of the electrical properties of these cells. Figure 24-1 on p. 384 shows the overall anatomy of the conduction system of the heart. Figure 25-1 illustrates some of the properties of this system from the standpoint of a single cardiac cell. Inside a resting cardiac cell, a net negative charge exists relative to the outside of the cell. This difference in the electronegative charge exists in all types of cardiac cells and is referred to as the resting membrane potential (RMP). The RMP results from an uneven distribution of ions (e.g., sodium, potassium, and calcium) across the cell membrane. This is known as *polarization*. Each ion moves through its own specific channel, which is a specialized protein molecule that sits across the cell membrane. These proteins work continuously to restore the specific intracellular and extracellular concentrations of each ion. At RMP, the ionic concentration gradient (distribution) is such that potassium ions are more highly concentrated intracellularly, whereas sodium and calcium ions are more highly concentrated extracellularly. For this reason, potassium is generally thought of as an intracellular ion, whereas sodium and calcium are generally thought of as extracellular ions. Negatively charged intracellular and extracellular ions such as chloride ($Cl^-$) and bicarbonate ($HCO_3^-$) also contribute to this uneven distribution of ions, which is known as a *polarized* state. This polarized distribution of ions is maintained by the sodium-potassium adenosine triphosphatase (ATPase) pump, an energy-requiring ionic pump. The energy that drives this pump comes from molecules of adenosine triphosphate (ATP), which are a major source of energy in cellular metabolism.

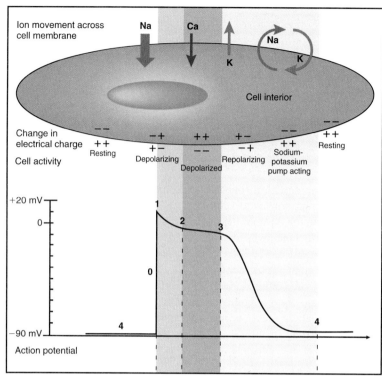

**FIGURE 25-1** Phases of the action potential of a cardiac cell. In resting phase (4), the cell membrane is polarized. The cell's interior has a net negative charge, and the membrane is more permeable to potassium ions (K) than to sodium ions (Na). When the cell is stimulated and begins to depolarize (0), sodium ions enter the cell, potassium leaves the cell, calcium (Ca) channels open, and sodium channels close. In its depolarized phase (1), the cell's interior has a net positive charge. In the plateau phase (2), calcium and other positive ions enter the cell and potassium permeability declines, which lengthens the action potential. Then (3), calcium channels close and sodium is pulled from the cell by the sodium-potassium pump. The cell's interior then returns to its polarized, negatively charged state (4). (From Monahan FD: *Phipps' medical-surgical nursing: health and illness perspectives,* ed 8, St Louis, 2007, Mosby.)

Cardiac cells become excited when there is a change in the baseline distribution of ions across their membranes (RMP) that leads to the propagation of an electrical impulse. This change is known as an action potential. Action potentials occur in a continuous and regular manner in the cells of the cardiac conduction system, such as the sinoatrial node (SA), atrioventricular node (AV), and His-Purkinje system. All of these tissues have the property of spontaneous electrical excitability known as *automaticity*. This excited state creates action potentials, which in turn generate electrical impulses that travel through the myocardium ultimately to create the heartbeat via contraction of cardiac muscle fibers.

An action potential has five phases. Phase 0 is also called the *upstroke* because it appears as an upward line on the graph of an action potential, as shown in Figure 25-2, *A* and *B*. Both of these figures graphically illustrate the cycle of electrical changes that create an action potential. Note the variation in the shape of the curve depending on the relative conduction speed of the specific tissue involved (SA node versus Purkinje fiber). A faster rate of conduction corresponds to a steeper slope on the graph.

During phase 0, the resting cardiac cell membrane suddenly becomes highly permeable to sodium ions, which rush from the outside of the cell membrane to the inside (influx) through what are known as *fast channels* or *sodium channels*. This disruption of the earlier polarized state of the membrane is known as depolarization. Depolarization can be thought of as a temporary equalization of positive and negative charges across the cell membrane. This releases electrochemical energy that drives the resulting electrical impulses through adjacent cells. Phase 1 of the action potential begins a rapid process of repolarization that continues through phases 2 and 3 to phase 4, which is the RMP. In phase 1, the sodium channels close and the concentrations of each ion begin to move back toward their ion-specific RMP levels. During phase 2, calcium influx occurs through the slow channels or calcium channels. They are called *slow channels* because the calcium influx occurs relatively more slowly than the earlier sodium influx. Potassium ions then flow from inside of the cell to outside (efflux) through specific potassium channels. This is done to offset the elevated positive charge caused by the influx of sodium and calcium ions. In the case of the Purkinje fibers, this causes a partial plateau (flattening on the graph) during which the overall membrane potential changes only slightly, as seen in Figure 25-2, *B*. In phase 3, the ionic flow patterns of phases 0 to 2 are changed by the sodium-potassium ATPase pump (or, more simply, the *sodium pump*). This reestablishes the baseline polarized state by restoring both intracellular and extracellular concentrations of sodium, potassium, and calcium (see Figure 25-1). As a result, the cell membrane is ultimately repolarized to its baseline level or RMP (phase 4). Note that this entire process occurs over roughly 400 milliseconds—that is, four hundred thousandths (less than one half) of one second.

There is some variation in this time period between different parts of the conduction system. As an example, Figure 25-3 illustrates the pattern of movement of sodium, potassium, and calcium ions into and out of a Purkinje cell during the four phases of the action potential. Note that there are several differences in the action potentials of SA nodal cells and Purkinje cells. The level of the RMP for a given type of cell is an important determinant of the rate of its impulse conduction to other cells. The less negative (i.e., the closer to zero) the RMP at the onset of phase 0 of the action potential, the slower the upstroke velocity of phase 0. The slope of phase 0 is directly related to the impulse velocity. An upstroke with a steeper slope indicates faster conduction velocity. Thus, in Purkinje cells, electrical conduction is relatively fast, and therefore electrical impulses are conducted quickly. These cells are referred to as *fast-response cells*, or *fast-channel cells*. Purkinje fibers can therefore be thought of as fast-channel tissue. Many antidysrhythmic drugs affect the RMP and sodium channels, which in turn influences the rate of impulse conduction.

In contrast to Purkinje fibers, the cells of the SA node have a slower upstroke velocity, or a slower phase 0. This is illustrated in Figure 25-2, *A*, as an upstroke curve that is less steep, which indicates a relatively slower rate of electrical conduction in these cells.

AV nodal cells are comparable to SA nodal cells in this regard. This slower upstroke in the SA and AV nodes is primarily dependent on the entry of calcium ions through the slow channels or calcium channels. This means that nodal action potentials are affected by calcium influx as early as phase 0. The nodes are therefore called *slow-channel tissue*, and conduction is slower than that in other parts of the conduction system. Drugs that affect calcium ion movement into or out of these cells (e.g., calcium channel blockers) tend to have significant effects on the SA and AV nodal conduction rates.

The interval between phase 0 and phase 4 is called the action potential duration (Figure 25-4). The period between phase 0 and midway through phase 3 is called the absolute or effective refractory period. During the effective refractory period, the cardiac cell cannot be restimulated to depolarize and generate another action potential. During the remainder of phase 3 and until the return to the RMP (phase 4), the cardiac cell *can* be depolarized again if it receives a powerful enough impulse (such as one induced by drug therapy or supplied by an electrical pacemaker). This period is referred to as the relative refractory

FIGURE 25-2 Action potentials. *RMP*, Resting membrane potential; *SA*, sinoatrial; *TP*, threshold potential.

FIGURE 25-3 Purkinje fiber action potential.

period. Figure 25-4 illustrates these various aspects of an action potential. Again, the actual shape of the action potential curve varies in different parts of the conduction system.

The RMP of certain cardiac cells gradually decreases (becomes less negative) over time in ongoing cycles. This is due to small changes in the flux of sodium and potassium ions. Depolarization eventually occurs when a certain critical voltage is reached (threshold potential). This process of spontaneous depolarization is referred to as *automaticity*, or *pacemaker activity*. It is normal when it occurs in the SA node (see Figure 24-1 on p. 384). When spontaneous depolarizations occur elsewhere, however, dysrhythmias often result.

The SA node, the AV node, and His-Purkinje cells all possess the property of automaticity. The SA node is the natural pacemaker of the heart because it spontaneously depolarizes the most frequently. The SA node has an intrinsic rate of 60 to 100 depolarizations or beats per minute; that of the AV node is 40 to 60 beats per minute; and that of the ventricular Purkinje fibers is 40 or fewer beats per minute. The action potentials and other properties in different areas of the heart are compared in Table 25-1.

As the pacemaker of the heart, the SA node, which is located near the top of the right atrium, generates the electrical impulse that ultimately produces the heartbeat. First, however, this impulse travels through the atria via specialized pathways called the internodal pathways (Bachmann bundle). This causes the atrial myocardial fibers to contract, which creates the first heart sound. Next, the impulse reaches the AV node, which is located near the bottom of the right atrium. The AV node slows this very fast moving electrical impulse just long enough to allow the ventricles to fill with blood. If the AV node did not slow the impulse in this way, ventricular contraction would overlap that of the atria, which would result in a smaller volume of ejected ventricular blood and reduced cardiac output.

Next, the AV nodal cells generate an electrical impulse that passes into the bundle of His (or His bundle). The bundle of His is a band of cardiac muscle fibers located between the right and left ventricles in what is called the *ventricular septum* (wall between the ventricles). The bundle of His distributes the impulse into both ventricles via the right and left bundle branches. Each branch terminates in the Purkinje fibers that are located in the myocardium of the ventricles. Stimulation of the Purkinje fibers causes ventricular contraction and ejection of blood from the ventricles. Blood from the right ventricle is pumped into the pulmonary circulation, whereas blood from the left ventricle is pumped into the systemic circulation to supply the rest of the body. The bundle of His and Purkinje fibers are so named for the medical scientists who first identified them. Together, they are often referred to in the literature as the *His-Purkinje system*. Any abnormality in cardiac automaticity or impulse conduction often results in some type of dysrhythmia.

## Electrocardiography

The electrophysiologic cardiac events described thus far in this chapter correspond more simply to the tracings of an electrocardiogram, abbreviated as ECG or EKG (Figure 25-5). The P wave corresponds to spontaneous impulse generation in the SA node followed immediately by depolarization of atrial myocardial fibers and their muscular contraction. This normally determines the heart rate. It is affected by the balance between sympathetic and parasympathetic nervous system tone, the intrinsic automaticity of the SA nodal tissue, the mechanical stretch of atrial fibers due to incoming blood volume, and cardiac drugs. The QRS complex (or QRS interval) corresponds to depolarization and contraction of ventricular fibers. The J point marks the start of the ST segment, which corresponds to the beginning of ventricular repolarization. The T wave corresponds to completion of the repolarization of these ventricular fibers. As an analogy, depolarization can be thought of as discharge or contraction of cardiac muscle fibers, whereas repolarization can be thought of as a relaxation of muscle fibers to prepare for the next contraction (heartbeat). Note that the repolarization of the atrial fibers is obscured on the ECG tracing by the QRS complex and thus has no corresponding deflection in the tracing. The U wave is

**FIGURE 25-4** Aspects of an action potential. *APD,* Action potential duration; *ERP,* effective refractory period; *RRP,* relative refractory period.

| TABLE 25-1 | COMPARISON OF ACTION POTENTIALS IN DIFFERENT CARDIAC TISSUE | | | | |
|---|---|---|---|---|---|
| TISSUE | ACTION POTENTIAL | SPEED OF RESPONSE | THRESHOLD POTENTIAL (mV) | CONDUCTION VELOCITY (m/sec) |
| SA node | | Slow | 260 | Less than 0.05 |
| Atrium | | Fast | 290 | 1 |
| AV node | | Slow | 260 | Less than 0.05 |
| His-Purkinje system | | Fast | 295 | 3 |
| Ventricle | | Fast | 290 | 1 |

*AV,* Atrioventricular; *SA,* sinoatrial.

not always present, and its physiologic basis is uncertain. When the U wave occurs, it is generally correlated with electrophysiologic events such as repolarization of Purkinje fibers. These events may be a source of dysrhythmias caused by a triggered automaticity. Prominent U waves are often associated with sinus bradycardia, hypokalemia, use of quinidine and other class Ia antidysrhythmics, and hyperthyroidism. Abnormal U waves (inverted) are associated with serious conditions such as MI, acute angina, coronary artery spasms, and ischemic heart disease. The PR and QT intervals and the ST segment are parts of the ECG tracing that are often altered by disease or by the adverse effects of certain types of drug therapy or drug interactions, as discussed in later sections of this chapter.

## Common Dysrhythmias

A variety of cardiac dysrhythmias are recognized. Some are easier to treat than others using drug therapy and/or interventional cardiology procedures such as pacemaker implantation, catheter ablation, cardioversion, and implantation of cardioverters-defibrillators. Dysrhythmias are subdivided into several broad categories depending on their anatomic site of origin in the heart. Supraventricular dysrhythmias originate above the ventricles in the SA or AV node or atrial myocardium. Ventricular dysrhythmias originate below the AV node in the His-Purkinje system or ventricular myocardium. Dysrhythmias that originate outside the conduction system (i.e., in atrial or ventricular cells) are known as *ectopic,* and their specific points of origin are called *ectopic foci* (*foci* is the plural of the Latin-derived word *focus*). Conduction blocks are dysrhythmias that involve disruption of impulse conduction between the atria and ventricles through the AV node, directly affecting ventricular function. They may also originate in the His-Purkinje system. Less commonly, impulse conduction between the SA and AV node is affected. Several of the most common dysrhythmias are described in Table 25-2, and corresponding ECG tracings are provided. They are also described further in the following text.

Among the supraventricular dysrhythmias, atrial fibrillation is a very common condition. It is characterized by rapid atrial contractions that incompletely pump blood into the

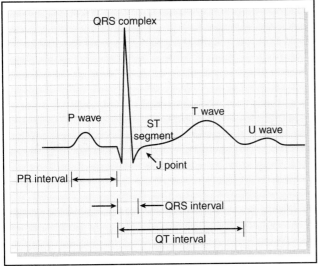

**FIGURE 25-5** The waves and intervals of a normal electrocardiogram. (From Goldberger AL: *Clinical electrocardiography: a simplified approach,* ed 7, St Louis, 2006, Mosby.)

| TABLE 25-2 | **COMMON DYSRHYTHMIAS** |
|---|---|
| **DYSRHYTHMIA** | **DESCRIPTION AND ECG TRACING** |
| Atrial flutter (AF) | Often progresses to atrial fibrillation (F = flutter waves) |
| Atrial fibrillation (AF) | Rapid, ineffective atrial contractions (f = fibrillation waves) |
| Paroxysmal supraventricular tachycardia (PSVT) | Heart rate of 180-200 beats/min or higher |

*Continued*

## TABLE 25-2 COMMON DYSRHYTHMIAS—cont'd

| DYSRHYTHMIA | DESCRIPTION AND ECG TRACING |
| --- | --- |

**Premature ventricular contractions (PVCs)**

Contractions generated by impulses arising from ectopic foci within ventricular myocardium

**Nonsustained ventricular tachycardia (NSVT)**

Relatively brief period (20 sec or less) in which ventricles contract rapidly on their own as well as in response to AV impulses

**Sustained ventricular tachycardia (SVT)**

Same as above but more prolonged

**Torsades de pointes (TdP)**

Rapid ventricular tachycardia preceded by QT interval prolongation (often progresses to ventricular fibrillation)

**Ventricular fibrillation (VF)**

Rapid, ineffective ventricular contractions (fatal if not reversed)

*ECG,* Electrocardiogram.

ventricles. Atrial fibrillation is notable in that it predisposes the patient to stroke. This is due to the fact that the blood tends to stagnate in the incompletely emptied atria and is therefore more likely to clot. If such blood clots manage to make their way into the left ventricle, they may be embolized to the brain and cause a stroke. Although there is a theoretically similar risk for pulmonary embolism, this seems to be of less clinical concern with atrial fibrillation than the risk for stroke. Patients with ongoing atrial fibrillation are often given anticoagulant therapy with warfarin (see Chapter 26) to reduce the likelihood of stroke.

AV nodal reentrant tachycardia (AVNRT) is a conduction disorder that often gives rise to a dysrhythmia known as *paroxysmal supraventricular tachycardia (PSVT)*. (The word *paroxysmal* means "sudden.") AVNRT occurs when electrical impulse transmission from the AV node into the His-Purkinje system of the ventricles is disrupted. As a result, some of the impulses circle backward (retrograde impulses) and reenter the atrial tissues to produce a tachycardic response. In Wolff-Parkinson-White syndrome, ectopic impulses that begin near the AV node actually bypass the AV node and reach the His-Purkinje system before the normal AV-generated impulses. This is one cause of ventricular tachycardia, although it is technically supraventricular in origin.

Varying degrees of AV block (often called *heart block*) involve different levels of disrupted conduction of impulses from the AV node and His-Purkinje system to the ventricles. Although first-degree AV block is often asymptomatic, third-degree block, or complete heart block, often requires use of a cardiac pacemaker to ensure adequate ventricular function. There can also be blocks within the His-Purkinje system of the ventricles, known as *bundle branch blocks*.

Premature ventricular contractions (PVCs) occur when impulses originate from ectopic foci within the ventricles (His-Purkinje system). PVCs probably occur periodically in many people; they become problematic when they occur frequently enough to compromise systolic blood volume. *Ventricular tachycardia* refers to a rapid heartbeat from impulses originating in the ventricles. It can be nonsustained (brief) or sustained, requiring definitive treatment. Worsening ventricular tachycardia can deteriorate into torsades de pointes, an intermediate dysrhythmia that often deteriorates into ventricular fibrillation. Ventricular fibrillation is fatal if not reversed, which most often requires electrical defibrillation. Interestingly, torsades de pointes often responds preferentially to intravenous magnesium sulfate.

## PHARMACOLOGY OVERVIEW

## ANTIDYSRHYTHMIC DRUGS

Numerous drugs are available to treat dysrhythmias. These drugs are categorized according to where and how they affect cardiac cells. Although other classifications are described in the literature, the most commonly used system for this purpose is still the Vaughan Williams classification. This system is based on the electrophysiologic effect of particular drugs on the action potential. This approach identifies four major classes of drugs: I (including Ia, Ib, and Ic), II, III, and IV. The various drugs in these four classes are listed in Table 25-3.

There is currently a gradual trend away from the use of class Ia drugs. The formerly available class Ic drug encainide was removed from the market after research indicated that the risk of fatal cardiac dysrhythmias associated with this drug overshadowed its dysrhythmia suppression effects. Class III drugs have emerged as among the most widely used antidysrhythmics at this time. The class IV drugs (calcium channel blockers) have limited usefulness in treating tachydysrhythmias (dysrhythmias involving tachycardia), unlike most of the other classes. The role of class II drugs (beta blockers) continues to grow in the field of cardiology, including in dysrhythmia management. Digoxin, the cardiac glycoside discussed in Chapter 24, still has a place in dysrhythmia management, especially in the prevention of dangerous ventricular tachydysrhythmias secondary to atrial fibrillation.

## Mechanism of Action and Drug Effects

Antidysrhythmic drugs work by correcting abnormal cardiac electrophysiologic function. They do this to varying degrees and by various mechanisms. Class I drugs are membrane-stabilizing drugs and exert their actions on the sodium (fast) channels. There are some slight differences in the actions of the drugs in this class, so they are divided into three subclasses. These subclasses are class Ia, Ib, and Ic drugs. The subclasses are based on the magnitude of the effects each drug has on phase 0, the action potential duration, and the effective refractory period. Class Ia drugs (quinidine, procainamide, and disopyramide) block the sodium channels; more specifically, they delay repolarization and increase the action potential duration. Class Ib drugs (phenytoin, lidocaine) also block the sodium

| TABLE 25-3 | VAUGHAN WILLIAMS CLASSIFICATION OF ANTIDYSRHYTHMIC DRUGS | |
|---|---|
| **FUNCTIONAL CLASS** | **DRUGS** |
| Class I: membrane-stabilizing drugs; fast sodium channel blockers | |
| Ia: ↑ blockade of sodium channel, delay repolarization, ↑ action potential duration | Quinidine, disopyramide, procainamide |
| Ib: ↑ blockade of sodium channel, accelerate repolarization, ± action potential duration | Lidocaine, phenytoin |
| Ic: ↑↑↑ blockade of sodium channel, ± repolarization; also suppress reentry | Flecainide, propafenone |
| Class II: beta-blocking drugs | All beta blockers |
| Class III: drugs whose principal effect on cardiac tissue is to ↑ action potential duration | Amiodarone, dronedarone, sotalol,* ibutilide, dofetilide |
| Class IV: calcium channel blockers | Verapamil, diltiazem |
| Other: antidysrhythmic drugs that have the properties of several classes and therefore cannot be placed in one particular class | Digoxin, adenosine |

↑, Increase; ±, increase or decrease.
*Sotalol also has class II properties.

channels, but unlike class Ia drugs, they accelerate repolarization and decrease the action potential duration. Phenytoin is more commonly used as an anticonvulsant (see Chapter 14) than as an antidysrhythmic drug. Class Ic drugs (flecainide, propafenone) have a more pronounced effect on the blockade of sodium channels but have little effect on repolarization or the action potential duration.

Class II drugs are the beta-adrenergic blockers (beta blockers; see Chapter 19), and they are commonly used as antihypertensives (see Chapter 22) and antianginal drugs (see Chapter 23). They work by blocking sympathetic nervous system stimulation to the heart and, as a result, the transmission of impulses in the heart's conduction system. This results in depression of phase 4 depolarization. These drugs mostly affect slower-conducting cardiac tissues.

Class III drugs (amiodarone, dronedarone, sotalol, ibutilide, and dofetilide) increase the action potential duration by prolonging repolarization in phase 3. They affect fast tissue and are most commonly used to manage dysrhythmias that are difficult to treat. They are usually reserved for patients for whom other therapies have failed. Sotalol actually has properties of both class II and class III drugs, and it may be listed as a member of either one or the other class, depending on the specific reference used.

Class IV drugs are the calcium channel blockers, which, like beta blockers, are also used as both antihypertensives (see Chapter 22) and antianginal drugs (see Chapter 23). As their name implies, they work specifically by inhibiting the calcium channels, which reduces the influx of calcium ions during action potentials. This results in depression of phase 4 depolarization. Diltiazem and verapamil are the calcium channel blockers most commonly used to treat cardiac dysrhythmias.

The mechanisms of action of the major classes of antidysrhythmics are summarized in Table 25-4. The effects of the various classes of antidysrhythmic drugs are presented in Box 25-1.

## Indications

Antidysrhythmic drugs are effective in treating a variety of cardiac dysrhythmias. The antidysrhythmic drugs and the most common indications for their use are listed in Table 25-5.

## Contraindications

As with all drugs, contraindications to the use of antidysrhythmic drugs include known drug allergy to a specific product. Other contraindications may include second- or third-degree AV block, bundle branch block, cardiogenic shock, sick sinus syndrome, and any other ECG changes depending on the clinical judgment of a cardiologist. The concurrent use of certain drugs that interact with antidysrhythmics is also considered. The reason for these concerns is that antidysrhythmic drugs can potentially worsen existing dysrhythmias (also termed *dysrhythmogenic*). The risk is greater in patients with structural heart damage (e.g., after MI). In patients with AV block and bundle branch block, there is a danger of drug-induced ventricular failure if a drug further compromises the

---

**BOX 25-1   EFFECTS OF ANTIDYSRHYTHMIC DRUGS**

**Class Ia (Disopyramide, Procainamide, Quinidine)**
- Depress myocardial excitability
- Prolong the effective refractory period
- Eliminate or reduce ectopic foci stimulation
- Decrease inotropic effect
- Have anticholinergic (vagolytic) activity

**Class Ib (Lidocaine, Phenytoin)**
- Decrease myocardial excitability in the ventricles
- Eliminate or reduce ectopic foci stimulation in the ventricles
- Have minimal effect on the SA node and automaticity
- Have minimal effect on the AV node and conduction
- Have minimal anticholinergic (vagolytic) activity

**Class Ic (Flecainide, Propafenone)**
- Produce dose-related depression of cardiac conduction, especially in the bundle of His–Purkinje system
- Have minimal effect on atrial conduction
- Eliminate or reduce ectopic foci stimulation in the ventricles
- Have minimal anticholinergic (vagolytic) activity
- Flecainide use now reserved for the most serious dysrhythmias

**Class II (Beta Blockers [e.g., Atenolol, Esmolol, Metoprolol])**
- Block beta-adrenergic cardiac stimulation
- Reduce SA nodal activity
- Eliminate or reduce atrial ectopic foci stimulation
- Reduce ventricular contraction rate
- Reduce cardiac output and blood pressure

**Class III (Amiodarone, Dronedarone, Sotalol,\* Ibutilide, Dofetilide)**
- Prolong the effective refractory period
- Prolong the myocardial action potential
- Block both alpha- and beta-adrenergic cardiac stimulation

**Class IV (Diltiazem, Verapamil)**
- Prolong AV nodal effective refractory period
- Reduce AV nodal conduction
- Reduce rapid ventricular conduction caused by atrial flutter

*AV,* Atrioventricular; *SA,* sinoatrial.
\*Sotalol also has class II properties.

---

**TABLE 25-4   ANTIDYSRHYTHMIC DRUGS: MECHANISMS OF ACTION**

| | **VAUGHAN WILLIAMS CLASS** | | | |
|---|---|---|---|---|
| | I | II | III | IV |
| Action | Blocks sodium channels, affects phase 0 | Decreases spontaneous depolarization, affects phase 4 | Prolongs action potential duration | Blocks slow calcium channels |
| Tissue | Fast | Slow | Fast | Slow |
| Effect on action potential | | | | |

## TABLE 25-5   ANTIDYSRHYTHMIC DRUGS: INDICATIONS

| DRUG CLASS | INDICATIONS |
|---|---|
| **Class Ia**<br>disopyramide<br>procainamide<br>quinidine | Atrial fibrillation, premature atrial contractions, premature ventricular contractions, ventricular tachycardia, Wolff-Parkinson-White syndrome |
| **Class Ib**<br>lidocaine | Ventricular dysrhythmias only (premature ventricular contractions, ventricular tachycardia, ventricular fibrillation) |
| phenytoin | Atrial and ventricular tachydysrhythmias caused by digitalis toxicity; long QT syndrome |
| **Class Ic**<br>flecainide<br>propafenone | Ventricular tachycardia and supraventricular tachycardia dysrhythmias, atrial fibrillation and flutter, Wolff-Parkinson-White syndrome |
| **Class II**<br>***Beta Blockers***<br>atenolol<br>esmolol<br>metoprolol | Both supraventricular and ventricular dysrhythmias (act as general myocardial depressants) |
| **Class III**<br>amiodarone<br>dronedarone<br>dofetilide<br>ibutilide<br>sotalol* | Life-threatening ventricular tachycardia or fibrillation<br>Atrial fibrillation or flutter resistant to other drug therapy |
| **Class IV**<br>***Calcium Channel Blockers***<br>diltiazem<br>verapamil | Paroxysmal supraventricular tachycardia; rate control for atrial fibrillation and flutter |

*Sotalol also has class II properties.

## TABLE 25-6   ANTIDYSRHYTHMIC DRUGS: COMMON ADVERSE EFFECTS

| CLASS | DRUG | ADVERSE EFFECTS |
|---|---|---|
| Ia | procainamide | Hypotension, rash, diarrhea, nausea, vomiting, agranulocytosis, SLE-like syndrome |
| | quinidine | Hypotension, QT prolongation, lightheadedness, diarrhea, bitter taste, anorexia, blurred vision, tinnitus, angina |
| Ib | lidocaine | Bradycardia, dysrhythmia, hypotension, anxiety, metallic taste |
| | phenytoin | Hypotension, bradycardia, thrombophlebitis, hypertrichosis, gingival hyperplasia |
| Ic | flecainide | Dizziness, visual disturbances, dyspnea, palpitations, nausea, vomiting, diarrhea, weakness |
| | propafenone | Prodysrhythmic effect, angina, tachycardia, syncope, AV block, dizziness, fatigue, dyspnea |
| II | Beta blockers | Bradycardia, hypotension, dizziness, fatigue, AV block, heart failure, hyperglycemia, hypoglycemia, bronchospasm, wheezing, dry mouth, impotence |
| III | amiodarone | Pulmonary toxicity, thyroid disorders, bradycardia, hypotension, SA node dysfunction, AV block, ataxia, QT prolongation, torsades de pointes, vomiting, constipation, photosensitivity, abnormal liver function test results, jaundice, visual disturbances, hyperglycemia or hypoglycemia, dermatologic reactions including rash, toxic epidermal necrolysis, vasculitis, blue-gray coloring of the skin (face, arms, neck) |
| | dofetilide | Headache, insomnia, ventricular tachycardia, chest pain, torsades de pointes, rash, back pain, nausea, diarrhea |
| | ibutilide | Nonsustained ventricular tachycardia, ventricular extrasystoles, tachycardia, hypotension, AV block, headache, nausea |
| | sotalol* | Bradycardia, chest pain, palpitations, fatigue, dizziness, lightheadedness, weakness, dyspnea |
| IV | Calcium channel blockers | Constipation, bradycardia, heart block, hypotension, dizziness, dyspnea |

*AV,* Atrioventricular; *SA,* sinoatrial; *SLE,* systemic lupus erythematosus.
*Sotalol also has class II properties.

already existing AV conduction delays. The safe prescribing of antidysrhythmic drugs is an area that requires especially strong clinical expertise and careful judgment on a case-by-case basis.

## Adverse Effects

Adverse effects common to most antidysrhythmics include hypersensitivity reactions, nausea, vomiting, and diarrhea. Other common effects include dizziness, headache, and blurred vision. In addition, many antidysrhythmics are themselves capable of producing new dysrhythmias (prodysrhythmic effect). Prolongation of the QT interval is a potentially severe adverse effect shared by many antidysrhythmics. The concern with QT prolongation is the potential for induction of torsades de pointes. As with any drug class, there are also cases of unpredictable or idiosyncratic (see Chapter 2) adverse effects that are not related to drug concentration in the body. Idiosyncratic reactions are unpredictable; however, it is thought that such effects will eventually be explained by genetic variations. Table 25-6 summarizes the most commonly reported adverse effects by specific drug.

### Toxicity and Management of Overdose

The main toxic effects of the antidysrhythmics involve the heart, circulation, and central nervous system (CNS). Specific antidotes are not available, and the management of an overdose involves maintaining adequate circulation and respiration

### TABLE 25-7 SELECTED ANTIDYSRHYTHMIC DRUGS: MANAGEMENT OF OVERDOSE

| DRUG | TOXIC EFFECT | MANAGEMENT |
|---|---|---|
| acebutolol | Bradycardia | Atropine 1-3 mg IV divided |
| | Bronchospasm | Beta$_2$-adrenergic or theophylline |
| | Cardiac failure | Digitalization |
| | Hypotension | Vasopressor |
| adenosine | Usually self-limiting due to a very short half-life | Competitive antagonists caffeine or theophylline |
| amiodarone | Bradycardia | Beta-adrenergic drug |
| | Hypotension | Positive inotropic drug or vasopressor |
| digoxin | Bradycardia | See Chapter 24 for more information |
| disopyramide | Loss of consciousness; cardiac and respiratory arrest | Neostigmine for anticholinergic effects, emesis induction, activated charcoal, and hemodialysis |
| esmolol | Same as for acebutolol | Same as for acebutolol |
| flecainide | Reduced heart rate | Dopamine or dobutamine; acidification of very alkaline urine |
| lidocaine | Convulsions | Diazepam or thiopental |
| moricizine | Hypotension, heart failure, myocardial infarction | Gastric evacuation and advanced life support measures |
| phenytoin | Circulatory and respiratory arrest, convulsions | Life support measures when required |
| procainamide | Cardiac depression | IV pressor drugs and supportive measures |
| | Convulsions | Diazepam and mechanically assisted respiration |
| propafenone | Same as for acebutolol | Same as for acebutolol |
| quinidine | Same as for acebutolol | Same as for acebutolol |
| sotalol* | Convulsions | Diazepam or short-acting barbiturate |
| verapamil | Cardiac failure | Dopamine or dobutamine |
| | Conduction problems | Cardiac pacing |
| | Hypotension | Vasopressors, 10% calcium chloride solution |

*IV,* Intravenous.
*Sotalol also has class II properties.

using general support measures and providing any required symptomatic treatment (Table 25-7).

## Interactions

Antidysrhythmics can interact with many different categories of drugs. The most serious drug interactions are those that can result in dysrhythmias, hypotension or hypertension, respiratory distress, or excessive therapeutic or toxic drug effects. Drug interactions occur when the presence of one drug strengthens or weakens the pharmacologic effects of another. This is most commonly seen when the first drug affects the activity of the enzymes that metabolize the second drug, either speeding or slowing its elimination. One particular interaction common to many antidysrhythmics is the potentiation of anticoagulant activity with warfarin (Coumadin) (see Chapter 26). Because many patients receiving antidysrhythmic therapy also need warfarin, the international normalized ratio (INR) must be closely monitored and necessary adjustments made to the warfarin dosage. This is especially true with amiodarone. The INR will increase by 50% in almost 100% of patients receiving amiodarone and warfarin. Grapefruit juice can also inhibit the metabolism of several antidysrhythmics such as amiodarone, disopyramide, and quinidine. Other common interactions are summarized in Table 25-8. To explain the mechanism for each interaction is beyond the scope of this text. Readers needing more detailed information are encouraged to consult other appropriate references.

## Dosages

For dosage information on selected antidysrhythmic drugs, see the table on p. 407.

## DRUG PROFILES

The four classes of antidysrhythmics produce a variety of effects on the action potential of the cardiac cell and exert a major influence on cardiac electrophysiologic function. The diversity of therapeutic effects and adverse effects pose a special challenge to ensuring the safe and efficacious use of these drugs. Because the aspects of the nursing process that relate to the administration of these drugs differ for each of the four classes of drug, each group is discussed separately.

### CLASS Ia DRUGS

Class Ia drugs are considered membrane-stabilizing drugs because they possess local anesthetic properties. They stabilize the membrane and have depressant effects on phase 0 of the action potential. These drugs include procainamide, quinidine, and disopyramide.

#### procainamide

The electrophysiologic effect of procainamide (Pronestyl) is similar to that of quinidine. Procainamide is useful in the management of atrial and ventricular tachydysrhythmias, although it is not used frequently. Procainamide is chemically related to the local anesthetic procaine. Significant adverse effects include ventricular dysrhythmias and blood disorders. It can cause a

## TABLE 25-8 SELECTED ANTIDYSRHYTHMIC DRUGS: COMMON DRUG INTERACTIONS

| DRUG (CLASS) | INTERACTING DRUGS | EFFECTS* |
|---|---|---|
| quinidine (Ia) | Amiodarone, dronedarone, amitriptyline, erythromycin, haloperidol, sotalol, moxifloxacin | Additive QT prolongation |
| | Digoxin | Increase in digoxin levels by 50% |
| | HMG-CoA reductase inhibitors (statins) | Increased statin levels and toxicity |
| lidocaine (Ib) | Amiodarone, azole antifungals, beta blockers, erythromycin, verapamil, cimetidine, tolvaptan | Increased serum levels of lidocaine |
| propafenone (Ic) | Cimetidine, quinidine, conivaptan, pimozide | Increased propafenone levels; use is contraindicated |
| | Digoxin, warfarin, beta blockers | Increase in level of interacting drugs |
| | Class Ia and III antidysrhythmics, erythromycin | Prolonged QT interval |
| amiodarone (III) | Azole antifungals, clarithromycin, erythromycin, haloperidol, moxifloxacin, quinidine, procainamide | Prolonged QT interval |
| | Digoxin, diltiazem, verapamil, beta blockers | AV block |
| | Warfarin, digoxin | Increase in INR by 50% in almost 100% of patients, increase in digoxin levels by 50% |
| | Cyclosporine | Increased cyclosporine levels and toxicity |
| | HMG-CoA reductase inhibitors (statins) | Increased statin levels and toxicity |
| dofetilide (III) | Cimetidine, verapamil, hydrochlorothiazide (HCTZ), ketoconazole, trimethoprim | Increased dofetilide concentrations—use is contraindicated |
| | Bepridil, clarithromycin, erythromycin, tricyclic antidepressants, phenothiazines, moxifloxacin | Prolonged QT interval |
| sotalol (III)† | Calcium channel blockers | Additive effects on AV conduction, bradycardia |
| | Class I antidysrhythmics, erythromycin, bepridil, moxifloxacin, amiodarone | Prolonged QT interval, bradycardia |
| verapamil, diltiazem (IV) | Amiodarone, beta blockers, flecainide, digoxin | Bradycardia, decreased cardiac output, hypotension |
| | Azole antifungals, clarithromycin, erythromycin, isoniazid, HIV drugs | Increased verapamil effects |
| | HMG-CoA reductase inhibitors (statins) | Increased statin levels and toxicity |

*AV,* Atrioventricular; *HIV,* human immunodeficiency virus; *HMG-CoA,* hydroxymethylglutaryl–coenzyme A; *INR,* international normalized ratio.
*Note that enhanced activity of any antidysrhythmic drug may reach the level of drug toxicity, including potentially fatal cardiac dysrhythmias.
†Sotalol also has class II properties.

## DOSAGES

### *Selected Antidysrhythmic Drugs*

| DRUG NAME (PREGNANCY CATEGORY) | PHARMACOLOGIC CLASS | USUAL DOSAGE RANGE |
|---|---|---|
| **Class I** | | |
| quinidine (Quinidex [sulfate], Quinaglute, Dura-Tab [gluconate]) (C) | Class Ia antidysrhythmic | **Adult**<br>Gluconate<br>PO: 324-648 mg q8-12h<br>IM: 600 mg followed by 400 mg q2-6h or more if needed<br>IV: 200-750 mg infused at up to 10 mg/min<br>Sulfate<br>PO: 200-mg load; 100-600 mg q4-6h |
| ◆ lidocaine (Xylocaine) (B) | Class Ib antidysrhythmic | **Pediatric**<br>IV: bolus dose, 1 mg/kg; usual maintenance infusion rate, 20-50 mcg/kg/min<br>**Adult**<br>IV: Bolus dose 50-100 mg; may be repeated in 5 min; do not exceed 200-300 mg over 1 hr; usual maintenance infusion rate 1-4 mg/min |
| propafenone (Rythmol) (C) | Class Ic antidysrhythmic | **Adult**<br>PO: Start with 150 mg q8h and increase q3-4d; usual range, 450-900 mg/day divided |
| **Class II**<br>metoprolol (Lopressor) (D) | Beta₁ blocker (class II antidysrhythmic) | **Adult**<br>IV/PO: 3 bolus injections of 5 mg at 2-min intervals followed by 50 mg PO q6h for 48 hr, thereafter 50-100 mg bid<br>PO: 50-100 mg bid |

*Continued*

## DOSAGES—cont'd

### Selected Antidysrhythmic Drugs

| DRUG NAME (PREGNANCY CATEGORY) | PHARMACOLOGIC CLASS | USUAL DOSAGE RANGE |
|---|---|---|
| **Class III** | | |
| ◆ amiodarone (Cordarone) (D) | Class III antidysrhythmic | **Adult**<br>IV: 150 mg over 10 min, then 60 mg/hr for 6 hr, then 30 mg/hr as maintenance dose<br>PO: 800-1600 mg/day for 1-3 wk, reduced to 400-800 mg/day for 5 wk; usual maintenance dose 200-400 mg/day |
| ◆ dofetilide (Tikosyn) (C) | Class III antidysrhythmic | **Adult**<br>PO: 125-500 mg bid (note dose is individualized) |
| ibutilide (Corvert) (C) | Class III antidysrhythmic | **Adult**<br>IV: 1-mg infusion over 10 min (if less than 60 kg, then 0.1 mL/kg) |
| ◆ sotalol* (Betapace) (B) | Class III antidysrhythmic | **Adult**<br>PO: 160-320 mg/day divided into 2-3 doses |
| **Class IV** | | |
| ◆ diltiazem (Cardizem) | Calcium channel blocker (class IV antidysrhythmic) | **Adult**<br>IV: Bolus dose 0.25 mg/kg over 2 min, second dose 0.35 mg/kg over 2 min after 15 min as needed, then 5-10 mg/hr by continuous infusion<br>Oral: 120-360 mg daily |
| ◆ verapamil (Calan, Isoptin, Verelan) (C) | Calcium channel blocker (class IV antidysrhythmic) | **Pediatric**<br>IV: 1-15 yr: 0.1-0.3 mg/kg bolus over 2 min; do not exceed 5-mg dose; repeat dose not exceeding 10 mg may be given after 30 min<br>**Adult**<br>PO: Start with 80 mg tid-qid; daily range 240-480 mg<br>IV: 2.5-5 mg bolus over 2 min; repeat dose of 5-10 mg may be given after 30 min |
| **Unclassified** | | |
| adenosine (Adenocard) (C) | Unclassified antidysrhythmic | **Adult**<br>IV: 6-mg bolus over 1-2 sec; second rapid bolus of 12 mg as needed, which may be repeated a second time as needed |

*IM,* Intramuscular; *IV,* intravenous; *PO,* oral.
*Sotalol also has Class II properties.

systemic lupus erythematosus–like syndrome, which occurs in about 30% of patients on long-term therapy. It can also cause gastrointestinal effects such as nausea, vomiting, and diarrhea. Other adverse effects include fever, leukopenia, maculopapular rash, flushing, and torsades de pointes resulting from prolongation of the QT interval. Box 25-2 lists selected drugs known to prolong the QT interval. Use of procainamide is contraindicated in patients with a known hypersensitivity to it and in those with heart block and systemic lupus erythematosus. It is available in both oral and injectable forms.

### Pharmacokinetics

| Route | Onset of Action | Peak Plasma Concentration | Elimination Half-life | Duration of Action |
|---|---|---|---|---|
| IV/IM | 10-30 min | 10-60 min | 3 hr | 3 hr |
| PO | 0.5-1 hr | 1-2 hr | 3 hr | 3-8 hr |

### quinidine

Quinidine (Quinidex) has both a direct action on the electrical activity of the heart and an indirect (anticholinergic)

effect. Significant adverse effects of the drug include cardiac asystole and ventricular ectopic beats. Quinidine can cause cinchonism. Symptoms of mild cinchonism include tinnitus, loss of hearing, slight blurring of vision, and gastrointestinal upset. Contraindications to the use of the drug include hypersensitivity, thrombocytopenic purpura resulting from previous therapy, AV block, intraventricular conduction defects, and torsades de pointes. Quinidine is available in both oral and parenteral (injectable) forms and in three different salt forms. The oral preparations include sulfate and gluconate salts.

### Pharmacokinetics

| Route | Onset of Action | Peak Plasma Concentration | Elimination Half-life | Duration of Action |
|---|---|---|---|---|
| PO | 1-3 hr | 0.5-6 hr | 6-7 hr | 6-12 hr |

### CLASS Ib DRUGS

Class Ib drugs share many characteristics with class Ia drugs but act preferentially on ischemic myocardial tissue. They have little effect on conduction velocity in normal tissue. Class Ib drugs have a weak depressive effect on phase 0 depolarization, the action potential duration, and the effective refractory period. They include lidocaine and phenytoin.

### ◆ lidocaine

Lidocaine (Xylocaine) is the prototypical Ib drug. It is one of the most effective drugs for the treatment of ventricular dysrhythmias, but it can only be administered intravenously because it has an extensive first-pass effect (i.e., when it is taken orally, the liver metabolizes most of it to inactive metabolites). Because of its extensive hepatic metabolism, dosage reduction by 50% is recommended for patients with liver failure or cirrhosis. Dosage reductions may also be necessary in patients with renal impairment because of extensive excretion of the drug and its metabolites by the kidney.

Lidocaine exerts its effects on the conduction system of the heart by making it difficult for the ventricles to develop a dysrhythmia. This action is known as *raising the ventricular fibrillation threshold*. It occurs by decreasing the sensitivity of the cardiac cell membrane to impulses and decreasing the cell's ability to depolarize on its own (decreasing automaticity). Many of these effects are accomplished by blocking the fast sodium channels.

Significant adverse effects include CNS toxic effects such as twitching, convulsions, and confusion; respiratory depression or arrest; and the cardiovascular effects of hypotension, bradycardia, and dysrhythmias. Use of the drug is contraindicated in patients who are hypersensitive to it, who have severe SA or AV intraventricular block, or who have Stokes-Adams or Wolff-Parkinson-White syndrome. Lidocaine is available only in parenteral form for intramuscular or intravenous administration. Lidocaine is commonly used as a local anesthetic

(see Chapter 11); a transdermal form is also available for analgesia (see Chapter 10).

### Pharmacokinetics

| Route | Onset of Action | Peak Plasma Concentration | Elimination Half-life | Duration of Action |
|-------|-----------------|---------------------------|-----------------------|--------------------|
| IV | 2-15 min | 5-10 min | 8 min | 20 min–1.5 hr |

### CLASS Ic DRUGS

Class Ic drugs (flecainide, propafenone) produce a more pronounced blockade of the sodium channel than class Ia and Ib drugs but have little effect on repolarization or the action potential duration. These drugs significantly slow conduction in the atria, AV node, and ventricles. Because of their marked effect on conduction, class Ic drugs strongly suppress PVCs, reducing or eliminating them in a large number of patients.

### flecainide

Flecainide (Tambocor) is a chemical analogue of procainamide. Historically, clinicians have been hesitant to prescribe flecainide because of the findings of a large multicenter study called the Cardiac Arrhythmia Suppression Trial (CAST). This study showed that mortality and nonfatal cardiac arrest rates in patients treated with flecainide were actually comparable to or higher than those seen in patients who received the placebo. Because of these findings, the U.S. Food and Drug Administration (FDA) required that the labeling of flecainide be revised to indicate that its use is to be limited to the treatment of documented life-threatening ventricular dysrhythmias. However, since the findings of the CAST were initially published in 1992, there have been numerous studies showing that flecainide is safe and effective for the treatment of atrial fibrillation. In fact, according to the most current practice guidelines, flecainide is considered a first-line drug in the treatment of atrial fibrillation.

Flecainide is better tolerated than quinidine or procainamide. It has a negative inotropic effect and depresses left ventricular function. Less serious but more common noncardiac adverse effects include dizziness, visual disturbances, and dyspnea. Contraindications to its use include hypersensitivity, cardiogenic shock, second- or third-degree AV block, and non–life-threatening dysrhythmias. Flecainide is available only for oral use.

### Pharmacokinetics

| Route | Onset of Action | Peak Plasma Concentration | Elimination Half-life | Duration of Action |
|-------|-----------------|---------------------------|-----------------------|--------------------|
| PO | 3 hr | 1.5-3 hr | 11-12 hr | 12-27 hr |

### propafenone

Propafenone (Rythmol) is similar in action to flecainide. It reduces the fast inward sodium current in Purkinje fibers and to a lesser extent in myocardial fibers. Unlike other class I drugs, propafenone has mild beta-blocking effects. This may contribute to its overall effects on the conduction system. It is also believed to have calcium channel–blocking effects, which may contribute to its mild negative inotropic effects.

Until recently, propafenone's use was limited to the treatment of documented life-threatening ventricular dysrhythmias, as was flecainide. Recent findings suggest that it has benefit in the treatment of atrial fibrillation as well. Treatment is started while the patient is in the hospital. Unlike flecainide, however, propafenone can be given to patients with depressed left ventricular function and may be a better drug than disopyramide, procainamide, and quinidine in these patients. Propafenone must be used with caution in patients with heart failure, because it has some beta-blocking properties and dose-dependent negative inotropic effects.

Propafenone is generally well tolerated. The most commonly reported adverse reaction is dizziness. Patients may also complain of a metallic taste, constipation, and headache, along with nausea and vomiting. These gastrointestinal adverse effects may be reduced by taking propafenone with food. Propafenone use is contraindicated in patients with a known hypersensitivity to it and in those with bradycardia, bronchial asthma, significant hypotension, uncontrolled heart failure, cardiogenic shock, and various conduction disorders. It is available only for oral use.

### Pharmacokinetics

| Route | Onset of Action | Peak Plasma Concentration | Elimination Half-life | Duration of Action |
|---|---|---|---|---|
| PO | 2 hr | 3-5 hr | 2-10 hr | Unknown |

## CLASS II DRUGS

Class II antidysrhythmics are also known as *beta blockers* (see Chapter 19). They work by blocking sympathetic nervous system stimulation to the heart and the heart's conduction system. By doing this, beta blockers prevent catecholamine-mediated actions on the heart. This is known as a *cardioprotective* quality of beta blockers. The resulting cardiovascular effects include a reduced heart rate, delayed AV node conduction, reduced myocardial contractility, and decreased myocardial automaticity. The pharmacologic effects of the beta blockers are especially beneficial after an MI. Following an MI, many catecholamines are released that make the heart hyperirritable and predisposed to many types of dysrhythmias. Beta blockers offer protection from these potentially very dangerous complications. Several studies have demonstrated a significant reduction (on the average of 25%) in the incidence of sudden cardiac death after MI in patients treated with beta blockers on an ongoing basis.

Although there are several beta blockers, only a few are commonly used as antidysrhythmics. Those currently approved by the FDA for this purpose are acebutolol, esmolol, propranolol, and sotalol (which has both class II and class III properties). Selected drugs are described here. The class II drugs are classified as pregnancy category C drugs, excepting acebutolol, pindolol, and sotalol, which are all category B drugs.

### ◆ atenolol

Atenolol (Tenormin) is a cardioselective beta blocker, which means that it preferentially blocks the beta₁-adrenergic receptors that are located primarily in the heart. Noncardioselective beta blockers block not only the beta₁-adrenergic receptors in the heart but also the beta₂-adrenergic receptors in the lungs and therefore can exacerbate preexisting asthma or chronic obstructive pulmonary disease. In addition to having class II antidysrhythmic properties, atenolol is useful in the treatment of hypertension and angina. Its use is contraindicated in patients with severe bradycardia, second- or third-degree heart block, heart failure, cardiogenic shock, or a known hypersensitivity to it. This drug is available in oral form.

### Pharmacokinetics

| Route | Onset of Action | Peak Plasma Concentration | Elimination Half-life | Duration of Action |
|---|---|---|---|---|
| PO | 1 hr | 2-4 hr | 6-7 hr | 24 hr |

### esmolol

Esmolol (Brevibloc) is an ultra-short-acting beta blocker with pharmacologic and electrophysiologic effects on the heart's conduction system similar to those of atenolol. Esmolol is also a cardioselective beta blocker that preferentially blocks the beta₁-adrenergic receptors in the heart. It is used in the acute treatment of supraventricular tachydysrhythmias or dysrhythmias that originate above the ventricles. It is also used to control hypertension and tachydysrhythmias that develop after an acute MI. Use of esmolol is contraindicated in patients with a known hypersensitivity to it or those with severe bradycardia, second- or third-degree heart block, heart failure, cardiogenic shock, or severe asthma. It is available only in injectable form and is most commonly used in anesthesia.

### Pharmacokinetics

| Route | Onset of Action | Peak Plasma Concentration | Elimination Half-life | Duration of Action |
|---|---|---|---|---|
| IV | Immediate | 6 min | 9 min | 15-20 min |

### ◆ metoprolol

Metoprolol (Lopressor) is another cardioselective beta blocker commonly given after an MI to reduce the risk of sudden cardiac death. It is also used in the treatment of hypertension and angina. The contraindications to metoprolol use are the same as those for the use of atenolol and esmolol. It is available in both oral and injectable forms.

### Pharmacokinetics

| Route | Onset of Action | Peak Plasma Concentration | Elimination Half-life | Duration of Action |
|---|---|---|---|---|
| IV | 1 min | 20 min | 3-8 hr | 5-8 hr |
| PO | 1 hr | 2-4 hr | 3-8 hr | 10-20 hr |

## CLASS III DRUGS

Class III drugs consist of amiodarone, dronedarone, sotalol (which also has class II properties), ibutilide, and dofetilide. Amiodarone controls dysrhythmias by inhibiting repolarization and markedly prolonging refractoriness and the action potential duration. Ibutilide and dofetilide are both indicated for conversion of atrial fibrillation or flutter to a normal sinus rhythm. Amiodarone is indicated for the management of life-threatening ventricular tachycardia or ventricular fibrillation that is resistant to other drug therapy. This drug has also been very effective in the treatment of sustained ventricular tachycardias. Amiodarone has recently been used more frequently to treat atrial dysrhythmias as well.

Dronedarone (Multaq) is the newest antidysrhythmic drug. It is very similar to amiodarone and is thought to have less potential for causing the classic amiodarone adverse effects and less potential for drug interactions. However, as with any newly marketed drug, the true incidence of toxicity is not known until it is used in numerous patients. In 2011, the FDA issued an advisory regarding the potential for hepatotoxicity related to dronedarone. Later that year, they also issued a safety communication regarding an increased risk of death and serious cardiovascular events associated with its use.

### ◆ amiodarone

Amiodarone (Cordarone, Pacerone) markedly prolongs the action potential duration and the effective refractory period in all cardiac tissues. Besides exerting these dramatic effects, it is also known to block both the alpha- and beta-adrenergic receptors of the sympathetic nervous system. Clinically it is one of the most effective antidysrhythmic drugs for controlling supraventricular and ventricular dysrhythmias. It is indicated for the management of sustained ventricular tachycardia, ventricular fibrillation, and nonsustained ventricular tachycardia. It is reported to be effective in 40% to 60% of all patients with ventricular tachycardia. It is the drug of choice for ventricular dysrhythmias according to the Advanced Cardiac Life Support guidelines. Recently it has shown promise in the management of atrial dysrhythmias that are difficult to treat with other less toxic drugs.

Amiodarone has many unwanted adverse effects, and these can be attributed to its chemical properties. Amiodarone is very *lipophilic*, or fat loving. Therefore, it can penetrate and concentrate in the adipose tissue of any organ in the body. It also has iodine in its chemical structure. One organ that sequesters iodine from the diet is the thyroid gland. As a result, amiodarone can cause either hypothyroidism or hyperthyroidism. The package insert for amiodarone lists iodine allergy as a contraindication. However, evidence for avoiding amiodarone in patients with iodine hypersensitivity is extremely limited and does not appear to support its contraindication in patients with severe dysrhythmias.

Adverse reactions occur in approximately 75% of patients treated with this drug, but the incidence is higher and the severity greater with higher dosages (those exceeding 400 mg/day) and prolonged therapy. One of the most common adverse effects is corneal microdeposits, which may cause visual halos, photophobia, and dry eyes. This occurs in virtually all adults who take the drug for longer than 6 months. Photosensitivity is also very common, reported in 10% to 75% of patients taking amiodarone.

The most serious adverse effect is pulmonary toxicity, which is fatal in about 10% of patients and involves a clinical syndrome of progressive dyspnea and cough accompanied by damage to the alveoli. The result can be pulmonary fibrosis. Another serious complication of amiodarone therapy is that it not only may treat the dysrhythmias but also may provoke them.

Amiodarone has an exceptionally long half-life, approaching many days. As a result, the therapeutic as well as any adverse effects of amiodarone may linger long after the drug has been discontinued. In fact, it may take as long as 2 to 3 months after the drug has been stopped for some adverse effects to subside. Therapy is usually started in the hospital and is closely monitored until the patient's serum levels are within a therapeutic range.

Amiodarone has two very significant drug interactions, namely with digoxin and warfarin. It is reported that digoxin levels will increase by 50% and that the INR will increase by 50% in 100% of patients taking these drugs in combination with amiodarone. When amiodarone is started in patients who are already taking one of these drugs, the dose of digoxin or warfarin is recommended to be reduced by 50% at the start of amiodarone therapy.

Use of amiodarone is contraindicated in patients who have a known hypersensitivity to it and in those with severe sinus bradycardia or second- or third-degree heart block. For cases in which the patient is maintained on long-term oral amiodarone therapy after intravenous amiodarone administration is discontinued, recommended conversions are available (Table 25-9). This drug is marketed in both oral and injectable forms.

### Pharmacokinetics

| Route | Onset of Action | Peak Plasma Concentration | Elimination Half-life | Duration of Action |
|---|---|---|---|---|
| PO | 1-3 wk | 2-10 hr | 15-100 days | 10-150 days |

### ibutilide

Ibutilide (Corvert) is a class III antidysrhythmic drug. Unlike the other two class III antidysrhythmics, ibutilide is indicated for atrial dysrhythmias. Atrial fibrillation and atrial flutter cause irregular contractions of the heart and can lead to serious conditions such as decreased cardiac output, heart failure, low blood pressure, and stroke. Although other pharmacologic

| TABLE 25-9 | RECOMMENDATIONS FOR ORAL DOSAGE AFTER INTRAVENOUS INFUSION OF AMIODARONE | |
|---|---|
| **DURATION OF AMIODARONE IV INFUSION** | **INITIAL DAILY DOSE OF ORAL AMIODARONE** |
| Less than 1 wk | 800-1600 mg |
| 1-3 wk | 600-800 mg |
| More than 3 wk | 400 mg |

*IV,* Intravenous.

therapies are used to treat atrial fibrillation and flutter, ibutilide and dofetilide are the only drugs available for rapid conversion of these two conditions to normal sinus rhythm. The only other treatment that can produce rapid conversion is electrical cardioversion. Although it is effective, electrical cardioversion carries the risk, expense, and inconvenience of both the procedure itself and the anesthesia it requires.

Ibutilide is dosed based on patient weight. Use of ibutilide is contraindicated in patients who have previously demonstrated hypersensitivity to it. As with other antidysrhythmic drugs, ibutilide is to be used with caution, because it can itself produce dysrhythmias, most significantly ventricular tachycardia and torsades de pointes. Class Ia antidysrhythmic drugs (e.g., disopyramide, quinidine, and procainamide) and other class III drugs (e.g., amiodarone and sotalol) should not be administered with ibutilide, nor should they be given within 4 hours after infusion of ibutilide because of their potential to prolong refractoriness. Ibutilide is available only in injectable form.

### Pharmacokinetics

| Route | Onset of Action | Peak Plasma Concentration | Elimination Half-life | Duration of Action |
|---|---|---|---|---|
| IV | 10 min | 30 min | 6 hr | 4 hr |

#### ♦ dofetilide

Dofetilide (Tikosyn) is one of the newer antidysrhythmic drugs. Because dofetilide can cause serious toxicity, specifically torsades de pointes, only physicians who have received special training are allowed to prescribe it. Dofetilide therapy must be initiated in the hospital, and the patient must have continuous ECG monitoring for the first 3 days. Any dosage adjustment or re-initiation of therapy also requires hospitalization.

Dofetilide is contraindicated in patients with hypersensitivity to it, as well as patients with congenital or acquired long QT intervals or in whom the QT interval is longer than 440 msec. It is also contraindicated in patients with severe renal impairment and in those taking the following drugs: verapamil, cimetidine, hydrochlorothiazide, trimethoprim, itraconazole, ketoconazole, prochlorperazine, and megestrol. Other drugs that can prolong the QT interval must be used with great caution during dofetilide therapy. Dofetilide is also contraindicated in patients with hypokalemia and/or hypomagnesemia, because these two states predispose patients to toxicity.

The most common adverse effects are torsades de pointes, supraventricular dysrhythmias, headache, dizziness, and chest pain.

### Pharmacokinetics

| Route | Onset of Action | Peak Plasma Concentration | Elimination Half-life | Duration of Action |
|---|---|---|---|---|
| PO | 1 hr | 2-3 hr | 10 hr | 12 hr |

#### ♦ sotalol

Sotalol (Betapace) is a selective beta blocker that is used to treat dysrhythmias. It is unique in that it possesses antidysrhythmic

properties similar to those of the class III drugs (such as amiodarone) while simultaneously exerting beta blocker or class II effects on the conduction system of the heart. In addition, sotalol has prodysrhythmic properties similar to those of the class Ic drugs. This means that while patients are taking sotalol, it can cause serious dysrhythmias such as torsades de pointes or a new ventricular tachycardia or fibrillation. Like flecainide and propafenone, sotalol was historically reserved for the treatment of documented life-threatening ventricular dysrhythmias such as sustained ventricular tachycardia. However, recent data indicates it to be safe.

Contraindications to sotalol use include hypersensitivity to it, bronchial asthma, cardiogenic shock, and sinus bradycardia. Sotalol is available only in oral form.

### Pharmacokinetics

| Route | Onset of Action | Peak Plasma Concentration | Elimination Half-life | Duration of Action |
|---|---|---|---|---|
| PO | 1-2 hr | 2.5-4 hr | 12 hr | 8-16 hr |

### CLASS IV DRUGS

Class IV antidysrhythmic drugs are calcium channel blockers. Although more than nine such drugs are currently available, only a few are commonly used as antidysrhythmics. Besides being effective antidysrhythmics, calcium channel blockers are useful in the treatment of hypertension (see Chapter 22) and angina (see Chapter 23). Verapamil and diltiazem are the two calcium channel blockers most commonly used for the following:

- Treating dysrhythmias, specifically those that arise above the ventricles (PSVT)
- Controlling the ventricular response to atrial fibrillation and flutter by slowing conduction and prolonging refractoriness of the AV node (i.e., preventing the ventricles from beating as fast as the atria)

These drugs block the slow inward flow of calcium ions into the slow (calcium) channels in cardiac conduction tissue. The conduction effects of these drugs are limited to the atria and the AV node, where conduction is prolonged and the tissues are made more refractory to stimulation. These drugs have little effect on the ventricular tissues.

#### ♦ diltiazem

Diltiazem (Cardizem, others) is primarily indicated for the temporary control of a rapid ventricular response in patients with atrial fibrillation or flutter and PSVT. Its use is contraindicated in patients with hypersensitivity, acute MI, pulmonary congestion, Wolff-Parkinson-White syndrome, severe hypotension, cardiogenic shock, sick sinus syndrome, or second- or third-degree AV block. Diltiazem is available in both oral and parenteral forms.

### Pharmacokinetics

| Route | Onset of Action | Peak Plasma Concentration | Elimination Half-life | Duration of Action |
|---|---|---|---|---|
| PO | 0.5-1 hr | 2-3 hr | 3.5-9 hr | 4-12 hr |

## ◆ verapamil

Verapamil (Calan, others) has actions similar to those of diltiazem in that it also inhibits calcium ion influx across the slow calcium channels in cardiac conduction tissue. This results in dramatic effects on the AV node. Verapamil is used to prevent and convert recurrent PSVT and to control ventricular response in atrial flutter or fibrillation. It can also temporarily control a rapid ventricular response to these frequent atrial stimulations, usually decreasing the heart rate by at least 20%. Verapamil is not only used for the management of various dysrhythmias but is also used to treat angina, hypertension, and hypertrophic cardiomyopathy. The contraindications that apply to diltiazem apply to verapamil as well. It is also available in both oral and parenteral forms.

### Pharmacokinetics

| Route | Onset of Action | Peak Plasma Concentration | Elimination Half-life | Duration of Action |
|---|---|---|---|---|
| PO | 1-2 hr | 3 hr | 4.5-12 hr | 6-8 hr |

## UNCLASSIFIED ANTIDYSRHYTHMIC

### adenosine

Adenosine (Adenocard) is an unclassified antidysrhythmic drug. It slows the electrical conduction time through the AV node and is indicated for the conversion of PSVT to sinus rhythm. It is particularly useful when the PSVT has failed to respond to verapamil or when the patient has coexisting conditions such as heart failure, hypotension, or left ventricular dysfunction that limit the use of verapamil. Its use is contraindicated in patients with second- or third-degree heart block, sick sinus syndrome, atrial flutter or fibrillation, or ventricular tachycardia, as well as in those with a known hypersensitivity to it. It has an extremely short half-life of less than 10 seconds. For this reason, it is administered only intravenously and only as a fast intravenous push. It commonly causes asystole for a period of seconds. All other adverse effects are minimal because of its very short duration of action. Adenosine is available only in parenteral form.

### Pharmacokinetics

| Route | Onset of Action | Peak Plasma Concentration | Elimination Half-life | Duration of Action |
|---|---|---|---|---|
| IV | Immediate | Immediate | Less than 10 sec | Very brief |

## NURSING PROCESS

## ASSESSMENT

Before administering any *antidysrhythmic* to a patient, conduct a thorough nursing assessment and head-to-toe physical assessment, and complete a medical history and medication profile. Assess for contraindications, cautions, and drug interactions. Review any baseline ECGs and interpret the results, and measure the patient's vital signs with attention to blood pressure, postural blood pressure, heart sounds, and heart rate, rhythm, and quality. Other signs and symptoms to assess for related to decreased cardiac functioning (as a result of a dysrhythmia and decrease in cardiac output) include apical-radial pulse deficits, jugular vein distension, edema, prolonged capillary refill (longer than 5 seconds), decreased urinary output, activity intolerance, chest pain or pressure, dyspnea, and fatigue. Document any changes in level of alertness, increase in anxiety levels, syncope, or dizziness.

Laboratory studies generally include renal and hepatic function tests because abnormal functioning may call for a decrease in the drug dosage by the prescriber to prevent toxicity. Be sure to emphasize to the patient the interaction with grapefruit juice, which inhibits metabolism by cytochrome P-450 3A4 hepatic enzymes (see Chapter 2 for a more in-depth discussion of this topic). The interaction of grapefruit juice with *amiodarone, disopyramide,* and *quinidine* leads to an increased risk of toxicity and cinchonism (see Table 25-8). Other drug interactions with antidysrhythmics are presented in Table 25-8.

With the use of *lidocaine,* assess the cardiovascular system, with attention to heart rate and blood pressure. With amiodarone, assess respiratory, thyroid, hepatic, dermatologic, and/or hypertensive conditions due to possible drug related pulmonary toxicity, exacerbation of thyroid disorders, abnormal liver function tests, and rash. Further assessment for drug interactions (see Table 25-8) as well as contraindications and cautions is also needed.

---

### TEAMWORK AND COLLABORATION: PHARMACOKINETIC BRIDGE TO NURSING PRACTICE

A study of long-term oral amiodarone therapy for the treatment of dysrhythmias provides a different perspective on pharmacokinetics. To aid in evaluating the complex pharmacokinetic properties of amiodarone and developing an optimal dosing schedule for the drug in long-term oral drug therapy, serum concentrations of the drug and its metabolite, desethylamiodarone, were monitored in 345 Japanese patients receiving amiodarone. Serum concentrations of the drug and its metabolite were determined by an analysis called *chromatography.* In 245 participants who took fixed maintenance dosages of the drug for 6 months, there were small variations in the ratio of the serum level of the actual drug to the serum level of its metabolite. (The concept of metabolism as it relates to pharmacokinetics is discussed in Chapter 2.) Other pharmacokinetic properties of amiodarone included a slightly higher average clearance in women than in men, even though there were no differences between men and women with regard to age, dosage, or duration of action of the dose. Japanese patients showed little variation in the pharmacokinetics of the drug. From this study, one can see how important it is to understand basic pharmacokinetic parameters (e.g., dosing, clearance, drug metabolism, serum concentrations) and to recognize that they are very critical components of drug therapy and the nursing process. It is also important to note that culture, gender, age, and racial or ethnic group have an impact on how each person responds to a drug and how each drug may vary in its action.

*Antidysrhythmic Medications*

A 46-year-old patient, V.T., is admitted to the intensive care unit after going to the hospital with complaints of chest pain. He is diagnosed with coronary artery disease with a partial block of one of his coronary arteries and is awaiting an angioplasty procedure. He has a history of alcoholism but states that he has not had a drink for 2 years, thanks to Alcoholics Anonymous. In the intensive care unit, V.T.'s heart monitor indicates increased episodes of premature ventricular contractions. When a 20-second run of ventricular tachycardia is noted, the nurse decides to implement the standing orders for a lidocaine infusion. The standing order reads: "For episodes of ventricular tachycardia, give a loading dose of 75 mg of lidocaine intravenous (IV) push; repeat this dose in 5 minutes, and then begin a continuous infusion of 2 mg/min IV."

1. What factors will the nurse consider before beginning the lidocaine infusion?

2. What will the nurse monitor while V.T. is receiving this infusion?

Three days later, V.T. is ready for discharge. He has had the angioplasty procedure, which was deemed a success, and the lidocaine infusion was discontinued yesterday. He has been started on oral quinidine, 324 mg, every 6 hours. One month later, he calls the office and tells the nurse that he is hearing a "ringing sound" in his ears, even when the television and radio are turned off.

3. Is this ringing sound significant?

The physician decides to change V.T.'s medication to procainamide. V.T. asks the nurse, "What are the possible side effects of this drug? It seems that they all have bad side effects."

4. What is the nurse's best answer to this question?

For answers, see http://evolve.elsevier.com/Lilley.

## NURSING DIAGNOSES

1. Decreased cardiac output related to the pathology of the dysrhythmia
2. Ineffective peripheral tissue perfusion related to the physiologic impact of the dysrhythmia
3. Deficient knowledge related to lack of experience with medication therapy

## PLANNING

### GOALS

1. Patient experiences improved cardiac output.
2. Patient experiences improved peripheral perfusion/circulation.
3. Patient demonstrates adequate knowledge about the medication therapy.

### OUTCOME CRITERIA

1. Patient's symptoms of dysrhythmia and subsequent decreased cardiac output are decreased and/or alleviated.
2. Patient's peripheral pulses are equal, strong and regular bilaterally with warm, pink extremities.
3. Patient states rationale for taking medication as prescribed as well as its therapeutic effects and adverse effects.

- Patient experiences increase in energy and stamina and improved ability to carry out activities of daily living due to positive therapeutic outcomes from drug therapy.

## IMPLEMENTATION

When *antidysrhythmics* are administered, monitor vital signs, especially pulse rate and blood pressure; if pulse rate is lower than 60 beats/min, notify the prescriber. During the initiation of therapy, closely monitor the electrocardiogram and vital signs because of possible prolongation of the patient's QT interval by more than 50%. The end result may be the occurrence of a variety of conduction disturbances. Advise patients that oral dosage forms are generally better tolerated if taken with food and fluids to help minimize gastrointestinal upset, unless otherwise ordered. *Quinidine* comes in different salt forms, and these are not interchangeable. During treatment with quinidine (or with any of the antidysrhythmics), immediately report any patient complaint of angina, hypotension, lightheadedness, loss of appetite, tinnitus, or diarrhea to the prescriber. It is recommended that an infusion pump be used for intravenous dosing of any of the classes of antidysrhythmics, with proper solution and dilution.

With *lidocaine*, vials of clear solution are labeled as either for cardiac or *not* for cardiac use. This is important to remember when reading the vial's label so that the wrong drug is not given. It is also important to remember that lidocaine solutions need to be used with extreme caution and that it is the plain solution that is used to treat various cardiac conditions. Parenteral solutions of these drugs are usually stable only for 24 hours. Lidocaine is also used as an anesthetic, and so the different concentrations of the drug need to double-checked—if not triple-checked. In addition, lidocaine comes in a solution with epinephrine, a potent vasoconstrictor. This combined solution is indicated when the surgeon or physician is suturing or repairing wounds, with the lidocaine acting as an anesthetic and the epinephrine causing vasoconstriction of the local blood vessels and helping to control bleeding of the area, or in dental or oral situations. The solution with epinephrine must *never* be used intravenously, but only as a topical anesthetic! With lidocaine, document vital signs prior to initiation of and during therapy, and closely monitor the ECG. Often patients are in a cardiac step-down unit, telemetry unit, or intensive care setting when receiving this drug.

*Amiodarone* may lead to gastrointestinal upset, which may be prevented or decreased by taking the drug with food or a snack. Photosensitivity (sunburn and other exaggerated skin reactions to the sunlight) and photophobia (light sensitivity) are other concerns with this drug. With photosensitivity, protective clothing/hat and sunscreen are needed. Emphasize protection of the eyes, with wearing of sunglasses and/or tinted contact lenses, to patients taking this medication. Recommend consumption of a high-fiber diet and forcing of fluids to minimize the constipation that is a common adverse effect of antidysrhythmic drugs. When beta blockers are used with an antidysrhythmic, any shortness of breath, weight gain, changes in baseline blood glucose levels, or excess fatigue (see Chapters 19 and 25) must be reported to the prescriber immediately.

*Beta blockers, diltiazem,* and *verapamil* may all be used to manage abnormal rhythms and are to be given only after checking and documenting pulse rates and blood pressures. Contact the prescriber and withhold the drug—if supported by facility policy and the prescriber's guidelines—if the pulse rate is 60 beats/min or lower or 100 beats/min or higher and/or the systolic blood pressure is 90 mm Hg or lower.

With the use of *dofetilide,* continually monitor the patient for any changes in the ECG, especially over the first few days of treatment. This drug requires specialized monitoring once ordered by the prescriber, who must have received special prescription training. Encourage the patient to report any difficulty such as chest pain, nausea, or diarrhea to the prescriber

immediately. If a dosage amount requires adjustment, hospitalization may be necessary.

## EVALUATION

The monitoring of patients receiving all classes of antidysrhythmics is important to confirm the therapeutic effects as well as identify the adverse and toxic effects. Class I through class IV antidysrhythmics drugs have many overlapping therapeutic effects, adverse effects, and toxicities. Therapeutic effects, in general, include improved cardiac output; decreased chest discomfort; decreased fatigue; improved vital signs, skin color, and urinary output; and conversion of irregularities to normal rhythm. Adverse effects for the *class I antidysrhythmics* include hypotension, rash, diarrhea, SLE-like syndrome

---

### EVIDENCE-BASED PRACTICE

#### A Short-Term, Randomized, Double-Blind, Parallel-Group Study to Evaluate the Efficacy and Safety of Dronedarone Versus Amiodarone in Patients with Persistent Atrial Fibrillation: The DIONYSOS Study

**Review**

Atrial fibrillation (AF) is a major cause of morbidity, increasing the risk of stroke and death and other health concerns. Amiodarone is widely used for the maintenance of sinus rhythm in patients with atrial fibrillation but is associated with adverse effects such as pulmonary toxicity, thyroid disorders, and hepatic toxicity. These adverse effects may lead to discontinuation of this drug and/or cause serious complications in its long-term use. Dronedarone is pharmacologically related to amiodarone but has improved pharmacokinetics resulting in a shorter half-life, less accumulation in tissues, and absence of amiodarone-like organ toxicity. These two drugs were part of a study that compared their efficacy and safety in patients with persistent atrial fibrillation.

**Type of Evidence**

DIONYSOS, or a comparative, randomized, double-blind, parallel-group research study, was conducted in some 112 centers in 23 countries after approval from local independent ethics committees, institutional review boards, and the protocol developed with the Helsinki principles. All patients provided written informed consent before the study was initiated. Outcomes of the study included the following: (1) a measurement of efficacy, recurrence of AF or the premature study drug discontinuation for lack of efficacy; and (2) a safety/tolerability measurement. Once the study was initiated in patients with AF, treatment failure was defined as unsuccessful electrical cardioversion as well as no spontaneous cardioversion and no electrical cardioversion. The primary composite endpoint was the recurrence of AF or premature study discontinuation. The main safety endpoint (MSE) was the occurrence of thyroid, hepatic, pulmonary, neurologic, skin, eye, or gastrointestinal-specific events or prematurely withdrawing from the study after experiencing an adverse event. After exclusion criteria were applied, the final sample size was 504 patients. After a period of up to 30 days of screening, patients were then randomized in a 1:1 ratio to dronedarone or amiodarone for at least 6 months with electrical cardioversion performed between 10 and 28 days if the patient had not converted spontaneously to sinus rhythm. Follow-up occurred at the 6-month endpoint with scheduled assessments within this time frame. Heart rhythms were documented by scheduled or unscheduled 12-lead ECGs, and other parameters being evaluated included vital signs and systolic and diastolic blood pressure readings after resting for 3 minutes and then in the supine position. Laboratory studies assessed included hematology, serum

biochemistry, thyroid function levels, digoxin serum levels, and international normalized ratio (INR) in patients receiving oral anticoagulants.

**Results of Study**

All patients were randomized in this study to receive dronedarone 400 mg twice daily (sample size of 249) or amiodarone 600 mg every day for a period of 28 days then 200 mg every day (sample size of 255) over a total period of 6 months. Mean age was 64 ± 10.7 years, and about 20% of the patients were 75 years of age or older. The majority of patients were Caucasian (83.9%), and 15.3% were Asian. One-third of patients were female. Cardiovascular history included 66.9% with hypertension, 18% with coronary heart disease, and 16.5% with AF. Congestive heart failure was found distributed similarly in about one-third of the patients. The median treatment duration was 7 months and a maximum of 13.8 months in both treatment groups. The primary composite endpoint was 75.1% and 58.8% with dronedarone and amiodarone, respectively, at 12 months treatment. The main safety endpoint was 39.3% and 44.5% in the dronedarone and amiodarone groups, respectively, at 12 months treatment, and mainly driven by fewer thyroid, neurologic, and skin and eye events in the dronedarone group. AF recurrence after successful cardioversion was 36.5% and 24.3% with dronedarone and amiodarone, respectively. Premature drug discontinuation was less frequent with dronedarone.

**Link of Evidence to Nursing Practice**

This study is another example of how research may impact professional nursing practice by showing comparative evidence of efficacy of certain drugs for specific disorders such as AF. It is also studies like this one that look at different medical diagnoses with associated medical care, including pharmacologic advances. Mortality and morbidity issues are also brought forward for discussion within the health care arena, and specifically how certain therapeutic regimens may be helpful or not. Nurses not only gain knowledge about certain pharmacologic or nonpharmacologic measures but can always learn and gain from research findings to enhance nursing care delivery as well as facilitate further nursing research.

Reference: Le Heuzey AL, De Ferrari GM, Radzik D, et al. A short-term, randomized, double-blind, parallel-group study to evaluate the efficacy and safety of dronedarone versus amiodarone in patients with persistent atrial fibrillation: the DIONYSOS study, *J Cardiovasc Electrophysiol* 21(6):597-605, 2010.

(procainamide); ECG changes, bitter taste, anorexia, blurred vision, and tinnitus (quinidine); and gingival hyperplasia and decrease in blood pressure and pulse rate (phenytoin). *Class II beta blockers* may cause bradycardia, AV block, heart failure, bronchospasm, and changes in blood glucose levels.

*Amiodarone,* a class III drug, may lead to pulmonary toxicity, thyroid disorders, decrease in blood pressure and pulse rate, photosensitivity, and abnormal liver function. Calcium channel blockers or class IV drugs are associated with heart block, hypotension, constipation, dizziness, and dyspnea (see Table 25-6).

## ▮ PATIENT TEACHING TIPS

- Instruct patients not to crush or chew any oral dosage form that is identified as sustained-release, and not to alter the original dosage form of the drug in any way.
- Some dosage forms are delivered in a sustained-released tablet or capsule that may be composed of a wax matrix, and this matrix may be visible in the patient's stool. This extended-release dosage form provides for a slow release of the medicine, and the wax substance may then be passed out of the body through the stool. Advise patients that the passing of the matrix through the stool occurs after the drug has been absorbed, and although the matrix is often visible to the naked eye, it is of no major concern.
- If the use of an oral preparation is associated with continual and moderate or severe gastrointestinal upset, tell the patient to take the drug with food and to contact the prescriber if nausea and vomiting worsen.
- If an antacid is needed, it must be taken either 2 hours before or 2 hours after the drug to avoid interference with drug absorption.
- Recommend a well-balanced diet without an excess of alkaline ash foods (e.g., citrus fruits, vegetables, and milk). Encourage an increase in fluid intake of up to 8 glasses of water a day, unless contraindicated.
- Educate the patient to limit or avoid caffeine intake. Caffeine-containing foods and beverages include coffee (decaffeinated contains 2 to 4 mg caffeine per 8 oz versus caffeinated 65 to 120 mg per 8 oz.), tea, some soft drinks, chocolate, and high-energy drinks.
- Instruct the patient to take medications exactly as prescribed without doubling up or omitting doses. If the patient forgets a dose or is ill and cannot take a dose, contact the prescriber for further instructions.
- Provide written and verbal instructions and demonstrations on measuring pulse and blood pressure. The local fire department and/or rescue station will usually take blood pressure and pulse rates, if needed.
- Journaling is important to document how the patient feels each day. Advise the patient to record in the journal any worsening or improvement of symptoms, adverse effects, daily weights, activity tolerance, blood pressure readings, and pulse rate.
- Daily weights need to be measured at the same time every day and with the same amount of clothing.

- Contact the prescriber immediately if there is a weight gain of 2 pounds or more in 24 hours or 5 pounds or more in 1 week.
- Inform the patient that changing positions purposefully and with caution is important because of the common adverse effect of postural hypotension. Moving too quickly may lead to dizziness, syncope, and subsequent injury or falls.
- At the beginning of therapy and after any dosage increase, encourage the patient to avoid driving and other hazardous activities until sedating adverse effects have resolved.
- Dry mouth may be helped by frequent mouth care, drinking fluids, sucking on sugarless gum or candy, and/or eating ice chips. Artificial saliva and special toothpaste made specifically for dry mouth and its management is available over the counter. Encourage frequent dental visits.
- Counsel the patient to avoid exertion, hot temperatures, saunas, and hot tubs because of heat-induced vasodilation, leading to postural hypotension with dizziness and/or syncope and a subsequent risk for falls or injury. Alcohol intake may also lead to vasodilation and subsequent dizziness and syncope.
- Instruct the patient to carry a medical alert identification card on his or her person at all times. Medical alert jewelry is also available to provide information on medical diagnoses, allergies, and medications.
- Instruct the patient to report immediately to the prescriber any dizziness, shortness of breath, chest pain, and/or worsening of symptoms or occurrence of new symptoms.
- The patient must *never* stop taking these medications without specific instructions to do so; an abrupt discontinuation of these drugs may lead to severe or life-threatening complications.
- With amiodarone, photosensitivity is an adverse effect; advise the patient to avoid sun exposure and to wear sun-protective clothing and dark glasses when outside. Sunscreens are ineffective because they do not block ultraviolet B light, to which the patient may react while taking this medication. Instead, barrier sunblocks, such as zinc or titanium chloride, are recommended.
- With amiodarone, instruct the patient to immediately report any blue-gray discoloration of the skin (often after 1 year, and especially on the face, neck, and arms) as well as any jaundice, unusual rash or skin reactions, nausea, vomiting, or dizziness.

## KEY POINTS

- The SA node, AV node, and His-Purkinje system are all areas in which there is automaticity (cells can depolarize spontaneously). The SA node is the pacemaker because it can spontaneously depolarize easier and faster than the other areas.
- Any disturbance or abnormality in the normal pattern of the heartbeat and pulse rate is termed a *dysrhythmia.*
- Antidysrhythmic drugs are used to correct dysrhythmias; however, they may also cause dysrhythmias, and for this reason are said to be *prodysrhythmic.* The Vaughan Williams classification is the system most commonly used to categorize antidysrhythmic drugs. It classifies drugs into the following groups according to where and how they affect cardiac cells and what their mechanisms of action is:
  - *Class I:* membrane-stabilizing drugs (e.g., class Ia, quinidine; class Ib, lidocaine; class Ic, flecainide)
  - *Class II:* beta-adrenergic blockers that depress phase 4 depolarization (e.g., atenolol)
  - *Class III:* drugs that prolong repolarization in phase 3 (e.g., amiodarone and dofetilide)
  - *Class IV:* calcium channel blockers that depress phase 4 depolarization (e.g., verapamil)
- Nursing actions for the various antidysrhythmics include skillful nursing assessment and close monitoring of heart rate, blood pressure, heart rhythms, general well-being, skin color, temperature, and heart and breath sounds.
- The therapeutic responses to antidysrhythmics include a decrease in blood pressure in hypertensive patients, a decrease in edema, and restoration of a regular pulse rate or a pulse rate without major irregularities or with improved regularity compared with the irregularity that existed before therapy.

## NCLEX® EXAMINATION REVIEW QUESTIONS

1 A patient with a rapid, irregular heart rhythm is being treated in the emergency department with adenosine. During administration of this drug, the nurse will be prepared to monitor the patient for which effect?
   a Nausea and vomiting
   b Transitory asystole
   c Muscle tetany
   d Hypertension

2 When assessing a patient who has been taking amiodarone for 6 months, the nurse monitors for which potential adverse effect?
   a Hyperglycemia
   b Dysphagia
   c Photophobia
   d Urticaria

3 The nurse is assessing a patient who has been taking quinidine and asks about adverse effects. An adverse effect associated with the use of this drug includes:
   a muscle pain.
   b tinnitus.
   c chest pain.
   d excessive thirst.

4 A patient calls the family practice office to report that he has seen his pills in his stools when he has a bowel movement. How will the nurse respond?
   a "The pills are not being digested properly. You need to take them on an empty stomach."
   b "The pills are not being digested properly. You need to take them with food."
   c "What you are seeing is the waxy matrix that contained the medication, but the drug has been absorbed."
   d "This indicates that you are not tolerating this medication and will need to switch to a different form."

5 The nurse is administering lidocaine and considers which condition, if present in the patient, a caution for the use of this drug?
   a Tachycardia
   b Hypertension
   c Ventricular dysrhythmias
   d Renal dysfunction

6 When the nurse is teaching a patient about taking an antidysrhythmic drug, which statements by the nurse are correct? (Select all that apply.)
   a "Take the medication with an antacid if stomach upset occurs."
   b "Do not chew sustained-release capsules."
   c "If weight gain of 5 pounds within 1 week occurs, notify your physician at the next office visit."
   d "If you experience severe adverse effects, stop the drug and notify your physician."
   e "You may take the medication with food if stomach upset occurs."

7 A patient is in the emergency department with new-onset rapid rate atrial fibrillation. The nurse is about to add a continuous infusion of diltiazem (Cardizem) at 5 mg/hr, but must first give a bolus of 0.25 mg/kg over 2 minutes. The patient weighs 220 pounds. The medication comes in a vial of 5 mg/mL. How many milligrams will the patient receive, and how many milliliters will the nurse draw up for this dose?

1. b, 2. c, 3. b, 4. c, 5. d, 6. b, e, 7. 25 mg; 5 mL.

For Critical Thinking and Prioritization Questions, see http://evolve.elsevier.com/Lilley.

## OBJECTIVES

When you reach the end of this chapter, you will be able to do the following:

1. Briefly review the coagulation process and the impact of coagulation modifiers, including anticoagulants, antiplatelets, thrombolytics, and antifibrinolytics.
2. Compare the mechanisms of action, indications, cautions, contraindications, drug interactions, adverse effects, routes of administration, and dosages of the various anticoagulants, antiplatelets, thrombolytics, and antifibrinolytics.
3. Discuss the administration procedures and techniques as well as related standards of care for the various coagulation modifiers.

4. Identify any available antidotes for the coagulation modifiers.
5. Compare the laboratory tests used in conjunction with treatment with the various coagulation modifiers and their implications for therapeutic use of these drugs and monitoring for adverse reactions.
6. Develop a nursing care plan that includes all phases of the nursing process for patients receiving anticoagulants, antiplatelets, thrombolytics, and antifibrinolytics.

## DRUG PROFILES

- ♦ **alteplase, p. 432**
  **aminocaproic acid, p. 433**
  **argatroban, p. 427**
- ♦ **aspirin, p. 430**
- ♦ **clopidogrel, p. 430**
- ♦ **dabigatran p. 427**
  **desmopressin, p. 434**

- ♦ **enoxaparin, p. 425**
- ♦ **eptifibatide, p. 430**
- ♦ **fondaparinux, p. 427**
- ♦ **heparin, p. 426**
- ♦ **warfarin, p. 424**

_____

- ♦ *Key drug*

## KEY TERMS

**Anticoagulants** Substances that prevent or delay coagulation of the blood. (p. 421)

**Antifibrinolytic drugs** Drugs that prevent the lysis of fibrin and in doing so promote clot formation. (p. 421)

**Antiplatelet drugs** Substances that prevent platelet plugs from forming. (p. 421)

**Antithrombin III** A substance that inactivates ("turns off") three major activating factors of the clotting cascade: activated factor II (thrombin), activated factor X, and activated factor IX. (p. 422)

**Clot** Insoluble solid elements of blood (e.g., cells, fibrin threads) that have chemically separated from the liquid (plasma) component of the blood. (p. 419)

**Coagulation** The process of blood clotting. More specifically, the sequential process by which the multiple coagulation factors of the blood interact in the *coagulation* cascade, ultimately forming an insoluble fibrin clot. (p. 419)

**Coagulation cascade** The series of steps beginning with the *intrinsic* or *extrinsic* pathways of coagulation and proceeding through the formation of a *fibrin clot.* (p. 420)

**Deep vein thrombosis (DVT)** The formation of a thrombus in one of the deep veins of the body. The deep veins most commonly affected are the iliac and femoral veins. (p. 422)

**Embolus** A blood clot *(thrombus)* that has been dislodged from the wall of a blood vessel and is traveling throughout the bloodstream. Emboli that lodge in critical blood vessels can result in ischemic injury to a vital organ (e.g., heart, lung, brain) and result in disability or death. (p. 419)

**Enzyme** A protein molecule that catalyzes chemical reactions of other substances without being altered or destroyed in the process. (p. 424)

**Fibrin** A stringy, insoluble protein produced by the action of thrombin on fibrinogen during the clotting process; a major component of blood *clots* or *thrombi* (see *thrombus*). (p. 420)

**Fibrin specificity** The property of some thrombolytic drugs of activating the conversion of plasminogen to plasmin only in the presence of established clots having fibrin threads rather than inducing systemic plasminogen activation throughout the body. (p. 431)

**Fibrinogen** A plasma protein that is converted into fibrin by thrombin in the presence of calcium ions. (p. 428)

**Fibrinolysis** The continual process of fibrin decomposition produced by the actions of the enzymatic protein fibrinolysin. It is the normal mechanism for removing small fibrin clots and is stimulated by anoxia, inflammatory reactions, and other kinds of stress. (p. 421)

**Fibrinolytic system** An area of the circulatory system undergoing fibrinolysis. (p. 421)

**Hemophilia** A rare, inherited blood disorder in which the blood does not clot normally. (p. 421)

**Hemorheologic drugs** Drugs that alter the function of platelets without compromising their blood-clotting properties. (p. 421)

**Hemostasis** The arrest of bleeding, either by the physiologic properties of vasoconstriction and coagulation or by mechanical, surgical, or pharmacologic means. (p. 419)

**Hemostatic** Referring to any procedure, device, or substance that arrests the flow of blood. (p. 421)

**Plasmin** The enzymatic protein that breaks down fibrin into fibrin degradation products; it is derived from plasminogen. (p. 421)

**Plasminogen** A plasma protein that is converted to plasmin. (p. 421)

**Pulmonary embolism** The blockage of a pulmonary artery by foreign matter such as fat, air, a tumor, or a thrombus (which usually arises from a peripheral vein). (p. 422)

**Stroke** Occlusion of the blood vessels of the brain by an embolus, thrombus, or cerebrovascular hemorrhage, resulting in ischemia of the brain tissue. (p. 422)

**Thromboembolic events** Events in which a blood vessel is blocked by an embolus carried in the bloodstream from the site of its formation. The tissue supplied by an obstructed artery may tingle and become cold, numb, cyanotic, and eventually necrotic (dead). (p. 422)

**Thrombolytic drugs** Drugs that dissolve thrombi by functioning similarly to *tissue plasminogen activator.* (p. 421)

**Thrombus** The technical term for a blood clot (plural: *thrombi*); an aggregation of platelets, fibrin, clotting factors, and the cellular elements of the blood that is attached to the interior wall of a vein or artery, sometimes occluding the vessel lumen. (p. 419)

**Tissue plasminogen activator** A naturally occurring plasminogen activator secreted by vascular endothelial cells in the walls of blood vessels. Thrombolytic drugs are based on this blood component. (p. 420)

## ANATOMY, PHYSIOLOGY, AND PATHOPHYSIOLOGY OVERVIEW

Hemostasis is a general term for any process that stops bleeding. This can be accomplished by mechanical means (e.g., compression to the bleeding site) or surgical means (e.g., surgical clamping or cauterization of a blood vessel). When hemostasis occurs due to physiologic clotting of blood, it is called coagulation, which is the process of blood clot formation. The technical term for a blood clot is a thrombus. A thrombus that is not stationary but moves through blood vessels is called an embolus. Normal hemostasis involves the complex interaction of substances that promote clot formation and substances that either inhibit coagulation or dissolve the formed clot. Substances that promote coagulation include platelets, von Willebrand factor, activated clotting factors, and tissue thromboplastin. Substances that inhibit coagulation include prostacyclin, antithrombin III, and proteins C and S. In addition, tissue plasminogen activator is a natural substance that dissolves clots that are already formed.

The coagulation system is illustrated in Figures 26-1 and 26-2. It is called a *cascade* (or coagulation cascade) because each activated clotting factor serves as a catalyst that amplifies the next reaction. The result is a large concentration of a clot-forming substance called fibrin. The coagulation cascade is

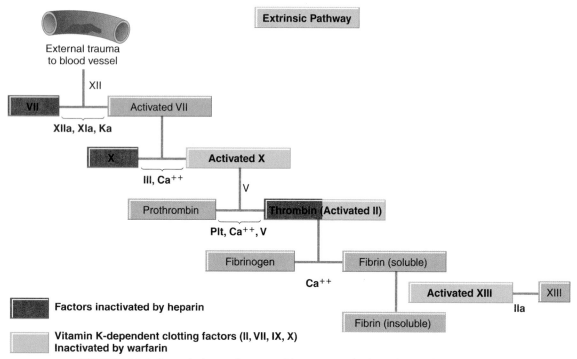

**FIGURE 26-1** Coagulation pathway and factors: extrinsic pathway. *Plt,* Platelets.

**FIGURE 26-2** Coagulation pathway and factors: intrinsic pathway. *HMW-K,* High molecular weight kininogen; *Plt,* platelets.

typically divided into the intrinsic and extrinsic pathways, and these pathways are activated by different types of injury. When blood vessels are damaged by penetration from the outside (e.g., knife or bullet wound), thromboplastin, a substance contained in the walls of blood vessels, is released. This initiates the extrinsic pathway by activating factors VII and X (see Figure 26-1). The components of the intrinsic pathway are present in the blood in their inactive forms (see Figure 26-2). This pathway is activated when factor XII comes in contact with exposed collagen on the inside of damaged blood vessels. Figures 26-1 and 26-2 illustrate the steps that occur in the extrinsic and intrinsic pathways, respectively, and the coagulation factors involved. They also illustrate the site of action of two commonly used anticoagulant drugs: warfarin and heparin.

Once a clot is formed and fibrin is present, the fibrinolytic system is activated. This system initiates the breakdown of clots and serves to balance the clotting process. Fibrinolysis is the reverse of the clotting process. It is the mechanism by which formed thrombi are lysed (broken down) to prevent excessive clot formation and blood vessel blockage. Fibrin in the clot binds to a circulating protein known as plasminogen. This binding converts plasminogen to plasmin. Plasmin is the enzymatic protein that eventually breaks down the fibrin thrombus into fibrin degradation products. This keeps the thrombus localized to prevent it from becoming an embolus that can travel to obstruct a major blood vessel in the lung, heart, or brain. Figure 26-3 illustrates the fibrinolytic system.

Hemophilia is a rare genetic disorder in which the previously mentioned natural coagulation and hemostasis factors are limited or absent. Hemophilia is categorized into two main types depending on which of the coagulation factors is absent (factor VII, factor VIII, and/or factor IX). Patients with hemophilia can bleed to death if coagulation factors are not given.

## PHARMACOLOGY OVERVIEW

Drugs that affect coagulation are some of the most dangerous drugs used today, and numerous factors can affect their action. These drugs are among the most commonly associated with adverse drug reactions. The Joint Commission, a hospital accreditation agency, has made safe use of these drugs a national patient safety goal. This goal requires hospitals to take steps to prevent adverse events associated with these drugs. Further information on this national patient safety goal may be found at www.jointcommission.org/standards_information/npsgs.aspx.

The drugs discussed in this chapter aid the body in reversing or achieving hemostasis, and they can be broken down into several main categories based on their actions. Anticoagulants inhibit the action or formation of clotting factors and therefore prevent clots from forming. Antiplatelet drugs prevent platelet plugs from forming by inhibiting platelet aggregation, which can be beneficial in preventing heart attacks and strokes. Hemorheologic drugs alter platelet function without preventing the platelets from working. Sometimes clots form and totally block a blood vessel. When this happens in one of the coronary arteries, a heart attack occurs, and the clot must be lysed to prevent or minimize damage to the myocardial muscle. Thrombolytic drugs lyse (break down) clots, or thrombi, that have already formed. This is a unique difference between thrombolytics and anticoagulants, which can only prevent the formation of a clot. Antifibrinolytic drugs, also known as hemostatic drugs, have the opposite effect of these other classes of drugs; they actually promote blood coagulation and are helpful in the management of conditions in which excessive bleeding would be harmful. The various drugs in each category of coagulation modifiers are listed in Table 26-1. Understanding the individual coagulation modifiers and their mechanisms of action requires a basic working knowledge of the coagulation pathway and coagulation factors, which is provided in the next section.

## ANTICOAGULANTS

Drugs that prevent the formation of a clot by inhibiting certain clotting factors are called *anticoagulants*. These drugs have no direct effect on a blood clot that has already formed. They

FIGURE 26-3 The fibrinolytic system.

**TABLE 26-1** **COAGULATION MODIFIERS: COMPARISON OF DRUG SUBCLASSES**

| TYPE OF COAGULATION MODIFIER AND MECHANISM OF ACTION | DRUG CLASS | INDIVIDUAL DRUGS |
|---|---|---|
| **Prevent Clot Formation** *Anticoagulant* | | |
| Inhibit clotting factors IIa (thrombin) and Xa | Heparins | Unfractionated heparin ("heparin") and low molecular weight heparins (enoxaparin [Lovenox], dalteparin [Fragmin]) |
| Inhibit vitamin K–dependent clotting factors II, VII, IX, and X | Coumarins | Warfarin (Coumadin) |
| Inhibit thrombin (factor IIa) | Direct thrombin inhibitors | Human antithrombin III (Thrombate), lepirudin (Refludan), argatroban (Argatroban), bivalirudin (Angiomax), dabigatran (Pradaxa) |
| Inhibit factor Xa | Selective factor Xa inhibitor | Fondaparinux (Arixtra), rivaroxaban (Xarelto) |
| **Antiplatelet Drugs** | | |
| Interfere with platelet function | Aggregation inhibitors | Cilostazol (Pletal), clopidogrel (Plavix), prasugrel (Effient) |
| | Aggregation inhibitors/vasodilators | Treprostinil (Remodulin) |
| | Glycoprotein IIb/IIIa inhibitors | Abciximab (ReoPro), eptifibatide (Integrilin), tirofiban (Aggrastat) |
| | Miscellaneous | Anagrelide (Agrylin), dipyridamole (Persantine) |
| **Lyse a Preformed Clot** *Thrombolytics* | | |
| Dissolve thrombi | Tissue plasminogen activators | Alteplase (Activase, Cathflo Activase), reteplase (Retavase), tenecteplase (TNKase) |
| **Promote Clot Formation** *Antifibrinolytics* | | |
| Prevent lysis of fibrin | Systemic hemostatics | Aminocaproic acid (Amicar), tranexamic acid (Cyklokapron) |
| **Reduce Blood Viscosity** *Reversal Drugs* | Hemorheologic | Pentoxifylline (Trental) |
| | Heparin antagonist | Protamine sulfate |
| | Warfarin antagonist | Vitamin K |

prevent intravascular thrombosis by decreasing blood coagulability. Their uses vary from preventing clot formation to preventing the extension of an established clot, or a thrombus.

Once a clot forms on the wall of a blood vessel, it may dislodge and travel through the bloodstream. This is referred to as an *embolus*. If it lodges in a coronary artery, it causes a myocardial infarction (MI); if it obstructs a brain vessel, it causes a stroke; if it goes to the lungs, it is a pulmonary embolism; and if it goes to a vein in the leg, it is a deep vein thrombosis (DVT). Collectively, these complications are called thromboembolic events, because they involve a thrombus that becomes an embolus and causes an adverse cardiovascular "event." Anticoagulants can prevent these from occurring if used in the correct manner. Both orally and parenterally administered anticoagulants are available, and each drug has a slightly different mechanism of action and indications. All of them have their own risks, mainly the risk for causing bleeding. The mechanisms of action of the anticoagulants vary depending on the drug. Drug classes of anticoagulants include older drugs such as unfractionated heparin and warfarin. There are also several newer drug classes, including low molecular weight heparins (LMWHs), direct thrombin inhibitors, and selective factor Xa inhibitors. For dosage information on anticoagulants, see the table on p. 426.

## Mechanism of Action and Drug Effects

Anticoagulants are also called *antithrombotic drugs* because they work to prevent the formation of a clot or thrombus, a condition known as *thrombosis*. All anticoagulants work in the clotting cascade but do so at different points. As shown in Figures 26-1 and 26-2, heparin works by binding to a substance called antithrombin III, which turns off three main activating factors: activated factor II (also called *thrombin*), activated factor X, and activated factor IX. (Factors XI and XII are also inactivated but do not play as important a role as the other three factors.) Of these, thrombin is the most sensitive to the actions of heparin. Antithrombin III is the major natural inhibitor of thrombin in the blood. The overall effect of heparin is that it turns off the coagulation pathway and prevents clots from forming. However, it cannot lyse a clot. The drug name *heparin* usually refers to unfractionated heparin, which is a relatively large molecule and is derived from various animal sources. In contrast, low molecular weight heparins are synthetic and have a smaller molecular structure. These include enoxaparin (Lovenox) and dalteparin (Fragmin). Both drugs work similarly to heparin. Heparin primarily binds to activated factors II, X, and IX, whereas the LMWHs differ from heparin in that they are much more specific for activated factor X (Xa) than for activated factor II (IIa, or thrombin). This property gives LMWHs a much more predictable anticoagulant response. As a result, frequent laboratory monitoring of bleeding times using tests such as activated partial thromboplastin time (aPTT), which is imperative with unfractionated heparin, is not required with LMWHs. When heparin is used for flushing catheters (10-100 units/mL), no monitoring is needed.

Warfarin (Coumadin) works by inhibiting vitamin K synthesis by bacteria in the gastrointestinal tract. This, in turn, inhibits production of clotting factors II, VII, IX, and X. These four factors are normally synthesized in the liver and are known as *vitamin K–dependent clotting factors.* As with heparin, the final effect is the prevention of clot formation. Figures 26-1 and 26-2 show where in the clotting cascade this occurs.

Fondaparinux (Arixtra) inhibits thrombosis by its specific action against factor Xa alone. Rivaroxaban (Xarelto) is a new oral acting factor Xa inhibitor that was approved in 2011. It is approved for DVT prophylaxis and atrial fibrillation. There are many new anticoagulants similar to rivaroxaban in the last stages of development, such as apixaban (Eliquis), which is anticipated to be approved in 2012. There are also currently five antithrombin drugs that inhibit the thrombin molecules directly, one natural and four synthetic. The natural drug is human antithrombin III (Thrombate), which is isolated from the plasma of human donors. The synthetic drugs are lepirudin (Refludan), argatroban (Argatroban), bivalirudin (Angiomax), and dabigatran (Pradaxa). Dabigatran is a new oral direct thrombin inhibitor that was approved in 2010. All of these drugs work similarly to inhibit thrombus formation by inhibiting thrombin.

## Indications

The ability of anticoagulants to prevent clot formation is of benefit in certain settings in which there is a high likelihood of clot formation. These include MI, unstable angina, atrial fibrillation, use of indwelling devices such as mechanical heart valves, and conditions in which blood flow may be slowed and blood may pool, such as major orthopedic surgery or prolonged periods of immobilization like hospitalization or even long plane rides. The ultimate consequence of a clot can be a stroke or a heart attack, DVT, or PE; therefore, the prevention of these serious events is the ultimate benefit of these drugs. Warfarin is indicated for prevention of any of these events, whereas unfractionated heparins, LMWHs, direct thrombin inhibitors, and factor Xa inhibitors are used for both prevention and treatment. Patients at risk for clots are given DVT prophylaxis while in the hospital and after major surgery. LMWHs, especially enoxaparin, are also routinely used as anticoagulant bridge therapy in situations in which a patient must stop warfarin for surgery or other invasive medical procedures. The term *bridge therapy* refers to the fact that enoxaparin acts as a bridge to provide anticoagulation while the patient must be off of his or her warfarin therapy. The remainder of the antithrombotic drugs have similar but more restricted indications, which are listed in the Dosages table for anticoagulants.

## Contraindications

Contraindications to the use of anticoagulants are similar for all of the different drugs. They include known drug allergy to a specific product and usually include any acute bleeding process

| TABLE 26-2 | ANTICOAGULANTS: COMMON ADVERSE EFFECTS |
| --- | --- |
| **DRUG SUBCLASS** | **ADVERSE EFFECTS** |
| Heparins (unfractionated heparin, low molecular weight heparin) | Bleeding, hematoma, anemia, thrombocytopenia |
| Direct thrombin inhibitors (lepirudin, argatroban, bivalirudin, dabigatran) | Bleeding, dizziness, shortness of breath, fever, urticaria |
| Selective factor Xa inhibitor (fondaparinux, rivaroxaban) | Bleeding, hematoma, dizziness, rash, gastrointestinal distress, anemia |
| warfarin (Coumadin) | Bleeding, lethargy, muscle pain, purple toes |

or high risk for such an occurrence, as well as thrombocytopenia. Warfarin is strongly contraindicated in pregnancy, whereas the other anticoagulants are rated in lower pregnancy categories (B or C). LMWHs are contraindicated in patients with an indwelling epidural catheter; they can be given 2 hours after the epidural is removed. This is very important to remember, because giving an LMWH with an epidural has been associated with epidural hematoma.

## Adverse Effects

Bleeding is the main complication of anticoagulation therapy, and the risk increases with increasing dosages. Such bleeding may be localized (e.g., hematoma at the site of injection) or systemic. It also depends on the nature of the patient's underlying clinical disorder and is increased in patients taking high doses of aspirin or other drugs that impair platelet function. One particularly notable adverse effect of heparin is *heparin-induced thrombocytopenia (HIT),* which is also called *heparin-associated thrombocytopenia.* There are two types of HIT. Type I is characterized by a more gradual reduction in platelets. In this type, heparin therapy can generally be continued. In contrast, in type II HIT there is an acute fall in the number of platelets (more than 50% reduction from baseline). Heparin therapy must be discontinued in patients with type II HIT. The greatest risk to the patient with HIT is the paradoxical occurrence of thrombosis, something that heparin normally prevents or alleviates. Thrombosis that occurs in the presence of HIT can be fatal. The incidence of this disorder ranges from 5% to 15% of patients and is higher with *bovine* (cow-derived) than with *porcine* (pig-derived) heparins. The direct thrombin inhibitors lepirudin and argatroban are both specifically indicated for treatment of HIT. Warfarin can cause skin necrosis and "purple toes" syndrome. Other adverse effects are listed in Table 26-2.

### Toxicity and Management of Overdose

Treatment of the toxic effects of anticoagulants is aimed at reversing the underlying cause. Although the toxic effects of heparin, LMWH, and warfarin are hemorrhagic in nature, the management is different for each drug. Symptoms that may be attributed to toxicity or an overdose of anticoagulants are hematuria, melena (blood in the stool), petechiae, ecchymoses, and gum or mucous membrane bleeding. In the event of heparin or warfarin toxicity, the drug is to be stopped immediately.

In the case of heparin, stopping the drug alone may be enough to reverse the toxic effects because of the drug's short half-life (1 to 2 hours). In severe cases or when large doses have been given intentionally (i.e., during cardiopulmonary bypass for heart surgery), IV injection of protamine sulfate is indicated. This drug is a specific heparin antidote and forms a complex with heparin, completely reversing its anticoagulant properties. This occurs in as few as 5 minutes. In general, 1 mg of protamine can reverse the effects of 100 units of heparin. Protamine may also be used to reverse the effects of LMWHs. A 1-mg dose of protamine is administered for each milligram of LMWH given, (e.g., 1 mg protamine for 1 mg enoxaparin). If the heparin overdose has resulted in a large blood loss, replacement with packed red blood cells may be necessary.

In the event of warfarin toxicity or overdose, the first step is to discontinue the warfarin. As with heparin, the toxicity associated with warfarin is an extension of its therapeutic effects on the clotting cascade. However, because warfarin inactivates the vitamin K–dependent clotting factors and because these clotting factors are synthesized in the liver, it may take 36 to 42 hours before the liver can resynthesize enough clotting factors to reverse the warfarin effects. Giving vitamin $K_1$ (phytonadione) can hasten the return to normal coagulation. The dose and route of administration of the vitamin K depend on the clinical situation and its acuity (i.e., how quickly the warfarin-induced effects must be reversed and whether the patient is having significant bleeding). High doses of vitamin K (10 mg) given IV will reverse the anticoagulation within 6 hours. Current recommendations are to use the lowest amount of vitamin K possible, based on the clinical situation. This is because once vitamin K is given, warfarin resistance will occur for up to 7 days; thus the patient cannot be anticoagulated by warfarin during this period. In such cases, either heparin or an LMWH may need to be added to provide adequate anticoagulation. In acute situations in which bleeding is severe and the time it would take for the vitamin K to take effect is too long, it may be necessary to administer transfusions of human plasma or clotting factor concentrates. Depending on the clinical situation, oral vitamin K is usually the preferred route. However, when the international normalized ratio (INR) is very elevated and/or the patient is bleeding, vitamin K is given IV. There is a risk of anaphylaxis when it is given by the IV route. The risk is diminished by diluting it and giving it over 30 minutes. Some institutions allow it to be given via IV push. Vitamin K is available in 5-mg tablets and in 10-mg and 1-mg injections. It is common to give the injectable form orally.

Transfusions may be indicated for overdoses of direct thrombin inhibitors and the selective factor Xa inhibitor fondaparinux, which both lack specific antidotes. These drugs may also be removed with hemodialysis.

## Interactions

Drug interactions involving the oral anticoagulants are profound and complicated. The main interaction mechanisms responsible for increasing anticoagulant activity include the following:
- Enzyme inhibition of metabolism
- Displacement of the drug from inactive protein-binding sites

- Decrease in vitamin K absorption or synthesis by the bacterial flora of the large intestines
- Alteration in the platelet count or activity

The drugs that interact with warfarin and heparin are listed in Table 26-3. More specifics on significant drug interactions are discussed under the drug profiles. Although both aspirin and warfarin increase the risk of bleeding when given with heparin, they are commonly given together in clinical practice. In fact, when a patient is placed on IV heparin, it is recommended that warfarin be started at the same time. Heparin is continued until the warfarin effect is therapeutic for at least 2 days.

## Dosages

For dosage information on selected anticoagulants, see the table on p. 426.

## DRUG PROFILES

Of the anticoagulants, warfarin, dabigatran, and rivaroxaban are used orally. The rest are given by IV and/or subcutaneous injection only. Intramuscular (IM) injection of these drugs is contraindicated due to their propensity to cause large hematomas at the site of injection.

### ◆ warfarin

Warfarin sodium (Coumadin) is a pharmaceutical derivative of the natural plant anticoagulant known as *coumarin*. Warfarin is the most commonly prescribed oral anticoagulant and is available oral and IV; however, it is used almost exclusively in the oral form. Use of this drug requires careful monitoring of the prothrombin time/international normalized ratio (PT/INR), which is a standardized measure of the degree to which a patient's blood coagulability has been reduced by the drug. A normal INR (without warfarin) is 1.0, whereas a therapeutic INR (with warfarin) ranges from 2 to 3.5, depending on the indication for use of the drug (e.g., atrial fibrillation, thromboprevention, prosthetic heart valve). Patients older than 65 years of age may have a lower INR threshold for bleeding complications and may need to be monitored accordingly. Elderly patients should be started on lower dosages initially. Recently, it has been shown that about one third of patients receiving warfarin metabolize it differently than expected, based on variations in certain genes, *CYP2CP* and *VKORC1*. Genetic testing for these genes is helpful in determining the appropriate initial dosage of warfarin. The maintenance dosage is still determined by the INR.

Warfarin has significant interactions with many drugs, including amiodarone, fluconazole, erythromycin, metronidazole, sulfonamide antibiotics, and cimetidine. Although many more drugs can interact with warfarin, the aforementioned are by far the most common. Combining warfarin and amiodarone will lead to a 50% increase in the INR. When amiodarone is added to warfarin therapy, it is recommended that the warfarin dose be cut in half.

Because warfarin inhibits vitamin K–dependent clotting factors, foods that are high in vitamin K may reduce warfarin's ability to prevent clots. Common foods rich in vitamin K include leafy green vegetables (kale, spinach, collard greens).

## TABLE 26-3   DRUG INTERACTIONS

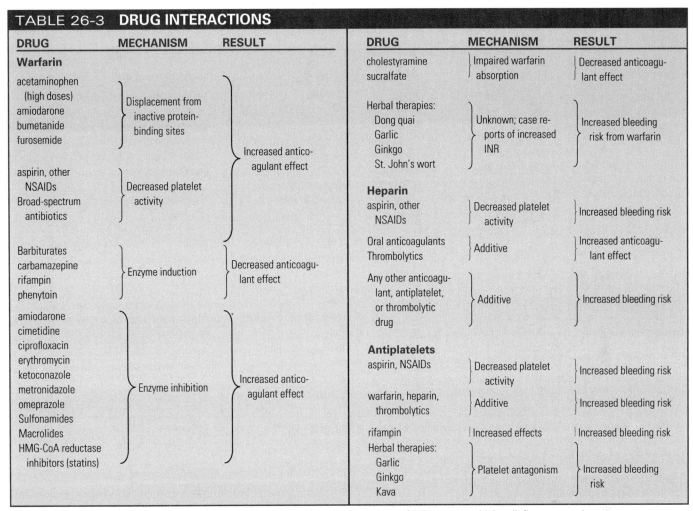

| DRUG | MECHANISM | RESULT |
|---|---|---|
| **Warfarin** | | |
| acetaminophen (high doses) | | |
| amiodarone | Displacement from inactive protein-binding sites | |
| bumetanide | | Increased anticoagulant effect |
| furosemide | | |
| aspirin, other NSAIDs | Decreased platelet activity | |
| Broad-spectrum antibiotics | | |
| Barbiturates | | |
| carbamazepine | Enzyme induction | Decreased anticoagulant effect |
| rifampin | | |
| phenytoin | | |
| amiodarone | | |
| cimetidine | | |
| ciprofloxacin | | |
| erythromycin | | |
| ketoconazole | | |
| metronidazole | Enzyme inhibition | Increased anticoagulant effect |
| omeprazole | | |
| Sulfonamides | | |
| Macrolides | | |
| HMG-CoA reductase inhibitors (statins) | | |

| DRUG | MECHANISM | RESULT |
|---|---|---|
| cholestyramine sucralfate | Impaired warfarin absorption | Decreased anticoagulant effect |
| **Herbal therapies:** Dong quai Garlic Ginkgo St. John's wort | Unknown; case reports of increased INR | Increased bleeding risk from warfarin |
| **Heparin** | | |
| aspirin, other NSAIDs | Decreased platelet activity | Increased bleeding risk |
| Oral anticoagulants Thrombolytics | Additive | Increased anticoagulant effect |
| Any other anticoagulant, antiplatelet, or thrombolytic drug | Additive | Increased bleeding risk |
| **Antiplatelets** | | |
| aspirin, NSAIDs | Decreased platelet activity | Increased bleeding risk |
| warfarin, heparin, thrombolytics | Additive | Increased bleeding risk |
| rifampin | Increased effects | Increased bleeding risk |
| Herbal therapies: Garlic Ginkgo Kava | Platelet antagonism | Increased bleeding risk |

*HMG-CoA,* Hydroxymethylglutaryl–coenzyme A; *INR,* international normalized ratio; *NSAIDs,* nonsteroidal antiinflammatory drugs.

The most important aspect of these food-drug interactions is consistency in diet. Educate patients to maintain consistency in their intake of leafy green vegetables. Many patients are under the misconception that they must avoid all leafy green vegetables. However, this is not true. Once their maintenance warfarin dose is established, patients may still eat greens, but they need to be consistent in their intake of green vegetables, because increasing or decreasing their intake can affect the INR. Herbal products that interact with warfarin and result in increased risk of bleeding include dong quai, garlic, ginkgo, and St. John's wort.

### Pharmacokinetics

| Route | Onset of Action | Peak Plasma Concentration | Elimination Half-life | Duration of Action |
|---|---|---|---|---|
| PO | 24-72 hr | 4 hr | 0.5-3 days | 2-5 days |

### ♦ enoxaparin
Enoxaparin (Lovenox) is the prototypical LMWH and is obtained by enzymatically cleaving large unfractionated heparin molecules into small fragments. These smaller fragments of heparin have a greater affinity for factor Xa than for factor IIa and have a higher degree of bioavailability and a longer elimination half-life than unfractionated heparin. Laboratory monitoring, as done with heparin therapy, is not necessary when enoxaparin is given because of its greater affinity for factor Xa. It is available only in injectable form. Other anticoagulants with comparable pharmacology and indications include danaparoid and dalteparin. Enoxaparin is the most frequently used LMWH and is commonly given for both prophylaxis and treatment. All LMWHs have a distinct advantage over heparin in that it does not require any laboratory monitoring and can be given at home for the treatment of DVT or pulmonary embolism. This allows patients to be discharged from the hospital sooner. It is also used at home after major orthopedic surgery.

A potentially deadly medication error is to give heparin in combination with enoxaparin (or any LMWH, dabigatran, or rivaroxaban). Always double-check that enoxaparin and heparin are never given to the same patient.

## DOSAGES

### Selected Anticoagulant Drugs

| DRUG (PREGNANCY CATEGORY) | PHARMACOLOGIC CLASS | USUAL DOSAGE RANGE | INDICATIONS/USES |
|---|---|---|---|
| argatroban (Argatroban) (B) | Synthetic direct thrombin inhibitor | **Adult**<br>IV: 2 mcg/kg/min until aPTT in desired range | Thromboprevention and treatment of HIT and with PCI in patients at risk for HIT |
| ◆ enoxaparin (Lovenox) (B) | LMWH | **Adult**<br>Subcut: 30-40 mg every 12 hr for prophylaxis or 1 mg/kg every 12 hr for treatment | Prevention and treatment of thromboembolic and ischemic processes in unstable angina and postoperative and post-MI situations |
| ◆ heparin (generic only) (C) | Natural anticoagulant | **Pediatric**<br>IV: Initial 50 units/kg, then 12-25 units/kg/hr, increased by 2-4 units/kg/hr q6-8h prn<br>**Adult**<br>Subcut: 5000 units q8-12hr for prophylaxis<br>IV infusion: 20,000-40,000 units/day usually given as 80 unit/kg bolus then 18 units/kg/hr (depending on indication)<br>aPTT determines maintenance dosage | Thrombosis/embolism, coagulopathies (e.g., DIC), DVT and PE prophylaxis, clotting prevention (e.g., open heart surgery, dialysis) |
| dabigatran (Pradaxa) (C) | Synthetic direct thrombin inhibitor | **Adult**<br>Oral: 75-150 mg bid (depending on renal function) | Prevention of strokes and thrombosis in patients with nonvalvular atrial fibrillation |
| fondaparinux (Arixtra) (B) | Factor Xa inhibitor | Prophylaxis: 2.5 mg subcut daily<br>Treatment: less than 50 kg: 5 mg daily<br>50-100 kg: 7.5 mg daily<br>Over 100 kg: 10 mg daily | Prevention and treatment of DVT and PE |
| ◆ warfarin (X) | Coumarin anticoagulant | INR determines maintenance dose, usually 1-10 mg/day orally | Thromboprevention and treatment of DVT, PE, atrial fibrillation, post-MI status |

*aPTT*, Activated partial thromboplastin time; *DIC*, disseminated intravascular coagulation; *DVT*, deep vein thrombosis; *HIT*, heparin-induced thrombocytopenia; *INR*, international normalized ratio; *IV*, intravenous; *LMWH*, low molecular weight heparin; *MI*, myocardial infarction; *PCI*, percutaneous coronary intervention; *PE*, pulmonary embolism; *subcut*, subcutaneous.

### Pharmacokinetics (enoxaparin)

| Route | Onset of Action | Peak Plasma Concentration | Elimination Half-life | Duration of Action |
|---|---|---|---|---|
| Subcut | 3-5 hr | 4-5 hr | 4-5 hr | 12 hr |

### ◆ heparin

Heparin is a natural mucopolysaccharide anticoagulant obtained from the lungs, intestinal mucosa, or other suitable tissues primarily of pigs. One brand name for some of the commonly used heparin products is Hep-Lock. This brand name refers only to small vials of heparin IV flush solutions used to maintain the patency of heparin-lock IV insertion sites. Because of the risk for the development of HIT, however, most institutions routinely use normal saline (0.9% sodium chloride) as a flush for heparin-lock IV ports and have moved away from using heparin flush solutions for this purpose. Heparin flushes are still used for central catheters. When used for flushing purposes, there is no need for monitoring.

Heparin is commonly used for DVT prophylaxis in a dose of 5000 units two or three times a day given subcutaneously, and it does not need to be monitored when used for prophylaxis. When heparin is used therapeutically (for treatment), it is given by continuous IV infusion or, rarely, by subcutaneous injection. Most hospitals have weight-based protocols for heparin administration. Because the dosage is based on the patient's weight in kilograms, ensure that the appropriate weight is recorded and that only kilograms are used, not

pounds. A potential double-dose medication error can occur if pounds and kilograms are mixed. This is also true for enoxaparin, because it is dosed on body weight when used therapeutically. When heparin is given by IV infusion, monitoring by frequent measurement of aPTT (usually every 6 hours until therapeutic effects are seen) is necessary. Because the required monitoring is very time-consuming, many institutions now use enoxaparin in place of heparin.

Other drugs that affect the coagulation cascade can have additive effects with heparin, which may lead to bleeding. Even though warfarin can cause additive effects, it is combined with IV heparin therapy. In fact, it is usually started within the first day or two of heparin infusion.

Heparin is available only in injectable form in multiple strengths ranging from 10 to 40,000 units/mL. The vials of different strengths of heparin are very similar and look very much alike. In fact, several newborns have died when a vial of more concentrated heparin was mistaken for a more dilute solution. Take great care in checking and double-checking the concentration of heparin before administering it.

### Pharmacokinetics

| Route | Onset of Action | Peak Plasma Concentration | Elimination Half-life | Duration of Action |
|---|---|---|---|---|
| IV | Immediate | Immediate | 1-2 hr | Dependent on infusion duration |
| Subcut | 20-30 min | 2-4 hr | 1-2 hr | 8-12 hr |

### dabigatran

Dabigatran (Pradaxa) is the first oral direct thrombin inhibitor that is approved for prevention of strokes and thrombosis in patients with nonvalvular atrial fibrillation. Dabigatran is a prodrug that becomes activated in the liver. It specifically and reversibly binds to both free and clot-bound thrombin. Dabigatran is excreted extensively in the kidneys, and the dose is dependent upon renal function. The normal dose is 150 mg twice daily, but it must be reduced to 75 mg twice daily if creatinine clearance is less than 30 mL/min. There is no antidote to dabigatran, and the most common and serious side effect is bleeding. No coagulation monitoring is required for dabigatran. Drug interactions include phenytoin (decreased effect) and amiodarone (increased effect). Information about storage and handling is discussed in the Nursing Process section later in the chapter.

#### Pharmacokinetics

| Route | Onset of Action | Peak Plasma Concentration | Elimination Half-life | Duration of Action |
|---|---|---|---|---|
| PO | 2-3 hr | 2 hr | 12-17 hr | 12 hr |

### fondaparinux

Fondaparinux (Arixtra) is a selective inhibitor of factor Xa, which is indicated for prophylaxis or treatment of DVT or PE. In 2009, the FDA required changes in the prescribing information to highlight potential adverse reactions and contraindications. It is contraindicated with known allergy or in patients with a creatinine clearance less than 30 mL/min or a body weight of less than 50 kg. Bleeding is the most common and serious adverse reaction. Thrombocytopenia has also been reported, and therapy should be stopped if platelet count falls below 100,000 platelets per microliter. It should not be given for at least 6 to 8 hours after surgery and should be used with caution in conjunction with warfarin or other anticoagulants. Other side effects include anemia, increased wound drainage, postoperative hemorrhage, hematoma, confusion, urinary tract infection, hypotension, dizziness, and hypokalemia. There is no antidote for fondaparinux, and its effect cannot be measured by standard anticoagulant tests. Fondaparinux is given only by subcutaneous injection. The dose for prophylaxis is 2.5 mg daily. The dose for acute DVT/PE treatment is 5 to 10 mg daily, depending on body weight.

#### Pharmacokinetics

| Route | Onset of Action | Peak Plasma Concentration | Elimination Half-life | Duration of Action |
|---|---|---|---|---|
| Subcut | 2 hr | 2-3 hr | 17-21 hr | 24 hr |

### argatroban

Argatroban, which has the same trade name, is a synthetic direct thrombin inhibitor that is derived from the amino acid L-arginine. It is indicated both for treatment of active HIT and for *percutaneous coronary intervention* procedures in patients at risk for HIT (i.e., those with a history of the disorder). It is given only by the IV route. A lower dosage must be used in patients with severe hepatic dysfunction.

#### Pharmacokinetics

| Route | Onset of Action | Peak Plasma Concentration | Elimination Half-life | Duration of Action |
|---|---|---|---|---|
| IV | Immediate | 1-3 hr | 30-50 min | Dependent on infusion duration |

## ANTIPLATELET DRUGS

Another class of coagulation modifiers that prevent clot formation is the antiplatelet drugs. The anticoagulants work in the clotting cascade. In contrast, antiplatelet drugs work to prevent platelet adhesion at the site of blood vessel injury, which actually occurs before the clotting cascade.

Platelets normally flow through blood vessels without adhering to their surfaces. Blood vessels can be injured by a disruption of blood flow, trauma, or the rupture of plaque from a vessel wall. When such events occur, substances such as collagen and fibronectin, which are present in the walls of blood vessels, become exposed. Collagen is a potent stimulator of platelet adhesion, as is a prevalent component of the platelet membranes called *glycoprotein IIb/IIIa (GP IIb/IIIa)*. Once platelet adhesion occurs, stimulators (compounds such as adenosine diphosphate [ADP], thrombin, thromboxane $A_2$ [$TXA_2$], and prostaglandin $H_2$) are released from the activated platelets. These cause the platelets to *aggregate* (accumulate) at the site of injury. Once at the site of vessel injury, the platelets change shape and release their contents, which include ADP, serotonin, and platelet factor IV. The hemostatic function of these substances is twofold. First, they act as platelet recruiters, attracting additional platelets to the site of injury; second, they are potent vasoconstrictors. Vasoconstriction limits blood flow to the damaged blood vessel to reduce blood loss.

A platelet plug that has formed at a site of vessel injury is not stable and can be dislodged. The clotting cascade is then stimulated to form a more permanent *fibrin* plug (blood clot). The role of platelets and their relationship to the clotting cascade are illustrated in Figure 26-4.

## Mechanism of Action and Drug Effects

Many of the antiplatelet drugs affect the *cyclooxygenase* pathway, which is one of the common final enzymatic pathways in the complex *arachidonic acid* pathway that operates within platelets and on blood vessel walls. This pathway as it functions in both platelets and blood vessel walls is illustrated in Figure 26-5.

Aspirin is widely used for its analgesic, antiinflammatory, and antipyretic (antifever) properties (see Chapter 44). Aspirin also has antiplatelet effects. Aspirin (acetylsalicylic acid) acetylates and inhibits cyclooxygenase in the platelet irreversibly so that the platelet cannot regenerate this enzyme. Therefore, the effects of aspirin last the lifespan of a platelet, or 7 days. This irreversible inhibition of cyclooxygenase in the platelet prevents the formation of $TXA_2$, a substance that causes blood vessels to constrict

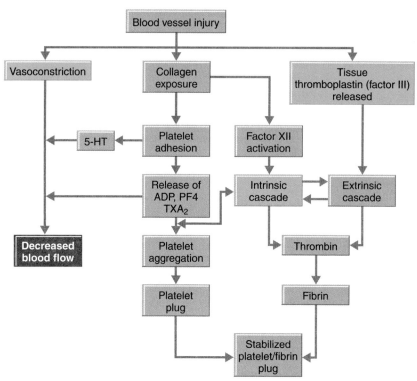

**FIGURE 26-4** Relationship between platelets and the clotting cascade. *ADP,* Adenosine diphosphate; *5-HT,* serotonin; *PF4,* platelet factor IV; *TXA₂,* thromboxane A₂.

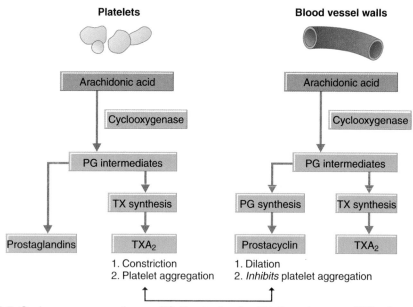

**FIGURE 26-5** Cyclooxygenase pathway. *PG,* Prostaglandin; *TX,* thromboxane; *TXA₂,* thromboxane A₂.

and platelets to aggregate. Thus, by preventing $TXA_2$ formation, aspirin prevents these actions, which results in dilation of the blood vessels and prevention of platelets from aggregating or forming a clot.

Dipyridamole, another antiplatelet drug, also works to inhibit platelet aggregation by preventing the release of ADP, platelet factor IV, and $TXA_2$, all substances that stimulate platelets to aggregate or form a clot. Figure 26-4 shows how these substances accomplish this. Dipyridamole may also directly

stimulate the release of prostacyclin and inhibit the formation of $TXA_2$ (see Figure 26-5).

Clopidogrel is a drug that belongs to the class of antiplatelet drugs called the ADP inhibitors. Its use has largely superseded that of the original ADP inhibitor ticlopidine. Its mechanism of action is entirely different from that of aspirin in that it inhibits platelet aggregation by altering the platelet membrane so that it can no longer receive the signal to aggregate and form a clot. This signal is in the form of **fibrinogen** molecules, which attach to glycoprotein receptors (GP IIb/IIIa) on the surface of the platelet. Clopidogrel inhibits the activation of this receptor. Clopidogrel has been shown to be somewhat better than aspirin at reducing the number of heart attacks, strokes, and vascular deaths in patients at risk. The combination of aspirin and clopidogrel has been shown to be effective in patients with known cardiovascular disease, but not in patients who only have risk factors. Prasugrel (Effient) is a newer antiplatelet drug, similar to clopidogrel, that is used primarily after interventional cardiac procedures and for patients who do not respond to clopidogrel. The newest antiplatelet drug is ticagrelor (BRILINTA), which was approved in 2011. It is indicated for patients with acute coronary syndrome. It must be avoided in patients taking more than 100 mg of aspirin daily.

Pentoxifylline, another antiplatelet drug, is a methylxanthine derivative with properties similar to those of other methylxanthines, such as caffeine and theophylline (see Chapter 37). It was one of the earliest antiplatelet drugs but is now much less commonly used. It reduces the viscosity of blood by increasing the flexibility of red blood cells and reducing the aggregation of platelets. It is sometimes referred to as a *hemorheologic* drug, or a drug that alters the fluid dynamics of the blood. The antiplatelet effects of pentoxifylline are attributed to its inhibition of ADP, serotonin, and platelet factor IV (see Figure 26-4). Pentoxifylline also stimulates the synthesis and release of prostacyclin from blood vessels (see Figure 26-5). In addition, it may have effects on the fibrinolytic system by raising the plasma concentrations of tissue plasminogen activator (see Figure 26-3).

Cilostazol is another antiplatelet drug, which works through inhibition of type 3 phosphodiesterase in the platelets and primarily lower-extremity blood vessels. Its effects are to reduce platelet aggregation and promote vasodilation.

Another class of antiplatelet drugs is the GP IIb/IIIa inhibitors. They work by blocking the receptor protein by the same name that occurs in the platelet wall membranes. This protein plays a role in promoting the aggregation of platelets in preparation for fibrin clot formation. There are currently three available drugs in this class: tirofiban (Aggrastat), eptifibatide (Integrilin), and abciximab (ReoPro). The GP IIb/IIIa inhibitors are available only for IV infusion.

## Indications

The therapeutic effects of the antiplatelet drugs depend on the particular drug. Aspirin has multiple therapeutic effects, but many of them vary depending on the dosage. Aspirin is officially recommended for stroke prevention by the American Stroke Society in daily doses of 50 to 325 mg. (However, in clinical practice, dosages may vary.) Clopidogrel is given to reduce the risk for fatal and nonfatal thrombotic stroke, and is used for prophylaxis against transient ischemic attacks as well for post-MI prevention of thrombosis. Dipyridamole is used as an adjunct to warfarin in the prevention of postoperative thromboembolic complications. It is also used to decrease platelet aggregation in various other thromboembolic disorders. The GP IIb/IIIa inhibitors are used to treat acute unstable angina and MI, and are given during percutaneous coronary intervention procedures, such as angioplasty. Their purpose is to prevent

| TABLE 26-4 | SELECTED ANTIPLATELET DRUGS: ADVERSE EFFECTS |
|---|---|
| **BODY SYSTEM** | **ADVERSE EFFECTS** |
| **Aspirin** | |
| Central nervous | Drowsiness, dizziness, confusion, flushing |
| Gastrointestinal | Nausea, vomiting, gastrointestinal bleeding, diarrhea |
| Hematologic | Thrombocytopenia, agranulocytosis, leukopenia, neutropenia, hemolytic anemia, bleeding |
| **Clopidogrel** | |
| Cardiovascular | Chest pain, edema |
| Central nervous | Flulike symptoms, headache, dizziness, fatigue |
| Gastrointestinal | Abdominal pain, diarrhea, nausea |
| Miscellaneous | Epistaxis, rash, and pruritus (itching) |
| **Glycoprotein IIb/IIIa Inhibitors** | |
| Cardiovascular | Bradycardia, hypotension, edema |
| Central nervous | Dizziness |
| Hematologic | Bleeding, thrombocytopenia |

the formation of thrombi. This is known as *thromboprevention.* This treatment approach is based on the fact that *prevention* of thrombus formation is easier and less risky overall from a pharmacologic standpoint than is lysing a formed thrombus. Pentoxifylline is indicated for peripheral vascular disease, whereas cilostazol is indicated specifically for *intermittent claudication* (pain and cramping in the calf muscles associated with walking). Cilostazol has been shown to be superior to pentoxifylline in improving exercise tolerance in elderly patients.

## Contraindications

Contraindications to the use of antiplatelet drugs include known drug allergy to a specific product, thrombocytopenia, active bleeding, leukemia, traumatic injury, gastrointestinal ulcer, vitamin K deficiency, and recent stroke.

## Adverse Effects

The potential adverse effects of the various antiplatelet drugs can be serious, and they all pose a risk for inducing a serious bleeding episode. The most common adverse effects are listed in Table 26-4.

## Interactions

Some potentially dangerous drug interactions can occur with antiplatelet drugs. The use of dipyridamole with clopidogrel, aspirin, and/or other nonsteroidal antiinflammatory drugs (NSAIDs) produces additive antiplatelet activity and increased bleeding potential. The combined use of steroids or nonaspirin NSAIDs with aspirin can increase the ulcerogenic effects of aspirin. The combined use of aspirin and heparin with GP IIb/IIIa inhibitors also further enhances antiplatelet activity and increases the likelihood of a serious bleeding episode. In spite of all of these interactions, it is not uncommon to see patients

## DOSAGES

### Selected Antiplatelet Drugs

| DRUG (PREGNANCY CATEGORY) | PHARMACOLOGIC CLASS | USUAL DOSAGE RANGE | INDICATIONS/USES |
|---|---|---|---|
| ◆ aspirin (C/D) | Salicylate antiplatelet | **Adult**<br>PO: 81-325 mg once daily<br>PO: 40-325 mg once daily | MI prophylaxis<br>TIA prophylaxis |
| ◆ clopidogrel (Plavix) (B) | ADP inhibitor | **Adult**<br>PO: 75 mg once daily; 300 mg may be given as a one-time loading dose after coronary stent implantation | Reduction of atherosclerotic events; acute coronary syndrome without ST segment elevation |
| ◆ eptifibatide (Integrilin) (B) | GP IIb/IIIa inhibitor | IV: Single bolus followed by continuous infusion; specific doses are based on patient weight from 37 to more than 121 kg* | Unstable angina, MI, percutaneous coronary procedures |

*ADP*, Adenosine diphosphate; *GP*, glycoprotein; *IV*, intravenous; *MI*, myocardial infarction; *PO*, oral; *TIA*, transient ischemic attack.
*See table in package insert for specific dose.

taking daily maintenance doses of aspirin for thrombopreventive purposes, sometimes in combination with other antiplatelet drugs. The most commonly used dose is the "baby aspirin" dose of 81 mg (the standard adult dose is 325 mg). Even though GP IIb/IIIa and heparin have additive therapeutic effects when given concurrently and are listed as interacting drugs, it is very common to see both used together. However, the therapeutic goal of heparin treatment, and thus the dose, is lower when used with a GP IIb/IIIa inhibitor.

## Dosages

For dosage information on selected antiplatelet drugs, see the table on this page.

## DRUG PROFILES

Antiplatelet drugs are extremely useful in the management of thromboembolic disorders. Each has unique pharmacologic properties, and therefore they all are somewhat different from one another.

### ◆ aspirin

Aspirin is available in many combinations with other prescription and nonprescription drugs and goes by many product names. One unique contraindication for aspirin is flulike symptoms in children and teenagers. The use of aspirin in this situation is associated with the occurrence of Reye's syndrome, a rare, acute, and sometimes fatal condition involving hepatic and central nervous system damage (see Chapter 44). There is also allergic cross-reactivity between aspirin and other NSAIDs. Patients with documented aspirin allergy must not receive NSAIDs. Aspirin is available in both oral and rectal forms. A combination form of aspirin and dipyridamole (Aggrenox) is used for antiplatelet purposes.

### Pharmacokinetics

| Route | Onset of Action | Peak Plasma Concentration | Elimination Half-life | Duration of Action |
|---|---|---|---|---|
| PO | 15-30 min | 0.25-2 hr | 2-3 hr | 4-6 hr |

### ◆ clopidogrel

Clopidogrel (Plavix) is currently the most widely used ADP inhibitor on the market. It has superseded ticlopidine (Ticlid) due to the associated serious adverse reactions to the latter drug, including life-threatening neutropenia and agranulocytosis. It was initially believed that clopidogrel might be free from such adverse effects. However, some case reports are emerging of clopidogrel-associated hematologic adverse effects. It is available only for oral use. Prasugrel (Effient) and ticagrelor (BRILINTA) are similar to clopidogrel.

### Pharmacokinetics

| Route | Onset of Action | Peak Plasma Concentration | Elimination Half-life | Duration of Action |
|---|---|---|---|---|
| PO | 1-2 hr | 1 hr | 8 hr | 7-10 days |

### ◆ eptifibatide

Eptifibatide (Integrilin) is a GP IIb/IIIa inhibitor, along with tirofiban (Aggrastat) and abciximab (ReoPro). These drugs are usually administered in intensive care or cardiac catheterization laboratory settings where continuous cardiovascular monitoring is the norm. All are available only for IV use.

### Pharmacokinetics

| Route | Onset of Action | Peak Plasma Concentration | Elimination Half-life | Duration of Action |
|---|---|---|---|---|
| IV | 1 hr | Unknown | 2-2.5 hr | 4 hr |

## THROMBOLYTIC DRUGS

Thrombolytics are coagulation modifiers that lyse thrombi in the blood vessels that supply the heart with blood, the coronary arteries. This reestablishes blood flow to the blood-starved heart muscle. If the blood flow is reestablished early, the heart muscle and left ventricular function can be saved. If blood flow is not reestablished early, the affected area of the heart muscle becomes ischemic, and eventually necrotic and nonfunctional.

Thrombolytic therapy made its debut in 1933 when a substance that broke down fibrin clots was isolated from a patient's blood. This substance was determined to be produced by certain bacteria growing in the patient's blood. The bacteria were found to be *beta-hemolytic streptococci (group A),* and the substance was eventually called *streptokinase.*

Streptokinase was first used in a patient in 1947 to dissolve a clotted hemothorax, but it was not until 1958 that it was given to a patient with an acute MI. In 1960, a naturally occurring human plasminogen activator called urokinase, which was found to exert fibrinolytic effects on pulmonary emboli (clots in the lungs), became available. However, the results of the early thrombolytic trials conducted during the 1960s and 1970s that enrolled patients who had had an acute MI were not taken seriously by the medical community. In the 1980s, the underlying cause of acute MI was determined to be due to coronary artery occlusion. This marked the start of rapid growth in the use of thrombolytic drugs for the early treatment of acute MI. Since that time, several new thrombolytics have become available for this and other clinical uses. *Tissue plasminogen activator (t-PA)* and *anisoylated plasminogen streptokinase activator complex (APSAC)* are two of these drugs. Following the advent of these new thrombolytics came the results of several large landmark thrombolytic research studies. These studies showed that early thrombolytic therapy could bring about a 50% reduction in mortality, a reduction in the infarct size, an improvement in left ventricular function, and a reduction in the incidence and severity of congestive heart failure. These findings and developments, along with a better understanding of the pathogenesis of acute MI, have led the way to the advancements made in the treatment of acute MI. However, the use of thrombolytics has almost completely been replaced by interventional cardiologic procedures, such as percutaneous coronary intervention. Thrombolytics are still a viable option in hospitals that do not offer percutaneous coronary intervention. Currently available thrombolytic drugs include t-PAs (anistreplase [Eminase], alteplase [Activase], reteplase [Retavase], and tenecteplase [TNKase]). For dosage information on thrombolytics, see the table on p. 432.

## Mechanism of Action and Drug Effects

There is a fine balance between the formation and dissolution of a clot. The coagulation system is responsible for forming clots, whereas the fibrinolytic system is responsible for dissolving clots. The natural fibrinolytic system within the blood takes several days to break down a clot (thrombus). This is of little value in the case of a clotted blood vessel that supplies blood to the heart muscle. Necrosis of the myocardium would not be prevented by these natural means, but thrombolytic drug therapy activates the fibrinolytic system to break down the thrombus in the blood vessel quickly so that the delivery of blood to the heart muscle via the coronary arteries is quickly reestablished. This prevents myocardial tissue (heart muscle) and heart function from being destroyed. Thrombolytics accomplish this by activating the conversion of plasminogen to plasmin, which breaks down, or lyses, the thrombus (see Figure 26-3). Plasmin is a proteolytic enzyme, which means that it breaks down proteins.

It is a relatively nonspecific serine protease that is capable of degrading proteins such as fibrin, fibrinogen, and other procoagulant proteins like factors V, VIII, and XII. In other words, the substances that form clots are destroyed by plasmin. Essentially, thrombolytic drugs work by mimicking the body's own process of clot destruction. Although the individual thrombolytic drugs are somewhat diverse in their actions, they all have this common result.

*Streptokinase,* the original thrombolytic enzyme, and the naturally occurring urokinase have been removed from the U.S. market, primarily due to their adverse effects—namely, they were not fibrin specific. The newer thrombolytics have chemical specificity for fibrin threads (fibrin specificity) and work primarily at the site of a clot. They still carry some bleeding risk, but much less than that of the thrombolytic enzymes.

Tissue plasminogen activator is a naturally occurring plasminogen activator secreted by vascular endothelial cells (the walls of blood vessels). However, the amount secreted naturally is not sufficient to dissolve a coronary thrombus quickly enough to restore circulation to the heart and save the heart muscle. Recombinant DNA techniques are now used to produce t-PA, and thus it can be administered in quantities sufficient to dissolve a coronary thrombus quickly. It is fibrin specific (clot specific); that is, only the fibrin clot stimulates t-PA to convert plasminogen to plasmin. Therefore, it has a lower propensity to induce a systemic thrombolytic state, compared to the thrombolytic enzymes.

## Indications

The purpose of all the thrombolytic drugs is to activate the conversion of plasminogen to plasmin, the enzyme that breaks down a thrombus. The presence of a thrombus that interferes significantly with normal blood flow on either the venous or the arterial side of the circulation is an indication for the use of thrombolytic therapy. An exception may be a thrombus that has formed in blood vessels that connect directly with the central nervous system. The indications for thrombolytic therapy include acute MI, arterial thrombosis, DVT, occlusion of shunts or catheters, pulmonary embolism, and acute ischemic stroke.

## Contraindications

Contraindications to the use of thrombolytic drugs include known drug allergy to the specific product and any preservatives, and concurrent use of other drugs that alter clotting.

## Adverse Effects

The most common undesirable effect of thrombolytic therapy is internal, intracranial, and superficial bleeding. Other problems include hypersensitivity, anaphylactoid reactions, nausea, vomiting, and hypotension. These drugs can also induce cardiac dysrhythmias.

## Toxicity and Management of Overdose

Acute toxicity primarily causes an extension of the adverse effects of the thrombolytic drug. Treatment is symptomatic and

*Selected Thrombolytic Drugs*

| DRUG (PREGNANCY CATEGORY) | PHARMACOLOGIC CLASS | USUAL DOSAGE RANGE | INDICATIONS |
|---|---|---|---|
| ◆ alteplase (Activase) (C) | Tissue plasminogen activator | **Adult** | |
| | | IV: 100 mg over 90 min given as a 15-mg IV bolus, then 50 mg over 30 min, then 35 mg over 60 min | Acute myocardial infarction |
| | | IV: 100 mg over 2 hr or 30-50 mg over 1.5-2 hr via pulmonary artery | Pulmonary embolism |
| | | IV: 0.9 mg/kg (total dose not to exceed 90 mg); 10% given as an IV bolus over 1 min, remainder over 60 min; must be given within 3 hr of onset of symptoms | Acute ischemic stroke |

*IV,* Intravenous.

supportive, because thrombolytic drugs have a relatively short half-life and no specific antidotes.

## Interactions

The most common effect of drug interactions is an increased bleeding tendency resulting from the concurrent use of anticoagulants, antiplatelets, or other drugs that affect platelet function.

A laboratory test interaction that can occur with thrombolytic drugs is a reduction in the plasminogen and fibrinogen levels.

## Dosages

For dosage information on alteplase, see the table on this page.

## DRUG PROFILE

All thrombolytic drugs exert their effects by activating plasminogen and converting it to plasmin, which is capable of digesting fibrin, a major component of clots.

### ◆ alteplase

Alteplase (Activase) is a pharmaceutically available t-PA made through recombinant DNA techniques. It is fibrin specific and therefore does not produce a systemic lytic state. In addition, because it is present in the human body in a natural state, its administration for therapeutic use does not induce an antigen-antibody reaction. Therefore, it can be re-administered immediately in the event of reinfarction. The drug t-PA has a very short half-life of 5 minutes. It is believed to open the clogged artery rapidly, but its action is short-lived. Therefore, it is given with heparin to prevent reocclusion of the affected blood vessel. Alteplase is available only in parenteral form. There is also a smaller dosage form known as Cathflo Activase that is used to flush clogged IV or arterial lines. Tenecteplase (TNKase) is a newer form of alteplase that is given by IV push after MI. Alteplase is also used in ischemic stroke.

### Pharmacokinetics

| Route | Onset of Action | Peak Plasma Concentration | Elimination Half-life | Duration of Action |
|---|---|---|---|---|
| IV | 30 min | 60 min | 26-50 min | Dependent on infusion duration |

## ANTIFIBRINOLYTIC DRUGS

The individual antifibrinolytic drugs have varying mechanisms of action, but all prevent the lysis of fibrin. Fibrin is the substance that helps make a platelet plug insoluble and anchors the clot to the damaged blood vessel (see Figures 26-1 and 26-2). The term *antifibrinolytic* refers to what these drugs do, which is to prevent the lysis of fibrin; in doing so, they actually *promote* clot formation. For this reason, they are also called *hemostatic* drugs. Their effects are opposite to those of anticoagulant and antiplatelet drugs, which *prevent* clot formation. Three synthetic antifibrinolytics are available—aminocaproic acid, tranexamic acid, and desmopressin. Dosages, indications, and other information appear in the associated Dosages table. There are also hemostatic drugs that are used *topically* (on the skin or tissue surface) in surgical settings to stop excessive bleeding. These include topical thrombin, microfibrillar collagen, absorbable gelatin, and oxidized cellulose.

Although not technically antifibrinolytic drugs, there are three drugs used for the treatment of hemophilia. These are produced by recombinant DNA technology, which eliminates the risk associated with obtaining them from human blood. Products currently available include rVII, rVIII, and rIX. As mentioned earlier, factors VII, VIII, and IX are important in the coagulation pathway. Warfarin also inhibits these factors. These products are used in patients with hemophilia and are also used in patients with severe bleeding due to warfarin therapy.

## Mechanism of Action and Drug Effects

The antifibrinolytic drugs vary in several ways. The various antifibrinolytic drugs and their proposed mechanisms of action are described in Table 26-5.

| TABLE 26-5 | ANTIFIBRINOLYTICS: MECHANISMS OF ACTION |
|---|---|
| **ANTIFIBRINOLYTIC DRUG** | **MECHANISM OF ACTION** |
| aminocaproic acid (Amicar) and tranexamic acid (Cyklokapron) | Form a reversible complex with plasminogen and plasmin. By binding to the lysine-binding site of plasminogen, these drugs displace plasminogen from the surface of fibrin. This prevents plasmin from lysing the fibrin clot. Therefore, these drugs can work only if a clot has formed. |
| desmopressin (DDAVP) | Works by increasing the level of factor VII (von Willebrand factor), which anchors platelets to damaged vessels via the glycoprotein Ib platelet receptor. It appears that desmopressin acts as a general endothelial stimulant, promoting the release of factor VIII, prostaglandin I2, and plasminogen activator. |

| TABLE 26-6 | ANTIFIBRINOLYTICS: ADVERSE EFFECTS |
|---|---|
| **BODY SYSTEM** | **ADVERSE EFFECTS** |
| Cardiovascular | Dysrhythmias, orthostatic hypotension, bradycardia |
| Central nervous | Headache, dizziness, fatigue, hallucinations, convulsions |
| Gastrointestinal | Nausea, vomiting, abdominal cramps, diarrhea |

The drug effects of the antifibrinolytics are very specific and limited. They do not have many effects outside of their hematologic ones. Aminocaproic acid and tranexamic acid inhibit the breakdown of fibrin, which prevents the destruction of the formed platelet clot. Desmopressin causes a dose-dependent increase in the concentration of plasma factor VIII (von Willebrand factor), along with an increase in the plasma concentration of tissue plasminogen activator. The overall effect of this is increased platelet aggregation and clot formation. This drug is also an analogue of antidiuretic hormone and is discussed further in Chapter 30.

## Indications

Antifibrinolytics are useful in both the prevention and treatment of excessive bleeding resulting from systemic hyperfibrinolysis or surgical complications. They have also proved successful in arresting excessive oozing from surgical sites such as chest tubes as well as in reducing the total blood loss and the duration of bleeding in the postoperative period.

Desmopressin may also be used in patients who have hemophilia A or type I von Willebrand disease. As stated earlier, recombinant factors VII, VIII, and IX are used to treat hemophilia or to stop the bleeding from excessive warfarin therapy.

## Contraindications

Contraindications to the use of antifibrinolytic drugs include known drug allergy to a specific product and disseminated intravascular coagulation, which could be worsened by these drugs.

## Adverse Effects

The adverse effects of antifibrinolytic drugs occur uncommonly and are mild. However, there have been rare reports of these drugs causing thrombotic events, such as acute cerebrovascular thrombosis and acute MI. The common adverse effects of antifibrinolytics are listed in Table 26-6.

## Interactions

When drugs such as estrogens or oral contraceptives are used concurrently with aminocaproic acid or tranexamic acid, additive effects may occur, resulting in increased coagulation. Few specific interactions have been reported for desmopressin, although use caution when giving to patients receiving lithium, large doses of epinephrine, heparin, or alcohol. Drugs such as chlorpropamide and fludrocortisone may potentiate the antidiuretic response, which may lead to edema.

## Dosages

For dosage information on aminocaproic acid and desmopressin, see the table on this page.

## DRUG PROFILES

### aminocaproic acid
Aminocaproic acid (Amicar) is a synthetic antifibrinolytic drug used to prevent and control the excessive bleeding that can result from surgery or overactivity of the fibrinolytic system. It is available in both oral and parenteral preparations.

## DOSAGES

### Selected Antifibrinolytic Drugs

| DRUG (PREGNANCY CATEGORY) | PHARMACOLOGIC CLASS | USUAL DOSAGE RANGE | INDICATIONS/USES |
|---|---|---|---|
| aminocaproic acid (Amicar) (C) | Hemostatic | **Adult**<br>IV infusion: 4-5 g during first hour, then 1 g at 1-hr intervals up to a daily max of 30 g | Excessive bleeding caused by systemic hyperfibrinolysis or urinary fibrinolysis |
| desmopressin (DDAVP) (B) | Synthetic posterior pituitary hormone | **Adult**<br>IV: 0.3 mcg/kg infused over 15-30 min; preoperative use: drug is administered 30 min before surgery | Surgical and postoperative hemostasis and management of bleeding in patients with hemophilia A or type I von Willebrand disease |

*IV,* Intravenous.

**Pharmacokinetics (aminocaproic acid)**

| Route | Onset of Action | Peak Plasma Concentration | Elimination Half-life | Duration of Action |
|-------|----------------|--------------------------|----------------------|-------------------|
| IV | Unknown | 1.2 hr | 2 hr | 3 hr |

### desmopressin

Desmopressin (DDAVP) is a synthetic polypeptide. It is structurally very similar to vasopressin, which is antidiuretic hormone, the natural human posterior pituitary hormone (see Chapter 30). Because of these physical characteristics, it is most often used to increase the resorption of water by the collecting ducts in the kidneys to prevent or control polydipsia, polyuria, and dehydration in patients with diabetes insipidus due to a deficiency of endogenous posterior pituitary vasopressin or in patients with polyuria and polydipsia resulting from trauma or surgery in the pituitary region.

Desmopressin also causes a dose-dependent increase in plasma factor VIII (von Willebrand factor), along with an increase in tissue plasminogen activator, which results in increased platelet aggregation and clot formation; thus it is often used to stop bleeding. Desmopressin is contraindicated in patients with a known hypersensitivity to it and in those with nephrogenic diabetes insipidus. It is available in both injectable and intranasal dosage forms. Desmopressin nasal spray is used for primary nocturnal enuresis.

**Pharmacokinetics**

| Route | Onset of Action | Peak Plasma Concentration | Elimination Half-life | Duration of Action |
|-------|----------------|--------------------------|----------------------|-------------------|
| IV | 15-30 min | 1-2 hr | 2 hr | Unknown |

## NURSING PROCESS

Coagulation modifiers have a variety of uses, including the following: (1) prevention or elimination of clotting in a peripherally inserted catheter (PIC, or PICC—a peripherally inserted central catheter), (2) maintenance of patency (without clotting) of central venous catheters, (3) clot prevention in coronary artery bypass grafting, (4) prevention of clotting after major vessel injury, (5) treatment of thrombophlebitis to prevent venous and/or arterial thromboembolism, and (6) prevention of clotting with use of prosthetics (e.g., heart valve replacements) and in atrial fibrillation. The drugs that are used for these different indications are varied in their mechanisms of action, and the related general and specific nursing process issues will be discussed.

## ASSESSMENT

Begin the nursing assessment associated with the use of all *coagulation-modifying* drugs by taking a thorough patient health history. This includes the following: any drug or food allergies, current medical problems, underlying systemic disease processes, past and present medical history, family health history, dietary habits, changes in body weight over time, ability to perform activities of daily living, level of exercise and/or degree of sedentary lifestyle, employment activities, success of previous treatment regimens, blood pressure, pulse rate, respirations, body weight, height, dietary intake, and fluid intake. A medication history is also needed and should include a listing of all drugs the patient takes on a daily basis such as prescription drugs, over-the-counter medications, herbal products, and dietary supplements, as well as nicotine, alcohol, and intake of other substances. Perform a thorough patient assessment to identify the presence of the following risk factors: immobility; history of limited activity or prolonged bed rest (e.g., generally for longer than 3 to 5 days); dehydration; obesity; smoking; congestive heart failure; mitral or aortic stenosis; coronary heart disease with documented atherosclerosis or arteriosclerosis; peripheral vascular disease; pelvic, gynecologic-genitourinary, abdominal, orthopedic, or vascular major surgery; history of thrombophlebitis, DVT, thromboembolism including pulmonary embolism, myocardial infarct, atrial fibrillation; edema of the periphery; trauma to the lower extremities; use of oral contraceptives; and/or recent extended airline travel time. If the patient has a history of clotting disorders and/or thromboembolism, assess and document the following: presenting signs and symptoms of thrombophlebitis of the leg such as calf edema; pain, warmth, or redness directly over the vessel (more indicative of a superficial clot); increased diameter of the calf of the affected leg; pain in the calf with dorsiflexion (often called the Homans sign; however, this is a very controversial method of assessment) or pain upon gentle compression of the calf muscle against the tibial bone; and presenting signs and symptoms of pulmonary embolism such as chest pain, cough, dyspnea, tachypnea, drop in oxygen saturation (by oximetry or blood gas measurement), hemoptysis, tachycardia, drop in blood pressure, and possible shock. All contraindications, cautions, and drug interactions also need to be assessed (see pharmacology discussion) and documented.

Because of the effects of *anticoagulants,* it is also important to assess the skin, oral mucous membranes, gums, urine, and stool for any evidence of bleeding. Assess patients for any blood in the urine or stool, easy bruising, excessive bleeding from tooth brushing or shaving, or unexplained nosebleeds while receiving these medications, and report any such findings. Laboratory tests performed before and during therapy with these drugs usually include, but are not limited to, baseline complete blood counts, hemoglobin level, hematocrit, lipoprotein fractionation, triglyceride and cholesterol levels, various clotting studies, and liver function tests. The serum laboratory tests that are usually ordered with anticoagulant therapy are presented in the Safety: Laboratory Values Related to Drug Therapy box.

With *heparin* and *LMWHs,* it is critical to patient safety to continually assess the skin to identify potential subcutaneous injection sites. For these injection sites, *avoid* any area within 2 inches of the umbilicus, open wounds, scars, open or abraded areas, incisions, drainage tubes, stomas, or areas of bruising or oozing. These sites would be at higher risk for further tissue damage with injection of the anticoagulant. Appropriate sites for injection of subcutaneous heparin and LMWHs include the upper, outer area of the arms, the thigh, and the subcutaneous fatty area across the lower abdomen and between the iliac crests (see Chapter 9 for more information).

With use of the *parenteral anticoagulant heparin*, to ensure patient safety and prevent injury, assess for allergies, contraindications, cautions, and drug interactions (see pharmacology discussion). Severe hypertension, ulcer disease, ulcerative colitis, aneurysms, malignant hypertension, alcoholism, and head injuries are all conditions in which a bleed is potential and possibly precipitated by parenteral anticoagulation. An important caution for heparin use is pregnancy or lactation; however, if there is a need for an anticoagulant during pregnancy, heparin is the drug of choice, not warfarin. Other information is presented in Table 26-1.

It is crucial to patient safety to remember that heparin is *not* interchangeable unit for unit with drugs in another class of anticoagulants, the LMWHs. It is important to know that heparin sodium contains benzyl alcohol; therefore, assess for allergy to this additional component. Although the use of *LMWHs* leads to fewer adverse reactions in some patients, these drugs are still associated with specific contraindications, cautions, and drug interactions (see previous discussion). When assessing the medication profile, remember that a potentially deadly medication error is to give heparin in combination with enoxaparin (or any LMWH). Always double-check that enoxaparin and heparin are never given to the same patient! The same assessment parameters discussed earlier for heparin are also appropriate for LMWHs. In addition, LMWHs contain sulfites and benzyl alcohol, and so assess the patient for allergies to these substances. It is important to note again that the LMWHs differ from standard heparin and also from each other and, for this reason, they are not interchangeable. LMWHs may be used for outpatient anticoagulant therapy because these drugs usually require less close monitoring than standard heparin. Assess the results of clotting studies prior to therapy.

The *oral anticoagulant* warfarin and its related contraindications, cautions, and drug interactions have been discussed earlier in this chapter. All of the previously mentioned assessment parameters are applicable to warfarin. Because of the drug's action, withdraw warfarin (as with all drugs altering bleeding/clotting)—as ordered—before the patient undergoes any dental procedures or if there is any evidence of tissue necrosis, gangrene, diarrhea, intestinal flora imbalances, or steatorrhea. Important to emphasize with this drug is the fact that warfarin is indicated for prophylaxis and long-term treatment of a variety of thromboembolic disorders (see previous pharmacology discussion), and constant and skillful assessment of the patient and clotting results is required. Most prescribers use standard protocols for warfarin to assist in dosing the drug based on PT/INR (the standardized measures of blood coagulability). The most common starting dosage for warfarin is 5 mg daily. However, the dose can range from 1 to 10 mg, and occasionally even higher (e.g., 12 mg) depending on individual patient response. In most situations, the dosage for adults is between 1 and 5 mg orally every day. In addition, it is important to understand the pharmacokinetics of warfarin, because it takes about 3 days for the drug to reach a steady state. Patients taking heparin may receive warfarin before discontinuation of heparin for anticoagulation.

Dabigatran (Pradaxa), although an anticoagulant, is the first oral *direct thrombin inhibitor*. Additional assessment parameters include renal function studies. No coagulation monitoring is needed for this drug. Assess for drug interactions with phenytoin and amiodarone. With fondaparinux (Arixtra), carefully assess renal function. As with dabigatran, its effect cannot be measured by standard anticoagulant tests. Liver function tests need to be assessed prior to the use of argatrobon.

With *antiplatelet* drugs, obtain a thorough nursing history and medication history as well as a physical assessment before beginning drug therapy. Possible drug interactions, cautions, and contraindications have been discussed, but close assessment of any bleeding is most important to patient safety. Because aspirin, other NSAIDs, and other antiplatelet drugs alter bleeding times, withhold these drugs as ordered for 5 to 7 days before the patient undergoes surgical procedures. Specific guidelines are generally given by the prescriber to avoid the concurrent use of other anticoagulants, antiplatelets, and fibrinolytics. See Chapter 44 for more information on aspirin. Perform a baseline cardiovascular assessment with clopidogrel and document any preexisting chest pain, edema, headache, dizziness, epistaxis, or flulike symptoms. Laboratory values usually include complete blood count, hemoglobin level and hematocrit, platelet counts, and PT and INR values. These laboratory values provide baseline levels with which therapy values can be compared. If platelet counts are at or fall below 80,000 cells/mm$^3$, notify the prescriber; antiplatelet therapy most likely will not be initiated (or will be discontinued).

In addition, it is important to patient safety to reemphasize the fact that aspirin is not to be used in children and teenagers, in patients with any bleeding disorder, in pregnant or lactating women, or in patients with vitamin K deficiency or peptic ulcer disease. These are situations in which major consequences could occur if aspirin were used; for example, Reye's syndrome in children and teenagers, teratogenic effects in pregnant women, and ulcers or bleeding tendencies in patients with vitamin K deficiency or peptic ulcer disease. Know how each of the drugs works in the body so that a sound knowledge base exists for critical thinking and decision making: for example, the decision to call the prescriber and not to administer two antiplatelets at the same time or not to give a thrombolytic with heparin, warfarin, or aspirin or other NSAIDs. This type of critical drug information is very important to make sure the patient receives the safest and most appropriate care during all phases of the nursing process.

The *GP IIb/IIIa inhibitors* (e.g., eptifibatide, tirofiban, and abciximab) require the same baseline assessment information (e.g., vital signs, medical history, history of chest pain or cardiac disease, complete blood counts, hemoglobin level, hematocrit, renal function tests, platelet counts) as well as assessment for any edema, bradycardia, and/or leg pain. Before or during therapy, if the platelet count is below 90,000/mm$^3$, contact the prescriber for further orders.

*Thrombolytics* require similar assessments, including attention to baseline complete blood counts and results of clotting studies. Additional concerns include a history of hypotension and cardiac dysrhythmias. The use of alteplase and other thrombolytics always carries major concerns/cautions, contraindications, and drug interactions (see previous pharmacology discussion). Constantly assess any arterial punctures, venous cut-down sites, peripherally inserted central catheter sites, and central infusion ports or sites for bleeding. Do not use IM injections in any situation, as they pose problems with bleeding. As with any drugs that alter clotting and platelet activity, the thrombolytics are associated with the risk of bleeding from wounds or from the gastrointestinal, genitourinary, or respiratory tract, so assess any drainage, urine, stool, emesis, sputum, and secretions for the presence of blood.

*Antifibrinolytics* require the same skillful assessment of baseline parameters and laboratory testing; however, there are additional concerns for patients with dysrhythmias, hypotension, bradycardia, convulsive disorders, nausea, vomiting, and abdominal pain or diarrhea. These are possible adverse effects and situations in which the prescriber may need to decrease the dosage of medication.

## NURSING DIAGNOSES

1. Deficient knowledge related to the new medication regimen and the need for altered lifestyle
2. Risk for ineffective cerebral tissue perfusion related to the clotting disorder, such as thrombus and subsequent embolus formation
3. Risk for injury related to possible adverse reactions to drugs altering blood clotting

## PLANNING

### GOALS

1. Patient demonstrates adequate knowledge regarding medication therapy and its potential adverse effects as well as the need for lifestyle changes.

2. Patient exhibits improved blood flow/tissue perfusion as a result of the therapeutic effects of the anticoagulant.
3. Patient remains free from injury resulting from either the disease or the medication being taken.

### OUTCOME CRITERIA

1. Patient states the adverse effects of the drug therapy, ways to monitor for complications of the anticoagulants, the importance of scheduling follow-up appointments with the prescriber and of frequent laboratory studies, and the circumstances under which to contact the prescriber to prevent complications such as hemorrhage.
   - Patient states the nature of and rationale for the lifestyle changes needed, such as improved diet, exercise, and avoidance of smoking.
2. Patient shows evidence of improved cerebral circulation with maintaining alertness, orientation and stable neurological status.
   - Patient's remains free of evidence of peripheral clotting with maintaining of pink, warm extremities with strong pedal pulses and/or experiences a return to his or her pre-disease state of maximal tissue perfusion.
3. Patient is free from bruising, bleeding problems, and any other injury to self because of safe medication use.

## IMPLEMENTATION

Routinely monitor vital signs, heart sounds, peripheral pulses, and neurologic status in all patients during and immediately after anticoagulant therapy. The various laboratory values to be monitored are presented in the Safety: Laboratory Values Related to Drug Therapy box on p. 440. If there is any change in pulse rate or rhythm, blood pressure, or level of consciousness, and/or unexplained restlessness occurs, contact the prescriber immediately. These changes may indicate bleeding or hemorrhage.

Knowledge of the proper techniques of administration is crucial for the safe and effective use of *heparin* and the *LMWHs* (see Box 26-1 for other dosing and route information). Heparin

## CASE STUDY

### Heparin Therapy

In the past 2 years, Mr. L., a 56-year-old architect, has experienced three episodes of deep vein thrombosis. All occurred without complications, and all were treated successfully with anticoagulant therapy and bed rest. He now arrives at the urgent care center because of increased pain and swelling in his left calf that has lasted for the past 3 days. Initially he is given 5000 units of heparin IV. On admission to the hospital for anticoagulant therapy, he is started on a continuous infusion of 25,000 units of heparin in 1000 mL of 0.9% sodium chloride.

1. What nursing actions should be implemented to ensure the accuracy and safety of the continuous heparin infusion?

2. What patient findings would indicate a therapeutic response to the heparin therapy?

   During Mr. L.'s hospital stay, the physician orders an extra bolus of 10,000 units of heparin, IV push, because the results of Mr. L.'s laboratory tests indicated that his activated partial thromboplastin time (aPTT) was not at a therapeutic level. After giving the dose, the nurse notices that a dose of 50,000 units was given instead of 10,000 units.

3. What will the nurse do first, and what subsequent orders will the nurse prepare to carry out?
4. How could this error have been prevented?

For answers, see http://evolve.elsevier.com/Lilley.

## BOX 26-1   ANTICOAGULATION THERAPY AND RELATED NURSING CONSIDERATIONS

### Subcutaneous Heparin and Low Molecular Weight Heparin Injections

- After thoroughly checking the prescriber's order, assess the patient for any allergies, contraindications, cautions, or drug interactions.
- Always begin by performing hand hygiene and maintain Standard Precautions. Gloves must be worn. Prefilled syringes are available. When the medication is not available in a prefilled or premeasured syringe use a ½ to ⅝ inch, 25 to 28 gauge needle. Check the site for bleeding or bruising, and do *not* massage/rub the site before or after the injection. *Do not aspirate* before injecting to prevent hematoma formation. See Chapter 9 for more information on the technique associated with heparin and LMWH injections.
- Make sure the patient is comfortable, and then remove gloves and wash hands. Document the medication given on the medication record, and monitor the patient for a therapeutic response as well as for adverse reactions.

### Intravenous Heparin Administration

- Always double-check the specific prescriber's order for dosage and rate of infusion before beginning therapy. Always follow the "Six Rights" of medication administration to prevent overdosing or erroneous dosing. Make sure the proper diluent is used. Check the compatibility of solutions or other drugs before beginning the infusion.
- For continuous intravenous (IV) administration of heparin, an IV pump must be used to ensure a precise rate of infusion.
- Continuous dosing is preferred over intermittent dosing because continuous dosing helps maintain blood levels of the drug and because intermittent IV dosing is associated with a higher risk for bleeding abnormalities.
- Treatment by continuous IV infusion generally begins with a loading dose and is followed by a maintenance dose. Be aware that dosage adjustments are made exactly as ordered. The patient's activated partial thromboplastin time (aPTT) and/or results of other related clotting studies are used as parameters for dosing of standard heparin.
- For intermittent infusions, a heparin lock was used in the past. Heparin locks are now referred to as *intermittent infusion locks* or *saline locks* (because the

locks are flushed with isotonic saline and not with heparin). The exception is with PICC lines and central lines in which heparin is still used as a flush.
- Intermittent infusions of heparin are usually ordered to be given every 4 to 6 hours because of heparin's short half-life. Needleless systems are used for intermittent infusions and all other types of IV infusions.
- Regardless of the type of IV infusion (e.g., intermittent or continuous IV infusion), it is crucial to check the site to determine whether infiltration has occurred so that hematoma formation may be prevented. If infiltration is suspected, remove the lock and replace at a new site before the next scheduled infusion. Document appropriately.
- The therapeutic dosage of heparin is guided by aPTT with a targeted level of 1.5 to 2.5 times the control (normal) value. The aPTT is measured within 24 hours of beginning therapy, 24 to 48 hours after therapy starts, and 1 to 2 times weekly for about 3 to 4 weeks on average. With long-term therapy, aPTT is monitored 1 to 2 times per month.

### Oral Anticoagulant Administration

- It is important to recheck the prescriber's orders and the patient's medication and medical history before administering any coagulation modifying drug. Always check to make sure the patient has no known hypersensitivity to the drug.
- Scored tablets may be crushed and may be given with or without food.
- Many more drugs can interact with oral anticoagulants than with heparin, especially those that are highly protein bound (see Table 26-3). Always check the patient's medication list before initiating therapy with warfarin.
- Dosages of warfarin are calculated based on international normalized ratio (INR) blood values. INRs are also used to monitor the effectiveness of therapy. Remember, however, that dosing is highly individualized!
- Oral anticoagulants are to be administered at the same time every day to maintain steady blood levels.
- Document the dose, time of administration, and any other pertinent facts with these and all other medications.

---

may be given by the subcutaneous or IV routes but *not* IM. You can easily avoid inadvertent IM injection if you use only subcutaneous syringes, which are usually made available in prefilled syringes that include a ½-inch (1.5-cm) 25- to 28-gauge needle. No major harm would result if a subcutaneous dose were inadvertently administered IV. If rapid anticoagulation is needed, IV heparin by continuous or intermittent infusion may be prescribed. Whether the drug is given by IV infusion or subcutaneous injection, monitor daily clotting study results, and perform these studies as ordered for therapeutic doses (monitoring is not done for prophylactic treatment).

The drug effects of heparin can be reversed with the IV administration of protamine sulfate. With subcutaneous heparin, several doses of protamine sulfate may be needed to reverse the anticoagulant effect because of the variable rates of absorption of this dosage form. See Box 26-1 for the procedure for the intermittent or continuous IV administration of heparin.

Administer *LMWHs* by subcutaneous injection deep into the injection site (see previous discussion) using the same techniques as for heparin. Rotate sites frequently. Avoid aspiration with subcutaneous injections to prevent hematoma formation and tissue injury. To avoid bruising, do not massage the site

after the injection. Prefilled syringes of LMWHs are available for inpatient use and for at-home treatment. Solutions may be clear to pale yellow. The usual length of therapy is approximately 5 to 10 days, and it is important to constantly be aware of any bleeding problems while the patient is taking this or other clotting-altering drugs. Complete blood counts, platelet counts, and stool tests for occult blood are tests that will probably be performed during therapy for monitoring purposes. Tests for occult blood in the stool can be done simply if occult blood test paper and developer are available. Blood in the stool may occur as an adverse effect of LMWHs or any clotting-altering drug.

When the *oral anticoagulant warfarin* is prescribed, therapy is often initiated while the patient is still receiving heparin. This overlapping is done purposefully to allow time for the blood levels of warfarin to rise, so that when the heparin is eventually discontinued, therapeutic anticoagulation levels of warfarin will have been achieved. The full therapeutic effect of warfarin does not occur until 4 to 5 days after the first dose. This overlap of activity is required in patients who have been receiving heparin for anticoagulation and are to be switched to warfarin so that prevention of clotting is continuous. Monitoring results of the various clotting studies is still of utmost priority, as is watching for any clotting or bleeding problems. The administration procedures for warfarin are outlined in Box 26-1.

For conversion from heparin to an oral anticoagulant such as warfarin, the dose of the oral drug is the usual initial dosage amount, with the prescriber using the PT/INR levels to determine the next appropriate dosage of warfarin. Once there is continuous therapeutic anticoagulation coverage and warfarin has reached therapeutic levels, the heparin or LMWH may be discontinued without tapering. If uncontrolled bleeding occurs with any of these medications, take action to control bleeding, institute emergency measures to stabilize the patient's condition, and contact the prescriber immediately.

The anticoagulant *dabigatran* (Pradaxa) is given orally. Important safety information about dabigatran (Pradaxa) from the U.S. Food and Drug Administration (FDA) includes that it is to be stored in and dispensed from its original bottle. This is important because if not stored properly and with the desiccant-drying agent (which absorbs moisture) in the packaging cap, the substance in the drug is easily broken down and a loss of potency occurs. This would result in less therapeutic effectiveness. This storage information is not widely disseminated and so it is important to be aware of these precautions. Additionally, the FDA is also alerting consumers that even though the label says to discard the drug after 30 days of opening the original container, recent data suggests that it can maintain its potency for up to 60 days if the cap is closed tightly after each use and the bottle is kept away from excessive moisture, heat, and/or cold. More information is to be released from the FDA once they complete further review of this product. The FDA suggests that Pradaxa be kept in the original bottle or blister package; not stored or placed in any other type of container; opened one bottle at a time; closed tightly after the capsule is removed; not used after 60 days; and have the blister package opened at time of use and not have the blister punctured prior to the use/administration of the drug. For more information, see www.consumermedsafety.org/alerts. *Fondaparinux* (Aristra) is given subcutaneously and, as with dabigatran, has no standard anticoagulant tests for monitoring.

Of benefit to counter the toxic effects of *anticoagulants* is the use of antidotes. The antidote to hemorrhage or uncontrolled bleeding resulting from heparin or LMWH therapy is protamine sulfate. For heparin, 1 mg of protamine sulfate given intravenously neutralizes 100 units of heparin. For the LMWHs, 1 mg of protamine sulfate neutralizes 1 mg of each LMWH given. It is important to note that too-rapid an infusion may lead to acute hypotensive episodes, bradycardia, dyspnea, and transient feelings of warmth and flushing. If the heparin overdose has resulted in a large blood loss, replacement with packed red blood cells may be necessary.

The aPTT ranges and hematocrit levels are generally used as ordered to monitor bleeding, clotting, and risk for bleeding. Always monitor the patient, especially for any changes in blood pressure and pulse rate. The antidote to oral anticoagulant (warfarin sodium) therapy is vitamin K. See the pharmacology section for more discussion on dosing and reversibility of vitamin K on the effects of warfarin. When given IV, vitamin K may lead to anaphylaxis with resultant dyspnea, dizziness, rapid or weak pulse, chest pain, and hypotension, which may progress to shock and cardiac arrest. Always check facility policy and the prescriber's order on the specific dosage and route of administration. Continual monitoring of the patient's vital signs, cardiac parameters, and bleeding times and other clotting study results are very important.

Constantly monitor the patient being treated with *antiplatelet* drugs (or any clotting-altering drug) for signs and symptoms of bleeding during and after their use, including epistaxis, hematuria, hematemesis, easy or excessive bruising, blood in the stools, and bleeding of the gums. If invasive procedures must be performed or injections given, apply appropriate pressure to bleeding sites, and closely watch all areas of venous or arterial catheter insertion for bleeding. Advise patients to take extended-release dosage forms in their entirety and without chewing or crushing. Enteric-coated aspirin is best taken with 6 to 8 oz of water and with food to help decrease gastrointestinal upset. To avoid irritation to the esophagus, instruct the patient to remain upright and not lie down for up to 30 minutes after the dose of aspirin. If the aspirin has a strong, vinegar-like odor, discard the drug. Interventions with clopidogrel therapy are similar to those for aspirin. Advise the patient to report the following if they occur: aches in the joints, back pain, dizziness, severe headache, dyspepsia, flulike signs and symptoms, and epigastric pain. These drugs are often discontinued for 7 days prior to surgery, as ordered. However, some surgical procedures (e.g., cardiovascular surgery) may warrant that the patient remain in an anticoagulated state intraoperatively. Oral forms of dipyridamole are recommended to be taken on an empty stomach; however, if this is not tolerated, the patient can take the drug with food. If nausea occurs, cola, unsalted crackers, or dry toast may help to alleviate this adverse effect. In addition, it may take up to 2 to 3 months of continuous therapy for the drug to reach therapeutic levels. Encourage patients to change positions slowly and to take their time in going from lying to sitting to standing because of the adverse effects of dizziness and postural hypotension with antiplatelets.

Nursing considerations associated with the *GP IIb/IIIa inhibitors,* such as abciximab, eptifibatide, and tirofiban, include some similar, yet different, nursing actions. Close monitoring of all vital signs, electrocardiogram readings, peripheral pulses, heart sounds, skin color, and temperature are an important part of nursing care during and after the use of these drugs. Because these drugs are used in combination with heparin to treat individuals suspected of having acute coronary syndrome or those undergoing percutaneous transluminal coronary angioplasty (PTCA), there is always concern for the stability of the patient as well as a high risk for serious bleeding and/or extension of an acute MI. The patient in this situation is at risk for other medical complications, and this risk may be intensified by the drug. Avoid further invasive procedures while the patient is taking these drugs to help prevent bleeding. If invasive procedures are required, constantly monitor for bleeding and measure all vital parameters before, during, and after the procedure. Protect IV tirofiban from light. Discard any unused solutions 24 hours after an infusion has been started. Do NOT give any other drugs with this drug except for heparin, which may be administered through the same IV line. For PCTA, abciximab can be given by bolus or by continuous infusion; closely monitor infusion rates. Manufacturer guidelines call for the use of a sterile, nonpyrogenic, low protein-binding 0.2- or 0.22-micron filter, and while the vascular shield is in position, keep the patient on complete bed rest with the head of the bed elevated 30 degrees. Maintain the affected extremity in a straight position, and constantly monitor peripheral pulses and the color and temperature of the distal extremities. Once the sheath is removed, apply pressure to the femoral artery for at least 30 minutes, either by manual or mechanical pressure. Apply a pressure dressing once bleeding has stopped. Closely monitor the site for any oozing or bleeding.

If serious bleeding occurs, discontinue the GP IIb/IIIa inhibitor and heparin (the usual protocol for PTCA) immediately, monitor the patient closely, and notify the prescriber immediately for initiation of emergency treatment. Always move and handle these patients with caution and avoid unnecessary trauma because of the risk for hematoma formation or bleeding. Do *not* take blood pressures in the lower extremities, but keep a close and constant watch on the patient's blood pressure (for hypotension) and pulse rate (for tachycardia). Also closely monitor the patient for any complaints of abdominal or back pain, severe headache, and any other signs or symptoms of hemorrhage. When adhesive or sticky tape is removed, take care to avoid tearing or ripping the skin, which would lead to tissue trauma and further risk for bleeding. Monitor aPTT levels after the procedure, and observe for bleeding, with attention to IM injection sites, arterial or venous puncture sites, and bleeding from nasogastric tubes and/or urinary catheters. Avoid such invasive procedures, if at all possible, during and immediately after the angioplasty.

Nursing considerations related to *thrombolytics* are very similar to those for the other drugs already discussed. Specifically, carry out the preparation for their IV administration per manufacturer guidelines and per protocol. Avoid invasive procedures during the use of these drugs. Avoid simultaneous use of anticoagulants or antiplatelets. Frequently monitor IV infusion sites for bleeding, redness, and pain. IM injections of other drugs are contraindicated to prevent tissue damage and bleeding. Report any bleeding from gums or mucous membranes or the occurrence of epistaxis or increased pulse (higher than 100 beats/min) to the prescriber immediately, and frequently monitor all vital signs. Other nursing considerations include monitoring for hypotension, restlessness, and a decrease in hemoglobin level or hematocrit, which are to be reported to the prescriber immediately (indicating possible shock). Advise patients to report pink, red, or cloudy urine; black, tarry stools or frank red blood in the stools; abdominal or chest pain; dizziness; or severe headache. The drug requires reconstitution for IV dosing with sodium chloride or 5% dextrose in water. Gently roll, not shake, the solutions to mix to maintain a stable solution. Continually monitor the INR, aPTT, platelet counts, and fibrinogen levels, beginning no later than 2 to 3 hours after the administration of thrombolytics. Measure the patient's fibrinogen level to check for the occurrence of fibrinolysis. With the breakdown

of fibrin (or fibrinolysis), INR will increase and aPTT will be prolonged. If bleeding occurs, the prescriber will most likely discontinue the drug and replace fibrinogen through infusions of whole blood plasma or cryoprecipitate. The antifibrinolytics, aminocaproic acid and tranexamic acid, may also be given. See the Patient Teaching Tips.

With *antifibrinolytics,* it is important to understand the reasons for the use of these drugs, such as to stop bleeding from overdosages of thrombolytic drugs or to control bleeding during cardiac surgery. Aminocaproic acid and tranexamic acid are usually given IV until bleeding is controlled. Because of the possibility of drug-induced internal, intracranial, and superficial bleeding, closely monitor the patient, and if there is any change in motor strength or level of consciousness, notify the prescriber immediately. You must apply your knowledge of certain adverse effects of drugs like these to prevent complications, maintain safety, and return the patient to a healthier state. It is also important to monitor heart rate and blood pressure with attention to the quality and strength of peripheral pulses. For the patient with hemophilia, tranexamic acid may be used to help decrease bleeding from dental extractions.

## EVALUATION

Monitoring for the therapeutic and adverse effects of coagulation modifier drugs is crucial for safe administration. Because these drugs are used for a variety of purposes, therapeutic responses vary. Some of the therapeutic effects include decreased chest pain and a decrease in dizziness, as well as in other neurologic symptoms. Adverse effects of *anticoagulants* include bleeding and hematoma formation (heparin); thrombocytopenia (heparin and LWMHs); bleeding, dizziness, shortness of breath, and fever (direct thrombin inhibitors); bleeding, hematoma, dizziness, and gastrointestinal distress (selective factor Xa inhibitors); and bleeding, lethargy, and muscle pain (warfarin). Early signs of drug overdose for any of the clotting-altering drugs (i.e., anticoagulants) include bleeding of the gums while brushing the teeth, unexplained nosebleeds or bruising, and heavier-than-usual menstrual bleeding. Abdominal pain, back pain, bloody or tarry stools, bloody urine, constipation, blood in the sputum, severe or continuous headaches, and the vomiting of frank red blood or a coffee ground–like substance (old blood) are all possible indications of internal bleeding.

Therapeutic effects of clopidogrel and other *antiplatelet drugs* include a decrease in the occurrence of clotting events such as transient ischemic attacks and strokes. The adverse effects of aspirin, as an antiplatelet drug, include dizziness, confusion, nausea, vomiting, gastrointestinal bleeding, diarrhea, thrombocytopenia, agranulocytosis, leukopenia, and neutropenia. Adverse effects of clopidogrel include chest pain, edema, flulike symptoms, headache, dizziness, fatigue, abdominal pain, diarrhea, and epistaxis. Therapeutic levels of anticoagulants and other clotting-altering drugs or coagulation modifier drugs are also monitored by laboratory studies such as aPTT, PT, and INR, which are described in the Safety: Laboratory Values Related to Drug Therapy box on p. 440. Remember, however, that aPTT levels are measured with heparin, whereas PT and INR are measured with warfarin. Once the level of the particular drug stabilizes and maintenance therapy is ongoing, the clotting studies may be performed at 1- to 4-week intervals, depending on the specific drug, the patient's response, and the patient's overall physical condition. If a heparin or LMWH overdose occurs, the antidote is protamine sulfate, whereas vitamin K, or phytonadione, is the antidote to oral anticoagulant overdose.

Continuous monitoring of the patient for the signs and symptoms of internal or external bleeding is critical during both the initiation and maintenance of therapy. Therapeutic effects of *thrombolytics* include improvement in cardiac status during an acute MI, improved blood flow from resolution of DVT, and improved neurologic status. Adverse effects include bleeding, hypotension, and cardiac dysrhythmias. Therapeutic effects of *antifibrinolytics* include the arrest of oozing of blood from a surgical site or a decrease in blood loss. Adverse effects to monitor for with the antifibrinolytics include orthostatic hypotension, dysrhythmias, headache, dizziness, fatigue, convulsions, nausea, vomiting, abdominal cramps, and diarrhea. Because of the complexity and life-threatening nature of the conditions for which these drugs are used, continually monitor and reevaluate the patient's response to the treatment, document this response accordingly, and always keep goals and outcome criteria within the plan of care to serve as a benchmark. From the evaluation phase, the patient will hopefully emerge experiencing full therapeutic effects and minimal adverse and/or toxic effects related to drug therapy.

## SAFETY: LABORATORY VALUES RELATED TO DRUG THERAPY

### Anticoagulants

| LABORATORY TEST | NORMAL RANGES | RATIONALE FOR ASSESSMENT |
|---|---|---|
| Activated partial thromboplastin time (aPTT), partial thromboplastin time (PTT)* | With heparin therapy, aPTT values need to fall between 1.5 and 2.5 times the control or baseline value. Normal control values are 25 to 35 seconds (sec). Target therapeutic level of anticoagulation is between 45 and 70 sec. | Therapeutic levels of aPTT indicate decreased levels of clotting factors and subsequent clotting activity and is the more sensitive part of PTT (and often replaces it). It is used to determine whether there are deficiencies in the patient's intrinsic coagulation pathway and to monitor heparin therapy. aPTT is sensitive to changes in blood clotting factors, except for factor VII. Therefore, it is used to assess for normal blood coagulation. With continuous IV infusions of heparin, blood samples for aPTT testing can be drawn at any time, but with intermittent infusions the blood sample is to be drawn approximately 1 hr before a dose of heparin is scheduled to be given. Monitoring of aPTT is not done for prophylactic doses (i.e., 5000 units every 12 hours subcut). |
| Prothrombin time (PT) | The normal control PT value ranges from 11 to 13 sec; target therapeutic level of anticoagulation is 1.5 times the control value, or about 18 sec. | Prothrombin is a vitamin K–dependent protein and a major component of the clotting process. It reflects clotting activity and is used to monitor the effectiveness of warfarin therapy. PT values vary for each laboratory center and are based on the specifics of the testing procedure. |
| International normalized ratio (INR) | Target levels of INR range from 2 to 3 or an average of 2.5. For individuals taking warfarin for treatment of recurring systemic clots or emboli and those with mechanical heart valves, the target INR may be 2.5 to 3.5, with a middle value of 3. | INR determination is a routine test to evaluate coagulation while patients are taking warfarin. When the therapy is initiated, the INR and PT are measured daily until a stable daily dose is reached (the dose maintains the PT and INR within therapeutic ranges and does not cause bleeding). INR values actually reflect the dose of warfarin given 36 to 72 hr prior to the testing. Advantages of INR testing include the fact that there is more consistency among laboratories and a more consistent warfarin dosage is achieved. Some laboratories report INR and PT together. |

*IV,* Intravenous.
*These terms are used interchangeably.

## ▮ PATIENT TEACHING TIPS

• The use of coagulation-modifying drugs to prevent serious complications related to clotting, such as strokes, heart attacks, clot formation (deep vein thrombosis of the legs) with heart valve replacements, and mini-strokes/TIAs (transient ischemic attacks), requires frequent and close monitoring. Educate the patient that a healthy lifestyle is an important part of therapy and will most likely include eating the right foods, weight reduction if needed, smoking cessation, control of blood pressure, and stress reduction. Advise the patient to provide a listing of all medications to all possible prescribers (e.g., dentists).

• Direct the patient to take all of the clotting-altering drugs exactly as prescribed because too little of the drug may lead to clot formation and too much of the drug may lead to bleeding. Regular follow-up appointments are an important part of patient care, with frequent blood tests to monitor for therapeutic effects and adverse effects of the medication. The results of the blood tests will help the prescriber determine the proper dosage.

• The patient must carry an identification card or wear a medical alert bracelet or necklace at all times stating allergies, medical diagnosis, list of drugs, prescriber's name and phone number, as well as an emergency contact name and number.

## PATIENT TEACHING TIPS—cont'd

- Home heparin therapy may require injections for a period of time, and LMWHs are generally used. If there is a switch from heparin to warfarin (Coumadin), there may be an overlap period of approximately 3 to 5 days during which both drugs are taken to allow therapeutic levels of the oral warfarin to be reached before the heparin is discontinued. This process may occur in the hospital or at home. Provide complete and thorough instructions to the patient, and use return demonstrations to evaluate learning (see Chapter 9).
- Advise the patient to report to the prescriber any unusual bleeding from anywhere on the body or the occurrence of a severe headache, blurred vision, vomiting of blood, dizziness, fainting, fever, muscular or limb weakness, rash, nosebleeds, or excessive vaginal or menstrual bleeding.
- With dabigatran (Pradaxa), educate the patient to protect the original bottle from moisture. Once a bottle is opened, it must be used within 60 days; this needs to be written on the bottle/label with the date of expiration. Instruct the patient to remove only 1 capsule from the opened bottle at the time of use and that the bottle needs to be immediately and tightly closed. Encourage the patient to take the medication with food if dyspepsia occurs. These capsules are *not* to be repackaged or placed in other pillboxes/organizers. For more information, visit www.pradaxapro.com.
- Journal keeping by the patient with daily notation of how the patient is feeling as well as how the patient is tolerating the medication and any adverse effects is beneficial to ensure safe, effective treatment.
- To reduce risk factors for cardiovascular disease, the prescriber may recommend consumption of a low-fat, low-cholesterol diet; cholesterol-lowering drug therapy; weight reduction; control of blood pressure if hypertension is present; avoidance of smoking; management of stress; and regular exercise.
- Teach the patient about clot-preventive measures, including situations to minimize sluggish circulation (e.g., avoid tight-fitting clothing, minimize sitting for prolonged periods of time, avoid crossing the legs at the knees and wearing of tight-fitting socks/stockings, avoid prolonged bed rest, make stops during long trips to walk around every 1 to 2 hours, keep well hydrated).
- When taking any of the anticoagulants (oral drugs and/or heparin or LMWHs) or clotting-altering drugs, encourage the patient to avoid brushing the teeth with a hard-bristled toothbrush, shaving with a straight razor, and/or engaging in any activity that would increase the risk for tissue injury. Always caution the patient when shaving, nail trimming, gardening, and/or participating in rough or contact sports.
- Instruct the patient to avoid ingesting large amounts of foods high in vitamin K (e.g., broccoli, Brussels sprouts, collard greens, kale, lettuce, mustard greens, tomatoes) while taking an anticoagulant to minimize food/drug interactions.
- Capsicum (red pepper), feverfew, garlic, ginger, ginkgo, and St. John's wort are some herbals that have potential interactions, especially with warfarin. Educate the patient about these and other interactions.
- Report any decrease in urine output; constant ringing in the ears; swelling of the feet, ankles, or legs; dark urine; clay-colored stools; abdominal pain; rash (use needs to be discontinued as ordered if rash occurs); and/or blurred vision to the prescriber immediately.
- If doses of medications are omitted, advise the patient to contact the prescriber for further instructions.
- Oral dosage forms of any of these medications are to be taken with at least 8 oz of water and/or with food to help minimize stomach upset.
- Keep all medication containers out of the reach of children, and use childproof tops. All syringes, needles, and other equipment must be kept out of the reach of children and other individuals as well.

## KEY POINTS

- Coagulation modifiers work by preventing/promoting clot formation, lysing a preformed clot, and/or reversing the action of anticoagulants. Coagulation modifiers include anticoagulants, antiplatelets, thrombolytics, antifibrinolytics, and reversal drugs.
- Warfarin prevents clot formation by inhibiting vitamin K–dependent clotting factors (factors II, VII, IX, and X) and is used prophylactically to prevent clots from forming; it cannot lyse preformed clots.
- The degree of anticoagulation (for any of these medications) is monitored by the PT.
- Heparin, given IV or subcutaneously, prevents clot formation by binding to antithrombin III, which turns off certain activating factors. The overall effect is to inactivate the coagulation pathway and prevent clots from forming. Heparin does not lyse (break down) a clot. Antiplatelet drugs prevent clot formation by preventing platelet involvement in clot formation.
- Thrombolytics are able to break down or lyse preformed clots in blood vessels such as those that supply the heart with blood. Therapeutic effects for which to monitor include improved tissue perfusion, decreased chest pain, and prevention of further myocardial damage. The therapeutic effects of most coagulation modifier drugs include improved circulation, improved tissue perfusion, decreased pain, and prevention of further tissue damage. Before giving these drugs, a thorough physical assessment should be performed as well as checking of pertinent laboratory values (e.g., INR, aPTT, PT).
- Antifibrinolytics prevent the lysis of fibrin, thus promoting clot formation, and have an effect opposite to that of the anticoagulants. Nursing care is very individualized and is based on the characteristics of the patient, thorough assessment data, existing medical conditions, and the specific drug.

## NCLEX® EXAMINATION REVIEW QUESTIONS

1 The nurse is monitoring a patient who is receiving antithrombolytic therapy in the emergency department because of a possible MI. Which adverse effect would be of the greatest concern at this time?
   a Dizziness
   b Blood pressure of 130/98 mm Hg
   c Slight bloody oozing from the IV insertion site
   d Irregular heart rhythm

2 A patient is receiving instructions regarding warfarin therapy and asks the nurse about what medications she can take for headaches. The nurse will tell her to avoid which type of medication?
   a Opioids
   b acetaminophen (Tylenol)
   c NSAIDs
   d There are no restrictions while taking warfarin.

3 The nurse is teaching a patient about self-administration of enoxaparin (Lovenox). Which statement should be included in this teaching session?
   a "We will need to teach a family member how to give this drug in your arm."
   b "This drug is given in the folds of your abdomen, but at least 2 inches away from your navel."
   c "This drug needs to be taken at the same time every day with a full glass of water."
   d "Be sure to massage the injection site thoroughly after giving the drug."

4 A patient is receiving dabigatran (Pradaxa), 150 mg twice daily, as part of treatment for atrial fibrillation. Which condition, if present, would be a concern if the patient were to receive this dose?
   a Asthma
   b Renal impairment
   c History of myocardial infarction
   d Elevated liver enzymes

5 A patient has received a double dose of heparin during surgery and is bleeding through the incision site. While the surgeons are working to stop the bleeding at the incision site, the nurse will prepare to take what action at this time?
   a Give IV vitamin K as an antidote
   b Give IV protamine sulfate as an antidote
   c Call the blood bank for an immediate platelet transfusion
   d Obtain an order for packed red blood cells

6 A patient is starting warfarin (Coumadin) therapy as part of treatment for atrial fibrillation. The nurse will follow which principles of warfarin therapy? (Select all that apply.)
   a Teach proper subcutaneous administration
   b Administer the oral dose at the same time every day
   c Assess carefully for excessive bruising or unusual bleeding
   d Monitor laboratory results for a target INR of 2 to 3
   e Monitor laboratory results for a therapeutic aPTT value of 1.5 to 2.5 times the control value

7 The order for enoxaparin (Lovenox) reads: Give 1 mg/kg subcut every 12 hours. The patient weighs 242 lb, and the medication is available in an injection form of 120 mg/0.8 mL. How many milligrams will this patient receive? How many milliliters will the nurse draw up for the injection? (Round to hundredths.)

1. d, 2. c, 3. b, 4. b, 5. b, 6. b, c, d, 7. 110 mg; 0.73 mL

For Critical Thinking and Prioritization Questions, see http://evolve.elsevier.com/Lilley.

# Antilipemic Drugs

**e**volve WEBSITE

*http://evolve.elsevier.com/Lilley*

- Animations
- Answer Key—Textbook Case Studies
- Critical Thinking and Prioritization Questions

- Key Points—Downloadable
- Review Questions for the NCLEX® Examination
- Unfolding Case Studies

## OBJECTIVES

When you reach the end of this chapter, you will be able to do the following:

1 Explain the pathology of primary and secondary hyperlipidemia, including causes and risk factors.
2 Discuss the different types of lipoproteins and their role in cardiovascular diseases and in hyperlipidemia.
3 List the overall drug classes and specific drugs that are used to treat hyperlipidemia.

4 Compare the various drugs used to treat hyperlipidemia with regard to the rationale for treatment, indications, mechanisms of action, dosages, routes of administration, adverse effects, toxicity, cautions, contraindications, and associated drug interactions.
5 Develop a nursing care plan that includes all phases of the nursing process for patients receiving antilipemic drugs.

## DRUG PROFILES

- ♦ **atorvastatin, p. 450**
- ♦ **cholestyramine, p. 451**
  **ezetimibe, p. 453**
  **gemfibrozil, p. 453**

- ♦ **niacin, p. 452**
- ♦ **simvastatin p. 450**

—————————
- ♦ *Key drug*

## KEY TERMS

**Antilipemic drugs** Drugs that reduce lipid levels. (p. 444)
**Apolipoproteins** The protein components of lipoproteins. (p. 444)
**Cholesterol** A fat-soluble steroid found in animal fats, oils, and egg yolk and widely distributed in the body, especially in the bile, blood, brain tissue, liver, kidneys, adrenal glands, and myelin sheaths of nerve fibers. (p. 444)
**Chylomicrons** Microscopic droplets made up of fat and protein that are produced by cells in the small intestine and released into the bloodstream. Their main purpose is to carry fats to the tissues throughout the body, primarily the

liver. Chylomicrons consist of about 90% triglycerides and small amounts of cholesterol, phospholipids, and proteins. (p. 445)
**Exogenous lipids** Lipids originating outside the body or an organ (e.g., dietary fats). (p. 445)
**Foam cells** The characteristic initial lesion of atherosclerosis, also known as a *fatty streak.* (p. 446)
**Hydroxymethylglutaryl–coenzyme A (HMG–CoA) reductase inhibitors** A class of cholesterol-lowering drugs that work by inhibiting the rate-limiting step in cholesterol synthesis; also commonly referred to as *statins.* (p. 448)

**KEY TERMS — cont'd**

**Hypercholesterolemia** A condition in which higher than normal amounts of cholesterol are present in the blood. High levels of cholesterol and other lipids may lead to the development of atherosclerosis and serious illnesses such as coronary heart disease. (p. 445)

**Lipoprotein** A conjugated protein synthesized in the liver that contains varying amounts of triglycerides, cholesterol, phospholipids, and protein; classified according to its composition and density. (p. 444)

**Statins** A class of cholesterol-lowering drugs that are more formally known as *HMG–CoA reductase inhibitors.* (p. 447)

**Triglycerides** Compounds that consist of fatty acids and a type of alcohol known as *glycerol.* Triglycerides make up most animal and vegetable fats and are the principal lipids in the blood, where they circulate bound to a protein, forming high-density and low-density lipoproteins (HDLs and LDLs). (p. 444)

## ANATOMY, PHYSIOLOGY, AND PATHOPHYSIOLOGY OVERVIEW

Key to understanding the use of antilipemic drugs is a working knowledge of the pathology of lipid abnormalities and their contribution to coronary heart disease (CHD). It is also important to understand, at the cellular level, the transporting and use of cholesterol and triglycerides in the human body. Lipoproteins, apolipoproteins, receptors, and enzyme systems are all integral parts of these processes. Armed with this knowledge, you can develop and implement a rational approach to treatment using both nonpharmacologic and pharmacologic interventions. See to the Safety: Herbal Therapies and Dietary Supplements boxes below and on p. 446 for information on some common dietary supplements patients may use to control hyperlipidemia.

## LIPIDS AND LIPID ABNORMALITIES

### Primary Forms of Lipids

Triglycerides and cholesterol are the two primary forms of lipids in the blood. Triglycerides function as an energy source and are stored in adipose (fat) tissue. Cholesterol is primarily used to make steroid hormones, cell membranes, and bile acids. Triglycerides and cholesterol are both water-insoluble fats that must be bound to specialized lipid-carrying proteins called apolipoproteins. The combination of triglycerides and cholesterol with an apolipoprotein is referred to as a lipoprotein.

## SAFETY: HERBAL THERAPIES AND DIETARY SUPPLEMENTS

### *Garlic* (Allium sativum)

**Overview**
Garlic obtains its pharmacologic effects from the active ingredient allicin.

**Common Uses**
Antispasmodic, antiseptic, antibacterial and antiviral, antihypertensive, antiplatelet, lipid reducer

**Adverse Effects**
Dermatitis, vomiting, diarrhea, anorexia, flatulence, antiplatelet activity

**Potential Drug Interactions**
May inhibit iodine uptake. May interact with warfarin, diazepam, protease inhibitors. Use with nonsteroidal antiinflammatory drugs may enhance bleeding.

**Contraindications**
Contraindicated in patients who will undergo surgery within 2 weeks and in patients with human immunodeficiency virus infection or diabetes.
Follow manufacturer directions on the bottle or box for use of specific preparations.

## SAFETY: HERBAL THERAPIES AND DIETARY SUPPLEMENTS

### *Flax*

**Overview**
Flax is a flowering annual found in Europe, Canada, and the United States. Both the seed and the oil of the plant are used medicinally.

**Common Uses**
Atherosclerosis, hypercholesterolemia, hypertriglyceridemia, gastrointestinal distress (especially constipation), menopausal symptoms, and bladder inflammation, among other uses

**Adverse Effects**
Diarrhea, allergic reactions

**Potential Drug Interactions**
Antidiabetic drugs: Theoretically can potentiate hypoglycemic effects
Anticoagulant drugs: Theoretically can potentiate anticoagulant effects by reducing platelet aggregation and prolonging bleeding time

**Contraindications**
Pregnancy (more information needed), bowel obstruction; use with caution in diabetes and cardiovascular disease
Follow manufacturer directions on the bottle or box for use of specific preparations.

Lipoproteins transport lipids via the blood. The various types of lipoproteins are classified according to their density and the type of apolipoproteins they contain. The lipoproteins and their classifications are presented in Table 27-1.

## Cholesterol Homeostasis

Cholesterol homeostasis involves a complex array of biochemical factors. Figure 27-1 summarizes the major concepts. Fats are taken into the body through the diet and are broken down in the small intestine to form triglycerides. Triglycerides are then incorporated into chylomicrons in the cells of the intestinal wall and are absorbed into the lymphatic system. The primary purpose of chylomicrons is to transport lipids obtained from dietary sources (exogenous lipids) from the intestines to the liver to be used to make steroid hormones, lipid structural components for peripheral body cells, and bile acids.

The liver is the major organ where lipid metabolism occurs. The liver produces very-low-density lipoprotein (VLDL) from both endogenous and exogenous sources. The major role of VLDL is the transport of endogenous lipids to peripheral cells. Once VLDL is circulating, it is enzymatically cleaved by lipoprotein lipase and then loses triglycerides. This creates intermediate-density lipoprotein (IDL), which is soon also cleaved by lipoprotein lipase to create low-density lipoprotein (LDL). Cholesterol is almost all that remains in LDL after this process. Any tissues that require LDL, such as endocrine cells, have LDL receptors. LDL and about half of IDL are reabsorbed from the circulation into the liver by means of LDL receptors on the liver.

High-density lipoprotein (HDL) is produced in the liver and intestines and is also formed when chylomicrons are broken down. Lipids that are not used by peripheral cells are transferred as cholesterol esters to HDL. HDL then transfers the cholesterol esters to IDL to be returned to the liver. HDL is responsible for the "recycling" of cholesterol. HDL is sometimes referred to as the *good lipid* (or good cholesterol) because it is believed to be cardioprotective.

If the liver has an excess amount of cholesterol, the number of LDL receptors on the liver decreases, which results in an accumulation of LDL in the blood. One explanation for hypercholesterolemia (cholesterol in the blood), therefore, is downregulation (reduced production) of hepatic LDL receptors. A major function of the liver is to manufacture cholesterol,

| TABLE 27-1 | LIPOPROTEIN CLASSIFICATION | |
| --- | --- | --- |
| LIPID CONTENT | LIPOPROTEIN CLASSIFICATION | PROTEIN CONTENT |
| Most | Chylomicron | Least |
| ↓ | VLDL | ↑ |
| | LDL | |
| | IDL | |
| Least | HDL | Most |

*HDL,* High-density lipoprotein; *IDL,* intermediate-density lipoprotein; *LDL,* low-density lipoprotein; *VLDL,* very-low-density lipoprotein.

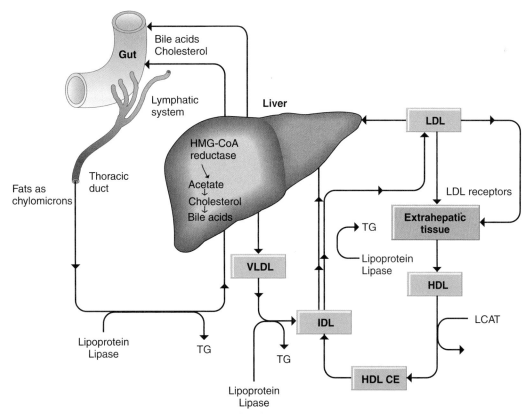

**FIGURE 27-1** Cholesterol homeostasis. *CE,* Cholesterol ester; *HDL,* high-density lipoprotein; *HMG-CoA,* hydroxymethylglutaryl-coenzyme A; *IDL,* intermediate-density lipoprotein; *LCAT,* lecithin cholesterol acetyltransferase; *LDL,* low-density lipoprotein; *TG,* triglyceride; *VLDL,* very-low-density lipoprotein.

a process that requires acetyl coenzyme A (CoA) reductase. Inhibition of this enzyme thus results in decreased cholesterol production by the liver.

## ATHEROSCLEROTIC PLAQUE FORMATION

Lipids and lipoproteins participate in the formation of atherosclerotic plaque, which subsequently leads to the development of CHD. When serum cholesterol levels are elevated, circulating monocytes adhere to the smooth endothelial surfaces of the coronary vasculature. These monocytes burrow into the next layer of the blood vessel (subendothelial tissue) and change into macrophage cells, which then take up cholesterol from circulating lipoproteins until they become filled with fat. Soon they become what are known as foam cells, the characteristic precursor lesion of atherosclerosis, also known as a *fatty streak*. Once this process is established, it is usually present throughout the coronary and systemic circulation.

## CHOLESTEROL AND CORONARY HEART DISEASE

Numerous epidemiologic trials have shown that as blood cholesterol levels increase, the incidence of death and disability related to CHD also increases. The risk for CHD in patients with cholesterol levels of 300 mg/dL is three to four times greater than that in patients with levels of less than 200 mg/dL. The incidence of CHD is lower in premenopausal women. This is thought to be secondary to the effects of estrogen, because the risk for CHD climbs considerably in postmenopausal women. However, there is controversy regarding this longstanding belief, because two major trials of estrogen replacement therapy (ERT) did not demonstrate prevention of cardiovascular events in women receiving ERT. Other experimental studies that looked for any benefits of low-dose estrogen therapy in male patients also failed to demonstrate significant cardioprotective efficacy.

Statistics show that half of all Americans, both male and female, will die of a heart attack. Thus, the goals of treatment are two-pronged: primary prevention of cardiac events in patients with risk factors and secondary prevention of subsequent cardiac events in individuals who have previously experienced a cardiac event (e.g., myocardial infarction). The benefits of cholesterol reduction for primary prevention have been illustrated in a number of trials. Results of some of the larger investigations support the view that, in patients with known risk factors for CHD, therapy with an antilipemic drug can reduce the occurrence of CHD. Drug therapy can also reduce first-time heart attack and death caused by heart disease. Benefits of cholesterol reduction for secondary prevention have been illustrated in a variety of trials as well. In patients with documented CHD, treatment with a cholesterol-lowering drug has many positive outcomes; decreased coronary events, regression of coronary atherosclerotic lesions, and prolonged survival.

Measures taken early in life to reduce and maintain cholesterol levels in a desirable range can have a dramatic effect in terms of preventing CHD. These include lifestyle modifications related to diet, weight, and activity level. Diets lower in

saturated fat and higher in fiber and plant chemicals known as *sterols* and *stanols,* and possibly the substitution of soy-based proteins for animal proteins, appear to promote healthier lipid profiles. These are among the dietary recommendations made by the National Cholesterol Education Program (NCEP) Adult Treatment Panel III (ATP III) of the National Institutes of Health. The consumption of fatty fish or dietary supplements containing omega-3 fatty acids appears to have beneficial effects on triglyceride and HDL levels and is currently recommended by the American Heart Association (AHA). The AHA also strongly emphasizes the substantial therapeutic benefits of even modest weight reduction and exercise in both improvement of lipid profiles and reduction of the likelihood of heart disease.

---

### SAFETY: HERBAL THERAPIES AND DIETARY SUPPLEMENTS

#### *Omega-3 Fatty Acids*

**Overview**
Omega-3 fatty acids are essential fatty acids, most commonly supplied as fish oil products. Several over-the-counter products are available, as well as one prescription product, known as Lovaza. Lovaza was originally named Omacor, but because of look-alike sound-alike errors that occurred with Amicar (aminocaproic acid, described in Chapter 26), the manufacturer agreed to change the name to Lovaza.

**Common Uses**
Cholesterol reduction

**Adverse Effects**
Rash, burping, allergic reactions, possible increase in total cholesterol or LDL levels in those patients with a combined hyperlipidemia, weight gain

**Potential Drug Interactions**
Anticoagulant drugs: May prolong bleeding time. There is a theoretical risk of increased bleeding with anticoagulant drugs, but the studies to date are inconclusive.

**Contraindications**
Pregnancy (more information is needed), allergy to fish oil
Follow manufacturer directions on the bottle or box for use of specific preparations.

---

## HYPERLIPIDEMIAS AND TREATMENT GUIDELINES

The decision to prescribe antilipemic drugs as an adjunct to dietary therapy in patients with an elevated cholesterol level is based on the patient's clinical profile. This includes the patient's age, sex, menopausal status for women, family history, and response to dietary treatment, as well as the presence of risk factors (other than hyperlipidemia) for premature CHD and the cause, duration, and phenotypic pattern of the patient's hyperlipidemia.

A major source of guidance for antilipemic treatment in the United States has been the NCEP, which is developed in close cooperation with major professional organizations such as the AHA. This program has two main focuses, both aimed at reducing the total risk for CHD. One is focused on the entire population and consists of general guidelines for the prevention of CHD. It emphasizes the appropriate dietary intake of total cholesterol and saturated fat, weight control, physical activity, and the control of other lifestyle risk factors. The other focus is on the management of individual patients who are at increased risk for CHD. The original guidelines for the detection, evaluation, and treatment of high serum cholesterol levels in adults were published in 1988 and 2001. They were updated again in July 2004 and will be updated in 2012.

The selection of dietary and drug therapy options is determined by the presence of certain risk factors. The latest guidelines are the first to include CHD risk equivalents. CHD risk equivalents have been statistically calculated to equate a person's 10-year risk for a major coronary event (e.g., myocardial infarction) for those patients who do not currently have CHD, but may have other diseases such as diabetes. These risk factors and risk equivalents are listed in Box 27-1.

When the decision to institute drug therapy has been made, the choice of drug is determined by the specific lipid profile of the patient. Five patterns or phenotypes of hyperlipidemia have been identified, and these are defined by the plasma (serum) concentrations of total cholesterol, triglycerides, and lipoprotein fractions (i.e., HDL, LDL, IDL, VLDL). The various types of hyperlipidemia are listed in Table 27-2. The process of characterizing a patient's specific lipid profile in this way is referred to as *phenotyping*.

One of the basic tenets of the NCEP guidelines is that all reasonable nonpharmaceutical means of controlling the blood cholesterol level (e.g., diet, exercise) are to be tried for at least 6 months and found to fail before drug therapy is considered. This is because the drug treatment for hyperlipidemias entails a long-term commitment to the therapy. Factors to be considered before the initiation of therapy are the type and magnitude of dyslipidemia, the age and lifestyle of the patient, the relative indications and contraindications of different drugs, potential drug interactions, adverse effects, and the overall cost of therapy. The 2004 NCEP guidelines recommend that all patients with LDL cholesterol levels exceeding 190 mg/dL and those with LDL cholesterol levels between 160 and 190 mg/dL who have CHD or two or more risk factors for heart disease be considered for drug therapy after an adequate trial of dietary and other nondrug therapies has proved ineffective. The treatment decisions made based on the LDL cholesterol levels are listed in Table 27-3. The updated guidelines also recommend optional use of drug therapy to reduce LDL to less than 70 mg/dL in patients at very high risk and to less than 100 mg/dL in patients at moderately high risk. "Very high risk" patients include those with active cardiovascular disease with other major risk factors such as diabetes, continued smoking, or *metabolic syndrome*. Metabolic syndrome is a set of risk factors associated with obesity, including hypertriglyceridemia and low HDL level. "Moderately high risk" patients include those without cardiovascular disease but with two or more risk factors. Box 27-2 lists the identifying features of metabolic syndrome.

There are currently four established classes of drugs used to treat dyslipidemia: hydroxymethylglutaryl–coenzyme A (HMG–CoA) reductase inhibitors (statins), bile acid sequestrants, the B vitamin niacin (vitamin $B_3$, also known as *nicotinic acid*), and the fibric acid derivatives (fibrates). In addition, a cholesterol absorption inhibitor, ezetimibe (Zetia), is also available. Vytorin is an example of a combination tablet that contains both the statin drug simvastatin and ezetimibe.

---

### BOX 27-1   CORONARY HEART DISEASE: RISK FACTORS

**Positive Risk Factors**
- Age: Males: 45 years or older
- Family history: History of premature CHD (e.g., MI or sudden death before 55 years of age in father or other male first-degree relative, or before 65 years of age in mother or other female first-degree relative)
- Current cigarette smoking
- Hypertension: blood pressure higher than 140/90 mm Hg or current antihypertensive drug therapy
- Low HDL cholesterol level: lower than 40 mg/dL
- Diabetes mellitus

**Negative Risk Factor**
- High HDL cholesterol: 60 mg/dL or higher—if the HDL cholesterol is 60 mg/dL or higher, subtract one risk factor

*CHD*, Coronary heart disease; *HDL*, high-density lipoprotein; *MI*, myocardial infarction.

---

### TABLE 27-2   TYPES OF HYPERLIPIDEMIAS

| | | LIPID COMPOSITION | |
| --- | --- | --- | --- |
| **PHENOTYPE** | **LIPOPROTEIN ELEVATED** | **CHOLESTEROL (mg/dL)** | **TRIGLYCERIDE** |
| I | Chylomicrons | Greater than or equal to 300 | Greater than 3000 |
| IIa | LDL | Greater than 300 | Normal ≈ 148 |
| IIb | LDL, VLDL | Greater than 300 | Normal ≈ 148 |
| III | IDL | Greater than 400 | Greater than 600 (1-3 times higher than cholesterol) |
| IV | VLDL | Normal or mildly elevated approximately equal to 250 | Greater than 400 |
| V | VLDL, chylomicrons | Greater than 300 | Greater than 2000 |

≈, Approximately equal to; *IDL*, intermediate-density lipoprotein; *LDL*, low-density lipoprotein; *VLDL*, very-low-density lipoprotein.

## TABLE 27-3 TREATMENT DECISIONS BASED ON LDL CHOLESTEROL LEVEL

| PATIENT CATEGORY | INITIATION LEVEL | LDL GOAL |
| --- | --- | --- |
| **Dietary Therapy** | | |
| Without CHD and with less than 2 risk factors (low risk) | Greater than or equal to 160 mg/dL (4.1 mmol/L) | Less than 160 mg/dL (4.1 mmol/L) |
| Without CHD and with greater than or equal to 2 risk factors (moderately high risk) | Greater than or equal to 130 mg/dL (3.4 mmol/L) | Less than 130 mg/dL (3.4 mmol/L) |
| With CHD (high or very high risk) | Greater than or equal to 100 mg/dL (2.6 mmol/L) | Less than 100 mg/dL (2.6 mmol/L) |
| **Drug Therapy** | | |
| Without CHD and with less than 2 risk factors (low risk) | Greater than or equal to 190 mg/dL (4.9 mmol/L) | Less than 160 mg/dL (4.1 mmol/L) |
| Without CHD and with greater than or equal to 2 risk factors (moderately high risk) | Greater than or equal to 160 mg/dL (4.1 mmol/L) | Less than 130 mg/dL (3.4 mmol/L) |
| With CHD (high or very high risk) | Greater than or equal to 130 mg/dL (3.4 mmol/L) | Less than 100 mg/dL (2.6 mmol/L) |

*CHD,* Coronary heart disease; *LDL,* low-density lipoprotein.

### BOX 27-2 METABOLIC SYNDROME: IDENTIFYING FEATURES

- Waist circumference greater than 40 inches in men or 30 inches in women
- Serum triglyceride level of 150 mg/dL or more
- High-density lipoprotein cholesterol level of less than 40 mg/dL in men or less than 50 mg/dL in women
- Blood pressure of 130/85 mm Hg or higher
- Fasting serum glucose level higher than 110 mg/dL

## PHARMACOLOGY OVERVIEW

### HYDROXYMETHYLGLUTARYL–COENZYME A REDUCTASE INHIBITORS

The rate-limiting enzyme in cholesterol synthesis is known as HMG–CoA reductase. The class of medications that competitively inhibit this enzyme, called the hydroxymethylglutaryl–coenzyme A (HMG–CoA) reductase inhibitors, are the most potent of the drugs available for reducing plasma concentrations of LDL cholesterol. Lovastatin was the first drug in this class to be approved for use, which occurred in 1987. Since that time, six other HMG–CoA reductase inhibitors have become available on the U.S. market: pravastatin, simvastatin, atorvastatin, fluvastatin, rosuvastatin, and pitavastatin. Because of the shared suffix of their generic names, these drugs are often collectively referred to as *statins.* Lipid levels may not be lowered to their maximum extent until 6 to 8 weeks after the start of therapy. Few direct comparisons of the statins have been reported in the literature. The following doses of drugs are considered to be "therapeutically equivalent," meaning they produce the same therapeutic effect: simvastatin 20 mg, pravastatin 40 mg, lovastatin 40 mg, atorvastatin 10 mg, fluvastatin 80 mg, rosuvastatin 5 mg, and pitavastatin 2 mg.

### Mechanism of Action and Drug Effects

Statins lower the blood cholesterol level by decreasing the rate of cholesterol production. The liver requires HMG–CoA reductase to produce cholesterol. It is the rate-limiting enzyme in the reactions needed to make cholesterol. The statins inhibit this enzyme, thereby decreasing cholesterol production. When less cholesterol is produced, the liver increases the number of LDL receptors to recycle LDL from the circulation back into the liver, where it is needed for the synthesis of other required substances such as steroids, bile acids, and cell membranes. Lovastatin and simvastatin are administered as inactive drugs or prodrugs that must be biotransformed into their active metabolites in the liver. In contrast, pravastatin is administered in its active form.

### Indications

The statins are recommended as first-line drug therapy for hypercholesterolemia (especially elevated levels of LDL cholesterol), the most common and dangerous form of dyslipidemia. More specifically, they are indicated for the treatment of type IIa and IIb hyperlipidemia and have been shown to reduce the plasma concentrations of LDL cholesterol by 30% to 40%. Their cholesterol-lowering properties are dose dependent; that is, the larger the dose, the greater the cholesterol-lowering effects. A 10% to 30% decrease in the concentrations of plasma triglycerides has also been observed in patients receiving these drugs. Another very important therapeutic effect of the statins is an overall tendency for the HDL cholesterol level to increase by 2% to 15%, a known beneficial factor that reduces risk (i.e., a negative risk factor) for cardiovascular disease.

These drugs appear to be equally effective in their ability to reduce LDL cholesterol concentrations. However, simvastatin, atorvastatin, and pitavastatin are more potent on a milligram basis. Atorvastatin appears to be more effective in lowering triglyceride levels than other HMG–CoA reductase inhibitors. Combined drug therapy with more than one class of antilipemic drug may be necessary for desired results. The statins are often combined with niacin or fibrates for this purpose, though this combination can increase the risk of adverse drug effects (see Adverse Effects).

### Contraindications

Contraindications to the use of HMG–CoA reductase inhibitors (statins) include known drug allergy and pregnancy. Other contraindications may include liver disease or elevation of liver enzyme levels.

| TABLE 27-4 | HMG-COA REDUCTASE INHIBITORS: ADVERSE EFFECTS |
|---|---|
| BODY SYSTEM | ADVERSE EFFECTS |
| Central nervous | Headache, dizziness, blurred vision, fatigue, insomnia |
| Gastrointestinal | Constipation, diarrhea, nausea |
| Other | Myalgias, skin rashes |

*HMG-CoA,* Hydroxymethylglutaryl–coenzyme A.

| TABLE 27-5 | HMG-COA REDUCTASE INHIBITORS: DRUG INTERACTIONS | | |
|---|---|---|---|
| DRUG | MECHANISM | EFFECT | |
| warfarin | Inhibit warfarin metabolism | Increased risk of bleeding | |
| erythromycin, azole antifungals, quinidine, verapamil, amiodarone, grapefruit juice, HIV and hepatitis C protease inhibitors, cyclosporine, clarithromycin, diltiazem, amlodipine | Inhibit statin metabolism | Increased risk of myopathy | |
| gemfibrozil | Potentiation | Increased risk of myopathy | |

## Adverse Effects

The HMG–CoA reductase inhibitors are generally well tolerated, and significant adverse effects are fairly uncommon. However, mild, transient gastrointestinal disturbances, rash, and headache are the most common problems and tend to be underreported in clinical trials. These and other less common adverse effects are listed in Table 27-4. Elevations in liver enzyme levels may also occur, and patients need to be monitored for excessive elevations, which may indicate the need for alternative drug therapy. Dose-dependent elevations in liver enzyme levels to values of more than three times the upper limit of normal have been noted in 0.4% to 1.9% of patients taking HMG–CoA reductase inhibitors. Serum creatine phosphokinase concentrations may be increased to more than 10 times the normal level in patients receiving these drugs. Most of these patients have remained asymptomatic, however.

A clinically important adverse effect is myopathy (muscle pain), which may progress to a serious condition known as *rhabdomyolysis.* The U.S. Food and Drug Administration (FDA) has issued public health advisories regarding reports of myopathy and rhabdomyolysis associated with the use of statins. Rhabdomyolysis is the breakdown of muscle protein accompanied by myoglobinuria, which is the urinary elimination of the muscle protein myoglobin. This abnormal urinary excretion of protein can place a severe strain on the kidneys, possibly leading to acute renal failure and even death. It appears to be dose dependent and is more common in patients receiving a statin in combination with cyclosporine, niacin, gemfibrozil (a fibrate), or erythromycin. Advise patients receiving statin therapy to immediately report to the prescriber any unexplained muscular pain or discomfort. When recognized reasonably early, rhabdomyolysis is usually reversible with discontinuation of the statin drug. Risk factors for myopathy include: age older than 65 years, hypothyroidism, renal insufficiency, and concurrent use of the immunosuppressant drug cyclosporine or the antihyperlipidemic drug gemfibrozil. Although these adverse effects are relatively uncommon, and although much benefit is often derived from the use of statin drugs, prescribers are advised to use minimal effective doses, with regular laboratory blood monitoring of liver and kidney function (every 3 to 6 months). Educate patients regarding these serious adverse drug effects, and instruct them to immediately report any signs of toxicity, including muscle soreness, changes in urine color, fever, malaise, nausea, or vomiting. In 2011, the FDA imposed new restrictions on simvastatin, which are discussed in detail in its Drug Profile. In 2012, the FDA required added warnings including memory loss, confusion, increase in blood glucose levels and glycosylated hemoglobin (HbA-1c) levels, dosage limitations to lovastatin, and drug interactions with HIV and hepatits C medications.

## Toxicity and Management of Overdose

Very limited data are available on the nature of toxicity and overdose in patients taking HMG–CoA reductase inhibitors. Treatment, if needed, is supportive and based on presenting symptoms.

## Interactions

Drug interactions with the HMG–CoA reductase inhibitors are listed in Table 27-5. They are to be used cautiously in patients taking oral anticoagulants. In addition, the coadministration of the statins with drugs that are metabolized by cytochrome P-450 enzyme 3A4 (CYP3A4) (see Chapter 2), such as erythromycin, azole antifungals, verapamil, diltiazem, HIV and hepatitis C protease inhibitors, amiodarone, and grapefruit juice, may lead to the development of rhabdomyolysis. Patients are advised to limit grapefruit juice to less than 1 quart daily, which is probably more than most people drink. The mechanism for most significant drug interactions involves inhibition of the metabolic protein CYP3A4. The following example involving grapefruit juice illustrates the interaction. Components in grapefruit juice inactivate CYP3A4 in both the liver and intestines. This enzyme plays a key role in statin metabolism. The presence of grapefruit juice in the body results in sustained levels of unmetabolized statin drug, which increases the risk for major drug toxicity (e.g., rhabdomyolysis). Pravastatin and fluvastatin inhibit CYP3A4 to a much smaller degree than the other statins, whereas lovastatin and simvastatin are the most potent inhibitors of this enzyme. The use of gemfibrozil and statins together is not generally recommended due to increased risk of rhabdomyolysis.

## Laboratory Test Interactions

Laboratory interactions that can occur include increases in ALT levels and activated clotting time, thrombocytopenia, and transient eosinophilia.

## Dosages

For dosage information on atorvastatin, see the table on p. 450.

## DOSAGES

### Selected Antilipemic Drugs

| DRUG (PREGNANCY CATEGORY) | PHARMACOLOGIC CLASS | USUAL DOSAGE RANGE | INDICATIONS |
|---|---|---|---|
| ♦ atorvastatin (Lipitor) (X) | HMG–CoA reductase inhibitor | **Adult**<br>PO: 10-80 mg/day | |
| ♦ cholestyramine (Questran) (C) | Bile acid sequestrant | **Adult**<br>PO: 4-16 g/day | |
| ezetimibe (Zetia) (C) | Cholesterol absorption inhibitor | **Adult**<br>PO: 10 mg 1×/day | Hyperlipidemia |
| gemfibrozil (Lopid) (C) | Fibric acid derivative | **Adult**<br>PO: 600 mg bid 30 min ac in AM and PM | |
| ♦ niacin (nicotinic acid, vitamin $B_3$) (A; C if dose exceeds RDA) | B vitamin | **Adult**<br>PO: 1.5 to 6 g/day in 2-4 divided doses. | |
| simvastatin (Zocor) (X) | HMG–CoA reductase inhibitor | **Adult**<br>PO: 5-40 mg daily | |

*HMG–CoA,* Hydroxymethylglutaryl–coenzyme A; *PO,* oral; *RDA,* recommended daily allowance.

## DRUG PROFILES

The HMG–CoA reductase inhibitors, or statins, are all potent inhibitors of the enzyme that catalyzes the rate-limiting step in the synthesis of cholesterol. Seven statins are currently on the market in the United States: atorvastatin (Lipitor), fluvastatin (Lescol), lovastatin (Mevacor), pravastatin (Pravachol), simvastatin (Zocor), rosuvastatin (Crestor), and pitavastatin (Livalo). There are some minor differences between drugs in this class of antilipemics; the most dramatic difference is that of potency. All statins are prescription-only drugs and are contraindicated in those with active liver dysfunction or elevated serum transaminase levels of unknown cause. They are classified as pregnancy category X drugs and are to be avoided during pregnancy and lactation. There is little evidence to recommend one drug over another.

### ♦ atorvastatin

Atorvastatin (Lipitor) has become one of the most commonly used drugs in this class of cholesterol-lowering drugs. It is used to lower total and LDL cholesterol levels as well as triglyceride levels. Atorvastatin has also been shown to raise levels of "good" cholesterol, the HDL component. All statins are dosed once daily, usually with the evening meal or at bedtime. One particular advantage of atorvastatin is that it can be dosed at any time of day. However, bedtime dosing provides peak drug levels in a time frame that correlates better with the natural *diurnal* (daytime) rhythm of cholesterol production in the body. The recommended dosage for atorvastatin is 10 to 80 mg daily. It is available only in tablet form in strengths of 10, 20, 40, and 80 mg. It is classified as a pregnancy category X drug.

### Pharmacokinetics

| Route | Onset of Action | Peak Plasma Concentration | Elimination Half-life | Duration of Action |
|---|---|---|---|---|
| PO | 0.5 hr | 1-2 hr | 7-14 hr | Unknown |

### ♦ simvastatin

Simvastatin (Zocor) was the one of the first statins to become generic and is one of the most commonly used drugs in this class. As with all statins, it is used primarily to lower total and LDL cholesterol levels as well as triglyceride levels. It can also modestly raise levels of HDL, the "good" cholesterol. The recommended dosage for simvastatin is 5 to 40 mg daily. It is available only in tablet form in strengths of 10, 20, 40, and 80 mg. It is classified as a pregnancy category X drug. In 2011, the FDA imposed new prescribing restrictions on simvastatin, stating "Physicians should limit using the 80-mg dose unless the patient has already been taking the drug for 12 months and there is no evidence of myopathy. Simvastatin 80 mg should not be started in new patients, including patients already taking lower doses of the drug." In addition, simvastatin is not to be used with certain other drugs including itraconazole, ketoconazole, posaconazole, erythromycin, clarithromycin, telithromycin, HIV protease inhibitors, nefazodone, femfibrozil, cyclosporine, and danazol. In patients taking verapamil and diltiazem, the dose of simvastatin is not to exceed 10 mg. In patients taking amiodarone, amlodipine, and ranolazine, the dose is not to exceed 20 mg.

### Pharmacokinetics

| Route | Onset of Action | Peak Plasma Concentration | Elimination Half-life | Duration of Action |
|---|---|---|---|---|
| PO | 3 days | 1.3-2.4 hr | Unknown | Unknown |

## BILE ACID SEQUESTRANTS

Bile acid sequestrants, also called *bile acid–binding resins* and *ion-exchange resins,* include cholestyramine, colestipol, and colesevelam. The first two of these drugs have been used widely for more than 20 years and have been evaluated extensively in well-controlled clinical trials. They have proven efficacy, but their powdered forms are somewhat inconvenient to use.

Colestipol is also available in tablet form. Colesevelam has a similar mechanism of action and is available only in tablet form. These drugs are considered second-line drugs after the more potent statins. They are suitable alternatives for patients intolerant of the statins. Generally these drugs lower the plasma concentrations of LDL cholesterol by 15% to 30%. They also increase the HDL cholesterol level by 3% to 8% and increase hepatic triglyceride and VLDL production, which may result in a 10% to 50% increase in the triglyceride level.

## Mechanism of Action and Drug Effects

Bile acid sequestrants bind bile and prevent the resorption of the bile acids from the small intestine. An insoluble bile acid and resin (drug) complex is formed and then excreted in the bowel movement. Bile acids are necessary for the absorption of cholesterol from the small intestine and are also synthesized from cholesterol by the liver. This is one natural way that the liver excretes cholesterol from the body. The more that bile acids are excreted in the feces, the more the liver converts cholesterol to bile acids. This reduces the level of cholesterol in the liver and thus in the circulation as well. The liver then attempts to compensate for the loss of cholesterol by increasing the number of LDL receptors on its surface. Circulating LDL molecules bind to these receptors to be taken up into the liver, which has the benefit of reducing circulating LDL in the bloodstream.

## Indications

Bile acid sequestrants may be used as primary or adjunct drug therapy in the management of type II hyperlipoproteinemia. A common strategy is to use them along with statins for an additive drug effect in reducing LDL cholesterol levels. In addition, cholestyramine is used to relieve the pruritus associated with partial biliary obstruction. Colesevelam may be better tolerated by higher-risk patients who are intolerant of other antilipemic therapy, including organ transplant recipients and those with serious liver or kidney disease.

## Contraindications

Contraindications to the use of bile acid sequestrants include known drug allergy, biliary or bowel obstruction, and phenylketonuria (PKU).

## Adverse Effects

The adverse effects of colestipol, cholestyramine, and colesevelam are similar; however, colesevelam is reported to have fewer gastrointestinal adverse effects and drug interactions. Constipation is a common problem and may be accompanied by heartburn, nausea, belching, and bloating. These adverse effects tend to disappear over time. Many patients require extra education and support to help them deal with the gastrointestinal effects and comply with the medication regimen. It is important that therapy be initiated with low dosages and that patients be instructed to take the drugs with meals to reduce the adverse effects. Increasing dietary fiber intake or taking a fiber supplement such as psyllium (Metamucil and others), as well as increasing fluid intake, may relieve constipation and bloating. These drugs may also cause mild increases in triglyceride levels.

| TABLE 27-6 | BILE ACID SEQUESTRANTS: ADVERSE EFFECTS |
|---|---|
| **BODY SYSTEM** | **ADVERSE EFFECTS** |
| Gastrointestinal | Constipation, nausea, belching, bloating |
| Other | Headache, tinnitus, burnt odor of urine |

The most common adverse effects of the bile acid sequestrants are listed in Table 27-6.

### Toxicity and Management of Overdose

Because the bile acid sequestrants are not absorbed, an overdose can cause obstruction of the gastrointestinal tract. Therefore, treatment of an overdose involves restoring gut motility.

### Interactions

The significant drug interactions associated with the use of bile acid sequestrants are limited to effects on the absorption of concurrently administered drugs. All drugs must be taken at least 1 hour before or 4 to 6 hours after the administration of bile acid sequestrants. In addition, high doses of a bile acid sequestrant decrease the absorption of fat-soluble vitamins (A, D, E, and K).

### Dosages

For dosage information on a selected bile acid sequestrant, see the table on p. 450.

## DRUG PROFILE

The bile acid sequestrants cholestyramine, colestipol, and colesevelam are indicated for the treatment of type IIa and IIb hyperlipidemia. They lower the cholesterol level, in particular the LDL cholesterol level, by increasing the destruction of LDL. However, their use may result in increases in the VLDL cholesterol level. Because of the high incidence of gastrointestinal adverse effects, adherence to the prescribed dosage schedules is often poor. However, educating patients about the purpose and expected adverse effects of therapy can foster improved adherence. Warn patients not to take bile acid sequestrants at the same time as other drugs because of reduced absorption. Other drugs must be taken at least 1 hour before or 4 to 6 hours after the bile sequestrant. This requirement cannot be overemphasized.

#### ◆ cholestyramine

Cholestyramine (Questran) is a prescription-only drug that is contraindicated in patients with a known hypersensitivity to it and in those who have complete biliary obstruction or PKU. It may interfere with the distribution of proper amounts of fat-soluble vitamins to the fetus or nursing infant of a pregnant or nursing woman taking the drug. Cholestyramine is now being used for its constipating effect, often given as needed for loose bowel movements.

## NIACIN

Niacin, or nicotinic acid, is not only a very unique lipid-lowering drug, it is also a vitamin. Much larger doses of the drug are required for its lipid-lowering effects than are commonly

## TABLE 27-7 NIACIN (NICOTINIC ACID): ADVERSE EFFECTS

| BODY SYSTEM | ADVERSE EFFECTS |
| --- | --- |
| Gastrointestinal | Abdominal discomfort |
| Integumentary | Cutaneous flushing, pruritus |
| Other | Blurred vision, glucose intolerance, hepatotoxicity |

given when it is used as a vitamin. Niacin is a B vitamin, specifically vitamin $B_3$. It is an effective and inexpensive medication that exerts favorable effects on the plasma concentrations of all lipoproteins. Niacin is often given in combination with other antilipemic drugs to enhance the lipid-lowering effects.

## Mechanism of Action and Drug Effects

Although the exact mechanism of action of niacin is unknown, the beneficial effects are believed to be related to its ability to inhibit lipolysis in adipose tissue, decrease esterification of triglycerides in the liver, and increase the activity of lipoprotein lipase. The drug effects are primarily limited to reduction of the metabolism or catabolism of cholesterol and triglycerides. Niacin decreases the LDL levels moderately (10% to 20%), decreases the triglyceride levels (30% to 70%), and increases the HDL levels moderately (20% to 35%). Niacin is also a vitamin needed for many bodily processes. In large doses, it may produce vasodilatation that is limited to the cutaneous vessels. This effect seems to be induced by prostaglandins. Niacin also causes the release of histamine, which results in an increase in gastric motility and acid secretion. Niacin may also stimulate the fibrinolytic system to break down fibrin clots.

## Indications

Niacin has been shown to be effective in lowering lipid levels, including triglyceride, total serum cholesterol, and LDL cholesterol levels. It also increases HDL cholesterol levels. Niacin may also lower the levels of lipoprotein (a), except in patients with severe hypertriglyceridemia. It has been shown to be effective in the treatment of type IIa, IIb, III, IV, and V hyperlipidemia. Niacin's effects on triglyceride levels begin to be noticed after 1 to 4 days of therapy, with the maximum effects seen after 3 to 5 weeks of continuous therapy.

## Contraindications

Contraindications to the use of niacin include known drug allergy and may include liver disease, hypertension, peptic ulcer, and the presence of any active hemorrhagic process.

## Adverse Effects

Niacin can cause flushing, pruritus, and gastrointestinal distress. Small doses of aspirin or nonsteroidal antiinflammatory drugs (NSAIDs) may be taken 30 minutes before the niacin dose to minimize the cutaneous flushing. These undesirable effects can also be minimized by starting patients on a low initial dosage and increasing it gradually, and by having patients take the drug with meals. The most common adverse effects associated with niacin therapy are listed in Table 27-7.

## Interactions

Drug interactions associated with niacin are minimal. However, when niacin is taken with an HMG–CoA reductase inhibitor, the likelihood of myopathy development is greatly increased, although it is not uncommon to see these drugs used together.

## Dosages

For dosage information on niacin, see the table on p. 450.

## DRUG PROFILE

### ♦ niacin

Used alone or in combination with other lipid-lowering drugs, niacin (nicotinic acid, vitamin $B_3$) (Nicobid) is a very effective, inexpensive medication that has beneficial effects on LDL cholesterol, triglyceride, and HDL cholesterol levels. Drug therapy is usually initiated at a small daily dose taken with or after meals to minimize the adverse effects. Liver dysfunction has been observed in individuals taking sustained-release forms of niacin, but not immediate-release forms. Extended-release dosage forms, which dissolve more slowly than the immediate-release but faster than the sustained-release forms, appear to have better adverse effect profiles, including less hepatotoxicity and flushing of the skin. Niacin is contraindicated in patients who have shown a hypersensitivity to it; in those with peptic ulcer, hepatic disease, hemorrhage, or severe hypotension; and in lactating women. It is also not recommended for patients with gout. Niacin is available over the counter and by prescription.

### Pharmacokinetics

| Route | Onset of Action | Peak Plasma Concentration | Elimination Half-life | Duration of Action |
| --- | --- | --- | --- | --- |
| PO | Rapid | 30-60 min | 45 min | Unknown |

## FIBRIC ACID DERIVATIVES

Current fibric acid derivatives include gemfibrozil and fenofibrate. These drugs primarily affect the triglyceride levels but may also lower the total cholesterol and LDL cholesterol levels and raise the HDL cholesterol level. They are often collectively referred to as *fibrates*.

## Mechanism of Action and Drug Effects

Fibric acid drugs are believed to work by activating lipoprotein lipase, an enzyme responsible for the breakdown of cholesterol. This enzyme usually cleaves off a triglyceride molecule from VLDL or LDL, leaving behind lipoproteins. Fibric acid derivatives also suppress the release of free fatty acid from adipose tissue, inhibit the synthesis of triglycerides in the liver, and increase the secretion of cholesterol into bile. They have been shown to reduce triglyceride levels and serum VLDL and LDL concentrations. Independent of their lipid-lowering actions, fibric acid derivatives can also induce changes in blood coagulation. This involves a tendency toward a decrease in platelet adhesiveness. They can also increase plasma fibrinolysis, the process that causes fibrin, and therefore clots, to be broken down.

| TABLE 27-8 | FIBRIC ACID DERIVATIVES: ADVERSE EFFECTS |
|---|---|
| **BODY SYSTEM** | **ADVERSE EFFECTS** |
| Gastrointestinal | Nausea, vomiting, diarrhea, gallstones |
| Genitourinary | Impotence, decreased urine output, hematuria |
| Other | Drowsiness, dizziness, rash, pruritus, vertigo |

## Indications

The fibric acid derivatives gemfibrozil and fenofibrate decrease the triglyceride level and increase the HDL cholesterol level by as much as 25%. Both decrease the LDL concentrations in patients with type IIa and IIb hyperlipidemia but increase the LDL levels in patients with type IV and V hyperlipidemia. They are indicated for the treatment of type III, IV, and V hyperlipidemia, and in some cases the type IIb form, although other classes of antilipemics are usually tried first.

## Contraindications

Contraindications to the use of fibrates include known drug allergy and may include severe liver or kidney disease, cirrhosis, and gallbladder disease.

## Adverse Effects

The most common adverse effects of the fibric acid derivatives are abdominal discomfort, diarrhea, nausea, headache, blurred vision, increased risk for gallstones, and prolonged prothrombin time. Liver function tests may also show increased enzyme levels. The more common adverse effects are listed in Table 27-8.

### Toxicity and Management of Overdose

The management of fibrate overdose, which is uncommon, is supportive care based on presenting symptoms.

## Interactions

Gemfibrozil can enhance the action of oral anticoagulants, thus careful adjustment of the dosage of warfarin is required. The risk for myositis, myalgias, and rhabdomyolysis is increased when either gemfibrozil or fenofibrate is given with a statin. Combining gemfibrozil with a statin is generally not recommended due to an increased risk of rhabdomyolysis. Laboratory test interactions that can occur in patients taking gemfibrozil include a decrease in the hemoglobin level, hematocrit value, and white blood cell count. In addition, the aspartate aminotransferase level, activated clotting time, lactate dehydrogenase level, and bilirubin level can be increased.

Fenofibrate may raise the blood level of ezetimibe if the two are taken concurrently.

## Dosages

For dosage information on gemfibrozil, see the table on p. 450.

## DRUG PROFILES

### FIBRIC ACID DERIVATIVES (FIBRATES)

The fibric acid derivatives gemfibrozil and fenofibrate are prescription-only drugs and are the only two drugs available in this class. They are both classified as pregnancy category C drugs and are contraindicated in patients with a known hypersensitivity, preexisting gallbladder disease, significant hepatic or renal dysfunction, and primary biliary cirrhosis. Both drugs decrease the triglyceride levels and increase the HDL levels by as much as 25%. They are good drugs for the treatment of mixed hyperlipidemias.

#### gemfibrozil

Gemfibrozil (Lopid) is a fibric acid derivative that decreases the synthesis of apolipoprotein B and lowers the VLDL level. It can also increase the HDL level. It is highly effective for lowering plasma triglyceride levels. In a landmark study reported in 1987 in the *New England Journal of Medicine,* known as the Helsinki study, the triglyceride levels of the group receiving gemfibrozil were reduced by as much as 43% compared with those in the control group. Total cholesterol and LDL cholesterol levels were reduced by 11% and 10%, respectively, and the HDL level was increased by 10%. Gemfibrozil is indicated for the treatment of type IV and V hyperlipidemia, and, in some cases, the type IIb form. Recommended dosages are given in the table on p. 450.

#### Pharmacokinetics

| Route | Onset of Action | Peak Plasma Concentration | Elimination Half-life | Duration of Action |
|---|---|---|---|---|
| PO | Several days | 1-2 hr | 1.3-1.5 hr | Unknown |

### CHOLESTEROL ABSORPTION INHIBITOR

#### ezetimibe

Ezetimibe (Zetia) is currently the only cholesterol absorption inhibitor available. Ezetimibe has a novel mechanism of action in that it selectively inhibits absorption of cholesterol and related sterols in the small intestine. The result is a reduction in several blood lipid parameters: total cholesterol level, LDL cholesterol level, apolipoprotein B level, and triglyceride level. Serum levels of HDL cholesterol, the so-called *good* cholesterol, have been shown to increase with the use of ezetimibe. Beneficial effects of ezetimibe appear to be further enhanced when given with a statin drug. Ezetimibe may also be used as monotherapy. Recent studies have shown that, although the combination of ezetimibe and a statin is effective in reducing LDL, the rate of atherosclerotic progression is no different than when a statin is given alone. A large multicenter trial is currently underway that will provide further information in defining the role of ezetimibe. Until the results are available, current recommendations are to reserve ezetimibe for patients who have not responded to or are intolerant of other therapy. In 2011, the FDA expanded the use of ezetimibe in patients with moderate to severe chronic kidney disease, as studies showed it was effective in reducing the risk of vascular events in such patients.

Ezetimibe levels are increased by the fibric acid derivatives (fibrates). It is not known whether this is harmful, but concurrent use of ezetimibe and fibrates is not recommended. The use of ezetimibe with bile acid sequestrants has been shown to reduce the serum level of ezetimibe by 55% to 80%. Ezetimibe is contraindicated in those with a known hypersensitivity to it and in those with active liver disease or unexplained elevations in serum liver enzyme levels. It may be taken with or without food, and for patient convenience it may be dosed at the same time as a statin drug, if prescribed.

Pharmacokinetics

| Route | Onset of Action | Peak Plasma Concentration | Elimination Half-life | Duration of Action |
|-------|-----------------|---------------------------|------------------------|--------------------|
| PO | Unknown | 4-12 hr | 22 hr | Unknown |

# NURSING PROCESS

## ASSESSMENT

Before initiating therapy with any *antilipemic* drug, obtain a thorough health and medication history with a listing of allergies and any prescription drugs, over-the-counter drugs, herbals, or supplements the patient is taking. Assess the patient's dietary patterns, exercise program and frequency, weight, height, and vital signs, and document these parameters—especially food intake—over time, such as for several weeks. Also, document the patient's use of tobacco, alcohol, and/or social drugs, along with information about frequency, amount, and duration of use. Some lipid disorders are hereditary; therefore, perform a thorough assessment of family history. Positive risk factors for CHD for which the patient needs to be assessed include the following: (1) males 45 years of age or older; (2) family history: history of premature CHD (e.g., myocardial infarction or sudden death before 55 years of age in father or other male first-degree relative, or before 65 years of age in mother or other female first-degree relative); (3) current cigarette smoking; (4) hypertension with a blood pressure higher than 140/90 mm Hg or current antihypertensive drug therapy; (5) low HDL cholesterol level: lower than 40 mg/dL; and, (6) diabetes mellitus.

Perform an assessment to identify any cautions, contraindications, and potential drug interactions before initiating use of any of the antilipemics. Also assess serum lipid values and lipoprotein levels (see the Safety: Laboratory Values Related to Drug Therapy box on p. 457). With the use of cholestyramine, which contains aspartame, it is of particular interest to know if there is a history of PKU. Patients with PKU cannot properly process the amino acid phenylalanine, a component of protein. It is known that high levels of phenylalanine lead to behavioral, cognitive, and learning dysfunction as early as 3 weeks of age in such patients. Dietary restrictions must continue throughout life. Adult patients require monthly testing of phenylalanine levels. Because of the aspartame in cholestyramine, another class of antilipemics would be indicated, as ordered, to prevent further complications from this disorder.

*HMG–CoA reductase inhibitors* (the statins) are not to be used in patients with liver disease or who have increased liver enzymes. Other contraindications, cautions, and drug interactions have been previously discussed in the pharmacology section of this chapter. With the use of the statins and all antilipemics, assess the patient's intake of alcohol, including the amount consumed and the period of time that alcohol has been used, because of the potential for liver dysfunction associated with the majority of lipid-lowering drugs. The statins may have more adverse effects on an already damaged liver. Monitor levels of liver enzymes that are indicative of liver function, including AST, CPK, and/or ALT. Review lipid and lipoprotein levels before, during, and after drug therapy with the statins as well as with other antilipemic drugs. Assess the patient for any musculoskeletal problems or complaints due to the possible adverse effect of myopathy. If AST or ALT blood levels increase or signs and symptoms of myopathy or rhabdomyolysis occur (i.e., muscle soreness, changes in urine color, fever, malaise, nausea, or vomiting), the drug will most likely be discontinued by the prescriber. It is always important to assess for cultural practices because of the impact of one's beliefs on dietary restrictions. Cultural practices may also include herbal or homeopathic therapies that may pose as contraindications to use of statins and other antilipemics.

Use of *bile acid sequestrants* requires careful assessment of possible contraindications such as a patient history of biliary or bowel obstructions and PKU. Drug interactions are numerous (see previous discussion) because of the decreased absorption of drugs by the bile acid sequestrants. With *niacin*, patient assessment includes noting contraindications such as liver disease, peptic ulcer disease, gout, hypertension, and any active bleeding. Liver function studies are usually ordered for baseline and comparative levels with the majority of antilipemics. *Fibric acid derivatives* are not used in patients with liver, kidney, or gallbladder disease, and so assessment for these disorders is critical to patient safety. With *ezetimibe* (Zetia), assess for liver disease and liver enzyme elevation before initiation of therapy.

## NURSING DIAGNOSES

1. Imbalanced nutrition, more than body requirements, related to poor dietary habits of high fat intake
2. Deficient knowledge related to a lack of information about the disease, related complications, and lack of information about drug therapy
3. Risk for impaired liver function related to potential adverse and toxic effects of drug therapy

## PLANNING

### GOALS

1. Patient maintains healthy nutritional intake with appropriate restrictions.
2. Patient demonstrates adequate knowledge of disease process and its associated drug therapeutic regimens.
3. Patient maintains baseline liver function during drug therapy.

## CASE STUDY

### Antilipemic Drug Therapy

S.P., a 49-year-old mayor, lives a busy life but manages to exercise regularly and tries to follow a healthy lifestyle, including watching her diet. She is a nonsmoker and is not overweight. Recently S.P. had a medical checkup and, to her surprise, was told that her lipid levels are elevated. She has no history of diabetes mellitus, and her blood pressure is within normal limits. Her nurse practitioner has recommended that she start the HMG–CoA reductase inhibitor (statin) drug atorvastatin (Lipitor) at a dosage of 20 mg every evening.

1. S.P. says, "Isn't there something else I can do instead of taking this medicine? I really don't like taking pills." What alternatives may be available to her?
2. After 4 months, S.P.'s lipid levels are not improved. The nurse practitioner discusses S.P.'s risk factors, including the fact that her father died at 54 years of age of a myocardial infarction. What other risk factors need to be considered?
3. S.P. agrees to take the medication and schedules a follow-up appointment for 3 months. Two months later, she wakes up with some pain in her legs and feels extremely tired. She thinks she is suffering the effects of a new workout program that she started the previous day. But when she goes to work, the pain gets worse, and she calls the office nurse to describe her symptoms. What could be happening?
4. S.P. asks whether she will just be switched to another "statin" drug. How will the nurse respond?

For answers, see http://evolve.elsevier.com/Lilley.

## OUTCOME CRITERIA

1. Patient states the importance of dietary restrictions with emphasis on low-fat, low-cholesterol, high-fiber, and low-calorie (if appropriate) diet as prescribed.
   - Patient has nutritional/dietary consult for implementation of changes in lifestyle and dietary intake to help decrease cholesterol and triglyceride levels.
   - Patient follows guidelines as designated by the Adult Treatment Panel III of the National Cholesterol Education Program such as decrease in saturated and trans fat intake; boosting intake of polyunsaturated and monounsaturated fats; and low-carbohydrate and/or low-fat diet.
   - Patient implements regular aerobic exercise for 2 hours or more per week as prescribed.
2. Patient demonstrates adequate knowledge about disease process and the need for lifelong treatment with drug therapy.
   - Patient states the rationale for antilipemic drug therapy (decrease in lipid levels).
   - Patient states the importance of taking the medication exactly as prescribed.
   - Patient states the various adverse effects, such as gastrointestinal upset, changes in liver function tests, and belching, as related to the specific drug prescribed.
   - Patient returns for follow-up care for monitoring of lipid levels and for adverse effects.
3. Patient demonstrates knowledge of the risk for liver dysfunction associated with antilipemic therapy.
   - Patient states the conditions that may arise of which the prescriber must be notified, such as jaundice and abdominal pain.
   - Patient states the importance of follow-up care with the prescriber to monitor for changes in liver function and monitoring of liver function tests.

## IMPLEMENTATION

Patients who are taking *antilipemics* for a long period may have altered levels of the fat-soluble vitamins and may then require supplementation of vitamins A, D, and K. Antilipemics may also cause problems with the liver and biliary systems and may cause gastrointestinal tract problems such as constipation. Appropriate actions need to be taken to avoid or minimize constipation, such as increasing intake of fiber and fluids. Monitoring the results of blood studies per the prescriber's instructions often includes reviewing levels of serum transaminases and results of other tests of liver function.

With the *HMG-CoA reductase inhibitors* or statin drugs, serum levels of the aforementioned components are often measured every 6 to 8 weeks for the first 6 months of statin therapy and then every 3 to 6 months, depending on the prescriber and the patient situation. If a lipid profile is ordered, instruct the patient to fast for 12 to 14 hours before the blood sample is drawn. Also, inform patients of the desired laboratory levels to achieve (see Table 27-3). Because severe cardiovascular diseases and cerebral vascular accidents (also known as *strokes*) are associated with very high cholesterol levels, it is critical to the maintenance of health and the prevention of complications that the patient continue with any prescribed nonpharmacologic and/or pharmacologic therapies, regardless of the specific antilipemic used. Another aspect to consider when administering these medications, specifically simvastatin (Zocor), is dosage amount. The FDA has imposed new prescribing restrictions on simvastatin 80-mg dosage forms (see pharmacology discussion). The FDA also recommends that the 80-mg dose of simvastatin "not be started in new patients, including patients already taking lower doses of the drug." There are additional concerns about simvastatin and other medications that have been discussed in the pharmacology section of this chapter.

*Bile acid sequestrants* often come in powder form and must be mixed thoroughly with food or fluids (at least 4 to 6 oz of fluid). The powder may not mix completely at first, but patients need to be sure to mix the dose as much as possible and then dilute any undissolved portion with additional fluid. The powder needs to be dissolved for at least 1 full minute. Powder and/or granule dosage forms are *never* to be taken in dry form. It is important that colestipol and any of these drugs be taken 1 hour before or 4 to 6 hours after any other oral medication or meals because of the high risk for drug-drug and drug-food interactions. Bile acid sequestrants do interfere

### Post-Stroke Statins Improve Patient Outcomes

**Review**

A prospective population-based analysis of ischemic stroke patients participating in the North Dublin Populations Stroke Study was performed to examine the relationship between acute treatment with statins (after ischemic stroke) and an improvement in survival and functional outcome.

**Type of Evidence**

The main researcher and her colleagues of Mater University Hospital in Dublin compared a statin to a no-statin group in 418 patients who had ischemic strokes. A prospective population-based analysis of these patients was done mainly because of the time and expense that would have been involved in the conducting of a randomized clinical trial for the same research purpose. Additionally, researchers assessed patients using the modified Rankin scale (mRS). The mRS is a commonly used scale for measuring the degree of disability or dependence in activities of daily living of people who have had a stroke. This scale ranges from 0 (no symptoms) to 6 (death), with 3 representing moderate disability and requiring some help but able to walk unassisted.

**Results of Study**

Of the total sample size, 30% of the patients had been on a statin drug before experiencing a stroke, and 87.3% of them continued to take their statin drug after the stroke. Forty-four percent of the sample size began taking statins within 72 hours of their stroke. Seventy-one percent of the group in all took a statin drug acutely after the stroke. Atorvastin was the specific statin in 87% of the patients. Researchers assessed the patients using the mRS and fatality at 1 week, 28 days, 90 days, and 1 year poststroke. Those patients who were taking statins after having the stroke, regardless of the fact that the drug was being taken beforehand or not, were more likely to have good outcomes or have an mRS score of 0 to 2 as compared to those who were not taking statins. Fatality risk was also significantly reduced among the patients on statins poststroke at every time point. It was also found that patients taking atorvastatin who increased their dose poststroke were more likely to have good outcomes. There was, however, no relationship between poststroke statin therapy and risk of having a recurrent stroke. Recurrent strokes did occur in 1.8% of the patients.

**Link of Evidence to Nursing Practice**

The results of this population-based prospective study emphasize the importance of initiation of preventative drug therapy (in this study, statins) in patients with the onset of a stroke. Specifically, it was found that statin therapy at the onset of stroke and newly begun statins were associated with improved early and late outcomes. With study results such as these, there is support for more research in the area of improving early and late outcomes with stroke patients. Dr. Ni Chroinin and her colleagues stated that randomized trials of statin for therapy in acute stroke patients are needed. Although the benefits of statins are known, there are still many patients at risk that could benefit from them. Nurses play a major role in performing assessments and interventions for patients with cardiovascular disorders, including strokes, as well as in monitoring pharmacologic management of these same disorders. Nurses also continue to play an important part in research clinical trials and in the education of patients about risk factors, new therapies, and lifestyle management associated with stroke and other cardiovascular diseases.

Reference: Ni Chroinin D et al: Association between acute statin therapy, survival, and improved functional outcome after ischemic stroke: the North Dublin Population Stroke Study, *Stroke* 42(4):1021-1029, 2011. The Modified Rankin Scale can be found at www.strokecenter.org/trials/scales/rankin.html.

with the absorption of other medications. Colestipol is also available in tablet form. Cholestyramine is to be taken just before meals or with meals, and it must never be given to a patient with PKU because it contains aspartame (see previous discussion). Constipation may be prevented with high fiber and increase in fluid intake.

With *niacin,* flushing of the face may occur; educate the patient on this adverse effect. To minimize gastrointestinal upset, advise the patient to take this medication with meals. Of the different dosage forms available, the extended-release dosage forms, which dissolve more slowly than the immediate-release forms but faster than the sustained-release forms, appear to be associated with less flushing of the skin. Other actions that may help to minimize flushing of the skin include titrating the drug dosage or taking a small dose of aspirin or NSAIDs 30 minutes before the niacin is taken, but only as ordered or recommended by the prescriber. Educate patients that *fibric acid derivatives* are to be taken as prescribed. Frequently monitor liver/kidney function tests and prothrombin times with these drugs. The *cholesterol absorption inhibitor* ezetimibe (Zetia) may be taken with or without food and may be taken with statin drugs.

# EVALUATION

Evaluation of goals and outcome criteria is the best place to begin when trying to evaluate for the therapeutic versus adverse effects of these medications. In addition, cholesterol and triglyceride levels are used to monitor the patient's response to the medication regimen, and specific target levels are listed in Table 27-3. While taking *antilipemics,* patients remain on a low-fat, low-cholesterol diet as an integrated part of a change in lifestyle. Monitor patients receiving antilipemic drugs for therapeutic and adverse effects during their therapy. The therapeutic effects of both nonpharmacologic and pharmacologic measures are evidenced by a decrease in cholesterol and triglyceride levels to within normal ranges (see previous serum laboratory values). Nonpharmacologic measures include a low-fat, low-cholesterol diet; supervised, moderate exercise; weight loss; cessation of smoking and drinking; and relaxation therapy. Adverse effects for which to monitor include gastrointestinal upset, increased liver enzyme levels, hepatomegaly, myalgias, and other effects mentioned earlier in the chapter. Closely monitor patients' renal and liver function before and throughout treatment to detect the development of liver or renal dysfunction.

## SAFETY: LABORATORY VALUES RELATED TO DRUG THERAPY

### Coronary Heart Disease

| LABORATORY TEST | NORMAL RANGES* | RATIONALE FOR ASSESSMENT |
|---|---|---|
| Serum lipid panel with cholesterol, triglycerides, and various lipids | Serum cholesterol level: less than or equal to 200 mg/dL (less than 5.17 mmol/L)<br>Triglyceride level: less than 150 mg/dL<br>Low-density lipoprotein (LDL) cholesterol level: less than 100 mg/dL (less than 2.6 mmol/L)<br>High-density lipoprotein (HDL) cholesterol level: greater than or equal to 60 mg/dL (1.56 mmol/L[CB8])<br>Very-low-density lipoprotein (VLDL) level: less than 130 mg/dL (less than 3.4 mmol/L) | A lipid panel is a serum test that measures the levels of lipids, fats, and fatty substances used as a source of energy in the body. Lipids include cholesterol, triglycerides, HDL, and LDL. When a lipid panel is ordered, the levels of all of the following are reported: total cholesterol, triglycerides, HDL, LDL, VLDL, ratio of total cholesterol to HDL, and ratio of LDL to HDL. Lipid levels are important to health status and are indicators of health; if there are abnormalities (e.g., high cholesterol, triglyceride, VLDL, and LDL levels and low HDL level), the individual is at increased risk for heart disease and stroke. Dietary and other lifestyle changes may be implemented to help decrease the levels of "bad" cholesterols (LDL and VLDL) and elevate the levels of "good" cholesterol (HDL). Medical treatment protocols may also be implemented to help prevent heart attack and strokes. |

*The values in this table are from the National Cholesterol Education Program of the National Institutes of Health.

## PATIENT TEACHING TIPS

• Notify the prescriber if there are any new or troublesome symptoms or if there is persistent gastrointestinal upset, constipation, gas, bloating, heartburn, nausea, vomiting, abnormal or unusual bleeding, or yellow discoloration of the skin. Another symptom to report is muscle pain.

• Advise the patient to keep these and all medications out of the reach of children and protected with childproof lids.

• Encourage a diet that is plentiful in raw vegetables, fruit, and bran. Forcing fluids (up to 3000 mL/day unless contraindicated) may also help prevent the constipation associated with these medications.

• Advise the patient to inform health care providers about all medications he or she is taking, including antilipemics. These drugs are highly protein bound and are therefore associated with many drug interactions, including drugs that a dentist may prescribe. In addition, these drugs may alter clotting if taken on a long-term basis. This information is also important for the patient to share with the dentist.

• Educate patients that exercise is to be done in moderation and often with supervision as indicated.

• Alert the patient to concerns regarding the use of 80-mg doses of simvastatin.

• When taking an HMG–CoA reductase inhibitor or statin drug, it is best taken with at least 6 oz of water or with meals to help minimize gastric upset. It takes several weeks before therapeutic results are seen. Monitor liver and renal function laboratory studies every 3 to 6 months.

• Drug and food interactions associated with the statin drugs that must be avoided include oral anticoagulants, erythromycin, verapamil, some antifungal drugs, and grapefruit juice.

• With the HMG-CoA reductase inhibitors or statin drugs, any muscle soreness, change in color of the urine, fever, nausea, vomiting, and/or malaise must be reported to the prescriber immediately.

• If taking a bile acid sequestrant, advise the patient to take the medication with meals to decrease gastrointestinal upset. Other drugs must be taken 1 hour before or 4 to 6 hours after taking a bile acid sequestrant.

• Niacin is contraindicated in those with liver disease, peptic ulcer disease, gout, hypertension, or active bleeding. Instruct patients to take niacin with meals to decrease gastrointestinal upset.

## KEY POINTS

• There are two primary forms of lipids: triglycerides and cholesterol. Triglycerides function as an energy source and are stored in adipose (fat) tissue. Cholesterol is primarily used to make steroid hormones, cell membranes, and bile acids.

• Lipids and lipoproteins participate in the formation of atherosclerotic plaque, which leads to CHD, and it is important to understand the pathology of this disease process so that appropriate patient education may be delivered.

• When plaque forms in the blood vessels that supply the heart with needed oxygen and nutrients, the lumens of these blood vessels will eventually decrease in size and the amount of oxygen and nutrients that can reach the heart (and major organs) will be reduced.

• Antilipemic drugs are used to lower the high levels of lipids in the blood (triglycerides and cholesterol).

• The major classes of antilipemics include HMG–CoA reductase inhibitors, bile acid sequestrants, niacin, fibric acid derivatives, and cholesterol absorption inhibitors, with each having their own mechanism of action.

• While taking a history, it is important to assess the patient for any possible cautions, contraindications, and drug interactions.

## KEY POINTS — cont'd

- Fat-soluble vitamins may need to be prescribed for patients taking these medications for long periods because the antilipemics have long-term effects on the liver's production of these vitamins.
- Monitoring for adverse effects of the antilipemics includes periodic liver and renal function studies.

- The statins have gained much attention for their adverse effects of muscle aches and pain due to breakdown of muscle tissue. Some patients experience irreversible renal damage and severe pain and may have to alter dosages or change drugs as ordered by the prescriber.

## NCLEX® EXAMINATION REVIEW QUESTIONS

1 A nurse administering niacin would implement which action to help to reduce adverse effects?
   a Give the medication with grapefruit juice.
   b Administer a small dose of aspirin or an NSAID 30 minutes before the niacin dose.
   c Administer the medication on an empty stomach.
   d Have the patient increase dietary fiber intake.

2 When administering niacin, the nurse needs to monitor for which adverse effect?
   a Cutaneous flushing
   b Muscle pain
   c Headache
   d Constipation

3 Which point will the nurse emphasize to a patient who is taking an antilipemic medication in the "statin" class?
   a The drug needs to be taken on an empty stomach before meals.
   b A low-fat diet is not necessary while taking these medications.
   c It is important to report muscle pain immediately.
   d Improved cholesterol levels will be evident within 2 weeks.

4 A patient is being assessed before a newly ordered antilipemic medication is given. Which condition would be a potential contraindication?
   a Diabetes insipidus
   b Pulmonary fibrosis
   c Liver cirrhosis
   d Myocardial infarction

5 A patient is currently taking a statin. The nurse considers that the patient may have a higher risk of developing rhabdomyolysis when also taking which product?
   a NSAIDs
   b A fibric acid derivative
   c Orange juice
   d Fat soluble vitamins

6 The nurse is administering cholestyramine (Questran), a bile acid sequestrant. Which nursing intervention(s) is appropriate? (Select all that apply.)
   a Administering the drug on an empty stomach
   b Administering the drug with meals
   c Instructing the patient to follow a low-fiber diet while taking this drug
   d Instructing the patient to take a fiber supplement while taking this drug
   e Increasing fluid intake
   f Not administering this drug at the same time as other drugs

7 The medication order reads: niacin, 500 mg PO, every evening. The medication is available in 250-mg tablets. How many tablets will the patient receive per dose?

1. b, 2. a, 3. c, 4. c, 5. b, 6. b, d, e, f, 7. 2 tablets

For Critical Thinking and Prioritization Questions, see http://evolve.elsevier.com/Lilley

# Diuretic Drugs

## OBJECTIVES

When you reach the end of this chapter, you will be able to do the following:

1 Describe the normal anatomy and physiology of the renal system.
2 Briefly discuss the impact of the renal system on blood pressure regulation.
3 Describe how diuretics work in the kidneys and how they lower blood pressure.

4 Distinguish among the different classes of diuretics with regard to mechanisms of action, indications, dosages, routes of administration, adverse effects, toxicity, cautions, contraindications, and drug interactions.
5 Develop a nursing care plan that includes all phases of the nursing process for patients receiving diuretics.

## DRUG PROFILES

acetazolamide, p. 462
amiloride, p. 466
♦ furosemide, p. 484
♦ hydrochlorothiazide, p. 467
♦ mannitol, p. 465

metolazone, p. 468
♦ spironolactone, p. 466
triamterene, p. 466

_____

♦ *Key drug*

## KEY TERMS

Afferent arterioles The small blood vessels approaching the glomerulus (proximal part of the nephron). (p. 460)

Aldosterone A mineralocorticoid steroid hormone produced by the adrenal cortex that regulates sodium and water balance. (p. 461)

Ascites Intraperitoneal accumulation of fluid (defined as a volume of 500 mL or more) containing large amounts of protein and electrolytes. (p. 464)

Collecting duct The most distal part of the nephron between the distal convoluted tubule and the ureters, which lead to the urinary bladder. (p. 461)

Distal convoluted tubule The part of the nephron immediately distal to the ascending loop of Henle and proximal to the collecting duct. (p. 460)

Diuretics Drugs or other substances that tend to promote the formation and excretion of urine. (p. 460)

Efferent arterioles The small blood vessels exiting the glomerulus. At this point blood has completed its filtration in the glomerulus. (p. 460)

Filtrate The material that passes through a filter. In the case of the kidney, the filter is the glomerulus and the filtrate is the material extracted from the blood (normally liquid) that becomes urine. (p. 461)

**Glomerular capsule** The open, rounded, and most proximal part of the proximal convoluted tubule that surrounds the glomerulus and receives the filtrate from the blood. (p. 460)

**Glomerular filtration rate (GFR)** An estimate of the volume of blood that passes through the glomeruli of the kidney per minute. (p. 460)

**Glomerulus** The cluster of kidney capillaries that marks the beginning of the nephron and is immediately proximal to the proximal convoluted tubule. (p. 460)

**Loop of Henle** The part of the nephron between the proximal and distal convoluted tubules. (p. 460)

**Nephron** The functional filtration unit of the kidney, consisting of (in anatomic order from proximal to distal) the glomerulus, proximal convoluted tubule, loop of Henle, distal convoluted tubule, and collecting duct, which empties urine into the ureters. There are approximately 1 million nephrons in each kidney. (p. 460)

**Open-angle glaucoma** A condition in which pressure is elevated in the eye because of obstruction of the outflow of aqueous humor. (p. 461)

**Proximal convoluted (twisted) tubule** The part of the nephron that is immediately distal to the glomerulus and proximal to the loop of Henle. (p. 460)

## ANATOMY, PHYSIOLOGY, AND PATHOPHYSIOLOGY OVERVIEW

**Diuretics** are drugs that accelerate the rate of urine formation via a variety of mechanisms. The result is the removal of sodium and water from the body. Diuretics were discovered by accident when it was noticed that a mercury-based antibiotic had a very potent diuretic effect. All the major classes of diuretic drugs in use today were developed between 1950 and 1970, and they remain among the most commonly prescribed drugs in the world.

*The Seventh Report of the Joint National Committee on Prevention, Detection, Evaluation, and Treatment of High Blood Pressure* reaffirmed the role of diuretics, especially the thiazides, as first-line drugs in the treatment of hypertension. The hypotensive activity of diuretics is due to many different mechanisms. They cause direct arteriolar dilation, which decreases peripheral vascular resistance. They also reduce extracellular fluid volume, plasma volume, and cardiac output, which may account for the decrease in blood pressure. They have long been the mainstay of therapy not only for hypertension but also for heart failure. Two of their advantages are their relatively low cost and their favorable safety profile. The main problem with their use is the metabolic adverse effects that can result from excessive fluid and electrolyte loss. These effects are usually dose related and are controllable with dosage *titration* (careful adjustment).

This chapter reviews the essential properties and actions of the following important classes of diuretic drugs: carbonic anhydrase inhibitors, loop diuretics, osmotic diuretics, potassium-sparing diuretics, and thiazide and thiazide-like diuretics. All diuretics work primarily in the kidney.

The kidney plays a very important role in the day-to-day functioning of the body. It filters out toxic waste products from the blood while simultaneously conserving essential substances. This delicate balance between elimination of toxins and retention of essential chemicals is maintained by the **nephron**. The nephron is the main structural unit of the kidney, and each kidney contains approximately 1 million nephrons. Diuretics exert their effect in the nephron. The initial filtering of the blood takes place in the **glomerulus**, a cluster of capillaries surrounded by the **glomerular capsule**. The rate at which this filtering occurs is referred to as the **glomerular filtration rate (GFR)**, and it is used as a gauge of how well the kidneys are functioning as filters. The GFR can be estimated mathematically by calculating creatinine clearance. This is typically calculated by hospital pharmacists and is used to adjust drugs based on the patient's renal function. Normally about 180 L of blood are filtered through the nephrons every day.

The GFR, which can also be thought of as the rate at which blood flows into and out of the glomerulus, is regulated by the small blood vessels approaching the glomerulus (**afferent arterioles**) and the small blood vessels exiting the glomerulus (**efferent arterioles**). A mnemonic (memory aid) for remembering which arteriole is which is "*A* for *approach* and *afferent*" and "*E* for *exit* and *efferent*." Alterations in blood flow such as those that occur in a patient in shock can therefore have a dramatic effect on kidney (renal) function. Diuretics may have diminished effects in situations of low blood flow, because the kidney receives less blood, and therefore less diuretic reaches the site of action.

The **proximal convoluted (twisted) tubule** or, more simply, the *proximal tubule,* follows the glomerulus anatomically and returns 60% to 70% of the sodium and water from the filtered fluid back into the bloodstream. Blood vessels surround the nephrons and allow substances to be directly resorbed from or secreted into the bloodstream. This process is one of active transport that requires energy in the form of adenosine triphosphate (ATP) molecules. The active transport of sodium and potassium ions back into the blood causes the passive resorption of chloride and water. The chloride ions ($Cl^-$) and water passively follow the sodium ions ($Na^+$) and, to a lesser extent, potassium ions ($K^+$) by osmosis. Another 20% to 25% of sodium is resorbed back into the bloodstream in the ascending **loop of Henle.** Chloride is actively resorbed in the loop of Henle, and sodium passively follows it.

The remaining 5% to 10% of sodium resorption takes place in the **distal convoluted tubule,** often called the *distal tubule,* which anatomically follows the ascending loop of Henle. In the distal tubule, sodium is actively filtered in exchange for potassium or hydrogen ions, a process regulated by the

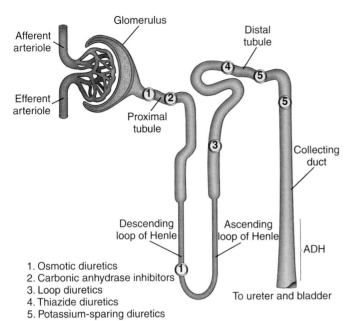

1. Osmotic diuretics
2. Carbonic anhydrase inhibitors
3. Loop diuretics
4. Thiazide diuretics
5. Potassium-sparing diuretics

FIGURE 28-1 The nephron and diuretic sites of action. *ADH,* Antidiuretic hormone.

| TABLE 28-1 | CLASSIFICATION OF DIURETICS |
|---|---|
| **CLASS** | **DRUGS** |
| Carbonic anhydrase inhibitors | Acetazolamide |
| Loop diuretics | Bumetanide, ethacrynic acid, furosemide, torsemide |
| Osmotic diuretics | Mannitol |
| Potassium-sparing diuretics | Amiloride, spironolactone, triamterene |
| thiazide and thiazide-like diuretics | Chlorthalidone, chlorothiazide, hydrochlorothiazide, indapamide, metolazone |

hormone aldosterone. The collecting duct is the final common pathway for the filtrate that started in the glomerulus. It is here that antidiuretic hormone acts to increase the absorption of water back into the bloodstream, thereby preventing it from being lost in the urine. The entire nephron, along with the sites of action of the different classes of diuretics, is shown in Figure 28-1.

## PHARMACOLOGY OVERVIEW

The various diuretics are classified according to their sites of action within the nephron, their chemical structure, and their diuretic potency. The sites of action of the various diuretics are determined by the way in which they affect the various solute (electrolyte) and water transport systems located along the nephron (see Figure 28-1). The commonly used classes of drugs and the individual drugs in these classes are listed in Table 28-1. The most potent diuretics are the loop diuretics, followed by mannitol, metolazone (a thiazide-like diuretic), the thiazides, and the potassium-sparing diuretics. The potency of these diuretics is a function of where they work in the nephron to inhibit sodium and water resorption. The more sodium and water they inhibit from resorption, the greater the amount of diuresis and therefore the greater the potency.

## CARBONIC ANHYDRASE INHIBITORS

Carbonic anhydrase inhibitors (CAIs) are chemical derivatives of sulfonamide antibiotics. As their name implies, CAIs inhibit the activity of the enzyme carbonic anhydrase, which is found in the kidneys, eyes, and other parts of the body. The CAIs work at the location of the carbonic anhydrase enzyme system along the nephron, primarily in the proximal tubule. Acetazolamide is the CAI most commonly used today.

## Mechanism of Action and Drug Effects

The carbonic anhydrase system in the kidney is located just distal to the glomerulus in the proximal tubules, where roughly two thirds of all sodium and water is resorbed into the blood. In the proximal tubules, there is an active transport system that exchanges sodium for hydrogen ions. For sodium and water to be resorbed back into the blood, hydrogen must be exchanged for it. Without hydrogen, this cannot occur, and the sodium and water will be eliminated with the urine. Carbonic anhydrase makes hydrogen ions available for this exchange. When its actions are inhibited by a CAI such as acetazolamide, little sodium and water can be resorbed into the blood and they are eliminated with the urine. The CAIs reduce the formation of hydrogen ($H^+$) and bicarbonate ($HCO_3^-$) ions from carbon dioxide and water through the noncompetitive, reversible inhibition of carbonic anhydrase activity. This results in a reduction in the availability of the ions, mainly hydrogen, for use by active transport systems.

The reduction in the formation of bicarbonate and hydrogen ions can have effects on other parts of the body. CAIs can induce respiratory and metabolic acidosis. Both respiratory and metabolic acidosis can increase oxygenation during hypoxia by increasing ventilation, cerebral blood flow, and the dissociation of oxygen from oxyhemoglobin. These actions are usually beneficial to the patient. An undesirable effect of CAIs is elevation of the blood glucose level and glycosuria in diabetic patients. This may be due in part to CAI-enhanced potassium loss through the urine.

## Indications

Therapeutic applications of CAIs include the treatment of glaucoma, edema, and high-altitude sickness.

CAIs are used as adjunct drugs in the long-term management of open-angle glaucoma that cannot be controlled by topical miotic drugs or epinephrine derivatives alone (see Chapter 57). Glaucoma is caused by the obstruction of the outflow of aqueous humor. When CAIs are given, an increase in the outflow of aqueous humor results. They are also used short term in conjunction with miotics to lower intraocular pressure in preparation for ocular surgery and as an adjunct in the treatment of secondary glaucoma.

Acetazolamide is also used to manage edema secondary to heart failure that has become resistant to other diuretics.

However, as a class, CAIs are much less potent diuretics than loop diuretics or thiazides, and the metabolic acidosis they induce diminishes their diuretic effect in 2 to 4 days.

Acetazolamide is also effective in both the prevention and treatment of the symptoms of high-altitude sickness. These symptoms include headache, nausea, shortness of breath, dizziness, drowsiness, and fatigue.

## Contraindications

Contraindications to the use of CAIs include known drug allergy, hyponatremia, hypokalemia, severe renal or hepatic dysfunction, adrenal gland insufficiency, and cirrhosis.

## Adverse Effects

Common undesirable effects of CAIs are metabolic abnormalities such as acidosis and hypokalemia. Drowsiness, anorexia, paresthesias, hematuria, urticaria, photosensitivity, and melena (blood in the stool) can also occur.

## Interactions

Because CAIs can cause hypokalemia, an increase in digoxin toxicity may occur when they are combined with digoxin. Use with corticosteroids may also cause hypokalemia. The effects of amphetamines, carbamazepine, cyclosporine, phenytoin, and quinidine may be increased when these drugs are taken concurrently with CAIs.

## Dosages

The usual dose of acetazolamide is 250 to 500 mg per day, which may be given orally or IV.

## DRUG PROFILE

### acetazolamide

Use of acetazolamide (Diamox) is contraindicated in patients who have shown a hypersensitivity to it as well as in those with significant liver or kidney dysfunction, low serum potassium or sodium levels, acidosis, or adrenal gland failure. Acetazolamide is available in both oral and parenteral forms. It is classified as a pregnancy category C drug.

**Pharmacokinetics**

| Route | Onset of Action | Peak Plasma Concentration | Elimination Half-life | Duration of Action |
|-------|-----------------|---------------------------|-----------------------|---------------------|
| PO | 1 hr | 2-4 hr | 10-15 hr | 8-12 hr |

## LOOP DIURETICS

Loop diuretics (bumetanide, ethacrynic acid, furosemide, and torsemide) are very potent diuretics. Bumetanide, furosemide, and torsemide are chemically related to the sulfonamide antibiotics. Because they are structurally related to the sulfonamides, they are often listed as contraindicated in sulfa-allergic patients. However, analysis of the literature indicates that cross-reaction is unlikely to occur. Loop diuretics are commonly given to patients with sulfa allergy with no problems; however, always be aware of the potential of allergy.

## Mechanism of Action and Drug Effects

Loop diuretics have renal, cardiovascular, and metabolic effects. These drugs act primarily along the thick ascending limb of the loop of Henle, blocking chloride and, secondarily, sodium resorption. They are also thought to activate renal prostaglandins, which results in dilatation of the blood vessels of the kidneys, the lungs, and the rest of the body (i.e., reduction in renal, pulmonary, and systemic vascular resistance). The hemodynamic effects of loop diuretics are a reduction in both the preload and central venous pressures (which are the filling pressures of the ventricles). These actions make them useful in the treatment of the edema associated with heart failure, hepatic cirrhosis, and renal disease.

Loop diuretics are particularly useful when rapid diuresis is needed, because of their rapid onset of action. The diuretic effect lasts at least 2 hours. Loop diuretics have a distinct advantage over thiazide diuretics in that their diuretic action continues even when creatinine clearance decreases below 25 mL/min. This means that even when kidney function diminishes, loop diuretics can still work. Because of their potent diuretic effect and the duration of action, loop diuretics are usually effective when given in a single daily dose. This allows the renal tubule time to partially compensate for the potassium depletion and other electrolyte derangements that often accompany around-the-clock diuretic therapy. Despite this, the major adverse effect of loop diuretics is electrolyte disturbances. Prolonged administration of high dosages can also result in hearing loss stemming from ototoxicity, although this is rare.

### Summary of Major Drug Effects of Loop Diuretics

Loop diuretics produce a potent diuresis and subsequent loss of fluid. The resulting decreased fluid volume leads to a decreased return of blood to the heart, or decreased filling pressures. This has the following cardiovascular effects:
- Reduces blood pressure
- Reduces pulmonary vascular resistance
- Reduces systemic vascular resistance
- Reduces central venous pressure
- Reduces left ventricular end-diastolic pressure

The metabolic effects of the loop diuretics are secondary to the electrolyte losses resulting from the potent diuresis. Major electrolyte losses include loss of sodium and potassium and, to a lesser extent, calcium. Changes in the plasma levels of insulin, glucagon, and growth hormone have also been observed in association with loop diuretic therapy.

## Indications

Loop diuretics are used to manage the edema associated with heart failure and hepatic or renal disease, to control hypertension, and to increase the renal excretion of calcium in patients with hypercalcemia. As with certain other classes of diuretics, they may also be indicated in cases of heart failure resulting from diastolic dysfunction.

## Contraindications

Contraindications to the use of loop diuretics include known drug allergy, hepatic coma, and severe electrolyte loss. Although allergy to sulfonamide antibiotics is listed as a contraindication, analysis of the literature indicates that cross-reaction with the loop diuretics is unlikely to occur. Loop diuretics are commonly given to such patients in clinical practice.

## Adverse Effects

Common undesirable effects of the loop diuretics are listed in Table 28-2. Hypokalemia is of serious clinical importance. To prevent hypokalemia, patients often receive potassium supplements along with furosemide. Furosemide can produce erythema multiforme, exfoliative dermatitis, photosensitivity, and in rare cases aplastic anemia. Torsemide may rarely cause blood disorders, including thrombocytopenia, agranulocytosis, leukopenia, and neutropenia. It may also cause a severe skin disorder called Stevens-Johnson syndrome.

### Toxicity and Management of Overdose

Electrolyte loss and dehydration, which can result in circulatory failure, are the main toxic effects of loop diuretics that require attention. Treatment involves electrolyte and fluid replacement.

## Interactions

Loop diuretics exhibit both neurotoxic and nephrotoxic properties, and they produce additive effects when given in combination with drugs that have similar toxicities. The drug interactions are summarized in Table 28-3.

Loop diuretics also affect certain laboratory results. They cause increases in the serum levels of uric acid, glucose, alanine aminotransferase, and aspartate aminotransferase. Their combined use with a thiazide (especially metolazone) results in the blockade of sodium and water resorption at multiple sites in the nephron, a property referred to as *sequential nephron blockade*, which increases their effects. Nonsteroidal antiinflammatory drugs (NSAIDs) may diminish the reduction in vascular resistance induced by loop diuretics because these two drug classes have opposite effects on prostaglandin activity.

## Dosages

For dosage information on loop diuretics, see the table on this page.

## DRUG PROFILE

The currently available loop diuretics are bumetanide, ethacrynic acid, furosemide, and torsemide. Ethacrynic acid is rarely used clinically. As a class they are very potent diuretics, but

| TABLE 28-2 | LOOP DIURETICS: COMMON ADVERSE EFFECTS | |
|---|---|---|
| **BODY SYSTEM** | **ADVERSE EFFECTS** | |
| Central nervous | Dizziness, headache, tinnitus, blurred vision | |
| Gastrointestinal | Nausea, vomiting, diarrhea | |
| Hematologic | Agranulocytosis, thrombocytopenia, neutropenia | |
| Metabolic | Hypokalemia, hyperglycemia, hyperuricemia | |

| TABLE 28-3 | LOOP DIURETICS: COMMON DRUG INTERACTIONS | |
|---|---|---|
| **INTERACTING DRUG** | **MECHANISM** | **RESULTS** |
| Aminoglycosides vancomycin | Additive effect | Increased neurotoxicity, especially ototoxicity |
| Corticosteroids digoxin | Hypokalemia | Additive hypokalemia Increased digoxin toxicity |
| lithium | Decrease in renal excretion | Increased lithium toxicity |
| NSAIDs | Inhibition of renal prostaglandins | Decreased diuretic activity |

*NSAIDs,* Nonsteroidal antiinflammatory drugs.

## DOSAGES

### Selected Loop Diuretics and Osmotic Diuretics

| DRUG | PHARMACOLOGIC CLASS | USUAL DOSAGE RANGE | INDICATIONS |
|---|---|---|---|
| ◆ furosemide (Lasix) | Loop diuretic | **Pediatric** IM/IV/PO: 1-2 mg/kg/dose; do not exceed 6 mg/kg/day **Adult** IM/IV: 20-40 mg/dose; max 600 mg/day; administer high-dose IV therapy as a controlled infusion at a rate of 4 mg/mL or less PO: 20-120 mg/day as a single dose | Heart failure, hypertension, renal failure, pulmonary edema, cirrhosis |
| ◆ mannitol (Osmitrol) | Osmotic diuretic | **Adult** IV infusion: 20-200 g/day, over a 24-hr period 1-2 g/kg over 30-60 min followed by 0.25-1 g/kg infusion 50-200 g IV given at a rate to induce urine output of 100-500 mL/hr | Renal failure High intraocular or intracranial pressure Drug intoxication (to induce diuresis) |

*IM,* Intramuscular; *IV,* intravenous; *PO,* oral.

potency varies for the different drugs. The equipotent doses of the drugs are as follows:

| bumetanide | ethacrynic acid | furosemide | torsemide |
|---|---|---|---|
| 1 mg | 50 mg | 40 mg | 10-20 mg |

#### ◆ furosemide

Furosemide (Lasix) is by far the most commonly used loop diuretic in clinical practice and the prototypical drug in this class. It has all the therapeutic and adverse effects of the loop diuretics mentioned earlier. It is used in the management of pulmonary edema and the edema associated with heart failure, liver disease, nephrotic syndrome, and ascites. It has also been used in the treatment of hypertension, usually that caused by heart failure.

Furosemide use is contraindicated in patients who have shown a hypersensitivity to it or to the sulfonamides (see previous discussion regarding sulfonamide allergy) and in patients with anuria, hypovolemia, or electrolyte depletion. It is available in oral form as a solution, tablets, and an injectable form. It is classified as a pregnancy category C drug. Recommended dosages are given in the table on p. 463.

#### Pharmacokinetics

| Route | Onset of Action | Peak Plasma Concentration | Elimination Half-life | Duration of Action |
|---|---|---|---|---|
| IV | 5 min | 15 min | 1-2 hr | 2 hr |
| PO | 30-60 min | 1-2 hr | 1-2 hr | 6-8 hr |

## OSMOTIC DIURETICS

The osmotic diuretics include mannitol, urea, organic acids, and glucose. Mannitol, a nonabsorbable solute, is the most commonly used of these drugs.

### Mechanism of Action and Drug Effects

Mannitol works along the entire nephron. Its major site of action, however, is the proximal tubule and descending limb of the loop of Henle. Because it is nonabsorbable, it increases osmotic pressure in the glomerular filtrate, which in turn pulls fluid, primarily water, into the renal tubules from the surrounding tissues. This process also inhibits the tubular resorption of water and solutes, which produces a rapid diuresis. Ultimately, this reduces cellular edema and increases urine production, causing diuresis. However, it produces only a slight loss of electrolytes, especially sodium. Therefore, mannitol is not indicated for patients with peripheral edema because it does not promote sufficient sodium excretion.

Mannitol may induce vasodilation and in doing so increase both glomerular filtration and renal plasma flow. This makes it an excellent drug for preventing kidney damage during acute renal failure. It is also often used to reduce intracranial pressure and cerebral edema resulting from

head trauma. In addition, mannitol treatment may be tried when elevated intraocular pressure is unresponsive to other drug therapies.

### Indications

Mannitol is the osmotic diuretic of choice. It is commonly used in the treatment of patients in the early, oliguric phase of acute renal failure. For it to be effective in this setting, however, enough renal blood flow and glomerular filtration must still remain to enable the drug to reach the renal tubules. Increased renal blood flow resulting from the dilatation of blood vessels supplying blood to the kidneys is another therapeutic benefit of mannitol. It can also be used to promote the excretion of toxic substances, reduce intracranial pressure, and treat cerebral edema. In addition, it can be used as a genitourinary irrigant in the preparation of patients for transurethral surgical procedures and as supportive treatment in patients with edema induced by other conditions.

### Contraindications

Contraindications to the use of mannitol normally include known drug allergy, severe renal disease, pulmonary edema (loop diuretics are used instead), and active intracranial bleeding.

### Adverse Effects

Significant undesirable effects of mannitol include convulsions, thrombophlebitis, and pulmonary congestion. Other less significant effects are headaches, chest pains, tachycardia, blurred vision, chills, and fever.

## Interactions

There are no drugs that interact significantly with mannitol.

## Dosages

For dosage information on mannitol, see the table on p. 463.

## DRUG PROFILE

♦ **mannitol**

Mannitol (Osmitrol) is the prototypical osmotic diuretic. Its use is contraindicated in patients with a hypersensitivity to it as well as in those with anuria, severe dehydration, pulmonary congestion, or cerebral hemorrhage. Treatment is terminated if severe cardiac or renal impairment develops after the initiation of therapy. It is available only in parenteral form as 5%, 10%, 15%, 20%, and 25% solutions for intravenous injection. The volume infused differs based on the concentration of mannitol provided. Calculations may need to performed to determine the volume to be used. Mannitol may crystallize when exposed to low temperatures. This is more likely to occur when concentrations exceed 15%. Because of this, mannitol is always administered intravenously through a filter, and vials of the drug are often stored in a warmer. Before administering mannitol, visually inspect the mannitol container for precipitants. Mannitol is classified as a pregnancy category C drug. Recommended dosages are given in the table on p. 463.

### Pharmacokinetics

| Route | Onset of Action | Peak Plasma Concentration | Elimination Half-life | Duration of Action |
|-------|-----------------|---------------------------|-----------------------|--------------------|
| IV | 0.5-1 hr | 0.25-2 hr | 1.5 hr | 6-8 hr |

## POTASSIUM-SPARING DIURETICS

The currently available potassium-sparing diuretics are amiloride, spironolactone, and triamterene. These diuretics are also referred to as *aldosterone-inhibiting diuretics* because they block the aldosterone receptors. Spironolactone is a competitive antagonist of aldosterone, and for this reason it causes sodium and water to be excreted while potassium is retained. It is the most commonly used of the three drugs.

## Mechanism of Action and Drug Effects

Potassium-sparing diuretics work in the collecting ducts and distal convoluted tubules, where they interfere with sodium-potassium exchange. Spironolactone competitively binds to aldosterone receptors and therefore blocks the resorption of sodium and water that is induced by aldosterone secretion. These receptors are found primarily in the distal tubule. Amiloride and triamterene do not bind to aldosterone receptors. However, they inhibit both aldosterone-induced and basal sodium reabsorption, working in both the distal tubule and collecting ducts. They are often prescribed for children with heart failure, because pediatric cardiac problems are frequently accompanied by an excess secretion of aldosterone.

The potassium-sparing diuretics are relatively weak compared with the thiazide and loop diuretics. When diuresis is

| TABLE 28-4 | POTASSIUM-SPARING DIURETICS: COMMON ADVERSE EFFECTS |
|------------|------------------------------------------------------|
| **BODY SYSTEM** | **ADVERSE EFFECTS** |
| Central nervous | Dizziness, headache |
| Gastrointestinal | Cramps, nausea, vomiting, diarrhea |
| Other | Urinary frequency, weakness, hyperkalemia |

needed, they are generally used as adjuncts to thiazide treatment. This combination is beneficial in two respects. First, the drugs have synergistic diuretic effects; second, the two drugs counteract the adverse metabolic effects of one another. The thiazide diuretics cause potassium, magnesium, and chloride to be lost in the urine, and the potassium-sparing diuretics counteract this by elevating the potassium and chloride levels.

## Indications

Therapeutic applications of the potassium-sparing diuretics vary depending on the particular drug. Spironolactone and triamterene are used to treat hyperaldosteronism and hypertension and to reverse the potassium loss caused by the potassium-wasting (e.g., loop, thiazide) diuretics. One common feature of heart failure is a hyperactive renin-angiotensin-aldosterone system. Research has identified this hyperactivity as a causative factor in permanent ventricular myocardial wall damage, known as *remodeling*, following myocardial infarction. Various clinical trials have demonstrated a cardioprotective benefit of spironolactone in preventing this remodeling process, due to its aldosterone-inhibiting activity. The uses for amiloride are similar to those for spironolactone and triamterene, but amiloride is less effective in the long term. It may be more effective than spironolactone or triamterene in the treatment of metabolic alkalosis, however. It is primarily used in the management of heart failure. As with certain other classes of diuretics, potassium-sparing diuretics may also be indicated in cases of heart failure due to diastolic dysfunction.

## Contraindications

Contraindications to the use of potassium-sparing diuretics include known drug allergy, hyperkalemia (i.e., serum potassium level exceeding 5.5 mEq/L), and severe renal failure or anuria. Triamterene use may also be contraindicated in cases of severe hepatic failure.

## Adverse Effects

Potassium-sparing diuretics have several common undesirable effects, which are listed in Table 28-4. There are also some significant adverse effects that are specific to individual drugs. Spironolactone can cause gynecomastia, amenorrhea, irregular menses, and postmenopausal bleeding. Triamterene may reduce folic acid levels and cause the formation of kidney stones and urinary casts. It may also precipitate megaloblastic anemia. However, adverse effects from triamterene are rare. Hyperkalemia may occur when potassium-sparing diuretics are used in combination with each other and/or with other potassium-sparing drugs such as angiotensin-converting enzyme (ACE) inhibitors (see Chapter 22, as well as the Interactions section to follow).

## Interactions

Concurrent use of potassium-sparing diuretics and lithium, ACE inhibitors, or potassium supplements can result in significant drug interactions. The administration of ACE inhibitors or potassium supplements in combination with potassium-sparing diuretics can result in hyperkalemia. When lithium and potassium-sparing diuretics are given together, lithium toxicity can result. NSAIDs can inhibit renal prostaglandins, which decreases blood flow to the kidneys and therefore decreases the delivery of diuretic drugs to this site of action. This in turn can lead to a diminished diuretic response.

## Dosages

For dosage information on potassium-sparing diuretics, see the table below.

## DOSAGES

### Selected Potassium-Sparing Diuretic Drugs

| DRUG | USUAL DOSAGE RANGE | INDICATIONS |
|---|---|---|
| amiloride (Midamor) | **Adult** PO: 5-20 mg/day | Edema, heart failure (as an adjunct to loop diuretics) |
| ◆ spirono-lactone (Aldactone) | **Pediatric** PO: 3.3 mg/kg/day in single or divided doses **Adult** PO: 25-200 mg/day; given once or divided twice daily | Edema, hypertension, heart failure, ascites |
| triamterene (Dyrenium) | **Adult** PO: 50-100 mg bid; do not exceed 300 mg/day | |

*PO,* Oral.

## DRUG PROFILES

### amiloride

Amiloride (Midamor) is generally used in combination with a thiazide or loop diuretic in the treatment of heart failure. Hyperkalemia may occur in as many as 10% of the patients who take amiloride alone. It should be used with caution in patients who have renal impairment or diabetes mellitus and in elderly patients. It has only weak antihypertensive properties. Amiloride is available only in oral form. It is also available in combination with hydrochlorothiazide. Amiloride is classified as a pregnancy category B drug. Recommended dosages are given in the table on this page.

### Pharmacokinetics

| Route | Onset of Action | Peak Plasma Concentration | Elimination Half-life | Duration of Action |
|---|---|---|---|---|
| PO | 2 hr | 6-10 hr | 6-9 hr | 24 hr |

### ◆ spironolactone

Spironolactone (Aldactone) is a synthetic steroid that blocks aldosterone receptors. It is used in high dosages for the treatment of ascites, a condition commonly associated with cirrhosis of the liver. Monitor serum potassium levels frequently in patients who have impaired renal function or who are currently taking potassium supplements, because hyperkalemia is a common complication of spironolactone therapy. It is the potassium-sparing diuretic most commonly prescribed for children who have heart failure. Recently spironolactone has been shown to reduce morbidity and mortality in patients with severe heart failure when added to standard therapy. Of the three commonly used potassium-sparing diuretics, spironolactone has the greatest antihypertensive activity. It is available only in oral form. It also is available in combination with hydrochlorothiazide. Spironolactone is classified as a pregnancy category D drug. Recommended dosages are given in the table on this page.

### Pharmacokinetics

| Route | Onset of Action | Peak Plasma Concentration | Elimination Half-life | Duration of Action |
|---|---|---|---|---|
| PO | 1-3 days | 2-3 days | 13-24 hr | 2-3 days |

### triamterene

The pharmacologic properties of triamterene (Dyrenium) are similar to those of amiloride. Like amiloride, triamterene acts directly on the distal renal tubule of the nephron to depress the resorption of sodium and the excretion of potassium and hydrogen. It has little or no antihypertensive effect. Triamterene is available only in oral form and is also available in combination with hydrochlorothiazide. It is classified as a pregnancy category D drug. Recommended dosages are given in the table on this page.

### Pharmacokinetics

| Route | Onset of Action | Peak Plasma Concentration | Elimination Half-life | Duration of Action |
|---|---|---|---|---|
| PO | 2-3 hr | 6-8 hr | 2-3 hr | 12-16 hr |

## THIAZIDES AND THIAZIDE-LIKE DIURETICS

Thiazide and thiazide-like diuretics are considered equivalent in their effects. Thiazide diuretics, like several of the loop diuretics, are benzothiadiazines, chemical derivatives of sulfonamide antibiotics. The thiazide diuretics include chlorothiazide and hydrochlorothiazide. Hydrochlorothiazide is the most commonly prescribed and the least expensive of the thiazide diuretics. Hydrochlorothiazide is included in numerous combination products with antihypertensive drugs. The thiazide-like diuretics are very similar to the thiazides and include chlorthalidone, indapamide, and metolazone. Metolazone may be more effective than other drugs in this class in the treatment of patients with renal dysfunction.

## Mechanism of Action and Drug Effects

The primary site of action of thiazides and thiazide-like diuretics is the distal convoluted tubule, where they inhibit the resorption of sodium, potassium, and chloride. This results in osmotic water loss. Thiazides also cause direct relaxation of the arterioles (small blood vessels), which reduces peripheral vascular resistance (afterload). Decreased preload (filling pressures) and decreased afterload (the force the ventricles must overcome to eject the volume of blood they contain) are beneficial hemodynamic effects. This makes them very effective for the treatment of both heart failure and hypertension.

As renal function decreases, the efficacy of thiazides diminishes, because delivery of the drug to the site of activity is impaired. Thiazides are not to be used if creatinine clearance is less than 30 to 50 mL/min. Normal creatinine clearance is 125 mL/min, depending on age of the patient. However, metolazone remains effective to a creatinine clearance of 10 mL/min, and thus is used in cases of renal failure. The major adverse effects of the drugs stem from the electrolyte disturbances they produce. They are noted for precipitating hypokalemia and hypercalcemia, as well as metabolic disturbances such as hyperlipidemia, hyperglycemia, and hyperuricemia.

## Indications

The thiazide and thiazide-like diuretics are used in the treatment of edema of various origins, idiopathic hypercalciuria, and diabetes insipidus, in addition to hypertension. They are also used as adjunct drugs in the management of heart failure and hepatic cirrhosis. Any of these drugs can be used either as monotherapy or in combination with other drugs. As with certain other classes of diuretics, they may also be indicated in cases of heart failure due to diastolic dysfunction.

## Contraindications

Contraindications to the use of thiazides and thiazide-like diuretics include known drug allergy, hepatic coma (metolazone), anuria, and severe renal failure.

## Adverse Effects

Major adverse effects of the thiazide and thiazide-like diuretics relate to the electrolyte and metabolic disturbances they cause—mainly reduced potassium levels and elevated levels of calcium, lipids, glucose, and uric acid. Other effects, such as gastrointestinal disturbances, skin rashes, photosensitivity, thrombocytopenia, pancreatitis, and cholecystitis, are less common. Dizziness and vertigo are common adverse effects of metolazone therapy and are attributed to sudden shifts in the plasma volume brought about by the drug. Headache, impotence, and decreased libido are other important adverse effects of these drugs. Many of these adverse effects are dose related and are seen at higher doses, especially those above 25 mg. The more common adverse effects of the thiazide and thiazide-like diuretics are listed in Table 28-5.

### Toxicity and Management of Overdose

An overdose of these drugs can lead to an electrolyte imbalance resulting from hypokalemia. Symptoms include anorexia, nausea, lethargy, muscle weakness, mental confusion, and hypotension. Treatment involves electrolyte replacement.

### TABLE 28-5   THIAZIDE AND THIAZIDE-LIKE DIURETICS: POTENTIAL ADVERSE EFFECTS

| BODY SYSTEM | ADVERSE EFFECTS |
| --- | --- |
| Central nervous | Dizziness, headache, blurred vision |
| Gastrointestinal | Anorexia, nausea, vomiting, diarrhea |
| Genitourinary | Impotence |
| Hematologic | Jaundice, leukopenia, agranulocytosis |
| Integumentary | Urticaria, photosensitivity |
| Metabolic | Hypokalemia, hyperglycemia, hyperuricemia, hypochloremic alkalosis |

### TABLE 28-6   THIAZIDE AND THIAZIDE-LIKE DIURETICS: COMMON DRUG INTERACTIONS

| INTERACTING DRUG | MECHANISM | RESULTS |
| --- | --- | --- |
| Antidiabetic drugs | Antagonism | Reduced therapeutic hypoglycemic effect (i.e., increased blood glucose levels) |
| Corticosteroids | Additive effect | Hypokalemia |
| digoxin | Hypokalemia | Increased digoxin toxicity |
| lithium | Decreased clearance | Increased lithium toxicity |
| NSAIDs | Inhibition of renal prostaglandins | Decreased diuretic activity |

NSAIDs, Nonsteroidal antiinflammatory drugs.

## Interactions

Thiazides and related drugs interact with corticosteroids, diazoxide, digitalis, and oral hypoglycemics. The mechanisms and results of these interactions are summarized in Table 28-6. Excessive consumption of licorice can lead to an additive hypokalemia in patients taking these drugs.

## Dosages

For dosage information on thiazides and thiazide-like diuretics, see the table on p. 468.

## DRUG PROFILES

### ♦ hydrochlorothiazide

Hydrochlorothiazide (HydroDIURIL), which is considered the prototypical thiazide diuretic, is a very commonly prescribed and inexpensive thiazide diuretic. It is also a very safe and effective diuretic. Hydrochlorothiazide is used in combination with many other drugs, including methyldopa, propranolol, spironolactone, triamterene, hydralazine, ACE inhibitors, beta blockers, and labetalol. Dosages exceeding 50 mg/day rarely produce additional clinical results and may only increase drug toxicity. This property is known as a *ceiling effect*. However, doses up to 100 mg/day are not uncommon.

Hydrochlorothiazide is available only in oral form. It is classified as a pregnancy category B drug. Recommended dosages are given in the table on p. 468.

## DOSAGES

### Selected Thiazide and Thiazide-Like Diuretic Drugs

| DRUG | PHARMACOLOGIC CLASS | USUAL DOSAGE RANGE | INDICATIONS |
|------|---------------------|--------------------|-------------|
| ♦ hydrochlorothiazide (HydroDIURIL) | Thiazide diuretic | **Pediatric**<br>Younger than 6 mo: 2-4 mg/kg/day<br>Older than 6 mo: 2-3 mg/kg/day<br>**Adult**<br>25-100 mg/day, usually divided<br>**Elderly**<br>12.5-25 mg/day | Edema, heart failure (as an adjunct to loop diuretics) |
| metolazone (Zaroxolyn) | Thiazide-like diuretic | **Adult**<br>PO: 2.5-20 mg/day | |

*PO, Oral.*

### Pharmacokinetics (hydrochlorothiazide)

| Route | Onset of Action | Peak Plasma Concentration | Elimination Half-life | Duration of Action |
|-------|-----------------|---------------------------|----------------------|--------------------|
| PO | 2 hr | 4-6 hr | 5-15 hr | 6-12 hr |

### metolazone

Metolazone (Zaroxolyn) is a thiazide-like diuretic that appears to be more potent than the thiazide diuretics. This greater potency becomes important in patients with renal dysfunction. It remains effective to a creatinine clearance as low as 10 mL/min. It may also be given in combination with loop diuretics to produce diuresis in patients with moderate to severe symptoms of heart failure. Metolazone is more efficacious when given 30 minutes before loop diuretics. It is available only in oral form. Metolazone is classified as a pregnancy category B drug. Recommended dosages are given in the table on this page.

### Pharmacokinetics

| Route | Onset of Action | Peak Plasma Concentration | Elimination Half-life | Duration of Action |
|-------|-----------------|---------------------------|----------------------|--------------------|
| PO | 1 hr | 1-2 hr | 6-20 hr | 24 hr |

## NURSING PROCESS

## ASSESSMENT

Before giving a patient any type of diuretic, obtain a complete patient history and thorough medication history. Perform a physical assessment and document all findings, with emphasis on the body systems affected by the disease process or indication for the diuretic as well as by potential drug-related adverse effects. This would most likely include assessing baseline breath sounds, heart sounds, neurologic status, as well as checking skin turgor (for edema), moisture levels of mucus membranes, and capillary refill. Because fluid volume levels and electrolyte concentrations are affected by diuretics, assess and document the patient's baseline fluid volume status (as indicated by vital signs, weight, and intake-output measurements). Assess postural blood pressures (e.g., lying, sitting, standing) before and during drug therapy because

of diuretic-induced fluid volume loss, which may lead to postural or orthostatic hypotension. Postural or orthostatic hypotension is a drop in blood pressure of 20 mm Hg or more upon standing.

In addition, assess specific laboratory values associated with renal and hepatic functioning; for example, BUN level (normal range, 8 to 25 mg/100 mL) and creatinine level (normal range, 0.6 to 1.5 mg/100 mL) for renal function, and ALP (normal range, 13 to 39 units/L), AST (normal range, 8 to 46 units/L in males, 7 to 34 units/L in females), and LDH (normal range, 45 to 90 units/L) for hepatic function. It is important to note, however, that normal ranges of these laboratory values may vary somewhat from facility to facility. Serum electrolyte levels are also critical to assess before and during diuretic therapy because of the subsequent loss of electrolytes through the urine and their relationship to fluid volume status. Specifically, obtain and document serum potassium, sodium, chloride, magnesium, calcium, uric acid, and creatinine levels, as ordered. Arterial blood gas levels may also be ordered.

*Carbonic anhydrase inhibitors* require close assessment of sodium and potassium levels. These drugs are not to be used in patients with a history of renal or liver dysfunction. As with any diuretic that results in loss of potassium (excluding potassium-sparing diuretics), if these drugs are given concurrently with digoxin, there is increased risk for digoxin toxicity (because of the hypokalemia).

*Loop diuretics* are more potent than thiazide diuretics, combination products, and potassium-sparing diuretics. These drugs may pose more problems for the elderly or those with severe electrolyte loss and liver failure. An additional and significant concern for patients taking loop diuretics is their interaction with other medications that are neurotoxic or ototoxic (see Table 28-3). Cross-sensitivity has been documented in patients who are allergic to sulfonamide antibiotics (see pharmacology discussion). Loop diuretics may also cause severe skin reactions (i.e., exfoliative dermatitis with furosemide, Steven Johnsons syndrome with torsemide), so a thorough assessment of the patient's skin prior to administration is important. With torsemide, assess baseline complete blood counts and clotting studies, if ordered, because of the adverse effects of leukopenia, neutropenia, and thrombocytopenia. Additionally, with loop diuretics, potential

## PATIENT-CENTERED CARE: LIFESPAN CONSIDERATIONS FOR THE ELDERLY PATIENT

### Diuretic Therapy

- Before and during diuretic drug therapy, measure the patient's height, weight, intake and output, blood pressure, pulse rate, respiratory rate, and temperature. Assess breath and heart sounds and edematous areas. Monitor serum sodium, potassium, and chloride levels.
- Emphasize to the elderly patient that diuretics need to be taken at the same time every day. These drugs are generally ordered to be taken in the morning to help prevent nocturia (voiding at night), which can result in lack of sleep. More importantly, nocturia can lead to injury if the individual needs to get out of bed to void, becomes dizzy and/or confused, and falls. A bedside commode may be used to decrease the risk of injury.
- If the elderly patient is living alone and has minimal or no assistance with the medication regimen, visits from a home health aide or other health care professional may help ensure safety, efficacy, and compliance not only in taking the medication but also in following all aspects of the therapeutic regimen.
- Exercise caution in administering diuretics to the elderly, because they are more sensitive to the therapeutic effects of these drugs (often reacting to smaller dosages of medication than are required by other patients) and are

also more likely to experience the adverse effects of diuretics such as dehydration, electrolyte loss, dizziness, and syncope.
- Encourage the patient to change positions slowly because of the risk of orthostatic hypotension and subsequent falls and injury. Emphasize the importance of daily recording of weight, blood pressure, and overall well-being.
- Advise patients to carry a card containing a brief medical history, blood pressure readings, names and telephone numbers of contact persons, and a list of medications to ensure safety and minimize complications. The card can be formatted so that it may fit in a wallet. A copy may also be placed in the kitchen on the refrigerator door or in another visible location so that it will be easily available to emergency personnel. Copies of the card may be given to the caregiver(s), family members, significant others, prescribers, dentist, and relevant health care personnel. The card then needs to be updated at regular intervals by the patient or another adult, caregiver, or prescriber involved in the patient's care. Such a card can be made easily using standard card stock or an index card. It can be placed in a wallet sleeve and information entered using an erasable pen or pencil. The following sample shows suggested headings and content for such a card:

Name:_____ Age:_____ Allergies (drug/food):_____ Medical history (place X to the right of all that apply; write in any not listed): Anemia__ Asthma__ Bleeding problems__ Blood clots__ Breathing problems__ Cancer__ Depression__ Diabetes__ Difficulty swallowing__ Heart problems__ High blood pressure__ Low blood pressure__ Nerve problems__ Pacemaker or defibrillator device__ Recent weight gain__ Recent weight loss__ Stroke__ Thyroid problems__ Others:_____

Surgery (list all with date, type of surgery, purpose, any complications):_____
_____

Prosthetics used:_____ Dentures/ dental problems:_____ Assistive devices: Glasses __ Hearing aids_____
Mobility assistance_____

Contact names and phone numbers:_____
_____

Current medications (prescription drugs; over-the-counter drugs; herbals, vitamins, others)
Name(s) _____
Dosage (s) _____
Frequency of doses _____
Why taking the drug _____

drug-laboratory value interactions include increased serum uric acid and glucose levels.

With *potassium-sparing diuretics,* hyperkalemia may be an adverse effect; therefore, assess the patient's serum levels of potassium. Additionally, because of the potassium-sparing effect, contraindications include drugs or conditions that may result in hyperkalemia. Thus, potassium supplements, ACE inhibitors, and severe renal failure are contraindications. Lithium toxicity may occur if given with these diuretics because of the hyperkalemia. See the pharmacology section of this chapter for further discussion of additional cautions, contraindications, and drug interactions associated with diuretic use.

## NURSING DIAGNOSES

1. Decreased cardiac output related to drug effects and adverse effects of diuretics (e.g., fluid and electrolyte loss)

2. Deficient fluid volume related to drug effects and adverse effects of diuretics
3. Risk for injury related to postural hypotension and dizziness

## PLANNING

### GOALS

1. Patient regains and maintains balanced cardiac output.
2. Patient regains and maintains balanced fluid volume status.
3. Patient remains free from injury.

### OUTCOME CRITERIA

1. Patient continues to show normal cardiac output while receiving diuretic therapy, as evidenced by vital signs, adequate intake, and output within normal limits (pulse between 60 and 100 beats/min; blood pressure 120/80 mm Hg or within normal parameters; urine output 30 mL/hr or higher).

- Patient has strong pedal pulses and warm, pink extremities with rapid capillary refill.
2. Patient regains balanced fluid volume status without dehydration or overhydration.
   - Patient's skin is pliable and with firm turgor.
   - Patient's laboratory values return within normal limits for urine specific gravity, serum sodium, chloride, and potassium.
3. Patient takes diuretic therapy as directed and with adequate fluid intake while avoiding hypotensive episodes.
   - Patient changes positions slowly and with purpose while on diuretic therapy.
   - Patient reports excessive dizziness, lightheadedness, palpitations, tingling of fingers and toes, confusion, disorientation, and/or any fainting episodes.

## IMPLEMENTATION

Measure and record blood pressure, pulse rate, intake and output, and daily weights during diuretic therapy. Changes from the initial baseline assessment data that alert you to possible problems with the drug therapy include the presence of dizziness, fainting, lightheadedness on standing or changing positions, weakness, fatigue, tremor, muscle cramping, changes in mental status, or cold clammy skin. Diuretic therapy may also precipitate cardiac irregularities or palpitations; therefore, continue to monitor heart rate and rhythm. Fluid loss from the action of the diuretic may lead to the adverse effect of constipation, so preventative measures are needed, such as increased intake of fluids and fiber (unless contraindicated) and/or the use of natural bulk-forming products. If constipation continues, the prescriber may need to provide alternatives to psyllium-based bulk-forming laxatives. Always give diuretics exactly as directed but with consideration of the patient's age and related needs. Dosing and timing of the drugs are often very important to enhance therapeutic effects and minimize adverse effects. Because diuretics taken late in the afternoon or evening may lead to nocturia (urination at night) and subsequent loss in sleep, these medications are usually scheduled for morning dosing. Safety concerns exist with nocturia, especially in the elderly, because possible confusion and dizziness associated with getting up in the middle of the night may create the potential for falls and injury.

*Loop diuretics* (if taken at high dosages as ordered) may put patients at greater risk for fluid volume and electrolyte depletion (e.g., hypokalemia, hyponatremia, dehydration). Monitoring of therapy includes frequent assessment of blood pressure and pulse rate, including orthostatic blood pressures and pulse rates (supine and standing), hydration status, and capillary refill, as well as daily measurement of weight. Acute hypotensive episodes may occur with higher dosages of loop diuretics and precipitate syncope and falls; therefore, educate the patient about safety measures to prevent falls. Hypokalemia is the most commonly encountered electrolyte imbalance and may be very dangerous. Symptoms include anorexia, nausea, lethargy, muscle weakness, mental confusion, and hypotension. If intravenous dosage forms are given, it is crucial to check for proper diluents, drug incompatibilities, and intactness of the intravenous site. Double-check rates of infusion and use an infusion pump as deemed necessary.

With *potassium-sparing diuretics*, potassium is reabsorbed and not excreted (as previously discussed), so hyperkalemia, rather than hypokalemia, may become problematic. Signs and symptoms of hyperkalemia include nausea, vomiting, and diarrhea (see Chapter 29), with toxic levels manifested by cardiac rhythm abnormalities. Any of the signs and symptoms of hyperkalemia need to be reported immediately. See the Patient Teaching Tips for more information.

## EVALUATION

The therapeutic effects of *diuretics* include the resolution of or reduction in edema, fluid volume overload, heart failure, or hypertension, or a return to normal intraocular pressures (if used for that purpose, as with the CAIs). Monitor the patient for the occurrence of adverse reactions to the diuretics, such as hypotension (from volume loss), electrolyte imbalances,

## CASE STUDY

### *Hydrochlorothiazide Therapy*

Dr. G., a 62-year-old university professor, has been diagnosed with primary hypertension and will be taking 50 mg of hydrochlorothiazide (HCTZ) daily. There is no evidence of renal insufficiency or cardiac damage at this time, nor is there evidence of retinopathy or other signs and symptoms of end-organ disease. She is anxious because the fall semester is starting and she has a heavy teaching load but is willing to take the steps needed for better health.

At her 1-month follow-up appointment, Dr. G. complains of "feeling so tired" and asks whether the medication causes sleepiness. When questioned, she says that she takes the HCTZ at dinnertime because she is afraid it will "interfere with her classes."

1. What do you suspect is happening with Dr. G., and what would you recommend?
2. During this follow-up appointment, you ask Dr. G. if she is eating foods high in potassium. She looks embarrassed and answers, "I lost that pamphlet about the foods with potassium, but I try to drink orange juice every day." What foods should she eat for the potassium content?
3. The report on Dr. G.'s potassium levels comes back from the laboratory, and the results are 3.4 mEq/L. She asks, "Am I going to be put on a potassium pill too?" What is your answer?
4. Six months later, Dr. G. is diagnosed with type 2 diabetes mellitus and is started on oral hypoglycemic therapy. What will you teach her about managing her diabetes while taking the HCTZ?

For answers, see http://evolve.elsevier.com/Lilley.

metabolic acidosis (arterial blood gas values may need to be measured), drowsiness (with *CAIs*), hypokalemia, tachycardia (less significant with *mannitol*), and hyperkalemia *(potassium-sparing diuretics)*. Hypokalemia may be manifested by anorexia, nausea, lethargy, muscle weakness, mental confusion, and

hypotension. With potassium-sparing diuretics, hyperkalemia may be the adverse effect for which to monitor and is manifested by nausea, vomiting, and diarrhea (see Chapter 29), and cardiac rhythm abnormalities with severe hyperkalemia. Review all goals and outcome criteria in the evaluation process.

## PATIENT TEACHING TIPS

- Patients taking diuretics need to maintain proper nutritional intake and fluid volume and eat potassium-rich foods, except when contraindicated or when potassium-sparing diuretics are used. Foods high in potassium include bananas, oranges, apricots, dates, raisins, broccoli, green beans, potatoes, tomatoes, meats, fish, wheat bread, and legumes.
- Potassium supplementation may be recommended by a prescriber, depending on the symptoms the patient presents and the serum levels. Normal serum potassium levels are 3.5-5 mEq/L (see Chapter 29).
- Frequent laboratory tests may be indicated at the beginning of and during therapy with diuretics. These tests may include measurement of electrolytes, uric acid, and blood gases.
- Encourage patients to change positions slowly and to rise slowly after sitting or lying to prevent dizziness and possible fainting (syncope).
- Forcing of fluids may be needed (if not contraindicated) to prevent dehydration and minimize constipation. Increased consumption of fiber may also help with constipation.
- Any unusual adverse effects or problems, such as excessive dizziness, syncope, weakness, or muscle aches, need to be reported immediately to the prescriber.
- Advise the patient to keep a daily journal; entries should include weight, how the patient feels each day, dosage of diuretic, and any other important information related to the diagnosis and medical treatment.
- Educate the patient about the signs and symptoms of hypokalemia, such as anorexia, nausea, lethargy, muscle weakness, mental confusion, and hypotension. In addition, emphasize the importance of being cautious with hot climates, excessive sweating, fever, and the use of saunas or hot tubs. Heat raises core body temperature and causes further loss of potassium, sodium, and water through sweat, which may increase the risk of more problems with hypotension and fluid-electrolyte imbalances. Fluid volume and electrolyte loss may also occur with vomiting and diarrhea.
- If the patient is taking a diuretic along with digoxin, educate the patient, family members, and anyone involved in the patient's care about how to monitor pulse rate. The warning signs and symptoms of digoxin toxicity include headache, dizziness, confusion, nausea, visual disturbances, and bradycardia. A pulse rate of 60 beats/min or lower is often used as a guideline, but always check facility policy or guidelines.
- Educate patients with diabetes who are also taking thiazide and/or loop diuretics about the need for close monitoring of blood glucose levels.

## KEY POINTS

- The five main types of diuretics are CAIs, loop, osmotic, potassium-sparing, and thiazide and thiazide-like diuretics.
- The loop, potassium-sparing, and thiazide diuretics are the most commonly used. Remember that the loop diuretics are more potent than the thiazides, combination diuretics, and potassium-sparing diuretics.
- It is important to have a thorough knowledge of renal anatomy and physiology and how it relates to the action of the various diuretics; for example, if a loop diuretic is given, its
site of action is the loop of Henle and it causes the excretion of sodium, potassium, and chloride into the urine.
- Methods for monitoring excess and deficit fluid volume states include assessment of skin and mucous membranes, blood pressure, pulse rate, intake and output, and daily weights.
- With diuretics, always be concerned about the more vulnerable patient populations, such as the elderly, those with chronic illnesses, and patients with altered renal or liver function.

## NCLEX® EXAMINATION REVIEW QUESTIONS

1 The nurse is reviewing the medications that have been ordered for a patient for whom a loop diuretic has just been prescribed. The loop diuretic may have a possible interaction with which of the following?
   a Vitamin D
   b warfarin
   c Penicillins
   d NSAIDs

2 When monitoring laboratory test results for patients receiving loop and thiazide diuretics, the nurse knows to look for
   a decreased serum levels of potassium.
   b increased serum levels of calcium.
   c decreased serum levels of glucose.
   d increased serum levels of sodium.

3 When the nurse is checking the laboratory data for a patient taking spironolactone (Aldactone), which result would be a potential concern?
   a Serum sodium level of 140 mEq/L
   b Serum calcium level of 10.2 mg/dL
   c Serum potassium level of 5.8 mEq/L
   d Serum magnesium level of 2.0 mg/dL

4 Which statement needs to be included when the nurse provides patient education for a patient with heart failure who is taking daily doses of spironolactone (Aldactone)?
   a "Be sure to eat foods that are high in potassium."
   b "Avoid foods that are high in potassium."
   c "Avoid grapefruit juice while taking this medication."
   d "A low-fiber diet will help prevent adverse effects of this medication."

5 A patient with diabetes has a new prescription for a thiazide diuretic. Which statement will the nurse include when teaching the patient about the thiazide drug?
   a "There is nothing for you to be concerned about when you are taking the thiazide diuretic."
   b "Be sure to avoid foods that are high in potassium."
   c "You need to take the thiazide at night to avoid interactions with the diabetes medicine."
   d "Monitor your blood glucose level closely, because the thiazide diuretic may cause the levels to increase."

6 An elderly patient has been discharged following treatment for a mild case of heart failure. He will be taking a loop diuretic. Which instruction(s) from the nurse are appropriate? (Select all that apply.)
   a "Take the diuretic at the same time each morning."
   b "Take the diuretic only if you notice swelling in your feet."
   c "Be sure to stand up slowly because the medicine may make you feel dizzy if you stand up quickly."
   d "Drink at least 8 glasses of water each day."
   e "Here is a list of foods that are high in potassium—you need to avoid these."
   f "Please call your doctor immediately if you notice muscle weakness or increased dizziness."

7 The order reads: Give mannitol 0.5 g/kg IV now, over 2 hours. The patient weighs 165 lb, and you have a 100-mL vial of 20% mannitol. How many grams will the patient receive? How many milliliters of mannitol will you prepare for this infusion?

1. d, 2. a, 3. c, 4. b, 5. d, 6. a, c, f, 7. 37.5 g, 187.5 mL.

For Critical Thinking and Prioritization Questions, see http://evolve.elsevier.com/Lilley.

# Fluids and Electrolytes

## OBJECTIVES

When you reach the end of this chapter, you will be able to do the following:

1 Review the function of fluid volume and compartments within the body as well as the role of each of the major electrolytes in maintaining homeostasis.
2 Identify the various electrolytes, and give normal serum values for each.
3 Briefly discuss the various fluid and electrolyte disorders that commonly occur in the body with attention to fluid volume and/or electrolyte deficits and excesses.
4 Identify the fluid and electrolyte solutions commonly used to correct states of deficiency or excess.

5 Discuss the mechanisms of action, indications, dosages, routes of administration, contraindications, cautions, adverse effects, toxicity, and drug interactions of the various fluid and electrolyte solutions.
6 Compare the various solutions used to expand and/or decrease a patient's fluid volume and electrolytes with regard to how they work, why they are used, and specific antidotes available to counter any toxic effects.
7 Develop a nursing care plan that includes all phases of the nursing process for patients receiving fluid and electrolyte solutions.

## DRUG PROFILES

albumin, p. 478
conivaptan, p. 483
dextran, p. 479
fresh frozen plasma, p. 480

packed red blood cells, p. 480
potassium, p. 482
sodium chloride, pp. 477, 483
sodium polystyrene sulfonate (potassium exchange resin), p. 482

## KEY TERMS

**Blood** The fluid that circulates through the heart, arteries, capillaries, and veins, carrying nutriment and oxygen to the body cells. It consists of plasma, its liquid component, plus three major solid components: erythrocytes (red blood cells or RBCs), leukocytes (white blood cells or WBCs), and platelets. (p. 474)

**Colloids** Protein substances that increase the colloid oncotic pressure (p. 478)

**Colloid oncotic pressure** Another name for oncotic pressure. It is a form of osmotic pressure exerted by protein in blood plasma that tends to pull water into the circulatory system. (p. 475)

**Crystalloids** Substances in a solution that diffuse through a semipermeable membrane. (p. 476)

## KEY TERMS—cont'd

**Dehydration** Excessive loss of water from the body tissues. It is accompanied by an imbalance in the concentrations of essential electrolytes, particularly sodium, potassium, and chloride. (p. 475)

**Edema** The abnormal accumulation of fluid in interstitial spaces. (p. 475)

**Extracellular fluid (ECF)** That portion of the body fluid comprising the interstitial fluid and blood plasma. (p. 475)

**Extravascular fluid (EVF)** Fluid in the body that is outside the blood vessels. (p. 474)

**Gradient** A difference in the concentration of a substance on two sides of a permeable barrier. (p. 476)

**Hydrostatic pressure (HP)** The pressure exerted by a liquid. (p. 475)

**Hyperkalemia** An abnormally high potassium concentration in the blood, most often due to defective renal excretion but also caused by excessive dietary potassium or certain drugs, such as potassium-sparing diuretics or ACE inhibitors. (p. 480)

**Hypernatremia** An abnormally high sodium concentration in the blood; may be due to defective renal excretion but is more commonly caused by excessive dietary sodium or replacement therapy. (p. 482)

**Hypokalemia** A condition in which there is an inadequate amount of potassium, the major intracellular cation, in the bloodstream. (p. 480)

**Hyponatremia** A condition in which there is an inadequate amount of sodium, the major extracellular cation, in the bloodstream, caused either by inadequate excretion of water or by excessive water intake. (p. 482)

**Interstitial fluid (ISF)** The extracellular fluid that fills in the spaces between most of the cells of the body. (p. 474)

**Intracellular fluid (ICF)** The fluid located within cell membranes throughout most of the body. It contains dissolved solutes that are essential to maintaining electrolyte balance and healthy metabolism. (p. 474)

**Intravascular fluid (IVF)** The fluid inside blood vessels. (p. 474)

**Isotonic** Having the same concentration of a solute as another solution and hence exerting the same osmotic pressure as that solution, such as an isotonic saline solution that contains an amount of salt equal to that found in the intracellular and extracellular fluid. (p. 475)

**Osmotic pressure** The pressure produced by a solution necessary to prevent the osmotic passage of solvent into it when the solution and solvent are separated by a semipermeable membrane. (p. 475)

**Plasma** The watery, straw-colored fluid component of lymph and blood in which the leukocytes, erythrocytes, and platelets are suspended. (p. 474)

**Serum** The clear, cell-free portion of the blood from which fibrinogen has also been separated during the clotting process, as typically carried out with a laboratory sample. (p. 474)

## ANATOMY, PHYSIOLOGY, AND PATHOPHYSIOLOGY OVERVIEW

Fluid and electrolyte management is one of the cornerstones of patient care. Most disease processes, tissue injuries, and surgical procedures greatly influence the physiologic status of fluids and electrolytes in the body. Understanding fluid and electrolyte management requires knowledge of the extent and composition of the various body fluid compartments.

Approximately 60% of the adult human body is water. This is referred to as the *total body water (TBW)*, and it is distributed in the three main compartments in the following proportions: intracellular fluid (ICF), 67%; interstitial fluid (ISF), 25%; and plasma volume, 8%. This distribution is illustrated in Figure 29-1. The actual volume of fluid that would normally be in each compartment in an average 70-kg man with a TBW content of 60% is shown in Table 29-1.

The terms used to identify the various spaces within which the TBW is distributed can be quite confusing, and there are two basic approaches to distinguishing among the locations of the fluid. The TBW can be described as being in or out of the blood vessels (vasculature). If this point of reference is used, then the term intravascular fluid (IVF) is used to describe the fluid inside the blood vessels and the term extravascular

fluid (EVF) is used to refer to the fluid outside the blood vessels. Examples of EVF include lymph and cerebrospinal fluid. As these concepts are learned, it is important to remember the difference between the prefixes *intra-* (inside), *inter-* (between), and *extra-* (outside). The term plasma is used to describe the fluid that flows through the blood vessels (intravascular fluid). Serum is a closely related term (see Key Terms). The interstitial fluid (ISF) is the fluid that is in the space between cells, tissues, and organs. When discussing blood *vessels*, the term extra*vascular* volume is used; extravascular volume is made up of plasma and interstitial fluid (ISF). When discussing *cells*, the term

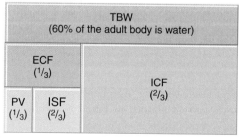

**FIGURE 29-1** Distribution of total body water (TBW). *ECF,* Extracellular fluid; *ICF,* intracellular fluid; *ISF,* interstitial fluid; *PV,* plasma volume.

extra*cellular* volume is used; extracellular volume is composed of ISF and intracellular fluid (ICF). These terms are often confused and misused. Table 29-1 lists these definitions for further clarity and understanding.

Extracellular fluid (ECF) consists of both plasma and ISF. There is one big difference between the plasma and the ISF. Plasma has a protein concentration four times greater than that of the ISF, composed primarily of albumin. The reason for this higher intravascular concentration of protein is that these solutes (proteins) have a very large molecular weight, which makes them too large to pass through the walls of the blood vessels. Because of the difference in the concentration, fluid flows from the area of low concentration in the interstitial compartment to the area of high concentration inside the blood vessel, trying to create an isotonic environment on either side of the blood vessel wall. (*Isotonic* means an equal concentration of solutes across a membrane.) The protein in the blood vessels exerts a constant osmotic pressure that prevents the leakage of too much plasma through the capillaries into the tissues. Because proteins suspended in plasma are in a *colloidal* state, this particular pressure is called colloid oncotic pressure, and normally it is 24 mm Hg. The opposing pressure, that exerted by the interstitial fluid (ISF), is called hydrostatic pressure (HP), and normally it is 17 mm Hg—which is less than the colloid oncotic pressure. The phenomenon of colloid oncotic pressure is illustrated in Figure 29-2.

| TABLE 29-1 | FLUID LOCATION: DESCRIPTIVE TERMS AND ACTUAL VOLUMES | |
|---|---|---|
| **TERM** | **LOCATION** | **ACTUAL VOLUMES (IN A 70-kg MAN WITH A TBW CONTENT OF 60% OF TOTAL BODY WEIGHT)** |
| **If the Point of Reference Is the Cells, These Terms Are Used** | | |
| Intracellular fluid (ICF) | Inside of cells | 28,000 mL |
| Extracellular fluid (ECF) | Outside of cells | 14,000 mL (composed of both intravascular plasma and interstitial fluid) |
| **If the Point of Reference Is the Blood Vessels, These Terms Are Used** | | |
| Intravascular fluid or plasma volume (PV) | In blood vessels | 3500 mL |
| Extravascular fluid (EVF) | Out of blood vessels | 38,500 mL |
| **If the Point of Reference Is the Tissues, These Terms Are Used** | | |
| Interstitial fluid (ISF) | In the spaces between cells, tissues, and organs but not in the plasma or the cells | 10,500 mL |

*TBW,* Total body water.

This regulation of the volume and composition of body water is essential for life, because body water is the medium in which all metabolic reactions occur. The body maintains the volume and composition remarkably constant by preserving the balance between intake and excretion. The amount of water gained each day is kept roughly equal to the amount of water lost. When the body cannot maintain this equilibrium, therapy with various agents is necessary. If the amount of water gained exceeds the amount of water lost, a water excess or overhydration occurs. Such fluid excesses often accumulate in interstitial spaces, such as in the pericardial sac, intrapleural space, peritoneal cavity, joint capsules, and lower extremities. This is referred to as edema. In contrast, if the quantity of water lost exceeds that gained, a water deficit, or dehydration, occurs. Death often occurs when 20% to 25% of TBW is lost.

Dehydration leads to a disturbance in the balance between the amount of fluid in the extracellular compartment and that in the intracellular compartment. Sodium is the principle extracellular electrolyte and plays a primary role in maintaining water concentration due to its highly osmotic chemistry. In the initial stages of dehydration, water is lost first from the extracellular compartments. The amount of further fluid losses, colloid oncotic pressure changes, or both determines the type of clinical dehydration that develops (Table 29-2). Clinical conditions that can result in dehydration and fluid loss, as well as the symptoms of dehydration and fluid loss, are presented in Table 29-3. When fluid that has been lost must be replaced, there are three categories of agents that can be used to accomplish this: crystalloids, colloids, and blood products. The clinical situation dictates which category of agents is most appropriate.

Acid-base balance is also important to normal bodily functions and is regulated by the respiratory system and the kidney. An *acid* is a substance that can donate or release hydrogen ions, such as carbonic acid or hydrochloric acid. A *base* is a substance that can accept hydrogen ions, such as bicarbonate. The *pH* is a measure of the degree of acidosis and alkalinity and is inversely related to hydrogen ion concentration. For example, when hydrogen ion concentration

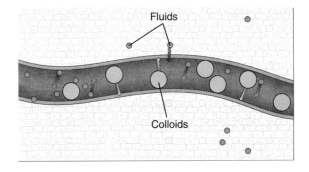

**FIGURE 29-2** Colloid osmotic pressure (oncotic pressure). As shown, the colloids inside the blood vessel are too large to pass through the vessel wall. The resulting oncotic pressure exerted by the colloids draws fluid from the surrounding tissues and other extravascular spaces into the blood vessels and also keeps fluid inside the blood vessel.

increases, the pH decreases and leads to acidity. As hydrogen ion concentration decreases, the pH increases, leading to more alkalinity. With the normal pH ranging from 7.35 to 7.45, acidosis occurs when there is an excess of hydrogen or carbon dioxide ($CO_2$) and the pH falls below 7.35. Conversely, alkalosis occurs when there is a hydrogen or $CO_2$ deficit and the pH rises above 7.45.

Regulation of the acid-base balance requires healthy functioning of the respiratory and renal systems. The respiratory system compensates for metabolic problems and pH imbalances by regulation of $CO_2$. In acidosis, $CO_2$ can be exhaled to try to normalize the lower pH; however, in alkalosis, carbon dioxide will be retained by the respiratory system to try and elevate the pH. The kidney also compensates by reabsorbing and generating bicarbonate and excreting hydrogen ions in acidosis to normalize the low pH. Conversely, the kidney can excrete bicarbonate and retain hydrogen ions to normalize the high pH seen with alkalosis. Certain drugs, such as the diuretic acetazolamide (see Chapter 28) and sodium bicarbonate (tablets or injection), can also be used to correct metabolic acid-base disturbances.

## PHARMACOLOGY OVERVIEW

### CRYSTALLOIDS

Crystalloids are fluids given by intravenous (IV) injection that supply water and sodium to maintain the osmotic gradient between the extravascular and intravascular compartments. Their plasma volume–expanding capacity is related to their sodium concentration. The different crystalloids are listed in Table 29-4.

### Mechanism of Action and Drug Effects

Crystalloid solutions contain fluids and electrolytes that are normally found in the body. They do not contain proteins (colloids), which are necessary to maintain the colloid oncotic pressure and prevent water from leaving the plasma compartment. In fact, the administration of large quantities of crystalloid solutions for fluid resuscitation decreases the colloid oncotic pressure, due to a dilutional effect. Crystalloids are distributed faster into the interstitial and intracellular compartments than colloids. This makes crystalloids better for treating dehydration than for expanding the plasma volume alone, such as in hypovolemic shock.

### Indications

Crystalloid solutions are most commonly used as maintenance fluids. They are used to compensate for insensible fluid losses, to replace fluids, and to manage specific fluid and electrolyte disturbances. Crystalloids also promote urinary flow. They are much less expensive than colloids and blood products. In addition, there is no risk for viral transmission or anaphylaxis and no alteration in the coagulation profile associated with their

| TABLE 29-2 | TYPES OF DEHYDRATION |
|---|---|
| **TYPE OF DEHYDRATION** | **CHARACTERISTICS** |
| Hypertonic | Occurs when water loss is greater than sodium loss, which results in a concentration of solutes outside the cells and causes the fluid inside the cells to move to the extracellular space, thus dehydrating the cells. Example: Elevated temperature resulting in perspiration. |
| Hypotonic | Occurs when sodium loss is greater than water loss, which results in higher concentrations of solute inside the cells and causes fluid to be pulled from outside the cells (plasma and interstitial spaces) into the cells. Examples: Renal insufficiency and inadequate aldosterone secretion. |
| Isotonic | Caused by a loss of both sodium and water from the body, which results in a decrease in the volume of extracellular fluid. Examples: Diarrhea and vomiting. |

| TABLE 29-3 | CONDITIONS LEADING TO FLUID LOSS OR DEHYDRATION AND ASSOCIATED CORRESPONDING SYMPTOMS* |
|---|---|
| **CONDITION** | **ASSOCIATED SYMPTOMS** |
| Bleeding | Tachycardia and hypotension |
| Bowel obstruction | Reduced perspiration and mucous secretions |
| Diarrhea | Reduced urine output (oliguria) |
| Fever | Dry skin and mucous membranes |
| Vomiting | Reduced lacrimal (tears) and salivary secretions |

*There may be overlap involving more than one of the symptoms depending on the patient's specific condition.

| TABLE 29-4 | CRYSTALLOIDS | | | | | | | |
|---|---|---|---|---|---|---|---|---|
| | **COMPOSITION (mEq/L)** | | | | | | | |
| **PRODUCT** | **Na** | **Cl** | **K** | **Ca** | **Mg** | **LACTATE** | **VOLUME (mL)** | **COST*** |
| NS | 154 | 154 | 0 | 0 | 0 | 0 | 1000 | 1 |
| Hypertonic saline | 513 | 513 | 0 | 0 | 0 | 0 | 500 | 1 |
| Lactated Ringer's | 130 | 109 | 4 | 3 | 0 | 28 | 1000 | 2.5 |
| D₅W | 0 | 0 | 1 | 0 | 0 | 0 | 1000 | 2 |

*Ca*, Calcium; *Cl*, chloride; *D₅W*, 5% dextrose in water; *K*, potassium; *Mg*, magnesium; *Na*, sodium; *NS*, normal saline.
*Relative cost compared with the cost of normal saline; for example, D₅W is two times the cost of normal saline.

use, unlike with blood products. The choice of whether to use a crystalloid or a colloid depends on the severity of the condition. The following are the common indications for either crystalloid or colloid replacement therapy:

- Acute liver failure
- Acute nephrosis
- Adult respiratory distress syndrome
- Burns
- Cardiopulmonary bypass
- Hypoproteinemia
- Reduction of the risk for deep vein thrombosis
- Renal dialysis
- Shock

## Contraindications

Contraindications to the use of crystalloids include known drug allergy to a specific product and hypervolemia, and may include severe electrolyte disturbance, depending on the type of crystalloid used.

## Adverse Effects

Crystalloids are a very safe and effective means of replacing needed fluid. They do, however, have some unwanted effects. Because they contain no large particles, such as proteins, they do not stay within the blood vessels and can leak out of the plasma into the tissues and cells. This may result in edema anywhere in the body. Peripheral edema and pulmonary edema are two common examples. Crystalloids also dilute the proteins that are in the plasma, which further reduces the colloid oncotic pressure. To be effective, large volumes (liters of fluid) are usually required. As a result, prolonged infusions may worsen acidosis or alkalosis, or adversely affect central nervous system function, due to fluid overload. Another disadvantage of crystalloids is that their effects are relatively short-lived.

## Interactions

Interactions with crystalloid solutions are rare because they are very similar if not identical to normal physiologic substances. Certain electrolytes contained in lactated Ringer's solution may be incompatible with other electrolytes, forming a chemical precipitate. Phenytoin precipitates if mixed with dextrose.

## Dosages

For the dosage information on crystalloids, see Table 29-5.

## DRUG PROFILE

The most commonly used crystalloid solutions are normal saline (NS or 0.9% sodium chloride) and lactated Ringer's solution. The available crystalloid solutions and their compositions are summarized in Table 29-4. Sodium chloride is also discussed briefly in the section on electrolytes and in the Nursing Process section under electrolytes.

### sodium chloride

Sodium chloride (NaCl) is available in several concentrations, the most common being 0.9%. This is the physiologically normal concentration of sodium chloride, and it is referred to as *normal saline* (NS). Other concentrations are 0.45% ("half-normal"), 0.25% ("quarter-normal"), 3% (hypertonic saline), and 5% (hypertonic saline). These solutions have different indications and are used in different situations, depending on how urgently fluid volume restoration is needed and/or the extent of the sodium loss.

Sodium chloride is a physiologic electrolyte that is present throughout the body's water. Thus, there are no hypersensitivity reactions to it. It is safe to administer it during any stage of pregnancy, but it is contraindicated in patients with hypernatremia and/or hyperchloremia. Hypertonic saline injections (3% and 5%) are contraindicated in the presence of increased, normal, or only slightly decreased serum electrolyte concentrations. Hypertonic saline is considered a high-risk drug because deaths have occurred when it is infused inappropriately. Correcting sodium too rapidly with hypertonic saline can lead to *osmotic demyelination syndrome,* which is potentially fatal. Conversely, infusing hypotonic saline (0.25% NaCl) is not recommended because it can cause hemolysis of the red blood cells. Adding potassium to hypotonic solutions makes them isotonic and safe to give. Sodium chloride is also available as a 650-mg tablet.

The dose of sodium chloride administered depends on the clinical situation. The volume of crystalloid or colloid needed to expand the plasma volume by 1 L (1000 mL) is given in Table 29-5, and this can be used as a general guide to dosing.

### Pharmacokinetics

| Plasma Volume Expansion* | Colloid Oncotic Pressure | Duration of Expansion |
|---|---|---|
| 60-70 mL | 30 mm Hg | A few hours |

*500 mL of normal saline will expand the plasma volume by 60 to 70 mL.

---

| TABLE 29-5 | CRYSTALLOIDS AND COLLOIDS: DOSING GUIDELINES |
|---|---|

| **CRYSTALLOIDS AND COLLOIDS** | | | |
|---|---|---|---|
| **0.9% SALINE** | **3% SALINE*** | **5% COLLOID†** | **25% COLLOID‡** |
| **To Raise Plasma Volume by 1 L, Administer:** | | | |
| 5-6 L | 1.5-2 L | 1 L | 0.5 L |
| **Compartment to Which Fluid Is Distributed:** | | | |
| Plasma 25% | 25% | 100% | 200%-300% |
| Interstitial space 75% | 75% | 0 | Decreased fluid levels |
| Intracellular space 0 | 0 | 0 | Decreased fluid levels |

*Hypertonic saline is a high-risk drug and should not be given faster than 100 mL/hr for short periods. Frequent monitoring of serum levels is required.
†Iso-oncotic solutions such as 5% albumin, dextran 70, and hetastarch.
‡Hyperoncotic solutions such as 25% albumin.

## COLLOIDS

Colloids are protein substances that increase the colloid oncotic pressure and move fluid from the interstitial compartment to the plasma compartment by pulling the fluid into the blood vessels. Normally, this task is performed by the three blood proteins: albumin, globulin, and fibrinogen. The total protein level must be in the range of 7.4 g/dL. If this level falls below 5.3 g/dL, fluid shifts out of blood vessels into the tissues. When this happens, colloid replacement therapy is required to reverse this process by increasing the colloid oncotic pressure. Colloid oncotic pressure decreases with age and also with hypotension and malnutrition. The commonly used colloids are listed in Table 29-6.

### Mechanism of Action and Drug Effects

The mechanism of action of colloids is related to their ability to increase the colloid oncotic pressure. Because the colloids cannot pass into the extravascular space, there is a higher concentration of colloid solutes (solid particles) inside the blood vessels (intravascular space) than outside the blood vessels. Fluid thus moves from the extravascular space into the blood vessels in an attempt to make it isotonic. As such, colloids increase the blood volume, and they are sometimes called *plasma expanders*. They also make up part of the total plasma volume.

Colloids increase the colloid oncotic pressure and move fluid from outside the blood vessels to inside the blood vessels. They can maintain the colloid oncotic pressure for several hours. They are naturally occurring products and consist of proteins (albumin), carbohydrates (dextrans or starches), fats (lipid emulsion), and animal collagen (gelatin). Usually they contain a combination of both small and large particles. The small particles are eliminated quickly and promote diuresis and perfusion of the kidneys; the larger particles maintain the plasma volume. Albumin is the one exception in that it contains particles that are all the same size.

### Indications

Colloids are used to treat a wide variety of conditions (see the list on p. 477). Clinically, colloids are superior to crystalloids because of their ability to maintain the plasma volume for a longer time. However, crystalloids are less expensive and are less likely to promote bleeding. Crystalloids are more likely to cause edema because of the larger volumes needed to achieve the desired clinical effect. Crystalloids are better than colloids for emergency short-term plasma volume expansion.

### Contraindications

Contraindications to the use of colloids include known drug allergy to a specific product and hypervolemia, and may include severe electrolyte disturbance.

### Adverse Effects

Colloids are relatively safe agents, although there are some disadvantages to their use. They have no oxygen-carrying ability and contain no clotting factors, unlike blood products. Because of this, they can alter the coagulation system through a dilutional effect, which results in impaired coagulation and possibly bleeding. They may also dilute the plasma protein concentration, which in turn may impair platelet function. Rarely, dextran therapy causes anaphylaxis or renal failure.

### Interactions

No drug interactions occur with colloids.

### Dosages

For dosage information on colloids, see Table 29-5.

## DRUG PROFILES

The specific colloid used for replacement therapy varies from institution to institution. The three most commonly used are 5% albumin, dextran 40, and hetastarch. They all have a very rapid onset of action as well as a long duration of action. They are metabolized in the liver and excreted by the kidneys. Albumin is the one exception; it is metabolized by the reticuloendothelial system and excreted by the kidneys and the intestines. Hetastarch is a synthetic colloid with properties similar to those of albumin and dextran.

### albumin

Albumin is a natural protein that is normally produced by the liver. It is responsible for generating approximately 70% of the colloid oncotic pressure. Human albumin is a sterile solution of serum albumin that is prepared from pooled blood, plasma, serum, or placentas obtained from healthy human donors. It is pasteurized (heated at 140° F [60° C] for 10 hours) to destroy any contaminants. Unfortunately, because it is derived from human donors, the supply is limited. Many institutions have specific indications for the use of albumin.

Albumin is contraindicated in patients with a known hypersensitivity to it and in those with heart failure, severe anemia, or renal insufficiency. Albumin is available only in parenteral form in concentrations of 5% and 25%. It is classified as a pregnancy category C drug. See Table 29-5 for dosing guidelines.

#### Pharmacokinetics

| Route | Onset of Action | Peak Plasma Concentration | Elimination Half-life | Duration of Action |
|---|---|---|---|---|
| IV | Less than 1 min | Unknown | 16 hr | Less than 24 hr |

| TABLE 29-6 | COMMONLY USED COLLOIDS | | | |
|---|---|---|---|---|
| | **COMPOSITION (mEq/L)** | | | |
| **PRODUCT** | **Na** | **Cl** | **VOLUME (mL)** | **COST\*** |
| Dextran 70† | 154 | 154 | 500 | 1 |
| Dextran 40† | 154 | 154 | 500 | 2 |
| Hetastarch | 154 | 154 | 500 | 5 |
| 5% Albumin | 145 | 145 | 500 | 10 |
| 25% Albumin | 145 | 145 | 100 | 10 |

*Cl*, Chloride; *Na*, sodium.
\*Relative cost compared with the cost of dextran 70.
†Dextran is available in NaCl, which has 154 mEq/L of both Na and Cl. It is also available in 5% dextrose in water, which contains no Na or Cl.

## dextran

Dextran is a solution of glucose. It is available in three concentrations, dextran 40 and the more concentrated dextran 70 and dextran 75, and it has a molecular weight similar to that of albumin. Dextran 40 is the more commonly used of the two. It is a derivative of sugar that has actions similar to those of human albumin in that it expands the plasma volume by drawing fluid from the interstitial space to the intravascular space.

Dextran is contraindicated in patients with a known hypersensitivity to it and in those with heart failure, renal insufficiency, and extreme dehydration. It is available only in parenteral form in either a 5% dextrose solution or a 0.9% sodium chloride solution. It is classified as a pregnancy category C drug. See Table 29-5 for dosing guidelines.

### Pharmacokinetics

| Route | Onset of Action | Peak Plasma Concentration | Elimination Half-life | Duration of Action |
|-------|-----------------|---------------------------|-----------------------|--------------------|
| IV | 5 min | Unknown | 2-6 hr | 4-6 hr |

## BLOOD PRODUCTS

Blood products can be thought of as biologic drugs. All of them can augment the plasma volume. Red blood cell (RBC)–containing products can also improve tissue oxygenation, as well as augment plasma volume. Blood products are more expensive than crystalloids and colloids and are less available because they are natural products and require human donors. The available blood products are listed in Table 29-7. They are most often indicated when a patient has lost 25% or more blood volume.

### Mechanism of Action and Drug Effects

The mechanism of action of blood products is related to their ability to increase the colloid oncotic pressure, and hence the plasma volume. They do so in the same manner as colloids and crystalloids, by pulling fluid from the extravascular space to the intravascular space. Because of this they are also considered plasma expanders. RBC products also have the ability to carry oxygen. They can maintain the colloid oncotic pressure for several hours to days. Because they come from human donors, they have all the benefits (and hazards) that human blood products have. They are administered when a person's body is deficient in these products.

| TABLE 29-7 | BLOOD PRODUCTS | |
|------------|----------------|---|
| **PRODUCT** | **DOSAGE** | **COST*** |
| Cryoprecipitate | 1 unit | 1 |
| FFP | 1 unit | 1.7 |
| PRBCs | 1 unit | 2.2 |
| PPF | 1 unit | 1 |
| Whole blood | 1 unit | 3.33 |

*FFP*, Fresh frozen plasma; *PPF*, plasma protein fraction; *PRBCs*, packed red blood cells.
*Relative cost compared with the cost of cryoprecipitate.

## Indications

Blood products are used to treat a wide variety of clinical conditions, and the blood product used depends on the specific indication. The available blood products and the specific conditions they are used to treat are listed in Table 29-8.

## Contraindications

There are no absolute contraindications to the use of blood products. However, because there is a risk for transfer of infectious disease, although remote, their use needs to be based on careful clinical evaluation of the patient's condition.

## Adverse Effects

Blood products can produce undesirable effects, some potentially serious. Because these products come from other humans, they can be incompatible with the recipient's immune system. These incompatibilities are tested for before their administration by determining the respective blood types of the donor and recipient and by performing cross-matching tests to screen for incompatibility between selected blood proteins. This helps reduce the likelihood that the recipient will reject the blood product, which would precipitate transfusion reactions and anaphylaxis. These products can also transmit pathogens from the donor to the recipient. Examples of such pathogens are hepatitis virus and human immunodeficiency virus. Various preparation techniques are now used to reduce the risk for pathogen transmission, and these have resulted in a drastic reduction in the incidence of such problems.

## Interactions

As with crystalloids and colloids, blood products are very similar if not identical to normal physiologic substances; therefore, they are involved in very few interactions. Calcium and aspirin, which normally affect coagulation, may interact with these

| TABLE 29-8 | BLOOD PRODUCTS: INDICATIONS |
|------------|------------------------------|
| **BLOOD PRODUCT** | **INDICATION** |
| Cryoprecipitate and PPF | To manage acute bleeding (over 50% blood loss slowly or 20% rapidly) |
| FFP | To increase clotting factor levels in patients with a demonstrated deficiency |
| PRBCs | To increase oxygen-carrying capacity in patients with anemia, in patients with substantial hemoglobin deficits, and in patients who have lost up to 25% of their total blood volume |
| Whole blood | Same as for PRBCs, except that whole blood is more beneficial in cases of extreme (over 25%) loss of blood volume because whole blood also contains plasma, the chief fluid volume of the blood; it also contains plasma proteins, the chief osmotic component, which help draw fluid back into blood vessels from surrounding tissues |

*FFP*, Fresh frozen plasma; *PPF*, plasma protein fraction; *PRBCs*, packed red blood cells.

| TABLE 29-9 | SUGGESTED GUIDELINES FOR BLOOD PRODUCTS: MANAGEMENT OF BLEEDING |
|---|---|
| **AMOUNT OF BLOOD LOSS** | **FLUID OF CHOICE** |
| 20% or less (slow loss) | Crystalloids |
| 20%-50% (slow loss) | Nonprotein plasma expanders (dextran and hetastarch) |
| Over 50% (slow loss) or 20% (acutely) | Whole blood or PRBCs, and/or PPF and FFP |
| 80% or more | As above, but for every 5 units of blood given, administer 1 to 2 units of FFP and 1 to 2 units of platelets to prevent the hemodilution of clotting factors and bleeding |

*FFP,* Fresh frozen plasma; *PPF,* plasma protein fraction; *PRBCs,* packed red blood cells.

substances when infused in the body in much the same way that they interact with the body's own blood components. Blood must not be administered with any solution other than normal saline.

## Dosages

For dosage information on blood products, see Table 29-9.

## DRUG PROFILES

Packed red blood cells (PRBCs) and fresh frozen plasma (FFP) are among the most commonly used blood products. All of the blood products are derived from pooled blood from human donors. Other less commonly used, but still important, blood products are whole blood, plasma protein fraction, cryoprecipitate, and platelets.

### packed red blood cells

Packed red blood cells (PRBCs) are obtained by the centrifugation of whole blood and the separation of RBCs from plasma and the other cellular elements. The advantage of PRBCs is that their oxygen-carrying capacity is better than that of the other blood products, and they are less likely to cause cardiac fluid overload. Their disadvantages include high cost, limited shelf life, and fluctuating availability, as well as their ability to transmit viruses, trigger allergic reactions, and cause bleeding abnormalities. The suggested guidelines for their use are given in Table 29-9.

### fresh frozen plasma

Fresh frozen plasma (FFP) is obtained by centrifuging whole blood and thereby removing the cellular elements. The resulting plasma is then frozen at −0.4° F (−18° C). FFP is not recommended for routine fluid resuscitation, but it may be used as an adjunct to massive blood transfusion in the treatment of patients with underlying coagulation disorders. The plasma-expanding capability of FFP is similar to that of dextran but slightly less than that of hetastarch. The disadvantage of FFP use is that it can transmit pathogens. The suggested guidelines for use are given in Table 29-9.

## PHYSIOLOGY OF ELECTOLYTE BALANCE

The chemical composition of the fluid compartments varies. The principal electrolytes in the extracellular fluid are sodium cations ($Na^+$) and chloride anions ($Cl^-$). The major electrolyte in the intracellular fluid (ICF) is the potassium cation ($K^+$). Other important electrolytes are calcium, magnesium, and phosphorus. These different chemical components are vital to the normal function of all body systems. They are controlled by the renin-angiotensin-aldosterone system, antidiuretic hormone system, and sympathetic nervous system. When these neuroendocrine systems are out of balance, adverse electrolyte imbalances commonly result. Patients who receive diuretics (see Chapter 28) are at risk of electrolyte abnormalities.

## POTASSIUM

Potassium is the most abundant cationic (positively charged) electrolyte inside cells (the intracellular space), where the normal concentration is approximately 150 mEq/L. Approximately 95% of the potassium in the body is intracellular. In contrast, the amount of potassium outside the cells in the plasma ranges from 3.5 to 5 mEq/L. These plasma levels are critical to normal body function.

Potassium is obtained from a variety of foods, the most common being fruit and juices, vegetables, fish, and meats. It has been estimated that for normal body functions to be maintained, a person must consume 5 to 10 mEq of potassium per day. Fortunately, the average daily diet usually provides 35 to 100 mEq of potassium, which is well above the required daily amount. Excess dietary potassium is usually excreted by the kidneys in the urine. However, if the kidneys lose their ability to filter and secrete waste products, potassium can accumulate. Excessive potassium can precipitate ventricular fibrillation and cardiac arrest. Hyperaldosteronism and use of potassium-sparing diuretics can alter normal potassium balance as well. Hyperkalemia is the term for an excessive serum potassium level and is defined as a serum potassium level exceeding 5.5 mEq/L. There are several causes of hyperkalemia, including the following:

- Angiotensin-converting enzyme (ACE) inhibitor use
- Burns
- Excessive loss from cells
- Infections
- Metabolic acidosis
- Potassium supplementation
- Potassium-sparing diuretic use
- Renal failure
- Trauma

The opposite of hyperkalemia is hypokalemia, or a deficiency of potassium. Hypokalemia is defined as a serum potassium level of less than 3.5 mEq/L. This condition is more often the result of excessive potassium loss than of poor dietary intake, however. As with hyperkalemia, there are many clinical conditions and other situations that can cause it. These include the following:

- Alkalosis
- Increased secretion of mineralocorticoids (hormones of the adrenal cortex)

## BOX 29-1 SYMPTOMS OF HYPOKALEMIA

| Early | Late |
|-------|------|
| Anorexia | Cardiac dysrhythmias |
| Hypotension | Neuropathy |
| Lethargy | Paralytic ileus |
| Mental confusion | Secondary alkalosis |
| Muscle weakness | |
| Nausea | |

- Burns*
- Corticosteroid use
- Crash diets
- Diarrhea
- Hyperaldosteronism
- Ketoacidosis
- Consumption of large amounts of licorice
- Loop diuretic use
- Malabsorption
- Prolonged laxative misuse
- Thiazide or thiazide-like diuretic use
- Vomiting

A low serum potassium level can increase the toxicity associated with digoxin, and this can precipitate serious ventricular dysrhythmias.

The early detection of hypokalemia is important to prevent the serious, life-threatening consequences of this metabolic disturbance if it goes untreated. The key to early detection is recognizing its early symptoms, which are generally mild and can easily go unnoticed. Both the early (mild) symptoms and late (severe) symptoms of hypokalemia are listed in Box 29-1. Treatment involves both identifying and treating the cause and restoring the serum potassium levels to normal (higher than 3.5 mEq/L). The consumption of potassium-rich foods can usually correct mild hypokalemia, but clinically significant hypokalemia requires the oral or parenteral administration of a potassium supplement, which usually contains potassium chloride.

### Mechanism of Action and Drug Effects

The importance of potassium as the primary intracellular electrolyte is highlighted by the number of life-sustaining physiologic functions that require it. Muscle contraction, the transmission of nerve impulses, and the regulation of heartbeats (the pacemaker function of the heart) are just a few of these functions.

Potassium is also essential for the maintenance of acid-base balance, isotonicity, and the electrodynamic characteristics of the cell. It plays a role in many enzymatic reactions, and it is an essential component in gastric secretion, renal function, tissue synthesis, and carbohydrate metabolism.

### Indications

Potassium replacement therapy is indicated in the treatment or prevention of potassium depletion in patients whenever dietary measures prove inadequate. Potassium salts commonly used for this purpose include potassium chloride, potassium phosphate, and potassium acetate. The chloride is required to correct the hypochloremia (low level of chloride in the blood) that commonly accompanies potassium deficiency, and the phosphate is used to correct hypophosphatemia. The acetate salt may be used to raise the blood pH in acidotic conditions.

Other therapeutic effects of potassium are related to its role in the contraction of muscles and the maintenance of the electrical characteristics of cells. Potassium salts may be used to stop irregular heartbeats (dysrhythmias) and to manage the tachy-dysrhythmias that can occur after cardiac surgery.

### Contraindications

Contraindications to potassium replacement products include known allergy to a specific drug product, hyperkalemia from any cause, severe renal disease, acute dehydration, untreated Addison's disease, severe hemolytic disease, and conditions involving extensive tissue breakdown (e.g., multiple trauma, severe burns).

### Adverse Effects

The adverse effects of oral potassium are primarily limited to the gastrointestinal (GI) tract, including diarrhea, nausea, and vomiting. More significant effects include GI bleeding and ulceration. The parenteral administration of potassium usually produces pain at the injection site. Cases of phlebitis have been associated with IV administration. The generally accepted maximum concentration for peripheral infusion is 20 to 40 mEq/L and up to 60 mEq/L for a central line. Excessive administration of potassium salts can lead to hyperkalemia and toxic effects. If IV potassium is administered too rapidly, cardiac arrest may occur. IV potassium must not be given faster than 10 mEq/hr to patients who are not on cardiac monitors. For critically ill patients on cardiac monitors, rates of 20 mEq/hr or more may be used.

### Toxicity and Management of Overdose

The toxic effects of potassium are the result of hyperkalemia. Symptoms include muscle weakness, paresthesia, paralysis, cardiac rhythm irregularities that can result in ventricular fibrillation, and cardiac arrest. The treatment instituted depends on the degree of the hyperkalemia and ranges from reversal of life-threatening problems to simple dietary restrictions. In the event of severe hyperkalemia, the IV administration of sodium bicarbonate, calcium gluconate or chloride, or dextrose solution with insulin is often required. These drugs correct severe hyperkalemia by causing a rapid intracellular shift of potassium ions, which reduces the serum potassium concentration. Such interventions are often followed with orally or rectally administered sodium polystyrene sulfonate (Kayexalate) or hemodialysis to eliminate the extra potassium from the body. Less critical levels can be reduced with dietary restrictions.

### Interactions

Concurrent use of potassium-sparing diuretics and ACE inhibitors can produce a hyperkalemic state. Concurrent use of

---

*Burn patients can exhibit either hyperkalemia or hypokalemia.

non–potassium-sparing diuretics, amphotericin B, and mineralocorticoids can produce a hypokalemic state.

## Dosages

Fluid and electrolyte therapy involves replacing any deficits or losses and/or providing maintenance levels for specific patient requirements. Accordingly, specific dosage amounts of fluids or electrolytes depend on several clinical factors, including the following:

- Specific patient losses
- Efficacy of patient physiologic systems involved in fluid and electrolyte metabolism, especially adrenal, cardiovascular, and kidney functions
- Current drug therapy for pathologic conditions that complicate the amount and duration of replacement
- Selection of oral or parenteral replacement formulations

Suggested dosage guidelines for potassium with subsequent adjustments are 10 to 20 mEq administered orally several times a day or parenteral administration of 30 to 60 mEq every 24 hours.

## DRUG PROFILES

### potassium

Potassium supplements are administered either to prevent or to treat potassium depletion. The acetate, bicarbonate, chloride, citrate, and gluconate salts of potassium are available for oral administration, including tablets, solutions, elixirs, and powders for solution. The parenteral salt forms of potassium for IV administration are acetate, chloride, and phosphate. The dosage of potassium supplements is usually expressed in milliequivalents of potassium and depends on the requirements of the individual patient. Different salt forms of potassium deliver varying milliequivalent amounts of potassium.

Potassium is contraindicated in patients with severe renal disease, severe hemolytic disease, or Addison's disease and in those with hyperkalemia, acute dehydration, or extensive tissue breakdown stemming from multiple traumas. It is classified as a pregnancy category A drug.

### Pharmacokinetics

| Route | Onset of Action | Peak Plasma Concentration | Elimination Half-life | Duration of Action |
|-------|-----------------|---------------------------|----------------------|--------------------|
| IV | Immediate | Rapid | Variable | Variable |

### sodium polystyrene sulfonate (potassium exchange resin)

Sodium polystyrene sulfonate (Kayexalate) is known as a *cation exchange resin* and is used to treat hyperkalemia. It is usually administered orally via nasogastric tube or as an enema. It works in the intestine, where potassium ions from the body are exchanged for sodium ions in the resin. Although the drug effects in each case are unpredictable, approximately 1 mEq of potassium is lost from the body per gram of resin administered. It can cause disturbances in electrolytes other than potassium, such as calcium and magnesium. For this reason, patients' electrolytes are closely monitored during treatment with sodium polystyrene sulfonate. In 2011, the FDA required safety labeling changes to state that cases of intestinal or colonic necrosis and other serious GI adverse events (bleeding, ischemic colitis, perforation) had been reported. Kayexalate should not be used in patients who do not have normal bowel function and should be discontinued in patients who develop constipation. It should not be used concurrently with sorbitol. Concurrent use of sorbitol with kayexelate has been implicated in cases of intestinal colonic necrosis. This condition may be fatal. Other adverse effects include hypernatremia, hypokalemia, hypocalcemia, hypomagnesemia, nausea, and vomiting. Drug interactions include antacids and laxatives, which should be avoided. It is typically dosed in multiples of 15 to 30 grams until the desired effect on serum potassium occurs. Onset of action varies from 2 to 12 hours and is generally faster with the oral route than with rectal administration. It is available in 15 g/60 mL suspensions and in a powder for reconstitution. It is classified as a pregnancy category C drug.

## SODIUM

Although sodium was discussed under colloids, it is also presented in the electrolyte section because it is most commonly given for replenishing purposes. Sodium is the counterpart of potassium, in that potassium is the principal cation inside cells, whereas sodium is the principal cation outside cells. The normal concentration of sodium outside cells is 135 to 145 mEq/L, and it is maintained through the dietary intake of sodium in the form of sodium chloride, which is obtained from salt, fish, meats, and other foods flavored, seasoned, or preserved with salt.

Hyponatremia is a condition of sodium loss or deficiency and occurs when the serum levels decrease less than 135 mEq/L. It is manifested by lethargy, hypotension, stomach cramps, vomiting, diarrhea, and seizures. Some of the same conditions that cause hypokalemia can also cause hyponatremia, and these are listed on pp. 480-481. Other causes of hyponatremia are excessive perspiration, occurring during hot weather or physical work; prolonged diarrhea or vomiting, especially in young children; renal disorders; and adrenocortical impairment.

Hypernatremia is the condition of sodium excess and occurs when the serum levels of sodium exceed 145 mEq/L. The most common cause is poor renal excretion stemming from kidney malfunction. Inadequate water consumption and dehydration are other causes. Symptoms of hypernatremia include red, flushed skin; dry, sticky mucous membranes; increased thirst; temperature elevation; water retention (edema); hypertension; and decreased or absent urination.

## Mechanism of Action and Drug Effects

As one of the body's electrolytes, sodium performs many physiologic roles necessary for the normal function of the body. It is the major cation in extracellular fluid and is involved in the control of water distribution, fluid and electrolyte balance, and osmotic pressure of body fluids. Sodium also participates along with both chloride and bicarbonate in the regulation of acid-base balance. Chloride, the major extracellular anion (negatively charged substance), closely complements the physiologic action of sodium. Sodium is also capable of causing diuresis.

## Indications

Sodium is primarily administered for the treatment or prevention of sodium depletion when dietary measures have proved inadequate. Sodium chloride is the primary salt used for this purpose. Mild hyponatremia is usually treated with the oral administration of sodium chloride tablets and/or fluid restriction. Pronounced sodium depletion is treated with IV normal saline or lactated Ringer's solution. These drugs were discussed earlier in this chapter.

Hypertonic saline (3% NaCl) is sometimes used to correct severe hyponatremia. It is considered a high-risk drug because giving it too rapidly or in too high of a dose can cause a syndrome known as *central pontine myelinolysis,* also known as *osmotic demyelination syndrome.* This can cause irreversible brainstem damage.

A new class of drugs for the treatment of euvolemic (normal fluid volume) hyponatremia is the dual arginine vasopressin (AVP) V1A and V2 receptor antagonists. These drugs are conivaptan (Vaprisol) and tolvaptan (Samsca). This class of drugs is often referred to as *vaptans.* Specific information on conivaptan is listed under its drug profile.

## Contraindications

The only usual contraindications to the use of sodium replacement products are known drug allergy to a specific product and hypernatremia.

## Adverse Effects

The oral administration of sodium chloride can cause gastric upset consisting of nausea, vomiting, and cramps. Venous phlebitis can be a consequence of its parenteral administration.

### Toxicity and Management of Overdose

Hypernatremia leads to hypertension, edema, thirst, tachycardia, weakness, convulsions, and possibly coma. Treatment consists of increased fluid intake and dietary restrictions. In more serious cases, diuretics may be required to enhance urinary sodium excretion. IV administration of dextrose in water solution (e.g., 5% dextrose in water [$D_5W$] or 10% dextrose in water [$D_{10}W$]) may also be helpful by producing both intravascular sodium dilution and enhanced urine volume output.

## Interactions

Sodium is not known to interact significantly with any drugs with the exception of the antibiotic Synercid (quinupristin and dalfopristin), with which it is incompatible.

## Dosages

Fluid and electrolyte therapy involves replacing any deficit losses and/or providing maintenance levels for specific patient requirements. Accordingly, specific dosage amounts of fluids or electrolytes depend on several clinical factors, as follows:
- Specific patient losses
- Efficacy of patient physiologic systems involved in fluid and electrolyte metabolism, especially adrenal, cardiovascular, and kidney functions
- Current drug therapy for pathologic conditions that complicate the amount and duration of replacement
- Selection of oral or parenteral replacement formulations

Suggested dosage guidelines for sodium chloride with subsequent adjustments are 1 to 2 g administered orally several times a day or parenteral administration of 1 L of sodium chloride injection (NS).

## DRUG PROFILES

### sodium chloride

Sodium chloride is primarily used as a replacement electrolyte for either the prevention or treatment of sodium loss. It is also used as a diluent for the infusion of compatible drugs and in the assessment of kidney function after a fluid challenge. Sodium chloride is contraindicated in patients who are hypersensitive to it. It is available in many IV preparations and in oral form as 650-mg tablets. It is classified as a pregnancy category C drug.

**Pharmacokinetics**

| Route | Onset of Action | Peak Plasma Concentration | Elimination Half-life | Duration of Action |
|---|---|---|---|---|
| IV | Immediate | Rapid | Unknown | Variable |

### conivaptan

Conivaptan (Vaprisol) is a nonpeptide dual arginine vasopressin (AVP) V1A and V2 receptor antagonist. It inhibits the effects of arginine vasopressin, also known as *antidiuretic hormone,* on receptors in the kidneys. It is specifically indicated for the treatment of hospitalized patients with euvolemic hyponatremia, or low serum sodium levels at normal water volumes. Conivaptan is available for IV infusion. The recommended regimen is a loading dose of 20 mg delivered via a 30-minute infusion, followed by an additional infusion of 20 mg continuously over 24 hours. Subsequent infusions can be administered every 1 to 3 days at 20 mg/day via continuous infusion. Dose may be titrated up to 40 mg/day if response is not sufficiently rapid.

Adverse events associated with the use of Vaprisol may include infusion site reactions (e.g., phlebitis, pain), thirst, headache, hypokalemia, vomiting, diarrhea, and polyuria. Closely monitor serum sodium levels during treatment, as overly rapid increases in serum sodium levels have been associated with potentially permanent adverse events, including osmotic demyelination syndrome. Several potential drug-drug interactions have been identified. Conivaptan is metabolized by the hepatic enzyme CYP3A4; co-administration drugs that inhibit this enzyme (including but not limited to ketoconazole, itraconazole, clarithromycin, ritonavir, and indinavir) may increase serum levels. Tolvaptan (Samsca) is an oral version of conivaptan. It is available at 15-mg and 30-mg tablets.

**Pharmacokinetics**

| Route | Onset of Action | Peak Plasma Concentration | Elimination Half-life | Duration of Action |
|---|---|---|---|---|
| IV | Immediate | Rapid | 6.7-8.6 hr | 12 hr after infusion is stopped |

# NURSING PROCESS

## ASSESSMENT

For fluid replacement, a patient's needs vary. Any medications or solutions ordered must be given exactly as prescribed and without substitution. However, never take the prescriber's order at face value without confirming any medication order against authoritative resources (e.g., current drug reference guides, *Physician's Desk Reference,* nursing pharmacology textbook, manufacturer's drug insert) or speaking with a pharmacist. Important to remember is that you are responsible for making sure that the drug therapy administration process— beginning with the assessment phase of the nursing process and through to evaluation—is accurate and safe, and meets professional standards of care.

To assist in the development of a thorough assessment, a brief review of the various solutions is needed. Parenterally administered hydrating and hypotonic solutions include 0.25% NaCl and 0.45% NaCl/$D_5$W. These are used mainly for the prevention and/or treatment of dehydration. $D_5$W alone in an IV bag is considered isotonic but acts as a hypotonic solution once in the bloodstream. Isotonic solutions (e.g., 0.9% NaCl [normal saline] and lactated Ringer's solution) are customarily used to augment extracellular volume in patients experiencing blood loss and/or severe vomiting. Isotonic NaCl is also used as diluting fluid for blood transfusions because $D_5$W results in hemolysis of red blood cells (in transfusions). Hypertonic solutions (e.g., 3% or 5% sodium chloride) are used for replacement of fluids and electrolytes in specific situations (see pharmacology discussion).

Because of the potential risks related to the use of these solutions, they are rarely administered outside of the hospital setting. After verifying all prescriber orders and checking for accuracy and completeness (as with all drugs), assess the solution or product, the patient, and the IV site (if applicable). Also assess the following for IV infusions of fluids and/or electrolytes: the solution to be infused, infusion equipment, infusion rate of the solution, concentration of the parenteral solution, related mathematical calculations, laboratory values (e.g., sodium, chloride, potassium), and parenteral compatibilities. More specific assessment of the patient who is to receive a parenteral replacement solution needs to focus on gathering information about the patient's medical history, including diseases of the GI, renal, cardiac, and/or hepatic systems. Obtain a medication history, including a list of prescription drugs, over-the-counter medications, supplements, and herbals. Also take a dietary history including specific dietary habits and recall of all foods consumed during the previous 24 hours. Assess fluid volume and electrolyte status (through laboratory testing and measurement of urinary specific gravity, vital signs, and intake and output). The skin and mucous membranes also reflect a patient's hydration status; assess skin turgor and/or rebound elasticity of skin over the top of the hand and other areas over the body. Document the findings as "immediate" rebound or "delayed" rebound. You count the number of seconds that the patient's skin stays in the pinched-up position, with normal return being immediately or within 3 to 5 seconds.

Potassium is presented first in the discussion of electrolytes, and one important place to begin assessment is knowledge of the normal range, usually 3.5 to 5 mEq/L. Serum potassium levels below 3.5 mEq/L, or hypokalemia, may result in a variety of problems, such as cardiac irregularities and muscle weakness. Early symptoms of hypokalemia include anorexia, hypotension, lethargy, mental confusion, muscle weakness, and nausea. Late symptoms of hypokalemia include cardiac irregularities, neuropathies, and paralytic ileus. Avoid potassium supplementation or use with extreme caution in patients taking ACE inhibitors or potassium-sparing diuretics (such as spironolactone). These drugs are associated with adverse effects of hyperkalemia and, if given with potassium supplementation, could worsen hyperkalemia and possibly result in severe cardiac dysrhythmias. Other concerns regarding contraindications with potassium include severe renal disease, untreated Addison's disease, severe tissue trauma, and acute dehydration. Oral potassium supplements are irritants and may be ulcerogenic; thus, perform a thorough GI tract assessment. If the patient has a history of ulcers or GI bleeding and oral supplementation is prescribed, contact the prescriber for further instructions.

The range of serum potassium levels defined as normal often varies depending on the institution and/or the prescriber. For identification and treatment of hyperkalemia, the normal range of potassium must be established. Realize that potassium levels of 5.3 mEq/L may be identified as abnormally high by some laboratories, whereas other laboratories may categorize 5.0 mEq/L as being abnormally high. Be sure to check hospital policy and laboratory guidelines for normal ranges and report any elevations (or decreases) in serum potassium. However, a serum level exceeding 5.5 mEq/L is considered by most sources to be toxic and dangerous to the patient; report this finding to the prescriber immediately. With close monitoring of patients, the dangerous effects of hyperkalemia (i.e., cardiac dysrhythmias) will hopefully be prevented or at least identified early and treated appropriately to prevent potentially life-threatening complications.

Venous access is an important issue with parenteral potassium supplementation because the vein can be irritated if infiltration occurs or if the solution has not been mixed thoroughly. The following are some important considerations regarding assessment and peripheral venous access (for potassium, sodium, fluid, and any other type of medication given by the IV route): (1) Assess the overall condition of the veins prior to selecting a site. (2) Try to use distal veins first as the IV site. (3) Know the purpose of administering potassium and other electrolytes. (4) Calculate and set the rate, as ordered, for the infusion. (5) Know the anticipated duration of therapy. (6) Know the restrictions imposed by the patient's history. For example, in post-mastectomy patients with lymph node dissection, the affected arm must not be used. The affected arm of a patient with a stroke must not be used. Limb circulation may be inadequate in these

## SAFETY: LABORATORY VALUES RELATED TO DRUG THERAPY

### Serum Potassium

| LABORATORY TEST | NORMAL RANGES | RATIONALE FOR ASSESSMENT |
|---|---|---|
| Serum potassium | 3.5-5 mEq/L | The main function of potassium is the regulation of water and electrolyte content in the cell. Potassium also assists in the cellular metabolism of carbohydrates and proteins. A decrease is generally considered to be a level less than 5.5 mEq/L. A serum level less than 3.5 mEq/L is known as hypokalemia and a small decrease in potassium levels may have profound effects with lethargy, muscle weakness, hypotension, and cardiac dysrhythmias. A serum potassium level greater than 5 mEq/L is known as hyperkalemia and is manifested by muscle weakness, paresthesia, paralysis, and cardiac rhythm abnormalities. Knowing the normal ranges allows quicker identification of abnormalities and thus more timely management. |

situations and lead to edema and other complications if used as a venous access site.

Sodium is another electrolyte that is an ingredient in various IV replacement solutions. Hyponatremia, or serum sodium level below 135 mEq/L, if not resolved with dietary and/or oral intake, may need to be treated with parenteral infusions. Signs and symptoms of hyponatremia include lethargy, hypotension, stomach cramps, vomiting, and diarrhea. Carefully assess venous access sites because of possible irritation of the vein and subsequent phlebitis. If replacement to correct hyponatremic states is overzealous, the result may be hypernatremia with fluid overload, edema, and dyspnea. Assess baseline vital signs. Continually monitor vital signs, hydration status of the skin and mucous membranes, and level of consciousness for safe replacement and prevention of further complications. Contraindications to sodium replacement include elevated serum sodium levels, edema, and hypertension.

Hypernatremia also requires careful assessment. Manifestations of hypernatremia include red, flushed skin; dry, sticky mucous membranes; increased thirst; temperature elevation; water retention (edema), hypertension; and decreased or absent urination. Identifying any precipitating events, medical concerns, and risk-prone patient situations is important to finding early solutions for treatment. The populations at risk for hypernatremia include the elderly, those with renal and cardiovascular diseases, patients who are receiving sodium supplements or who have increased sodium intake, and those with decreased fluid intake. Perform an assessment of cautions, contraindications, and drug interactions.

Albumin and other colloids (e.g., dextran) have associated cautions, contraindications, and drug interactions that need to be assessed. Contraindications include patients with heart failure, severe anemia, and renal insufficiency. The rationale is that these products cause fluids to shift from interstitial to intravascular spaces. This places more strain on the patient's cardiac and respiratory systems. Assess the patient's hematocrit, hemoglobin levels, and serum protein levels. Assess the patient's blood pressure, pulse rate, respiratory status, and intake and output.

Document and report any abnormal assessment findings (e.g., dyspnea, edema) immediately.

Fluid infusions may also include the giving of blood or blood components. Obtain a thorough history regarding any transfusions received previously and the patient's response. Report any history of adverse reactions to blood transfusions or problems with PRBCs and/or FFP to the prescriber, and document the nature of these reactions. Assess the status of venous access areas. Check the patient's laboratory values (e.g., hematocrit, hemoglobin, white blood cells [WBCs], RBCs, platelets, and clotting factors). Note baseline vital signs, blood pressure, pulse rate, respiratory rate, and temperature before infusing the blood or blood product. Even the general appearance of the patient, energy levels, ability to carry out activities of daily living, and color of extremities are important to note. Assess for any potential drug interactions, specifically aspirin and calcium, as these may potentially alter clotting. During the infusion of blood components, constantly assess for the occurrence of fever and blood in the urine. Both of these findings are indicative of a reaction requiring immediate medical attention.

In summary, safety and caution are top priorities when patients receive any drug, and fluid and electrolyte replacements are no exception. Deficient and/or excess fluid and electrolyte levels may pose tremendous risks to patients. A thorough assessment is critical to patient safety. In addition, because so many patients receive therapies in the home setting, there is even more accountability and responsibility for performing skillful and thorough assessment before, during, and after therapy.

## NURSING DIAGNOSES

1. Risk for falls related to fluid and electrolyte losses
2. Risk for imbalanced fluid volume related to drug-induced fluid and electrolyte deficits and/or excesses.
3. Risk for injury related to complications of the transfusion or infusion of blood products, blood components, or related agents

# PLANNING

## GOALS

1. Patient remains free from falls and injury.
2. Patient regains balanced fluid volume status.
3. Patient remains free from injury related to complications of blood product infusion.

## OUTCOME CRITERIA

1. Patient minimizes risk for falls through careful actions.
   - Patient changes positions slowly and ambulates with assistance until symptoms (e.g., dizziness, lightheadedness) have subsided.
2. Patient regains fluid volume status through replacement of at least 8 to 10 glasses/day or up to 3 L/day of water, unless contraindicated.
   - Patient receives adequate fluid volume infusions with improvement of fluid and electrolyte status.
   - Patient's urinary output is at least 30 mL/hr.
   - Patient reports any dizziness, lethargy, confusion, disorientation, muscle weakness, irregular heart rhythm, and/or abdominal cramping.
3. Patient remains free from injury during infusion of blood products/components.
   - Patient reports any shortness of breath, irregular heart rate or palpitations, or feeling of increased body temperature.
   - Patient's laboratory values (e.g., hemoglobin, hematocrit, RBCs) return to normal levels.

# IMPLEMENTATION

Continued monitoring of the patient during fluid or electrolyte therapy is crucial to ensure safe and effective treatment. It is also important to continue monitoring to identify adverse effects early and to prevent complications of overzealous treatment and/or undertreatment. During replacement therapy, serum electrolyte levels need to remain within normal ranges. Educate patients at risk for volume deficits (especially the elderly) about this risk and about the effect of a hot, humid environment on physiologic functioning and the danger of exacerbation by excessive perspiration. Water is at the crux of every metabolic reaction that occurs within the body, and deficits will negatively impact physiologic reactions and alter the composition of fluids and electrolytes. For any age group, staying hydrated at all times is a preventive measure.

With parenteral dosing, you must monitor infusion rates as well as the appearance of the fluid or solution (i.e., potassium and saline solutions are clear, whereas albumin is brown, clear, and viscous). Frequently monitor the IV site, as per facility policy and nursing standards of care, for evidence of infiltration (e.g., swelling, coolness of skin to the touch around IV site, no or decreased flow rate, and no blood return from IV catheter) or thrombophlebitis (e.g., swelling, redness, heat, and pain at IV site). Volume overload, drug toxicity, fever, infection, and emboli are other complications of IV therapy. With the administration of any of these drugs per the IV route, maintain a steady and even flow rate to prevent complications. Ensure that infusion rates follow the prescriber's orders, and recheck all calculations for accuracy. Check the IV site, tubing, IV bag, and fluids or solutions as well as expiration dates. Always behave in a prudent, safe, and thorough manner when administering fluids and electrolyte solutions. Remember that elderly and/or pediatric patients have an increased sensitivity to fluids and electrolytes.

With the various IV solutions, knowing their osmolality and concentrations is important to their safe use. Administration of *isotonic solutions* (e.g., 0.9% sodium chloride, lactated Ringer's solution) requires constant monitoring during and after therapy with vital signs and observation for possible fluid overload, especially in those at risk, or those with heart failure. *Hypertonic solutions* are used rarely because of the risk of cellular dehydration and vascular volume overload. These solutions are also associated with phlebitis and spasm if IV infiltration and/or extravasation occur in the peripheral veins. Therefore, if ordered, administer these solutions through a larger bore vein (e.g., central line), but only with close monitoring of the patient's vital signs and cardiac status.

For the patient who is at risk for hypokalemia, provide educational materials and patient teaching to encourage consumption of certain foods high in potassium. The minimal daily requirement for potassium is between 40 and 50 mEq for adults and 2 to 3 mEq/kg of body weight for infants. Share a list of foods containing potassium with the patient. Two medium-sized bananas or an 8-oz glass of orange juice contains 45 mEq; 20 large dried apricots contain 40 mEq; and a level teaspoon of salt substitute (KCl) contains 60 mEq of potassium. Conversely, if the patient is already hyperkalemic, advise the patient to avoid these food items (see the Patient Teaching Tips for more information). If potassium levels do not increase with dietary changes, supplementation may be needed. Oral preparations of *potassium*, rather than parenteral dosage forms, are preferred whenever possible. Prepare the oral dosage forms per the manufacturer's insert or per policy and standard of care. Generally, oral forms of potassium should be taken with food to minimize gastric distress or irritation. Prepare powder or effervescent forms according to the package guidelines, and mix thoroughly with at least 4 to 6 oz of fluid before administering the medication. Enteric-coated and sustained-release forms may still result in gastric upset and lead to ulcer development (ulcerogenic). With oral supplementation, the safest and most effective intervention is frequent and close monitoring for complaints of nausea, vomiting, abdominal pain, or bleeding (such as the occurrence of melena or blood in the stool and/or hematemesis or blood in the vomitus). If abnormalities are noted, continue to monitor vital signs and other parameters, and report findings to the prescriber immediately. Monitor serum levels of potassium during therapy as well.

Hyperkalemia is treated with *sodium polystyrene sulfonate* (Kayexalate). It is used only under very specific situations and under very close monitoring of the patient and his or her serum potassium, sodium, calcium, and magnesium levels (see Pharmacology discussion). If Kayexalate is given orally (or via nasogastric tube), elevate the head of the patient's bed to prevent aspiration. The FDA issued a warning in 2011 regarding cases of intestinal necrosis associated with the use of Kayexalate (see pharmacology discussion). Never give Kayexelate with sorbitol because of the connection of these two drugs with the potentially fatal condition of colonic intestinal necrosis. If oral Kayexelate is given, do not give it with antacids or laxatives. Administer each dose as a suspension in a small quantity of water for improved palatability. Follow directions regarding the amount of water to use; it generally ranges from 20 to 100 mL, depending on the dose. If given per the rectal route, a retention enema is used. Follow the medication orders carefully, and expect that more than one dose may be needed. The enema must be retained as long as possible and followed by a physician-prescribed cleansing enema. Usually an initial cleansing enema is prescribed, and then the resin solution is administered. If leakage occurs, elevating the patient's hips on a pillow or placing the patient in a knee-chest position may be helpful.

*Potassium chloride* is the salt customarily used for IV infusions. The concern and caution with potassium chloride use is to avoid overdosage, because it can lead to cardiac arrest. *IV dosage forms of potassium must always be given in a DILUTED form. There is no use or place for undiluted potassium because undiluted potassium is associated with cardiac arrest!* Therefore, parenteral forms of potassium need to be diluted properly. Nowadays, most pharmacies premix the infusion; however, it is still imperative to double-check the order, amount of diluent, and concentration of potassium to diluent. Never assume that what was premixed is 100% correct, because you are ultimately responsible for whatever you administer. Additionally, *only give diluted potassium when there is adequate urine output of at least 30 mL/hr* (to prevent toxicity). Toxicity or overdosage of potassium (hyperkalemia) is manifested by cardiac rhythm irregularities, muscle spasms, paresthesia, and possible cardiac arrest. Most policy protocols recommend that IV solutions be given at concentrations of less than 40 mEq/L of potassium and a rate not exceeding 20 mEq/hr. As previously discussed, IV potassium is to be given no faster than 10 mEq/hr to those patients not on cardiac monitoring. In patients who are critically ill and on cardiac monitors, a rate of 20 mEq/hr or more may be used. Avoid adding potassium chloride to an already existing IV solution because the exact concentration cannot be accurately calculated and overdosage or toxicity may result. Make sure that all IV fluids are labeled appropriately and documented, as with any medication. If the IV fluid rate must be monitored very closely, an infusion pump may be used. *There is no place for IV push or IV bolus potassium replacement!* Treatment of severe hyperkalemia caused by IV administration is through use of IV sodium bicarbonate, calcium gluconate or chloride, or dextrose solution with insulin. These drugs work by leading to a rapid shifting of potassium ions intracellularly, thereby reducing the serum potassium concentration.

Replacement of sodium carries the same concern regarding dosing and route of administration. When the patient is only mildly depleted, an increase in oral intake of sodium needs to be tried. Food items high in sodium include catsup, mustard, cured meats, cheeses, potato chips, peanut butter, popcorn, and table salt. In some situations, salt tablets may be necessary. If the patient is given salt tablets, advise him or her to take plenty of fluids, up to 3000 mL/24 hr, unless contraindicated. If the sodium deficit requires IV replacement, venous access issues and drip rate are as important as with volume and potassium infusions (see previous discussion regarding IV infusion and IV sites). *Hypertonic saline* (3% NaCl) is sometimes used for severe hyponatremia but is considered to be a high risk due to the possible occurrence of osmotic demyelination syndrome. This occurs if the 3% NaCl is given too fast or in too high amounts. It results in irreversible brainstem damage. Other treatment of hyponatremia includes the use of either IV *conivaptan* (Vaprisol) or orally administered *tolvaptan* (Samsca). These drugs are indicated for euvolemic hyponatremia (see pharmacology discussion). Administer these drugs as ordered while monitoring serum sodium levels. Hypernatremia is treated with increased fluid intake and dietary restrictions, so you must provide thorough and complete patient education. Intravenous dextrose in water ($D_5W$ or $D_{10}W$) may be indicated and helps by creating intravascular sodium dilution and enhanced urine volume output with sodium excretion.

Always carry out IV infusion of *albumin* and other colloids slowly and cautiously. Carefully monitor the patient to prevent fluid overload and potential heart failure, especially in patients who are at particular risk. Fluid overload is evidenced by shortness of breath, crackles at the bases of the lungs, decreased pulse oximeter readings, edema of dependent areas, and increase in weight (see previous parameters). Determine serum hematocrit and hemoglobin values in advance of therapy—as well as during and after therapy—so that any dilutional effects can be determined. For example, if a patient has received albumin and other colloids too quickly, and hypervolemia results, the patient's hemoglobin and hematocrit may actually be decreased. This decrease would be from a caused by dilutional factor because of too much volume in relation to the concentration of solutes. Clinically, the patient would appear to be anemic but in fact the deficit would be attributable to the increase in volume. It is also important to remember that albumin is to be given at room temperature.

For infusion of blood, always check the expiration date of *blood* and/or *blood components* to make sure that the blood is not outdated. *Under NO circumstances is outdated blood to be used!* Policies at most hospitals and other health care agencies require that blood and blood products be double-checked by another registered nurse BEFORE the blood is hung and infused. This is important to prevent a mix-up in blood types. Blood types must always be a major concern because of the possible complications that can occur, some life-threatening, if the wrong blood type is given or if the blood is given to the wrong person. The "Six Rights" of drug administration remain critical in all that you do with medications, and administering blood is no exception.

When blood and blood products are infused, it is important to patient safety to document all vital signs and related parameters before, during, and after administration of the blood product, component (e.g., PRBCs, FFP), or solution. Monitor vital signs, and frequently record during and after administration. A transfusion reaction would most likely be manifested by the occurrence of the following: apprehension, restlessness, flushed skin, increased pulse and respirations, dyspnea, rash, joint or lower back pain, swelling, fever and chills (a febrile reaction beginning 1 hour after the start of administration and possibly lasting up to 10 hours), nausea, weakness, and jaundice. Report these signs and symptoms to the prescriber immediately, and (regardless of when the reaction occurs), stop the blood or product, and keep the IV line patent with isotonic NS solution infusing at a slow rate. Monitor patient and vital signs closely. Always follow the facility's protocol for transfusion reactions.

In summary, encourage patients receiving any type of fluid or electrolyte substance, colloid, or blood component to immediately report unusual adverse effects to their prescriber. Such complaints may include chest pain, dizziness, weakness, and shortness of breath.

## EVALUATION

The therapeutic response to *fluid, electrolyte,* and *blood* or *blood component* therapy includes normalization of fluid volume and laboratory values, including RBC and WBC counts, hemoglobin level, hematocrit, and sodium and potassium levels. In addition to review of these laboratory values, evaluation of the patient's cardiac, respiratory, musculoskeletal, and GI functioning is also important. Therapeutic effects include improved energy levels and tolerance of activities of daily living. Skin color will improve, and there will be improved shortness of breath as well as minimal to no chest pain, weakness, or fatigue. Correct treatment of blood volume problems will be evidenced by a return of laboratory values to the normal range, improved vital signs, an increase in energy, and near-normal oxygen saturation levels. The therapeutic response to albumin therapy includes an elevation of blood pressure, decreased edema, and increased serum albumin levels. Frequently monitor for adverse effects of any of these drugs and/or solutions, and check for distended neck veins; shortness of breath; anxiety; insomnia; expiratory crackles; frothy, blood-tinged sputum; and cyanosis (indicative of fluid volume overload).

---

### CASE STUDY
#### *Fluid and Electrolyte Replacement*

M.S., an 85-year-old retired engineer, seemed somewhat confused when his daughter came home from work. When she brings him to the emergency department, his blood pressure is 90/62 mm Hg, his heart rate is 114 beats/min, and his skin is dry but cool. His daughter says that he seems "much weaker" than usual, and he is unable to answer questions clearly. His daughter reports that he has "lost his appetite" lately and has not taken in much food or drink. The nurse starts an IV infusion of 0.9% sodium chloride (NS) at 100 mL/hr via a gravity drip infusion.

1. What do you think is M.S.'s main medical problem at this time?

   The emergency department is very busy, and when the nurse returns, she is shocked to see that almost the entire 500-mL bag of NS has infused within an hour's time.

2. What will the nurse do first? What will the nurse watch for at this time?
3. When monitoring M.S.'s fluid status, which indicators will the nurse consider the most reliable?

   Twenty-four hours after his admission, M.S. is much less confused and is able to move to a chair for lunch without much difficulty. He is receiving 5% dextrose/½ NS with 20 mEq of potassium chloride at a rate of 75 mL/hr via an infusion pump. His daughter notices that the area above the IV insertion site is red, and M.S. complains that the area is "very sore."

4. What is the possible problem with the IV line? What needs to be done at this time?

For answers, see http://evolve.elsevier.com/Lilley.

---

## PATIENT TEACHING TIPS

- As needed, educate the patient about the difference in the signs and symptoms of hyponatremia and hypernatremia. Hyponatremia is manifested by lethargy, hypotension, stomach cramps, vomiting, diarrhea, and seizures. Some of the causes of hyponatremia include excessive perspiration, occurring during hot weather or physical work, and prolonged diarrhea or vomiting.
- Hypernatremia is associated with symptoms of water retention (edema); hypertension; red, flushed skin; dry, sticky mucous membranes; increased thirst; temperature elevation; and decreased or absent urination. The most common cause is poor renal excretion as a result of kidney malfunction. Inadequate water consumption and dehydration are other causes.

- Educate the patient about the early symptoms of hypokalemia, such as anorexia, hypotension, lethargy, mental confusion, nausea, and muscle weakness. Late symptoms include cardiac dysrhythmias (the patient may feel palpitations or shortness of breath), neuropathies, and paralytic ileus.
- Share the symptoms of hyperkalemia with the patient, including muscle weakness, paresthesia, paralysis, and cardiac rhythm abnormalities.
- Provide the patient with adequate and appropriate information about how to take oral potassium chloride. In the directions, include the fact that the powdered or liquid solutions require thorough mixing in at least 4 to 8 oz of cold water/juice before drinking the mixture slowly. Encourage the patient to take oral doses with food or a snack, and tell

## PATIENT TEACHING TIPS—cont'd

patients taking potassium supplements to report to the prescriber immediately any GI upset or abdominal pain (indicative of gastric irritation from the oral potassium). Educate the patient about potential drug interactions such as potassium-sparing diuretics and ACE inhibitors because their concurrent use may produce hyperkalemia.

- Educate patients on foods high in potassium, including bananas, oranges, apricots, dates, raisins, broccoli, green beans, potatoes, tomatoes, meats, fish, wheat bread, and legumes.
- Advise patients that sustained-release potassium capsules and tablets must be swallowed whole and should not be crushed, chewed, or allowed to dissolve in the mouth.
- Encourage the patient to report any difficulty in swallowing, painful swallowing, or feeling that the capsule or tablet is getting stuck in the throat. Other serious adverse effects that need to be reported include vomiting of coffee ground–like material, stomach or abdominal pain or swelling, and black tarry stools.
- Educate the patient that extended-release dosage forms of potassium need to be taken in full. Each prescribed dose is to be taken with meals and full glass of water. If the patient has difficulty swallowing the whole tablet, and if approved by the prescriber, the patient can break the tablet in half and take each half separately, drinking half a glass of water (4 oz) with each half and taking the entire dose within a few minutes. The patient must take the full dose and not save partial dosages of potassium for later. Another option is to take the extended-release dosage form and place the whole tablet in 4 ounces of water. Instruct the patient to allow 2 minutes for the tablet to dissolve in the recommended 4 ounces of water, stir for 30 seconds, and then drink immediately. Adding 1 oz of water to the glass, swirling it, and then drinking the residual will allow adequate dosing. Water is recommended as the fluid for mixing the extended-release dosage form. A straw may be used.
- Instruct the patient to dissolve effervescent potassium tablets, as directed. At least 3 ounces of cold water needs to be used per tablet. The patient needs to take the dose as soon as it is fully dissolved, sipping the mixture over 5 to 10 minutes and taking the dose after food to minimize GI upset.
- Educate the patient that salt substitutes contain potassium. Another alternative must be recommended if the patient is hyperkalemic.
- If receiving IV potassium, tell the patient to report any feelings of irritation (e.g., burning) at the IV site.
- Educate the patient about the safe use of salt tablets, and instruct him or her to take them as prescribed. Salt tablets must be taken with adequate fluid intake.

## KEY POINTS

- Total body water (TBW) is divided into intracellular (inside the cell) and extracellular (outside the cell) compartments. Fluid volume outside the cells is either in the plasma (intravascular volume) or between the tissues, cells, or organs.
- Colloids are large protein particles that cannot leak out of the blood vessels. Because of their greater concentration inside blood vessels, fluid is pulled into the blood vessels. Examples of colloids include albumin, hetastarch, and dextran. Administer albumin with caution because of the high risk for hypervolemia and possible heart failure. Monitor intake and output, weights, heart and breath sounds, and appropriate laboratory values.
- Blood products are the only fluids that are able to carry oxygen because they are the only fluids that contain hemoglobin. Patients will hopefully begin to show improved energy and increasing tolerance for activities of daily living as a result of the treatments with blood products. Pulse oximeter readings will also show improved readings.
- Dehydration may be hypotonic, resulting from the loss of salt; hypertonic, resulting from fever with perspiration; or isotonic, resulting from diarrhea or vomiting. Each form of dehydration is treated differently. Carefully assess intake and output as well as skin turgor, urine specific gravity, and blood levels of potassium, sodium, and chloride.

- Hypertonic solutions must be used very cautiously and given slowly because of the risk for hypervolemia from overzealous replacement.
- Early symptoms of hypokalemia include anorexia, hypotension, lethargy, mental confusion, nausea, and muscle weakness. Late symptoms include cardiac dysrhythmias (the patient may feel palpitations or shortness of breath), neuropathies, and paralytic ileus.
- Symptoms of hyperkalemia include muscle weakness, paresthesia, paralysis, and cardiac rhythm abnormalities.
- Hyponatremia is manifested by lethargy, hypotension, stomach cramps, vomiting, diarrhea, and seizures. Hypernatremia is associated with symptoms of water retention (edema), hypertension, red, flushed skin; dry, sticky mucous membranes; increased thirst; temperature elevation; and decreased or absent urination.
- With administration of blood products, measurement of vital signs and frequent monitoring of the patient before, during, and after infusions are critical to patient safety. Blood products must be given only with normal saline (0.9% sodium chloride), because the solution of $D_5W$ results in hemolysis of red blood cells.

## NCLEX® EXAMINATION REVIEW QUESTIONS

1 Which action by the nurse is most appropriate for the patient receiving an infusion of packed red blood cells?
   a Flush the IV line with normal saline before the blood is added to the infusion.
   b Flush the IV line with dextrose before the blood is added to the infusion.
   c Check the patient's vital signs once the infusion is completed.
   d Anticipate that flushed skin and fever are expected reactions to a blood transfusion.

2 When preparing an IV solution that contains potassium, the nurse knows that a contraindication to the potassium infusion would be
   a diarrhea.
   b serum sodium level of 145 mEq/L.
   c serum potassium level of 5.6 mEq/L.
   d dehydration.

3 When assessing a patient who is about to receive an albumin infusion, the nurse knows that a contraindication for albumin would be
   a acute liver failure.
   b heart failure.
   c severe burns.
   d fluid-volume deficit.

4 The nurse is preparing an infusion for a patient who has a deficiency in clotting factors. Which type of infusion is most appropriate?
   a Albumin 5%
   b Packed RBCs
   c Whole blood
   d Fresh frozen plasma

5 While monitoring a patient who is receiving an infusion of a crystalloid solution, the nurse will monitor for which potential problem?
   a Bradycardia
   b Hypotension
   c Decreased skin turgor
   d Fluid overload

6 The nurse is administering an IV solution that contains potassium chloride to a patient in the critical care unit who has a severely decreased serum potassium level. Which action(s) by the nurse are appropriate? (Select all that apply.)
   a Administer the potassium by slow IV bolus.
   b Administer the potassium at a rate no faster than 20 mEq/hr.
   c Monitor the patient's cardiac rhythm with a heart monitor.
   d Use an infusion pump for the administration of IV potassium chloride.
   e Administer the potassium IV push.

7 The order reads: "Infuse 1000 mL of normal saline over the next 8 hours." The IV tubing has a drop factor of 15 gtt/mL. Calculate the mL/hour rate, and calculate the drops/minute setting for the IV tubing with this gravity infusion.

1. a, 2. c, 3. b, 4. d, 5. d, 6. b, c, d, 7. 125 mL/hr; 31 gtt/min

For Critical Thinking and Prioritization Questions, see http://evolve.elsevier.com/Lilley

### PART 5

# Drugs Affecting the Endocrine System

## QUESTIONING STRATEGY

One of the most important activities for learning is to become actively involved with the text. The best way to achieve this involvement is to develop the habit of asking questions. These questions can be generated using a number of different cues and elements that are part of the part and chapter structure. Some of what you anticipate as related material will not be correct, so you will adjust your expectations as you read the material. For now, focus on asking a lot of questions and making use of everything you know, which can help start the process of answering your questions.

### Part Title

As you begin each new part, ask a question to focus your attention, seeking to learn what all the chapters in this part have in common. In Part 5, this question is, "What is the endocrine system?" This same question could be asked of Parts 2 through 9 by simply replacing *endocrine* with the appropriate system for the specific part. Looking at the chapter titles in the part tells you that the endocrine system has to do with the pituitary drugs, thyroid and antithyroid drugs, antidiabetic drugs, adrenal drugs, women's health drugs, and men's health drugs. Although this answer is far too general to demonstrate any real understanding of the endocrine system, it is a beginning and helps keep you aware of what you need to learn from each chapter.

### Chapter Titles

Chapter titles provide the first mechanism that can be used to generate questions. The first question to ask about each chapter is a very basic one, involving what the chapter is about. That question is also answered immediately. "What is Chapter 30 about?" It is about pituitary drugs.

The next question is equally obvious but also extremely important. The question to ask next is, "To what do pituitary (see Chapter 30), thyroid and antithyroid (see Chapter 31), antidiabetic (see Chapter 32), adrenal (see Chapter 33), women's health (see Chapter 34), and men's health (see Chapter 35) refer?" Take the chapter title and state it as a question. What do you know about these subjects?

### Chapter Objectives

To enhance your study, turn each chapter objective into one or more questions. Here are some possible questions using the objectives from Chapter 32.

*Objective 1:* Discuss the normal functions of the pancreas.
- What are the normal functions of the pancreas?

*Objective 2:* Contrast age of onset, signs and symptoms, pharmacologic and nonpharmacologic treatment, incidence, and etiology of type 1 and type 2 diabetes mellitus.
- What is type 1 diabetes mellitus?
- What is type 2 diabetes mellitus?
- How do types 1 and 2 diabetes mellitus differ in age of onset, signs and symptoms, treatment, incidence, and etiology?

Because the objectives tell you what the authors expect you to know at the end of the chapter, starting out with questions based on the objectives will improve your learning and probably save you time.

## Chapter Headings

The same principle can be applied to each of the topic headings set out in the chapter. Continuing to use Chapter 32 as a model, here are some samples of questions that might be useful as preparation for reading.

### Type 1 Diabetes Mellitus
- What is type 1 diabetes?
- What is mellitus?

As you start to process the chapter headings, you should also notice that they begin to answer some of the questions from the chapter objectives. This is a good time to begin setting up vocabulary cards.

### Mechanism of Action and Drug Effects
- What is the mechanism of action of insulin?
- Is there more than one mechanism?
- What are the most important drug effects of insulin?
- Where do these effects take place?
- What is the evidence of these effects?

The idea is to focus on the major content of the chapter and establish a guide for learning as you read.

## Print Conventions within the Body of the Chapter

Print conventions are useful in this study skills strategy. The use of *italics*, **bold**, underlining, and multiple colors of ink are examples of print conventions. They are designed to catch your attention. Use them as a basis for questions.

In the first paragraph of Chapter 32, the first obvious print convention is the word insulin. It is printed in bold and in the color blue. If you let your

eyes float down the page and do not read anything, this word stands out. It must be important.
- What is insulin?
- What is the relationship between insulin and type 1 diabetes mellitus?

There are more words on the first page of the chapter text that are in the same print style. Apply the same procedure to these terms. Also, notice that two of the terms, glycogen and glycogenolysis, must have some direct relationship, because the second term contains the first term. The basic question in each case is, "What does the term mean?" However, there should be more to your questions than just the basics. *Glycogenolysis* seems to mean that there is some operation or activity taking place. Ask yourself the following:
- What happens in glycogenolysis?
- Where does glycogenolysis occur?
- When does glycogenolysis occur?
- How does it relate to type 1 diabetes mellitus?

## Chapter Tables

Tables serve as a summary of information discussed in the chapter. You can learn a great deal from tables if you take the time.

Look at Table 32-2. The table summarizes characteristics of type 1 and type 2 diabetes. There are two obvious questions for each type.
- What is type 1 (and type 2) diabetes?
- What are its characteristics?

Use these questions to study Table 32-2 and you will find that all the information you need for responding to these questions is found here. It may be useful to make a first pass through the chapter, focusing only on the tables before you begin to read. You will learn a great deal about some of the topics, and you will have established background information that will help you ask better questions and read with better understanding.

The time you spend asking questions makes the reading and learning go more quickly. Another benefit is that some of the questions you ask may appear on tests. These questions will be easy for you to answer. This promotes test-taking confidence, and better test scores result in better grades. If you have not been using questioning strategy up to this point in your text, begin now. After you use the strategy for two or three chapters, you will find that the benefits far outweigh the time it takes.

# Pituitary Drugs

## OBJECTIVES

When you reach the end of this chapter, you will be able to do the following:

1  Describe the normal function of the anterior and posterior lobes of the pituitary gland and the impact of the pituitary gland on the human body.
2  Compare the various pituitary drugs with regard to their indications, mechanisms of action, dosages, routes of administration, adverse effects, cautions, contraindications, and drug interactions.
3  Develop a nursing care plan that includes all phases of the nursing process for patients receiving pituitary drugs, such as desmopressin, vasopressin, octreotide, and somatropin.

## DRUG PROFILES

- ♦ **octreotide, p. 496**
- ♦ **somatropin, p. 497**

- ♦ **vasopressin, p. 497**
  _____
- ♦ *Key drug*

## KEY TERMS

**Hypothalamus**  The gland above and behind the pituitary gland and the optic chiasm. Both glands are suspended beneath the middle area of the bottom of the brain. The hypothalamus secretes the hormones vasopressin and oxytocin, which are stored in the posterior pituitary gland. The hypothalamus also secretes several hormone-releasing factors that stimulate the anterior pituitary gland to secrete a variety of hormones that control many body functions. (p. 494)

**Negative feedback loop**  A system in which the production of one hormone is controlled by the levels of a second hormone in a way that reduces the output of the first hormone. A gland produces a hormone that stimulates a second gland to produce a second hormone. In response to the increased levels of the second hormone, the source gland of the first hormone reduces production of that hormone, until blood levels of the second hormone fall below a certain minimum level needed; then the cycle begins again. (p. 494)

**Neuroendocrine system**  The system that regulates the reactions to both internal and external stimuli and involves the integrated activities of the endocrine glands and nervous system. (p. 494)

**Pituitary gland**  An endocrine gland that is suspended beneath the brain and supplies numerous hormones that control many vital processes. (p. 494)

## ANATOMY, PHYSIOLOGY AND PATHOPHYSIOLOGY OVERVIEW

### ENDOCRINE SYSTEM

Maintenance of physiologic stability is the main goal of the endocrine system. The endocrine system must accomplish this task despite constant changes in the internal and external environments. Every cell and organ in the body comes under the influence of the endocrine system. It communicates with the nearly 50 million target cells in the body using a chemical "language" called *hormones*. Hormones are a large group of natural substances that cause highly specific physiologic effects in the cells of their target tissues. They are secreted into the bloodstream in response to the body's needs and travel through the blood to their site of action—the target cell.

For decades, the pituitary gland was believed to be the master gland that regulated and controlled the other endocrine glands. However, evidence now suggests that the central nervous system (CNS), specifically the hypothalamus, controls the pituitary gland. The hypothalamus and pituitary gland are now viewed as functioning together as an integrated unit, with the primary direction coming from the hypothalamus. For this reason, these structures are now commonly referred to as the neuroendocrine system. In fact, the endocrine system can be considered in much the same way as the CNS. Each is basically a system for signaling, and each operates in a stimulus-and-response manner. Together these two systems essentially govern all bodily functions.

The pituitary gland is made up of two distinct lobes—the anterior pituitary gland (adenohypophysis) and posterior pituitary gland (neurohypophysis). They are individually linked to and communicate with the hypothalamus, and each lobe secretes its own different set of hormones. These various hormones are listed in Box 30-1 and shown in Figure 30-1.

Hormones are either water- or lipid-soluble. The water-soluble hormones are protein-based substances such as the catecholamines norepinephrine and epinephrine. The lipid-soluble hormones consist of the steroid and thyroid hormones.

The activity of the endocrine system is regulated by a system of surveillance and signaling usually dictated by the body's ongoing needs. Hormone secretion is commonly regulated by a negative feedback loop. This is best explained using a fictional example: When gland X releases hormone X, this stimulates target cells to release hormone Y. When there is an excess of hormone Y, gland X senses this excess and decreases its release of hormone X.

---

| BOX 30-1 | **HORMONES OF THE ANTERIOR AND POSTERIOR PITUITARY GLAND** |
|---|---|

**Anterior Pituitary Gland (Adenohypophysis)**
Adrenocorticotropic hormone (ACTH)
Follicle-stimulating hormone (FSH)
Growth hormone (GH)
Luteinizing hormone (LH)
Prolactin (PH)
Thyroid-stimulating hormone (TSH)

**Posterior Pituitary Gland (Neurohypophysis)**
Antidiuretic hormone (ADH)
Oxytocin

---

## PHARMACOLOGY OVERVIEW

### PITUITARY DRUGS

A variety of drugs affect the pituitary gland. They are generally used either as replacement drug therapy to make up for a hormone deficiency or as diagnostic aids to determine the status of the patient's hormonal functions. The currently identified anterior and posterior pituitary hormones and the drugs that mimic or antagonize their actions are listed in Table 30-1.

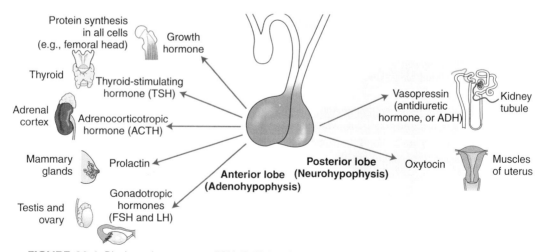

**FIGURE 30-1** Pituitary hormones. *FSH,* Follicle-stimulating hormone; *LH,* luteinizing hormone. (Adapted from McKenry LM, Tessier E, Hogan MA: *Mosby's pharmacology in nursing,* ed 22, St Louis, 2006, Mosby.)

The anterior pituitary drugs discussed in this chapter are cosyntropin, somatropin, and octreotide; the posterior pituitary drugs discussed in this chapter are vasopressin and desmopressin.

## Mechanism of Action and Drug Effects

The mechanisms of action of the various pituitary drugs differ depending on the drug, but overall they either augment or antagonize the natural effects of the pituitary hormones. Exogenously administered corticotropin elicits all of the same pharmacologic responses as those elicited by endogenous corticotropin (also known as adrenocorticotropic hormone, or ACTH). Intravenous exogenous corticotropin is no longer manufactured; however, an intramuscular/subcutaneous injection, known as H.P. Acthar Gel, is available. The intravenous corticotropin has been replaced by cosyntropin (Cortrosyn). Cosyntropin travels to the adrenal cortex, located just above the kidney, and stimulates the secretion of cortisol (the drug form of which is hydrocortisone [Solu-Cortef]). Cortisol has many antiinflammatory effects, including reduction of inflammatory leukocyte functions and scar tissue formation. Cortisol also promotes renal retention of sodium, which can result in edema and hypertension.

The drugs that mimic growth hormone (GH) are somatropin and somatrem. These drugs promote growth by stimulating various anabolic (tissue-building) processes, liver glycogenolysis (to raise blood sugar levels), lipid mobilization from body fat stores, and retention of sodium, potassium, and phosphorus. Both drugs promote linear growth in children who lack normal amounts of the endogenous hormone.

Octreotide is a drug that antagonizes the effects of natural GH. It does so by inhibiting GH release. Octreotide is a synthetic polypeptide that is structurally and pharmacologically similar to GH release–inhibiting factor, which is also called *somatostatin*. It also reduces plasma concentrations of vasoactive intestinal polypeptide (VIP), a protein secreted by a type of tumor known as a *VIPoma* that causes profuse watery diarrhea (see Chapter 46).

The drugs that affect the posterior pituitary gland, such as vasopressin and desmopressin, mimic the actions of the naturally occurring antidiuretic hormone (ADH). They increase water resorption in the distal tubules and collecting ducts of the nephrons, and they concentrate urine, reducing water excretion by up to 90%. Vasopressin is also a potent vasoconstrictor in larger doses and is therefore used in certain hypotensive emergencies, such as vasodilatory shock (septic shock). It is also used in the Advanced Cardiac Life Support (ACLS) guidelines for treatment of pulseless cardiac arrest. Vasopressin is also used to stop bleeding of esophageal varices. Desmopressin causes a dose-dependent increase in the plasma levels of factor VIII (antihemophilic factor), von Willebrand factor (acts closely with factor VIII), and tissue plasminogen activator. These properties make it useful in treating certain blood disorders. Desmopressin is also used for management of nocturnal enuresis. The drug form of oxytocin mimics the endogenous hormone, thus promoting uterine contractions (see Chapter 34).

## Indications

Cosyntropin is used in the diagnosis of adrenocortical insufficiency. Upon diagnosis, the actual drug treatment generally

---

### TABLE 30-1   ANTERIOR AND POSTERIOR PITUITARY HORMONES AND DRUGS

| HORMONE | FUNCTION AND MIMICKING DRUG |
| --- | --- |
| **Anterior Pituitary Gland** | |
| Adrenocorticotropic hormone (ACTH) | Targets adrenal gland; mediates adaptation to physical and emotional stress and starvation; redistributes body nutrients; promotes synthesis of adrenocortical hormones (glucocorticoids, mineralocorticoids, androgens); involved in skin pigmentation |
| | Cosyntropin: Used for diagnosis of adrenocortical insufficiency |
| Follicle-stimulating hormone (FSH) | Stimulates oogenesis and follicular growth in females and spermatogenesis in males |
| | Menotropins: Same pharmacologic effects as FSH; many of the other gonadotropins also stimulate FSH (see Chapter 34) |
| Growth hormone (GH) | Regulates anabolic processes related to growth and adaptation to stressors; promotes skeletal and muscle growth; increases protein synthesis; increases liver glycogenolysis; increases fat mobilization |
| | Somatropin, somatrem: Human GH for treatment of hypopituitary dwarfism |
| | Octreotide: A synthetic polypeptide structurally and pharmacologically similar to GH release–inhibiting factor; inhibits GH |
| Luteinizing hormone (LH) | Stimulates ovulation and estrogen release by ovaries in females; stimulates interstitial cells in males to promote spermatogenesis and testosterone secretion |
| | Pergonal and clomiphene: Increase LH levels and the chance of pregnancy |
| Prolactin | Targets mammary glands; stimulates lactogenesis and breast growth in females; purpose in males is poorly understood |
| | Bromocriptine: Inhibits action of prolactin and therefore inhibits lactogenesis (see Chapter 15) |
| Thyroid-stimulating hormone (TSH) | Stimulates secretion of thyroid hormones $T_3$ and $T_4$ by the thyroid gland |
| | Thyrotropin: Increases the production and secretion of thyroid hormones (see Chapter 31) |
| **Posterior Pituitary Gland** | |
| Antidiuretic hormone (ADH) | Increases water resorption in distal tubules and collecting duct of nephron; concentrates urine; causes potent vasoconstriction |
| | Vasopressin: ADH; performs all the physiologic functions of ADH |
| | Desmopressin: A synthetic vasopressin |
| Oxytocin | Targets mammary glands; stimulates ejection of milk and contraction of uterine smooth muscle |
| | Pitocin: Has all the physiologic actions of oxytocin (see Chapter 34) |

$T_3$, Triiodothyronine; $T_4$, thyroxine.

involves replacement hormonal therapy using drug forms of the deficient corticosteroid hormones. These drugs are discussed in more detail in Chapter 33. Somatropin and somatrem are human GH produced by recombinant technology. They are effective in stimulating skeletal growth in patients with an inadequate secretion of normal endogenous GH, such as those with hypopituitary dwarfism, and are also used for wasting associated with human immunodeficiency virus infection (HIV). Octreotide is useful in alleviating certain symptoms of carcinoid tumors stemming from the secretion of VIP, including severe diarrhea and flushing and potentially life-threatening hypotension associated with a carcinoid crisis. It is also used for the treatment of esophageal varices. Vasopressin and desmopressin are used to prevent or control polydipsia (excessive thirst), polyuria, and dehydration in patients with diabetes insipidus caused by a deficiency of endogenous ADH. Because of their vasoconstrictor properties, they are useful in the treatment of various types of bleeding, in particular gastrointestinal hemorrhage. Desmopressin is useful in the treatment of hemophilia A and type I von Willebrand's disease because of its effects on various blood-clotting factors.

## Contraindications

Contraindications for the use of pituitary drugs vary with each individual drug and are listed in each of the drug profiles included in this chapter. Because even small amounts of these drugs can initiate major physiologic changes, all of them should be used with special caution in patients with acute or chronic illnesses such as migraine headaches, epilepsy, and asthma.

## Adverse Effects

Most of the adverse effects of the pituitary drugs are specific to the individual drug. Those drugs possessing similar hormonal effects generally have similar adverse effects. The most common adverse effects of the pituitary drugs described here are listed in Tables 30-2 to 30-4.

## Interactions

Selected interactions involving pituitary drugs are summarized in Table 30-5.

## Dosages

For dosage information on pituitary drugs, see the table on p. 497.

## DRUG PROFILES

♦ **octreotide**

Octreotide (Sandostatin) is useful in alleviating certain symptoms of carcinoid tumors stemming from the secretion of VIP, including severe diarrhea and flushing and potentially life-threatening hypotension associated with a carcinoid crisis. It is also used for the treatment of esophageal varices. It is contraindicated in patients who have shown a hypersensitivity to it or any of its components. Octreotide may impair gallbladder function and needs to be used with caution in patients with renal impairment. It may affect glucose regulation, and severe hypoglycemia may occur in patients with type 1 diabetes. It may cause hyperglycemia in patients with type 2

| TABLE 30-3 | DESMOPRESSIN AND VASOPRESSIN: COMMON ADVERSE EFFECTS | |
|---|---|---|
| **BODY SYSTEM** | **ADVERSE EFFECTS** | |
| Cardiovascular | Increased blood pressure | |
| Central nervous | Fever, vertigo, headache | |
| Gastrointestinal | Nausea, heartburn, cramps | |
| Genitourinary | Uterine cramping | |
| Other | Nasal irritation and congestion, tremor, sweating | |

| TABLE 30-4 | GROWTH HORMONE ANALOGUES: COMMON ADVERSE EFFECTS | |
|---|---|---|
| **BODY SYSTEM** | **ADVERSE EFFECTS** | |
| Central nervous | Headache | |
| Endocrine | Hyperglycemia, hypothyroidism | |
| Genitourinary | Hypercalciuria | |
| Other | Rash, urticaria, development of antibodies to growth hormone, inflammation at injection site, flulike syndrome | |

| TABLE 30-2 | OCTREOTIDE: COMMON ADVERSE EFFECTS | |
|---|---|---|
| **BODY SYSTEM** | **ADVERSE EFFECTS** | |
| Central nervous | Fatigue, malaise, headache | |
| Endocrine | Increase or decrease in blood glucose levels | |
| Gastrointestinal | Diarrhea, nausea, vomiting | |
| Respiratory | Dyspnea | |
| Musculoskeletal | Arthralgia | |
| Cardiovascular | Conduction abnormalities | |

| TABLE 30-5 | PITUITARY DRUGS: SELECTED DRUG INTERACTIONS | |
|---|---|---|
| **PITUITARY DRUG** | **INTERACTING DRUG** | **POTENTIAL RESULT** |
| desmopressin | carbamazepine | Enhanced desmopressin effects |
| | lithium, alcohol, demeclocycline | Reduced desmopressin effects |
| octreotide | cyclosporine | Case report of transplant rejection |
| | thioridazine, Ciprofloxacin | Prolongation of QT interval |
| somatropin | Glucocorticoids | Reduction of growth effects |
| vasopressin | carbamazepine, fludrocortisone | Enhanced antidiuretic effect |
| | demeclocycline, norepinephrine, lithium | Reduced antidiuretic effect |

## DOSAGES

### Selected Pituitary Drugs

| DRUG | PHARMACOLOGIC CLASS | USUAL DOSAGE RANGE | INDICATIONS/USES |
|------|---------------------|--------------------|------------------|
| ◆ octreotide (Sandostatin, Sandostatin LAR Depot) | Somatostatin (GH inhibitor) analogue | **Adult***<br>IV/subcut: Initial dose of 50 mcg bid-tid; may titrate up to 500 mcg tid<br>IV/subcut: 100-750 mcg/day divided bid-qid<br>Depot IM: 10-30 mg q4wk | Acromegaly<br>Metastatic carcinoid tumor (to control flushing and diarrhea symptoms)<br>VIPoma<br>Small bowel fistula<br>Esophageal varices |
| ◆ somatropin (Humatrope, others) | Anterior pituitary hormone | **Pediatric**<br>0.35mg/kg/week IM or subcut | Growth hormone deficiency |
| ◆ vasopressin (Pitressin) | Natural or synthetic ADH | **Adult**<br>IM/subcut: 5-10 units bid-qid<br>**Pediatric**<br>IV: 2.5-10 units bid-qid | Diabetes insipidus |
|  |  | **Adult**<br>IV: 0.01-0.04 units/min<br>**Pediatric**<br>IV: 0.3-0.4 milliunits/kg/min | Vasodilatory shock (septic shock) |
|  |  | **Adult**<br>IV: 0.2-0.4 unit/min<br>**Pediatric**<br>IV: 0.002-0.005 units/kg/min | GI hemorrhage<br>Esophageal varices |

*ADH,* Antidiuretic hormone; *GH,* growth hormone; *GI,* gastrointestinal; *IM,* intramuscular; *IV,* intravenous; *subcut,* subcutaneous; *VIPoma,* vasoactive intestinal peptide–producing tumor.
*Normally used only in adults.

diabetes or in patients without diabetes. Octreotide may enhance the toxic effects of drugs that prolong the QT interval. Ciprofloxacin may enhance the QT-prolonging effects of octreotide. Octreotide can be given intravenously (IV), intramuscularly (IM), or subcutaneously. It is classified as a pregnancy category B drug. Recommended dosages are given in the table on this page.

### Pharmacokinetics

| Route | Onset of Action | Peak Plasma Concentration | Elimination Half-life | Duration of Action |
|-------|-----------------|---------------------------|-----------------------|--------------------|
| PO | Rapid | 0.4-1 hr | 1.7-1.9 hr | 6-12 hr |

### ◆ somatropin

Somatropin (Humatrope, Nutropin, Serostim, others) is a growth hormone that is indicated in the treatment of growth failure due to inadequate endogenous growth hormone secretion. It is also used for patients with HIV infection with wasting or cachexia in conjunction with antiviral therapy. It is classified as a pregnancy category B or C drug, depending on the manufacturer. Somatropin is contraindicated in patients with hypersensitivity to any component of the product and in children with closed growth plates, patients with tumors, and patients with acute illnesses. Adverse effects include headache, injection site reactions, muscle pain, hypoglycemia, or hyperglycemia. It is important not to shake the product. It is generally given subcutaneously; however, some manufactured products can be given intramuscularly. Check the specific prescribing information before administering.

### Pharmacokinetics

| Route | Onset of Action | Peak Plasma Concentration | Elimination Half-life | Duration of Action |
|-------|-----------------|---------------------------|-----------------------|--------------------|
| Subcut or IM | Not available | 2-6 hr | 2-4 hr (subcut) | 18-20 hr |

### ◆ vasopressin

Vasopressin (Pitressin) and desmopressin (DDAVP) are used to prevent or control polydipsia (excessive thirst), polyuria, and dehydration in patients with diabetes insipidus caused by a deficiency of endogenous ADH. Vasopressin is also used to control various types of bleeding (in particular gastrointestinal hemorrhage) and in pulseless arrest and vasodilatory shock. Desmopressin is also useful in the treatment of hemophilia A and type I von Willebrand's disease because of its effects on various blood-clotting factors. Vasopressin is contraindicated in patients with known hypersensitivity. It is classified as a pregnancy category C drug. It should be used with caution in patients with seizure disorders, asthma, cardiovascular disease, and renal disease. IV infiltration may lead to severe vasoconstriction and localized tissue necrosis. Watch the IV site closely for any signs of infiltration, and use a central venous access device when possible. Vasopressin is available as a nasal spray or injection for IM or IV use. When used to treat septic shock, it is given by continuous IV infusion. Both drugs can be given via the nasal route. Vasopressin nasal is used topically to nasal membranes and must not be inhaled. Desmopressin is given via nasal pump.

Pharmacokinetics (vasopressin)

| Route | Onset of Action | Peak Plasma Concentration | Elimination Half-life | Duration of Action |
|-------|-----------------|---------------------------|-----------------------|--------------------|
| IV | Rapid | 1 hr | 0.5 hr | 2-8 hr |

# NURSING PROCESS

## ASSESSMENT

Before administering any of the pituitary drugs, perform a thorough assessment and document the findings. Assess the patient's height, weight, and vital signs. Take a complete medication history with notation of allergies, prescription drug use, and use of over-the-counter drugs and herbals. With octreotide, the prescriber may order an electrocardiogram prior to use because of the adverse effect of conduction abnormalities. Assess baseline glucose levels and note respiratory status with *octreotide acetate* use. Patients taking octreotide may require special dosing if they have decreased liver and kidney function; therefore, assess and record baseline liver and kidney function tests. It is also important to be sure that assessment includes steps to prevent medication errors and awareness of concerns regarding look-alike sound-alike drugs. Specifically, octreotide acetate, or Sandostatin and Sandostatin LAR are not to be confused with Sandimmune (cyclosporine) or Sandoglobulin (IV immune globulin).

With *desmopressin,* check vital signs and assess for a history of seizures, asthma, or cardiovascular disease. These conditions require cautious use with careful monitoring of vital signs, heart sounds, and breath sounds. If *vasopressin* is being administered for shock, close monitoring in an intensive care setting is needed with ECG, vital signs, and other possibly invasive monitoring methods (e.g., arterial lines, central venous pressure lines, arterial blood gases). Obtain baseline thyroid, glucose, and calcium levels in patients receiving *growth hormones* due to the potential side effects of hyperglycemia, hypothyroidism, and hypercalciuria. Specifically, use of *somatropin* requires attention to the growth, motor skills, height, and weight of the pediatric patient. Additionally, with all of the pituitary drugs, always perform a thorough assessment of cautions, contraindications, and drug interactions prior to their administration.

## NURSING DIAGNOSES

1. Disturbed body image related to the specific disease process and/or drug adverse effects and their impact on the patient's physical characteristics
2. Acute pain related to gastrointestinal adverse effects associated with the use of various pituitary drugs
3. Deficient knowledge related to lack of information and experience with pituitary drug treatment

## PLANNING

### GOALS

1. Patient maintains positive body image while receiving drug therapy.

2. Patient experiences little to no pain related to medication-induced gastrointestinal upset or epigastric distress.
3. Patient gains increased knowledge about drug therapy.

### OUTCOME CRITERIA

1. Patient openly verbalizes fears, anxieties, and concerns to health care professionals regarding changes in body image related to disease process and the adverse effects of drug therapy.
2. Patient experiences minimal gastrointestinal upset and gastric distress by taking medication with food or at mealtimes.
3. Patient states specific rationale for drug therapy as well as adverse effects.
   - Patient states the importance of keeping follow-up appointments with the prescriber.

## CASE STUDY

### Octreotide for VIPoma-Related Diarrhea

J.R., a 56-year-old beautician, has been diagnosed with a VIPoma (vasoactive intestinal peptide–producing tumor). She was scheduled for surgery but developed severe diarrhea. She has been hospitalized because she became dehydrated after 2 days of profuse, watery diarrhea. She has not eaten for several days. In addition to having diarrhea, she is nauseated, has facial flushing, and has lost 5 pounds in 2 days. Intravenous fluid replacement with normal saline has been started, and she will be receiving octreotide (Sandostatin). She had her gallbladder removed 8 years ago but has no history of other illnesses.

1. How does the octreotide work to control the VIPoma-related diarrhea?
2. As J.R. begins therapy with octreotide, the nurse should continue to assess what parameters?

   After 2 days of treatment, the episodes of diarrhea have become less frequent. However, the nurse notes that J.R.'s blood glucose levels are elevated.
3. What is the best explanation for this elevation?

For answers, see http://evolve.elsevier.com/Lilley.

## IMPLEMENTATION

*Octreotide* must be given as ordered with attention to the route of administration. To avoid giving the wrong medication, be careful not to confuse octreotide acetate injection with the injectable depot suspension dosage form. Use only clear solutions, and always check for incompatibilities. Make sure patients understand the importance of immediately reporting to the prescriber any abdominal distress such as diarrhea, nausea, or vomiting if not manageable. Stress the importance of follow-up appointments for laboratory testing during treatment with this drug. Monitor glucose levels during therapy, especially if patients are already diabetic. Octreotide may cause alterations in blood glucose levels; closely monitor blood glucose during drug therapy.

Administer *desmopressin* per the prescriber's orders because dosage and route may vary with the indication. Dosage forms include oral, IV, intranasal, and subcutaneous. For desmopressin and somatropin, rotate subcutaneous injection sites (also given IM, in ventral gluteal site) to avoid tissue damage. Mix injectable solutions by gently swirling the liquid, using only clear solutions. Intranasal use may lead to changes in the nasal mucosa with unpredictable absorption. Instruct the patient to contact the prescriber immediately if the condition worsens. If used in patients diagnosed with diabetes insipidus, fluid intake may be adjusted according to the predicted risk of water intoxication and sodium deficit. See the Patient Teaching Tips for more information on dosage administration.

*Vasopressin* is available as a nasal spray or as an injection for IM or IV use. Always check the clarity of parenteral solutions before administering the medication, and discard the solution if there are visible particles or any fluid discoloration. Be alert to the adverse effects of elevated blood pressure, fever, nausea, abdominal cramping, or diarrhea. If these worsen or persist, notify the prescriber immediately.

## EVALUATION

Once goals and outcome criteria have been reviewed, evaluate the therapeutic responses to these drugs. With *octreotide*, therapeutic effects include improved symptoms related to carcinoid tumors, VIPoma, or esophageal varices. With *vasopressin*, an improvement in diabetes insipidus, esophageal varices, or vasodilatory shock is expected. With *somatropin*, increased growth is expected for whom it is indicated. Adverse effects to evaluate for include fatigue, headache, altered blood glucose levels, diarrhea, nausea, vomiting, conduction disorders, and dyspnea. Adverse effects associated with desmopressin and vasopressin include increased blood pressure, fever, headache, abdominal cramps, and nausea. *Growth hormones* may lead to headache, hyperglycemia, hypothyroidism, hypercalciuria, and flulike syndrome.

## PATIENT TEACHING TIPS

- Carefully discuss routes and techniques of administration with the patient and anyone else involved in the patient's care. With pediatric patients, demonstrate the technique of administration to the family or caregiver before discharge, and evaluate comprehension with return demonstrations. Provide written instructions to the patient, if age-appropriate, but also to the parents or caregiver. Keeping a journal about how the drug is being tolerated may prove to be beneficial. As for any medication or illness, the patient should keep a medical alert bracelet, necklace, or wallet card on his or her person at all times.
- Intranasal dosage forms of desmopressin are to be given only after the nasal passages have been cleared. The pump must be primed prior to use. Instruct the patient to prime the nasal pump by pressing down the pump four times. The spray pump delivers 10 mcg of drug each time it is pressed. To administer a 10-mcg dose as ordered, place the spray nozzle in the nostril (for a child, have a parent/adult/caregiver administer the dose) and press the spray pump once. If a higher dose has been prescribed, half the dose is to be

administered in each nostril. The pump cannot deliver doses smaller than 10 mcg. Once completed, replace the cap on the bottle. The pump will stay primed for up to 1 week. After 1 week, the pump will require re-priming. Carefully monitor the level of drug left in the pump so that there is always enough medication on hand. The pump may not have enough medication left after 25 doses (at 150 mcg per spray) or 50 doses (at 10 mcg per spray).
- Vasopressin is given topically to the nasal membranes and is not to be inhaled.
- Educate parents about the fact that children with endocrine disorders may have an increased risk of bone problems. Instruct parents that if they notice their child limping, this needs to be evaluated by the prescriber. Closely monitor the diabetic patient for changes in serum glucose levels if he or she is taking ocreotide.
- Water intake amounts may need to be monitored closely in patients with diabetes insipidus. Exact amounts may be prescribed or determined for each patient.

## KEY POINTS

- The pituitary gland is composed of two distinct lobes: anterior and posterior. Each lobe secretes its own set of hormones: *anterior:* thyroid-stimulating hormone (TSH), GH, ACTH, prolactin, follicle-stimulating hormone (FSH), luteinizing hormone; *posterior:* ADH, oxytocin.
- Pituitary drugs are used to either mimic or antagonize the action of endogenous pituitary hormones.
- Drugs that mimic the action of endogenous pituitary hormones include cosyntropin, somatropin, somatrem, vasopressin, and desmopressin. A drug that antagonizes the actions of endogenous pituitary hormones is octreotide.

- In the assessment of patients receiving pituitary hormones, measure baseline vital signs, review blood glucose levels, and measure weight.
- For patients receiving somatropin, constantly monitor levels of thyroid hormones and growth hormones. Include measurement of vital signs, intake/output, and weight in the assessment.

## NCLEX® EXAMINATION REVIEW QUESTIONS

1 A patient is experiencing severe diarrhea, flushing, and life-threatening hypotension associated with carcinoid crisis. The nurse will prepare to administer which drug?
   a  octreotide (Sandostatin)
   b  vasopressin (Pitressin)
   c  somatropin (Humatrope)
   d  cosyntropin (Cortrosyn)

2 A patient is suspected of having adrenocortical insufficiency. The nurse expects to administer which drug to aid in the diagnosis of this condition?
   a  octreotide (Sandostatin)
   b  vasopressin (Pitressin)
   c  somatropin (Humatrope)
   d  cosyntropin (Cortrosyn)

3 The nurse is reviewing the medication list for a patient who will be starting therapy with somatropin. Which type of drug would raise a concern that needs to be addressed before the patient starts the somatropin?
   a  Nonsteroidal antiinflammatory drug for arthritis
   b  Antidepressant drug
   c  Penicillin
   d  Glucocorticoid

4 A patient who is about to be given octreotide is also taking a diuretic, IV heparin, ciprofloxacin (Cipro), and an opioid as needed for pain. The nurse will monitor for what possible interaction?
   a  Hypokalemia due to an interaction with the diuretic
   b  Decreased anticoagulation due to an interaction with the heparin
   c  Prolongation of the QT interval due to an interaction with ciprofloxacin
   d  Increased sedation if the opioid is given

5 When monitoring for the therapeutic effects of intranasal desmopressin (DDAVP) in a patient who has diabetes insipidus, which assessment finding will the nurse look for as an indication that the medication therapy is successful?
   a  Increased insulin levels
   b  Decreased diarrhea
   c  Improved nasal patency
   d  Decreased thirst

6 Which drugs have an action similar to that of the naturally occurring hormone ADH? (Select all that apply.)
   a  cosyntropin (Cortrosyn)
   b  desmopressin (DDAVP)
   c  somatropin (Humatrope)
   d  vasopressin (Pitressin)
   e  octreotide (Sandostatin)

7 The order reads: "Give ocreotide (Sandostatin) 50 mcg subcut twice a day." The medication is available in an injectable form of 0.05 mg/mL. How many milliliters will the nurse draw up for the ordered dose?

1. a, 2. d, 3. d, 4. c, 5. d, 6. b, d, 7. 1 mL.

For Critical Thinking and Prioritization Questions, see http://evolve.elsevier.com/Lilley.

# Thyroid and Antithyroid Drugs

## OBJECTIVES

When you reach the end of this chapter, you will be able to do the following:

1  Briefly describe the normal anatomy and physiology of the thyroid gland.
2  Discuss the various functions of the thyroid gland and related hormones.
3  Describe the differences in the diseases resulting from the hyposecretion and hypersecretion of thyroid gland hormones.
4  Identify the various drugs used to treat the hyposecretion and hypersecretion states of the thyroid gland.

5  Discuss the mechanisms of action, indications, dosages, routes of administration, contraindications, cautions, drug interactions, and adverse effects of the various drugs used to treat hypothyroidism and hyperthyroidism.
6  Develop a nursing care plan that includes all phases of the nursing process for patients receiving thyroid replacement therapy as well as for patients receiving antithyroid drugs.

## DRUG PROFILES

♦ **levothyroxine, p. 504**
♦ **propylthiouracil, p. 506**

_____

♦  *Key drug*

## KEY TERMS

**Euthyroid**  Referring to normal thyroid function. (p. 503)

**Hyperthyroidism**  A condition characterized by excessive production of the thyroid hormones. A severe form of this disorder is called *thyrotoxicosis.* (p. 502)

**Hypothyroidism**  A condition characterized by diminished production of the thyroid hormones. (p. 502)

**Thyroid-stimulating hormone (TSH)**  An endogenous substance secreted by the pituitary gland that controls the release of thyroid gland hormones and is necessary for the growth and function of the thyroid gland (also called *thyrotropin*). (p. 502)

**Thyroxine ($T_4$)**  The principle thyroid hormone that influences the metabolic rate. (p. 502)

**Triiodothyronine ($T_3$)**  A secondary thyroid hormone that also affects body metabolism. (p. 502)

## ANATOMY, PHYSIOLOGY, AND PATHOPHYSIOLOGY OVERVIEW

### THYROID FUNCTION

The thyroid gland lies across the larynx in front of the thyroid cartilage ("Adam's apple"). Its lobes extend laterally on both sides of the front of the neck. It is responsible for the secretion of three hormones essential for the proper regulation of metabolism: thyroxine ($T_4$), triiodothyronine ($T_3$), and calcitonin (see Chapter 34). It is located close to and communicates with the parathyroid glands, which lie just above and behind it. The parathyroid glands are two pairs of bean-shaped glands. These glands are made up of encapsulated cells, which are responsible for maintaining adequate levels of calcium in the extracellular fluid, primarily by mobilizing calcium from bone.

Thyroxine ($T_4$) and triiodothyronine ($T_3$) are produced in the thyroid gland through the coupling of iodine and the amino acid tyrosine. The iodide ($I^-$, which is the ionized form of iodine) needed for this process is acquired from the diet. One mg of iodide is needed per week. This iodide is absorbed from the blood and then sequestered by the thyroid gland, where it is concentrated to 20 times its blood level. Here it is also converted to iodine ($I_2$), which is combined with tyrosine to make diiodotyrosine. The combination of two molecules of diiodotyrosine causes the formation of thyroxine, which therefore has four iodine molecules in its structure ($T_4$). Triiodothyronine is formed by the coupling of one molecule of diiodotyrosine with one molecule of monoiodotyrosine; thus it has three iodine molecules in its structure ($T_3$). The biologic potency of $T_3$ is about four times greater than that of $T_4$, but $T_4$ is present in much greater quantities. After the synthesis of these two thyroid hormones, they are stored in the follicles in the thyroid gland in a complex with thyroglobulin (a protein that contains tyrosine and an amino acid) called the *colloid*. When the thyroid gland is signaled to do so, the thyroglobulin–thyroid hormone complex is enzymatically broken down to release $T_3$ and $T_4$ into the circulation. This entire process is triggered by thyroid-stimulating hormone (TSH), also called *thyrotropin*. Its release from the anterior pituitary gland is stimulated when blood levels of $T_3$ and $T_4$ are low.

The thyroid hormones are involved in a wide variety of bodily processes. They regulate the basal metabolic rate and lipid and carbohydrate metabolism, are essential for normal growth and development, control the heat-regulating system (thermoregulatory center in the brain), and have various effects on the cardiovascular, endocrine, and neuromuscular systems. Therefore, hyperfunction or hypofunction of the thyroid gland can lead to a wide range of serious consequences.

### PATHOPHYSIOLOGY OF HYPOTHYROIDISM

There are three types of hypothyroidism. Primary hypothyroidism stems from an abnormality in the thyroid gland itself. It occurs when the thyroid gland is not able to perform one of its many functions, such as releasing the thyroid hormones from their storage sites, coupling iodine with tyrosine, trapping iodide, converting iodide to iodine, or any combination of these defects. Primary hypothyroidism is the most common of the three types of hypothyroidism. Secondary hypothyroidism begins at the level of the pituitary gland and results from reduced secretion of thyroid stimulating hormone (TSH). TSH is needed to trigger the release of the $T_3$ and $T_4$ stored in the thyroid gland. Tertiary hypothyroidism is caused by a reduced level of the thyrotropin-releasing hormone from the hypothalamus. This reduced level, in turn, reduces TSH and thyroid hormone levels. Symptoms of hypothyroidism include cold intolerance, unintentional weight gain, depression, dry brittle hair and nails, and fatigue.

Hypothyroidism can also be classified by when it occurs in the lifespan. Hyposecretion of thyroid hormone during youth may lead to cretinism. Cretinism is characterized by low metabolic rate, retarded growth and sexual development, and possible mental retardation. Hyposecretion of thyroid hormone as an adult may lead to myxedema. Myxedema is a condition manifested by decreased metabolic rate, but it also involves loss of mental and physical stamina, weight gain, hair loss, firm edema, and yellow dullness of the skin.

Some forms of hypothyroidism may result in the formation of a goiter, which is an enlargement of the thyroid gland resulting from its overstimulation by elevated levels of TSH. The TSH level is elevated because there is little or no thyroid hormone in the circulation. Certain drugs can cause hypothyroidism, with amiodarone (see Chapter 25) being the most common. Interestingly, amiodarone can also cause hyperthyroidism.

### PATHOPHYSIOLOGY OF HYPERTHYROIDISM

Excessive secretion of thyroid hormones, or hyperthyroidism, may be caused by several different diseases. Diseases known to cause hyperthyroidism include Graves' disease, which is the most common cause; Plummer's disease, also known as *toxic nodular disease*, which is the least common cause; multinodular disease; and thyroid storm, which is a severe and potentially life-threatening exacerbation of the symptoms of hyperthyroidism that is usually induced by stress or infection.

Hyperthyroidism can affect multiple body systems, resulting in an overall increase in metabolism. Commonly reported symptoms are diarrhea, flushing, increased appetite, muscle weakness, fatigue, palpitations, irritability, nervousness, sleep disorders, heat intolerance, and altered menstrual flow.

## PHARMACOLOGY OVERVIEW

### THYROID REPLACEMENT DRUGS

Hypothyroidism is treated with thyroid hormone replacement using various thyroid preparations. These drugs can be either natural or synthetic in origin. The natural thyroid preparations are derived from the thyroid glands of animals such as cattle and hogs. Currently only one natural preparation is available in the United States, and it is called simply *thyroid* or *thyroid, desiccated*. *Desiccation* is the term for the drying process used to prepare this drug form. All natural preparations are standardized for their iodine content. The synthetic thyroid preparations are levothyroxine ($T_4$), liothyronine ($T_3$), and liotrix (which contains a combination of $T_4$ and $T_3$ in a 4:1 ratio). The approximate clinically equivalent doses of the drugs are given in Table 31-1. This information is useful for guiding dosage adjustments when a patient is switched from one thyroid hormone to another. Monitoring of serum TSH and free thyroid hormone levels are required to determine the appropriate dose of thyroid replacement drugs.

## Mechanism of Action and Drug Effects

Thyroid drugs work in the same manner as the endogenous thyroid hormones, affecting many body systems. At the cellular level, they work to induce changes in the metabolic rate, including the rate of protein, carbohydrate, and lipid metabolism, and to increase oxygen consumption, body temperature, blood volume, and overall cellular growth and differentiation. They also stimulate the cardiovascular system by increasing the number of myocardial beta-adrenergic receptors. This, in turn, increases the sensitivity of the heart to catecholamines and ultimately increases cardiac output. In addition, thyroid hormones increase renal blood flow and the glomerular filtration rate, which results in a diuretic effect.

## Indications

Thyroid preparations are given to replace what the thyroid gland itself cannot produce to achieve normal thyroid hormone levels (euthyroid condition). Levothyroxine is the preferred thyroid drug because its hormonal content is standardized and its effect is predictable. Thyroid drugs can also be used for the diagnosis of suspected hyperthyroidism (as in a TSH-suppression test) and in the prevention or treatment of various types of goiters. They are also used for replacement hormonal therapy in patients whose thyroid glands have been surgically removed or destroyed by radioactive iodine in the treatment of thyroid cancer or hyperthyroidism. Hypothyroidism during pregnancy is treated with dosage adjustments every 4 weeks to maintain the TSH level at the lower end of the normal range. Fetal growth may be retarded if maternal hypothyroidism remains untreated during pregnancy.

## Contraindications

Contraindications to thyroid preparations include known drug allergy, recent myocardial infarction, adrenal insufficiency, and hyperthyroidism.

## Adverse Effects

The adverse effects of thyroid medications are usually the result of overdose. The most significant adverse effect is cardiac dysrhythmia with the risk for life-threatening or fatal irregularities. Other more common undesirable effects are listed in Table 31-2.

## Interactions

Thyroid drugs may enhance the activity of oral anticoagulants, the dosages of which may need to be reduced. Taking thyroid preparations concurrently with digitalis glycosides may decrease serum digitalis levels. Cholestyramine binds to thyroid hormone in the gastrointestinal tract, which possibly reduces the absorption of both drugs. Diabetic patients taking a thyroid drug may require increased dosages of their hypoglycemic drugs. In addition, the use of thyroid preparations with epinephrine in patients with coronary disease may induce coronary insufficiency. See Table 31-3 for more drug interactions.

## Dosages

For dosage information on the thyroid drugs, see the table on p. 504.

### DRUG PROFILE

The most commonly used thyroid replacement drugs are the synthetic drugs levothyroxine and liotrix. Some patients experience better results with the animal-derived products. Although the thyroid drugs differ chemically, their therapeutic actions are all the same. Factors to be considered before the initiation of drug therapy with a thyroid drug include the desired ratio of

| TABLE 31-2 | THYROID DRUGS: COMMON ADVERSE EFFECTS | |
|---|---|
| **BODY SYSTEM** | **ADVERSE EFFECTS** |
| Cardiovascular | Tachycardia, palpitations, angina, dysrhythmias, hypertension |
| Central nervous | Insomnia, tremors, headache, anxiety |
| Gastrointestinal | Nausea, diarrhea, cramps |
| Other | Menstrual irregularities, weight loss, sweating, heat intolerance, fever |

| TABLE 31-1 | THYROID DRUGS: CLINICALLY EQUIVALENT DOSES | |
|---|---|
| **THYROID DRUG** | **APPROXIMATE EQUIVALENT DOSE** |
| **Natural Thyroid Preparation** | |
| thyroid | 60-65 mg (1 grain) |
| **Synthetic Thyroid Preparations** | |
| levothyroxine | 100 mcg or more |
| liothyronine | 25 mcg |
| liotrix | 50 mcg/12.5 mcg ($T_4$/$T_3$) |

$T_3$, Triiodothyronine; $T_4$, thyroxine.

| TABLE 31-3 | THYROID DRUGS: INTERACTIONS | |
|---|---|
| **DRUG** | **ACTION** |
| insulin | Decreased efficacy of insulin (resulting in increased blood glucose levels) |
| Antidiabetic oral drugs | Decreased efficacy of antidiabetic drugs (resulting in increased blood glucose levels) |
| estrogen | Reduced thyroid drug activity |
| digoxin | Decreased digoxin effectiveness |
| phenytoin and fosphenytoin | Reduced levothyroxine effectiveness |
| phenobarbital | Reduced levothyroxine effectiveness |

## DOSAGES

### Selected Thyroid Drugs

| DRUG (PREGNANCY CATEGORY) | PHARMACOLOGIC CLASS | USUAL DOSAGE RANGE | INDICATIONS |
|---|---|---|---|
| ◆ levothyroxine (Synthroid, Levoxyl, others) (A) | Synthetic thyroid hormone ($T_4$) | **Adult**<br>PO: 25-200 mcg/day<br>IM/IV: 50% of oral dose<br>IV: 300-500 mcg in a single dose; repeat next day 100-300 mcg if necessary<br>**Pediatric 0-12 yr**<br>PO: 25-150 mcg/day | Hypothyroidism<br><br>Myxedema coma<br><br>Congenital hypothyroidism |
| liotrix (Thyrolar) | Synthetic thyroid hormone ($T_4$: $T_3$ in a 4:1 ratio) | **Adult**<br>PO: 30-120 mg/day<br>**Pediatric**<br>Dose varies depending on age | Hypothyroidism |
| thyroid, dessicated (Armour Thyroid, Westhroid) | Desiccated thyroid | **Adult**<br>PO: 60-120 mg/day<br>**Pediatric**<br>Dose varies depending on age | Hypothyroidism |

*IM,* Intramuscular; *IV,* intravenous; *PO,* oral.

$T_3$ to $T_4$, the cost, and the desired duration of effect. Thyroid hormone replacement drugs are classified as pregnancy category A drugs. They are all contraindicated in patients who have had a hypersensitivity reaction to them in the past and in those with adrenal insufficiency, previous myocardial infarction, or hyperthyroidism.

### ◆ levothyroxine

Levothyroxine (Levoxyl, Levothroid, Synthroid, others), or $T_4$, is the most commonly prescribed synthetic thyroid hormone and is generally considered the drug of choice. One advantage it has over the natural thyroid preparations is that it is chemically pure, being 100% $T_4$ (thyroxine); this makes its effects more predictable than other thyroid preparations. Its half-life is long enough that it only needs to be administered once a day. It is available in oral form and in parenteral form. It is classified as a pregnancy category A drug.

Switching between different brands of levothyroxine during treatment can destabilize the course of treatment. Thyroid function test results need to be monitored more carefully when switching products. Recommended dosages are given in the table on this page. Levothyroxine is dosed in micrograms. A common medication error is to write the intended dose in milligrams instead of micrograms. If not caught, this error would result in a thousandfold overdose. Doses higher than 200 mcg need to be questioned in case this error has occurred. Levothyroxine is available in an intravenous form. The intravenous dose is generally 50% of the oral dose.

### Pharmacokinetics

| Route | Onset of Action | Peak Plasma Concentration | Elimination Half-life | Duration of Action |
|---|---|---|---|---|
| PO | 3-5 days | 24 hr | 6-10 days | 24 hr |

### ⚡ SAFETY AND QUALITY IMPROVEMENT: PREVENTING MEDICATION ERRORS

#### Giving IV Doses of Levothyroxine

Care must be taken when preparing IV doses of levothyroxine for infusions. The medication comes in vials for reconstitution, either in 200-mcg or 500-mcg vials. The vials must be reconstituted with 5 mL of 0.9% NaCl to provide a concentration of 40 mcg/mL (the 200-mcg vial) or 100 mcg/mL (the 500-mcg vial).

Problems occur when pharmacy computer systems profile the dose as "X amount of the *vial*" instead of calculating the dose based on the diluted strength. For example, for a dose of 120 mcg, the computer may list the dose as 120 mcg/0.755 vials, when actually the nurse needs to draw up 3 mL (40 mcg/mL) for the 120-mcg dose.

Other errors have occurred when the final volume was miscalculated using 10 mL (the size of the vial), which yields an incorrect concentration of 50 mcg/mL. As a result, the patient received too much medication.

It is essential to remember that the vial must be diluted FIRST, and then the dose is calculated upon the concentration of the reconstituted medication, not the size of the vial.

Data from Institute for Safe Medication Practices (ISMP): ISMP Medication Safety Alert, September 6, 2000, available at www.ismp.org/Newsletters/acutecare/articles/20000906_2.asp. Accessed Sept 2, 2011.

## ANTITHYROID DRUGS

Treatment of hyperthyroidism is aimed at treating either the primary cause or the symptoms of the disease. Antithyroid drugs, iodides, ionic inhibitors, surgery, and radioactive isotopes of iodine are used to treat the underlying cause, and drugs such as beta blockers are used to treat the symptoms. The focus of the discussion here is on the antithyroid drugs called *thioamide derivatives,* namely methimazole and propylthiouracil. In addition to the thioamides, radioactive iodine (iodine 131) and potassium iodide may be used to treat hyperthyroidism. Radioactive iodine works by destroying the thyroid gland, in a process known as *ablation*. It does this by emitting destructive beta rays once it is taken up into the follicles of the thyroid gland. It is a commonly used treatment for both hyperthyroidism and thyroid cancer. Potassium iodide is also used as prophylaxis for radiation exposure (see Chapter 49). Thyroid surgery involves removal of part or all of the thyroid gland. It is usually a very effective way to treat hyperthyroidism, but lifelong hormone replacement therapy is normally required after thyroid surgery.

## Mechanism of Action and Drug Effects

Methimazole and propylthiouracil act by inhibiting the incorporation of iodine molecules into the amino acid tyrosine, a process required to make the precursors of $T_3$ and $T_4$. By doing so, these drugs impede the formation of thyroid hormone. Propylthiouracil has the added ability to inhibit the conversion of $T_4$ to $T_3$ in the peripheral circulation. Neither drug can inactivate already existing thyroid hormone, however.

The drug effects of methimazole and propylthiouracil are primarily limited to the thyroid gland, and their overall effect is a decrease in the thyroid hormone level. Administration of these medications to patients with hyperthyroidism lowers the high levels of thyroid hormone, thereby normalizing the overall metabolic rate.

## Indications

Antithyroid drugs are used to treat hyperthyroidism and to prevent the surge in thyroid hormones that occurs after the surgical treatment of or during radioactive iodine therapy for hyperthyroidism or thyroid cancer. In some types of hyperthyroidism, such as that seen in Graves' disease, the long-term administration of these drugs (for several years) may induce a spontaneous remission. Surgical resection of the thyroid gland (thyroidectomy) is often used both in patients who are intolerant of antithyroid drug therapy and in pregnant women, in whom both antithyroid drugs and radioactive iodine therapy are usually contraindicated.

## Contraindications

The only usual contraindications to the use of the two antithyroid drugs is known drug allergy. Their use in pregnancy, although necessary, is somewhat controversial. Per the U.S. Food and Drug Administration (FDA), propythiouracil is to be used during the first trimester only, and then methimazole is used for the remainder of the pregnancy. However, there are case reports of scalp abnormalities when methimazole is used. The choice of how to treat pregnant patients is physician specific. Both drugs are classified as pregnancy category D drugs.

## Adverse Effects

The most damaging or serious adverse effects of the antithyroid medications are liver and bone marrow toxicity. These and the more common adverse effects of methimazole and propylthiouracil are listed in Table 31-4.

## Interactions

Drug interactions that occur with antithyroid drugs include additive leukopenic effects when they are taken in conjunction with other bone marrow depressants and an increase in the activity of oral anticoagulants.

## Dosages

For dosage information on propylthiouracil, see the table on this page.

| TABLE 31-4 | ANTITHYROID DRUGS: COMMON ADVERSE EFFECTS |
|---|---|
| **BODY SYSTEM** | **ADVERSE EFFECTS** |
| Central nervous | Drowsiness, headache, vertigo, paresthesia |
| Gastrointestinal | Nausea, vomiting, diarrhea, hepatitis, loss of taste |
| Genitourinary | Smoky urine, decreased urine output |
| Hematologic | Agranulocytosis, leukopenia, thrombocytopenia, hypothrombinemia, lymphadenopathy, bleeding |
| Integumentary | Rash, pruritus |
| Musculoskeletal | Myalgia, arthralgia |
| Renal | Increased blood urea nitrogen and serum creatinine levels |
| Other | Enlarged thyroid gland, nephritis |

## DOSAGES

### Selected Antithyroid Drugs

| DRUG (PREGNANCY CATEGORY) | PHARMACOLOGIC CLASS | USUAL DOSAGE RANGE | INDICATIONS |
|---|---|---|---|
| ♦ propylthiouracil* (generic only) (D) | Antithyroid | **Adult** 300-900 mg/day **Pediatric 6-10 yr** PO: 50-150 mg/day **Pediatric older than 10 yr** PO: 150-300 mg/day | Hyperthyroidism |
| methimazole (Tapazole) | Antithyroid | **Adult** 15-60 mg/day **Pediatric** 0.2 mg/kg/day with a maximum of 30 mg/day | Hyperthyroidism |

*PO*, Oral.
*Often abbreviated PTU.

## DRUG PROFILE

### ♦ propylthiouracil

Propylthiouracil (PTU) is a thioamide antithyroid drug and is classified as a pregnancy category D drug. Approximately 2 weeks of therapy with propylthiouracil may be necessary before symptoms improve. It is available only in oral form as a 50-mg tablet. Methimazole is the only alternative drug in this class and is rarely used clinically. Recommended dosages are given in the table on p. 505.

### Pharmacokinetics

| Route | Onset of Action | Peak Plasma Concentration | Elimination Half-life | Duration of Action |
|-------|-----------------|---------------------------|-----------------------|--------------------|
| PO | 24-36 hr | 1 hr | 1.5-5 hr | 2-3 hr |

## NURSING PROCESS

## ASSESSMENT

In assessing the patient taking *thyroid replacement drugs* for hypothyroidism, include baseline vital signs for comparative purposes. Assess levels of $T_3$, $T_4$, and TSH before and during drug therapy, as ordered. It is also important to thoroughly assess and document any past and present medical problems or concerns with a thorough physical assessment. Take a medication history that includes drug allergies and a list of all prescription drugs, over-the-counter drugs, herbals, and supplements the patient is taking. Cautions, contraindications, and drug interactions associated with the use of thyroid hormone have been previously discussed; thoroughly assess the patient for these before giving the medication. Review baseline vital signs with increased attention to a history of cardiac dysrhythmias because of the possible adverse effects of cardiac irregularities. These may be life-threatening. For the female patient, perform a thorough assessment of the reproductive system due to the impact of thyroid hormones on this system.

It is also important to remember that certain thyroid hormones may work faster than others because of their dosage form and properties (see the Teamwork and Collaboration: Pharmacokinetic Bridge to Nursing Practice box). Drug interactions that deserve emphasis because of their importance for patient safety and because they involve commonly used medications include interactions with oral anticoagulants (increased activity of the oral anticoagulants), digitalis glycosides (decrease in digitalis levels), cholyestyramine, and oral hypoglycemic drugs. See Table 31-3 for a more detailed listing of drug interactions. If the patient is taking an oral anticoagulant, monitor blood levels of the anticoagulant closely. Lifespan considerations include increased sensitivity to the effects of thyroid medications in elderly patients. Individualization of drug therapy is important with thyroid replacement, because different patients may respond very differently to the same drug and/or dosage.

For *antithyroid drugs,* such as propylthiouracil and methimazole, first measure vital signs and assess for signs and symptoms of thyroid crisis, or what is often called *thyroid storm.* Thyroid storm is manifested by exacerbation of hyperthyroidism symptoms (see pharmacology discussion) and is potentially life-threatening.

### TEAMWORK AND COLLABORATION: PHARMACOKINETIC BRIDGE TO NURSING PRACTICE

Thyroid replacement drugs possess very specific pharmacokinetic characteristics, as do many drugs. You must understand the pharmacokinetics to think your way critically through clinical situations involving patients who are taking thyroid replacement drugs. For levothyroxine (Synthroid, Levothroid, Levoxyl), the pharmacokinetic characteristics include an onset of action of 3 to 5 days, peak plasma concentrations within 24 hours, elimination half-life of 6 to 10 days, and a duration of action of 24 hours. Due to the prolonged half-life of this drug, there is an increased risk of toxicity. Toxicity is manifested by the following: weight loss, tachycardia, nervousness, tremors, hypertension, headache, insomnia, menstrual irregularities, and cardiac irregularities or palpitations. Another important pharmacokinetic property is that the drug is protein bound. A highly protein-bound drug acts like a biologic sustained-release drug and remains in the body longer, with increased risk of more interactions with other highly protein-bound drugs as well as greater potential for toxicity. This is yet another example of how important a current and thorough knowledge base about drugs—and specifically about their pharmacokinetics—is to their safe and efficient administration.

### PATIENT-CENTERED CARE: LIFESPAN CONSIDERATIONS FOR THE ELDERLY PATIENT

#### Thyroid Hormones

- Elderly patients are much more sensitive to thyroid hormone replacement drugs (as they are to most drugs). They are also more likely to experience adverse reactions to thyroid hormones than are patients in any other age group.
- Elderly patients experience more negative consequences related to drug therapy because their hepatic and renal functioning is decreased.
- Thyroid hormone replacement requirements are approximately 25% lower in patients 60 years of age and older than in younger patients. Dosage in elderly patients may therefore need to be adjusted or titrated downward.
- Elderly patients must contact the prescriber immediately if they experience palpitations, chest pain, stumbling, falling, depression, incontinence, sweating, shortness of breath and/or aggravated heart disease, cold intolerance, or weight gain.
- Drug therapy for elderly patients must be initiated with caution and with very individualized dosages. If higher dosages are necessary, increases must be made with the prescriber's guidance and done gradually.

Assessing for thyroid storm also means assessing for potential causes, such as stress or infection. Related cautions and contraindications have been discussed previously, but some important drug interactions to reemphasize include the interactions with oral anticoagulants (which can cause an increase in anticoagulation and thus risk for bleeding) and any medications that may lead to bone marrow suppression or cause leukopenia (antithyroid drugs may cause additive effects or worsening of bone marrow suppression).

## NURSING DIAGNOSES

1. Noncompliance due to lack of experience/education regarding thyroid hormone replacement and the need for everyday self-administration.

2. Ineffective health management due to lack of experience/ education about the use of thyroid medication
3. Risk for infection related to the bone marrow depression caused by antithyroid medication

## PLANNING

### GOALS

1. Patient remains compliant with daily administration of thyroid hormone replacement therapy.
2. Patient demonstrates improvement in health management behaviors through more experience/education about the rationale for use of the thyroid drug and related adverse effects.
3. Patient remains free from infection while receiving antithyroid medication.

### OUTCOME CRITERIA

1. Patient states the importance of taking thyroid hormone replacement therapy daily as ordered.
   - Patient takes thyroid hormone replacement therapy upon awakening in the morning and on an empty stomach to maximize therapeutic effects.
   - Patient takes medication in a single daily dose before breakfast and does not stop the medication unless consulting with the prescriber.
   - Patient understands the fact that replacement therapy is lifelong in most situations.
2. Patient states the importance of taking the medication as prescribed as well as the rationale for its use (e.g., lifelong replacement therapy).
   - Patient states adverse effects associated with thyroid replacement therapy that need to be reported to the prescriber (i.e., cardiac dysrhythmias [felt as palpitations]).
   - Patient reports adverse effects that may indicate the need for re-regulation of dosage such as signs and symptoms of hyperthyroidism (i.e., irregular heartbeat, palpitations).
3. Patient states ways to decrease the risk for infection while receiving an antithyroid medication, such as avoiding persons with infections, eating a proper diet, getting adequate rest, and increasing fluid intake.

## IMPLEMENTATION

When *thyroid drugs* are administered, it is important that the drug be given at the same time every day to help maintain consistent blood levels of the drug. Emphasize to the patient that it is best to administer thyroid drugs once daily in the morning, if possible, to decrease the likelihood of insomnia, which may result from evening dosing and the subsequent increase in energy level. Patients must also avoid interchanging brands because of problems with the bioequivalence of drugs from different manufacturers. If needed, patients may crush tablets. If the patient is scheduled to undergo radioactive iodine isotope studies, the thyroid medication is usually

discontinued about 4 weeks before the test, but only as prescribed. Elderly patients may require alteration of the dosage amount, with a decrease of up to 25% for patients 60 years of age and older.

Educate the patient taking the *antithyroid drug* propylthiouracil about dosing the medication with meals to help decrease stomach upset. Any fever, sore throat, mouth ulcers or sores, or skin eruptions, as well as any unusual bleeding or bruising needs to be reported to the prescriber immediately. These symptoms may indicate problems of liver and bone marrow toxicity and possible leukopenia. Further educate patients to avoid the use of iodized salt or eating shellfish because of their potential for altering the drug's effectiveness. Advise patients to be aware of the signs and symptoms of hypothyroidism, including unexplained weight gain, loss of mental and physical stamina, hair loss, firm edema, and yellow dullness of the skin (indicative of myxedema or a decrease in metabolic rate). If these occur, patients must report them immediately to the prescriber. Frequently monitor complete blood counts to watch for potential problems with leukopenia. It is also important to monitor the results of liver function studies during follow-up visits with the prescriber.

## EVALUATION

A therapeutic response to *thyroid drugs* is manifested by the disappearance of the symptoms of hypothyroidism; the patient would demonstrate improved energy levels as well as improved mental and physical stamina. Adverse effects to monitor for include cardiac dysrhythmia (see Table 31-2). Clues that a patient is possibly receiving inadequate doses of the thyroid medication include a return of the symptoms of hypothyroidism (see previous discussion).

A therapeutic response to *antithyroid medications* includes a return to normal status with little to no evidence of hyperthyroid.

Adverse effects include the possibility of leukopenia, which may be manifested by fever, sore throat, lesions, or other signs of infection. Clues that a patient is not receiving adequate doses include continued signs and symptoms of hyperthyroidism (see previous discussion).

## PATIENT TEACHING TIPS

- Thyroid replacement drugs are best taken ½ to 1 hour before breakfast on an empty stomach to enhance their absorption orally, maintain constant hormone levels, and help prevent insomnia.
- These medications are not to be abruptly discontinued. Life-long therapy is usually the norm.
- Emphasize to the patient the importance of keeping follow-up visits so the prescriber can monitor thyroid hormone levels, complete blood counts, and results of liver function studies.
- Brands of thyroid replacement drugs cannot be interchanged. Advise patients to always check that the pharmacy has provided the correct brand of thyroid replacement drug.
- Signs and symptoms associated with hypothyroidism include myxedema with decreased metabolic rate, loss of mental/physical stamina, weight gain, hair loss, firm edema, and yellow dullness of the skin. Share this information with the patient.
- Instruct the patient taking thyroid replacement drugs to immediately report any of the following to the prescriber: chest pain, weight loss, palpitations, tremors, sweating, nervousness, shortness of breath, or insomnia. These may indicate toxicity.
- Encourage the patient to keep a daily journal, with notations about how the patient is feeling, energy levels, appetite, and any adverse effects.

- Advise the patient that it may take up to 3 to 4 weeks to see the full therapeutic effects of thyroid drugs.
- All thyroid tablets must be protected from light.
- Signs and symptoms of hyperthyroidism include increased metabolic rate, diarrhea, flushing, increased appetite, muscle weakness, fatigue, palpitations, irritability, nervousness, sleep disorders, heat intolerance, and altered menstrual flow. Patients with this disorder and on drug therapy need to be aware of these signs and symptoms.
- Antithyroid medications are better tolerated when taken with meals or a snack. These drugs must also be given at the same time every day to maintain consistent blood levels of the drug. They must never be withdrawn abruptly.
- Instruct patients taking thyroid or antithyroid drugs not to take any over-the-counter medications without first consulting with the prescriber or pharmacist and to read all drug labels thoroughly.
- Patients taking antithyroid medications must avoid eating foods high in iodine, such as tofu and other soy products, turnips, seafood, iodized salt, and some breads. These foods may interfere with the effectiveness of the antithyroid drug.

## KEY POINTS

- T₄ and T₃ are the two hormones produced by the thyroid gland; thyroid hormones are made by iodination and coupling with the amino acid tyrosine.
- Thyroid hormone replacement is generally carried out carefully by the prescriber with frequent monitoring of serum levels until stabilization appears to have occurred. Monitor and review laboratory values to be sure that serum levels are within normal limits to avoid possible toxicity.
- Hyperthyroidism is caused by excessive secretion of thyroid hormone by the thyroid gland and may be caused by different diseases (Graves' disease, Plummer's disease, and multinodular disease) or drugs. Always assess and document important information about the patient's medical history appropriately.

- Patients receiving levothyroxine need to report the occurrence of excitability, irritability, or palpitations to the prescriber because these symptoms may indicate toxicity.
- Adverse effects associated with thyroid drugs include tachycardia, palpitations, angina, dysrhythmias, hypertension, insomnia, tremors, headache, anxiety, nausea, diarrhea, cramps, menstrual irregularities, weight loss, sweating, fever, and heat intolerance.
- Adverse effects associated with antithyroid drugs include drowsiness, headache, vertigo, nausea, vomiting, diarrhea, loss of taste, bleeding, leukopenia, rash, myalgia, and arthralgia.

# NCLEX® EXAMINATION REVIEW QUESTIONS

1 When monitoring the laboratory values of a patient who is taking antithyroid drugs, the nurse knows to watch for
   a increased platelet counts.
   b decreased white blood cell counts.
   c decreased blood urea nitrogen level.
   d increased blood glucose levels.

2 The pharmacy has called a patient to notify her that the current brand of thyroid replacement hormone is on back order. The patient calls the clinic to ask what to do. Which is the best response by the nurse?
   a "Go ahead and take the other brand that the pharmacy has available for now."
   b "You can stop the medication until your current brand is available."
   c "You can split the thyroid pills that you have left so that they will last longer."
   d "Let me ask your physician what needs to be done; we will need to watch how you do if you switch brands."

3 When assessing the elderly patient, the nurse keeps in mind that certain nonspecific symptoms may represent hypothyroidism in these patients, such as:
   a leukopenia, anemia
   b loss of appetite, polyuria
   c weight loss, dry cough
   d cold intolerance, depression

4 To help with the insomnia associated with thyroid hormone replacement therapy, the nurse will teach the patient to
   a take half the dose at lunchtime and the other half 2 hours later.
   b use a sedative to assist with falling asleep.
   c take the dose upon awakening in the morning.
   d reduce the dosage as needed if sleep is impaired.

5 The nurse is teaching a patient who has a new prescription for the antithyroid drug propylthiouracil (PTU). Which statement by the nurse is correct?
   a "There are no food restrictions while on this drug."
   b "You need to avoid foods high in iodine, such as iodized salt, seafood, and soy products."
   c "This drug is given to raise the thyroid hormone levels in your blood."
   d "Take this drug in the morning on an empty stomach."

6 When teaching a patient who has a new prescription for thyroid hormone, the nurse will instruct the patient to notify the physician if which adverse effects are noted? (Select all that apply.)
   a Palpitations
   b Weight gain
   c Angina
   d Fatigue
   e Cold intolerance

7 The nurse is giving an intravenous dose of levothyroxine (Synthroid). The order reads: "Give 0.1 mg IV push now." What is the ordered dose in micrograms?

1. b, 2. d, 3. d, 4. c, 5. b, 6. a, c, 7. 100 mcg

For Critical Thinking and Prioritization Questions, see http://evolve.elsevier.com/Lilley.

**WEBSITE**

*http://evolve.elsevier.com/Lilley*

- Animations
- Answer Key—Textbook Case Studies
- Critical Thinking and Prioritization Questions

- Key Points—Downloadable
- Review Questions for the NCLEX® Examination
- Unfolding Case Studies

## OBJECTIVES

When you reach the end of this chapter, you will be able to do the following:

1  Discuss the normal functions of the pancreas.
2  Contrast age of onset, signs and symptoms, pharmacologic and nonpharmacologic treatment, incidence, and etiology of type 1 and type 2 diabetes mellitus.
3  Differentiate gestational diabetes from type 1 and type 2 diabetes mellitus.
4  Discuss the various factors influencing blood glucose level in nondiabetic individuals and in patients with diabetes mellitus.
5  Identify the various drugs used to manage type 1 and type 2 diabetes mellitus.

6  Discuss the mechanisms of action, indications, contraindications, cautions, drug interactions, and adverse effects of insulin, oral antidiabetic drugs, and injectable antidiabetic drugs.
7  Compare rapid-, short-, intermediate-, and long-acting insulins with regard to their onset of action, peak effects, and duration of action.
8  Compare the signs and symptoms of hypoglycemia and hyperglycemia and their related treatments.
9  Develop a nursing care plan that includes all phases of the nursing process for patients with type 1 or type 2 diabetes with a focus on drug therapies.

## DRUG PROFILES

acarbose, p. 523
♦ glipizide, p. 523
♦ insulin glargine and insulin detemir, p. 519
insulin isophane suspension (NPH), p. 519
insulin lispro, p. 518
♦ metformin, p. 523

♦ pioglitazone, p. 523
♦ regular insulin, p. 518
♦ repaglinide, p. 524
♦ sitagliptin, p. 524

_____

♦ *Key drug*

## KEY TERMS

**Diabetes mellitus** A complex disorder of carbohydrate, fat, and protein metabolism resulting from the lack of insulin secretion by the beta cells of the pancreas or from defects of the insulin receptors; it is commonly referred to simply as *diabetes.* There are two major types of diabetes: type 1 and type 2. (p. 512)

**Diabetic ketoacidosis (DKA)** A severe metabolic complication of uncontrolled diabetes that, if untreated, leads to diabetic coma and death. (p. 513)

**Gestational diabetes** Diabetes that develops during pregnancy. It may resolve after pregnancy but may also be a precursor of type 2 diabetes in later life. (p. 515)

**Glucagon**  A hormone produced by the alpha cells in the islets of Langerhans that stimulates the conversion of glycogen to glucose in the liver. (p. 511)

**Glucose**  One of the simple sugars that serves as a major source of energy. It is found in foods (e.g., fruits, refined sweets) and also is the final breakdown product of complex carbohydrate metabolism in the body; it is commonly referred to as *dextrose*. (p. 511)

**Glycogen**  A polysaccharide that is the major carbohydrate stored in animal cells. (p. 511)

**Glycogenolysis**  The breakdown of glycogen to glucose. (p. 511)

**Hemoglobin A1C (A1C)**  Hemoglobin molecules to which glucose molecules are bound; blood levels of hemoglobin A1C are used as a diagnostic measure of average daily blood glucose levels in the monitoring and diagnosing of diabetes; it is also called *glycosylated hemoglobin* and most commonly referred to as *A1C*. (p. 515)

**Hyperglycemia**  A fasting blood glucose level of 126 mg/dL or higher or a nonfasting blood glucose level of 200 mg/dL or higher. (p. 512)

**Hyperosmolar nonketotic syndrome (HNKS)**  A metabolic complication of uncontrolled type 2 diabetes, similar in severity to diabetic ketoacidosis but without ketosis and acidosis. (p. 514)

**Hypoglycemia**  A blood glucose level of less than 50 mg/dL, or above 50 mg/dL with signs and symptoms of hypoglycemia. (p. 525)

**Impaired fasting glucose level**  A fasting glucose level of at least 100 mg/dL but lower than 126 mg/dL; it defines a prediabetic state that is sometimes called *prediabetes*. (p. 515)

**Insulin**  A naturally occurring hormone secreted by the beta cells of the islets of Langerhans in the pancreas in response to increased levels of glucose in the blood. (p. 511)

**Ketones**  Organic chemical compounds produced through the oxidation of secondary alcohols (e.g., fat molecules), including dietary carbohydrates. (p. 512)

**Polydipsia**  Chronic excessive intake of water; it is a common symptom of uncontrolled diabetes. (p. 512)

**Polyphagia**  Excessive eating; it is a common symptom of uncontrolled diabetes. (p. 512)

**Polyuria**  Increased frequency or volume of urinary output; it is a common symptom of diabetes. (p. 512)

**Type 1 diabetes mellitus**  Diabetes mellitus that is a genetically determined autoimmune disorder characterized by a complete or nearly complete lack of insulin production; it most commonly arises in children or adolescents. (p. 513)

**Type 2 diabetes mellitus**  A type of diabetes mellitus that most commonly presents in adults and is becoming more common in children and adolescents due to inactivity and weight gain. The disease may be controlled by lifestyle modifications, oral drug therapy, and/or insulin, but patients are not necessarily dependent on insulin therapy. (p. 514)

## ANATOMY, PHYSIOLOGY, AND PATHOPHYSIOLOGY OVERVIEW

### PANCREAS

The pancreas is a large, elongated organ that is located behind the stomach. It is both an exocrine gland (secreting digestive enzymes through the pancreatic duct) and an endocrine gland (secreting hormones directly into the bloodstream and not through a duct). The endocrine functions of the pancreas are the focus of this chapter. Two main hormones that are produced by the pancreas are insulin and glucagon. Both hormones play an important role in the regulation of glucose homeostasis, specifically the use, mobilization, and storage of glucose by the body. Glucose is one of the primary sources of energy for the cells of the body. It is also the simplest form of carbohydrate (sugar) found in the body and is often referred to as *dextrose*. There is a normal amount of glucose that circulates in the blood to meet requirements for quick energy. When the quantity of glucose in the blood is sufficient, the excess is stored as glycogen in the liver and, to a lesser extent, in skeletal muscle tissue, where it remains until the body needs it. Glucose is also stored in adipose tissue as triglyceride body fat. When more circulating glucose is needed, glycogen—primarily that stored in the liver—is converted back to glucose through a process called glycogenolysis. The hormone responsible for initiating this process is glucagon. Glucagon has only minimal effects on muscle glycogen and adipose tissue triglyceride stores.

Glucagon is a protein hormone consisting of a single chain of amino acids (polypeptide chain). Its molecules are about half the size of those of insulin. Glucagon is released from the alpha cells of the islets of Langerhans in the pancreas. Insulin is secreted from the beta cells of these same islets. Insulin is a protein hormone composed of two amino acid chains (acidic A chain and basic B chain) joined by a disulfide linkage. There is a continuous homeostatic balance in the body between the actions of insulin and those of glucagon. This natural balance serves to maintain optimal blood glucose levels, which normally range between 70 and 100 mg/dL. Because of the critical role of the pancreas in producing and maintaining these two hormones, the drastic measures of pancreatic or islet cell transplant are sometimes undertaken to treat type 1 diabetes that has not been successfully controlled by other means. Another common treatment is continuous insulin administration via a mechanized insulin pump, which may be used to treat type 1 or type 2 diabetes.

Insulin serves several important metabolic functions in the body. It stimulates carbohydrate metabolism in skeletal and cardiac muscle and in adipose tissue by facilitating the transport of glucose into these cells. In the liver, insulin facilitates the phosphorylation of glucose to glucose-6-phosphate, which is then converted to glycogen for storage. By causing glucose to be stored in the liver as glycogen, insulin keeps the kidney free of glucose. Without insulin, blood glucose levels rise; when the kidneys are unable to reabsorb this excess glucose, they excrete large amounts of glucose (a critical body nutrient and energy source), ketones, and other solutes into the urine. This loss of nutrient energy sources eventually leads to polyphagia, weight loss, and malnutrition. The presence of these solutes in the distal renal tubules and collecting ducts also draws large volumes of water into the urine through osmotic diuresis, which leads to polyuria, dehydration, and polydipsia.

Insulin also has a direct effect on fat metabolism. It stimulates lipogenesis and inhibits lipolysis and the release of fatty acids from adipose cells. In addition, insulin stimulates protein synthesis and promotes the intracellular shift of potassium and magnesium into the cells, thereby temporarily decreasing elevated blood concentrations of these electrolytes. Other substances such as cortisol, epinephrine, and growth hormone work synergistically with glucagon to counter the effects of insulin and cause increases in the blood glucose level.

## PATHOPHYSIOLOGY OF DIABETES MELLITUS

Hyperglycemia is a state involving excessive concentrations of glucose in the blood and results when the normal counterbalancing actions of glucagon and insulin fail to maintain normal glucose homeostasis (i.e., serum levels of 70 to 100 mg/dL). Complications in protein and fat metabolism (*dyslipidemia*; see Chapter 27) are also involved. The current key diagnostic criterion for diabetes mellitus is hyperglycemia with a fasting plasma glucose level of higher than 126 mg/dL or a hemoglobin A1C (A1C) level greater than or equal to 6.5%. Diagnostic indicators are described in more detail in Box 32-1. It is important to note that the diagnostic definition of diabetes established by the American Diabetes Association (ADA) differs from that issued

by the American College of Endocrinology. This text uses the ADA as a reference.

Diabetes mellitus, more commonly referred to simply as *diabetes*, is primarily a disorder of carbohydrate metabolism that involves either a deficiency of insulin, a resistance of tissue (e.g., muscle, liver) to insulin, or both. Whatever the cause of the diabetes, the result is hyperglycemia. Uncontrolled hyperglycemia correlates strongly with serious long-term macrovascular and microvascular complications. Macrovascular complications are usually secondary to large vessel damage caused by deposition of atherosclerotic plaque. This compromises both central and peripheral circulation. In contrast, microvascular complications are secondary to damage to the capillary vessels, which impairs peripheral circulation and damages eyes and kidneys. In addition, both autonomic and somatic nerve damage occur, caused primarily by the metabolic changes themselves and to a lesser degree by the compromised circulation. Table 32-1 lists the common long-term complications of diabetes.

Diabetes mellitus has been recognized since 1550 BC, when Egyptians wrote of a malady they called *honeyed urine*. The first step toward identifying the cause of diabetes mellitus occurred in 1788 when Thomas Cawley, an English physician, voiced his suspicion that the source of the illness lay in the pancreas. However, it took over a century to prove this conjecture correct, and it took even longer to discover the active substance, insulin, that is secreted from the pancreas. Not until the early 1920s was insulin finally isolated. Its discovery is now considered one of the greatest triumphs of twentieth-century medicine, and its

| BOX 32-1 | CRITERIA FOR DIAGNOSIS OF DIABETES |
|---|---|

Fasting plasma glucose level of 126 mg/dL or higher, or A1C greater than 6.5%. "Fasting" is defined as no caloric intake for at least 8 hours.
OR
Symptoms of diabetes plus casual plasma glucose level of 200 mg/dL or higher. "Casual" means measured at any time of day without regard to time since last meal. The classic symptoms of hyperglycemia include polyuria, polydipsia, and unexplained weight loss.
OR
Two-hour plasma glucose level of 200 mg/dL or higher during an oral glucose tolerance test (OGTT). The glucose load should contain the equivalent of 75 gm of glucose dissolved in water. Note that the OGTT is not recommended for routine clinical use.

Any positive finding for the above assessments should be confirmed by repeat testing on a different day.

Data from American Diabetes Association: Diagnosis and classification of diabetes mellitus, *Diabetes Care* 35(Suppl 1): S64-S71, 2012.

| TABLE 32-1 | MAJOR LONG-TERM CONSEQUENCES OF TYPE 1 AND TYPE 2 DIABETES |
|---|---|
| **PATHOLOGY** | **POSSIBLE CONSEQUENCES** |
| **Macrovascular (Atherosclerotic Plaque)** | |
| Coronary arteries | Myocardial infarction |
| Cerebral arteries | Stroke |
| Peripheral vessels | Peripheral vascular disease (e.g., neuropathies [see below], foot ulcers, possible amputations) |
| **Microvascular (Capillary Damage)** | |
| Retinopathy (retinal damage) | Partial or complete blindness |
| Neuropathy (autonomic and somatic nerve damage, due to both metabolic alterations and compromised circulation) | Autonomic nerve damage: Example: diabetic gastroparesis, bladder dysfunction, unawareness of hypoglycemia, sexual dysfunction Somatic nerve damage: Example: diabetic foot ulcer and/or leg or foot amputation (resulting from undetected injuries due to loss of sensation and also from compromised circulation) |
| Nephropathy (kidney damage) | Proteinuria (microalbuminuria), chronic renal failure (may require dialysis or kidney transplantation) |

Data from American Diabetes Association: Executive summary: standards of medical care in diabetes, *Diabetes Care* 35(Suppl 1): S4-S10, 2012.

use in the treatment of diabetes mellitus has proved to be life saving for millions of people affected by the disease.

Diabetes mellitus actually is not a single disease, but a group of progressive diseases. For this reason, it is often regarded as a syndrome rather than a disease. In some cases, diabetes is caused by a relative or absolute lack of insulin that is believed to result from the destruction of beta cells in the pancreas. As a result, insulin cannot be produced. However, hyperglycemia can also be caused by defects in insulin receptors that result in insulin resistance. The proteins that serve as insulin receptors are attached to the surface of cells in the liver, muscle, and adipose tissue. These receptor proteins are stimulated by insulin molecules to move glucose from blood to cells. When insulin receptors become defective, they no longer respond normally to insulin molecules. Although serum insulin and glucose levels are both elevated, they do not respond and transport glucose into the cell where it is needed. The result is that glucose molecules remain in the blood, rather than being used in the cell or stored in the tissues.

Two major types of diabetes mellitus are currently recognized and designated by the ADA: type 1 and type 2. Type 1 diabetes was previously called *insulin-dependent diabetes mellitus (IDDM)* or *juvenile-onset diabetes.* Type 2 diabetes was previously called *non–insulin-dependent diabetes mellitus (NIDDM)* or *adult-onset diabetes.* The numeric designations for both conditions were adopted by the ADA as the preferred terms in 1995. The previous designations were abandoned for several reasons. One reason is that many patients with type 2 diabetes do eventually become dependent on insulin therapy for control of their illness. A second reason is that the current epidemic of both child and adult obesity in the United States is increasing the incidence of type 2 diabetes in children, adolescents, and young adults. Obesity is one of the major risk factors for the development of type 2 diabetes. Nonwhite ethnic groups, including African Americans, Asian Americans, Hispanic Americans, and Native Americans, are all at higher risk for the disease than are whites.

The usual differences between type 1 and type 2 diabetes mellitus are listed in Table 32-2. Interestingly, approximately 10% of patients with type 2 diabetes have circulating antibodies that suggest an autoimmune origin for the disease. This condition is known as *latent autoimmune diabetes in adults (LADA)* and is basically a more slowly progressing form of type 1 diabetes.

The most common signs and symptoms of diabetes are elevated blood glucose level (fasting glucose level higher than 126 mg/dL) and polyuria, polydipsia, polyphagia, glucosuria, weight loss, blurred vision, and fatigue.

## Type 1 Diabetes Mellitus

Type 1 diabetes mellitus is characterized by a lack of insulin production or by the production of defective insulin, which results in acute hyperglycemia. Affected patients require exogenous insulin to lower the blood glucose level and prevent diabetic complications. It is believed that a genetically determined autoimmune reaction gradually destroys the insulin-producing beta cells of the pancreatic islets of Langerhans (Figure 32-1). The preclinical phase of beta cell destruction may be prolonged,

possibly lasting several years. At some critical point, a rapid transition from preclinical to clinical type 1 diabetes occurs. This transition is believed to be triggered by a specific event such as an acute illness or major emotional stress. An unidentified viral infection is also strongly suspected as an environmental trigger. Those stressors trigger the release of the counter-regulatory hormones cortisol and epinephrine. These hormones then mobilize glucagon to release glucose from the storage sites in the liver. This further increases the already rising levels of glucose in the blood secondary to islet cell damage. At some point during this critical cascade of events, an autoimmune reaction may be initiated that destroys the insulin-producing beta cells of the pancreatic islets of Langerhans. The result is essentially a complete lack of endogenous insulin production by the pancreas, which necessitates long-term insulin replacement therapy. Fortunately, type 1 diabetes accounts for fewer than 10% of all diabetes cases. Uncontrolled type 1 diabetes is often referred to as *brittle diabetes,* and these patients have large fluctuations in their blood glucose levels.

### Acute Diabetic Complications: Diabetic Ketoacidosis and Hyperosmolar Nonketotic Syndrome

When blood glucose levels are high but no insulin is present to allow glucose to be used for energy production, the body may break down fatty acids for fuel, producing ketones as a metabolic by-product. If this occurs to a sufficient degree, diabetic ketoacidosis (DKA) may result. DKA is a complex multisystem

| TABLE 32-2 | CHARACTERISTICS OF TYPE 1 AND TYPE 2 DIABETES | |
|---|---|---|
| **CHARACTERISTIC** | **TYPE 1** | **TYPE 2** |
| Etiology | Autoimmune destruction of beta cells in the pancreas | Multifactorial genetic defects; strong association with obesity and insulin resistance resulting from a reduction in the number or activity of insulin receptors |
| Incidence | 10% of cases | 90% of cases |
| Onset | Juvenile onset, usually younger than 20 yr | Previously maturity onset, age older than 40 yr; now increasingly seen in younger adults and even adolescents—attributed to obesity epidemic |
| Endogenous insulin | Little or none | Normal or high levels in early disease; reduced later in disease |
| Insulin receptors | Normal | Decreased or defective |
| Body weight | Usually nonobese | Obese (80% of cases) |
| Treatment | Insulin | Weight loss, diet and exercise, and oral hypoglycemics; only about one third of all patients need insulin. Earlier use of insulin is associated with improved outcomes. |

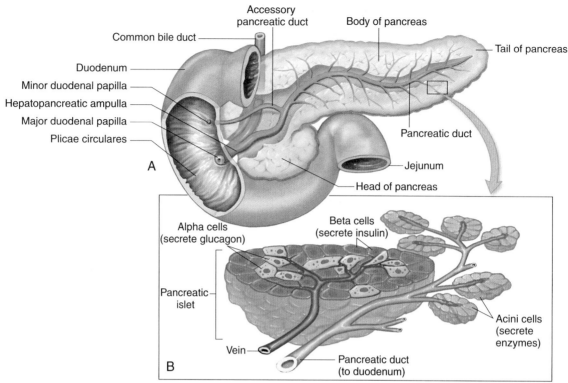

**FIGURE 32-1** The pancreas. **A,** Pancreas dissected to show main and accessory ducts. **B,** Exocrine glandular cells (around small pancreatic ducts) and endocrine glandular cells of the pancreatic islets (adjacent to blood capillaries). Exocrine pancreatic cells secrete pancreatic enzymes, alpha endocrine cells secrete glucagon, and beta endocrine cells secrete insulin. (From Patton KT, Thibodeau GA: *Anatomy and physiology,* ed 7, St Louis, 2010, Mosby.)

complication of uncontrolled diabetes. Without treatment, DKA will lead to coma and death. DKA is characterized by extreme hyperglycemia, the presence of ketones in the serum, acidosis, dehydration, and electrolyte imbalances. Approximately 25% to 30% of patients with newly diagnosed type 1 diabetes mellitus present with DKA. Another complication of comparable severity that is also triggered by extreme hyperglycemia is hyperosmolar nonketotic syndrome (HNKS). The most common precipitator of DKA and HNKS is some type of physical or emotional stress. It was formerly believed that DKA occurred only in type 1 diabetes and HNKS occurred only in type 2 diabetes. However, it is now recognized that both disorders can occur with diabetes of either type, and this overlap is increasingly common with the rapidly decreasing age of patients with type 2 diabetes.

Table 32-3 describes the subtle differences between DKA and HNKS. Treatment for either complication involves fluid and electrolyte replacement as well as intravenous insulin therapy (more common for DKA).

## Type 2 Diabetes Mellitus

Type 2 diabetes mellitus is by far the most common form of diabetes, accounting for at least 90% of all cases of diabetes mellitus and affecting over 23 million people in the United States. Because this form of diabetes does not always require insulin therapy, there are many common and dangerous misconceptions regarding type 2 diabetes mellitus: that it is a mild diabetes;

| TABLE 32-3 | COMPARISON OF FEATURES OF DIABETIC KETOACIDOSIS AND HYPEROSMOLAR NONKETOTIC SYNDROME | |
|---|---|---|
| | **CONDITION** | |
| **FEATURE** | **DIABETIC KETOACIDOSIS** | **HYPEROSMOLAR NONKETOTIC SYNDROME** |
| Age of patient | Younger than 40 yr | Older than 40 yr |
| Duration of symptoms | Less than 2 days | More than 5 days |
| Serum glucose level | Lower than 800 mg/dL | Higher than 800 mg/dL |
| Serum Na level | Normal or low | Normal or high |
| Serum HCO₃ level | Low | Normal |
| Ketone bodies | At least 4+ | Less than 2+ |
| pH | Low | Normal |
| Serum osmolality | Less than 350 mOsm/kg | Greater than 350 mOsm/kg |
| Prognosis | 3% to 10% mortality | 10% to 20% mortality or more |
| Subsequent course | Insulin therapy required in all cases | Insulin therapy not required in many cases after initial treatment |

Adapted from Harmel AP, Mathur R: *Davidson's diabetes mellitus: diagnosis and treatment,* ed 5, Philadelphia, 2004, Saunders.

that it is easy to treat; and that tight metabolic control is unnecessary because these patients, who are mostly older adults, will die before diabetic complications develop. The clinical realities of this disease demonstrate otherwise.

Type 2 diabetes mellitus is caused by both insulin resistance and insulin deficiency, but there is no absolute lack of insulin as in type 1 diabetes. One of the normal roles of insulin is to facilitate the uptake of circulating glucose molecules into tissues to be used as energy. In type 2 diabetes, all of the main target tissues of insulin (i.e., muscle, liver, and adipose tissue) are hyporesponsive (resistant) to the effects of the hormone. Not only is the absolute number of insulin receptors in these tissues reduced, but their individual sensitivity and responsiveness to insulin is decreased as well. Therefore, it is possible for a patient with type 2 diabetes mellitus to have normal or even elevated levels of insulin yet still have high blood glucose levels. These processes also result in impaired postprandial (after a meal) glucose metabolism, which is another problematic feature of type 2 diabetes that contributes to the hazardous hyperglycemic state.

In addition to the reduction in the number and sensitivity of insulin receptors in type 2 diabetes, there is often reduced insulin secretion by the pancreas. This insulin deficiency results from a loss of the normal responsiveness of the beta cells in the pancreas to elevated blood glucose levels. When the beta cells do not recognize glucose, they do not secrete insulin, and the normal insulin-facilitated transport of glucose into cells of muscle, liver, and adipose tissue does not occur.

Type 2 diabetes is a multifaceted disorder. Although loss of blood glucose control is its primary hallmark, several other significant conditions are strongly associated with the disease. These include obesity, coronary heart disease, dyslipidemia, hypertension, microalbuminuria (spilling of protein into the urine), and an increased risk for thrombotic (blood clotting) events. For patients with type 2 diabetes, the ADA recommends the use of aspirin for prevention of coronary artery (heart) disease and antihyperlipidemic drug therapy (see Chapter 27), when indicated, in addition to any necessary antidiabetic drug therapy. These comorbidities are strongly associated with the development of type 2 diabetes and are collectively referred to as *metabolic syndrome* (also known as *insulin-resistance syndrome* and *syndrome X*). Roughly 80% of patients with diabetes are obese at the time of initial diagnosis. Obesity serves only to worsen the insulin resistance, because adipose tissue is often the site of a large proportion of the body's defective insulin receptors. The goal for patients with diabetes is a blood pressure less than 130/80 mm Hg and a low-density lipid (LDL) less than 100 mg/dL.

## Gestational Diabetes

Gestational diabetes is a type of hyperglycemia that develops during pregnancy. Relatively uncommon, it occurs in about 2% to 10% of pregnancies. Many patients are well controlled with diet, but the use of insulin may be necessary to decrease the risk of birth defects, hypoglycemia in the newborn, and high birth weight. In most cases, gestational diabetes subsides after delivery. However, as many as 30% of patients who experience gestational diabetes are estimated to develop type 2 diabetes within 10 to 15 years.

All pregnant women need to have blood glucose screenings at regular prenatal visits. Women who develop gestational diabetes need to be screened for lingering diabetes 6 to 8 weeks postpartum and be advised of their increased risk for recurrent diabetes and of the importance of regular medical checkups and weight control. Women who are known to be diabetic before pregnancy should have detailed prepregnancy counseling and prenatal care from a prescriber who is experienced in managing pregnancies in diabetic women. Specific drug therapy issues pertaining to gestational diabetes are discussed further in the section on insulins.

## Prevention and Screening

Both macrovascular and microvascular problems are now recognized to occur at fasting plasma glucose (FPG) levels as low as 126 mg/dL. *Fasting* is defined loosely as an 8-hour or an overnight fast (no food from midnight until after the blood sample is taken in the morning). Impaired fasting glucose level is defined as an FPG level higher than or equal to 100 mg/dL but less than 126 mg/dL. This condition often proves to be a precursor to diabetes and is therefore referred to as *prediabetes*. The 2012 ADA guidelines renamed *prediabetes* as "categories of increased risk for diabetes" and define it as impaired fasting glucose and hemoglobin A1C of 5.7% to 6.4%. Another recognized prediabetic condition is impaired glucose tolerance, which is identified using an oral glucose challenge test (see Box 32-1). The ADA, the National Institute of Diabetes and Digestive and Kidney Diseases, and the Centers for Disease Control and Prevention recommend that all adults 45 years of age and older be screened for elevated FPG levels every 3 years. Several preventive measures are also recommended. Reducing alcohol consumption is helpful, because alcohol is broken down in the body to simple carbohydrates, which leads to increases in blood glucose levels. Regular exercise, in addition to having beneficial effects on weight and high blood pressure, also lowers blood glucose levels by increasing insulin receptor sensitivity.

## Nonpharmacologic Treatment Interventions

Patients diagnosed with type 1 diabetes always require insulin therapy. For patients with new-onset type 2 diabetes, lifestyle changes should be initiated as a first step in treatment. Weight loss not only lowers the blood glucose and lipid levels of these patients, but it also reduces another common comorbidity, hypertension. Other recommended lifestyle changes include improved dietary habits (e.g., consumption of a diet higher in protein and lower in fat and carbohydrates), smoking cessation, reduced alcohol consumption, and regular physical exercise. Cigarette smoking doubles the risk of cardiovascular disease in diabetic patients, largely because of its effects on peripheral vascular circulation and respiratory function. In fact, smoking cessation would probably save far more lives than antihypertensive, antilipemic, and antidiabetic drug treatment combined!

## Glycemic Goal of Treatment

The glycemic goal recommended by the ADA for diabetic patients is a hemoglobin A1C (A1C) level of less than 7%. The A1C test measures the percentage of hemoglobin A that is irreversibly glycosylated. A1C is an indicator of glycemic control in a patient over the preceding 2 to 3 months (the average lifespan of a red blood cell) and is not affected by recent fluctuations in blood glucose levels. The ADA recommended a fasting blood glucose goal for diabetic patients of 70 to 130 mg/dL.

## PHARMACOLOGY OVERVIEW

The major classes of drugs used to treat diabetes mellitus are the insulins and the oral antidiabetic drugs. Several new classes of injectable drugs with unique mechanisms of action have been developed that may be used in addition to insulins or oral antidiabetic drugs to treat resistant diabetes. All of these drugs are referred to as *antidiabetic drugs,* and they are aimed at producing a normoglycemic or euglycemic (normal blood glucose) state.

## INSULINS

Insulin is required in patients with type 1 diabetes. Patients with type 2 diabetes are not generally prescribed insulin until other measures (i.e., lifestyle changes and oral drug therapy) no longer provide adequate glycemic control. Currently insulin is synthesized in laboratories using recombinant deoxyribonucleic acid (DNA) technology and is referred to as *human insulin.* Insulin was originally isolated from cattle or pigs, but bovine (cow) and porcine (pig) insulins are associated with a higher incidence of allergic reactions and insulin resistance than human insulin and are no longer available in the U.S. market. Recombinant insulin is produced by bacteria or yeast that have been altered to contain the genetic information necessary for them to reproduce an insulin that is like human insulin. The pharmacokinetic properties of insulin (onset of action, peak effect, and duration of action) can be altered by making various minor modifications to either the insulin molecule itself or the drug formulation (final product). This practice has led to the development of many different insulin preparations, including several combination insulin products that contain more than one type of insulin in the same solution. Chemical manipulation of insulin activity in this way helps to meet the individual meal-related metabolic demands of patients with diabetes. Further modifications can be accomplished by mixing compatible insulin preparations in the syringe before administration. The latest syringe compatibility data for currently available insulin products are given in Table 32-4. Thoroughly educate patients regarding how, when, and whether they can (or cannot) mix different types of insulin. Some combinations are chemically incompatible and can result in an undesirable alteration of glycemic effects.

## Mechanism of Action and Drug Effects

Exogenous insulin functions as a substitute for the endogenous hormone. It serves to replace the insulin that is either not made or is made defectively in a diabetic patient. The drug effects of exogenously administered insulin involve many body systems. They are the same as those of normal endogenous insulin. That is, exogenous insulin restores the patient's ability to metabolize carbohydrates, fats, and proteins; to store glucose in the liver; and to convert glycogen to fat stores. Unfortunately, exogenous insulin does not reverse defects in insulin receptor sensitivity. Insulin pumps are a very attractive way to administer insulin to

### TABLE 32-4 INSULIN MIXING COMPATIBILITIES

| TYPE OF INSULIN | COMPATIBLE WITH |
|---|---|
| Regular insulin (Humulin R, Novolin R) | All insulins except glargine, and glulisine |
| Insulin glulisine (Apidra) | NPH only |
| Insulin lispro (Humalog), insulin aspart (NovoLog) | Regular, NPH insulins |
| Insulin detemir (Levemir) | Must be given alone |
| Insulin glargine (Lantus) | Must be given alone due to low pH of diluent |
| NPH 70% and regular insulin 30% (Humulin 70/30, Novolin 70/30) | Premixed; do not mix with other insulins |
| NPH 50% and regular insulin 50% (Humulin 50/50) | |
| Insulin aspart protamine suspension 75% and insulin aspart 25% (NovoLog Mix 75/25) | |
| Insulin lispro protamine suspension 75% and insulin lispro 25% (Humalog Mix 75/25) | |

patients. The insulin pump provides an alternative to multiple daily subcutaneous injections and allows patients to match their insulin intake to their lifestyle. When an insulin pump is used, insulin is administered constantly over a 24-hour period, and the patient is then allowed to give bolus injections based on the amount of food ingested. Insulin pumps are described further in the Nursing Process section.

## Indications

All insulin preparations can be used to treat both type 1 and type 2 diabetes, but each patient requires careful customization of the dosing regimen for optimal glycemic control. Additional therapeutic approaches such as lifestyle modifications (e.g., dietary and exercise habits) are also indicated and, for type 2 diabetes, oral drug therapy as well.

## Contraindications

Contraindications to the use of all insulin products include known drug allergy to the specific product. Insulin is never to be administered to an already hypoglycemic patient. Blood glucose must always be tested prior to administration.

## Adverse Effects

Hypoglycemia resulting from excessive insulin dosing can result in brain damage, shock, and possible death. This is the most immediate and serious adverse effect of insulin. Other adverse effects of insulin therapy include weight gain, lipodystrophy at the site of repeated injections, and in rare cases allergic reactions. Because weight gain is a common and often undesirable adverse effect, insulin therapy is usually delayed in type 2 patients until other agents and lifestyle changes have failed to bring the blood glucose to target levels.

## Interactions

Drug interactions that can occur with the insulins are significant; they are listed in Table 32-5.

## TABLE 32-5  SELECTED DRUG INTERACTIONS WITH ANTIDIABETIC DRUGS

| DRUG | INTERACTING DRUG | MECHANISM | RESULT |
|---|---|---|---|
| insulin | Corticosteroids, niacin, diuretics, sympathomimetic drugs, thyroid drugs | Antagonizes insulin effect | Increased blood glucose levels |
| | Alcohol, anabolic steroids, sulfa antibiotics, clofibrate, MAOIs, salicylates | Increases the hypoglycemic effects of insulin | Decreased blood glucose levels |
| | Nonselective beta blockers | Masks the tachycardia from hypoglycemia | Risk of not noticing hypoglycemic symptoms |
| metformin | Hypoglycemic drugs | Additive effects | Additive hypoglycemia |
| | Cimetidine | Inhibits metabolism | Increased metformin effects |
| | Diuretics, steroids | Additive effects | Additive hypoglycemia |
| | Contrast media | Decreases excretion | Lactic acidosis |
| glipizide | Alcohol, antacids, cimetidine, clofibrate, fluconazole, NSAIDs, sulfonamide antibiotics, garlic, ginger, ginseng | Enhanced effects | Increased hypoglycemia |
| | Carbamazepine, phenobarbital, phenytoin, rifampin | Increases metabolism | Decreased effectiveness |

*MAOI,* Monoamine oxidase inhibitor; *NSAID,* nonsteroidal antiinflammatory drug

## DOSAGES

### Selected Human-Based Insulin Products

| DRUG (PREGNANCY CATEGORY) | PHARMACOLOGIC CLASS | USUAL DOSAGE RANGE | INDICATIONS |
|---|---|---|---|
| **Rapid Acting** insulin lispro (Humalog) (B) | Human recombinant rapid-acting insulin analogue | Subcut: 0.5-1 unit/kg/day; doses are highly individualized to desired glycemic control; rapid-acting insulins are best given 15 min before a meal. May be given per sliding scale or as basal/bolus; may also be given via continuous subcutaneous infusion pump | Diabetes mellitus type 1 and type 2 |
| **Short Acting** ◆ regular insulin (Humulin R, Novolin R) (B) | Human recombinant short-acting insulin | Subcut: Same dosage as insulin lispro; subcut doses of regular insulin are best given 30 min before a meal. Regular insulin may also be given per sliding scale or basal/bolus and is the insulin usually given IV as a continuous infusion | |
| **Long Acting** insulin glargine (Lantus) (C) | Human recombinant long-acting insulin analogue | Subcut only: Same dosage as others but is approved only for once- or twice-daily dosage (basal dosing) | |

*IV,* Intravenous; *Subcut,* subcutaneous.

## Dosages

For dosage information on the various insulin products, see the table above. The concentration of insulin is expressed as the number of units of insulin per milliliter. For example, U-100 insulin has 100 units in 1 milliliter. Insulin is usually given by subcutaneous injection or via a subcutaneous infusion pump. In emergency situations requiring prompt insulin action, regular insulin can be given intravenously.

## Insulin Use in Special Populations

Two special patient populations for whom careful attention is required during insulin therapy are pediatric patients and pregnant women. Insulin dosages for both are calculated by weight as they are for the general adult population. The usual dosage range is 0.5 to 1 units/kg/day as a total daily dose. Be aware that there are a few important differences regarding the use of some insulin products in pediatric populations. The rapid-acting insulin lispro is approved for use in children older than 3 years of age. However, the combination lispro product Humalog 75/25, which contains 75% insulin lispro protamine (an intermediate-acting insulin) and 25% insulin lispro (a rapid-acting insulin), is not currently approved for use in children younger than 18 years of age. Children need age-appropriate education and supervision by health care professionals and parents, which includes a safe and gradual transfer of responsibility for self-management of their illness, as appropriate.

Pregnant women also require special care with regard to diabetes management. Although most of these mothers will

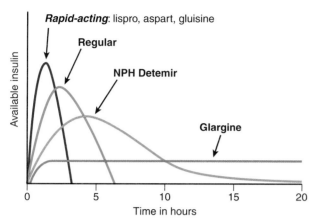

**FIGURE 32-2** Comparison of the pharmacokinetics of various insulins. (From Messinger-Rapport BJ, Thomas DR, Gammack JK: Clinical update on nursing home medicine: 2008, *J Am Med Dir Assoc* 9(7):460-475, 2008.)

return to a normal glycemic state after pregnancy, they are at risk of developing diabetes again in later life. All currently available oral and injectable antidiabetic drugs are classified as pregnancy category B or C drugs. Oral medications are generally not recommended for pregnant patients because of a lack of firm safety data. For this reason, insulin therapy is the only currently recommended drug therapy for pregnant women with diabetes. Roughly 15% of women who develop gestational diabetes require insulin therapy during pregnancy. Insulin does not normally cross the placenta. Effective glycemic control during pregnancy is essential because infants born to women with gestational diabetes have a twofold to threefold greater risk of congenital anomalies. In addition, the incidence of stillbirth is directly related to the degree of maternal hyperglycemia. Weight reduction is generally not advised for these women, because it can jeopardize fetal nutritional status. Women with gestational diabetes tend to have babies that weigh more, and these children may have low blood sugar postnatally. Insulin is excreted into human milk. It is currently unknown whether insulin glargine is excreted in breast milk, and thus it is to be avoided in breast-feeding women. It is very important that insulin therapy and diet be well controlled for a nursing mother, because inadequate or excessive glycemic control may reduce milk production.

## DRUG PROFILES

There are currently four major classes of insulin, as determined by their pharmacokinetic properties: rapid acting, short acting, intermediate acting, and long acting. The duration of action ranges from several hours to over 24 hours depending on the insulin class (Figure 32-2). The insulin dosage regimen for all diabetic patients is highly individualized and may consist of one or more classes of insulin administered at either fixed dosages or variable dosages in response to self-measurements of blood glucose level or the number of grams of carbohydrate consumed. With the use of insulins, clarity, color, and appearance are important to understand for patient safety and for the prevention of adverse effects and complications. Several insulins are clear, colorless solutions. These include regular insulin, insulin lispro (Humalog), and insulin glargine (Lantus). Other

insulins, such as NPH insulin (insulin isophane), are white opaque (cloudy) solutions. This issue is discussed further in the Implementation section under Nursing Process.

### RAPID-ACTING INSULINS
#### insulin lispro

There are currently three insulin products that are classified as rapid acting: insulin lispro (Humalog), insulin aspart (Novo-Log), and the most recently developed, insulin glulisine (Apidra). These have the most rapid onset of action (roughly 15 minutes) as well as a shorter duration of action than other insulin categories. The effect of insulin lispro is most like that of the endogenous insulin produced by the pancreas in response to a meal. After, or during a meal, the glucose that is ingested stimulates the pancreas to secrete insulin. This insulin then facilitates the uptake of the excess glucose at hepatic insulin receptor sites for storage in the liver as glycogen. In people with diabetes, the insulin response to meals is often impaired; therefore, a rapid-acting insulin product is often used within 15 minutes of mealtime. This corresponds to the time required for the onset of action of these products. It is essential that patients with diabetes eat a meal after injection. Otherwise profound hypoglycemia may result. Insulin lispro was approved by the U.S. Food and Drug Administration (FDA) in 1996, becoming the first new insulin product to appear in the U.S. market in 14 years.

**Pharmacokinetics**

| Route | Onset of Action | Peak Plasma Concentration | Elimination Half-life | Duration of Action |
|---|---|---|---|---|
| Subcut | 15 min | 1-2 hr | 80 min | 3-5 hr |

### SHORT-ACTING INSULIN
#### ♦ regular insulin

Regular insulin (Humulin R) is currently the only insulin that is classified as a short-acting insulin. Regular insulin can be given via intravenous bolus, intravenous infusion, or even intramuscularly. These routes, especially the intravenous infusion route, are often used in cases of DKA or coma associated with uncontrolled type 1 diabetes.

Regular insulin solution was the first medicinal insulin product developed. It was originally isolated from bovine and porcine sources, but it is now made primarily from human insulin sources using recombinant DNA technology.

There are some differences between regular insulin and the newer rapid-acting drugs. Both insulin lispro and insulin aspart are human insulin analogues. This means that they are insulin molecules with synthetic alterations to their chemical structures that alter their onset or duration of action. Both insulins have a faster onset of action and a shorter time to peak plasma level, but they also have a shorter duration of action than does regular insulin.

**Pharmacokinetics**

| Route | Onset of Action | Peak Plasma Concentration | Elimination Half-life | Duration of Action |
|---|---|---|---|---|
| Subcut | 30-60 min | 2.5 hr | Unknown | 6-10 hr |

## INTERMEDIATE-ACTING INSULINS
### insulin isophane suspension (NPH)

Insulin isophane suspension (also known as *NPH insulin*) is the only available intermediate-acting insulin product. NPH is an acronym for *neutral protamine Hagedorn insulin,* the original name of this type of insulin. NPH insulin is a sterile suspension of zinc insulin crystals and protamine sulfate in buffered water for injection. The suspension appears cloudy or opaque. NPH insulin has a slower onset and longer duration of action than regular insulin, but not as long as the long-acting insulins. NPH insulin is often combined with regular insulin to reduce the number of insulin injections per day.

### Pharmacokinetics

| Route | Onset of Action | Peak Plasma Concentration | Elimination Half-life | Duration of Action |
|---|---|---|---|---|
| Subcut | 1-2 hr | 4-8 hr | Unknown | 10-18 hr |

## LONG-ACTING INSULINS
### ♦ insulin glargine and insulin detemir

Two long-acting insulin products are now available: insulin glargine (Lantus) and insulin detemir (Levemir). Insulin glargine is normally a clear, colorless solution with a pH of 4.0. Once it is injected into subcutaneous tissue at physiologic pH, it forms microprecipitates that are slowly absorbed over the next 24 hours. It is a recombinant DNA–produced insulin analogue and is unique in that it provides a constant level of insulin in the body. This enhances its safety because blood levels do not rise and fall as with other insulins. Insulin glargine is usually dosed once daily, but the drug may be dosed every 12 hours, depending on the patient's glycemic response. Because insulin glargine provides a more prolonged, consistent blood glucose level, it is sometimes referred to as a *basal insulin.*

Often for those being switched from twice-daily NPH to insulin glargine, the initial daily glargine dose is reduced to 80% of the previous total NPH dose. Insulin detemir has a different mechanism of action from insulin glargine, and the two insulins are not considered interchangeable. The duration of action of insulin detemir is dose dependent, so that lower doses require twice-daily dosing and higher doses may be given once daily.

## FIXED-COMBINATION INSULINS

Currently available fixed-combination insulin products include Humulin 70/30, Humulin 50/50, Novolin 70/30, Humalog Mix 75/25, Humalog 50/50, and NovoLog 70/30. Each of these products contains two different insulins, one intermediate-acting type and either one rapid-acting type (Humalog, NovoLog) or one short-acting type (Humulin). The numeric designations indicate the percentages of each of the two components in the product. For example, Novolin 70/30 has 70% short-acting and 30% intermediate-acting insulin. Notice that the numbers add up to 100 (percent). These products were developed to more closely simulate the varying levels of endogenous insulin that occur normally in nondiabetic people. In most insulin regimens, patients take a combination of a rapid-acting insulin to deal with the surges in glucose that occur after meals and an intermediate- or long-acting insulin for the period between meals when glucose levels are lower. However, this requires the mixing and administration of different types of insulins. Fixed-combination products were developed in an attempt to simplify the dosing process. The insulin lispro protamine component of Humalog Mix 75/25 is a modified insulin lispro molecule with a longer duration of action. These combinations allow for twice daily dosing but often result in glycemic control that is not as tight as daily dosing with meals. Patients who cannot afford frequent glucose monitoring or who refuse more than two injections per day may insist on using a combination insulin with twice daily dosing.

### Pharmacokinetics

| Route | Onset of Action | Peak Plasma Concentration | Elimination Half-life | Duration of Action |
|---|---|---|---|---|
| Subcut | 1-2 hr | None | Unknown | 24 hr |

## BASAL-BOLUS AND SLIDING-SCALE INSULIN DOSING

Historically, sliding scale insulin was used to correct blood glucose levels. In this method, subcutaneous doses of rapid-acting (lispro or aspart) or short-acting (regular) insulin are adjusted according to blood glucose test results. This method was typically used in treating hospitalized diabetic patients, whose insulin requirements may vary drastically because of stress (e.g., infections, surgery, acute illness), inactivity, or variable caloric intake, including receipt of total parenteral nutrition (TPN), enteral nutrition, or time spent with a "nothing by mouth" (NPO) diet. Other hospital diets that result in high numbers of carbohydrates consumed are full liquid and clear liquid diets.

When an individual is on a sliding-scale insulin regimen, blood glucose concentrations are determined several times a day (e.g., before meals and at bedtime) for patients on normal meal schedules, or every 4 to 6 hours around the clock for patients receiving TPN or enteral tube feedings. Subcutaneously administered regular or rapid insulin is then given in an amount that increases with the rise in blood glucose level. The disadvantage of sliding-scale dosing is that, because it delays insulin administration until hyperglycemia occurs, it does not meet basal insulin requirements and results in large swings in glucose control. Current research does not support the use of sliding scales or insulin without basal insulin, and many institutions are moving away from sliding-scale coverage. Nonetheless, sliding-scale dosing is still commonly used.

Basal-bolus insulin therapy is now the preferred method of treatment for hospitalized diabetic patients. Basal-bolus therapy is the attempt to mimic a healthy pancreas by delivering basal insulin constantly as a basal and then as needed as a bolus. The basal insulin is a long-acting insulin (insulin glargine) administered constantly to keep the blood glucose from fluctuating due to the normal release of glucose from the liver. Bolus insulin (insulin lispro or insulin aspart) mimics the burst secretions of the pancreas in response to increases in blood glucose levels. Bolus insulin is broken up into meal and correction boluses. Meal boluses are given to reduce blood glucose with the intake of carbohydrates. Correction boluses are any boluses taken to bring blood glucose back to normal. Blood glucose levels are monitored frequently when using basal-bolus insulin. This method of treatment is far superior to the traditional sliding scale. Still, patients who need to receive nothing by mouth for therapeutic or diagnostic reasons are not good candidates for basal insulin due to the risk of hypoglycemia and the unpredictability of insulin needed for glucose control while not eating.

## ORAL ANTIDIABETIC DRUGS

Type 2 diabetes is a very complex illness. Effective treatment involves several elements, including lifestyle modifications (e.g., diet control, exercise, smoking cessation, nutrition therapy), careful monitoring of blood glucose levels, and therapy with one or more drugs. In addition, the treatment of associated comorbid conditions (such as high cholesterol and high blood pressure) is a necessity that serves to further complicate the entire process. The goal blood pressure for patients with diabetes is less than 130/80 mm Hg, and the goal LDL (low-density lipid) level is less than 100 mg/dL.

The consensus statement from the ADA in 2011 recommends that new-onset type 2 diabetes be treated with both lifestyle interventions and the oral biguanide drug metformin, if there are no contraindications to the drug. In some past statements, only lifestyle changes were recommended as initial treatment. The consensus recognizes the reality that lifestyle changes, although essential, usually are not effective enough alone to lower blood glucose to the desired levels. If lifestyle modifications and the maximum tolerated metformin dose do not achieve the recommended A1C goals after 2 to 3 months, additional treatment with basal insulin or either a sulfonylurea or a thiazolidinedione is recommended. Studies have shown that metformin and the sulfonylureas (available in generic form) were either similar to or superior to the more expensive thiazolidinediones, glinides, and alpha-glucosidase inhibitors. Although not a traditional oral antidiabetic agent, bromocriptine (Cycloset), a dopamine agonist (see Chapter 15), is now being marketed for the treatment of diabetes. The exact mechanism of action is not known, but it has been shown to lower A1C levels in patients with type 2 diabetes.

## BIGUANIDE

### Mechanism of Action and Drug Effects

Metformin is currently the only drug classified as a biguanide. It is considered a first-line drug, especially for patients with a body mass index over 25, and is the most commonly used oral drug for the treatment of type 2 diabetes. It is not used for type 1 diabetes. Metformin works by decreasing glucose production by the liver. It may also decrease intestinal absorption of glucose and improve insulin receptor sensitivity. This results in increased peripheral glucose uptake and use, and decreased hepatic production of triglycerides and cholesterol. Unlike sulfonylureas, metformin does not stimulate insulin secretion

and therefore is not associated with weight gain and significant hypoglycemia when used alone.

### Indications

The ADA guidelines recommend metformin as the initial oral antidiabetic drug for treatment of newly diagnosed type 2 diabetes if no contraindications exist. Because it may also cause moderate weight loss, it is particularly useful for the many patients with type 2 diabetes who are overweight or obese. Metformin may be used as monotherapy or in combination with other oral antidiabetic drugs if single-drug therapy is unsuccessful. For this reason, it is available in combination products containing either sulfonylureas, thiazolidinediones, or incretin mimetics. Metformin may also be combined with insulin. It is also used in prediabetic patients.

### Contraindications

Metformin is contraindicated in patients with renal disease or renal dysfunction (serum creatinine level higher than 1.5 mg/dL in males or higher than 1.4 mg/dL in females). Because metformin is primarily excreted by the kidneys, it can accumulate in these individuals, increasing the risk of development of lactic acidosis. Other contraindications include alcoholism, metabolic acidosis, hepatic disease, heart failure, and other conditions that predispose to tissue hypoxia and increase the risk of lactic acidosis.

### Adverse Effects

The most common adverse effects of metformin are gastrointestinal. Metformin can cause abdominal bloating, nausea, cramping, a feeling of fullness, and diarrhea, especially at the start of therapy. Some research attributes the weight loss experienced early in the course of treatment with these side effects. These effects are all usually self-limiting and can be lessened by starting with low dosages, titrating up slowly, and taking the medication with food. Less common adverse effects with metformin are a metallic taste, hypoglycemia, and a reduction in vitamin $B_{12}$ levels after long-term use. Lactic acidosis is an extremely rare complication with metformin, but the risk increases with very high blood glucose levels and/or clinical conditions predisposing to hypoxemia. Lactic acidosis is lethal in up to 50% of cases. Symptoms of lactic acidosis include hyperventilation, cold and clammy skin, muscle pain, abdominal pain, dizziness, and irregular heartbeat.

### Interactions

Drug interactions with metformin are listed in Table 32-5. In addition, the use of metformin with iodinated (iodine-containing) radiologic contrast media has been associated with both acute renal failure and lactic acidosis. For these reasons, metformin therapy is to be discontinued the day of the test and for at least 48 hours after the patient undergoes any radiologic study that requires the use of such contrast media.

### Dosages

For dosage information on metformin, see the table on p. 521.

### Selected Oral Antidiabetic Drugs

| DRUG (PREGNANCY CATEGORY) | PHARMACOLOGIC CLASS | USUAL DOSAGE RANGE | INDICATIONS |
|---|---|---|---|
| acarbose (Precose) (B) | Alpha-glucosidase inhibitor | PO: 25-100 mg three times daily, taken with first bite of meal | |
| ♦ glipizide (Glucotrol, Glucotrol XL) (C) | Second-generation sulfonylurea | PO: 5-10 mg daily (max daily dose 20 mg) | |
| glimepiride (Amaryl) (C) | Second-generation sulfonylurea | PO: 1-4 mg daily (max daily dose 8 mg) | |
| ♦ metformin (Glucophage, Glucophage XR) (B) | Biguanide | PO: 1000 mg twice daily or 850 mg twice daily; max daily dose 2550 mg for adults and 2000 mg for pediatric patients age 10-16 yr | |
| ♦ pioglitazone (Actos) (C) | Thiazolidinedione | PO: 15-45 mg once daily | |
| ♦ repaglinide (Prandin) (C) | Meglitinide | PO: 0.5-4 mg three times daily; best taken 15 min before a meal | Diabetes mellitus type 2 |
| sitagliptin (Januvia) (B) | DPP-IV Inhibitor | PO: 100 mg daily | |
| **Combination Oral Drugs** | | | |
| glipizide/metformin (Metaglip) (C) | Combination sulfonylurea/biguanide | PO: 1-2 tabs twice daily | |
| pioglitazone/metformin (ACTOplus Met) (C) | Combination thiazolidinedione/biguanide | PO: 1 tab twice daily | |
| sitagliptin/metformin (Janumet) (C) | Combination incretin mimetic/biguanide | PO: 1 tab twice daily | |
| saxagliptin/metformin (Kombiglyze) (C) | Combination incretin mimetic/biguanide | PO: 1 tab twice daily | |

## SULFONYLUREAS

### Mechanism of Action and Drug Effects

The sulfonylureas are the oldest group of oral antidiabetic drugs. The drugs currently used are considered second-generation drugs and have a better potency and adverse effect profile than first-generation drugs (e.g., acetazolamide and tolbutamide), which are no longer used clinically. Second-generation drugs include glipizide (Glucotrol), glyburide (Diabeta), and glimepiride (Amaryl). Sulfonylureas bind to specific receptors on beta cells in the pancreas to stimulate the release of insulin. In addition, sulfonylureas appear to secondarily decrease the secretion of glucagon. For this class of drugs to be effective, the patient must still have functioning beta cells in the pancreas. Thus, these drugs work best during the early stages of type 2 diabetes and are not used in type 1 diabetes.

### Indications

The ADA guidelines currently recommend sulfonylureas as second-step drugs for patients with type 2 diabetes whose A1C levels remain elevated after metformin is initiated. Because they have different mechanisms of action, sulfonylureas can be used in conjunction with metformin and thiazolidinediones. Sulfonylureas should not be used in patients with advanced diabetes dependent on insulin administration, because the beta cells in such patients are no longer able to produce insulin. Once insulin is started, sulfonylurea medication is stopped.

### Contraindications

Contraindications include hypoglycemia or conditions that can predispose to hypoglycemia, such as reduced caloric intake (e.g., NPO), ethanol use, or advanced age. There is a potential for cross-allergy in patients who are allergic to sulfonamide antibiotics. Although such an allergy is listed as a contraindication by the manufacturer, most clinicians will prescribe sulfonylureas

for such patients. However, be aware of the potential for cross-allergy, and inform patients of the possibility.

### Adverse Effects

The most common adverse effect of the sulfonylureas is hypoglycemia, the degree to which depends on the dose, eating habits, and presence of hepatic or renal disease. Another predictable adverse effect is weight gain because of the stimulation of insulin secretion. Other adverse effects include skin rash, nausea, epigastric fullness, and heartburn.

### Interactions

Drug interactions with the second-generation sulfonylureas are listed in Table 32-5.

### Dosages

For dosage information on sulfonylureas, see the table on this page.

## GLINIDES

### Mechanism of Action and Drug Effects

Repaglinide (Prandin) and nateglinide (Starlix) are currently the only two drugs in the glinide class. They are structurally different from the sulfonylureas but have a similar mechanism of action in that they also increase insulin secretion from the pancreas. However, they have a much shorter duration of action and must be given with each meal.

### Indications

Like the sulfonylureas, the glinides are indicated for treatment of type 2 diabetes. They may be particularly useful for diabetic patients with high postprandial glucose levels who have low levels of circulating insulin. Glinides can be used along with metformin and thiazolidinediones, but not combined with sulfonylureas, because they share a similar mechanism of action.

## Contraindications

Contraindications are similar to those for the sulfonylureas.

## Adverse Effects

The most commonly reported adverse effect of the glinides is hypoglycemia, which can occur particularly if food is not eaten after a dose. Weight gain is also commonly reported.

## Interactions

Drug interactions with the glinides are similar to those with the sulfonylureas.

## Dosages

For dosage information on the glinides, see the table on p. 521.

## THIAZOLIDINEDIONES (GLITAZONES)

### Mechanism of Action and Drug Effects

The third major drug category to emerge for the oral treatment of type 2 diabetes mellitus is the thiazolidinediones, most commonly referred to as *glitazones*. This class of drugs acts by regulating genes involved in glucose and lipid metabolism. The first drug in this class to be used in the United States was troglitazone (Rezulin). In 2000, it was removed from the market because of concerns about liver toxicity. In 2011, rosiglitazone (Avandia) was essentially removed from the market due to cardiac problems. It is no longer available in retail pharmacies. It can only be obtained through specialized manufacturer programs. Pioglitazone (Actos) is the only glitazone currently available and is widely used.

Glitazones are referred to as *insulin-sensitizing drugs.* They work to decrease insulin resistance by enhancing the sensitivity of insulin receptors. These drugs are also known to directly stimulate peripheral glucose uptake and storage, as well as to inhibit glucose and triglyceride production in the liver. Because glitazones affect gene regulation, they have a slow onset of activity over several weeks, and maximal activity may not be evident for several months. Some amount of preservation of beta cell function has also been reported with glitazone administration, thereby slowing disease progression in type 2 diabetes.

### Indications

Thiazolidinediones (glitazones) are indicated for the management of type 2 diabetes. Because of their cost, adverse effect profile, and slow onset of action, they are usually reserved for patients who cannot tolerate or cannot achieve glucose control with metformin or the sulfonylureas. They may also be combined with metformin or a sulfonylurea for a synergistic effect. Pioglitazone can be used with insulin.

### Contraindications

Thiazolidinediones are contraindicated for use in patients with New York Heart Association class III or IV heart failure and are to be used with caution in patients with liver or kidney disease.

### Adverse Effects

The glitazones increase the risk of heart failure and are not recommended for use in patients with symptoms of heart failure. The glitazones also commonly cause peripheral edema and weight gain. The weight gain may be due to both water retention and an increase in adipose tissue. Their use has also been associated with reduced bone mineral density and an increased risk of fractures.

### Interactions

Pioglitazone is partly metabolized by cytochrome P-450 enzyme 3A4 (CYP3A4). Serum concentrations of pioglitazone may be increased if the drug is taken concurrently with a CYP3A4 inhibitor such as ketoconazole or erythromycin.

### Dosages

For dosage information on thiazolidinediones, see the table on p. 521.

## ALPHA-GLUCOSIDASE INHIBITORS

### Mechanism of Action and Drug Effects

Less commonly used oral drugs are the alpha-glucosidase inhibitors, acarbose (Precose) and miglitol (Glyset). As the name implies, these drugs work by reversibly inhibiting the enzyme alpha-glucosidase that is found in small intestine. This enzyme is responsible for the hydrolysis of oligosaccharides and disaccharides to glucose. When this enzyme is blocked, glucose absorption is delayed. The timing of administration of the alpha-glucosidase inhibitors is important, and they must be taken with food. When an alpha-glucosidase inhibitor is taken with a meal, excessive postprandial blood glucose elevation (a glucose "spike") can be prevented or reduced, making these medications impractical for directly lowering fasting blood glucose.

### Indications

The alpha-glucosidase inhibitors are used to treat type 2 diabetes, usually in combination with another oral hypoglycemic drug. They may be particularly effective in controlling high postprandial glucose levels.

### Contraindications

Because of their adverse gastrointestinal effects, alpha-glucosidase inhibitors are not recommended for use in patients with inflammatory bowel disease, malabsorption syndromes, or intestinal obstruction.

### Adverse Effects

These drugs can cause a high incidence of flatulence, diarrhea, and abdominal pain. At high dosages, they may also elevate levels of hepatic enzymes (transaminases). Unlike sulfonylureas, they do not cause hypoglycemia or weight gain. In the rare instance that a patient develops hypoglycemia from these drugs, complex carbohydrates cannot be used because alpha-glucosidase is blocked; IV or oral glucose must be administered.

### Interactions

The bioavailability of digoxin, ranitidine, and propranolol may be reduced when they are taken with alpha-glucosidase inhibitors.

## Dosages

For dosage information on alpha-glucosidase inhibitors, see the table on p. 521.

## DIPEPTIDYL PEPTIDASE IV (DPP-IV) INHIBITORS

### Mechanism of Action and Drug Effects

Dipeptidyl peptidase-IV (DPP-IV) inhibitors work by delaying the breakdown of incretin hormones (see Incretin Mimetics) by inhibiting the enzyme DPP-IV. Incretin hormones are released throughout the day and are increased after a meal. When blood glucose concentrations are normal or high, the incretin hormones increase insulin synthesis and lower glucagon secretion. By inhibiting the enzyme responsible for incretin breakdown (DPP-IV), the DPP-IV inhibitors reduce fasting and postprandial glucose concentrations. Currently there are three DPP-IV inhibitors: sitagliptin (Januvia), saxagliptin (Onglyza), and linagliptin (Tradjenta). There are several DPP-IV inhibitors currently under investigation. This class of drugs is commonly referred to as the *gliptins*.

### Indications

The DPP-IV inhibitors are indicated as an adjunct to diet and exercise to improve glycemic control in adults with type 2 diabetes mellitus.

### Contraindications

The DPP-IV inhibitors are contraindicated in patients with known drug allergy.

### Adverse Effects

The most common effects are upper respiratory tract infection, headache, and diarrhea. Hypoglycemia can occur and is more common if used in conjunction with a sulfonylurea. Cases of pancreatitis have been reported.

### Interactions

Sitagliptin may increase digoxin levels. Concurrent use of sulfonylureas and insulin may increase the risk of hypoglycemia. The metabolism of saxagliptin is inhibited by strong CYP4A inhibitors. Rifampin may decrease the efficacy of linagliptin.

### Dosages

The recommended dosage of sitagliptin is 100 mg daily; saxagliptin is 5 mg daily; and linagliptin is 5 mg daily.

### DRUG PROFILES

#### acarbose

Acarbose (Precose) is one of the two currently available alpha-glucosidase inhibitors. The other drug in this drug category is miglitol (Glyset). These drugs work by blunting the elevation of blood glucose levels after a meal. To work optimally, they are to be taken with the first bite of each meal. They also may be taken along with sulfonylurea drugs or with metformin. Acarbose use is contraindicated in patients with a hypersensitivity to alpha-glucosidase inhibitors, DKA, cirrhosis, inflammatory

bowel disease, colonic ulceration, partial intestinal obstruction, or chronic intestinal disease.

#### Pharmacokinetics

| Route | Onset of Action | Peak Plasma Concentration | Elimination Half-life | Duration of Action |
|---|---|---|---|---|
| PO | 1-1.5 hr | 2 hr | 2-3 hr | Unknown |

#### ◆ glipizide

Glipizide (Glucotrol) is a second-generation sulfonylurea drug. In contrast to another second-generation sulfonylurea, glimepiride, it has a very rapid onset and short duration of action, with no active metabolites. The rapid onset of action allows it to function much like the body normally does in response to meals when greater levels of insulin are required rapidly to deal with the increased glucose in the blood. When a patient with type 2 diabetes mellitus takes glipizide, it rapidly stimulates the pancreas to release insulin. This, in turn, facilitates the transport of excess glucose from the blood into the cells of the muscles, liver, and adipose tissues.

Glipizide use is contraindicated in cases of known drug allergy as well as in type 1 or brittle type 2 diabetes. Unlike most other oral antidiabetic drugs, it is not contraindicated in patients with severe renal failure. It works best if given 30 minutes before meals, usually before breakfast. This allows the timing of the insulin secretion induced by the glipizide to correspond with the elevation in blood glucose level induced by the meal in much the same way as endogenous insulin levels are raised in a person without diabetes. The extended-release dosage form of glipizide can be given once daily.

#### Pharmacokinetics

| Route | Onset of Action | Peak Plasma Concentration | Elimination Half-life | Duration of Action |
|---|---|---|---|---|
| PO | 1 hr | 1-3 hr | 2-5 hr | 6-8 hr |

#### ◆ metformin

Metformin (Glucophage) is currently the only biguanide oral antidiabetic drug. It works primarily by inhibiting hepatic glucose production and increasing the sensitivity of peripheral tissue to insulin. Because its mechanism of action differs from that of sulfonylurea drugs, it may be given along with these drugs.

Metformin use is contraindicated in patients with a known hypersensitivity to biguanides, hepatic or renal disease, alcoholism, or cardiopulmonary disease.

#### Pharmacokinetics

| Route | Onset of Action | Peak Plasma Concentration | Elimination Half-life | Duration of Action |
|---|---|---|---|---|
| PO | Less than 1 hr | 1-3 hr | 1.5-5 hr | 24 hr |

#### ◆ pioglitazone

Pioglitazone (Actos) is classified as a glitazone or thiazolidinedione derivative. It is marketed for the treatment of patients with type 2 diabetes. Pioglitazone is used alone or with a sulfonylurea, metformin, or insulin. It works by decreasing insulin resistance. It can worsen or precipitate heart failure and is best avoided in patients with cardiac disease. The safety of these drugs for use in pregnant women and children has not been established.

### Pharmacokinetics

| Route | Onset of Action | Peak Plasma Concentration | Elimination Half-life | Duration of Action |
|---|---|---|---|---|
| PO | Delayed | 2 hr | 3-7 hr | Unknown |

#### ◆ repaglinide

Repaglinide (Prandin) is one of two antidiabetic drugs classified as *glinides,* the other being nateglinide (Starlix). These drugs have a mechanism of action similar to that of the sulfonylureas in that they also stimulate the release of insulin from pancreatic beta cells. They are especially helpful in the treatment of patients who have erratic eating habits, because the drug dose is skipped when a meal is missed. Contraindications include known drug allergy.

### Pharmacokinetics

| Route | Onset of Action | Peak Plasma Concentration | Elimination Half-life | Duration of Action |
|---|---|---|---|---|
| PO | 15-60 min | 1 hr | 2-3 hr | 4-6 hr |

#### ◆ sitagliptin

Sitagliptin (Januvia) was the first DPP-IV inhibitor approved. It is an oral drug that selectively inhibits the action of DPP-IV, thus increasing concentrations of the naturally occurring incretins GLP-1 and GIP. Sitagliptin is indicated for management of type 2 diabetes, either as monotherapy or in combination with metformin, a sulfonylurea, or a glitazone, but not with insulin. Clinical trials have demonstrated A1C reductions of 0.6% to 0.8%, which is less than the reductions seen with traditional oral antidiabetic drugs. Significant hypoglycemia may occur when the drug is combined with a sulfonylurea. There have been no significant adverse effects. However, in September 2009, the FDA received postmarketing cases of acute pancreatitis and advised health care providers to monitor patients closely for the development of pancreatitis after both initiation and dose increases. Sitagliptin is given once daily as a 100-mg tablet with or without food. It is classified as a pregnancy category B drug.

### Pharmacokinetics

| Route | Onset of Action | Peak Plasma Concentration | Elimination Half-life | Duration of Action |
|---|---|---|---|---|
| PO | 15-30 min | 1 hr | 12 hr | Unknown |

## INJECTABLE ANTIDIABETIC DRUGS
### AMYLIN AGONISTS

### Mechanism of Action and Drug Effects

Amylin is a natural hormone secreted by the beta cells of the pancreas along with insulin in response to food. It functions to decrease postprandial plasma glucose levels, which it accomplishes in the following three ways:
1. Slows gastric emptying
2. Suppresses glucagon secretion and hepatic glucose production
3. Increases satiety (sense of having eaten enough)

When given before major meals, the amylin agonists work by mimicking the action of the natural hormone amylin.

### Indications

Pramlintide (Symlin; pregnancy category C) is the only available amylin agonist. It is available only as a subcutaneous injection. It is indicated for use in patients with type 1 or type 2 diabetes receiving mealtime insulin who failed to achieve optimal glucose control with insulin. Pramlintide was the first drug approved for use in type 1 diabetes since insulin was discovered in the early twentieth century.

### Contraindications

Pramlintide is contraindicated in patients with gastroparesis or those taking drugs that alter gastrointestinal motility.

### Adverse Effects

Adverse effects include nausea, vomiting, anorexia, and headache.

### Interactions

Pramlintide itself does not cause hypoglycemia, but if the patient is taking any preprandial rapid- or short-acting insulin product, the insulin dose usually needs to be reduced by 50%. It can delay the oral absorption of any drug taken at the same time and needs to be given at least 1 hour before other medications.

### Dosages

Recommended dosage ranges are from 15 to 60 mcg for management of type 1 diabetes and 60 to 120 mcg for management of type 2 diabetes, taken before any major meal.

### INCRETIN MIMETICS

### Mechanism of Action and Drug Effects

Incretins are hormones released by the gastrointestinal tract in response to food. Incretins do the following:
1. Stimulate insulin secretion
2. Reduce postprandial glucagon production
3. Slow gastric emptying
4. Increase satiety

The most important incretin hormones that have been identified so far are glucagon-like peptide 1 (GLP-1) and gastric inhibitory peptide (GIP). These hormones are rapidly deactivated by the enzyme DPP-IV. The incretin mimetics enhance glucose-dependent insulin secretion, suppress elevated glucagon secretion, and slow gastric emptying. Currently, there are two incretin mimetics: exenatide and liraglutide.

## Indications

Exenatide (Byetta; pregnancy category C) was approved by the FDA in 2005 as the first incretin mimetic drug. Exenatide is a long-acting analogue of GLP-1 that was initially derived from the salivary gland of the Gila monster. This drug is available only as a subcutaneous injection and is indicated only for patients with type 2 diabetes who have been unable to achieve blood glucose control with metformin, a sulfonylurea, and/or a glitazone. It cannot be used with insulin. It is best given 60 minutes before a meal. Liraglutide (Victoza) is similar to exenatide.

## Contraindications

These drugs are contraindicated in patients who are allergic to either drug.

## Adverse Effects

Adverse effects include nausea, vomiting, and diarrhea. Rare cases of hemorrhagic or necrotizing pancreatitis have also been reported. Patients may experience weight loss of 5 to 10 pounds.

## Interactions

The incretin mimetics can delay absorption of other orally administered drugs by slowing gastric emptying. In patients taking sulfonylurea drugs, the dose may need to be reduced if hypoglycemia appears on initiation of exenatide therapy.

## Dosages

The usual starting dosage of exenatide is 5 mcg within 1 hour of both the morning and evening meals. If necessary, the dosage may be increased after 1 month to 10 mcg twice daily before meals. The dose of liraglutide is 0.6 mg titrated up to 1.2 or 1.8 mg daily.

## GLUCOSE-ELEVATING DRUGS

Hypoglycemia is an abnormally low blood glucose level (generally below 50 mg/dL). When the cause is organic and the effects are mild, treatment usually consists of dietary modifications (a higher intake of protein and lower intake of carbohydrates), to prevent a rebound postprandial hypoglycemic effect. Hypoglycemia is also a common adverse effect of many antidiabetic drugs when their pharmacologic effects are greater than expected. Because the brain needs a constant amount of glucose to function, early symptoms of hypoglycemia include the central nervous system (CNS) manifestations of confusion, irritability, tremor, and sweating. Later symptoms include hypothermia and seizures. Without adequate restoration of normal blood and CNS glucose levels, coma and death will occur.

Oral forms of concentrated glucose are available for patients to use in the event of a hypoglycemic crisis. Dosage forms include rapidly dissolving buccal tablets and semisolid gel forms designed for oral use and rapid mucosal absorption. Table sugar, which is sucrose, will not produce as rapid an effect as the glucose products intended for use by diabetic patients. This is because sucrose is a disaccharide (two-molecule) sugar that must first be digested in the body to yield glucose as a monosaccharide (one-molecule) by-product. In the hospital setting or when the patient is unconscious, intravenous glucose is an obvious option to treat hypoglycemia. Concentrations of up to 50% dextrose in water ($D_{50}W$) are most often used for this purpose.

In addition to oral and/or intravenous glucose, glucagon, a natural hormone secreted by the pancreas, is available as a subcutaneous injection to be given when a quick response to severe hypoglycemia is needed. Because glucagon injection may induce vomiting, roll an unconscious patient onto his or her side before injection. Glucagon is useful in the unconscious hypoglycemic patient without established intravenous access.

---

### TEAMWORK AND COLLABORATION: PHARMACOKINETIC BRIDGE TO NURSING PRACTICE

Continuous subcutaneous insulin infusion has been used in patients with type 1 diabetes for over a quarter of a century and is increasing. Provision of insulin therapy by continuous subcutaneous insulin infusion (CSII) is becoming an option for selected diabetic patients in an attempt to minimize the risks and complications of the disease. One previously used option for achieving tight control of blood glucose levels was multiple daily injections of insulin (MDI). With CSII, normal serum glucose levels are maintained by the continuous delivery of basal insulin, and then with food intake—primarily carbohydrate consumption—bolus doses of insulin are given. Use of an insulin pump (i.e., CSII) leads to a more rapid, consistent absorption of the drug and a reduction in the occurrence of hypoglycemia. Research has also shown that use of an insulin pump helps to decrease the occurrence of elevated pre-breakfast serum glucose levels, often called the *dawn phenomenon* (referring to the dawn of the day). Because the insulin pump delivers insulin through the subcutaneous route and the infusion is a continuous one, fewer problems occur than with once- or twice-daily injections. Patients using CSII achieve mean serum glucose and A1C levels that remain somewhat lower than those associated with MDI, so that the risk for hypoglycemia is decreased. Understanding new and different drugs and their pharmacokinetic properties allows you to help patients achieve better quality of life, minimize risks, and maximize wellness.

---

## NURSING PROCESS

## ASSESSMENT

Before administering any type of antidiabetic drug, assess the patient's knowledge about the disease and recommended treatment. Complete a head-to-toe physical assessment, medication history taking, and nursing assessment and document the findings. With *insulin*, as well as other antidiabetic drugs, a thorough medication history includes a list of the patient's current medications, including over-the-counter drugs, herbals, and supplements. Review the appropriate laboratory test results (e.g., fasting blood glucose level, A1C level) for any abnormalities compared with baseline levels. Assess the prescriber's order for insulin, so that the correct drug, route, type of insulin (i.e., rapid acting, short acting, intermediate acting, short- and intermediate-acting mixtures, long acting), and dosage are implemented correctly. Assess the specific insulin, paying additional attention to the specific pharmacokinetics such as onset of action, peak, and duration of action. Knowing this information prior to giving the insulin is key to patient safety because these drug properties actually define parameters within which reactions, adverse effects, or problems versus therapeutic effects potentially occur. With insulin, it is also important to assess the prescriber's order for type of insulin. If more than one insulin type is prescribed, mixing of insulins may be ordered. It is important for you to know the chemically compatible combinations (see Table 32-4) so as to avoid an undesirable altered glycemic effect. Additionally, with all insulin orders, perform a second check of the prepared insulin dosage against the medication order with another registered nurse, or perform per facility policy and document.

Assess blood glucose levels prior to administering insulin to avoid giving the drug to a patient who is already hypoglycemic. The 2012 ADA guidelines identify the key diagnostic criterion for diabetes as being a fasting plasma glucose of greater than 126 mg/dL or a hemoglobin AIC greater than 6.5% (see Box 32-1). Furthermore, the ADA recommends the following control criteria for the diabetic patient: fasting blood glucose within the range of 70 to 130 mg/dL and/or a hemoglobin A1C less than 7%. Keep in mind that allergic reactions are less likely to occur with recombinant human insulins because of their similarity with endogenous insulin; however, allergies may still occur and have to be considered in the assessment. Contraindications and cautions associated with insulin have been previously discussed. Significant drug interactions are presented in Table 32-5, but it is important to remember the drugs that work against the effect of insulin, include corticosteroids, thyroid drugs, and diuretics. Drugs that increase the hypoglycemic effects of insulin include, alcohol, sulfa antibiotics, and salicylates.

*Oral antidiabetic drugs* also require close assessment for contraindications, cautions, and drug interactions, so obtain a thorough medication and patient history. Make sure to know the patient's history because type 2 diabetes can be treated with oral antidiabetic drugs, most of which require functioning beta cells in the pancreas. Functioning beta cells are not present in type 1 diabetes. With *biguanides*, be aware that elderly or malnourished patients may react adversely to this group of drugs. Contraindications, cautions, and interactions for this drug class have been previously discussed, but it is important to patient safety to emphasize the interaction between metformin and the iodine-containing radiologic contrast media used for certain diagnostic purposes (e.g., computed tomography with contrast). This interaction is associated with an increased risk for acute renal failure and lactic acidosis. If the patient is taking *metformin*, closely assess and monitor for this scenario so that the metformin may be discontinued the day of the test and for at least 48 hours afterwards. See Table 32-5 for more drug interactions associated with the oral antidiabetic drugs.

With *sulfonylureas*, it is important to know baseline glucose levels as well as conditions that may predispose the patient to hypoglycemia, such as a drop in caloric intake, alcohol use, or advanced age. Assessment of allergic reaction to sulfonamide antibiotics is important, as well, because of a potential for cross-allergic reactions. With *glinides*, cautions, contraindications, and drug interactions are similar to those for sulfonylureas. With *thiazolidinediones (glitazones)*, a major contraindication is with class III or IV heart failure (as per the New York Heart Association classification); the FDA has essentially removed rosiglitazone (Avandia) from the market due to these cardiac problems. It is only available through specialized manufacturing programs. With *alpha-glucosidase inhibitors* (e.g., acarbose and miglitol), assess for contraindications, such as inflammatory bowel disease or malabsorption syndromes. With *second-generation sulfonylureas*, assess the patient's type of diabetes because these drugs are contraindicated in type 1 diabetes.

Newer antidiabetic drugs include the *amylin mimetics* (see pharmacology section). These drugs are contraindicated in patients with gastroparesis or in patients who are taking medications that alter GI motility. Assessing for the type of diabetes is important because the drug pramlintide is indicated for both patients with type 1 or type 2 diabetes with particular mealtime needs and who are not able to achieve optimal blood glucose level control with insulin. Exenatide, an *incretin mimetic*, requires assessment of the patient's diagnosis because the drug is used for patients with type 2 diabetes and an inability to control blood glucose levels with metformin, a sulfonylurea, and/or a glitazone. It should not be used with insulin.

With diabetes mellitus, unstable serum glucose levels require immediate attention, so assess the patient for any signs and symptoms of hypoglycemia (e.g., acute onset of confusion, irritability, tremor, and sweating, with progression to possible hypothermia and seizures, and blood glucose level of less than 50 mg/dL) or of hyperglycemia (e.g., polyuria, polydipsia, polyphagia, glucosuria, weight loss, and fatigue, with a fasting blood glucose levels of 126 mg/dL or higher or a nonfasting blood glucose level of 200 mg/dL or higher). Assessment is even more critical for a diabetic patient who is also under stress, has an infection or is ill, is pregnant or lactating, or is experiencing trauma or any serious change in health status. With treatment, diabetic patients are at risk of hypoglycemia with the potential danger of loss of consciousness; therefore, constantly assess serum glucose levels and neurologic status. Along with assessment of the therapeutic regimen and patient adherence to treatment, note any cultural factors, socioeconomic factors, and family support, and follow throughout therapy.

*Glucose-elevating drugs* are to be given only after thorough assessment of the patient's presenting clinical picture and a thorough collection of data, including laboratory values, medication and patient history, as well as a list of current medications. Assess for level of consciousness as well, because glucagon injection may induce vomiting and precautions must be implemented to prevent aspiration.

## CASE STUDY

### Diabetes Mellitus: Lispro Insulin

B.G., age 58, was diagnosed with type 2 adult-onset diabetes mellitus 10 years ago. Although he has type 2 diabetes mellitus, he has needed to take insulin for the last 2 years. He has been recovering, without complications, from a laparoscopic cholecystectomy, but his blood glucose levels have shown some wide fluctuations over the past 24 hours. The physician has changed his insulin from regular to lispro (Humalog) to see if it will provide better control of his blood glucose levels.

1. Before his surgery, B.G.'s hemoglobin A1C level was 9%. What does this value imply regarding his glycemic control?
2. While reviewing the instructions for the lispro insulin, B.G. states, "I took my regular insulin shots about 30 minutes before my meals. Hopefully I can keep that same routine." How will the nurse respond to this statement?
3. After his discharge, B.G. wakes up one morning feeling nauseated. He gives himself the lispro insulin injection, but then after eating breakfast he vomits and cannot keep any food down. What must he do at this time?

For answers, see http://evolve.elsevier.com/Lilley.

## NURSING DIAGNOSES

1. Imbalanced nutrition, less than body requirements, related to the body's inability to use glucose (for type 1)
2. Ineffective family therapeutic regimen management related to lack of experience with a significant daily treatment regimen of diabetes mellitus
3. Risk for unstable glucose due to recent onset of possible signs and symptoms of diabetes mellitus

## PLANNING

### GOALS

1. Patient maintains adequate and balanced nutrition with stable weight and improved dietary habits in the overall management of diabetes.
2. Patient and family state the importance of adherence to medication regimens, lifestyle changes, dietary restrictions, and avoidance of high-risk behaviors.
3. Patient begins to understand the etiology of unstable glucose levels and its management.

### OUTCOME CRITERIA

1. Patient adheres to the diet recommended by the ADA or other dietary advisor per the orders of the prescriber or nutritional consultant.
   - Patient eats a healthy diet, gets sufficient rest and relaxation, and notifies the prescriber if any unusual problems occur when customary activities are changed.
2. Patient and family report increase in therapeutic regimen management as noted by support (by family), keeping all scheduled appointments with the prescriber to monitor therapeutic effectiveness, diet, and lifestyle change implementation and awareness for the complications of therapy.
3. Patient takes medication as scheduled, monitors blood glucose levels as prescribed, and watches for any signs and symptoms of hyperglycemia or hypoglycemia.
   - Patient's fasting blood glucose (fasting is considered to be no food/meals/snacks for 8 hours) goal is to be within the range of 70 to 130 mg/dL and/or hemoglobin A1C less than 7%.

## IMPLEMENTATION

With any patient who is taking *insulin* (or *oral antidiabetic drugs*), always check serum glucose levels (and other related laboratory values, as ordered) before giving the drug so that accurate baseline glucose levels are obtained and documented. Do not shake NPH (cloudy) and premixed insulin mixtures, but roll between the hands before administering the prescribed dose. The rolling helps to avoid air in the syringe and inaccurate dose administration. Administer insulins at room temperature. Insulin may be stored at room temperature if used within 1 month; otherwise, refrigeration is needed. Refrigeration is also recommended in warm or hot climates and with any major changes in environmental temperatures from cold to hot. Never use expired or discolored insulin. For information about the handling, mixing, storage, and administration of insulin, see Box 32-2.

Administer *insulin* subcutaneously at a 90-degree angle unless the patient is emaciated, in which case you may give the insulin at a 45-degree angle. Only regular insulin may be administered intravenously and is often used in intensive care settings. Only use insulin syringes for subcutaneous injections or when drawing up insulin dosage amounts. These syringes are easy to identify because of their orange caps and calibration in units, not milliliters. These syringes have preattached needles that are 29 gauge and ½ inch in length. When insulins are mixed (if ordered), withdraw the regular or rapid-acting insulin (unmodified and clear) first, followed by withdrawing the intermediate-acting or NPH insulin (modified and cloudy). Only do this after the appropriate amount of air has been injected into the vials. The amount of air to inject into the vials equals the prescribed number of units. Inject air into the intermediate-acting insulin vial first. Next, inject air into the regular or rapid- or short-acting insulin vial. This technique helps keep the intermediate-acting insulin from contaminating the rapid-acting insulin vial. This contamination would lead to a change in the regular, short-acting, unmodified insulin by the NPH, intermediate-acting, modified insulin. The net effect is an interference of the activity of the regular insulin (no longer considered modified), thus impacting its effect in the patient (see Table 32-4 and Chapter 9).

Understanding the action of the insulin and its related pharmacokinetics (e.g., onset, peak, duration) is critical for safe care and patient education. For example, it is important to know that the rapid-acting insulins (insulin lispro, insulin aspart, and insulin glulisine) have an onset of action of about 15 minutes and must be given 15 minutes before meals, compared with 30 minutes before meals for regular insulin or a short-acting insulin, which has an onset of action of 30 to 60 minutes. If lispro insulin is to be mixed with NPH (intermediate-acting) insulin, give the combination 15 minutes before meals. Always double-check

## BOX 32-2 ADMINISTRATION, HANDLING, AND STORAGE OF INSULIN

### Dosages, Storage, Handling, and Mixing

1. Individualize insulin dosages, and monitor closely for adequate control of hypoglycemia and hyperglycemia. Follow guidelines for basal/bolus insulin therapy or sliding scale, depending on specific regimen identified in the hospital setting.
2. Adjust dosages, as ordered, to achieve the prescriber's specific fasting blood glucose level for the patient. Using the ADA 2012 guidelines, this would be a fasting blood glucose level of 70 to 130 mg/dL and/or hemoglobin A1C less than 7% for the diabetic patient.
3. Store insulin for current use at room temperature. Avoid extreme temperatures and exposure to sunlight, because the insulin's protein structure will be permanently denatured. Extra vials not in use may be kept in the refrigerator. Vials being used in high environmental temperatures need to be stored in the refrigerator, but never give cold insulin. Never freeze insulin. To maintain drug stability, only store insulin for up to 1 month at room temperature or up to 3 months in the refrigerator.
4. Discard unused vials if they have not been used for several weeks (or follow hospital policy). Do not use any insulin that does not have the proper clarity or color (e.g., clear for regular, cloudy for NPH).
5. Store prefilled insulin syringes in the refrigerator for up to 1 week.
6. Always check expiration dates of insulin and all equipment.

### Administration

1. Administer insulin subcutaneously (see Chapter 9); however, regular insulin may be given intravenously in special situations (e.g., intravenous drip in patient with diabetic ketoacidosis; in postoperative patients), if ordered.
2. Roll the cloudy drug vial gently between the hands without shaking to avoid bubble formation in the vial, which may lead to inaccurate dosage withdrawal.

Give freshly mixed insulins within 5 minutes of mixing to avoid binding of the solution and subsequent altered activity of the drugs.
3. Administer insulin at the recommended times, but always with meals or meal trays ready. Give insulin lispro and other rapid-acting insulins approximately 15 minutes before meals (it has a quicker onset of action) and only after monitoring the patient's fasting serum glucose level (as with all insulin administration). Give regular insulin (short-acting insulin) 30 minutes before meals, and NPH intermediate insulin 30 to 60 minutes before meals.
4. When giving regular and NPH insulin at the same time (if ordered), mix the two appropriately (see discussion of mixing insulins in the Implementation subsection under Nursing Process).
5. Administer insulin subcutaneously at a 90-degree angle. However, if the patient is emaciated, the injection may be given at a 45-degree angle. Only use insulin syringes (see text discussion and Chapter 9).
6. Instruct patients using insulin injections to rotate sites within the same general location for about 1 week before moving to a new location (e.g., all injections for a week in the upper right thigh before moving a little lower on the right thigh). This technique allows for better insulin absorption. Each injection site should be at least ½ to 1 inch away from the previous injection site. If this practice is followed, it will be approximately 6 weeks before the patient will have to rotate to a totally new area of the body. Note the following sites for subcutaneous insulin injections: thigh areas (front and back), outer areas of the upper arm (middle third of the upper arm between the shoulder and the elbow), and the abdominal area using the iliac crests as landmarks and using the fatty part of the abdomen, but not within 2 inches of umbilicus or incision/stoma (see Chapter 9).
7. Continuous subcutaneous insulin infusion and/or multiple daily injections may be ordered for tight glucose control.

---

the prescriber's orders for clarification of the dosage and drug as well as of any change in dietary intake, such as a possible increase in carbohydrates and decrease in fat to avoid postprandial hypoglycemia. A meal high in fat can delay carbohydrate absorption while rapid-acting insulin is already in its peak action.

Regardless of the specific type of recombinant human insulin used, understanding the peak, onset, and duration of action of the insulin to be used (e.g., rapid acting versus short acting versus intermediate acting versus long acting) will help determine when food or meals are to be given. The intermediate-acting insulin (NPH) has an onset of action of 1 to 2 hours, so serve meals at least 30 to 45 minutes prior to its administration. Many combination products of rapid- and short-acting with intermediate-acting insulin are available; give these combination insulins 15 to 30 minutes before meals. In the hospital setting, be sure that meal trays have arrived on the unit before giving insulin to avoid time lapses and subsequent hypoglycemic episodes. Also be sure that other forms of allowed foods are available to the patient in case meals are delayed and insulin has already been administered.

Patients may require dosing by a sliding-scale or a basal-bolus method in a hospital setting. Sliding scale has historically been the method for administering subcutaneous regular insulin doses adjusted according to serum glucose test results. Although controversial (see previous pharmacology discussion), sliding-scale dosing may be used for hospitalized diabetic patients experiencing drastic changes in serum glucose levels due to physical and/or emotional stress, infections, surgery, acute illness, inactivity, or variable caloric intake, as well as for

patients needing intensive insulin therapy or patients—even if nondiabetic—receiving total parenteral nutrition (TPN) with a high glucose concentration. When this insulin regimen is used, measure blood glucose levels several times per day (e.g., every 4 hours, every 6 hours, or at specified times such as 7 AM, 11 AM, 4 PM, and midnight) to obtain fasting and/or premeal blood glucose values. The newer method, basal-bolus insulin dosing, is now the preferred method of treatment for hospitalized diabetic patients; orders for the dosages and frequency will be issued by the prescriber. A long-acting insulin (insulin glargine) is used to mimic the basal secretion of a healthy pancreas and constant delivery of an amount of insulin, and then the bolus is used (insulin lispro or insulin apart) to control increases in daily blood glucose levels. Bolus insulin is divided into meal and correction boluses (see pharmacology discussion). Monitor blood glucose levels frequently when using these methods.

*Oral antidiabetic drugs* are usually given at least 30 minutes before meals, as ordered. With any antidiabetic drug or insulin, it is important for both you and the patient to know what to do if symptoms of hypoglycemia occur—for example, the patient needs to take glucagon; eat glucose tablets or gel, corn syrup, or honey; drink fruit juice or a nondiet soft drink; or eat a small snack such as crackers or half a sandwich. If the patient receiving metformin is to undergo diagnostic studies with contrast dye, the prescriber will need to discontinue the drug prior to the procedure and restart it after the tests, but only after reevaluation of the patient's renal status. During therapy with metformin, the risk of lactic acidosis is possible, so it is important to monitor for and then report hyperventilation, cold and clammy skin, muscle pain, abdominal pain, dizziness, and irregular heartbeat. Some of the sulfonylureas are to be taken with breakfast; the alpha-glucosidase inhibitors are always taken with the first bite of each main meal, and the thiazolidinediones are given once daily or in two divided doses. Always check the exact timing of the dose against the prescriber's order and with consideration of the drug's onset of action.

It is critical to the safe and efficient use of oral antidiabetics to be sure that food will be or is being tolerated before the dose is given. If the oral drug is taken and no meal is consumed or it is consumed at a later time than usual, hypoglycemia may be problematic and result in negative health consequences and even unconsciousness. Because the glitazones (e.g., rosiglitazone and pioglitazone) may both cause moderate weight gain and edema, it is important to weigh the patient daily at the same time every day and in the same amount of clothing. Several combination oral antidiabetic drug products are available (see the pharmacology discussion) and need to be given exactly as prescribed. Pramlintide needs to be given before any major meal. Exenatide is given by subcutaneous injection in patients with type 2 diabetes and cannot be used with insulin. Sitagliptin is not to be used with insulin and may be taken with or without food.

In special situations, such as when the patient has been ordered to have nothing by mouth (NPO status) and is taking either an oral antidiabetic drug or insulin, it is crucial to follow the prescriber's orders regarding drug administration. If there are no written orders about this situation, contact the prescriber for further instructions. If a patient is on NPO status but is receiving an intravenous solution of dextrose, the prescriber may still order insulin, but always clarify this (with the prescriber). Contact the prescriber if a patient becomes ill and unable to take the usual dosage of an oral antidiabetic drug (or insulin). Encourage the patient to always wear a medical alert bracelet or necklace giving the diagnosis, list of medications, and emergency contact information.

It is also very important to stay informed and up to date about the latest research on diabetes and to keep patients and family members well informed. For example, as previously discussed in the pharmacology section, macrovascular and microvascular problems are now being recognized to occur at fasting blood glucose levels as low as 126 mg/dL. See the Evidence-Based Practice box for more information on specific nursing research.

In summary, there are many nursing considerations related to drug therapy in patients with diabetes mellitus. Patient education is also very important and needs to begin the moment the patient has entered into the health care system or upon diagnosis. Instruction that is tailored to the patient's educational level and that uses appropriate teaching-learning concepts and teaching aids is important to patient adherence with the treatment regimen. In addition, be sure that all necessary resources are made available to patients (e.g., financial assistance, visual assistance, dietary plans, daily menus, ADA information, transportation assistance, and Meals on Wheels and other community services). See the Patient Teaching Tips for more information.

## EVIDENCE-BASED PRACTICE

### Sensor-Augmented Insulin Pump Therapy Trumps Multiple Daily Injections

**Review**

In patients with type 1 diabetes and poor glycemic control, a sensor-augmented insulin pump is significantly improving glycated hemoglobin levels as compared with regimens with multiple daily insulin injections. This research was presented at the American Diabetes Association 70th Scientific Session on June 29, 2010. Research has confirmed that the use of these pumps has demonstrated more effective control than the use of multiple daily injections.

**Type of Evidence**

Some 329 adults and 156 children were randomly assigned to either pump therapy with the MiniMed Paradigm REAL-Time system (Medtronic) or to continue with their regimen of multiple daily injections under close supervision for the duration of the study that lasted for one year. Patients in the study received intensive diabetes management education and training including carbohydrate counting and the administration of correction doses of insulin. Once patients were randomized to insulin pump therapy, they were placed on it for 2 weeks. After they had become comfortable with the pump, the glucose sensor was added. This group used the insulin aspart, and the injection therapy group used both insulin aspart and insulin glargine. All patients were seen at 3, 6, 9, and 12 months and used Carelink, which is a diabetes-management software program. This program was used to relay the patients' glucose data to communicate with their health care providers from home. It is important to know that the sensor-augmented pump therapy uses the two technologies of an insulin pump and continuous glucose monitoring all in one system. This pump allows patients and their physicians to monitor treatment and their response through Internet-based software. The patients needed to have computer access to participate in the study.

**Results of Study**

At 1 year, the researchers found that the patients on pump therapy had hemoglobin A1C levels that were significantly lower than the injection-therapy group. The baseline mean glycated hemoglobin level, which was 8.3% in the two groups, decreased to 7.5% in the pump therapy group as compared to 8.1% in the injection therapy group. Among the adults, the absolute reduction in the mean glycated hemoglobin level was 1.0% ± 0.7% in the pump-therapy group and 0.4% ± 0.8% in the injection-therapy group. The between-group difference in the pump-therapy group was −0.6%. The occurrence of hypoglycemia and diabetic ketoacidosis were similar in both groups. There was no significant weight gain in adult or child participants.

**Link of Evidence to Nursing Practice**

This study has been identified as one of the longest and largest randomized controlled study of sensor-augmented insulin pump therapy in type 1 diabetic patients. Another significant point to this study was the comparison of two therapeutic approaches. For nursing and for the care of diabetic patients, the impact of this study is important in that patients may be able to achieve better control of their diabetes with improved outcomes and safety. Having the positive results without the occurrence of increased hypoglycemia represents even larger breakthroughs in the care of these patients as well as the possibility of increased adherence to treatment. This study holds great promise in the treatment of type 1 diabetic patients and for evidenced-based nursing practice. The possibility of enhanced quality of life and prevention of complications in the treatment of patients with chronic illnesses, such as type 1 diabetes, is truly exciting and promising.

Reference: Bergenstal RM, Tamborlane VV, Ahmann A, et al: Effectiveness of sensor-augmented insulin-pump therapy in type 1 diabetes, *N Engl J Med* 363(4):311-320, 2010.

# EVALUATION

It is important to understand current therapeutic guidelines. The prevailing key diagnostic criterion for diabetes mellitus is hyperglycemia with a fasting blood glucose level of 126 mg/dL or higher or a nonfasting blood glucose level of 200 mg/dL or higher; however, the therapeutic response to insulin and any of the oral antidiabetic drugs is a decrease in blood glucose to the level prescribed by the prescriber or to near-normal levels. Most often, fasting blood glucose levels are used to measure the degree of glycemic control. To provide a picture of the patient's adherence to the therapy regimen for the previous several months, the level of A1C is measured. This value reflects how well the patient has been doing with diet and drug therapy.

Patients with diabetes need to be monitored frequently by their prescribers (as well as at home) to make sure they are adhering to the therapy regimen as evidenced by normalization of blood test results. It is important to monitor the patient for indications of hypoglycemia or hyperglycemia and insulin allergy as well. With short-acting insulins such as lispro, the onset of action is more rapid than with regular insulin and the duration of action is shorter, so monitor blood glucose levels very closely until the dosage is regulated and blood glucose is at the level the prescriber desires. If a patient is switched from one insulin or oral antidiabetic drug to another, advise the patient that glucose levels must be monitored very closely at home or by the prescriber. Always evaluate whether identified goals and outcome criteria are being met, and plan nursing care accordingly.

# PATIENT TEACHING TIPS

- Encourage the patient to keep medical alert jewelry or a medical alert card on his or her person at all times and to keep medical information in clear view on the refrigerator at home.
- Provide instructions and demonstrations regarding the proper storage of insulin, the equipment needed for administration, the drawing up and mixing of insulins (if ordered), technique for insulin injections, and rotation of subcutaneous insulin injection sites. Provide the opportunity for return demonstrations from the patient, including rotation of sites. (see Chapter 9 for more information about insulin injections). Emphasize that insulin may be stored at room temperature unless the heat is extreme or the patient is traveling.
- Encourage the keeping of a daily dietary intake and blood glucose journal.
- Educate about the need to have serum glucose levels monitored. Emphasize instructions that are specific to the patient's glucometer. Stress the importance of exercise, hygiene, foot care, dietary plan, and weight control in the management of diabetes.
- Pay attention to and assess the patient's economic situation when teaching about the frequency of blood glucose monitoring. If the patient must pay for supplies, each blood glucose check costs over $1. This expense can add up quickly, especially for those who are economically disadvantaged.
- Advise the patient to avoid smoking and alcohol consumption (with oral antidiabetic drugs) and maintain strict adherence to dietary instructions. Instruct the patient to avoid skipping meals or skipping doses of insulin or oral antidiabetic drugs, and to contact the prescriber for further instructions when needed.
- Explain the difference between hypoglycemia and hyperglycemia (see earlier discussion for specific signs and symptoms), with emphasis on the treatment of each (e.g., having on hand quick sources of glucose, such as candy, sugar packets, over-the-counter glucose tablets, sugar cubes, honey, corn syrup, orange juice, or nondiet soda beverages for hypoglycemia, and having more insulin on hand for hyperglycemia, as ordered). Encourage the patient to keep quick dosage forms of glucose in possession at all times!

- Educate the patient about situations or conditions that lead to altered serum glucose levels, such as fever, illness, stress, increased activity or exercise, surgery, and emotional distress. Encourage the patient to contact the prescriber for any questions or concerns about maintaining glucose control.
- Educate about the importance of knowing premeal serum glucose levels before taking insulin and the importance of timing meals related to the type of insulin.
- Emphasize the importance of having adequate supplies of insulin and equipment at all times and planning ahead for vacations. Instruct the patient to keep all medications and related equipment out of the reach of children. If needed, magnifying attachments are available for syringes and vials. Specialized syringes are available for those with impaired vision. Patients using these types of syringes learn to rely on the sound the syringe makes when a dosage is selected; for example, with Novologpen, 5 clicks equals 5 units.
- Encourage the diabetic patient to report any yellow discoloration of the skin, dark urine, fever, sore throat, weakness, or unusual bleeding or easy bruising.
- Emphasize the importance of A1C monitoring (e.g., at least two times per year for those with good glycemic control and quarterly for patients who are not at target values, have changed their therapy, or are not adhering to the therapy regimen) (Table 32-6). Review with the patient lifestyle modifications, including weight control and glucose level maintenance with diet, exercise, and/or drug therapy. Patients with type 2 diabetes have a greater therapeutic response to diet and exercise and glucose level control than patients with type 1 diabetes. ADA recommendations for fasting serum glucose level measurement need to be followed. Educate the patient about the importance of engaging in supervised exercise, as prescribed, and as a lifelong lifestyle change. A nutritional consult with specific menu planning may help the patient with changes in intake (e.g., low-fat diet with 160 to 300 g of carbohydrates). The ADA has also encouraged the "Create Your Plate" method of meal planning. (Visit www.diabetes.org/food-and-fitness/food/planning-meals/create-your-plate/ for specific information.) The

| TABLE 32-6 | **DIABETES CARE: CORRELATION OF GLYCOSYLATED HEMOGLOBIN LEVELS WITH MEAN SERUM GLUCOSE LEVELS** | |
|---|---|---|
| **HEMOGLOBIN A1C (%)** | **MEAN SERUM GLUCOSE LEVEL (mg/dL)** | **MEAN SERUM GLUCOSE LEVEL (mmol/L)** |
| 6 | 126 | 7.0 |
| 7 | 154 | 8.6 |
| 8 | 183 | 10.2 |
| 9 | 212 | 11.8 |
| 10 | 240 | 13.4 |
| 11 | 269 | 14.9 |
| 12 | 298 | 16.5 |

Data from American Diabetes Association: Executive summary: standards of medical care in diabetes, *Diabetes Care* 35(Suppl 1): S4-S10, 2012.

"Create Your Plate" method has six simple steps as a means of getting larger portions of nonstarchy vegetables and smaller portions of starchy foods. An imaginary line is drawn down the middle of the plate, creating two sections. One side is split into two equal smaller sections so there are now three total sections on the plate. The largest section (one side of the plate) is filled with nonstarchy vegetables. One of the small sections is filled with starchy foods. The other small section is filled with meat or meat substitutes. An 8-oz glass of nonfat or low-fat milk is also added.

- Emphasize the importance of the American Heart Association recommendations for diabetic patients, including 30 minutes of exercise daily with use of a treadmill, prolonged walking, swimming or aquatic aerobics, bicycling, rowing, chair exercises, arm exercises, and non–weight-bearing exercises. It is recommended to use a pedometer and to exercise for 150 minutes per week.
- Emphasize that therapy will be lifelong and that strict blood glucose control, drug therapy, and lifestyle changes are critical to reducing complications.
- Stress the need for strict foot care to the patient and those involved in the patient's care. Begin with the need for a daily basic assessment of the feet and toes to check for sores, lesions, cuts, bruises, ingrown toenails, and any other changes. Foot care is needed to enhance circulation and prevent infections. It may include soaking the feet daily or as ordered in lukewarm water (the temperature of the water must be checked) and then adequate drying of the feet and application of moisturizing lotion; checking the feet and legs for abnormal changes in color (e.g., purplish or reddish discoloration), cool temperature of the feet to the touch, swelling of the extremities or feet, and the appearance of any drainage. Emphasize the importance of contacting the prescriber for further instructions if there is suspicion of any type of wound or alteration in skin integrity. Frequent pedicures and nail trimming by a podiatrist or other licensed, certified individual may be indicated.
- Some of the oral antidiabetic drugs cause photosensitivity, so instruct the patient on wearing protective sunscreen and proper clothing when exposed to the sun. Advise against the use of tanning beds.

## KEY POINTS

- Insulin normally facilitates removal of glucose from the blood and its storage as glycogen in the liver.
- Type 1 diabetes mellitus was formerly known as *insulin-dependent diabetes* or *juvenile-onset diabetes*. Little or no endogenous insulin is produced by individuals with type 1 diabetes. It is much less common than type 2 diabetes and affects only about 10% of all diabetic patients. Patients with type 1 diabetes usually are not obese. Because insulin therapy is required for type 1 diabetics, type 1 patients who have the cognitive and financial ability need to be encouraged to consider adding an insulin pump with continuous glucose monitoring as part of their therapy.
- The primary treatment for type 1 diabetes mellitus is insulin therapy. Patients with type 2 diabetes are managed with lifestyle changes (dietary changes, exercise, smoking cessation) and oral drug therapy (one or more drugs). If normal blood glucose levels are not achieved after 2 to 3 months of lifestyle changes, treatment with oral antidiabetic drugs is often added to the regimen.
- Insulin was originally isolated from cattle and pigs, but bovine and porcine insulins are associated with a higher incidence of allergic reactions and insulin resistance than human insulin and are no longer available in the U.S. market.

- Complications associated with diabetes include retinopathy, neuropathy, nephropathy, hypertension, cardiovascular disease, and coronary artery disease. Annual screening with an ophthalmologist specializing in retinopathies is needed in the care of diabetic patients for screening purposes. Because of the renal complications (e.g., nephropathies), annual urinalysis screening and renal function studies are also recommended for diabetic patients.
- All rapid-acting, short-acting, and long-acting insulin preparations are clear solutions. Intermediate-acting insulins are cloudy solutions. Mixtures of short- and intermediate-acting insulin still look uniformly cloudy. The cloudy appearance of these mixtures is due to the presence of the intermediate-acting insulin. Insulin vials are to be rolled in the hands instead of shaken, when used.
- Always carefully check the exact timing of the dose of insulin or oral antidiabetic drug against the prescriber's order. Take into consideration the drug's pharmacokinetics, including onset peak, and duration of action.
- Nursing care must be individualized with patient education focused on the patient's needs and learning abilities. Include pertinent and age-appropriate information on the disease process, drug therapy, and lifestyle modifications.

## NCLEX® EXAMINATION REVIEW QUESTIONS

1 Which is the most appropriate timing regarding the nurse's administration of a rapid-acting insulin to a hospitalized patient?
   a Give it 15 minutes before the patient begins a meal.
   b Give it ½ hour before a meal.
   c Give it 1 hour after a meal.
   d The timing of the insulin injection does not matter with insulin lispro.

2 Which statement is appropriate for the nurse to include in patient teaching regarding type 2 diabetes?
   a "Insulin injections are never used with type 2 diabetes."
   b "You don't need to measure your blood glucose levels because you are not taking insulin injections."
   c "A person with type 2 diabetes still has functioning beta cells in his or her pancreas."
   d "Patients with type 2 diabetes usually have better control over their diabetes than those with type 1 diabetes."

3 The nurse monitoring a patient for a therapeutic response to oral antidiabetic drugs will look for
   a fewer episodes of diabetic ketoacidosis (DKA).
   b weight loss of 5 pounds.
   c hemoglobin A1C levels of less than 7%.
   d glucose levels of 150 mg/dL.

4 A patient with type 2 diabetes is scheduled for magnetic resonance imaging (MRI) with contrast dye. The nurse reviews the orders and notices that the patient is receiving metformin (Glucophage). Which action by the nurse is appropriate?
   a Proceed with the MRI as scheduled.
   b Notify the radiology department that the patient is receiving metformin.
   c Expect to hold the metformin the day of the test and for 48 hours after the test is performed.
   d Call the prescriber regarding holding the metformin for 2 days before the MRI is performed.

5 A patient with type 2 diabetes has a new prescription for repaglinide (Prandin). After 1 week, she calls the office to ask what to do, because she keeps missing meals. "I work right through lunch sometimes, and I'm not sure whether I need to take it. What do I need to do?" What is the nurse's best response?
   a "You need to try not to skip meals, but if that happens, you will need to skip that dose of Prandin."
   b "We will probably need to change your prescription to insulin injections because you can't eat meals on a regular basis."
   c "Go ahead and take the pill when you first remember that you missed it."
   d "Take both pills with the next meal, and try to eat a little extra to make up for what you missed at lunchtime."

6 When checking a patient's fingerstick blood glucose level, the nurse obtains a reading of 42 mg/dL. The patient is awake but states he feels a bit "cloudy-headed." After double-checking the patient's glucose level and getting the same reading, which action by the nurse is most appropriate?
   a Administer two packets of table sugar.
   b Administer oral glucose in the form of a semisolid gel.
   c Administer 50% dextrose IV push.
   d Administer the morning dose of lispro insulin.

7 A patient is taking metformin for new-onset type 2 diabetes mellitus. When reviewing potential adverse effects, the nurse will include information about: (Select all that apply.)
   a Abdominal bloating
   b Nausea
   c Diarrhea
   d Headache
   e Weight gain
   f Metallic taste

1. a, 2. c, 3. c, 4. c, 5. a, 6. b, 7. a, b, c, f

For Critical Thinking and Prioritization Questions, see http://evolve.elsevier.com/Lilley.

# Adrenal Drugs

## OBJECTIVES

When you reach the end of this chapter, you will be able to do the following:

1 Discuss the normal anatomy, physiology, and related functions of the adrenal glands, including specific hormones released from the glands.

2 Briefly compare the hormones secreted by the adrenal medulla with those secreted by the adrenal cortex.

3 Contrast Cushing's syndrome, Addison's disease, and addisonian crisis.

4 Compare the glucocorticoids and mineralocorticoids with regard to the roles they perform in normal bodily func-

tions, the diseases that alter them, how they are used in pharmacotherapy, and their basic properties.

5 Contrast the mechanisms of action, indications, dosages, routes of administration, cautions, contraindications, drug interactions, and adverse effects of glucocorticoids, mineralocorticoids, and antiadrenal drugs.

6 Develop a nursing care plan that includes all phases of the nursing process for patients taking adrenal and antiadrenal drugs.

## DRUG PROFILES

♦ **aminoglutethimide, p. 539**
♦ **fludrocortisone, p. 538**
  **methylprednisolone, p. 538**

♦ **prednisone, p. 538**

_____

♦ *Key drug*

## KEY TERMS

**Addison's disease** A potentially life-threatening condition caused by partial or complete failure of adrenocortical function, with resulting decrease in glucocorticoid, mineralocorticoid, and androgenic hormones. It is a chronic disease of hyposecretion of steroids. (p. 535)

**Adrenal cortex** The outer portion of the adrenal gland. (p. 534)

**Adrenal crisis** An acute, life-threatening state of profound adrenocortical insufficiency requiring immediate medical management. It is characterized by glucocorticoid deficiency, a drop in extracellular fluid volume, hyponatremia, and hyperkalemia. (p. 540)

**Adrenal medulla** The inner portion of the adrenal gland. (p. 534)

**Aldosterone** A mineralocorticoid hormone produced by the adrenal cortex that acts on the renal tubule to regulate sodium and potassium balance in the blood. (p. 534)

**Cortex** The general anatomic term for the outer layers of a body organ or other structure. (p. 534)

**Corticosteroids** Any of the natural or synthetic adrenocortical hormones; those produced by the cortex of the adrenal gland (adrenocorticosteroids). (p. 534)

**Cushing's syndrome** A metabolic disorder characterized by abnormally increased secretion of the adrenocorticosteroids. (p. 534)

**Epinephrine** An endogenous hormone secreted into the bloodstream by the adrenal medulla; also a synthetic drug that is an adrenergic vasoconstrictor and also increases cardiac output. (p. 534)

**Glucocorticoids** A major group of corticosteroid hormones that regulate carbohydrate, protein, and lipid metabolism and inhibit the release of adrenocorticotropic hormone (corticotropin). (p. 534)

**Hypothalamic-pituitary-adrenal (HPA) axis** A negative feedback system involved in regulating the release of corticotropin-releasing hormone by the hypothalamus, adrenocorticotropic hormone (corticotropin) by the pituitary gland, and corticosteroids by the adrenal glands. Suppression of the HPA may lead to Addison's disease and possible adrenal crisis or addisonian

crisis. This suppression results from chronic disease or exogenous sources, such as long-term glucocorticoid therapy. (p. 534)

**Medulla** A general anatomic term for the most interior portions of an organ or structure. (p. 534)

**Mineralocorticoids** A major group of corticosteroid hormones that regulate electrolyte and water balance; in humans the primary mineralocorticoid is aldosterone. (p. 534)

**Norepinephrine** An adrenergic hormone, also secreted by the adrenal medulla, that increases blood pressure by causing vasoconstriction but does not appreciably affect cardiac output; it is the immediate metabolic precursor to epinephrine. (p. 534)

# ANATOMY, PHYSIOLOGY, AND PATHOPHYSIOLOGY OVERVIEW

## ADRENAL SYSTEM

The adrenal gland is an endocrine organ that sits on top of the kidney like a cap. It is composed of two distinct parts called the adrenal cortex and the adrenal medulla; both are structurally and functionally different from one another. In general, the term cortex refers to the outer layers of various organs (e.g., cerebral cortex), whereas the term medulla refers to the most internal layers. The adrenal cortex composes roughly 80% to 90% of the entire adrenal gland; the remainder is the medulla. The adrenal cortex is made up of regular endocrine tissue (hormone driven). The adrenal medulla is made up of neurosecretory endocrine tissue (driven by both hormones and peripheral autonomic nerve impulses). Therefore, the adrenal gland actually functions as two different endocrine glands, each secreting different hormones.

The adrenal medulla secretes two important hormones, both of which are catecholamines. These are epinephrine, which accounts for about 80% of the secretion, and norepinephrine, which accounts for the other 20%. (Both of these hormones are discussed in Chapter 18 and are not described further in this chapter in any detail.) Characteristics of the adrenal cortex and the adrenal medulla and the various hormones secreted by each are presented in Table 33-1.

The hormones secreted by the adrenal cortex, which are the focus of this chapter, are broadly referred to as corticosteroids. They arise from the cortex and are made from the steroid known as *cholesterol*. There are two types of corticosteroids— glucocorticoids and mineralocorticoids. They are secreted by two different layers, or zones, of the cortex. The *zona glomerulosa*, which is the outer layer, secretes the mineralocorticoids, and the *zona fasciculata*, which lies under the zona glomerulosa, secretes the glucocorticoids. A third, inner layer, the *zona reticularis*, secretes small amounts of sex hormones. All the hormones secreted by the adrenal cortex are steroid hormones; that is, they have the steroid chemical structure.

The mineralocorticoids get their name from the fact that they play an important role in regulating mineral salts (electrolytes) in the body. In humans, the only physiologically important mineralocorticoid is aldosterone. Its primary role is to maintain normal levels of sodium in the blood (sodium homeostasis) by causing sodium to be resorbed from the urine back into the blood in exchange for potassium and hydrogen ions. In this way aldosterone not only regulates blood sodium levels but also influences the potassium levels in the blood and blood pH.

The corticosteroids are necessary for many vital bodily functions. Some of the more important ones are listed in Box 33-1. Without these hormones, life-threatening consequences may arise.

Adrenal corticosteroids are synthesized as needed; the body does not store them as it does other hormones. The body levels of these hormones are regulated by the hypothalamic-pituitary-adrenal (HPA) axis in much the same way that the levels of hormones secreted by the pancreas, thyroid, and pituitary are regulated. As the name implies, this axis consists of a very organized system of communications between the adrenal gland, the pituitary gland, and the hypothalamus. As is the case for the other endocrine glands, it uses hormones as the messengers and a negative feedback mechanism as the controller and maintainer of the process. This feedback mechanism operates as follows: When the level of a particular corticosteroid is low, corticotropin-releasing hormone is released from the hypothalamus into the bloodstream and travels to the anterior pituitary gland, where it triggers the release of adrenocorticotropic hormone (ACTH; also called *corticotropin*). The ACTH is then transported in the blood to the adrenal cortex, where it stimulates the production of the corticosteroids. Corticosteroids are then released into the bloodstream. When they reach peak levels, a signal (negative feedback) is sent to the hypothalamus, and the HPA axis is inhibited until the level of corticosteroids again falls below physiologic threshold, whereupon the axis is stimulated once again.

The oversecretion (hypersecretion) of adrenocortical hormones can lead to a group of signs and symptoms called Cushing's syndrome. This hypersecretion of glucocorticoids results in

## TABLE 33-1 ADRENAL GLAND: CHARACTERISTICS

| TYPE OF TISSUE | TYPE OF HORMONE SECRETED | HORMONES SECRETED AND RELATED DRUGS |
|---|---|---|
| **Adrenal Cortex** | | |
| Endocrine | Glucocorticoids | Adrenocorticotropic hormone, betamethasone, cortisone, dexamethasone, hydrocortisone, methylprednisolone, prednisolone, triamcinolone |
| | Mineralocorticoids | Aldosterone, desoxycorticosterone, fludrocortisone |
| **Adrenal Medulla** | | |
| Neuroendocrine | Catecholamines | Epinephrine, norepinephrine |

## BOX 33-1 ADRENAL CORTEX HORMONES: BIOLOGIC FUNCTIONS

**Glucocorticoids**
Antiinflammatory actions
Carbohydrate and protein metabolism
Fat metabolism
Maintenance of normal blood pressure
Stress effects

**Mineralocorticoids**
Blood pressure control
Maintenance of serum potassium levels
Maintenance of pH levels in the blood
Sodium and water resorption

## TABLE 33-2 AVAILABLE SYNTHETIC CORTICOSTEROIDS

| TYPE OF HORMONE | METHOD OF ADMINISTRATION | INDIVIDUAL DRUGS |
|---|---|---|
| Adrenal steroid inhibitor | Systemic | Aminoglutethimide |
| Glucocorticoid | Topical | Alclometasone, betamethasone, clobetasol dexamethasone, fluocinolone, halobetasol hydrocortisone, mometasone, triamcinolone |
| | Systemic | Betamethasone, cortisone, dexamethasone, hydrocortisone, methylprednisolone, prednisolone, prednisone, triamcinolone |
| | Inhaled | Beclomethasone, dexamethasone, flunisolide, triamcinolone, fluticasone |
| | Nasal | Beclomethasone, dexamethasone, flunisolide, triamcinolone, fluticasone |
| Mineralocorticoid | Systemic | Fludrocortisone |

the redistribution of body fat from the arms and legs to the face, shoulders, trunk, and abdomen, which leads to the characteristic "moon face." Such a glucocorticoid excess can be due to several causes, including ACTH-dependent adrenocortical hyperplasia or tumor, ectopic ACTH-secreting tumor, or excessive administration of steroids. The hypersecretion of aldosterone, or primary aldosteronism, leads to increased retention of water and sodium, which causes muscle weakness due to the potassium loss.

The undersecretion (hyposecretion) of adrenocortical hormones causes a condition known as Addison's disease. It is associated with decreased blood sodium and glucose levels, increased potassium levels, dehydration, and weight loss. The combination of a mineralocorticoid (fludrocortisone) and a glucocorticoid (prednisone or some other suitable drug) is used for treatment.

## PHARMACOLOGY OVERVIEW

### ADRENAL DRUGS

All of the naturally occurring corticosteroids are available as exogenous drugs. There are also higher-potency synthetic analogues. The adrenal glucocorticoids are an extremely large group of steroids and can be categorized in various ways. They can be classified by whether they are a natural or synthetic corticosteroid, by the method of administration (e.g., systemic, topical), by their salt and water retention potential (mineralocorticoid activity), by their duration of action (i.e., short, intermediate, or long acting), or by some combination of these methods. The only corticosteroid drug with exclusive mineralocorticoid activity is fludrocortisone. Its uses are much more specific than those of the glucocorticoids and are discussed in the drug profile for fludrocortisone. The currently available synthetic adrenal hormones and adrenal steroid inhibitors are listed in Table 33-2.

## Mechanism of Action and Drug Effects

The action of the corticosteroids is related to their involvement in the synthesis of specific proteins. There are several steps to this process. Initially the steroid hormone binds to a receptor on the surface of a target cell to form a steroid-receptor complex, which is then transported through the cytoplasm to the nucleus of that target cell. Once inside the nucleus, the complex stimulates the cell's deoxyribonucleic acid (DNA) to produce messenger ribonucleic acid (mRNA), which is then used as a template for the synthesis of a specific protein. It is these proteins that exert specific effects.

Most of the corticosteroids exert their effects by modifying enzyme activity; therefore, their role is more intermediary than direct. The naturally occurring mineralocorticoid aldosterone affects electrolyte and fluid balance by acting on the distal renal tubule. It promotes sodium resorption from the nephron into the blood, which pulls water and fluid along with it. In doing so, it causes fluid and water retention, which leads to edema and hypertension. It also increases urinary excretion of potassium and hydrogen via the kidney.

The glucocorticoid drugs hydrocortisone (called *cortisol* in its naturally occurring form) and cortisone have some mineralocorticoid activity and therefore have some of the same effects as aldosterone (i.e., fluid and water retention). However, their main effect is the inhibition of inflammatory and immune responses. Glucocorticoids inhibit or help control the inflammatory response by stabilizing the cell membranes of inflammatory cells called *lysosomes,* decreasing the permeability of capillaries to the inflammatory cells, and decreasing the migration of white blood cells into already inflamed areas. They may lower fever by reducing the release of interleukin-1 from white blood cells. They also stimulate the *erythroid cells* that eventually become red blood cells. The glucocorticoids also promote the breakdown (catabolism) of protein, the production of glycogen in the liver (glycogenesis), and the redistribution of fat from peripheral to central areas of the body. In addition, they have the following effects on various bodily functions: increasing levels of blood sugar, increasing the breakdown of proteins to amino acids, inducing lipolysis, stimulating bone demineralization, and stabilizing mast cells.

## Indications

All of the systemically administered glucocorticoids have a similar clinical efficacy but differ in their potency and duration of action and in the extent to which they cause salt and water retention (Table 33-3). These drugs have broad indications, including the following:

- Adrenocortical deficiency
- Adrenogenital syndrome
- Bacterial meningitis (particularly in infants)
- Cerebral edema
- Collagen diseases (e.g., systemic lupus erythematosus)
- Dermatologic diseases (e.g., exfoliative dermatitis, pemphigus)
- Endocrine disorders (thyroiditis)
- Gastrointestinal (GI) diseases (e.g., ulcerative colitis, regional enteritis)
- Exacerbations of chronic respiratory illnesses such as asthma and chronic obstructive pulmonary disease
- Hematologic disorders (reduce bleeding tendencies)
- Ophthalmic disorders (e.g., nonpyogenic inflammations)

- Organ transplantation (decrease immune response to prevent organ rejection)
- Leukemias and lymphomas (palliative management)
- Nephrotic syndrome (remission of proteinuria)
- Spinal cord injury

Glucocorticoids are also administered by inhalation for the control of steroid-responsive bronchospastic states. However, glucocorticoid inhalers are not used as rescue inhalers for acute bronchospasm. Nasally administered glucocorticoids are used to manage rhinitis and to prevent the recurrence of polyps after surgical removal (see Chapter 36). Topical steroids are used in the management of inflammation of the eye, ear, and skin. Prednisone is the most commonly used oral drug, followed by dexamethasone. Methylprednisolone is the most commonly used injectable glucocorticoid, followed by hydrocortisone and dexamethasone. Betamethasone is the drug of choice for women in premature labor to accelerate fetal lung maturation.

## Contraindications

Contraindications to the administration of glucocorticoids include drug allergy and may include cataracts, glaucoma, peptic ulcer disease, mental health problems, and diabetes mellitus. The adrenal drugs may intensify these diseases. For example, one common adverse effect seen in hospitalized patients is an increase in blood glucose levels, often requiring insulin. This is not to say that diabetic patients who require glucocorticoids should not receive them, but be aware of the potential increases in blood glucose levels. Because of their immunosuppressant properties, glucocorticoids are often avoided in the presence of any serious infection, including septicemia, systemic fungal infections, and varicella. One exception is tuberculous meningitis, for which glucocorticoids may be used to prevent inflammatory central nervous system damage. Caution is emphasized in treating any patient with gastritis, reflux disease, or ulcer disease because of the potential of these drugs to cause gastric perforation, as well as any patient with cardiac, renal, and/or liver dysfunction because of the associated alterations in elimination.

## Adverse Effects

The potent metabolic, physiologic, and pharmacologic effects of the corticosteroids can influence every body system, so these drugs can produce a wide variety of significant undesirable

## TABLE 33-3 SYSTEMIC GLUCOCORTICOIDS: A COMPARISON

| DRUG | ORIGIN | DURATION OF ACTION | EQUIVALENT DOSE (mg)* | SALT AND WATER RETENTION POTENTIAL |
|---|---|---|---|---|
| betamethasone | Synthetic | Long | 0.75 | Very low |
| cortisone | Natural | Short | 25 | High |
| dexamethasone | Synthetic | Long | 0.75 | Very low |
| hydrocortisone | Natural | Short | 20 | High |
| methylprednisolone | Synthetic | Intermediate | 4 | Low |
| prednisolone | Synthetic | Intermediate | 5 | Low |
| prednisone | Synthetic | Intermediate | 5 | Low |
| triamcinolone | Synthetic | Intermediate | 4 | Very low |

*Drugs with higher potency require smaller milligram doses than those with lower potency. This column lists the approximate dose equivalency between different drugs that is expected to achieve a comparable therapeutic effect.

effects. The more common of these are summarized in Table 33-4. Moon facies is a very common adverse effect of long-term use. Two of the adverse effects most commonly seen in hospitalized patients are hyperglycemia and psychosis. The most serious adverse effect of glucocorticoids is adrenal (or HPA) suppression, which is discussed in the drug profiles. Glucocorticoids should be used with caution in patients with heart failure, due to their ability to cause fluid retention.

## Interactions

Systemically administered corticosteroids can interact with many drugs:

- Their use with non–potassium-sparing diuretics (e.g., thiazides, loop diuretics) can lead to severe hypocalcemia and hypokalemia.
- Their use with aspirin, other nonsteroidal antiinflammatory drugs, and other ulcerogenic drugs produces additive GI effects and an increased chance of gastric ulcer development.
- Their use with anticholinesterase drugs produces weakness in patients with myasthenia gravis.
- Their use with immunizing biologics inhibits the immune response to the biologic.
- Their use with antidiabetic drugs may reduce the hypoglycemic effects of the latter and result in elevated blood glucose levels.

Many other drugs can interact with glucocorticoids, including thyroid hormones and antifungal drugs (such as fluconazole), which can decrease renal clearance of the adrenal drug. Barbiturates and hydantoins can increase the metabolism of prednisone and similar drugs. Oral anticoagulants interact with adrenal drugs in ways that can affect the international normalized ratio. Oral contraceptives can increase the half-life of adrenal drugs. Various other drug interactions may be possible between adrenal drugs and over-the-counter drugs and herbals.

## Dosages

For dosage information on adrenal drugs, see the table below.

## DRUG PROFILES
### CORTICOSTEROIDS

The systemic corticosteroids consist of 13 chemically different but pharmacologically similar hormones. They all exert varying degrees of glucocorticoid and mineralocorticoid effects.

### TABLE 33-4 CORTICOSTEROIDS: COMMON ADVERSE EFFECTS

| BODY SYSTEM | ADVERSE EFFECTS |
|---|---|
| Cardiovascular | Heart failure, edema, hypertension—all due to electrolyte imbalances (e.g., hypokalemia, hypernatremia) |
| Central nervous | Convulsions, headache, vertigo, mood swings, psychic impairment, nervousness, insomnia |
| Endocrine | Growth suppression, Cushing's syndrome, menstrual irregularities, carbohydrate intolerance, hyperglycemia, hypothalamic-pituitary-adrenal axis suppression |
| Gastrointestinal | Peptic ulcers with possible perforation, pancreatitis, ulcerative esophagitis, abdominal distension |
| Integumentary | Fragile skin, petechiae, ecchymosis, facial erythema, poor wound healing, hirsutism, urticaria |
| Musculoskeletal | Muscle weakness, loss of muscle mass, osteoporosis |
| Ocular | Increased intraocular pressure, glaucoma, cataracts |
| Other | Weight gain |

## DOSAGES
### Selected Antiadrenal and Corticosteroid Drugs

| DRUG | PHARMACOLOGIC CLASS | USUAL DOSAGE RANGE | INDICATIONS |
|---|---|---|---|
| ◆ aminoglutethimide | Adrenal corticosteroid inhibitor (antiadrenal drug) | **Adult** PO: 250 mg q6h; titrate in increments of 250 mg to a max daily dose of 2000 mg | Cushing's syndrome |
| ◆ fludrocortisone (Florinef) | Synthetic mineralocorticoid | **Adult and pediatric** (including infant) PO: 0.05-0.2 mg q24h | Addison's disease; salt-losing adrenogenital syndrome |
| methylprednisolone (Solu-Medrol) | Systemic corticosteroid | **Adult** IV: 10-120 mg every 6 hr **Pediatric** IV: 0.5 mg/kg every 6 hr | Wide variety of endocrine disorders (including adrenocortical insufficiency) and rheumatic, collagen, dermatologic, allergic, ophthalmic, respiratory, hematologic, neoplastic, GI, and nervous system disorders; edematous states |
| ◆ prednisone (Deltasone, Sterapred, Liquid Pred, others) | Synthetic intermediate-acting glucocorticoid | **Adult** PO: 5-60 mg/day **Pediatric** PO: 0.05-2 mg/kg/day divided daily qid | Wide variety of endocrine disorders (including adrenocortical insufficiency) and rheumatic, collagen, dermatologic, allergic, ophthalmic, respiratory, hematologic, neoplastic, GI, and nervous system disorders; edematous states |

*GI,* Gastrointestinal; *IV,* intravenous; *PO,* oral.

Their differences are due to slight changes in their chemical structures.

Corticosteroid drugs can cross the placenta and produce fetal abnormalities. For this reason, they are classified as pregnancy category C drugs. They can also be secreted in breast milk and cause abnormalities in the nursing infant. Their use is contraindicated in patients who have exhibited hypersensitivity reactions to them in the past as well as in patients with fungal or bacterial infections. Short- or long-term use can lead to a condition known as *steroid psychosis*. One very important point about long-term use of steroids is that they must not be stopped abruptly. These drugs require a tapering of the daily dose, because the administration of these drugs causes the endogenous (body's own) production of the hormones to stop. This is referred to as *HPA* or *adrenal suppression*. This suppression can cause impaired stress response and place the patient at risk of developing hypoadrenal crisis (shock, circulatory collapse) in times of increased stress (i.e., surgery, trauma). Adrenal suppression can occur as early as 1 week after a corticosteroid is started. HPA suppression typically does not occur in patients taking prednisone 5 mg/day (or equivalent) or less. Tapering of daily doses allows the HPA axis the time to recover and to start stimulating the normal production of the endogenous hormones. Patients on long-term steroid therapy who are taking at least 10 mg/day (or equivalent) of prednisone and who undergo trauma or require surgery will need replacement doses of steroids (also known as *stress doses*).

### ♦ fludrocortisone

Fludrocortisone (Florinef) is the most commonly prescribed mineralocorticoid. It is used as partial replacement therapy for adrenocortical insufficiency in Addison's disease and in the treatment of salt-losing adrenogenital syndrome. It is contraindicated in cases of systemic fungal infection. Adverse effects generally relate to water retention and include heart failure, hypertension, and elevated intracerebral pressure (e.g., leading to seizures). Other potential adverse effects involve several body systems and include skin rash, menstrual irregularities, peptic ulcer, hyperglycemia, hypokalemia, muscle pain and weakness, compression bone fractures, glaucoma, and thrombophlebitis, among others. Drugs with which fludrocortisone interacts include anabolic steroids (increased edema); barbiturates, hydantoins, and rifamycins (increased fludrocortisone clearance); estrogens (reduced fludrocortisone clearance); amphotericin B and thiazide and loop diuretics (hypokalemia); anticoagulants (enhanced or reduced anticoagulant activity); antidiabetic drugs (reduced activity leading to hyperglycemia); digoxin (increased risk for dysrhythmias due to fludrocortisone-induced hypokalemia); salicylates (reduced efficacy); and vaccines (increased risk of neurologic complications). Fortunately, adverse effects and serious drug interactions secondary to fludrocortisone therapy are uncommon due to the relatively small dosages of the drug that are normally prescribed. This drug is available only in oral form as a 0.1-mg tablet. It is classified as a pregnancy category C drug. Recommended dosages are given in the table on p. 537.

## Pharmacokinetics

| Route | Onset of Action | Peak Plasma Concentration | Elimination Half-life | Duration of Action |
|---|---|---|---|---|
| PO | 10-20 min | 1.7 hr | 18-36 hr | Unknown |

### ♦ prednisone

Prednisone is one of the four intermediate-acting glucocorticoids; the others are methylprednisolone, prednisolone, and triamcinolone. These drugs have half-lives that are more than double those of the short-acting corticosteroids (2 to 5 hours), and therefore they have longer durations of action. Prednisone is the preferred oral glucocorticoid for antiinflammatory or immunosuppressant purposes. Along with methylprednisolone and prednisolone, it is also used to treat exacerbations of chronic respiratory illnesses such as asthma and chronic bronchitis. Prednisone has only minimal mineralocorticoid properties and therefore alone is inadequate for the management of adrenocortical insufficiency (Addison's disease).

Prednisolone, a prednisone metabolite, is also the liquid drug form of prednisone. Prednisone itself comes in solid form. It is classified as a pregnancy category C drug. Recommended dosages are given in the table on p. 537.

## Pharmacokinetics

| Route | Onset of Action | Peak Plasma Concentration | Elimination Half-life | Duration of Action |
|---|---|---|---|---|
| PO | Unknown | 1-2 hr | 18-36 hr | 36 hr |

### methylprednisolone

Methylprednisolone (Solu-Medrol) is the most commonly used injectable glucocorticoid drug. It is used primarily as an antiinflammatory or immunosuppressant drug. It is usually given intravenously. It is available in a long-acting (depot) formulation as well. Like prednisone, it is classified as a pregnancy category C drug. Most injectable formulations contain a preservative (benzyl alcohol) that cannot be given to children younger than 28 days of age.

## Pharmacokinetics

| Route | Onset of Action | Peak Plasma Concentration | Elimination Half-life | Duration of Action |
|---|---|---|---|---|
| IV | Immediate | 30 min | 3-4 hr | 24-36 hr |

## ANTIADRENAL DRUG

Aminoglutethimide is an adrenal steroid inhibitor. Aminoglutethimide obstructs the normal actions of the adrenal cortex by inhibiting the conversion of cholesterol into adrenal corticosteroids. Aminoglutethimide is indicated for the treatment of Cushing's syndrome, which results from an overproduction of corticosteroids by the adrenal gland. Use of antiadrenals is contraindicated in patients who have shown a previous hypersensitivity reaction to them. The most common adverse effects are nausea, anorexia, dizziness, and skin rash. Adverse effects for which to monitor include jaundice, skin lesions, hypotension, headache, lethargy, weakness, GI upset, and hepatotoxicity.

## ◆ aminoglutethimide

Aminoglutethimide is used in the treatment of Cushing's syndrome, metastatic breast cancer, and adrenal cancer (see Chapters 45 and 46). It is available only in oral form. Aminoglutethimide is classified as a pregnancy category D drug. Recommended dosages are given in the table on p. 537.

### Pharmacokinetics

| Route | Onset of Action | Peak Plasma Concentration | Elimination Half-life | Duration of Action |
|---|---|---|---|---|
| PO | Unknown | Unknown | 9 hr | Unknown |

### ⚡ SAFETY AND QUALITY IMPROVEMENT: PREVENTING MEDICATION ERRORS

#### Look-Alike/Sound-Alike Drugs: Solu-Cortef and Solu-Medrol

Be careful about sound-alike, look-alike drugs! Medication errors often occur when drug names are similar.

Solu-Cortef is a trade name for hydrocortisone; Solu-Medrol is a trade name for methylprednisolone. Both are commonly used glucocorticoids and are given intravenously. However, 4 mg of Solu-Medrol is equivalent to 20 mg of Solu-Cortef; therefore, Solu-Medrol is five times stronger than Solu-Cortef. Despite the similar names, these drugs are not interchangeable!

## NURSING PROCESS

### ASSESSMENT

Before administering any of the *adrenal* or *antiadrenal drugs,* perform a thorough physical assessment to determine the patient's baseline nutritional, hydration, and immune statuses as well as document baseline weight, intake and output, vital signs (especially blood pressure ranges), and the patient's skin condition (noting bruising, fragility, turgor, and color). Assess important baseline laboratory values, including serum sodium, serum potassium, and serum glucose. These specific laboratory tests are important because of the potential drug-related adverse effects (see Table 33-4). For instance, serum potassium levels usually decrease and blood glucose levels increase when a glucocorticoid (e.g., prednisone) is given. In addition, assess and document the patient's muscle strength and body stature. In your assessment, include the identification of potential contraindications, cautions, and drug interactions including interactions with prescription drugs, over-the-counter drugs, and herbals.

For *adrenal drugs,* lifespan considerations include concern about their use during pregnancy and lactation. Growth suppression may occur in children who are receiving long-term adrenal drug therapy (e.g., glucocorticoids) if the epiphyseal plates of the long bones have not closed. However, there may be situations in which the benefits to the therapy outweigh the risks of the drug's adverse effects. Perform and document baseline height and weight measurements in pediatric patients. Elderly patients are more prone to adrenal suppression with prolonged adrenal therapy and may require dosage alterations by the prescriber to minimize the impact of the drug on muscle mass, blood pressure,

and serum glucose and electrolyte levels. Adrenal drugs may exacerbate muscle weakness; produce fatigue; worsen or precipitate osteoporosis, peptic ulcer disease, glaucoma, and cataracts; and increase intraocular pressure. Additionally, because adrenal drugs are associated with the adverse effects of sodium retention, closely assess patients for exacerbation of any preexisting edema and/or cardiac disease. Aminoglutethimide, an antiadrenal drug, requires assessment for contraindications such as noted allergic reaction to the drug. Because of the adverse effects (see previous pharmacology discussion), it is important to assess for history of liver disorders.

### NURSING DIAGNOSES

1. Disturbed body image related to the physiologic effects of diseases of the adrenal gland on the body or the cushingoid appearance caused by glucocorticoid therapy (e.g., prednisone)
2. Excess fluid volume related to the fluid retention associated with glucocorticoid and mineralocorticoid use
3. Risk for infection related to the antiinflammatory, immunosuppressive, metabolic, and dermatologic effects of long-term glucocorticoid therapy

### PLANNING

#### GOALS

1. Patient experiences minimal body image disturbances.
2. Patient exhibits normal fluid volume status during management with glucocorticoid and/or mineralocorticoid therapy.
3. Patient is free from infection during adrenal drug therapy.

#### OUTCOME CRITERIA

1. Patient openly verbalizes fears about body image disturbances and other changes to health care providers, family, and significant others.
2. Patient experiences minimal problems with fluid volume excess and experiences minimal to no edema.
   - Patient performs and records daily weights.
   - Patient reports to the prescriber an increase in weight of more than 2 pounds in 24 hours or 5 pounds or more in 1 week.
3. Patient notifies the prescriber if body temperature is higher than 100° F (38° C).
   - Patient performs frequent mouth and skin care to prevent infections.

### IMPLEMENTATION

It is important to understand how *glucocorticoids* work in the body so that the patient may receive adequate explanations and education to maximize the drug's therapeutic effects and minimize adverse effects. Remember the following points when giving these drugs: (1) Hormone production by the adrenal gland is influenced by time of day and follows a diurnal (daily or 24-hour) pattern with peak levels occurring early in the morning between 6 AM and 8 AM, a decrease during the day,

## CASE STUDY

### Glucocorticoid Drug Therapy

Mr. J., a 68-year-old farmer, has been in the hospital for 1 week because of an exacerbation of chronic emphysema, which was aggravated by dust from the fall harvesting. He has a history of diabetes mellitus type 2. He says that he stopped smoking "4 years ago" and tries to "watch what I eat." He has no history of drug allergies. He is receiving oxygen at 1 L/min through a nasal cannula. At this time, he is breathing more easily and hopes to be going home soon. His medication orders include the following, among others:

- metformin/glipizide (Metaglip) 500 mg/5 mg twice a day by mouth (PO)
- prednisone (Deltasone), 20 mg, every morning PO
- albuterol (Ventolin) inhaler, 2 puffs every 4 hours

Mr. J. is complaining of a headache. When you check the medication sheet, you see two orders:

- acetaminophen (generic), 650 mg PO every 4 hours as needed for pain
- ibuprofen (generic), 200 mg PO every 6 hours as needed for pain

1. Which medication will you choose to give to Mr. J.? Explain your answer.

In the morning, while assessing Mr. J., you notice that he now has increased edema around his ankles, measured at 2+ bilaterally. When you listen to his lungs, you hear scattered rhonchi but no crackles, and his weight has increased since yesterday by 1 kg. When you call his physician, you receive orders for furosemide (Lasix) 40 mg intravenously now, then 20 mg every morning PO. When you check Mr. J.'s fasting fingerstick blood glucose level, the result is 236 mg/dL. Mr. J. is surprised at this result.

2. Considering Mr. J.'s medications, what could be contributing to this elevated glucose level? What other laboratory values need to be monitored closely during this time?

One week later, Mr. J. is discharged. His prednisone prescription contains instructions for tapering the dose over the next 2 weeks. You provide patient teaching for his medication management, and both Mr. and Mrs. J. demonstrate that they understand the information. However, 3 days later, Mr. J. is back in the emergency department with severe nausea, vomiting, and fatigue. His blood pressure is 92/56 mm Hg, and the results of his stat laboratory tests reflect hyponatremia and hyperkalemia. His wife says that he hates the way the "prednisone makes him look and feel" but she thinks he has been taking his medicine.

3. What do you expect happened to cause these symptoms?
4. What nursing diagnoses are appropriate for Mr. J.?

For answers, see http//evolve.elsevier.com/Lilley.

and a lower peak in the late afternoon between 4 PM and 6 PM. (2) Cortisol levels increase in response to both emotional and physiologic stress. (3) Cortisol levels increase when endogenous levels decrease due to a physiologic negative feedback system. (4) When exogenous glucocorticoids are given, endogenous levels decrease; for endogenous production to resume, exogenous levels must be decreased gradually so that hormone output responds to the negative feedback system. (5) The best time to give exogenous glucocorticoids, if at all possible, is early in the morning (6 AM to 9 AM), to minimize the amount of adrenal suppression. It is important to remember, however, that the patient must not alter dosing or abruptly discontinue medication without consulting with the prescriber.

*Prednisone*, a synthetic glucocorticoid, and *fludrocortisone*, a synthetic mineralocorticoid, are given orally. It is recommended that oral dosage forms be given with milk and/or food to help minimize GI upset. Another option is for the prescriber to order an $H_2$ receptor antagonist or a proton pump inhibitor to prevent ulcer formation because these drugs are ulcerogenic. Emphasize to patients the importance of avoiding alcohol, caffeine, and aspirin and other nonsteroidal antiinflammatory drugs to minimize gastric irritation and possible gastric bleeding from the compounding ulcerogenic effects. In long-term therapy, alternate-day dosing of glucocorticoids, if possible, will help minimize the adrenal suppression. Because of delayed wound healing, monitor patients taking these drugs for flulike symptoms, sore throat, and fever. Methylprednisolone, a systemic corticosteroid, is given intravenously. Mix all parenteral forms per manufacturer guidelines, with intravenous doses administered over the recommended time period and in the proper diluent.

With oral and all other forms of glucocorticoids that are given short and/or long term, abrupt withdrawal must be avoided. Abrupt withdrawal of adrenal drugs (e.g., prednisone, methylprednisolone) may lead to a sudden decrease in or no production of endogenous glucocorticoids, resulting in adrenal insufficiency. Signs and symptoms of partial or complete adrenal insufficiency or Addison's disease include fatigue, nausea, vomiting, and hypotension. If left untreated, this condition may lead to an adrenal crisis or a life-threatening state of profound adrenocortical insufficiency requiring immediate medical management. Signs and symptoms include a drop in extracellular fluid volume, hyponatremia, and hyperkalemia. This is also referred to as addisonian crisis.

Other adrenal drug dosage forms include those for intraarticular, intrabursal, intradermal, intralesional, and intrasynovial administration (see Table 33-3). Do not overuse intraarticular injections, and if a joint is injected with medication, the patient needs to rest that area for up to 48 hours after the injection is given. Application of cold packs over the injected area may be indicated for up to the first 24 hours to help minimize the discomfort associated with intraarticular injections. Topical dosage forms (e.g., for skin, eye, or inhalation into the bronchial tree) are also available and must be given exactly as ordered. For dermatologic use, clean and dry the skin before application. Wear gloves and apply the medication with either a sterile tongue depressor or a cotton-tipped applicator. Use sterile technique if the skin is not intact. Nasally administered glucocorticoids (e.g., beclomethasone) must also be used exactly as ordered (see Chapter 36). Any written instructions that come with the product must be read and followed carefully. Before using the nasal sprays (see Chapter 9 for more information), the patient needs to first clear the nasal passages and then use the spray per instructions. After the nasal passages are cleared, the container is placed gently inside the nasal passage and the medication is released at the same time that the patient breathes in through the nose, one nasal passage at a time or as ordered. Instructions for use must be followed exactly.

Glucocorticoid inhalers (e.g., beclomethasone, dexamethasone, flunisolide, triamcinolone, fluticasone) are to be used strictly as ordered; explain the negative consequences of overuse to the patient. Use of these inhaled glucocorticoids may lead to fungal infections (candidiasis) of the oral mucosa and oral cavity, larynx, and pharynx. Therefore, the patient must rinse the mouth and oral mucous membranes with lukewarm water after each use to help prevent fungal overgrowth and further complications. In addition to fungal infections, hoarseness, throat irritation, and dry mouth are also possible adverse effects associated with the use of inhaled glucocorticoids. Occurrence of any of these conditions needs to be reported to the prescriber. See Chapter 9 and Patient Teaching Tips for more information on inhaled dosage forms.

If a patient is receiving long-term maintenance glucocorticoid therapy and requires surgery, recognize the importance of reviewing the patient's medical records for laboratory values, cautions, contraindications, and drug interactions. If the preoperative orders do not include the maintenance dosage of glucocorticoid therapy, contact the surgeon and/or other prescriber and ensure that he or she is aware of the situation and the possible need for a rapid-acting corticosteroid. After surgery, the dosage of steroid may well be increased, with a gradual decrease in dosage over several days until the patient returns to baseline. In addition, you must be constantly aware of the decrease in wound healing in patients taking these drugs on a long-term basis.

In summary, because of their suppressed immune systems, patients taking corticosteroids need to avoid contact with people with known infections and report any fever, increased weakness and lethargy, or sore throat. Monitoring nutritional status, weight, fluid volume, electrolyte status, skin turgor, and glucose levels during therapy is very important to ensure safe and effective therapy. The prescriber needs to be notified if there is any edema, shortness of breath (possible heart failure), joint pain, fever, mood swings, or other unusual symptoms.

## EVALUATION

A therapeutic response to *glucocorticoids* includes a resolution of the underlying manifestations of the disease or pathology, such as a decrease in inflammation, increased feeling of well-being, less pain and discomfort in the joints, decrease in lymphocytes, or other improvement in the condition for which the medication was ordered. Adverse effects include weight gain; increased blood pressure; sodium increase and potassium loss; mental status changes such as mood swings, psychic impairment, and nervousness; abdominal distension; ulcer-related symptoms; and changes in vision. Cushing's syndrome occurs with prolonged or frequent use of glucocorticoids and is characterized by moon face, obesity of the trunk area (often referred to as *belly fat*), increase in blood glucose and sodium levels, loss of serum potassium, wasting of muscle mass, buffalo hump, and other features previously discussed. Cataract formation and osteoporosis may also occur with long-term use. Rapid drops in cortisol levels (e.g., from abrupt withdrawal of medication) may lead to Addison's disease and addisonian crisis (see previous discussions). Therapeutic responses to *aminoglutethimide* include a decrease in the size of the tumor and a decrease in Cushing's syndrome. Adverse effects for which to monitor include nausea, anorexia, dizziness, and skin rash. Other adverse effects to report include jaundice, skin lesions, hypotension, lethargy, weakness, GI upset, and liver toxicity.

## PATIENT TEACHING TIPS

- Gluccocorticoids are to be taken exactly as ordered and never abruptly discontinued. Contact the prescriber if there are situations that prevent proper dosing. Abrupt withdrawal may precipitate adrenal crisis or Addison's disease and/or possible addisonian crisis.
- If a once-a-day dose of glucocorticoids is missed, the patient needs to take the dose as soon as possible after remembering that the dose was missed. If the patient does *not* remember until close to the time for the next dose, then he or she is usually instructed to skip the dose and resume dosing on the next day without doubling up. If any questions arise, the patient needs to clarify with the prescriber. Educate the patient about the adverse effects of long-term therapy, such as changes in body appearance including acne, buffalo hump, obesity of the trunk area, moon face, and thinning of the extremities.
- With glucocorticoid therapy, emphasize the importance of bone health and ways to prevent falls due to the possibility of osteoporosis with long-term use. Foods high in vitamin D include cod liver oil (amount to be recommended by health care provider) and salmon. Foods high in calcium include milk, cheese, yogurt, and ice cream. Fortified dairy products are high in both vitamin D and calcium. The prescriber may suggest a daily supplement of oral calcium and vitamin D.

- Contact the prescriber immediately if any signs and symptoms of acute adrenal insufficiency appear, such as decreased serum sodium and glucose levels, increased potassium levels, dehydration, and weight loss.
- Fludrocortisone, a mineralocorticoid, is better tolerated if taken with food or milk to minimize GI upset. With any of the adrenal drugs, weight gain of 2 pounds or more in 24 hours or 5 pounds or more in 1 week needs to be reported to the prescriber immediately.
- Encourage the patient to keep a journal to document responses to treatment, blood pressure readings, daily weight measurements, mood changes, and any adverse effects.
- Emphasize the importance of follow-up appointments with the prescriber so that electrolyte levels and adverse effects may be monitored. Also, stress the importance of maintaining a low-sodium and high-potassium diet, if ordered.
- Encourage the patient to wear a medical alert identification bracelet or necklace with the diagnosis and a list of medications and allergies. A medical card with important relevant information needs to be kept on the person at all times and updated frequently.

## KEY POINTS

- The adrenal gland is an endocrine organ that is located on top of the kidney and is composed of two distinct tissues: the adrenal cortex and the adrenal medulla. The adrenal medulla secretes two important hormones: epinephrine and norepinephrine; the adrenal cortex secretes two classes of hormones known as *corticosteroids:* glucocorticoids and mineralocorticoids.
- The biologic functions of glucocorticoids include antiinflammatory actions; maintenance of normal blood pressure; carbohydrate, protein, and fat metabolism; and stress effects. The biologic functions of mineralocorticoids include sodium and water resorption, blood pressure control, and maintenance of potassium levels and pH of the blood.
- Patients taking adrenal drugs may receive them by various routes, such as orally, intramuscularly, intravenously, intranasally, intraarticularly, and by inhalation.
- Glucocorticoid inhaled dosage forms are only to be used as prescribed and only after adequate patient education. Rinsing of the mouth after each use is needed to avoid oral fungal infections (oral candidiasis) and oral-pharyngeal irritation.
- Long-term or frequent glucocorticoid use produces increased levels of glucocorticoids, which can lead to Cushing's syndrome. Abrupt withdrawal of glucocorticoids leads to adrenal insufficiency and negative effects on the patient's homeostasis.
- With once-a-day dosing of these drugs, adrenal suppression from corticosteroid therapy can be minimized if the dose is given between 6 AM and 9 AM, but it needs to be given only as ordered.

## NCLEX® EXAMINATION REVIEW QUESTIONS

1 When monitoring for a therapeutic response to aminoglutethimide, the nurse will look for which potential outcomes?
   a Increase in Cushing's syndrome characteristics
   b Decrease in Cushing's syndrome characteristics
   c Increased lymphocyte levels
   d Growth suppression

2 The nurse has provided teaching about oral corticosteroid therapy to a patient. Which statement by the patient shows a need for more teaching?
   a "I will report any fever or sore throat symptoms."
   b "I will stay away from anyone who has a cold or infection."
   c "I can stop this medication if I have severe adverse effects."
   d "I will take this drug with food or milk."

3 During long-term corticosteroid therapy, the nurse will monitor the patient for Cushing's syndrome, which is manifested by
   a weight loss.
   b moon face.
   c hypotension.
   d thickened hair growth.

4 When teaching a patient who has been prescribed a daily dose of prednisone (Deltasone), the nurse knows that the patient will be told to take the medication at which time of day to help reduce adrenal suppression?
   a In the morning
   b At lunchtime
   c At dinnertime
   d At bedtime

5 Which teaching is appropriate for a patient who is taking an inhaled glucocorticoid for asthma?
   a "Exhale while pushing in on the canister of the inhaler."
   b "Blow your nose after taking the medication."
   c "Rinse your mouth thoroughly after taking the medication."
   d "Do not eat immediately after taking the medication."

6 During long-term corticosteroid therapy, the nurse will monitor the patient's laboratory results for adverse effects, such as: (Select all that apply.)
   a Increased serum potassium levels
   b Decreased serum potassium levels
   c Increased sodium levels
   d Decreased sodium levels
   e Hyperglycemia
   f Hypoglycemia

7 The order reads: "Give methylprednisolone (Solu-Medrol) 100 mg IV every 6 hours." The drug is available in vials of 80 mg/mL. How many mL will the nurse draw up for each dose?

1. b, 2. c, 3. b, 4. a, 5. c, 6. b, c, e, 7. 1.25 mL.

For Critical Thinking and Prioritization Questions, see http://evolve.elsevier.com/Lilley.

# Women's Health Drugs

## evolve WEBSITE

*http://evolve.elsevier.com/Lilley*

- Animations
- Answer Key—Textbook Case Studies
- Critical Thinking and Prioritization Questions

- Key Points—Downloadable
- Review Questions for the NCLEX® Examination
- Unfolding Case Studies

## OBJECTIVES

When you reach the end of this chapter, you will be able to do the following:

1 Discuss the normal anatomy and physiology of the female reproductive system.
2 Describe the normal hormonally mediated feedback system that regulates the female reproductive system.
3 Briefly describe the variety of disorders affecting women's health and the drugs used to treat them.
4 Discuss the rationale for use, indications, adverse effects, cautions, contraindications, drug interactions, dosages, and

routes of administration for estrogen, progestins, uterine motility–altering drugs, and osteoporosis drugs.
5 Develop a nursing care plan that includes all phases of the nursing process for patients receiving any of the drugs related to women's health (e.g., estrogens, progestins, uterine mobility–altering drugs, and osteoporosis drugs).

## DRUG PROFILES

- ♦ **alendronate, p. 553**
  **calcitonin, p. 554**
  **clomiphene, p. 555**
  **contraceptive drugs, p. 551**
- ♦ **dinoprostone, p. 556**
- ♦ **estrogen, p. 547**

- ♦ **medroxyprogesterone, p. 549**
  **megestrol, p. 550**
- ♦ **methylergonovine, p. 556**
- ♦ **oxytocin, p. 557**
  **raloxifene, p. 554**

---

♦ *Key drug*

## KEY TERMS

**Chloasma** Hyperpigmentation from the melanin in the skin, characterized by brownish macules on the cheeks, forehead, lips, and/or neck; a common dermatologic adverse effect of female hormonal medications (also called *melasma*). (p. 547)

**Corpus luteum** The structure that forms on the surface of the ovary after every ovulation and acts as a short-lived endocrine organ that secretes progesterone. (p. 545)

**Endocrine glands** Glands that secrete one or more hormones directly into the blood. (p. 544)

**Estrogens** The term for a major class of female sex steroid hormones; of the estrogens, estradiol is responsible for most estrogenic physiologic activity. (p. 544)

**Fallopian tubes** The passages through which ova are carried from the ovary to the uterus. (p. 544)

**Gonadotropin** The hormone that stimulates the testes and ovaries. (p. 544)

**Hormone replacement therapy (HRT)** The term used to describe any replacement of natural body hormones with hormonal drug dosage forms. Most commonly, HRT refers to estrogen replacement therapy for treating symptoms associated with menopause-related estrogen deficiency. It is also referred to as simply hormone therapy. (p. 547)

**Implantation** The attachment to, penetration of, and embedding of the fertilized ovum in the lining of the uterine wall; it is one of the first stages of pregnancy. (p. 545)

**Menarche** The first menses in a young woman's life and the beginning of cyclic menstrual function. (p. 545)

**Menopause** The cessation of menses for 12 consecutive months that marks the end of a woman's childbearing capability. (p. 545)

**Menses** The normal flow of blood that occurs during menstruation. (p. 544)

**Menstrual cycle** The recurring cycle of changes in the endometrium in which the decidual layer is shed, regrows, proliferates, is maintained for several days, and is shed again at menstruation unless a pregnancy begins. Also referred to as the *uterine cycle*. (p. 544)

**Nucleic acids** The term used for specific molecules in the cell that are composed of strings of repeating units that serve to encode information. The two most common ones are DNA and RNA whose functions have to do with the storage and expression of genetic information. (p. 546)

**Osteoporosis** A condition characterized by the progressive loss of bone density and thinning of bone tissue; it is associated with increased risk of fractures. (p. 551)

**Ova** Female reproductive or germ cells (singular: *ovum;* also called *eggs*). (p. 544)

**Ovarian follicles** The location of egg production and ovulation in the ovary; the follicle is the precursor to the corpus luteum. (p. 544)

**Ovaries** The pair of female gonads located on each side of the lower abdomen beside the uterus. They store the *ova* (eggs) and release ova during the ovulation phase of the menstrual cycle. (p. 544)

**Ovulation** The rupture of the ovarian follicle, which results in the release of an unfertilized ovum into the peritoneal cavity, from which it normally enters the fallopian tube. (p. 544)

**Progesterone** A sex hormone that is produced by the corpus luteum and serves to prepare the uterus for possible implantation. (p. 544)

**Progestins** Synthetic or natural substances that have properties similar to progesterone, but are not considered to be the naturally occurring progesterone that is present in the human female body. (p. 549)

**Puberty** The period of life when the ability to reproduce begins. (p. 544)

**Uterus** The hollow, pear-shaped female organ in which the fertilized ovum is implanted (see *implantation*) and the fetus develops. (p. 544)

**Vagina** The part of the female genitalia that forms a canal from its external orifice through its vestibule to the uterine cervix. (p. 544)

## ANATOMY, PHYSIOLOGY, AND PATHOPHYSIOLOGY OVERVIEW

### FEMALE REPRODUCTIVE FUNCTIONS

The female reproductive system consists of the ovaries, fallopian tubes, uterus, vagina, and the external structure known as the *vulva*. The development of these primary sex structures, initiation of their subsequent reproductive functions (starting at puberty), and their maintenance are controlled by pituitary gonadotropin hormones and the female sex steroid hormones—estrogens and progesterone. Pituitary gonadotropins include follicle-stimulating hormone (FSH) and luteinizing hormone (LH). Both play a primary role in hormonal communication between the pituitary gland (see Chapter 30) and the ovaries in the continuous regulation of the menstrual cycle from month to month.

Estrogens are also responsible for stimulating the development of secondary female sex characteristics, including the characteristic breast, skin, and bone development and distribution of body fat and hair. Progesterone helps create optimal conditions for pregnancy in the endometrium just after

ovulation and also promotes the start of menses in the absence of a fertilized ovum.

The ovaries (female gonads) are paired glands located on each side of the uterus. They function both as endocrine glands and as reproductive glands. As reproductive glands, they produce mature ova within ovarian follicles, which are then ovulated or released into the space in the peritoneal cavity between the ovary and the fallopian tube. Fingerlike projections known as *fimbriae* lie adjacent to each ovary and catch the released ovum and guide it into the fallopian tube. Once inside the fallopian tube, the ovum is moved through its lumen to the uterus. This movement is accomplished through the muscular contractions of the tube walls and the actions of ciliated cells inside the lumen of the tube, which "beat" in the direction of the uterus. Fertilization of the ovum, when it occurs, takes place in the fallopian tube.

As endocrine glands, the ovaries are responsible for producing the two sex steroid hormones, estrogen and progesterone. Chemically speaking, the estrogens and progestational hormones include several distinct substances. However, only two of these hormones occur in significant amounts, and have the greatest physiologic activity. These are the estrogen estradiol and the progestational hormone progesterone. Estradiol is the principal secretory product of the ovary and has several estrogenic effects. One of these effects is the regulation of gonadotropin (FSH and LH) secretion via negative feedback to the pituitary gland. Others include promotion of the development of women's secondary sex characteristics, monthly endometrial growth, thickening of the vaginal mucosa, thinning of the cervical mucus, and growth of the ductal system of the breasts. Progesterone is the principle secretory product of the corpus luteum and has progestational effects. These include promotion of tissue growth and secretory activity in the endometrium following the estrogen-driven *proliferative phase* of the menstrual cycle. This important secretory process is required for endometrial egg implantation and maintenance of pregnancy. Other progestational effects include induction of menstruation when fertilization has not occurred and, during pregnancy, inhibition of uterine contractions, increase in the viscosity of cervical mucus (which protects the fetus from external contamination), and growth of the alveolar glands of the breasts.

The uterus consists of three layers: the outer protective *perimetrium*, the muscular *myometrium*, and the inner mucosal layer known as the *endometrium*. The myometrium provides the powerful smooth muscle contractions needed for childbirth. The endometrium is the site of the following:

- Implantation of a fertilized ovum and subsequent development of the fetus
- Initiation of labor and birthing of the infant
- Menstruation

The vagina serves as a common passageway for birthing and menstrual flow. In addition, it is a receptacle for the penis during sexual intercourse and for the sperm after male ejaculation.

The menstrual cycle usually takes roughly 1 month to complete. Menstrual cycles begin during puberty with the first menses (menarche) and cease at menopause, which in most women occurs between 45 and 55 years of age. The hormonally controlled menstrual cycle consists of four distinct but interrelated phases that occur in overlapping sequence. Phase names correspond to activity in either the ovarian follicle or the endometrium (Table 34-1).

- **Phase 1:** the *menstruation phase* (uterine cycle), which initiates the cycle and lasts from 5 to 7 days.
- **Phase 2:** the *follicular phase* (ovarian cycle), during which a mature ovum develops from an ovarian follicle. This phase is also called the *proliferative* or *preovulatory phase* and is characterized by rising estrogen secretion from the ovary and LH secretion from the pituitary gland. It terminates on or about day 14 of the cycle.

- **Phase 3:** the *ovulation phase*, which involves release of the unfertilized ovum from the ovary. This process occurs over a roughly 24- to 48-hour period starting at about day 14. Both estrogen and LH levels peak near this time.
- **Phase 4:** the final phase of the cycle, called the *luteal* or *postovulatory phase*. It is also known as the *secretory phase*. It occurs when the corpus luteum forms from the ruptured ovarian follicle. The corpus luteum is a mass of secretory cells on the surface of the ovary. Its primary function is to produce progesterone, which helps to optimize the endometrial mucosa for implantation of a fertilized ovum. The corpus luteum also serves as an initial source of the progesterone needed during early pregnancy. This function is later assumed by the developing placenta. If fertilization does not occur, the corpus luteum then degenerates causing a fall in progesterone levels. The menstrual cycle begins again on or about day 28.

Figure 34-1 illustrates the sequence of hormone secretions and related events that take place during the menstrual cycle.

## PHARMACOLOGY OVERVIEW

## FEMALE SEX HORMONES
### ESTROGENS

There are three major endogenous estrogens: estradiol, estrone, and estriol. All are synthesized from cholesterol in the ovarian follicles and have the basic chemical structure of a steroid, known as the *steroid nucleus*. For this reason, they are sometimes referred to as *steroid hormones*. Estradiol is the principal and most active of the three and represents the end product of estrogen synthesis.

Exogenous estrogenic drugs, those used as drug therapy, were developed because most of the endogenous estrogens are inactive when taken orally. These synthetic drugs fall into two categories: steroidal and nonsteroidal. Nonsteroidal estrogen products are no longer available in the United States because major adverse effects occurred when one of them, diethylstilbestrol (DES), was used in obstetrics. Box 34-1 describes this important episode in medical history. The estrogenic drugs currently in use are as follows:

- Conjugated estrogens (Premarin)
- Esterified estrogens (Estratab)
- Estradiol transdermal (Estraderm, Climara, Vivelle)
- Estradiol cypionate (Depo-Estradiol, DepoGen)
- Estradiol valerate (Delestrogen)
- Ethinyl estradiol (Estinyl)
- Estradiol vaginal dosage forms (Vagifem, Estrace Vaginal Cream)
- Estrone (Estrone Aqueous)
- Estropipate (Ogen, Ortho-Est)

The most widely used estrogen product is an estrogen mixture known as *conjugated estrogens*. This mixture contains a combination of natural estrogen compounds equivalent to the average estrogen composition of the urine of pregnant mares, hence its brand name of Premarin. A nonanimal source for this conjugated estrogen mixture is also available. Cenestin is

| | OVARIAN FOLLICLE | ENDOMETRIUM |
|---|---|---|
| **PHASE** | **ACTIVITY** | **ACTIVITY** |
| Phase 1 | Menstruation | Menstruation |
| Phase 2 | Follicular phase (preovulatory) | Proliferative phase |
| Phase 3 | Ovulation | Ovulation |
| Phase 4 | Luteal phase (postovulatory) | Secretory phase |

**TABLE 34-1   PHASES OF THE MENSTRUAL CYCLE**

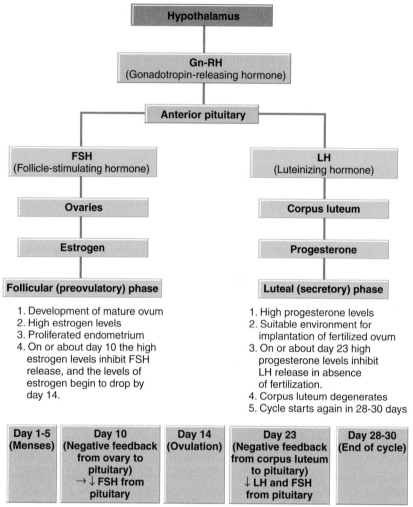

**FIGURE 34-1** Hormonal activity during the monthly menstrual cycle. Gonadotropin-releasing hormone (Gn-RH) from the hypothalamus stimulates the pituitary gland, causing it to secrete follicle-stimulating hormone (FSH) early in the cycle (coinciding with the menses) and later luteinizing hormone (LH). FSH stimulates the ovaries to produce estrogen (primarily estradiol). Later in the cycle, the combined surges in the levels of estrogen, Gn-RH, FSH, and LH stimulate ovulation. The corpus luteum then secretes estrogen and progesterone, which provide negative feedback to the hypothalamus and pituitary gland to reduce Gn-RH, FSH, and LH secretions. If the ovum (egg) is not fertilized by a spermatozoon, levels of estrogen and progesterone then fall to their monthly lows, Gn-RH and FSH rise again, and the onset of menses begins a new cycle.

---

### BOX 34-1    DIETHYLSTILBESTROL

Between 1940 and 1971, an estimated 6 million mothers and their fetuses were exposed to diethylstilbestrol (DES). The drug was used to prevent reproductive problems such as miscarriage, premature delivery, intrauterine fetal death, and toxemia. This use resulted in significant complications of the reproductive system in both female and male offspring. Two large groups have been established to monitor these complications: the Registry for Research on Hormonal Transplacental Carcinogenesis and the National Cooperative Diethylstilbestrol Adenosis (DESAD) Project.

---

composed of various conjugated estrogens obtained from soy and yam plants. This product was developed in response to consumer demand from women who wanted an alternative to an animal-derived product (see the Safety: Herbal Therapies and Dietary Supplements box on p. 547). Some women obtain other natural estrogen products from naturopathic prescribers and prefer these to standard prescription drugs such as Premarin.

Patients report varying degrees of satisfaction with the numerous products available, and it can take both time and patience to find the best choice for a given individual. Ethinyl estradiol is one of the more potent estrogens and is most commonly found in oral contraceptive drugs. Another commonly used form of estrogen is the patch formulation. Several patches exist, all of which are dosed differently, thus patient education is necessary to ensure proper use. The most commonly used patch is Climara (estradiol).

## Mechanism of Action and Drug Effects

The binding of estrogen to intracellular estrogen receptors stimulates the synthesis of nucleic acids (deoxyribonucleic acid [DNA] and ribonucleic acid [RNA]) and proteins, which

## SAFETY: HERBAL THERAPIES AND DIETARY SUPPLEMENTS

### Soy (Glycine max)

**Overview**
Soy is a bean commonly grown throughout the world. The isoflavones in soy are chemically similar to the female hormone estradiol. Some studies have shown soy to be useful in the prevention of menopausal symptoms in perimenopausal women. Estrasorb is a new form of estrogen therapy that is a soy-based emulsion applied like a lotion. Other studies have found that soy reduces both low-density lipoprotein and total cholesterol levels.

**Common Uses**
Reduction of cholesterol level, relief of menopause symptoms (alternative to hormonal therapy), osteoporosis prevention

**Adverse Effects**
Nausea, bloating, diarrhea, abdominal pain (ingested forms), and hypersensitivity reaction have been reported from soy. When Estrasorb is used, it has been found that estradiol is still present on the skin up to 8 hours after application and can transfer to men, which results in increased estradiol levels.

**Potential Drug Interactions**
Orally administered soy may interfere with thyroid hormone absorption (avoid concurrent use).

**Contraindications**
Allergy to soy products; Estrasorb shares the same contraindications as other estrogen products
Follow manufacturer directions on the label for use of specific preparations.

are the building blocks for all living tissue. Estrogens are also required at puberty for the development and maintenance of the female reproductive system and the development of female secondary sex characteristics, a process known as *feminization.*

Estrogens produce their effects in estrogen-responsive tissues, which have a large number of estrogen receptors. These tissues include the female genital organs, the breasts, the pituitary gland, and the hypothalamus. At the time of puberty, the production of estrogen increases greatly. This causes initiation of the menses, breast development, redistribution of body fat, softening of the skin, and other feminizing changes. Estrogens play a role in the shaping of body contours and development of the skeleton. For instance, long bones are usually inhibited from growing, with the result that females are usually shorter than males.

## Indications

Estrogens are used in the treatment or prevention of a variety of disorders that result primarily from estrogen deficiency. These conditions are listed in Box 34-2. Hormone replacement therapy (HRT) to counter such estrogen deficiency is most commonly known for its benefits in treating menopausal symptoms (e.g., hot flashes).

## Contraindications

Contraindications for estrogen administration include known drug allergy, any estrogen-dependent cancer, undiagnosed

### BOX 34-2   INDICATIONS FOR ESTROGEN THERAPY

- Atrophic vaginitis (shrinkage of the vagina and/or urethra)
- Hypogonadism
- Oral contraception (in combination with a progestin)
- Ovarian failure or castration (or removal of ovaries)
- Uterine bleeding
- Breast or prostate cancer (palliative treatment of advanced inoperable cases)
- Osteoporosis (treatment and prophylaxis)
- Vasomotor symptoms of menopause (e.g., hot flashes)

abnormal vaginal bleeding, pregnancy, and active thromboembolic disorder (e.g., stroke, thrombophlebitis) or a history of such a disorder.

## Adverse Effects

The most serious adverse effects of the estrogens are thromboembolic events. The most common undesirable effect of estrogen use is nausea. Photosensitivity also may occur with estrogen therapy. One common dermatologic effect of note is chloasma. Chloasma consists of brownish, macular spots that often occur on the forehead, cheeks, lips, and neck. This and other adverse effects are listed in Table 34-2.

## Interactions

Estrogens can decrease the activity of the oral anticoagulants, and the concurrent administration of rifampin and St. John's wort can decrease their estrogenic effect. Their use with tricyclic antidepressants may promote toxicity of the antidepressant. Smoking should be avoided during estrogen therapy, because this, too, can diminish the estrogenic effect and add to the risk for thrombosis.

## Dosages

For dosage information on some of the many available estrogen products, see the table on p. 548.

## DRUG PROFILE

### ◆ estrogen

Estrogen is indicated for the treatment of many clinical conditions, primarily those resulting from estrogen deficiency (see Box 34-2). Many of these conditions occur around menopause, when the endogenous estradiol level is declining. Any estrogen capable of binding to the estrogen receptors in target organs can alleviate menopausal symptoms. As a general rule, the smallest dosage of estrogen that relieves the symptoms or prevents the condition is used. Although many women receive estrogen or estrogen-progestin therapy for many months or years, some clinicians (and patients) may prefer that the patient be weaned from such therapy in light of the known adverse effects.

Two studies that were performed as part of the Women's Health Initiative (WHI), a large research program sponsored by the National Institutes of Health, demonstrated the possible detrimental effects of estrogen and estrogen-progestin therapy.

## DOSAGES

### Selected Estrogenic Drugs

| DRUG (PREGNANCY CATEGORY) | PHARMACOLOGIC CLASS | USUAL DOSAGE RANGE | INDICATIONS |
|---|---|---|---|
| ◆ conjugated estrogens (Cenestin, Premarin) (X) and esterified estrogens (Estratab, Menest) (X) | Estrogenic hormone mixture | PO: 0.3-1.25 mg/day<br>PO: 0.625-1.25 mg/day<br><br>PO: 1.25 mg/day cyclically, 3 wk on, 1 wk off<br>PO: 0.3-0.625 mg/day cyclically<br>PO: 1.25 mg q4h × 24 hr, then 1.25 mg daily × 7-10 days | Atrophic vaginitis<br>Vasomotor symptoms of menopause<br><br>Female castration, ovarian failure<br>Female hypogonadism<br>Abnormal uterine bleeding |
| estradiol (Estrace) (X) | Estrogenic hormone | 1-2 mg daily<br><br>PO: 0.5 mg daily cyclically | Vasomotor symptoms of menopause, female castration, ovarian failure<br>Osteoporosis prophylaxis |
| estradiol transdermal (Estraderm, FemPatch, Vivelle, Climara, Menostar) (X) | Estrogenic hormone | Transdermal patch: 1 patch applied once or twice weekly to lower abdomen (not breast) ranging from 0.025 to 0.1 mg (instructions may vary by product) | Vasomotor symptoms of menopause |

*PO*, Oral.

| TABLE 34-2 | ESTROGENS: COMMON ADVERSE EFFECTS |
|---|---|
| **BODY SYSTEM** | **ADVERSE EFFECTS** |
| Cardiovascular | Hypertension, thrombophlebitis, edema |
| Gastrointestinal | Nausea, vomiting, diarrhea, constipation |
| Genitourinary | Amenorrhea, breakthrough uterine bleeding, enlarged uterine fibromyomas |
| Dermatologic | Chloasma (facial skin discoloration; also called *melasma*), hirsutism, alopecia |
| Other | Tender breasts, fluid retention, decreased carbohydrate tolerance, headaches |

Both studies attempted to determine the value of HRT, if any, in preventing diseases and conditions commonly affecting older women, including breast cancer, heart disease, stroke, and hip fracture. The WHI was launched in 1991 under the direction of the National Heart, Lung, and Blood Institute (NHLBI). In one of the WHI studies of HRT, research subjects who took a certain estrogen-progestin combination product were found to have an increased risk of breast cancer, heart disease, stroke, and blood clots, although their risk of hip fractures and colon cancer was reduced. These preliminary results were so alarming that this study of combined estrogen-progestin therapy was discontinued in 2002.

A part of the WHI investigation focusing on cognitive function, the WHI Memory Study, also identified adverse cognitive effects in women receiving combination estrogen-progestin therapy. These patients showed an increased risk of developing dementia and demonstrated reduced performance on tests of cognitive function. A second HRT study was begun in which women who had undergone hysterectomy received estrogen alone without progestin. In March 2004, however, these participants were advised to stop taking their assigned medication, because the estrogen-only therapy appeared to be associated with an increased risk of stroke. The data also indicated that

estrogen therapy had no effect on the rates of coronary heart disease or breast cancer but was associated with a reduced rate of hip fracture.

Since publication of the WHI studies, much confusion and controversy has arisen. One of the biggest challenges to the WHI study is that the majority of the women studied were at least 10 years postmenopause. Recent data have suggested that the use of estrogen in women who are younger is beneficial. Follow-up of the WHI study subjects began in 2010. The North American Menopause Society (NAMS) also updated its position statement in 2010 regarding estrogen use in perimenopausal and postmenopausal women. The updated recommendations support the initiation of HT (hormonal therapy) around the time of menopause to treat menopause-related symptoms and to treat or reduce the risk of certain disorders, such as osteoporosis or fractures. The benefit-risk ratio for menopausal HT is favorable for women who initiate HT close to menopause but decreases in older women and with time since menopause. Hormone replacement is not recommended for women with histories of endometrial cancer. In women with breast cancer, estrogen therapy has not been proven safe and might raise recurrence risk. When hormone therapy is discontinued after several years of use, assess bone-mineral density and begin treatment if indicated. Because this is a topic about which views are so rapidly changing, the reader is referred to the website of the North American Menopause Society at www.menopause.org for the latest position statements.

The pharmacologic effects of all estrogens are similar because there are only slight differences in their chemical structures. These differences yield drugs of different potencies, which in turn make them useful for a variety of indications. They also allow the drugs to be given by different routes of administration and at often highly customized dosages.

Many fixed estrogen-progestin combination products have been developed over the years. Their use is commonly referred to as *continuous combined hormone replacement therapy.* The use of estrogen therapy alone has been associated with an increased risk of endometrial hyperplasia, a possible precursor of endometrial cancer. The addition of continuously administered progestin to an estrogen regimen reduces the incidence of endometrial hyperplasia associated with unopposed estrogen therapy. Examples of these fixed combinations are conjugated estrogens with medroxyprogesterone, norethindrone acetate with ethinyl estradiol, and estradiol with norethindrone.

## PROGESTINS

Available progestational medications, or progestins, include both natural and synthetic drugs. Progesterone is the most active natural progestational hormone and is the primary progestin component in most drug formulations. It is produced by the corpus luteum after each ovulation and during pregnancy by the placenta. In addition, there are two other major natural progestational hormones. The first is 17-hydroxyprogesterone, an inactive metabolite of progesterone. The second is pregnenolone, a chemical precursor to all steroid hormones that is synthesized from cholesterol in the ovary. Because orally administered progesterone is relatively inactive and parenterally administered progesterone causes local reactions and pain, chemical derivatives were developed that are effective orally and are also more potent. Their actions are also more specific and of longer duration. The following are some of the most commonly used progestins:

- Hydroxyprogesterone (Hylutin)
- Levonorgestrel (Plan B)
- Medroxyprogesterone (Provera, Depo-Provera)
- Megestrol (Megace)
- Norethindrone acetate (Aygestin)
- Norgestrel (Ovrette, Ovral)
- Progesterone (Prometrium)
- Etonogestrel implant (Implanon)

### Mechanism of Action and Drug Effects

All of the progestin products produce the same physiologic responses as those produced by progesterone itself. These responses include induction of secretory changes in the endometrium, including diminished endometrial tissue proliferation; an increase in the basal body temperature; thickening of the vaginal mucosa; relaxation of uterine smooth muscle; stimulation of mammary alveolar tissue growth; feedback inhibition (negative feedback) of the release of pituitary gonadotropins (FSH and LH); and alterations in menstrual blood flow, especially in the presence of estrogen.

### Indications

Progestins are useful in the treatment of functional uterine bleeding caused by a hormonal imbalance, fibroids, or uterine cancer; in the treatment of primary and secondary amenorrhea; in the adjunctive and palliative treatment of some cancers and endometriosis; and, alone or in combination with estrogens, in the prevention of conception. They may also be helpful in preventing a threatened miscarriage and alleviating the symptoms of premenstrual syndrome. Medroxyprogesterone

| TABLE 34-3 | PROGESTINS: COMMON ADVERSE EFFECTS | |
|---|---|
| **BODY SYSTEM** | **ADVERSE EFFECTS** |
| Gastrointestinal | Nausea, vomiting |
| Genitourinary | Amenorrhea, spotting |
| Other | Edema, weight gain or loss, rash, pyrexia, somnolence or insomnia, depression |

is the one most commonly used. Norethindrone and norgestrel are commonly used alone or in combination with estrogens as contraceptives. Megestrol is commonly used as adjunct therapy in the treatment of breast and endometrial cancers. When estrogen replacement therapy is initiated after menopause, progestins are often included to decrease the endometrial proliferation that can be caused by unopposed estrogen in women with an intact uterus. Formulations of progesterone itself are also used to treat female infertility (see Dosages table on p. 550).

### Contraindications

Contraindications for progestin are similar to those for estrogens.

### Adverse Effects

The most serious undesirable effects of progestin use include liver dysfunction, commonly manifested as jaundice, thrombophlebitis, and thromboembolic disorders such as pulmonary embolism. The more common adverse effects are listed in Table 34-3.

### Interactions

There are reports of possible decreases in glucose tolerance when progestins are taken with antidiabetic drugs, and the dosage of the antidiabetic drug may need to be adjusted. The concurrent use of medroxyprogesterone or norethindrone and aminoglutethimide or rifampin induces increased metabolism of the progestin.

### Dosages

For recommended dosages of selected progestins, see the Dosages table on p. 550.

## DRUG PROFILES

### ◆ medroxyprogesterone

Medroxyprogesterone (Provera, Depo-Provera) inhibits the secretion of pituitary gonadotropins, which prevents follicular maturation and ovulation, stimulates the growth of mammary tissue, and has an antineoplastic action against endometrial cancer. Medroxyprogesterone is used to treat uterine bleeding, secondary amenorrhea, endometrial cancer, and renal cancer and is also used as a contraceptive. Its most common use is to prevent endometrial cancer caused by estrogen replacement therapy. It is also sometimes used as adjunct therapy in certain types of cancer (see Chapter 46). Medroxyprogesterone is available in both oral and parenteral preparations. It is also available in a long-acting injection formulation called Depo-Provera.

## DOSAGES

*Selected Progestational Drugs*

| DRUG (PREGNANCY CATEGORY) | PHARMACOLOGIC CLASS | USUAL DOSAGE RANGE | INDICATIONS |
|---|---|---|---|
| ◆ medroxyprogesterone acetate (Provera, others) (X) | Progestin | PO: 5-10 mg/day for set number of days or cyclically (smaller doses may be given on a continuous daily basis) | Amenorrhea, uterine bleeding |
| | | PO: 5-10 mg/day on last 10-13 days of each month to accompany estrogen dosing | Vasomotor symptoms of menopause |
| megestrol (Megace) (X) | | 400-800 mg/day | Severe weight loss in male and female patients with HIV/AIDS |
| | | PO: 40 mg bid-qid | Uterine bleeding |

*AIDS,* Acquired immunodeficiency syndrome; *HIV,* human immunodeficiency virus (infection); *PO,* oral.

Depo-Provera is used for birth control, and one shot protects the woman for 3 months. There is concern about its use in women younger than 25 years of age and use for longer than 2 years due to the potential for bone density loss.

### Pharmacokinetics

| Route | Onset of Action | Peak Plasma Concentration | Elimination Half-life | Duration of Action |
|---|---|---|---|---|
| IM | Unknown | 2-7 hr | 14.5 hr | 3 mo |

### megestrol

Megestrol (Megace) is a synthetic progestin that is structurally very similar to progesterone. Although megestrol shares the actions of the progestins, it is primarily used in the palliative management of recurrent, inoperable, or metastatic endometrial or breast cancer. Because it can cause appetite stimulation and weight gain, it is also used in the management of anorexia, cachexia, or unexplained substantial weight loss in patients with acquired immunodeficiency syndrome (AIDS) and in patients with cancer. It is available only for oral use.

### Pharmacokinetics

| Route | Onset of Action | Peak Plasma Concentration | Elimination Half-life | Duration of Action |
|---|---|---|---|---|
| PO | 6-8 wk | 1-3 hr | 13-105 hr | 4-10 mo |

## CONTRACEPTIVE DRUGS

Contraceptive drugs are medications used to prevent pregnancy. Contraceptive devices are nondrug methods of pregnancy prevention such as intrauterine devices, male and female condoms, cervical diaphragms, and others, which are beyond the scope of a pharmacology text. Patients must be informed, for their own safety, of the fact that contraceptive drug therapy serves only to prevent pregnancy and does not protect them from sexually transmitted diseases, including human immunodeficiency virus (HIV) infection/AIDS. This includes even spermicidal drugs such as the over-the-counter (OTC) foams for intravaginal use. These products most often contain the spermicide nonoxynol-9, which does kill sperm cells to prevent

pregnancy but does not necessarily kill microbes capable of causing sexually transmitted diseases, including HIV infection.

Aside from sexual abstinence, oral contraceptives are the most effective form of birth control currently available. Estrogen-progestin combinations, often referred to as "the pill," are oral contraceptives that contain both estrogenic and progestational steroids. The most common estrogenic component is ethinyl estradiol, a semisynthetic steroidal estrogen. The most common progestin component is norethindrone.

The currently available oral contraceptives may be *biphasic, triphasic,* or *monophasic,* in terms of the doses taken at different times of the menstrual cycle. The newest are the extended-cycle oral contraceptives. The biphasic drugs contain a fixed estrogen dose combined with a low progestin dose for the first 10 days and a higher dose for the rest of the cycle and are available in 21- or 28-day dosage packages. The triphasic oral contraceptives contain three different estrogen-progestin dose ratios that are administered sequentially during the cycle and are provided in 21- or 28-day dosage packages. The triphasic products most closely duplicate the normal hormonal levels of the female cycle. These contraceptives also come in monophasic forms, in which the estrogen and progestin doses are the same throughout the cycle. There are also oral contraceptives that are progestin-only drugs. The monophasic and triphasic oral contraceptives are the most numerous on the market and the most widely prescribed. The extended-cycle oral contraceptives differ from the traditional 21 days on, 7 days off pills by decreasing or eliminating the hormone-free dosing interval. Consecutive days of hormonal therapy may extend to 84 to 365 days. Reasons for switching to an extended-cycle product include improved efficacy in women who forget to restart the pill and patient preference to decrease the frequency of menstrual bleeding. Some patients (e.g., those with menstrual irregularities) may require special assistance in selecting drug products with their prescribers. Three other important contraceptive medications are a long-acting injectable form of medroxyprogesterone, a transdermal contraceptive patch, and, most recently, an intravaginal contraceptive ring.

## Mechanism of Action and Drug Effects

Contraceptive drugs prevent ovulation by inhibiting the release of gonadotropins and by increasing uterine mucous viscosity, which results in (1) decreased sperm movement and fertilization of the ovum, and (2) possible inhibition of implantation (nidation) of a fertilized egg (zygote) into the endometrial lining.

Oral contraceptives have many of the same hormonal effects as those normally produced by endogenous estrogens and progesterone. The contraceptive effect results mainly from the suppression of the hypothalamic-pituitary system, which in turn prevents ovulation. Other incidental benefits to their use are that they improve menstrual cycle regularity and decrease blood loss during menstruation. A decreased incidence of functional ovarian cysts and ectopic pregnancies has also been associated with their use.

## Indications

Oral contraceptive drugs are primarily used to prevent pregnancy. In addition, they are used to treat endometriosis and hypermenorrhea and to produce cyclic withdrawal bleeding in patients with amenorrhea. Occasionally combination oral contraceptives are used to provide postcoital emergency contraception. Emergency contraception pills are not effective if the woman is already pregnant (i.e., egg implantation has occurred). They should therefore be taken within 72 hours of unprotected intercourse with a follow-up dose 12 hours after the first dose. They are intended to prevent pregnancy after known or suspected contraceptive failure or unprotected intercourse. Preven, Plan B, Alesse, and Ella are drugs used for this indication. One oral contraceptive of note is Seasonale (extended cycle), which includes both estrogen and progestin components. It is sold in packages containing 3 months' worth of medication, including 1 week's worth of nonhormonal tablets. This is because Seasonale reduces a woman's menstrual cycles to once every 3 months.

## Contraindications

Contraindications to the use of oral contraceptives include known drug allergy to a specific product, pregnancy, and known high risk for or history of thromboembolic events such as myocardial infarction, venous thrombosis, pulmonary embolism, or stroke.

## Adverse Effects

Common adverse effects associated with the use of oral contraceptives are listed in Table 34-4. These effects include hypertension, thromboembolism, alterations in carbohydrate and lipid metabolism, increases in serum hormone concentrations, and alterations in serum metal and plasma protein levels. It is the estrogen component that appears to be the source of most of these metabolic effects.

## Interactions

Several drugs and drug classes can potentially reduce the effectiveness of oral contraceptives, which can possibly result in an unintended pregnancy. Educate patients about the need to use alternative birth control methods for at least 1 month during and after taking any of the following drugs: antibiotics (especially penicillins and cephalosporins), barbiturates, isoniazid, and rifampin. The effectiveness of other drugs,

| TABLE 34-4 | ORAL CONTRACEPTIVES: COMMON ADVERSE EFFECTS |
|---|---|
| **BODY SYSTEM** | **ADVERSE EFFECTS** |
| Cardiovascular | Hypertension, edema, thromboembolism, pulmonary embolism, myocardial infarction |
| Central nervous | Dizziness, headache, migraines, depression, stroke |
| Gastrointestinal | Nausea, vomiting, diarrhea, anorexia, cramps, constipation, increased weight, cholestatic jaundice |
| Genitourinary | Amenorrhea, cervical erosion, breakthrough bleeding, dysmenorrhea, breast changes |

such as anticonvulsants, beta-blockers, hypnotics, antidiabetic drugs, warfarin, theophylline, tricyclic antidepressants, and vitamins, may be reduced when they are taken with oral contraceptives.

## Dosages

For the recommended dosages of oral contraceptives, see the Dosages table on p. 552.

## DRUG PROFILE
### CONTRACEPTIVE DRUGS

The Dosages table on p. 552 provides selected examples of the many contraceptive drugs available. All work in similar fashion to prevent pregnancy. They are classified as pregnancy category X drugs by the U.S. Food and Drug Administration (FDA). Drugs that are intended for termination of pregnancy are known as *abortifacients* and are discussed later in this chapter.

## DRUGS FOR OSTEOPOROSIS

Approximately 8 million women in the United States are currently affected by osteoporosis, or low bone mass with increased risk of fracture. Nearly 40% of U.S. women over 50 years of age will develop an osteoporotic fracture, and the annual costs to society equal nearly $11 billion. Risk factors for postmenopausal osteoporosis include white or Asian descent, slender body build, early estrogen deficiency, smoking, alcohol consumption, low-calcium diet, sedentary lifestyle, and family history of osteoporosis. Although osteoporosis is primarily a disorder that affects women, up to 20% of individuals with this condition are men.

Supplementation with calcium and vitamin D are thought to play a role in the prevention of this common bone disorder. Current recommendations are that women, especially those older than age 60, *consider* taking calcium and vitamin D supplements for bone health.

Several drug classes are used for the treatment of existing osteoporosis: the bisphosphonates, the selective estrogen receptor modulators (SERMs), the hormones calcitonin and teriparatide, and most recently, denosumab. Currently available bisphosphonates used for osteoporosis prevention and treatment include alendronate, ibandronate, risedronate, and the once-a-year injection zoledronic acid. Raloxifene and tamoxifen

## DOSAGES

### *Selected Contraceptive Drugs*

| DRUG (PREGNANCY CATEGORY) | PHARMACOLOGIC CLASS | USUAL DOSAGE RANGE | INDICATIONS/USES |
|---|---|---|---|
| **Oral Contraceptives** | | | |
| norethindrone and ethinyl estradiol (Ortho-Novum, Necon, Jenest, others) (X) | Biphasic: fixed estrogen–variable progestin 21- or 28-day products | For the most reliable contraceptive action, the patient must take all preparations according to instructions from prescriber or patient information product insert, at intervals not to exceed 24 hr | |
| norethindrone and ethinyl estradiol (Loestrin, Modicon, Necon, others) (X) | Monophasic: fixed estrogen-progestin combinations; 21- or 28-day products; 28-day products contain 7 inert tabs | | |
| norethindrone and ethinyl estradiol (Ortho-Novum 7/7/7, Estrostep, Tri-Norinyl, others) (X) | Triphasic: 3 or 4 monthly phases of variable estrogen and progestin combinations; 21- or 28-day products; 28-day products contain 7 inert tabs | | |
| levonorgestrel and ethinyl estradiol (Seasonale, Yaz, Lybrel, others) | Extended-cycle products | | Prevention of pregnancy |
| **Injectable Contraceptives (Depot)** | | | |
| medroxyprogesterone (Depo-Provera) (X) | Progestin-only injectable contraceptive | IM: 150 mg q3mo | |
| **Transdermal Contraceptives** | | | |
| norelgestromin and ethinyl estradiol (X) | Fixed-combination estrogen-progestin transdermal contraceptive | Transdermal patch: 1 patch applied weekly × 3 wk each month, scheduled around menses in wk 4 | |
| **Intravaginal Contraceptives** | | | |
| etonogestrel–ethinyl estradiol vaginal ring (NuvaRing) (X) | Fixed-combination estrogen-progestin intravaginal contraceptive | 1 ring inserted into vagina by patient and left in place for 3 wk, followed by removal for 1 wk; new ring is then inserted | |

*IM,* Intramuscular.

are the currently available SERMs. Tamoxifen is primarily used in oncology settings and is discussed further in Chapter 46. Raloxifene is indicated for use in the prevention and treatment of osteoporosis. A drug form of the hormone calcitonin is also commonly used. Teripartide stimulates bone formation, while denosumab (Prolia) prevents bone resorption.

## Mechanism of Action and Drug Effects

### Bisphosphonates

The bisphosphonates work by inhibiting osteoclast-mediated bone resorption, which in turn indirectly enhances bone mineral density. *Osteoclasts* are bone cells that break down bone, causing calcium to be reabsorbed into the circulation; this resorption eventually leads to osteoporosis if not controlled or countered by adequate new bone formation. Strong clinical evidence indicates reversal of lost bone mass and reduction of facture risk, and, as a result, these drugs are considered drugs of choice for this condition.

### Selective Estrogen Receptor Modulators

Raloxifene helps prevent osteoporosis by stimulating estrogen receptors on bone and increasing bone density in a manner similar to that of the estrogens themselves.

### Calcitonin

Like the natural thyroid hormone, calcitonin directly inhibits osteoclastic bone resorption.

### Teriparatide

In contrast to the other therapies described thus far, which inhibit bone resorption, teriparatide is the first and currently the only drug available that acts by stimulating bone formation. It is a derivative of parathyroid hormone and works to treat osteoporosis by modulating the body's metabolism of calcium and phosphorus in a manner similar to that of the natural parathyroid hormone.

### Denosumab

Denosumab (Prolia) is a monoclonal antibody that blocks osteoclast activation, thereby preventing bone resorption. It is given as a subcutaneous injection once every 6 months along with daily calcium and vitamin D. Denosumab is used in the treatment of osteoporosis and bone metastases.

## Indications

Raloxifene is primarily used for the prevention of postmenopausal osteoporosis. The bisphosphonates are used in both the prevention and treatment of osteoporosis. Teriparatide is used primarily for the subset of osteoporosis patients at highest risk of fracture (e.g., those with prior fracture), and calcitonin is used for treatment of osteoporosis.

## Contraindications

### Bisphosphonates

Contraindications to bisphosphonate use include drug allergy, hypocalcemia, esophageal dysfunction, and the inability to sit or stand upright for at least 30 minutes after taking the medication.

### Selective Estrogen Receptor Modulators

The use of SERMs is contraindicated in women with a known allergy to these drugs, in women who are or may become pregnant, and in women with a venous thromboembolic disorder, including deep vein thrombosis, pulmonary embolism, and retinal vein thrombosis, or with a history of such a disorder.

### Calcitonin

Contraindications to calcitonin use include drug allergy or allergy to salmon (the drug is salmon derived).

### Teriparatide

Contraindications to the use of teriparatide include drug allergy.

### Denosumab

Contraindications to the use of denosumab are hypocalcemia, renal impairment or failure, and infection.

## Adverse Effects

The primary adverse effects of SERMs are hot flashes and leg cramps. They can increase the risk of venous thromboembolism and are teratogenic. Leukopenia may also occur and predispose the patient to various infections. The most common adverse effects of bisphosphonates are headache, gastrointestinal (GI) upset, and joint pain. However, the bisphosphonates are usually well tolerated. There is a risk of esophageal burns with these medications if they become lodged in the esophagus before reaching the stomach. For this reason the patient must take these medications with a full glass of water and must remain sitting upright or standing for at least 30 minutes afterward. Several case reports of osteonecrosis of the jaw in patients taking bisphosphonates have been released. The FDA issued a public health advisory in January 2008 alerting practitioners to the possible association between bisphosphonate use and the development of severe (possibly incapacitating) bone, muscle, and/or joint pain, as well as low energy fractures when taking bisphosphates for long periods. Common adverse effects of calcitonin include flushing of the face, nausea, diarrhea, and reduced appetite. Common adverse effects of teriparatide include chest pain, dizziness, hypercalcemia, nausea, and arthralgia. Infections occur more frequently in those taking denosumab.

## Interactions

Cholestyramine and ampicillin decrease the absorption of raloxifene, and raloxifene can decrease the effects of warfarin. Calcium supplements and antacids can interfere with the absorption of the bisphosphonates, and therefore they need to be spaced 1 to 2 hours apart to avoid this interaction. Calcium supplements, although often needed by patients with osteoporosis, are also more likely to cause hypercalcemia in patients receiving calcitonin. Aspirin and other nonsteroidal antiinflammatory drugs (NSAIDs) have the potential for additive GI irritation if taken with bisphosphonates.

## Dosages

For the recommended dosages of osteoporosis drugs, see the Dosages table on this page.

## DRUG PROFILES

### ♦ alendronate

Alendronate (Fosamax) is an oral bisphosphonate and the first nonestrogen nonhormonal option for preventing bone loss. This drug works by inhibiting and/or reversing osteoclast-mediated bone resorption. Recall that *osteoclasts* are the bone cells that cause breakdown or *resorption* of bone tissue as part of their normal physiologic action. However, unchecked osteoclastic activity often leads to osteoporosis if not managed, so this drug class represents a major breakthrough in the treatment of osteoporosis. It is indicated for the prevention and treatment of osteoporosis in men and in postmenopausal women. It is also indicated for the treatment of glucocorticoid-induced osteoporosis in men and for the treatment of Paget disease in women.

Data show that alendronate therapy may reduce the risk of hip fracture by 51%, of spinal fracture by 47%, and of wrist fracture by 48%. Take precautions in patients with dysphagia, esophagitis,

### DOSAGES

#### Selected Drugs Used Specifically for Osteoporosis

| DRUG (PREGNANCY CATEGORY) | PHARMACOLOGIC CLASS | USUAL DOSAGE RANGE | INDICATIONS/USES |
|---|---|---|---|
| ♦ alendronate (Fosamax) (C) | Bisphosphonate | PO: 5 mg/day or 35 mg/wk<br>PO: 10 mg/day or 70 mg/wk | Osteoporosis prevention<br>Osteoporosis treatment |
| calcitonin, salmon (Calcimar, Miacalcin, others) (C) | Calcitonin hormonal substitute derived from salmon | IM/subcut: 100 units/day<br>Nasal spray: 200 units (1 spray)/day | Osteoporosis treatment |
| raloxifene (Evista) (X) | Selective estrogen receptor modulator | PO: 60 mg/day | Osteoporosis prevention and treatment |

*IM*, Intramuscular; *PO*, oral; *subcut*, subcutaneous.

esophageal ulcer, or gastric ulcer, because the drug can be very irritating. Case reports of esophageal erosions have been published. It is recommended that alendronate be taken with an 8-oz glass of water immediately upon arising in the morning and that the patient not lie down for at least 30 minutes after taking it. When patients whose condition has been stabilized on alendronate are hospitalized and cannot comply with these recommendations, the medication is often withheld. Alendronate has an extremely long half-life, so going several days without taking a dose will do little to reduce the therapeutic efficacy of the drug. There is debate on how long a woman should remain on bisphosphonate therapy, with most experts recommending roughly 5 years.

### Pharmacokinetics

| Route | Onset of Action | Peak Plasma Concentration | Elimination Half-life | Duration of Action |
|---|---|---|---|---|
| PO | 3 wk | Unknown | Longer than 10 yr due to storage in bone tissue | Unknown |

**raloxifene**

Raloxifene (Evista) is a SERM. It is used primarily for the prevention of postmenopausal osteoporosis. Interestingly, raloxifene has positive effects on cholesterol level, but it is not normally used specifically for this purpose. It may not be the best choice for women near menopause, because use of the drug is associated with the adverse effect of hot flashes. It is available only for oral use.

### Pharmacokinetics

| Route | Onset of Action | Peak Plasma Concentration | Elimination Half-life | Duration of Action |
|---|---|---|---|---|
| PO | 8 wk | Unknown | 28 hr | Unknown |

**calcitonin**

Calcitonin, in its drug forms, is derived from salmon (fish) sources. Although it is available in both injectable form and nasal spray, the nasal spray (Miacalcin) is now more commonly used.

### Pharmacokinetics

| Route | Onset of Action | Peak Plasma Concentration | Elimination Half-life | Duration of Action |
|---|---|---|---|---|
| Inhalation (nasal spray) | Unknown | 30-40 min | 43 min | Unknown |

## DRUGS RELATED TO PREGNANCY, LABOR, DELIVERY, AND THE POSTPARTUM PERIOD
### FERTILITY DRUGS

Infertility in women is often the result of absence of ovulation (anovulation), which is normally due to various imbalances in female reproductive hormones. Such imbalances can occur at the level of the hypothalamus, the pituitary gland, the ovary, or any combination of these. Exogenous administration of estrogens or progestins may be used to fortify the blood levels of these hormones when ovarian output is inadequate. The use of drug forms of these hormones was described earlier in this chapter.

Hormone deficiencies at the hypothalamic and pituitary levels are often treated with gonadotropin ovarian stimulants. These drugs stimulate increased secretion of gonadotropin-releasing hormone (Gn-RH) from the hypothalamus, which then results in increased secretion of FSH and LH from the pituitary gland. These hormones, in turn, stimulate the development of ovarian follicles and ovulation. They also stimulate ovarian secretion of the estrogens and progestins that are part of the normal ovulatory cycle. Proper selection and dosage adjustment of fertility drugs often requires the expertise of a fertility specialist. The various medical techniques used in the treatment of infertility, including drug therapy, are now collectively referred to as assisted reproductive technology. One particularly common specific technique is in vitro fertilization, during which a woman's ovum is fertilized with her partner's sperm in a laboratory and the fertilized ovum is then medically implanted into the woman's uterus. Infants born through the use of this technique used to be referred to as "test tube babies." The success of such fertilization techniques may be further aided with the use of medications such as those described earlier. Representative examples of ovulation stimulants include the drugs clomiphene, menotropins, and choriogonadotropin alfa.

## Mechanism of Action and Drug Effects

Clomiphene is a nonsteroidal ovulation stimulant that works by blocking estrogen receptors in the uterus and brain. This results in a false signal of low estrogen levels to the brain. The hypothalamus and pituitary gland then increase their production of Gn-RH (from the hypothalamus) and FSH and LH (from the pituitary), which stimulates the maturation of ovarian follicles. Ideally this leads to ovulation and increases the likelihood of conception in a previously infertile woman.

Menotropins is the drug name for a standardized mixture of FSH and LH that is derived from the urine of postmenopausal women. The FSH component stimulates the development of ovarian follicles, which leads to ovulation. The LH component stimulates the development of the corpus luteum, which supplies female sex hormones (estrogens and progesterone) during the first trimester of pregnancy. Choriogonadotropin alfa is a recombinant form (i.e., developed using recombinant DNA technology) of the hormone human chorionic gonadotropin. This hormone is naturally produced by the placenta during pregnancy and can be isolated from the urine of pregnant women. It is an analogue of LH and can provide a substitute for the natural LH surge that promotes ovulation. It does this by binding to LH receptors in the ovary and stimulating the rupture of mature ovarian follicles and the subsequent development of the corpus luteum. Human chorionic gonadotropin also maintains the viability of the corpus luteum during early pregnancy. This is critical, because the corpus luteum provides the supply of estrogens and progesterone necessary to support the first trimester of pregnancy until the placenta assumes this role. Choriogonadotropin alfa is often given in a carefully timed fashion after FSH-active therapy such as menotropins or clomiphene therapy, when patient monitoring indicates sufficient maturation of ovarian follicles.

## Indications

These drugs are used primarily for the promotion of ovulation in anovulatory female patients. They may also be used to promote spermatogenesis in infertile men. As was mentioned in the section on progestins, progesterone formulations are also used to treat female infertility.

## Contraindications

Contraindications to the use of the ovarian stimulants include known drug allergy to a specific product and may also include primary ovarian failure, uncontrolled thyroid or adrenal dysfunction, liver disease, pituitary tumor, abnormal uterine bleeding, ovarian enlargement of uncertain cause, sex hormone–dependent tumors, and pregnancy.

## Adverse Effects

The most common adverse effects of the ovulation stimulants are listed in Table 34-5.

## Interactions

Few drugs interact with fertility drugs. The most notable are the tricyclic antidepressants, the butyrophenones (e.g., haloperidol), the phenothiazines (e.g., promethazine), and the antihypertensive drug methyldopa. When any of these drugs is taken with the fertility drugs, prolactin concentrations may be increased, which may impair fertility.

| TABLE 34-5 | FERTILITY DRUGS: MOST COMMON ADVERSE EFFECTS |
|---|---|
| **BODY SYSTEM** | **ADVERSE EFFECTS** |
| Cardiovascular | Tachycardia, deep vein thrombosis, hypovolemia |
| Central nervous | Dizziness, headache, flushing, depression, restlessness, anxiety, nervousness, fatigue |
| Gastrointestinal | Nausea, bloating, constipation, vomiting, anorexia |
| Other | Urticaria, ovarian hyperstimulation, multiple pregnancy (twins or more), blurred vision, diplopia, photophobia, breast pain |

## Dosages

For recommended dosages of clomiphene, see the Dosages table on this page.

## DRUG PROFILE

### clomiphene

Clomiphene (Clomid) is primarily used to stimulate the production of pituitary gonadotropins, which in turn induces the maturation of the ovarian follicle and eventually ovulation. It is currently available only for oral use.

### Pharmacokinetics

| Route | Onset of Action | Peak Plasma Concentration | Elimination Half-life | Duration of Action |
|---|---|---|---|---|
| PO | 4-12 days | Unknown | 5 days | 30 days |

## UTERINE STIMULANTS

A variety of medications are used to alter the dynamics of uterine contractions either to promote or to prevent the start or progression of labor. In the immediate postpartum period, medications may be used to promote rapid shrinkage (involution) of the uterus to reduce the risk of postpartum hemorrhage.

Four types of drugs are used to stimulate uterine contractions: ergot derivatives, prostaglandins, the progesterone antagonist mifepristone (RU-486), and the hormone oxytocin. These drugs all act on the uterus, a highly muscular organ that has a complex network of smooth muscle fibers and a large blood supply. These drugs are often collectively referred to as *oxytocics*, after the naturally occurring hormone oxytocin, whose action they mimic. The uterus undergoes several changes during normal gestation and childbirth that at different times make it either resistant or susceptible to various hormones and drugs. Oxytocin is one of the two hormones secreted by the posterior lobe of the pituitary gland. The other is vasopressin, which is also known as *antidiuretic hormone* (see Chapter 30).

## Mechanism of Action and Drug Effects

The uterus of a woman who is not pregnant is relatively insensitive to oxytocin, but during pregnancy the uterus becomes more sensitive to this hormone and is most sensitive at term (the end of gestation).

During childbirth, oxytocin stimulates uterine contraction, and during lactation it promotes the movement of milk

## DOSAGES

### Selected Fertility Drugs

| DRUG (PREGNANCY CATEGORY) | PHARMACOLOGIC CLASS | USUAL DOSAGE RANGE | INDICATIONS |
|---|---|---|---|
| clomiphene (Clomid, Serophene) (X) | Ovulation stimulant | PO: 50-100 mg daily × 5 days; repeatable cycle depending on response | Female infertility in selected patients |

*PO*, Oral.

from the mammary glands to the nipples. Another class of oxytocic drugs is the prostaglandins, natural hormones involved in regulating the network of smooth muscle fibers of the uterus. This network is known as the myometrium. The prostaglandins cause very potent contractions of the myometrium and may also play a role in the natural induction of labor. When the prostaglandin concentrations increase during the final few weeks of pregnancy, mild myometrial contractions, commonly known as Braxton Hicks contractions, are stimulated. The third major class of oxytocic drugs is the ergot alkaloids, which are also potent simulators of uterine muscle. These drugs increase the force and frequency of uterine contractions. One of the most politically charged prescription drug approvals ever made by the FDA was approval of the progesterone antagonist mifepristone (Mifeprex), also known as the "abortion pill." This drug also stimulates uterine contractions and is used to induce elective termination of pregnancy.

## Indications

Oxytocin is available in a synthetic injectable form (e.g., Pitocin). This drug is used to induce labor at or near full-term gestation and to enhance labor when uterine contractions are weak and ineffective. Oxytocin is also used to prevent or control uterine bleeding after delivery, to induce completion of an incomplete abortion (including miscarriages), and to promote milk ejection during lactation.

The prostaglandins may be used therapeutically to induce labor by softening the cervix (cervical ripening) and enhancing uterine muscle tone. They may also be used to stimulate the myometrium to induce abortion during the second trimester when the uterus is resistant to oxytocin. Examples of these drugs are dinoprostone and misoprostol. Misoprostol is an oral tablet and is also used as a stomach protectant (see Chapter 45). Misoprostol is used off-label for cervical ripening and is administered orally or intravaginally. It offers the advantage of costing pennies as opposed to the hundreds of dollars paid for dinoprostone. Because of this, misoprostol is widely used in third-world countries as well as throughout the United States. Be aware that the prescribing information states that misoprostol should not be used in this way; however it is common to see it used clinically.

Ergot alkaloids are used after delivery of the infant and placenta to prevent postpartum uterine atony (lack of muscle tone) and hemorrhage.

Mifepristone is used to induce abortion and is often given with the synthetic prostaglandin drug misoprostol for this purpose.

## Contraindications

Contraindications to the use of labor-inducing uterine stimulants include known drug allergy to a specific product and may include pelvic inflammatory disease, cervical stenosis, uterine fibrosis, high-risk intrauterine fetal positions before delivery, placenta previa, hypertonic uterus, uterine prolapse, or any condition in which vaginal delivery is contraindicated (e.g., increased bleeding risk). Contraindications to the use of abortifacients include known drug allergy as well as the presence of an intrauterine device, ectopic pregnancy, concurrent anticoagulant therapy or bleeding disorder, inadequate access to emergency health care, or the inability to understand or comply with follow-up instructions.

## Adverse Effects

The most common undesirable effects of oxytocic drugs are listed in Table 34-6.

## Interactions

Few clinically significant drug interactions occur with the oxytocic drugs. The most common and important of these involve sympathomimetic drugs. Combining drugs that produce vasoconstriction, such as sympathomimetics, with the oxytocic drugs can result in severe hypertension.

## Dosages

For the recommended dosages of selected oxytocic drugs, see the Dosages table on p. 557.

## DRUG PROFILES

### ◆ dinoprostone

Dinoprostone (Prostin $E_2$, Cervidil, Prepidil) is a synthetic derivative of the naturally occurring hormone prostaglandin $E_2$. It is used for the termination of pregnancy from the twelfth through the twentieth gestational weeks, for evacuation of the uterine contents in the management of missed abortion or intrauterine fetal death up to 28 weeks of gestational age, for the management of nonmetastatic gestational trophoblastic disease, and for ripening of an unfavorable cervix in pregnant women at or near term when there is a medical or obstetric need for labor induction. It is available only for vaginal use in various dosage forms.

### Pharmacokinetics

| Route | Onset of Action | Peak Plasma Concentration | Elimination Half-life | Duration of Action |
|---|---|---|---|---|
| Topical gel | Rapid | 30-45 min | Unknown | Not available |

### ◆ methylergonovine

The ergot alkaloid methylergonovine (Methergine) is used primarily in the immediately postpartal period to enhance myometrial tone and reduce the likelihood of postpartum uterine hemorrhage. Its use is contraindicated in patients with a known hypersensitivity to ergot medications and in those with pelvic

| TABLE 34-6 | OXYTOCIC DRUGS: MOST COMMON ADVERSE EFFECTS |
|---|---|
| **BODY SYSTEM** | **ADVERSE EFFECTS** |
| Cardiovascular | Hypotension or hypertension, chest pain |
| Central nervous | Headache, dizziness, fainting |
| Gastrointestinal | Nausea, vomiting, diarrhea |
| Genitourinary | Vaginitis, vaginal pain, cramping |
| Other | Leg cramps, joint swelling, chills, fever, weakness, blurred vision |

## DOSAGES

### Selected Uterine Stimulants

| DRUG (PREGNANCY CATEGORY)* | PHARMACOLOGIC CLASS | USUAL DOSAGE RANGE | INDICATIONS/USES |
|---|---|---|---|
| ◆ dinoprostone (Prostin E₂, Prepidil, Cervidil) (X) | Prostaglandin E₂ abortifacient and cervical ripening drug | Vaginal suppository (Prostin E₂): 1 suppository (20 mg) into vagina at 3-5 hr intervals until uterine evacuation | Termination of pregnancy; uterine evacuation in cases of miscarriage or benign hydatidiform mole |
| | | Cervical gel (Prepidil): 0.5 mg into cervical canal at 6-hr dosing intervals (max 1.5 mg/24 hr) | Cervical ripening for induction of labor |
| | | Vaginal suppository (Cervidil): 10 mg into posterior vaginal fornix (space behind cervix) × 1 dose | Cervical ripening for induction of labor |
| ◆ methylergonovine (Methergine) (X) | Oxytocic ergot alkaloid | IM/IV: 0.2 mg after delivery of placenta, repeatable at 2-4 hr intervals | Postpartum uterine atony and hemorrhage |
| | | PO: 0.2 mg tid-qid for up to 7 days postpartum | |
| ◆ oxytocin (Pitocin) (X) | Oxytocic hypothalamic hormone | IV infusion: 0.5-20 milliunits/min, titrated to effect | Labor induction |
| | | IV infusion: 10-40 units in 1 L of D₅LR titrated to effect | Postpartum uterine atony and hemorrhage |
| | | IM: 10 units in a single dose after delivery of placenta | |

*D₅LR*, Dextrose 5% in lactated Ringer's solution; *IM*, intramuscular; *IV*, intravenous; *PO*, oral.
*Use of these medications is contraindicated in pregnancy (pregnancy category X) unless needed for the indications listed.

inflammatory disease. It should be used with caution in patients with hypertension. It is not to be used for augmentation of labor, before delivery of the placenta, during a spontaneous abortion, or given to patients with pregnancy induced hypertension. Methylergonovine is available in both oral and injectable forms.

### Pharmacokinetics

| Route | Onset of Action | Peak Plasma Concentration | Elimination Half-life | Duration of Action |
|---|---|---|---|---|
| PO | 5-15 min | 30 min | 2 hr | 3 hr |

### ◆ oxytocin

The drug oxytocin (Pitocin, Syntocinon) is the synthetic form of the endogenous hormone oxytocin and has all of its pharmacologic properties.

### Pharmacokinetics

| Route | Onset of Action | Peak Plasma Concentration | Elimination Half-life | Duration of Action |
|---|---|---|---|---|
| IV | Immediate | Immediate | 3-5 min | 1 hr |

## DRUGS FOR PRETERM LABOR MANAGEMENT

*Preterm labor* is defined as substantial uterine contractions which could progress to delivery and occur prior to the 37th week of pregnancy. When contractions of the uterus begin before term, it may be desirable to stop labor, because premature birth increases the risk of neonatal death. Postponing delivery increases the likelihood of the infant's survival. However, this measure is generally employed only between weeks 20 to 37 of gestation, because spontaneous labor occurring before

the twentieth week is commonly associated with a nonviable fetus and thus is usually not interrupted.

The nonpharmacologic treatment of premature labor includes bed rest, sedation, and hydration. Drugs given to inhibit labor and maintain the pregnancy are called *tocolytics*. Terbutaline is a beta-adrenergic drug (see Chapter 18) and used to be the drug of choice for preterm labor. It works by directly relaxing uterine smooth muscle. In 2011, the FDA stated that terbutaline should not be used to prevent preterm labor or for prolonged treatment due to maternal and fetal safety risks. Concentrated solutions of the electrolyte magnesium sulfate are also used intravenously for this purpose. The efficacy of magnesium sulfate is questionable; however, it is still used clinically by some physicians. Magnesium sulfate is also used in pregnancy induced hypertension. Calcium gluconate must be readily available to reverse magnesium toxicity if it occurs.

The current recommendations for the management of preterm labor include the use of the nonsteroidal antiinflammatory agent, indomethacin (see Chapter 44), and the calcium channel blocker, nifedipine (see Chapter 23). Indomethacin is the most effective tocolytic currently available and works by inhibiting prostaglandin activity. Nifedipine inhibits myometrial activity by blocking calcium influx. The dose of indomethacin is 100 mg load followed by 50 mg every 8 hours. It is given in along with sucralfate (Carafate), which acts to protect the stomach (see Chapter 50). Nifedipine (immediate-release formulation) is dosed as 20 mg, followed by 20 mg after 30 minutes, and if contractions persist, 20 mg every 3 to 8 hours for 48 to 72 hours can be given, with a maximum dose of 160 mg/day. If after 72 hours, maintenance is still required, the sustained-release formulation can be used at doses of 30 to 60 mg daily. When these treatments are ineffective and delivery is proceeding, corticosteroids (betamethasone or dexamethasone) (see Chapter 33) are given to the mother to promote lung maturity in the fetus between 24 to 34 weeks of gestation.

## TEAMWORK AND COLLABORATION: PHARMACOKINETIC BRIDGE TO NURSING PRACTICE

Estrasorb is a form of estrogen that is FDA approved to help ease the severity of postmenopausal hot flashes by increasing estrogen levels when these are found to be deficient in the patient. Estrasorb contains estradiol, which is identical to the estrogen produced in the woman's body. The absorption of the topical emulsion dosage form results in measurable levels of estradiol on the skin for up to 8 hours after application. It is important to fully understand this pharmacokinetic property, because the transfer of the drug to another individual may result. In fact, traces of Estrasorb have been found on other individuals from such transfer for up to a 2-day period. This transfer of medication to other individuals may be reduced by allowing the dosage form to fully dry and then covering it with clothing before having contact with another individual. Although no specific investigation of the tissue distribution of the estradiol absorbed from Estrasorb in humans has been conducted, it is known that the distribution of exogenous estrogens is similar to that of endogenous estrogens. The metabolism of exogenous estrogens is also similar to that of endogenous estrogens, with biotransformation taking place mainly in the liver and excretion in the urine. The specific dosage form of an emulsion is desirable because it may be applied easily, once daily to the thighs and/or calves. One dose is contained in two separate foil pouches, and patients need to be fully aware of the application instructions. For example, sunscreen products are not to be applied at the same time, because sunscreen reduces the absorption of Estrasorb.

Knowing the pharmacokinetic properties of Estrasorb is necessary for safe and efficient administration of the drug. It is also important to understand all the pharmacokinetic properties of this drug to be able to fully educate patients about the drug, its effect on the body, and the subsequent implications for its absorption, distribution, metabolism, and excretion.

# NURSING PROCESS

## ASSESSMENT

In this section, estrogenic and progestational medications (progestins/progesterone drugs) are discussed first, followed by the major drug classes used in treatment of osteoporosis. Next, information on fertility drugs, uterine stimulants, and preterm labor management drugs is discussed. Before initiating therapy with any of the hormonal drugs (e.g., estrogens, progestins) or other women's health-related drugs, obtain the patient's blood pressure and weight and document the findings. Assess and document drug allergies, contraindications, cautions, and drug interactions. Include a thorough medication history, medical history, and menstrual history in your patient assessment. Note the results of the patient's last physical examination, clinician-performed breast examination, and gynecologic examination as well.

*Estrogen-only* hormones are to only be given after the following disorders and conditions have been ruled out: any estrogen-dependent cancer, undiagnosed abnormal vaginal bleeding, active thromboembolic disorders such as stroke or thrombophlebitis, or a history of these disorders. Include questions about breast examination, breast self-examination practices, and dates of last complete physical examination and Papanicolaou (Pap) smear in the assessment. It is important to assess for potential drug interactions such as with tricyclic antidepressants, which may reach toxic levels if given with estrogens. Advise patients to avoid smoking because of the

risk of thrombosis. It has been documented that smoking also decreases the effectiveness of estrogen; hence, take a thorough smoking history. Question about the number of packs smoked per day and the number of years the patient has smoked. Other drug interactions to assess for include oral anticoagulants (decreased effectiveness) as well as rifampin and St. John's wort (decreased estrogen effectiveness). If being used for hormonal replacement therapy for menopausal symptoms, recent changes to older recommendations from the North American Menopause Society include the following: hormonal replacement is not recommended for women with histories of endometrial cancer; in women with breast cancer, estrogen therapy has not been proved safe and may raise recurrence risk. Therefore, perform a thorough assessment for history or diagnosis of endometrial and/or breast cancer. Bone density may also be impacted once hormonal therapy is discontinued; further assessment is needed in these particular patients.

Assess the patient's knowledge about the use of hormones (e.g., estrogens and progestins), whether for contraception or replacement therapy. Also assess the patient's readiness to learn, educational level, and degree of adherence to other medication regimens. The success of treatment with oral contraceptives, hormone replacement medication, and other therapies depends heavily on the patient's understanding instructions. With *oral contraceptive drugs* (e.g., combination estrogen-progestin drugs), perform a pregnancy test and assess for history of vascular and/or thromboembolic disorders (such as myocardial infarction, venous thrombosis, stroke), malignancies of the reproductive tract, and abnormal vaginal bleeding. Closely monitor patients with the following: hypertension, migraine headaches, alterations in lipid and/or carbohydrate metabolism, fluid retention or edema, hair loss, amenorrhea, breakthrough vaginal/uterine bleeding, and uterine fibroids. The concern is for exacerbation of these conditions and the potential for subsequent complications. Closely monitor patients who smoke because of the increased risk of complications (increased risk of thrombosis) with estrogens. Assess for drug interactions, such as with drugs leading to decreased effectiveness of oral contraception—antibiotics (especially penicillins and cephalosporins), barbiturates, isoniazid, and rifampin. Drugs that may have their therapeutic effects decreased if taken concurrently with oral contraceptives include antiepileptic drugs, beta blockers, hypnotics, antidiabetic drugs, warfarin, theophylline, tricyclic antidepressants, and vitamins. When combination oral contraceptives are used in emergency situations for postcoital conception, the same contraindications, cautions, and drug interactions apply, even if the drug is for one-time use.

The chemically derived progestins, such as medroxyprogesterone and megestrol, have the same contraindications as estrogens. Additionally, with progestins, assess for a history of liver/gallbladder disease, thrombophlebitis, and thromboembolic disorders due to possible adverse effects (see Table 34-3). Be mindful that a significant drug interaction occurs with the antidiabetic drugs. Look thoroughly at the patient's medical history in reference to the specific condition for which the progestin is ordered. Some of these include prevention of endometrial cancer caused by estrogen therapy, palliative management of recurrent endometrial or breast cancer, as well as management of anorexia and cachexia in those with AIDS or cancer.

With the osteoporosis drug class of *bisphosphonates*, there are many contraindications, cautions, and drug interactions. Assessment of the following is therefore important to patient safety: drug allergy, esophageal dysfunction, hypocalcemia, and the inability to sit or stand upright for at least 30 minutes after taking the medication. Selective estrogen receptor modulators (SERMs) are not to be used in patients who are or may become pregnant and in women with thromboembolic disorders including deep vein thrombosis. Assess for allergies to salmon with the use of calcitonin because the drug is derived from this fish. Drug interactions to assess for include ampicillin and cholestyramine because they decrease the absorption of raloxifene. Raloxifene also decreases the effects of warfarin. Assess patients for the drug interaction between bisphosphonates and calcium supplements and/or antacids (decreased absorption) as well as aspirin and NSAIDs (potential for additive GI irritation).

Use of *clomiphene* requires assessment of the patient's medical and medication history with attention to the patient's menstrual history. Medical history is critical, especially reproductive and uterine status, because use of the drug may result in multiple pregnancy (twins or more) and compromise maternal health status. Assess family stability and economic status because of the additional family and financial stressors associated with a multiple birth. Assess thoroughly for possible contraindications such as primary ovarian failure, adrenal and/or thyroid dysfunction, liver disease, and abnormal uterine bleeding. Assess also for potential drug interactions with tricyclic antidepressants, haloperidol, phenothiazines, and methyldopa (an antihypertensive drug). Fertility may be impaired if clomiphene is given with these drugs.

Before administering *uterine stimulants* (e.g., oxytocin or prostaglandins), assess and document the patient's blood pressure, pulse, and respiration. Also determine the fetal heart rate and contraction-related fetal heart rates and document findings. Contraindications to the use of labor-inducing uterine stimulants in early pregnancy include the presence of an intrauterine device for birth control, ectopic pregnancy, use of anticoagulants, bleeding disorders, and inability to understand and then comply with instructions. Assess for the concurrent use of sympathomimetics because of enhanced vasoconstrictive effects, possibly leading to severe hypertension. For labor and delivery, the patient's cervix must be ready for induction. (Consult a current maternal child health or obstetric nursing textbook for more information on the rating of the cervix.) Perform continuous monitoring of maternal blood pressure, pulse, contractions, and fluid status, as well as fetal heart rate. Oxytocin is *not* used during the first trimester except in some cases of spontaneous or induced abortion.

With the ergot alkaloid methylergonovine maleate, assess the medication order after vital signs and note that the first dose is given after delivery of the placenta to help stimulate the uterus to contract and decrease blood loss after delivery in special situations. Continue to assess blood pressure during the drug's administration. Assess for contraindications such as pregnancy, labor, liver/renal disease, cardiac disease, and pregnancy induced hypertension. Assess for any history of seizures. If this drug is given to hypertensive women, it may precipitate seizures or a stroke. The use of dinoprostone or other *prostaglandin E$_2$* drugs is indicated in specific situations requiring termination of pregnancy. Question the patient about the presence of any contraindications, cautions, and drug interactions. Misoprostol is also used intravaginally in an "off label" use for cervical ripening.

*Terbutaline* was formerly the drug of choice for the management of preterm labor but has been identified as having maternal and fetal risks. Instead, patients may receive indomethacin (see Chapter 44), nifedipine (see Chapter 23), or magnesium sulfate. Take baseline maternal vital signs, and assess fetal heart rate prior to administering any drug indicated for preterm labor. Assess the maternal history for estimated gestation as these medications are generally used between weeks 20 to 37. Spontaneous labor before the twentieth week is commonly associated with a nonviable fetus, and the labor is not interrupted. With indomethacin, additional concerns to assess for include a history of coagulation disorders, chronic hypertension, heart failure, impaired liver function, and cardiovascular disease. With nifedepine, a history of hypotension and cardiovascular problems are contraindications.

### 🌐 PATIENT-CENTERED CARE: CULTURAL IMPLICATIONS

#### *Racial Disparities between Black Women and White Women in the Incidence, Treatment, and Prognosis of Endometrial Cancer*

An estimated 40,100 new cases of uterine cancer were diagnosed in 2008, with the majority of the cases occurring in white women. The incidence of endometrial cancer was at 33% in black women and thought to be due partially to an underestimation of the cancer in this population. Over 7400 women with endometrial cancer died of their disease in 2008, with the mortality rate about 80% higher in black women (with the cancer) as compared with white women. Some 14% of endometrial cancer–related deaths occur in black women, while only 7% of newly diagnosed patients with endometrial cancer are black. Even though the number of new cases presenting each year has remained relatively stable, the number of deaths per year, especially among blacks, is increasing. A survey of recent literature published in the English language was performed by Allard and Maxwell (2009). This survey of literature serves as the basis of this information regarding racial disparities. The cause of racial disparity among black women with endometrial cancer appears to be multifaceted and most likely the result of barriers to the access of care, increasing incidence of co-morbidities among black women, inequalities in their surgical care/radiation and/or adjuvant chemotherapy, and biological or genetic differences associated with more aggressive cancerous tumors developing in black women.

Data from Allard JE, Maxwell GL: Race disparities between black and white women in the incidence, treatment and prognosis of endometrial cancer, *Cancer Control* 16(1): 53-56, 2009.

## ▎NURSING DIAGNOSES

1. Decisional conflict related to the risks versus benefits of postmenopausal estrogen replacement therapy
2. Acute pain related to adverse effects and improper dosing of SERM
3. Noncompliance related to lack of information and experience with daily dosing of oral contraceptives

# PLANNING

## GOALS

1. Patient makes informed decision regarding the use of estrogen replacement therapy.
2. Patient experiences minimal pain (epigastric) associated with SERMs.
3. Patient remains compliant with oral contraceptive therapy.

## OUTCOME CRITERIA

1. Patient correctly self-administers estrogen replacement therapy daily after decision to opt for pharmacologic treatment.
2. Patient remains without esophageal pain after taking SERM as ordered and with the full ability to sit or stand upright for at least 30 minutes after taking the oral dosage form to avoid/prevent esophageal irritation/erosion.
3. Patient is compliant with oral contraceptive therapy, states rationale for daily use (effectiveness based on taking medication daily), and contacts health care provider with any high incidence of adverse effects.

# IMPLEMENTATION

When administering *estrogens,* directions need to be followed exactly. Provide precise and thorough instructions to patients when self-administration of the hormone is ordered. Oral dosage forms are best taken at the same time every day and with meals or a snack to minimize GI upset.

It is also important to understand the indication and rationale for the use of estrogen so that accurate facts about the drug are given to the patient. If estradiol is being given, vasomotor symptoms of menopause are generally the indication, and the drug is to be given daily at the same time. If the estradiol transdermal patch is given, it is to be applied as ordered, which is usually one patch applied once or twice weekly to the lower abdomen and not to the breast and chest areas. See the Patient Teaching Tips for more information.

Use of *progestins* is indicated for birth control, such as the use of Depo-Provera with one IM injection every 3 months. Depo-Provera, however, remains controversial in women of any reproductive age because of the associated bone density loss. Give these injections in deep muscle mass and rotate sites. Oral forms of medroxyprogesterone acetate are used for amenorrhea and uterine bleeding. Doses are to be taken exactly as ordered, such as for a specific number of days or cyclically. Megestrol, a synthetic progestin, is often indicted for palliative reasons or for management of anorexia, cachexia, or weight loss that is unexplained in AIDS patients. It is given orally as ordered and given to maximize appetite. It is recommended, however, that the lowest dosage possible of either *estrogens* and/or *progestins* be used and titrated as needed, but only as ordered.

Oral contraception is available in various formulations based on doses that are taken at different times of the menstrual cycle (see pharmacology discussion). Progestin-only oral contraceptive pills are taken daily. It is important for the patient to take this oral contraceptive at the same time every day so that effective hormone serum levels are maintained. Because use of the progestin-only pill leads to a higher incidence of ovulatory cycles, there is an increased rate and risk of contraceptive failure if not taken as per instructions. Be aware that this type of pill is usually prescribed for those women who cannot tolerate estrogens or for whom estrogens are contraindicated. Often it is more effective in women who are older than 35 years of age and women who are breastfeeding. Combination estrogen-progestin pills contain low doses of the hormones. Biphasic forms contain fixed estrogen and variable progestin for 21- or 28-day products. The low-dose monophasic (fixed estrogen-progestin combination) types are provided as 21 or 28 days of pills, with the 28-day products containing 7 inert tablets. Triphasic products offer 3 or 4 phases of variable estrogen and progestin combinations, and there are also new extended-cycle products available. Make sure the patient fully understands how to take the medication. Emphasize that the reduction in the level of estrogen has been associated with a decrease in adverse effects and a decrease in the risk for complications; however, more breakthrough bleeding may occur.

The success of therapy with *bisphosphonates* depends on providing thorough patient teaching and ensuring that the patient understands all aspects of the drug regimen. With oral bisphosphonates, emphasize the need to take the medication upon rising in the morning with a full glass (6 to 8 oz) of water at least 30 minutes before the intake of any food, other fluids, or other medication. In addition, emphasize that the patient remain upright in either a standing or sitting position for approximately 30 minutes after taking the drug to help prevent esophageal erosion or irritation. Inform the patient taking the *SERM* raloxifene that the drug must be discontinued 72 hours before and during prolonged immobility. Therapy may be resumed, as ordered, once the patient becomes fully ambulatory. See the Patient Teaching Tips for more information.

*Fertility drugs* (e.g., clomiphene) are often self-administered. Provide specific instructions regarding how to administer the drug at home and how to monitor drug effectiveness to improve the success of treatment. Journal tracking of the medication regimen is helpful to those involved in the care of the infertile patient or couple. See the Patient Teaching Tips for more information.

With *tocolytics,* either indomethacin (Indocin) or nifedipine (Procardia) will be used. It is important to note, however, that magnesium sulfate may also be used. Follow the dosing and routes exactly as determined by the prescriber. Long-term dosing of indomethacin is not recommended due to birth defects. Nifedipine may lead to potentially life-threatening maternal-fetal problems. Discontinue both medications, as ordered, once contractions cease. Monitor vital signs and fetal heart rates closely with these drugs. Placement of the patient in the left lateral recumbent position minimizes hypotension, increases renal blood flow, and increases blood flow to the fetus.

Administer *oxytocin* only as ordered, and strictly follow any instructions or protocols. The cervix must be ripe (see earlier discussion). *Prostaglandin $E_2$* may be instilled vaginally to help accomplish this if the mother's cervix is not ripe or at a Bishop score of 5 or higher. Because oxytocin has vasopressive and antidiuretic properties, the patient is at risk for hypertensive episodes as well as fluid retention; continuously monitor maternal blood

### Bisphosphonate Drug Therapy for Osteoporosis

 Mrs. S. is a relatively healthy 73-year-old retired clerk who has recently been diagnosed with postmenopausal osteoporosis. She has been prescribed treatment with ibandronate (Boniva), 150 mg each month. She has many questions, and you are reviewing the drug and its use with her.

1. Mrs. S. tells you that she likes to have breakfast, take her morning medicines, then lie down on the couch to read the morning newspaper. She asks whether the ibandronate will fit into her routine. What will you tell her?
2. Mrs. S. calls the clinic to ask what to use for headaches. "I have several different types of headache pills, so aren't they all the same?" How will you respond?
3. A few months later, Mrs. S. comes in for a follow-up visit. She tells you that she is due for her next osteoporosis pill next week, but she has been having some jaw pains ever since she went to the dentist 2 weeks earlier to have a tooth pulled. She is worried that her osteoporosis has affected her jaw. What could be the reason for this pain? What do you think will be done about it?

For answers, see http://evolve.elsevier.com/Lilley.

pressure and pulse rate as well as fetal heart rate. Report any of the following to the prescriber immediately if they occur: strong contractions, edema, and any changes in fetal heart rate. Administer intravenous infusions (via infusion pump) of oxytocin with the proper dilutional fluid and at the proper rate. To minimize the adverse effects of the drug, intravenous piggyback dosing is often ordered so that the diluted oxytocin solution can be discontinued immediately if maternal and/or fetal decline occurs while an intravenous line with hydration is maintained. Doses are generally titrated as ordered and are based on the progress of labor and degree of fetal tolerance of the drug. If the labor progresses at 1 cm/hr, oxytocin may no longer be needed. This decision is made by the prescriber and on an individual basis. Generally speaking, with oxytocin therapy, if there are hypertensive responses or major changes in the maternal vital signs *or* if the fetal heart rate shows any indication of fetal intolerance of labor, contact the prescriber immediately. Hyperstimulation may also occur. If contractions are more frequent than every 2 minutes and last longer than 1 minute (and are accompanied by changes in other parameters), stop the infusion and contact the prescriber immediately. If this does occur, place the patient in a side-lying position, maintain administration of intravenous fluids, give oxygen as ordered (generally via tight face mask at 10 to 12 L/min), and monitor patient and fetus closely. If there is concern about overstimulation, discuss concerns with the prescriber and document actions thoroughly.

When misoprostol is used, give orally or intravaginally for cervical ripening and only as ordered.

*Dinoprostone* is given by vaginal suppository to patients who are 12 to 20 weeks pregnant and are seeking termination and/or to those in whom evacuation of the uterus is needed for the management of incomplete spontaneous abortion or intrauterine fetal death (up to 28 weeks). Give the drug exactly as ordered and monitor the patient closely.

## EVALUATION

Measure therapeutic responses to the various drugs discussed in this chapter by evaluating whether goals and outcome criteria have been met. Many drugs have been discussed, often with several indications for use; thus, the therapeutic response will be the occurrence of the indicated therapeutic effect. Monitor the patient for adverse effects and/or toxicity as well.

Therapeutic effects of *estrogens* may range from prevention of pregnancy to a decrease in menopausal symptoms to a reduction in the size of a tumor. Adverse effects of estrogens may include hypertension, thromboembolism, edema, amenorrhea, nausea, vomiting, facial skin discoloration, hirsutism, breast tenderness, and headaches. Therapeutic responses to *progestins* include a decrease in abnormal uterine bleeding and the disappearance of menstrual disorders (e.g., amenorrhea). The adverse effects of progestins include jaundice, thrombophlebitis, liver dysfunction, and thromboembolic disorders. Adverse effects associated with oral contraceptives include hypertension, edema, thromboembolism, headaches, migraines, depression, stroke, nausea, vomiting, amenorrhea, and breakthrough bleeding.

Therapeutic effects of oxytocin and other *uterine stimulants* include stimulation of labor and control of postpartum bleeding. Adverse effects may include hypotension or hypertension, chest pain, nausea, vomiting, blurred vision, and fainting. The primary therapeutic effect of tocolytics includes absence of preterm labor. Adverse maternal effects may include vasodilation and increase in heart rate, and fetal side effects include possible intrauterine growth retardation.

The therapeutic effects of *fertility drugs* include successful conception. Adverse reactions include tachycardia, deep vein thrombosis, hypovolemia, CNS depression, nausea, vomiting, ovarian hyperstimulation, blurred vision, and photophobia. Therapeutic effects of *osteoporosis drugs* include increased bone density and prevention or management of osteoporosis. Adverse effects of SERMs are hot flashes, leg cramps, leukopenia, headache, GI upset, joint pain, and esophageal burns if the drug is lodged in the esophagus before reaching the stomach.

## PATIENT TEACHING TIPS

- Hormonal drugs are better tolerated if taken with food or milk to minimize GI upset.
- With the use of oral contraceptives as well as any form of hormonal replacement therapy (HRT) with estrogens and/or progestins, encourage the patient to openly discuss concerns about the medications. Assure the patient that, although risks may be associated with HRT, the prescriber will weigh each case individually and make a recommendation based on the benefits versus risks, but with the ultimate decision resting with the patient.
- With estrogens and progestins, advise the patient to report the following conditions to the prescriber immediately: hypertension, edema, thromboembolism, migraines, depression, and breakthrough bleeding.
- Instruct the patient to report a weight gain of 2 pounds or more in 24 hours or 5 pounds or more in 1 week, as well as any breakthrough bleeding or a change in menstrual flow.
- Instruct the patient to take oral contraceptives exactly as ordered and to keep all appointments for follow-up examinations (e.g., pelvic examination, Pap smear, and practitioner-performed breast examination).
- Instruct the patient on the importance of and technique for monthly breast self-examinations during the ideal time—that is, 7 to 10 days after the start of menstruation or 2 to 5 days after menses ends. Stress the need for follow-up appointments and annual examinations by a health care provider.
- Hormones make the patient sensitive to sunlight and tanning beds. Emphasize that the patient must use the appropriate sun protection at all times.
- If the patient is using progesterone-only intravaginal gel with other gels, advise the patient to be sure to insert the other gels at least 6 hours before or after the progesterone-based product.
- Slow-release progesterone intrauterine devices are placed in the uterine cavity by a health care provider. Provide thorough education that inserts are left in place for 5 years (after insertion) and then must be replaced. Advise the patient to report abnormal uterine bleeding, cramping, abdominal pain, or amenorrhea immediately.
- Instruct the patient using an estrogen/progestin vaginal ring for contraception on what to expect with its insertion. Use of this contraceptive device requires thorough teaching and follow-up, including instruction on insertion and removal techniques and a return demonstration before the patient leaves the prescriber's office. Inform the patient that menstruation will follow in 2 to 3 days after the ring is removed and to replace the used ring in its foil pouch and discard it in the trash rather than flushing it down the commode.
- Oral contraceptive hormones must be taken at the same time every day and exactly as prescribed. If one dose is missed, advise the patient to take the dose as soon as it is remembered; however, if it is close to the next dose time, advise the patient not to double up and to use a backup form of contraception in these situations. Provide more specific instructions regarding the omission of more than one pill and/or 1 day's dose depending on the specific oral contraceptive drug prescribed.

These specific instructions will most likely include the following: If the patient misses one "active" tablet in weeks 1, 2, or 3, the tablet needs to be taken as soon as she remembers. If the patient misses two "active" tablets in week 1 or week 2, the patient needs to take two tablets the day she remembers and two tablets the next day, then continue taking one tablet a day until the pack is finished. The patient needs to be instructed to use a backup method of birth control such as condoms if she has sex in the 7 days after missing pills. If the patient misses two "active" tablets in the third week or misses three or more "active" tablets in a row, the patient needs to throw out the rest of the pack and start a new pack that same day. Instruct the patient to use a backup method of birth control if she has sex in the seven 7 days after missing pills.
- Stress the importance of using condoms with oral contraception to prevent sexually transmitted diseases.
- Emphasize to the patient that backup contraception (e.g., condom use) is needed when antibiotics, barbiturates, griseofulvin, isoniazid, rifampin , or St. John's wort is taken with oral contraceptives. These drugs and herbs diminish the effectiveness of oral contraception.
- Estrasorb is generally applied once daily to the thighs and calves, as ordered, with one dose provided in two separate pouches. Do not apply sunscreen and other lotions at the same time because they interfere with the drug. To reduce the chance of transfer of this medication to other individuals, allow the application areas to dry completely before covering them with clothing. The drug contained in this dosage form, estradiol, has been found to be present on the skin up to 8 hours after application.
- Conjugated estrogens are used for menopausal symptoms and are given orally every day; however, other uses of these estrogens may require different doses and a different dosage schedule/regimen. Emphasize the expected adverse effects such as edema, nausea, diarrhea/constipation, breakthrough uterine bleeding, chloasma (facial skin discoloration), hirsutism, tender breasts, and headaches. Encourage the patient to report the following conditions: elevated blood pressure, severe headaches with changes in vision and vomiting, abdominal pain, and edema.
- Bisphosphonates (e.g., alendronate) are to be taken exactly as prescribed; that is, the drug is taken at least 30 minutes before the first morning beverage, food, or other medication and with at least 6 to 8 oz of water. Emphasize the importance of remaining upright for at least 30 minutes after taking the medication to prevent esophageal and GI adverse effects. Esophageal irritation, dysphagia, severe heartburn, and retrosternal pain must be reported to the prescriber immediately to help prevent severe reactions.
- Patients taking bisphosphonates may also require supplemental calcium and vitamin D, as ordered by the prescriber.
- Educate the patient about making lifestyle changes as recommended, such as engaging in weight-bearing exercise (e.g., walking), stopping smoking, and limiting or eliminating alcohol intake. These measures will help encourage fewer adverse effects of oral contraception and/or drug therapy with hormones.

## KEY POINTS

- Three major estrogens are synthesized in the ovaries: estradiol (the principal estrogen), esterone, and estriol. Exogenous estrogens can be classified into two main groups: steroidal estrogens (e.g., conjugated estrogens, esterified estrogens, estradiol) and nonsteroidal estrogens (e.g., chlorotrianisene, dienestrol, diethylstilbestrol).
- Progestins have a variety of uses, including treatment of uterine bleeding and amenorrhea and adjunctive and palliative treatment of some cancers.
- Oral contraceptives containing a combination of estrogens and progestins are the most effective forms of reversible contraception currently available.

- Uterine stimulants (sometimes called *oxytocic drugs*) include ergot derivatives, prostaglandins, and oxytocin.
- Uterine relaxants (often called *tocolytic drugs*) are used to stop preterm labor and maintain pregnancy by halting uterine contractions.
- A thorough nursing assessment is necessary to ensure the safe and effective use of female reproductive drugs. Obtain information on the patient's past medical problems, history of menses and problems with the menstrual cycle, medications taken (prescribed and OTC), number of pregnancies and miscarriages, last menstrual period, and any related surgical or medical treatments.

## NCLEX® EXAMINATION REVIEW QUESTIONS

1 The nurse is assessing a patient who is to receive dinoprostone (Prostin E$_2$). Which condition would be a contraindication to the use of this drug?
   a Pregnancy at 15 weeks' gestation
   b GI upset or ulcer disease
   c Ectopic pregnancy
   d Incomplete abortion

2 When teaching a patient who is taking oral contraceptive therapy for the first time, the nurse relates that adverse effects may include which of the following?
   a Dizziness
   b Nausea
   c Tingling in the extremities
   d Polyuria

3 The nurse is reviewing the use of obstetric drugs. Which situation is an indication for an oxytocin (Pitocin) infusion?
   a Termination of a pregnancy at 12 weeks
   b Hypertonic uterus
   c Cervical stenosis in a patient who is in labor
   d Induction of labor at full term

4 The nurse has provided patient education regarding therapy with the SERM raloxifene (Evista). Which statement from the patient reflects a good understanding of the instruction?
   a "When I take that long flight to Asia, I will need to stop taking this drug at least 3 days before I travel."
   b "I can continue this drug even when traveling as long as I take it with a full glass of water each time."
   c "After I take this drug, I must sit upright for at least 30 minutes."
   d "One advantage of this drug is that it will reduce my hot flashes."

5 The nurse is discussing therapy with clomiphene (Clomid) with a husband and wife who are considering trying this drug as part of treatment for infertility. It is important that they be informed of which possible effect of this drug?
   a Increased menstrual flow
   b Increased menstrual cramping
   c Multiple pregnancy (twins or more)
   d Sedation

6 A patient calls the clinic because she realized she missed one dose of an oral contraceptive. Which statement from the nurse is appropriate? (Select all that apply.)
   a "Go ahead and take the missed dose now, along with today's dose."
   b "Don't worry, you are still protected from pregnancy."
   c "Please come to the clinic for a reevaluation of your therapy."
   d "Wait 7 days, and then start a new pack of pills."
   e "You will need to use a backup form of contraception concurrently for 7 days."

7 The order reads: "Give calcitonin (Miacalcin) 50 international units subcut daily." The medication is available in a vial that contains 200 international units/mL. How many milliliters will the nurse draw up in the syringe for this dose?

1. c, 2. b, 3. d, 4. a, 5. c, 6. a, e, 7. 0.25 mL

For Critical Thinking and Prioritization Questions, see http://evolve.elsevier.com/Lilley

# Men's Health Drugs

## ⊖volve WEBSITE

*http://evolve.elsevier.com/Lilley*

- Animations
- Answer Key—Textbook Case Studies
- Critical Thinking and Prioritization Questions

- Key Points—Downloadable
- Review Questions for the NCLEX® Examination
- Unfolding Case Studies

## OBJECTIVES

When you reach the end of this chapter, you will be able to do the following:

1 Discuss the normal anatomy, physiology, and functions of the male reproductive system.
2 Compare the various men's health drugs, with discussion of their rationale for use, dosages, and dosage forms.
3 Describe the mechanisms of action, dosages, adverse effects, cautions, contraindications, drug interactions, and routes of administration for the various men's health drugs.

4 Develop a nursing care plan that includes all phases of the nursing process for patients receiving men's health drugs for treatment of benign prostatic hyperplasia, sexual dysfunction, hormone deficiency, or prostate cancer.

## DRUG PROFILES

**finasteride, p. 568**
♦ **sildenafil, p. 569**

♦ **testosterone, p. 569**
_____

♦ *Key drug*

## KEY TERMS

**Anabolic activity** Any metabolic activity that promotes the building up of body tissues, such as the activity produced by testosterone that causes the development of bone and muscle tissue; also called *anabolism*. (p. 565)

**Androgenic activity** The activity produced by testosterone that causes the development and maintenance of the male reproductive system and male secondary sex characteristics. (p. 565)

**Androgens** Male sex hormones responsible for mediating the development and maintenance of male sex characteristics. Chief among these are testosterone and its various biochemical precursors. (p. 565)

**Benign prostatic hyperplasia (BPH)** (also called *hypertrophy*) Nonmalignant (noncancerous) enlargement of the prostate gland. (p. 566)

**Catabolism** The opposite of anabolic activity; any metabolic activity that results in the breakdown of body tissues. Examples of conditions in which catabolism occurs are debilitating illnesses such as end-stage cancer and starvation. (p. 565)

**Erythropoietic effect** The effect of stimulating the production of red blood cells (erythropoiesis). (p. 565)

**Prostate cancer** A malignant tumor within the prostate gland. (p. 566)

**Testosterone** The main androgenic hormone. (p. 565)

## ANATOMY, PHYSIOLOGY, AND PATHOPHYSIOLOGY OVERVIEW

### MALE REPRODUCTIVE SYSTEM

The male reproductive system consists of several structures; two of these structures, the testes and seminiferous tubules, produce the primary male hormones. The *testes,* a pair of oval glands located in the scrotal sac, are the male gonads. The testes produce male sex hormones. The *seminiferous tubules,* which are channels in the testes, are the site of spermatogenesis, which is the process by which mature sperm cells are produced.

Androgens are the group of male sex hormones (primarily testosterone) that mediate the normal development and maintenance of the primary and secondary male sex characteristics. Secondary male sex characteristics include advanced development of the prostate, seminal vesicles (two glands adjacent to the prostate), penis, and scrotum, as well as male hair distribution, laryngeal enlargement, thickening of the vocal cords, and male body musculature and fat distribution. Androgens must be secreted in adequate amounts for these characteristics to appear. The most important androgen is testosterone, which is produced from clusters of interstitial cells located between the seminiferous tubules. Besides having androgenic activity, testosterone is also involved in the development of bone and muscle tissue; inhibition of protein catabolism (metabolic breakdown); and retention of nitrogen, phosphorus, potassium, and sodium. These functions contribute to its anabolic activity. The hormone initiates the synthesis of specific proteins needed for androgenic and anabolic activity by binding to chromatin (strands of deoxyribonucleic acid [DNA]) in the nuclei of interstitial cells. In addition, testosterone appears to have an erythropoietic effect in that it stimulates the production of red blood cells (see Chapter 54).

## PHARMACOLOGY OVERVIEW

### ANDROGENS AND OTHER DRUGS PERTAINING TO MEN'S HEALTH

Testosterone deficiency is treated with exogenous testosterone. There are several synthetic derivatives of testosterone that have improved pharmacokinetic and pharmacodynamic characteristics over the naturally occurring hormone. This is accomplished by combining various esters with testosterone, which prolongs the duration of action of the hormone. For example, testosterone propionate is formulated as an oily solution, and its hormonal effects last for 2 to 3 days; the effects of testosterone cypionate and testosterone enanthate in oil last for up to 2 to 4 weeks. Orally administered testosterone has very poor absorption, because most of the dose is metabolized and destroyed by the liver before it can reach the circulation (first-pass effect; see Chapter 2). To circumvent this problem, researchers developed methyltestosterone (Android) and fluoxymesterone (Halotestin). Both are synthetic dosage forms (tablets or capsules) designed to be effective following oral administration. Methyltestosterone is also available in a

buccal tablet, which is dissolved in the buccal cavity (the space in the mouth between the cheek and teeth) and in an injectable form. Transdermal dosage forms of testosterone, including skin patches and a gel, have provided another way to circumvent the first-pass effect that occurs with oral administration of this hormone.

There are other chemical derivatives of testosterone known as *anabolic steroids.* These are synthetic drugs that closely resemble the natural hormone but possess high anabolic activity. Currently three anabolic steroid drug products are commercially available. These include oxymetholone (Anadrol-50), oxandrolone (Oxandrin), and nandrolone (Deca-Durabolin). Approved indications include anemia, hereditary angioedema, and metastatic breast cancer. Unlabeled (non–FDA-approved) uses for oxandrolone include treatment of human immunodeficiency virus (HIV)–associated wasting syndrome (debilitation related to disease-induced nutritional malabsorption) and alcoholic hepatitis. Oxandrolone is also used in hospitalized patients to stimulate weight gain. Anabolic steroids have a great potential for misuse by athletes, especially bodybuilders and weight lifters, because of their muscle-building properties. Improper use of these substances can have many serious consequences, such as sterility, cardiovascular diseases, and even liver cancer. For this reason, anabolic steroids are currently classified as Schedule III controlled substances by the U.S. Drug Enforcement Administration. This classification implies that misuse of these drugs can lead to psychological or physical dependence or both.

Another synthetic androgen is danazol (Danocrine). Its labeled uses include treatment of hereditary angioedema, and, in women, endometriosis and fibrocystic breast disease.

### Mechanism of Action and Drug Effects

The natural and synthetic androgens and the synthetic anabolic steroids have effects similar to those of the endogenous androgens. These include stimulation of the normal growth and development of the male sex organs (primary sex characteristics) and development and maintenance of the secondary sex characteristics. Androgens stimulate the synthesis of ribonucleic acid (RNA) at the cellular level, thereby promoting cellular growth and reproduction. They also retard the breakdown of amino acids. These properties contribute to an increased synthesis of body proteins, which aids in the formation and maintenance of muscle tissue. Another potent anabolic effect of androgens is the retention of nitrogen, also essential for protein synthesis. Nitrogen also promotes the storage of inorganic phosphorus, sulfate, sodium, and potassium, all of which have important metabolic roles, including protein synthesis, nerve impulse conduction, and muscular contractions. All of these effects result in weight gain and an increase in muscular strength. Finally, androgens also stimulate the production of erythropoietin by the kidney, which leads to enhanced erythropoiesis (red blood cell synthesis; see Chapter 54). However, the administration of exogenous androgens causes the release of endogenous testosterone to be inhibited as a result of the feedback inhibition of pituitary luteinizing hormone. Large doses of exogenous androgens may also suppress sperm production as a result of the feedback inhibition of pituitary follicle-stimulating hormone, which leads to infertility.

Androgen inhibitors block the effects of naturally occurring (endogenous) androgens. This is accomplished via inhibition of a specific enzyme, 5-alpha reductase. For this reason, these drugs are also called *5-alpha reductase inhibitors*. For unknown reasons, normal male physiology often results in an enlargement of the prostate known as benign prostatic hyperplasia (BPH). This process begins as early as 30 years of age and is present in at least 85% of men by 80 years of age. The most troubling symptom is usually varying degrees of obstructed urinary outflow. Although surgical treatment by *transurethral resection of the prostate (TURP)* is a common strategy, BPH is also often treatable with a 5-alpha reductase inhibitor. There are currently two such drugs: finasteride and dutasteride. Finasteride (Proscar), the prototypical drug for this class, works by inhibiting this enzyme, which normally converts testosterone to 5-alpha dihydrotestosterone (DHT). DHT is a more potent type of testosterone and is the principal androgen responsible for stimulating prostatic growth, as well as the expression of other male primary and secondary sex characteristics. Finasteride can dramatically lower the prostatic DHT concentrations, which helps to reduce the size of the prostate to ease the passage of urine. Fortunately, finasteride does not cause antiandrogen adverse effects that might be expected, such as loss of muscle strength, and fertility.

The effects of finasteride are limited primarily to the prostate, but this drug may also affect 5-alpha reductase–dependent processes elsewhere in the body, such as in the hair follicles, skin, and liver. Research has demonstrated that the pharmacologic inhibition of 5-alpha reductase prevents the thinning of hair caused by increased levels of DHT. It has been noted that men taking finasteride experience increased hair growth. Therefore, finasteride is also indicated for the treatment of male-pattern baldness as Propecia. Finasteride is indicated for the treatment of baldness only in men, not in women. Finasteride can be teratogenic in pregnant women, and its use in women of any age (pregnant or not) is not recommended. Women need to wear gloves when handling finasteride. Another medication, minoxidil (Rogaine), can be used topically to treat baldness in both men and women. It is discussed in more detail in Chapter 56.

Another class of drugs that may be used to help alleviate the symptoms of obstruction due to BPH are the alpha$_1$-adrenergic blockers. These drugs are discussed in greater detail in Chapter 19. The alpha$_1$-adrenergic blockers that are most commonly used for symptomatic relief of obstruction secondary to BPH are terazosin (Hytrin), doxazosin (Cardura), tamsulosin (Flomax), alfuzosin (Uroxatral), and silodosin (Rapaflo). Tamsulosin, alfuzosin, and silodosin appear to have a greater specificity for the alpha$_1$-receptors in the prostate and thus may cause less hypotension. These drugs have clinical effects of prostate shrinkage immediately, as opposed to the 5-alpha reductase inhibitors, which may take up to 6 months of continual therapy.

There are also two other classes of androgen inhibitors. The first includes the androgen receptor blockers flutamide (Eulexin), nilutamide (Nilandron), and bicalutamide

(Casodex). These drugs work by blocking the activity of androgen hormones at the level of the receptors in target tissues (e.g., prostate). For this reason, these drugs are used in the treatment of prostate cancer (see Chapter 46). The second class is the gonadotropin-releasing hormone (Gn-RH) analogues, including leuprolide (Lupron), goserelin (Zoladex), and triptorelin (Trelstar). These drugs work by inhibiting the secretion of pituitary gonadotropin, which eventually leads to a decrease in testosterone production. Both androgen receptor blockers and Gn-RH analogues are used most commonly to treat prostate cancer and are discussed in further detail in Chapter 46.

---

### 🌐 PATIENT-CENTERED CARE: CULTURAL IMPLICATIONS

#### *Men's Health Concerns: Prostate Cancer and Its Occurrence and Mortality*

It is estimated that 217,730 men will be diagnosed in 2010 with prostate cancer and 32,050 will die of the cancer. During the years 2004 to 2008, the median age at diagnosis for prostate cancer was 67 years of age. Incidence rates by race per 100,000 men are as follows (from cases diagnosed from 2004 to 2008): 156 per 100,000 for all races, 149.5 for whites, 233.8 for African Americans, 88.3 for Asians and Pacific Islanders, 75.3 for Native Americans and Alaska Natives, and 107.4 per 100,000 for Hispanics. Prostate cancer is the most common nonskin malignancy in men and the second leading cause of cancer-related death in men in the United States. African-American men have a higher incidence and at least double the mortality rates as compared with men from other racial ethnic groups.

Data from Howlader N, Noone AM, Krapcho M, et al, editors: *SEER cancer statistics review, 1975-2008,* Bethesda, MD, 2011, National Cancer Institute, available at http://seer.cancer.gov/csr/1975_2008/. Accessed May 25, 2011; National Cancer Institute at the National Institutes of Health: Prostate cancer, available at www.cancer.gov/cancertopics/types/prostate. Accessed May 25, 2011.

---

Phosphodiesterase inhibitors are used in the treatment of erectile dysfunction. Sildenafil (Viagra) was the first oral drug approved for the treatment of erectile dysfunction. Sildenafil works by inhibiting the action of the enzyme phosphodiesterase. This in turn allows the buildup in the penis of the chemical cyclic guanosine monophosphate, which causes relaxation of the smooth muscle in the corpora cavernosa (erectile tubes) of the penis and permits the inflow of blood. Nitric oxide is also released inside the corpora cavernosa during sexual stimulation and contributes to the erectile effect. Two drugs that are similar but have a longer duration of action are vardenafil (Levitra) and tadalafil (Cialis). Collectively, these drugs are referred to as *erectile dysfunction drugs*. Sildenafil is also used to treat pulmonary hypertension (see Chapter 22) under the trade name Revatio.

A second type of drug used to treat erectile dysfunction is the prostaglandin alprostadil (Caverject). This drug must be given by injecting it directly into the erectile tissue of the penis or pushing a suppository form of the drug into the urethra.

A list of all of the men's health drugs mentioned in the chapter appears in Box 35-1. More information on selected drugs can be found in the Drug Profiles section.

## BOX 35-1 CURRENTLY AVAILABLE MEN'S HEALTH DRUGS

**Alpha₁-Adrenergic Blockers**
doxazosin
tamsulosin
terazosin
alfuzosin

**Anabolic Steroids**
nandrolone
oxandrolone
oxymetholone

**Other Androgens**
danazol
fluoxymesterone
methyltestosterone
testosterone

**Antiandrogens**
bicalutamide
flutamide
nilutamide

**5-Alpha Reductase Inhibitors**
finasteride
dutasteride

**Gonadotropin-Releasing Hormone Analogues**
goserelin
leuprolide
triptorelin

**Peripheral Vasodilator**
minoxidil

**Drugs for Erectile Dysfunction**
sildenafil
tadalafil
vardenafil
alprostadil

## PATIENT-CENTERED CARE: LIFESPAN CONSIDERATIONS FOR THE ELDERLY PATIENT

### Sildenafil: Use and Concerns

- One in 10 men in the world has erectile dysfunction (ED). Some 30 million men in the U.S. have erectile dysfunction. Fifty percent of men with diabetes experience erectile dysfunction. The incidence of ED increases with age, with 39% at 40 years of age and 65% older than 65 years of age.
- Sildenafil (Viagra) is a prescription medication that is commonly ordered to treat ED, but it is not without concerns and cautions for the patient. This is especially true for elderly patients who generally have other medical conditions (e.g., renal disorders, hypertension, diabetes) and are usually taking more than one other prescribed medication.
- Liver function declines with age; therefore, drugs may not be metabolized as effectively in older adults as they are in younger adults. In addition, sildenafil is highly protein bound, which causes it to stay in the body longer and thus increases the possibility for drug interactions and toxicity.
- A decreased dosage of sildenafil is generally indicated for patients older than 65 years of age and for those with liver or renal impairment.
- Adverse effects to be concerned about in all patients, particularly older patients, include headache, flushing, and dyspepsia.
- Sildenafil must be used cautiously in patients who have cardiac disease and angina, because these patients are at greater risk for complications, especially if they are taking nitrates for their cardiovascular disease. Severe hypotension may occur.
- Discussing topics of a sexual nature may be comfortable for some patients but very anxiety producing for others. Be aware of cultural and gender differences in how individuals perceive their own sexuality and how they generally deal with sexual performance issues. Be respectful of each individual's beliefs and feelings and their sexual beliefs and practices. This requires knowledge, sensitivity, and objectivity.

## TABLE 35-1 MEN'S HEALTH DRUGS: INDICATIONS

| DRUG | INDICATION |
|---|---|
| danazol and stanozolol | Hereditary angioedema |
| finasteride | Benign prostatic hyperplasia |
| | Male androgenetic alopecia |
| fluoxymesterone and methyltestosterone | Male hypogonadism, inoperable breast cancer |
| methyltestosterone | Postpubertal cryptorchidism |
| minoxidil | Hypertension |
| | Female and male androgenetic alopecia |
| oxandrolone | Weight gain |
| sildenafil, tadalafil, vardenafil | Erectile dysfunction |
| testosterone | Primary or secondary hypogonadism |

## Indications

The primary use for androgens is as hormone replacement therapy. Indications for other types of drugs discussed in this chapter are listed in Table 35-1.

## Contraindications

Contraindications to the use of androgenic drugs include known androgen-responsive tumors. Use of sildenafil, vardenafil, and tadalafil is also contraindicated in men with major cardiovascular disorders, especially if they use nitrate medications such as nitroglycerin. Concurrent use of erectile dysfunction drugs and nitrates may cause severe hypotension, which may not respond to treatment. Use of finasteride is contraindicated in women (especially pregnant women) and children.

## Adverse Effects

Although rare, some of the most devastating effects of androgenic steroids occur in the liver, where they cause the formation of blood-filled cavities, a condition known as *peliosis of the liver.* This condition is a possible consequence of the long-term administration of androgenic anabolic steroids and can be life-threatening. Other serious hepatic effects are hepatic neoplasms (liver cancer), cholestatic hepatitis, jaundice, and abnormal liver function. Fluid retention is another undesirable effect of androgens and may account for some of the weight gain seen. The serious adverse effects that can be caused by the androgens far outweigh the advantages to be gained from their use by those seeking improved athletic ability. Other less serious adverse effects of androgens are listed in Table 35-2.

Sildenafil, vardenafil, and tadalafil appear to have relatively favorable adverse effect profiles. In patients with preexisting cardiovascular disease, especially those taking nitrates (e.g., nitroglycerin, isosorbide mononitrate, or dinitrate), these drugs can lower blood pressure substantially, potentially leading to more serious adverse events. Headache, flushing, and dyspepsia are the most common adverse effects reported. *Priapism* or abnormally prolonged penile erection is a relatively uncommon, but possible, adverse effect of both the erectile dysfunction drugs

## TABLE 35-2    MEN'S HEALTH DRUGS: SELECTED ADVERSE EFFECTS

| DRUG CLASS | ADVERSE EFFECTS |
|---|---|
| Alpha$_1$-adrenergic blockers | Tachycardia, hypotension, syncope, depression, drowsiness, rash, impotence, urinary frequency, dyspnea, visual changes, headache |
| Androgens (including anabolic steroids) | Headache, changes in libido, anxiety, depression, acne, male pattern baldness, hirsutism, nausea, abnormal liver function test results, priapism, elevated cholesterol level |
| 5-Alpha reductase inhibitors | Reduced libido, hypotension, dizziness, drowsiness |
| Peripheral vasodilator (topical minoxidil) | With topical route, usually limited to localized dermatologic reactions, including erythema, dermatitis, eczema, pruritus |
| Drugs for erectile dysfunction | Dizziness, headache, muscular pain, chest pain, hypertension or hypotension, rash, dry mouth, nausea, vomiting, diarrhea, priapism |

and the androgens. This condition is a medical emergency and warrants urgent medical attention. It is simply due to an excessive therapeutic drug response. Phosphodiesterase inhibitors can also cause unexplained visual loss.

Finasteride has been reported to cause loss of libido, loss of erection, ejaculatory dysfunction, hypersensitivity reactions, gynecomastia, and severe myopathy. The drug has also caused a 50% decrease in prostate-specific antigen (PSA) concentrations. Pregnant women must not handle crushed or broken tablets on a regular basis because of the possibility of topical absorption, which can lead to teratogenic effects.

## Interactions

Androgens, when used with oral anticoagulants, can significantly increase or decrease anticoagulant activity (see Chapter 26). Concurrent use of androgens with cyclosporine (see Chapter 48) increases the risk of cyclosporine toxicity and is not recommended. Sildenafil, vardenafil, and tadalafil may cause severe hypotension when given together with nitrates such as nitroglycerin, isosorbide mononitrate, or isosorbide dinitrate (see Chapter 23). Alpha blockers can cause additive hypotension when given with other drugs that lower blood pressure (see Chapter 22). Effects of tamsulosin may be increased when it is taken with azole antifungal drugs, erythromycin and clarithromycin (see Chapter 38), cardiac drugs such as propranolol and verapamil (see Chapters 19 and 25), and protease inhibitors (see Chapter 40).

## Dosages

For dosage information on the men's health drugs, see the table below.

## DRUG PROFILES

### finasteride

Finasteride (Proscar) is available in two tablet forms of 1- and 5-mg strengths. The lower strength is indicated for androgenetic alopecia in men. The higher strength is indicated for BPH, with clinical effects of prostate shrinkage in approximately 3 to 6 months of continual therapy. A similar drug, dutasteride (Avodart), is also indicated for BPH and is currently available in 0.5-mg capsule form. Both drugs are contraindicated in patients who have shown hypersensitivity and in pregnant women and children. It is considered potentially dangerous for a pregnant woman even to handle crushed or broken tablets. Both drugs are classified as pregnancy category X. Recommended dosages are given in the table on this page.

## DOSAGES

### Selected Men's Health Drugs

| DRUG | PHARMACOLOGIC CLASS | USUAL DOSAGE RANGE | INDICATIONS |
|---|---|---|---|
| finasteride (Propecia, Proscar) | 5-Alpha reductase inhibitor | **Adult**<br>PO: 1 mg daily (Propecia)<br>PO: 5 mg daily (Proscar) | Androgenetic alopecia (baldness) (males only)<br>Benign prostatic hyperplasia |
| ◆ sildenafil (Viagra) | Phosphodiesterase inhibitor | **Adult (males only)**<br>PO: 25-100 mg 1 hr before intercourse, no more than once daily | Erectile dysfunction |
| ◆ testosterone cypionate (Depo-Testosterone) | Androgenic hormone | **Adult and adolescent**<br>IM: 50-400 mg q2-4wk | Delayed puberty or hypogonadism (in males) |
| ◆ testosterone, transdermal (Testoderm, Androderm, AndroGel) | Androgenic hormone | **Adult and adolescent**<br>Testoderm patch (applied only to scrotal skin): 4-6 mg/day<br>Androderm patch (applied to skin of back, abdomen, upper arms, or thighs): 2.5-5 mg/day<br>AndroGel (applied to shoulders, arms, or abdominal skin): 5 g daily (delivers 50 mg of testosterone) | Male hypogonadism |

*IM,* Intramuscular; *PO,* oral.

## Pharmacokinetics (finasteride)

| Route | Onset of Action | Peak Plasma Concentration | Elimination Half-life | Duration of Action |
|-------|-----------------|---------------------------|----------------------|--------------------|
| PO | 3-12 mo | 8 hr | 4-15 hr | Unknown |

#### ◆ sildenafil

Sildenafil (Viagra) is approved for the treatment of erectile dysfunction. Other erectile dysfunction drugs with longer durations of action include vardenafil and tadalafil. Sildenafil potentiates the physiologic sexual response, causing penile erection after sexual arousal by relaxing smooth muscle and increasing blood flow into the penis.

Sildenafil use is contraindicated in patients with a known hypersensitivity to it. Sildenafil can potentiate the hypotensive effects of nitrates, and its administration to patients who are using organic nitrates in any form, either regularly or intermittently, is therefore contraindicated. Recommended dosages are given in the table on p. 568.

## Pharmacokinetics

| Route | Onset of Action | Peak Plasma Concentration | Elimination Half-life | Duration of Action |
|-------|-----------------|---------------------------|----------------------|--------------------|
| PO | 0.5-1 hr | 1 hr | 4 hr | 4-6 hr |

#### ◆ testosterone

Testosterone (Androderm) is a naturally occurring anabolic steroid. It is used for primary and secondary hypogonadism but may also be used to treat oligospermia in men as well as inoperable breast cancer in women, where its purpose is to counteract tumor-enhancing estrogen activity. When it is used as hormone replacement therapy, a transdermal product is desirable. There are presently two transdermal patch formulations. They attempt to mimic the normal circadian variation in testosterone concentration seen in young healthy men, in whom the maximum testosterone levels occur in the early morning hours and the minimum concentrations occur in the evening. Of the two available transdermal delivery systems, Testoderm is always applied to the scrotal skin, whereas Androderm is always applied to skin elsewhere on the body and never to the scrotal skin. Educate patients to wash their hands and cover the area where testosterone is applied, as transfer to others can occur.

Testosterone use is contraindicated in patients with severe renal, cardiac, or hepatic disease; male breast cancer; prostate cancer; hypersensitivity; or genital bleeding, as well as in pregnant or lactating women. Testosterone is considered a Schedule III controlled substance under the Anabolic Steroids Control Act. It is available as intramuscular injections, transdermal gel, transdermal patches, and even implantable pellets. It is classified as a pregnancy category X drug. Recommended dosages are given in the table on p. 568.

## Pharmacokinetics

| Route | Onset of Action | Peak Plasma Concentration | Elimination Half-life | Duration of Action |
|-------|-----------------|---------------------------|----------------------|--------------------|
| Topical | 1-2 hr | 2-4 hr | 10-100 min | 2-4 wk |

### TEAMWORK AND COLLABORATION: PHARMACOKINETIC BRIDGE TO NURSING PRACTICE

Drugs used to manage erectile dysfunction (e.g., sildenafil) essentially work in the same way as the body to assist the male patient in achieving an erection. The related pharmacokinetics must be understood so that the drug is taken safely and effectively. Sildenafil is a rapidly absorbed drug with onset of action within 1 hour, peak plasma concentrations within 1 hour, and duration of action of up to 4 to 6 hours. If the drug is taken with a high-fat meal, absorption will be delayed, and it may take an additional 60 minutes for the drug to reach peak levels. This is yet another example of how specific drug pharmacokinetics may be affected by variables in a patient's everyday life, such as eating habits. Another pharmacokinetic consideration is that patients who are 65 years of age or older have reduced clearance of sildenafil and may experience increased plasma concentrations of free (or pharmacologically active) drug. This could possibly lead to drug accumulation and/or toxicity.

## NURSING PROCESS

### ASSESSMENT

Before any drug is given to a male patient for the treatment of benign or malignant diseases of the male reproductive tract, thoroughly assess presenting symptoms and obtain a complete history of past and present medical diseases or conditions. In addition, assess the patient's urinary elimination patterns and any difficulties, and document the findings. The health care provider usually performs a rectal examination to palpate for enlargement of the prostate or for other possible pathology. If enlargement exists, a serum PSA test will most likely be ordered, especially prior to any treatment, and the test may also be ordered during treatment. PSA levels may be increased in pathologic conditions such as prostate cancer. Monitor levels for baseline and comparative reasons. PSA levels are expected to decrease with effective therapeutic regimens. More recent research encourages the use of a PSA value of less than 2.5 or 3 ng/mL as the criterion for normal levels, especially for younger patients.

With *testosterone* and related drugs, assess the patient for liver disease because formation of blood-filled cavities may occur. This condition, also called *peliosis,* is associated with long-term therapy and may be life-threatening. Perform liver function studies (e.g., LDH, CPK, and bilirubin levels) as ordered to monitor for the possible adverse effect of abnormal liver function and jaundice. Because edema is also a problem with these drugs, recording baseline weights, intake and output, and history of any cardiovascular diseases is important. Another contraindication to assess for is that of a history of known androgen-responsive tumors.

*Finasteride* requires baseline assessment of urinary patterns with attention to frequency, urgency, and flow of urine with micturation. As the tissue responds to the drug and there is a reduction in the size of the prostate gland and thus improvement in the symptoms of BPH, urinary flow will be increased. With potentially teratogenic drugs such as finasteride, follow special handling precautions and advise any pregnant caregiver or partner to do the same. Finasteride is not to be given in women. Assessment of the patient's sexual functioning and libido is important due to possible interference from the drug.

Before *drugs for erectile dysfunction* are given, the prescriber will perform a physical examination. You will need to perform a thorough nursing assessment including vital signs, and obtain a thorough medication history. Take a thorough cardiac history and assess for contraindications with the use of phosphodiesterase inhibitors (e.g., sildenafil, vardenafil [Levitra], and tadalafil [Cialis]), such as major cardiovascular disorders or the use of nitrate medications (nitroglycerin, isosorbide mononitrate, or dinitrate). The erectile dysfunction drugs and nitrates may lead to severe hypotension that may not respond to treatment.

## NURSING DIAGNOSES

1. Decreased cardiac output related to drug interaction between erectile dysfunction drug and nitrates
2. Ineffective sexuality pattern related to the effects of treatment with androgen and/or therapy with phosphodiesterase inhibitors
3. Deficient knowledge related to lack of information about drug therapy and disease process of BPH as well as drug interactions with finasteride

## PLANNING

### GOALS
1. Patient maintains normal and adequate cardiac output.
2. Patient maintains or regains effective sexual patterns and functioning.
3. Patient displays adequate knowledge regarding disease process and recommended drug therapy.

### OUTCOME CRITERIA
1. Patient maintains blood pressure within normal limits with at least 120/80 mmHg readings.
   - Patient experiences minimal drop in systolic and diastolic blood pressure during drug therapy with erectile dysfunction drugs or androgens.
   - Patient avoids potential interactions with medication regimen (e.g., nitrates not to be taken with erectile dysfunction drugs) as well as situations that may exacerbate hypotension, such as saunas, alcohol, and hot climates.
   - Patient reports continued low blood pressure readings, dizziness, or feelings of lightheadedness to prescriber.
2. Patient openly verbalizes feelings of inadequacies associated with changes in libido or sexual functioning and seeks out help from health care provider.
   - Patient takes medication as prescribed to minimize adverse effects and maximize therapeutic effects.
   - Patient implements suggestions for improving libido and sexual functioning as recommended by prescriber.
   - Patient verbalizes the ability to sustain and maintain an erection or complete the act of coitus.
3. Patient states understanding of the rationale for drug therapy.

## IMPLEMENTATION

The therapeutic effects of *testosterone* are maximized when the drug is taken as ordered and at regular intervals so that steady levels are maintained. If the drug is being used for hypogonadism or induction of puberty, dosages may be managed differently, so that at the end of the growth spurt the patient is placed on maintenance dosages. Instruct patients to apply Testoderm transdermal patches as ordered, which is usually to clean, dry scrotal skin that has been shaved for optimal skin contact and replaced every day. Advise the patient to follow instructions for application and time of duration per prescriber's orders. Educate patients that Androderm patches are to be applied to clean, dry skin on the back, abdomen, upper arms, or thighs; the scrotum and bony areas (shoulder, hip) are not to be used with this particular drug. Be sure the proper patch is being used and that drugs are not confused. AndroGel is to be applied to shoulders, arms, or abdominal skin as ordered. If testosterone is being given intramuscularly, it is usually given every 2 to 4 weeks as prescribed. Mix the vial of medication thoroughly by agitating it before withdrawing the prescribed amount of medication.

*Finasteride* may be given orally without regard to meals. When used for treatment of the urinary symptoms of BPH, finasteride and related drugs may be ordered for approximately 3 to 6 months with a reevaluation of the condition at that time. Advise the patient to protect the drug from exposure to light and heat. Due to the teratogenic effects of finasteride, emphasize that it must not be handled in any form by a pregnant woman. Recommend that female nurses/members of the health care team wear gloves when handling this medication. Women need to wear gloves when handling this medication.

## SAFETY: HERBAL THERAPIES AND DIETARY SUPPLEMENTS

### Saw Palmetto (Serenoa repens, Sabal serrulata)

**Overview**
Saw palmetto comes from a tree that is also known as the American dwarf palm. The therapeutically active part of the tree is its ripe fruit. Saw palmetto is believed to inhibit dihydrotestosterone and 5-alpha reductase. A prostatic-specific antigen test and digital rectal examination should be performed before initiation of treatment with saw palmetto for benign prostatic hyperplasia.

**Common Uses**
Diuretic, urinary antiseptic, treatment of benign prostatic hyperplasia, treatment of alopecia

**Adverse Effects**
Gastrointestinal upset, headache, back pain, dysuria

**Potential Drug Interactions**
Nonsteroidal antiinflammatory drugs, hormones such as estrogen replacement therapy and oral contraceptives, immunostimulants

**Contraindications**
None

It is recommended that women of any age do not take this medication. See the Safety: Herbal Therapies and Dietary Supplements box for a description of saw palmetto, an herbal supplement that is often taken to relieve symptoms of an enlarged prostate.

For patients taking *erectile dysfunction drugs,* alert them to the drug interaction-related serious adverse effect of severe drops in blood pressure if taken with nitrates. When taking sildenafil, vardenafil, or tadalafil, priapism, which is the abnormally prolonged erection of the penis, may occur; it is considered a medical emergency and requires immediate and urgent medical attention. See the Patient Teaching Tips for more information.

# EVALUATION

The therapeutic effects of drugs related to the male reproductive tract include improvement of the condition and/or signs and symptoms for which the patient is being treated, such as hypogonadism, sexual dysfunction, erectile dysfunction, and urinary elimination problems caused by BPH. The therapeutic effects of some drugs (e.g., finasteride) may not be seen for 3 to 6 months, so it is important to observe and monitor the patient for the intended effects of the drugs. In addition, evaluate for the adverse effects of these medications (see the pharmacology section for specific adverse effects). Always evaluate goals and outcome criteria to see if the patient's needs have been met.

---

## CASE STUDY

### *Erectile Dysfunction Drugs*

Mr. S., a 63-year-old college professor, is in the office for a yearly checkup. He feels he is generally healthy, and he does not take any medications. He does say that he has one problem that he wants to discuss with the physician. During his physical examination, he tells the physician, "I have something embarrassing to ask. I want to try one of those drugs that can help my sex life." The physician reassures Mr. S. that he does not need to be embarrassed to ask about this. The physician then assesses Mr. S.'s sexual difficulties. At the end of the examination and assessment, Mr. S. is given a prescription for sildenafil (Viagra).

1. What teaching is important for Mr. S. before he starts this medication?
2. Eleven months later, Mr. S. is admitted to the emergency department with chest pains. After a thorough examination, including a cardiac catheterization,

he is diagnosed with mild coronary artery disease and is started on isosorbide dinitrate, sustained-release, 40 mg every 12 hours. He is given a follow-up appointment with his physician in 1 week. What specific teaching is important at this time?

3. Mr. S. comes to the office for the follow-up appointment and tells the nurse that he wants to try saw palmetto for his prostate health. He has a neighbor who takes it and has no problems with it, and he has noticed that he has had a slight increase in difficulty with urination. He is also upset about what he was told in the hospital about his medications. How will the nurse respond to Mr. S., and what assessments are needed at this time?

For answers, see http://evolve.elsevier.com/Lilley.

---

## PATIENT TEACHING TIPS

- With finasteride, provide education at the patient's educational level about the drug's therapeutic effects as well as adverse effects (see the pharmacology discussion for more information). Educate female family members, significant others, and caregivers who are pregnant or of childbearing age about the need to avoid exposure during handling of this drug, including *not* touching any broken or crushed tablets, which could result in exposure to the drug and the risk of teratogenic effects. Emphasize the need to wear gloves when handling the medication.
- Finasteride may be given orally without regard to meals. Instruct patients to protect the drug from exposure to light and heat.
- Sildenafil is usually prescribed to be taken about 1 hour before sexual activity. This drug, and other drugs for erectile dysfunction, should not be taken with nitrates because it

may lead to significant hypotensive consequences that could be life-threatening.
- Inform the patient that drug therapy for erectile dysfunction is not effective without sexual stimulation and arousal.
- With testosterone, educate the patient about all therapeutic and adverse effects. Emphasize the importance of follow-up appointments, which are crucial to evaluating the therapeutic effectiveness of the medication (as well as with any drugs discussed in this chapter).
- Prolonged erections (i.e., longer than 4 hours) must be reported immediately and are considered to be a medical emergency.
- Testosterone is not be withdrawn abruptly except under the supervision of the prescriber. Weaning is usually done over several weeks.

# KEY POINTS

- The most commonly used drugs related to male health and the male reproductive tract are finasteride, sildenafil, and testosterone. It is important to know the way these drugs work and their adverse effects, contraindications, cautions, and drug interactions to ensure their safe and effective use.
- Testosterone is responsible for the development and maintenance of the male reproductive system and secondary sex characteristics. Oral testosterone has very poor pharmacokinetic and pharmacodynamic characteristics, and therefore it is recommended that testosterone be administered via injection (parenteral route) or a transdermal patch.

- Methyltestosterone was developed to circumvent the problems associated with the oral administration of testosterone.
- Finasteride is usually indicated to stop growth of the prostate in men with BPH and to treat men with androgenic alopecia.
- Warn patients taking drugs for erectile dysfunction (e.g., sildenafil) about potential adverse effects, such as hypotension, headache, and heartburn.
- There are major concerns about heart-related deaths associated with concurrent use of nitrates and drugs used for erectile dysfunction. Focus patient education on the prevention of drug interactions and related adverse effects and complications.

# NCLEX® EXAMINATION REVIEW QUESTIONS

1. A patient has been taking finasteride (Proscar) for almost a year. The nurse knows that which is most important to evaluate at this time?
   a. Complete blood count
   b. PSA levels
   c. Blood pressure
   d. Fluid retention

2. The nurse is performing an assessment of a patient who is asking for a prescription for sildenafil (Viagra). Which finding would be a contraindication to its use?
   a. Age of 65 years
   b. History of thyroid disease
   c. Medication list that includes nitrates
   d. Medication list that includes saw palmetto

3. During a counseling session for a group of teenage athletes, the use of androgenic steroids is discussed. The nurse will explain that which problem is a rare but devastating effect of androgenic steroid use?
   a. Peliosis of the liver
   b. Bradycardia
   c. Kidney failure
   d. Tachydysrhythmias

4. The nurse is teaching a patient about the possible adverse effect of priapism, which may occur when taking erectile dysfunction drugs. The nurse emphasizes that, if this occurs, the most important action is to
   a. stay in bed until the erection ceases.
   b. apply an ice pack for 30 minutes.
   c. turn toward his left side and rest.
   d. seek medical attention immediately.

5. A patient is asking about the use of saw palmetto for prostate health. The nurse tells him that drugs that interact with saw palmetto include:
   a. acetaminophen (Tylenol).
   b. nitrates.
   c. nonsteroidal antiinflammatory drugs.
   d. antihypertensive drugs.

6. When the Testoderm form of testosterone is ordered to treat hypogonadism in a teenage boy, which instructions by the nurse are correct? (Select all that apply.)
   a. Place the patch on clean, dry skin on the back, upper arms, abdomen, or thighs.
   b. Place the patch on clean, dry scrotal skin that has been shaved.
   c. Place the patch on clean, dry scrotal skin, but do not shave the skin first.
   d. Place the patch on any clean, dry, nonhairy area of the body.
   e. Remove the old patch before applying a new patch.

7. A 16-year-old male is to receive testosterone cypionate (Depo-Testosterone), 50 mg IM every 2 weeks. The medication is available in 100-mg/mL containers. How many mL will the nurse draw up in the syringe to administer for each dose?

1. b, 2. c, 3. a, 4. d, 5. c, 6. b, e, 7. 0.5 mL per dose

For Critical Thinking and Prioritization Questions, see http://evolve.elsevier.com/Lilley.

# Drugs Affecting the Respiratory System

Study on the Run • PURR

## STUDY ON THE RUN, PURR

The basic approach in applying Study on the Run (SOTR) is to make use of small blocks of time that are otherwise nonproductive. Plan, Rehearse, and Review do not require that the entire chapter be covered in one study session. These steps produce their benefits by promoting repetition of learning.

### Where Is the Time?

SOTR time is everywhere. In the course of a single day, you might have an hour or more that can be used for SOTR activities. It is just a matter of becoming aware of little bits and pieces of your day that can ordinarily slip away without being productive. Small blocks of time are everywhere in your day; it just takes a little creativity on your part to become aware of them. Finishing an examination early, standing in the checkout line, waiting for the teakettle to boil, or even waiting for the washing machine to finish the last spin before you change loads can be time used for SOTR. Get creative and be flexible. Remember, every minute of time you use this way is a minute of time you will not have to find later.

### SOTR and Plan

Remember the importance of questioning as an essential component in Plan. Look at the chapter objectives for Chapter 37. There are five objectives presented for this chapter. Work on the questions for as many of these objectives as can be covered in the time you have. If you complete questions for only two objectives, do not look upon it as failure to complete something. Instead, learn to view what you have done as that much less to do later. The time you spend now frees up that much more time during your large blocks of study time for intense study reading.

Will you forget the questions you generated in this session before you have the opportunity to read the chapter? If you make it a habit to ask questions as a continuing part of all study, you will find that you remember the focus questions very well. If you have trouble remembering your own questions, write the questions in the margins of the text. Gradually you will find that questioning becomes such an automatic procedure that you will be able to dispense with writing questions. You will remember them.

### SOTR and Vocabulary

One of the most challenging aspects of a course like this is the almost overwhelming vocabulary load. If the new vocabulary load were not enough, there is also the need to keep reviewing previous parts and chapters because some term that was introduced three chapters ago has reappeared and you do not remember it clearly. Creating your own vocabulary cards is a perfect SOTR activity.

The basic card model is simple. The word, common form, prefix, or suffix appears on the card front. The back of the card may have just a little information (the minimum being a definition of what is on the front) or may contain considerable information. I recommend that you include part, chapter, and page number on the back so that you can locate the term quickly if the need arises. In addition, you may want to add a specific example from the text or of your own creation to help clarify the term. Put as much information on the back as you find useful.

### Creating Vocabulary Cards with SOTR

Use the time between classes to create several personal vocabulary cards. Grab your text and your blank note cards. Open to the next chapter you will be studying. Flip over to the key terms pages. Write the first word from the key terms on the front of a blank note card. Turn the card over. Write the part and chapter numbers and the page number for the key term on the card. Pick a standard location for this. Put these numbers in a top or bottom corner, but make sure you put them in the same corner every time. Eventually this becomes a habit and makes the preparation process faster. It also helps when you are making use of the cards, because you will know exactly what information you put on the card and where you put it. Put this card aside and repeat the process with the next term. In those few minutes before you go to class you can have completed the basic preparation for a full set of cards covering, for example, the 17 key terms in Chapter 36.

Notice that all I proposed was that you copy the term and the location information. I did not tell you to copy the definition listed in the key terms at this time. The term used in the context of a sentence and a paragraph may be much easier to understand. If, as you read the chapter, you feel that the glossary definition is also useful to have on this card, you can always flip back by using the location information you put on the card.

### SOTR and Vocabulary Review

Your vocabulary cards are ideal for SOTR action. Carry a pack of cards with you at all times. Whenever you have even a minute or two, you can pull out a stack of cards from previous chapters or the current chapter. Use the oral ask-and-answer method discussed in the *Study Guide*. For instance, the first key term in Chapter 37 is *allergen*. Ask yourself aloud, "What is an allergen?" Then try to answer the question aloud. Answer: "An allergen is a substance that produces an allergic reaction." It is not necessary to recall the exact answer presented in the key

terms and/or chapter. What is important is that you respond with a clear and meaningful answer. The answer given earlier is not exactly the same as that stated in the key terms, but the general concept is the same. Once you have stated your answer, turn the card over and check to make sure that you were correct. Each time you do this with a term, you are strengthening your long-term memory, and you will find that it takes less and less time to recall the terms you need.

Vocabulary cards can also be used with your study group. You may want to give oral quizzes to each other. This is one sure way to check that your answer is stated clearly.

### SOTR and Chapter Review

Chapter review can be overwhelming if you think that review means rereading the material and that you therefore need large blocks of uninterrupted time. There is a much more efficient way to review, and it works well in short time blocks, which makes it a perfect technique for SOTR.

Look at the first page of Chapter 36. You should instantly see a number of visible structures that make it easy to review key terms and concepts without rereading the entire block of material. First, there is the chapter title: Antihistamines, Decongestants, Antitussives, and Expectorants. What are antihistamines? This is a question you would have generated when you were engaged in the Plan step of PURR. Now that you have read the chapter, repeat the question and answer it aloud. Answer aloud because you will hear what you say and will either know the material or need to mark it to come back and reread. Now ask more complex questions: "What is the role of antihistamines? What do they do?" Now try to answer these questions. If you can, then you do not need to reread to find out what antihistamines are. Next, looking at p. 576, you will notice some terms in **bold blue print.** Apply the same process. Using these words and phrases as stimuli, ask questions and try to answer them to your own satisfaction. If you cannot develop a satisfactory answer, then you know that some rereading is needed. However, it should be very focused. You are not trying to reread everything on the page, but only the material right there that is associated with the term.

On p. 576 you will see a bulleted list. Look at the sentence preceding the list: "The release of excessive amounts of histamine can lead to anaphylaxis and severe allergic symptoms and may result in any or all of the following physiologic changes…" Ask questions. If you can answer them, no reading is necessary. If you cannot answer, you know that the answers are found immediately after this sentence in the bulleted list. Use the structures in the chapter to accomplish focused review. Comprehension is improved and long-term memory is strengthened, and your test grades will reflect this.

The benefits of SOTR are enormous. There are no drawbacks. You are using time that otherwise would be "wasted," and this time now becomes productive study time. The more active you become in looking for SOTR opportunities, the more you will find. The more SOTR time you spend, the better student you will become.

# Antihistamines, Decongestants, Antitussives, and Expectorants

## evolve WEBSITE

*http://evolve.elsevier.com/Lilley*
- Animations
- Answer Key—Textbook Case Studies
- Critical Thinking and Prioritization Questions
- Key Points—Downloadable
- Review Questions for the NCLEX® Examination
- Unfolding Case Studies

## OBJECTIVES

When you reach the end of this chapter, you will be able to do the following:
1 Provide specific examples of the drugs categorized as antihistamines (both sedating and nonsedating), decongestants, antitussives, and expectorants.
2 Discuss the mechanisms of action, indications, contraindications, cautions, drug interactions, adverse effects, dosages, and route of administration for antihistamines, decongestants, antitussives, and expectorants.
3 Develop a nursing care plan that includes all phases of the nursing process for patients taking any of the antihistamines, decongestants, antitussives, and/or expectorants.

## DRUG PROFILES

benzonatate, p. 583
codeine, p. 583
♦ dextromethorphan, p. 583
♦ diphenhydramine, p. 580
♦ guaifenesin, p. 584

♦ loratadine, p. 580
naphazoline, p. 582

_____

♦ *Key drug*

## KEY TERMS

Adrenergics (sympathomimetics) Drugs that stimulate the sympathetic nerve fibers of the autonomic nervous system that use epinephrine or epinephrine-like substances as neurotransmitters. (p. 580)

Antagonists Drugs that exert an action opposite to that of another drug or compete for the same receptor sites. (p. 577)

Anticholinergics (parasympatholytics) Drugs that block the action of acetylcholine and similar substances at acetylcholine receptors, which results in inhibition of the transmission of parasympathetic nerve impulses. (p. 580)

Antigens Substances that are capable of inducing specific immune responses and reacting with the specific products of those responses, such as antibodies and specifically sensitized T lymphocytes. Antigens can be soluble (e.g., a foreign protein) or particulate or insoluble (e.g., a bacterial cell). (p. 577)

Antihistamines Substances capable of reducing the physiologic and pharmacologic effects of histamine. (p. 577)

Antitussive A drug that reduces coughing, often by inhibiting neural activity in the cough center of the central nervous system. (p. 582)

**Corticosteroids** Any of the hormones produced by the adrenal cortex, either in natural or synthetic drug form. They control many key processes in the body, such as carbohydrate and protein metabolism, the maintenance of serum glucose levels, electrolyte and water balance, and the functions of the cardiovascular system, skeletal muscle, kidneys, and other organs. (p. 580)

**Decongestants** Drugs that reduce congestion or swelling, especially of the upper or lower respiratory tract. (p. 580)

**Empiric therapy** A method of treating disease based on observations and experience, rather than a knowledge of the precise cause for the disorder. (p. 576)

**Expectorants** Drugs that increase the flow of fluid in the respiratory tract, usually by reducing the viscosity of secretions, and facilitate their removal by coughing. (p. 584)

**Histamine antagonists** Drugs that compete with histamine for binding sites on histamine receptors. (p. 577)

**Influenza** A highly contagious infection of the respiratory tract caused by a myxovirus and transmitted by airborne droplets. (p. 576)

**Nonsedating antihistamines** Medications that primarily work peripherally to block the actions of histamine and therefore do not generally have the central nervous system effects of many of the older antihistamines; also called *second-generation antihistamines* and *peripherally acting antihistamines.* (p. 580)

**Reflex stimulation** An irritation of the respiratory tract occurring in response to an irritation of the gastrointestinal tract. (p. 583)

**Rhinovirus** Any of about 100 serologically distinct ribonucleic acid (RNA) viruses that cause about 40% of acute respiratory illnesses. (p. 576)

**Sympathomimetic drugs** A class of drugs whose effects mimic those resulting from the stimulation of the sympathetic nervous system. (p. 581)

**Upper respiratory tract infection (URI)** Any infectious disease of the upper respiratory tract, including the common cold, laryngitis, pharyngitis, rhinitis, sinusitis, and tonsillitis. (p. 576)

## ANATOMY, PHYSIOLOGY, AND PATHOPHYSIOLOGY OVERVIEW

Common colds result from a viral infection, most often infection with a rhinovirus or an influenza virus. These viruses invade the tissues (mucosa) of the upper respiratory tract (nose, pharynx, and larynx) to cause an upper respiratory tract infection (URI). The inflammatory response elicited by these viruses stimulates excessive mucus production. This fluid drips behind the nose, down the pharynx, and into the esophagus and lower respiratory tract, which leads to symptoms typical of a cold: sore throat, coughing, and upset stomach. Irritation of the nasal mucosa often triggers the sneeze reflex and also causes the release of several inflammatory and vasoactive substances, which results in the dilation of the small blood vessels in the nasal sinuses and leads to nasal congestion. Treatment of the common symptoms of URI involves the combined use of antihistamines, nasal decongestants, antitussives, and expectorants.

In 2008, the U.S. Food and Drug Administration (FDA) issued recommendations that over-the-counter (OTC) cough and cold products not be given to children younger than 2 years of age. This followed numerous case reports of symptoms such as oversedation, seizures, tachycardia, and even death in toddlers. There is also evidence that such medications are simply not effective in small children, and parents are advised to consult their pediatrician on the best ways to manage these illnesses. A 2010 study showed a dramatic decrease in young children emergency room visits since the FDA recommendation.

Many antihistamines, nasal decongestants, antitussives, and expectorants are available without prescription. However, these drugs can only relieve the symptoms of a URI. They can do nothing to eliminate the causative pathogen. Antiviral drugs

are currently the only drugs that are effective; however, treatment with these mediations is often hampered by the fact that the viral cause cannot be readily identified. Because of this, the treatment rendered can only be based on what is believed to be the most likely cause, given the presenting clinical symptoms. Such treatment is called empiric therapy. Some patients seem to gain benefit from the use of herbal products and other supplements, such as vitamin C, to prevent the onset of cold signs and symptoms or at least to decrease their severity. Herbal products commonly used for colds are echinacea and goldenseal (see the Safety: Herbal Therapies and Dietary Supplements boxes on p. 577). There is limited research data regarding the efficacy of herbal products, and some can have significant drug-drug or drug-disease interactions.

## PHARMACOLOGY OVERVIEW
### ANTIHISTAMINES

Histamine is a substance that performs many functions. It is involved in nerve impulse transmission in the central nervous system (CNS), dilation of capillaries, contraction of smooth muscle, stimulation of gastric secretion, and acceleration of the heart rate. There are two types of cellular receptors for histamine. Histamine 1 ($H_1$) receptors mediate smooth muscle contraction and dilation of capillaries; histamine 2 ($H_2$) receptors mediate acceleration of the heart rate and gastric acid secretion. The release of excessive amounts of histamine can lead to anaphylaxis and severe allergic symptoms and may result in any or all of the following physiologic changes:

- Constriction of smooth muscle, especially in the stomach and lungs
- Increase in body secretions

## SAFETY: HERBAL THERAPIES AND DIETARY SUPPLEMENTS

### *Echinacea* (Echinacea)

**Overview**

The three species of echinacea used medicinally are *Echinacea angustifolia*, *Echinacea pallida*, and *Echinacea purpurea*. Echinacea has been shown in clinical trials to reduce cold symptoms and recovery time when taken early in the illness. This is believed to be due to its immunostimulant effects. At this time, there is no strong research evidence to warrant recommending the herb for urinary tract infections, wound healing, or prevention of colds; further study is needed to provide evidence of its therapeutic effects and indications.

**Common Uses**

Stimulation of the immune system, antisepsis, treatment of viral infections and influenza-like respiratory tract infections, promotion of healing of wounds, and chronic ulcerations

**Adverse Effects**

Dermatitis, upset stomach or vomiting, dizziness, headache, unpleasant taste

**Potential Drug Interactions**

Amiodarone, cyclosporine, phenytoin, methotrexate, ketoconazole, barbiturates; tolerance likely to develop if used for more than 8 weeks. Because some preparations have a high alcohol content, they may cause acetaldehyde syndrome in patients taking disulfiram (Antabuse) to prevent alcohol abuse (see Chapter 17).

**Contraindications**

Contraindicated for patients with acquired immunodeficiency syndrome, tuberculosis, connective tissue diseases, multiple sclerosis

## SAFETY: HERBAL THERAPIES AND DIETARY SUPPLEMENTS

### *Goldenseal* (Hydrastis canadensis)

**Overview**

Goldenseal is found in wooded areas from the northeastern to midwestern United States. It is the dried root of the plant that is most commonly used for its various biologically active alkaloids. These components have been shown to have antibacterial, antifungal, and antiprotozoal activity. The alkaloid berberine has both anticholinergic and antihistaminic activity.

**Common Uses**

Treatment of upper respiratory tract infections, allergies, nasal congestion, and numerous genitourinary, skin, ophthalmic, and otic conditions

**Adverse Effects**

Gastrointestinal (GI) distress, emotional instability, mucosal ulceration (e.g., when used as a vaginal douche)

**Potential Drug Interactions**

**Gastric acid suppressors** (including antacids, histamine $H_2$ blockers [e.g., ranitidine], proton pump inhibitors [e.g., omeprazole]): theoretically reduced effectiveness due to acid-promoting effect of herb

**Antihypertensives:** theoretically reduced effectiveness due to vasoconstrictive activity of herb

**Contraindications**

Acute or chronic GI disorders; pregnancy (has uterine stimulant properties); should be used with caution by those with cardiovascular disease

Data from Skidmore-Roth L: *Mosby's handbook of herbs and natural supplements*, ed 4, St Louis, 2010, Mosby.

• Vasodilatation and increased capillary permeability, which results in the movement of fluid out of the blood vessels and into the tissues and thus causes a drop in blood pressure and edema

**Antihistamines** are drugs that directly compete with histamine for specific receptor sites. For this reason, they are also called histamine antagonists. Antihistamines that compete with histamine for the $H_2$ receptors are called $H_2$ antagonists or $H_2$ blockers and include cimetidine (Tagamet), ranitidine (Zantac), famotidine (Pepcid), and nizatidine (Axid). Because they act on the gastrointestinal (GI) system, they are discussed in detail in Chapter 50. This chapter focuses on the $H_1$ antagonists (also called $H_1$ blockers); they are the drugs commonly known as *antihistamines*. They are very useful drugs, because approximately 10% to 20% of the general population is sensitive to various environmental allergens. Histamine is a major inflammatory mediator in many allergic disorders, such as allergic rhinitis (e.g., hay fever and mold, dust allergies), anaphylaxis, angioedema, drug fevers, insect bite reactions, and urticaria (itching).

$H_1$ antagonists include drugs such as diphenhydramine (Benadryl), chlorpheniramine (generic), fexofenadine (Allegra), loratadine (Claritin), and cetirizine (Zyrtec). They are of greatest value in the treatment of nasal allergies, particularly seasonal hay fever. They are also given to relieve the symptoms of the common cold, such as sneezing and runny nose. In this regard they are palliative, not curative; that is, they can help alleviate the symptoms of a cold but can do nothing to destroy the virus causing it.

The clinical efficacy of the different antihistamines is very similar, although they have varying degrees of antihistaminic, anticholinergic, and sedating properties. The particular actions and indications for a particular antihistamine are determined by its specific chemical makeup. All antihistamines compete with histamine for the $H_1$ receptors in the smooth muscle surrounding blood vessels and bronchioles. They also affect the secretions of the lacrimal, salivary, and respiratory mucosal glands, which are the primary anticholinergic actions of antihistamines. These drugs differ from each other in their potency and adverse effects, especially in the degree of drowsiness they produce. The antihistaminic, anticholinergic, and sedative properties of some of the more commonly used antihistamines are summarized in Figure 36-1. Because of their antihistaminic properties, they are indicated for the treatment of allergies. They are also useful for the treatment of problems such as vertigo, motion sickness, insomnia, and cough. Several classes of antihistamines are listed in Table 36-1, along with their various anticholinergic and sedative effects.

## Mechanism of Action and Drug Effects

During allergic reactions, histamine and other substances are released from mast cells, basophils, and other cells in response to antigens circulating in the blood. Histamine molecules then bind to and activate other cells in the nose, eyes, respiratory tract, GI tract, and skin, producing the characteristic allergic signs and symptoms. For example, in the respiratory tract histamine causes extravascular smooth muscle (e.g., in the bronchial tree) to contract, whereas antihistamines cause it to relax. Also, histamine causes pruritus by stimulating nerve endings. Antihistamines can prevent or alleviate this itching.

Circulating histamine molecules bind to histamine receptors on basophils and mast cells. This stimulates further release of histamine stored within these cells. Antihistamine drugs work by blocking the histamine receptors on the surfaces of basophils and mast cells, thereby preventing the release and actions of histamine stored within these cells. They do not push off histamine that is already bound to a receptor but compete with histamine for unoccupied receptors. Therefore, they are most beneficial when given early in a histamine-mediated reaction, before all of the free histamine molecules bind to cell membrane receptors. The binding of $H_1$ blockers to these receptors prevents the adverse consequences of histamine binding: vasodilation; increased GI, respiratory, salivary, and lacrimal secretions; and increased capillary permeability with resultant edema. The various drug effects of antihistamines are listed in Table 36-2.

## Indications

Antihistamines are indicated for the management of nasal allergies, seasonal or perennial allergic rhinitis (e.g., hay fever), and

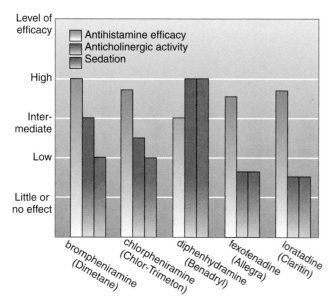

**FIGURE 36-1** Comparison of the efficacy and adverse effects of selected antihistamines.

### TABLE 36-2 ANTIHISTAMINES: DRUG EFFECTS

| BODY SYSTEM | HISTAMINE EFFECTS | ANTIHISTAMINE EFFECTS |
|---|---|---|
| Cardiovascular (small blood vessels) | Dilates blood vessels, increases blood vessel permeability (allows substances to leak into tissues) | Reduces dilation of blood vessels and increased permeability |
| Immune (release of various substances commonly associated with allergic reactions) | Released from mast cells along with several other substances, which results in allergic reactions | Does not stabilize mast cells or prevent the release of histamine and other substances, but does bind to histamine receptors and prevent the actions of histamine |
| Smooth muscle (on exocrine glands) | Stimulates salivary, gastric, lacrimal, and bronchial secretions | Reduces salivary, gastric, lacrimal, and bronchial secretions |

### TABLE 36-1 EFFECTS OF VARIOUS ANTIHISTAMINES

| CHEMICAL CLASS | ANTICHOLINERGIC EFFECTS | SEDATIVE EFFECTS | COMMENTS |
|---|---|---|---|
| **Alkylamines** | | | |
| brompheniramine | Moderate | Low | Cause less drowsiness and more CNS stimulation; suitable for daytime use. |
| chlorpheniramine | Moderate | Low | |
| dexchlorpheniramine | Moderate | Low | |
| **Ethanolamines** | | | |
| clemastine | High | Moderate | Substantial anticholinergic effects; commonly cause sedation; at usual dosages, drowsiness occurs in about 50% of patients; diphenhydramine and dimenhydrinate also used as antiemetics. |
| diphenhydramine | High | High | |
| dimenhydrinate | High | High | |
| **Phenothiazine** | | | |
| promethazine | High | High | Drugs in this class are principally used as antipsychotics; promethazine is useful as an antihistamine and antiemetic. |
| **Piperidines** | | | |
| cyproheptadine | Moderate | Low | Commonly used in the treatment of motion sickness; hydroxyzine is used as a tranquilizer, sedative, antipruritic, and antiemetic. |
| hydroxyzine | Moderate | Moderate | |
| **Miscellaneous** | | | |
| fexofenadine | Low to none | Low to none | Very few adverse anticholinergic or sedative effects; almost exclusively antihistaminic effects; can be taken during the day because no sedative effects occur; they are longer acting and have fewer adverse effects than other classes. |
| loratadine | Low | Low to none | |

*CNS,* Central nervous system; *GI,* gastrointestinal.

some of the typical symptoms of the common cold. They are also useful in the treatment of allergic reactions, motion sickness, Parkinson's disease (due to their anticholinergic effects), and vertigo. In addition, they are sometimes used as sleep aids.

## Contraindications

Use of antihistamines is contraindicated in cases of known drug allergy. They are not to be used as the sole drug therapy during acute asthmatic attacks. In such cases, a rapidly acting bronchodilator such as albuterol, or in extreme cases epinephrine, is the most urgently needed medication. Other contraindications may include narrow-angle glaucoma, cardiac disease, kidney disease, hypertension, bronchial asthma, chronic obstructive pulmonary disease, peptic ulcer disease, seizure disorders, benign prostatic hyperplasia, and pregnancy. Fexofenadine is not recommended for those with renal impairment. Desloratadine is not recommended for pediatric patients. Loratadine is not recommended for children younger than 2 years of age. Antihistamines should be used with caution in patients with impaired liver function or renal insufficiency, as well as in lactating mothers.

## Adverse Effects

Drowsiness is usually the chief complaint of people who take antihistamines, but the sedative effects vary from class to class (see Table 36-1). Fortunately, sedative effects are much less common, although still possible, with the newer "nonsedating" drugs. The anticholinergic (drying) effects of antihistamines can cause adverse effects such as dry mouth, changes in vision, difficulty urinating, and constipation. Reported adverse effects of the antihistamines are listed in Table 36-3.

## Interactions

Drug interactions of antihistamines are listed in Table 36-4. An allergist will usually recommend discontinuation of antihistamine drug therapy at least 4 days prior to allergy testing.

## Dosages

For dosage information on selected antihistamines, see the table on this page.

### TABLE 36-3 ANTIHISTAMINES: REPORTED ADVERSE EFFECTS

| BODY SYSTEM | ADVERSE EFFECTS |
| --- | --- |
| Cardiovascular | Dysrhythmias, hypotension, palpitations, syncope |
| Central nervous | Sedation, dizziness, muscular weakness, paradoxical excitement, restlessness, nervousness, seizures |
| Gastrointestinal | Nausea, vomiting, diarrhea, constipation, hepatitis |
| Other | Dryness of mouth, nose, and throat; urinary retention; vertigo; visual disturbances; tinnitus; headache |

### TABLE 36-4 ANTIHISTAMINES: DRUG INTERACTIONS

| DRUG | INTERACTING DRUG | MECHANISM | RESULT |
| --- | --- | --- | --- |
| fexofenadine | Erythromycin and other CYP450 inhibitors | Inhibit metabolism | Increased fexofenadine levels |
| | Phenytoin | Increased metabolism | Decreased fexofenadine levels |
| loratadine | Ketoconazole, cimetidine, erythromycin | Inhibit metabolism | Increased loratadine levels |
| diphenhydramine, cetirizine | Alcohol, MAOIs, CNS depressants | Additive effects | Increased CNS depression |

*CNS*, Central nervous system; *CYP450*, cytochrome P-450; *MAOI*, monoamine oxidase inhibitor.

## DOSAGES

### Selected Antihistamines

| DRUG (PREGNANCY CATEGORY) | PHARMACOLOGIC CLASS | USUAL DOSAGE RANGE | INDICATIONS |
| --- | --- | --- | --- |
| **Nonsedating Antihistamine** | | | |
| ◆ loratadine (Claritin) (B) | H$_1$ antihistamine | **Adult and pediatric 6 yr and older** PO: 10 mg once daily **Pediatric 2-5 yr** PO: 5 mg once daily | Allergic rhinitis, chronic urticaria |
| **Traditional Antihistamine (More Commonly Associated with Sedation)** | | | |
| ◆ diphenhydramine (Benadryl) (B) | H$_1$ antihistamine | **Pediatric more than 10 kg** PO/IM/IV: 12.5-25 mg tid-qid | Allergic disorders, nighttime insomnia, motion sickness |
| | | **Adult and pediatric 12 yr and older** PO: 25-50 mg qhs | Nighttime insomnia |
| | | **Adult only** PO/IM/IV: 25-50 mg tid-qid | Allergic disorders, PD symptoms |
| | | **Adult only** PO: 25-50 mg tid-qid | Motion sickness |

*IM*, Intramuscular; *IV*, intravenous; *PD*, Parkinson's disease; *PO*, oral.

# DRUG PROFILES

Although some antihistamines are prescription drugs, most are available over the counter. Antihistamines are available in many dosage forms to be administered orally, intramuscularly, intravenously, or topically.

## NONSEDATING ANTIHISTAMINES

A major advance in antihistamine therapy occurred with the development of the nonsedating antihistamines loratadine, cetirizine, and fexofenadine. These drugs were developed to eliminate many of the unwanted adverse effects (mainly sedation) of the older antihistamines. These drugs work peripherally to block the actions of histamine and therefore have significantly less of the CNS effects of many older antihistamines. For this reason, these drugs are also called *peripherally acting antihistamines* because they do not readily cross the blood-brain barrier, unlike their traditional counterparts. Another advantage of the nonsedating antihistamines is that they have longer durations of action, which allow for once daily dosing. This increases patient adherence to therapy. The original nonsedating antihistamines terfenadine and astemizole were withdrawn from the U.S. market in the 1990s following the occurrence of several cases of fatal drug-induced cardiac dysrhythmias. Fexofenadine is the active metabolite of terfenadine but is not associated with such severe cardiac effects, nor are loratadine or cetirizine.

### ◆ loratadine

Loratadine (Claritin) is a nonsedating antihistamine and is taken only once a day. It is structurally similar to cyproheptadine, but it does not readily distribute into the CNS, which diminishes the sedative effects associated with traditional antihistamines. However, at higher doses, central side effects such as drowsiness, headache, and fatigue can be seen. Loratadine is used to relieve the symptoms of seasonal allergic rhinitis (e.g., hay fever) as well as chronic urticaria. Loratadine has recently been converted to OTC status. However, a drug containing its primary active metabolite, desloratadine is currently available only by prescription.

Drug allergy is the only contraindication to the use of loratadine. The drug is available in oral form as a 10-mg tablet, as a 1-mg/mL syrup, as a 10-mg rapidly disintegrating tablet, and in a combination tablet with the decongestant pseudoephedrine. It is classified as a pregnancy category B drug. Recommended dosages are given in the table on p. 579.

### Pharmacokinetics

| Route | Onset of Action | Peak Plasma Concentration | Elimination Half-life | Duration of Action |
|-------|-----------------|---------------------------|----------------------|--------------------|
| PO | 1-3 hr | 8-12 hr | 8-24 hr | 24 hr |

## TRADITIONAL ANTIHISTAMINES

The traditional antihistamines are older drugs that work both peripherally and centrally. They also have anticholinergic effects, which in some cases make them more effective than nonsedating antihistamines. Some of the commonly used older drugs are diphenhydramine, brompheniramine, chlorpheniramine, dimenhydrinate, meclizine, and promethazine. They are used either alone or in combination with other drugs in the symptomatic relief of many disorders ranging from insomnia to motion sickness. Many patients respond to and tolerate the older drugs quite well, and because many are generically available, they are much less expensive. These drugs are available both OTC and by prescription.

### ◆ diphenhydramine

Diphenhydramine (Benadryl) is a traditional antihistamine that works both peripherally and centrally. It also has anticholinergic and sedative effects. In fact, it is used as a hypnotic drug because of its sedating effects. Its use is not generally advised in elderly patients, however, because of the "hangover" effect and increased potential for falls. Diphenhydramine is one of the most commonly used antihistamines, in part because of its excellent safety profile and efficacy. It has the greatest range of therapeutic indications of any antihistamine available. It is used for the relief or prevention of histamine-mediated allergies, motion sickness, the treatment of Parkinson's disease (due to its anticholinergic effects; see Chapter 15), and the promotion of sleep (see Chapter 12). It is also used in conjunction with epinephrine in the management of anaphylaxis and in the treatment of acute dystonic reactions.

Diphenhydramine is classified as a pregnancy category B drug, and its use is contraindicated in patients with a known hypersensitivity to it. It is to be used with caution in nursing mothers, neonates, and patients with lower respiratory tract symptoms. It is available in oral, parenteral, and topical preparations. In oral form, diphenhydramine is available as capsules, tablets, and liquid, as well as in several combination products that contain other cough and cold medications. It is also available as an injection. In topical form, diphenhydramine is available as a cream, gel, and spray. It also is available in combination with several other drugs that are commonly given topically, such as calamine, camphor, and zinc oxide. These combination preparations come in the form of aerosols, creams, gels, and lotions. Recommended dosages for the oral and injectable forms are given in the table on p. 579.

### Pharmacokinetics

| Route | Onset of Action | Peak Plasma Concentration | Elimination Half-life | Duration of Action |
|-------|-----------------|---------------------------|----------------------|--------------------|
| PO | 15-30 min | 2-4 hr | 2-7 hr | 4 hr |

# DECONGESTANTS

Nasal congestion is due to excessive nasal secretions and inflamed and swollen nasal mucosa. The primary causes of nasal congestion are allergies and URIs, especially the common cold. There are three separate groups of nasal decongestants: adrenergics (sympathomimetics), which are the largest group; anticholinergics (parasympatholytics), which are somewhat less commonly used; and selected topical corticosteroids (intranasal steroids).

Decongestants can be taken orally to produce a systemic effect, can be inhaled, or can be administered topically to the nose. Each method of administration has its advantages and disadvantages. Decongestants administered by the oral route include pseudoephedrine, which is available OTC. A commonly used nasal decongestant spray is phenylephrine, which is also OTC.

Drugs administered by the oral route produce prolonged decongestant effects, but the onset of action is more delayed and the effect less potent than for decongestants applied topically. However, the clinical problem of rebound congestion associated with topically administered drugs is almost nonexistent with oral dosage forms. Rebound congestion occurs because of the very rapid absorption of drug through mucous membranes followed by a more rapid decline in therapeutic activity. This rebound congestion can cause overuse and dependence to the nasal spray, as patients take it frequently due to the rapid decline in activity. This is in contrast to oral dosage forms, which provide a more gradual increase and decline in pharmacologic activity due to the time required for GI absorption. Decongestants suitable for nasal inhalation include ephedrine, oxymetazoline, phenylephrine, and tetrahydrozoline.

Inhaled intranasal steroids and anticholinergic drugs are not associated with rebound congestion and are often used prophylactically to prevent nasal congestion in patients with chronic upper respiratory tract symptoms. Commonly used intranasal steroids include the following:

- beclomethasone dipropionate (Beconase)
- budesonide (Rhinocort)
- flunisolide (Nasalide)
- fluticasone (Flonase)
- triamcinolone (Nasacort)
- ciclesonide (Omnaris)

The only intranasal anticholinergic drug in use is ipratropium nasal spray (Atrovent).

## Mechanism of Action and Drug Effects

Nasal decongestants are most commonly used for their ability to shrink engorged nasal mucous membranes and relieve nasal stuffiness. Adrenergic drugs (e.g., ephedrine, oxymetazoline) accomplish this by constricting the small arterioles that supply the structures of the upper respiratory tract, primarily the blood vessels surrounding the nasal sinuses. When these blood vessels are stimulated by alpha-adrenergic drugs, they constrict. Once these blood vessels shrink, the nasal secretions in the swollen mucous membranes are better able to drain, either externally through the nostrils or internally through reabsorption into the bloodstream or lymphatic circulation. Because stimulation of the sympathetic nervous system produces the same effect, these drugs are also referred to as *sympathomimetics*.

Nasal steroids are aimed at the inflammatory response elicited by invading organisms (viruses and bacteria) or other antigens (e.g., allergens). The body responds to these antigens by producing inflammation in an effort to isolate or wall off the area and by attracting various cells of the immune system to consume and destroy the offending antigens. Steroids exert their antiinflammatory effect by causing these cells to be turned off or rendered unresponsive. The goal is *not* complete immunosuppression of the respiratory tract but rather to reduce the inflammatory symptoms to improve patient comfort and air exchange. The drug effects of intranasal steroids are discussed in more detail in Chapter 33.

## Indications

Nasal decongestants reduce the nasal congestion associated with acute or chronic rhinitis, the common cold, sinusitis, and hay fever or other allergies. They may also be used to reduce swelling of the nasal passages and to facilitate visualization of the nasal and pharyngeal membranes before surgery or diagnostic procedures.

## Contraindications

Contraindications to the use of decongestants include drug allergy. Adrenergic drugs are contraindicated in narrow-angle glaucoma, uncontrolled cardiovascular disease, hypertension, diabetes, hyperthyroidism, and prostatitis. They are also contraindicated in situations in which the patient is unable to close his or her eyes (such as after a cerebrovascular accident), as well as in patients with a history of cerebrovascular accident or transient ischemic attacks, cerebral arteriosclerosis, long-standing asthma, benign prostatic hyperplasia, or diabetes.

## Adverse Effects

Adrenergic drugs are usually well tolerated. Possible adverse effects of these drugs include nervousness, insomnia, palpitations, and tremor. The most common adverse effects of intranasal steroids are localized and include mucosal irritation and dryness.

Although a topically applied adrenergic nasal decongestant can be absorbed into the bloodstream, the amount absorbed is usually too small to cause systemic effects at normal dosages. Excessive dosages of these medications are likely to cause systemic effects elsewhere in the body. These may include cardiovascular effects such as hypertension and palpitations and CNS effects such as headache, nervousness, and dizziness. These systemic effects are the result of alpha-adrenergic stimulation of the heart, blood vessels, and CNS.

## Interactions

There are few significant drug interactions with nasal decongestants. Systemic sympathomimetic drugs and sympathomimetic nasal decongestants are likely to cause drug toxicity when given together. Monoamine oxidase inhibitors (MAOIs) may result in additive pressor effects (e.g., raising of the blood pressure) when given with sympathomimetic nasal decongestants. Other interacting drugs include methyldopa and urinary acidifiers and alkalinizers.

## Dosages

For dosage information on naphazoline, see the table on p. 582.

## DRUG PROFILE

Many of the decongestants are OTC drugs, but the more potent drugs that can cause serious adverse effects are available only by prescription. Although nasal steroids are relatively safe, their use is also contraindicated in some circumstances, including in patients with nasal mucosal infections (because of their ability

## DOSAGES

### Selected Decongestant, Expectorant, and Antitussive Drugs

| DRUG (PREGNANCY CATEGORY) | PHARMACOLOGIC CLASS | USUAL DOSAGE RANGE | INDICATIONS |
|---|---|---|---|
| naphazoline (Privine) (C) | Alpha-adrenergic vasoconstrictor | **Adult and pediatric 12 yr and older**<br>1 or 2 drops or sprays in each nostril q6h prn, usually for no more than 3-5 days | Nasal congestion |
| benzonatate (Tessalon Perles) (C) | Nonopioid antitussive | **Adult and pediatric older than 10 yr**<br>PO: 100-200 mg tid | Cough |
| codeine (as part of a combination product such as Dimetane-DC, Tussar SF, Novahistine DH, Robitussin A-C, others) (C) | Opioid antitussive | **Adult and pediatric older than 12 yr**<br>PO: 10-20 mg q4-6h, max 120 mg/24 hr<br>**Pediatric 6-12 yr**<br>PO: 5-10 mg q4-6h, max 60 mg/24 hr<br>**Pediatric 2-5 yr**<br>PO: 2.5-5 mg q4-6h, max 30 mg/24 hr | Cough |
| ◆ dextromethorphan (as part of a combination product such as Vicks Formula 44, Robitussin DM, others) (C) | Nonopioid antitussive | **Adult and pediatric older than 12 yr**<br>PO: 10-30 mg q4-8h, max 120 mg/24 hr<br>**Pediatric 6-12 yr**<br>PO: 5-10 mg q4h or 15 mg q6-8h, max 60 mg/24 hr<br>**Pediatric 2-6 yr**<br>PO: 2.5-7.5 mg q4-8h, max 30 mg/24 hr | Cough |
| ◆ guaifenesin (glyceryl guaiacolate) (Guiatuss, Humibid, Robitussin, Mucinex, others) (C) | Expectorant | **Adult and pediatric 12 yr and older**<br>PO: 100-400 mg q4h, max 2400 mg/24 hr<br>**Pediatric 6-12 yr**<br>PO: 100-200 mg q4h, max 1200 mg/24 hr<br>**Pediatric 2-6 yr**<br>PO: 50-100 mg q4h, max 600 mg/24 hr | Respiratory congestion, cough |

to depress the body's immune response as part of their antiinflammatory effect) or known drug allergy.

Many inhaled corticosteroids (e.g., beclomethasone, dexamethasone, flunisolide) are discussed in greater detail in Chapter 33. The adrenergic drugs (e.g., naphazoline) are discussed in this chapter. Both of these drug categories are generally first-line drugs for the treatment of chronic nasal congestion.

### naphazoline

Naphazoline (Privine) is chemically and pharmacologically similar to the other sympathomimetic drugs oxymetazoline and tetrahydrozoline. During a cold, the blood vessels that surround the nasal sinus are dilated and engorged with plasma, white blood cells, mast cells, histamines, and many other blood components that are involved in fighting infections of the respiratory tract. This swelling, or dilation, blocks the nasal passages, which results in nasal congestion. When these drugs are administered intranasally, they cause dilated arterioles to constrict, which reduces nasal blood flow and congestion. Naphazoline is classified as a pregnancy category C drug and has the same contraindications as the other nasal decongestants. Naphazoline for nasal administration is available as a 0.05% solution and is meant to be instilled into each nostril. Recommended dosages are given in the table on this page.

### Pharmacokinetics

| Route | Onset of Action | Peak Plasma Concentration | Elimination Half-life | Duration of Action |
|---|---|---|---|---|
| Intranasal | 5-10 min | Unknown | Unknown | 2-6 hr |

## ANTITUSSIVES

Coughing is a normal physiologic function and serves the purpose of removing potentially harmful foreign substances and excessive secretions from the respiratory tract. The cough reflex is stimulated when receptors in the bronchi, alveoli, and pleura (lining of the lungs) are stretched. This causes a signal to be sent to the cough center in the medulla of the brain, which in turn stimulates the cough. Most of the time coughing is a beneficial response; however, there are times when it is not useful and may even be harmful (e.g., after a surgical procedure such as hernia repair or in cases of nonproductive or "dry" cough). In these situations, the use of an antitussive drug may enhance patient comfort and reduce respiratory distress. There are two main categories of antitussive drugs: opioid and nonopioid.

Although all opioid drugs have antitussive effects, only codeine and its semisynthetic derivative hydrocodone are used as antitussives. Both drugs are effective in suppressing the cough reflex, and if they are taken in the prescribed manner, their use does not generally lead to dependency. These two drugs are commonly incorporated into various combination formulations with other respiratory drugs and are rarely used alone for the purpose of cough suppression.

Nonopioid antitussive drugs are less effective than opioid drugs and are available either alone or in combination with other drugs in an array of OTC cold and cough preparations. Dextromethorphan is the most widely used of the nonopioid antitussive drugs and is a derivative of the synthetic opioid levorphanol. Benzonatate is another nonopioid antitussive.

## Mechanism of Action and Drug Effects

The opioid antitussives codeine and hydrocodone suppress the cough reflex through direct action on the cough center in the CNS (medulla). Opioid antitussives also provide analgesia and have a drying effect on the mucosa of the respiratory tract, which increases the viscosity of respiratory secretions. This helps to reduce symptoms such as runny nose and postnasal drip. The nonopioid cough suppressant dextromethorphan works in the same way. Because it is not an opioid, however, it does not have analgesic properties, nor does it cause CNS depression. Another nonopioid antitussive is benzonatate. Its mechanism of action is entirely different from that of the other drugs. Benzonatate suppresses the cough reflex by anesthetizing (numbing) the stretch receptor cells in the respiratory tract, which prevents reflex stimulation of the medullary cough center.

## Indications

Although they have other properties, such as analgesic effects for the opioid drugs, antitussives are used primarily to stop the cough reflex when the cough is nonproductive and/or harmful.

## Contraindications

The only absolute contraindication to the antitussives is drug allergy. Relative contraindications include opioid dependency (for opioid antitussives) and high risk for respiratory depression (e.g., in frail elderly patients). Patients with these conditions are often able to tolerate lower medication dosages and still experience some symptom relief.

Additional contraindications and cautions include the following:

- Benzonatate: no known contraindications but cautious use in those with productive cough
- Dextromethorphan: contraindications of hyperthyroidism, advanced cardiac and vessel disease, hypertension, glaucoma, and use of MAOIs within the past 14 days
- Diphenhydramine: see antihistamines
- Codeine and hydrocodone: contraindicated with alcohol use; cautious use required with CNS depression, anoxia, high serum levels of carbon dioxide (hypercapnia), and respiratory depression; increased intracranial pressure, impaired renal function, liver diseases, benign prostatic hyperplasia, Addison's disease, and chronic obstructive pulmonary disease

## Adverse Effects

The following are the common adverse effects of selected antitussive drugs:

- Benzonatate: dizziness, headache, sedation, nausea, constipation, pruritus, and nasal congestion
- Codeine and hydrocodone: sedation, nausea, vomiting, lightheadedness, and constipation
- Dextromethorphan: dizziness, drowsiness, and nausea
- Diphenhydramine: sedation, dry mouth, and other anticholinergic effects

## Interactions

Very few drug interactions occur with benzonatate. Opioid antitussives (codeine and hydrocodone) may potentiate the effects of other opioids, general anesthetics, tranquilizers, sedatives and hypnotics, tricyclic antidepressants, alcohol, and other CNS depressants.

## Dosages

For dosage information on selected antitussive drugs, see the table on p. 582.

## DRUG PROFILES

Antitussives come in many oral dosage forms and are available both with and without a prescription. Most of the opioid antitussives are available only by prescription because of the associated abuse potential. Dextromethorphan is the most popular nonopioid antitussive available OTC.

### benzonatate

Benzonatate (Tessalon Perles) is a nonopioid antitussive drug that is thought to work by anesthetizing or numbing the cough receptors. It is available in oral form as a 100- and 200-mg capsules. Its use is contraindicated in patients with a known hypersensitivity to it. It is classified as a pregnancy category C drug. Recommended dosages are given in the table on p. 582.

#### Pharmacokinetics

| Route | Onset of Action | Peak Plasma Concentration | Elimination Half-life | Duration of Action |
|-------|-----------------|---------------------------|-----------------------|--------------------|
| PO | 15-20 min | Unknown | Unknown | 3-8 hr |

### codeine

Codeine is a popular opioid antitussive drug. It is used in combination with many other respiratory medications to control coughs. Because it is an opioid, it is potentially addictive and can depress respirations as part of its CNS depressant effects. For this reason, codeine-containing cough suppressants are controlled substances. Many states allow persons over 18 years of age to purchase at least one oral liquid combination product without a prescription. However, most codeine antitussive products are obtained with a prescription. Codeine alone, without being combined with other drugs, is a Schedule II drug. Codeine-containing cough suppressants are Schedule V. They are available in many oral dosage forms: solutions, tablets, capsules, and suspensions. Their use is contraindicated in patients with a known hypersensitivity to opiates and in those who have respiratory depression, increased intracranial pressure, seizure disorders, or severe respiratory disorders. It is classified as a pregnancy category C drug. Recommended dosages are given in the table on p. 582.

#### Pharmacokinetics

| Route | Onset of Action | Peak Plasma Concentration | Elimination Half-life | Duration of Action |
|-------|-----------------|---------------------------|-----------------------|--------------------|
| PO | 15-30 min | 34-45 min | 2.5-4 hr | 4-6 hr |

### ◆ dextromethorphan

Dextromethorphan is a nonopioid antitussive that is available alone or in combination with many other cough and cold preparations. It is widely used because it is safe and nonaddicting and does not cause respiratory or CNS depression when used in recommended dosages. Dextromethorphan has become a popular drug of abuse and is discussed in detail in Chapter 17. Its use is contraindicated in cases of drug allergy, asthma or emphysema, or persistent headache. Dextromethorphan is available as lozenges, solution, liquid-filled capsules, granules, tablets (chewable, extended-release, and film-coated), and extended-release suspension. It is classified as a pregnancy category C drug. Recommended dosages are given in the table on p. 582.

### Pharmacokinetics

| Route | Onset of Action | Peak Plasma Concentration | Elimination Half-life | Duration of Action |
|---|---|---|---|---|
| PO | 15-30 min | 2.5 hr | Unknown | 3-6 hr |

## EXPECTORANTS

Expectorants aid in the expectoration (i.e., coughing up and spitting out) of excessive mucus that has accumulated in the respiratory tract by breaking down and thinning out the secretions. They are administered orally either as single drugs or in combination with other drugs to facilitate the flow of respiratory secretions by reducing the viscosity of secretions. The clinical effectiveness of expectorants is somewhat questionable. Placebo-controlled clinical evaluations have failed to confirm that expectorants reduce the viscosity of sputum. Despite this, expectorants are popular drugs, are contained in most OTC cold and cough preparations, and provide symptom relief for many users. The most common expectorant in OTC products is guaifenesin.

## Mechanism of Action and Drug Effects

Expectorants have one of two different mechanisms of action, depending on the drug. The first is reflex stimulation, in which loosening and thinning of respiratory tract secretions occurs in response to an irritation of the GI tract produced by the drug. Guaifenesin is the only such drug currently available. The second mechanism of action is direct stimulation of the secretory glands in the respiratory tract.

## Indications

Expectorants are used for the relief of productive cough commonly associated with the common cold, bronchitis, laryngitis, pharyngitis, pertussis, influenza, and measles. They may also be used for the suppression of coughs caused by chronic paranasal sinusitis. By loosening and thinning sputum and the bronchial secretions, they may also indirectly diminish the tendency to cough.

## Contraindications

Guaifenesin is contraindicated if drug allergy is present.

## Adverse Effects

The adverse effects of expectorants are minimal. Guaifenesin may cause nausea, vomiting, and gastric irritation.

## Interactions

There are no known significant interactions involving guaifenesin.

## Dosages

For dosage information on guaifenesin, the only expectorant profiled, see the table on p. 582.

## DRUG PROFILE

### ♦ guaifenesin

Guaifenesin (Mucinex) is a commonly used expectorant that is available in several different oral dosage forms: capsules, tablets, solutions, and granules. It is used in the symptomatic management of coughs of varying origin. It is beneficial in the treatment of productive coughs because it thins mucus in the respiratory tract that is difficult to cough up. There are few published pharmacokinetic data on guaifenesin, but its half-life is estimated to be approximately 1 hour. This short half-life helps to explain why it is usually dosed several times throughout the day. However, there are sustained-release products that are given once or twice daily. Although this drug remains popular, there is some evidence in the literature to suggest that it has no greater therapeutic activity than water in terms of loosening respiratory tract secretions. It is classified as a pregnancy category C drug. For dosage information on guaifenesin, see the table on p. 582.

## NURSING PROCESS

## ASSESSMENT

When the patient is to be given drugs to treat symptoms related to the respiratory tract, begin the assessment by gathering data about the condition and determining if symptoms are caused by an allergic reaction. Obtaining the patient's medical history and medication profile, completing a thorough head-to-toe physical assessment, and taking a nursing history are critical to understanding possible causes, risks, or links to diseases or conditions such as allergy, a cold, or flu. For example, if an allergic reaction to a drug, food, or substance has occurred, the patient may be experiencing signs and symptoms such as hives, wheezing or bronchospasm, tachycardia, or hypotension (requiring immediate medical attention). However, if the cause is a cold or flu, the symptoms are different and treated completely differently. The drug of choice is then selected based on the type and severity of the symptoms.

Most *nonsedating antihistamines* (e.g., fexofenadine, loratadine, cetirizine) are contraindicated in those with known allergies to the drugs. Remember with the traditional and nontraditional antihistamines that if allergy testing is to be performed, these medications are usually discontinued at least 4 days before the testing, but only on a prescriber's order and as directed. Assess for the following possible drug interactions that need to be avoided: fexofenadine given with erythromycin and other CYP450 inhibitors, leading to increased antihistamine levels; fexofenadine and phenytoin, leading to decreased fexofenadine levels; loratadine given with some antifungals, cimetidine, and erythromycin, leading to increased antihistamine levels; and diphenhydramine and cetirizine given with alcohol, MAOIs, and CNS depressants, leading to increased CNS depression.

Before administering the *traditional antihistamines* such as diphenhydramine, chlorpheniramine, or brompheniramine, ensure that the patient has no allergies to this group of medications, even though these drugs are used for allergic reactions. Assess contraindications, cautions, and drug interactions with these and all other drugs. Use of these antihistamines is of concern in patients who are experiencing an acute asthma attack and in those who have lower respiratory tract disease or are at risk for pneumonia. The rationale for not using these drugs in these situations is that antihistamines (and nonsedating antihistamines) dry up secretions; if the patient cannot expectorate the secretions, the secretions may become viscous (thick), occlude airways, and lead to atelectasis, infection, or occlusion of the bronchioles. It is also important to know that these drugs may lead to paradoxical reactions in elderly patients, with subsequent irritability as well as dizziness, confusion, sedation, and hypotension.

Use of *decongestants* requires assessment of contraindications, cautions, and drug interactions. Because decongestants are available in oral, nasal drop and spray, and eyedrop dosage forms, any condition that could affect the functional structures of the eye or nose may be a possible caution or contraindication. Decongestants may increase blood pressure and heart rate, so assess and document the patient's blood pressure, pulse, and other vital parameters. Because so many of these drugs are found in OTC cough and cold products and have been associated with numerous cases of oversedation, seizures, tachycardia, and even in death, their use warrants extreme caution. Contraindications to the use of decongestants include drug allergy, narrow-angle glaucoma, uncontrolled cardiovascular disease, hypertension, diabetes, and prostatitis. Topically applied adrenergic nasal decongestants may be absorbed into the circulation; however, the dosage amount absorbed is usually too small to cause systemic effects. If there are excessive dosages (e.g., excessive use or amounts), these may precipitate cardiovascular effects such as increase in blood pressure and CNS stimulation with headache, nervousness, or dizziness. Some drug interactions include the use of systemic sympathomimetics and sympathomimetic nasal decongestants with possible toxicity when given together. Other drug interactions to assess for with nasal decongestants include their use with MAOIs.

*Inhaled intranasal steroids* are contraindicated in situations in which the patient is experiencing a nasal mucosal infection or drug allergy. Chapter 33 discusses some of the inhaled corticosteroids. With the use of any decongestant, always perform a thorough assessment of signs and symptoms before and after use of these drugs. Include description of cough, secretions, and breath sounds in this assessment.

With *antitussive* therapy, assessment is tailored to the patient and the specific drug. Most of these drugs result in sedation, dizziness, and drowsiness, so assessment of the patient's safety is very important. Complete an assessment for allergies, contraindications, cautions, and drug interactions, and document the findings. In the respiratory assessment (as for all of the drugs in this chapter), include rate, rhythm and depth, as well as breath sounds, presence of cough, and description of cough and sputum if present. For individuals with chronic respiratory disease, the prescriber may order further studies to determine the safety of using these drugs without causing further respiratory concerns or depression. Pulse oximetry readings with measurement of vital signs may be used to provide more information. Assess

for potential drug interactions including alcohol, MAOIs, and antihistamines. With use of codeine and hydrocodone antitussives, there are contraindications with alcohol and other opioid drugs; these drugs must be used cautiously with CNS depression, anoxia, hypercapnia, respiratory depression, and impaired renal function and in those with chronic obstructive pulmonary disease such as emphysema. With the nonopioid antitussive dextromethorphan, monitor its use carefully because it is a popular drug of abuse (see Chapter 17).

*Expectorants* are generally tolerated well, and the only contraindication is with drug allergy. There are no known drug interactions to assess for with use of the expectorant guaifenesin (Mucinex).

## NURSING DIAGNOSES

1. Impaired gas exchange related to the disorder, condition, or disease affecting the respiratory system and various respiratory-related signs and symptoms
2. Ineffective airway clearance related to diminished ability to cough and/or a suppressed cough reflex (with antitussives)
3. Deficient knowledge related to the effective use of cold medications and other related products due to lack of information and patient teaching

## PLANNING

### GOALS

1. Patient experiences improved gas exchange with drug therapy.
2. Patient has improved airway clearance and relief of symptoms.
3. Patient displays improved knowledge about drug therapy.

### OUTCOME CRITERIA

1. Patient experiences improved oxygen exchange and breath sounds and a return to normal respiratory rate and rhythm.
2. Patient takes medications exactly as prescribed to enhance airway clearance.
   - Patient increases fluid intake to thin secretions and increase expectoration of mucus.

- Patient's breath sounds clear with expectoration of secretions and return to a respiratory rate of 12 to 20 breaths/min.
- Patient reports to the prescriber immediately the following symptoms: increase in cough, congestion, shortness of breath, chest pain, fever (above 100.4° F or 38° C), or any change in sputum production or color (i.e., if not clear or if a change from baseline).
3. Patient states rationale for therapy as well as adverse effects to expect while on drug therapy.
   - Patient remains compliant with the antihistamine, antitussive, decongestant, or expectorant medication regimen until symptoms are resolved or the prescriber orders discontinuation.

## IMPLEMENTATION

If patients are receiving a *nonsedating antihistamine,* advise them to take the drug as directed. Reduced dosages may be needed for patients who are elderly or have decreased renal function. The $H_1$ receptor antagonist drugs do not cross the blood-brain barrier as readily as do older antihistamines and are therefore less likely to cause sedation. They are generally very well tolerated with minimal adverse effects.

Instruct patients taking *traditional antihistamines* (e.g., diphenhydramine) to take the medications as prescribed. Most of these medications, including the OTC antihistamines, are best tolerated when taken with meals. Although food may slightly decrease absorption of these drugs, it has the benefit of minimizing the GI upset these drugs may cause. Encourage patients who experience dry mouth to chew or suck on candy (sugar-free if needed) or OTC throat, cough, or cold lozenges, or to chew gum, as well as to perform frequent mouth care to ease the dryness and related discomfort. Other OTC or prescribed cold or cough medications must not be taken with antihistamines unless they were previously approved or ordered by the prescriber because of the potential for serious drug interactions. Dosage amounts and routes may vary depending on whether the patient is elderly, an adult, or younger than 12 years of age, so encourage proper dosing and usage. Monitor blood pressure and other vital signs

as needed. Monitor the elderly and children for any paradoxical reactions, which are common with these drugs.

Patients taking *decongestants* are generally using the drugs for nasal decongestion. These drugs come in oral dosage forms, including sustained-release and chewable forms. Educate patients that all dosage forms are to be taken as instructed and with an increase in fluid intake of up to 3000 mL per day, unless contraindicated. The fluid helps to liquefy secretions, assists in breaking up thick secretions, and makes it easier to cough up secretions. Counsel patients to use nasal decongestant dosage forms exactly as ordered and with no increase in frequency. Excessive use of decongestant nasal sprays/drops may lead to rebound congestion. See the Patient Teaching Tips for further information.

With *antitussives,* instruct patients that the various dosage forms of the drugs are to be used exactly as ordered. Drowsiness or dizziness may occur with the use of antitussives; therefore, caution patients against driving a car or engaging in other activities that require mental alertness until they feel back to normal. If the antitussive contains codeine, the CNS depressant effects of the narcotic opiate may further depress breathing and respiratory effort. Other antitussives, such as dextromethorphan, as well as the codeine-containing drugs are to be given at evenly spaced intervals so that the drug reaches a steady state.

## EVALUATION

A therapeutic response to drugs given to treat respiratory conditions, such as *antihistamines, decongestants, antitussives,* and *expectorants,* includes resolution of the symptoms for which the drugs were originally prescribed or taken. These symptoms may include cough; nasal, sinus, or chest congestion; nasal, salivary, and lacrimal gland hypersecretion; motion sickness; sneezing; watery, red, or itchy eyes; itchy nose; allergic rhinitis; and allergic symptoms. Monitor for the adverse effects of excessive dry mouth, nose, and throat; urinary retention; drowsiness; oversedation; dizziness; paradoxical excitement; nervousness; restlessness; dysrhythmias; palpitations; nausea; diarrhea or constipation; and headache, depending on the drug prescribed.

## PATIENT TEACHING TIPS

- Provide the patient with education about the sedating effects of traditional antihistamines. The patient needs to avoid activities that require mental alertness until tolerance to sedation occurs or until he or she accurately judges that the drug has no impact on motor skills or responses to motor activities. Include a list of drugs the patient must avoid, such as alcohol and CNS depressants.
- With traditional and nonsedating antihistamines, a humidifier may be needed to help liquefy secretions, making expectoration of sputum easier. Encourage intake of fluids, unless contraindicated.
- Educate patients with upper or lower respiratory symptoms or disease processes of the impact of the environment on their symptoms or condition, and instruct patients to avoid dry air, smoke-filled environments, and allergens.

- Encourage the patient to always check for possible drug interactions because of the many OTC and prescription drugs that could lead to adverse effects if taken concurrently with any of the antihistamines, decongestants, antitussives, or expectorants.
- Advise the patient to take the medication with food to avoid GI upset.
- Any difficulty breathing, palpitations or unusual adverse effects must be reported to the prescriber immediately.
- Instruct the patient to take antitussives with caution and to report to the prescriber any fever, chest tightness, change in sputum from clear to colored, difficult or noisy breathing, activity intolerance, or weakness.
- With decongestants, emphasize the importance of only taking the medication as ordered and adhering to

## PATIENT TEACHING TIPS—cont'd

instructions regarding dose and frequency. Emphasize that frequent, long-term, or excessive use of decongestants (whether oral forms or nasal inhaled forms) may lead to rebound congestion in which the nasal passages become more congested as the effects of the drug wear off. When this occurs, the patient generally uses more of the drug, precipitating a vicious cycle with more congestion. Advise the patient to report to the prescriber any excessive dizziness, heart palpitations, weakness, sedation, or excessive irritability.

- Patients taking expectorants must avoid alcohol and products containing alcohol and should not use these medications for longer than 1 week. If cough or symptoms continue, the patient should contact the prescriber for further instructions or assessment. Encourage intake of fluids, unless contraindicated, to help thin secretions for easier expectoration.
- Decongestants and expectorants are recommended to treat cold symptoms, but the patient must report a fever of higher than 100.4° F (38° C), cough, or other symptoms lasting longer than 3 to 4 days.

## KEY POINTS

- There are two types of histamine blockers: $H_1$ blockers and $H_2$ blockers. $H_1$ blockers are the drugs to which most people are referring when they use the term *antihistamine*. $H_1$ blockers prevent the harmful effects of histamine and are used to treat seasonal allergic rhinitis, anaphylaxis, reactions to insect bites, and so forth. $H_2$ blockers are used to treat gastric acid disorders, such as hyperacidity or ulcer disease.
- Educate the patient about the purposes of the medication regimen, the expected adverse effects, and any drug interactions. A list of all medications (prescription, over-the-counter, and herbal) needs to be provided to all health care providers.

- Decongestants work by causing constriction of the engorged and swollen blood vessels in the sinuses, which decreases pressure and allows mucous membranes to drain. It is important to understand the action of these drugs and know other important information such as significant adverse effects, including cardiac and CNS-stimulating effects.
- Nonopioid antitussive drugs may also cause sedation, drowsiness, or dizziness. Patients should not drive a car or engage in other activities that require mental alertness if these adverse effects occur. Codeine-containing antitussives may lead to CNS depression; these drugs are to be used cautiously and are not to be mixed with anything containing alcohol.

## NCLEX® EXAMINATION REVIEW QUESTIONS

1 When assessing a patient who is to receive a decongestant, the nurse will recognize that a potential contraindication to this drug would be which condition?
   a Glaucoma
   b Fever
   c Peptic ulcer disease
   d Allergic rhinitis

2 When giving decongestants, the nurse must remember that these drugs have alpha-adrenergic–stimulating effects that may result in which effect?
   a Fever
   b Bradycardia
   c Hypertension
   d CNS depression

3 The nurse is reviewing a patient's medication orders for prn (as necessary) medications that can be given to a patient who has bronchitis with a productive cough. Which drug will the nurse choose?
   a An antitussive
   b An expectorant
   c An antihistamine
   d A decongestant

4 The nurse knows that an antitussive cough medication would be the best choice for which patient?
   a A patient with a productive cough
   b A patient with chronic paranasal sinusitis

   c A patient who has had recent abdominal surgery
   d A patient who has influenza

5 A patient is taking a decongestant to help reduce symptoms of a cold. The nurse will instruct the patient to observe for which possible symptom, which may indicate an adverse effect of this drug?
   a Increased cough
   b Dry mouth
   c Slower heart rate
   d Heart palpitations

6 The nurse is giving an antihistamine and will observe the patient for which side effects? (Select all that apply.)
   a Hypertension
   b Dizziness
   c "Hangover" effect
   d Drowsiness
   e Tachycardia
   f Dry mouth

7 The order for a 4-year-old patient reads: "Give guaifenesin, 80 mg PO, every 4 hours as needed for cough. Maximum of 600 mg/24 hours." The medication comes in a bottle that has 100 mg/5 mL. How many milliliters will the nurse give per dose?

1. a, 2. c, 3. b, 4. c, 5. d, 6. b, c, d, f, 7. 4 mL.

For Critical Thinking and Prioritization Questions, see http://evolve.elsevier.com/Lilley.

# Respiratory Drugs

## OBJECTIVES

When you reach the end of this chapter, you will be able to do the following:

1. Describe the anatomy and physiology of the respiratory system.
2. Discuss the impact of respiratory drugs on various lower and upper respiratory tract diseases and conditions.
3. List the classifications of drugs used to treat diseases and conditions of the respiratory system, and provide specific examples.
4. Discuss the mechanisms of action, indications, contraindications, cautions, drug interactions, dosages, routes of administration, adverse effects, and toxic effects of the bronchodilators and other respiratory drugs.
5. Develop a nursing care plan that includes all phases of the nursing process for patients who use bronchodilators and other respiratory drugs.

## DRUG PROFILES

- ♦ **albuterol, p. 593**
  **fluticasone propionate, p. 599**
  **ipratropium, p. 594**
  **methylprednisolone, p. 599**
- ♦ **montelukast, p. 597**

- ♦ **salmeterol, p. 593**
  **theophylline, p. 595**

  _____

- ♦ *Key drug*

## KEY TERMS

**Allergen** Any substance that evokes an allergic response. (p. 589)

**Allergic asthma** Bronchial asthma caused by hypersensitivity to an allergen or allergens. (p. 589)

**Alveoli** Microscopic sacs in the lungs where oxygen is exchanged for carbon dioxide; also called *air sacs.* (p. 589)

**Antibodies** Immunoglobulins produced by lymphocytes in response to bacteria, viruses, or other antigenic substances. (p. 590)

**Antigen** A substance (usually a protein) that causes the formation of an antibody and reacts specifically with that antibody. (p. 590)

**Asthma attack** The onset of wheezing together with difficulty breathing. (p. 589)

**Bronchial asthma** The general term for recurrent and reversible shortness of breath resulting from narrowing of the bronchi and bronchioles; it is often referred to simply as *asthma.* Key characteristics are inflammation, bronchial smooth muscle spasticity, and sputum production; inflammation is the most important. (p. 589)

**Bronchodilators** Medications that improve airflow by relaxing bronchial smooth muscle cells (e.g., xanthines, adrenergic agonists). (p. 591)

**Chronic bronchitis** Chronic inflammation and low-grade infection of the bronchi. (p. 589)

**Emphysema** A condition of the lungs characterized by enlargement of the air spaces distal to the bronchioles. (p. 589)

**Immunoglobulins** Proteins belonging to any of five structurally and antigenically distinct classes of antibodies present in the serum and external secretions of the body; they play a major role in immune responses; *immunoglobulin* is often abbreviated *Ig.* (p. 590)

**Lower respiratory tract (LRT)** The division of the respiratory system composed of organs located almost entirely within the chest. (p. 589)

**Status asthmaticus** A prolonged asthma attack. (p. 589)

**Upper respiratory tract (URT)** The division of the respiratory system composed of organs located outside the chest cavity (thorax). (p. 589)

## ANATOMY, PHYSIOLOGY, AND PATHOPHYSIOLOGY OVERVIEW

The main function of the respiratory system is to deliver oxygen to, and remove carbon dioxide from, the cells of the body. To perform this deceptively simple task requires a very intricate system of tissues, muscles, and organs called the respiratory system. It consists of two divisions or tracts: the upper and lower respiratory tracts. The upper respiratory tract (URT) is composed of the structures that are located outside of the chest cavity or thorax. These are the nose, nasopharynx, oropharynx, laryngopharynx, and larynx. The lower respiratory tract (LRT) is located almost entirely within the thorax and is composed of the trachea, all segments of the bronchial tree, and the lungs. The URT and LRT have four main accessory structures that aid in their overall function. These are the oral cavity (mouth), the rib cage, the muscles of the rib cage (intercostal muscles), and the diaphragm. The upper and lower respiratory tracts together with the accessory structures make up the respiratory system. Elements of this system are in constant communication with each other as they perform the vital function of respiration and the exchange of oxygen for carbon dioxide.

The air we breathe is a mixture of many gases. During inhalation, oxygen molecules from the air diffuse across the semipermeable membranes of the alveoli, where they are exchanged for carbon dioxide molecules, which are then exhaled. The lungs also filter, warm, and humidify the air. Oxygen is then delivered to the cells by the blood vessels of the circulatory system, where the respiratory system transfers the oxygen it has extracted from inhaled air to the hemoglobin protein molecules contained within red blood cells. Also within the circulatory system, the cellular metabolic waste product carbon dioxide is collected from the tissues by the red blood cells. This waste is then transported back to the lungs via the circulatory system, where it diffuses back across the alveolar membranes and is then exhaled into the air. The respiratory system also plays a central role in speech, smell, and regulation of pH (acid-base balance).

## PATHOPHYSIOLOGY OF DISEASES OF THE RESPIRATORY SYSTEM

Several diseases impair the function of the respiratory system. Those that affect the URT include colds, rhinitis, and hay fever.

These conditions and the drugs used to treat them are discussed in Chapter 36. The major diseases that impair the function of the LRT include asthma, emphysema, and chronic bronchitis. All of these diseases have one feature in common; they all involve the obstruction of airflow through the airways. Chronic obstructive pulmonary disease (COPD) is the name applied collectively to emphysema and chronic bronchitis, because the obstruction is relatively constant. Asthma that is persistent and present most of the time despite treatment is also considered a COPD. Cystic fibrosis and infant respiratory distress syndrome are other disorders that affect the LRT, but they are not a focus of discussion in this chapter because treatment for them places more emphasis on nonpharmacologic than on pharmacologic measures.

### Asthma

Bronchial asthma is defined as a recurrent and reversible shortness of breath and occurs when the airways of the lung (bronchi and bronchioles) become narrow as a result of bronchospasm, inflammation and edema of the bronchial mucosa, and the production of viscous (sticky) mucus. The alveolar ducts and alveoli distal to the bronchioles remain open, but the obstruction to the airflow in the airways prevents carbon dioxide from getting out of the air spaces and oxygen from getting in. Symptoms include wheezing and difficulty breathing. When an episode has a sudden and dramatic onset, it is referred to as an asthma attack. Most asthma attacks are short, and normal breathing is subsequently recovered. However, an asthma attack may be prolonged and may not respond to typical drug therapy. This is a condition known as status asthmaticus and requires hospitalization. The onset of asthma occurs before 10 years of age in 50% of patients and before 40 years of age in about 80% of patients.

There are different types of asthma: intrinsic (occurring in patients with no history of allergies), extrinsic (occurring in patients exposed to a known allergen), exercise induced, and drug induced. Allergic asthma, or extrinsic asthma, is caused by a hypersensitivity to an allergen or allergens in the environment. An allergen is any substance that elicits an allergic reaction. In patients with seasonal asthma, the allergen is a substance such as pollen or mold, which is present only periodically (seasonally). The offending allergens in patients with nonseasonal asthma are substances such as dust, mold, and

---

**BOX 37-1    STEPS INVOLVED IN AN ATTACK OF ALLERGIC ASTHMA**

1. The offending allergen provokes the production of hypersensitive antibodies (most commonly immunoglobulin E [IgE]) that are specific to the allergen. This immunologic response initiates patient sensitivity.
2. The IgE antibodies are homocytotropic and collect on the surface of mast cells, thus sensitizing the patient to the allergen.
3. Subsequent allergen contact provokes the antigen-antibody reaction on the surface of mast cells.
4. Mast cell integrity is then violated, and these cells release chemical mediators stored in the cell. They also synthesize and then release other chemical mediators. These mediators include bradykinin, eosinophil chemotactic factor of anaphylaxis, histamine, prostaglandins, and slow-reacting substance of anaphylaxis (SRS-A).
5. The released chemical mediators, especially histamine and SRS-A, trigger bronchial constriction and an asthma attack.

---

**BOX 37-2    CLASSIFICATIONS OF DRUGS USED TO TREAT ASTHMA**

**Long-Term Control**
Leukotriene receptor antagonists
Mast cell stabilizers
Inhaled corticosteroids
Anticholinergic agents
Long-acting beta$_2$ agonists (LABA)
theophylline
Long-acting beta$_2$ agonists in combination with inhaled corticosteroids

**Quick Relief**
Intravenous systemic corticosteroids
Short-acting inhaled beta$_2$ agonists (rescue agents)

---

**TABLE 37-1    STEPWISE THERAPY FOR THE MANAGEMENT OF ASTHMA**

| STEP | DRUG CLASSIFICATION |
|---|---|
| Step 1 | Short-acting inhaled beta$_2$ agonist as needed |
| Step 2 | Preferred: low-dose inhaled corticosteroid (ICS) |
| | Alternative: cromolyn, nedocromil, leukotriene receptor antagonist (LTRA), or theophylline |
| Step 3 | Preferred: low-dose ICS and long-acting beta$_2$ agonist (LABA) or medium-dose ICS |
| | Alternative: low-dose ICS and either LTRA, theophylline, or zileuton |
| Step 4 | Preferred: medium-dose ICS plus LABA |
| | Alternative: medium-dose ICS plus either LTRA, theophylline, or zileuton |
| Step 5 | High-dose ICS and LABA, and consider omalizumab for patients with allergies |
| Step 6 | High-dose ICS and LABA and oral corticosteroid, and consider omalizumab for patients with allergies |

Adapted from National Institutes of Health: Expert Panel Report 3: guidelines for the diagnosis and management of asthma, 2007, U.S. Department of Health and Human Services, available at www.nhlbi.nih.gov/guidelines/asthma. Accessed December 3, 2011.

---

animal dander, which are present in the environment throughout the year. Cigarette smoke, from either smoking or exposure to secondhand smoke, is another common allergen. Examples of common food allergens include nuts, eggs, and corn. Exposure to the offending allergen in a patient with allergic asthma causes an immediate allergic reaction in the form of an asthma attack. This attack is mediated by antibodies already present in the patient's body that chemically recognize the allergen to be a foreign substance, or antigen. These antibodies are specialized immune system proteins known as immunoglobulins. The antibody in individuals with asthma is usually immunoglobulin E (IgE), which is one of the five types of antibodies in the body (the others are IgG, IgA, IgM, and IgD). On exposure to the allergen, the patient's body responds by mounting an immediate and potent antigen-antibody reaction (immune response). This reaction occurs on the surfaces of cells such as mast cells that are rich in histamines, leukotrienes, and other substances involved in the immune response. These substances are collectively known as inflammatory mediators, and they are released from the mast cells as part of the immune response. This in turn, as described in Chapter 36, triggers the mucosal swelling and bronchoconstriction that are characteristic of an allergic asthma attack. The sequence of events that occurs in a patient with allergic asthma is shown in Box 37-1.

The specific cause of intrinsic, or idiopathic, asthma is unknown. It is not mediated by IgE, and there is often no family history of allergies in affected patients. However, certain factors have been noted to precipitate asthma attacks in these patients, including respiratory infections, stress, and cold weather. Patients with exercise-induced asthma have bronchospasm at the beginning of exercise, and symptoms stop when exercise is halted. Drug-induced asthma can be the result of different drugs including NSAIDs (see Chapter 44), beta blockers (see Chapters 22 and 24), sulfites, or certain foods. Patients with any type of asthma who know their suspected "triggers," whether an allergen, the weather, or another factor, are advised to avoid these triggers as much as is feasible as part of managing their disease. When it is not feasible or advisable to avoid a certain trigger (e.g., exercise), patients need to work with their prescribers to prevent the response to these triggers through appropriate drug therapy (e.g., use of a bronchodilator inhaler before exercise or other strenuous activity).

The National Asthma Education and Prevention Panel (NAEPP) of the National Heart, Lung, and Blood Institute has maintained ongoing guidelines for the diagnosis and management of asthma since 1989. The current guideline revision was published in 2007. In general, these guidelines classify asthma medications as either for long-term symptom control or rapid symptom relief. The specific drugs in each classification are listed in Box 37-2. The guidelines advocate the use of a stepwise approach in the treatment of asthma. The particular steps and recommended drug classifications for treatment at each step are listed in Table 37-1.

## Chronic Bronchitis

Chronic bronchitis is a continuous inflammation and low-grade infection of the bronchi. The inflammation in the associated bronchioles (smaller bronchi) is responsible for most of the airflow obstruction. Chronic bronchitis involves the excessive secretion of mucus and certain pathologic changes in the bronchial structure. The disease can arise as a result of repeated episodes of acute bronchitis or in the context of chronic generalized diseases. It is usually precipitated by prolonged exposure to bronchial irritants. One of the most common is cigarette smoke. Some patients acquire the disease because of other predisposing factors such as viral or bacterial pulmonary infections during childhood. Others may have mild impairment of the ability to inactivate proteolytic (protein-destroying) enzymes, which then damage the airway mucosal tissues. Unknown genetic characteristics may be responsible as well.

## Emphysema

Emphysema is a condition in which the air spaces enlarge as a result of the destruction of the alveolar walls. This appears to be caused by the effect of proteolytic enzymes released from leukocytes in response to alveolar inflammation. Because the alveolar walls are partially destroyed, the surface area available for oxygen and carbon dioxide exchange is reduced, which impairs effective respiration. As with chronic bronchitis, cigarette smoke appears to be the primary irritant responsible for precipitating the underlying inflammation that leads to the development of emphysema. There is also an associated genetic deficiency of the enzyme $alpha_1$-antitrypsin.

## TREATMENT OF DISEASES OF THE LOWER RESPIRATORY TRACT

In the past, the treatment of asthma and other COPDs was focused primarily on the use of drugs that cause the airways to dilate. Now there is a greater understanding of the pathophysiology of these diseases. The emphasis of research has shifted from the bronchoconstriction component of the disease to the inflammatory component. This is also reflected in the various medication classes used to treat COPDs, although bronchodilators still play an important role. A synopsis of the mechanisms of action of the various classes of antiasthmatic drugs is provided in Table 37-2. Figure 37-1 gives an overview of the various drugs used in asthma.

### PHARMACOLOGY OVERVIEW

## BRONCHODILATORS

Bronchodilators are an important part of the pharmacotherapy for all respiratory diseases. These drugs relax bronchial smooth muscle, which causes dilation of the bronchi and bronchioles that are narrowed as a result of the disease process. There are three classes of such drugs: beta adrenergic agonists, anticholinergics, and xanthine derivatives.

## BETA-ADRENERGIC AGONISTS

The beta adrenergic agonists are a group of drugs that are commonly used during the acute phase of an asthmatic attack to quickly reduce airway constriction and restore airflow to

| TABLE 37-2 | MECHANISMS OF ANTIASTHMATIC DRUG ACTION |
|---|---|
| **ANTIASTHMATIC** | **MECHANISM IN ASTHMA RELIEF** |
| Anticholinergics | Block cholinergic receptors, thus preventing the binding of cholinergic substances that cause bronchoconstriction and increase secretions |
| Leukotriene receptor antagonists | Modify or inhibit the activity of leukotrienes, which decreases arachidonic acid–induced inflammation and allergen-induced bronchoconstriction |
| Beta agonists and xanthine derivatives | Raise intracellular levels of cyclic adenosine monophosphate, which in turn produces smooth muscle relaxation and dilates the constricted bronchi and bronchioles |
| Corticosteroids | Prevent the inflammation commonly provoked by the substances released from mast cells |
| Mast cell stabilizers (cromolyn and nedocromil) | Stabilize the cell membranes of the mast cells in which the antigen-antibody reactions take place, thereby preventing the release of substances such as histamine that cause constriction |

normal. They are agonists, or stimulators, of the adrenergic receptors in the sympathetic nervous system. The beta and alpha adrenergic receptors are discussed in Chapters 18 and 19. The beta agonists imitate the effects of norepinephrine on beta receptors. For this reason, they are also called *sympathomimetic* bronchodilators. The beta agonists are categorized by their onset of action. Short-acting beta agonist (SABA) inhalers include albuterol (Ventolin), levalbuterol (Xopenex), pirbuterol (Maxair), terbutaline (Brethine), and metaproterenol (Alupent). Long-acting beta agonist (LABA) inhalers include arformoterol (Brovana), formoterol (Foradil, Perforomist), and salmeterol (Serevent). Because the LABAs have a longer onset of action, they must never be used for acute treatment. Patients must be taught to use the SABAs as rescue treatment.

## Mechanism of Action and Drug Effects

The beta agonists dilate airways by stimulating the $beta_2$-adrenergic receptors located throughout the lungs.

There are three subtypes of these drugs, based on their selectivity for $beta_2$ receptors:

1. Nonselective adrenergic drugs, which stimulate the beta, $beta_1$ (cardiac), and $beta_2$ (respiratory) receptors. Example: epinephrine. (NOTE: Epinephrine inhalers were taken off the market in 2012 because they did not comply with FDA requirements; they may return to the market in the future.) Epinephrine is available as a prefilled syringe for elf-administration by patients with severe allergic reactions and is called Epipen (Figure 37-2.)
2. Nonselective beta-adrenergic drugs, which stimulate both $beta_1$ and $beta_2$ receptors. Example: metaproterenol.
3. Selective $beta_2$ drugs, which primarily stimulate the $beta_2$ receptors. Example: albuterol.

ALLERGENS such as dust, wool blankets, feather pillows, pollen, etc., in hypersensitive persons with IgE antibodies stimulate mast cells in lungs to release histamine (H) and slow-reacting substance of anaphylaxis (SRS-A).

HISTAMINE stimulates larger bronchi to cause smooth muscle spasms, inflammation, and edema.

SRS-A stimulates small bronchi to cause smooth muscle swelling.

Result is spasms of smooth bronchial muscle, increased mucus secretions, swollen mucosa, hyperinflation of alveoli eventually leading to loss of elasticity and collapsed alveoli.

LEUKOTRIENE ANTAGONISTS block the release of leukotrienes in the lungs. Inflammation causes an increase in leukotrienes, substances that constitute the slow-reacting substance of anaphylaxis (SRS-A).

THEOPHYLLINE increases cyclic AMP to inhibit breakdown of sensitized mast cells that stimulate the release of histamine, serotonin, and SRS-A.

MAST CELL STABILIZERS inhibit the release of histamine from mast cells to reduce allergic effects.

SYMPATHETIC AGONISTS stimulate sympathetic systems to decrease mucus secretions and relax bronchial muscle spasms.

CORTICOSTEROIDS produce an antiinflammatory effect and reduce mucus secretions and tissue histamine.

**FIGURE 37-1** Overview of the effects of various antiasthmatic medications. (From McKenry LM, Tessier E, Hogan M: *Mosby's pharmacology in nursing,* ed 22, St Louis, 2006, Mosby.)

**FIGURE 37-2** The EpiPen Auto-Injector (epinephrine) is used for immediate treatment of anaphylaxis (allergic emergencies). The EpiPen is given into the outer thigh, through the clothing. Anaphylactic emergencies also require emergency medical services in addition to the EpiPen. Additional information is available at www.epipen.com. (Copyright Mylan Specialty, L.P. Used with permission.)

| TABLE 37-3 | BETA AGONIST BRONCHODILATORS | | |
|---|---|---|---|
| DRUG | TYPE | TRADE NAMES | ADMINISTRATION |
| **Short Acting** | | | |
| albuterol | Beta$_2$ | Proventil, Ventolin | PO, inhalation |
| ephedrine | Alpha/beta | None (various generic) | IM, IV, subcut |
| epinephrine | Alpha/beta | Adrenalin | Subcut, IM |
| metaproterenol | Beta$_1$/beta$_2$ | Alupent | PO, inhalation |
| levalbuterol | Beta$_2$ | Xopenex | Inhalation |
| metaproterenol | Beta$_1$/beta$_2$ | Alupent, Metaprel | PO, inhalation |
| pirbuterol | Beta$_2$ | Maxair | Inhalation |
| terbutaline | Beta$_2$ | Brethine | PO, subcut, inhalation |
| **Long Acting** | | | |
| salmeterol | Beta$_2$ | Serevent, Serevent Diskus | Inhalation |
| formoterol | Beta$_2$ | Foradil, Performist | Inhalation |
| arformoterol | Beta$_2$ | Brovana | Inhalation |

*IM,* Intramuscular; *IV,* intravenous; *PO,* oral; *subcut,* subcutaneous.

These drugs can also be categorized according to their routes of administration as oral, injectable, or inhaled. The various beta agonist bronchodilators are listed in Table 37-3.

The bronchioles are surrounded by smooth muscle. When the smooth muscle contracts, the airways are narrowed and the amount of oxygen and carbon dioxide exchanged is reduced. The action of beta agonist bronchodilators begins at the specific receptor stimulated and ends with the dilation of the airways. However, many reactions must take place at the cellular level

for this bronchodilation to occur. When a beta$_2$-adrenergic receptor is stimulated by a beta agonist, adenylate cyclase is activated and produces cyclic adenosine monophosphate (cAMP). Adenylate cyclase is an enzyme needed to make cAMP. The increased levels of cAMP cause bronchial smooth muscles to

## DOSAGES

### Bronchodilators

| DRUG (PREGNANCY CATEGORY) | PHARMACOLOGIC CLASS | USUAL DOSAGE RANGE | INDICATIONS |
|---|---|---|---|
| ◆ albuterol (Proventil, Proventil Repetabs, Ventolin, others) (C) | Short-acting beta₂ agonist (SABA) | **Pediatric 2-6 yr**<br>PO: 0.1-0.2 mg/kg 3 times daily<br>**Pediatric 7-11 yr**<br>PO: 2 mg 3-4 times daily<br>**Adult and pediatric 12 yr and older**<br>PO: 2-4 mg 3-4 times daily<br>**Adult and pediatric 4 yr and older**<br>MDI: 2 puffs q4-6h<br>Inhalation solution: 2.5 mg 3-4 times daily | Asthma, bronchospasm |
| ipratropium (Atrovent) (B) | Anticholinergic | **Adult and pediatric 12 yr and older**<br>MDI: 2 puffs 4 times daily<br>Nasal spray, 0.03%: 2 sprays 2-3 times daily<br>Nasal spray, 0.06%: 2 sprays 3-4 times daily<br>Inhalation solution: 500 mcg 3-4 times daily | |
| ◆salmeterol* (Severent) (C) | Long-acting beta₂ agonist (LABA) | **Adult**<br>1 puff twice a day | Asthma, COPD |

*IM*, Intramuscular; *IV*, intravenous; *MDI*, metered-dose inhaler; *PO*, oral.
*Long-acting beta agonists are no longer recommended to be used alone; they need to be combined with an asthma controlling medication such as an inhaled corticosteroid (e.g., Advair inhaler [fluticasone and salmeterol]).

relax, which results in bronchial dilation and increased airflow into and out of the lungs.

Nonselective adrenergic agonist drugs such as epinephrine also stimulate alpha-adrenergic receptors, causing constriction within the blood vessels. This vasoconstriction reduces the amount of edema or swelling in the mucous membranes and limits the quantity of secretions normally produced by these membranes. In addition, these drugs stimulate beta₁ receptors, which results in cardiovascular adverse effects such as an increase in heart rate, force of contraction, and blood pressure, as well as central nervous system (CNS) effects such as nervousness and tremor.

Drugs such as albuterol that predominantly stimulate the beta₂ receptors have more specific drug effects and cause less adverse effects. By primarily stimulating the beta₂-adrenergic receptors of the bronchial and vascular smooth muscles, they cause bronchodilation and may also have a dilating effect on the peripheral vasculature, which results in a decrease in diastolic blood pressure.

## Indications

The primary therapeutic effect of the beta agonists is the prevention or relief of bronchospasm related to bronchial asthma, bronchitis, and other pulmonary diseases. However, they are also used for effects outside the respiratory system. Because some of these drugs have the ability to stimulate both beta₁- and alpha-adrenergic receptors, they may be used to treat hypotension and shock (see Chapter 18).

## Contraindications

Contraindications include known drug allergy, uncontrolled hypertension or cardiac dysrhythmias, and high risk of stroke (because of the vasoconstrictive drug action).

## Adverse Effects

Mixed alpha/beta agonists produce the most adverse effects because they are nonselective. These include insomnia, restlessness, anorexia, cardiac stimulation, hyperglycemia, tremor, and vascular headache. The adverse effects of the nonselective beta agonists are limited to beta-adrenergic effects, including cardiac stimulation, tremor, anginal pain, and vascular headache. The beta₂ drugs can cause both hypertension and hypotension, vascular headaches, and tremor. Overdose management may include careful administration of a beta blocker while the patient is under close observation due to the risk of bronchospasm. Because the half-life of most adrenergic agonists is relatively short, the patient may just be observed while the body eliminates the medication.

## Interactions

When nonselective beta blockers are used with the beta agonist bronchodilators, the bronchodilation from the beta agonist is diminished. The use of beta agonists with monoamine oxidase inhibitors and other sympathomimetics is best avoided because of the enhanced risk for hypertension. Patients with diabetes may require an adjustment in the dosage of their hypoglycemic drugs, especially patients receiving epinephrine, because of the increase in blood glucose levels that can occur.

## Dosages

For dosage information on selected beta agonists, see the table on this page.

## DRUG PROFILES

### ◆ albuterol

Albuterol (Proventil) is a short-acting beta₂-specific bronchodilating beta agonist. Other similar drugs include bitolterol

(Tornalate), levalbuterol (Xopenex), pirbuterol (Maxair), and terbutaline (Brethine). Albuterol is the most commonly used drug in this class. If albuterol is used too frequently, dose-related adverse effects may be seen, because albuterol loses its beta$_2$-specific actions, especially at larger dosages. As a consequence, the beta$_1$ receptors are stimulated, which causes nausea, increased anxiety, palpitations, tremors, and an increased heart rate.

Albuterol is available for both oral and inhalational use. Inhalational dosage forms include metered-dose inhalers (MDIs) as well as solutions for inhalation. The levorotatory isomeric form of albuterol, levalbuterol, is sometimes prescribed as an albuterol alternative for patients with certain risk factors (e.g., tachycardia, including tachycardia associated with albuterol treatment).

Pharmacokinetics

| Route | Onset of Action | Peak Plasma Concentration | Elimination Half-life | Duration of Action |
|---|---|---|---|---|
| Inhalation | Immediate | 10-25 min | 3-4 hr | 3-4 hr |

♦ **salmeterol**

Salmeterol (Serevent) is a long-acting beta$_2$ agonist bronchodilator. Other long-acting inhalers include formoterol (Foradil, Perforomist) and arformoterol (Brovana). The long-acting inhalers are never to be used for acute treatment. Salmeterol is used for the maintenance treatment of asthma and COPD and is used in conjunction with an inhaled corticosteroid. It is given twice daily for maintenance treatment only. In 2006, a large randomized clinical trial showed that use of salmeterol was associated with an increase in asthma-related deaths (when added to usual asthma therapy). The risk appears to be higher in African-American patients. Adverse effects include immediate hypersensitivity reactions, headache, hypertension, and neuromuscular and skeletal pain. Salmeterol should never be given more than twice daily nor should the maximum daily dose (one puff twice daily) be exceeded. It is available as a powder for inhalation either alone (Serevent Diskus) or combined with a corticosteroid (Advair). The long-acting inhalers, including salmeterol, are not to be used alone, but in combination with other drugs such as the inhaled corticosteroids. Advair (salmeterol and fluticasone) is a very popular inhaler for COPD. Symbicort, a newer inhaler consisting of the corticosteroid budesonide and the bronchodilator formoterol, is similar to Advair.

Pharmacokinetics

| Route | Onset of Action | Peak Plasma Concentration | Elimination Half-life | Duration of Action |
|---|---|---|---|---|
| Inhalation | Asthma: 30-48 min COPD: 2 hr | Asthma: 2-4 hr COPD: 3-4.5 hr | 5.5 hr | 12 hr |

## ANTICHOLINERGICS

Currently there are two anticholinergic drugs used in the treatment of COPD: ipratropium (Atrovent) and tiotropium (Spiriva).

## Mechanism of Action and Drug Effects

On the surface of the bronchial tree are receptors for acetylcholine (ACh), the neurotransmitter for the parasympathetic nervous system (PSNS). When the PSNS releases ACh from its nerve endings, it binds to the ACh receptors on the surface of the bronchial tree, which results in bronchial constriction and narrowing of the airways. Anticholinergic drugs block these ACh receptors to prevent bronchoconstriction. This indirectly causes airway dilation. Anticholinergic agents also help reduce secretions in COPD patients.

## Indications

Because their actions are slow and prolonged, anticholinergics are used for prevention of the bronchospasm associated with chronic bronchitis or emphysema and not for the management of acute symptoms.

## Contraindications

The only usual contraindication to the use of bronchial anticholinergic drugs is drug allergy, including allergy to atropine or to soy lecithin (found in some of the inhalational formulations), or allergy to related food products such as peanut oils, peanuts, soybeans, and other legumes (beans). There have been reported cases of severe anaphylactic reactions to ipratropium inhalers in patients with peanut allergy, and such use is to be avoided. Caution is necessary in patients with acute narrow-angle glaucoma and prostate enlargement.

## Adverse Effects

The most commonly reported adverse effects of ipratropium and tiotropium therapy are related to the drugs' anticholinergic effects and include dry mouth or throat, nasal congestion, heart palpitations, gastrointestinal (GI) distress, urinary retention, increased intraocular pressure, headache, coughing, and anxiety. Ipratropium is classified as a pregnancy category B drug; tiotropium is classified as pregnancy category C.

## Drug Interactions

Possible additive toxicity may occur when anticholinergic bronchodilators are taken with other anticholinergic drugs.

## Dosages

For dosage information on anticholinergic drugs, see the table on p. 593.

## DRUG PROFILE

### ipratropium

Ipratropium (Atrovent) is the oldest and most commonly used anticholinergic bronchodilator. It is pharmacologically very similar to atropine (see Chapter 21). It is available both as a liquid aerosol for inhalation and as a multidose inhaler; both forms are usually dosed twice daily. Tiotropium (Spiriva) is a similar drug but is formulated for once-daily dosing. Many patients also benefit from taking both a beta$_2$ agonist and an anticholinergic drug, with the most popular combination being albuterol and ipratropium. Although many patients receive the two drugs separately, two combination products are available containing both of these drugs: Combivent (an MDI) and DuoNeb (an inhalation solution).

## DOSAGES

### *Theophylline Salts*

| DRUG (PREGNANCY CATEGORY) | PHARMACOLOGIC CLASS | USUAL DOSAGE RANGE | INDICATION |
|---|---|---|---|
| theophylline (Elixophyllin, Theo-Dur, Uniphyl, others) (C) | Xanthine-derived bronchodilator | **Adult**<br>PO: 400-600 mg/day in 1-4 divided doses | Asthma |

### Pharmacokinetics (ipratropium)

| Route | Onset of Action | Peak Plasma Concentration | Elimination Half-life | Duration of Action |
|---|---|---|---|---|
| Inhalation | 5-15 min | 1-2 hr | 1.6 hr | 4-5 hr |

## XANTHINE DERIVATIVES

The natural xanthines consist of the plant alkaloids caffeine, theobromine, and theophylline, but only theophylline and caffeine are currently used clinically. Synthetic xanthines include aminophylline and dyphylline. Caffeine, which is actually a metabolite of theophylline, has other uses described later.

### Mechanism of Action and Drug Effects

Xanthines cause bronchodilation by increasing the levels of the energy-producing substance cAMP. They do this by competitively inhibiting phosphodiesterase, the enzyme responsible for breaking down cAMP. In patients with COPD, cAMP plays an integral role in the maintenance of open airways. Higher intracellular levels of cAMP contribute to smooth muscle relaxation and also inhibit IgE-induced release of the chemical mediators that drive allergic reactions (histamine, slow-reacting substance of anaphylaxis, and others).

Theophylline is metabolized to caffeine in the body, whereas aminophylline is metabolized to theophylline. Theophylline and other xanthines also stimulate the CNS, but to a lesser degree than caffeine. This stimulation of the CNS has the beneficial effect of acting directly on the medullary respiratory center to enhance respiratory drive. In large doses, theophylline may stimulate the cardiovascular system, which results in both an increased force of contraction (positive inotropy) and an increased heart rate (positive chronotropy). The increased force of contraction raises cardiac output and hence blood flow to the kidneys. This, in combination with the ability of the xanthines to dilate blood vessels in and around the kidney, increases the glomerular filtration rate, which produces a diuretic effect.

### Indications

Xanthines are used to dilate the airways in patients with asthma, chronic bronchitis, or emphysema. They may be used in mild to moderate cases of acute asthma and as an adjunct drug in the management of COPD. Xanthines are now deemphasized as treatment for milder asthma because of their greater potential for drug interactions and the greater interpatient variability in therapeutic drug levels in the blood. Because of their relatively slow onset of action, xanthines are more often used for the prevention of asthmatic symptoms than for the relief of acute asthma attacks. However, they are also used as adjunct bronchodilators for patients with chronic bronchitis or emphysema.

Caffeine is used without prescription as a CNS stimulant, or analeptic (see Chapter 13), to promote alertness (e.g., for long-duration driving or studying). It is also used as a cardiac stimulant in infants with bradycardia and for enhancement of respiratory drive in infants in neonatal intensive care units. It is not normally used clinically in adults for these purposes, although theoretically it would have similar effects.

### Contraindications

Contraindications to therapy with xanthine derivatives include known drug allergy, uncontrolled cardiac dysrhythmias, seizure disorders, hyperthyroidism, and peptic ulcers.

### Adverse Effects

The common adverse effects of the xanthine derivatives include nausea, vomiting, and anorexia. In addition, gastroesophageal reflux has been observed to occur during sleep in patients taking these drugs. Cardiac adverse effects include sinus tachycardia, extrasystole, palpitations, and ventricular dysrhythmias. Transient increased urination and hyperglycemia are other possible adverse effects. Overdose and other toxicity of xanthine derivatives are usually treated by the repeated administration of doses of activated charcoal.

### Interactions

The use of xanthine derivatives with any of the following drugs causes an increase in the serum level: allopurinol, cimetidine, macrolide antibiotics (e.g., erythromycin), quinolones (e.g., ciprofloxacin), influenza vaccine, and oral contraceptives. Their use with sympathomimetics, or even caffeine, can produce additive cardiac and CNS stimulation. Rifampin increases the metabolism of theophylline, which results in decreased theophylline levels. St. John's wort (*Hypericum perforatum*) enhances the rate of xanthine drug metabolism; thus, higher dosages of theophylline and other xanthine derivatives may be needed. Cigarette smoking has a similar effect because of the enzyme-inducing effect of nicotine. Interacting foods include charcoal-broiled, high-protein, and low-carbohydrate foods. These foods may reduce serum levels of xanthines through various metabolic mechanisms.

### Dosages

For dosage information on selected theophylline salts, see the table on this page.

## DRUG PROFILE

### theophylline

Theophylline is the most commonly used xanthine derivative, albeit not often used. It is available in oral, rectal, injectable (as aminophylline), and topical dosage forms. Besides theophylline, which occurs in various salt forms, the other xanthine bronchodilator used clinically for the treatment of bronchoconstriction is aminophylline. Aminophylline is a prodrug of theophylline; it is metabolized to theophylline in the body. Aminophylline is sometimes given intravenously to patients with status asthmaticus who have not responded to fast-acting beta agonists such as epinephrine.

The beneficial effects of theophylline can be maximized by maintaining blood levels within a certain target range. If these levels become too high, unwanted adverse effects can occur. If the levels become too low, the patient receives little therapeutic benefit. Although the optimal level may vary from patient to patient, most standard references have suggested that the therapeutic range for theophylline blood level is 10 to 20 mcg/mL. However, most clinicians now advise levels between 5 and 15 mcg/mL. Laboratory monitoring of drug blood levels is common to ensure adequate dosage, especially in the hospital setting.

### Pharmacokinetics

| Route | Onset of Action | Peak Plasma Concentration | Elimination Half-life | Duration of Action |
|-------|-----------------|---------------------------|-----------------------|--------------------|
| PO    | Unknown         | 1-2 hr                    | 7-9 hr                | 12 hr              |

## NONBRONCHODILATING RESPIRATORY DRUGS

Bronchodilators (beta-adrenergic agonists and xanthines) are just one type of drug used to treat asthma, chronic bronchitis, and emphysema. There are also other drugs that are effective in suppressing the various underlying causes of some of these respiratory illnesses. These include leukotriene receptor antagonists (montelukast, zafirlukast, and zileuton) and corticosteroids (beclomethasone, budesonide, dexamethasone, flunisolide, fluticasone, ciclesonide, and triamcinolone). Another drug class known as *mast cell stabilizers* is now rarely used. However, these drugs are still listed in the national guidelines as *alternative* therapy and include cromolyn and nedocromil; they are sometimes used for exercise-induced asthma. As their class name implies, they work by stabilizing the cell membranes of mast cells to prevent the release of inflammatory mediators such as histamine.

## LEUKOTRIENE RECEPTOR ANTAGONISTS

When they became available in the 1990s, the leukotriene receptor antagonists (LTRAs) were the first new class of asthma medications to be introduced in the United States in more than 20 years.

Before the development of LTRAs, most asthma treatments focused on relaxing the contraction of bronchial muscles with bronchodilators. More recently, researchers have begun to understand how asthma symptoms are caused by the immune system at the cellular level. A chain reaction starts when a trigger allergen, such as cat hair or dust, initiates a series of chemical reactions in the body. Several substances are produced, including a family of molecules known as *leukotrienes*. In people with asthma, leukotrienes cause inflammation, bronchoconstriction, and mucus production. This in turn leads to coughing, wheezing, and shortness of breath.

## Mechanism of Action and Drug Effects

Currently two subclasses of LTRAs are available. These subclasses differ in the mechanism by which they block the inflammatory process in asthma. The first subclass of LTRAs acts by an indirect mechanism and inhibits the enzyme 5-lipoxygenase, which is necessary for leukotriene synthesis. Zileuton (Zyflo) is the only drug of this type currently available. Drugs in the second subclass of LTRAs act more directly by binding to the $D_4$ leukotriene receptor subtype in respiratory tract tissues and organs. These drugs include montelukast (Singulair) and zafirlukast (Accolate).

The drug effects of LTRAs are primarily limited to the lungs. As their name implies, LTRAs prevent leukotrienes from attaching to receptors located on circulating immune cells (e.g., lymphocytes in the blood) as well as local immune cells within the lungs (e.g., alveolar macrophages). This alleviates asthma symptoms in the lungs by reducing inflammation. They prevent smooth muscle contraction of the bronchial airways, decrease mucus secretion, and reduce vascular permeability (which reduces edema) through their reduction of leukotriene synthesis. Other antileukotriene effects of these drugs include prevention of the mobilization and migration of such cells as neutrophils and lymphocytes into the lungs. This also serves to reduce airway inflammation.

## Indications

The LTRAs montelukast, zafirlukast, and zileuton are used for the prophylaxis and long-term treatment and prevention of asthma in adults and children 12 years of age and older. Because it is dosed once daily, montelukast is the most widely used of these drugs and has also been approved for treatment of allergic rhinitis, a condition discussed in Chapter 36. These drugs are not meant for the management of acute asthmatic attacks. Improvement with their use is typically seen in about 1 week.

## Contraindications

Known drug allergy or other previous adverse drug reaction is the primary contraindication to the use of these drugs. Allergy to povidone, lactose, titanium dioxide, or cellulose derivatives is also important to note, because these are inactive ingredients in these drugs.

## Adverse Effects

The adverse effects of LTRAs differ depending on the specific drug. The most commonly reported adverse effects of zileuton include headache, nausea, dizziness, and insomnia. The most common adverse effects of zafirlukast include headache, nausea, and diarrhea. Both drugs may also lead to liver dysfunction. For this reason, monitor liver enzyme levels regularly in patients taking these drugs, especially early in the course of therapy.

## Interactions

Montelukast has fewer drug interactions than zafirlukast or zileuton. Phenobarbital and rifampin, both of which are enzyme

## DOSAGES

### Selected Antileukotriene Drug

| DRUG (PREGNANCY CATEGORY) | PHARMACOLOGIC CLASS | USUAL DOSAGE RANGE | INDICATIONS |
|---|---|---|---|
| ◆ montelukast (Singulair) (B) | Leukotriene receptor antagonist | **Pediatric 2-5 yr**<br>4 mg daily in evening<br>**Pediatric 6-14 yr**<br>5 mg daily in evening<br>**Adult and pediatric 15 yr and older**<br>10 mg daily in evening | Asthma (prophylaxis and maintenance treatment) |

inducers, decrease montelukast concentrations. For information on the drugs that interact with zafirlukast and zileuton, see Table 37-4.

## Dosages

For dosage information on montelukast, see the table on this page.

## DRUG PROFILE

LTRAs are used primarily for oral prophylaxis and long-term treatment of asthma. The three drugs currently available are zileuton, zafirlukast, and montelukast. These drugs are not recommended for treatment of acute asthma attacks.

### ◆ montelukast

Montelukast (Singulair) belongs to the same subcategory of LTRAs as zafirlukast. Montelukast and zafirlukast work by blocking leukotriene $D_4$ receptors to augment the inflammatory response. Montelukast offers the advantage of being approved for use in children 2 years of age and older. It also has fewer adverse effects and drug interactions than zafirlukast. Use of montelukast is contraindicated in patients with a known hypersensitivity to it. It is available only for oral use. It is classified as a pregnancy category B drug. Recommended dosages are given in the table on this page.

### Pharmacokinetics

| Route | Onset of Action | Peak Plasma Concentration | Elimination Half-life | Duration of Action |
|---|---|---|---|---|
| PO | 30 min | 3-4 hr | 2.7-5 hr | 24 hr |

## CORTICOSTEROIDS

Corticosteroids, also known as *glucocorticoids,* are either naturally occurring or synthetic drugs used in the treatment of pulmonary diseases for their antiinflammatory effects. All have actions similar to those of the natural steroid hormone cortisol, which is chemically the same as the drug hydrocortisone. Synthetic steroids are more commonly used in drug therapy. They can be given by inhalation, orally, or even intravenously in severe cases of asthma. Corticosteroids administered by inhalation have an advantage over orally administered corticosteroids in that their action is relatively limited to the topical

site in the lungs. This generally limits, although does not totally prevent, systemic effects. The chemical structures of the corticosteroids given by inhalation have also been slightly altered to limit their systemic absorption from the respiratory tract. The corticosteroids administered by inhalation include the following:

- beclomethasone dipropionate (Beclovent)
- budesonide (Pulmicort Turbuhaler)
- dexamethasone sodium phosphate (Decadron Phosphate Respihaler)
- flunisolide (AeroBid)
- fluticasone (Flovent)
- triamcinolone acetonide (Azmacort)
- ciclesonide (Omnaris)

The systemic use of corticosteroids was described in Chapter 33. The systemic corticosteroids most commonly used for respiratory illness include the following:

- prednisone (oral)
- methylprednisolone (intravenous or oral)

### TABLE 37-4 DRUG INTERACTIONS: LEUKOTRIENE RECEPTOR ANTAGONISTS

| DRUG | INTERACTING DRUGS | MECHANISM | RESULT |
|---|---|---|---|
| montelukast (Singulair) | phenobarbital, rifampin | Increased metabolism | Decreased montelukast levels |
| zafirlukast (Accolate) | aspirin | Decreased clearance | Increased zafirlukast levels |
| | erythromycin | Decreased bioavailability | Decreased zafirlukast levels |
| | warfarin | Decreased clearance | Increased warfarin levels |
| zileuton (Zyflo) | propranolol | Decreased clearance | Increased propranolol levels |
| | theophylline | Decreased clearance | Increased theophylline levels |
| | warfarin | Decreased clearance | Increased warfarin levels |

| TABLE 37-5 | WHITE BLOOD CELLS (LEUKOCYTES) | |
|---|---|---|
| **WBC TYPE\*** | **ROLE IN INFLAMMATION** | **CORTICOSTEROID EFFECT** |
| **Granulocytes** | | |
| Neutrophils (65%) | Contain powerful lysosomes (very small bodies that hold cellular digestive enzymes); release chemicals that destroy invading organisms and also attack other WBCs | Stabilize cell membranes so that inflammation-causing substances are not released |
| Eosinophils (2%-5%) | Function mainly in allergic reactions and protect against parasitic infections; ingest inflammatory chemicals and antigen-antibody complexes | Little effect if any |
| Basophils (0.5%-1%) | Contain histamine, an inflammation-causing substance, and heparin, an anticoagulant | Stabilize cell membranes so that histamine is not released |
| **Agranulocytes** | | |
| Lymphocytes (25%) | Two types: T lymphocytes and B lymphocytes; T cells attack infecting microbial or cancerous cells; B cells produce antibodies against specific antigens | Decrease activity of the lymphocytes |
| Monocytes (3%-5%) | Produce macrophages, which can migrate out of the bloodstream to such places as mucous membranes, where they are capable of engulfing large bacteria or virus-infected cells | Inhibit macrophage accumulation in already inflamed areas, thus preventing more inflammation |

*WBC*, White blood cell.
\*Value in parentheses is the percentage of all leukocytes represented by the given type.

## Mechanism of Action and Drug Effects

Although the exact mechanism of action of the corticosteroids has not been determined, it is thought that they have the dual effect of both reducing inflammation and enhancing the activity of beta agonists. The corticosteroids produce their antiinflammatory effects through a complex sequence of actions. The overall effect is to prevent various nonspecific inflammatory processes. These include the accumulation of inflammatory mediators as well as altered vascular permeability (which causes edema).

Corticosteroids essentially work by stabilizing the membranes of cells that normally release bronchoconstricting substances. These cells include leukocytes, which is another name for white blood cells (WBCs). There are five different types of WBC, each with its own specific characteristics. The five types of WBC, their role in the inflammatory process, and the way in which corticosteroids inhibit their normal action, combat inflammation, and produce bronchodilation are summarized in Table 37-5. Inflammatory mediators are primarily released by lymphocytes in the circulation as well as by mast cells and alveolar macrophages. These latter two cell types are stationary (noncirculating) inflammatory cells that remain localized in the various tissues and organs of the respiratory tract.

Corticosteroids have also been shown to restore or increase the responsiveness of bronchial smooth muscle to beta-adrenergic receptor stimulation, which results in more pronounced stimulation of the beta$_2$ receptors by beta agonist drugs such as albuterol. It may take several weeks of continuous therapy before the full therapeutic effects of the corticosteroids are realized.

## Indications

Inhaled corticosteroids are used for the primary treatment of bronchospastic disorders to control the inflammatory responses that are believed to be the cause of these disorders; they are indicated for persistent asthma. They are often used concurrently with the beta-adrenergic agonists. In respiratory illnesses, systemic corticosteroids are generally used only to treat acute exacerbations, or severe asthma. Their long-term use is associated with adverse effects (see later). The NAEPP recommends long-term use in cases of truly disabling illness (Step 6 of the recommended therapeutic approach) in which the benefits of this drug therapy arguably outweigh the adverse effects. When a more pronounced antiinflammatory effect is needed, however, as in an acute exacerbation of asthma or other COPD, intravenous corticosteroids (e.g., methylprednisolone) are often used.

## Contraindications

Drug allergy is the primary contraindication and is usually due to other ingredients in the drug formulation. These drugs are not intended as sole therapy for acute asthma attacks. Inhaled corticosteroids are contraindicated in patients who are hypersensitive to glucocorticoids, in patients whose sputum tests positive for *Candida* organisms, and in patients with systemic fungal infection, as the corticosteroids can suppress the immune system.

## Adverse Effects

The main undesirable local effects of typical doses of inhaled corticosteroids in the respiratory system include pharyngeal irritation, coughing, dry mouth, and oral fungal infections. Instruct patients to rinse their mouths after use of an inhaled corticosteroid. Most of the drug effects of inhaled corticosteroids are limited to their topical site of action in the lungs. Because of the chemical structure of these inhaled dosage forms, there is relatively little systemic absorption of the drugs when they are administered by inhalation at normal therapeutic dosages. However, the degree of systemic absorption is more likely to be increased in patients who require higher inhaled dosages. When there is significant

## DOSAGES

### Selected Corticosteroids

| DRUG (PREGNANCY CATEGORY) | PHARMACOLOGIC CLASS | USUAL DOSAGE RANGE | INDICATIONS |
|---|---|---|---|
| fluticasone propionate (Flovent, Flonase) (C) | Synthetic glucocorticoid | **Adult and pediatric 12 yr and older**<br>Flovent MDI, 3 strengths available: 88-880 mcg twice daily<br>**Pediatric 4-11 yr**<br>Flovent inhalation powder, 3 strengths available: 50-100 mcg twice daily<br>**Adult and pediatric 12 yr and older**<br>Flovent inhalation powder, 3 strengths available: 100-1000 mcg twice daily | Asthma (prophylaxis and maintenance treatment)<br><br><br><br>Seasonal allergic rhinitis |
| methylprednisolone (Solu-Medrol injection, Medrol tablets) (C) | Synthetic glucocorticoid | Dosage varies as above, but usually 40-125 mg IV, 1-3 times daily, usually tapered down<br>Oral taper: usually from 24 to 2 mg daily | Exacerbations of asthma or COPD |

*COPD*, Chronic obstructive pulmonary disease; *IV*, intravenous; *MDI*, metered-dose inhaler.

systemic absorption, which is most likely with high-dose intravenous or oral administration, corticosteroids can affect any of the organ systems in the body. Some of these systemic drug effects include adrenocortical insufficiency, increased susceptibility to infection, fluid and electrolyte disturbances, endocrine effects, CNS effects (insomnia, nervousness, seizures), and dermatologic and connective tissue effects, including brittle skin, bone loss, osteoporosis, and Cushing's syndrome (see Chapter 33).

It is important to remember that when patients are switched to inhaled corticosteroids after receiving systemic corticosteroids, especially at high dosages for an extended period, adrenal suppression (Addisonian crisis) may occur when the systemically administered corticosteroid is not tapered slowly. Patient deaths have been reported due to adrenal gland failure in such cases when the switch to inhaled corticosteroids is made quickly and the dosage of systemic corticosteroids is not reduced gradually. Prevention of this occurrence requires careful monitoring with slow tapering of systemic drug dosages. The patient who is dependent on systemic corticosteroids may need up to 1 year of recovery time after discontinuation of systemic therapy. There is evidence that bone growth is suppressed in children and adolescents taking corticosteroids. This suppression is more apparent in children receiving larger systemic (versus inhaled) dosages over longer treatment durations. Growth needs to be tracked (e.g., with standardized charts) and medications reevaluated if growth suppression becomes evident. In some cases, supplemental growth hormone may be prescribed.

## Interactions

Drug interactions are more likely to occur with systemic (versus inhaled) corticosteroids. These drugs may increase serum glucose levels, possibly requiring adjustments in dosages of antidiabetic drugs. Because of interactions related to metabolizing enzymes, they may also raise blood

levels of the immunosuppressants cyclosporine and tacrolimus. Likewise, the antifungal drug itraconazole may reduce clearance of the steroids, whereas phenytoin, phenobarbital, and rifampin may enhance clearance. There is also greater risk for hypokalemia with concurrent use of potassium-depleting diuretics such as hydrochlorothiazide and furosemide.

## Dosages

For dosage information on selected corticosteroids, see the table on this page.

## DRUG PROFILES

### fluticasone propionate

Fluticasone is administered intranasally (Flonase) (one inhalation in each nostril daily) and by oral inhalation (Flovent) (usually one inhalation by mouth twice daily). Fluticasone is also available in a combination formulation with the bronchodilator salmeterol (Advair). Advair is one of the most commonly used inhalers, but because it contains a long-acting beta agonist, it must never be used for acute treatment.

### Pharmacokinetics

| Route | Onset of Action | Peak Plasma Concentration | Elimination Half-life | Duration of Action |
|---|---|---|---|---|
| Inhalation | Unknown | Unknown | 3 hr | Up to 24 hr |

### methylprednisolone

Methylprednisolone is a systemic corticosteroid available in both oral (Medrol) and injectable (Solu-Medrol) forms.

### Pharmacokinetics

| Route | Onset of Action | Peak Plasma Concentration | Elimination Half-life | Duration of Action |
|---|---|---|---|---|
| IV | Immediate | 30 min | 3-4 hr | 24-36 hr |

### Bronchodilators and Corticosteroids for COPD

Ms. B. is a 73-year-old woman who worked in the local traffic tunnel for about 25 years and has had chronic obstructive pulmonary disease (COPD) for 10 years, caused by exposure to environmental pollutants while on the job and by cigarette smoking. She is now retired and is frequently admitted to the hospital for treatment of her condition. She quit smoking about 8 years ago. Ms. B. is now in the hospital for treatment of an acute exacerbation of her COPD and an upper respiratory tract infection. The physician has ordered the following: Oxygen per nasal cannula at 2 L/min, methylprednisolone (Solu-Medrol), 125 mg IVPB, then 80 mg IVPB every 6 hours; Advair 50 mcg/250 mcg, 1 puff every 12 hours; albuterol (Accuneb) 2.5 mg by nebulizer every 4 hours for 2 days, then every 4 hours as needed; piperacillin/tazobactam (Zosyn) antibiotic therapy, 3.375 g intravenously every 6 hours; measurement of intake and output; daily weight measurement; assessment of vital signs with breath sounds and pulse oximetry every 2 hours until stable; chest physiotherapy twice a day and as needed.

1. What is in Advair, and what does the "50 mcg/250 mcg" mean? Explain the class and purposes of the drug(s) it contains.

Within 2 days, Ms. B's condition stabilizes, and the methylprednisolone dose is gradually reduced. After 1 week, the IV corticosteroid is discontinued and she is started on oral prednisone (generic) 40 mg daily. Her discharge medications include the following:

prednisone (generic) 40 mg PO daily for 3 days, then taper and discontinue by reducing the dose by 5 mg daily. (Prescription calls for 5-mg tablets.)

Advair 50 mcg/250 mcg, 1 puff every 12 hours

albuterol (Proventil HFA) metered-dose inhaler, 90 mcg/spray, every 4 hours as needed

2. What is the reason for tapering the methylprednisolone and prednisone before they are discontinued?

3. Ms. B states, "This is confusing! How do I know how many tablets to take? It's different each day!" What can you do to help her with the tapering dosage of prednisone?

4. While going over the medications, Ms. B asks you, "So which inhaler do I take if I feel short of breath? The Advair or the albuterol? Aren't they the same thing?" What is the nurse's best response?

For answers, see http://evolve.elsevier.com/Lilley.

## PHOSPHODIESTERASE-4 INHIBITOR

In 2011, the FDA approved roflumilast (Daliresp), which is a selective inhibitor of the enzyme called *phophodiesterase type 4 (PDE4)*. It is indicated to prevent coughing and excess mucus from worsening and to decrease the frequency of life-threatening COPD exacerbations. It is not intended to treat acute bronchospasm. The most commonly reported adverse effects include nausea, diarrhea, headache, insomnia, dizziness, weight loss, and psychiatric symptoms. The FDA requires a medication guide that informs patients of the potential risk of psychiatric adverse effects. Further information can be found at www.daliresp.com.

## MONOCLONAL ANTIBODY ANTIASTHMATIC

Omalizumab (Xolair) is the newest antiasthmatic medication to become available. It is a monoclonal antibody that selectively binds to the immunoglobulin IgE, which in turn limits

the release of mediators of the allergic response. Omalizumab is given by injection and has the potential for producing anaphylaxis. Patients receiving omalizumab must be monitored closely for hypersensitivity reactions.

## NURSING PROCESS

### ASSESSMENT

The net drug effect of beta agonists, xanthine derivatives, anticholinergics, LTRAs, and corticosteroids is improved airflow in airway passages and increased oxygen supply. Thoroughly assess for cautions, contraindications, and drug interactions. Before administering these drugs, assess the patient's skin color, temperature, respiration rate (at a rate of 12-24 breaths/min) respiration depth and rhythm, breath sounds, blood pressure, and pulse rate. Determine if the patient is having problems with cough, dyspnea, orthopnea, or hypoxia, or has other signs or symptoms of respiratory distress. If a cough is present, assess its character, frequency, presence or absence of sputum, as well as the color of the sputum. Assess the patient for presence of any of the following: sternal retractions, cyanosis, restlessness, activity intolerance, cardiac irregularities, palpitations, hypertension, tachycardia, and use of accessory muscles to breathe, indicating significant respiratory compromise. Determine the anterior-posterior diameter of the thorax. Note pulse oximetry reading to determine oxygen saturation levels.

Obtain a complete medication history that includes information about prescription and over-the-counter (OTC) drugs, herbal products, alternative therapies, use of nebulizers and/or humidifiers, use of a home air conditioner, and intactness of the heating and air conditioning system. Collect information about environmental allergies such as to dust, mold, pollen, mildew, seasonal allergies, as well as food allergies. Note the characteristics of any respiratory symptoms (e.g., seasonally induced, exercise- or stress-induced) and any family history of respiratory diseases. Identify any environmental exposures, such as to chemicals or irritants, as well as precipitating and alleviating factors for any respiratory symptoms and/or disease processes. Assess smoking habits because smoking exacerbates respiratory symptoms, and nicotine interacts with many respiratory drugs.

Cardiac status may be compromised due to respiratory distress and respiratory illnesses; thus closely assess the patient's blood pressure, pulse rate, heart sounds, and electrocardiogram, as ordered. Blood gas analysis may be indicated with attention to the patient's pH, oxygen, carbon dioxide, and serum bicarbonate levels. Assess nail beds for abnormalities (e.g., clubbing, cyanosis) and the area around the lips for cyanotic changes. Restlessness is often the first sign of hypoxia, so frequent assessment before, during, and after drug treatment is needed. If hypoxia present, it needs to be reported to the prescriber. If chest radiographs, scans, or magnetic resonance images have been ordered, review the findings. Along with a physical assessment, perform a psychosocial and emotional assessment, because anxiety, stress, and fear may only further compromise the patient's respiratory status and oxygen levels. Be sure to note the age of the patient because of increased drug sensitivity in the very young and the elderly.

For the *beta agonists* (e.g., albuterol and salmeterol), cautions, contraindications, and drug interactions associated with these drugs must be noted. A respiratory assessment is needed to assess for allergies to the fluorocarbon propellant in inhaled dosage forms. Assess for the contraindications in patients with dysrhythmias and those at risk for stroke. Assess the patient's intake of caffeine (e.g., chocolate, tea, coffee, candy, and sodas) and use of OTC medications containing caffeine (e.g., appetite suppressants, pain relievers). The intake of caffeine is important to determine, because of its sympathomimetic effects and possible potentiation of adverse effects along with albuterol and other beta agonists (e.g., restlessness, cardiac stimulation, tremor, hyperglycemia and vascular headache; hypotension/hypertension with $beta_2$ drugs). Assess the patient's medication history because these drugs are not to be taken with monoamine oxidase inhibitors because of the enhanced risk for hypertension. Assess educational level and readiness to learn.

With use of the nonselective adrenergic agonist drug EpiPen (0.3 mg epinephrine) or EpiPen Jr (0.15 mg epinephrine) Auto-Injectors, assess for the main indication (which is emergency use with severe allergic reactions caused by allergens, exercise, and unknown triggers) and for those individuals who are considered at increased risk for these reactions.

Specific to the use of *anticholinergics* is the need to assess for allergies to atropine, soy lecithin, peanut oils, peanuts, soybeans, and other legumes, as there have been reported cases of severe anaphylactic reactions to ipratropium inhalers in patients with these type of allergies. In your assessments for patients taking anticholinergics, include any history of heart palpitations, GI distress, benign prostatic hyperplasia and/or urinary retention, and glaucoma due to the adverse effects of the drugs, leading to potentiation of these conditions or symptoms. Ipratropium and its aerosol forms have been associated with bronchospasm, so assess for any preexisting problems with the use of MDIs. If a combination product containing both ipratropium and albuterol is prescribed, perform an assessment appropriate to the use of both of these drugs.

In patients taking *xanthine derivatives* (e.g., theophylline), identify any contraindications and cautions. Perform a careful cardiovascular assessment, noting heart rate, blood pressure, and history of cardiac disease. This is important because of the adverse effects of sinus tachycardia and palpitations. GI reflux may also occur with these drugs. Assess bowel patterns and for preexisting disease, such as gastroesophageal reflux and/or ulcers. Because of possible drug-induced transient urinary frequency, conduct a baseline assessment of urinary patterns. Assessment needs to also include the patient's medication history to assess for possible drug interactions such as with allopurinol, cimetidine, erythromycin, ciprofloxacin, oral contraceptives, caffeine, and sympathomimetics. Perform a dietary assessment, including questions about consumption of a low-carbohydrate, high-protein diet and intake of charcoal-broiled meat. These dietary practices may lead to increased theophylline elimination and decrease the therapeutic levels of the drug. Note caffeine-containing foods, beverages, prescription drugs, OTC drugs, and herbals because of additional interactions.

With *LTRAs*, assess for contraindications, cautions, and drug interactions. Determine liver functioning because of specific concerns about the use of these drugs in patients with altered hepatic function. As with other medications, elderly patients are more sensitive to these drugs.

## PATIENT-CENTERED-CARE: LIFESPAN CONSIDERATIONS FOR THE ELDERLY PATIENT

### Xanthine Derivatives

- Administer xanthine derivatives cautiously with careful monitoring in the elderly because sensitivity to these drugs is increased in this patient population due to decreased drug metabolism.
- Assess for signs and symptoms of xanthine toxicity, which include nausea, vomiting, restlessness, insomnia, irritability, and tremors. Discriminating the cause of restlessness (e.g., hypoxia versus drug toxicity) is important to patient safety.
- Instruct elderly patients to never chew or crush sustained-released dosage forms and to remain aware of drug interactions, especially interactions with other asthma-related drugs/bronchodilators. Advise elderly patients to avoid omitting and/or doubling up on doses. If a dose is missed, the prescriber must be contacted for further instructions.
- Monitoring of serum levels during follow-up visits is important to avoid possible toxicity and ensure therapeutic blood levels.
- Lower dosages may be necessary initially in elderly patients, not only because of their increased sensitivity to the drug but also because of the possibility of decreased liver and renal functioning. Close monitoring for adverse effects and toxicity should be part of everyday therapy. Note and report any palpitations and increased blood pressure (from cardiovascular and central nervous system stimulation).

With *corticosteroids* (also known as *glucocorticoids*), perform a baseline assessment of vital signs, breath sounds, and heart sounds. Assessment for underlying adrenal disorders is important because of the adrenal suppression that occurs with the use of these medications. Age is important to consider because corticosteroids may be problematic for the pediatric patient if long-term therapy and/or high dosage amounts are used. The systemic impact on the pediatric patient is suppressed growth (see the Pharmacology Overview section for further discussion). As with the other drugs in this chapter, awareness of basic information about these drugs, especially their action, is very important for safe use and prevention of medication errors. For example, glucocorticoids are used for their antiinflammatory effects, beta agonists and xanthines for their bronchodilating effects, and anticholinergics for their blockage of cholinergic receptors. Knowing what drugs do and why they are used helps to prevent or decrease medication errors and adverse effects. Significant drug interactions to assess for, especially with systemic versus inhaled corticosteroids, include antidiabetic drugs, antifungals, phenytoin, phenobarbital, rifampin, and potassium-sparing diuretics. See Chapter 33 for more information on these antiinflammatory adrenal drugs.

With the *PDE4 inhibitors,* assess for presenting symptoms as well as any baseline psychiatric issues or disorders. Note that these drugs are not for acute bronchospasms. Omalizumab, a *monoclonal antibody antiasthmatic drug,* requires additional assessment of known risks associated with certain malignancies. Taking a thorough nursing history will help identify any of these risks. Assess also for signs and symptoms of hypersensitivity due to an increased incidence.

---

### ⚡ SAFETY AND QUALITY IMPROVEMENT: PREVENTING MEDICATION ERRORS

#### *Oral Ingestion of Capsules for Inhalation Devices*

Some inhalation products use capsules and a device that pierces the capsules to allow the powdered medication to be inhaled with a special inhaler. Two products, Foradil Aerolizer (formoterol fumarate inhalation powder) and Spiriva HandiHaler (tiotropium bromide inhalation powder) contain such capsules. Even though these capsules are packaged with inhaler devices, they closely resemble oral capsules. The U.S. Food and Drug Administration (FDA) has received reports that the capsules have been taken orally by patients, which can potentially result in adverse effects. If the capsules are swallowed instead of taken using the inhalation device, the medication's onset of action may be delayed, the efficacy is reduced, and as a result the patient receives inadequate drug delivery. The FDA has taken steps to work with the drug manufacturers to mark the packaging clearly. Be certain to instruct patients on the proper use and correct route of administration for these inhaled drugs to prevent their confusion with oral products.

Data from FDA: Public health advisory: important information on the correct use of Spiriva and Foradil capsules, 2008, available at www.fda.gov/Drugs/DrugSafety/PostmarketDrugSafetyInformationfor PatientsandProviders/DrugSafetyInformationforHeathcareProfessionals/ PublicHealthAdvisories/ucm051132.html. Accessed March 13, 2012.

### ▌NURSING DIAGNOSES

1. Impaired gas exchange related to pathophysiologic changes caused by respiratory disease
2. Fatigue related to the disease process and lack of oxygen saturation
3. Noncompliance with the medication regimen related to undesirable adverse effects of drug therapy

### ▌PLANNING

#### ▌GOALS

1. Patient experiences improved gas exchange due to improved disease process and symptomatology.
2. Patient exhibits improved energy and less fatigue.
3. Patient remains compliant with the medication regimen and with the nonpharmacologic therapies.

#### ▌OUTCOME CRITERIA

1. Patient briefly describes measures to improve gas exchange such as use of deep breathing, use of medications as described, and avoiding precipitating factors.

- Patient shows evidence of improved oxygen levels with an $SpO_2$ greater than or equal to 95% (depending on pathology).
2. Patient is well rested and allows time for frequent rest periods during activities of daily living while minimizing oxygen demands.
3. Patient states the importance of taking the medication as prescribed, the reasons for not increasing or decreasing the dosage of the drug, and the importance of not stopping the drug therapy abruptly to prevent complications and exacerbations of the disease.
- Patient takes medication(s) as prescribed to improve oxygenation and prevent exacerbation of symptoms.

### ▌IMPLEMENTATION

Nursing interventions that apply to patients with respiratory disease processes (e.g., COPD, asthma, other upper and lower respiratory tract disorders) include patient education and an emphasis on compliance and prevention, in addition to the specific actions related to the prescribed drug therapy. Emphasize measures that help to prevent, relieve, or decrease the manifestations of the disease. A resource that provides excellent information as well as photographs and slideshows can be found at http://www.medicinenet.com/asthma.

*Bronchodilators* and other respiratory drugs must be given exactly as prescribed and by the prescribed route (e.g., parenterally, orally, by intermittent positive pressure breathing, or by inhalation). Demonstrate the proper method for administering the inhaled forms of these drugs to the patient (see Chapter 9). Provide time for a return demonstration. Emphasize the importance of taking only the prescribed dose of the *beta agonists, anticholinergics, xanthines, LTRAs,* and *other respiratory drugs* because of the possible adverse effects, such as cardiac stimulation, hypertension or hypotension, vascular headaches, heart palpitations, GI distress, urinary retention, gastroesophageal reflux, dysrhythmias, nausea, and dizziness.

The use of MDIs requires coordination to inhale the medication correctly and to obtain approximately 10% of drug delivery to the lungs. If a second puff of the same drug is ordered, instruct the patient to wait 1 to 2 minutes between puffs. If a second type of inhaled drug is ordered, instruct the patient to wait 2 to 5 minutes between the medications or to take as prescribed. Use of a spacer may be indicated to increase the amount of drug delivered. See the Teamwork and Collaboration: Legal and Ethical Principles box for information concerning the environmental hazards associated with MDIs. Dry powder inhalers are small handheld devices that deliver a specific amount of dry micronized powder with each inhaled breath. A nebulizer dosage form delivers small amounts of misted droplets of the drug to the lungs through a small mouthpiece or mask. Although a nebulizer may take a longer time to deliver the drug to the lungs than the inhalers, the nebulizer dosage form may be more effective for some patients. See Chapter 9 for more information on these dosage routes.

## TEAMWORK AND COLLABORATION: LEGAL AND ETHICAL PRINCIPLES

### Inhaled Medications and the Environment

A method of delivery or route of administration for inhalers poses concern for the environment. These inhaled medications are often used by people who have asthma or other breathing problems, such as chronic obstructive pulmonary disease. Traditionally, many inhalers have contained chlorofluorocarbons (CFCs), a propellant that damages the protective ozone layer. However, these CFC inhalers are being phased out and replaced with more environmentally friendly inhalers. Depending on the specific type of product being used and where one lives geographically, inhalers and aerosol products may be thrown into household trash or recyclables, or may be considered hazardous waste and require special handling. Read the handling instructions on the label, as some inhalers should not be punctured or thrown into a fire or incinerator. To ensure safe disposal, contact your local trash and recycling facility. For more information, visit www.fda.gov.

Modified from the U.S. Food and Drug Administration: How to dispose of unused medications, *FDA Consumer Updates*, April 14, 2011, available at www.fda.gov/forconsumers/consumerupdates/ucm101653. htm. Accessed March 13, 2012.

*Beta agonists* must be taken exactly as prescribed because overdosage may be life-threatening. Educate patients not to crush or chew oral sustained-release tablets and to take them with food to decrease GI upset. Instructions for inhaled dosage forms are presented in Chapter 9. See Figure 37-2 for instructions for use of the EpiPen Auto-Injector. Reassess the respiratory status and breath sounds before, during, and after therapy with these drugs to determine therapeutic effectiveness.

*Anticholinergic drugs* used for respiratory diseases (e.g., ipratropium) are to be taken daily as ordered and with appropriate use of the MDI. See the Patient Teaching Tips for more information on the administration of these drugs. It is important that the patient waits from 1 to 2 minutes (or as prescribed) before inhaling the second dose of the drug to allow for maximal lung penetration. Encourage rinsing the mouth with water immediately after use of any inhaled or nebulized drug to help prevent mucosal irritation and dryness.

*Xanthine derivatives* are also to be given exactly as prescribed. If they are to be administered parenterally, determine the correct diluent, compatibility, and rate of administration. Use intravenous infusion pumps to ensure dosage accuracy and help prevent toxicity. Too rapid an infusion may lead to profound hypotension with possible syncope, tachycardia, seizures, and even cardiac arrest. Oral forms are to be taken with food to decrease GI upset. To prevent a sudden increase in drug release and irritating effects on the gastric mucosa, instruct patients not to crush or chew timed-release preparations. Educate patients that suppository forms of the drug need to be refrigerated, and to notify the prescriber if rectal burning, itching, or irritation occurs. Continue to monitor the patient for respiratory status and improvement in baseline condition during drug therapy.

The *LTRAs*, specifically zileuton, montelukast, and zafirlukast, are given orally. Of most concern are the montelukast chewable tablets, which contain aspartame and approximately 0.842 mg of phenylamine per 5-mg tablet. Some patients may need to avoid these substances. Emphasize that these drugs are indicated for treatment of chronic, not acute, asthma attacks. Stress that these drugs are to be taken as ordered and on a continuous schedule, even if symptoms improve. Increase fluid intake, as with all the respiratory drugs, to help in decreasing the viscosity of secretions.

Inhaled *corticosteroids* (glucocorticoids) are yet another group of drugs that must be used as prescribed and with cautions regarding overuse. Advise the patient to take the medication as ordered every day, regardless of whether or not he or she is feeling better. Often these drugs (e.g., flunisolide) are used as maintenance drugs and are taken twice daily for maximal response. An inhaled beta$_2$ agonist may be used before the inhaled corticosteroid to provide bronchodilation before administration of the antiinflammatory drug. The bronchodilator inhaled drug is generally taken 2 to 5 minutes (or as ordered) before the corticosteroid aerosol. Stress the importance of keeping all equipment (inhalers or nebulizers) clean, cleaning and changing filters (nebulizers), and maintaining it in good working condition. Use of a spacer may be indicated, especially if success with inhalation is limited. Recommend rinsing the mouth immediately after use of the inhaler or nebulizer dosage forms of corticosteroids to help prevent overgrowth of oral fungi and subsequent development of oral candidiasis (thrush). Pediatric patients may need a prescriber's order to have these medications on hand, at school, and during athletic events or physical education. Peak flow meter use is also encouraged to help patients of all ages better regulate their disease. A peak flow meter is a handheld device used to monitor a patient's ability to breath out air and reflects the airflow through the bronchi and thus the degree of obstruction in the airways. Encourage journaling to record peak flow levels, signs and symptoms of the disease, any improvement, and the occurrence of adverse effects associated with therapy. For pediatric patients, use of systemic forms of corticosteroids is a concern. Specifically in children, the use of systemic forms of these drugs may lead to suppression of the hypothalamic-pituitary-adrenal axis and subsequent growth stunting. However, the benefits are considerable when compared to the risks. Inhaled forms are often combined with short-term systemic therapy in pediatric patients. Continue to monitor the patient's condition during therapy with a focus on the respiratory, cardiac, and central nervous systems.

With *PDE4 inhibitor drugs*, educate the patient about the importance of reporting any change in psychiatric status to the prescriber immediately. The *monoclonal antibody antiasthmatic drug* omalizumab is to be taken exactly as ordered. Since it is given as a subcutaneous injection, instruct the patient in self-injection, or alert the patient that frequent visits to the prescriber, nurse, or other health care provider to receive the injection are necessary. This drug is usually given every 2 to 4 weeks. Omalizumab is not indicated for acute asthma attacks, and it may be used in conjunction with other acute-acting asthma medications. Closely monitor the patient for any allergic or hypersensitivity reactions.

## ▌EVALUATION

The therapeutic effects of any of the drugs used to improve the control of acute or chronic respiratory diseases and to treat or help prevent respiratory symptoms include the following: decreased dyspnea, wheezing, restlessness, and anxiety; improved respiratory patterns with return to normal rate and quality; improved oxygen saturation levels; improved activity tolerance and arterial blood gas levels; improved quality of life; and decreased severity and incidence of respiratory symptoms. The therapeutic effects of *bronchodilators* (e.g., *xanthines, beta agonists*) include decreased symptoms and increased ease of breathing. Blood levels of theophylline need to be between 5 and 15 mcg/mL and need to be frequently monitored. Peak flow meters are easy to use and help reveal early decreases in peak flow caused by bronchospasm. They also aid in monitoring

treatment effectiveness. Other respiratory drugs produce therapeutic effects as related to the specific drug. Adverse effects for which to monitor during therapy include the following: *beta agonists*—headache, insomnia, cardiac stimulation, and tremor; *anticholinergics*—headache, GI distress, urinary retention, and increased intraocular pressure; *xanthines*—nausea, vomiting, or palpitations; *LTRAs*—dyspepsia, headaches, and insomnia; and *corticosteroids*—adrenocortical insufficiency, increased susceptibility to infection, fluid and electrolyte disturbances, and insomnia. With corticosteroids, adrenal suppression may occur with high doses for an extended period of time. See the previous discussion for a complete listing of adverse effects.

## PATIENT TEACHING TIPS

### Beta Agonists
- Educate the patient about any potential drug interactions.
- Encourage patients with asthma, bronchitis, or COPD to avoid precipitating events such as exposure to conditions or situations that may lead to bronchoconstriction and/or worsening of the disorder (e.g., allergens, stress, smoking, and/or air pollutants).
- Provide instructions about the proper use and care of MDIs, dry powder inhalers, and other such devices. See Chapter 9 for more specific information.
- Emphasize the importance of not overusing the medication due to the risk of rebound bronchospasm.

### Xanthines
- Educate the patient about the interaction between smoking and xanthines (e.g., smoking decreases the blood concentrations of aminophylline and theophylline). Xanthines also interact with charcoal-broiled foods and may lead to decreased serum levels of xanthine drugs.
- Instruct patients about food and beverage items that contain caffeine (e.g., chocolate, coffee, cola, cocoa, tea), because their consumption can exacerbate CNS stimulation.
- Encourage the patient that he or she needs to take medications around the clock to maintain steady-state drug levels. Extended-released dosage forms and other oral dosage forms are not to be crushed or chewed. Advise patients that any worsening of adverse effects, such as epigastric pain, nausea, vomiting, tremors, and headache, must be reported immediately.
- Encourage the patient to keep follow-up appointments because of the importance in monitoring therapeutic levels of medications and therapeutic effectiveness.
- Some patients may need to learn to take their own pulse rate. Demonstrate proper technique.

### Anticholinergics
- Educate patients that ipratropium is used prophylactically to decrease the frequency and severity of asthma and must be taken as ordered and generally year round

for therapeutic effectiveness. This drug must be avoided in patients with existing allergy to soybeans, peanuts, or other legumes.
- Encourage forcing fluids, unless contraindicated, to decrease the viscosity of secretions and increase the expectoration of sputum.
- When inhaled forms of these drugs (and other respiratory drugs) are used, instruct the patient to take the prescribed number of puffs of the inhaler and no more than two puffs with one dosing or as ordered. Educate the patient about how to properly use an MDI with or without a spacer, how to use a dry powder inhaler, and how to properly clean and store the equipment (see Chapter 9). Instruct the patient to wait 2 to 5 minutes (or as prescribed) before using additional different inhaled medications.

### Leukotriene Receptor Antagonists
- Educate the patient about the action and purpose of LTRAs and how they work differently by preventing leukotriene formation and thus preventing/decreasing inflammation, bronchoconstriction, and mucus production. Emphasize that these drugs are indicated for prevention, not treatment, of acute asthmatic attacks.

### Corticosteroids (Glucocorticoids)
- In addition to adhering to the specified dose and frequency of these drugs, if inhaled forms are used, the patient must practice good oral hygiene (e.g., rinsing of the mouth) after the last inhalation. Rinsing the mouth with water is appropriate and necessary to prevent oral fungal infections. Instruct the patient about keeping the inhaler clean, including weekly removing of the canister from the plastic casing and washing the casing in warm, soapy water. Once the casing is dry, the canister and mouthpiece may be put back together and the cap applied. The glucocorticoid may predispose the patient to oral fungal overgrowth. Provide implicit instructions for mouth care after each use and for the cleaning of inhaled devices.
- Instruct the patient to keep track of the doses left in the MDI. Many inhalers have built-in counters, but if not, the patient can do the following: Divide the number of doses in the canister by

## PATIENT TEACHING TIPS—cont'd

the number of puffs used per day. For example, assume that two puffs are taken four times a day, and the inhaler has a capacity of 200 inhalations. Two puffs four times a day equals eight inhalations per day. Eight divided into 200 yields 25; that is, the inhaler will last approximately 25 days. The MDI may then be marked with the date it will be empty and a refill obtained a few days before that date. Note that using extra doses will alter the refill date. Advise the patient to always check expiration dates.

• Stress the importance of journaling, which should include notation of how the patient feels, medications being taken, adverse effects, and precipitators/alleviators/symptoms of the asthma/illness.

• Counsel the patient to wear a medical alert bracelet or necklace at all times and to keep a medical card with the diagnoses and list of medications and allergies on his or her person at all times. Emergency contact persons and phone numbers must also be listed.

• With intranasal dosage forms, instruct the patient to clear nasal passages before administration. The patient needs to tilt his or her head slightly forward and insert the spray tip into one nostril and point toward the inflamed nasal turbinates. Instruct the patient to pump the medication into the nasal passage as the patient sniffs inward while holding the other nostril closed. This procedure may then be repeated in the other nostril. It is recommended to discard any unused portion after 3 months or by the expiration date.

• Educate the patient about the fact that excess levels of systemic corticosteroids may lead to Cushing's syndrome with symptoms such as moon face, acne, an increase in fat pads, and swelling. Although use of inhaled forms helps to minimize this problem, education about it remains important to patient safety. As noted previously, the risk of occurrence of these signs and symptoms is higher when these drugs are given systemically (e.g., oral or parenteral dosage forms).

• Educate the patient about the possibility of Addisonian crisis, which may occur if a systemic corticosteroid is abruptly discontinued. These drugs require weaning prior to discontinuation of the medication. Addisonian crisis may be manifested by nausea, shortness of breath, joint pain, weakness, and fatigue, and the patient must contact the prescriber immediately if these occur.

• Educate the patient about the importance of reporting to the prescriber any weight gain of 2 pounds or more in 24 hours or 5 pounds or more in 1 week.

### Phosphodiesterase-4 Inhibitor

• Emphasize that the patient report any change in mood or emotions to the prescriber immediately.

### Monoclonal Antibody Antiasthmatic Drugs

• Omalizumab is used for the treatment of moderate to severe asthma and not for aborting acute asthma attacks. The patient needs to provide return demonstrations of subcutaneous injection techniques. Instruct the patient to keep medications and needles, syringes, and other equipment out of the reach of children and to use puncture-proof needle waste containers. Each needle is used for only one injection.

## KEY POINTS

• The beta agonists stimulate beta$_1$ and beta$_2$ receptors. The beta$_2$ agonists are specific for the lungs.

• Xanthines, such as theophylline, help to relax the smooth muscles of the bronchioles by inhibiting phosphodiesterase. Phosphodiesterase breaks down cAMP, which is needed to relax smooth muscles.

• Anticholinergic drugs are used for maintenance and not for relief of acute bronchospasm and work by blocking the bronchoconstrictive effects of ACh.

• Corticosteroids (e.g., beclomethasone, dexamethasone, flunisolide, triamcinolone) have many indications and work by stabilizing the membranes of cells that release harmful bronchoconstricting substances.

• The LTRAs, such as zileuton and zafirlukast, are given orally. Adverse effects include headache, dizziness, insomnia, and dyspepsia.

• Omalizumab, a monoclonal antibody antiasthmatic drug, works by preventing the release of mediators that lead to allergic responses. It is given for preventative purposes.

## NCLEX® EXAMINATION REVIEW QUESTIONS

1 A patient who has a history of asthma is experiencing an acute episode of shortness of breath and needs to take a medication for immediate relief. The nurse will choose which medication that is appropriate for this situation?
   a  A beta agonist, such as albuterol
   b  An leukotriene receptor antagonist, such as montelukast
   c  A corticosteroid, such as fluticasone
   d  An anticholinergic, such as ipratropium

2 After a nebulizer treatment with the beta agonist albuterol, the patient complains of feeling a little "shaky," with slight tremors of the hands. The patient's heart rate is 98 beats/min, increased from the pretreatment rate of 88 beats/min. The nurse knows that this reaction is an
   a  expected adverse effect of the medication.
   b  allergic reaction to the medication.

c indication that he has received an overdose of the medication.

d idiosyncratic reaction to the medication.

3 A patient has been receiving an aminophylline (xanthine derivative) infusion for 24 hours. The nurse will assess for which adverse effect when assessing the patient during the infusion?

a CNS depression

b Sinus tachycardia

c Increased appetite

d Temporary urinary retention

4 During a teaching session for a patient who will be receiving a new prescription for the LTRA montelukast (Singulair), the nurse will tell the patient that the drug has which therapeutic effect?

a Improves the respiratory drive

b Loosens and removes thickened secretions

c Reduces inflammation in the airway

d Stimulates immediate bronchodilation

5 After the patient takes a dose of an inhaled corticosteroid, such as fluticasone (Flovent), what is the most important action the patient needs to do next?

a Hold the breath for 60 seconds.

b Rinse out the mouth with water.

c Follow the corticosteroid with a bronchodilator inhaler, if ordered.

d Repeat the dose in 15 minutes if the patient feels short of breath.

6 The nurse is teaching a patient about the inhaler Advair (salmeterol/fluticasone). Which statements by the patient indicate a correct understanding of this medication? Select all that apply.

a "I will rinse my mouth with water after each dose."

b "I need to use this inhaler whenever I feel short of breath, but not less than 4 hours between doses."

c "This medication is taken twice a day, every 12 hours."

d "I can take this inhaler if I get short of breath while exercising."

e "I will call my doctor if I notice white patches inside my mouth."

7 A patient has been given an MDI of albuterol and is instructed to take two puffs three times a day, with doses 6 hours apart. The inhaler contains 200 actuations, but does not have a dose counter. Calculate how many days the inhaler will deliver this ordered dose.

1. a 2. a 3. b 4. c 5. b 6. a, c, e 7. Approximately 33 days (6 puffs/day divided into 200)

For Critical Thinking and Prioritization Questions, see http://evolve.elsevier.com/Lilley.

# Antiinfective and Antiinflammatory Drugs

## STUDY SKILLS TIPS

Nursing Process • Assessment • Nursing Diagnoses • Evaluation

### NURSING PROCESS

This study model focuses on the Nursing Process section in Chapter 38. Since there is a Nursing Process section at the end of each chapter, the discussion of the example in Chapter 38 is applicable to all chapters.

### ASSESSMENT

What is the purpose of this section? Each time you begin to read the Nursing Process section of a chapter, you need to ask this question. What are you supposed to learn? What are you supposed to know? What are you supposed to be able to do? All these questions relate to your role as a nurse. Consider the following sentence from this section in Chapter 38.

*In general, before the administration of any antibiotic, it is crucial to gather data regarding a history of or symptoms indicative of hypersensitivity or allergic reactions (from mild reactions with rash, pruritus, or hives to severe reactions with laryngeal edema, bronchospasm, hypotension, and possible cardiac arrest).*

Assessment clearly has to do with patient care. You are assessing the patient in relation to the pharmacologic interventions that this chapter discusses.

Notice the use of the word *crucial* in the first line. Something is so important at this point that it cannot be ignored. Immediately the questioning process should be activated. What is crucial? The answer follows immediately in the sentence. You must assess for history of or symptoms indicative of hypersensitivity or allergic reactions. The sentence goes on to identify the kind of data that should be available, and the sentence makes it clear that these data must be obtained *before the administration* of any drug. Each of the data factors is important, and each relates to other parts and chapters in this text. The next item to notice is hypersensitivity. Some individuals are *allergic* to certain antibiotics. It would be dangerous and possibly fatal, however, to administer an antibiotic to a patient if he or she is hypersensitive.

Another data item specifies *rash, pruritus, or hives* and *laryngeal edema, bronchospasms, hypotension, and possible cardiac arrest*. As you read this, you should instantly think of the reactions to which they refer. Then you should try to recall information from this chapter that related the specific antibiotics to these reactions. Learning is cumulative. The Nursing Process section assumes you have read and understood what was presented earlier in the chapter.

Often you will encounter standard medical abbreviations. As you read on in the Assessment section, you find this sentence:

> Also determine the patient's age, weight, and baseline vital signs with body temperature. Examine the results of any laboratory tests that have been ordered, such as liver function studies (AST and ALT levels), kidney function studies (usually BUN and creatinine levels), cardiac function studies (pertinent laboratory tests, electrocardiogram), ultrasonography (if indicated), culture and sensitivity tests, CBC, and platelet and clotting tests.

In earlier Study Skills Tips, it has been suggested that you prepare vocabulary cards for these abbreviations to help you in a situation such as this. When you see abbreviations such as AST, ALT, BUN, and CBC, you may refer to the Abbreviations for Diagnostic and Laboratory Tests table on the inside back cover of this text. However, you need to know what these abbreviations mean, what they measure, and how they relate to appropriate and effective administration of antibiotics. If these letters are not meaningful to you, then you will not be able to link what you know about the antibiotics with what you must know about administering them as a nurse. Many test questions on nursing examinations use the standard abbreviations, and you must know them instantly and be able to relate them to the situation covered. As you look at antibiotic administration and CBC, think what a test question might ask about this data element in a real application in patient care. This is what the nursing process is all about.

## NURSING DIAGNOSES

The same first question applies here as in every other section. What am I supposed to learn? Since the focus is on administration of antibiotics, the expectation you should bring to this is an awareness of your role in diagnosis. What should you look for in working with patients that affects the administration of antibiotics?

This same procedure should be applied to the Planning, Goals, Outcome Criteria, and Implementation sections. Consider what each of these headings suggests about the nursing process, and read and evaluate the information, relating it to

what you have already learned. Also consider the implications of the information as possible test questions that may ask you to do more than recall specific facts. As an example, consider the following case:

> Patient A, age 23, has bronchitis and a fever of 100.8° F (38.2° C). She was admitted yesterday and delivered a healthy infant 8 hours ago. She is breastfeeding the newborn. What antibiotics might be administered for the bronchitis? What specific antibiotics should be used with caution or eliminated from consideration?

This case demonstrates the need to read and think critically. Not only do you need to remember the specific facts from the chapter, but you should also be able to take a case study example and apply those facts to that specific situation.

## EVALUATION

Evaluation is the final section under Nursing Process. What are you supposed to evaluate?

> Include monitoring of goals, outcome criteria, therapeutic effects, and adverse effects in the evaluation. Therapeutic effects of antibiotics include a decrease in the signs and symptoms of the infection; a return to normal vital signs, including temperature; negative results on culture and sensitivity tests; normal results for CBC; and improved appetite, energy level, and sense of well-being. Evaluation for adverse effects includes monitoring for specific drug-related adverse effects (see each drug profile).

First you should look for the positive responses (therapeutic effects) set forth in the preceding text sample that indicate the patient is responding favorably to the treatment. However, then you read, "Evaluation for adverse effects includes…." This says that part of your role in evaluation is to monitor the patient for negative responses and be prepared to educate the patient about the effects he or she is experiencing and possible steps to help alleviate the symptoms.

The Nursing Process section in each chapter should be read carefully and thoughtfully, because it is in this section where you begin to see how the complex pharmacologic material presented earlier in the chapter fits into your role as a nurse. This material should be read with the same concern and care that you have given to the highly complex material earlier in the chapter, because this is the section in which you must think about *application* of all you have learned. Your thinking process may be stimulated when you review this section with your study group. Each person brings his or her understanding and experience to the discussion. The insights can be richer and the learning more complete as you exchange ideas. Apply the PURR model with a study group or alone and be an active questioner and reader, and you will be successful in working with the Nursing Process section in each chapter.

# Antibiotics Part 1

## OBJECTIVES

When you reach the end of this chapter, you will be able to do the following:

1. Discuss the general principles of antibiotic therapy.
2. Explain how antibiotics work to rid the body of infection.
3. Briefly compare the characteristics and uses of antiseptics and disinfectants.
4. List the most commonly used antiseptics and disinfectants.
5. Discuss any nursing-related considerations associated with the environmental use of antiseptics and disinfectants.
6. Discuss the pros and cons of antibiotic use with attention to the overuse or abuse of antibiotics and the development of drug resistance.
7. Classify the various antibiotics by general category, including sulfonamides, penicillins, cephalosporins, macrolides, and tetracyclines.
8. Discuss the mechanisms of action, indications, cautions, contraindications, routes of administration, and drug interactions for the sulfonamides, penicillins, cephalosporins, macrolides, and tetracyclines.
9. Identify drug-specific adverse effects and toxic effects of each of the antibiotic classes listed earlier, and cite measures to decrease their occurrence.
10. Briefly discuss superinfection, including its etiology and prevention.
11. Develop a nursing care plan that includes all phases of the nursing process for patients receiving drugs in each of the following classes of antibiotic: sulfonamides, penicillins, cephalosporins, macrolides, and tetracyclines.

## DRUG PROFILES

- **amoxicillin, p. 619**
  ampicillin, p. 619
- **azithromycin and clarithromycin, p. 625**
  aztreonam, p. 623
- **cefazolin, p. 620**
  cefepime, p. 622
- **cefoxitin, p. 621**
  ceftazidime, p. 622
- **ceftriaxone, p. 622**
  cefuroxime, p. 622

- **cephalexin, p. 621**
  demeclocycline, p. 627
- **doxycycline, p. 627**
- **erythromycin, p. 625**
- **imipenem/cilastatin, p. 623**
  nafcillin, p. 618
- **penicillin G and penicillin V potassium, p. 618**
  sulfamethoxazole/trimethoprim (co-trimoxazole), p. 616
  tigecycline, p. 627

  ---

- *Key drug*

## KEY TERMS

**Antibiotic** Having the ability to destroy or interfere with the development of a living organism. The term is used most commonly to refer to antibacterial drugs. (p. 611)

**Antiseptic** One of two types of topical antimicrobial agents; a chemical that inhibits the growth and reproduction of microorganisms without necessarily killing them. Antiseptics are also called *static agents*. (p. 612)

**Bactericidal antibiotics** Antibiotics that kill bacteria. (p. 616)

**Bacteriostatic antibiotics** Antibiotics that do not actually kill bacteria but rather inhibit their growth. (p. 614)

**Beta-lactam** The designation for a broad class of antibiotics that includes four subclasses: penicillins, cephalosporins, carbapenems, and monobactams; so named because of the beta-lactam ring that is part of the chemical structure of all drugs in this class. (p. 616)

**Beta-lactamase** Any of a group of enzymes produced by bacteria that catalyze the chemical opening of the crucial beta-lactam ring structures in beta-lactam antibiotics. (p. 616)

**Beta-lactamase inhibitors** Medications combined with certain penicillin drugs to block the effect of beta-lactamase enzymes. (p. 616)

**Colonization** The establishment and growth of microorganisms on the skin, open wounds, or mucous membranes, or in secretions without causing an infection. (p. 611)

**Community-associated infection** An infection that is acquired by persons who have not been hospitalized or had a medical procedure recently. (p. 611)

**Definitive therapy** The administration of antibiotics based on known results of culture and sensitivity testing identifying the pathogen causing infection. (p. 612)

**Disinfectant** One of two types of topical antimicrobial agents; a chemical applied to nonliving objects to kill microorganisms. Also called *cidal agents*. (p. 612)

**Empiric therapy** The administration of antibiotics based on the practitioner's judgment of the pathogens most likely to be causing an apparent infection; it involves the presumptive treatment of an infection to avoid treatment delay before specific culture information has been obtained. (p. 612)

**Glucose-6-phosphate dehydrogenase (G6PD) deficiency** An inherited disorder in which the red blood cells are partially or completely deficient in glucose-6-phosphate dehydrogenase, a critical enzyme in the metabolism of glucose. Certain medications can cause hemolytic anemia in patients with this disorder. This is an example of a host factor related to drug therapy. (p. 614)

**Health care–associated infection** An infection that is acquired during the course of receiving treatment for another condition in a health care facility. The infection is not present or incubating at the time of admission; also known as a *nosocomial infection*. (p. 611)

**Host factors** Factors that are unique to a particular patient that affect the patient's susceptibility to infection and response to various antibiotic drugs. Examples include a low neutrophil count or a lack of immunoglobulins in the blood that carry antibodies. (p. 613)

**Infections** Invasions and multiplications of microorganisms in body tissues. (p. 611)

**Microorganisms** Microscopic living organisms (also called *microbes*). (p. 610)

**Prophylactic antibiotic therapy** Antibiotics taken before anticipated exposure to an infectious organism in an effort to prevent the development of infection. (p. 612)

**Pseudomembranous colitis** A potentially-necrotizing inflammatory bowel condition that is often associated with antibiotic therapy; often caused by the bacteria *Clostridium difficile*. A more general term that is also used is *antibiotic-associated colitis*. (p. 613)

**Slow acetylation** A common genetic host factor in which the rate of metabolism of certain drugs is reduced. (p. 614)

**Subtherapeutic** Generally refers to blood levels below therapeutic levels due to insufficient dosing. Also refers to antibiotic treatment that is ineffective in treating a given infection. Possible causes include inappropriate drug therapy, insufficient drug dosing, and bacterial drug resistance. (p. 612)

**Superinfection** (1) An infection occurring during antimicrobial treatment for another infection, resulting from overgrowth of an organism not susceptible to the antibiotic used. (2) A secondary microbial infection that occurs in addition to an earlier primary infection, often due to weakening of the patient's immune system function by the first infection. (p. 613)

**Teratogens** Substances that can interfere with normal prenatal development and cause one or more developmental abnormalities in the fetus. (p. 614)

**Therapeutic** Referring to antibiotic therapy that is given in sufficient doses so that the concentration of the drug in the blood or other tissues renders it effective against specific bacterial pathogens. (p. 612)

## ANATOMY, PHYSIOLOGY, AND PATHOPHYSIOLOGY OVERVIEW

### MICROBIAL INFECTION

Microorganisms are everywhere, both in the external environment and in parts of the internal environment of our bodies. They can be harmful to humans, or they can be beneficial under normal circumstances but become harmful when conditions are altered in some way. A person is normally able to remain healthy and resistant to infectious microorganisms because of the existence of certain host defenses. These defenses include actual physical barriers, such as intact skin or the ciliated respiratory mucosa, or physiologic defenses, such as the gastric acid

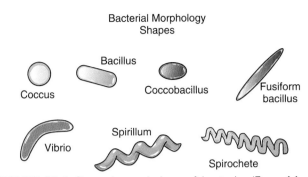

FIGURE 38-1 General morphology of bacteria. (From Murray PR, Rosenthal KS, Pfaller MA: *Medical microbiology*, ed 6, St Louis, 2009, Mosby.)

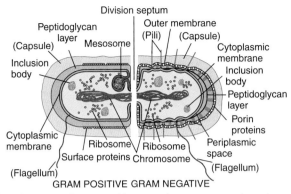

FIGURE 38-2 Gram-positive and gram-negative bacteria. A gram-positive bacterium has a thick layer of peptidoglycan *(left)*. A gram-negative bacterium has a thin peptidoglycan layer and an outer membrane *(right)*. Structures in parentheses are not found in all bacteria. (From Murray PR, Rosenthal KS, Pfaller MA: *Medical microbiology,* ed 6, St Louis, 2009, Mosby.)

in the stomach and immune factors such as antibodies. Other defenses are the phagocytic cells (macrophages and polymorphonuclear neutrophils) that are part of the mononuclear phagocyte system.

Every known major class of microbes contains organisms that can infect humans. This includes bacteria, viruses, fungi, and protozoans. The focus of this chapter is common bacterial infections.

Recall from microbiology that bacteria may take a number of different shapes. This property of bacteria is called their morphology (Figure 38-1), and they are often grouped based on this property. Bacteria may also be grouped according to other common recognizable characteristics. One of the most important ways of categorizing different bacteria is on the basis of their response to the Gram stain procedure. Bacterial species that stain purple with Gram staining are classified as *gram-positive* organisms. Bacteria that stain red are classified as *gram-negative* organisms. This seemingly simple difference proves to be very significant in guiding the choice of antibiotic therapy.

Gram-positive organisms have a very thick cell wall, known as peptidoglycan, and they also have a thick outer capsule. Gram-negative organisms have a cell wall structure that is more complex, with a smaller outer capsule and peptidoglycan layer and two cell membranes: an outer and an inner membrane (Figure 38-2). These differences usually make gram-negative bacterial infections more difficult to treat, because the drug molecules have a harder time penetrating the more complex cell walls of gram-negative organisms.

When the normal host defenses are somehow compromised, that person becomes susceptible to infection. The microorganisms invade and multiply in the body tissues, and if the infective process overwhelms the body's defense system, the infection becomes clinically apparent. The patient usually manifests some of the following classic signs and symptoms of infection: fever, chills, sweats, redness, pain and swelling, fatigue, weight loss, increased white blood cell (WBC) count, and the formation of pus. Not all patients will exhibit signs of the infection. This is especially true in elderly and immunocompromised patients.

To help the body and its normal host defenses combat an infection, antibiotic therapy is often required. Antibiotics are most effective when their actions are combined with functioning bodily defense mechanisms. Oftentimes patients will

become colonized with bacteria. Although bacteria are present in open wounds, in secretions, on mucous membranes, or on the skin, these patients do not have any overt signs of infection. Colonization does not require antibiotic treatment. However, it is not uncommon for these colonizations to be treated, which may be one way in which drug-resistant organisms emerge.

## Health Care–Associated Infection

A community-associated infection is defined as an infection that is acquired by a person who has not recently (within the past year) been hospitalized or had a medical procedure (e.g., dialysis, surgery, catheterization). A health care–associated infection, previously known as a *nosocomial infection,* is defined as an infection that a patient acquires during the course of receiving treatment for another condition in a health care facility. The infection was not present or incubating at the time of admission but occurs greater than 48 hours after admission. Health care–associated infections are one of the top ten leading causes of death in the United States. They tend to be more difficult to treat because the causative microorganisms have been exposed to strong antibiotics in the past and are the most drug resistant and the most virulent. The particular organisms that cause hospital-associated infections have changed over time, with methicillin-resistant *Staphylococcus aureus* (MRSA) now being the most common. Other serious pathogens include *Enterococcus, Klebsiella, Acinetobacter,* and *Pseudomonas aeruginosa.* Most of these microorganisms are now resistant to many of the commonly used antibiotics.

Health care–associated infections develop in approximately 10% of hospitalized patients, and the cost of treating these infections amounts to $4 to $11 billion annually. Most of these infections (70% or more) are either urinary tract infections (UTIs) or postoperative wound infections. Often they are acquired from various devices, such as mechanical ventilators, intravenous (IV) infusion lines, catheters, and dialysis equipment. Areas of the hospital associated with the greatest risk for acquiring a hospital-associated infection are the critical care, dialysis, oncology, transplant, and burn units. This is because the host

## TABLE 38-1 ANTISEPTICS VERSUS DISINFECTANTS

| | ANTISEPTICS | DISINFECTANTS |
|---|---|---|
| Where used | Living tissue | Nonliving objects |
| Potency | Lower | Higher |
| Activity against organisms | Primarily inhibits growth (bacteriostatic) | Kills (bactericidal) |

defenses of the patients in these areas are typically compromised, which makes them more vulnerable to infection. Over 70% of hospital-associated infections are preventable. The most common mode of transmitting hospital-associated infections is by direct contact. Handwashing is the single most important thing health care professionals can do to prevent the spread of these potentially deadly infections. Because health care–associated infections cause numerous deaths and cost billions of dollars, The Joint Commission has made the prevention of health care associated–infections a national patient safety goal. In addition, they have added prevention of catheter-associated UTIs as a 2012 national patient safety goal.

Other methods of reducing hospital-associated infections include the use of disinfectants and antiseptics. A disinfectant is able to kill organisms and is used only on nonliving objects to destroy organisms that may be present. Disinfectants are sometimes called *cidal agents*. An antiseptic generally only inhibits the growth of microorganisms but does not necessarily kill them and is applied exclusively to living tissue. Antiseptics are also called *static agents*. The differences between antiseptics and disinfectants in a clinical sense are summarized in Table 38-1. Topical antimicrobial drugs are discussed further in Chapter 56.

## PHARMACOLOGY OVERVIEW

The selection of antimicrobial drugs requires clinical judgment and detailed knowledge of pharmacologic and microbiologic factors. Antibiotics have three general uses: empiric therapy, definitive therapy, and prophylactic or preventative therapy. Antibiotic drug therapy begins with a clinical assessment of the patient to determine whether he or she has the common signs and symptoms of infection. The patient is assessed during and after antibiotic therapy to evaluate the effectiveness of the drug therapy, monitor for adverse drug effects, and make sure the infection is not recurring.

Often the signs and symptoms of an infection appear long before a causative organism can be identified. When this happens and the risk of life-threatening or severe complications is high (e.g., suspected acute meningitis), an antibiotic is given to the patient immediately. The antibiotic selected is one that can best kill the microorganisms known to be the most common causes of the infection. This is called empiric therapy. Before the start of empiric antibiotic therapy, specimens are obtained from suspected areas of infection to be cultured in an attempt to identify a causative organism. It must be emphasized that culture specimens must be obtained before drug therapy is

initiated whenever possible. Otherwise, the presence of antibiotics in the tissues may result in misleading culture results. However, sometimes it is not possible to obtain a sample (especially sputum) in a reasonable amount of time, and antibiotic therapy is begun without a sample in that situation. If an organism is identified in the laboratory, it is then tested for susceptibility to various antibiotics. The results of these tests can confirm whether the empiric therapy chosen is appropriate for eradicating the organism identified. If not, therapy can be adjusted to optimize its efficacy against the specific infectious organism(s). Once the results of culture and sensitivity testing are available (usually in 48 to 72 hours), the antibiotic therapy is then tailored to treat the identified organism by using the most narrow-spectrum, least toxic drug based on sensitivity results. This is known as definitive therapy. Broad-spectrum antibiotics are those that are active against numerous organisms (gram-positive, gram-negative, and anaerobic). Narrow-spectrum antibiotics are effective against only a few organisms. Once the results of culture and sensitivity testing are available, it is always better to use an antibiotic that targets the specific organism identified (i.e., a narrow-spectrum antibiotic). Overuse of broad-spectrum antibiotics contributes to resistance. The goal of therapy is to use the most narrow-spectrum drug when possible based on sensitivity results.

Antibiotics are also given for prophylaxis. This is often the case when patients are scheduled to undergo a procedure (i.e., surgery) in which the likelihood of dangerous microbial contamination is high during or after the procedure. Prophylactic antibiotic therapy is used to prevent an infection. The risk of infection varies depending on the procedure being performed. For example, the risk of infection in a patient undergoing coronary artery bypass surgery (with standard preoperative cleansing of the body) is relatively low compared with that in a person undergoing intraabdominal surgery for the treatment of injuries sustained in a motor vehicle accident. In the latter case, contamination with bacteria from the gastrointestinal (GI) tract is more likely to be present in the abdominal cavity. This would constitute a contaminated or "dirty" surgical field, and therefore the likelihood of clinically serious infection would be much higher. Antibiotic therapy would likely be required for a longer period after the procedure. To be effective, prophylactic antibiotics need to be given before the procedure, generally 30 minutes before the incision to ensure adequate tissue penetration. The Surgical Care Improvement Project (SCIP) is a national performance improvement project that provides hospitals with evidence-based recommendations on the administration of prophylactic antibiotics. More information can be found at www.jointcommission.org/surgical_care_improvement_project/.

To optimize antibiotic therapy, the patient is continuously monitored for both therapeutic efficacy and adverse drug effects. A therapeutic response to antibiotics is one in which there is a decrease in the specific signs and symptoms of infection compared with the baseline findings (e.g., fever, elevated WBC count, redness, inflammation, drainage, pain). Antibiotic therapy is said to be subtherapeutic when these signs and symptoms do not improve. This can result from use of an incorrect route of drug administration, inadequate drainage of an abscess, poor drug penetration to the infected area, insufficient serum levels of the drug, or bacterial resistance to the drug. Antibiotic therapy is considered toxic when the serum levels of the antibiotic are too high or when the patient has an allergic or other major adverse reaction to the drug. These reactions include rash, itching, hives, fever, chills, joint pain, difficulty breathing, or wheezing. Relatively minor adverse drug reactions such as nausea, vomiting, and diarrhea are quite common with antibiotic therapy and are usually not severe enough to require drug discontinuation.

Superinfection can occur when antibiotics reduce or completely eliminate the normal bacterial flora, which consist of certain bacteria and fungi that are needed to maintain normal function in various organs. When these bacteria or fungi are killed by antibiotics, other bacteria or fungi are permitted to take over and cause infection. An example of a superinfection caused by antibiotics is the development of a vaginal yeast infection when the normal vaginal bacterial flora is reduced by antibiotic therapy and yeast growth is no longer kept in balance. Antibiotic use is strongly associated with the potential for the development of diarrhea. Antibiotic-associated diarrhea is a common adverse effect of antibiotics. However, it becomes a serious superinfection when it causes antibiotic-associated colitis, also known as pseudomembranous colitis or simply *C. difficile infection*. This happens because antibiotics disrupt the normal gut flora and can cause an overgrowth of *Clostridium difficile*. The most common symptoms of *C. difficile* colitis are watery diarrhea, abdominal pain, and fever. Whenever a patient who was previously treated with antibiotics develops watery diarrhea, the patient needs to be tested for *C. difficile* infection. If the results are positive, the patient will need to be treated for this serious superinfection. Infections with *C. difficile* are increasingly becoming resistant to standard therapy.

Another type of superinfection occurs when a second infection closely follows the initial infection and comes from an external source (as opposed to normal body flora). A common example is a case in which a patient who has a viral respiratory infection develops a secondary bacterial infection. This is likely due to weakening of the patient's immune system function by the primary viral infection. Although the viral infection will not respond to antibiotic therapy, antibiotics may be needed to treat the secondary bacterial infection. This situation calls for some diagnostic finesse on the part of the prescriber, who needs to avoid prescribing unnecessary antibiotics for a viral infection. The presence of colored sputum (e.g., green or yellow) may or may not be a sign of a bacterial superinfection during a viral respiratory illness. Patients will often expect to receive an antibiotic prescription even when they show no signs of a bacterial superinfection. From their perspective, they know they are "sick" and want "some medicine" to expedite their recovery from illness. This can create both diagnostic confusion and an emotional dilemma for the prescriber.

Over the decades, many easily treatable bacterial infections have become resistant to antibiotic therapy. One major cause of this phenomenon is considered to be the overprescribing of antibiotics, often in the clinical situations described earlier.

Antibiotic resistance is now considered one of the world's most pressing public health problems. Another factor that contributes to this problem is the tendency of many patients not to complete their antibiotic regimen. Patients must be counseled to take the entire course of prescribed antibiotic drugs, even if they feel that they are no longer ill.

Food-drug and drug-drug interactions are common problems when antibiotics are taken. One of the more common food-drug interactions is that between milk or cheese and tetracycline, which results in decreased GI absorption of tetracycline. An example of a drug-drug interaction is that between quinolone antibiotics and antacids or multivitamins with iron, which leads to decreased absorption of quinolones. This is especially important, as will be discussed later, because quinolone antibiotics are used orally to treat serious infections. If they are not absorbed, treatment failure is likely to ensue.

Other important factors that must be understood to use antibiotics appropriately are host-specific factors, or host factors. These are factors that pertain specifically to a given patient, and they can have an important bearing on the success or failure of antibiotic therapy. Some of these host factors are age, allergy history, kidney and liver function, pregnancy status, genetic characteristics, site of infection, and host defenses.

Age-related host factors are those that apply to patients at either end of the age spectrum. For example, infants and children may not be able to take certain antibiotics such as tetracyclines, which affect developing teeth or bones; quinolones, which may affect bone or cartilage development in children; and sulfonamides, which may displace bilirubin from albumin and precipitate kernicterus (hyperbilirubinemia) in neonates. The aging process affects the function of various organ systems. As people age, there is a gradual decline in the function of the kidneys and liver, the organs primarily responsible for metabolizing and eliminating antibiotics. Therefore, depending on the level of kidney or liver function of a given older adult, dosage adjustments may be necessary. Pharmacists often play a role in evaluating the dosages of antibiotics and other medications to ensure optimal dosing for a given patient's level of organ function.

A patient history of allergic reaction to an antibiotic is important in the selection of the most appropriate antibiotic. Penicillins and sulfonamides are two broad classes of antibiotic to which many people have allergic anaphylactic reactions. Symptoms of anaphylaxis include flushing, itching, hives, anxiety, fast irregular pulse, and throat and tongue swelling. The most dangerous such reaction is anaphylactic shock, in which a patient can suffocate from drug-induced respiratory arrest. Although this outcome is the most extreme, the potential for it does underscore the importance of consistently assessing patients for drug allergies and documenting any known allergies clearly in the medical record. All reported drug allergies are to be taken seriously and investigated further before a final decision is made about whether to administer a given drug. Many patients will say that they are "allergic" to a medication when in fact what they experienced was a common mild adverse effect such as stomach upset or nausea. Patients who report drug allergies need to be asked open-ended questions to elicit descriptions of prior allergic reactions so that the actual severity of the reaction can be assessed. The most common severe reactions to any medication that need to be noted in the patient's chart are any difficulty breathing; significant rash, hives, or other skin reaction; and severe GI intolerance. Although some antibiotics are ideally taken on an empty stomach, eating a small amount of food with the medication may be sufficient to help the patient tolerate it and realize its therapeutic benefits.

Pregnancy-related host factors are also important to the selection of appropriate antibiotics, because several antibiotics can pass through the placenta and cause harm to the developing fetus. Drugs that cause development abnormalities in the fetus are called teratogens. Their use by pregnant women can result in birth defects.

Some patients also have certain genetic abnormalities that result in various enzyme deficiencies. These conditions can adversely affect drug actions in the body. Two of the most common examples of such genetic host factors are glucose-6-phosphate dehydrogenase (G6PD) deficiency and slow acetylation. The administration of antibiotics such as sulfonamides, nitrofurantoin, and dapsone to a person with G6PD deficiency may result in the *hemolysis*, or destruction, of red blood cells. Patients who are slow acetylators have a physiologic makeup that causes certain drugs to be metabolized more slowly than usual in a chemical step known as *acetylation*. This can lead to toxicity from drug accumulation (see Chapter 4).

The anatomic site of the infection is a very important host factor to consider when deciding not only which antibiotic to use but also the dosage, route of administration, and duration of therapy. Some antibiotics do not penetrate into the site of infection, such as the lung or bone or abscesses, which can lead to treatment failures.

Consideration of these host factors helps prescribers and pharmacists to ensure optimal drug selection for each individual patient. Continued patient assessment and proper monitoring of antibiotic therapy increase the likelihood that this therapy will be safe and effective.

## ANTIBIOTICS

Antibiotics are classified into broad categories based on their chemical structure. The common categories include sulfonamides, penicillins, cephalosporins, macrolides, quinolones, aminoglycosides, and tetracyclines. In addition to chemical structure, other characteristics that distinguish classes of drugs include antibacterial spectrum, mechanism of action, potency, toxicity, and pharmacokinetic properties. The four most common mechanisms of antibiotic action are: (1) interference with bacterial cell wall synthesis, (2) interference with protein synthesis, (3) interference with replication of nucleic acids (deoxyribonucleic acid [DNA] and ribonucleic acid [RNA]), and (4) antimetabolite action that disrupts critical metabolic reactions inside the bacterial cell. Figure 38-3 portrays these mechanisms in combating bacterial infections and indicates which mechanism is used by several major antibiotic classes.

Perhaps the greatest challenge in understanding antimicrobial therapy is remembering the types and species of microorganisms against which a given drug can act. The list of microorganisms that a given drug has activity against can be

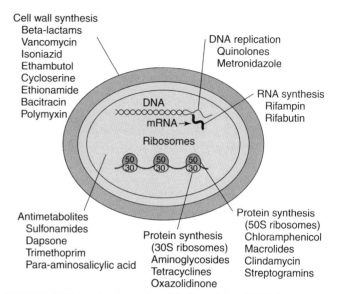

**FIGURE 38-3** Basic sites of antibiotic activity. *DNA*, Deoxyribonucleic acid; *mRNA*, messenger ribonucleic acid; *RNA*, ribonucleic acid. (From Murray PR, Rosenthal KS, Pfaller MA: *Medical microbiology*, ed 6, St Louis, 2009, Mosby.)

quite extensive and can seem daunting to the inexperienced practitioner. Most antimicrobials have activity against only one type of microbe (e.g., bacteria, viruses, fungi, protozoans). However, a few drugs do have activity against more than one class of organisms.

The field of infectious disease treatment is continually evolving, largely because of the continual emergence of resistant bacterial strains. For this reason, drug indications change frequently, often from year to year, as various bacterial species become resistant to previously effective antiinfective therapy. It is always appropriate to check the most current reference materials or consult with colleagues (e.g., nurses, pharmacists, prescribers) when questions remain. Pharmacists are excellent resources regarding antibiotics. Many hospitals now have pharmacists who are specially trained in the treatment of infectious diseases.

## SULFONAMIDES

Sulfonamides were one of the first groups of drugs used as antibiotics. Although there are many compounds in the sulfonamide family, only sulfamethoxazole combined with trimethoprim (a nonsulfonamide antibiotic), known as Bactrim, Septra, or co-trimoxazole and often abbreviated as SMX-TMP, is used commonly in clinical practice. Sulfisoxazole combined with erythromycin (a macrolide antibiotic) is occasionally used in pediatrics. Sulfasalazine, another sulfonamide, is used to treat ulcerative colitis and rheumatoid arthritis and is not used as an antibiotic.

### Mechanism of Action and Drug Effects

Sulfonamides do not actually destroy bacteria but rather inhibit their growth. For this reason, they are considered bacteriostatic antibiotics. They inhibit the growth of susceptible bacteria by preventing bacterial synthesis of folic acid. Folic acid is a B-complex vitamin that is required for the proper synthesis of purines, one of the chemical components of nucleic acids (DNA and RNA). Chemical components of folic acid include paraaminobenzoic acid (PABA), pteridine, and glutamic acid. Specifically, in a process known as competitive inhibition, sulfonamides compete with PABA for the bacterial enzyme tetrahydropteroic acid synthetase, which incorporates PABA into the folic acid molecule. Because sulfonamides are capable of blocking a specific step in a biosynthetic pathway, they are also considered antimetabolites. Microorganisms that require exogenous folic acid (not synthesized by the bacterium itself) are not affected by sulfonamide antibiotics. Therefore, these drugs do not affect folic acid metabolism in human cells. Trimethoprim, although not a sulfonamide, works via a similar mechanism, inhibiting dihydrofolic acid reduction to tetrahydrofolate, which results in inhibition of the enzymes of the folic acid pathway.

## Indications

Sulfonamides have a broad spectrum of antibacterial activity, including activity against both gram-positive and gram-negative organisms. These antibiotics achieve very high concentrations in the kidneys, through which they are eliminated. Therefore, sulfamethoxazole/trimethoprim is often used in the treatment of UTIs. The combination of these two drugs allows for a synergistic (see Chapter 2) antibacterial effect. Commonly susceptible organisms include strains of *Enterobacter* species (spp.), *Escherichia coli, Klebsiella* spp., *Proteus mirabilis, Proteus vulgaris,* and *S. aureus.* Unfortunately, however, resistant bacterial strains are a growing problem, as is the case with other antibiotic classes. Results of culture and sensitivity testing help to optimize drug selection in individual cases. This combination drug is also used for respiratory tract infections. However, it is now less effective against streptococci infecting the upper respiratory tract and pharynx. Another specific use for sulfamethoxazole/trimethoprim is prophylaxis and treatment of opportunistic infections in patients with human immunodeficiency virus (HIV) infection, especially infection by *Pneumocystis jirovecii,* a common cause of HIV-associated pneumonia. Sulfamethoxazole/trimethoprim is also a drug of choice for infection caused by the bacterium *Stenotrophomonas maltophilia.* Sulfamethoxazole/trimethoprim has become common treatment for outpatient *Staphylococcus* infections, due to the high rate of community-acquired methicillin-resistant *S. aureus* (MRSA) infections. MRSA and other resistant organisms are discussed in Chapter 39.

## Contraindications

Use of sulfonamides is contraindicated in cases of known drug allergy to sulfonamides. Chemically related drugs such as the sulfonylureas (used to treat diabetes; see Chapter 32), thiazide and loop diuretics (see Chapter 28), and carbonic anhydrase inhibitors (see Chapter 28) are generally considered relatively safe in a patient who has a sulfonamide allergy. However, the cyclooxygenase-2 inhibitor celecoxib (Celebrex) should not be used (see Chapter 44) in patients with a known sulfonamide allergy. It is important to differentiate between sulfites and

| TABLE 38-2 | SULFONAMIDES: REPORTED ADVERSE EFFECTS |
|---|---|
| **BODY SYSTEM** | **ADVERSE EFFECTS** |
| Blood | Agranulocytosis, aplastic anemia, hemolytic anemia, thrombocytopenia |
| Gastrointestinal | Nausea, vomiting, diarrhea, pancreatitis, hepatotoxicity |
| Integumentary | Epidermal necrolysis, exfoliative dermatitis, Stevens-Johnson syndrome, photosensitivity |
| Other | Convulsions, crystalluria, toxic nephrosis, headache, peripheral neuritis, urticaria, cough |

sulfonamides. Sulfites are commonly used as preservatives in everything from wine to food to injectable drugs. A person allergic to sulfonamide drugs may or may not also be allergic to sulfite preservatives. The use of sulfonamides is also contraindicated in pregnant women at term and in infants younger than 2 months of age.

## Adverse Effects

Sulfonamide drugs are a common cause of allergic reaction. Patients will sometimes refer to this as "sulfa allergy" or even "sulfur allergy." Although immediate reactions can occur, sulfonamides typically cause delayed cutaneous reactions. These reactions frequently begin with fever followed by a rash (morbilliform eruptions, erythema multiforme, or toxic epidermal necrolysis). Photosensitivity reactions are another type of skin reaction that is induced by exposure to sunlight during sulfonamide drug therapy. In some cases, such reactions can result in severe sunburn. Such reactions are also common with the tetracycline class of antibiotics discussed later in this chapter, as well as with various other drug classes and may occur immediately or have a delayed onset. Other reactions to sulfonamides include mucocutaneous, GI, hepatic, renal, and hematologic complications, all of which may be fatal in severe cases. It is believed that sulfonamide reactions are immune mediated and involve the production of reactive drug metabolites in the body. Reported adverse effects of the sulfonamides are listed in Table 38-2.

## Interactions

Sulfonamides can have clinically significant interactions with a number of other medications. Sulfonamides may potentiate the hypoglycemic effects of sulfonylureas in diabetes treatment, the toxic effects of phenytoin, and the anticoagulant effects of warfarin, which can lead to hemorrhage. Sulfonamides may increase the likelihood of cyclosporine-induced nephrotoxicity. Patients receiving any of the above drug combinations may require more frequent monitoring. Sulfonamides, and all antibiotics, may also reduce the efficacy of oral contraceptives. Instruct patients taking these drugs to use additional contraceptive methods.

## Dosages

For dosage information on selected sulfonamides, see the table on p. 616.

## DOSAGES

### Selected Sulfonamide Combination Drug Products

| DRUG (PREGNANCY CATEGORY) | PHARMACOLOGIC CLASS | USUAL DOSAGE RANGE* | INDICATIONS |
|---|---|---|---|
| Sulfamethoxazole/trimethoprim (co-trimoxazole, SMX-TMP, SMZ-TMP) (Bactrim, Septra) (C) | Sulfonamide and folate antimetabolite | **Adult and pediatric** IV/PO: 8-20 mg/kg/day divided twice a day (dose is in terms of trimethoprim component) | UTI, shigellosis enteritis; higher doses for nocardiosis and *Pneumocystis jirovecii* infection |
| | | **Adult** PO: 160 mg TMP/800 mg SMX twice daily (every 12 hr) | *P. jirovecii* prophylaxis, acute exacerbation of chronic bronchitis |
| | | **Pediatric** PO: 6-10 mg/kg/day (trimethoprim component) | Otitis media |

*IV*, Intravenous; *PO*, oral; *TMP*, trimethoprim; *UTI*, urinary tract infection.
*Dosage ranges are typical but are not necessarily exhaustive due to space limitations. Clinical variations may occur. Check current drug handbook for exact dosages for specific indications.

## DRUG PROFILE

Sulfonamides work by interfering with bacterial synthesis of the essential nutrient folic acid. Most sulfonamide therapy today uses the combination drug sulfamethoxazole/trimethoprim.

### sulfamethoxazole/trimethoprim (co-trimoxazole)

Co-trimoxazole (Bactrim) is a fixed-combination drug product containing a 5:1 ratio of sulfamethoxazole to trimethoprim. It is available in both oral and injectable dosage forms.

### Pharmacokinetics

| Route | Onset of Action | Peak Plasma Concentration | Elimination Half-life | Duration of Action |
|---|---|---|---|---|
| PO | Variable | 2-4 hr | 7-12 hr | 12 hr |

## BETA-LACTAM ANTIBIOTICS

The beta-lactam antibiotics are very commonly used drugs. They are so named because of the beta-lactam ring that is part of their chemical structure (Figure 38-4). This broad group of drugs includes four major subclasses: penicillins, cephalosporins, carbapenems, and monobactams. They share a common structure and mechanism of action: they inhibit the synthesis of the bacterial peptidoglycan cell wall.

Some bacterial strains produce the enzyme beta-lactamase. This enzyme provides a mechanism for bacterial resistance to these antibiotics. The enzyme can break the chemical bond between the carbon (C) and nitrogen (N) atoms in the structure of the beta-lactam ring. When this happens, all beta-lactam drugs lose their antibacterial efficacy. Because of this, additional drugs known as beta-lactamase inhibitors are added to several of the penicillin antibiotics to make the drug more powerful against beta-lactamase–producing bacterial strains. Each of the four classes of beta-lactam antibiotics is examined in detail in the following sections.

FIGURE 38-4 Chemical structure of penicillins showing the beta-lactam ring. **R,** Variable portion of drug chemical structure.

## PENICILLINS

The penicillins are a very large group of chemically related antibiotics that were first derived from a mold (fungus) often seen on bread or fruit. The penicillins can be divided into four subgroups based on their structure and the spectrum of bacteria they are active against: natural penicillins, penicillinase-resistant penicillins, aminopenicillins, and extended-spectrum penicillins. Examples of antibiotics in each subgroup and a brief description of their characteristics are given in Table 38-3.

Penicillins are bactericidal antibiotics, meaning they kill a wide variety of gram-positive and some gram-negative bacteria. However, some bacteria have acquired the capacity to produce enzymes capable of destroying penicillins. These enzymes are called *beta-lactamases*, and they can inactivate the penicillin molecules by opening the beta-lactam ring. The beta-lactamases that specifically inactivate penicillin molecules are called *penicillinases*. Bacterial strains that produce these drug-inactivating enzymes were a therapeutic obstacle until drugs were synthesized that inhibit these enzymes. Three of these beta-lactamase inhibitors are clavulanic acid (also called *clavulanate*), tazobactam, and sulbactam. These drugs bind with the beta-lactamase enzyme itself to prevent the enzyme from breaking down the penicillin molecule, although they are not always effective. The following are examples of currently available combinations of a penicillin and a beta-lactamase inhibitor:
- ampicillin/sulbactam (Unasyn)
- amoxicillin/clavulanic acid (Augmentin)

**TABLE 38-3 CLASSIFICATION OF PENICILLINS**

| SUBCLASS | GENERIC DRUG NAMES | DESCRIPTION |
|---|---|---|
| Natural penicillins | penicillin G, penicillin V | Although many modifications of the original natural (mold-produced) structure have been made, these are the only two in current clinical use. Penicillin G is the injectable form for IV or IM use; penicillin V is a PO dosage form (tablet and liquid). |
| Penicillinase-resistant drugs | cloxacillin, dicloxacillin, nafcillin, oxacillin | Stable against hydrolysis by most staphylococcal penicillinases (enzymes that normally break down the natural penicillins). |
| Aminopenicillins | amoxicillin, ampicillin | Have an amino group attached to the basic penicillin structure that enhances their activity against gram-negative bacteria compared with natural penicillins. |
| Extended-spectrum drugs | piperacillin, ticarcillin, carbenicillin, piperacillin/tazobactam | Have wider spectra of activity than do all other penicillins. |

*IM,* Intramuscular; *IV,* intravenous; *PO,* oral.

- ticarcillin/clavulanic acid (Timentin)
- piperacillin/tazobactam (Zosyn)

## Mechanism of Action and Drug Effects

The mechanism of action of penicillins involves the inhibition of bacterial cell wall synthesis. Once distributed by the patient's bloodstream to infected areas, penicillin molecules slide through bacterial cell walls to get to their site of action. Some penicillins, however, are too large to pass through the openings in the cell walls, and because they cannot get to their site of action they cannot kill the bacteria. Some bacteria make the openings in their cell walls small so that the penicillin cannot get through to kill them. The penicillin molecules that do gain entry into the bacterium must then find the appropriate binding sites. These are known as *penicillin-binding proteins*. By binding to these proteins, the penicillin molecules interfere with normal cell wall synthesis, causing the formation of defective cell walls that are unstable and easily broken down (see Figure 38-3). Bacterial death usually results from lysis (rupture) of the bacterial cells due to this drug-induced disruption of cell wall structure.

## Indications

Penicillins are indicated for the prevention and treatment of infections caused by susceptible bacteria. The microorganisms most commonly destroyed by penicillins are gram-positive bacteria, including *Streptococcus* spp., *Enterococcus* spp., and *Staphylococcus* spp. Most natural penicillins have little if any ability to kill gram-negative bacteria. However, the extended-spectrum penicillins (i.e., piperacillin/tazobactam [Zosyn]) have excellent gram-positive, gram-negative, and anaerobic coverage. Because of this, the extended-spectrum penicillins are used to treat many hospital-associated infections, including pneumonia, intraabdominal infections, and sepsis.

## Contraindications

Penicillins are usually safe and well-tolerated medications. The only usual contraindication is known drug allergy. It is very important to obtain an accurate history regarding the type of reaction that occurs in patients who state they are allergic to penicillins. It is also important to note that often drugs are referred to by their trade names, and these don't always end in *"cillin"* (e.g., Zosyn, Augmentin). Many medication errors have occurred when a penicillin drug called by its trade name is given

to a patient with a penicillin allergy (see the Safety and Quality Improvement: Preventing Medication Errors box).

### ⚡ SAFETY AND QUALITY IMPROVEMENT: PREVENTING MEDICATION ERRORS

#### *Do You Know Your Penicillins?*

Medication errors have occurred when nurses gave penicillin products to patients who were allergic to penicillin. In these cases, the drugs were referred to by their trade names, which lack the *"cillin"* suffix. Examples of these drugs are Zosyn and Unasyn. Both drugs contain a form of penicillin and a beta-lactamase inhibitor. Zosyn is a combination of piperacillin and tazobactam; Unasyn is a combination of ampicillin and sulbactam. Analysis of these errors revealed that the person administering the drug did not realize that the drug with the non-*"cillin"* name was a penicillin.

These errors illustrate why is it important to use both trade and generic names when ordering medications for patients. It is essential to know what you are administering to your patients! Be sure to check both names of the medications you give, and check the patient's allergies.

## Adverse Effects

Allergic reactions to the penicillins occur in 0.7% to 4% of treatment courses. The most common reactions are urticaria, pruritus, and angioedema. A wide variety of idiosyncratic (unpredictable) drug reactions can occur, such as maculopapular eruptions, eosinophilia, Stevens-Johnson syndrome, and exfoliative dermatitis. Maculopapular rash occurs in about 2% of treatment courses with natural penicillin and 5.2% to 9.5% of those with ampicillin. Anaphylactic reactions are much less common, occurring in 0.004% to 0.015% of patients. Severe reactions are much more common with injected than with orally administered penicillin, as is the case with most antibiotics. Patients who are allergic to penicillins have an increased risk of allergy to other beta-lactam antibiotics. The incidence of cross-reactivity between cephalosporins and penicillins is reported to be between 1% and 4%. Patients reporting penicillin allergy need to describe their prior allergic reaction. It is very important to document the type of reaction. The decision to treat with cephalosporin therapy in such cases is often a matter of clinical judgment, based on the severity of reported prior reactions to penicillin drugs, the nature of the infection, the drug susceptibility of the infective organism if known, and the availability and patient tolerance of other alternative antibiotics. Generally speaking, only those patients with a history of throat swelling or hives from penicillin should not receive cephalosporins. Some patients may require skin testing and desensitization.

Penicillins are generally well tolerated and associated with very few adverse effects. As with many drugs, the most common adverse effects involve the GI system. The intravenous (IV) formulations of some penicillins contain large amounts of sodium and/or potassium. Doses must be adjusted for patients with renal dysfunction. The most common adverse effects of the penicillins are listed in Table 38-4.

## Interactions

Many drugs interact with penicillins; some have positive effects, and others have harmful effects. The most common and clinically significant drug interactions associated with penicillin use are listed in Table 38-5.

## Dosages

For dosage information on selected penicillins, see the table on p. 619.

## DRUG PROFILES

Penicillins are classified as pregnancy category B drugs. They are very safe antibiotics. Their use is contraindicated in patients with a hypersensitivity to them, but because of their relatively good adverse effects profile, there are otherwise very few contraindications to their use.

### NATURAL PENICILLINS

♦ **penicillin G and penicillin V potassium**

Penicillin G has three salt forms: benzathine, procaine, and potassium. All of these forms are given by injection, either IV or intramuscularly (IM). The benzathine and procaine salts are used as longer-acting IM injections. They are formulated into a thick, white, pastelike material that is designed for prolonged

dissolution and absorption from the IM site of injection. Never give these preparations IV, however, because their consistency is too thick for IV administration, and such use can be fatal. The IM formulations can be especially helpful for treating the sexually transmitted disease syphilis, because often only one injection is needed. Penicillin G potassium is formulated for IV use. Penicillin V potassium is available only for oral use.

### Pharmacokinetics

| Route | Onset of Action | Peak Plasma Concentration | Elimination Half-life | Duration of Action |
|---|---|---|---|---|
| PO | Variable | 30-60 min | 30 min | 4-6 hr |
| IV | Variable | 30 min | 24-54 min | 4-6 hr |

### PENICILLINASE-RESISTANT PENICILLINS
#### nafcillin

Nafcillin is one of the four currently available penicillinase-resistant penicillins; the other three are cloxacillin, dicloxacillin, and oxacillin. Nafcillin is available only in injectable form, whereas cloxacillin and dicloxacillin are available only in oral form. Oxacillin is available in both oral and injectable forms. The penicillinase-resistant penicillins are able to resist breakdown by the penicillin-destroying enzyme (penicillinase) commonly produced by bacteria such as staphylococci. For this reason, they may also be referred to as *antistaphylococcal penicillins*. The chemical structure of these drugs features a large, bulky side chain near the beta-lactam ring. This side chain serves as a barrier to the penicillinase enzyme, preventing it from breaking the beta-lactam ring, which would inactivate the drug. There are, however, certain strains of staphylococci, specifically *S. aureus,* that are resistant to these drugs. Such bacteria therefore require alternative antibiotic regimens.

### Pharmacokinetics

| Route | Onset of Action | Peak Plasma Concentration | Elimination Half-life | Duration of Action |
|---|---|---|---|---|
| IV | Variable | 15-30 min | 30-60 min | 6 hr |

### AMINOPENICILLINS

There are two aminopenicillins: amoxicillin and ampicillin. They are so named because of the presence of a free amino group ($-NH^2$) in their chemical structure. This structural feature gives aminopenicillins enhanced activity against gram-negative bacteria against which the natural and penicillinase-resistant

| TABLE 38-4 | **PENICILLINS: REPORTED ADVERSE EFFECTS** |
|---|---|
| **BODY SYSTEM** | **ADVERSE EFFECTS** |
| Central nervous | Lethargy, anxiety, depression, seizures |
| Gastrointestinal | Nausea, vomiting, diarrhea, taste alterations, oral candidiasis |
| Hematologic | Anemia, bone marrow depression, granulocytopenia |
| Metabolic | Hyperkalemia, hypernatremia, alkalosis |
| Skin | Pruritus, hives, rash |

| TABLE 38-5 | **PENICILLINS: DRUG INTERACTIONS** | |
|---|---|---|
| **DRUG INTERACTING WITH PENICILLINS** | **MECHANISM** | **RESULT** |
| Aminoglycosides (IV) and clavulanic acid | Additivity | More effective killing of bacteria |
| methotrexate | Decreased renal elimination of methotrexate | Increased methotrexate levels |
| NSAIDs | Compete for protein binding | More free and active penicillin (may be beneficial) |
| Oral contraceptives | Uncertain | May decrease efficacy of the contraceptive |
| probenecid | Competes for elimination | Prolongs the effects of penicillins |
| rifampin | Inhibition | May inhibit the killing activity of penicillins |
| warfarin | Reduced vitamin K from gut flora | Enhanced anticoagulant effect of warfarin |

*IV,* Intravenous; *NSAIDs,* nonsteroidal antiinflammatory drugs.

## DOSAGES

### Selected Penicillins

| DRUG (PREGNANCY CATEGORY) | PHARMACOLOGIC CLASS | USUAL DOSAGE RANGE | INDICATIONS |
|---|---|---|---|
| ◆ amoxicillin (Amoxil, generics) (B) | Aminopenicillin | **Pediatric** PO: 45-90 mg/kg/day divided q8-12h **Adult** PO: 250-500 mg q8h | Otitis media; sinusitis; various susceptible respiratory, skin, and urinary tract infections; dental prophylaxis for bacterial endocarditis; *Helicobacter pylori* infection |
| ampicillin (generic only) (B) | Aminopenicillin | **Adult** PO/IV/IM: 1-12 g/day divided q4-6h **Pediatric** 25-50 mg/kg/day divided q6h (doses up to 300 mg/kg/day may be required for meningitis and other serious infections) | Primarily infection with gram-negative organisms such as *Shigella, Salmonella, Escherichia, Haemophilus, Proteus,* and *Neisseria* spp.; infection with some gram-positive organisms |
| nafcillin (generic only) (B) | Penicillinase-resistant penicillin | **Adult** IV/IM: 500-1000 mg q4-6h **Pediatric** IV/IM: 50-200 mg/kg/day divided q6h | Infection with penicillinase-producing staphylococci |
| ◆ penicillin V potassium (Pen-Vee K) (B) | Natural penicillin | **Adult and pediatric** PO: 125-500 mg q6-8h | Primarily infection with gram-positive organisms such as Streptococcus (including *Streptococcus pneumoniae*) |

*IM,* Intramuscular; *IV,* intravenous; *PO,* oral; *spp.,* species.

penicillins are relatively ineffective. The aminopenicillins are also effective against some gram-positive organisms. Amoxicillin is an analogue of ampicillin.

### ◆ amoxicillin

Amoxicillin is a very commonly prescribed aminopenicillin. Amoxicillin is used to treat infections caused by susceptible organisms in the ears, nose, throat, genitourinary tract, skin, and skin structures. Pediatric dosages are sometimes higher than in the past because of the development of increasingly resistant *Streptococcus pneumoniae* organisms. The drug is available only for oral use and can be given with or without food.

### Pharmacokinetics

| Route | Onset of Action | Peak Plasma Concentration | Elimination Half-life | Duration of Action |
|---|---|---|---|---|
| PO | 0.5-1 hr | 1-2 hr | 1-1.5 hr | 6-8 hr |

### ampicillin

Ampicillin is available in three different salt forms: anhydrous, trihydrate, and sodium. The different salt forms are administered by different routes. Ampicillin anhydrous and trihydrate are both administered orally, whereas ampicillin sodium is given parenterally. This drug is still currently available, although it is now used less frequently than before because of resistance.

### Pharmacokinetics

| Route | Onset of Action | Peak Plasma Concentration | Elimination Half-life | Duration of Action |
|---|---|---|---|---|
| PO | Variable | 1-2 hr | 1-1.5 hr | 4-6 hr |
| IV | Variable | 5 min | 1-1.8 hr | 6-8 hr |

### EXTENDED-SPECTRUM PENICILLINS

By making a few changes in the basic penicillin structure, drug developers produced another generation of penicillins that have a wider spectrum of activity than that possessed by either of the other two classes of semisynthetic penicillins (penicillinase-resistant penicillins and aminopenicillins) or by the natural penicillins. Currently three extended-spectrum penicillins are available: carbenicillin, piperacillin, and ticarcillin; however, they are rarely used by themselves. Both ticarcillin and piperacillin are available in fixed-combination products that include beta-lactamase inhibitors. The ticarcillin fixed-combination product (Timentin) includes clavulanate potassium. Piperacillin is available in combination with tazobactam (a combination called Zosyn). These beta-lactamase–inhibiting products allow for enhanced multiorganism coverage, especially against anaerobic organisms that are common in intestinal infections and *Pseudomonas* spp., which are common in hospital-acquired infections. Zosyn is commonly used in hospitalized patients with suspected or documented serious infections. Because of its broad spectrum of activity (gram positive, gram negative, and anaerobic), it is often used as empiric therapy. Zosyn and Timentin are available only by injection.

## CEPHALOSPORINS

Cephalosporins are semisynthetic antibiotics widely used in clinical practice. They are structurally and pharmacologically related to the penicillins. Like penicillins, cephalosporins are bactericidal and work by interfering with bacterial cell wall synthesis. They also bind to the same penicillin-binding proteins inside bacteria that were described earlier for the penicillins. Although there are a variety of such proteins, they are collectively referred to as penicillin binding regardless of the type of beta-lactam drug involved.

## TABLE 38-6 CEPHALOSPORINS: PARENTERAL AND ORAL PREPARATIONS

| FIRST GENERATION | | SECOND GENERATION | | THIRD GENERATION | | FOURTH GENERATION | FIFTH GENERATION |
|---|---|---|---|---|---|---|---|
| IV | PO | IV | PO | IV | PO | IV | IV |
| cefazolin | cefadroxil | cefoxitin | cefaclor | cefotaxime | cefpodoxime | cefepime | ceftaroline |
| cephradine | cephalexin | cefuroxime | cefuroxime axetil* | ceftizoxime | ceftibuten | | |
| | cephradine | cefotetan | cefprozil | ceftriaxone | cefdinir | | |
| | | loracarbef | | ceftazidime | | | |

*IV*, Intravenous; *PO*, oral.
*Prodrug salts that aid in drug delivery into the gastrointestinal tract.

## TABLE 38-7 CEPHALOSPORINS: DRUG INTERACTIONS

| INTERACTING DRUG | MECHANISM | RESULT |
|---|---|---|
| Ethanol (alcohol) | Accumulation of acetaldehyde metabolite of ethanol | Acute alcohol intolerance (disulfiram-like reaction) after drinking alcoholic beverages within 72 hr of taking cefotetan. Symptoms include stomach cramps, nausea, vomiting, diaphoresis, pruritus, headache, and hypotension. |
| Antacids, iron | Decreased absorption of certain oral cephalosporins (cefdinir, cefditoren) | Decreased effectiveness of drug |
| probenecid | Decreased renal excretion | Increased cephalosporin levels |
| Oral contraceptives (OCs) | Enhanced OC metabolism | Increased risk for unintended pregnancy |

Cephalosporins can destroy a broad spectrum of bacteria, and this ability is directly related to the chemical changes that have been made to their basic cephalosporin structure. Modifications to this chemical structure by pharmaceutical scientists have given rise to five generations of cephalosporins. Depending on the generation, these drugs may be active against gram-positive, gram-negative, or anaerobic bacteria. They are not active against fungi and viruses. The different drugs of each generation have certain chemical similarities, and thus they can kill similar spectra of bacteria. In general, the level of gram-negative coverage increases with each successive generation. The first-generation drugs have the most gram-positive coverage, and the later generations have the most gram-negative coverage. Anaerobic coverage is found only with the second-generation drugs. Cefepime, cefdinir, and cefditoren pivoxil are the oral third-generation cephalosporins. Ceftaroline, the newest cephalosporin, often referred as the fifth generation, has a broad spectrum and covers gram-positive (including MRSA) and gram-negative organisms. The currently available parenteral and oral cephalosporin antibiotics are listed in Table 38-6. As is often the case, injectable drugs produce higher serum concentrations than drugs administered by the oral route and thus are used to treat more serious infections.

The safety profiles, contraindications, and pregnancy ratings of the cephalosporins are very similar to those of the penicillins. The most commonly reported adverse effects are mild diarrhea, abdominal cramps, rash, pruritus, redness, and edema. Because cephalosporins are chemically very similar to penicillins, a person who has had an allergic reaction to penicillin may also have an allergic reaction to a cephalosporin. This is referred to as cross-sensitivity. Various investigators have observed that the incidence of cross-sensitivity between penicillins and cephalosporins is between 1% and 4%. However, only those patients who have had a serious anaphylactic reaction to penicillin must not be given cephalosporins. As a class, the cephalosporins are very safe and effective antibiotics.

Penicillins and cephalosporins are practically identical in their mechanism of action, drug effects, therapeutic effects, and adverse effects. For this reason, this information is not repeated for the cephalosporins, and the reader is referred to the pertinent discussions in the section on the penicillin drugs. Cephalosporins of all generations are very safe drugs that are classified as pregnancy category B drugs. Their use is contraindicated in patients who have shown a hypersensitivity to them and in any patient with a history of life-threatening allergic reaction to penicillins. Drug interactions are listed in Table 38-7.

## Dosages

For the dosage information on selected cephalosporins, see the table on p. 621.

## DRUG PROFILES

### FIRST-GENERATION CEPHALOSPORINS

First-generation cephalosporins are usually active against gram-positive bacteria and have limited activity against gram-negative bacteria. They are available in both parenteral and oral forms. Currently available first-generation cephalosporins include cefadroxil, cefazolin, cephalexin, and cephradine.

### ♦ cefazolin

Cefazolin (Ancef) is a prototypical first-generation cephalosporin. As with all first-generation cephalosporins, it provides excellent coverage against gram-positive bacteria but limited coverage against gram-negative bacteria. It is available only for

## DOSAGES

### *Selected Cephalosporins*

| DRUG (PREGNANCY CATEGORY) | PHARMACOLOGIC CLASS | USUAL DOSAGE RANGE | INDICATIONS |
|---|---|---|---|
| ◆ cefazolin (Kefzol, Ancef) (B) | First-generation cephalosporin | **Adult** IV/IM: 500-2000 mg q8h **Pediatric** IV/IM: 25-100 mg/kg/day divided q6-8h | Infections due to gram positive organisms, some penicillinase-producing organisms, and some gram-negative organisms; preoperative and postoperative surgical prophylaxis |
| ◆ cefoxitin (Mefoxin) (B) | Second-generation cephalosporin | **Adult** IV/IM: 3-12 g/day divided q6-8h **Pediatric** IV/IM: 80-160 mg/kg/day divided q4-6h, not to exceed 12 g/day | Infections; less coverage of gram-positive organisms, greater coverage of gram-negative and anaerobic organisms |
| cefuroxime (Kefurox, Zinacef); cefuroxime axetil* (Ceftin, tablet form) (B) | Second-generation cephalosporin | **Adult** PO (tabs): 125-500 mg bid IV/IM: 750-1500 mg q8h **Pediatric** PO: 20-30 mg/kg/day divided bid IV/IM: 50-150 mg/kg/day, divided q8h | Comparable to those for cefazolin, and provides more coverage of gram-negative organisms |
| ceftazidime (Fortaz, Tazidime) (B) | Third-generation cephalosporin | **Adult** IV/IM: 250-2000 mg q6-12h **Pediatric** IV/IM: 30-50 mg/kg/day divided q8-12h | Infections; more extensive coverage of gram-negative organisms, including *Pseudomonas* spp. |
| ◆ ceftriaxone (Rocephin) (B) | Third-generation cephalosporin | **Adult** IV/IM: 1-2 g given once daily except for meningitis, for which it is given twice daily **Pediatric** IV/IM: 50-100 mg/kg/day divided daily-bid (as above) | Comparable to those for ceftazidime |
| cefepime (Maxipime) (B) | Fourth-generation cephalosporin | **Adult** IV/IM: 250-2000 mg daily-bid **Pediatric** IV/IM: 50 mg/kg q12h | Infections; provides more extensive coverage of gram-negative organisms and better gram-positive coverage than third generation, including organisms causing intraabdominal infections |

*IM,* Intramuscular; *IV,* intravenous; *PO,* oral; *spp.,* species.
*Cefuroxime axetil and cefditoren pivoxil are both prodrugs for PO use that are hydrolyzed into the active ingredient in the fluids of the gastrointestinal tract.

parenteral use. It is used commonly for surgical prophylaxis and for susceptible staphylococcal infections.

### Pharmacokinetics

| Route | Onset of Action | Peak Plasma Concentration | Elimination Half-life | Duration of Action |
|---|---|---|---|---|
| IV | Variable | 5 min | 1.2-2.5 hr | 8 hr |

### ◆ cephalexin

Cephalexin (Keflex) is a prototypical oral first-generation cephalosporin. It also provides excellent coverage against gram-positive bacteria but limited coverage against gram-negative bacteria. It is available only for oral use. Cephradine is another oral first-generation cephalosporin.

### Pharmacokinetics

| Route | Onset of Action | Peak Plasma Concentration | Elimination Half-life | Duration of Action |
|---|---|---|---|---|
| PO | Variable | 1 hr | 0.6-2 hr | 6-12 hr |

## SECOND-GENERATION CEPHALOSPORINS

Second-generation cephalosporins have coverage against gram-positive organisms similar to that of the first-generation cephalosporins but have enhanced coverage against gram-negative bacteria. Both parenteral and oral formulations are available. Currently available second-generation cephalosporins include cefaclor, cefoxitin, cefuroxime, cefotetan, cefprozil, and loracarbef. These drugs differ slightly with regard to their antibacterial coverage. Cefoxitin and cefotetan are often referred to as *cephamycins* and have better coverage against various anaerobic bacteria such as *Bacteroides fragilis, Peptostreptococcus* spp., and *Clostridium* spp. than the other drugs in this class.

### ◆ cefoxitin

Cefoxitin (Mefoxin) is a parenteral second-generation cephalosporin. It provides excellent gram-positive coverage and better gram-negative coverage than the first-generation drugs. Cefoxitin has been used extensively as a prophylactic antibiotic in patients undergoing abdominal surgery because it can effectively kill intestinal bacteria, including anaerobes. Normal intestinal flora include gram-positive, gram-negative, and anaerobic bacteria.

## Pharmacokinetics

| Route | Onset of Action | Peak Plasma Concentration | Elimination Half-life | Duration of Action |
|-------|-----------------|---------------------------|----------------------|---------------------|
| IV | Variable | 0.5 hr | 1 hr | 8 hr |

## cefuroxime

Cefuroxime sodium (Zinacef) is the parenteral form of this second-generation cephalosporin. The oral form is a different salt, cefuroxime axetil (Ceftin). It has more activity against gram-negative bacteria than first-generation cephalosporins but a narrower spectrum of activity against gram-negative bacteria than third-generation cephalosporins. It differs from the cephamycins such as cefoxitin in that it does not kill anaerobic bacteria. Cefuroxime axetil is a prodrug. It has little antibacterial activity until it is hydrolyzed in the liver to its active cefuroxime form. It is available only for oral use. Cefuroxime sodium is available only in injectable form.

## Pharmacokinetics

| Route | Onset of Action | Peak Plasma Concentration | Elimination Half-life | Duration of Action |
|-------|-----------------|---------------------------|----------------------|---------------------|
| PO | Variable | 2-3 hr | 1.3 hr | 6-8 hr |
| IV | Variable | 30 min | 1-2 hr | 6-8 hr |

## THIRD-GENERATION CEPHALOSPORINS

The available third-generation cephalosporins include cefotaxime, cefpodoxime, ceftazidime, ceftibuten, cefdinir, ceftizoxime, and ceftriaxone. These are the most potent of the first three generations of cephalosporins in fighting gram-negative bacteria, but they generally have less activity than first- and second-generation drugs against gram-positive organisms.

Because of specific changes in the basic cephalosporin structure, ceftazidime has activity against *Pseudomonas* spp. However resistance is beginning to limit its usefulness. Cefpodoxime, cefdinir, and ceftibuten are currently the only third-generation cephalosporins available for oral use. All the other third-generation drugs are available only in parenteral forms.

## ◆ ceftriaxone

Ceftriaxone (Rocephin) is an extremely long-acting third-generation drug that can be given only once a day for the treatment of most infections. It also has the unique characteristic of being able to pass easily through the blood-brain barrier. For this reason, it is one of the few cephalosporins that is indicated for the treatment of meningitis, an infection of the meninges of the brain. The spectrum of activity of ceftriaxone is similar to that of the other third-generation drugs cefotaxime and ceftizoxime. It can be given both IV and IM. In some cases of infection, one IM injection can eradicate the infection. Ceftriaxone is 93% to 96% bound to plasma protein, a proportion higher than that of many of the other cephalosporins. This drug is

also unique in that it is metabolized in the intestine after biliary excretion. Ceftriaxone is not given to hyperbilirubinemic neonates or to patients with severe liver dysfunction. It should not be administered with calcium infusions. Ceftriaxone is available only for injection.

## Pharmacokinetics

| Route | Onset of Action | Peak Plasma Concentration | Elimination Half-life | Duration of Action |
|-------|-----------------|---------------------------|----------------------|---------------------|
| IV | Variable | 1.5-4 hr | 4.3-8.7 hr | 24 hr |

## ceftazidime

Ceftazidime (Ceptaz, Fortaz, Tazidime) is a parenterally administered third-generation cephalosporin with activity against difficult-to-treat infections with gram-negative bacteria such as *Pseudomonas* spp. It is the third-generation cephalosporin of choice for many indications because of its excellent spectrum of activity and safety profile; however, resistance is beginning to limit its usefulness, and it is generally given in combination with an aminoglycoside (discussed in Chapter 39). Ceftazidime is available only in injectable form.

## Pharmacokinetics

| Route | Onset of Action | Peak Plasma Concentration | Elimination Half-life | Duration of Action |
|-------|-----------------|---------------------------|----------------------|---------------------|
| IV/IM | Variable | 1 hr | 2 hr | 8-12 hr |

## FOURTH-GENERATION CEPHALOSPORINS

### cefepime

Cefepime (Maxipime) is the prototypical fourth-generation cephalosporin. Cefepime is a broad-spectrum cephalosporin that most closely resembles ceftazidime in its spectrum of activity. It differs from ceftazidime in that it has increased activity against many *Enterobacter* spp. (gram-negative) as well as gram-positive organisms. Cefepime is indicated for the treatment of uncomplicated and complicated UTIs, uncomplicated skin and skin structure infections, and pneumonia. It is available only in injectable form.

## Pharmacokinetics

| Route | Onset of Action | Peak Plasma Concentration | Elimination Half-life | Duration of Action |
|-------|-----------------|---------------------------|----------------------|---------------------|
| IV | 0.5 hr | 0.5-1.5 hr | 2 hr | 8-12 hr |

## FIFTH-GENERATION CEPHALOSPORINS

Cefaroline (Teflaro) is the newest cephalosporin. It has a broader spectrum of activity than the current cephalosporins. It is effective against a wide variety of organisms, including methicillin-resistant *S. aureus* (MRSA), making it the only cephalosporin that treats MRSA. Cefaroline is indicated for acute skin and skin structure infections and community-acquired pneumonia. The dose needs to be adjusted for decreased renal function. It is available only in injectable form.

## CARBAPENEMS

Carbapenems have the broadest antibacterial action of any antibiotics to date. They are bactericidal and inhibit cell wall synthesis. Because of this, they are often reserved for complicated body cavity and connective tissue infections in acutely ill hospitalized patients. They are also effective against many gram-positive organisms. One hazard of carbapenem use is drug-induced seizure activity, which occurs in a relatively small percentage of patients. However, the risk of seizures can be reduced by proper dosage adjustment in impaired patients. There is a small risk of cross-allergenicity in patients with penicillin allergies. Only those patients with anaphylactic-type reactions to penicillins must not receive a carbapenem. Currently available carbapenems include imipenem/cilastatin, meropenem, ertapenem, and doripenem. Carbapenems must be infused over 60 minutes.

### DRUG PROFILE

#### ♦ imipenem/cilastatin

Imipenem/cilastatin (Primaxin) is a fixed combination of imipenem, which is a semisynthetic carbapenem antibiotic similar to beta-lactam antibiotics, and cilastatin, an inhibitor of an enzyme that breaks down imipenem. Imipenem has a wide spectrum of activity against gram-positive and gram-negative aerobic and anaerobic bacteria. Cilastatin is a unique drug in that it inhibits an enzyme in the kidneys called *dehydropeptidase*, which would otherwise quickly break down the imipenem. Cilastatin also blocks the renal tubular secretion of imipenem, which impairs imipenem from being excreted by the kidneys, the primary route of elimination of the drug.

Imipenem/cilastatin exerts its antibacterial effect by binding to penicillin-binding proteins inside bacteria, which in turn inhibits bacterial cell wall synthesis. Unlike many of the penicillins and cephalosporins, imipenem/cilastatin is very resistant to the antibiotic-inhibiting actions of beta-lactamases. Drugs with which it potentially interacts include cyclosporine, ganciclovir, and probenecid, all of which may potentiate the central nervous system (CNS) adverse effects (including seizures) of imipenem. The most serious adverse effect associated with imipenem/cilastatin therapy is seizures, which have been reported in up to 1.5% of patients receiving less than 500 mg every 6 hours. In patients receiving high dosages of the drug (more than 500 mg every 6 hours), however, there is a 10% incidence of seizures. Seizures are more likely in elderly and renally impaired patients. Seizures have been associated with all of the carbapenems, but the data suggest that they are most likely to occur with imipenem/cilastatin.

Imipenem/cilastatin is indicated for the treatment of bone, joint, skin, and soft-tissue infections; bacterial endocarditis caused by *S. aureus*; intraabdominal bacterial infections; pneumonia; UTIs and pelvic infections; and bacterial septicemia caused by susceptible bacterial organisms. The IM form of imipenem/cilastatin contains lidocaine, and its use is therefore contraindicated in patients with a known drug allergy to lidocaine or related local anesthetics. All dosage forms contain the same number of milligrams of both imipenem and cilastatin.

Meropenem (Merrem) is the second drug in the carbapenem class of antibiotics. Compared with imipenem/cilastatin, meropenem appears to be somewhat less active against gram-positive organisms, more active against *Enterobacteriaceae*, and equally active against *P. aeruginosa*. However, meropenem is the only carbapenem currently indicated for treatment of bacterial meningitis. Ertapenem (Invanz) has a spectrum of activity comparable to that of imipenem/cilastatin, although it is not active against *Enterococcal* or *Pseudomonas* spp. Doripenem (Doribax) is the newest carbapenem. It has less seizure potential than imipenem/cilastatin. It is indicated for intraabdominal infections, pyelonephritis, UTIs, and pneumonia. Recommended dosages of imipenem/cilastatin are given in the table on p. 624.

**Pharmacokinetics**

| Route | Onset of Action | Peak Plasma Concentration | Elimination Half-life | Duration of Action |
|---|---|---|---|---|
| IV | Variable | 2 hr | 2-3 hr | 6-8 hr |

## MONOBACTAMS

### DRUG PROFILE

#### aztreonam

Aztreonam (Azactam) is the only monobactam antibiotic to be developed thus far. It is a synthetic beta-lactam antibiotic that is primarily active against aerobic gram-negative bacteria, including *E. coli*, *Klebsiella* spp., and *Pseudomonas* spp. Aztreonam is a bactericidal antibiotic. It destroys bacteria by inhibiting bacterial cell wall synthesis, which results in lysis. Aztreonam is indicated for the treatment of moderately severe systemic infections and UTIs. It is often combined with other antibiotics for the treatment of intraabdominal and gynecologic infections. Aztreonam is available only in injectable form. Its use is contraindicated in patients with a known drug allergy, although it is believed to have less allergic cross-reactivity with other beta-lactam antibiotics. Common adverse effects include rash, nausea, vomiting, and diarrhea. Recommended dosages for this monobactam are given in the table on p. 624.

**Pharmacokinetics**

| Route | Onset of Action | Peak Plasma Concentration | Elimination Half-life | Duration of Action |
|---|---|---|---|---|
| IV/IM | Variable | 1 hr | 1.5-2.1 hr | 6-12 hr |

## MACROLIDES

The macrolides are a large group of antibiotics that first became available in the early 1950s with the introduction of erythromycin. Macrolides are considered bacteriostatic; however, in high enough concentrations they may be bactericidal to some susceptible bacteria. There are three macrolide antibiotics: azithromycin, clarithromycin, and erythromycin. Azithromycin and clarithromycin are currently the most widely used of the macrolides. Although the spectra of antibacterial activity of both azithromycin and clarithromycin are similar to that of

## DOSAGES

### Selected Carbapenems and Monobactams

| DRUG (PREGNANCY CATEGORY) | PHARMACOLOGIC CLASS | USUAL DOSAGE RANGE | INDICATIONS |
|---|---|---|---|
| aztreonam (Azactam) (B) | Monobactam | **Adult**<br>IV/IM: 500-2000 mg q6-12h<br>**Pediatric**<br>IV/IM: 30 mg/kg q6-8 hr | Primarily UTI caused by gram-negative organisms, severe systemic infections |
| ◆ imipenem/cilastatin (Primaxin) (C) | Carbapenem | **Adult**<br>IV: 250-500 mg q6-8h<br>IM: 500-750 mg q12h<br>**Pediatric**<br>15-25 mg/kg q6 hr | Infection with gram-positive, gram-negative, and aerobic bacteria, including *Pseudomonas aeruginosa*; includes infections of bone, joint, skin, or soft tissue and endocarditis, pneumonia, UTI, intraabdominal and pelvic infections, and septicemia |

*IM,* Intramuscular; *IV,* intravenous; *UTI,* urinary tract infection.

erythromycin, the former have longer durations of action than erythromycin, which allows them to be given less often. They produce fewer and milder GI tract adverse effects than erythromycin, and azithromycin is usually dosed over a shorter length of time than many of the erythromycin products. Azithromycin and clarithromycin also exhibit better efficacy in eradicating various bacteria and are capable of better tissue penetration. Because erythromycin has a bitter taste and is quickly degraded by the acidity of the stomach, several salt forms and many dosage formulations were developed to circumvent these problems. Fidaxomicin (Dificid) is the newest macrolide antibiotic. It is indicated only for the treatment of *Clostridium difficile*–associated diarrhea. The most common adverse effects are nausea, vomiting, and GI bleed. It is pregnancy category B. It has minimal absorption and, as such, there are known drug interactions.

## Mechanism of Action and Drug Effects

Macrolide antibiotics are bacteriostatic drugs that inhibit protein synthesis by binding reversibly to the 50S ribosomal subunits of susceptible microorganisms. Macrolides are effective in the treatment of a wide range of infections. These include various infections of the upper and lower respiratory tract, skin, and soft tissue caused by some strains of *Streptococcus* and *Haemophilus;* spirochetal infections such as syphilis and Lyme disease; gonorrhea; and *Chlamydia, Mycoplasma,* and *Corynebacterium* infections. Gonorrheal infections have become increasingly difficult to treat with macrolide monotherapy, so these drugs are sometimes used in combination with other antibiotics such as cephalosporins. Macrolides are also somewhat unique among antibiotics in that they are especially effective against several bacterial species that often reproduce inside host cells instead of just in the bloodstream or interstitial spaces. Common examples of such bacteria, some of which were previously listed, are *Listeria, Chlamydia, Legionella* (one species of which causes Legionnaires' disease), *Neisseria* (one species of which causes gonorrhea), and *Campylobacter.*

## Indications

Infections caused by *Streptococcus pyogenes* (group A beta-hemolytic streptococci) are inhibited by macrolides, as are mild to moderate upper and lower respiratory tract infections caused by

*Haemophilus influenzae.* Spirochetal infections that are treated with erythromycin and other macrolides are syphilis and Lyme disease. Various forms of gonorrhea and *Chlamydia* and Mycoplasma infections are also susceptible to the effects of macrolides.

A therapeutic effect of erythromycin outside its antibiotic actions is its ability to irritate the GI tract, which stimulates smooth muscle and GI motility. This may be of benefit to patients who have decreased GI motility, such as delayed gastric emptying in diabetic patients (known as *diabetic gastroparesis*). It has also been shown to be helpful in facilitating the passage of feeding tubes from the stomach into the small bowel. Azithromycin and clarithromycin are approved for the prevention and treatment of *Mycobacterium avium-intracellulare (MAC)* complex infections. This is a common *opportunistic infection* often associated with HIV infection/acquired immunodeficiency syndrome (AIDS) (see Chapter 40). Clarithromycin also has been approved for use in combination with omeprazole and amoxicillin for the treatment of patients with active ulcer associated with *Helicobacter pylori* infection.

## Contraindications

The only usual contraindication to macrolide use is known drug allergy. Macrolides are often used as alternative drugs for patients with allergies to beta-lactam antibiotics.

## Adverse Effects

Erythromycin formulations cause many GI-related adverse effects, especially nausea and vomiting. Azithromycin and clarithromycin seem to be associated with a lower incidence of these GI tract complications. Reported adverse effects are listed in Table 38-8.

## Interactions

There are a number of potential drug interactions with the macrolides. The macrolides possess two properties that can cause drug interactions: they are highly protein bound and they are metabolized in the liver. For drugs metabolized in the liver, drug interactions arise from competition between the different drugs for metabolic enzymes, specifically the enzymes known as the *cytochrome P-450 complex* (see Chapter 2). Such

## TABLE 38-8 MACROLIDES: REPORTED ADVERSE EFFECTS

| BODY SYSTEM | ADVERSE EFFECTS |
|---|---|
| Cardiovascular | Palpitations, chest pain, QT prolongation |
| Central nervous | Headache, dizziness, vertigo |
| Gastrointestinal | Nausea, hepatotoxicity, heartburn, vomiting, diarrhea, flatulence, cholestatic jaundice, anorexia, abnormal taste |
| Integumentary | Rash, urticaria, phlebitis at intravenous site |
| Other | Hearing loss, tinnitus |

enzymatic effects generally lead to more pronounced drug interactions than competition for protein binding. The result is a delay in the metabolic clearance of one or more interacting drugs and thus a prolonged and possibly toxic drug effect. Examples of some especially common drugs that compete for hepatic metabolism with the macrolides are carbamazepine, cyclosporine, theophylline, and warfarin. When macrolides are given with these drugs, the results are enhanced effects and possible toxicity of the latter drugs, and patients must be monitored. Macrolides can also reduce the efficacy of oral contraceptives. Clarithromycin and erythromycin are not to be used with moxifloxacin, pimozide, thioridazine, or other drugs that prolong the QT interval, because malignant dysrhythmias can occur. Concurrent use of simvastatin or lovastatin with clarithromycin or erythromycin is not recommended. Azithromycin is not as prone to such interactions as are the other macrolides, because of its minimal effects on the cytochrome P-450 enzymes.

## Dosages

For dosages information on selected macrolide antibiotics, see the table below.

## DRUG PROFILES

Macrolide antibiotics are used to treat a variety of infections. Azithromycin and clarithromycin have fewer adverse effects and a better pharmacokinetics profile than erythromycin.

Macrolide use is contraindicated in patients with known drug allergy. Because these drugs are significantly protein bound and are metabolized in the liver, they may interact with other drugs that are also highly protein bound or hepatically metabolized.

### ◆ erythromycin

Erythromycin, which goes by many product names, was for many years the most commonly prescribed macrolide antibiotic. However, other macrolides are now more commonly used. The drug is available in several different salt and dosage forms for oral use that were developed to circumvent some of the drawbacks it has chemically. An injectable form is also available for IV use. Erythromycin is also available in topical forms for dermatologic use (see Chapter 56) and in ophthalmic dosage forms (see Chapter 57). The absorption of oral erythromycin is enhanced if it is taken on an empty stomach, but because of the high incidence of stomach irritation associated with its use, many of these drugs are taken with a meal or snack.

### ◆ azithromycin and clarithromycin

Azithromycin (Zithromax) and clarithromycin (Biaxin) are semisynthetic macrolide antibiotics that differ structurally from erythromycin and as a result have advantages over it. These include better adverse effect profiles, including less GI tract irritation, and more favorable pharmacokinetic properties. Both have very similar spectra of activity that differ only slightly from that of erythromycin. The two drugs are used for the treatment of both upper and lower respiratory tract and skin structure infections.

## DOSAGES

### Selected Macrolides

| DRUG (PREGNANCY CATEGORY) | PHARMACOLOGIC CLASS | USUAL DOSAGE RANGE | INDICATIONS |
|---|---|---|---|
| ◆ azithromycin (Zithromax) (B) | Semisynthetic macrolide | **Adult**<br>PO: 500 mg × 1 dose, then 250 mg daily × 4 days<br>IV: 500 mg q day<br>**Pediatric**<br>PO: 5-12 mg/kg once a day × 4 days or as 30 mg/kg single dose (max dose 500 mg)<br>IV: 10 mg/kg × 1 day then 5 mg/kg/day × 4 days | Comparable to those for erythromycin, but especially GU and respiratory tract infections, including MAC infections |
| ◆ clarithromycin (Biaxin) (C) | Semisynthetic macrolide | **Adult**<br>PO: 500 mg twice daily<br>**Pediatric**<br>PO: 7.5 mg/kg bid (max 500 mg/dose) | Comparable to those for erythromycin, but especially GU and respiratory tract infections, including MAC infections |
| ◆ erythromycin (E-mycin, EryPed, Eryc, E.E.S., many others) (B) | Natural macrolide | **Adult***<br>PO: 250-500 mg qid<br>**Pediatric***<br>25-50 mg/kg/day divided qid | Infections of respiratory and GI tracts and skin caused by various gram-positive, gram-negative, and miscellaneous organisms |

*GI*, Gastrointestinal; *GU*, genitourinary; *IV*, intravenous; *MAC, Mycobacterium avium-intracellulare* complex; *PO*, oral.
*There are many dosage forms, and dosages may vary from those listed.

Azithromycin has excellent tissue penetration, so that it can reach high concentrations in infected tissues. It also has a long duration of action, which allows it to be dosed once daily. It is usually given in a regimen of 500 mg on day 1 and then 250 mg/day for four days. Taking the drug with food decreases both the rate and extent of GI absorption. The drug is available in oral and injectable forms.

Clarithromycin is given orally twice daily in adults and children older than 6 months of age. It can be given with or without food. The extended-release preparation must not be crushed.

**Pharmacokinetics (azithromycin)**

| Route | Onset of Action | Peak Plasma Concentration | Elimination Half-life | Duration of Action |
|---|---|---|---|---|
| PO | Variable | 2.5-4 hr | 60-70 hr | Up to 24 hr |

**Pharmacokinetics (clarithromycin)**

| Route | Onset of Action | Peak Plasma Concentration | Elimination Half-life | Duration of Action |
|---|---|---|---|---|
| PO | Variable | 2-4 hr | 3-7 hr | Up to 12 hr |

## KETOLIDES

Telithromycin (Ketek) is currently the only drug in a new class known as ketolides. It is derived from erythromycin A and has better acid stability and better antibacterial coverage than the macrolides. Its mechanism of action is also similar to that of the macrolides. However, telithromycin has been associated with severe liver damage, and its use is very limited.

## TETRACYCLINES

The tetracyclines are bacteriostatic drugs that inhibit bacterial protein synthesis by binding to the 30S bacterial ribosome. The three naturally occurring tetracyclines are demeclocycline, oxytetracycline, and tetracycline. The two semisynthetic tetracyclines are doxycycline and minocycline. The newest tetracycline antibiotic is tigecycline (Tygacil). Tigecycline is indicated for skin and soft-tissue infections, intraabdominal infections, and pneumonia. It is effective against many resistant bacteria. The available tetracycline antibiotics are listed in Box 38-1.

Tetracyclines are chemically and pharmacologically similar to one another. The most significant chemical characteristic of these drugs is their ability to bind to (chelate) divalent ($Ca^{+++}$, $Mg^{++}$) and trivalent ($Al^{+++}$) metallic ions to form insoluble complexes. Therefore, their coadministration with milk, antacids, or iron salts causes a considerable reduction in the oral absorption of the tetracycline. In addition, their strong affinity for calcium usually precludes their use in pediatric patients younger than 8 years of age, because it can result in significant tooth discoloration. These drugs must be avoided in pregnant women and nursing mothers. The drugs do pass into breast milk, and this can be another route of exposure leading to tooth discoloration in nursing children.

Tetracyclines primarily differ from one another in the following ways:
- *Oral absorption:* All except tigecycline are adequately absorbed, but doxycycline and minocycline have the best absorption.
- *Body tissue penetration:* Doxycycline and minocycline possess the best penetration potential (brain and cerebrospinal fluid).
- *Half-life and resulting dosage schedule:* See the Dosages table on p. 627 and pharmacokinetics information in the Drug Profiles section.

## Mechanism of Action and Drug Effects

Tetracyclines work by inhibiting protein synthesis in susceptible bacteria. They inhibit the growth of and kill a very wide range of *Rickettsia, Chlamydia,* and *Mycoplasma* organisms, as well as a variety of gram-negative and gram-positive bacteria. They are also useful in the treatment of spirochetal infections, such as syphilis and Lyme disease, and pelvic inflammatory disease. Demeclocycline possesses a unique drug effect in that it inhibits the action of antidiuretic hormone, which makes it useful in the treatment of the syndrome of inappropriate secretion of antidiuretic hormone (SIADH).

## Indications

Tetracyclines have a wide range of activity, and all drugs in this class are effective against essentially the same spectrum of microbes. They inhibit the growth of many gram-negative and gram-positive organisms and even of some protozoans. Traditionally used to treat acne in adolescents and adults, they are also considered the drugs of choice for the treatment of the following infections caused by susceptible organisms:
- *Chlamydia:* lymphogranuloma venereum, psittacosis, and nonspecific endocervical, rectal, and urethral infections
- *Mycoplasma: Mycoplasma* pneumonia
- *Rickettsia:* Q fever, rickettsial pox, Rocky Mountain spotted fever, and typhus
- *Other bacteria:* acne, brucellosis, chancroid, cholera, granuloma inguinale, shigellosis, spirochetal relapsing fever, Lyme disease, *H. pylori* infections associated with peptic ulcer disease (used as part of the treatment regimen), syphilis (used as an alternative drug to treat patients with penicillin allergy); tetracyclines are now unreliable in treating gonorrhea due to the development of resistant bacterial strains
- *Protozoa:* balantidiasis

## Contraindications

The only usual contraindication is known drug allergy. However, tetracyclines must be avoided in pregnant and nursing women and not given to children younger than 8 years of age.

**BOX 38-1   AVAILABLE TETRACYCLINE ANTIBIOTICS**

demeclocycline
oxytetracycline
tetracycline
doxycycline
minocycline
tigecycline

## DOSAGES

### Selected Tetracyclines

| DRUG (PREGNANCY CATEGORY) | PHARMACOLOGIC CLASS | USUAL DOSAGE RANGE | INDICATIONS |
|---|---|---|---|
| demeclocycline (Declomycin) (D) | Tetracycline | **Adult** PO: 150 mg qid or 300 mg bid **Pediatric older than 8 yr\*** 7-13 mg/kg divided bid-qid | Infections; provides broad antibacterial coverage, including treatment of skin infections and respiratory, GI, and GU tract infections |
| ◆ doxycycline (Vibramycin, others) (D) | Tetracycline | **Adult** PO: 100 mg bid first day, then 100 mg daily thereafter **Pediatric older than 8 yr\*** PO/IV: 2.2-4.4 mg/kg/day in 1-2 divided doses | Comparable to those for demeclocycline |
| tigecycline (Tygacil) (D) | Glycylcycline | **Adult** IV: 100 mg × 1, then 50 mg q12h | Skin and skin structure infections, MRSA infections, intraabdominal infections |

*GI*, Gastrointestinal; *GU*, genitourinary; *IV*, intravenous; *MRSA*, methicillin-resistant *Staphylococcus aureus*; *PO*, oral.
\*Use of tetracyclines is contraindicated in children younger than 8 years of age and in pregnant women because of the risk of significant tooth discoloration in children.

## Adverse Effects

All tetracyclines cause similar adverse effects. They can cause discoloration of the permanent teeth and tooth enamel hypoplasia in both fetuses and children and possibly retard fetal skeletal development if taken during pregnancy. Other clinically significant undesirable effects include photosensitivity, which is most frequent in patients taking demeclocycline; alteration of the intestinal and vaginal flora, which can result in diarrhea or vaginal candidiasis; reversible bulging fontanelles in neonates; thrombocytopenia, possible coagulation irregularities, and hemolytic anemia; and exacerbation of systemic lupus erythematosus. Other effects include gastric upset, enterocolitis, and maculopapular rash.

## Interactions

There are several significant drug interactions associated with the use of tetracyclines. When tetracyclines are taken with antacids, antidiarrheal drugs, dairy products, calcium, enteral feedings, or iron preparations, the oral absorption of the tetracycline is reduced. Tetracyclines can potentiate the effects of oral anticoagulants, which necessitates more frequent monitoring of anticoagulant effect and possible dosage adjustment. They can also antagonize the effects of bactericidal antibiotics and oral contraceptives. In addition, depending on the dosage, they can cause blood urea nitrogen levels to be increased.

## Dosages

For dosage information on selected tetracyclines, see the table on this page.

## DRUG PROFILES

Tetracyclines were one of the first classes of antibiotic capable of providing coverage against a broad spectrum of microorganisms. Their use is contraindicated in patients who have had hypersensitivity reactions to them in the past and in lactating women. Resistance to one tetracycline implies resistance to all tetracyclines.

### demeclocycline

Demeclocycline (Declomycin) is a naturally occurring tetracycline antibiotic that is derived from strains of *Streptomyces*. It is used both for its antibacterial action and for its ability to inhibit the action of antidiuretic hormone in SIADH. Demeclocycline has all the characteristics of this class of tetracyclines. It is available only for oral use.

### ◆ doxycycline

Doxycycline (Doryx) is a semisynthetic tetracycline antibiotic. It is useful in the treatment of rickettsial infections such as Rocky Mountain spotted fever, chlamydial and mycoplasmal infections, spirochetal infections, and many infections with gram-negative organisms. It can also be used for the prevention and treatment of anthrax and malaria. Doxycycline may also be used in the treatment of acne. It is available in both oral and injectable forms.

### Pharmacokinetics

| Route | Onset of Action | Peak Plasma Concentration | Elimination Half-life | Duration of Action |
|---|---|---|---|---|
| PO | Variable | 1.5-4 hr | 14-24 hr | Up to 10-12 hr |

### tigecycline

Tigecycline (Tygacil) is the newest tetracycline, referred to as a *glycylcycline*. It differs from other tetracyclines in that it is effective against many organisms resistant to others in its class. It is indicated for the treatment of complicated skin and skin structure infections caused by susceptible organisms, including MRSA and vancomycin-sensitive *Enterococcus faecalis*, and for the treatment of complicated intraabdominal infections. Tigecycline is given by injection only. Nausea and vomiting are the most common adverse effects, occurring in 20% to 30% of patients.

### Pharmacokinetics

| Route | Onset of Action | Peak Plasma Concentration | Elimination Half-life | Duration of Action |
|---|---|---|---|---|
| IV | Immediate | Immediate after infusion | 27 hr | 12 hr |

The remaining antibiotic classes are discussed in Chapter 39.

# NURSING PROCESS

## ASSESSMENT

In general, before the administration of any *antibiotic,* it is crucial to gather data regarding a history of or symptoms indicative of hypersensitivity or allergic reactions (from mild reactions with rash, pruritus, or hives to severe reactions with laryngeal edema, bronchospasm, hypotension, and possible cardiac arrest). Also, determine the patient's age, weight, and baseline vital signs with body temperature. Examine the results of any laboratory tests that have been ordered, such as liver function studies (AST and ALT levels), kidney function studies (usually BUN and creatinine levels), cardiac function studies (pertinent laboratory tests, electrocardiogram), ultrasonography (if indicated), culture and sensitivity tests, CBC, and platelet and clotting tests. Assess intake and output measurements, if appropriate (e.g., more than 30 mL/hr or 600 mL/day). Record baseline neurologic assessment findings because of the possibility of CNS adverse effects from the various antibiotics. Assess bowel sounds and patterns because of potential antibiotic-related GI tract adverse effects. Further assessment needs to include checking for contraindications, cautions, and drug interactions. Obtain a complete list of all medications, including over-the-counter drugs, herbals, and dietary supplements. Cultural assessment is also important because of the well-documented variations in responses among different racial and ethnic groups as well as some patients' use of folk remedies or alternative therapies to try and alleviate infections. Assess learning preparedness, willingness to learn, and educational level because of the importance of patient education to safe medication administration. Note baseline findings from assessment of the oral mucosa, respiratory tract, GI tract, and genitourinary tract because of the risk of superinfection in these areas. Superinfections are often evidenced by fever, lethargy, mouth sores, perineal itching, and other system-related symptoms. Because antibiotic resistance is so prevalent, pose questions about long-term use, overuse, or abuse of antibiotics to the patient or caregiver. Assessment information related to each group of antibiotics is presented in the following paragraphs.

For patients taking *sulfonamides,* a careful assessment for drug allergies to sulfa-type drugs and/or sulfites, such as oral sulfonylureas (antidiabetic drugs) and thiazide diuretics, is important to patient safety (see pharmacology discussion). Perform a thorough skin assessment during drug therapy because of the potential for occurrence of the adverse effect of Stevens-Johnson syndrome (see Table 38-2). Assess red blood cell count before beginning sulfonamide therapy because of the possibility of drug-related anemias. With frequent or long-term therapy, assess renal function due to the potential for drug-related crystalluria. Check the patient's medication and medical history for any manifestations of G6PD and slow acetylation (see Chapters 2 and 4).

With *penicillins,* because of the high incidence of hypersensitivity, determine if there are drug allergies before initiation

of therapy. Potential drug interactions are presented in Table 38-5. In addition, assess the patient for a history of asthma, sensitivity to multiple allergens, aspirin allergy, and sensitivity to cephalosporins, because these are associated with a higher risk for penicillin allergy. If procaine penicillin is to be given, also assess for procaine hypersensitivity. Note results of culture and sensitivity testing as soon as they are available to confirm the appropriateness of therapy. Because of possible CNS and/or GI adverse effects, complete a thorough neurologic, abdominal, and bowel assessment. Especially important for patients with electrolyte disturbances, cardiac disease, and/or renal disease is assessment of serum sodium and potassium levels, primarily because of the high sodium and potassium ion concentrations in some penicillin preparations. For example, penicillin G contains 1.7 mEq of potassium ion per million units and 2 mEq of sodium ion per million units. With these particular preparations, if a patient has heart failure, fluid overload, or cardiac dysrhythmias, a high sodium or potassium level (hypernatremia or hyperkalemia) can lead to exacerbation of these problems. With any dosage form of the penicillins, it is important to patient safety to assess for the possibility of an immediate, accelerated, or delayed allergic reaction. Also, assess the medication order and be aware that many times these drugs are referred to by their trade names and don't always end in *"cillin,"* such as with Zosyn and Augmentin (see the Safety and Quality Improvement: Preventing Medication Errors box).

With *cephalosporins,* conduct a thorough assessment of allergies, including allergy to penicillins, because of possible cross-sensitivity. Because of the similarity in their mechanism of action to penicillins, assessment data is also similar. Obtain information about the specific drug and note the generation of cephalosporins to which it belongs. Each of the five drug generations has distinctive adverse effects and/or complications in addition to commonalities with the other groups.

*Carbapenems* are used when there are complicated connective tissue infections in acutely ill patients who are hospitalized. Assess patients for a history of seizure activity because of the potential seizure-type, drug-induced reaction.

With *macrolides,* assessment of baseline cardiac function with documentation of vital signs is important because these drugs may lead to palpitations, chest pain, and ECG changes. Note baseline hearing status because of drug-induced hearing loss and tinnitus. Assess liver function and history of liver disease due to possible hepatotoxicity and jaundice. Drug interactions have been discussed previously, but special consideration should be given to concurrent use of a macrolide with warfarin, digoxin, or theophylline, resulting in possible toxicity of the latter drugs. Macrolides also reduce the effectiveness of oral contraceptives.

With *tetracyclines,* carefully assess culture and sensitivity reports as with all antibiotic therapy. There is concern regarding the use of these drugs in patients younger than 8 years of age because of the problem of permanent mottling and discoloration of the teeth. Use of these drugs in pregnancy may also pose problems for the fetus. Assess for any whitish sore patches on the oral

| BOX 38-2 | **BRIEF SUMMARY OF NURSING CONSIDERATIONS FOR ANTISEPTICS AND DISINFECTANTS** |
|---|---|

- Check for allergies to any of the chemicals or compounds contained in the antiseptic or disinfectant before use. These include alcohol, chlorine, and hydrogen peroxide.
- If the agent is iodine based (e.g., povidone-iodine), be sure to ask about any allergies to iodine or seafood. If allergies exist, then the agent must not be used. There is a higher risk for reactions to antiseptics if there have been previous allergic reactions to antibacterial topical drugs. Use of disinfectants may also be associated with allergic reactions.
- Research the product or chemical and be aware of specific instructions and application technique.
- Always follow Standard Precautions. Dispose of any soiled bandages in a biohazard bag.
- With antiseptics, always research the product and any special application instructions or directions. If the skin is intact, nonsterile gloves are recommended for use unless otherwise indicated. If integrity is broken and the skin is not intact, use sterile gloves and/or sterile technique.
- With antiseptics, cleanse the site of any debris (e.g., pus, drainage) and any residual medication. Use normal saline or lukewarm soap and water for cleansing. Use a tongue blade, cotton-tipped applicator, or gloved finger to apply the antiseptic solution or product. Document any unusual findings at the site of use, such as swelling, redness, or drainage.
- Always follow the instructions related to each specific disinfectant agent.
- Adverse effects of antiseptics may include excessive dryness of the skin, burns to the skin or mucous membranes, blistering, and skin staining.
- Instruct patients to report any increase in redness, drainage, pain, swelling, and/or fever associated with the use of antiseptics, as deemed appropriate.

mucosa (due to candidiasis or yeast infection) as well as any vaginal itching, pain, and/or cottage cheese–like discharge (due to vaginal candidiasis) for early identification and early treatment of superinfections (see previous discussion). Assess for significant drug interactions, including simultaneous use of antacids, antidiarrheal drugs, dairy products, calcium, enteral feedings, and iron preparations. These medications may lead to reduced absorption of the tetracycline. Tetracyclines may also decrease the effectiveness of oral contraceptives. Assess the patient taking oral anticoagulants more closely due to possible potentiation of bleeding.

Antiseptics and disinfectants have also been put in this chapter. See Box 38-2 for a brief summary of nursing-related considerations for these agents.

# NURSING DIAGNOSES

1. Noncompliance with the treatment regimen related to lack of information and/or inability to pay for and obtain the necessary medication
2. Deficient knowledge related to lack of information about the disease process and the medication regimen
3. Risk for infection related to the patient's possible development of a compromised immune status (due to use of sulfonamides)

# PLANNING

## GOALS

1. Patient remains compliant with the antibiotic therapy regimen for the full duration of treatment.
2. Patient demonstrates an increase in knowledge and information about the disease process and related drug therapy.
3. Patient maintains homeostasis and a healthy immune system, and is free from risk for infection.

## OUTCOME CRITERIA

1. Patient describes the rationale for the specific antibiotic therapeutic regimen, associated adverse effects, as well as measures to decrease these adverse effects.
   - Patient takes specific antibiotic with attention to instructions about whether to take with meals and/or increased fluids and foods, medications, and beverages to avoid while on antibiotic regimen.
   - Patient briefly describes the importance to therapeutic effectiveness of taking the antibiotic for the duration of therapy and as prescribed.
2. Patient takes medication exactly as prescribed and for the full time prescribed.
   - Patient understands the importance to therapeutic effectiveness of taking the medication exactly as prescribed and until the full prescription is taken.
   - Patient reports adverse effects that are unresolved and are of concern such as jaundice, excessive fatigue, elevated temperature, increase in pain associated with the infection, and severe GI distress, nausea, or diarrhea.

3. Patient remains free of elevated WBC count and maintains temperature, pulse rate, and respiratory rate within normal ranges with negative culture and sensitivity reports.

# IMPLEMENTATION

General nursing interventions that apply to antibiotics include the following: (1) Give oral antibiotics within the recommended time frames and fluids/foods as indicated. (2) All medication is to be taken as ordered and in full and around the clock to maintain effective blood levels unless otherwise instructed by the prescriber. (3) Doses are not to be omitted or doubled up. (4) Oral antibiotics are not to be given at the same time as antacids, calcium supplements, iron products, laxatives containing magnesium, or some of the antilipemic drugs (see pharmacology listing of drug interactions). (5) Herbal products and dietary supplements are to be used only if they do not interact with the antibiotic. (6) Continually monitor for hypersensitivity reactions past the initial assessment phase because immediate reactions may not occur for up to 30 minutes, accelerated reactions may occur within 1 to 72 hours, and delayed responses may occur after 72 hours. These are characterized by wheezing; shortness of breath; swelling of the face, tongue, or hands; itching; or rash. (7) If there are signs of a possible hypersensitivity reaction, the first thing to do is stop the dosage form immediately (if IV, stop the infusion), contact the prescriber, and monitor the patient closely.

*Sulfonamides* need to be avoided in patients with G6PD and slow acetylation. Encourage forcing of fluids (2000 to 3000 mL/24 hr) to prevent drug-related crystalluria. Oral dosage forms are to be taken with food to minimize GI upset. Encourage patients to immediately report the following to the prescriber: worsening abdominal cramps, stomach pain, diarrhea, blood in the urine, severe or worsening rash, shortness of breath, and fever. These may indicate adverse reactions to these drugs; remember that the mucocutaneous, GI, hepatic, and hematologic complications may be of a fatal nature.

With *penicillins,* as with other antibiotics, the natural flora in the GI tract may be killed off by the antibiotic. Unaffected GI bacteria such as *C. difficile* may overgrow (see pharmacology discussion for more information). This process may be prevented by the consumption of probiotics, such as products containing *Lactobacillus,* supplements, or cultured dairy products like yogurt, buttermilk, and kefir. Kefir is prepared using milk from sheep, goats, and cows. Soy milk kefirs are now also commercially available. Keep in mind the following important points when giving various penicillin formulations: (1) Advise patients to take oral penicillins with at least 6 oz of water (not juices); juices are acidic fluids and may nullify the drug's antibacterial action. (2) Penicillin V, amoxicillin, and amoxicillin/clavulanate are given with water and 1 hour before or 2 hours after meals to maximize absorption; however, because of GI upset, these medications may need to be taken with a snack or meals. (3) Procaine and benzathine salt penicillins are thick solutions; give them as ordered IM, using at least a 21-gauge needle, and into a large muscle mass, rotating sites as needed. (4) Reconstitute IM imipenem/cilastatin in sterile saline, with plain lidocaine—as ordered and if the patient has no allergy to it—give into a large muscle

mass. (5) With IV penicillins (e.g., ampicillin), as with any IV therapy, use the proper diluent and infuse the medication over the recommended time. Monitor the IV site frequently for swelling, tenderness, heat, redness, leaking, and pain. Calculate IV rates to deliver the prescribed amount per minute/hour. Change IV sites per facility protocol. (6) Check for compatibilities of IV fluids and drugs prior to infusion. (7) If the patient experiences an anaphylactic reaction to a penicillin (or any drug), give epinephrine and other emergency drugs as ordered, and have supportive treatment (e.g., oxygen) available at all times.

Orally administered *cephalosporins* may be given with food to decrease GI upset. Alcohol and alcohol-containing products are to be avoided due to the potentiation of a disulfiram-like reaction (known as *acute alcohol intolerance*) with some of the cephalosporins. This may occur up to 72 hours after taking cefotetan. Symptoms that may occur include stomach cramping, nausea, vomiting, headache, diaphoresis, pruritus, and hypotension. With the newer cephalosporins, as with many drug groups, check the drug names carefully to ensure patient safety. Many drug names sound alike, and this could lead to medication errors.

*Macrolides* need to be administered with the same precautions as used with other antibiotics. Macrolides are *not* to be given with or immediately before or after fruit juices to avoid interaction with the drug. Inform the patient about the many drug interactions (discussed in the pharmacology section), including those with over-the-counter drugs, herbal products, and dietary supplements. Encourage patients to report the following to their prescriber immediately: chest pain, palpitations, dizziness, jaundice, rash, and hearing loss.

*Tetracyclines* cause photosensitivity, so advise the patient to take precautions to avoid sun exposure and tanning bed use. Encourage the patient to take oral doses with at least 8 oz of fluids and food to minimize GI upset. However, warn the patient *not* to take tetracyclines with calcium, magnesium, and iron. These chemicals *chelate* or bind with the tetracycline, leading to a significant reduction in the oral absorption, and thus the effectiveness, of this group of antibiotics. Therefore, concurrent use of dairy products, antacids, or iron needs to be avoided. The patient may take these interacting foods and drugs 2 hours before or 3 hours after the tetracycline to avoid this interaction. IV doxycycline is very irritating to the veins, so check the IV infusion site frequently. Remember that tetracyclines can cause discoloration of the permanent teeth and tooth enamel in fetuses and children. They may also retard fetal skeletal growth if taken during pregnancy. Continually monitor for diarrhea or vaginal yeast infections due to altered intestinal and/or vaginal flora.

# EVALUATION

Include monitoring of goals, outcome criteria, therapeutic effects, and adverse effects in the evaluation. Therapeutic effects of *antibiotics* include a decrease in the signs and symptoms of the infection; a return to normal vital signs, including temperature; negative results on culture and sensitivity tests; normal results for CBC; and improved appetite, energy level, and sense of well-being. Evaluation for adverse effects includes monitoring for specific drug-related adverse effects (see each drug profile).

## PATIENT TEACHING TIPS

- Provide the patient with a list of foods and beverages that may interact negatively with antibiotics, such as alcohol, acidic fruit juices, and dairy products.
- Advise the patient to report severe adverse effects to the prescriber and to keep any follow-up visits so that the effectiveness of therapy may be monitored. Laboratory tests (e.g., CBC) may also be performed at these visits.
- Foods that may help prevent superinfections (e.g., vaginal yeast infections) include yogurt, buttermilk, and kefir. New yogurts, termed *probiotics*, are available for reestablishing the natural flora of the GI tract.
- Educate patients who are taking oral contraceptives for birth control, about the interactions between them and certain antibiotics. This is because the effectiveness of oral contraceptives may be decreased with certain antibiotics. Reliable backup methods of contraception must be used in addition to the oral contraception during antibiotic use.
- Recommend wearing of a medical alert bracelet or necklace if there are drug allergies, especially if anaphylactic in nature. It is recommended that drug allergy information and a listing of medical diagnoses and list of all medications be kept on the patient's person at all times.
- For *sulfonamides*, the medication is to be taken with plenty of fluids (2000 to 3000 mL/24 hr) and taken with food to decrease GI adverse effects.
- For *penicillins*, medications are to be taken exactly as prescribed and for the full duration indicated, as with all antibiotics. Doses are to be spaced at regularly scheduled intervals. Instruct the patient to take oral dosage forms with water, avoiding the following beverages: caffeine-containing beverages, citrus fruit, cola beverages, fruit juices, and tomato juice (decrease effectiveness of the antibiotic). If the patient must take a penicillin drug four times a day, encourage the patient to set up a reminder system (with cell phone alarms or a watch) so that blood levels remain steady.
- For *cephalosporins*, advise the patient to report unresolved GI upset, such as diarrhea and nausea. Alcohol must be avoided.
- For *tetracyclines*, advise patients to avoid exposure to tanning beds and direct sunlight or to use sunscreen and/or wear protective clothing because of drug-related photosensitivity. These photosensitive effects may be noticed within a few minutes to hours after taking the drug and may last up to several days after the drug has been discontinued.
- For *macrolides*, instruct the patient to take the drug as directed, and check for interactions with other drugs being taken at the same time, especially interactions between erythromycin and other medications. For some drugs in this class (e.g., azithromycin), newer dosage forms are available in 3-day and 1-day dose packs rather than the 5-day dose pack. Always be sure that the patient knows the proper dosage and instructions for the drug the patient is taking.

## KEY POINTS

- Antibiotics are either bacteriostatic or bactericidal. Bacteriostatic antibiotics inhibit the growth of bacteria but do not directly kill them. Bactericidal antibiotics directly kill the bacteria.
- Most antibiotics work by inhibiting bacterial cell wall synthesis in some way. Bacteria have survived over the ages because they can adapt to their surroundings. If a bacterium's environment includes an antibiotic, over time it can mutate in such a way that it can survive an attack by the antibiotic. The production of beta-lactamases is one way in which bacteria can fend off the effects of antibiotics.
- Be aware of the most common adverse effects of antibiotics, which include nausea, vomiting, and diarrhea. Inform patients that antibiotics should be taken for the prescribed length of time.
- Each class of antibiotics is associated with specific cautions, contraindications, drug interactions, and adverse effects that must be carefully assessed for and monitored by the nurse.
- Because normally occurring bacteria are killed during antibiotic therapy, superinfections may arise during treatment. These may be manifested by the following signs and symptoms: fever, perineal itching, oral lesions, vaginal irritation and discharge, cough, and lethargy.

## NCLEX® EXAMINATION REVIEW QUESTIONS

1  A patient is scheduled for colorectal surgery tomorrow. He does not have sepsis, his WBC count is normal, he has no fever, and he is otherwise in good health. However, there is an order to administer an antibiotic on call before he goes to surgery. The nurse knows that the rationale for this antibiotic order is to
   a   provide empiric therapy.
   b   provide prophylactic therapy.
   c   treat for a superinfection.
   d   reduce the number of resistant organisms.

2  A teenage patient is taking a tetracycline drug as part of treatment for severe acne. When the nurse teaches this patient about drug-related precautions, which is the most important information to convey?
   a   When the acne clears up, the medication may be discontinued.
   b   This medication needs to be taken with antacids to reduce GI upset.
   c   The patient needs to use sunscreen or avoid exposure to sunlight, because this drug may cause photosensitivity.
   d   The teeth should be observed closely for signs of mottling or other color changes.

3  A newly admitted patient reports a penicillin allergy. The prescriber has ordered a second-generation cephalosporin as part of the therapy. Which nursing action is appropriate?
   a   Call the prescriber to clarify the order because of the patient's allergy.
   b   Give the medication, and monitor for adverse effects.
   c   Ask the pharmacy to change the order to a first-generation cephalosporin.
   d   Administer the drug with a nonsteroidal antiinflammatory drug to reduce adverse effects.

4  During patient education regarding an oral macrolide such as erythromycin, the nurse will include which information?
   a   If GI upset occurs, the drug will have to be stopped.
   b   The drug needs to be taken with an antacid to avoid GI problems.
   c   The patient needs to take each dose with a sip of water.
   d   The patient may take the drug with a small snack to reduce GI irritation.

5  A woman who has been taking an antibiotic for a UTI calls the nurse practitioner to complain of severe vaginal itching. She has also noticed a thick, whitish vaginal discharge. The nurse practitioner suspects that
   a   this is an expected response to antibiotic therapy.
   b   the UTI has become worse instead of better.
   c   a superinfection has developed.
   d   the UTI is resistant to the antibiotic.

6  The nurse is reviewing the orders for wound care, which include use of an antiseptic. Which statements best describe the use of antiseptics? (Select all that apply.)
   a   Antiseptics are appropriate for use on living tissue.
   b   Antiseptics work by sterilizing the surface of the wound.
   c   Antiseptics are applied to nonliving objects to kill microorganisms.
   d   The patient's allergies must be assessed before using the antiseptic.
   e   Antiseptics are used to inhibit the growth of microorganisms on the wound surface.

7  The order for a child reads: "Give cefoxitin (Mefoxin) 160 mg/kg/day, IVPB, divided into doses given every 6 hours." The child weighs 55 lb. How much will the patient receive each day? For each dose?

1. b, 2. c, 3. a, 4. d, 5. c, 6. a, d, e, 7. 4000 mg/day; 1000 mg/dose

For Critical Thinking and Prioritization Questions, see http://evolve.elsevier.com/Lilley.

# Antibiotics Part 2

## OBJECTIVES

When you reach the end of this chapter, you will be able to do the following:

1 Review the general principles of antibiotic therapy and all of the antibiotics covered previously in Chapter 38 in preparation for discussion of the following antibiotics or antibiotic classes: aminoglycosides, quinolones, clindamycin, metronidazole, nitrofurantoin, vancomycin, and several other miscellaneous antibiotics.

2 Describe the advantages and disadvantages associated with the use of antibiotics, including overuse and abuse of antibiotics, development of drug resistance, superinfections, and antibiotic-associated colitis.

3 Discuss the indications, cautions, contraindications, mechanisms of action, adverse effects, toxic effects, routes of administration, and drug interactions for the aminoglycosides, fluoroquinolones, clindamycin, metronidazole, nitrofurantoin, vancomycin, and miscellaneous antibiotics.

4 Develop a nursing care plan that includes all phases of the nursing process for the patient receiving antibiotics.

## DRUG PROFILES

amikacin, p. 638
♦ ciprofloxacin, p. 640
♦ clindamycin, p. 640
colistimethate, p. 643
daptomycin, p. 643
♦ gentamicin, p. 638
levofloxacin, p. 640
linezolid, p. 641

♦ metronidazole, p. 642
neomycin, p. 638
nitrofurantoin, p. 642
quinupristin/dalfopristin, p. 642
telavancin, p. 644
tobramycin, p. 638
♦ vancomycin, p. 643

♦ *Key drug*

## KEY TERMS

**Concentration-dependent killing** A property of some antibiotics, especially aminoglycosides, whereby achieving high plasma drug concentrations, even if briefly, results in the most effective bacterial kill (compare *time-dependent killing*). (p. 635)

**Extended-spectrum beta-lactamases (ESBLs)** A group of beta-lactamase enzymes produced by some organisms that makes the organism resistant to all beta-lactam antibiotics (penicillins and cephalosporins) and aztreonam. Patients who are infected by such organisms must be in contact isolation;

proper handwashing is key to preventing the spread of these organisms. (p. 634)

***Klebsiella pneumoniae* carbapenemase (KPC)** An enzyme first found in isolates of the bacterium *Klebsiella pneumoniae* that renders the organism resistant to all carbapenem antibiotics as well as beta-lactam antibiotics and monobactams. Such organisms produce a very serious resistant infection. (p. 634)

**Methicillin-resistant *Staphylococcus aureus* (MRSA)** A strain of *Staphylococcus aureus* that is resistant to the beta-lactamase penicillin known as *methicillin*. Originally, the abbreviation MRSA referred exclusively to methicillin-resistant *S. aureus*. It is now used more commonly to refer to strains of *S. aureus* that are resistant to several drug classes, and therefore, depending on the context or health facility, it may also stand for "multidrug-resistant *S. aureus*." (p. 634)

**Microgram** One millionth of a gram. Be careful not to confuse it with milligram (one thousandth of a gram), which is one thousand times greater than 1 microgram. Confusion of these two units sometimes results in drug dosage errors. (p. 635)

**Minimum inhibitory concentration (MIC)** A laboratory measure of the lowest concentration of a drug needed to kill a certain standardized amount of bacteria. (p. 635)

**Multidrug-resistant organisms** Bacteria that are resistant to one or more classes of antimicrobial drugs. These include multidrug-resistant *Staphylococcus aureus*, extended-spectrum beta-lactamase–producing organisms, and *Klebsiella pneumoniae* carbapenemase–producing organisms. (p. 634)

**Nephrotoxicity** Toxicity to the kidneys, often drug induced and manifesting as compromised renal function; usually reversible upon withdrawal of the offending drug. (p. 635)

**Ototoxicity** Toxicity to the ears, often drug induced and manifesting as varying degrees of hearing loss that is likely to be permanent. (p. 635)

**Postantibiotic effect** A period of continued bacterial suppression that occurs after brief exposure to certain antibiotic drug classes, especially aminoglycosides (discussed in this chapter) and carbapenems (see Chapter 38). The mechanism of this effect is uncertain. (p. 636)

**Pseudomembranous colitis** A necrotizing inflammatory bowel condition that is often associated with antibiotic therapy. Some antibiotics (e.g., clindamycin) are more likely to produce it than others. More commonly referred to as *antibiotic-associated colitis* or *Clostridium difficile diarrhea* or *C. difficile infection*. (p. 641)

**Synergistic effect** Drug interaction in which the bacterial killing effect of two antibiotics given together is greater than the sum of the individual effects of the same drugs given alone. (p. 636)

**Therapeutic drug monitoring** Ongoing monitoring of plasma drug concentrations and dosage adjustment based on these values as well as other laboratory indicators such as kidney and liver function test results; it is often carried out by a pharmacist in collaboration with medical, nursing, and laboratory staff. (p. 635)

**Time-dependent killing** A property of most antibiotic classes whereby prolonged high plasma drug concentrations are required for effective bacterial kill (compare *concentration-dependent killing*). (p. 635)

**Vancomycin-resistant *Enterococcus* (VRE)** *Enterococcus* species that are resistant to beta-lactam antibiotics and vancomycin. Most commonly refers to *Enterococcus faecium*. (p. 634)

---

This chapter is a continuation of Chapter 38 and focuses on additional classes of antibiotics, which are used for more serious and harder-to-treat infections. Most of the drugs discussed in this chapter are given by the *parenteral* (injection) route only, a route generally reserved for treating more clinically serious infections. Also included are miscellaneous drugs that are unique in their class, as well as newer drugs and drug classes. This chapter also focuses on multidrug-resistant organisms, specifically methicillin-resistant *Staphylococcus aureus* (MRSA), vancomycin-resistant *Enterococcus* (VRE), organisms producing extended-spectrum beta-lactamases (ESBLs), and organisms producing *Klebsiella pneumoniae* carbapenemase (KPC).

## PATHOPHYSIOLOGY OF RESISTANT INFECTIONS

Organisms that are resistant to one or more classes of antimicrobial drugs are referred to as multidrug-resistant organisms. These include MRSA, VRE, and ESBL- and KPC-producing

organisms. MRSA has been around for many years, and fortunately new antibiotics have been developed to treat MRSA. However, the threat of MRSA becoming resistant to all antibiotics currently available is all too real. MRSA is no longer seen just in hospitals; it has spread to the community setting, and approximately 50% of staphylococcal infections contracted in the community involve MRSA, depending on location. Local community and hospital MRSA strains vary. VRE is usually seen in urinary tract infections. Some newer antibiotics have been developed to successfully treat VRE, as well as MRSA. Unfortunately, ESBL- and KPC-producing bacteria are the newest players in this saga. Organisms that produce ESBL are resistant to all beta-lactam antibiotics and aztreonam, and can be treated only with carbapenems or sometimes quinolones. In our noble effort to treat infection with ESBL-producing organisms, the use of carbapenems increased, and unfortunately in response, bacteria created a new means of resistance, namely, the ability to produce KPC. When patients become infected with KPC-producing bacteria, there are only two known antibiotics that can be used, tigecycline and colistimethate. Reports of resistance to these antibiotics have been described, which leaves the patient untreatable. Multidrug-resistant organisms are one of the world's top health problems. When patients become infected with such an organism, they must be placed in contact isolation. Many hospitals are placing all patients infected with KPC-producing bacteria in one area, and some hospitals have been shut down due to this organism. Proper handwashing is of the utmost importance. These organisms are spread by contact, so all health care professionals must wash their hands before and after all patient contact. Some research indicates that patterns of antibiotic resistance for a certain class of antibiotics are influenced by the prescription of antibiotics in other, previously-assumed unrelated classes. (For example, quinolone use may influence the emergence of resistance to other antibiotic classes.)

## PHARMACOLOGY OVERVIEW

### AMINOGLYCOSIDES

The aminoglycosides are a group of natural and semisynthetic antibiotics that are classified as bactericidal drugs (see Chapter 38). They are potent antibiotics, which makes aminoglycosides the drugs of choice for the treatment of particularly virulent infections. The aminoglycoside antibiotics available for clinical use are listed in Table 39-1. These drugs can be given by several different routes, but they are not given orally because of their poor oral absorption. An exception to this is neomycin (see Drug Profiles). The three aminoglycosides most commonly used for the treatment of systemic infections are amikacin, gentamicin, and tobramycin. Serum levels of these drugs are routinely monitored in patients' blood samples. Dosages are adjusted to maintain known optimal levels that maximize drug efficacy and minimize the risk for toxicity. This process is known as therapeutic drug monitoring. Aminoglycoside therapy is monitored in this way due to the nephrotoxicity and ototoxicity associated with these drugs. Most commonly, dosing is adjusted to the patient's level of renal function, based on estimates of creatinine clearance calculated from serum creatinine values. This task is often carried out by a hospital pharmacist, consulting for the prescriber. Not only are serum levels measured to prevent toxicity, but it has been shown that for the aminoglycosides to be effective, the serum level needs to be at least eight times higher than the minimum inhibitory concentration (MIC). The MIC for any antibiotic is a measure of the lowest concentration of drug needed to kill a certain standard amount of bacteria. This value is determined *in vitro* (in the laboratory) for each drug. It has been shown that other classes of antibiotics, such as beta-lactams, act through time-dependent killing, that is, the amount of time the drug is above the MIC is critical for maximal bacterial kill. However, aminoglycosides work primarily through concentration-dependent killing; that is, achieving a drug plasma concentration that is a certain level above the MIC, even for a brief period of time, results in the most effective bacterial kill. For this reason, although these drugs were originally given in three daily intravenous doses, the current predominant practice is once-daily aminoglycoside dosing. Dosages of 5 to 7 mg/kg/day are used. Several clinical studies have shown that once-daily dosing provides a sufficient plasma drug concentration for bacterial kill, along with equal or lower risk for toxicity compared with multiple daily dosing regimens. Use of a once-daily regimen instead of the traditional three-times-daily regimen also reduces the nursing care time required and often allows for outpatient or even home-based aminoglycoside drug therapy.

Peak (highest) drug levels for once-daily regimens are usually not measured as it is assumed that the peak level for a single daily dose will be short lived and will drop within a reasonable time frame. However, trough (lowest) levels are routinely measured to ensure adequate renal clearance of the drug and avoid toxicity. For dosage information on selected aminoglycosides, see the table on p. 637. Dosage regimens and ranges for serum levels may vary for different institutions.

With once-daily dosing, the blood sample for trough measurement is drawn at least 8 to 12 hours after completion of dose administration. The therapeutic goal is a trough concentration at or below 1 mcg/mL (which is considered undetectable). Trough levels above 2 mcg/mL are associated with greater risk for both *ototoxicity* and *nephrotoxicity*. Ototoxicity (toxicity to the ears) often manifests as some degree of temporary or permanent hearing loss. Nephrotoxicity (toxicity to the kidneys) manifests as varying degrees of reduced renal function. This is generally indicated by laboratory test results such as serum creatinine level. A rising serum creatinine level suggests reduced creatinine clearance by the kidneys and is indicative of declining renal function. Trough levels are normally monitored initially, and then once every 5 to 7 days until drug therapy is discontinued. The patient's serum creatinine level is measured at least every 3 days as an index of renal function,

| SERUM DRUG LEVELS | PEAK | | TROUGH | |
|---|---|---|---|---|
| | MULTIPLE DAILY DOSING* | ONCE-DAILY DOSING | MULTIPLE DAILY DOSING | ONCE-DAILY DOSING |
| amikacin | 15-30 mcg/mL† | Usually not measured | 5-10 mcg/mL | Less than 10 mcg/mL |
| gentamicin and tobramycin | 4-10 mcg/mL | Usually not measured | 1-2 mcg/mL | Less than 1 mcg/mL |

**TABLE 39-1  AMINOGLYCOSIDE ANTIBIOTICS**

*q8h or q12h.
†*mcg, microgram*; note that 1 microgram = 1/1000 (one thousandth) of a milligram or 1/1,000,000 (one millionth) of a gram. Also note that microgram is abbreviated *mcg*, while milligram is abbreviated *mg*.

and drug dosages are adjusted as needed for any changes in renal function.

Traditional dosing of aminoglycosides (i.e., three times a day) can still be used. When an aminoglycoside is given in this manner, both peak and trough levels are measured. Samples for measurement of peak levels are drawn 30 minutes after a 30-minute infusion, and samples for measurement of trough levels are drawn just before the next dose. Pharmacists can adjust the dose based on a pharmacokinetic evaluation of these levels. When the drug is given in the traditional manner, the desired peak levels vary depending on the type of organism and the site of infection. Higher levels are needed when treating pneumonia, as opposed to treating a urinary tract infection. Because the aminoglycosides are eliminated by the kidney, the drug concentrates in the urine, so lower dosages can be used to treat urinary tract infections. Regardless of the infection being treated, however, it is desirable to keep the trough levels below 2 mcg/mL. Table 39-1 lists the traditional desired drug levels for these drugs.

## Mechanism of Action and Drug Effects

Aminoglycosides work in a way that is similar to that of the tetracyclines in that they bind to ribosomes, specifically the 30S ribosome, and thereby prevent protein synthesis in bacteria (see Figure 38-3). Aminoglycosides are most often used in combination with other antibiotics such as beta-lactams or vancomycin in the treatment of various infections, because the combined effect of the two antibiotics is greater than the sum of the effects of each drug acting separately. This is known as a synergistic effect. When aminoglycosides are used in combination with beta-lactam antibiotics (i.e., penicillins, cephalosporins, monobactams [see Chapter 38]), the beta-lactam antibiotic is given first. This is because the beta-lactams break down the cell wall of the bacteria and allow the aminoglycoside to gain access to the ribosomes where they work. Aminoglycosides also have a property known as the postantibiotic effect. This is a period of continued bacterial growth suppression that occurs *after* short-term antibiotic exposure, as in once-daily aminoglycoside dosing (see earlier). Carbapenems are another antibiotic class with a postantibiotic effect. The postantibiotic effect is enhanced with higher peak drug concentrations and concurrent use of beta-lactam antibiotics.

As is the case with most antibiotic drug classes, various bacterial mechanisms of resistance to aminoglycosides have emerged among both gram-positive and gram-negative species previously more susceptible to these drugs. The prevalence and strength of such resistance varies for different drugs, organisms, patient populations, disease states, and geographic prescribing patterns.

## Indications

The toxicity associated with aminoglycosides limits their use to treatment of serious gram-negative infections and specific conditions involving gram-positive cocci, in which case gentamicin is usually given in combination with a penicillin. Gram-negative infections commonly treated with aminoglycosides include those caused by *Pseudomonas* species (spp.) and several organisms belonging to the Enterobacteriaceae family (facultatively anaerobic gram-negative rods), including *Escherichia coli*, *Proteus* spp., *Klebsiella* spp., and *Serratia* spp. Such infections are often treated with a suitable aminoglycoside and an extended-spectrum penicillin, third-generation cephalosporin, or carbapenem. Gram-positive infections treated with aminoglycosides may include infections due to *Enterococcus* spp. and *S. aureus,* and bacterial endocarditis, which is usually streptococcal in origin. A regimen of three daily doses is more common when treating gram-positive infections, because this often enhances synergy with other antibiotics that are used. Aminoglycosides are never used alone to treat gram-positive infections. Aminoglycosides are also used for prophylaxis in procedures involving the gastrointestinal (GI) or genitourinary (GU) tract, because such procedures carry a high risk for enterococcal bacteremia. They are also commonly given in combination with either ampicillin or vancomycin (for penicillin-allergic patients) to surgical patients with a history of valvular heart disease, because diseased heart valves are also more prone to enterococcal infection.

Aminoglycosides are to be administered with caution in premature and full-term neonates. Because of the renal immaturity of these patients, prolonged actions of the aminoglycosides and a greater risk for toxicities may result. Serious pediatric infections for which aminoglycosides are used include pneumonia, meningitis, and urinary tract infections. Drug selection for both pediatric and adult patients is based on the susceptibility of the causative organism. Refer to Table 39-2 for more information on the antibacterial spectra of specific aminoglycosides. A few aminoglycosides have more specific indications. Streptomycin is active against *Mycobacterium* spp. (see Chapter 41), whereas paromomycin is used to treat amebic dysentery, a protozoal intestinal disease (see Chapter 43).

| TABLE 39-2 | AMINOGLYCOSIDES: COMPARATIVE SPECTRA OF ANTIMICROBIAL ACTIVITY | |
|---|---|
| **AMINOGLYCOSIDE** | **SPECTRUM OF ACTIVITY** |
| amikacin | *Acinetobacter* spp., *Enterobacter aerogenes*, *Escherichia coli*, *Klebsiella pneumoniae*, *Proteus* spp., *Providencia* spp., *Pseudomonas* spp., *Serratia* spp., *Staphylococcus* |
| gentamicin | *E. aerogenes*, *E. coli*, *K. pneumoniae*, *Proteus* spp., *Pseudomonas* spp., *Salmonella* spp., *Serratia* spp. (nonpigmented), *Shigella* spp. |
| neomycin | Toxicity limits use to gastrointestinal tract (hepatic coma, *E. coli* diarrhea, and antisepsis) and as a topical antibacterial |
| streptomycin | *Klebsiella granulomatis* (granuloma inguinale), *Yersinia pestis* (plague), *Francisella tularensis* (tularemia), *Mycobacterium tuberculosis* (tuberculosis), *Streptococcus* spp. (nonhemolytic endocarditis) |
| tobramycin | *Citrobacter* spp., *Enterobacter* spp., *E. coli*, *Klebsiella* spp., *Proteus* spp., *Providencia* spp., *P. aeruginosa*, *Serratia* spp. |

*GI,* Gastrointestinal; *spp.,* species.

Aminoglycosides are inactive against fungi, viruses, and most anaerobic bacteria.

## Contraindications

The only usual contraindication is known drug allergy. The pregnancy categories of these drugs range from C to D. Aminoglycosides have been shown to cross the placenta and cause fetal harm when administered to pregnant women. There have been several case reports of total irreversible bilateral congenital deafness in the children of women receiving aminoglycosides during pregnancy. Therefore, aminoglycosides are used in pregnant women only in the event of life-threatening infections when safer drugs are ineffective. These drugs are also distributed in breast milk. They should not be used by lactating women to avoid the risk of drug toxicity in nursing infants.

## Adverse Effects

Aminoglycosides are very potent antibiotics and are capable of potentially serious toxicities, especially to the kidneys (nephrotoxicity) and to the ears (ototoxicity), in which they can affect hearing and balance functions. Duration of drug therapy needs to be as short as possible, based on sound clinical judgment and monitoring of the patient's progress. Nephrotoxicity typically occurs in 5% to 25% of patients and is usually manifested by urinary casts (visible remnants of destroyed renal cells), proteinuria, and increased blood urea nitrogen (BUN) and serum creatinine levels. It is usually reversible, but the patient's renal function test results must be monitored throughout therapy. In contrast, ototoxicity is less common, occurring in 3% to 14% of patients, and often is not reversible. It can result in varying degrees of permanent hearing loss, depending on the dosage and duration of drug therapy. It is believed to result from injury to the eighth cranial nerve (CN VIII, also called the *cochleovestibular nerve* or *auditory nerve*) and involves both cochlear damage (hearing loss) and vestibular damage (disrupted sense of balance). Symptoms include dizziness, tinnitus, a sense of fullness in the ears, and hearing loss. Other less common effects include headache, paresthesia, vertigo, skin rash, fever, overgrowth of nonsusceptible organisms, and neuromuscular paralysis (very rare and reversible). The risk for these toxicities is greatest in patients with preexisting renal impairment, patients already receiving other renally toxic drugs, and patients receiving high-dose or prolonged aminoglycoside therapy.

## Interactions

The risk for nephrotoxicity can be increased with concurrent use of other nephrotoxic drugs such as vancomycin, cyclosporine, and amphotericin B. Concurrent use with loop diuretics increases the risk for ototoxicity. In addition, because aminoglycosides, like many other antibiotics, kill intestinal bacterial flora, they also reduce the amount of vitamin K produced by these gut bacteria. These normal flora normally serve to balance the effects of oral anticoagulants such as warfarin (Coumadin). Therefore, aminoglycosides can potentiate warfarin toxicity. Concurrent use with neuromuscular blocking drugs may prolong the duration of action of the neuromuscular blockade.

## Dosages

For dosages information on selected aminoglycosides, see the table on this page.

## DOSAGES

### Selected Aminoglycosides

| DRUG (PREGNANCY CATEGORY) | USUAL DOSAGE RANGE | INDICATIONS/USES |
|---|---|---|
| amikacin (generic only) (D) | **Adult and pediatric**<br>IV: 15 mg/kg/day divided 2-3 times daily or 15-20 mg/kg once daily<br>**Neonatal***<br>IV: 10 mg/kg load, then 7.5 mg/kg q12h | Primarily infection with gentamicin- and tobramycin-resistant gram-negative organisms along with severe staphylococcal infections |
| ♦ gentamicin (generic only) (C) | **Adult**<br>IV/IM: 2-6 mg/kg/day divided 1-4 times daily or 5-7 mg/kg once daily<br>**Pediatric and neonatal**<br>IV/IM: 2-2.5 mg/kg q8h | Primarily gram-negative infections along with severe staphylococcal infections |
| neomycin (C) | **Adult**<br>PO/PR: 3000-9000 mg divided between 3-9 doses | Preoperative bowel cleansing (also used with different dosage regimens for hepatic encephalopathy) |
| tobramycin (generic, TOBI) (D) | **Adult**<br>IV/IM: 3-6 mg/kg/day divided 1-3 times daily or 5-7 mg/kg once daily<br>**Pediatric**<br>IV/IM: 6-7.5 mg/kg/day divided 3-4 times daily<br>**Neonatal***<br>IV/IM: 3 mg/kg q24h or 2 mg/kg q12h | Primarily gram-negative infections along with severe staphylococcal infections |

*IM*, Intramuscular; *IV*, intravenous; *PO*, oral; *PR*, rectal.
*Dosing and frequency vary depending on age of patient.

## DRUG PROFILES

Historically, the aminoglycoside antibiotics were used primarily to treat gram-negative infections. However, they are now used as a synergistic drug in the treatment of gram-positive infections as well. They are normally given intravenously or intramuscularly, but neomycin is administered only orally, rectally, or topically. Topical dosage forms of both gentamicin and tobramycin are also available for dermatologic (see Chapter 56) and ophthalmic (see Chapter 57) use. Currently available aminoglycosides include amikacin, gentamicin, kanamycin, neomycin, streptomycin, and tobramycin. Dosage and other information are given in the table on p. 637.

### ♦ amikacin

Amikacin is a semisynthetic aminoglycoside antibiotic that is often used to treat infections that are resistant to gentamicin or tobramycin. It is available only in injectable form.

Pharmacokinetics

| Route | Onset of Action | Peak Plasma Concentration | Elimination Half-life | Duration of Action |
|---|---|---|---|---|
| IV | Variable | 1 hr | 2-3 hr | 8-12 hr |
| IM | Variable | 30 min-2 hr | 2-3 hr | 8-12 hr |

### ♦ gentamicin

Gentamicin is the most commonly used aminoglycoside in clinical practice today. It can be given either intravenously or intramuscularly, and the dosage is the same for both routes. It is indicated for the treatment of infection with several susceptible gram-positive and gram-negative bacteria. Gentamicin is available in several dosage forms, including injections, topical ointments, and ophthalmic drops and ointments.

Pharmacokinetics

| Route | Onset of Action | Peak Plasma Concentration | Elimination Half-life | Duration of Action |
|---|---|---|---|---|
| IV | Variable | 30 min | 2-3 hr | Up to 24 hr |
| IM | Variable | 30-90 min | 2-3 hr | Up to 24 hr |

### tobramycin

Tobramycin has dosages, routes of administration, and indications that are comparable to those for gentamicin for generalized infections. In addition, it is commonly used to treat recurrent pulmonary infections in patients with cystic fibrosis by both injectable and inhaled dosing. When used for inhalation, it goes by the trade name of TOBI. It is also available in topical and ophthalmic dosage forms.

Pharmacokinetics

| Route | Onset of Action | Peak Plasma Concentration | Elimination Half-life | Duration of Action |
|---|---|---|---|---|
| IV | Variable | 30 min | 2-3 hr | Up to 24 hr |
| IM | Variable | 30-90 min | 2-3 hr | Up to 24 hr |

### neomycin

Neomycin is most commonly used for bacterial decontamination of the GI tract before surgical procedures, and it is given both orally and rectally (as an enema) for this purpose. Other uses include topical application for skin infections, bladder irrigation, and treatment of E. coli diarrhea, hepatic encephalopathy, and eye infections. In hepatic encephalopathy, the drug helps reduce the number of ammonia-producing bacteria in the GI tract. The subsequent reduced blood ammonia levels sometimes result in improvement of neurologic symptoms of the hepatic illness. This drug is not available in injectable form but instead is available in tablets, solutions, and powders for oral, topical, or irrigation administration.

Pharmacokinetics

| Route | Onset of Action | Peak Plasma Concentration | Elimination Half-life | Duration of Action |
|---|---|---|---|---|
| PO | Variable | 1-4 hr | 3 hr | Up to 24 hr |

## QUINOLONES

Quinolones, sometimes referred to as *fluoroquinolones,* are very potent bactericidal broad-spectrum antibiotics. Currently available quinolone antibiotics include norfloxacin, ciprofloxacin, levofloxacin, and moxifloxacin. With the exception of norfloxacin, these antibiotics have excellent oral absorption. In most cases, the extent of oral absorption is comparable to that of intravenous injection.

### Mechanism of Action and Drug Effects

Quinolone antibiotics destroy bacteria by altering their deoxyribonucleic acid (DNA) (see Figure 38-3). They accomplish this by interfering with the bacterial enzymes DNA gyrase and topo-isomerase IV. Quinolones do not inhibit the production of human DNA.

The quinolones kill susceptible strains of mostly gram-negative and some gram-positive organisms. Some quinolones are also believed to diffuse into and concentrate themselves in human neutrophils, killing bacteria such as *S. aureus, Serratia marcescens,* and *Mycobacterium fortuitum* that sometimes accumulate in these cells. Bacterial resistance to quinolone antibiotics has been identified among several bacterial species, including *Pseudomonas aeruginosa, S. aureus, Pneumococcus* spp., *Enterococcus* spp., and the broad Enterobacteriaceae family that includes *E. coli.*

### Indications

Quinolones are active against a wide variety of gram-negative and selected gram-positive bacteria. Most are excreted primarily by the kidneys as unchanged drug. This characteristic, together with the fact that they have extensive gram-negative coverage, makes them suitable for treating complicated urinary tract infections. They are also commonly used to treat respiratory, skin, GI, and bone and joint infections.

Ciprofloxacin (Cipro) was the first quinolone to enjoy widespread use. Resistance was soon seen in *Pseudomonas*

## BOX 39-1 OVERVIEW OF QUINOLONE-SUSCEPTIBLE ORGANISMS

- Gram-positive: *Streptococcus* (including *Streptococcus pneumoniae*), *Staphylococcus, Enterococcus, Listeria monocytogenes*
- Gram-negative: *Neisseria gonorrhea, Neisseria meningitidis, Haemophilus influenzae, Haemophilus parainfluenzae*, Enterobacteriaceae (including *Escherichia coli, Enterobacter, Klebsiella, Proteus mirabilis, Salmonella, Shigella*), *Acinetobacter, Pseudomonas aeruginosa, Pasteurella multocida, Legionella, Mycoplasma pneumoniae, Chlamydia*
- Anaerobes: *Bacteroides fragilis, Peptococcus, Peptostreptococcus* (moxifloxacin is strongest)
- Other: *Rickettsia* (ciprofloxacin only)

and some *Streptococcus* spp. Ciprofloxacin and levofloxacin are available both orally and by injection and are both available in generic form, which means that it costs significantly less than brand name quinolones. Levofloxacin (Levaquin) is somewhat more active than ciprofloxacin against gram-positive organisms such as *Streptococcus pneumoniae*, including penicillin-resistant strains, as well as *Enterococcus* and *S. aureus*. Moxifloxacin is also effective against *S. pneumoniae* as well as some strains of *S. aureus* and enterococci. However, MRSA and VRE are generally also resistant to moxifloxacin. The activity of moxifloxacin against many enteric gram-negative bacteria and *P. aeruginosa* is similar to that of levofloxacin and less than that of ciprofloxacin. Moxifloxacin often has stronger anaerobic bacterial coverage. Norfloxacin has limited oral absorption and is available only in oral form, and its use is limited to GU tract infections. Quinolones are often combined with aminoglycosides to treat *P. aeruginosa* infections. Moxifloxacin also has some *in vitro* activity against anaerobes.

The use of quinolones in prepubescent children is not generally recommended, because these drugs have been shown to affect cartilage development in laboratory animals. However, more recent evidence suggests that judicious use in children might be less of a risk than previously thought, and in fact these drugs are used commonly in children with cystic fibrosis. Box 39-1 lists selected microbes commonly susceptible to quinolone therapy in general, but there is some variation in spectra among drugs. Table 39-3 gives common indications for individual drugs.

## Contraindications

The only true contraindication is known drug allergy.

## Adverse Effects

Quinolones are capable of causing a variety of adverse effects, the most common of which are listed in Table 39-4. Bacterial overgrowth is another possible complication of quinolone therapy, but this is more commonly associated with long-term use. More worrisome is a cardiac effect that involves prolongation of the QT interval on the electrocardiogram (ECG). Dangerous cardiac dysrhythmias are more likely to occur when quinolones are taken by patients who are also receiving class Ia and class III antidysrhythmic drugs, such as disopyramide and amiodarone.

## TABLE 39-3 QUINOLONES: COMMON INDICATIONS FOR SPECIFIC DRUGS

| GENERIC NAME (TRADE NAME, YEAR OF FDA APPROVAL) | ANTIBACTERIAL SPECTRUM | COMMON INDICATIONS |
|---|---|---|
| norfloxacin (Noroxin, 1986) | Extensive gram-negative and selected gram-positive coverage | Urinary tract infections, prostatitis, STIs |
| ciprofloxacin (Cipro, 1987) | Comparable to that of norfloxacin | Anthrax (inhalational, post-exposure); respiratory, skin, urinary tract, prostate, intraabdominal, GI, bone, and joint infections; typhoid fever; selected nosocomial pneumonias |
| levofloxacin (Levaquin, 1996) | Comparable to that of ciprofloxacin with better gram-positive coverage | Respiratory and urinary tract infections; prophylaxis in various transrectal and transurethral prostate surgical procedures |
| moxifloxacin (Avelox, 1999) | Comparable to that of levofloxacin plus anaerobic coverage | Respiratory and skin infections; CAP caused by PRSP; anaerobic infections |
| gemifloxacin (Factive, 2004) | Comparable to ciprofloxacin | CAP, exacerbation of COPD |

*CAP,* Community-acquired pneumonia; *COPD,* chronic obstructive pulmonary disease; *FDA,* U.S. Food and Drug Administration; *GI,* gastrointestinal; *PRSP,* penicillin-resistant streptococcal pneumonia; *STI,* sexually transmitted infection.

## TABLE 39-4 QUINOLONES: REPORTED ADVERSE EFFECTS

| BODY SYSTEM | ADVERSE EFFECTS |
|---|---|
| Central nervous | Headache, dizziness, insomnia, depression, restlessness, convulsions |
| Gastrointestinal | Nausea, constipation, increased AST and ALT levels, flatulence, heartburn, vomiting, diarrhea, oral candidiasis, dysphagia |
| Integumentary | Rash, pruritus, urticaria, flushing |
| Other | Ruptured tendons and tendonitis (black box warning added in 2008), fever, chills, blurred vision, tinnitus |

*ALT,* Alanine aminotransferase; *AST,* aspartate aminotransferase.

For this reason, such drug combinations are best avoided. A black box warning is required by the U.S. Food and Drug Administration for all quinolones because of the increased risk of tendinitis and tendon rupture with use of these drugs. This effect is more common in elderly patients, patients with renal failure, and those receiving concurrent glucocorticoid therapy (e.g., prednisone). Central nervous system stimulation (i.e., seizures) has been reported. Quinolones must be infused over 1 to 1.5 hours.

## DOSAGES

### Selected Quinolones

| DRUG | PHARMACOLOGIC CLASS | USUAL DOSAGE RANGE | INDICATION/USES |
|------|--------------------|--------------------|-----------------|
| ♦ ciprofloxacin (Cipro) (C) | Fluoroquinolone | **Adult\*** IV: 200-400 mg q12h PO: 250-750 mg q8-12h | Broad gram-positive and gram-negative coverage for infections throughout the body |
| levofloxacin (Levaquin) (C) | | **Adult only** IV/PO: 250-750 mg once daily | Various susceptible bacterial infections |

*IV*, Intravenous; *PO*, oral.

*Not normally recommended for children younger than 18 years of age due to finding of adverse musculoskeletal effects in studies of immature animals.

## Interactions

There are several drugs that interact with quinolones. Concurrent use of quinolones with antacids, calcium, magnesium, iron, zinc preparations or sucralfate causes a reduction in the oral absorption of the quinolone. Patients need to take the interacting drugs at least 1 hour before or after taking quinolones. Dairy products also reduce the absorption of quinolones and should be separated as stated previously for interacting drugs. Enteral tube feedings can also reduce the absorption of quinolones. Probenecid can reduce the renal excretion of quinolones. Nitrofurantoin (which is discussed later in the chapter) can antagonize the antibacterial activity of the quinolones, and oral anticoagulants are to be used with caution in patients receiving quinolones because of the antibiotic-induced alteration of the intestinal flora, which affects vitamin K synthesis.

## Dosages

For dosage information on selected quinolones, see the table on this page.

## DRUG PROFILES

### ♦ ciprofloxacin

Ciprofloxacin (Cipro) was one of the first of the broad-coverage, potent quinolones to become available. It was first marketed in an oral form but is also available in injectable, ophthalmic (see Chapter 57), and otic (see Chapter 58) formulations. Because of its excellent bioavailability, it can work orally as well as many intravenous antibiotics. It is capable of killing a wide range of gram-negative bacteria and is even effective against traditionally difficult-to-kill gram-negative bacteria such as *Pseudomonas*. Some anaerobic bacteria as well as atypical organisms such as *Chlamydia, Mycoplasma,* and *Mycobacterium* can also be killed by ciprofloxacin. It is also a drug of choice for the treatment of anthrax (infection with *Bacillus anthracis*).

### Pharmacokinetics

| Route | Onset of Action | Peak Plasma Concentration | Elimination Half-life | Duration of Action |
|-------|-----------------|---------------------------|-----------------------|--------------------|
| IV | 30 min | 1 hr | 3-4.8 hr | Up to 12 hr |
| PO | Variable | 1-2 hr | 3-4.8 hr | Up to 12 hr |

### levofloxacin

Levofloxacin (Levaquin) is one of the most widely used quinolones. It has a broad spectrum of activity similar to that of ciprofloxacin, but it has the advantage of once-daily dosing. Levofloxacin is available in both oral and injectable forms.

### Pharmacokinetics

| Route | Onset of Action | Peak Plasma Concentration | Elimination Half-life | Duration of Action |
|-------|-----------------|---------------------------|-----------------------|--------------------|
| IV | Variable | 1-2 hr | 6-8 hr | Up to 24 hr |
| PO | Variable | 2 hr | 6-8 hr | Up to 24 hr |

## MISCELLANEOUS ANTIBIOTICS

There are a number of antibiotics that do not fit into any of the previously described broad categories. Most have somewhat unique indications or are especially preferred for a particular type of infection. Although they may not be used as commonly as drugs from the other major classes, they are still of clinical importance. Several of these drugs are described individually in the following drug profiles. Dosage information for these drugs is given in the table on p. 641.

## DRUG PROFILES

### ♦ clindamycin

Clindamycin (Cleocin) is a semisynthetic antibiotic. Clindamycin can be either bactericidal or bacteriostatic (see Chapter 38), depending on the concentration of the drug at the site of infection and on the infecting bacteria. It inhibits protein synthesis in bacteria (see Figure 38-3). It is indicated for the treatment of chronic bone infections, GU tract infections, intraabdominal infections, anaerobic pneumonia, septicemia caused by streptococci and staphylococci, and serious skin and soft-tissue infections caused by susceptible bacteria. Most gram-positive bacteria, including staphylococci, streptococci, and pneumococci, are susceptible to clindamycin's actions. It also has the special advantage of being active against several anaerobic organisms and is most often used for this purpose. However, resistant strains of gram-positive, gram-negative, and anaerobic organisms do exist. Also, all Enterobacteriaceae are resistant to clindamycin.

## DOSAGES

### Selected Miscellaneous Antibiotics

| DRUG (PREGNANCY CATEGORY) | PHARMACOLOGIC CLASS | USUAL DOSAGE RANGE | INDICATIONS |
|---|---|---|---|
| ◆ clindamycin (Cleocin) (B) | Lincosamide | **Adult** <br> IV/PO: 300-900 mg bid-qid <br> **Pediatric** <br> IV/PO: 8-20 mg/kg/day divided tid-qid | Anaerobic infections; streptococcal and staphylococcal infections of bone, skin, respiratory, and GU tract |
| colistimethate (Colisitin) (C) | Polypeptide | 2.5-5 mg/kg/day; infuse over 3-5 min | Treatment of KPC-producing organisms; renal and neurotoxicity common |
| daptomycin (Cubicin) (B) | Lipopeptide | **Adult only** <br> IV: 4-6 mg/kg once daily × 7-14 days | Complicated skin and soft-tissue infections |
| linezolid (Zyvox) (C) | Oxazolidinone | **Adult only** <br> IV/PO: 600 mg q12h | VRE infections; skin and respiratory infections caused by various *Staphylococcus* and *Streptococcus* spp. |
| ◆ metronidazole (Flagyl) (B) | Nitroimidazole | **Adult\*** <br> IV/PO: 250-500 mg q6-12h | Primarily anaerobic and gram-negative infections of abdominal cavity, skin, bone, and respiratory and GU tracts |
| nitrofurantoin (Macrodantin, Furadantin) (B) | Nitrofuran | **Adult** <br> PO: 50-100 mg qid <br> **Pediatric** <br> PO: 1-2 mg/kg/day | Primarily UTIs caused by gram-negative organisms and *Staphylococcus aureus* |
| quinupristin/dalfopristin (Synercid) (B) | Streptogramins | **Adult and pediatric** <br> IV: 7.5 mg/kg q8-12h | VRE infections; skin infections caused by streptococcal and staphylococcal infections |
| telavancin (Vibativ) (C) | Lipoglycopeptides | **Adult** <br> IV: 7.5 mg/kg/day | Serious gram-positive infections caused by MRSA and VRE |
| vancomycin (Vancocin, Vancoled) (B, oral; C injection) | Tricyclic glycopeptide | **Adult** <br> IV: 15 mg/kg/day (frequency dependent on renal function) <br> PO†: 500 mg q6h <br> **Pediatric‡** <br> IV/PO†:10-15 mg/kg q6h | Severe staphylococcal infections, including MRSA infections; other serious gram-positive infections, including streptococcal infections |

*GU*, Genitourinary; *IV*, intravenous; *KPC*, *Klebsiella pneumoniae* carbapenemase; *MRSA*, methicillin-resistant *Staphylococcus aureus*; *PO*, oral; *spp.*, species; *UTI*, urinary tract infection; *VRE*, vancomycin-resistant *Enterococcus*.
\*Not normally used in children except to treat amebiasis.
†Oral is not absorbed and is used only for *C. difficile* diarrhea.
‡Dosing varies depending on age of patient.

Clindamycin is contraindicated in patients with a known hypersensitivity to it, those with ulcerative colitis or enteritis, and infants younger than 1 month of age. GI tract adverse effects are the most common and include nausea, vomiting, abdominal pain, diarrhea, pseudomembranous colitis, and anorexia. Pseudomembranous colitis (also known as antibiotic-associated colitis, *C. difficile* diarrhea, or *C. difficile* infection) is a necrotizing inflammatory bowel condition that is often associated with antibiotic therapy, especially clindamycin therapy. Clindamycin is available in oral, injectable, and topical (see Chapter 56) forms.

Clindamycin is also known to have some neuromuscular blocking properties that may enhance the actions of neuromuscular drugs used in perioperative and intensive care settings, such as vecuronium (see Chapter 11). Patients receiving both drugs need to be monitored for excessive neuromuscular blockade and respiratory paralysis, and appropriate ventilatory support provided as needed.

### Pharmacokinetics

| Route | Onset of Action | Peak Plasma Concentration | Elimination Half-life | Duration of Action |
|---|---|---|---|---|
| PO | 30 min | 45 min | 2-3 hr | 6 hr |
| IM/IV | Variable | IM: 3 hr | 2-3 hr | IM: 8-12 hr |

### linezolid

Linezolid (Zyvox) is the first antibacterial drug in a new class of antibiotics known as oxazolidinones. This drug works by inhibiting bacterial protein synthesis. Linezolid was originally developed to treat infections associated with vancomycin-resistant *Enterococcus faecium,* more commonly referred to as VRE. VRE infection is notoriously difficult to treat and often occurs as a *nosocomial* (hospital-acquired) infection. Linezolid is commonly used to treat hospital-acquired pneumonia; complicated skin and skin structure infections, including cases caused by MRSA; and gram-positive infections in infants and children. MRSA is a virulent organism and stands for "methicillin-resistant *S. aureus*." However, methicillin, a penicillinase-resistant penicillin, has recently been removed from the U.S. market. Nonetheless, *MRSA* is still the term used, although oxacillin is now the test drug for this organism. To confuse things even further, oxacillin is rarely used for therapy, and nafcillin is the most commonly used drug for methicillin-susceptible *S. aureus*. MRSA is notorious for causing serious infections, especially in the hospital setting. Linezolid is also approved for treatment of community-acquired pneumonia and uncomplicated skin and skin structure infections.

The most commonly reported adverse effects attributed to linezolid are headache, nausea, diarrhea, and vomiting. It has also been shown to decrease platelet count. Linezolid is contraindicated in patients with a known hypersensitivity to it. It is available in oral and injectable forms. It has excellent oral absorption, which allows patients to continue oral therapy at home for serious infections that would otherwise require hospitalization. With regard to drug interactions, linezolid has the potential to strengthen the vasopressor (prohypertensive) effects of various vasopressive drugs (see Chapter 18) such as dopamine by an unclear mechanism. Also, there have been postmarketing case reports of this drug causing serotonin syndrome when used concurrently with serotonergic drugs such as the selective serotonin reuptake inhibitor (SSRI) antidepressants (see Chapter 16). It is recommended that the SSRI be stopped while the patient is receiving linezolid therapy; however, oftentimes this is not realistic and patients must be watched carefully for signs of serotonin syndrome. Finally, tyramine-containing foods such as aged cheese or wine, soy sauce, smoked meats or fish, and sauerkraut can interact with linezolid to raise blood pressure.

### Pharmacokinetics

| Route | Onset of Action | Peak Plasma Concentration | Elimination Half-life | Duration of Action |
|---|---|---|---|---|
| PO | Variable | 1-2 hr | 5 hr | 12 hr |
| IV | Variable | Immediate | 6-7 hr | 8-12 hr |

### ◆ metronidazole

Metronidazole (Flagyl) is an antimicrobial drug of the class nitroimidazole. It has especially good activity against anaerobic organisms and is widely used to treat intraabdominal and gynecologic infections that are caused by such organisms. Examples of the anaerobes against which it is active are *Peptostreptococcus* spp., *Eubacterium* spp., *Bacteroides* spp., and *Clostridium* spp. Metronidazole is also indicated for the treatment of protozoal infections such as amebiasis and trichomoniasis (see Chapter 43). It works by interfering with microbial DNA synthesis, and in this regard is similar to the quinolones (see Figure 38-3). It is used orally to treat antibiotic-associated colitis; however, resistance is being noted. Metronidazole is contraindicated in cases of known drug allergy. It is available in both oral and injectable forms. Metronidazole is classified as a pregnancy category B drug, although it is not recommended for use during the first trimester of pregnancy. Adverse effects include dizziness, headache, GI discomfort, nasal congestion, and reversible neutropenia and thrombocytopenia. Drug interactions include acute alcohol intolerance when it is taken with alcoholic beverages, due to the accumulation of acetaldehyde, the principal alcohol metabolite. Patients must avoid alcohol for 24 hours before initiation of therapy and for at least 36 hours after the last dose of metronidazole. Metronidazole may also increase the toxicity of lithium, benzodiazepines, cyclosporine, calcium channel blockers, various antidepressants (e.g., venlafaxine), warfarin, and other drugs. In contrast, phenytoin and phenobarbital may reduce the effects of metronidazole. These interactions occur because of various enzymatic effects involving the cytochrome P-450 liver enzymes that result in altered drug metabolism when these drugs are taken concurrently with metronidazole.

### Pharmacokinetics

| Route | Onset of Action | Peak Plasma Concentration | Elimination Half-life | Duration of Action |
|---|---|---|---|---|
| PO | Variable | 1-2 hr | 8 hr | Unknown |
| IV | Variable | 1 hr | 8 hr | Unknown |

### nitrofurantoin

Nitrofurantoin (Macrodantin) is an antibiotic drug of the class nitrofuran. It is indicated primarily for urinary tract infections caused by *E. coli*, *S. aureus*, *Klebsiella* spp., and *Enterobacter* spp. It works by interfering with the activity of enzymes that regulate bacterial carbohydrate metabolism and also by disrupting bacterial cell wall formation. It is contraindicated in cases of known drug allergy and also in cases of significant renal function impairment, because the drug concentrates in the urine. The drug is available only for oral use. Adverse effects include GI discomfort, dizziness, headache, skin reactions (mild to severe reported), blood dyscrasias, ECG changes, possibly irreversible peripheral neuropathy, and hepatotoxicity. Although hepatotoxicity is rare, it is often fatal. Interacting drugs are few and include probenecid, which can reduce renal excretion of nitrofurantoin, and antacids, which can reduce the extent of its GI absorption. The dose must be reduced for elderly patients or those with decreased renal function. Another drug that is approved for urinary tract infections is fosfomycin (Monurol). It is given as a one-time dose and maintains high concentrations in the urine for up to 48 hours.

### Pharmacokinetics

| Route | Onset of Action | Peak Plasma Concentration | Elimination Half-life | Duration of Action |
|---|---|---|---|---|
| PO | 2.5-4.5 hr | 30 min | 0.5-1 hr | 5-8 hr |

### quinupristin/dalfopristin

Quinupristin and dalfopristin (Synercid) are two streptogramin antibacterials marketed in a 30:70 fixed combination. The combination drug is approved for intravenous treatment of bacteremia and life-threatening infection caused by VRE and for treatment of complicated skin and skin structure infections caused by *S. pyogenes* and *S. aureus,* including MRSA.

Common adverse effects are arthralgias and myalgias, which may become severe. Adverse effects related to the infusion site, including pain, inflammation, edema, and thrombophlebitis, have developed in approximately 75% of patients treated through a peripheral intravenous line. The drug is contraindicated in patients with a known hypersensitivity to it. It is available only in injectable form. Drug interactions are limited, the most serious being potential increase in levels of cyclosporine. Quinupristin/dalfopristin must be infused with 5% dextrose in water ($D_5W$) only and cannot be mixed with saline or heparin, including heparinized flushes.

Pharmacokinetics (quinupristin/dalfopristin)

| Route | Onset of Action | Peak Plasma Concentration | Elimination Half-life | Duration of Action |
|-------|-----------------|---------------------------|-----------------------|--------------------|
| IV    | 1-2 hr          | 3-4 hr                    | 1-3 hr                | 8-12 hr            |

### ◆ vancomycin

Vancomycin is a natural bactericidal antibiotic that is structurally unrelated to any other commercially available antibiotics. It destroys bacteria by binding to the bacterial cell wall, producing immediate inhibition of cell wall synthesis and death (see Figure 38-3). This mechanism differs from that of the beta-lactam antibiotics.

Vancomycin is the antibiotic of choice for the treatment of MRSA infection and infections caused by many other gram-positive bacteria. It is not active against gram-negative bacteria, fungi, or yeast. Oral vancomycin is indicated for the treatment of antibiotic-induced colitis (*Clostridium difficile*) and for the treatment of staphylococcal enterocolitis. Because the oral formulation is poorly absorbed from the GI tract, it is used for its local effects on the surface of the GI tract. The parenteral form is indicated for the treatment of bone and joint infections and bacterial bloodstream infections caused by *Staphylococcus* spp. Resistance to vancomycin has been noted with increasing frequency in patients with infections caused by *Enterococcus* organisms. These strains have been isolated most often from GI tract infections but have also been isolated from skin, soft tissue, and bloodstream infections. Resistance to MRSA has been rarely reported to occur with vancomycin.

Vancomycin is contraindicated in patients with a known hypersensitivity to it. It should be used with caution in those with preexisting renal dysfunction or hearing loss, as well as in elderly patients and neonates. Vancomycin is similar to the aminoglycosides in that there are very specific drug levels in the blood that are safe. If the levels are too low (less than 5 mcg/mL), the dosage may be subtherapeutic with reduced antibacterial efficacy. If the blood levels are too high (over 50 mcg/mL), toxicities may result, the two most severe of which are ototoxicity (hearing loss) and nephrotoxicity (kidney damage). Nephrotoxicity is more likely to occur with concurrent therapy with other nephrotoxic drugs such as aminoglycosides, cyclosporine, and contrast media used for CT scans. Vancomycin can also cause additive neuromuscular blocking effects in patients receiving neuromuscular blockers. Another common adverse effect that is bothersome but usually not harmful is known as *red man syndrome*. This syndrome is characterized by flushing and/or itching of the head, face, neck, and upper trunk area. It is most commonly seen when the drug is infused too rapidly. It can usually be alleviated by slowing the rate of infusion of the dose to at least 1 hour. Rapid infusions may also cause hypotension. Optimal blood levels of vancomycin are a peak level of 18 to 50 mcg/mL and a trough level of 10 to 20 mcg/mL. Measurement of peak levels is no longer routinely recommended, and only trough levels are commonly monitored. Blood samples for measurement of trough levels are drawn immediately before administration of the next dose. Because of the increase in resistant organisms, many clinicians use a trough level of 15 to 20 mcg/mL as their goal.

Pharmacokinetics

| Route | Onset of Action | Peak Plasma Concentration | Elimination Half-life | Duration of Action |
|-------|-----------------|---------------------------|-----------------------|--------------------|
| IV    | Variable        | 1 hr                      | 4-6 hr                | Up to 24 hr Longer in renal dysfunction |

### daptomycin

Daptomycin (Cubicin) is currently the only drug of the new class known as *lipopeptides*. Its mechanism of action is not completely known, but it binds to gram-positive cells in a calcium-dependent process and disrupts the cell membrane potential. It is used to treat complicated skin and soft-tissue infections caused by susceptible gram-positive bacteria, including MRSA and VRE. It can also be used to treat vancomycin-intermediate or vancomycin-resistant strains of MRSA. This drug is contraindicated in cases of known drug allergy. It is available only in injectable form. Adverse reactions include hypotension or hypertension (low incidence for both), headache, dizziness, rash, GI discomfort, elevated liver enzyme levels, local injection site reaction, renal failure, dyspnea, and fungal infection. The precise mechanisms for these reactions are uncertain, but all occur in a relatively small percentage of patients (fewer than 5%). Major drug interactions have yet to be identified; however, there is a theoretical risk of increased myopathy when daptomycin is given in conjunction with hydroxymethylglutaryl–coenzyme A (HMG-CoA) reductase inhibitors, commonly referred to as *statins*.

Pharmacokinetics

| Route | Onset of Action | Peak Plasma Concentration | Elimination Half-life | Duration of Action |
|-------|-----------------|---------------------------|-----------------------|--------------------|
| IV    | Unknown         | 30 min                    | 8-9 hr                | Unknown            |

### colistimethate

Colistimethate (Coly-Mycin) is a polypeptide antibiotic that penetrates and disrupts the bacterial membrane of susceptible strains of gram-negative bacteria. It is commonly referred to as *colistin*. It is an old drug that fell out of clinical use when newer, less toxic drugs became available. Unfortunately, due to the emergence of infections with KPC-producing organisms, it is now being used again, often as one of the only drugs available to treat KPC. Colistin is available for intravenous, intramuscular, and inhalational administration. It has serious adverse effects, including renal failure and neurotoxic effects such as paresthesia, numbness, tingling, vertigo, dizziness, and impairment of speech. It can cause acute respiratory failure when administered by inhalation. Colistin crosses the placenta and needs to be used with caution in pregnant women. Colistin is infused over 3 to 5 minutes.

Pharmacokinetics

| Route | Onset of Action | Peak Plasma Concentration | Elimination Half-life | Duration of Action |
|-------|-----------------|---------------------------|-----------------------|--------------------|
| IV    | Unknown         | 10 min                    | 2-3 hr                | 8-12 hr            |

**telavancin**

Telavancin (Vibativ) is a new drug and the only one in the class called the *lipoglycopeptides*. It is indicated for the treatment of skin and skin structure infections caused by susceptible gram-positive organisms. It is effective against MRSA and VRE. It must not be used in pregnant women, and the dose needs to be adjusted for renal dysfunction. Most common adverse effects include renal toxicity, infusion-related reactions, and QT prolongation.

### Pharmacokinetics

| Route | Onset of Action | Peak Plasma Concentration | Elimination Half-life | Duration of Action |
|-------|-----------------|---------------------------|-----------------------|--------------------|
| IV | Variable | 1 hr | 8-9 hours | Up to 24 hr |

## NURSING PROCESS

## ASSESSMENT

Many of the antibiotics discussed in this chapter, in contrast to those in Chapter 38, are the types of drugs that are often reserved for treatment of more potent infections and are mainly administered by parenteral routes; thus, they demand more skillful and thorough assessment of the patient and the specific drug. These antibiotics all require a critical assessment for any history of or current symptoms indicative of hypersensitivity or allergic reactions, with symptoms ranging from mild reactions with rash, pruritus, or hives to severe reactions with laryngeal edema, bronchospasm, hypotension to possible cardiac arrest. Further assessment associated with these groups of antibiotics in general includes conducting a nursing physical examination and recording age, weight, and baseline vital sign values. Diagnostic and laboratory studies that may be ordered include the following: (1) AST and ALT levels for assessing liver function; (2) urinalysis, BUN, and serum creatinine levels for assessing renal function; (3) ECG, echocardiography, ultrasonography, and/or cardiac enzyme levels for assessing cardiac function; (4) culture and sensitivity of infected tissue or blood samples for assessing sensitivity of the bacteria to the antibiotic; and (5) white blood cell (WBC) count, hemoglobin level, hematocrit, RBC count, platelet count, and clotting values for baseline blood count levels. In the baseline neurologic assessment, note baseline sensory and motor intactness and/or assessment of any alterations in neurologic functioning—for example, altered sensorium and level of consciousness—because of the potential for central nervous system adverse effects. Baseline abdominal and GI assessments are important, with a focus on bowel patterns and bowel sounds because of the possibility of GI adverse effects. Note contraindications, cautions, and drug interactions, and obtain a complete list of the patient's medications, including over-the-counter drugs, herbals, and dietary supplements. Perform a cultural assessment because of the various responses of certain racial and ethnic groups to specific drugs as well as the potential use of alternative healing practices.

With any antibiotic, assess for *superinfection,* or a secondary infection that occurs with the destruction of normal flora during antibiotic therapy (see Chapter 38). Fungal superinfections may be evidenced by fever, lethargy, perineal itching, and other anatomically related symptoms. Assess the patient's immune system status and overall condition because if there is a deficiency (e.g., in patients with cancer, autoimmune disorders such as lupus, acquired immunodeficiency syndromes, and any chronic illness), the patient's ability to physically resist infection may be diminished. Antibiotic resistance is a continual concern with antibiotic drug therapy, especially in pediatrics and in large health care institutions and long-term care facilities. You must consider this possibility of resistance to certain antibiotics when assessing patients for symptoms of infection and superinfection.

With *aminoglycosides,* assess for hypersensitivity and preexisting conditions. Obtain a list of all medications the patient is taking because of the many cautions, contraindications, and drug interactions associated with these drugs. The aminoglycosides are known for their ototoxicity and nephrotoxicity; therefore, if deemed appropriate, perform baseline hearing tests and assessment of vestibular function. Nephrotoxicity is at an increased risk with the use of other nephrotoxic drugs, such as cyclosporine and the intravenous contrast used for CT scan. For patients requiring a CT scan with contrast who are also on a nephrotoxic medication, alert the prescriber to the situation so that the dose may be adjusted and additional fluids and/or medications ordered. Additionally, perform renal function studies (BUN level, urinalysis, serum and urine creatinine levels), as ordered, and document all results. If renal baseline functioning is decreased the prescriber may need to adjust the dosage amounts because of the risk of nephrotoxicity. Complete a thorough neuromuscular assessment because of the potential for drug-related neurotoxicity and higher risk for complications in those with impaired neurologic functioning. For example, patients with myasthenia gravis or Parkinson's disease may experience worsening of muscle weakness because of the drug's neuromuscular blockade. Neonates (because of the immaturity of the nervous and renal systems) and the elderly (because of decreased neurologic and renal functioning) are also at higher risk for nephrotoxicity, neurotoxicity, and ototoxicity and require careful assessment before and during drug therapy. Assess hydration status. The toxicities of these drugs are greater in those with preexisting renal impairment, those receiving other renal toxic drugs, and in those patients taking the aminoglycoside for a long period of time or on high-dose therapy.

*Quinolones,* such as ciprofloxacin, require careful assessment for preexisting central nervous system conditions (e.g., seizure or stroke disorders) that may be exacerbated by the concurrent use of these drugs. Assess for a cardiac history, and note if the patient is taking certain antidysrhythmics because of the potential for dangerous cardiac irregularities. Significant drug interactions include antacids, iron, zinc preparations, and sucralfate as they affect the absorption of the quinolone.

Oral anticoagulants also interact with and alter the antibacterial activity of quinolones (see pharmacology discussion).

If *clindamycin* is being used, assess for hypersensitivity to the drug or related compounds. Clindamycin is not to be used in patients with ulcerative colitis or in those younger than 1 month of age. Perform a thorough assessment of GI disorders because of the possibility of drug-induced pseudomembranous colitis, vomiting, and diarrhea (see pharmacology discussion). Assess bowel sounds as well as bowel patterns prior to giving this drug. Preoperatively, or if the patient is in an intensive care setting and receiving clindamycin, assess for the concurrent use of neuromuscular blocking drugs because of clindamycin's excessive blockade of neuromuscular functioning and respiratory paralysis. These patients, if in need of clindamycin, would need ventilator support.

*Linezolid* is used to treat hospital-acquired infections, pneumonia, and complicated skin infections, including MRSA. Use of methicillin (removed from the market) and oxacillin are no longer options for treatment, so this drug offers another pharmacotherapeutic option. Assess for the concurrent use of serotonergic drugs (e.g., SSRIs [antidepressants]) because of drug-induced serotonin syndrome (see Chapter 17). Additionally, assess for intake of tyramine-containing foods (e.g., aged cheese or wine, soy sauce, and smoked fish or meat) because of the risk of elevated blood pressure.

Assess patients taking *metronidazole* for allergy to the drug and to other nitroimidazole derivatives. As with all medications, assess for contraindications, cautions, and drug interactions, and document the findings (see the pharmacology discussion). It is important for patient safety to review culture and sensitivity reports before therapy is initiated. However, it may be necessary to start the medication regimen (due to clinical presentation) prior to results being obtained and then medications can be changed as dictated by the culture and sensitivity results. Baseline assessments are needed of the neurologic system (noting any dizziness, numbness, tingling, and other sensory and motor abnormalities), GI system (checking bowel sounds, problems, and patterns), and GU system (documenting urinary patterns, color of urine, and intake and output). Inquire about alcohol intake because of the interaction of alcohol with the drug and subsequent acute alcohol intolerance. Assess for potential drug interactions, such as with benzodiazepines, calcium channel blockers, various antidepressants, and warfarin.

Assessment of drug allergies is important with *nitrofurantoin*. Renal and liver functions are also important to assess due to the possibility of hepatotoxic adverse effects and the need for a decrease in dosage amounts in the elderly with renal function impairment. Complete a baseline assessment of any sensory or motor problems because of the possible adverse effect of peripheral neuropathy, which may be irreversible. Assess the patient's skin color, turgor, intactness, and presence of rash due to the possibility of drug-related mild to severe skin reactions. With *quinupristin/dalfopristin*, assess vital signs as well as for any muscular aches and pains due to drug-induced arthralgia and myalgia.

With *vancomycin*, ask questions about other medications the patient is taking, especially drugs that are nephrotoxic or ototoxic. Assess the patient for a history of preexisting renal disease or hearing loss due to the possibility of nephrotoxicity or ototoxicity. Note the baseline hearing status because of the risk of hearing loss. Part of the prescriber's order will be to order trough levels of vancomycin. These labs will be drawn immediately before the next dose. Assessment of these levels will be important to patient safety. Peak levels are no longer utilized. The color of the patient's skin is important to assess because of the risk for red man syndrome. This syndrome is bothersome but usually not harmful, and is characterized by flushing of the face, head, neck, and upper trunk areas. Red man syndrome is seen when infusions are administered too rapidly, so always assess and monitor IV rates to be sure the drug is administered over at least 1 hour. Assess vital signs with attention to blood pressure because too rapid infusions may precipitate hypotension. Because of multiple drug and diluent incompatibilities, as with several of the other parenteral antibiotics mentioned previously in this chapter, always assess for potential fluid and medication interactions.

*Daptinomycin* is a drug now indicated for complicated cases of skin and soft tissue infections caused by MRSA. Assess vital signs and blood pressure prior to and during infusion of this drug.

With the emergence of multidrug-resistant organisms (e.g., MRSA, VRE, and ESBL- and KPC-producing organisms), ensure that proper handwashing techniques are used by health care providers and caregivers.

## CASE STUDY

### *Vancomycin*

Mr. M., a 45-year-old quadriplegic, is being treated for an infected stage IV sacral pressure ulcer. The wound cultures have indicated the presence of multidrug-resistant *Staphylococcus aureus* (MRSA). The physician has ordered intravenous vancomycin to be given every 12 hours, application of wet-to-dry dressings (twice a day) as part of the treatment, as well as a referral to the enterostomal therapist. In addition, Mr. M. is placed on contact precautions because of the MRSA.

1. What will you assess before starting the vancomycin infusion?
2. Two days later, Mr. M. complains of feeling "hot" in his face and neck, and itching in those same areas. His face and neck are flushed. What do you suspect is happening?
3. What can you do to minimize complications during vancomycin infusions?
4. The physician orders measurement of vancomycin blood levels. What is the therapeutic goal when vancomycin levels are monitored?
5. What is the single best action you can take to prevent the spread of Mr. M.'s MRSA infection?

For answers, see http://evolve.elsevier.com/Lilley.

## NURSING DIAGNOSES

1. Deficient knowledge related to lack of information and experience with the medication regimen
2. Risk for infection related to the patient's compromised immune status before and during treatment
3. Risk for injury (compromised organ function) related to adverse effects of medications (e.g., ototoxicity and nephrotoxicity) and weakened physical state

## PLANNING

### GOALS

1. Patient demonstrates adequate knowledge base about the antibiotic therapeutic regimen.
2. Patient remains free from infection and has improved immune status during antibiotic therapy.
3. Patient remains free from injury.

### OUTCOME CRITERIA

1. Patient states action and rationale for use of antibiotic therapy.
   - Patient understands the need to take the antibiotic exactly as ordered and for the duration of therapy.
2. Patient experiences an increased sense of well-being and improved immune status while taking antibiotics.
   - Patient remains without fever, pain, and malaise.
   - Patient experiences increased comfort and improved energy levels.
   - Patient experiences minimal adverse effects of antibiotic therapy.
3. Patient remains free from injury as related to adverse effects such as minimal to no problems with GI upset, diarrhea, nausea, and hearing loss.
   - Patient states measures to minimize adverse effects associated with antibiotic therapy, such as taking medications with yogurt, increasing fluids, eating well-balanced meals, and following instructions associated with safe use of the specific antibiotic.

## IMPLEMENTATION

*Aminoglycosides,* as well as any antibiotics, need to be given exactly as ordered and with adequate hydration. Encourage fluid intake of up to 3000 mL/day unless contraindicated, especially with oral dosage forms. Parenteral dosage forms are the most commonly used. Neomycin is the only oral dosage form available for this class of antibiotic. Oral neomycin is generally used in special situations such as preoperative bowel preparation, treatment of diarrhea caused by *E. coli,* and treatment of hepatic encephalopathy. It is to be given exactly as ordered. Because of the potential for nephrotoxicity and ototoxicity, determine and monitor the patient's renal function during therapy. Dosing is adjusted based on estimates of creatinine clearance calculated from the patient's serum creatinine level. This assists in keeping a close watch on the patient's renal function and thus helps to prevent toxicity. Also monitor BUN levels and glomerular filtration rate (GFR) during therapy. Alteration in auditory, vestibular, or renal function may indicate the need for a possible dosage adjustment or withdrawal of the drug. Consumption of yogurt or buttermilk may help prevent antibiotic-induced superinfections (see Chapter 38).

With *aminoglycosides,* instruct the patient to report to the prescriber any changes in hearing, ringing in the ears (tinnitus), or a full feeling in the ears. Nausea, vomiting with motion, ataxia, nystagmus, and dizziness should also be reported immediately and may indicate issues with the vestibular nerve. With ophthalmic dosage forms, redness, burning, and itching of the eyes may indicate an adverse reaction to ophthalmic forms, and redness over the skin area may indicate an adverse reaction to topical forms. Check intramuscular administration sites for induration. If noted, report it immediately to the prescriber, and do not reuse the site. Monitor intravenous sites for heat, swelling, redness, pain, or red streaking over the vein (phlebitis), and initiate measures as per institutional protocol or policy. Keep in mind the following special considerations for gentamicin: (1) Intramuscular: Give deeply and slowly into muscle mass (ventrogluteal) to minimize discomfort; and (2) Intravenous: Check for incompatibilities with other drugs, and give only clear or very slightly yellow solutions that have been diluted with either normal saline (NS) or $D_5W$, infusing at the correct rate.

*Quinolones,* as with any antibiotics that are self-administered, are to be taken exactly as prescribed and for the full course of treatment. Instruct the patient not to take these medications with antacids, iron, zinc preparations, multivitamins, or sucralfate because the absorption of the antibiotic will be decreased. If the patient needs to take calcium or magnesium, instruct the patient to take it 1 hour before or after the quinolone. Forcing of fluids is recommended, unless contraindicated. See the Patient Teaching Tips for more information.

With *clindamycin,* instruct the patient to take the medication as ordered. Oral dosage forms are to be taken with 8 oz of water or other fluid. With topical forms, advise patients to avoid the simultaneous use of peeling or abrasive acne products, soaps, or alcohol-containing cosmetics to prevent cumulative effects; however, some products combine clindamycin with anti-acne medications (e.g., Acayna). Topical forms are to be applied in a thin layer to the affected area. Infuse intravenous dosage forms by piggyback technique and as ordered. Most references state *never* to give these drugs via parenteral intravenous push. Dilute doses of the drug, and infuse per manufacturer guidelines. Too rapid intravenous infusion can lead to severe hypotension and possible cardiac arrest. Give intramuscular dosage forms deep into a large muscle mass (see Chapter 9).

*Linezolid* is generally given orally or intravenously, which makes it advantageous for those requiring an antibiotic with a spectrum similar to vancomycin for an extended period or on an outpatient basis. Oral doses are to be evenly spaced around the clock, as ordered, and given with food or milk to decrease the possibility of GI upset. Oral suspension forms must be used within 21 days of reconstitution. Protect intravenous doses from light, and infuse over 30 to 120 minutes; do not mix with any other medication. Foods that may increase blood pressure while taking linezolid and need to be avoided include aged cheeses, wine, soy sauce, smoked meats or fish, and sauerkraut due to their tyramine content.

Oral forms of *metronidazole* need to be given with food or meals to help decrease GI upset. Educate patients not to chew extended-release dosage. Intravaginal doses are recommended to be administered at bedtime. Topical creams, ointments, or lotions are to be applied thinly to the affected area. An applicator should be used for intravaginal dosages. Gloves are worn to protect from undue exposure to the medication and as a part of Standard Precautions. Do not apply topical forms close to the eyes to avoid irritation. Store intravenous dosage forms, which are supplied in a ready-to-use infusion bag, at room temperature.

*Nitrofurantoin* is available in oral forms and should be given with plenty of fluids, food, or milk to decrease GI upset. Do not crush tablets to help prevent tooth staining and GI upset. Because of the risk for superinfection, hepatotoxicity, and peripheral neuropathy (which may be irreversible), constantly monitor for signs and symptoms of these adverse effects and document the findings. Be aware that jaundice, itching, rash, and liver enlargement may indicate toxic effects to the liver, whereas numbness and tingling may occur with peripheral neuropathy.

For *quinupristin/dalfopristin,* only intravenous dosage forms are available. Reconstitute the drug using only $D_5W$. Use a gentle swirling action instead of shaking to mix the drug (to help minimize foaming). A diluted infusion bag of the drug is stable for up to 6 hours, or 54 hours if refrigerated. These characteristics are important to know to help prevent untoward complications. Infusions are generally given over at least 60 minutes. Implement the same measures, as with other antibiotics, to monitor for superinfection.

*Vancomycin* may be used orally but is poorly absorbed by this route, and is only used to treat microbes in the GI tract (e.g., staphylococcal enterocolitis). Parenteral dosage forms must be used to treat infection outside of the intima of the GI tract. Reconstitute intravenous dosage forms as recommended (e.g., with either $D_5W$ or NS) and infuse over at least 60 minutes. Too rapid an infusion of vancomycin or administration by intravenous push may lead to severe hypotension and red man syndrome. Extravasation may cause local skin irritation and damage, so frequently monitor the infusion, and in particular the intravenous site. Constant monitoring for drug-related neurotoxicity, nephrotoxicity, ototoxicity, and superinfection remain critical to patient safety. In addition, adequate hydration (at least 2 L of fluids every 24 hours unless contraindicated) is important to prevent nephrotoxicity. Trough levels need to be ordered prior to the third or fourth dose; peak levels are no longer used (see the pharmacology discussion for more information).

If the new drug *telavancin* is ordered, use it very carefully and as ordered, especially if the patient has renal dysfunction. When this drug is infused, give it exactly as ordered while also watching for ECG changes, such as changes in the QT segment.

Because of the significant issue of multidrug-resistant organisms, encourage patients and family members not to abuse or overuse antibiotics and to report immediately to the prescriber any signs and symptoms of an infection that is not resolving or responding to antibiotic therapy. Regardless of drug management, in today's health care settings (acute and long-term facilities, medical offices, urgent care centers, emergency departments) as well as in the home setting and abroad, teach and demonstrate proper and thorough handwashing technique. Handwashing must be performed often, especially during cold and flu season, before and after preparing food, and after engaging in any of the following activities: going to the bathroom or changing diapers; touching bare human body parts; coughing, sneezing, or using a handkerchief or disposable tissue; eating or drinking; using tobacco; using the telephone; shaking hands; and playing with pets. The Centers for Disease Control and Prevention (CDC) recommend the following as the proper handwashing technique: Wash hands with warm running water and soap; lather well by rubbing hands vigorously for at least 15 to 20 seconds; pay attention to the wrist area, backs of the hands, areas between the fingers, and under the fingernails; and rinse well. Allow the water to run while drying hands with a paper towel and then use a dry paper towel as a barrier between the faucet and clean hands while turning off the water. If soap and water are not available and hands are not visibly soiled, gel hand sanitizers or alcohol-based hand wipes containing at least 60% ethyl alcohol or isopropanol may be used. Once the gel is applied and all surfaces covered, rub hands until gel is dry and do not towel gel off. It is also imperative to educate patients and family members as well as the community at large that taking antibiotics excessively and when not needed may lead to problems of antibiotic resistance!

# EVALUATION

Once antibiotic therapy has been initiated, evaluation that is focused on goals, outcome criteria, therapeutic effects, and adverse effects must always be ongoing. Ask patients to report a decrease in symptoms (e.g., infection) as well as absence of injury to self and a decrease in pain. Therapeutic goals include a return to normal of all blood counts and vital signs, negative results on culture and sensitivity testing, and improved appetite, energy level, and sense of well-being. Signs and symptoms of the infection will begin to resolve once therapeutic levels of antibiotics are achieved. Another aspect of evaluation is monitoring for adverse effects of therapy such as superinfections, antibiotic-associated colitis, nephrotoxicity, ototoxicity, neurotoxicity, hepatotoxicity, and other drug-specific adverse effects.

## ■ PATIENT TEACHING TIPS

### Aminoglycosides

- Educate the patient about the drug, its purpose, and its adverse effects, including the risk of hearing loss, which may occur after completion of therapy. Advise the patient to report to the prescriber any change in hearing.
- Forcing fluids up to 3000 mL/day, unless contraindicated, is important with any medication but especially with antibiotics to maximize absorption of oral doses, minimize some of the adverse effects, and ensure adequate hydration.
- Instruct the patient to report to the prescriber any persistent headache, nausea, or vertigo. Educate the patient about the signs and symptoms of superinfection, such as diarrhea; vaginal discharge; stomatitis; loose and foul-smelling stools; and cough.

### Quinolones

- Educate about the importance of avoiding exposure to the sun and tanning beds. Recommend the use of sunglasses and sunscreen protection.
- Advise the patient to report to the prescriber any headache, dizziness, restlessness, diarrhea, vomiting, oral candidiasis, flushing of the face, and/or inflammation of the tendons.
- Educate about drug interactions that may occur with the following drugs: calcium, magnesium, probenecid, nitrofurantoin, oral anticoagulants, antacids, iron, sucralfate, and zinc preparations. Instruct the patient to take calcium and magnesium supplements at least 1 hour before or after taking the quinolone. Probenecid may reduce the excretion of the antibiotic and cause toxicity. Since quinolones may alter the intestinal flora and thus vitamin K synthesis, oral anticoagulants must be used with caution in patients taking these antibiotics.
- Instruct the patient to take ciprofloxacin and levofloxacin, both quinolones, exactly as ordered.

### Clindamycin

- Instruct the patient not to use topical forms near the eyes or near any abraded areas to avoid irritation.
- When vaginal dosage forms are used, the patient needs to be advised not to engage in sexual intercourse for the duration of therapy. The full course of antibiotics are to be taken as ordered to obtain maximal therapeutic benefit.

- If cream dosage forms get into the eyes accidentally, instruct the patient to rinse the eyes immediately with copious amounts of cool tap water.

### Linezolid

- Instruct the patient to continue therapy for the full prescribed length of treatment (as with all antibiotics).
- Educate the patient to avoid tyramine-containing foods (e.g., red wine, aged cheeses) while taking the drug.
- Instruct the patient to report to the prescriber immediately any severe abdominal pain, fever, severe diarrhea, and/or worsening of signs and symptoms of infection.

### Metronidazole

- Caution the patient to avoid alcohol and any alcohol-containing products (e.g., cough preparations and elixirs) while taking the drug because of the risk for a disulfiram-like reaction (e.g., severe vomiting).
- Educate the patient about the purpose of the drug, such as its use as either an antibacterial or an antifungal medication, because this knowledge is crucial to achieving therapeutic effects and preventing adverse effects.

### Nitrofurantoin

- Advise the patient to report to the prescriber any abdominal cramping, dizziness, severe skin reactions, or jaundice.

### Vancomycin

- Instruct the patient to report any changes in hearing such as ringing in the ears or a feeling of fullness in the ears. Any nausea, vomiting, unsteady gait, dizziness, generalized tingling (usually after intravenous dosing), chills, fever, rash, and/or hives must also be reported.
- Monitor therapeutic serum levels throughout therapy; this monitoring is key to prevention of toxicity. Trough levels are usually monitored throughout therapy. Stress to the patient that follow-up appointments are important for monitoring serum drug levels and identifying possible toxic effects.

## KEY POINTS

- Over the years, bacteria have developed enzymes and mechanisms to interact with antibiotics and render the antibiotic ineffective. Multidrug resistance is a significant health issue, and such resistant organisms include ESBL- and KPC-producing bacteria, MRSA, and VRE.
- The aminoglycosides are a group of natural and semisynthetic antibiotics that are classified as *bactericidal* drugs, are very potent, and are capable of potentially serious toxicities (e.g., nephrotoxicity, ototoxicity).
- Quinolones are very potent, bactericidal, broad-spectrum antibiotics and include norfloxacin, ciprofloxacin, levofloxacin, and moxifloxacin.
- Clindamycin is a semisynthetic derivative of lincomycin, an older antibiotic.
- Linezolid is an antibacterial drug used to treat infections associated with vancomycin-resistant *Enterococcus faecium,* more commonly referred to as VRE. VRE is a difficult infection to treat and often occurs as a *nosocomial* (hospital-acquired) infection.
- Metronidazole (Flagyl) is an antimicrobial drug of the class nitroimidazole, has good activity against anaerobic organisms, and is widely used for intraabdominal and gynecologic infections; it is also used to treat protozoal infections (e.g., amebiasis, trichomoniasis).

- Nitrofurantoin (Macrodantin) is an antibiotic drug of the class *nitrofuran.* It is indicated primarily for urinary tract infections caused by *E. coli, S. aureus, Klebsiella* spp., and *Enterobacter* spp.
- Quinupristin and dalfopristin (Synercid) are two streptogramin antibacterials approved for intravenous treatment of bacteremia and life-threatening infection caused by VRE and for treatment of complicated skin and skin structure infections caused by *S. aureus* and *S. pyogenes.*
- Daptomycin (Cubicin) is used to treat complicated skin and soft-tissue infections. Telavancin is a newer drug that is effective against MRSA and VRE and is indicated in the treatment of skin and skin structure infections.
- Use of these antibiotics requires a critical assessment for any history or current symptoms indicative of hypersensitivity or allergic reactions (from mild reactions with rash, pruritus, and hives to severe reactions with laryngeal edema, bronchospasm, hypotension, and possible cardiac arrest).
- With use of any antibiotic, it is important to assess for superinfection, or a secondary infection that occurs because of the destruction of normal flora during antibiotic therapy. Superinfections may occur in the mouth, respiratory tract, GI and GU tracts, and on the skin. Fungal infections are evidenced by fever, lethargy, perineal itching, and other anatomically related symptoms.

## NCLEX® EXAMINATION REVIEW QUESTIONS

1  While assessing a woman who is receiving an antibiotic for community acquired pneumonia, the nurse notes that the patient has a thick, white vaginal discharge. The patient is also complaining about perineal itching. The nurse suspects that the patient has
   a  resistance to the antibiotic.
   b  an adverse effect of the antibiotic.
   c  a superinfection.
   d  an allergic reaction.

2  A patient has been admitted for treatment of an infected leg ulcer and will be started on intravenous linezolid. The nurse is reviewing the list of the patient's current medications. Which type of medication, if listed, would be of most concern if taken with the linezolid?
   a  Beta blocker
   b  Oral anticoagulant
   c  Selective serotonin reuptake inhibitor antidepressant
   d  Thyroid replacement hormone

3  When administering vancomycin, the nurse knows that which of these is most important to assess before giving the medication?
   a  Renal function
   b  WBC count
   c  Liver function
   d  Platelet count

4  During therapy with an intravenous aminoglycoside, the patient calls the nurse and says, "I'm hearing some odd sounds, like ringing, in my ears." What is the nurse's priority action at this time?

   a  Reassure the patient that these are expected adverse effects.
   b  Reduce the rate of the intravenous infusion.
   c  Increase the rate of the intravenous infusion.
   d  Stop the infusion immediately.

5  When giving intravenous quinolones, the nurse needs to keep in mind that these drugs may have serious interactions with which drugs?
   a  Selective serotonin reuptake inhibitor antidepressants
   b  Nonsteroidal antiinflammatory drugs
   c  Oral anticoagulants
   d  Antihypertensives

6  The nurse is administering an intravenous aminoglycoside to a patient who has had gastrointestinal surgery. Which nursing measures are appropriate? (Select all that apply.)
   a  Report a trough drug level of 0.8 mcg/mL, and hold the drug.
   b  Enforce a strict fluid restriction.
   c  Monitor serum creatinine levels.
   d  Instruct the patient to report dizziness or a feeling of fullness in the ears.
   e  Warn the patient that the urine may turn darker in color.

7  The order reads: "Give vancomycin, 1250 mg in 250 mL NS, IVPB, every 12 hours. Infuse over 90 minutes." The nurse will set the infusion pump to what setting for mL/hour?

1. c, 2. c, 3. a, 4. d, 5. c, 6. c, d, 7. 167 mL/hour

For Critical Thinking and Prioritization Questions, see http://evolve.elsevier.com/Lilley.

## OBJECTIVES

When you reach the end of this chapter, you will be able to do the following:

1  Discuss the effects of the immune system with attention to the various types of immunity.
2  Describe the effects of viruses in the human body.
3  List specific drugs categorized as non–human immunodeficiency virus (HIV) antivirals and HIV antivirals or antiretrovirals.
4  Discuss the process of immunosuppression in patients with viral infections, specifically those with HIV infection.

5  Describe the stages of acquired immunodeficiency syndrome (AIDS) and various drugs used to manage the illness.
6  Discuss the mechanism of action, indications, contraindications, cautions, routes, adverse effects, and toxic effects of the various non-HIV antiviral and HIV antiviral drugs.
7  Develop a nursing care plan that includes all phases of the nursing process for patients receiving non-HIV and HIV antiviral drugs.

## DRUG PROFILES

- ♦ acyclovir, p. 657
  amantadine and rimantadine, p. 656
  enfuvirtide, p. 664
- ♦ ganciclovir, p. 658
- ♦ indinavir, p. 665
- ♦ nevirapine, p. 666
  maraviroc, p. 665

  oseltamivir and zanamivir, p. 658
  raltegravir, p. 666
  ribavirin, p. 658
  tenofovir, p. 666
- ♦ zidovudine, p. 666

♦ *Key drug*

## KEY TERMS

**Acquired immunodeficiency syndrome (AIDS)** Infection caused by the *human immunodeficiency virus (HIV)*, which weakens the host's immune system, giving rise to opportunistic infections. (p. 652)

**Antibodies** Immunoglobulin molecules that have an antigen-specific amino acid sequence and are produced by the humoral immune system (antibodies produced from B lymphocytes) in response to exposure to a specific antigen, the purpose of which is to attack and destroy molecules of this antigen. (p. 652)

**Antigen** A substance, usually a protein, that is foreign to a host and causes the formation of an antibody that reacts specifically with that antibody. Examples of antigens include bacterial exotoxins, viruses, and allergens. An allergen (e.g., dust, pollen, mold) is a specific type of antigen that causes allergic reactions (see Chapter 36). (p. 652)

**Antiretroviral drugs** A specific term for antiviral drugs that work against retroviruses such as HIV. (p. 654)

## KEY TERMS—cont'd

**Antiviral drugs** A general term for drugs that destroy viruses, either directly or indirectly by suppressing their replication. (p. 653)

**Cell-mediated immunity** One of two major parts of the immune system. It consists of nonspecific immune responses mediated primarily by T lymphocytes (T cells) and other immune system cells (e.g., monocytes, macrophages, neutrophils) but not by antibody-producing cells (B lymphocytes). (p. 652)

**Deoxyribonucleic acid (DNA)** A nucleic acid composed of nucleotide units that contain molecules of the sugar deoxyribose, phosphate groups, and purine and pyrimidine bases. DNA molecules transmit genetic information and are found primarily in the nuclei of cells. (Compare with *ribonucleic acid [RNA]*.) (p. 651)

**Fusion** The process by which viruses attach themselves to, or fuse with, the cell membranes of host cells, in preparation for infecting the cell for purposes of viral replication. (p. 651)

**Genome** The complete set of genetic material of any organism; it may consist of multiple chromosomes (groups of DNA or RNA molecules) in higher organisms; a single chromosome, as in bacteria; or one or two DNA or RNA molecules, as in viruses. (p. 651)

**Herpesviruses** Several different types of viruses belonging to the family Herpesviridae that cause various forms of herpes infection. (p. 653)

**Host** Any organism that is infected with a microorganism, such as bacteria or viruses. (p. 651)

**Human immunodeficiency virus (HIV)** The retrovirus that causes AIDS. (p. 652)

**Humoral immunity** One of two major parts of the immune system. It consists of specific immune responses in the form of antigen-specific antibodies produced from B lymphocytes. (p. 653)

**Immunoglobulins** Synonymous with immune globulins. Glycoproteins produced and used by the humoral immune system to attack and kill any substance (antigen) that is foreign to the body. An immunoglobulin with an antigen-specific amino acid sequence is called an antibody and is able to recognize and inactivate molecules of a specific antigen. (p. 653)

**Influenza viruses** The viruses that cause influenza, an acute viral infection of the respiratory tract. There are three types of influenza virus: A, B, and C. Currently, medications are available only to treat types A and B. (p. 653)

**Nucleic acids** A general term referring to DNA and RNA. These complex biomolecules contain the genetic material of all living organisms, which is passed to future generations during reproduction. (p. 652)

**Nucleoside** A structural component of nucleic acid molecules (DNA or RNA) that consists of a purine or pyrimidine base attached to a sugar molecule. (p. 654)

**Nucleotide** A nucleoside that is attached to a phosphate unit, which makes up the side chain "backbone" of a DNA or an RNA molecule. (p. 654)

**Opportunistic infections** Infections caused by any type of microorganism that occur in an immunocompromised host but normally would not occur in an immunocompetent host. (p. 653)

**Protease** An enzyme that breaks down the amino acid structure of protein molecules by chemically cleaving the peptide bonds that link together the individual amino acids. (p. 659)

**Replication** Any process of duplication or reproduction, such as that involved in the duplication of nucleic acid molecules (DNA or RNA) during the reproduction processes of all living organisms. This is also the term used most often to describe the entire process of viral reproduction, which occurs only inside the cells of an infected host organism. (p. 652)

**Retroviruses** Viruses belonging to the family Retroviridae. These viruses contain RNA (as opposed to DNA) as their genome and replicate using the enzyme reverse transcriptase. Currently the most clinically significant retrovirus is HIV. (p. 653)

**Reverse transcriptase** An RNA-directed DNA polymerase enzyme. It promotes the synthesis of a DNA molecule from an RNA molecule, which is the reverse of the usual process. HIV replicates in this manner. (p. 659)

**Ribonucleic acid (RNA)** A nucleic acid composed of nucleotide units that contain molecules of the sugar ribose, phosphate groups, and purine and pyrimidine bases. RNA molecules transmit genetic information and are found in both the nuclei and cytoplasm of cells. (Compare with deoxyribonucleic acid [DNA].) (p. 651)

**Virion** A mature virus particle. (p. 651)

**Viruses** The smallest known class of microorganisms; viruses can only replicate inside host cells. (p. 651)

## ANATOMY, PHYSIOLOGY, AND PATHOPHYSIOLOGY OVERVIEW

### GENERAL PRINCIPLES OF VIROLOGY

**Viruses** are very small microorganisms, usually many times smaller than bacteria. Unlike bacteria, viruses can replicate only inside the cells of their host. In this respect, all viruses are obligate intracellular parasites. It must be emphasized that viruses are not cells, per se, but instead are particles that infect and replicate inside of cells. A mature virus particle is known as a virion. Compared with other organisms, virions have a relatively simple structure that consists of the genome, the capsid, and the envelope. The genome is the inner core of the virion, which is composed of single- or double-stranded deoxyribonucleic acid (DNA) or ribonucleic acid (RNA) molecules, but not both.

Viruses are the simplest of all organisms. The cells of more complex organisms have much larger nucleic acid strands or multiple strands, which make up chromosomes. The viral capsid is a protein coat that surrounds and protects the genome. It also plays a role in the process of fusion between the virions

1. Attachment to host cell
2. Uncoating of virus, and entry of viral nucleic acid into host cell nucleus
3. Control of DNA, RNA, and/or protein production
4. Production of viral subunits
5. Assembly of virions
6. Release of virions

**FIGURE 40-1** Virus replication. Some viruses integrate into host chromosome and enter a period of latency. *mRNA,* Messenger RNA. (Modified from Brody TM, Larner J, Minneman KP: *Human pharmacology: molecular to clinical,* ed 5, St Louis, 2010, Mosby.)

and the host cells. Fusion occurs when virions attach themselves to host cells in preparation for infecting the cells. The envelope is the outermost layer of the virion and is present in some, but not all, viruses. It has a lipoprotein structure containing viral antigens that are often chemically specific for various proteins on the surface of the host cell membranes. This biochemical specificity, when present, also facilitates the fusion process. The human immunodeficiency virus (HIV), which causes acquired immune deficiency syndrome (AIDS), functions in this manner.

Viruses can enter the body through at least four routes: inhalation through the respiratory tract, ingestion via the gastrointestinal (GI) tract, transplacentally via mother to infant, and inoculation via skin or mucous membranes. The inoculation route can take several forms, including sexual contact, blood transfusions, sharing of syringes or needles, organ transplantation, and bites (including human, animal, insect, spider, and others). Once inside the body, the virus particles, or virions, begin to attach themselves to the outer membranes of host cells (cell membranes or plasma membranes) as illustrated in Figure 40-1.

The viral genome then passes through the plasma membrane into the cytoplasm of the host cell. It later enters the cell nucleus, where the replication process begins. The virion may use its own or host enzymes (or both) to direct the replication process. In the host cell nucleus, the viral genome uses the cell's genetic material (the nucleic acids RNA and DNA) to synthesize viral nucleic acids and proteins. These are then used to construct complete new virions. These new virions then exit the infected host cell by budding through the plasma membrane and go on to infect other host cells, where the replication process continues. The changes in the cell associated with viral replication are known as the *cytopathic effect* and usually result in the destruction of the host cell. Repeated over time, host cell destruction gives rise to the pathologic effects of the virus, which can eventually impair or even kill the host organism.

Although this cytopathic effect is the most common outcome, there are other possible outcomes of viral infection. One is viral transformation, which involves mutation of the host cell DNA or RNA and can result in malignant (cancerous) host cells. Viruses that can induce cancer in this way are known as oncogenic viruses. More common is latent, or dormant, infection in which the virions remain inside host cells but do not actively replicate to any significant degree. For example, HIV infection may have a lengthy dormant phase of 10 years or longer before giving rise to AIDS in an infected person. HIV infection is discussed in greater detail later in the chapter in the section on retroviruses.

Viruses are ubiquitous (widespread) in the environment, and most viral infections may not even be noticed before they are eliminated by the host's immune system. These are referred to as "silent" viral infections. Although the host's immune system acts to neutralize viral infection, it can become overwhelmed, depending on how virulent the virus is and how rapidly it replicates inside host cells. In most cases, however, a person's immune system is able to arrest and eliminate the virus. Host immune responses to viral infections are classified as either *nonspecific* or *specific.* Nonspecific immune responses include phagocytosis (eating) of viral particles by leukocytes such as neutrophils, macrophages, monocytes, and T lymphocytes (T cells). Another nonspecific immune response is the release of cytokines from these leukocytes. Cytokines are biochemical substances (e.g., histamine, tumor necrosis factor) that stimulate other protective immune functions. In addition, these activated immune system cells may also phagocytize infected host cells to curb the growth and spread of infection. These types of immune responses are collectively referred to as cell-mediated immunity. Cell-mediated immunity is nonspecific in the sense that it does not involve antibodies that are specific for a given antigen. In contrast, specific immune responses include the production of antibodies from B lymphocytes (B cells). These are immune-system proteins (immunoglobulins) that are chemically specific for viral antigens. This type of immune response is also called humoral immunity. Immune system function is discussed in more detail in Chapters 48 and 49.

## OVERVIEW OF VIRAL ILLNESSES AND THEIR TREATMENT

There are at least 6 classes of DNA viruses and at least 14 classes of RNA viruses that are known to infect humans. Some of the more prominent viral illnesses include smallpox (poxviruses), sore throat and conjunctivitis (adenoviruses), warts (papovaviruses), influenza (orthomyxoviruses), respiratory infections (coronaviruses, rhinoviruses), gastroenteritis (rotaviruses, Norwalk-like viruses), HIV/AIDS (retroviruses), herpes (herpesviruses), and hepatitis (hepadnaviruses). Effective drug therapy is currently available only for a relatively small number of active viral infections. The drug therapy for hepatitis is discussed further in Chapter 47. HIV belongs to the relatively unique viral class known as *retroviruses* and is discussed in more detail in a separate section of this chapter.

Fortunately, many viral illnesses are survivable (e.g., chickenpox), albeit bothersome and uncomfortable. The incidence of some of these illnesses has been reduced by the development of effective vaccines (e.g., vaccines for polio, smallpox, measles, chickenpox). Vaccines are discussed in more detail in Chapter 49. However, many other viral illnesses are either fatal or have much more severe long-term outcomes (e.g., hepatitis, HIV infection).

Antiviral drugs are chemicals that kill or suppress viruses by either destroying virions or inhibiting their ability to replicate. Even the best medications currently available never fully eradicate a virus completely from its host. However, the body's immune system has a better chance of controlling or eliminating a viral infection when the ability of the virus to replicate itself is suppressed. Drugs that actually destroy virions include various disinfectants and immunoglobulins. Disinfectants such as povidone-iodine (Betadine) are virucides and are commonly used to disinfect medical equipment. Such drugs are discussed further in Chapter 38.

Immunoglobulins are concentrated antibodies that can attack and destroy viruses. They are isolated and pooled from human or animal blood. Their activity may be either nonspecific (e.g., human gamma globulin) or specific (e.g., rabies immunoglobulin, varicella-zoster immunoglobulin). Although such substances can technically be considered as antiviral drugs, they are more commonly thought of as immunizing drugs and are therefore discussed in more detail in Chapter 49. A few antiviral drugs, such as the interferons, stimulate the body's immune system to kill the virions directly. These drugs are discussed in Chapter 47.

The current antiviral drugs are all synthetic compounds that work indirectly by inhibiting viral replication as opposed to directly by destroying mature virions themselves. Only relatively few of the known viruses can be controlled by current drug therapy. Some of the viruses in this group are the following:

- Cytomegalovirus (CMV)
- Hepatitis viruses
- Herpesviruses

- HIV
- Influenza viruses ("flu" viruses)
- Respiratory syncytial virus

Active viral infections are usually more difficult to eradicate than those caused by bacteria. One reason is that viruses replicate only inside host cells rather than replicating independently in the bloodstream or in other tissues. Most antiviral drugs must therefore enter these cells to disrupt viral replication. The need to develop antiviral drugs that are not overly toxic to host cells is one reason that there are relatively few effective antiviral medications on the market. However, the HIV/AIDS epidemic that began in the early 1980s strongly boosted antiviral drug research. This has increased the number of available antiviral drugs to treat HIV and other viral infections such as influenza, CMV infection, and varicella-zoster virus (VZV) infection. Many drugs for the treatment of HIV are approved by the U.S. Food and Drug Administration (FDA) via an accelerated process, which means that they are approved faster than other drugs, because of the nature of the illness. Because of the rapid addition of HIV drugs to the market, it is beyond the scope of this book to list every available drug. The reader is referred to the FDA website on approved AIDS drugs at www.fda.gov/For Consumers/byAudience/ForPatientAdvocates/HIVandAIDS Activities/ucm118915.html for the most recently approved AIDS drugs.

Another reason viral illnesses are difficult to treat is that the virus has often replicated itself many thousands or even millions of times before symptoms of illness appear. Therefore, one goal in the field of infectious disease is to be able to diagnose viral illnesses before an infecting virus has undergone widespread replication in a human host. This would theoretically allow the dual benefit of both early drug therapy and easier elimination of the virus by the host's immune system. This has happened to some degree with HIV infection, with relatively early diagnosis made possible by blood tests to screen for HIV antibodies. Of course, the patient must also be alerted of the need to seek medical care before serious illness develops.

Recall that for a virus to replicate, virions must first attach themselves to host cell membranes in a process known as *fusion*. Once inside the cell, the viral genome makes nucleic acids and proteins, which are then used to build new viral particles, or virions (see Figure 40-1). All virions contain a genome that consists of either DNA or RNA, but not both. Antiviral drugs inhibit this replication process in various ways. Most antiviral drugs enter the same cells that the viruses enter. Once inside, these antiviral drugs interfere with viral nucleic acid synthesis. Other antiviral drugs work by preventing the fusion process itself.

The best responses to antiviral drug therapy are usually seen in patients with competent immune systems. The immune system can work synergistically with the drug to eliminate or suppress viral activity. Patients who are immunocompromised (have weakened immune systems) are at greater risk for opportunistic infections, which are infections caused by organisms that would not normally harm an immunocompetent person. The most common examples of immunocompromised patients are cancer patients, organ transplant recipients, and patients with AIDS. These patients are prone to frequent and often severe opportunistic infections of many types, including those caused by other (non-HIV) viruses, bacteria, fungi, and protozoans. Such infections often require long-term prophylactic antiinfective drug therapy to control the infection and prevent its recurrence because of compromised host immune functions.

Recall that there are two types of nucleic acid found in living organisms: DNA and RNA. There are also five organic bases that are the structural components of these nucleic acids. DNA consists of long chains of deoxyribose sugar molecules, phosphate groups, and purine (adenine or guanine) and pyrimidine (cytosine or thymine) bases. RNA consists of long chains of ribose sugar molecules linked to phosphate groups, together with purine (adenine or guanine) and pyrimidine (cytosine or uracil) bases. A nucleoside is a single unit consisting of a base and its attached sugar molecule. Nucleosides have names similar to their bases with minor spelling modifications (e.g., adenosine, guanosine, cytidine, thymidine). A nucleotide is a nucleoside plus its attached phosphate molecule. Most antiviral drugs are synthetic purine or pyrimidine nucleoside or nucleotide analogues. Some pharmacology texts categorize the antiviral drugs based on their nucleoside-nucleotide activity. However, for ease of learning, this book divides antiviral drugs into drugs that treat HIV infections and those that treat non-HIV viral infections. Antiretroviral drugs are indicated specifically for the treatment of infections caused by HIV, the virus that causes AIDS. The effectiveness of antiviral drugs varies widely among patients and even over time in the same patient.

## HERPES SIMPLEX VIRUS AND VARICELLA-ZOSTER VIRUS INFECTIONS

The family of viruses known as Herpesviridae includes those viruses that cause all kinds of herpes infection. There are several specific types of such viruses. Herpes simplex virus type 1 (HSV-1) causes mucocutaneous herpes—usually in the form of perioral blisters ("fever blisters" or "cold sores"). Herpes simplex virus type 2 (HSV-2) causes genital herpes. Human herpesvirus 3 (HHV-3) causes both chickenpox and shingles. This virus is more commonly known as *herpes zoster virus* or *varicella-zoster virus (VZV)*. Human herpesvirus 4 (HHV-4), more frequently known as Epstein-Barr virus, is associated with illnesses such as infectious mononucleosis ("mono") and chronic fatigue syndrome. Human herpesvirus 5 (HHV-5) is more commonly known as *cytomegalovirus (CMV)* and is the cause of CMV retinitis (a serious viral infection of the eye) and CMV disease, which is most commonly seen in immunocompromised patients. Human herpesviruses 6 and 7 are not especially clinically significant, and infection with these viruses may be more likely to occur in immunocompromised patients. Human herpesvirus 8, also known as *Kaposi's sarcoma herpesvirus*, is an oncogenic (cancer-inducing) virus believed to cause Kaposi's sarcoma, an AIDS-associated cancer. All of these viruses occur, often asymptomatically, in varying percentages of the population. Types 3 through 7 normally do not cause diseases that require medication, except in the case of immunocompromised patients. However, the HSVs (types 1 and 2) and VZV (HHV-3) commonly cause illnesses that are now routinely treated with prescription medications.

## Herpes Simplex Viruses

Although there can be anatomic overlap between the two types of herpesviruses, HSV-1 infection is most commonly associated with perioral blisters and is therefore often thought of as *oral herpes*. In contrast, HSV-2 infection is most commonly associated with blisters on both male and female genitalia and is therefore commonly referred to as *genital herpes*. Although they usually do not cause serious or life-threatening illness, both infections are annoying and highly transmissible through close physical contact (e.g., kissing, sexual intercourse). Outbreaks of painful skin lesions occur intermittently, with periods of latency (no sores or other symptoms) occurring between acute outbreaks. Although antiviral medications are not always required and are *not* curative, they can speed up the process of remission and reduce the duration of painful symptoms. This is especially true if the medications are started early in a given outbreak. Patients may be prescribed an ongoing lower dose of antiviral drug for prophylaxis of outbreaks. HSV infections can become serious, even life-threatening, when the patient is immunocompromised or a newborn infant. Neonatal herpes is often a life-threatening infection, and babies with this disease are often treated in neonatal intensive care units with intravenous antiviral drugs. However, treatments may fail, causing infant death and/or permanent disability. Therefore, the best strategy is to prevent transmission to the newborn infant. For this reason, obstetricians will usually recommend delivery by cesarean section ("C-section") for any mother with active genital herpes lesions.

## Varicella-Zoster Virus

Varicella-zoster virus (VZV) is a type of herpesvirus (HHV-3) that most commonly causes chickenpox (varicella) in childhood, remains dormant for many years, and can then reemerge in later adulthood as painful herpes zoster lesions known as *shingles*.

Chickenpox is usually an uncomfortable but self-limiting disease of childhood. However, it is highly contagious and easily spread by either direct contact with weeping lesions or via droplet inhalation. It may also lead to significant scarring. The serious condition known as *Reye's syndrome* (fatty liver damage with encephalopathy) may also complicate varicella, as can other viral infections such as influenza. Herpes zoster, more commonly known as shingles, is caused by the reactivation of VZV from its dormant state, often decades after a case of childhood chickenpox. It is also referred to simply as *zoster*. Its most common manifestation is in the form of skin lesions that follow nerve tracts, known as *dermatomes*, along the skin surface. The most common site of these lesions is around the side of the trunk, although they can appear in other areas (e.g., along trigeminal nerve dermatomes of the face). Zoster lesions are often quite painful, and some patients even require opioids for pain control. In addition, postherpetic neuralgias (long-term nerve pain) remain following shingles outbreaks in up to 50% of elderly patients. Early administration of antiviral drugs such as acyclovir may speed recovery, but this effect is usually not dramatic. The best results are generally seen when the antiviral drug is started within 72 hours of symptom onset.

Active childhood varicella (chickenpox) infections are usually self-limiting and are not normally treated with antiviral drugs, except in high-risk (e.g., immunocompromised) pediatric patients. The varicella virus vaccine was approved in 1995 and is now routinely recommended for healthy children older than 1 year of age who have not had chickenpox. A new vaccine, Zostavax, is available for prevention of herpes shingles in patients 50 years of age or older (see Chapter 49).

In a small percentage of shingles cases, skin lesions may progress beyond the usual dermatome regions, and the virus can cause solid organ infections such as pneumonitis, hepatitis, encephalitis, and optic neuritis (infection of the optic nerve). Such infections are uncommon, with elderly and immunocompromised patients being the most vulnerable. Rarely, these serious infections can be caused by first-time exposure to varicella (chickenpox). In general, these more serious infections require intravenous antiviral drugs, especially in high-risk patients. Intravenous acyclovir is the most commonly used drug, and it may prevent fatalities or disability. Less serious infections are usually treated orally with acyclovir, valacyclovir, or famciclovir. Topical dosage forms of some of these drugs are also available and are discussed further in Chapter 56. Although VZV reactivation is comparable in pathology to that of HSV (e.g., oral or genital herpes lesions), VZV reactivation occurs much less regularly than does HSV reactivation because of a lack of reactivation genes. Secondary bacterial infections (e.g., group A *Streptococcus* skin infection) are common with VZV exacerbations, so antibiotics may also be needed. This is especially true in cases of ophthalmic involvement.

## PHARMACOLOGY OVERVIEW

## ANTIVIRALS (NON-HIV)

The drugs discussed in this section include those used to treat non-HIV viral infections such as those caused by influenza viruses, HSV, VZV, and CMV. There are also antiviral drugs used to treat infections with hepatitis A, B, and C viruses. However, hepatitis treatment is covered in detail in Chapter 47 because it involves some additional unique drug therapy.

### Mechanism of Action and Drug Effects

Most of the current antiviral drugs work by blocking the activity of a polymerase enzyme that normally stimulates the synthesis of new viral genomes. The result is impaired viral replication, which results in viral concentrations low enough to allow elimination of the virus by the patient's immune system. If this does not occur, the virus may either enter a dormant state or remain at a low level of replication with continuous drug therapy.

### Indications

The antivirals discussed in this section are those used to treat HSV, VZV, and CMV infections and are listed in Table 40-1.

| TABLE 40-1 | EXAMPLES OF ANTIVIRAL DRUGS (NON-HIV) |
|---|---|
| **DRUG** | **INDICATIONS** |
| **Drugs to Treat Herpesviruses** | |
| acyclovir, valacyclovir | Herpes simplex types 1 and 2, herpes zoster, chickenpox |
| trifluridine | Herpes simplex keratitis |
| **Drugs to Treat Influenza Viruses** | |
| amantadine | Influenza A |
| rimantadine | Influenza A |
| zanamivir, oseltamivir | Influenza A and B |
| **Miscellaneous Antivirals** | |
| ribavirin | Respiratory syncytial virus infection |
| cidofovir | Cytomegalovirus infection |
| foscarnet | Cytomegalovirus infection, acyclovir herpes simplex infections |

*HIV,* Human immunodeficiency virus.

### Contraindications

Most of the antiviral drugs used to treat non-HIV viral infections are surprisingly well tolerated. The only usual contraindication for most of these drugs is known severe drug allergy. However, a small number of contraindications are listed for a few of the antiviral drugs. Amantadine is contraindicated in lactating women, children younger than 12 months of age, and patients with an eczematous rash. Famciclovir is contraindicated in cases of allergy to the drug itself or to a similar drug called *penciclovir,* which is used topically to treat herpes labialis (perioral sores). Cidofovir has a strong propensity for renal toxicity, and it is contraindicated in patients who already have severely compromised renal function as well as those receiving concurrent drug therapy with other highly nephrotoxic drugs. It is also contraindicated in cases of allergy to probenecid, because probenecid is recommended as concurrent drug therapy with cidofovir to help alleviate its nephrotoxicity. Ribavirin also has additional specific contraindications besides drug allergy. Because of the drug's teratogenic potential, it is also contraindicated in pregnant women and even in their male sexual partners. The aerosol form must not be used by pregnant women or by women who may become pregnant during exposure to the drug. This includes health care providers administering the drug in aerosol form, because of the potential for second-hand inhalation on the part of the health care provider.

### Adverse Effects

The adverse effects of the antiviral drugs are as different as the drugs themselves. Each has its own specific adverse effect profile. Because viruses reproduce in human cells, selective killing is difficult, and consequently many healthy human cells, in addition to virally infected cells, may be killed in the process, which results in more serious toxicities for these drugs. However, this effect is usually not as pronounced as in cancer chemotherapy, which often kills many more healthy cells. The more serious adverse effects are listed by drug in Table 40-2.

## TABLE 40-2 SELECTED ANTIVIRAL DRUGS: ADVERSE EFFECTS

| DRUG | ADVERSE EFFECTS |
|---|---|
| acyclovir | Nausea, diarrhea, headache, burning when topically applied |
| amantadine, rimantadine | Insomnia, nervousness, lightheadedness, anorexia, nausea, anticholinergic effects, orthostatic hypotension, blurred vision |
| didanosine | Pancreatitis, peripheral neuropathies, seizures |
| foscarnet | Headache, seizures, electrolyte disturbances, acute renal failure, bone marrow suppression, nausea, vomiting, diarrhea |
| ganciclovir | Bone marrow toxicity, nausea, vomiting, headache, seizures |
| indinavir | Nausea; abdominal, back, or flank pain; headache; diarrhea; vomiting; weakness; taste changes; acid regurgitation; nephrolithiasis |
| nevirapine | Rash, fever, nausea, headache, elevation in liver enzyme levels |
| ribavirin | Rash, conjunctivitis, anemia, mild bronchospasm |
| trifluridine | Ophthalmic effects: burning, swelling, stinging, photophobia, pain |
| vidarabine | Ophthalmic effects: burning, lacrimation, keratitis, foreign body sensation, pain, photophobia, uveitis |
| zalcitabine | Peripheral neuropathy, rash, ulcers |
| zidovudine | Bone marrow suppression, nausea, headache |

## Interactions

Significant drug interactions that occur with the antiviral drugs arise most often when they are administered via systemic routes such as intravenously and orally. Many of these drugs are also applied topically to the eye or body, however, and the incidence of drug interactions associated with these routes of administration is much lower. Selected common drug interactions for both antiviral and antiretroviral drugs are listed in Table 40-3.

## Dosages

For dosage information on some of the commonly used antiviral drugs, see the table on this page.

## DRUG PROFILES

### amantadine and rimantadine

Amantadine (Symmetrel), one of the earliest antiviral drugs, has a narrow antiviral spectrum in that it is active only against influenza A viruses. It has been used both prophylactically and therapeutically. However, the most recent guidelines of the Centers for Disease Control and Prevention (CDC) do not recommend the use of amantadine or rimantadine to prevent or

## DOSAGES

### Antiviral Drugs (Non-HIV)

| DRUG (PREGNANCY CATEGORY) | PHARMACOLOGIC CLASS | USUAL DOSAGE RANGE | INDICATIONS |
|---|---|---|---|
| ◆ acyclovir (Zovirax) (B) | Antiherpesvirus | **Pediatric younger than 12 yr**<br>IV: 10-20 mg/kg q8h × 7-10 days<br>**Pediatric 12 yr to adult**<br>IV: 5-10 mg/kg q8h × 7-10 days<br>PO: 200-800 mg q4h 5 times daily × 7-10 days<br>PO: 20 mg/kg (max 800 mg/dose) 5 times daily × 5 days | HSV-1 and HSV-2 infection, including genital herpes, mucocutaneous herpes, herpes encephalitis; herpes zoster (shingles); higher-dose therapy for acute episodes; lower-dose therapy for viral suppression<br>Chickenpox (varicella) |
| amantadine (Symmetrel) (C) | Antiinfluenza | **Pediatric 1-9 yr**<br>4.4-8.8 mg/kg/day divided once or twice daily<br>**Pediatric 9-12 yr**<br>100 mg twice daily<br>**Adolescent and adult 13-64 yr**<br>200 mg/day or divided bid<br>**Adult older than 65 yr**<br>100 mg daily | Influenza A |
| ganciclovir (Cytovene) (C) | Antiviral | **Adult**<br>IV: 5-10 mg/kg/day<br>PO: 1000 mg tid | CMV retinitis treatment or maintenance |
| oseltamivir (Tamiflu) (C) | Antiinfluenza | **Pediatric 1-12 yr***<br>30-60 mg twice daily, depending on weight<br>**More than 40 kg or 13 yr to adult**<br>75 mg twice daily | Influenza A or B |
| ribavirin (Virazole) (X) | Anti-RSV | **Pediatric**<br>Aerosol: 6 g reconstituted to 20 mg/mL via continuous aerosol 12-18 hr/day for 3-7 days | Severe RSV infection in hospitalized infants and toddlers |
| zanamivir (Relenza) (C) | Antiinfluenza | **Pediatric 7 yr to adult**<br>Inhalation*: 10 mg (two 5-mg powder doses) twice daily; first day's doses must be at least 2 hr apart and q12h thereafter | Influenza A or B |

NOTE: When pediatric dosages are not provided, dosing guidelines for pediatric patients are not firmly established for the drug in question and are based on the careful clinical judgment of a qualified prescriber.

*HIV*, Human immunodeficiency virus; *HSV-1, HSV-2,* herpes simplex virus types 1 and 2; *IV*, intravenous; *PO,* oral; *RSV,* respiratory syncytial virus.
*Use bronchodilator inhaler first if applicable.

## TABLE 40-3   SELECTED ANTIVIRAL DRUGS: INTERACTIONS

| DRUG | INTERACTING DRUGS | INTERACTION |
|---|---|---|
| **Non-HIV Drugs** | | |
| acyclovir | interferon | Additive antiviral effects |
| | probenecid | Increased acyclovir levels due to decreasing renal clearance |
| | zidovudine | Increased risk for neurotoxicity |
| amantadine | Anticholinergic drugs | Increased adverse anticholinergic effects |
| | CNS stimulants | Additive CNS stimulant effects |
| ganciclovir | foscarnet | Additive or synergistic effect against CMV and HSV type 2 |
| | imipenem | Increased risk for seizures |
| | zidovudine | Increased risk for hematologic toxicity (i.e., bone marrow suppression) |
| ribavirin | Nucleoside reverse transcriptase inhibitors | Increased risk for hepatotoxicity and lactic acidosis |
| **HIV Drugs** | | |
| indinavir | Drugs metabolized by the CYP3A4 hepatic microsomal enzyme system (azole antifungals, clarithromycin, doxycycline, erythromycin, isoniazid, nefazodone, nicardipine, protease inhibitors, quinidine, statins, telithromycin, and verapamil) | Competition for metabolism resulting in elevated blood levels and potential toxicity |
| | rifabutin and ketoconazole | Increased plasma concentrations of rifabutin and ketoconazole |
| | rifampin | Increased metabolism of indinavir |
| nevirapine | Drugs metabolized by the CYP3A4 hepatic microsomal enzyme system (see indinavir) | Increased metabolism of these drugs |
| | Oral contraceptives | Decreased plasma concentrations of oral contraceptives |
| | Protease inhibitors | Decreased plasma concentrations of protease inhibitors |
| | rifampin and rifabutin | Decreased nevirapine serum concentration |
| tenofovir | acyclovir, cidofovir, ganciclovir, valacyclovir | May increase serum concentrations of tenofovir |
| | Protease inhibitors | Increased serum concentrations of tenofovir |
| maraviroc | CYP3A4 inhibitors (see indinavir) | May increase maraviroc toxicity |
| | CYP3A4 inducers (phenytoin, carbamazepine, rifampin) | May decrease effects of maraviroc |
| | St. John's wort | May decrease effects of maraviroc |
| raltegravir | atazanavir (with or without ritonavir) | May increase effects of raltegravir |
| | rifampin | May decrease effects of raltegravir |
| zidovudine | acyclovir | Increased neurotoxicity |
| | interferon beta | Increased serum levels of zidovudine |
| | Cytotoxic drugs | Increased risk for hematologic toxicity |
| | didanosine and zalcitabine | Additive or synergistic effect against HIV |
| | ganciclovir and ribavirin | Antagonize the antiviral action of zidovudine |

*CMV*, Cytomegalovirus; *CNS*, central nervous system; *CYP3A4*, cytochrome P-450 enzyme 3A4; *HIV*, human immunodeficiency virus.

treat the flu. The recommendations on the use of amantadine change yearly based on the type of influenza that is prevalent. The reader is referred to www.cdc.gov/flu/professionals/antivirals/ for the latest recommendations.

Rimantadine is a structural analogue of amantadine that has the same spectrum of activity, mechanism of action, and clinical indications. However, it differs from amantadine in that it has a longer half-life and causes fewer central nervous system adverse effects such as dizziness and blurred vision. Rimantadine has GI adverse effects similar to those of amantadine. Both medications may be used in children. Both drugs are available only for oral use.

## Pharmacokinetics

| Route | Onset of Action | Peak Plasma Concentration | Elimination Half-life | Duration of Action |
|---|---|---|---|---|
| PO | Within 48 hr | 1-4 hr | 17 hr | 12-24 hr |

### ♦ acyclovir

Acyclovir (Zovirax) is a synthetic nucleoside analogue that is used mainly to suppress the replication of HSV-1, HSV-2, and VZV. Acyclovir is considered the drug of choice for the treatment of both initial and recurrent episodes of these viral infections.

Acyclovir is available in oral, topical, and injectable formulations. Its topical use is discussed in Chapter 56. Other similar antiviral drugs include valacyclovir and famciclovir. However, these latter two drugs are currently available only for oral use and are indicated for the treatment of less serious infections. Note the slight inconsistencies in the spelling of these drug names. Valacyclovir is a prodrug that is metabolized to acyclovir in the body. It has the advantage of greater oral bioavailability and less frequent dosing (three times daily versus five times daily for acyclovir). It may also provide more effective relief of pain from zoster lesions.

Pharmacokinetics (acyclovir)

| Route | Onset of Action | Peak Plasma Concentration | Elimination Half-life | Duration of Action |
|-------|-----------------|---------------------------|-----------------------|--------------------|
| PO | 1.5-2 hr | 1.5-2 hr | 2-3 hr | 10-15 hr |
| IV | Variable | 1 hr | 3 hr | 8 hr |

#### ♦ ganciclovir

Like acyclovir, ganciclovir (Cytovene) is a synthetic nucleoside analogue of guanosine, but it has a much different spectrum of antiviral activity. It is indicated for the treatment of infections caused by CMV. CMV is carried by up to 50% of the adult population and normally causes no harm. However, in immunocompromised patients (including premature infants), it can cause life-threatening or disabling opportunistic infections. Valganciclovir (Valcyte), foscarnet (Foscavir), and cidofovir (Vistide) are three other antiviral drugs that are used in the treatment of CMV infection. Of these three antiviral drugs, ganciclovir is the one most often used for this purpose. A common site of CMV infections in the immunocompromised patient is the eye, and it can result in CMV retinitis, a devastating viral infection that can lead to blindness. Ganciclovir is most commonly administered intravenously or orally. However, there is also an ophthalmic form (Vitrasert) for treating active CMV retinitis, which must be surgically inserted. Ganciclovir is also administered to prevent CMV disease (generalized infection) in high-risk patients, such as those receiving organ transplants.

The dose-limiting toxicity of ganciclovir treatment is bone marrow suppression, whereas that of foscarnet and cidofovir is renal toxicity. These toxicities must be kept in mind when deciding which drug is more appropriate in a particular patient. For example, a heart transplant recipient who contracts CMV retinitis is immunocompromised because of immunosuppressant drug therapy and is most likely taking cyclosporine, which is nephrotoxic. Therefore, using foscarnet in this patient may be more dangerous than using ganciclovir. On the other hand, a patient who contracts a CMV infection and is immunocompromised because of a bone marrow transplant might be better treated using foscarnet.

Valganciclovir is a prodrug of ganciclovir, formulated for oral use, that is metabolized to ganciclovir in the body. As in the case described previously for valacyclovir and acyclovir, the prodrug provides greater oral bioavailability and allows less frequent daily dosing. Cidofovir and foscarnet are available only in injectable form.

Pharmacokinetics

| Route | Onset of Action | Peak Plasma Concentration | Elimination Half-life | Duration of Action |
|-------|-----------------|---------------------------|-----------------------|--------------------|
| PO | Unknown | 24 hr | 4.8 hr | Variable |

#### oseltamivir and zanamivir

Oseltamivir (Tamiflu) and zanamivir (Relenza) belong to one of the newest classes of antiviral drugs known as *neuraminidase inhibitors*. These drugs are active against influenza virus types A and B. They are indicated for the treatment of uncomplicated acute illness caused by influenza infection in adults. They have been shown to reduce the duration of influenza infection by several days. The neuraminidase enzyme enables budding virions to escape from infected cells and spread throughout the body. Neuraminidase inhibitors are designed to stop this process in the body, speeding recovery from infection.

The most commonly reported adverse events with oseltamivir are nausea and vomiting; those with zanamivir are diarrhea, nausea, and sinusitis. Oseltamivir is available only for oral use. The drug is indicated for prophylaxis and treatment of influenza infection. Zanamivir is available in dry powder for inhalation. It is currently indicated only for treatment of active influenza illness. Treatment with oseltamivir and zanamivir needs to begin within 2 days of symptom onset.

Pharmacokinetics (oseltamivir)

| Route | Onset of Action | Peak Plasma Concentration | Elimination Half-life | Duration of Action |
|-------|-----------------|---------------------------|-----------------------|--------------------|
| PO | Unknown | 1-2 hr | 1-3 hr | 5-15 hr |

Pharmacokinetics (zanamivir)

| Route | Onset of Action | Peak Plasma Concentration | Elimination Half-life | Duration of Action |
|-------|-----------------|---------------------------|-----------------------|--------------------|
| PO | Unknown | 1-2 hr | 2-5 hr | 10-24 hr |

#### ribavirin

Ribavirin (Virazole) is a synthetic nucleoside analogue of guanosine, as are many of the other antiviral drugs, but it has a spectrum of antiviral activity that is broader than that of other currently available antiviral drugs. It interferes with both RNA and DNA synthesis and as a result inhibits both protein synthesis and viral replication overall.

The inhalational form (Virazole) is used primarily in the treatment of hospitalized infants with severe lower respiratory tract infections caused by respiratory syncytial virus. This drug was first available only in inhalational form. More recently, oral dosage forms have become available for use in the treatment of hepatitis C; these are discussed in Chapter 47.

Pharmacokinetics

| Route | Onset of Action | Peak Plasma Concentration | Elimination Half-life | Duration of Action |
|-------|-----------------|---------------------------|-----------------------|--------------------|
| Inhalation | Unknown | End of inhalation | 1.4-2.5 hr | Variable |
| PO | Unknown | 2-3 hr | 120-170 hr | Unknown |

## PATHOPHYSIOLOGY OVERVIEW

### HIV INFECTION AND AIDS

The first U.S. cases of acquired immune deficiency syndrome (AIDS) were recognized in 1981 in 31 previously healthy homosexual men in Los Angeles and New York City. These first patients mysteriously developed *Pneumocystis carinii* pneumonia

### Look-Alike/Sound-Alike Drugs: Zostrix and Zovirax

An incident was reported that involved the confusion of the two similarly named drugs Zostrix and Zovirax. A physician prescribed Zostrix cream with the directions, "Apply to affected area four times a day." There were no other specific instructions for the medication. The pharmacist mistakenly entered "Zovirax" into the pharmacy computer, and the nursing staff did not catch the error. The next day, the physician saw the tube of Zovirax in the patient's room instead of Zostrix. The sound-alike drug names can be easily confused.

Zostrix is capsaicin, derived from hot chili peppers, and is used topically for the treatment of arthritic pain, muscle strains, and joint sprains. In this case, it was ordered for neuralgic pain. Zovirax 5% ointment is a topical form of acyclovir, an antiviral medication, and is used for the management of initial genital herpes.

This incident illustrates how important it is to clarify the instructions in a medication order (e.g., application to a *specific* site) and how the use of generic names can help to avoid a medication error. In addition, it shows how important it is for nurses to be familiar with the indications of the drugs they are administering.

Data from ISMP Medication Safety Alert, *Nurse Advise-ERR,* May 2004, Volume 2, Issue 5, available at http://www.ismp.org/newsletters/nursing/issues/nurseadviseerr200405.pdf. Accessed April 12, 2012.

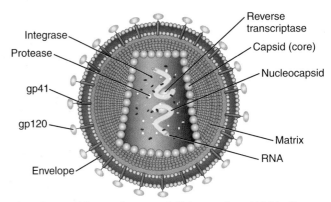

**FIGURE 40-2** Human immunodeficiency virus. Within the core capsid, the diploid, single-stranded, positive-sense RNA is complexed to nucleoprotein. *gp,* Glycoprotein. (From *Dorland's illustrated medical dictionary,* ed 32, Philadelphia, 2012, Saunders.)

(PCP) or Kaposi's sarcoma, both normally extremely rare illnesses. (PCP is now known as *Pneumocystis jirovecii* pneumonia). Within months, similar disease patterns were recognized in intravenous drug users and in hemophiliac patients who had been transfused with blood-derived clotting factors. Other cases began to occur in hospitalized patients transfused with a variety of blood-derived products. In 1983 human T-cell lymphotropic virus type 3 (HTLV-3) was isolated from a patient with lymphadenopathy (swollen lymph nodes), and in 1984 this virus was demonstrated to be the cause of AIDS. The virus was later renamed *human immunodeficiency virus (HIV),* a member of the retrovirus family. There are two recognized types of HIV: human immunodeficiency virus type 1 (HIV-1) and human immunodeficiency virus type 2 (HIV-2). Both cause AIDS, but HIV-2 is primarily localized in western Africa, with HIV-1 causing the majority of the HIV pandemic in the rest of the world. By 1985, a laboratory technique known as *enzyme-linked immunosorbent assay (ELISA)* was developed. This technique allowed the detection of HIV exposure based on the presence of human antibodies to the virus in blood samples. This diagnostic breakthrough led to an appreciation of the enormity of HIV prevalence both in U.S. high-risk groups and as an emerging world pandemic, especially in developing countries. This laboratory screening technique also helped to restore the safety of the transfusion blood supply, although it is not 100% reliable.

The retrovirus family got its name upon discovery of a unique feature of its replication process. Retroviruses are all RNA viruses and are unique in their use of the enzyme reverse transcriptase during their replication process. This enzyme promotes the synthesis of complementary (mirror image) DNA molecules from the viral RNA genome. A second enzyme, integrase, promotes the integration of this viral DNA into the host

cell DNA. This hybrid DNA complex is known as a *provirus.* It produces new viral RNA genomes and proteins, which in turn combine to make mature HIV virions that infect other host cells. Another important enzyme is protease, which serves to chemically separate the new viral RNA from viral protein molecules. These components are initially synthesized into one large macromolecular strand, and the protease enzyme carefully breaks up this strand into its key components. Figure 40-2 shows the major structural features of the HIV virion, and Figure 40-3 illustrates the steps in its replication process. Reverse transcriptase is not normally found in host cells—both reverse transcriptase and integrase are carried by the virus itself. "Reversal" of the usual replication processes led to the name *reverse transcriptase* for this enzyme and also to the name *retrovirus* for this family of viruses. Furthermore, the fact that retroviruses synthesize DNA from viral RNA molecules is also a reversal of the norm, because in most other organisms, RNA molecules are synthesized from DNA molecules as part of the reproductive process. Reverse transcriptase has a high rate of errors when stringing together the purine and pyrimidine bases during transcription of the viral RNA genome into a DNA molecule in the replication process. This allows more frequent genetic mutations among HIV virions and often results in viral strains that are resistant to both medications and the patient's immune system. Such mutations also hamper the development of an effective vaccine against the virus. Drugs used to treat HIV are called *antiretrovirals.*

The most common routes of transmission of HIV are sexual activity, intravenous drug use, and perinatal transfer from mother to child. According to the most recent data, over 33 million people worldwide are infected with HIV, with 2.7 million cases newly diagnosed in 2008. Transmission was most common in homosexual or bisexual men followed by high-risk heterosexual intercourse and intravenous drug use for 12% of cases. African-American males and females had a rate of HIV infection seven times higher than that seen in white Americans. Cases of sexual transmission via oral mucosa have also been documented. However, no solid evidence to date confirms transmission of HIV by more casual contact, including hugging, kissing, coughing, sneezing, swimming in pools, and sharing of food, water, eating utensils, or toilet facilities. HIV

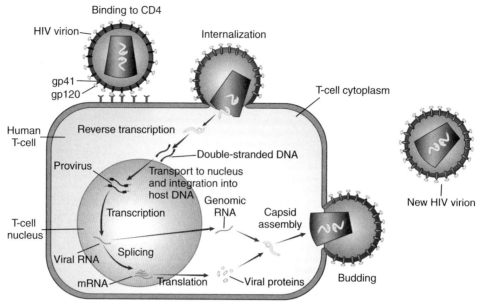

**FIGURE 40-3** Life cycle of the human immunodeficiency virus (HIV). The extracellular envelope protein gp120 binds to CD4 on the surface of T lymphocytes or mononuclear phagocytes, while the transmembrane protein gp41 mediates the fusion of the viral envelope with the cell membrane. *gp,* Glycoprotein; *mRNA,* messenger RNA. (From *Dorland's illustrated medical dictionary,* ed 32, Philadelphia, 2012, Saunders.)

also is not transmitted by insect bites, unlike some other viral illnesses. Although HIV can be isolated from almost any body fluid, including tears, sweat, saliva, and urine, its concentrations in these fluids are much lower than those in blood and genital secretions. In approximately 6% of cases, specific risk factors cannot be determined. The risk for transmission to health care workers via percutaneous (needlestick) injuries is currently calculated at approximately 0.3%. Performing hand hygiene and maintaining Standard Precautions to avoid contact with all body fluids during patient care dramatically reduces the risk for caregiver infection (see Box 9-1).

The rate of new infections is rising more rapidly in minority populations, especially among African Americans and Hispanics. Patients in underdeveloped countries often lack access to adequate drug therapy. Untreated HIV-infected pregnant women transmit the virus to their infants in 15% to 30% of pregnancies. This can occur transplacentally, causing infection in utero, or during birth. When the first antiretroviral drugs were developed in the 1980s, it was feared that they would be too toxic and even teratogenic if given to pregnant women. However, prophylactic antiretroviral treatment of infected mothers has been shown to reduce infant infection by at least two thirds and is not normally harmful to either mother or infant. Medication may also be given prophylactically to the newborn infant, typically for the first 6 weeks of life. Infants and children with established HIV infection must usually continue taking medication indefinitely. Breast milk can transmit the virus to the infant in 10% to 20% of cases, and therefore breastfeeding is contraindicated in developed countries. In developing countries, however, breastfeeding may be the only available source of nutrition for the infant and therefore worth the risk. Box 40-1 summarizes the key epidemiologic concepts related to HIV/AIDS.

---

**BOX 40-1  EPIDEMIOLOGY OF HIV INFECTION**

**Disease Viral Factors**
- Developed virus is easily inactivated and must be transmitted in body fluids
- Disease has a long prodromal or incubation period
- Virus can be shed before development of identifiable symptoms

**Transmission**
- Virus is present in blood, semen, and vaginal secretions

**Groups at Risk**
- Intravenous drug abusers; sexually active people with many partners (homosexual and heterosexual); prostitutes; newborns of HIV-positive mothers
- Blood and organ transplant recipients and hemophiliacs: before 1985 (before screening programs)

**Geographic Factors**
- Continuously expanding epidemic worldwide
- No particular seasonal pattern of infection (i.e., unlike influenza)

**Modes of Control**
- Antiviral drugs limit progression of disease.
- Vaccines for prevention and treatment are in trials.
- Monogamous sex using safe sexual practices helps limit spread.
- Sterile injection needles need to be used.
- Large-scale screening programs have been developed to test blood for transfusions, organs for transplantation, and clotting factors given to hemophiliacs.

Data from U.S. Department of Health and Human Services: AIDSinfo (AIDS information website), available at www.aidsinfo.nih.gov. *HIV,* Human immunodeficiency virus.

HIV infection that is untreated or treatment resistant eventually leads to severe immune system failure, with death occurring secondary to opportunistic infections. AIDS often progresses over a period of several years. Various health organizations, including the CDC and the World Health Organization (WHO), have published classification systems describing the various "stages" of this infection. The most recent WHO model lists four stages as follows:

- Stage 1: asymptomatic infection
- Stage 2: early, general symptoms of disease
- Stage 3: moderate symptoms
- Stage 4: severe symptoms, often leading to death

Stage 1 refers to the first few weeks or months after initial exposure to the virus. Patients may be asymptomatic but may show signs of persistent generalized lymphadenopathy or swollen lymph nodes ("swollen glands"). Persistent generalized lymphadenopathy is more specifically defined as inflammation of the lymph nodes in at least two sites outside the inguinal (groin) area that lasts for some months. During this time, the virus is present in the blood at low levels and has a low rate of replication. An important measure of immune function, the CD4 count, is usually still within normal limits at 350 cells/mm$^3$ of blood. CD4 refers to the protein on the cell surface of helper T lymphocytes, to which HIV virions attach themselves. Helper T cells normally function by releasing cytokines. Cytokines are chemicals that activate and modulate cell-mediated immunity, which is a general term for all immune system actions other than those involving antibodies. Immune system function is described further in Chapters 47 to 49. Helper T cells circulate in the blood and are the primary target cells for HIV. It is ultimately through widespread destruction of these helper T cells in the blood that HIV infection weakens the patient's immune system.

Stage 2 involves continued lymphadenopathy along with other symptoms, including fever, rash, sore throat, night sweats, malaise, diarrhea, idiopathic thrombocytopenia, oral candidiasis, and herpes zoster (shingles). In the early years of the epidemic (early 1980s), this stage was also known as AIDS-related complex or ARC. These symptoms may actually resolve spontaneously about the time of seroconversion, which is when the patient's own antibodies to the virus (HIV antibodies) begin to appear in blood samples. Seroconversion usually occurs 3 weeks to 3 months after exposure. At this point, the patient is said to be HIV positive. However, the patient may not have further progression of symptoms for 1 to 10 years. During this stage, the CD4 T-cell count begins to drop, and HIV antibody levels rise as part of an attempt by the patient's own immune system to neutralize the virus. The virus begins to multiply in the body but does not necessarily produce disabling symptoms. This stage is often the first presenting sign of HIV infection, and stage 1 may not have been noticed or reported by the patient.

During stage 3, the infection progresses to a moderately symptomatic state. Weight loss, chronic diarrhea, and fever continue, and CD4 counts continue to drop. Opportunistic infections begin, including severe bacterial pneumonias and pulmonary tuberculosis (TB). Pulmonary TB is usually more severe in persons with AIDS and is currently the leading cause of death worldwide for HIV-infected patients. Opportunistic infections are so named because the destruction by HIV of the patient's immune system gives the "opportunity" for normally harmless microorganisms in the body to proliferate to cause serious infections. These infections may become life-threatening or produce significant disability (e.g., blindness from CMV retinitis).

In stage 4, viral replication increases dramatically, which results in increasing destruction of helper T cells and a corresponding decrease in CD4 counts. At this point, there is a major decline in immune system function, and the illness begins to seriously affect the entire body. When the CD4 count drops below 200 cells/mm$^3$, fever, night sweats, and malaise resume and are now accompanied by increasingly severe opportunistic infections, such as *Mycobacterium avium-intracellulare* complex infection and *Pneumocystis jirovecii* pneumonia. Other common opportunistic infections include parasitic infections such as cryptosporidial diarrhea and toxoplasmosis encephalitis; viral infections such as HSV mouth ulcers, disseminated extrapulmonary tuberculosis, esophagitis, pneumonitis, CMV pneumonia, and CMV retinitis; and fungal infections, such as candidiasis of the GI and respiratory tracts, and invasive aspergillosis of the lungs. Similarly opportunistic disorders are HIV-associated neoplasms. The most common of these are Kaposi's sarcoma and various types of lymphoma. There is also some evidence that cervical cancer is more likely to be diagnosed in advanced stages in HIV-infected women. HIV wasting syndrome is yet another defining condition of the disease and involves major weight loss, chronic diarrhea, more frequent or even constant fever, and chronic fatigue. In addition to attacking helper T cells and macrophages, the HIV virus can also cause pathologic changes in organs such as the brain (HIV-induced encephalopathy and dementia), bone marrow, lungs (recurrent pneumonia), and skin. Death is most likely when the CD4 count falls below 50 cells/mm$^3$. The viral load, which is measured as the number of viral RNA copies per milliliter of blood, also continues to rise uncontrollably. If this condition persists, death often ensues. All of these manifestations are said to be the defining conditions of AIDS. Box 40-2 lists several such conditions.

Figure 40-4 illustrates events that roughly correlate with these four stages of HIV infection. This figure shows the hypothetical natural course of the disease through the previously described stages in patients *without* treatment. Patients who are effectively treated with drug therapy usually do not progress through all of these stages, or at least such progression is slowed considerably (by years). In fact, advances in antiretroviral drug therapy have given rise to increasingly greater numbers of long-term survivors of HIV infection. Highly active antiretroviral therapy (HAART) refers to combinations of antiretroviral drugs ("cocktails") that are now standard for treating HIV-infected patients. This combination therapy (HAART) is normally begun immediately upon confirmation of HIV infection. Opportunistic infections are treated with infection-specific antimicrobial drugs (see corresponding chapters) as they arise. Prophylactic treatment for opportunistic infections is also common and is most frequently given when a patient's

## BOX 40-2   INDICATOR DISEASES OF AIDS

**Opportunistic Infections**

*Protozoal*
- Toxoplasmosis of the brain
- Cryptosporidiosis with diarrhea
- Isosporiasis with diarrhea

*Fungal*
- Candidiasis of the esophagus, trachea, and lungs
- *Pneumocystis jirovecii* pneumonia
- Cryptococcosis (extrapulmonary)
- Histoplasmosis (disseminated)
- Coccidioidomycosis (disseminated)

*Viral*
- Cytomegalovirus disease
- Herpes simplex virus infection (persistent or disseminated)
- Progressive multifocal leukoencephalopathy
- Hairy leukoplakia caused by Epstein-Barr virus

*Bacterial*
- *Mycobacterium avium-intracellulare* complex infection (disseminated)
- Any atypical mycobacterial disease
- Extrapulmonary tuberculosis
- *Salmonella* septicemia (recurrent)
- Pyogenic bacterial infections (multiple or recurrent)

**Opportunistic Neoplasias**
- Kaposi's sarcoma
- Primary lymphoma of the brain
- Other non-Hodgkin's lymphomas

**Others**
- HIV wasting syndrome
- HIV encephalopathy
- Lymphoid interstitial pneumonia

*AIDS,* Acquired immunodeficiency syndrome; *HIV,* human immuno-deficiency virus.
Data from Mandell GL, Bennett JE, Dolin R, et al: *Mandell, Douglas, and Bennett's principles and practices of infectious diseases,* ed 7, Philadelphia, 2010, Churchill Livingstone.

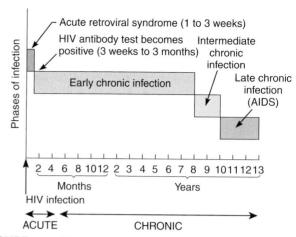

**FIGURE 40-4** Timeline for the spectrum of untreated HIV infection. The timeline represents the course of untreated illness from the time of infection to clinical manifestations of disease. (From Lewis SL, Dirksen SR, Heitkemper MM, et al: *Medical-surgical nursing: assessment and management of clinical problems,* ed 8, Philadelphia, 2011, Elsevier.)

CD4 count falls below 200 cells/mm³. Opportunistic malignancies, such as Kaposi's sarcoma and lymphomas, are also treated with specific antineoplastic medications, which are discussed in Chapters 45 and 46, as well as with radiation and/or surgery as indicated. Long-term survival is defined as living with HIV infection for at least 10 to 15 years after infection. Some particularly remarkable patients have lived for several years with CD4 counts remaining at levels considered fatal. Improved drug therapy against both HIV and opportunistic infections is believed to play an important role in these unusual cases. Other remarkable patients are the long-term nonprogressors. These are long-term survivors who have maintained normal CD4 counts and low HIV viral loads despite not receiving *any* anti-HIV drug treatment. These patients are usually able to mount especially strong cell-mediated and humoral immune responses that prevent progression of the viral infection. They are also the subject of much research to identify the mechanisms of their survival and hopefully to find ways to share these advantages

with other patients. Research attempts to develop an effective anti-HIV vaccine are also underway throughout the world. Human clinical trials have been conducted since 1990, primarily in non–HIV-infected research volunteers. However, vaccines are also being studied in HIV-positive patients. Despite encouraging data regarding potential benefits, the design of an effective HIV vaccine continues to remain elusive.

## PHARMACOLOGY OVERVIEW

### DRUGS USED TO TREAT HIV INFECTION

Much has happened in medical science since the AIDS virus was first identified in the early 1980s. The increasing urgency and public awareness of the HIV epidemic have stimulated much research in the fields of immunology and pharmacology. This has resulted in the development of several effective antiretroviral drugs, as well as of antiviral drugs in general. Although new drug combinations have prolonged lives, these medications often carry significant toxicities. Furthermore, HIV/AIDS is still not considered to be a curable disease. There are currently five classes of antiretroviral drugs, including the reverse transcriptase inhibitors, the protease inhibitors, the fusion inhibitors, and the newest classes, the entry inhibitor–CCR5 co-receptor antagonists and the HIV integrase strand transfer inhibitors. There are currently two subclasses of reverse transcriptase inhibitors: nucleoside reverse transcriptase inhibitors (NRTIs) and the nonnucleoside reverse transcriptase inhibitors (NNRTIs). Drugs from many of these drug classes are combined together into a single drug dosage form for ease of use. Table 40-4 lists these drugs and their respective classes. In 2012, the FDA approved Truvada for the prevention of HIV in high-risk patients. HIV drug therapy is rapidly changing, and the reader is referred to various websites including the FDA's website at www.fda.gov/ForConsumers/byAudience/ForPatientAdvocates/HIVandAIDSActivities/ucm118915.htm for the most up-to-date listing.

| TABLE 40-4 | **EXAMPLES OF ANTI-RETROVIRALS USED TO TREAT HIV** |
|---|---|

| GENERIC NAME | TRADE NAME |
|---|---|
| **Nucleoside Reverse Transcriptase Inhibitors** | |
| abacavir | Ziagen |
| abacavir/lamivudine | Epzicom |
| abacavir/zidovudine/lamivudine | Trizivir |
| didanosine (enteric coated) | Videx EC |
| didanosine (dideoxyinosine) | Videx |
| emtricitabine | Emtriva |
| lamivudine | Epivir |
| stavudine (d4t) | Zerit |
| tenofovir | Viread |
| tenofovir/emtricitabine | Truvada |
| zalcitabine | Hivid |
| zidovudine | Retrovir |
| | |
| **Nonnucleoside Reverse Transcriptase Inhibitors** | |
| delavirdine | Rescriptor |
| efavirenz | Sustiva |
| etravirine | Intelence |
| nevirapine | Viramune |
| | |
| **Protease Inhibitors** | |
| amprenavir | Agenerase |
| atazanavir | Reyataz |
| darunavir | Prezista |
| fosamprenavir | Lexiva |
| indinavir | Crixivan |
| lopinavir/ritonavir | Kaletra |
| nelfinavir | Viracept |
| ritonavir | Norvir |
| saquinavir mesylate | Invirase |
| tipranavir | Aptivus |
| | |
| **Fusion Inhibitor** | |
| Enfuvirtide | Fuzeon |
| | |
| **Entry Inhibitor–CCR5 Coreceptor Antagonist (Also Known as CCR5 Kntagonist)** | |
| maraviroc | Selzentry |
| | |
| **HIV Integrase Strand Transfer Inhibitor (Also Known as Integrase Inhibitor)** | |
| raltegravir | Isentress |
| | |
| **Multiclass Combination Products** | |
| efavirenz/emtricitabine/tenofovir | Atripla |
| abacavir/lamivudine/zidovudine | Trizivir |
| lamivudine/zidovudine | Combivir |
| lopinavir/ritonavir | Kaletra |

*CCR5,* Chemokine receptor 5; *HIV,* human immunodeficiency virus.

## Mechanism of Action and Drug Effects

Although HIV/AIDS is a very complex illness, the mechanisms of action of the various drug classes are fortunately straightforward and distinct. The name of each class of medication provides a reminder of its role in suppressing the viral replication process. Thus, reverse transcriptase inhibitors work by blocking activity of the enzyme reverse transcriptase. Reverse transcriptase promotes the synthesis of new viral DNA molecules from the RNA genome. The protease inhibitors work by inhibiting the protease retroviral enzyme. This enzyme promotes the breakup of chains of protein molecules at designated points, a process necessary for viral replication. There is also one combination protease inhibitor that includes both lopinavir and ritonavir. Both medications are protease inhibitors. The ritonavir component also serves to inhibit cytochrome P-450–mediated enzymatic metabolism of the lopinavir component. There is currently one fusion inhibitor. This compound works by inhibiting viral fusion. This is the process by which an HIV virion attaches to (fuses with) the membrane of a host cell (T lymphocyte) before infecting it in preparation for viral replication. The entry inhibitor–CCR5 co-receptor antagonists, or CCR5 antagonists, work by selectively and reversibly binding to the type 5 chemokine co-receptors located on the CD4 cells that are used by the HIV virion to gain entry to the cells. The integrase strand transfer inhibitors, also referred to as *integrase inhibitors,* work by inhibiting the catalytic activity of the enzyme integrase thus preventing integration of the proviral gene into human DNA.

Single-drug therapy was most common in the early years of the HIV epidemic, partly due to a lack of treatment options. However, both the development of multiple antiretroviral drugs and the emergence of resistant viral strains have given rise to combination drug therapy as the current standard of care. This is the most effective treatment to date and is referred to as highly active antiretroviral therapy (HAART). HAART usually includes at least three medications. The most commonly recommended drug combinations include two or three NRTIs; two NRTIs plus one or two protease inhibitors; or an NRTI plus an NNRTI with one or two protease inhibitors. Despite the effectiveness of HAART, prescribers may still need to alter a given patient's drug regimen in cases of major drug intolerance (see Adverse Effects) or drug resistance. A given patient's HIV strain can still evolve and mutate over time, which allows it to become resistant to any drug therapy, especially when that therapy is used for a prolonged period of time. Evidence of drug resistance includes a falling CD4 count and/or increased viral load in a patient in whom a given drug regimen previously kept these parameters under control.

All antiretroviral drugs have similar therapeutic effects in that they reduce the viral load. A viral load of less than 50 copies/mL is considered to be an undetectable viral load and is a primary goal of antiretroviral therapy. HIV-infected patients need to be followed by practitioners with extensive training and specialization in drug therapy for infectious diseases. These practitioners must often make careful choices and changes in drug therapy over time, based on a given patient's clinical response and severity of any drug-related toxicity. When effective, treatment leads to a significant reduction in mortality and incidence of opportunistic infections, improves patient's physical performance, and significantly increases T-cell counts.

**TABLE 40-5    RECOMMENDATIONS FOR OCCUPATIONAL HIV EXPOSURE CHEMOPROPHYLAXIS**

| TYPE OF EXPOSURE | SOURCE | PROPHYLAXIS | THERAPY |
|---|---|---|---|
| Percutaneous | Blood | Recommended | zidovudine + lamivudine + indinavir; OR |
| | Fluid containing visible blood or other potentially infectious fluid or tissue | | zidovudine + lamivudine ± indinavir |
| Mucous membrane | Blood | Offer | zidovudine + lamivudine |
| | Fluid containing visible blood or other potentially infectious fluid or tissue | Offer | zidovudine + lamivudine ± indinavir; OR zidovudine ± lamivudine |
| Skin (i.e., prolonged contact, extensive area, area without skin integrity) | Blood | Offer | zidovudine + lamivudine ± indinavir |

NOTE: Recommendations vary and change often, and the reader is referred to the CDC website (www.cdc.gov) for updated guidelines.
*HIV,* Human immunodeficiency virus.

## Indications

The only usual indication for all of the current antiretroviral drugs is active HIV infection. Prophylactic therapy is also given to individuals such as health care workers and high-risk infants with a known potential exposure to HIV (e.g., via needlestick injuries in hospitals [Table 40-5]).

## Contraindications

Because of the potentially fatal outcome of HIV infection, the only usual contraindication to a given medication is known severe drug allergy or other intolerable toxicity. Most of the current antiretroviral drug classes have several alternative drugs to choose from, if a patient is especially intolerant of a given drug.

## Adverse Effects

Common adverse effects of selected antiretroviral drugs are listed in Table 40-2. The need to modify drug therapy because of adverse effects is not uncommon. The goal is to find the regimen that will best control a given patient's infection and that has as tolerable an adverse effect profile as possible. Different patients vary widely in their drug tolerance, and their tolerance may change over time. Thus, medication regimens often must be strategically individualized and evolve with the course of the patient's illness.

Approximately 25% of HIV-infected patients in the United States are also infected with hepatitis C virus (HCV), which tends to cause more severe disease in HIV patients. Hepatitis C is the most important cause of chronic liver disease in the United States and is the most common reason for liver transplantation. Unfortunately, HAART is strongly correlated with increased mortality from HCV-induced liver disease, because the anti-HIV drugs produce strain on the liver as these drugs are metabolized via the liver.

A major adverse effect of protease inhibitors is lipid abnormalities, including lipodystrophy, or redistribution of fat stores under the skin. This condition often results in cosmetically undesirable outcomes for the patient, such as a "hump" at the posterior base of the neck and also a skeletonized (bony) appearance of the face. In addition, dyslipidemias such as hypertriglyceridemia can occur, and insulin resistance and type 2 diabetes symptoms can result. It is reported that in these cases, switching a patient from a protease inhibitor to an NNRTI may help to reduce such symptoms without decreasing antiretroviral efficacy.

The increase in long-term antiretroviral drug therapy due to prolonged disease survival has led to the emergence of another long-term adverse effect associated with these medications—bone demineralization and possible osteoporosis. When this condition occurs, it may require treatment with standard medications for osteoporosis, such as calcium, vitamin D, and bisphosphonates (see Chapter 34).

## Interactions

Common selected drug interactions involving both antiretrovirals and other antivirals are listed in Table 40-3.

## Dosages

Because of rapidly changing antiviral drug therapy and the complexity of dosing and the disease state, only selected dosages are listed in this book (see the Dosages table on p. 665). Refer to an up-to-date drug information handbook for specifics on dosing.

## DRUG PROFILES

### enfuvirtide

Enfuvirtide (Fuzeon) is the only medication in one of the newest classes of antiretroviral drugs, called *fusion inhibitors.* It works by suppressing the fusion process whereby a virion is attached to the outer membrane of a host T cell before entry into the cell and subsequent viral replication. This mechanism of action serves as yet another example of how antiretroviral drugs are strategically designed to interfere with specific steps of the viral replication process. The use of combinations of drugs that work by different mechanisms improves a patient's chances for continued survival by reducing the likelihood of viral resistance to the drug therapy regimen. Enfuvirtide is indicated for treatment of HIV infection in combination with other antiretroviral drugs. Adult and pediatric patients have shown comparable tolerance of the drug in clinical trials thus far. Use of this drug in combination with other standard antiretroviral drugs has been associated with markedly reduced viral loads, compared with drug regimens that did not include this drug. The drug is currently available only in injectable form.

## DOSAGES

### HIV/AIDS Drugs

| DRUG (PREGNANCY CATEGORY) | PHARMACOLOGIC CLASS | USUAL DOSAGE RANGE |
|---|---|---|
| enfuvirtide (Fuzeon) (B) | Fusion inhibitor | **Pediatric 6-16 yr**<br>Subcut: 2 mg/kg twice daily<br>**17 yr to adult**<br>Subcut: 90 mg twice daily |
| ◆ indinavir (Crixivan) (C) | Protease inhibitor | **Adult**<br>PO: 800 mg q8h |
| maraviroc (Selzentry) (B) | CCR5 antagonist | **Adults and children older than 16 yr**<br>300 mg twice daily |
| ◆ nevirapine (NVP) (Viramune) (C) | Nonnucleoside reverse transcriptase inhibitor | **Pediatric 2 mo-8 yr**<br>PO: 4 mg/kg daily × 14 days, then 7 mg/kg twice daily<br>**8 yr to adult**<br>PO: 4 mg/kg daily × 14 days, then 4 mg/kg twice daily<br>**Adult**<br>PO: 200 mg daily × 14 days, then twice daily |
| raltegravir (Isentress) (C) | Integrase inhibitor | **Adults and children older than 16 yr**<br>400 mg twice daily |
| tenofovir (Viread) (B) | Nucleotide reverse transcriptase inhibitor | **Adult**<br>PO: 300 mg once daily |
| ◆ zidovudine (AZT, ZDV) (Retrovir) (C) | Nucleoside reverse transcriptase inhibitor | **Pediatric 0-3 mo***<br>PO: 2 mg/kg q6h starting within 12 hr after birth and through 6 wk of age<br>IV: 1.5 mg/kg q6h<br>**Pediatric 6 wk-12 yr**<br>PO: 160 mg/m² q8h (max 200 mg/dose)<br>**Adult**<br>PO: 300 mg twice a day<br>IV: 1 mg/kg over 1 hr; 5-6 times daily<br>**Pregnant women**<br>PO: 100 mg 5 times daily during pregnancy until start of labor, then give IV bolus dose of 2 mg/kg over 1 hr followed by an IV infusion of 1 mg/kg/hr until the umbilical cord is clamped |

NOTE: Where pediatric dosages are not provided, dosing guidelines for pediatric patients are not firmly established for the drug in question and are based on the careful clinical judgment of a qualified prescriber.

AIDS, Acquired immunodeficiency syndrome; CCR5, chemokine receptor 5; HIV, human immunodeficiency virus; IV, intravenous; PO, oral; subcut, subcutaneous.

*Drug needs to be continued either IV or PO through at least 6 wk of age.

### Pharmacokinetics (enfuvirtide)

| Route | Onset of Action | Peak Plasma Concentration | Elimination Half-life | Duration of Action |
|---|---|---|---|---|
| Subcut | Unknown | 4-8 hr | 4 hr | Unknown |

### ◆ indinavir

Indinavir (Crixivan) belongs to the *protease inhibitor* class of antiretroviral drugs. Others include ritonavir (Norvir), nelfinavir (Viracept), amprenavir (Agenerase), fosamprenavir (Lexiva), atazanavir (Reyataz), tipranavir (Aptivus), ritonavir (Norvir), darunavir (Prezista), and the combination product lopinavir/ritonavir (Kaletra). Indinavir can be taken in combination with other anti-HIV therapies or alone. This drug is best dissolved and absorbed in an acidic gastric environment, and the presence of high-protein and high-fat foods reduces its absorption. Therefore, it is recommended that it be administered in a fasting state. Indinavir therapy produces increases in CD4 cell counts and significant reductions in viral load.

Protease inhibitors are commonly given in combination with two reverse transcriptase inhibitors to maximize efficacy and decrease the likelihood of viral drug resistance. Indinavir is relatively well tolerated in most patients. Nephrolithiasis (kidney stones) occur in approximately 4% of patients. Patients who take indinavir are encouraged to drink at least 48 oz of liquids every day to maintain hydration and help avoid nephrolithiasis. Indinavir and all other protease inhibitors are available only for oral use.

### Pharmacokinetics

| Route | Onset of Action | Peak Plasma Concentration | Elimination Half-life | Duration of Action |
|---|---|---|---|---|
| PO | 2 wk to therapeutic effect | 0.5-1 hr | 1.5-2.5 hr | 6 mo |

### maraviroc

Maraviroc (Selzentry) is the only drug available in a new class of antiretrovirals called *CCR5 antagonists*. Maraviroc works by selectively and reversibly binding to the chemokine co-receptors located on the CD4 cells. It is used in treatment-experienced patients with evidence of viral replication and HIV-1 strains resistant to multiple antiretroviral therapies. Patients must receive an FDA-approved medication guide before this drug is dispensed. Hepatotoxicity with allergic-type features has been reported. Drug interactions of significance include interactions with cytochrome P-450 3A4 (CYP3A4) inhibitors (azole antifungals, clarithromycin, doxycycline, erythromycin, isoniazid, nefazodone, nicardipine, protease inhibitors, quinidine, telithromycin, and verapamil), which may increase maraviroc toxicity. CYP3A4 inducers, including phenytoin, carbamazepine, nafcillin, and rifampin, may decrease maraviroc's effects. Maraviroc is available only for oral use.

**Pharmacokinetics**

| Route | Onset of Action | Peak Plasma Concentration | Elimination Half-life | Duration of Action |
|---|---|---|---|---|
| PO | Unknown | 0.5-4 hr | 14-18 hr | Unknown |

### ◆ nevirapine

Nevirapine (Viramune) is an NNRTI. This is the second class of antiviral drugs indicated for the treatment of HIV infection. Other currently available NNRTIs include delavirdine (Rescriptor), efavirenz (Sustiva), and etravirine (Intelence). These drugs are often used in combination with NRTIs.

Nevirapine is well tolerated compared with other therapies for HIV. The most common adverse events associated with nevirapine therapy are rash, fever, nausea, headache, and abnormal liver function test results. Nevirapine and the other NNRTIs are available only for oral use.

**Pharmacokinetics**

| Route | Onset of Action | Peak Plasma Concentration | Elimination Half-life | Duration of Action |
|---|---|---|---|---|
| PO | 2 hr | 2-4 hr | 25-30 hr | 24 hr |

### raltegravir

Raltegravir (Isentress) is the only drug in the new class called *integrase inhibitors*. Raltegravir works by inhibiting the activity of the integrase enzyme, thus preventing integration of the proviral gene into human DNA. Raltegravir is used in treatment-experienced patients with virus that shows multidrug resistance and active replication. Myopathy and rhabdomyolysis have been reported, as well as an immune reconstitution syndrome, which may result in an inflammatory response to a residual opportunistic infection. Raltegravir does not interact with CYP3A4 inducers or inhibitors (as do many other AIDS drugs).

**Pharmacokinetics**

| Route | Onset of Action | Peak Plasma Concentration | Elimination Half-life | Duration of Action |
|---|---|---|---|---|
| PO | Unknown | 3 hr | 9 hr | Unknown |

### tenofovir

Tenofovir (Viread) is one of many NRTIs. Others in this class include emtricitabine (Emtriva), lamivudine (Epivir), stavudine (Zerit), and abacavir (Ziagen), as well as many combination products. Lactic acidosis and severe hepatomegaly have been reported with this drug and others in its class. Tenofovir is indicated for use against HIV infection in combination with other antiretroviral drugs. It is currently available only for oral use.

**Pharmacokinetics**

| Route | Onset of Action | Peak Plasma Concentration | Elimination Half-life | Duration of Action |
|---|---|---|---|---|
| PO | 4-8 days for therapeutic effect | 1 hr | 10-14 hr | 7 days |

### ◆ zidovudine

Zidovudine (Retrovir), also known as azidothymidine or AZT, is a synthetic nucleoside analogue of thymidine that has had an enormous impact on the treatment and quality of life of patients who have AIDS. It was the very first and, for a long time, the only anti-HIV medication. Zidovudine, along with various other antiretroviral drugs, is given to HIV-infected pregnant women and even to newborn babies to prevent maternal transmission of the virus to the infant.

The major dose-limiting adverse effect of zidovudine is bone marrow suppression, and this is often the reason a patient with HIV infection must be switched to another anti-HIV drug such as zalcitabine or didanosine. Some patients may receive a combination of two of these drugs, in lower dosages, to maximize their combined actions. This strategy may reduce the likelihood of toxicity. Zidovudine is available in both oral and injectable formulations.

**Pharmacokinetics**

| Route | Onset of Action | Peak Plasma Concentration | Elimination Half-life | Duration of Action |
|---|---|---|---|---|
| PO | At least 6 mo for therapeutic effect | 0.4-1.5 hr | 0.8-2 hr | 3-5 hr |

## PATHOPHYSIOLOGY OVERVIEW
### OTHER VIRAL INFECTIONS

There are numerous other viral infections; however, four of recent significance include avian flu, West Nile virus (WNV) infection, severe acute respiratory syndrome (SARS), and the novel influenza virus (H1N1).

In 1999, the first North American cases of WNV infection occurred in New York City. WNV is a member of the arbovirus family and is transmitted to humans by mosquitoes. It also infects animals, primarily birds, and has been detected in horses and cows. In humans, WNV infection can lead to meningitis and encephalitis. In 2001, an epidemic occurred with more than 4000 documented human cases, including 284 deaths. Organ transplant patients constituted one of the key groups infected. The virus can also be transmitted through blood transfusions and has been detected in breast milk. It is currently being investigated to determine whether maternal-fetal transmission can occur during pregnancy. In July 2003, national blood banks began screening blood donations for WNV using newly developed laboratory techniques. There are currently no specific antiviral medications or vaccines available for treatment of human WNV infection. Prevention focuses on reducing mosquito reproduction by eliminating unneeded pools of water near residential environments.

November 2002 marked the emergence of a new, serious viral illness known as severe acute respiratory syndrome (SARS). A large outbreak later occurred in Singapore in March 2003. This outbreak was eventually traced to a traveler returning from Hong Kong. Cases later appeared in Europe and North America. SARS can range from a mild to a life-threatening respiratory illness. The disease usually resolves on its own within 3 to 4 weeks. However, 10% to 20% of patients required mechanical ventilation and intensive care support, and the overall fatality rate is 3%. Although standard antiviral drugs, including oseltamivir, have been used to treat SARS, no specific drug therapy has proved to be definitively helpful. The cause of SARS has been determined to be a coronavirus, which was named the *SARS coronavirus*. Coronaviruses commonly cause mild to moderate upper respiratory tract illnesses in humans, including the common cold.

Avian influenza or "bird flu" is an influenza virus infection that has been shown to infect birds in Europe and both birds and humans in Asia. This disease is caused by an influenza A virus known as *avian influenza A, subtype H5N1*. The virus is carried in the intestines of many wild birds worldwide, often without causing any serious illness. However, more serious infections can be fatal and spread rapidly among an entire flock of birds. Usually, these viruses do not infect humans. However, since 1997, there have been cases of human infection, mostly following contact with infected birds or their secretions or excrement (e.g., in poultry workers). Most of these cases have occurred in Europe and Asia. There have also been one documented case in New York and one in Virginia of infection with H7N2 virus, another avian influenza virus subtype. Human-to-human transmission has been especially rare. Symptoms in humans have ranged from typical flulike symptoms such as fever, cough, sore throat, and muscle aches, to eye infections and acute respiratory illness, sometimes with life-threatening complications. This virus is resistant to amantadine and rimantadine, although it is believed (but remains to be confirmed) that zanamivir and oseltamivir would likely offer some therapeutic benefit for this condition.

Many health experts fear a flu pandemic caused by this virus, if it mutates to a more easily transmissible form. This occurs frequently with influenza viruses in general, which is why a new seasonal flu vaccine must be developed each year. Although no one can predict if and when such a pandemic might occur with this virus, the WHO and other health agencies, including the CDC, are continuously monitoring activity patterns as well as the virus's resistance to other antiviral drugs. Some countries, including the United States, have also implemented a ban on the import of birds from countries where avian influenza has been shown to be prevalent.

In 2009, the WHO signaled that a pandemic was underway with the new influenza virus H1N1 (originally called *swine flu*). The H1N1 virus spreads person to person, much the same way the regular seasonal influenza virus spreads. Symptoms include fever, cough, sore throat, body aches, chills, and fatigue. Severe illness and death have occurred with H1N1. A vaccine was developed and made available in October 2009. Antiviral medications such as oseltamivir or zanamivir are recommended for all patients with suspected or confirmed influenza requiring hospitalization. Prophylactic treatment is considered for patients at high risk for complications.

# NURSING PROCESS

## ASSESSMENT

Before administering an antiviral drug, perform a thorough head-to-toe physical assessment and take a medical and medication history. Document any known allergies. Assess the patient's nutritional status and baseline vital signs because of the profound effects of viral illnesses on physiologic status, especially if the patient is immune-compromised. Assess for any contraindications, cautions, and drug interactions.

In your assessment related to the use of *non-HIV antivirals,* inquire about the patient's allergy to medications. Ask for a listing of any prescription and over-the-counter drugs, herbals, and dietary supplements. Before initiation of therapy, assess energy levels, any weight loss, vital signs, and the characteristics of any visible lesions. Document the findings for baseline comparison. Age is also important to assess, because amantadine is not to be used in children younger than 12 months of age. Cidofovir requires assessment of renal function and is contraindicated in those with renal compromise or with use of other nephrotoxic drugs. Ribavirin is contraindicated in pregnant women and in their male sexual partners due to its teratogenic properties; it must also not be handled by health care personnel who are or might be pregnant. With ribavirin, analysis of respiratory secretions via sputum specimen will most likely be ordered for diagnostic purposes prior to initiation of drug therapy. With respiratory illness, also assess and document breath sounds, respiratory rate and patterns, cough, sputum production, and vital signs including temperature. A dose-limiting toxicity of ganciclovir treatment is bone marrow suppression; thus, perform a close review of the patient's CBC; CBC includes RBCs, WBCs, and platelets. With foscarnet and cidofovir, assess renal function because of the potential for renal toxicity.

Before giving acyclovir, assess vital signs and take a thorough medication history. Assess pain levels associated with the zoster lesions prior to giving the medication because relief of pain is expected with use of the drug. See Chapter 56 for more information on the topical form of acyclovir.

Famciclovir also requires assessment of allergies. Oseltamivir and zanamivir, useful against influenza virus types A and B, must be given as ordered within 2 days of the onset of flu symptoms. Ganciclovir is associated with bone marrow suppression; therefore, assess blood counts prior to and during use.

With use of *HIV antivirals* or *antiretrovirals,* closely assess allergies, cautions, contraindications, and drug interactions. Because of the severity of HIV infections and potential for a fatal outcome, the main contraindication includes severe drug allergy and other toxicities. Use of protease inhibitors requires assessment of the patient's medical history, vital signs, baseline weight, allergies, medication history, and results of baseline laboratory tests, such as CBC and renal and liver function studies. These laboratory tests are also generally ordered during the different phases of treatment; document results appropriately. A major adverse effect of the protease inhibitors is lipid abnormalities with redistribution of fat stores under the skin, leading to undesirable cosmetic outcomes for the patient. Assess emotional status and support systems due to the impact of this adverse effect on body image. Bone demineralization is yet another adverse effect with long-term use, so assessment of calcium and vitamin D levels is crucial to patient safety before, during, and after therapy.

The antiretroviral drug maraviroc requires assessment of allergies and liver function as well as review of the list of medications the patient is taking because of many interacting drugs. Raltegravir is associated with myopathies and breakdown of muscle cells; thus, baseline notation of skeletal muscle functioning and pain level is crucial to patient safety. Perform a baseline measurement, and frequently monitor vital signs, including temperature, due to the possibility of opportunistic infections. The prescriber may also order CBCs and other laboratory studies before, during, and after therapy. Avoid tenofovir in patients with liver disorders. Bone marrow suppression is a dose-limiting adverse effect of zidovudine, so review blood cell counts and results of clotting studies before and during therapy.

With any of the drugs presented in this chapter, especially those used for the management of HIV infection, assessment of the patient's knowledge about the illness and the need for long-term and often lifelong therapy is crucial. In addition, an assessment of the patient's knowledge about the illness as well as his or her educational level, reading level, the way in which he or she learns best, and familiarity with community resources is important in implementing patient education effectively. Be sure to assess mental status and emotional state because of the psychological impact of chronic illness. Value systems, social patterns, hobbies, support systems, and spiritual beliefs need to also be documented. Perform an assessment of financial status and resources as well. Many patients may need to be referred to social services because of lack of health care insurance and because many of these drugs are lifelong. For patients with chronic illnesses, the synthesis of this information will help ensure the development of a nursing care plan that is complete and holistic.

## NURSING DIAGNOSES

1. Activity intolerance related to weakness secondary to decreased energy from pathology of viral infections
2. Deficient knowledge related to the lack of information about and experience with long-term medication therapy and lack of information about the viral infection, its transmission, and its treatment
3. Risk for injury related to the immunosuppressive effects of viral disease processes and their treatment

## PLANNING

### GOALS

1. Patient experiences improved energy and activity level while receiving therapy.
2. Patient demonstrates improved knowledge base about the disease process and the need for lifelong therapy.
3. Patient remains free from injury while taking medication for viral disease.

### OUTCOME CRITERIA

1. Patient experiences increased periods of comfort with greater participation in care and activities of daily living as a result of successful treatment of viral infection.
   - Patient's energy levels improve to a level greater than what was experienced before antiviral therapy.
2. Patient states the rationale for the treatment regimen and the possibility of lifelong therapy with HIV illnesses.
   - Patient understands the need for taking the medication exactly as prescribed.
   - Patient identifies possible adverse effects associated with the HIV antiviral drugs such as GI upset.
   - Patient identifies financial resources to pay for lifelong medication therapy.
3. Patient states the physical impact of a viral infection on the patient's overall state of health (e.g., compromised

immune system) and the effect of appropriate therapy with either non-HIV antivirals and/or HIV antivirals (antiretrovirals).

- Patient takes appropriate precautions during antiviral therapy such as avoiding others who are ill and staying away from crowds.

## IMPLEMENTATION

Nursing interventions pertinent to patients receiving *non-HIV antivirals* include use of the appropriate technique when applying or administering ointments, aerosol powders, and intravenous or oral forms of medication. Wear gloves and wash hands thoroughly before and after the administration of medication to prevent contamination of the site and spread of infection. It is important to the safety of both the patient and you to always begin by performing hand hygiene and maintain Standard Precautions (see Box 9-1). The use of non-HIV antivirals as well as HIV antivirals or antiretrovirals may lead to superimposed infection or superinfection, so constantly monitor for such infections and implement measures for their prevention (see Chapters 38 and 39).

Instruct the patient to take *oral antivirals* with meals to help minimize GI upset. Also advise the patient to store capsules at room temperature and not to crush or break the capsules. Acyclovir is available in various dosage forms, and there are slight inconsistencies in the spelling of the drug names so be sure to double-check the specific drug and dosage form ordered. Topical dosage forms (e.g., acyclovir) must be applied using a finger cot or gloves to prevent autoinoculation. Eye contact must also be avoided. Intravenous acyclovir is stable for 12 hours at room temperature and will often precipitate when refrigerated. Dilute intravenous infusions as recommended (e.g., with 5% dextrose in water or normal saline), and infuse with caution. Infusion over longer than 1 hour is suggested to avoid the renal tubular damage seen with more rapid infusions. Encourage adequate hydration during the infusion and for several hours afterward to prevent drug-related crystalluria. Carefully monitor the intravenous site. Document and report to the prescriber any redness, heat, pain, swelling, or red streaks that may indicate possible phlebitis. Document the characteristics of any lesions. Implement appropriate isolation for individuals with chickenpox or herpes zoster, and give analgesics for comfort, as ordered. Some of the more common adverse effects of acyclovir include nausea, diarrhea, and headache. Comfort measures may need to be implemented.

Amantadine and other antivirals need to be taken for the entire course of therapy, and, if a dose is missed, instruct the patient to take the dose as soon as it is remembered or contact the prescriber for further instructions. If dry mouth occurs due to anticholinergic effects, sucking on sugarless candy or chewing gum might be helpful. Encourage daily mouth care, including the use of dental floss, and regular dental preventive visits. Saliva substitutes may be needed, and if dry mouth continues for longer than 2 weeks, contact the prescriber for further management. Orthostatic hypotension may occur, so it is important to monitor vital signs with postural blood pressures during therapy. If given intravenously, dilute ganciclovir with 5% dextrose in water or normal saline to a concentration and in a time frame

indicated by the prescriber and authoritative sources. Administration into large veins is recommended to provide the dilution needed to minimize the risk for vein irritation. When the solution of ganciclovir is being handled, avoid exposure of the eyes, mucous membranes, and skin to the drug, and use latex gloves and safety glasses for handling and preparation. If the drug comes in contact with these areas, flush the eyes with plain water and thoroughly wash other affected areas with soap and water. Laboratory values including blood counts will most likely be monitored during therapy due to possible bone marrow toxicity. Ribavirin may be given by nasal or oral inhalation, but the drug is not to be administered to pregnant women or handled by a health care provider who is (or may be) pregnant. Continually monitor for possible altered breath sounds, as wheezing may occur due to mild bronchospasm. When certain antivirals are given, always check the order closely against the drug being administered, because other drugs are spelled similarly or sound alike. For example, acyclovir may be mistaken for valacyclovir and famciclovir. When the patient is taking oseltamivir and other non-HIV antivirals for influenza, it is important to remember that this medication must be prescribed and is most effective if started within 2 days of the onset of flu symptoms.

Aerosol generators are available from the drug manufacturer. Discard reservoir solutions if levels are low or empty and change every 24 hours. For patients taking ribavirin and similar drugs for treatment of respiratory syncytial virus via a small particle aerosol generator (SPAG) device, provide clear and precise instructions to on how to properly mix and administer the drug. Be sure to reconstitute the drug (e.g., ribavirin powder) as instructed in the manufacturer guidelines. Discard old solutions left in the equipment before adding fresh medication. Drugs given using SPAG equipment are usually administered 12 to 18 hours daily for up to 7 days beginning within 3 days of the onset of symptoms. Much controversy exists about the use of this drug in patients on ventilators, and it is to be administered by only health care providers who are specially trained in this drug and its use. Frequently empty any "rain out" in the tubing of the ventilator, and continually monitor breath sounds in patients receiving inhaled forms of this drug, whether they are receiving artificial ventilation or not. Zanamivir is administered by inhalation using a Diskhaler device. Be sure that the patient exhales completely first; then, while holding the mouthpiece between the teeth with lips snug around it and tongue down and out of the way, the patient needs to inhale deeply through the mouth and then hold the breath as long as possible before exhaling the drug and the breath. Encourage rinsing of the mouth with water to prevent irritation and dryness, and instruct the patient to never exhale into the Diskhaler.

*HIV antivirals,* or *antiretrovirals,* include numerous drugs. With regard to dosage forms, there are special administration and handling guidelines for some of these drugs. With zidovudine, monitor for the adverse effects of bone marrow suppression by checking RBCs, WBCs, platelets, and other blood counts. If the patient experiences signs and symptoms of an opportunistic infection (e.g., respiratory signs and symptoms, fever, changes in oral mucosa), the prescriber needs to be contacted immediately. The patient may experience headaches; therefore, provide the appropriate form of analgesia, as ordered. See Table 40-2 for a listing of more adverse effects associated with the various antiviral drugs.

With film-coated oral dosage forms, advise the patient not to alter the drugs in any way. Patients may improve the taste of ritonavir by mixing it with chocolate milk or a nutritional beverage within 1 hour of its dosing. Emphasize to patient and family that ritonavir's dosage form needs to be protected from light. Absorption of oral dosage forms of zidovudine is not impeded by taking the drug with food or milk, but instruct the patient to remain upright or with the head of the bed elevated while administering the medication and for up to 30 minutes afterward to prevent esophageal ulceration. Give intravenous doses only if the solution is clear and does not contain any particulate matter. Be sure to use the appropriate dosage, diluents, and infusion time. Because these drugs often come in oral dosage forms, it is usually recommended that they be given with food. Generally, administer zidovudine and other antiretrovirals at evenly spaced intervals around the clock—as ordered—to ensure steady-state levels. With all oral and parenteral dosage forms of antiretrovirals, observe the patient for nausea and vomiting as well as any changes in weight, anorexia, or changes in bowel activity and patterns. Maraviroc and tenofovir are available for oral dosing and are to be given as prescribed.

Throughout therapy, always remember that the goal of treatment is to find the regimen that provides the best control of the individual patient's infection with the most tolerable adverse effects possible. Because patients vary greatly in their drug tolerance, carefully individualize medication regimens. Other nursing interventions associated with these drugs include: (1) Continually monitor for adverse effects throughout therapy with a focus on the various organ systems, such as GI, neurologic, renal, and hepatic. (2) With oral forms of indinavir and nevirapine, encourage forcing of fluids (unless contraindicated) of at least 6 to 8 glasses of water daily to maintain adequate hydration and help prevent nephrolithiasis. (3) Nevirapine, zidovudine, and similar drugs may be associated with a rash; however, if the rash is accompanied by blistering, fever, malaise, myalgias, oral lesions, swelling or edema, or conjunctivitis, contact the prescriber immediately. (4) If drug therapy results in worsening of signs and symptoms, notify the prescriber immediately. The drug may be discontinued. (5) Continually monitor laboratory testing (e.g., CBC, renal/liver function studies, HIV RNA levels), and report abnormalities to the prescriber. See the Patient Teaching Tips for more information.

## EVALUATION

The therapeutic effects of *non-HIV antivirals* and *HIV antivirals* or *antiretrovirals* include elimination of the virus or a decrease in the symptoms of the viral infection. There may be a delayed progression of HIV infection and AIDS as well as a decrease in flulike symptoms and/or the frequency of herpetic flare-ups and other lesion breakouts. With successful therapy, herpetic lesions will crust over, and the frequency of recurrence will decrease. In addition, constantly evaluate for the occurrence of adverse effects and toxicity associated with specific antiviral and antiretroviral drugs. These specific adverse effects are listed in Table 40-2. Continually reevaluate the nursing care plan to ensure that the goals and outcome criteria have been met. Remain constantly attentive in reviewing reports from the CDC, other federal and state health care agencies, and public health care organizations regarding new strains of viruses and flu syndromes (see earlier discussion).

## PATIENT TEACHING TIPS

• Alert the patient to the adverse effect of dizziness, and instruct him or her to use caution while driving or participating in activities requiring alertness while taking antiviral drugs. Advise the patient to take all medications exactly as prescribed and for the full course of therapy.
• Inform the patient of all possible drug interactions including over-the-counter medications.
• Advise immunocompromised patients to avoid crowds and persons with infections.
• Advocate standard precautions and safe sex practices for all patients but especially those with sexually transmitted viral diseases, such as HIV-positive individuals. Condom use is a necessity for prevention of these viral infections and other sexually transmitted diseases. The presence of genital herpes requires sexual abstinence.
• It is generally recommended that female patients with genital herpes undergo a Papanicolaou smear test (Pap test) every 6 months or as ordered by the prescriber to monitor the virus and effectiveness of therapy.
• Instruct the patient to report the following adverse reactions to the prescriber: decreased urinary output, seizure activity, syncope, jaundice, wheezing, abnormal sensations in the hands and feet, vomiting, or diarrhea.

• Provide the patient with adequate demonstrations, teaching aids, and instructions for special application procedures (e.g., instillation of ophthalmic drops, use of finger cots or gloves when applying medication to lesions, use of respiratory inhalation forms). Explain that gloves or finger cots are needed for medication application and cleansing to prevent the spread of lesions.
• Encourage forcing fluids up to 3000 mL/24 hr unless contraindicated.
• Educate the patient about the fact that these drugs suppress but do not cure the viral infection.
• Inform the patient that therapy is to be started as prescribed but at the first sign (as with valacyclovir or other antivirals) of a recurrent episode of genital herpes or herpes zoster. In addition, explain that early treatment within 24 to 48 hours of symptom onset is needed to achieve full therapeutic results.
• Instruct the patient to report to the prescriber immediately any difficulty breathing; drastic changes in blood pressure; bleeding; new symptoms; worsening of infection, fever, or chills; or other unusual problems.
• Emphasize the importance of follow-up appointments.

# KEY POINTS

- Viruses are difficult to kill and to treat because they live inside human cells, and most antiviral drugs work by inhibiting replication of the virus. In this chapter, antiviral drugs are categorized as either non-HIV antivirals or HIV antivirals (antiretrovirals).
- Non-HIV antivirals include amantadine, rimantadine, acyclovir, ganciclovir, oseltamivir, zanamivir, and ribavirin. HIV antivirals include enfuvirtide, indinavir, maraviroc, nevirapine, raltegravir, tenofovir, and zidovudine.

- Administer antiretroviral drugs only after the prescriber's orders are read and understood and after performing a thorough nursing assessment that includes a review of the patient's nutritional status, weight, baseline vital sign values, and renal and hepatic functioning as well as an assessment of heart sounds, neurologic status, and GI tract functioning.
- Comfort measures and supportive nursing care are to accompany drug therapy. Patients need to drink plenty of fluids and to space medications around the clock, as ordered, to maintain steady blood levels of the drug.

# NCLEX® EXAMINATION REVIEW QUESTIONS

1 During treatment with zidovudine, the nurse needs to monitor for which potential adverse effect?
  a Retinitis
  b Deep vein thromboses
  c Kaposi's sarcoma
  d Bone marrow suppression

2 After giving an injection to a patient with HIV infection, the nurse accidentally receives a needlestick from a too-full needle disposal box. Recommendations for occupational HIV exposure may include the use of which drug(s)?
  a didanosine
  b lamivudine and enfuvirtide
  c zidovudine, lamivudine, and indinavir
  d acyclovir

3 When the nurse is teaching a patient who is taking acyclovir for genital herpes, which statement by the nurse is accurate?
  a "This drug will help the lesions to dry and crust over."
  b "Acyclovir will eradicate the herpes virus."
  c "This drug will prevent the spread of this virus to others."
  d "Be sure to give this drug to your partner, too."

4 A patient who has been newly diagnosed with HIV has many questions about the effectiveness of drug therapy. After a teaching session, which statement by the patient reflects a need for more education?
  a "I will be monitored for side effects and improvements while I'm taking this medicine."
  b "These drugs do not eliminate the HIV, but hopefully the amount of virus in my body will be reduced."
  c "There is no cure for HIV."
  d "These drugs will eventually eliminate the virus from my body."

5 After surgery for organ transplantation, a patient is receiving ganciclovir, even though he does not have a viral infection. Which statement best explains the rationale for this medication therapy?
  a Ganciclovir is used to prevent potential exposure to the HIV virus.
  b This medication is given prophylactically to prevent influenza A infection.
  c Ganciclovir is given to prevent CMV infection.
  d The drug works synergistically with antibiotics to prevent superinfections.

6 The nurse is reviewing the use of multidrug therapy for HIV with a patient. Which statements are correct regarding the reason for using multiple drugs to treat HIV? (Select all that apply.)
  a The combination of drugs has fewer associated toxicities.
  b The use of multiple drugs is more effective against resistant strains of HIV.
  c Effective treatment results in reduced T-cell counts.
  d The goal of this treatment is to reduce the viral load.
  e This type of therapy reduces the incidence of opportunistic infections.

7 The order for an 11-year-old child who has chickenpox reads: "Give acyclovir (Zovirax) 20 mg/kg PO daily × 5 days. The child weighs 99 pounds. How much is each dose? Is this dose safe for this child?

1. d, 2. c, 3. a, 4. d, 5. c, 6. b, d, e, 7. 900 mg; no, the dose exceeds the 800 mg maximum per dose

For Critical Thinking and Prioritization Questions, see http://evolve.elsevier.com/Lilley.

# 41

# Antitubercular Drugs

## evolve WEBSITE

*http://evolve.elsevier.com/Lilley*

- Animations
- Answer Key—Textbook Case Studies
- Critical Thinking and Prioritization Questions

- Key Points—Downloadable
- Review Questions for the NCLEX® Examination
- Unfolding Case Studies

## OBJECTIVES

When you reach the end of this chapter, you will be able to do the following:

1. Identify the various first-line and second-line drugs indicated for the treatment of tuberculosis.
2. Discuss the mechanisms of action, dosages, adverse effects, routes of administration, special dosing considerations, cautions, contraindications, and drug interactions of the various antitubercular drugs.

3. Develop a nursing care plan that includes all phases of the nursing process for patients receiving antitubercular drugs.
4. Develop a comprehensive teaching guide for patients and families impacted by the diagnosis and treatment of antitubercular drugs.

## DRUG PROFILES

ethambutol, p. 677
♦ isoniazid, p. 677
pyrazinamide, p. 678
rifabutin, p. 678
rifampin, p. 678

rifapentine, p. 678
streptomycin, p. 678

_____

♦ *Key drug*

## KEY TERMS

**Aerobic** Requiring oxygen for the maintenance of life. (p. 673)

**Antitubercular drugs** Drugs used to treat infections caused by *Mycobacterium* bacterial species. (p. 674)

**Bacillus** A rod-shaped bacterium. (p. 673)

**Granulomas** Small nodular aggregations of inflammatory cells (e.g., macrophages, lymphocytes); usually characterized by clearly delimited boundaries, as found in tuberculosis. (p. 673)

**Isoniazid** The primary and most commonly prescribed tuberculostatic drug. (p. 674)

**Multidrug-resistant tuberculosis (MDR-TB)** Tuberculosis that demonstrates resistance to two or more drugs. (p. 673)

**Slow acetylator** An individual with a genetic defect that causes a deficiency in the enzyme needed to metabolize isoniazid, the most widely used tuberculosis drug. (p. 677)

**Tubercle** The characteristic lesion of tuberculosis; a small round gray translucent granulomatous lesion, usually with a caseated (cheesy) consistency in its interior. (See *granuloma*.) (p. 673)

**Tubercle bacilli** Another common name for rod-shaped tuberculosis bacteria; essentially synonymous with *Mycobacterium tuberculosis*. (p. 673)

**Tuberculosis (TB)** Any infectious disease caused by species of *Mycobacterium*, usually *Mycobacterium tuberculosis* (adjectives: *tuberculous, tubercular*). (p. 673)

# ANATOMY, PHYSIOLOGY, AND PATHOPHYSIOLOGY OVERVIEW

## PATHOPHYSIOLOGY OF TUBERCULOSIS

Tuberculosis (TB) is the medical diagnosis for any infection caused by a bacterial species known as *Mycobacterium.* TB is most commonly characterized by granulomas in the lungs. These are nodular accumulations of inflammatory cells (e.g., macrophages, lymphocytes) that are delimited ("walled off" with clear boundaries) and have a center that has a cheesy or caseated consistency. (*Casein* is the name of a protein that is prevalent in cheese and milk.) Although there are two mycobacterial species that can cause TB, *Mycobacterium tuberculosis* and *Mycobacterium bovis,* infections caused by *M. tuberculosis* (abbreviated MTB) are the most common. There are also several other mycobacterial species, including *Mycobacterium leprae,* which causes leprosy, and *Mycobacterium avium-intracellulare* complex, which causes a disease that is similar to TB but often has gastrointestinal symptoms, both of which have varying susceptibility to different drugs used for TB. Infections with these bacteria are much less of a public health problem and hence are not the focus of this chapter.

MTB is an aerobic bacillus, which means that it is a rod-shaped microorganism (bacillus) that requires a large supply of oxygen to grow and flourish (aerobic). This bacterium's need for a highly oxygenated body site explains why *Mycobacterium* infections most commonly affect the lungs. Other common sites of infection are the growing ends of bones and the brain (cerebral cortex). Less common sites of infection include the kidney, liver, and genitourinary tract, as well as virtually every other tissue and organ in the body.

These tubercle bacilli (a common synonym for MTB) are transmitted from one of three sources: humans, cattle (adjective: *bovine,* hence the species name *M. bovis*), or birds (adjective: *avian*), although bovine and avian transmission are much less common than human transmission. Tubercle bacilli are conveyed in droplets expelled by infected people or animals during coughing or sneezing and then inhaled by the new host. After these infectious droplets are inhaled, the infection spreads to the susceptible organ sites by means of the blood and lymphatic system. MTB is a very slow-growing organism, which makes it more difficult to treat than most other bacterial infections. Many of the antibiotics used to treat TB work by inhibiting growth (bacteriostatic) rather than by directly killing the organism. The reason why microorganisms that grow slowly are more difficult to kill is because their cells are not as metabolically active as those of faster-growing organisms. Most bactericidal (cell-killing) drugs work by disrupting critical cellular metabolic processes in the organism. Therefore, the most drug-susceptible organisms are those with faster (not slower) metabolic activity.

The first infectious episode is considered the primary TB infection; reinfection represents the more chronic form of the disease. However, TB does not develop in all people who are exposed to the bacteria. In some cases, the bacteria become dormant and walled off by calcified or fibrous tissues. These patients may test positive for exposure but are not necessarily infectious because of this dormancy process. In immunocompromised patients, TB can inflict devastating and irreversible damage. The steps for diagnosis of TB are listed in Box 41-1.

TB cases have been reported on a national level in the United States beginning in 1953. Since that time, the TB incidence decreased in most years until about 1985. At that point, the epidemic of human immunodeficiency virus (HIV) infection was growing strongly, and the TB incidence began to rise for the first time in 20 years because of the development of TB in patients co-infected with HIV. Many cities were unprepared to handle this reemergence of TB. After an 18% increase in TB incidence between 1985 and 1991, a 50% decline was recorded from 1992 through 2002, and a 3.1% decline was seen from 2009 to 2010. In 2010, 11,182 new cases were reported in the United States. The rate in 2010 represented the lowest recorded number of cases since 1953. This is attributed to intensified public health efforts aimed at preventing, diagnosing, and treating TB as well as HIV infection, including more effective antiretroviral drug therapy (see Chapter 40). However, the rate of decline has now slowed, primarily due to one contributing factor: the number of multidrug-resistant tuberculosis (MDR-TB) cases. An upward trend in drug resistance, especially to isoniazid (abbreviated INH) and rifampin, has been observed since the 1970s. In the 1990s, one third of TB cases in New York City were resistant to at least one drug, and 20% to both isoniazid and rifampin. Fortunately, these numbers have since declined, which has been attributed to stronger TB-related public health efforts.

The prevalence and growth of TB continues to be greater in the larger global community, and TB infects one third of the world's population. It is currently second only to HIV infection in the number of deaths caused by a single infectious organism. MDR-TB is defined as TB that is resistant to both isoniazid and rifampin, according to the World Health Organization. Close contacts of patients with MDR-TB need to be treated as well. Extensively drug-resistant tuberculosis (XDR-TB) is a relatively rare type of MDR-TB. It is resistant to almost all drugs used to treat TB, including the two best first-line drugs, isoniazid and rifampin, as well as to the best second-line medications. Because XDR-TB is resistant to the most powerful first-line and second-line drugs, patients are left with treatment options that are much less effective and often have worse treatment outcomes. XDR-TB is of special concern for patients who have AIDS or are otherwise immunocompromised. Not only are these patients more likely to contract TB, they are also more likely to die of it. At this point, XDR-TB is rare.

---

**BOX 41-1  DIAGNOSIS OF TUBERCULOSIS**

**Step 1:** Tuberculin skin test (Mantoux test)
**Step 2:** If skin test results are positive, then chest radiograph
**Step 3:** If chest radiograph shows signs of tuberculosis, then culture of sputum* or stomach secretions

*The acid-fast bacillus smear test is performed on sputum as a quick method of determining whether tuberculosis treatment and precautions are needed until a more definite diagnosis is made.

Several factors have contributed to this health care crisis, but one very important source of the problem is the increasing numbers of people in groups that are particularly susceptible to the infection—the homeless, undernourished or malnourished individuals, HIV-infected persons, drug abusers, cancer patients, those taking immunosuppressant drugs, and those who live in crowded and poorly sanitized housing facilities. All of these circumstances also favor the acquisition of a drug-resistant infection. Members of racial and ethnic minority groups are at greater risk than white populations and account for two thirds of new cases. Asian and Hispanic immigrants are at particularly high risk, accounting for more than half of all U.S. cases of foreign-acquired TB.

## PHARMACOLOGY OVERVIEW

## ANTITUBERCULAR DRUGS

The drugs used to treat infections caused by all forms of *Mycobacterium* are called antitubercular drugs, and these drugs fall into two categories: primary or first-line drugs and secondary or second-line drugs. As these designations imply, primary drugs are those tried first, whereas secondary drugs are reserved for more complicated cases, such as those resistant to primary drugs. The antimycobacterial activity, efficacy, and potential adverse and toxic effects of the various drugs determine the class to which they belong. Isoniazid is a primary antitubercular drug and is the most widely used. It can be administered either as the sole drug in the prophylaxis of TB or in combination with other antitubercular drugs in the treatment of TB. The various first-line and second-line antibiotic drugs are listed in Box 41-2. There are also two miscellaneous TB-related injections—one diagnostic, the other a vaccine. These are described in Box 41-3.

An important consideration during drug selection is the likelihood of drug-resistant organisms and drug toxicity. Following are other key elements that are important in the planning and implementation of effective therapy:

- Drug-susceptibility tests are performed on the first *Mycobacterium* species that is isolated from a patient specimen (to prevent the development of MDR-TB).
- Before the results of the susceptibility tests are known, the patient is started on a four-drug regimen consisting of isoniazid, rifampin, pyrazinamide (PZA), and ethambutol or streptomycin, which together are 95% effective in combating the infection. The use of multiple medications reduces the possibility of the organism's becoming drug resistant.
- Once drug susceptibility results are available, the regimen is adjusted accordingly.
- Patient adherence to the prescribed drug regimen and any adverse effects of therapy need to be monitored closely, because the incidence of both patient nonadherence and adverse effects is high.
- Despite the availability of many drugs to combat TB and the efforts mounted to detect and treat victims of the disease, treatment has been made difficult by two problems previously mentioned: patient nonadherence with therapy and the growing incidence of drug-resistant organisms.

### BOX 41-2 FIRST-LINE AND SECOND-LINE ANTITUBERCULAR DRUGS

| First-Line Drugs | Second-Line Drugs |
|---|---|
| ethambutol | amikacin |
| isoniazid (INH) | capreomycin |
| pyrazinamide (PZA) | cycloserine |
| rifabutin | ethionamide |
| rifampin | kanamycin |
| rifapentine | levofloxacin |
| streptomycin | ofloxacin |
| | para-aminosalicylic acid (PAS) |

### BOX 41-3 TUBERCULOSIS-RELATED INJECTIONS

**Purified protein derivative (PPD):** A diagnostic injection given intradermally in doses of 5 tuberculin units (0.1 mL) to detect exposure to the tuberculosis (TB) organism. It is composed of a protein precipitate derived from TB bacteria. A positive result is indicated by induration (not erythema) at the site of injection and is known as the Mantoux reaction, named for the physician who described it.

**Bacille Calmette-Guérin (BCG):** A vaccine injection derived from an inactivated strain of *Mycobacterium bovis*. Although it is not normally administered in the United States because the risk is not as high, it is used in much of the world to vaccinate young children against tuberculosis. Although it does not prevent infection, evidence indicates that it reduces active tuberculosis by 60% to 80% and is even more effective at preventing more severe cases involving dissemination of infection throughout the body. The bacille Calmette-Guérin vaccine for tuberculosis can cause false-positive results on the tuberculin skin test.

## Mechanism of Action and Drug Effects

The mechanisms of action of the various antitubercular drugs vary depending on the drug. These drugs act on MTB by inhibiting protein synthesis, inhibiting cell wall synthesis, or various other mechanisms. The antitubercular drugs are listed in Table 41-1 by their mechanism of action. The major effects of drug therapy include reduction of cough and, therefore, reduction of the infectiousness of the patient. This normally occurs within 2 weeks of the initiation of drug therapy, assuming that the patient's TB strain is drug sensitive.

## Indications

Antitubercular medications are indicated for the treatment of TB infections, including both pulmonary and extrapulmonary TB. Most antitubercular drugs have not been fully tested for their effects in pregnant women. However, the combination of isoniazid and ethambutol has been used to treat pregnant women with clinically apparent TB without teratogenic complications. Rifampin is another drug that is usually safe during pregnancy and is a more likely choice for more advanced disease.

Besides being used for the initial treatment of TB, antitubercular drugs have also proved effective in the management of treatment failures and relapses. Infection with species of *Mycobacterium* other than *M. tuberculosis* and atypical mycobacterial

## TABLE 41-1   ANTITUBERCULAR DRUGS: MECHANISMS OF ACTION

| DRUGS | DESCRIPTION |
|---|---|
| **Inhibit Protein Synthesis** | |
| kanamycin, capreomycin, rifabutin, rifampin, streptomycin | Streptomycin and kanamycin work by interfering with normal protein synthesis and causing the production of faulty proteins. Rifampin and capreomycin act at different points in the protein synthesis pathway than streptomycin and kanamycin. Rifampin inhibits RNA synthesis and may also inhibit DNA synthesis. Human cells are not as sensitive as the mycobacterial cells and are not affected by rifampin except at high drug concentrations. Capreomycin inhibits protein synthesis by preventing translocation on ribosomes. |
| **Inhibit Cell Wall Synthesis** | |
| cycloserine, ethionamide, isoniazid | Cycloserine acts by inhibiting the amino acid (D-alanine) involved in the synthesis of cell walls. Isoniazid and ethionamide also act at least partly to inhibit the synthesis of wall components, but the mechanisms of these two drugs are still not clearly understood. |
| **Other Mechanisms** | |
| ethambutol, ethionamide, isoniazid, para-aminosalicylic acid, pyrazinamide | Isoniazid is taken up by mycobacterial cells and undergoes hydrolysis to isonicotinic acid, which reacts with cofactor NAD to form a defective NAD that is no longer active as a coenzyme for certain life-sustaining reactions in the *Mycobacterium tuberculosis* organism. Ethionamide directly inhibits mycolic acid synthesis, which eventually has the same deleterious effects on the TB organism as isoniazid. Ethambutol affects lipid synthesis, which results in the inhibition of mycolic acid incorporation into the cell wall and thus inhibits protein synthesis. Para-aminosalicylic acid acts as a competitive inhibitor of para-aminobenzoic acid in the synthesis of folate. The mechanism of action of pyrazinamide in the inhibition of TB is unknown. It can be either bacteriostatic or bactericidal, depending on the susceptibility of the particular *Mycobacterium* organism and the concentration of the drug attained at the site of infection. |

*NAD,* Nicotinamide adenine; *TB,* tuberculosis.

infections have also been successfully treated with these drugs. Nontuberculous *Mycobacteria* may also be susceptible to antitubercular drugs. However, in general, antitubercular drugs are not as effective against other species of *Mycobacterium* as they are against MTB. Some of these other species that may be of particular concern in immunocompromised patients such as AIDS patients are *M. avium-intracellulare* complex, *Mycobacterium flavescens*, *Mycobacterium marinum*, and *Mycobacterium kansasii*. Additional *Mycobacterium* infections that may respond to antitubercular drugs are those caused by *Mycobacterium fortuitum*, *Mycobacterium chelonae*, *Mycobacterium smegmatis*, *Mycobacterium xenopi*, and *Mycobacterium scrofulaceum*. Treatment regimens for these non-TB mycobacterial infections often include the macrolide antibiotics clarithromycin or azithromycin (see Chapter 38), either alone or in combination with one or more antitubercular drugs.

In summary, antitubercular drugs are primarily used for the prophylaxis or treatment of TB. The effectiveness of these drugs depends on the type of infection, adequate dosing, sufficient duration of treatment, adherence to the drug regimen, and selection of an effective drug combination. The indications of the different antitubercular drugs are listed in Table 41-2.

## Contraindications

Contraindications to the use of various antitubercular drugs include severe drug allergy and major renal or liver dysfunction. However, it must be recognized that the urgency of treating a potentially fatal infection may have to be balanced against any prevailing contraindications. In extreme cases, patients are sometimes given a drug to which they have some degree of allergy with supportive care that enables them at least to tolerate the medication. Examples of such supportive care are treatment with antipyretics (e.g., acetaminophen), antihistamines (e.g., diphenhydramine), or even corticosteroids (e.g., prednisone, methylprednisolone).

One relative contraindication to ethambutol is optic neuritis. Chronic alcohol use, especially when associated with major liver damage, may also be a contraindication to therapy with any antitubercular drug. Other contraindications for specific drugs, if any, can be found in the drug profiles presented later in the chapter.

## Adverse Effects

Antitubercular drugs are fairly well tolerated. Isoniazid, one of the mainstays of treatment, is noted for causing pyridoxine deficiency and liver toxicity. For this reason, supplements of pyridoxine (vitamin $B_6$; see Chapter 53) are often given concurrently with isoniazid, with a common oral dose of 50 mg daily. The most problematic drugs and their associated adverse effects are listed in Table 41-3.

## Interactions

The drugs that can interact with antitubercular drugs can cause significant effects. See Table 41-4 for a listing of selected interactions. Besides these drug interactions, isoniazid can cause false-positive readings on urine glucose tests (e.g., Clinitest) and an increase in the serum levels of the liver function enzymes alanine aminotransferase and aspartate aminotransferase.

## Dosages

For dosage information on selected antitubercular drugs, see the table on p. 677.

## TABLE 41-2    ANTITUBERCULAR DRUGS: CLINICAL USES

| DRUG | CLINICAL USES |
|---|---|
| amikacin, kanamycin | Used in combination with other antitubercular drugs in the treatment of clinical TB. Not intended for long-term use. |
| capreomycin | Used with other antitubercular drugs for the treatment of pulmonary TB caused by *Mycobacterium tuberculosis* after first-line drugs fail, drug resistance appears, or drug toxicity occurs. |
| cycloserine | Used with other antitubercular drugs for treatment of active pulmonary and extrapulmonary TB after failure of first-line drugs. |
| ethambutol | Indicated as a first-line drug for treatment of TB. |
| ethionamide | Used with other antitubercular drugs in treatment of clinical TB after failure of first-line drugs and for treatment of other types of mycobacterial infections. |
| isoniazid | Used alone or in combination with other antitubercular drugs in treatment and prevention of clinical TB. |
| para-aminosalicylic acid | Used in combination with other antitubercular drugs for treatment of pulmonary and extrapulmonary *M. tuberculosis* infection after failure of first-line drugs. |
| pyrazinamide | Used with other antitubercular drugs in treatment of clinical TB. |
| rifabutin | Used to prevent or delay development of *Mycobacterium avium-intracellulare* bacteremia and disseminated infections in patients with advanced HIV infection. |
| rifampin | Used with other antitubercular drugs in treatment of clinical TB. |
|  | Used in treatment of diseases caused by mycobacteria other than *M. tuberculosis*. |
|  | Used for preventive therapy in patients exposed to isoniazid-resistant *M. tuberculosis*. |
|  | Used to eliminate meningococci from the nasopharynx of asymptomatic *Neisseria meningitidis* carriers when risk for meningococcal meningitis is high. |
|  | Used for chemoprophylaxis in contacts of patients with HiB infection. |
|  | Used with at least one other antiinfective drug in the treatment of leprosy. |
|  | Used in the treatment of endocarditis caused by methicillin-resistant staphylococci, chronic staphylococcal prostatitis, and multiple-antiinfective–resistant pneumococci. |
| rifapentine | Used with other antitubercular drugs in the treatment of clinical TB. |
| streptomycin | Used in combination with other antitubercular drugs in the treatment of clinical TB and other mycobacterial diseases. |

*HiB,* Haemophilus influenzae type b; *HIV,* human immunodeficiency virus; *TB,* tuberculosis.

## TABLE 41-3    ANTITUBERCULAR DRUGS: COMMON ADVERSE EFFECTS

| DRUG | ADVERSE EFFECTS |
|---|---|
| amikacin, kanamycin | Ototoxicity, nephrotoxicity |
| capreomycin | Ototoxicity, nephrotoxicity |
| cycloserine | Psychotic behavior, seizures |
| ethambutol | Retrobulbar neuritis, blindness |
| ethionamide | GI tract disturbances, hepatotoxicity |
| isoniazid | Peripheral neuropathy, hepatotoxicity, optic neuritis and visual disturbances, hyperglycemia |
| para-aminosalicylic acid | GI tract disturbances, hepatotoxicity |
| pyrazinamide | Hepatotoxicity, hyperuricemia |
| rifabutin | GI tract disturbances; rash; neutropenia; red-orange-brown discoloration of urine, feces, saliva, sputum, sweat, tears, skin |
| rifampin | Hepatitis; hematologic disorders; red-orange-brown discoloration of urine, tears, sweat, sputum |
| rifapentine | GI upset; red-orange-brown discoloration of tears, sweat, skin, teeth, tongue, sputum, saliva, urine, feces, CSF |
| streptomycin | Ototoxicity, nephrotoxicity, blood dyscrasias |

*CSF,* Cerebrospinal fluid; *GI,* gastrointestinal.

## TABLE 41-4    SELECTED ANTITUBERCULAR DRUGS: DRUG INTERACTIONS

| DRUG | INTERACTING DRUGS | MECHANISM | RESULTS |
|---|---|---|---|
| isoniazid | Antacids | Reduce absorption | Decreased isoniazid levels |
|  | cycloserine, ethionamide, rifampin | Have additive effects | Increased central nervous system and hepatic toxicity |
|  | phenytoin, carbamazepine | Decrease metabolism | Increased phenytoin and carbamazepine effects |
| streptomycin | Nephrotoxic and neurotoxic drugs | Additive effects | Increased toxicity |
|  | Oral anticoagulants | Alter intestinal flora | Increased bleeding tendencies |
| rifampin | Beta blockers, benzodiazepines, cyclosporine, oral anticoagulants, oral antidiabetics, oral contraceptives, phenytoin, quinidine, sirolimus, theophylline | Increase metabolism | Decreased therapeutic effects of these drugs |

## DOSAGES

### Selected Antitubercular Drugs

| DRUG (PREGNANCY CATEGORY) | PHARMACOLOGIC CLASS | USUAL DOSAGE RANGE | INDICATIONS |
|---|---|---|---|
| ethambutol (Myambutol) (B) | Synthetic first-line antimycobacterial | **Adult and pediatric** <br> PO: 15-25 mg/kg/day; may also be divided in 2×/wk and 3×/wk dosage regimens with higher doses; no maximum dose listed | |
| ♦ isoniazid (INH), generic only (C) | Synthetic first-line antimycobacterial | **Adult** <br> PO: 5 mg/kg daily (max 300 mg) or 15 mg/kg 1-3×/wk (max 900 mg/dose) <br> **Pediatric** <br> PO: 10-20 mg/kg/day (max 300 mg) | |
| pyrazinamide (generic only) (C) | Synthetic first-line antimycobacterial | **Adult and pediatric** <br> PO: 15-30 mg/kg/day (max 2 g) | |
| rifabutin (Mycobutin) (B) | Semisynthetic first-line antimycobacterial antibiotic | **Adult only** <br> PO: 150-300 mg once daily | Active TB |
| rifampin (Rifadin, Rimactane) (C) | Semisynthetic first-line antimycobacterial antibiotic | **Adult** <br> PO/IV: 10 mg/kg up to 600 mg once daily <br> **Pediatric** <br> PO/IV*: 10-20 mg/kg/day or 2-3×/wk (max 600 mg/dose for all regimens) | |
| rifapentine (Priftin) (C) | Semisynthetic first-line antimycobacterial antibiotic | **Adult only** <br> PO: 600 mg 2×/wk for first 2 mo; then 1×/wk for 4 mo | |
| streptomycin (generic) (D) | Aminoglycoside antibiotic used in combination with other drugs for TB | **Adult** <br> Deep IM: 15 mg/kg/day <br> **Pediatric** <br> Deep IM: 20-40 mg/kg/day (Maximum dose: 1 g/day for all) | |

*IM*, Intramuscular; *IV*, intravenous; *PO*, oral; *TB*, tuberculosis.
*Use of intramuscular and subcutaneous injections is contraindicated due to soft-tissue toxicity.

## DRUG PROFILES

### ethambutol

Ethambutol (Myambutol) is a first-line bacteriostatic drug used in the treatment of TB. It works by diffusing into the mycobacteria and suppressing ribonucleic acid (RNA) synthesis, which thereby inhibits protein synthesis. Ethambutol is included with isoniazid, streptomycin, and rifampin in many TB combination-drug therapies. It may also be used to treat other mycobacterial diseases. It is contraindicated in patients with known optic neuritis, because it can both exacerbate and cause this condition, which can result in varying degrees of vision loss. Ethambutol is also contraindicated in children younger than 13 years of age. It is available only in oral form.

### Pharmacokinetics

| Route | Onset of Action | Peak Plasma Concentration | Elimination Half-life | Duration of Action |
|---|---|---|---|---|
| PO | Variable | 2-4 hr | 3.5 hr | 24 hr |

### ♦ isoniazid

Isoniazid (also called INH) is the mainstay in the treatment of TB and the most widely used antitubercular drug. It may be given either as a single drug for prophylaxis or in combination with other antitubercular drugs for the treatment of active TB. It is a bactericidal drug that kills the mycobacteria by disrupting cell wall synthesis and essential cellular functions. Isoniazid is metabolized in the liver through a process called *acetylation*, which requires a certain enzymatic pathway to break down the drug. However, some people have a genetic deficiency of the liver enzymes needed for this to occur. Such people are called slow acetylators. When isoniazid is taken by slow acetylators, the isoniazid accumulates, because there is not enough of the enzyme to break down the isoniazid. Therefore, the dosages of isoniazid may need to be adjusted downward in these patients.

Isoniazid is most commonly used in oral form, although an injection is available. There is also a combination oral formulation containing both isoniazid and rifampin (Rifamate). Another combination drug product, Rifater, contains rifampin, isoniazid, and pyrazinamide. Isoniazid is contraindicated in those with previous isoniazid-associated hepatic injury or any acute liver disease.

### Pharmacokinetics

| Route | Onset of Action | Peak Plasma Concentration | Elimination Half-life | Duration of Action |
|---|---|---|---|---|
| PO | Variable | 1-2 hr | 1-4 hr | 24 hr |

## pyrazinamide

Pyrazinamide (also called PZA) is an antitubercular drug that can be either bacteriostatic or bactericidal, depending on its concentration at the site of infection and the particular susceptibility of the mycobacteria. It is commonly used in combination with other antitubercular drugs for the treatment of TB. Its mechanism of action is unknown, but it is believed to work by inhibiting lipid and nucleic acid synthesis in the mycobacteria. Pyrazinamide is available only in generic oral form. It is contraindicated in patients with severe hepatic disease or acute gout. It is also not normally used in pregnant patients in the United States, due to a lack of teratogenicity data, although it is often used in pregnant patients in other countries.

### Pharmacokinetics

| Route | Onset of Action | Peak Plasma Concentration | Elimination Half-life | Duration of Action |
|---|---|---|---|---|
| PO | Variable | 2 hr | 9-10 hr | 24 hr |

## rifabutin

Rifabutin is one of three currently available *rifamycin* antibiotics. Although it is considered a first-line TB drug by some clinicians, it is more commonly used to treat infections caused by *M. avium-intracellulare* complex, which includes several non-TB mycobacterial species. This is also the case with the two other rifamycin-derived drugs, rifampin and rifapentine. A notable adverse effect of rifabutin, as well as rifampin (see later in the chapter), is that it can turn urine, feces, saliva, skin, sputum, sweat, and tears a red-orange-brown color. Rifabutin is currently available only for oral use.

### Pharmacokinetics

| Route | Onset of Action | Peak Plasma Concentration | Elimination Half-life | Duration of Action |
|---|---|---|---|---|
| PO | Variable | 2-4 hr | 16-69 hr | 1 to several days |

## rifampin

Rifampin (Rifadin) is the first of the rifamycin class of synthetic macrocyclic antibiotics, which also includes rifabutin and rifapentine. The term *macrocyclic* connotes the very large and complex hydrocarbon ring structure included in all three of the rifamycin compounds. Rifampin has activity against many *Mycobacterium* species, as well as against *Meningococcus, Haemophilus influenzae* type b, and *M. leprae*. It is a broad-spectrum bactericidal drug that kills the offending organism by inhibiting protein synthesis. Rifampin is used either alone in the prevention of TB or in combination with other antitubercular drugs in its treatment. It is available in both oral and parenteral formulations and in combination with isoniazid (Rifamate). Rifampin is contraindicated in patients with known drug allergy to it or to any other rifamycin (i.e., rifabutin, rifapentine). The drug is a potent enzyme inducer and is associated with many drug interactions (see Table 41-4.) Rifampin may cause urine, saliva, tears, and sweat to be red-orange colored.

### Pharmacokinetics

| Route | Onset of Action | Peak Plasma Concentration | Elimination Half-life | Duration of Action |
|---|---|---|---|---|
| PO | Variable | 2-4 hr | 3.5 hr | Up to 24 hr |

## rifapentine

Rifapentine (Priftin) is a derivative of rifampin. It offers advantages over rifampin in that it has a much longer duration of action and possibly better efficacy. It has been shown to have greater antimycobacterial efficacy and macrophage penetration. Its accumulation into tissue macrophages allows it to work synergistically against bacterial cells that are ingested by the macrophage during phagocytosis ("cell eating"). Rifapentine is available only for oral use.

### Pharmacokinetics

| Route | Onset of Action | Peak Plasma Concentration | Elimination Half-life | Duration of Action |
|---|---|---|---|---|
| PO | Unknown | 5-6 hr | 13-17 hr | 1 to several days |

## streptomycin

Streptomycin is an aminoglycoside antibiotic currently available only in generic form. Introduced in 1944, it was the very first drug available that could effectively treat TB. Because of its toxicities, it is used most commonly today in combination drug regimens for the treatment of MDR-TB infections. Streptomycin is currently available only in injectable form. It is classified as a pregnancy category D drug and is usually not given to pregnant patients.

### Pharmacokinetics

| Route | Onset of Action | Peak Plasma Concentration | Elimination Half-life | Duration of Action |
|---|---|---|---|---|
| IM | Variable | 1-2 hr | 2-3 hr | Up to 24 hr |

# NURSING PROCESS

## ASSESSMENT

Before administering any of the *antitubercular drugs*, and to ensure the safe and effective use of these medications, obtain a thorough medical history, medication profile, and nursing history. Perform a complete head-to-toe physical assessment. Note any specific history of diagnoses or symptoms of TB. Determine the results of the patient's last purified protein derivative (PPD) or tuberculin skin test and the reaction at the intradermal injection site. Review the most recent chest radiograph and results. Assess the results of liver function studies (e.g., bilirubin level, liver enzyme levels) and kidney function studies (e.g., blood urea nitrogen [BUN], creatinine clearance). As noted earlier, major liver and/or renal dysfunction are contraindications. These values also provide comparative baseline data throughout therapy.

Because some drugs may lead to peripheral neuropathies, note baseline neurologic functioning prior to therapy. Assess hearing status, especially when streptomycin is to be used, because of its drug-related ototoxicity. A gross eye examination is important due to the drug-induced adverse effect of visual disturbances and optic neuritis with isoniazid, levofloxacin, and ofloxacin. Blindness may occur with the use of ethambutol.

Assessment of age is also important because the likelihood of adverse reactions and toxicity is increased in elderly patients due to age-related liver and kidney dysfunction. Additionally, the safety of these drugs in children 13 years of age and younger has not been established. Assess the patient's complete blood count (CBC) prior to giving isoniazid, streptomycin, and rifampin because of the potential for drug-related hematologic disorders. Renal function studies, such as creatinine clearance and BUN, may be ordered prior to therapy with streptomycin due to the nephrotoxicity associated with its use. Document uric acid baseline levels with use of pyrazinamide due to the drug-induced adverse effect of hyperuricemia and symptoms of gout. Analysis of sputum specimens is usually ordered as well, to aid in determining the appropriate drug regimen. Contraindications, cautions, and drug interactions have been discussed previously.

## NURSING DIAGNOSES

1. Ineffective family therapeutic regimen management related to poor compliance with antitubercular drug therapy and lack of knowledge about long-term therapies
2. Deficient knowledge related to the disease process and treatment protocol
3. Risk for injury related to noncompliance with the drug therapy regimen and an overall poor health status

## PLANNING

### GOALS

1. Patient experiences improved therapeutic regimen management and compliance.
   • Patient, family, and others in home environment understand the disease/infectious process, methods of spread and the need for the patient to remain on therapy, as prescribed.
2. Patient gains increased knowledge about antitubercular medication therapy and takes medication regularly and for the length of time prescribed.
3. Patient remains free from injury related to noncompliance to antitubercular drugs.

### OUTCOME CRITERIA

1. Patient shows improvement of disease state with adherence to the drug regimen, including a decrease in cough, fever, and sputum production; return of laboratory values to normal ranges; and no spread of infection to those in the environment/home setting.
   • Patient reports family support and lack of spread of infection (to those in the environment/home setting) while on antitubercular drug therapy.

2. Patient states rationale for antitubercular drug therapy as well as anticipated adverse effects.
   • Patient takes medication as ordered and regularly with acknowledgement of more effective therapy and prevention of complications, relapses, or recurrences.
3. Patient takes antitubercular drugs as ordered and routinely, with stated goal of improved health status.
   • Patient minimizes adverse effects by taking medication as prescribed.
   • Patient reports the following to the prescriber immediately: fever, increase in cough/sputum, hearing loss, severe numbness/tingling of extremities, and altered vision.

### CASE STUDY

*Antitubercular Drugs*

M.C., a 59-year-old homemaker, lives on the farm with her husband, R.C. Recently she has been experiencing weight loss, night sweats, and a chronic cough. When she is given the purified protein derivative (PPD) test, the result is positive, and a chest radiograph indicates areas of consolidation characteristic of tuberculosis. She is hospitalized, and special precautions are initiated to prevent the spread to others.

1. What is the next step in diagnosing the disease?

   The physician orders that M.C. be started on a four-drug regimen consisting of isoniazid, rifampin, pyrazinamide, and ethambutol until the final results of testing are back.
2. What is the purpose of the multiple drugs in this order?
3. What needs to be assessed before M.C. begins this medication therapy?

   Two weeks later, M.C. is discharged and given a prescription for Rifamate (combination of rifampin and isoniazid). In addition, she is given instructions to take pyridoxine (vitamin B₆).
4. M.C. asks, "Can't I just take my regular multivitamin? Why do I need this one?" What is the nurse's best answer?

For answers, see http://evolve.elsevier.com/Lilley.

## IMPLEMENTATION

Because drug therapy is the mainstay of treatment for TB and often lasts for up to 24 months, patient education is critical, with a special emphasis on adherence to the drug regimen. Provide simple, clear, and concise instructions to the patient, with appropriate use of audiovisuals and take-home information. Include the fact that multiple drugs are often used to improve cure rates in the education. The patient needs to be able to state an understanding of all instructions. Because many of the patients affected by tuberculosis may be from other countries and cultures, it is important to have a translator available.

All *antitubercular drugs* need to be taken exactly as ordered and at the same time every day. Consistent use and dosing around the clock are critical to maintaining steady blood levels and minimizing the chances of resistance to the drug therapy. Always emphasize the need for strict adherence to the therapeutic regimen in the instructions to the patient. Additionally, emphasize that the entire prescription must be finished over the prescribed time and as ordered by a prescriber, even if the patient is feeling better.

Although many drugs are given without food for maximum absorption, antitubercular drugs may need to be taken with food to minimize gastrointestinal upset. Constantly monitor for any signs and symptoms of liver dysfunction such as fatigue, jaundice, nausea, vomiting, dark urine, and anorexia. If these occur, contact the prescriber immediately. Also monitor kidney functioning (e.g., BUN, creatinine), and notify the prescriber if levels are altered. If vision changes occur (e.g., altered color perception, changes in visual acuity), in particular with ethambutol use, these changes must be reported immediately to the prescriber. Monitor uric acid levels during therapy, and advise the patient to report any symptoms of gout such as hot, painful, or swollen joints of the big toe, knee, or ankle. In addition, the prescriber must be notified if there are signs and symptoms of peripheral neuropathy (e.g., numbness, burning, and tingling of extremities). Pyridoxine (vitamin $B_6$) may be beneficial for isoniazid-induced peripheral neuropathy. If the prescriber has ordered collection of a sputum specimen to test for acid-fast bacilli, it is best to obtain the sample early in the morning. The most common order is for three consecutive morning specimens and a repeat specimen several weeks later. All drugs are to be taken as ordered and without any omission of doses for maximal therapeutic results.

Follow-up visits to the prescriber are important for monitoring therapeutic effects and watching for adverse effects and toxicity. If intravenous dosing of an antitubercular drug is ordered, use the appropriate diluent and infuse over the recommended time. Monitor the intravenous site every hour during the infusion for extravasation with possible tissue inflammation (e.g., redness, heat, and swelling at the intravenous site). See the Patient Teaching Tips for more information on antitubercular drugs.

Cultural considerations associated with these drugs include the fact that when patients have active TB, thorough patient teaching of all family members is required, and some family members may need prophylactic therapy for up to 1 full year. Because some cultural practices include living in close-knit communities or close living quarters, this teaching is critical to make sure the spread of this highly communicable disease is adequately prevented. All family members or those in close contact with the patient must receive the same thorough instructions about maintaining health while taking their medications appropriately, with emphasis on adherence.

## EVALUATION

Always document a patient's response, or lack of, to the therapeutic regimen. A therapeutic response to *antitubercular* therapy is manifested by a decrease in the symptoms of TB, such as cough and fever, and by weight gain. The results of laboratory studies (culture and sensitivity tests) and the chest radiographic findings will aid in the confirmation of resolution of the infection along with improved clinical status. Continually evaluate the meeting of goals and outcome criteria to confirm that the infection is being adequately treated and that the drug therapy is providing therapeutic relief without complications or toxicity and with minimal adverse effects. Also monitor patients for the occurrence of adverse reactions to *antitubercular* drugs, such as hearing loss (ototoxicity); nephrotoxicity; seizure activity; altered vision; blindness; extreme GI upset; fatigue; nausea; vomiting; fever; jaundice; numbness, tingling, or burning of the extremities; abdominal pain; and easy bruising. Because of the need for long-term therapy and possible treatment of family or those in close contact, further evaluation of these individuals is important during and after completion of therapy.

## ▮ PATIENT TEACHING TIPS

- Educate the patient to take medications exactly as ordered by the prescriber with attention to long-term therapy and strict adherence to the drug regimen. Treatment may be ineffective if drugs are taken intermittently or stopped once the patient begins to feel better.
- Stress the importance of follow-up appointments with the prescriber or health clinic so that the infection and therapeutic effectiveness may be closely monitored.
- Instruct the patient to avoid certain medications while taking antitubercular drugs, such as antacids, phenytoin, carbamazepine, beta blockers, benzodiazepines, oral anticoagulants, oral antidiabetic drugs, oral contraceptives, and theophylline. Inform the patient of all drug interactions prior to beginning therapy.
- Pyridoxine (vitamin $B_6$) may be indicated to prevent isoniazid-precipitated peripheral neuropathies and numbness, tingling, or burning of the extremities.
- Educate the patient taking isoniazid about the occurrence of the following adverse effects: numbness/tingling of extremities, abdominal pain, jaundice, and visual changes.

- Advise the patient taking rifampin to report the occurrence of the following adverse effects to the prescriber immediately: fever, nausea, vomiting, loss of appetite, jaundice, and/or unusual bleeding. These may indicate the possible occurrence of the adverse effects of hepatitis and/or various hematologic disorders.
- Encourage the patient to wear sunscreen and protective clothing during therapy to avoid ultraviolet light exposure. Drug-related photosensitivity reactions may be avoided by preventing exposure to the sun.
- Women taking oral contraceptives who are prescribed rifampin must be switched to another form of birth control. Oral contraceptives become ineffective when given with rifampin.
- During initial periods of the illness, instruct the patient to make every effort to wash hands and cover the mouth when coughing or sneezing. Emphasize methods of proper disposal of secretions.
- Emphasize the importance of proper rest, good sleep habits, adequate nutrition, and maintenance of general health. Advise the patient to always keep antitubercular drugs and other medications out of the reach of children.

## PATIENT TEACHING TIPS—cont'd

- Recommend wearing of a medical alert tag or bracelet with a list of allergies, prescription drugs, and medical conditions at all times. Written medical information must also be kept on the patient's person at all times.
- Instruct the patient to contact the prescriber immediately upon any increase in fatigue, cough, sputum production, bloody sputum, chest pain, unusual bleeding, or yellow skin and/or eyes.

- Patients taking rifampin, rifabutin, or rifapentine may experience red-orange-brown discoloration of the skin, sweat, tears, urine, feces, sputum, saliva, and tongue as an adverse effect of the drug. The discoloration reverses with discontinuation of the drug; however, contact lenses may be permanently stained.

## KEY POINTS

- All antitubercular drugs are to be taken exactly as prescribed. Emphasize adherence to the therapeutic regimen and long-term dosing combined with healthy living practices.
- Therapeutic effects include resolution of pulmonary and extrapulmonary MTB infections.
- Vitamin $B_6$ is needed to combat the peripheral neuropathy associated with isoniazid.

- Counsel women taking oral contraceptive therapy who are prescribed rifampin on other forms of birth control because of the ineffectiveness of oral contraception when rifampin is taken.
- Educate the patient about the importance of strict adherence to the drug regimen for improvement or cure of the condition. Provide instructions in written and oral formats about drug interactions and the need to avoid alcohol while taking any of these medications.

## NCLEX® EXAMINATION REVIEW QUESTIONS

1 The nurse is teaching a patient who is starting antitubercular therapy with rifampin. Which adverse effects would the nurse expect to see?
  a Headache and neck pain
  b Gynecomastia
  c Reddish brown urine
  d Numbness or tingling of extremities

2 During antitubercular therapy with isoniazid, the patient received another prescription for pyridoxine. Which statement by the nurse best explains the rationale for this second medication?
  a "This vitamin will help to improve your energy levels."
  b "This vitamin helps to prevent neurologic adverse effects."
  c "This vitamin works to protect your heart from toxic effects."
  d "This vitamin helps to reduce gastrointestinal adverse effects."

3 The nurse is counseling a woman who is beginning antitubercular therapy with rifampin. The patient also takes an oral contraceptive. Which statement by the nurse is most accurate regarding potential drug interactions?
  a "You will need to switch to another form of birth control while you are taking the rifampin."
  b "Your birth control pills will remain effective while you are taking the rifampin."
  c "You will need to take a stronger dose of birth control pills while you are on the rifampin."
  d "You will need to abstain from sexual intercourse while on the rifampin to avoid pregnancy."

4 When counseling a patient who has been newly diagnosed with TB, the nurse will make sure that the patient realizes that he or she is contagious
  a during all phases of the illness.
  b any time up to 18 months after therapy begins.
  c during the postictal phase of TB.
  d during the initial period of the illness and its diagnosis.

5 While monitoring a patient, the nurse knows that a therapeutic response to antitubercular drugs would be:
  a The patient states that he or she is feeling much better.
  b The patient's laboratory test results show a lower white blood cell count.
  c The patient reports a decrease in cough and night sweats.
  d There is a decrease in symptoms, along with improved chest radiograph and sputum culture results.

6 The nurse is monitoring for liver toxicity in a patient who has been receiving long-term isoniazid therapy. Manifestations of liver toxicity include: (Select all that apply.)
  a Orange discoloration of sweat and tears
  b Darkened urine
  c Dizziness
  d Fatigue
  e Visual disturbances
  f Jaundice

7 The order for isoniazid (INH) reads: "Give 5 mg/kg PO daily." The patient weighs 275 pounds. What is the amount per dose? Is this a safe dose?

For answers see http://evolve.elsevier.com/Lilley.

1. c, 2. b, 3. a, 4. d, 5. d, 6. b, d, f, 7. 625 mg/dose; no, maximum dose is 300 mg

For Critical Thinking and Prioritization Questions, see http://evolve.elsevier.com/Lilley.

# Antifungal Drugs

## ⊖volve WEBSITE

*http://evolve.elsevier.com/Lilley*

- Animations
- Answer Key—Textbook Case Studies
- Critical Thinking and Prioritization Questions

- Key Points—Downloadable
- Review Questions for the NCLEX® Examination
- Unfolding Case Studies

## OBJECTIVES

When you reach the end of this chapter, you will be able to do the following:

1 Identify the various antifungal drugs.
2 Describe the mechanisms of action, indications, contraindications, routes of administration, adverse and toxic effects, and drug interactions of the various antifungal drugs.

3 Develop a nursing care plan that includes all phases of the nursing process for patients receiving antifungal drugs.

## DRUG PROFILES

- **amphotericin B, p. 686**
  **caspofungin, p. 686**
- **fluconazole, p. 687**
  **nystatin, p. 688**

**terbinafine, p. 688**
**voriconazole, p. 688**

⸻

- *Key drug*

## KEY TERMS

Antimetabolite  A drug that is a either a receptor antagonist or that resembles a normal human metabolite and interferes with its function in the body, usually by competing for the metabolite's usual receptors or enzymes. (p. 684)

Dermatophyte  One of several fungi that are often found in soil and infect the skin, nails, or hair of humans. (p. 683)

Ergosterol  The main sterol in fungal membranes. (p. 684)

Fungi  A very large, diverse group of eukaryotic microorganisms that require an external carbon source and that form a plant structure known as a *thallus*. Fungi consist of yeasts and molds. (p. 683)

Molds  Multicellular fungi characterized by long, branching filaments called *hyphae,* which entwine to form a complex branched structure known as a *mycelium.* (p. 683)

Mycosis  The general term for any fungal infection. (p. 683)

Pathologic fungi  Fungi that cause mycoses. (p. 683)

Sterols  Substances in the cell membranes of fungi to which polyene antifungal drugs bind. (p. 684)

Yeasts  Single-celled fungi that reproduce by *budding.* (p. 683)

## ANATOMY, PHYSIOLOGY, AND PATHOPHYSIOLOGY OVERVIEW

### FUNGAL INFECTIONS

Fungi are a very large and diverse group of microorganisms that include all yeasts and molds. Yeasts are single-celled fungi that reproduce by budding (in which a daughter cell forms by pouching out of and breaking off from a mother cell). These organisms have common practical uses in the baking of breads and the preparation of alcoholic beverages. Molds are multicellular and are characterized by long, branching filaments. Some fungi are part of the normal flora of the skin, mouth, intestines, and vagina.

An infection caused by a fungus is called a mycosis. A variety of fungi can cause clinically significant infections or mycoses. These are called pathologic fungi, and the infections they cause range in severity from mild infections with annoying symptoms (e.g., athlete's foot) to systemic mycoses that can become life-threatening. These infections are acquired by various routes: the fungi can be ingested orally; can grow on or in the skin, hair, or nails; and, if the fungal spores are airborne, can be inhaled. There are four general types of mycotic infection: *systemic, cutaneous, subcutaneous,* and *superficial.* The latter three are infections of various layers of the *integumentary* system (skin, hair, or nails). Fungi that cause integumentary infections are known as dermatophytes, and such infections are known as *dermatomycoses.* The most severe systemic fungal infections generally affect people whose host immune defenses are compromised. Commonly, these are patients who have received organ transplants and are taking immunosuppressive drug therapy, cancer patients who are immunocompromised as a result of their chemotherapy, and patients with acquired immunodeficiency syndrome (AIDS). In addition, the use of antibiotics, antineoplastics, or immunosuppressants such as corticosteroids may result in colonization of *Candida albicans,* followed by the development of a systemic infection. When the infection affects the mouth, it is referred to as oral *candidiasis,* or thrush. It is common in newborns and immunocompromised patients. Vaginal candidiasis, commonly called a *yeast infection,* often affects pregnant women, women with diabetes mellitus, women taking antibiotics, and women taking oral contraceptives. The characteristics of some of the systemic, cutaneous, and superficial mycotic infections are summarized in Table 42-1.

## PHARMACOLOGY OVERVIEW

### ANTIFUNGAL DRUGS

Drugs used to treat fungal infections are called *antifungal drugs.* Systemic mycotic infections and some cutaneous or subcutaneous mycoses are treated with oral or parenteral drugs. Antifungals are a fairly small group of drugs. There are few such drugs because the fungi that cause these infections have proved to be very difficult to kill, and research into new and improved drugs has occurred at a slow pace. One difficulty is that often the chemical concentrations required for experimental drugs to be effective cannot be tolerated by human beings. The drugs that proved successful in the treatment of systemic mycoses as well

### TABLE 42-1 MYCOTIC INFECTIONS

| MYCOSIS | FUNGUS | ENDEMIC LOCATION | RESERVOIR | TRANSMISSION | PRIMARY TISSUE AFFECTED |
|---|---|---|---|---|---|
| **Systemic Infections** | | | | | |
| Aspergillosis | *Aspergillus* spp. | Universal | Soil | Inhalation | Lungs |
| Blastomycosis | *Blastomyces dermatitidis* | North America | Soil, animal droppings | Inhalation | Lungs |
| Candidiasis | *Candida albicans, glabrata, krusei, tropicalisis, parapsilosis* | Universal | Humans | Direct contact, overgrowth in response to treatment with antibiotic to which it is nonsusceptible | Blood, lungs |
| Coccidioidomycosis | *Coccidioides immitis* | Southwestern United States | Soil, dust | Inhalation | Lungs |
| Cryptococcosis | *Cryptococcus neoformans* | Universal | Soil, bird and chicken droppings | Inhalation | Lungs, meninges of brain |
| Histoplasmosis | *Histoplasma capsulatum* | Universal | | Inhalation | Lungs |
| **Superficial/Topical Infections** | | | | | |
| Candidiasis | *Candida albicans* | Universal | Humans | Direct contact, overgrowth in response to treatment with antibiotic to which it is nonsusceptible | Mucous membrane, skin; disseminated (may be systemic) |
| Dermatophytosis, tinea | *Epidermophyton* spp. *Microsporum* spp. *Trichophyton* spp. | Universal | Humans | Direct and indirect contact with infected persons | Scalp, skin (e.g., groin, feet) |
| Tinea versicolor | *Malassezia furfur* | Universal | Humans | Unknown* | Skin |

*spp.,* Species.

*\**Malassezia* spp. are a usual part of the normal human flora and appear to cause infection in only select individuals.

as severe dermatomycoses include amphotericin B, caspofungin, fluconazole, flucytosine, griseofulvin, itraconazole, ketoconazole, micafungin, nystatin, terbinafine, posaconazole, anidulafungin, and voriconazole. These drugs are the focus of this chapter.

Topical antifungal drugs are the most commonly used drugs in this class and are often administered without prescription for the treatment of dermatomycoses as well as oral and vaginal mycoses. Although topical drug therapy is usually sufficient for these conditions, systemic oral medications are sometimes used, especially for more severe or recurrent cases. Antifungal drugs available for topical use are discussed further in Chapter 56. There is also a single antifungal drug (natamycin) for ophthalmic use (see Chapter 57).

Two antifungal drugs, flucytosine and griseofulvin, are individually listed and are not specifically classified according to their chemical structures. The remaining drugs currently include four specific chemical classes: *polyenes* (amphotericin B and nystatin), *imidazoles* (ketoconazole), *triazoles* (fluconazole, itraconazole, voriconazole, and posaconazole), and the *echinocandins* (caspofungin, micafungin, and anidulafungin). The imidazoles and triazoles are sometimes referred to by the more general term *azole antifungals*. Also included in some of these classes are drugs for topical use.

## Mechanism of Action and Drug Effects

The mechanisms of action of the various antifungal drugs differ between drug subclasses. Flucytosine, also known as *5-fluorocytosine (5-FC)*, acts in much the same way as the antiviral drugs. It is an antimetabolite, which is a drug that disrupts critical cellular metabolic pathways of the fungal cell. Once inside a susceptible fungal cell, the drug is deaminated by the enzyme *cytosine deaminase* to 5-fluorouracil (5-FU). Because human cells do not have this enzyme, they are not harmed by this antimetabolite. Once the 5-FU is generated inside the fungal cell, it interferes with fungal deoxyribonucleic acid (DNA) synthesis, which results in both inhibition of cell growth and reproduction, and cell death. 5-FU is also available as an antineoplastic (anticancer) drug and is discussed in more detail in Chapter 45.

Griseofulvin, like flucytosine, is one of the older types of antifungal drugs. It works by preventing susceptible fungi from reproducing. It enters the fungal cell through an energy-dependent transport system and inhibits fungal mitosis (cell division) by binding to key structures known as *microtubules*. It has also been proposed that griseofulvin causes the production of defective DNA, which is then unable to replicate. Although both griseofulvin and flucytosine are still currently available in the U.S. market, their use has been largely replaced by the newer antifungal drug classes.

The polyenes (amphotericin B and nystatin) act by binding to sterols in the cell membranes of fungi. The main sterol in fungal membranes is ergosterol. Human cell membranes have cholesterol instead of ergosterol. Because polyene antifungals have a strong chemical affinity for ergosterol instead of cholesterol, they do not bind to human cell membranes and therefore do not kill human cells. Once the polyene drug molecule binds to the ergosterol, a channel forms in the fungal cell membrane

that allows potassium and magnesium ions to leak out of the fungal cell. This loss of ions causes fungal cellular metabolism to be altered, which leads to death of the cell.

Imidazoles and triazoles (ketoconazole, fluconazole, itraconazole, voriconazole, and posaconazole) act as either fungistatic or fungicidal drugs, depending on their concentration in the fungus. They are most effective in combating rapidly growing fungi and work by inhibiting fungal cell cytochrome P-450 enzymes. These enzymes are needed to produce ergosterol. The allylamine terbinafine is believed to act by a similar mechanism. When the production of ergosterol is inhibited, other sterols called *methylsterols* are produced instead, which results in a defect similar to that caused by the polyene antifungals, namely, a leaky cell membrane that allows needed electrolytes to escape. The fungal cells die because they cannot carry on cellular metabolism.

The echinocandins (caspofungin, micafungin, and anidulafungin) act by preventing the synthesis of glucans, essential components of fungal cell walls that are not present in mammalian cells. This also contributes to fungal cell death. Some of the fungi that are susceptible to these drugs are the pathogens involved in the various mycoses listed in Box 42-1.

## Indications

Indications for the use of the various antifungal drugs are specific to the drug. The adverse effects of the newer antifungals are fewer and less serious than those of the older drugs. However, the drug of choice for the treatment of many severe systemic fungal infections remains one of the oldest antifungals, amphotericin B, which does have major adverse effects. Amphotericin B is effective against a wide range of fungi. It is sometimes given with flucytosine in the treatment of *Candida* and cryptococcal infections because of the synergy of the two drugs. Amphotericin B is also effective for treating aspergillosis, blastomycosis, candidiasis, coccidioidomycosis, cryptococcosis, fungal endocarditis, histoplasmosis, zygomycosis, fungal septicemia, and many other systemic fungal infections. The activity of nystatin is similar to that of amphotericin B, but its usefulness is limited because of its toxic effects when given in the dosages required to accomplish

| BOX 42-1 | FUNGAL SPECIES SUSCEPTIBLE TO CURRENT ANTIFUNGAL DRUGS |
|---|---|
| **Superficial/Topical Mycoses** | **Systemic Mycoses** |
| *Epidermophyton* spp. | *Absidia* spp. |
| *Malassezia furfur* (causes tinea versicolor) | *Aspergillus* spp. |
| | *Basidiobolus* spp. |
| *Microsporum* spp. | *Blastomyces dermatitidis* |
| *Sporothrix* spp. | *Candida* spp. |
| *Trichophyton* spp. | *Coccidioides immitis* |
| | *Conidiobolus* spp. |
| | *Cryptococcus neoformans* |
| | *Histoplasma capsulatum* |
| | *Mucor* spp. |
| | *Rhizopus* spp. |
| | *Scedosporium apiospermum* spp. |

the same antifungal actions as amphotericin B. It is also not available in parenteral form. Nystatin is most commonly used to treat oropharyngeal candidiasis, commonly referred to as *thrush*.

Fluconazole and itraconazole are synthetic azole antifungals. Fluconazole can pass into the cerebrospinal fluid (CSF) and inhibit the growth of cryptococcal fungi. This makes it effective in the treatment of cryptococcal meningitis. Both drugs are active against oropharyngeal and esophageal *Candida* infections. Itraconazole is capable of only poor CSF penetration but can be widely distributed throughout other areas of the body. It is indicated for the treatment of fungal infections in immunocompromised and nonimmunocompromised patients with disseminated candidiasis, histoplasmosis, blastomycosis, and aspergillosis. Ketoconazole, a systemic imidazole, inhibits many dermatophytes and fungi that cause systemic mycoses, but it is not active against *Aspergillus* organisms or *Phycomycetes* (common molds) such as *Mucor* species (spp.). Fortunately, the newest triazole antifungal drug, voriconazole, does have activity against some of these more tenacious fungi, including *Aspergillus* spp. causing invasive infection, *Scedosporium* spp., and *Fusarium* spp.

Of the azole antifungals, fluconazole is the most effective for combating infections with *Candida, Cryptococcus, Blastomyces,* and *Histoplasma* organisms. Fluconazole is very effective against vaginal candidiasis. One dose of 150 mg of fluconazole can cure many vaginal candidal infections.

Flucytosine inhibits *Cryptococcus neoformans, C. albicans,* and many *Cladosporium* and *Phialophora* spp. It does not inhibit *Aspergillus, Sporothrix, Blastomyces,* or *Histoplasma* spp. or *Coccidioides immitis.*

Griseofulvin inhibits dermatophytes of *Microsporum, Trichophyton,* and *Epidermophyton* spp. It has no effect on filamentous fungi such as *Aspergillus,* yeasts such as *Candida* spp., or dimorphic species such as *Histoplasma.* Terbinafine is a synthetic allylamine derivative used in a systemic oral form for treatment of onychomycoses—fungal infections of the fingernails or toenails. Topical forms of terbinafine are also used for various skin infections (see Chapter 56).

## Contraindications

Drug allergy, liver failure, kidney failure, and porphyria (for griseofulvin) are the most common contraindications for antifungal drugs. Itraconazole should not be used to treat onychomycoses in patients with severe cardiac problems. Voriconazole can cause fetal harm in pregnant women.

## Adverse Effects

The major adverse effects caused by antifungal drugs are encountered most commonly in conjunction with amphotericin B treatment. Drug interactions and hepatotoxicity are the primary concerns in patients receiving other antifungal drugs, but the intravenous administration of amphotericin B is associated with a multitude of adverse effects. The most common and problematic of the adverse effects of the various antifungal drugs are listed in Table 42-2. With amphotericin B treatment in particular, prescribers commonly order various premedications (including antiemetics, antihistamines, antipyretics, and corticosteroids) to prevent or minimize infusion-related reactions. The likelihood of such reactions can also be reduced by using longer-than-average drug infusion times (i.e., 2 to 6 hours) for this particular drug.

## Interactions

There are many important drug interactions associated antifungal drugs, some of which can be life-threatening. A common underlying source of the problem is that many of the antifungal drugs, as well as other drugs, are metabolized by the *cytochrome P-450 enzyme system.* The result of the coadministration of two drugs that are both broken down by this system is that they compete for the limited amount of enzymes, and one of the drugs ends up accumulating. Key drug interactions for the systemic antifungal drugs are summarized in Table 42-3.

## TABLE 42-2   SELECTED ANTIFUNGAL DRUGS: COMMON ADVERSE EFFECTS AND CAUTIONS

| BODY SYSTEM | ADVERSE EFFECTS | CAUTIONS |
|---|---|---|
| **Amphotericin B (Sy)** | | |
| Cardiovascular | Cardiac dysrhythmias | Recheck dosage and type of amphotericin B being administered |
| Central nervous | Neurotoxicity; tinnitus; visual disturbances; hand or feet numbness, tingling, or pain; convulsions | |
| Renal | Renal toxicity, potassium loss, hypomagnesemia | |
| Pulmonary | Pulmonary infiltrates | |
| Other (infusion related) | Fever, chills, headache, malaise, nausea, occasional hypotension, gastrointestinal upset, anemia | |
| **Fluconazole (Sy)** | | |
| Gastrointestinal | Nausea, vomiting, diarrhea, stomach pain | Use with caution in patients with renal or hepatic dysfunction |
| Other | Increased liver enzyme levels, dizziness | |
| **Caspofungin (Sy)** | | |
| Central nervous | Fever, chills, headache | Adjust dose for patients with hepatic dysfunction |
| Cardiovascular | Hypotension, peripheral edema, tachycardia | |
| Gastrointestinal | Nausea, vomiting, diarrhea, hepatotoxicity | |
| Hematologic | Decreased hemoglobin and hematocrit, leukopenia, anemia | |
| Integumentary | Rash, facial edema, itching | |

*Continued*

## TABLE 42-2    SELECTED ANTIFUNGAL DRUGS: COMMON ADVERSE EFFECTS AND CAUTIONS—cont'd

| BODY SYSTEM | ADVERSE EFFECTS | CAUTIONS |
|---|---|---|
| **Voriconazole (Sy)** | | |
| Central nervous | Hallucinations | |
| Gastrointestinal | Nausea, vomiting | |
| Hepatic | Increased liver enzyme levels | |
| Integumentary | Rash | |
| Other | Photophobia, hypokalemia | |
| **Nystatin (T)** | | |
| Gastrointestinal | Nausea, vomiting, diarrhea, cramps | Local irritation may occur |
| Integumentary | Rash, urticaria | |
| **Terbinafine (Sy, T)** | | |
| Central nervous | Headache, dizziness | Rarely causes irritation |
| Gastrointestinal | Nausea, vomiting, diarrhea | |
| Integumentary | Rash, pruritus | |
| Other | Alopecia, fatigue | |

*Sy*, Systemic; *T*, topical.

## TABLE 42-3    ANTIFUNGAL DRUGS: DRUG INTERACTIONS

| DRUG | POSSIBLE EFFECTS |
|---|---|
| **Amphotericin B** | |
| Digitalis glycosides | Amphotericin B–induced hypokalemia may increase the potential for digitalis toxicity |
| Nephrotoxic drug | Additive nephrotoxicity |
| Thiazide diuretics | Severe hypokalemia or decreased adrenal cortex response to corticotrophin |
| **Fluconazole, itraconazole** | |
| cyclosporine, phenytoin, sirolimus | Increased plasma concentrations of both drugs |
| Oral anticoagulants | Increased effects of anticoagulants |
| Oral hypoglycemics | Reduced metabolism of hypoglycemic drugs |
| Statins | Reduced metabolism of statins, increased toxicity |
| **Voriconazole** | |
| quinidine | Prolongation of QT interval on electrocardiogram |

## Dosages

For the dosage information on selected antifungal drugs, see the table on p. 687.

## DRUG PROFILES

### ◆ amphotericin B

Amphotericin B (Fungizone) remains one of the drugs of choice for the treatment of severe systemic mycoses. The main drawback of amphotericin B therapy is that the drug causes many adverse effects. Almost all patients given the drug intravenously experience fever, chills, hypotension, tachycardia, malaise, muscle and joint pain, anorexia, nausea and vomiting, and headache. For this reason, pretreatment with antipyretics, antihistamines, antiemetics, and coricosteroids is common to decrease the severity of the infusion-related reaction.

Lipid formulations of amphotericin B were developed in an attempt to decrease the incidence of its adverse effects and increase its efficacy. There are currently three lipid preparations of amphotericin B: amphotericin B lipid complex (Abelcet), amphotericin B cholesteryl complex (Amphotec), and liposomal amphotericin B (AmBisome). These lipid dosage forms have a much higher cost than conventional amphotericin B and for this reason are often used only when patients are intolerant of or have an infection refractory to nonlipid amphotericin B.

Amphotericin B is contraindicated in patients who have a known hypersensitivity to it and in those with severe bone marrow suppression or renal impairment. However, patients who have life-threatening fungal infections may still be treated with this drug if culture results indicate that no other drug will kill the causative organism. The drug is available in injectable, oral, and topical preparations. Often a 1-mg test dose is given over 20 to 30 minutes to see if the patient will tolerate the drug. Amphotericin has been used as a local irrigant (in bladder irrigation) for the treatment of candidal cystitis and has been used intrapleurally and intraperitoneally for the treatment of fungal infections in those body cavities.

### Pharmacokinetics

| Route | Onset of Action | Peak Plasma Concentration | Elimination Half-life | Duration of Action |
|---|---|---|---|---|
| IV | Variable | 1 hr | 1-15 days | 18-24 hr |

### caspofungin

Caspofungin (Cancidas) was the first echinocandin antifungal drug, approved in 2001. It is used for treatment of severe *Aspergillus* infection (invasive aspergillosis) in patients who are intolerant of or have infections refractory to other drugs. Caspofungin doses need to be reduced in patients with impaired liver function. The drug is available only in injectable form. In 2005, a second echinocandin known as micafungin (Mycamine) was approved, and in 2007, a third, anidulafungin (Eraxis), was approved.

### Pharmacokinetics

| Route | Onset of Action | Peak Plasma Concentration | Elimination Half-life | Duration of Action |
|---|---|---|---|---|
| IV | Unknown | 1 hr | 9-50 hr | Unknown |

## DOSAGES

### *Selected Antifungal Drugs*

| DRUG (PREGNANCY CATEGORY) | PHARMACOLOGIC CLASS | USUAL DOSAGE RANGE | INDICATIONS |
|---|---|---|---|
| ♦ amphotericin B (Amphocin, Fungizone) (B) | Polyene antifungal | IV: Initial daily dose, 0.25 mg/kg; titrate up to 0.5-1.5 mg/kg/day | Systemic infections with broad spectrum of fungi |
| | | Topical: apply cream or lotion 2-4 times daily | Topical candidiasis |
| amphotericin B lipid complex; dosages vary with product as follows: | Polyene antifungal | **Adult and pediatric** | Systemic fungal infections |
| Abelcet (B) | | IV: 5 mg/kg once daily, infused at 2.5 mg/kg/hr | |
| Amphotec (B) | | IV: 3-4 mg/kg/day, infused at 1 mg/kg/hr | |
| AmBisome (B) | | IV: 3-5 mg/kg/day, infused over 1-2 hr | |
| caspofungin (Cancidas) (C) | Echinocandin antifungal | **Adult only** IV: 70 mg loading dose on day 1, followed by 50 mg/day thereafter; infuse doses over 1 hr | Invasive aspergillosis in patients who do not tolerate or respond to other drugs |
| ♦ fluconazole (Diflucan) (C) | Synthetic triazole antifungal | **Adult** PO: 150 mg in a single dose | Vaginal candidiasis |
| | | **Adult** IV/PO: 100-400 mg/day × 2-5 wk (dose and duration dependent on severity of infection) | Oropharyngeal and esophageal candidiasis, systemic candidiasis |
| | | **Pediatric** IV/PO: 3-12 mg/kg, same guidelines as for adult | |
| | | **Adult** IV/PO: 200-400 mg/day × 10-12 wk after negative CSF culture results | Cryptococcal meningitis |
| | | **Pediatric** IV/PO: 3-12 mg/kg × 10-12 wk after negative CSF culture results | |
| nystatin (Nilstat, Mycostatin, Nystex) (C) | Polyene antifungal | **Infant** PO: 200,000 units (2 mL) oral suspension in oral cavity 4 times daily | Oral candidiasis |
| | | **Adult and pediatric** PO: 400,000-600,000 units (4-6 mL) oral suspension in oral cavity 4 times daily | |
| | | **Adult and pediatric** PO (troche): 200,000-400,000 units (1-2 troches dissolved in mouth) 4-5 times daily | |
| | | **Adult only** PO (tab): 500,000-1,000,000 units (1-2 tabs) 3 times daily | Intestinal candidiasis |
| | | Topical (cream, lotion, or powder): apply 2-3 times daily | Topical candidiasis |
| terbinafine (Lamisil) (B) | Synthetic allylamine antifungal | **Adult only** PO: 250 mg/day × 6 wk (fingernail) or × 12 wk (toenail) | Onychomycosis (fungal infection of fingernail or toenail) |
| | | Topical cream or solution: Apply twice daily to affected area × 1-4 wk | Athlete's foot *(tinea pedis)*, jock itch *(tinea cruris)*, or ringworm *(tinea corporis)* |
| voriconazole (Vfend) (D) | Synthetic triazole antifungal | **Adult only** PO: 200 mg q12h | Invasive aspergillosis; other major fungal infections in patients who do not tolerate or respond to other antifungal drugs |
| | | IV: 6 mg/kg q12h × 2 doses followed by 4 mg/kg q12h | |

*CSF*, Cerebrospinal fluid; *IV*, intravenous; *PO*, oral.

### ♦ fluconazole

Fluconazole (Diflucan) has proved to be a significant improvement in the area of antifungal treatment. It has a much better adverse effect profile than that of amphotericin B, and it also has excellent coverage against many fungi. In fact, it is often preferred to amphotericin B because of these qualities. Oral fluconazole has excellent bioavailability, which means that almost the entire dose administered is absorbed into the circulation. Fluconazole is available in both oral and injectable forms.

**Pharmacokinetics**

| Route | Onset of Action | Peak Plasma Concentration | Elimination Half-life | Duration of Action |
|---|---|---|---|---|
| PO | 1 hr | 1-2 hr | 22-30 hr | Variable |

### nystatin

Nystatin (Mycostatin) is a polyene antifungal drug that is often applied topically for the treatment of candidal diaper rash, taken orally as prophylaxis against candidal infections during periods of neutropenia in patients receiving immunosuppressive therapy, and used for the treatment of oral and vaginal candidiasis. It is not available in a parenteral form but does come in several oral and topical formulations.

### Pharmacokinetics

| Route | Onset of Action | Peak Plasma Concentration | Elimination Half-life | Duration of Action |
|---|---|---|---|---|
| PO | 24 hr | 2 hr | Unknown | Unknown |

### terbinafine

Terbinafine (Lamisil) is classified as an allylamine antifungal drug and is currently the only drug in its class. It is available in a topical cream, gel, and spray for treating superficial dermatologic infections, including *tinea pedis* (athlete's foot), *tinea cruris* (jock itch), and *tinea corporis* (ringworm). A tablet form is also available for systemic use and is used primarily to treat onychomycoses of the fingernails or toenails.

### Pharmacokinetics

| Route | Onset of Action | Peak Plasma Concentration | Elimination Half-life | Duration of Action |
|---|---|---|---|---|
| PO | Unknown | 1-2 hr | 22-26 hr | Unknown |

### voriconazole

Voriconazole (Vfend) is used for treating severe fungal infections caused by *Aspergillus* spp. (invasive aspergillosis). It is also used for a variety of other severe fungal infections, such as those caused by *Scedosporium* and *Fusarium* spp. Voriconazole is contraindicated in patients who have a known drug allergy to it and in patients who are taking certain other drugs metabolized by the cytochrome P-450 enzyme 3A4 (e.g., quinidine) because of the risk for induction of serious cardiac dysrhythmias. It is also the only antifungal drug contraindicated in pregnancy. The drug is available in oral and injectable forms.

### Pharmacokinetics

| Route | Onset of Action | Peak Plasma Concentration | Elimination Half-life | Duration of Action |
|---|---|---|---|---|
| PO | Unknown | 1-2 hr | Variable | Unknown |

## NURSING PROCESS

## ASSESSMENT

Although topical dosage forms are discussed in detail in Chapter 56, it is important to discuss all *antifungal* dosage forms and their related nursing process. Before initiation of therapy with antifungals, assess and document vital signs, weight, hemoglobin (Hgb) level, hematocrit (Hct), red blood cell (RBC) counts, complete blood counts (CBCs) with differential, liver and renal function test results and culture and sensitivity test results.

Before administering amphotericin B (or any other antifungal drug), identify any contraindications, cautions, and drug interactions (see Tables 42-2 and 42-3). Baseline renal function studies are generally ordered as well as hepatic function tests due to adverse effects of nephrotoxicity and hepatotoxicity. Avoid any concurrent administration of nephrotoxic drugs if at all possible. There is a risk for severe adverse reactions (e.g., cardiac dysrhythmias, headache, chills, malaise, nausea, hypotension, anemia, GI upset) with intravenous amphotericin B administration. Perform an assessment of any special premedication orders for antiemetics, antihistamines, antipyretics, and/or antiinflammatory drugs prior to giving amphotericin B. Bone marrow suppression is another contraindication to the use of amphotericin B.

Caspofungin use requires careful assessment of blood pressure, pulse rate, liver function, RBC counts, and WBC counts due to potential drug-induced adverse effects of hypotension, tachycardia, hepatotoxicity, decreased Hgb and Hct, and leukopenia. Fluconazole requires a close assessment of preexisting GI problems and of renal and/or hepatic functioning due to drug-induced adverse effects impacting these systems. Nystatin lozenges are generally not used in children younger than 5 years of age. See Tables 42-2 and 42-3 for more information about specific adverse effects and drug interactions for all antifungals.

## NURSING DIAGNOSES

1. Acute pain related to symptoms of the infectious process
2. Deficient knowledge related to lack of information and experience with the antifungal drug therapy
3. Risk for injury related to adverse effects of the medication treatment regimen

## CASE STUDY

### *Amphotericin B*

A.B., a 63-year-old retired delivery driver, has been hospitalized for pneumonia. Since his admission, he has been diagnosed with a severe systemic fungal infection, and an amphotericin B infusion will be started. Before beginning this medication, the nurse assesses the results of his renal and liver function laboratory studies, as well as his complete blood count. The patency of the intravenous line is verified, and the nurse gives A.B. a dose of acetaminophen (Tylenol) as well as an antihistamine before starting the infusion.

1. What is the purpose of the acetaminophen and antihistamine?
2. The nurse stays with the patient for the first 15 minutes of the infusion and monitors A.B.'s vital signs. Explain the rationale for these nursing actions.
3. One hour after the infusion is completed, A.B. calls the nurse and says that he feels as if he may vomit and has chills, yet feels hot at the same time. What does the nurse need to do next?
4. A.B. continues to feel "terrible" the rest of the night, and the next morning his physician, Dr. F., changes the order to liposomal amphotericin B (AmBisome). Why did the physician continue an antifungal medication? What is the rationale behind this order change?

For answers, see http://evolve.elsevier.com/Lilley.

# PLANNING

## GOALS

1. Patient has minimal to no pain after therapy has been initiated.
2. Patient gains increased knowledge about the antifungal drug, its use, and its adverse effects.
3. Patient experiences minimal to no injury to self as related to the adverse effects of antifungal therapy.

## OUTCOME CRITERIA

1. Patient is free of pain associated with the fungal infection once therapy is initiated.
   - Patient's fever and discomfort associated with the infection decreases with therapy.
   - Patient experiences improved health status/energy and well being.
2. Patient demonstrates adequate knowledge about medication regimen by following directions about when and how to take the antifungal drug.
   - Patient experiences minimal to no adverse effects and reports to the prescriber any nausea, vomiting, or gastrointestinal upset if they become unmanageable.
   - Patient remains compliant with the medication regimen, without skipping doses while experiencing relief from the infection, and experiences a return to normal vital signs and negative findings on culture and sensitivity tests after the full course of therapy.
   - Patient experiences improved appetite, energy level, and physical strength and stamina after taking the antifungal drugs for the prescribed period.
3. Patient experiences minimal to no injury to self and is able to manage adverse effects or contact prescriber if they become problematic.
   - Patient takes medication as prescribed.
   - Patient returns to the prescriber regularly as recommended by the prescriber for constant monitoring of the infection and of drug therapy with various blood tests (e.g., CBC with differential, RBC count, hemoglobin level, hematocrit, renal and liver function tests).

# IMPLEMENTATION

The nursing interventions appropriate for patients receiving *antifungal* drugs vary depending on the particular drug. With intravenous amphotericin B, do not administer solutions that are cloudy or have precipitates. Use of an intravenous infusion pump is recommended. Once the intravenous infusion has begun, monitor vital signs every 15 minutes, or as needed, to assess for adverse reactions such as cardiac dysrhythmias, visual disturbances, paresthesias (numbness or tingling of the hands or feet), respiratory difficulty, pain, fever, chills, and nausea (see Table 42-2 for a listing of adverse effects). If a severe reaction occurs (e.g., exacerbation of adverse effects and/or a decline in vital signs), discontinue the infusion while continuing to closely monitor the patient. Contact the prescriber immediately. Monitor the intravenous site for signs of phlebitis (e.g., heat, pain, and redness over the vein), as per hospital policy. Continually monitor all laboratory values during therapy (see earlier discussion). Document weight frequently, as indicated, with long-term or at-home therapy. A gain of 2 pounds or more in a 24-hour period or 5 pounds or more in 1 week may indicate possible medication-induced renal damage and the need for prompt medical attention. Follow manufacturer guidelines and the prescriber's order for specific solutions and rates of intravenous administration. See the Patient Teaching Tips for further information.

Only use clear solutions of caspofungin and dilute doses with the recommended amount of normal saline. Liver toxicity may occur, so monitor liver function tests during therapy as ordered. In addition, constantly monitor the patient for the occurrence of tachycardia, hypotension, fever, chills, or headache. Hemoglobin and hematocrit levels must also be monitored frequently because of the possibility of drug-induced anemias. Fluconazole may be given either orally or intravenously, with intravenous dosage forms used if there is a specific indication or if the oral dosage forms are poorly tolerated. Only administer intravenous dosage forms if solution is clear, and do not add other medications. If itching or a rash occurs, stop the infusion, take vital signs, and contact the prescriber immediately. Nystatin may be given orally in the form of lozenges or troches, which the patient should slowly and completely dissolve in the mouth for optimal effects; these should not be chewed or swallowed whole. If a suspension is used, instruct the patient to swish the medication solution thoroughly in the mouth for as long as possible before swallowing. Terbinafine may be given orally or topically. Local skin reactions that need to be reported include blistering, itching, oozing, redness, and swelling. Oral doses of voriconazole are to be given 1 hour before or 1 hour after a meal. Intravenous doses may be diluted with 5% dextrose in water or normal saline, with the accurate dose infused over the recommended time. Monitor visual acuity when this drug is given (especially if ordered for longer than 28 days), and report any visual changes to the prescriber.

# EVALUATION

The therapeutic effects of *antifungals* include improvement and eventual resolution of the signs and symptoms of the fungal infection if the patient has remained totally adherent to the therapy regimen. Improved energy levels and improvement in overall sense of well-being with a normal temperature and other vital sign values also indicate a therapeutic response. Specific adverse effects for which to monitor in patients receiving these drugs are listed in Table 42-2. Evaluate goals and outcome criteria in the context of the nursing care plan.

## PATIENT TEACHING TIPS

- Instruct female patients taking antifungal medications for the treatment of vaginal infection to abstain from sexual intercourse until the treatment is completed and the infection is resolved, and advise patients to continue to take the medication even if actively menstruating. Tell patients to notify the prescriber if symptoms persist after treatment is completed.
- Some patients receiving amphotericin B may need long-term treatment (i.e., over weeks to months). If so, possible adverse effects include tinnitus, blurred vision, burning and itching at the infusion site, headache, rash, fever, chills, hypokalemia, gastrointestinal upset, and various anemias.
- Instruct patients taking caspofungin to immediately report to the prescriber any problems with shortness of breath, itching, facial swelling, and/or a rash.

- Encourage the patient to practice good hand washing technique.
- Instruct the patient on the proper dosing instructions for nystatin (e.g., for oral solutions, swish and swallow). If vaginal troches are prescribed, use the appropriate applicator with a gloved hand and insert high into the vagina, followed by thorough hand washing (see Chapter 9).
- Encourage the patient to keep affected body areas clean and dry and to wear light and cool clothing. Avoid contact of the topical dosage form with the eyes, mouth, nose, or other mucous membranes.
- Voriconazole is to be taken 1 hour before or 1 hour after meals. Warn the patient about the adverse effect of photophobia with use of this drug.

## KEY POINTS

- Fungi are a very large and diverse group of microorganisms and consist of yeasts and molds. Yeasts are single-celled fungi that may be harmful (e.g., causing infections) or helpful (e.g., aiding in baking or brewing beer). Molds are multicellular and are characterized by long, branching filaments called *hyphae.*
- Candidiasis is an opportunistic fungal infection caused by *C. albicans* and occurs in patients taking broad-spectrum antibiotics, antineoplastics, or immunosuppressants, as well as in immunocompromised persons. When candidiasis occurs in the mouth, it is commonly called *oral candidiasis* or *thrush.* Oral candidiasis is more commonly seen in newborns or immunocompromised persons.
- Vaginal candidiasis is a yeast infection and occurs most commonly in individuals with diabetes mellitus, women taking oral contraceptives, and pregnant women.

- Antifungals may be administered either systemically or topically. Some of the most common systemic antifungals are amphotericin B and fluconazole; an example of a topical antifungal is nystatin.
- Before administering antifungals, thoroughly assess for allergies as well as interactions with other drugs patients are taking, including prescription drugs, over-the-counter drugs, and herbals.
- Amphotericin B must be properly diluted according to manufacturer guidelines and administered using an intravenous infusion pump. Tissue extravasation of fluconazole at the intravenous infusion site leads to tissue necrosis; therefore, check the site hourly and document the assessment.

## NCLEX® EXAMINATION REVIEW QUESTIONS

1 The nurse is assessing a patient who is about to receive antifungal drug therapy. Which problem would be of most concern?
   a Endocrine disease
   b Hepatic disease
   c Cardiac disease
   d Pulmonary disease

2 While monitoring a patient who is receiving intravenous amphotericin B, the nurse expects to see which adverse effect(s)?
   a Hypertension
   b Bradycardia
   c Fever and chills
   d Diarrhea and stomach cramps

3 When administering antifungal drug therapy, the nurse knows that an issue that contributes to many of the drug interactions with antifungals is the patient's
   a history of cardiac disease.
   b history of gallbladder surgery.
   c ethnic background.
   d cytochrome P-450 enzyme system.

4 During an infusion of amphotericin B, the nurse knows that which administration technique may be used to minimize infusion-related adverse effects?
   a Forcing of fluids during the infusion
   b Infusing the medication quickly
   c Infusing the medication over a longer period of time
   d Stopping the infusion for 2 hours after half of the bag has infused, then resuming 1 hour later

5 When teaching a patient who is taking nystatin lozenges for oral candidiasis, which instruction by the nurse is correct?
  a "Chew the lozenge carefully before swallowing."
  b "Dissolve the lozenge slowly and completely in your mouth."
  c "Dissolve the lozenge until it is half the original size, and then swallow it."
  d "These lozenges need to be swallowed whole with a glass of water."
6 When monitoring a patient who is receiving caspofungin, the nurse will look for which serious adverse effects? (Select all that apply.)
  a Blood dyscrasias
  b Hypotension
  c Pulmonary infiltrates
  d Tinnitus
  e Hepatotoxicity

7 The order reads, "Give nystatin (Mycostatin) suspension, 500,000 units by mouth (swish and swallow) 4 times a day for 1 week." The medication is available in a suspension of 100,000 units per mL. How many milliliters will the nurse give per dose?

1. b, 2. c, 3. d, 4. c, 5. b, 6. a, b, e, 7. 5 mL.

For Critical Thinking and Prioritization Questions, see http://evolve.elsevier.com/Lilley.

# CHAPTER

# 43

# Antimalarial, Antiprotozoal, and Anthelmintic Drugs

## evolve WEBSITE

*http://evolve.elsevier.com/Lilley*

- Animations
- Answer Key—Textbook Case Studies
- Critical Thinking and Prioritization Questions

- Key Points—Downloadable
- Review Questions for the NCLEX® Examination
- Unfolding Case Studies

## OBJECTIVES

When you reach the end of this chapter, you will be able to do the following:

1. Briefly discuss the infectious process associated with malaria, other protozoal infections, and helminth infections.
2. Compare the signs and symptoms of malarial, other protozoal, and helminthic infection processes.
3. Identify the more commonly used antimalarial, antiprotozoal, and anthelmintic drugs.

4. Discuss the mechanisms of action, indications, cautions, contraindications, adverse effects, dosages, drug interactions, and routes of administration of the antimalarial, antiprotozoal, and anthelmintic drugs.
5. Develop a nursing care plan that includes all phases of the nursing process for patients receiving antimalarial, antiprotozoal, or anthelmintic drugs.

## DRUG PROFILES

atovaquone, p. 700
♦ chloroquine and hydroxychloroquine, p. 696
♦ mefloquine, p. 697
♦ metronidazole, p. 700
pentamidine, p. 700
praziquantel, p. 702

♦ primaquine, p. 697
pyrantel, p. 702
pyrimethamine, p. 697

_____

♦ *Key drug*

## KEY TERMS

**Anthelmintic** A drug that destroys or prevents the development of parasitic worm (helminthic) infections. Also called *antihelmintic* or *vermicide;* notice that the terms for the drug categories are spelled with only one *h,* which appears in the second syllable of the term, whereas the term for worm infection *(helminthic)* is spelled with two *h*'s, appearing in both the first and third syllables of the term. (p. 700)

**Antimalarial drugs** Drugs that destroy or prevent the development of the malaria parasite *(Plasmodium* sp.) in humans. Antimalarial drugs are a subset of the broader category of antiprotozoal drugs. (p. 694)
**Antiprotozoal** A drug that destroys or prevents the development of protozoans in humans. (p. 698)
**Helminthic infections** Parasitic worm infections. (p. 700)

**KEY TERMS—cont'd**

**Malaria** A widespread protozoal infectious disease caused by four species of the genus *Plasmodium*. (p. 693)

**Parasite** Any organism that feeds on another living organism (known as a *host*) in a way that results in varying degrees of harm to the host organism. (p. 693)

**Parasitic protozoans** Harmful protozoans that live on or in humans or animals and cause disease in the process. (p. 693)

**Protozoans** Single-celled organisms that are the smallest and simplest members of the animal kingdom. (p. 693)

## ANATOMY, PHYSIOLOGY, AND PATHOPHYSIOLOGY OVERVIEW

There are more than 28,000 known types of protozoans, which are single-celled organisms. Those that live on or in humans are called parasitic protozoans. Billions of people worldwide are infected with these organisms, and, as a result, these infections are considered a serious public health problem. Some of the more common protozoal infections are malaria, leishmaniasis, trypanosomiasis, amebiasis, giardiasis, and trichomoniasis. They are relatively uncommon in the United States but are becoming increasingly prevalent in immunocompromised individuals, including those with acquired immunodeficiency syndrome (AIDS). Protozoal diseases are especially prevalent among people living in tropical climates because it is easier for protozoans to survive and be transmitted in environments that are warm and humid year round. Although the population of the United States is relatively free of many of these protozoal infections, international travel and the immigration of people from other countries where such infections are endemic are providing opportunities for increased exposure.

## PATHOPHYSIOLOGY OF MALARIA

The most significant protozoal disease in terms of morbidity and mortality is malaria. Worldwide, it is estimated that 350 to 500 million people are infected, with an annual death rate of 1 million to 2 million people. In Africa alone, malaria accounts for more than 1 million infant deaths per year. The geographic areas with the highest prevalence are sub-Saharan Africa, Southeast Asia, and Latin America. Approximately 1200 cases of malaria are reported in the United States annually, seen mostly in people who traveled to malaria-infested countries. Malaria is caused by a particular genus of protozoans called *Plasmodium,* and there are four species of organisms in this genus, each with its own characteristics and its own ability to resist being killed by antimalarial drugs. These four species are *Plasmodium vivax, Plasmodium falciparum, Plasmodium malariae,* and *Plasmodium ovale.* Although *P. vivax* is the most widespread of the four, *P. falciparum* is nearly as widespread and causes greater problems with drug resistance. The two remaining species are much less common and more geographically limited in their occurrence, but they can still cause serious malarial infections.

Most commonly, malaria is transmitted by the bite of an infected female anopheline mosquito. This type of mosquito is endemic to many tropical regions of the earth. Malaria can also be transmitted by blood transfusions, congenitally from mother to infant via an infected placenta, or through the use of contaminated needles. Despite the combined efforts of many countries to eradicate malaria, it remains one of the most devastating infectious diseases in the world. As is also the case with tuberculosis (see Chapter 41) and AIDS (see Chapter 40), many lives are lost to malaria, and the cost of treating and preventing the disease imposes a tremendous economic burden on the often poor countries where the disease is prevalent.

The *Plasmodium* life cycle is quite complex and involves many stages. The organism has two interdependent life cycles: the *sexual cycle,* which takes place inside the mosquito, and the *asexual cycle,* which occurs in the human host (Figure 43-1). In addition, the asexual cycle of the parasite consists of a phase outside the erythrocyte (primarily in liver tissues) called the *exoerythrocytic phase* (or the *tissue phase*) and a phase inside the erythrocyte called the *erythrocytic phase* (or the *blood phase*). The malarial parasite undergoes many changes during these two phases (Figure 43-2).

Malaria signs and symptoms are often described in terms of the *classic malaria paroxysm.* A *paroxysm* is a sudden recurrence or intensification of symptoms. Symptoms include chills and rigors, followed by fever of up to 104° F (40° C) and diaphoresis, frequently leading to extreme fatigue and prolonged sleep. This syndrome often repeats itself periodically in 48- to 72-hour cycles. Other common symptoms include headache, nausea, and joint pain.

## PHARMACOLOGY OVERVIEW

### ANTIMALARIAL DRUGS

Treatment for malaria is not initiated until the diagnosis has been confirmed by laboratory tests. Once confirmed, appropriate antimalarial treatment must be initiated immediately. Treatment is guided by three main factors: the infecting *Plasmodium* species, the clinical status of the patient, and the drug susceptibility of the infecting parasites as determined by the geographic area where the infection was acquired. Because the resistance patterns are constantly changing, depending on geographic location, the reader is referred to the website of the Centers for Disease Control and Prevention (CDC) at www.cdc.gov/malaria/ for the most up-to-date information. People traveling to different parts of the world may require antimalarial prophylaxis and need to check with their prescribers and/or the CDC website mentioned above for specific drug therapy.

Antimalarial drugs administered to humans cannot affect the parasite during its sexual cycle when it resides in the mosquito. Instead, these drugs work against the parasite during its asexual cycle, which takes place within the human body. Often these drugs are given in various combinations to achieve an additive or synergistic antimalarial effect. One example is the combination of the two antiprotozoal drugs atovaquone and proguanil (Malarone). The antibiotic combination of pyrimethamine and sulfadoxine (Fansidar) is also commonly used, especially in cases caused by drug-resistant organisms.

## Mechanism of Action and Drug Effects

The mechanisms of action of the various antimalarial drugs differ depending on the chemical family to which they belong. The *4-aminoquinoline derivatives* (chloroquine and hydroxychloroquine) work by inhibiting deoxyribonucleic acid (DNA) and ribonucleic acid (RNA) polymerase, enzymes essential to DNA and RNA synthesis by the parasite cells. Parasite protein synthesis is also disrupted, because protein synthesis is dependent on proper nucleic acid (DNA and RNA) function. These drugs also raise the pH within the parasite, which interferes with the parasite's ability to metabolize and use erythrocyte hemoglobin; this is one reason these drugs are ineffective during the

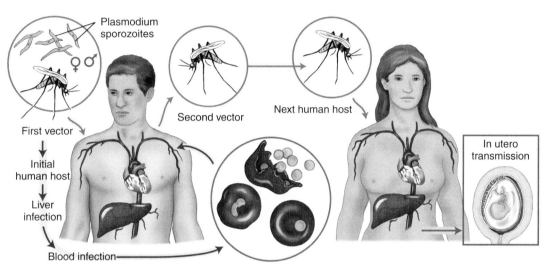

**FIGURE 43-1** An infected Anopheles mosquito carries parasites to humans, causing malaria. These parasites mature in the liver before entering the bloodstream and rupturing red blood cells. A pregnant woman infected with malaria may transmit the disease to her unborn child.

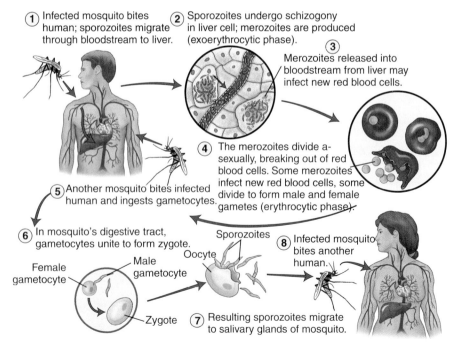

**FIGURE 43-2** Life cycle of the malarial parasite. (From Van Meter K, Hubert R: *Microbiology for the healthcare professional,* St Louis, 2010, Mosby.)

exoerythrocytic (tissue) phase of infection. All of these actions contribute to the destruction of the parasite. Quinine, quinidine, and mefloquine are thought to be similar to the 4-aminoquinoline derivatives in their actions in that all are also believed to raise the pH within the parasite.

The *diaminopyrimidines* (pyrimethamine and trimethoprim [see Chapter 38]) work by inhibiting dihydrofolate reductase, an enzyme that is needed for the production of certain vital substances in malarial parasites. Specifically, inhibiting this enzyme blocks the synthesis of tetrahydrofolate, which is a precursor of purines and pyrimidines (nucleic acid components) and certain amino acids (protein components) that are essential for the growth and survival of plasmodia parasites. These two drugs are effective only during the erythrocytic phase. Pyrimethamine and trimethoprim are often used with a sulfonamide (sulfadoxine or dapsone) because of the resulting synergistic effects exerted by such drug combinations. Tetracyclines such as doxycycline (see Chapter 38) and lincomycins such as clindamycin (see Chapter 39) may also be used in combination with some of the other antimalarial drugs because of the synergistic effects resulting from these drug combinations.

Primaquine, an *8-aminoquinoline* that is structurally similar to the 4-aminoquinolines, has the ability to bind to and alter parasitic DNA. It is one of the few drugs that is effective in the exoerythrocytic phase. Atovaquone/proguanil also works by interference with nucleic acid synthesis.

The drug effects of the antimalarial drugs are mostly limited to their ability to kill parasitic organisms, most of which are *Plasmodium* species (spp.). However, some of these drugs have other effects and therapeutic uses. Hydroxychloroquine also has antiinflammatory effects and is sometimes used in the treatment of rheumatoid arthritis and systemic lupus erythematosus. Quinine and quinidine can also decrease the excitability of both cardiac and skeletal muscles. Quinidine is still currently used to treat certain types of cardiac dysrhythmias (see Chapter 25).

## Indications

Antimalarial drugs are used to kill *Plasmodium* organisms, the parasites that cause malaria. The various antimalarial drugs work during different phases of the parasite's growth inside the human. The antimalarials that exert the greatest effect on all four *Plasmodium* organisms during the erythrocytic or blood phase are chloroquine, hydroxychloroquine, and pyrimethamine. Other drugs that are known to work during the blood phase are quinine, quinidine, and mefloquine. Because these drugs are ineffective during the exoerythrocytic phase, however, they cannot *prevent* infection. The most effective antimalarial drug for eradicating the parasite during the exoerythrocytic phase is primaquine, which actually works during both phases. Primaquine is indicated specifically for infection with *P. vivax*. Chloroquine and hydroxychloroquine (4-aminoquinolines) are the drugs of choice for the treatment of susceptible strains of malarial parasites. They are highly toxic to all *Plasmodium* spp., except resistant strains of *P. falciparum*.

Quinine is indicated for infection with chloroquine-resistant *P. falciparum*, which can cause a type of malaria that affects the brain. Quinine can be used alone but is more commonly given in combination with pyrimethamine, a sulfonamide, or a tetracycline (such as doxycycline). Pyrimethamine is another antimalarial antibiotic that is commonly used in combination with the sulfonamide antibiotic sulfadoxine (Fansidar) for prophylaxis against chloroquine-resistant *P. falciparum* and *P. vivax*. However, drug resistance in most locations has reduced its use for this purpose. Other antimalarial drugs are generally preferred for the treatment of active disease. Mefloquine is an antimalarial drug that may also be used for both prophylaxis and treatment of malaria caused by *P. falciparum* or *P. vivax*. The drug combination atovaquone and proguanil (Malarone) is also used for prevention and treatment of *P. falciparum* infection.

## Contraindications

Contraindications to various antimalarial drugs include drug allergy, tinnitus (ear ringing), and pregnancy (quinine). Severe renal, hepatic, or hematologic dysfunction may also be a contraindication to the use of antimalarial drugs. Other drug-specific contraindications are noted in the drug profiles that follow.

## Adverse Effects

Antimalarial drugs cause diverse adverse effects, and these are listed for each drug in Table 43-1.

| TABLE 43-1 | ANTIMALARIAL DRUGS: COMMON ADVERSE EFFECTS |
|---|---|
| **BODY SYSTEM** | **ADVERSE EFFECTS** |
| **Chloroquine and hydroxychloroquine** | |
| Gastrointestinal | Diarrhea, anorexia, nausea, vomiting |
| Central nervous | Dizziness, headache, seizure, personality changes |
| Other | Alopecia, rash, pruritus |
| **Mefloquine** | |
| Central nervous | Headache, fatigue, tinnitus |
| Gastrointestinal | Stomach pain, anorexia, nausea, vomiting |
| Other | Fever, chills, rash, myalgia |
| **Primaquine** | |
| Gastrointestinal | Nausea, vomiting, abdominal distress |
| Other | Headaches, pruritus, dark discoloration of urine, hemolytic anemia due to G6PD deficiency |
| **Pyrimethamine** | |
| Gastrointestinal | Anorexia; vomiting; taste disturbances; soreness, redness, swelling, or burning of tongue; diarrhea; throat pain; swallowing difficulties; sores, ulcerations, or white spots in mouth; sore throat |
| Other | Malaise, weakness, rash, abnormal skin pigmentation, hemolytic anemia resulting from G6PD deficiency, severe hypersensitivity reactions |
| **Quinine** | |
| Central nervous | Visual disturbances, dizziness, headaches, tinnitus |
| Gastrointestinal | Diarrhea, nausea, vomiting, abdominal pain |
| Other | Rash, pruritus, hives, photosensitivity, respiratory difficulties |

*G6PD,* Glucose-6-phosphate dehydrogenase.

## Interactions

Some common drug interactions associated with antimalarial drugs are listed in Table 43-2.

## Dosages

For dosage information on selected antimalarial drugs, see the table on this page.

| TABLE 43-2 | ANTIMALARIAL DRUGS: DRUG INTERACTIONS | |
|---|---|---|
| **DRUG** | **MECHANISM** | **RESULT** |
| **Chloroquine** | | |
| divalproex, valproic acid, anthelmintics, beta blockers | Decreased serum levels of target drug | Treatment failures of target drugs |
| digoxin | Increased serum levels of digoxin | Potential toxicity |
| **Mefloquine** | | |
| Beta blockers, calcium channel blockers, quinidine, quinine | Unknown | Increased risk of dysrhythmia, cardiac arrest, seizures |
| **Primaquine** | | |
| Other hemolytic drugs | Unknown | Increased risk for myelotoxic effects (monitor for muscle weakness) |

## DRUG PROFILES

The dosing instructions for several of the antimalarial drugs can be confusing, because tablet strengths listed on the medication packaging often indicate the strength of the tablet in terms of the entire salt form of the drug, not just the active ingredient itself, which is referred to as the *base ingredient*. However, dosing guidelines often list recommended dosages in terms of the base ingredient and not the entire salt. For example, as described later in the drug profile for chloroquine, the tablets come in 250-mg and 500-mg strengths of the salt form of the drug, but these tablets actually only have 150 mg and 300 mg, respectively, of the active ingredient or base. Be mindful of these distinctions.

### ◆ chloroquine and hydroxychloroquine

Chloroquine (Aralen) is a synthetic antimalarial drug that is chemically classified as a 4-aminoquinoline derivative. In addition to malaria, it is also indicated for treatment of other parasitic infections, such as amebiasis. Hydroxychloroquine is another synthetic 4-aminoquinoline derivative that differs from chloroquine by only one hydroxyl group ($^-OH$). Its efficacy in treating malaria is comparable to that of quinine. Both medications also possess antiinflammatory actions and have been used to treat rheumatoid arthritis and systemic lupus erythematosus since the 1950s. However, only hydroxychloroquine (Plaquenil) is now used for these indications.

Contraindications include visual field changes, optic neuritis, and psoriasis, but its use may still be warranted in urgent clinical situations, based on sound clinical judgment.

## DOSAGES

### Selected Antimalarial Drugs

| DRUG (PREGNANCY CATEGORY) | PHARMACOLOGIC CLASS | USUAL DOSAGE RANGE | INDICATIONS/USES |
|---|---|---|---|
| ◆ chloroquine (Aralen) (C) | Synthetic antimalarial and antiamebic | **Adult\*** PO: 300 mg base weekly, beginning 2 wk before and continuing for 8 wk after visiting endemic area | Malaria prophylaxis |
| | | PO: 600 mg base on day 1, followed by 300 mg 6 hr later and on days 2 and 3 | Malaria treatment |
| ◆ hydroxychloroquine (Plaquenil) (C) | Synthetic antimalarial | **Adult\*** PO: 310 mg base weekly, beginning 1-2 wk before and continuing through 4 wk after visiting endemic area | Malaria prophylaxis |
| | | PO: 620 mg base on day 1, followed by 310 mg 6 hr later and once daily on days 2 and 3 | Malaria treatment |
| mefloquine (Lariam) (C) | Synthetic antimalarial | **Adult and children weighing over 45 kg** PO: 250 mg weekly beginning 1-2 wk before travel and continuing until 4 wk after visiting endemic area | Malaria prophylaxis |
| | | **Pediatric** PO: Dosing varies based on weight. | |
| | | **Adult** PO: 1250 mg (5 tabs) in a single dose | Malaria treatment |
| | | **Pediatric** PO: 15-25 mg/kg in a single dose, not to exceed 1250 mg | |
| ◆ primaquine (generic only) (C) | Synthetic antimalarial | **Adult** 30 mg PO daily × 14 days after leaving endemic area. Doses vary if dealing with drug-resistant malaria. | Malaria prophylaxis |

## DOSAGES—cont'd

### Selected Antimalarial Drugs

| DRUG (PREGNANCY CATEGORY) | PHARMACOLOGIC CLASS | USUAL DOSAGE RANGE | INDICATIONS/USES |
|---|---|---|---|
| pyrimethamine (Daraprim) (C) | Folic acid antagonist, antimalarial, antitoxoplasmotic | **Adult**<br>PO: 15 mg base daily × 14 days<br>**Pediatric**<br>PO: 0.5 mg base/kg/day × 14 days | Malaria treatment |
| | | **Adult and pediatric older than 10 yr**<br>PO: 25 mg weekly<br>**Pediatric 4-10 yr**<br>PO: 12.5 mg weekly<br>**Pediatric infant to 3 yr**<br>PO: 6.25 mg weekly | Malaria prophylaxis |
| | | **Adult and pediatric older than 10 yr**<br>PO: 50 mg daily × 2 days<br>**Pediatric 4-10 yr**<br>PO: 25 mg daily × 2 days | Malaria treatment |

*PO,* oral.

*Only adult dosages are given. Pediatric dosages range from 5 to 10 mg/kg but not to exceed adult dosages.

Chloroquine and hydroxychloroquine are available only for oral use. Both drugs are classified as pregnancy category C drugs, but it is recommended that they be used in pregnant women only in truly urgent clinical situations. These drugs are also distributed into breast milk.

### Pharmacokinetics (chloroquine)

| Route | Onset of Action | Peak Plasma Concentration | Elimination Half-life | Duration of Action |
|---|---|---|---|---|
| PO | 8-10 hr | 1-2 hr | 3-5 days | Variable |

### Pharmacokinetics (hydroxychloroquine)

| Route | Onset of Action | Peak Plasma Concentration | Elimination Half-life | Duration of Action |
|---|---|---|---|---|
| PO | 4 hr | 2-3 hr | 32-50 days | Variable |

### mefloquine

Mefloquine (Lariam) is an analogue of quinine that is indicated for the management of mild to moderate acute malaria and for the prevention and treatment of malaria caused by chloroquine-resistant organisms. It is also used to treat multidrug-resistant strains of *P. falciparum,* which, as already noted, is a very difficult species of *Plasmodium* to kill. The drug is commonly used prophylactically by travelers to prevent malarial infection while visiting malaria-endemic areas. The tetracycline antibiotic doxycycline (see Chapter 38) is also commonly used for this purpose. Mefloquine is available only for oral use.

### Pharmacokinetics

| Route | Onset of Action | Peak Plasma Concentration | Elimination Half-life | Duration of Action |
|---|---|---|---|---|
| PO | Less than 24 hr | 7-24 hr | 21-22 days | Variable |

### ♦ primaquine

Primaquine is similar in chemical structure and antimalarial activity to the 4-aminoquinolines, but it is classified as an 8-aminoquinoline. It is one of the few antimalarial drugs that can destroy the malarial parasites while they are in their exoerythrocytic phase. Primaquine is indicated for curative therapy in acute cases of *P. vivax, P. ovale,* and to a lesser degree, *P. falciparum* infection.

Primaquine is contraindicated in patients with allergy or any disease states that may cause granulocytopenia (rheumatoid arthritis, systemic lupus erythematosus). Primaquine must be used with caution in patients with methemoglobinemia, porphyria, methemoglobin reductase deficiency, and glucose-6-phosphate dehydrogenase (G6PD) deficiency (see Chapter 2). It is available only for oral use.

### Pharmacokinetics

| Route | Onset of Action | Peak Plasma Concentration | Elimination Half-life | Duration of Action |
|---|---|---|---|---|
| PO | 2 hr | 1-3 hr | 4-10 hr | 24 hr |

### pyrimethamine

Pyrimethamine (Daraprim) is a synthetic antimalarial drug that is structurally related to trimethoprim (see Chapter 38). Both drugs are chemically subclassified as *diaminopyrimidines.* Fansidar is a commonly used fixed-combination drug product that contains 500 mg of sulfadoxine and 25 mg of pyrimethamine. Pyrimethamine is contraindicated in patients with megaloblastic anemia caused by folate deficiency. It is available only for oral use.

### Pharmacokinetics

| Route | Onset of Action | Peak Plasma Concentration | Elimination Half-life | Duration of Action |
|---|---|---|---|---|
| PO | 6 hr | 2-6 hr | 80-123 hours | Up to 2 wk |

| TABLE 43-3 | TYPES OF PROTOZOAL INFECTIONS AND COMMON DRUG THERAPY | |
|---|---|---|
| **INFECTION** | **DESCRIPTION** | **ANTIPROTOZOAL DRUG** |
| Amebiasis | Caused by the protozoal parasite *Entamoeba histolytica*. Infection mainly resides in the large intestine but can also migrate to other parts of the body, such as the liver. Usually transmitted in contaminated food or water. | chloroquine, metronidazole, paromomycin, iodoquinol |
| Giardiasis | Caused by *Giardia lamblia*. The most common intestinal protozoal infection, usually residing in the intestinal mucosa (most commonly the duodenum). May cause diarrhea, bloating, and foul-smelling stools. Transmitted in contaminated food or water or by contact with stool from infected persons. | metronidazole, nitazoxanide, quinacrine, furazolidone, albendazole, paromomycin |
| Pneumocystosis | Pneumonia caused by *Pneumocystis jirovecii** that occurs exclusively in immunocompromised individuals. Always fatal if left untreated. | trimethoprim/sulfamethoxazole, dapsone, atovaquone, primaquine, pentamidine, clindamycin |
| Toxoplasmosis | Caused by *Toxoplasma gondii*. Can produce systemic infection in both immunocompetent and immunocompromised hosts. Domesticated animals, usually cats, serve as intermediate host for parasites, passing infective oocysts in their feces. | sulfonamides with pyrimethamine, clindamycin, metronidazole |
| Trichomoniasis | Sexually transmitted disease caused by *Trichomonas vaginalis*. | metronidazole |

*\*Pneumocystis jirovecii* is now classified as a fungus.

## PATHOPHYSIOLOGY OVERVIEW

### OTHER PROTOZOAL INFECTIONS

There are several other common protozoal infections. These include amebiasis (caused by *Entamoeba histolytica*), giardiasis (caused by *Giardia lamblia*), toxoplasmosis (caused by *Toxoplasma gondii*), and trichomoniasis, (caused by *Trichomonas vaginalis*). These diseases are more prevalent in tropical regions. Pneumocystosis, which is caused by *Pneumocystis jirovecii* (formerly *Pneumocystis carinii*), used to be classified as a protozoal infection; however, it is now classified as fungal infection. It is a common infection that complicates HIV and AIDS. It will be discussed in this chapter as opposed to the antifungal chapter (see Chapter 42) because it is treated with drugs discussed in this chapter.

These protozoal infections can be transmitted in a number of ways: from person to person (e.g., via sexual contact), through the ingestion of contaminated water or food, through direct contact with the parasite, or by the bite of an insect (mosquito or tick). These infections can be systemic and occur throughout the body, or they can be localized to a specific region. For example, amebiasis most commonly affects the gastrointestinal tract (e.g., amebic dysentery), whereas pneumocystosis is predominantly a pulmonary infection.

The more common protozoal infections are described briefly in Table 43-3, and the antiprotozoal drugs commonly used in their treatment are listed. Only selected drugs are discussed here. Patients whose immune systems are compromised are at particular risk for acquiring a protozoal infection. Often such infections are fatal in these patients.

## PHARMACOLOGY OVERVIEW

### ANTIPROTOZOAL DRUGS

Several drugs used to treat malaria are also used to treat nonmalarial protozoal infections, including chloroquine, primaquine, pyrimethamine, and atovaquone. Other antiprotozoal drugs

| TABLE 43-4 | SELECTED ANTIPROTOZOAL DRUGS: MECHANISMS OF ACTION |
|---|---|
| **DRUG** | **MECHANISM OF ACTION** |
| atovaquone | Atovaquone selectively inhibits mitochondrial electron transport, reducing synthesis of adenosine triphosphate (required for cellular energy). Also inhibits nucleic acid synthesis. |
| metronidazole | Interferes with DNA, resulting in inhibition of protein synthesis and cell death in susceptible organisms. |
| pentamidine | Inhibits production of much-needed substances such as DNA and RNA. Can bind to and aggregate ribosomes. Is directly lethal to *Pneumocystis jirovecii** by inhibiting glucose metabolism, protein and RNA synthesis, and intracellular amino acid transport. |

*\*Pneumocystis jirovecii* is now classified as a fungus.

normally used against nonmalarial parasites include iodoquinol, metronidazole, paromomycin, and pentamidine.

### Mechanism of Action and Drug Effects

Antiprotozoal drugs work by several different mechanisms. The most commonly used of these drugs, together with brief descriptions of their mechanisms of action, are given in Table 43-4. Pyrimethamine and chloroquine were discussed earlier in this chapter in the section on malaria. The drug effects of antiprotozoal drugs are primarily limited to their ability to kill various forms of protozoal parasites.

### Indications

Antiprotozoal drugs are used to treat various protozoal infections, ranging from intestinal amebiasis to pneumocystosis. Indications for selected drugs are summarized in Table 43-5. Atovaquone and pentamidine are used for the treatment of

## TABLE 43-5 SELECTED ANTIPROTOZOAL DRUGS: INDICATIONS

| DRUG | INDICATIONS |
|---|---|
| atovaquone | Indicated for treatment of acute mild to moderately severe *Pneumocystis jirovecii* pneumonia in patients who cannot tolerate co-trimoxazole |
| iodoquinol | Indicated for treatment of intestinal amebiasis in asymptomatic carriers of *Entamoeba histolytica;* also has been used for treatment of *Giardia lamblia* and *Trichomonas vaginalis* infections |
| metronidazole | Indicated for treatment of bacterial (including anaerobic), protozoal, and helminthic infections |
| pentamidine | Indicated for treatment of *P. jirovecii** pneumonia |

**Pneumocystis jirovecii* is now classified as a fungus.

## TABLE 43-6 SELECTED ANTIPROTOZOAL DRUGS: ADVERSE EFFECTS

| BODY SYSTEM | ADVERSE EFFECTS |
|---|---|
| **Atovaquone** | |
| Hematologic | Anemia, neutropenia, leukopenia |
| Integumentary | Pruritus, urticaria, rash |
| Gastrointestinal | Anorexia, elevated liver enzymes, nausea, constipation |
| Central nervous | Dizziness, headache, anxiety, fever |
| Metabolic | Hyperkalemia, hypoglycemia, hyponatremia |
| Other | Cough |
| **Iodoquinol** | |
| Hematologic | Agranulocytosis |
| Integumentary | Rash; pruritus; discolored skin, hair, nails |
| Central nervous | Headache, agitation, peripheral neuropathy |
| Eyes, ears, nose, and throat | Blurred vision, sore throat, optic neuritis, blindness |
| Gastrointestinal | Anorexia, gastritis, nausea, vomiting, diarrhea |
| **Metronidazole** | |
| Central nervous | Headache, dizziness, confusion, fatigue, peripheral neuropathy, weakness |
| Eyes, ears, nose, and throat | Blurred vision, sore throat, dry mouth, metallic taste, glossitis |
| Gastrointestinal | Anorexia, vomiting, diarrhea, constipation |
| Genitourinary | Dysuria, cystitis |
| Hematologic | Neutropenia |
| Integumentary | Rash, pruritus, urticaria |
| **Paromomycin** | |
| Gastrointestinal | Stomach cramps, nausea, vomiting, diarrhea |
| Central nervous | Hearing loss, dizziness, tinnitus |
| **Pentamidine** | |
| Cardiovascular | Hypotension, chest pain, dysrythmias |
| Hematologic | Leukopenia, thrombocytopenia, neutropenia |
| Integumentary | Pain at injection site, pruritus, urticaria, rash |
| Genitourinary | Nephrotoxicity |
| Gastrointestinal | Increased liver enzyme levels, pancreatitis, metallic taste, nausea, vomiting, diarrhea |
| Respiratory | Cough, wheezing, dyspnea, pharyngitis |
| Metabolic | Hypoglycemia followed by hyperglycemia |
| Other | Fatigue, chills, night sweats |

## TABLE 43-7 ANTIPROTOZOAL DRUGS: DRUG AND LABORATORY TEST INTERACTIONS

| DRUG | MECHANISM | RESULT |
|---|---|---|
| atovaquone | Competition for binding on protein, resulting in free, active atovaquone | Highly protein-bound drugs (e.g., warfarin, phenytoin) may increase atovaquone drug concentrations and risk of adverse reactions |
| iodoquinol | Increase in protein-bound serum iodine concentrations, reflecting a decrease in iodine 131 uptake | May interfere with certain thyroid function test results |
| metronidazole | Decreased absorption of vitamin K from the intestines due to elimination of the bacteria needed to absorb vitamin K, increased plasma acetaldehyde concentration after ingestion of alcohol | Alcohol causes a disulfiram-like reaction; action of warfarin may be increased (increased bleeding risk) |
| pentamidine | Additive nephrotoxic effects | Use with an aminoglycoside, amphotericin B, colistin, cisplatin, or vancomycin may result in nephrotoxicity |

*P. jirovecii* infection. Iodoquinol, metronidazole, and paromomycin are all used to treat intestinal amebiasis. Metronidazole is effective against several forms of bacteria, including anaerobic bacteria (see Chapter 39), as well as against protozoans and helminths (parasitic worms). Worm infection (helminthiasis) is discussed later in the chapter.

## Contraindications

Contraindications to the use of antiprotozoal drugs include known drug allergy. Additional contraindications may include serious renal, liver, or other illnesses, with the seriousness of the infection weighed against the patient's overall condition.

## Adverse Effects

The adverse effects of antiprotozoal drugs vary greatly depending on the drug and are listed in Table 43-6.

## Interactions

The common drug and laboratory test interactions associated with the use of antiprotozoal drugs are listed in Table 43-7.

## Dosages

For dosage information for selected antiprotozoal drugs, see the table on p. 700.

## DOSAGES

### *Selected Antiprotozoal Drugs*

| DRUG (PREGNANCY CATEGORY) | PHARMACOLOGIC CLASS | USUAL DOSAGE RANGE | INDICATIONS/USES |
|---|---|---|---|
| atovaquone* (Mepron) (C) | Synthetic anti-*Pneumocystis* drug | **Adult and adolescent 13-16 yr**<br>PO: 1500 mg daily with meal × 21 days | Prophylaxis of PJP; treatment of active PJP |
| ◆ metronidazole (Flagyl) (X, first trimester; B, second and third trimesters) | Amebicide, antibacterial, trichomonacide | **Adult**<br>PO: 750 mg 3 times daily × 7-10 days<br>**Pediatric**<br>PO: 35-50 mg/kg (max 750 mg/dose) 3 times daily × 7-10 days | Amebiasis, including amebic liver abscess |
| | | **Adult 7-day treatment**<br>PO: 250 mg 3 times daily × 5-7 days | Trichomoniasis, giardiasis |
| | | **Pediatric 7-day treatment**<br>PO: 15 mg/kg/day in 3 divided doses × 5 days | |
| pentamidine (NebuPent, Pentam 300) (C) | Synthetic anti-*Pneumocystis*† drug | **Adult and pediatric**<br>Inhalation aerosol: 300 mg q4wk<br>IV/IM: 4 mg/kg daily × 14-21 days | Prophylaxis of PJP; treatment of active PJP |

*IM,* Intramuscular; *IV,* intravenous; *PO,* oral; *PJP, Pneumocystis jirovecii* pneumonia.
\*NOTE: A combination product containing atovaquone and the drug proguanil is also used against malaria.
†*Pneumocystis jirovecii* is now classified as a fungus.

## DRUG PROFILES

### atovaquone

Atovaquone (Mepron) is a synthetic antiprotozoal drug indicated for the treatment of mild to moderate *P. jirovecii* pneumonia in patients who cannot tolerate co-trimoxazole (trimethoprim/sulfamethoxazole [see Chapter 38]). It is available only for oral use.

#### Pharmacokinetics

| Route | Onset of Action | Peak Plasma Concentration | Elimination Half-life | Duration of Action |
|---|---|---|---|---|
| PO | 8-24 hr | 24-96 hr | 2-3 days | Unknown |

### ◆ metronidazole

Metronidazole (Flagyl) is an antiprotozoal drug that also has fairly broad antibacterial activity as well as anthelmintic activity. The therapeutic uses of metronidazole are many and range from the treatment of trichomoniasis, amebiasis, and giardiasis to the treatment of anaerobic bacterial infections and antibiotic-induced pseudomembranous colitis (see Chapters 38 and 39). Metronidazole is believed to directly kill protozoans by causing free-radical reactions that damage their DNA and other vital biomolecules. Tinidazole (Tindamax) is a newer, similar drug.

Metronidazole is contraindicated during the first trimester of pregnancy. It is available in both oral and injectable forms.

#### Pharmacokinetics

| Route | Onset of Action | Peak Plasma Concentration | Elimination Half-life | Duration of Action |
|---|---|---|---|---|
| PO | 1 hr | 1-2 hr | 8 hr | Variable |

### pentamidine

Pentamidine (NebuPent, Pentam 300) is an antiprotozoal drug that is used mainly for the management of *P. jirovecii* pneumonia (which is actually a fungal infection), although it is sometimes used to treat various protozoal infections. It works by inhibiting protein and nucleic acid synthesis. It is used for the treatment of active pneumocystosis and for prophylaxis of *P. jirovecii* pneumonia in patients at high risk for initial or recurrent *Pneumocystis* infection, such as patients with human immunodeficiency virus (HIV) infection and AIDS.

The only contraindication to pentamidine is known hypersensitivity to the drug. Hypersensitivity is more common when the drug is administered by inhalation. Due to the seriousness of the *Pneumocystis* infection, an allergic reaction to the inhalational form does not preclude its administration by either the intramuscular or intravenous route. The drug needs to be used with caution in patients with blood dyscrasias, hepatic or renal disease, diabetes mellitus, cardiac disease, hypocalcemia, or hypertension. Pentamidine is available as an oral inhalational solution and also in injectable form.

#### Pharmacokinetics

| Route | Onset of Action | Peak Plasma Concentration | Elimination Half-life | Duration of Action |
|---|---|---|---|---|
| Inhalation | 0.5-1 hr | Less than 1 hr | 6-9 hr | Variable |

## PATHOPHYSIOLOGY OVERVIEW

## HELMINTHIC INFECTIONS

Parasitic helminthic infections (worm infections) are a worldwide problem. It has been estimated that one third of the world's population is infected with these parasites, but persons

### TABLE 43-8 HELMINTHIC INFECTIONS

| INFECTION | ORGANISM AND OTHER FACTS |
|---|---|
| **Nematodes (Various Intestinal and Tissue Roundworms)** | |
| Ascariasis | Caused by *Ascaris lumbricoides* (giant round-worm); worm resides in small intestine; treated with pyrantel or albendazole |
| Enterobiasis | Caused by *Enterobius vermicularis* (pinworm); worm resides in large intestine; treated with pyrantel or albendazole |
| **Platyhelminthes (Intestinal Tapeworms or Flatworms)** | |
| Diphyllobothriasis | Caused by *Diphyllobothrium latum* (fish worm); acquired from fish; treated with paromomycin, praziquantel, or albendazole |
| Hymenolepiasis | Caused by *Hymenolepis nana* (dwarf tapeworm); treated with niclosamide, paromomycin, praziquantel, or albendazole |
| Taeniasis | Caused by *Taenia saginata* (beef tapeworm); acquired from beef; treated with paromomycin, praziquantel, or albendazole |
| | Caused by *Taenia solium* (pork tapeworm); acquired from pork; treated with paromomycin, praziquantel, or albendazole |

### TABLE 43-9 ANTHELMINTICS: CLASS OF WORMS KILLED

| ANTHELMINTIC DRUG | CESTODES | NEMATODES | TREMATODES |
|---|---|---|---|
| albendazole | Yes | Yes | Yes |
| ivermectin | No | Yes | No |
| piperazine and pyrantel | No | Yes (giant worm and pinworm) | No |
| praziquantel | Yes | No | Yes |

living in undeveloped countries where sanitary conditions are often poor are by far the most common victims. The incidence of worm infection in developed countries where sewage treatment is adequate is much lower, and usually only a few select helminthic diseases are the source of the problem. The most prevalent helminthic infection in the United States is enterobiasis, caused by one genus of roundworm, *Enterobius*.

Helminths that are parasitic in humans are classified in the following way:

- Platyhelminthes (flatworms)
- Cestodes (tapeworms)
- Trematodes (flukes)
- Nematodes (roundworms)

The characteristics of a few of the most common of the many helminthic infections are summarized in Table 43-8. These usually first infect the intestines of their host and reside there but can sometimes also migrate to other tissues.

## PHARMACOLOGY OVERVIEW

### ANTHELMINTIC DRUGS

Unlike protozoans, which are the single-celled members of the animal kingdom, helminths are larger and have complex multicellular structures. Anthelmintic drugs (also spelled *antihelmintic*) work to destroy these organisms by disrupting their structures. The currently available anthelmintic drugs are very specific with regard to the worms they can kill. For this reason, the causative worm in an infected host must be accurately identified before treatment is started. This can usually be done by analyzing samples of feces, urine, blood, sputum, or tissue from the infected host for the presence of ova or larvae of the particular parasite.

Several anthelmintics are commercially available in the United States. These include albendazole (Albenza), ivermectin (Stromectol), praziquantel (Biltricide), and pyrantel (Antiminth).

Other drugs, such as niclosamide and piperazine, may be available either in other countries or by special request from the CDC. Anthelmintics are very specific in their actions. Albendazole can be used to treat both tapeworms and roundworms. Praziquantel is a drug that can kill flukes (trematodes). The most commonly used anthelmintics and the specific class of worms they can effectively kill are summarized in Table 43-9.

### Mechanism of Action and Drug Effects

The mechanisms of action of the various anthelmintics vary greatly from drug to drug, although there are some similarities among the drugs used to kill similar types of worms. The various anthelmintic drugs and their respective mechanisms of action are listed in Table 43-10. The drug effects of the anthelmintic drugs are limited to their ability to kill various forms of worms and flukes.

### Indications

Anthelmintic drugs are used to treat roundworm, tapeworm, and fluke infections. Specific drugs are used to treat specific helminthic infections.

### Contraindications

The only usual contraindication to a specific anthelmintic drug product is known drug allergy. Pyrantel is contraindicated in patients with liver disease. Praziquantel is also contraindicated in patients with *ocular cysticercosis* (tapeworm infection of the eye).

### Adverse Effects

The anthelmintic drugs show a remarkable diversity in their drug-specific adverse effects. Common adverse effects are listed in Table 43-11.

### Interactions

The concurrent use of pyrantel with piperazine is not recommended, and pyrantel is used cautiously in patients with hepatic impairment. Pyrantel has also been shown to raise blood levels of theophylline in pediatric patients. Dexamethasone and the anthelmintic praziquantel may raise blood levels of albendazole.

## TABLE 43-10 ANTHELMINTICS: MECHANISMS OF ACTION

| DRUG | MECHANISM OF ACTION | INDICATION |
|------|---------------------|------------|
| albendazole | Cells of intestinal and tissue-dwelling larvae are selectively destroyed by degenerating cytoplasmic microtubules. This in turn causes secretory substances to accumulate intracellularly, which leads to impaired cholinesterase secretion and glucose. Glycogen becomes depleted, which leads to decreased ATP production and energy depletion, which immobilizes and kills the worm. | Neurocysticercosis, hydatid disease |
| ivermectin | Potentiates inhibitory signals in the CNS of nematodes, which leads to their paralysis. | Nondisseminated intestinal infection with *Strongyloides* (threadworms) |
| praziquantel | Increases permeability of the cell membrane of susceptible worms to calcium, which results in the influx of calcium. This causes the worms to be dislodged from their usual site of residence in the mesenteric veins to the liver; they are then killed by host tissue reactions. | Schistosomiasis, opisthorchiasis (liver fluke infection), clonorchiasis (infection with Chinese or Oriental liver fluke), diphyllobothriasis (fish worm infection), hymenolepiasis (dwarf tapeworm infection), neurocysticercosis |
| pyrantel | Blocks ACh at the neuromuscular junction, which results in paralysis of the worm. The paralyzed worm is then expelled from the GI tract by normal peristalsis. | Ascariasis, enterobiasis, other helminthic infections |
| thiabendazole | Inhibits the helminth-specific enzyme fumarate reductase. | Cutaneous larva migrans (creeping eruption), strongyloidiasis, trichinosis |

*ACh,* Acetylcholine; *ATP,* adenosine triphosphate; *CNS,* central nervous system; *GI,* gastrointestinal.

## TABLE 43-11 ANTHELMINTICS: COMMON ADVERSE EFFECTS

| BODY SYSTEM | ADVERSE EFFECTS |
|-------------|-----------------|
| **Primaquine** | |
| Gastrointestinal | Nausea, vomiting, abdominal distress |
| Other | Headaches, pruritus, dark discoloration of urine, hemolytic anemia due to glucose-6-phosphate dehydrogenase deficiency |
| **Pyrantel** | |
| Central nervous system | Headache, dizziness, insomnia |
| Dermatologic | Skin rash |
| Gastrointestinal | Anorexia, abdominal cramps, diarrhea, nausea, vomiting |
| **Praziquantel** | |
| Central nervous system | Dizziness, headache, drowsiness |
| Gastrointestinal | Abdominal pain, nausea |
| Other | Malaise |

Histamine $H_2$ antagonists (e.g., cimetidine, ranitidine) may also raise blood levels of praziquantel.

## Dosages

For dosage information on selected anthelmintic drugs, see the table on p. 703.

## DRUG PROFILES

Anthelmintics are available only as oral preparations and, with the exception of pyrantel, all require a prescription. Different drugs are selected to treat infection with different helminthic species.

### praziquantel

Praziquantel (Biltricide) is one of the primary anthelmintic drugs used for the treatment of various fluke infections. It is also useful against many species of tapeworm. It is contraindicated in patients with ocular worm infestation (*ocular cysticercosis*). It is available only for oral use.

### Pharmacokinetics

| Route | Onset of Action | Peak Plasma Concentration | Elimination Half-life | Duration of Action |
|-------|-----------------|---------------------------|-----------------------|---------------------|
| PO | 1 hr | 1-3 hr | 4-5 hr | Variable |

### pyrantel

Pyrantel (Pin-X) is a pyrimidine-derived anthelmintic drug that is indicated for the treatment of infection with intestinal roundworms, including ascariasis, enterobiasis, and other helminthic infections. It is the only anthelmintic available in the United States without a prescription. It is available only for oral use.

### Pharmacokinetics

| Route | Onset of Action | Peak Plasma Concentration | Elimination Half-life | Duration of Action |
|-------|-----------------|---------------------------|-----------------------|---------------------|
| PO | 1 hr | 1-3 hr | Unknown | Unknown |

## NURSING PROCESS

## ASSESSMENT

Before beginning treatment with an *antimalarial drug,* obtain a thorough medication history, perform a head-to-toe physical assessment and measure vital signs. Give special attention to assessment findings of any common manifestations of malaria, such as headache, nausea, and joint pain. Other symptoms include chills and rigors followed by fever of up to 104° F (40° C) frequently leading to extreme fatigue and prolonged sleep. Baseline visual acuity tests may be needed due to the contraindications of visual field problems and optic

## DOSAGES

### Selected Anthelmintic Drugs

| DRUG (PREGNANCY CATEGORY) | PHARMACOLOGIC CLASS | USUAL DOSAGE RANGE | INDICATIONS |
|---|---|---|---|
| praziquantel (Biltricide) (B) | Trematode anthelmintic | **Adult and pediatric**<br>PO: approx 20-25 mg/kg 3 times daily × 1 day | Fluke infections |
| pyrantel (Pin-X) (C) | Nematode anthelmintic | **Adult and pediatric**<br>PO: 11 mg/kg in a single dose (max dose 1 g) | Roundworm infections |

*PO*, oral.

neuritis with chloroquine, quinine, and hydroxychoroquine. Perform a skin assessment as well, because of the contraindication with those individuals with psoriasis. Other drugs, such as mefloquine and primaquine, require assessment of baseline hearing and (with primaquine as well as pryimethamine) assessment of G6PD deficiency due to drug-induced hemolytic anemia. Common drug interactions to assess for are listed in Table 43-2.

*Antiprotozoal drugs* and their contraindications, cautions, and drug interactions have been previously discussed. Assess baseline renal and liver function as well as overall health status. With atovaquone, determine baseline blood counts due to risk of drug-induced anemia/neutropenia and leukopenia. Assess serum potassium, sodium, and glucose levels as ordered. With iodoquinol, it is important to assess blood counts prior to its use as well as baseline vision and neurologic intactness (e.g., presence of normal sensations). Metronidazole requires assessment for allergy to any of the nitroimidazole derivatives as well as to parabens (for the topical dosage forms). Obtain appropriate specimens for analysis before treatment. Assess blood counts, presence of central nervous system disorders or abnormalities, and bladder function prior to use of metronidazole. Pentamidine is associated with serious cardiac, hematologic, skin, renal, GI, and respiratory adverse effects; therefore, documentation of a thorough assessment of each of these systems is critical to patient safety.

With any of the *anthelmintic drugs,* obtain a thorough history of the foods eaten, especially meat and fish, and their means of preparation. Also assess other individuals in the family household for helminth infection. Obtaining stool specimens is indicated. Assess the patient's energy level, ability to perform activities of daily living, weight, and appetite. Document the findings. Assess for contraindications, such as liver disease and drug allergy, and any cautions. Drug interactions to assess for include theophylline, antiepileptic drugs, and histamine $H_2$ antagonists.

## NURSING DIAGNOSES

1. Imbalanced nutrition, less than body requirements, related to the disease process and adverse effects of medication
2. Deficient knowledge related to the infection and its drug treatment
3. Ineffective family therapeutic regimen management related to poor compliance with treatment and/or lack of knowledge about the infection and its treatment

## CASE STUDY

### Metronidazole

T.J., a 28-year-old graduate student, just returned from an archeology internship in a third-world country. She has had severe diarrhea for several days and has been diagnosed with intestinal amebiasis. She will receive fluids for rehydration and metronidazole (Flagyl) as part of her treatment.

1. What specific laboratory test must be ordered before initiation of the metronidazole therapy? List other laboratory studies that will be performed.
2. T.J. is started on the intravenous piggyback infusions, and after a day she reports that her diarrhea has decreased and that she feels a little better. During afternoon rounds, she tells the nurse that she feels dizzy and tired, and has some nausea. She asks, "Is this because of my infection?" How will the nurse respond?
3. T.J. is discharged to home with a prescription to take the metronidazole for 2 more weeks. The nurse knows that one serious adverse effect is leukopenia. What symptoms will the nurse tell T.J. to report?
4. A week later, T.J. calls to tell the nurse that she went out to a bar with some friends and became very ill after having a drink. Explain what happened.

For answers, see http://evolve.elsevier.com/Lilley.

## PLANNING

### GOALS

1. Patient maintains balanced nutrition during drug therapy.
2. Patient, family, and significant others demonstrate adequate knowledge regarding the infection and its treatment.
3. Patient, family, and others in the home environment experience improved therapeutic regimen management and compliance.as well as with family and others in the household.

### OUTCOME CRITERIA

1. Patient states measures to enhance balanced nutrition with recommendations for increased caloric and protein intake.
   - Patient identifies menu planning with grocery lists appropriate to meet increased nutritional demands.
   - Patient lists foods to be included in the daily diet with use of MyPlate to improve overall nutritional status along with prescribed dietary changes.
2. Patient states the impact of infectious process on the human body and its daily functioning.
   - Patient states the various measures to prevent worsening of lesions and minimize tissue injury, such as washing hands

thoroughly; reporting worsening of lesions and/or drainage, fever, or joint pain; and taking medication as prescribed.

- Patient states the importance and need for reporting the worsening of symptoms of the infection, such as fever, lethargy, and loss of appetite.
- Patient states the rationale for staying on treatment for the prescribed length of time.
- Patient states the importance of effective family therapeutic management through compliance with therapy, returning for follow-up visits to the prescriber to monitor progress, checking for adverse reactions and reporting any new symptoms in members of the household/family.

## IMPLEMENTATION

With *antimalarials*, encourage adequate dietary and fluid intake while the patient is fighting the infection and taking the medications. Take oral doses with at least 6 to 8 oz of water or other fluid. Increase fluids unless contraindicated. Because antimalarials concentrate in the liver first, emphasize to the patient the importance of follow-up visits to the prescriber so that liver function may be monitored during therapy.

Chloroquine and hydroxychloroquine are administered orally and are to be taken exactly as prescribed. Follow dosing orders and instructions as prescribed, with specific attention to the loading doses, subsequent doses, and prophylactic dosing. Photosensitivity may occur with quinine; provide adequate teaching about the use of sunscreen and sun safety. Sun protection must include coverage against UVA and UVB rays. See the Patient Teaching Tips for more information.

Most of the *antiprotozoal drugs* (e.g., atovaquone, metronidazole) are given with food when taken orally. Infuse intravenous doses of metronidazole as ordered. Intravenous (IV) doses are to infuse over 30 to 60 minutes and are never given as an IV bolus. During use of this drug, report to the prescriber any changes in neurologic status (e.g., dizziness, confusion).

All *anthelmintic drugs* are to be administered as ordered and for the prescribed length of time. Warn patients that use of primaquine may lead to dark discoloration of the urine. Perform collection of stool specimens as ordered. The stool must not be in contact with water, urine, or chemicals because of the risk of destroying the parasitic worms and/or altering the test results. See the Patient Teaching Tips for more information on these drugs.

## EVALUATION

Monitor the patient for the therapeutic effects of the *antimalarials, antiprotozoals, and anthelmintic* drugs such as improved energy levels and decrease in and/or eventual resolution of all symptoms. Evaluation of proper hygiene and prevention of the spread of the infestation or infection is also important. With these three groups of drugs, evaluate for the adverse effects associated with each type of drug (see Tables 43-1, 43-6, and 43-11). Some *antimalarials and anthelmintics* may precipitate hemolysis in patients with G6PD deficiency (mostly African-American patients and those of Mediterranean ancestry); therefore, closely monitor such patients for this complication during the treatment protocol. See Chapter 2 for further discussion of G6PD deficiency.

## PATIENT TEACHING TIPS

- Antimalarials are known to cause gastrointestinal upset; however, this may be decreased if the medication is taken with food. Encourage the patient to contact the prescriber if there is unresolved nausea, vomiting, profuse diarrhea, or abdominal pain. Report immediately any visual disturbances, dizziness, or respiratory difficulties.
- Educate the patient about the need for prophylactic doses of antimalarials, as prescribed, before visiting malaria-infested countries as well as the need to obtain appropriate treatment upon return.
- Keep antimalarials, like all other medications, out of the reach of children.
- Instruct the patient to take the entire course of medication as directed.
- Oral dosage forms of metronidazole to be taken with food.

- Inform the patient taking metronidazole for a sexually transmitted disease to avoid sexual intercourse until the prescriber states otherwise.
- When the patient is taking metronidazole for amebiasis, include in your instructions how to check stool samples correctly and safely and how to dispose of samples properly.
- Apply topical forms of the drug with a finger cot or gloved hand and caution the patient to avoid contact of the drug with the eyes.
- Metronidazole may precipitate dizziness. Encourage the patient to be cautious in all activities until a response to the drug is noted and is consistent.
- Anthelmintics are to be taken exactly as prescribed; emphasize the importance of compliance with the drug regimen.

## KEY POINTS

- Malaria is caused by *Plasmodium,* a particular genus of protozoans, and is transmitted by the bite of an infected female mosquito. The drug primaquine attacks the parasite when it is outside the exoerythrocytic (tissue) phase.
- Other common protozoal infections are amebiasis, giardiasis, toxoplasmosis, and trichomoniasis. Protozoans are parasites that are transmitted by person-to-person contact, ingestion of contaminated water or food, direct contact with the parasite, and the bite of an insect (mosquito or tick). Pneumocystosis is now classified as a fungal infection, but it is treated with antiprotozoal drugs.
- Antiprotozoals include atovaquone and pentamidine. Metronidazole is an antibacterial, antiprotozoal, and anthelmintic. The drugs iodoquinol and paromomycin directly kill protozoans such as *Entamoeba histolytica.*
- Anthelmintics are drugs used to treat parasitic worm infections caused by cestodes (tapeworms), nematodes (roundworms), and trematodes (flukes).
- Nursing considerations with the use of any of the antimalarials, antiprotozoals, and anthelmintics include assessment for contraindications, cautions, and drug interactions.

## NCLEX® EXAMINATION REVIEW QUESTIONS

1 The nurse is reviewing the medication history of a patient who is taking hydroxychloroquine. However, the patient's chart does not reveal a history of malaria or travel out of the country. The patient is most likely taking this medication for
   a *Plasmodium.*
   b thyroid disorders.
   c roundworms.
   d rheumatoid arthritis.

2 Which teaching point would be appropriate to include when the nurse is informing a patient about the adverse effects of antimalarials?
   a The skin may turn blotchy while these medications are taken.
   b These medications may cause anorexia and abdominal distress.
   c These medications may cause increased urinary output.
   d The patient may experience periods of diaphoresis and chills.

3 When teaching a patient about the potential drug interactions with antiprotozoal drugs, the nurse will include information about
   a acetaminophen.
   b warfarin.
   c decongestants.
   d antibiotics.

4 Before administering antiprotozoal drugs, the nurse will review which baseline assessment?
   a Complete blood count
   b Serum magnesium level
   c Creatinine clearance
   d Arterial blood gas concentrations

5 The nurse knows that antimalarial drugs are used to treat patients with infections caused by which microorganism?
   a *Plasmodium* spp.
   b *Candida albicans*
   c *Pneumocystis jirovecii*
   d *Mycobacterium*

6 When giving metronidazole, the nurse implements appropriate administration techniques, including which of these? (Select all that apply.)
   a Giving oral forms with food
   b Giving oral forms on an empty stomach with a full glass of water
   c Infusing intravenous doses over 30 to 60 minutes
   d Administering intravenous doses by bolus over 5 minutes
   e Obtaining ordered specimens before starting the medication

7 A 5-year-old patient has been diagnosed with malaria after returning from a trip. The patient is to receive one dose of mefloquine (Lariam), 25 mg/kg PO. The child weighs 44 lb. How much mefloquine will this child receive? Is this a safe dose?

1. d, 2. b, 3. b, 4. a, 5. a, 6. a, c, e, 7. 500 mg; yes

For Critical Thinking and Prioritization Questions, see http://evolve.elsevier.com/Lilley.

# Antiinflammatory and Antigout Drugs

## OBJECTIVES

When you reach the end of this chapter, you will be able to do the following:

1 Discuss the inflammatory response and the part it plays in the generation of pain.
2 Compare the disease processes or pathologies that are inflammatory in nature with those of gout.
3 Discuss the mechanisms of action, indications, adverse effects, dosage ranges, routes of administration, cautions,

contraindications, drug interactions, and toxicities of the various antiinflammatory and antigout drugs.
4 Develop a nursing care plan that includes all phases of the nursing process for patients receiving antiinflammatory and/or antigout drugs.

## DRUG PROFILES

- ♦ **allopurinol, p. 713**
- ♦ **aspirin, p. 712**
- ♦ **celecoxib, p. 713**
- **colchicine, p. 714**
- ♦ **ibuprofen, p. 712**

- ♦ **indomethacin, p. 712**
- ♦ **ketorolac, p. 712**
- **probenecid, p. 715**

---

♦ *Key drug*

## KEY TERMS

**Done nomogram** A standard data graph, originally published in 1960 in the journal *Pediatrics,* for rating the severity of aspirin toxicity following overdose. Serum salicylate levels are plotted against time elapsed since ingestion. (p. 710)

**Gout** Hyperuricemia (elevated blood uric acid level); the arthritis caused by tissue buildup of uric acid crystals. (p. 713)

**Inflammation** A localized protective response stimulated by injury to tissues that serves to destroy, dilute, or wall off (sequester) both the injurious agent and the injured tissue. (p. 707)

**Nonsteroidal antiinflammatory drugs (NSAIDs)** A large and chemically diverse group of drugs that possess analgesic, antiinflammatory, and antipyretic (fever-reducing) activity. (p. 707)

**Salicylism** The syndrome of salicylate toxicity, including symptoms such as tinnitus (ringing sound in the ears), nausea, and vomiting. (p. 710)

## ANATOMY, PHYSIOLOGY, AND PATHOPHYSIOLOGY OVERVIEW

Inflammation is defined as a localized protective response stimulated by injury to tissues, which serves to destroy, dilute, or wall off (sequester) both the injurious agent and the injured tissue. Classic signs and symptoms of inflammation include pain, fever, loss of function, redness, and swelling. These symptoms result from arterial, venous, and capillary dilation; enhanced blood flow and vascular permeability; exudation of fluids, including plasma proteins; and leukocyte migration into the inflammatory focus. The inflammatory response is mediated by a host of endogenous compounds, including proteins of the complement system, histamine, serotonin, bradykinin, leukotrienes, and prostaglandins, the latter two being major contributors to the symptoms of inflammation.

Arachidonic acid is released from phospholipids in cell membranes in response to a triggering event (e.g., an injury). It is metabolized in either the prostaglandin pathway or the leukotriene pathway, both of which are branches of the arachidonic acid pathway, as shown in Figure 44-1. Both of these pathways lead to inflammation, edema, headache, and other pain characteristic of the body's response to injury or inflammatory illnesses such as arthritis.

In the prostaglandin pathway, arachidonic acid is converted by the enzyme cyclooxygenase into various prostaglandins. Prostaglandins mediate inflammation by inducing vasodilation and enhancing vasopermeability. These effects in turn potentiate the action of proinflammatory substances such as histamine and bradykinin in the production of edema and pain. These symptoms arise as a result of prostaglandin-induced hyperalgesia (excessive sensitivity). In this situation, stimuli that normally would not be painful, such as simply moving a joint through its natural range of motion, become painful because of the inflammatory process at work. Fever occurs when prostaglandin $E_2$ is synthesized in the preoptic hypothalamic region, the area of the brain that regulates temperature.

The leukotriene pathway utilizes lipoxygenases to metabolize the arachidonic acid and convert it into various leukotrienes. Although leukotrienes are more newly discovered than prostaglandins and not as well studied, they are also mediators of inflammation, promoting vasoconstriction, bronchospasm, and increased vascular permeability with resultant edema (see Chapter 37).

## PHARMACOLOGY OVERVIEW

### NONSTEROIDAL ANTIINFLAMMATORY DRUGS

Nonsteroidal antiinflammatory drugs (NSAIDs) are among the most commonly prescribed drugs. Every year, over 70 million prescriptions are written for these drugs. This represents more than 5% of all prescriptions. Currently more than 23 different NSAIDs are available in the United States. Some of these are used much more commonly than others. A given patient may respond better to one NSAID than to others, in terms of both symptom relief and adverse effects.

NSAIDs comprise a large and chemically diverse group of drugs that possess analgesic, antiinflammatory, and antipyretic (antifever) activity. They are also used for the relief of mild to moderate headaches, myalgia, neuralgia, and arthralgia; alleviation of postoperative pain; relief of the pain associated with arthritic disorders such as rheumatoid arthritis, juvenile arthritis, ankylosing spondylitis, and osteoarthritis; and treatment of

**FIGURE 44-1** Arachidonic acid pathway. *PGI2,* Prostaglandin I$_2$; *PLT,* platelet; *TXA$_2$,* thromboxane A$_2$.

BOX 44-1   CHEMICAL CATEGORIES OF NSAIDs

**Salicylates**
aspirin
diflunisal (Dolobid)
salsalate (Salistab)
choline salicylate (Arthropan)

**Acetic Acid Derivatives**
diclofenac sodium (Voltaren)
indomethacin (Indocin)
sulindac (Clinoril)
tolmetin (Tolectin)
etodolac (Lodine)
ketorolac (Toradol)
meclofenamate (generic only)
mefenamic acid (Ponstel)

**Cyclooxygenase-2 Inhibitors**
celecoxib (Celebrex)

**Enolic Acid Derivatives**
nabumetone (Relafen)
meloxicam (Mobic)
piroxicam (Feldene)

**Propionic Acid Derivatives**
fenoprofen (Nalfon)
flurbiprofen (Ansaid)
ibuprofen (Motrin, Advil, others)
ketoprofen (Orudis KT)
naproxen (Naprosyn, Aleve)
oxaprozin (Daypro)

*NSAID,* Nonsteroidal antiinflammatory drug.

BOX 44-2   NSAIDs: FDA-APPROVED INDICATIONS

- Acute gout
- Acute gouty arthritis
- Ankylosing spondylitis
- Bursitis
- Fever
- Juvenile rheumatoid arthritis
- Mild to moderate pain
- Osteoarthritis
- Primary dysmenorrhea
- Rheumatoid arthritis
- Tendinitis
- Various ophthalmic uses

*FDA,* U.S. Food and Drug Administration; *NSAID,* nonsteroidal antiinflammatory drug.

gout and hyperuricemia (discussed later in the chapter). Aspirin is used for its effect in inhibiting platelet aggregation, which has been shown to have protective qualities against certain cardiovascular events such as myocardial infarction and stroke. Corticosteroid antiinflammatory drugs (e.g., prednisone, dexamethasone) are also used for similar purposes and were discussed in Chapter 33. NSAIDs have a generally more favorable adverse effect profile than the corticosteroid antiinflammatory drugs.

In 1899, acetylsalicylic acid (ASA; aspirin) was marketed and rapidly became the most widely used drug in the world. The success of aspirin established the importance of drugs with antipyretic, analgesic, and antiinflammatory properties—the properties that all NSAIDs share. The widespread use of aspirin also yielded evidence of its potential for causing major adverse effects. Gastrointestinal intolerance, bleeding, and renal impairment became major factors limiting its long-term administration. As a result, efforts were mounted to develop drugs that did not have the adverse effects of aspirin. This led to the discovery of other NSAIDs, which in general are associated with a lower incidence of and less serious adverse effects and are often better tolerated than aspirin in patients with chronic diseases. If aspirin were to be a newly discovered drug today, it would require a prescription.

As a single class, NSAIDs constitute an exceptional variety of drugs, and they are used for an equally wide range of indications. Box 44-1 categorizes these drugs into a number of distinct chemical classes. The NSAIDs have been approved for a variety of indications and are considered the drug of choice for most of the conditions listed in Box 44-2. Almost all NSAIDs are used for the treatment of rheumatoid arthritis (see Chapter 47) and degenerative joint disease (osteoarthritis). Several of these drugs are available in sustained-release formulations. This allows once- or twice-daily dosing, which is known to improve patients' adherence to prescribed drug therapy regimens.

## Mechanism of Action and Drug Effects
The NSAIDs work through inhibition of the leukotriene pathway, the prostaglandin pathway, or both. More specifically,

NSAIDs relieve pain, headache, and inflammation by blocking the chemical activity of the enzyme called *cyclooxygenase (COX)*. It is now recognized that there are at least two types of cyclooxygenase. Cyclooxygenase-1 (COX-1) is the isoform of the enzyme that promotes the synthesis of prostaglandins, which have primarily beneficial effects on various body functions. One example is their role in maintaining an intact gastrointestinal mucosa. In contrast, the cyclooxygenase-2 (COX-2) isoform promotes the synthesis of prostaglandins that are involved in inflammatory processes. In 1998, the newest class of NSAIDs, the COX-2 inhibitors, was approved. These drugs work by specifically inhibiting the COX-2 isoform of cyclooxygenase and theoretically have limited or no effects on COX-1. Previous NSAIDs nonspecifically inhibited both COX-1 and COX-2 activity. This greater enzyme specificity of the COX-2 inhibitors allows for the beneficial antiinflammatory effects while reducing the prevalence of adverse effects associated with the nonspecific NSAIDs, such as gastrointestinal ulceration. The leukotriene pathway is inhibited by some antiinflammatory drugs, but not by salicylates.

All NSAIDs can be ulcerogenic and induce gastrointestinal bleeding due to their activity against tissue COX-1. One notable effect of aspirin is its inhibition of platelet aggregation, also known as its *antiplatelet activity.* Aspirin has the unique property among NSAIDs of being an irreversible inhibitor of COX-1 receptors within the platelets themselves. This in turn results in reduced formation of thromboxane $A_2$, a substance that normally promotes platelet aggregation. This antiplatelet action has made aspirin, along with thrombolytic drugs (see Chapter 26), a primary drug in the treatment of acute myocardial infarction and many other thromboembolic disorders. Other NSAIDs lack these antiplatelet effects.

## Indications
Some of the therapeutic uses of this broad class of drugs are listed in Table 44-1; however, NSAIDs are primarily used for their analgesic, antiinflammatory, and antipyretic effects, and for platelet inhibition. NSAIDs are also widely used for the treatment of rheumatoid arthritis (see Chapter 47) and osteoarthritis, as well as other inflammatory conditions, rheumatic

| TABLE 44-1 | SUGGESTED NSAIDs FOR PATIENTS WITH VARIOUS MEDICAL CONDITIONS |
| --- | --- |
| **MEDICAL CONDITION** | **RECOMMENDED NSAID** |
| Ankylosing spondylitis | indomethacin, diclofenac |
| Diabetic neuropathy | sulindac |
| Dysmenorrhea | Fenamates, naproxen, ibuprofen |
| Gout | indomethacin, naproxen, sulindac |
| Headaches | aspirin, naproxen, ibuprofen |
| Hepatotoxicity | tolmetin, naproxen, ibuprofen, piroxicam, fenamates |
| History of aspirin or NSAID allergy | Avoid if possible; if deemed necessary, consider a nonacetylated salicylate |
| Hypertension | sulindac, nonacetylated salicylate, ibuprofen, etodolac |
| Osteoarthritis | diclofenac, oxaprozin, indomethacin |
| Risk for gastrointestinal toxicity | COX-2 inhibitors (celecoxib), nonacetylated salicylate, enteric-coated aspirin, diclofenac, nabumetone, etodolac, ibuprofen, oxaprozin |
| Risk for nephrotoxicity | sulindac, nonacetylated salicylate, nabumetone, etodolac, diclofenac, oxaprozin |
| Warfarin therapy | sulindac, tolmetin, naproxen, ibuprofen, oxaprozin |

*COX,* Cyclooxygenase; *NSAID,* nonsteroidal antiinflammatory drug.

| TABLE 44-2 | NSAIDs: ADVERSE EFFECTS |
| --- | --- |
| **BODY SYSTEM** | **ADVERSE EFFECTS** |
| Cardiovascular | Moderate to severe noncardiogenic pulmonary edema |
| Gastrointestinal | Dyspepsia, heartburn, epigastric distress, nausea, vomiting, anorexia, abdominal pain, gastrointestinal bleeding, mucosal lesions (erosions or ulcerations) |
| Hematologic | Altered hemostasis through effects on platelet function |
| Hepatic | Acute reversible hepatotoxicity |
| Renal | Reduction in creatinine clearance, acute tubular necrosis with renal failure |
| Other | Skin eruption, sensitivity reactions, tinnitus, hearing loss |

*NSAID,* Nonsteroidal antiinflammatory drug.

fever, mild to moderate pain, and acute gout. They also have proved beneficial as adjunctive pain relief medications in patients with chronic pain syndromes, such as pain from bone cancer and chronic back pain. For the relief of pain, NSAIDs are sometimes combined with an opioid (see Chapter 10). They tend to have an opioid-sparing effect when given together with opioids, because the drugs attack pain using two different mechanisms. This often allows less opioids to be used. Unlike opioids, NSAIDs show a ceiling effect that limits their effectiveness; that is, any further increase in the dosage beyond a certain level increases the risk for adverse effects without a corresponding increase in the therapeutic effect. In contrast, opioid dosages may be titrated almost indefinitely to increasingly higher levels, especially in terminally ill patients with severe pain.

The appropriate selection of an NSAID is a clinical judgment based on consideration of the patient's history, including any previous medical conditions; the intended use of the drug; the patient's previous experience with NSAIDs; the patient's preference; and the cost.

## Contraindications

Contraindications to NSAIDs include known drug allergy and conditions that place the patient at risk for bleeding, such as rhinitis (risk for epistaxis [nosebleed]), vitamin K deficiency, and peptic ulcer disease. Patients with documented aspirin allergy must not receive NSAIDs. Other common contraindications are those that apply to most drugs and include severe renal or hepatic disease. NSAIDs are generally categorized as pregnancy category C drugs for use during the first two trimesters of pregnancy but are categorized as pregnancy category D (not recommended) for use during the third trimester. This is because NSAID use has been associated with both excessive maternal bleeding and neonatal toxicity during the perinatal period. These drugs also are not recommended for nursing mothers, because they are known to be excreted into human milk. Because of the potential of NSAIDs to increase bleeding, patients undergoing elective surgery need to stop taking NSAIDs at least 1 week prior to surgery.

## Adverse Effects

Although NSAIDs are the most widely used class of drugs, and some are available without prescription, their potential for serious adverse events has been underemphasized. Over 100,000 hospitalizations occur each year due to NSAID use, with over 16,000 deaths reported annually. One of the more common and potentially serious adverse effects of the NSAIDs is their effect on the gastrointestinal tract. Symptoms can range from mild symptoms such as heartburn to the most severe gastrointestinal complication, gastrointestinal bleeding. Most fatalities associated with NSAID use are related to gastrointestinal bleeding. In addition, acute renal failure is quite common with NSAID use, especially if the patient is dehydrated. The potential adverse effects of NSAIDs are listed in Table 44-2. Not all of the adverse effects necessarily apply to all drugs, but many do. In 2006, the U.S. Food and Drug Administration (FDA) began requiring a black box warning on all of the NSAIDs (see Box 44-3).

Many of the adverse effects of NSAIDs are secondary to their inactivation of protective prostaglandins that help maintain the normal integrity of the stomach lining. The drug misoprostol (Cytotec) (see Chapter 50) has proved successful in preventing the gastric ulcers and hence gastrointestinal bleeding that can occur in patients receiving NSAIDs. Misoprostol is a synthetic prostaglandin $E_1$ analogue that inhibits gastric acid secretion and also has a cytoprotective component, although the mechanism responsible for this action is unclear. This drug also has abortifacient properties, which were discussed in Chapter 34.

Renal function depends partly on prostaglandins. Disruption of prostaglandin function by NSAIDs is sometimes strong enough to precipitate acute or chronic renal failure, depending on the patient's current level of renal function. The use of NSAIDs can compromise existing renal function. Renal toxicity can occur in patients who are dehydrated, those with heart failure or liver dysfunction, and those taking diuretics or angiotensin-converting enzyme inhibitors.

## BOX 44-3 FDA REQUIRED WARNINGS ON ALL NSAIDs

The following black box warning must now be included in the packaging for all NSAIDs:

**Cardiovascular Risk**
- NSAIDs may cause an increased risk of serious cardiovascular thrombotic events, myocardial infarction, and stroke, which can be fatal. This risk may increase with duration of use. Patients with cardiovascular disease or risk factors for cardiovascular disease may be at greater risk.
- NSAIDs are contraindicated for the treatment of perioperative pain in the setting of coronary artery bypass graft surgery.

**Gastrointestinal Risk**
- NSAIDs cause an increased risk of serious gastrointestinal adverse events, including bleeding, ulceration, and perforation of the stomach or intestines, which can be fatal. These events can occur at any time during use and without warning symptoms. Elderly patients are at greater risk for serious gastrointestinal events.
- See Chapter 4 for more information on black box warnings.

*FDA,* U.S. Food and Drug Administration; *NSAID,* nonsteroidal antiinflammatory drug.

## TABLE 44-3 ACUTE OR CHRONIC SALICYLATE INTOXICATION: SIGNS AND SYMPTOMS

| BODY SYSTEM | SIGNS AND SYMPTOMS |
|---|---|
| Cardiovascular | Increased heart rate |
| Central nervous | Tinnitus, hearing loss, dimness of vision, headache, dizziness, mental confusion, lassitude, drowsiness |
| Gastrointestinal | Nausea, vomiting, diarrhea |
| Metabolic | Sweating, thirst, hyperventilation, hypoglycemia or hyperglycemia |

## Toxicity and Management of Overdose

Salicylate toxicity, usually from aspirin, is not as common as it was; however, there are both chronic and acute manifestations of salicylate toxicity. Chronic salicylate intoxication is also known as salicylism and results from either short-term administration of high dosages or prolonged therapy with high or even lower dosages. The most common signs and symptoms of acute or chronic salicylate intoxication are listed in Table 44-3.

The most common manifestations of chronic salicylate intoxication in adults are tinnitus and hearing loss. Those in children are hyperventilation and central nervous system (CNS) effects such as dizziness, drowsiness, and behavioral changes. Metabolic complications such as metabolic acidosis and respiratory alkalosis often occur to varying degrees in cases of chronic salicylate intoxication. Metabolic acidosis can also occur with acute intoxication, but it is usually less severe than that in patients with chronic intoxication. Hypoglycemia may also arise and can be life-threatening. The treatment of chronic intoxication is based on the presenting symptoms.

The signs and symptoms of acute salicylate toxicity are similar to those of chronic intoxication, but the effects are often more pronounced and occur more quickly. Acute salicylate overdose

## TABLE 44-4 ACUTE SALICYLATE INTOXICATION: TREATMENT

| SEVERITY | TREATMENT |
|---|---|
| Mild | 1. Dosage reduction or discontinuation of salicylates |
| | 2. Symptomatic and supportive therapy |
| Severe | 1. Discontinuation of salicylates |
| | 2. Intensive symptomatic and supportive therapy |
| | 3. Dialysis if: high salicylate levels, unresponsive acidosis (pH less than 7.1), impaired renal function or renal failure, pulmonary edema, persistent CNS symptoms (e.g., seizures, coma), progressive deterioration despite appropriate therapy |

*CNS,* Central nervous system.

usually results from the ingestion of a single toxic dose, and its severity can be judged based on the estimated amount ingested (in milligrams per kilogram of body weight), as follows:
- Little or no toxicity: less than 150 mg/kg
- Mild to moderate toxicity: 150 to 300 mg/kg
- Severe toxicity: 300 to 500 mg/kg
- Life-threatening toxicity: over 500 mg/kg

However, doses lower than 150 mg/kg have resulted in fatal toxicity. A serum salicylate concentration measured 6 hours or longer after the ingestion may be used in conjunction with the Done nomogram to estimate the severity of intoxication and help guide treatment. The Done nomogram is a graphic plot of serum salicylate level as a function of time since salicylate ingestion. It was first published in a 1960 issue of the journal *Pediatrics* and is still used today for gauging salicylate toxicity. This nomogram is intended for estimating only the severity of acute intoxications and not the severity of chronic salicylate intoxication. Table 44-4 describes, in general terms, the treatment for cases of varying severity. Treatment goals include removing salicylate from the gastrointestinal tract and/or preventing its further absorption; correcting fluid, electrolyte, and acid-base disturbances; and implementing measures to enhance salicylate elimination, including hemodialysis.

An acute overdose of nonsalicylate NSAIDs (e.g., ibuprofen) causes effects similar to those of salicylate overdose, but they are generally not as extensive or as dangerous. Symptoms include CNS toxicities such as drowsiness, lethargy, mental confusion, paresthesias (abnormal touch sensations), numbness, aggressive behavior, disorientation, and seizures, and gastrointestinal toxicities such as nausea, vomiting, and gastrointestinal bleeding. Intense headache, dizziness, cerebral edema, cardiac arrest, and death have also been known to occur in extreme cases. Treatment consists of the administration of activated charcoal, with supportive and symptomatic treatment initiated thereafter. Unlike in the case of salicylates, hemodialysis appears to be of no value in enhancing the elimination of nonsalicylate NSAIDs.

## Interactions

Drug interactions associated with the use of salicylates and other NSAIDs can result in significant complications and morbidity. Some of the more common of these are listed in Table 44-5.

## TABLE 44-5 SALICYLATES AND OTHER NSAIDs: DRUG INTERACTIONS

| INTERACTING DRUG | MECHANISM | RESULT |
|---|---|---|
| Alcohol | Additive effect | Increased gastrointestinal bleeding |
| Anticoagulants | Platelet inhibition, hypoprothrombinemia | Increased bleeding tendencies |
| aspirin and other salicylates with other NSAIDs | Reduction of NSAID absorption, additive gastrointestinal toxicities | Increased gastrointestinal toxicity with no therapeutic advantage |
| Bisphosphonates | Additive GI toxicities | Increased GI bleeding risk |
| Corticosteroids and other ulcerogenic drugs | Additive toxicities | Increased ulcerogenic effects |
| cyclosporine | Inhibition of renal prostaglandin synthesis | Increased nephrotoxic effects of cyclosporine, renal failure |
| Diuretics and ACE inhibitors | Inhibition of prostaglandin synthesis | Reduced hypotensive and diuretic effects |
| lithium | Increased lithium absorption | Increased lithium concentrations |
| Protein-bound drugs | Competition for binding | More pronounced drug actions |
| Uricosurics | Antagonism | Decreased uric acid excretion |
| Herbals: feverfew, garlic, ginger, gingko | Interference with platelet function | Increased bleeding risk |

*ACE*, Angiotensin-converting enzyme; *GI*, gastrointestinal; *NSAID*, nonsteroidal antiinflammatory drug.

## DOSAGES

### Most Commonly Used NSAIDs

| DRUG (PREGNANCY CATEGORY*) | PHARMACOLOGIC CLASS | USUAL DOSAGE RANGE | INDICATIONS |
|---|---|---|---|
| ◆ aspirin (ASA; many product names) (C/D) | Salicylate | **Adult**<br>PO/PR: 325-650 mg 4-6 times daily (max 4 g/day)<br>PO/PR: 3 g/day divided q4-6h<br>PO: 81-325 mg once daily<br>PO/PR: 90-130 mg/kg/day | Fever, pain<br>Arthritis<br>Thromboprevention<br>Juvenile rheumatoid arthritis |
| ◆ celecoxib (Celebrex) (C/D) | COX-2 inhibitor | **Adult and adolescent older than 15 yr**<br>PO: 100-200 mg/day given in 1 or 2 doses<br><br>**Pediatric**<br>Less than 25 kg: 50 mg twice daily<br>More than 25 kg: 100 mg twice daily | Arthritis, acute pain, primary dysmenorrhea<br><br>Juvenile rheumatoid arthritis |
| ◆ ibuprofen (Motrin, Advil, others) (C/D) | Propionic acid derivative | **Adult**<br>1200-3200 mg/day divided 3-4 times daily<br>**Pediatric**<br>30-40 mg/kg/day divided 3-4 times daily | Arthritis, fever, pain, dysmenorrhea |
| ◆ indomethacin (Indocin, Indocin SR) (C/D) | Acetic acid derivative | **Adult**<br>PO/PR: 25-50 mg 2-3 times daily (max 200 mg/day)<br>**Pediatric**<br>PO/PR: 1-2 mg/kg/day divided 2-4 times daily (max 200 mg/day) | Arthritis, including acute gouty arthritis, bursitis or tendonitis |
| ◆ ketorolac (Toradol) (C/D) | Acetic acid derivative | **Adult†**<br>PO‡: 10 mg q4-6h (max 40 mg/day)<br>IV/IM: 15-60 mg q6-12h (max 120 mg/day if younger than 65 yr; max 60 mg/day if 65 yr or older)<br>Maximum treatment 5 days | Acute painful conditions that would otherwise require opioid-level analgesia |

*ASA*, Acetylsalicylic acid; *COX*, cyclooxygenase; *IM*, intramuscular; *IV*, intravenous; *NSAID*, nonsteroidal antiinflammatory drug; *PO*, oral; *PR*, rectal; *SR*, sustained release.
*Pregnancy category C/D = C, first trimester; D, third trimester.
†Pediatric dosing guidelines are not as well established, but the recommended range for IV, IM, or PO use is 0.4 to 1 mg/kg as a single dose for acute conditions (e.g., sports injury).
‡PO form is recommended only when transitioning from injectable form to oral form of ketorolac.

NSAIDs can also interfere with laboratory test results. Specifically, salicylates can cause what are usually minor and transient elevations in the levels of liver enzymes (ALT, AST), but, unlike with acetaminophen (see Chapter 10), cases of severe hepatotoxicity are rare. Hematocrit, hemoglobin level, and RBC count can drop if any drug-induced gastrointestinal bleeding does occur, and bleeding time may be prolonged. NSAID-induced hyperkalemia or hyponatremia can also occur.

## Dosages

For dosage information on selected NSAIDs, see the table on this page.

# DRUG PROFILES

## SALICYLATES

Aspirin is the most commonly used of all salicylates. Although aspirin is available over the counter, many of the other salicylate drugs do require a prescription. These include diflunisal (Dolobid), choline magnesium trisalicylate (Trilisate), and salsalate (Salsitab). Salicylates are most commonly used in solid oral dosage forms (i.e., tablets, capsules). Other available dosage forms include a topical cream (Aspercreme), rectal suppositories, and oral liquids. Aspirin is also contained in many combination products, including aspirin/acetaminophen/caffeine combinations such as Excedrin and aspirin/antacid combinations (e.g., Bufferin). Aspirin also is available in special dosage forms, such as enteric-coated aspirin (Ecotrin), designed to protect the stomach mucosa by dissolving in the duodenum.

### ♦ aspirin

Aspirin is known chemically as acetylsalicylic acid (ASA). It is the prototype salicylate and NSAID and is the most widely used drug in the world. A daily aspirin tablet (81 mg or 325 mg) is now routinely recommended as prophylactic therapy for adults who have strong risk factors for developing coronary artery disease or stroke, even if they have no previous history of such an event. The 81-mg strength (which is traditionally thought of as "children's" aspirin) and the 325-mg strength appear to be equally beneficial for the prevention of thrombotic events. For this reason, the lower strength is often chosen for patients who have any elevated risk for bleeding, such as those with previous stroke history or history of peptic ulcer disease and those taking the anticoagulant warfarin (Coumadin). Aspirin is also often used to treat the pain associated with headache, neuralgia, myalgia, and arthralgia, as well as other pain syndromes resulting from inflammation. These include arthritis, pleurisy, and pericarditis. Patients with systemic lupus erythematosus may also benefit from aspirin therapy because of its antirheumatic effects. Aspirin is also used for its antipyretic action.

Aspirin and other salicylates all have one very specific contraindication. This drug class is contraindicated in children with flulike symptoms, because the use of these drugs has been strongly associated with Reye's syndrome. This is an acute and potentially life-threatening condition involving progressive neurologic deficits that can lead to coma and may also involve liver damage. It is believed to be triggered by viral illnesses such as influenza as well as by salicylate therapy itself, in the presence of a viral illness. Survivors of this condition may or may not suffer permanent neurologic damage.

### Pharmacokinetics

| Route | Onset of Action | Peak Plasma Concentration | Elimination Half-life | Duration of Action |
|-------|-----------------|---------------------------|------------------------|---------------------|
| PO | 15-30 min | 1-2 hr | 5-9 hr | 4-6 hr |

## ACETIC ACID DERIVATIVES

There are several acetic acid derivatives, and they are listed in Table 44-1. Indomethacin and ketorolac are the most commonly used.

### ♦ indomethacin

Like the other NSAIDs, indomethacin (Indocin) has analgesic, antiinflammatory, antirheumatic, and antipyretic properties. Its therapeutic actions are of particular use in the treatment of rheumatoid arthritis, osteoarthritis, acute bursitis or tendonitis, ankylosing spondylitis, and acute gouty arthritis. The drug is available for both oral and rectal use. An injectable form of the drug is also used intravenously (IV) to promote closure of patent ductus arteriosus, a heart defect that sometimes occurs in premature infants. It is also used for the treatment of preterm labor (see Chapter 34).

### Pharmacokinetics

| Route | Onset of Action | Peak Plasma Concentration | Elimination Half-life | Duration of Action |
|-------|-----------------|---------------------------|------------------------|---------------------|
| PO | 30 min | 2 hr | 4.5 hr | 4-6 hr |

### ♦ ketorolac

Ketorolac (Toradol) is somewhat unique in that, although it does have some antiinflammatory activity, it is used primarily for its powerful analgesic effects. Its analgesic effects are comparable to those of narcotic drugs such as morphine, which can make it a desirable choice for opiate-addicted patients who have acute pain control needs, because ketorolac lacks the addictive properties of the opioids. Ketorolac is indicated for the treatment of moderate to severe acute pain such as that resulting from orthopedic injuries or surgery. Ketorolac can be given orally or by injection, and there is also a dosage form for ophthalmic use (see Chapter 57). It is available only by prescription. It is indicated for short-term use (up to 5 days) to manage moderate to severe acute pain. It is not indicated for treatment of minor pain or chronic pain. The main adverse effects of ketorolac include renal impairment, edema, gastrointestinal pain, dyspepsia, and nausea. It is important to note that the drug can only be used for 5 days, because of its potential adverse effects on the kidney and gastrointestinal tract.

### Pharmacokinetics

| Route | Onset of Action | Peak Plasma Concentration | Elimination Half-life | Duration of Action |
|-------|-----------------|---------------------------|------------------------|---------------------|
| IV/IM | 0.5 hr | 1-2 hr | 5-7 hr | 4-6 hr |

## PROPIONIC ACID DERIVATIVES

### ♦ ibuprofen

Ibuprofen (Motrin, Advil) is the prototype NSAID in the propionic acid category, which also includes fenoprofen, flurbiprofen, ketoprofen, naproxen, and oxaprozin. Ibuprofen is the most commonly used of the propionic acid drugs because of the numerous indications for its use and because of its relatively safe adverse effect profile. It is often used for its analgesic effects in the management of rheumatoid arthritis, osteoarthritis, primary dysmenorrhea, gout, dental pain, and musculoskeletal disorders; in addition, it is used for its antipyretic actions. Naproxen is the second most commonly used NSAID, with a reportedly somewhat better adverse effect profile than ibuprofen, as well as fewer drug interactions with angiotensin-converting enzyme inhibitors given for hypertension. Both drugs are available for oral use in both over-the-counter and prescription strengths. In 2011, an injectable form of ibuprofen became available.

### Pharmacokinetics

| Route | Onset of Action | Peak Plasma Concentration | Elimination Half-life | Duration of Action |
|---|---|---|---|---|
| PO | 30-60 min (analgesic) 7 days (anti-inflammatory) | 1-2 hr | 2-4 hr | 4-6 hr |

### CYCLOOXYGENASE-2 INHIBITORS

The COX-2 inhibitors were developed primarily to decrease the gastrointestinal adverse effects characteristic of other NSAIDs because of their COX-2 selectivity. However, they are not totally devoid of gastrointestinal toxicity. Gastritis and upper gastrointestinal bleeding have been reported with their use, although much less frequently than with the older NSAIDs. Originally there were three COX-2 inhibitors; however, because the use of rofecoxib (Vioxx) and valdecoxib (Bextra) was found to be associated with an increased risk for adverse cardiovascular events, including myocardial infarction, stroke, and death, they were removed from the U.S. market.

#### ♦ celecoxib

Celecoxib (Celebrex) was the first COX-2 inhibitor and is the only one remaining on the market. It is indicated for the treatment of osteoarthritis, rheumatoid arthritis, acute pain symptoms, ankylosing spondylitis, and primary dysmenorrhea. It is available only for oral use. There is evidence that celecoxib may pose a risk of cardiovascular events similar to that associated with rofecoxib and valdecoxib. However, there is inconsistency in the literature regarding the true potential for these effects. Celecoxib currently remains on the U.S. market, although its use is now being monitored more closely by the FDA. Other adverse effects associated with celecoxib include headache, sinus irritation, diarrhea, fatigue, dizziness, lower extremity edema, and hypertension. COX-2 inhibitors have little effect on platelet function. Celecoxib is not to be used in patients with known sulfa allergy.

### Pharmacokinetics

| Route | Onset of Action | Peak Plasma Concentration | Elimination Half-life | Duration of Action |
|---|---|---|---|---|
| PO | 1 hr | 3 hr | 11 hr | 4-8 hr |

### ENOLIC ACID DERIVATIVES

The enolic acid derivatives include piroxicam, meloxicam, and nabumetone. Piroxicam and meloxicam are very potent drugs that are commonly used in the treatment of mild to moderate osteoarthritis, rheumatoid arthritis, and gouty arthritis. Both are available only in oral dosage formulations and have contraindications similar to those of the other NSAIDs.

Nabumetone (Relafen) is better tolerated than some of the others in terms of gastrointestinal adverse effects. It is relatively nonacidic compared with most of the other NSAIDs, which may account for its improved gastrointestinal tolerance. Currently it is indicated only for the treatment of osteoarthritis and rheumatoid arthritis.

## ANTIGOUT DRUGS

**Gout** is caused by the overproduction of uric acid or decreased uric acid excretion, or both. This overproduction and/or decreased excretion can often result in hyperuricemia (too much uric acid in the blood). Persons with gout either overproduce or underexcrete uric acid. When the body contains too much uric acid, deposits of uric acid crystals collect in tissues and joints. This causes an inflammatory response and extreme pain, because these crystals are like small needles that jab and stick into sensitive tissues and joints, which is an end product of purine metabolism. Purines are part of the normal dietary intake and are used to make the essential structural units of deoxyribonucleic acid (DNA) and ribonucleic acid (RNA). During purine metabolism, they are converted from hypoxanthine to xanthine and eventually to uric acid. The normal pathway for purine metabolism is depicted in Figure 44-2. This pathway is overactive in patients with gout and is reduced by antigout drug therapy. The goals of gout treatment are to decrease the symptoms of an acute attack and to prevent recurrent attacks.

## DRUG PROFILES

Although specific antigout drugs are available, the NSAIDs (described earlier) are considered first-line therapy for most patients with gout. The specific antigout drugs—allopurinol, febuxostat, colchicine, probenecid, and sulfinpyrazone—are targeted at the underlying defect in uric acid metabolism, which causes either overproduction or underexcretion of uric acid (see Figure 44-2). Both of these pathologic processes lead to tissue accumulations of uric acid crystalline deposits (gouty deposits) and symptoms of gout. Not all gouty deposits occur within joints. Gouty arthritis is the condition in which one or more joints are inflamed due to the collection of gouty deposits inside the joint anatomy. This is also called *articular gout*, whereas gout that occurs in tissues outside of the joints is called *abarticular gout.*

#### ♦ allopurinol

The beneficial effect of allopurinol (Zyloprim) in the relief of gout is the inhibition of the enzyme xanthine oxidase, which thereby prevents uric acid production. Allopurinol is indicated for patients whose gout is caused by the excess production of uric acid (hyperuricemia). Oxypurinol, a metabolite of allopurinol, also prevents uric acid production. Oxypurinol is available as an orphan drug for patients with hyperuricemia who are intolerant of allopurinol therapy. Allopurinol is also used to prevent acute tumor lysis syndrome (see Chapter 45).

Allopurinol is contraindicated in patients with a hypersensitivity to it. Significant adverse effects of the drug include agranulocytosis, aplastic anemia, and serious and potentially fatal

## PATIENT-CENTERED CARE: LIFESPAN CONSIDERATIONS FOR THE PEDIATRIC PATIENT

### Reye's Syndrome

Reye's syndrome is associated with the administration of aspirin to children and teenagers and is a potentially life-threatening illness. Encephalopathy and liver damage are two of the serious complications resulting from Reye's syndrome, which usually occurs after a viral infection such as chickenpox or influenza B, during which time aspirin is often given to decrease fever. To reduce the risk for Reye's syndrome, aspirin or medications that contain aspirin must not be given to children or teenagers to treat viral illnesses or fever. Other names for aspirin include acetylsalicylic acid, acetylsalicylate, salicylic acid, and salicylate. Other drugs that can be used instead of aspirin to reduce fever and relieve pain include acetaminophen and ibuprofen. Check the label on any medication that is to be given to a child, because aspirin is contained in many over-the-counter drugs, for example, Alka-Seltzer, some Excedrin products, and Pepto-Bismol.

### Signs and Symptoms of Reye's Syndrome
- Altered liver function
- Encephalopathy and fatty degeneration of the viscera, primarily in children and teenagers
- Changes in level of consciousness
- Coma, flaccid paralysis, loss of deep tendon reflexes
- Hypoglycemia
- Seizures
- Vomiting

### Medical Management
- Provide supportive treatment in intensive care unit
- Maintain life functions, restore metabolic balance, and control cerebral edema

- Administer intravenous glucose (10% or higher) for treatment of hypoglycemia
- Monitor blood glucose level; insulin may be needed
- Administer vitamin K for clotting problems
- Give fresh frozen plasma if needed for significant bleeding
- Provide prophylactic antiepileptic drugs
- Monitor intracranial pressure
- Initiate cautious fluid administration
- Administer osmotic diuretics with steroids if needed to treat cerebral edema

### Nursing Management
- Critical care setting often indicated for care of these patients
- Assess neurologic status, vital signs, and arterial and central venous pressures
- Monitor blood gas concentrations and intracranial pressure as ordered
- Control temperature to prevent elevations and increased $O_2$ demands
- Elevate the head of the bed
- Monitor intake and output
- Initiate hyperventilation (if patient is intubated and if ordered) to reduce intracranial pressure by lowering $CO_2$ levels and increasing $O_2$ levels
- Provide a quiet environment
- Handle gently
- Monitor for seizure activity
- Provide family support during critical phase of the illness
- Provide physical and emotional support for the child and family with recovery
- Ensure appropriate spiritual care
- Educate the public about Reye's syndrome and its life-threatening complications

Data from Mayo Foundation for Medical Education and Research: Reye's syndrome, September 17, 2011. Available at www.mayoclinic.com/health/reyes-syndrome/DS00142. Accessed October 14, 2011.

**FIGURE 44-2** Uric acid production. *XO*, Xanthine oxidase.

skin conditions such as exfoliative dermatitis, Stevens-Johnson syndrome, and toxic epidermal necrolysis. Azathioprine and mercaptopurine both significantly interact with allopurinol, and, as a result, their dosages may have to be adjusted. Allopurinol is available only for oral use. The usual recommended adult dosage is 200 to 600 mg/day, and the maximum dosage is 800 mg/day. It is categorized as a pregnancy category C drug.

The new drug febuxostat (Uloric) is non-purine selective inhibitor of xanthine oxidase. It is the first new drug approved for the treatment of gout since the 1960s. It is more selective for xanthine oxidase than allopurinol and may pose a greater risk of cardiovascular events than allopurinol. It is not to be given along with theophylline, azathioprine, or mercaptopurine. It is dosed as 40 to 80 mg/day, with a maximum dose of 120 mg/day.

### Pharmacokinetics

| Route | Onset of Action | Peak Plasma Concentration | Elimination Half-life | Duration of Action |
|---|---|---|---|---|
| PO | 1-2 wk | 30-120 min | 18-30 hr | Unknown |

### colchicine

Colchicine is the oldest available therapy for acute gout and is considered second-line therapy, after the NSAIDs. Colchicine appears to be effective in the treatment of gout by reducing the inflammatory response to the deposits of urate crystals in joint tissue. Its mechanism of action is not clearly defined, but it is thought to inhibit the metabolism, mobility, and chemotaxis of polymorphonuclear leukocytes. Chemotaxis is the chemical attraction of leukocytes to the site of inflammation, which worsens an inflammatory response.

Colchicine is a powerful inhibitor of cell mitosis and can cause short-term leukopenia. For this reason, it is generally used for the short-term treatment of acute attacks of gout. However, it may be used for prophylaxis of acute attacks in dosages of 0.6 mg once or twice a day. The more severe adverse effects can include bleeding into the gastrointestinal or urinary tracts, and the drug needs to be stopped if such effects appear. Colchicine is contraindicated in patients with a known hypersensitivity to it and in those with severe renal, gastrointestinal, hepatic, or cardiac disorders, and blood dyscrasias. There is no specific antidote for colchicine poisoning. The drug is available in oral forms only. Until 2008, it was also available in an injectable form, but at that time the FDA asked that it no longer be manufactured in or shipped to the United States, because of the potential for life-threatening adverse effects. In 2010, the FDA required the withdrawal of all "unapproved" colchicine products that had been used for decades. Currently, there is only one FDA-approved colchicine product, Colcrys, which is an oral tablet.

For acute gout, colchicine is given in an initial dose of 0.6 to 1.2 mg, followed by 0.6 mg/hr until pain is relieved, the patient develops severe nausea and diarrhea, or a total of 6 mg has been administered. Some clinicians choose to limit the cumulative dose to 3 mg. When colchicine is used for treatment of acute gout, 3 days must pass before a second course of therapy is initiated. Colchicine dosage must be reduced with renal impairment. It is categorized as a pregnancy category D drug.

## Pharmacokinetics

| Route | Onset of Action | Peak Plasma Concentration | Elimination Half-life | Duration of Action |
|---|---|---|---|---|
| PO | 12 hr | 0.5-2 hr | 12-30 min | 12 hr |

### probenecid

Probenecid (generic) inhibits the reabsorption of uric acid in the kidney and thus increases the excretion of uric acid. Drugs that promote uric acid excretion are known as *uricosurics*. In some patients, gout is due to the underexcretion of uric acid. Probenecid works by binding to the special transporter protein in the proximal convoluted renal tubule that takes uric acid from the urine and places it back into the blood. The probenecid is then reabsorbed back into the bloodstream while the uric acid remains in the urine and is excreted. Besides being used to treat the hyperuricemia associated with gout and gouty arthritis, it also has the ability to delay the renal excretion of penicillin, which increases the serum levels of penicillin and prolongs its effect (see Chapter 38). Probenecid is available as a 500-mg oral tablet. The usual adult dosage is 250 mg twice a day with food, milk, or antacids for 1 week, followed by 500 mg twice daily thereafter. This dosage may be adjusted as needed to maintain desirable serum uric acid levels. Contraindications include peptic ulcer disease and blood dyscrasias. Probenecid is ineffective and is not to be used in patients with renal impairment. It is categorized as a pregnancy category B drug.

## Pharmacokinetics

| Route | Onset of Action | Peak Plasma Concentration | Elimination Half-life | Duration of Action |
|---|---|---|---|---|
| PO | 1 hr | 3 hr | 3-17 hr | 8 hr |

# NURSING PROCESS

## ASSESSMENT

Prior to giving an *antiinflammatory, antigout,* and/or related drugs, it is critical to patient safety and drug effectiveness to assess for drug allergies, contraindications, cautions, and drug interactions associated with each drug in these major groups. Before administering antiinflammatory drugs, perform a thorough head-to-toe physical assessment, measure vital signs, perform a nursing assessment, and take a thorough medication history, noting any prescription, over-the-counter, herbal, and/or alternative drugs that the patient is taking. Analyze results of laboratory tests reflecting hematologic, renal, and hepatic functioning before initiation of therapy as ordered, especially if long-term use is indicated. These tests will most likely include RBC count, hemoglobin level, hematocrit, WBC count, platelet count, BUN level, and liver enzyme levels such as ALP, AST, and LDH. If NSAIDs are used short-term for other conditions (e.g., fever, acute pain), laboratory studies are not usually indicated since these drugs are available over the counter and are self-administered.

With aspirin, NSAIDs, other *antiinflammatory* drugs, and *antigout* drugs, assess and document the duration, onset, location, and type of inflammation and/or pain the patient is experiencing as well as any precipitating, exacerbating, or relieving factors. Note any interference of the symptoms with the patient's ability to perform activities of daily living (ADLs). Inspect all joints with attention to deformities, immobility or limitations in mobility, overlying skin condition, and presence of any heat or swelling over the joint. Age is important to assess because aspirin and many of the other NSAIDs are not to be used in children and teenagers due to the increased risk for Reye's syndrome (see the Patient-Centered Care: Lifespan Considerations for the Pediatric Patient box on p. 714). These drugs are to be used very cautiously in elderly patients. Assessing the odor of aspirin is also important because a vinegary odor is associated with a chemical breakdown of the drug. With aspirin, assess the patient for a history of asthma, wheezing, or other respiratory problems because of the increased incidence of allergic reactions to aspirin in these individuals. With aspirin, identify patients who have been diagnosed with what is called the *aspirin triad,* which includes asthma, nasal polyps, and rhinitis. These conditions are considered to put the patient at risk for reactions to aspirin. Other contraindications, cautions, and drug interactions for aspirin and other NSAIDs have been discussed previously. Remember that salicylic acid or aspirin and other NSAIDs have antiinflammatory, antipyretic, analgesic, and antiplatelet activity but also carry a risk for ulcerogenic and gastrointestinal bleeding adverse effects. NSAIDs carry the risk for acute reversible hepatotoxicity, renal

**SAFETY: HERBAL THERAPIES AND DIETARY SUPPLEMENTS**

### *Glucosamine and Chondroitin*

**Overview**
Glucosamine is chemically derived from glucose. Its chemical name is 2-amino-2-deoxyglucose sulfate.

Chondroitin is a protein usually isolated from bovine (cow) cartilage. To date, there are no reports of any type of disease transmission from cows to humans with chondroitin.

**Common Uses**
These two supplements are often used in combination, and sometimes individually, to treat pain from osteoarthritis. Although they are most commonly taken orally, injectable forms are commercially available (e.g., for administration by naturopathic prescribers).

**Adverse Effects**
**Glucosamine:** Usually mild adverse effects that are comparable to those of placebo in clinical studies, including gastrointestinal discomfort, drowsiness, headache, and skin reactions.
**Chondroitin:** No major ill effects in studies lasting from 2 months to 6 years. Gastrointestinal discomfort is the most common adverse effect but is usually well tolerated.

**Potential Drug Interactions**
**Both supplements:** May enhance the anticoagulant effects of warfarin. The patient's international normalized ratio needs to be measured more frequently during glucosamine/chondroitin therapy, and the warfarin dosage adjusted if indicated.
**Glucosamine:** May cause an increase in insulin resistance, necessitating the need for higher dosages of oral hypoglycemics or insulin.

**Contraindications**
**Both supplements:** No specific contraindications listed, but avoidance during pregnancy is recommended due to lack of firm safety data.

---

failure, hearing loss, and noncardiogenic pulmonary edema, so a review of the patient's history of pre-existing medical conditions is important.

In addition to patient assessment, the use of ketorolac requires assessment of the drug order because it is important to be sure the drug has been ordered for a short term (e.g., no more than 5 days) and for patients experiencing moderate to severe acute pain. Assess the patient for underlying signs of infection before the use of any NSAID or other antiinflammatory drug, because these drugs may mask symptoms. With use of celecoxib, document any cardiovascular disorders or symptoms because use of the drug, as with rofecoxib and valdecoxib, carries a risk of cardiovascular events.

With *antigout* drugs, perform a thorough assessment of hydration status and baseline serum uric acid levels. Closely assess urinary output prior to and during drug therapy to ensure an output of at least 30 to 60 mL/hr. Determine and assess renal function through monitoring of BUN and serum creatinine as well as liver function through monitoring of ALP, AST, ALT, and LDH. If receiving febuxostat (Uloric), assess the patient for a history of cardiovascular disease due to risk of adverse effects linked to the cardiac system. Additionally, drug interactions

may occur with theophylline, azathiaprine, or mercaptopurine. If the patient is taking allopurinol, assess the integrity of the skin due to potentially life-threatening skin adverse effects of exfoliative dermatitis, Stevens-Johnson syndrome, and toxic epidermal necrolysis. Assess blood counts because of the potential for aplastic anemia and agranulocytosis. With colchicine, conduct a thorough assessment for a history of gastrointestinal distress; ulcers; or cardiac, renal, or liver disease. When assessing the prescriber's order, remember that there is only one colchicine product available, Colcrys, because of FDA recall. Also worthy of mentioning for antigout drugs (e.g., allopurinol, Colycrys, probenecid) is that these drugs may be used for either their short-term or long-term effects. Therefore, assess the order and indication for the antigout drug to ensure that the patient is receiving the appropriate treatment. Also assess for all contraindications, cautions, and drug interactions (see earlier discussion).

## NURSING DIAGNOSES

1. Acute pain related to the disease process or injury to joints and other disease-affected areas
2. Deficient knowledge related to first-time drug therapy for treatment of a disease process
3. Risk for injury related to the effects of the disease and treatment on mobility and the performance of ADLs

## PLANNING

### GOALS

1. Patient experiences pain relief or relief of symptoms within the expected time frame.
2. Patient demonstrates increased knowledge about the disease process, medication regimen, and lifestyle changes.
3. Patient remains free from injury related to the disease process and/or drug regimen.

### OUTCOME CRITERIA

1. Patient remains pain free or near pain free with adequate drug and nondrug therapy.
   - Patient states that pain and changes in joints and mobility are characteristic of inflammation, injury, or related disease processes and will decrease with effective therapy.
   - Patient identifies factors that aggravate or alleviate pain, such as movement, activity, exercise, and change in the weather or atmosphere.
   - Patient states nonpharmacologic measures to use to promote comfort, increase joint function and mobility, and increase performance of ADLs (e.g., biofeedback, imagery, massage, application of hot or cold packs, physical therapy, relaxation therapy).
2. Patient describes disease process requiring treatment with NSAID or antigout drug therapy.
   - Patient states impact of effective and consistent drug therapy in the prevention of damage to the part of the musculoskeletal system being impacted by disease process of injury, gout, arthritis, and so on.

## PATIENT-CENTERED CARE: LIFESPAN CONSIDERATIONS FOR THE ELDERLY PATIENT

### NSAIDs

It is anticipated that by 2030 there will be more than 60 million Americans 65 years of age and older, exceeding 20% of the population. It is also anticipated that the use of over-the-counter NSAIDs will be widespread and increasing in this population and require special attention and education to prevent and/or minimize adverse effects. Understanding the physiologic changes of the elderly patient will help ensure safe and effective use of these medications.

The underlying pharmacokinetic characteristics and physical and biologic changes in elderly patients must be understood. Even if older patients have normal kidney and liver function, they have a reduced rate of drug metabolism and drug elimination compared with younger adults.

Patients 65 years of age and older do not have to be ill for NSAIDs to adversely affect them because of normal age-related physiologic changes. The presence of chronic or multiple illnesses may result in an increased incidence of adverse reactions.

Some changes noted in elderly patients that effect drug treatment include changes in renal elimination, protein binding, body composition, drug distribution, drug clearance, and sensitivity to drugs, as well as an increased incidence of adverse reactions to all types of medications.

Older patients who are at risk for renal insufficiency because of natural physiologic changes may experience changes in fluid balance as well as changes in drug reabsorption, excretion, and filtration processes. This may lead to drug toxicity.

Cardiac output decreases by 25% between 25 and 65 years of age, which results in decreased blood flow to the kidneys and, consequently, reduced glomerular filtration rate. There is also an overall decline in circulating blood volume, which may affect overall pharmacokinetics and lead to decreased drug absorption, distribution, metabolism, and excretion.

Many individuals older than 65 years of age become slow metabolizers of medications, which affects the way NSAIDs are handled by the liver. In addition, the liver decreases in size and weight with advancing age. Liver blood flow is also decreased. Drug metabolism is affected by these changes, resulting in the need to possibly decrease drug dosages and/or monitor very closely for toxicity.

Gastrointestinal functioning is impacted by aging, with a more acidic content of gastric juice and decreased gastric motility. This may lead to slower emptying of the stomach and result in decreased intestinal absorption and drug absorption. Serum levels of drugs, including NSAIDs, may be higher due to these changes, and the overall drug dosage may need to be decreased. It has also been documented that elderly individuals may be at increased risk for developing NSAID-related gastrointestinal problems.

Interventions to help decrease NSAID-related adverse reactions include asking questions, listing all drugs, teaching about all medications, and assessing the patient's gastrointestinal, cardiovascular, and neurologic systems, depending on patient complaints.

*NSAID,* Nonsteroidal antiinflammatory drug.
Data from Argoff CH: Optimal pain management in older patients, 2010, available at http://www.medscape.com/viewarticle/730074. Accessed July 2, 2011; Durrance S: Older adults and NSAIDs: avoiding adverse reactions, 2004, available at http://www.medscape.com/viewarticle/466796. Accessed July 2, 2011.

- Patient states adverse effects associated with NSAIDs or antigout therapy.
- Patient states symptoms to report to the prescriber immediately such as fever, increase in symptoms, joint pain, jaundice, changes in skin, severe rash, and so on.
3. Patient takes medication regimen as prescribed to prevent further damage and injury to self.
   - Patient contacts prescriber if lack of improvement in injury or disease process.
   - Patient maintains follow-up appointments with prescriber to enhance therapeutic effectiveness and minimize injury.

## IMPLEMENTATION

If *aspirin,* an antigout drug is used, the oral dosage forms are given with food, milk, or meals. Advise the patient that sustained-release or enteric-coated tablets are not to be crushed or broken. Monitor serum levels of aspirin if aspirin therapy is used for its antiarthritic effect; however, this indication is very rare. Because of the high risk of adverse effects that may be severe, aspirin is mainly used in lower doses (e.g., 81 mg) for cardioprotective reasons. If used in higher doses, monitor for clinical presentation as well as serum aspirin levels to help distinguish among mild, moderate, and severe toxicity (see pharmacology discussion). If aspirin is used in higher doses, it is important to be aware of signs and symptoms of toxicity such as gastrointestinal bleeding, other bleeding, and abdominal pain. If these occur, report the findings to the prescriber for immediate treatment. If

aspirin is used as an antipyretic, the patient's temperature generally begins to decrease within 1 hour. See the Patient Teaching Tips for more information on the safe use of aspirin.

*Non-aspirin NSAIDs* or other *antiinflammatory drugs* may also come in enteric-coated or sustained-release preparations; stress to the patient that these are not to be crushed or chewed. Oral dosage forms of these drugs—including ketorolac—may be taken with antacids or food to decrease gastrointestinal upset or irritation. Instruct the patient to report to the prescriber immediately any moderate to severe gastrointestinal upset, dyspepsia with nausea, vomiting, abdominal pain, or blood in the stool or vomitus. Advise the patient to avoid other ulcerogenic substances (e.g., alcohol, prednisone, aspirin-containing products, other NSAIDs) to help minimize the risk of gastrointestinal mucosal breakdown. During therapy with NSAIDs, continuously monitor the patient for bowel patterns, stool consistency, and any occurrence of gastrointestinal symptoms and/or dizziness, and document the findings. Monitor laboratory tests during high-dose or long-term treatment, including CBC; BUN levels; platelet counts; and serum bilirubin, ALP, AST, and ALT levels. Emphasize safe ambulation with NSAID use as well as with the use of any other antiinflammatory drugs and/or analgesics. With ketorolac, understand that dosing is not to exceed a 5-day period for either the oral, intramuscular, or IV dosage forms. Administer intramuscular injections slowly into a large muscle mass, and administer IV dosage forms over a period of no less than 15 seconds. Educate the patient to take celecoxib only as ordered and, as with the other NSAIDs, to avoid alcohol, aspirin, salicylates, and over-the-counter drugs containing any of these. Celecoxib may be taken without regard to meals; however, taking the drug with food and fluids may decrease any gastrointestinal upset. Instruct the patient to report immediately to the prescriber any stomach or abdominal pain, gastrointestinal problems, unusual bleeding, blood in the stool or vomitus, chest pain, edema, and/or palpitations.

The *antigout drugs* are somewhat different from the NSAIDs, with different mechanisms of action and also very different nursing considerations. Colchicine needs to be taken on an empty stomach for more complete absorption but is best tolerated if given with food. Educate the patient with gout on the importance of increasing fluid intake of up to 3 L/day, unless contraindicated. Advise the patient to avoid alcohol and any over-the-counter cold relief products that contain alcohol while this medication is being taken. In addition, instruct the patient with gout that adherence to the complete medical regimen—both pharmacologic and non-pharmacologic—is critical to successful treatment. If allopurinol is prescribed, it is to be given with meals to minimize the occurrence of gastrointestinal symptoms such as nausea, vomiting, and anorexia. If allopurinol is to be administered in conjunction with chemotherapy (in an attempt to decrease hyperuricemia associated with malignancy and cell death from successful treatment), it is recommended that it be given a few days before the antineoplastic therapy. Patients taking allopurinol must also increase fluid intake to 3 L/day. Patients need to avoid hazardous activities if dizziness or drowsiness occurs with the medication. Alcohol and caffeine must also be avoided because these drugs will increase uric acid levels and decrease the level of allopurinol.

# EVALUATION

*Aspirin* and *NSAIDs* may vary in their potency and antiinflammatory and analgesic effects. Therapeutic responses to NSAIDs include the following: decrease in acute pain; decrease in swelling, pain, stiffness, and tenderness of a joint or muscle area; improved ability to perform ADLs; improved muscle grip and strength; reduction in fever; return to normal laboratory values for CBC and sedimentation rate; and return to a less inflamed state as evidenced by improved sedimentation rates, radiographic

examination, computed tomographic scan, or magnetic resonance imaging. Monitoring for the occurrence of adverse effects and toxicity is essential to the safe and effective use of *antiinflammatory drugs* (aspirin, COX-II inhibitors, other NSAIDs) and *antigout drugs* (see Box 44-3 and Tables 44-2 and 44-3).

Therapeutic responses to the *antigout* drug colchicine include decreased pain in the affected joints and increased sense of well-being. Monitor the patient closely for any increased pain, blood in the urine, excessive fatigue and lethargy, or chills or fever, and contact the prescriber immediately should these occur. A therapeutic response to allopurinol, another antigout drug, includes a decrease in pain in the joints, a decrease in uric acid levels, and a decrease in stone formation in the kidneys.

# PATIENT TEACHING TIPS

- Instruct the patient that these drugs—if in sustained-release or enteric-coated dosage forms—are not to be crushed or chewed. Instruct the patient to report to the prescriber immediately any ringing in the ears, persistent gastrointestinal or abdominal pain, or easy bruising or bleeding.
- Educate the patient that the full antiinflammatory effect of the drug may not be apparent immediately, depending on the specific drug. For example, onset of full therapeutic antiinflammatory action may take 7 days for ibuprofen or 30 to 60 minutes for its analgesic effects.
- Advise the patient to share a list of all medications with all health care providers/dentists especially if the patient is taking high dosages of aspirin or has been taking aspirin or other NSAIDs for prolonged periods. Aspirin and other NSAIDs are generally discontinued 1 week before any type of surgery, including oral or dental surgery, per the prescriber's or surgeon's orders.

- Always keep aspirin and other drugs out of the reach of children. If a child (or adult) has consumed large or unknown quantities of aspirin or other NSAIDs, contact a poison control center and/or seek emergency medical attention immediately. Children and teenagers must never take aspirin because of the risk of Reye's syndrome (see the Patient-Centered Care: Lifespan Considerations for the Pediatric Patient box on p. 714). Acetaminophen in the recommended dosage range is usually preferred.
- Educate the patient about the adverse effects of aspirin, such as gastrointestinal upset, nausea, vomiting, diarrhea, dizziness, and tinnitus. Table 44-3 lists the signs and symptoms of acute or chronic salicylate intoxication. Instruct the patient to report to the prescriber immediately any black or tarry stools, bleeding around the gums, petechiae (very small red-brown spots), ecchymosis (easy bruising), or purpura (large red spots).

## PATIENT TEACHING TIPS—cont'd

- Inform the patient about the most common adverse effects of NSAIDs (see Table 44-2). Advise the patient to take NSAIDs with food, milk, or antacids to help minimize gastrointestinal distress.

- Educate the patient about the many drug interactions with aspirin, other NSAIDs, and antigout drugs.
- Alert the patient to look-alike sound-alike drugs, especially Celebrex (celecoxib), which may be confused with Celexa (citalopram) or Cerebyx (fosphenytoin).

## KEY POINTS

- Antiinflammatory drugs include aspirin, NSAIDs, and COX-2 inhibitors.
- NSAIDs are one of the most commonly prescribed categories of drugs.
- The first drug in this category to be synthesized was salicylic acid or aspirin. Aspirin is often identified as and included in discussion of antiinflammatory drugs. NSAIDs have analgesic, antiinflammatory, and antipyretic activity; aspirin also has antiplatelet activity. NSAIDs are often used in the treatment of gout, osteoarthritis, juvenile arthritis, rheumatoid arthritis, dysmenorrhea, and musculoskeletal injuries such as strains and sprains.
- The three main adverse effects of NSAIDs are gastrointestinal intolerance, bleeding (often gastrointestinal bleeding), and renal impairment. Misoprostol (Cytotec) may be given to prevent

gastrointestinal intolerance and ulcers resulting from NSAID use. It is classified as a prostaglandin analogue. There are also many contraindications to the use of NSAIDs, such as gastrointestinal tract lesions, peptic ulcers, and bleeding disorders.
- Most oral NSAIDs are better tolerated if taken with food to minimize gastrointestinal upset.
- When NSAIDs are used to decrease joint inflammation in arthritis patients, full therapeutic effects may not be experienced for 1 week or longer.
- Antigout drugs are indicated for either acute or chronic gout or gout prophylaxis. Diarrhea and abdominal pain are common adverse effects. Antigout drugs are often given to patients during cancer chemotherapy that causes cell death to avoid gout-like syndromes and pain.

## NCLEX® EXAMINATION REVIEW QUESTIONS

1 When a patient is receiving long-term NSAID therapy, which drug may be given to prevent the serious gastrointestinal adverse effects of NSAIDs?
   a misoprostol (Cytotec)
   b metoprolol (Lopressor)
   c metoclopramide (Reglan)
   d magnesium sulfate
2 The nurse recognizes that manifestations of NSAID toxicity include
   a constipation.
   b nausea and vomiting.
   c tremors.
   d urinary retention.
3 During a teaching session about antigout drugs, the nurse tells the patient that antigout drugs work by which mechanism?
   a Increasing blood oxygen levels
   b Decreasing leukocytes and platelets
   c Increasing protein and rheumatoid factors
   d Decreasing serum uric acid levels
4 When the nurse is teaching about antigout drugs, which statement by the nurse is accurate?
   a "Drink only limited amounts of fluids with the drug."
   b "This drug may cause limited movements of your joints."
   c "There are very few drug interactions with these medications."
   d "Colchicine is best taken on an empty stomach."

5 A mother calls the clinic to ask what medication to give her 5-year-old child for a fever during a bout of chickenpox. The nurse's best response would be:
   a "Your child is 5 years old, so it would be okay to use children's aspirin to treat his fever."
   b "Start with acetaminophen or ibuprofen, but if these do not work, then you can try aspirin."
   c "You can use children's dosages of acetaminophen or ibuprofen, but aspirin is not recommended."
   d "It is best to wait to let the fever break on its own without medication."
6 A 49-year-old patient has been admitted with possible chronic salicylate intoxication after self-treatment for arthritis pain. The nurse will assess for which symptoms of salicylate intoxication?
   a Tinnitus
   b Headache
   c Constipation
   d Nausea
   e Bradycardia
7 An order for a child reads: "Give ibuprofen suspension 30 mg/kg/day, divided into four doses, for pain." The child weighs 33 pounds. How many milligrams will this child receive per dose?

1. a, 2. b, 3. d, 4. d, 5. c, 6. a, b, d, 7. 112.5 mg per dose

For Critical Thinking and Prioritization Questions, see http://evolve.elsevier.com/Lilley.

# PART 8

# Immune and Biologic Modifiers and Chemotherapeutic Drugs

## STUDY SKILLS TIPS

Manage Time • Evaluate Prior Performance • Anticipate the Test • Plan for Distributed Study

## MANAGE TIME

The first step in preparing for a chapter or part exam is to plan for the time needed. Let us begin by assuming that the next test you have will cover the chapters in Part 8. First, examine the material to determine just how much there is to cover. Look at the objectives, the key terms, and the number of pages of text in each chapter. This will help you determine just how big a task you face. As you are doing this, also consider how much study time you have been devoting to these chapters in the days before the exam. If you have been doing regular study with frequent review sessions, then the demand on your time in the day or two just before the exam will be less than if you have to do a major "cram" session to try to catch up on study that has been put off. The basic question to answer here is a simple one: "How much time do I need to schedule for exam preparation?" The answer varies with each student. Some will need 6, 8, or more hours of preparation time in the 2 to 3 days before the exam. Others will find that 3, 4, or 5 hours will be adequate. You must assess your own learning and prior success to determine what time is necessary for you, but you must set time aside and use it effectively.

There is one thing that should play a major role in helping you determine how much time you will need to set aside. Evaluate your performance on prior exams. How have you been doing? How much time have you been spending to achieve that level? If you are not achieving according to your capabilities, then you should certainly consider spending more time preparing for the next exam. If you are achieving at a satisfactory level, then plan on devoting about the same amount of time to test preparation as you have devoted before.

The next step in preparing for an exam is to organize the time. Write down what you are going to study and when, as well as how much time you will spend. Consider the following example based on the materials in Chapters 47 and 49:

1. Review Chapter 47 objectives. Monday, 4:00 to 4:30 PM. Note objectives that are unclear for further review.
2. Question and answer review. Monday, 4:30 to 5:15 PM.
3. Self-test, Chapter 47 key terms. Monday, 6:30 to 7:00 PM. Note terms that need further review for mastery.
4. Review Chapter 49 objectives. Monday, 7:00 to 7:30 PM.
5. Question and answer review. Monday, 7:30 to 8:00 PM.
6. Self-test, Chapter 49 key terms. Monday, 8:00 to 8:30 PM.

The advantage to this test preparation model is that you now know where you must focus in the days before the exam.

## EVALUATE PRIOR PERFORMANCE

As you begin preparing to review for any exam, take some time to look back at previous exams. Evaluate your performance and use that evaluation to improve on subsequent tests. As you look at prior tests, consider the following factors.

### Did I Have Trouble with Questions That Required Mastery of Terminology?

As part of the evaluation of prior tests, also look at questions that demanded mastery of the terms from the chapters. If you missed more than one or two questions of that type, then you know you need to spend more time reviewing terminology.

### Did I Miss Concept Questions?

If the question asked you to apply a principle, evaluate a drug response, or in some other way apply knowledge from the course, you are dealing with concepts rather than facts. If you missed a number of concept questions, then you should spend more of your review time studying applications and principles than memorizing facts and terms. Working with a study group may help you to improve your responses to concept questions.

### Did I Make Errors Because I Did Not Know the Material?

This question focuses on the quality of your learning. If you miss one or two questions on an exam because you did not learn (or did not remember) the material, it is not a major problem. There will almost always be one or two questions that one does not remember. If you are analyzing past performance and find that there are several questions on which you guessed because you did not recall any information that seemed relevant to the question, it may be necessary to put more time into review. This may involve doing more oral rehearsal so that the material is stored in long-term memory. Whatever the cause, it is essential that you acknowledge to yourself that you have missed questions because you did not know the material. Once you have acknowledged the problem, take steps to correct it.

## ANTICIPATE THE TEST

Do not wait until exam time to find out what you should know. As you do your review, try to think like the instructor. Generate questions that you think might be a part of the test. This does not mean you need to try to write multiple-choice stems and choices, but you should be trying to focus your review in a way that will facilitate learning and long-term memory. The process of working with a study group to anticipate test questions and to quiz each other can help move concepts from short-term memory to long-term memory.

Here are some examples of questioning that you might use based on material found in Chapter 47.

1. What are biologic response modifiers?
2. What is the role of biologic response modifiers in the care of patients with cancer?
3. What is the role of the immune system in treating cancer?

These sample questions were drawn from just the first few pages of the chapter. Some questions may focus on literal comprehension and are relatively easy to generate. Being able to answer them is important, but if all of your questions are literal, it may be difficult to answer questions that require application of principles and concepts. For that reason, it is essential that some questions require analysis, synthesis, and/or evaluation of the material. A study group is helpful in creating this more complicated type of question. The process of discussion can generate ideas you may not develop on your own. Answers to these questions require the learner to put together the literal information and relate the terms to the concepts being explained.

## PLAN FOR DISTRIBUTED STUDY

One of the major problems that many students encounter when trying to review for a test is waiting too long to begin the review, which forces them into a review pattern of long hours of intensive study all packed into the last day or two before the exam. This is known as "cramming," and although cramming does work to some degree, it is not the most effective way to learn. A better model is to distribute the review over a period of several days with short study sessions of 30 minutes to 1 hour several times each day. Distributing practice in this way allows time for you to think about what you have been learning, and it fosters long-term memory. Studying with a group adds variety to your study time and provides another method of receiving and processing information.

One important consideration is spending more of the review time doing oral rehearsal ("ask and answer" sessions) and not simply rereading material. Oral rehearsal encourages active learning, which enhances your ability to concentrate, improves comprehension and memory, and thus improves test performance. Oral rehearsals work well in study groups, but if you are satisfied with the test results you get by reviewing alone, keep doing what works for you.

# Antineoplastic Drugs Part 1:
# Cancer Overview and
# Cell Cycle–Specific Drugs

## OBJECTIVES

When you reach the end of this chapter, you will be able to do the following:

1. Briefly describe the concepts related to carcinogenesis.
2. Define the different types of malignancy.
3. Discuss the purpose and role of the various treatment modalities in the management of cancer.
4. Define *antineoplastic.*
5. Discuss the role of antineoplastic therapy in the treatment of cancer.
6. Contrast the cell cycle of normal cells and malignant cells with regard to growth, function, and response of the cell to chemotherapeutic drugs and other treatment modalities.
7. Compare the characteristics of highly proliferating normal cells (including cells of the hair follicles, gastrointestinal tract, and bone marrow) with the characteristics of highly proliferating cancerous cells.
8. Briefly describe the specific differences between cell cycle–specific and cell cycle–nonspecific antineoplastic drugs (cell cycle–nonspecific drugs and miscellaneous other antineoplastics are discussed in Chapter 46).

9. Identify the drugs that are categorized as cell cycle specific, including mitotic inhibitors, topoisomerase inhibitors, and antineoplastic enzymes.
10. Describe the common adverse effects and toxic reactions associated with the various antineoplastic drugs, including the causes for their occurrence and methods of treatment, such as antidotes for toxicity.
11. Discuss the mechanisms of action, indications, dosages, routes of administration, cautions, contraindications, and drug interactions of cell cycle–specific drugs, including mitotic inhibitors, topoisomerase inhibitors, and antineoplastic enzymes.
12. Apply knowledge about the various antineoplastic drugs to the development of a comprehensive nursing care plan for patients receiving cell cycle–specific drugs, including mitotic inhibitors, topoisomerase inhibitors, and antineoplastic enzymes.

## DRUG PROFILES

- ♦ **asparaginase, p. 738**
- capecitabine, p. 734
- cladribine, p. 734
- ♦ **cytarabine, p. 734**
- ♦ **etoposide, p. 735**
- fludarabine, p. 734
- fluorouracil, p. 734
- gemcitabine, p. 734

- irinotecan, p. 737
- ♦ **methotrexate, p. 732**
- ♦ **paclitaxel, p. 736**
- pegaspargase, p. 738
- topotecan, p. 737
- ♦ **vincristine, p. 736**

---

♦ *Key drug*

## KEY TERMS

**Analogue** A chemical compound with a structure similar to that of another compound but differing from it with respect to some component. (p. 730)

**Anaplasia** The absence of the cellular differentiation that is part of the normal cellular growth process (see *differentiation;* adjective: *anaplastic*). (p. 728)

**Antineoplastic drugs** Drugs used to treat cancer. Also called *cancer drugs, anticancer drugs, cancer chemotherapy,* and *chemotherapy*. (p. 728)

**Benign** Denoting a neoplasm that is noncancerous and therefore not an immediate threat to life. (p. 724)

**Cancer** A malignant neoplastic disease, the natural course of which is fatal (see *neoplasm*). (p. 724)

**Carcinogen** Any cancer-producing substance or organism. (p. 726)

**Carcinomas** Malignant epithelial neoplasms that tend to invade surrounding tissue and metastasize to distant regions of the body. (p. 724)

**Cell cycle–nonspecific** Denoting antineoplastic drugs that are cytotoxic in any phase of the cellular growth cycle. (p. 728)

**Cell cycle–specific** Denoting antineoplastic drugs that are cytotoxic during a specific phase of the cellular growth cycle. (p. 729)

**Clone** A cell or group of cells that is genetically identical to a given parent cell. (p. 724)

**Differentiation** An important part of normal cellular growth in which immature cells mature into specialized cells. (p. 724)

**Dose-limiting adverse effects** Adverse effects that prevent an antineoplastic drug from being given in higher dosages, often restricting the effectiveness of the drug. (p. 729)

**Emetic potential** The potential of a drug to cause nausea and vomiting. (p. 729)

**Extravasation** The leakage of any intravenously or intraarterially administered medication into the tissue space surrounding the vein or artery. Such an event can cause serious tissue injury, especially with antineoplastic drugs. (p. 729)

**Gene expression** How a cell expresses a receptor or gene; the process in which information from a gene is used in the synthesis of a gene product. (p. 726)

**Growth fraction** The percentage of cells in mitosis at any given time. (p. 728)

**Intrathecal** A route of drug injection through the theca of the spinal cord and into the subarachnoid space. This route is used to deliver certain chemotherapy medications to kill cancer cells in the central nervous system. (p. 734)

**Leukemias** Malignant neoplasms of blood-forming tissues characterized by the replacement of normal bone marrow cells with leukemic blasts resulting in abnormal numbers and forms of immature white blood cells in the circulation. (p. 724)

**Lymphomas** Malignant neoplasms of lymphoid tissue. (p. 724)

**Malignant** Tending to worsen and cause death; anaplastic, invasive, and metastatic. (p. 724)

**Metastasis** The process by which a cancer spreads from the original site of growth to a new and remote part of the body (adjective: *metastatic*). (p. 724)

**Mitosis** The process of cell reproduction occurring in somatic (nonsexual) cells and resulting in the formation of two genetically identical daughter cells containing the diploid (complete) number of chromosomes characteristic of the species. (p. 727)

**Mitotic index** The number of cells per unit (usually 1000 cells) undergoing mitosis during a given time. (p. 728)

**Mutagen** A chemical or physical agent that induces or increases genetic mutations by causing changes in deoxyribonucleic acid (DNA). (p. 726)

**Mutation** A permanent change in DNA that is transmissible to future cellular generations. Mutations can transform normal cells into cancer cells. (p. 724)

**Myelosuppression** Suppression of bone marrow function, which can result in dangerously reduced numbers of red blood cells, white blood cells, and platelets. (p. 729)

**Nadir** Lowest point in any fluctuating value over time; for example, the lowest white blood cell count measured after the count has been depressed by chemotherapy. (p. 729)

**Neoplasm** Any new and abnormal growth, specifically growth that is uncontrolled and progressive; a synonym for *tumor*. A malignant neoplasm or tumor is synonymous with *cancer*. (p. 724)

**Nucleic acids** Molecules of DNA and ribonucleic acid (RNA) in the nucleus of every cell (hence the name *nucleic acid*). Chromosomes are made up of DNA and encode all of the genes necessary for cellular structure and function. (p. 726)

**Oncogenic** Cancer producing; often applied to tumor-inducing viruses. (p. 726)

**Paraneoplastic syndromes** Symptom complexes arising in patients with cancer that cannot be explained by local or distant spread of their tumors. (p. 725)

**Primary lesion** The original site of growth of a tumor. (p. 724)

**Sarcomas** Malignant neoplasms of the connective tissues arising in bone, fibrous, fatty, muscular, synovial, vascular, or neural tissue, often first presenting as painless swellings. (p. 724)

**Tumor** A new growth of tissue characterized by a progressive, uncontrolled proliferation of cells. Tumors can be solid (e.g., brain tumor) or circulating (e.g., leukemia or lymphoma), and benign (noncancerous) or malignant (cancerous). Circulating tumors are more precisely called *hematologic tumors* or *hematologic malignancies*. A tumor is also called a *neoplasm*. (p. 724)

**Tumor lysis syndrome** A common metabolic complication of chemotherapy for rapidly growing tumors. It is characterized by the presence of excessive cellular waste products and electrolytes, including uric acid, phosphate, and potassium, and by reduced serum calcium levels. (p. 731)

## ANATOMY, PHYSIOLOGY, AND PATHOPHYSIOLOGY OVERVIEW

Cancer is a broad term encompassing a group of diseases that are characterized by cellular transformation (e.g., by genetic mutation), uncontrolled cellular growth, possible invasion into surrounding tissue, and metastasis to other tissues or organs distant from the original body site. This cellular growth differs from normal cellular growth in that cancerous cells do not possess a growth control mechanism. Lack of cellular differentiation or maturation into specialized, productive cells is also a common characteristic of cancer cells. Figure 45-1 illustrates the multiple steps involved in the development of cancer. Cancerous cells will continue to grow and invade adjacent structures. They may break away from the original tumor mass and travel by means of the blood or lymphatic system to establish a new clone of cancer cells and create a metastatic growth elsewhere in the body. A clone is a cell or group of cells that is genetically identical to a given parent cell. For the remainder of this and the next chapter, the term *cancer* will generally be used to refer to any type of malignant neoplasm.

Metastasis refers to the spreading of a cancer from the original site of growth (primary lesion) to a new and remote part of the body (secondary or metastatic lesion). The terms *malignancy, neoplasm,* and *tumor* are often used as synonyms for *cancer.* A neoplasm ("new tissue") is a mass of new cells. It is another term for tumor. There are two types of tumors: benign and malignant. A benign tumor is of a uniform size and shape and displays no invasiveness (in terms of infiltrating other tissues) or metastatic properties. The terms *nonmalignant* and *benign* suggest that tumors may be harmless, which is true in most cases. However, a benign tumor can be lethal if it grows large enough to mechanically interrupt the normal function of a critical tissue or organ. Malignant neoplasms consist of cancer cells that invade (infiltrate) surrounding tissues and metastasize to other tissues and organs. Some of the various characteristics of benign and malignant neoplasms are listed in Table 45-1.

Over 100 types of cancer affect humans. Various tumor types based on tissue categories include sarcomas, carcinomas, lymphomas, leukemias, and tumors of nervous tissue origin. Examples of these common types of malignant tumors are presented in Table 45-2. It is important to know the tissue of origin, because this determines the type of treatment, the likely response to therapy, and the prognosis.

Carcinomas arise from epithelial tissue, which is located throughout the body. This tissue covers or lines all body surfaces, both inside and outside the body. Examples are the skin, the mucosal lining of the entire gastrointestinal (GI) tract, and the lining of the bronchial tree (lungs). The purpose of these epithelial tissues is to protect the body's vital organs.

Sarcomas are malignant tumors that arise primarily from connective tissues, but some sarcomas are tumors of epithelial cell origin. Connective tissue is the most abundant and widely distributed of all tissues and includes bone, cartilage, muscle, and lymphatic and vascular structures. Its purpose is to support and protect other tissues.

Lymphomas are cancers within the lymphatic tissues. Leukemias arise from the bone marrow and are cancers of blood and bone marrow. Leukemias differ from carcinomas and sarcomas in that the cancerous cells do not form solid tumors but are interspersed throughout the lymphatic or circulatory system and interfere with the normal functioning of these systems. For

| TABLE 45-1 | TUMOR CHARACTERISTICS: BENIGN AND MALIGNANT | |
|---|---|---|
| **CHARACTERISTIC** | **BENIGN** | **MALIGNANT** |
| Potential to metastasize | No | Yes |
| Encapsulated | Yes | No |
| Similar to tissue of origin | Yes | No |
| Rate of growth | Slow | Unpredictable and unrestrained |
| Recurrence after surgical removal | Rare | Common |

**FIGURE 45-1** Schematic model of multistep carcinogenesis. Genetic change refers to events such as the activation of protooncogenes or drug resistance genes or the inactivation of tumor suppressor genes, antimetastasis genes, or apoptosis (normal cell death). Genetic change may be relatively minimal, as with the translocations seen in various leukemias, or it may involve multiple sequential genetic alterations, as exemplified by the development of colon cancer. (From Haskell CM: *Cancer treatment,* ed 5, Philadelphia, 2001, Saunders.)

this reason, they are sometimes referred to as *circulating tumors,* although *hematologic malignancy* is a more precise term. Lymphomas can be quite bulky and are usually classified as solid tumors.

Cancer patients may also experience various groups of symptoms that cannot be directly attributed to the spread of a cancerous tumor. Such symptom complexes are referred to as paraneoplastic syndromes. They are estimated to occur in up to 15% of patients with cancer and may even be the first sign of malignancy. *Cachexia* (general ill health and malnutrition) is the most common such symptom complex. Examples of other common paraneoplastic syndromes are given in Table 45-3. These syndromes are believed to result from the effects of biologically or immunologically active substances, such as hormones and antibodies, secreted by the tumor cells. Many patients also exhibit more generalized symptoms, such as anorexia, weight loss, fatigue, and fever.

## ETIOLOGY OF CANCER

The etiology of cancer remains a mystery for the most part, and cancer researchers have made slow progress toward identifying possible causes. Certain etiologic factors have been identified, and some of these factors and the cancers with which they are causally associated are listed in Table 45-4. Causative factors that have been identified include age-related and sex-related characteristics; genetic and ethnic factors; oncogenic viruses; environmental and occupational factors; radiation; and immunologic factors.

### Age- and Sex-Related Differences

The probability that a neoplastic disease will develop generally increases with advancing age. A number of rare cancers, such as acute lymphocytic leukemia and Wilms tumor, occur predominantly in pediatric patients.

With the exception of cancers affecting the reproductive system, few cancers exhibit a sex-related difference in incidence. Lung and urinary cancers are more common in men than in women, but this may have more to do with exogenous factors such as smoking patterns and occupational exposure to environmental toxins than to sex-related characteristics. The incidence of colon, rectal, pancreatic, and skin cancers are comparable

| TABLE 45-2 | TUMOR CLASSIFICATION BASED ON SPECIFIC TISSUE OF ORIGIN | |
|---|---|---|
| **TISSUE OF ORIGIN** | **MALIGNANT TISSUE** | |
| **Epithelial = Carcinomas** | | |
| Glands or ducts | Adenocarcinomas | |
| Respiratory tract | Small and large cell carcinomas | |
| Kidney | Renal cell carcinoma | |
| Skin | Squamous cell, epidermoid, and basal cell carcinoma; melanoma | |
| **Connective = Sarcomas** | | |
| Fibrous tissue | Fibrosarcoma | |
| Cartilage | Chondrosarcoma | |
| Bone | Osteogenic sarcoma (Ewing's tumor) | |
| Blood vessels | Kaposi's sarcoma | |
| Synovia | Synoviosarcoma | |
| Mesothelium | Mesothelioma | |
| **Lymphatic = Lymphomas** | | |
| Lymph tissue | Lymphomas (e.g., Hodgkin's, non-Hodgkin's) | |
| Glia | Glioma | |
| Adrenal medulla nerves | Pheochromocytoma | |
| **Blood and Bone Marrow** | | |
| White blood cells | Leukemia | |
| Bone marrow | Multiple myeloma | |

| TABLE 45-3 | PARANEOPLASTIC SYNDROMES ASSOCIATED WITH SOME CANCERS |
|---|---|
| **PARANEOPLASTIC SYNDROME** | **ASSOCIATED CANCER** |
| Hypercalcemia, sensory neuropathies, SIADH | Lung |
| Disseminated intravascular coagulation | Leukemia |
| Cushing's syndrome | Lung, thyroid, testes, adrenal |
| Addison's syndrome | Adrenal, lymphoma |

*SIADH,* Syndrome of inappropriate secretion of antidiuretic hormone.

| TABLE 45-4 | CANCER: PROPOSED ETIOLOGIC FACTORS |
|---|---|
| **RISK FACTOR** | **ASSOCIATED CANCER** |
| **Environment** | |
| Radiation (ionizing) | Leukemia, breast, thyroid, lung |
| Radiation (ultraviolet) | Skin, melanoma |
| Viruses | Leukemia, lymphoma, nasopharyngeal |
| **Food** | |
| Aflatoxin | Liver |
| Dietary factors | Colon, breast, endometrial, gallbladder |
| **Lifestyle** | |
| Alcohol | Esophageal, liver, stomach, laryngeal, breast |
| Tobacco | Lung, oral, esophageal, laryngeal, bladder |
| **Medical Drugs** | |
| Diethylstilbestrol (DES) | Vaginal in offspring, breast, testicular, ovarian |
| Estrogens | Endometrial, breast |
| Alkylating drugs | Leukemia, bladder |
| **Occupational** | |
| Asbestos | Lung, mesothelioma |
| Aniline dye | Bladder |
| Benzene | Leukemia |
| Vinyl chloride | Liver |
| **Reproductive History** | |
| Late first pregnancy, early menses | Breast |
| No children | Ovarian |
| Multiple sexual partners | Cervical, uterine |

in men and women. A number of hematologic cancers have a slight male predominance.

## Genetic and Ethnic Factors

Few cancers have been confirmed to have a hereditary basis (some types of breast, colon, and stomach cancer are exceptions). The understanding of tumor biology has helped guide therapy tremendously. Two such advances are determination of hormone receptor status and identification of specific gene expression in various types of tumor cells. For example, some tumor cells express themselves on their cell membrane surfaces, either estrogen receptors or progesterone receptors, and some tumor cells express specific genes such as the *HER2/neu* gene. Because these indicators aid in classification of a patient's tumor, they also help in choosing appropriate drug therapy, predicting response to therapy, and anticipating prognosis. Discovery of the *BRCA1* and *BRCA2* genes has allowed identification of women who are at risk of breast cancer because they have a certain alteration in one of these *BRCA* genes. Many women with a family history of breast cancer choose to be tested for the presence of a *BRCA* gene mutation, which has led some women to undergo prophylactic breast removal. Tumors with identifiable gene expression patterns can show a familial pattern of inheritance. For example, Burkitt's lymphoma is more common in young African children and children of African descent. Another example of an ethnic predisposition is the high incidence of nasopharyngeal cancer in persons of Chinese descent. These associations with race are complicated by a well-recognized viral pathogenesis for both diseases.

## Oncogenic Viruses

Extensive research has indicated that there are cancer-causing (oncogenic) viruses that can affect most mammalian species. Examples include human papillomavirus, the various cat leukemia viruses, the Rous sarcoma virus in chickens, and the Shope papillomavirus in rabbits.

The herpesviruses are common examples of oncogenic viruses. Epstein-Barr virus is a type of herpesvirus. It is most commonly recognized as the cause of infectious mononucleosis (commonly referred to as "mono" or the "kissing disease"). However, it is also associated with the development of Burkitt's lymphoma and nasopharyngeal cancer. Infection with human papillomavirus (often abbreviated as HPV) has been linked to both cervical and anal cancer.

## Occupational and Environmental Carcinogens

A carcinogen is any substance that can cause cancer. In the nucleus of every cell are found molecules of nucleic acids, so named because of their location in the cell nucleus. The two types of nucleic acids are deoxyribonucleic acid (DNA) and ribonucleic acid (RNA). DNA molecules are the master molecules of genetic material within cells and contain the approximately 30,000 genes of the human genome. Genes are transcribed into messenger RNA molecules, which in turn are translated into protein molecules necessary for cellular structure and function. This process is discussed further in the section on alkylating drugs in Chapter 46. A mutagen is any substance or physical agent (e.g., radiation) that induces changes in DNA molecules. Mutations often transform normal cells into cancer cells. Thus, mutagenicity is associated with and often (but not always) leads to carcinogenicity. The U.S. Food and Drug Administration (FDA) mandates that carcinogenic studies be performed before any new drug is approved for use. However, no amount of clinical testing can fully reveal all of a drug's possible carcinogenic effects. Carcinogenic effects may not be observed in the laboratory animals on which the drug has been tested but may be reported when the drugs are used in human subjects. Given the relatively small numbers of patients tested in clinical research trials, the carcinogenic potential of a given drug may not be observed until after the drug is marketed for use in the general population. If patterns of carcinogenicity begin to emerge during this period of postmarketing surveillance (or postmarketing studies), the drug may be recalled from the market.

## Radiation

Radiation is a well-known and potent carcinogenic agent. There are two basic types of radiation: (1) ionizing, or high-energy, radiation, and (2) nonionizing, or low-energy, radiation. Both types can be carcinogenic. Ionizing radiation is very potent and can penetrate deeply into the body. It is called *ionizing* because it causes the formation of ions within living cells. This type of radiation (e.g., that used in radiographic studies) is also used to treat (irradiate) cancerous tumors (e.g., radium implants). Nonionizing radiation is much less potent and cannot penetrate deeply into the body. Ultraviolet light is an example of this type of radiation and is the cause of skin cancer. In contrast to chemotherapy, radiation therapy is considered to be a locoregional and not a systemic cancer treatment. Adverse effects of radiation therapy (e.g., radiation burns; nausea with GI tract irradiation) tend to be more localized to the site of treatment as well. Scientific specialists known as *radiation oncologists* are involved in the planning of radiation treatments, including calculation of the appropriate dose (dosimetry).

## Immunologic Factors

The immune system plays an important role in the body in terms of cancer surveillance and the elimination of neoplastic cells. Neoplastic cells are believed to develop in everyone; however, a healthy person's immune system recognizes them as abnormal and eliminates them by means of cell-mediated immunity (cytotoxic T lymphocytes; see Chapter 47). It has also been shown that the incidence of cancer is much higher in immunocompromised individuals. The relationship between cancer and a suppressed immune system has also been noted in cancer patients being treated with immunosuppressive drugs after organ transplantation. The higher rates of cancers such as skin cancer and lymphoma in transplant patients is a result of this aggressive use of drugs to prevent organ rejection.

## Cell Growth Cycle

Normal cells in the body divide (proliferate) in a controlled and organized fashion, and this growth is regulated by various mechanisms. In contrast, cancer cells lack such regulatory mechanisms and divide uncontrollably. Often the growth of

FIGURE 45-2  Cell life cycle and metabolic activity. Generation time is the period from M phase to M phase. Cells not in the cycle but capable of division are in the resting phase (G₀). (From Lewis SL, Dirksen SR, Heitkemper MM, et al: *Medical-surgical nursing: assessment and management of clinical problems,* ed 8, St. Louis, 2011, Mosby).

| TABLE 45-5 | CELL CYCLE PHASES |
|---|---|
| **PHASE** | **DESCRIPTION** |
| G₀: Resting phase | Most normal human cells exist predominantly in this phase. Cancer cells in this phase are not susceptible to the toxic effects of cell cycle–specific drugs. |
| G₁: First gap phase or postmitotic phase | Enzymes necessary for DNA synthesis are produced. |
| S: DNA synthesis phase | DNA synthesis takes place, from DNA strand separation to replication of each strand to create duplicate DNA molecules. |
| G₂: Second gap phase or premitotic phase | RNA and specialized proteins are made. |
| M: Mitosis phase | Divided into four subphases: prophase, metaphase, anaphase, and telophase; cell divides (reproduces) into two daughter cells. |

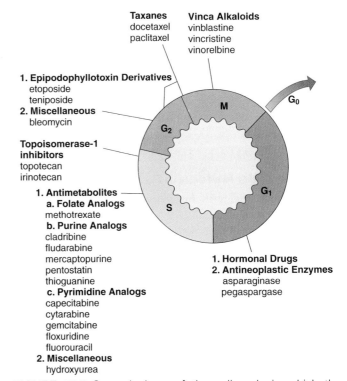

FIGURE 45-3  General phase of the cell cycle in which the various cell cycle–specific chemotherapeutic drugs have their greatest proportionate kill of cancer cells.

cancer cells is more constant or continuous than that of nonmalignant cells. Thus, one important growth index for malignant tumors is the time it takes for the tumor to double in size. This doubling time varies greatly for various types of cancers and is directly related to and important in determining the prognosis. Cancer treatment that cannot destroy every neoplastic cell does not prevent the regrowth of the tumor. The time it takes for regrowth to occur depends on the doubling time of the particular cancer. For instance, Burkitt's lymphoma has an extremely short doubling time. This shorter doubling time is associated with a tumor that, although it may be chemosensitive, is often difficult to cure due to rapid regrowth.

The cell growth characteristics of normal and neoplastic cells are similar. Both types of cells pass through five distinct gap phases: G₀, the resting phase, in which the cell is considered out of the cell cycle; G₁, the first gap phase; S, the synthesis phase; G₂, the second gap phase; and M, the mitosis phase (Figure 45-2). During mitosis, one cell divides into two identical daughter cells. Mitosis is further subdivided into four distinct

subphases related to the time periods before and during the alignment and separation of the chromosomes (DNA strands): prophase, metaphase, anaphase, and telophase. A complete cell cycle from one mitosis to the next is called the *generation time.* It is different for all tumors, ranging from hours to days. The cell growth cycle and the events that occur in the various phases are summarized in Table 45-5. Figure 45-3 shows where in the general phases of the cell cycle the various cell cycle–specific chemotherapeutic drugs show their greatest activity.

The growth activity in a mass of tumor cells has an important bearing on the killing power of chemotherapeutic drugs. The percentage of cells undergoing mitosis at any given time is called the growth fraction of the tumor. The actual number of cells that are in the M phase of the cell cycle is called the mitotic index. Chemotherapy is most effective when used in a rapidly dividing or highly proliferative tumor.

Hematopoietic stem cells are cells in the bone marrow that have the capacity for self-renewal and repopulation of the different types of blood and bone marrow cells. In the bone marrow, the hematopoietic stem cell divides asynchronously, regenerating itself while producing a cell that will go through a series of cell divisions to produce mature blood cells. Tumors in the bone marrow that affect a cell close to the stem cell are unable to mature and are considered poorly differentiated. The level of differentiation within a tumor, whether solid or circulating, becomes especially important in the treatment of neoplasms. This is because more highly differentiated tumors generally have a better therapeutic response (tumor shrinkage) to treatments such as chemotherapy and radiation. In contrast, some cancers, such as leukemia, involve proliferation of immature white blood cells (WBCs) known as *blast cells.* Cancers with a larger proportion of such undifferentiated cells are often less responsive to chemotherapy or radiation and therefore are more difficult to treat. Lack of normal cellular differentiation is known as anaplasia, and such undifferentiated cells are said to be *anaplastic* cells.

## PHARMACOLOGY OVERVIEW

## CANCER DRUG NOMENCLATURE

The more technical term for cancer is *malignant neoplasm.* Drugs used to treat cancer are therefore known as antineoplastic drugs but are also called *cancer drugs, anticancer drugs,* and, most commonly, *cytotoxic chemotherapy* or just *chemotherapy.* The nomenclature (naming system) of cancer drugs can be somewhat more complex and confusing than that for other drug classes. Cancer treatment is an intensively researched area in health care with many active research protocols. Multiple names are often used for the same drug, depending on its stage of development.

Recall from Chapter 2 that medications have a chemical name, a generic name, and a trade name. This section introduces yet another name for medications, especially cancer drugs: the investigational or protocol name. A drug's chemical name is used by the chemists who first discover and work with the drug. The generic name is frequently first assigned to a chemical compound after a pharmaceutical manufacturer has determined that it is worthy of continued clinical research. It is often at this point that the chemical compound becomes an investigational drug. The trade name is a marketing name used by the manufacturer of a given drug primarily to market the drug. During the time before marketing and while a given medication is undergoing clinical research, it is frequently referred to by its protocol name. The protocol name is often a code name that consists of a combination of letters and

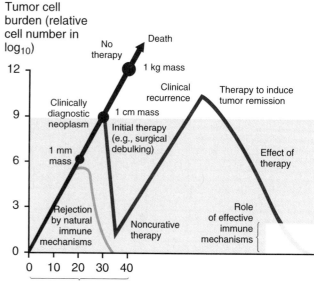

**FIGURE 45-4** Relationship between tumor cell burden and phases of cancer treatment. (From McCance KL: *Pathophysiology: The biologic basis for disease in adults and children,* ed 5, St Louis, 2006, Mosby.)

numbers separated by one or more dashes. Although investigational drugs for all disease classes usually have some kind of protocol name, protocol names tend to be used more commonly in patient care settings for cancer drugs than for other drug classes. Here are two typical examples that illustrate these concepts:

| Other Name | Generic Name | Trade Name |
| --- | --- | --- |
| STI-571 (protocol name) | imatinib | Gleevec |
| 5-fluorouracil* (chemical name) | fluorouracil | Adrucil |

*The "5" refers to the position of a fluorine atom in the cyclic ring structure of the uracil molecule.

## DRUG THERAPY

Cancer is normally treated using one or more of three major medical approaches: surgery, radiation therapy, and chemotherapy. The term *chemotherapy* is a general term that technically can refer to chemical (drug) therapy for any kind of illness. In practice, however, this term usually refers to the pharmacologic treatment of cancer.

Normal cells in the body divide (proliferate) in a controlled and organized fashion, and this growth is regulated by means of various mechanisms. In contrast, cancer cells lack regulatory mechanisms, and they proliferate uncontrollably. Figure 45-4 shows how various combinations of cancer treatment may succeed, or fail, over time.

Cancer chemotherapy drugs can be subdivided into two main groups based on where in the cell cycle they have their effects. Antineoplastic drugs that are cytotoxic (cell killing) in any phase of the cycle are called cell cycle–nonspecific drugs.

Those drugs that are cytotoxic during a specific cell cycle phase are called cell cycle–specific drugs. These are broad categories that describe the activity of a drug with regard to cell cycle. Individual drugs may have actions that fall into both of these categories. Regardless of the cell cycle characteristics of a drug, it is more effective on rapidly growing tumors. This chapter discusses the cell cycle–specific drugs. Chapter 46 focuses on cell cycle–nonspecific drugs as well as various miscellaneous antineoplastic drugs.

The ultimate goal of any anticancer regimen is to kill every neoplastic cell and produce a cure, but this goal is not achieved in most cases. Fortunately, some patients' immune systems may be able to clear the remaining tumor. Factors that affect the chances of cure and the length of patient survival include the cancer stage at time of diagnosis, the type of cancer and its doubling time, the efficacy of the cancer treatment, the development of drug resistance, and the general health of the patient. When total cure is not possible, the primary goal of therapy is to control the growth of the cancer while maintaining the best quality of life for the patient with the least possible level of discomfort and fewest treatment adverse effects.

It must be emphasized that cancer care and treatment involve many rapidly evolving medical sciences. Cancer is an intensively researched area, with the ultimate goals being to prevent cancer and to prevent premature death. Chemotherapy medications are often dosed as part of complex, specific treatment protocols that are subject to frequent revision by oncology clinicians and researchers. For these reasons, you must recognize that the drug dosing information provided in this chapter is intended only to be representative of current cancer treatment and is not absolute or comprehensive. Furthermore, the indications that are listed for each specific drug are the primary FDA-approved indications that are current at the time of this writing. These, too, may change unpredictably with time as a given drug is determined to be more (or less) effective for treating certain types of cancer. Also, in clinical practice, patients are often treated with one or more antineoplastic medications in "off-label" uses; that is, the drug is not currently approved for those particular uses by the FDA.

No antineoplastic drug is effective against all types of cancer. Most cancer drugs have a low therapeutic index, which means that a fine line exists between therapeutic and toxic levels. Clinical experience has shown that a combination of drugs is usually more effective than single-drug therapy. Because drug-resistant cells often develop, exposure to multiple drugs with multiple mechanisms and sites of action will destroy more subpopulations of cells. The delayed onset of resistance to a particular antineoplastic drug is one benefit of combination drug therapy. To be most effective, however, the drugs used in such a combination regimen would ideally possess the following characteristics:

- Some efficacy even as single drugs in the treatment of the particular type of cancer
- Different mechanisms of action so that the cytotoxic effect is maximized; this includes differences in cell cycle specificity
- No or minimal overlapping toxicities

One major drawback to the use of antineoplastic drugs is that nearly all of them cause adverse effects. These toxicities generally stem from the fact that chemotherapy drugs affect rapidly dividing cells—both harmful cancer cells and healthy, normal cells. Three types of rapidly dividing human cells are the cells of hair follicles, GI tract cells, and bone marrow cells. Because most of today's antineoplastic drugs cannot differentiate between cancer cells and healthy cells, the healthy cells are also destroyed, so hair loss, nausea and vomiting, and bone marrow toxicity are the undesirable consequences. Effects on the GI tract and bone marrow are often dose-limiting adverse effects; that is, the patient can no longer tolerate an increase in dosage that may be necessary to adequately treat the cancer and achieve good disease response.

Hair follicle cells are rapidly dividing cells. Cancer drugs that affect these cells often cause the adverse effect known as *alopecia*, or hair loss. Many patients, especially women, choose to wear wigs, hats, or scarves to disguise this adverse effect. Some antineoplastic drugs are more harmful to the epithelial cells of the stomach and intestinal tract, which often leads to diarrhea and mucositis, and may also increase the risk of nausea and vomiting. The likelihood that a given drug will produce vomiting is known as its emetic potential. Anticancer drugs cause nausea and vomiting by stimulating the cells of the chemoreceptor trigger zone. Several antiemetic drugs are used to prevent these symptoms and are described in Chapter 52. Box 45-1 lists the relative emetic potential of selected chemotherapy drugs.

Myelosuppression, also known as *bone marrow suppression* or *bone marrow depression,* is another unwanted adverse effect of certain antineoplastics. It commonly results from drug- or radiation-induced destruction of certain rapidly dividing cells in the bone marrow, primarily the cellular precursors of WBCs, red blood cells (RBCs), and platelets. This can also occur due to the disease processes of the cancer itself. Myelosuppression, in turn, leads to leukopenia, anemia, and thrombocytopenia. The cancer patient is often at greater risk for infection because of leukopenia (reduced WBC count) secondary to chemotherapy. Patients often need antibiotics intravenously (IV), either to prevent or to treat bacterial infections. Such patients are referred to as being neutropenic. Drug-induced anemia (reduced RBC count) often leads to hypoxia and fatigue, whereas thrombocytopenia (reduced platelet count) makes the patient more susceptible to bleeding. The lowest level of WBCs in the blood following chemotherapy (or radiation) treatment is called the nadir. The time until the nadir is reached in a given patient may become shorter and the recovery time for the bone marrow may become longer with multiple courses of antineoplastic treatment. The nadir normally occurs roughly 10 to 28 days after dosing, depending on the particular cancer drug or combination of drugs that is used to treat the patient. Anticipation of this nadir based on known cancer drug data can be used to guide the timing of prophylactic (preventative) administration of antibiotics and blood stimulants known as *hematopoietic growth factors* (see Chapter 47).

Common indications for various antineoplastic drugs are listed in the Dosages tables. Also provided in various locations in this chapter and in Chapter 46 are tables and boxes (Tables 45-8 and 46-2 and Boxes 46-1 and 46-2) containing drug-specific guidelines for the treatment of extravasation—unintended

## BOX 45-1 RELATIVE EMETIC POTENTIAL OF SELECTED ANTINEOPLASTIC DRUGS*

| Low (Less than 10% to 30%) | Moderate (30% to 60%) |
|---|---|
| asparaginase | altretamine |
| bleomycin | cyclophosphamide |
| busulfan | (less than 750 mg/m²) |
| capecitabine | dactinomycin |
| chlorambucil | daunorubicin (50 mg/m² or less) |
| cladribine | doxorubicin (20 to 60 mg/m²) |
| cytarabine (less than 1000 mg/m²) | epirubicin (less than 90 mg/m²) |
| daunorubicin, liposomal | idarubicin |
| docetaxel | ifosfamide (1500 mg/m² or less) |
| doxorubicin (less than 20 mg/m²) | irinotecan |
| doxorubicin, liposomal | methotrexate (250 to 1000 mg/m²) |
| estramustine | mitoxantrone (15 mg/m² or less) |
| etoposide | temozolomide |
| floxuridine | |
| fludarabine | **High (60% to More than 90%)** |
| fluorouracil (less than 1000 mg/m²) | carboplatin |
| gefitinib | carmustine |
| gemcitabine | cisplatin |
| hydroxyurea | cyclophosphamide (750 to more than 1500 mg/m²) |
| imatinib | cytarabine (more than 1000 mg/m²) |
| melphalan | dacarbazine |
| mercaptopurine | dactinomycin |
| methotrexate (less than 250 mg/m²) | daunorubicin (more than 50 mg/m²) |
| mitomycin | doxorubicin (more than 60 mg/m²) |
| paclitaxel | ifosfamide (more than 1500 mg/m²) |
| pegaspargase | lomustine |
| pentostatin | mechlorethamine |
| rituximab | methotrexate (more than 1000 mg/m²) |
| teniposide | mitoxantrone (more than 15 mg/m²) |
| thioguanine | oxaliplatin |
| thiotepa | procarbazine |
| topotecan | streptozocin |
| trastuzumab | |
| tretinoin | |
| vinblastine | |
| vincristine | |
| vinorelbine | |

*Drugs in this list not covered in this chapter are described in Chapter 46.

leakage of a chemotherapy drug (with vesicant potential) into the surrounding tissues outside of the IV line.

Because of the often severe toxicity of cancer medications, a current major focus of cancer drug research is the development of targeted drug therapy. Targeted drug therapy utilizes drugs that recognize a specific molecule involved in the growth of cancer cells, while mostly sparing healthy cells. One example of such targeted therapy is the newer class of cancer drugs known as *monoclonal antibodies* (see Chapter 47).

Pharmacokinetic data for antineoplastic medications is seldom used to guide dosing. Assay complexity coupled with a poor correlation between blood concentration and toxicity and efficacy limits its value. Only a handful of anticancer drugs benefit from therapeutic drug monitoring. For these reasons, pharmacokinetic data are not included with the drug profiles in this chapter.

In spite of their notorious toxicity, given the often fatal outcome of neoplastic diseases, most cancer drugs are only rarely considered to be absolutely contraindicated. Even if a patient has a known allergic reaction to an antineoplastic medication, the urgency of treating the patient's cancer necessitates administering the medication and treating any allergic symptoms with premedications such as antihistamines, corticosteroids, and acetaminophen. For these reasons, no specific contraindications are listed for any of the drugs in this chapter.

Common relative contraindications for cancer drugs include weakened status of the patient as manifested by indicators such as very low WBC count, ongoing infectious process, severe compromise in nutritional and hydration status, reduced kidney or liver function, or a decline in organ function in any system that may be further affected by the toxic effect of the drug being administered. These are situations in which chemotherapy treatment is commonly delayed until the patient's status improves. In general, most chemotherapy is held when the patient's absolute neutrophil count (ANC) is less than 500 cells/mm³ (severe neutropenia) (see Chapter 46). Alternatively, dosages are often reduced for frail elderly patients or others with significantly compromised organ system function, depending on the drugs used.

Reduction in fertility is a major concern in postpubertal patients. Cancer also complicates 1 in 1000 pregnancies. All chemotherapy drugs are classified as pregnancy category D. The choice to use chemotherapy in a pregnant woman is based on risk versus benefit. Both radiation and chemotherapy treatments can cause significant permanent fetal harm or death. The greatest risk is during the first trimester. Chemotherapy treatment during the second or third trimester is more likely to improve maternal outcome without significant fetal risk. However, radiation treatment poses great risk to the fetus throughout pregnancy and is reserved for the postpartum period if possible. Prepubertal patients are more resilient, however, and can have normal puberty and fertility.

In the elderly, *frailty* refers to loss of most of the patient's functional reserve and limited ability to tolerate even minimal physiologic stress (e.g., chemotherapy treatment). More robust elderly patients are certainly better candidates for cancer treatment, although frail patients often benefit as well, especially in terms of palliative (noncurative) symptom control.

## CELL CYCLE–SPECIFIC ANTINEOPLASTIC DRUGS

Cell cycle–specific drug classes include antimetabolites, mitotic inhibitors, alkaloid topoisomerase II inhibitors, topoisomerase I inhibitors, and antineoplastic enzymes. These drugs are collectively used to treat a variety of solid and/or circulating tumors, although some drugs have much more specific indications than others.

### ANTIMETABOLITES

A compound that is structurally similar to a normal cellular metabolite is known as an analogue of that metabolite. Analogues may have agonist or antagonist activity relative to the corresponding cellular compounds. An antagonist analogue is also known as an *antimetabolite*.

## Mechanism of Action and Drug Effects

Antineoplastic antimetabolites are cell cycle–specific analogues that work by antagonizing the actions of key cellular metabolites. More specifically, antimetabolites inhibit cellular growth by interfering with the synthesis or actions of compounds critical to cellular reproduction: the vitamin folic acid, purines, and pyrimidines. Purines and pyrimidines make up the bases contained in nucleic acid molecules (DNA and RNA). Antimetabolites work via two mechanisms: (1) by falsely substituting for purines, pyrimidines, or folic acid; and (2) by inhibiting critical enzymes involved in the synthesis or function of these compounds. Thus, they ultimately inhibit the synthesis of DNA, RNA, and proteins, all of which are necessary for cell survival. Antimetabolites work primarily in the S phase of the cell cycle, during which DNA synthesis is most active. The available antimetabolites and the metabolites they antagonize are as follows:

**Folate antagonists**
- methotrexate (MTX)
- pemetrexed
- pralatrexate

**Purine antagonists**
- cladribine
- fludarabine (F-AMP)
- mercaptopurine (6-MP)
- pentostatin
- thioguanine (6-TG)

**Pyrimidine antagonists**
- capecitabine
- cytarabine (ara-C)
- floxuridine (FUDR)
- fluorouracil (5-FU)
- gemcitabine

### Folic Acid Antagonism

The antimetabolite methotrexate is an analogue of folic acid. It inhibits the action of dihydrofolate reductase, an enzyme responsible for converting folic acid to its active form, folate, which is needed for the synthesis of DNA. The result is that DNA is not produced and the cell dies. In practice, the terms *folic acid* and *folate* are often used interchangeably. Pemetrexed is the name of a newer folate antagonist with a mechanism of action similar to that of methotrexate. Pralatrexate (Folotyn) is the newest dihydrofolate reductase inhibitor, specifically indicated for T-cell lymphoma.

### Purine Antagonism

The purine bases present in DNA and RNA are adenine and guanine (see the discussion in Chapter 46), and they are required for the synthesis of the purine nucleotides that are incorporated into the nucleic acid molecules. Mercaptopurine and fludarabine are synthetic analogues of adenine, and thioguanine is a synthetic analogue of guanine. Cladribine is a more general purine antagonist, whereas pentostatin inhibits the action of the critical enzyme adenosine deaminase. Cladribine is unique in that it actually lacks cell cycle specificity relative to other drugs in its class. It is included in this section because of its similar pharmacology and mechanism of action. All of these drugs work by ultimately interrupting the synthesis of both DNA and RNA.

Although allopurinol is chemically similar to purines, it does not disrupt DNA synthesis. Instead, it inhibits xanthine oxidase, which reduces serum and/or urinary levels of uric acid. Rasburicase is an enzyme that degrades uric acid to more soluble end products. Uric acid is a common waste product that often accumulates in the blood following lysis of tumor cells, part of a condition known as tumor lysis syndrome (see Adverse Effects).

### Pyrimidine Antagonism

The pyrimidine bases, cytosine and thymine, occur in the structure of DNA molecules, and cytosine and uracil are part of the structure of RNA molecules. These bases are essential for DNA and RNA synthesis. Floxuridine and fluorouracil are synthetic analogues of uracil, and cytarabine is a synthetic analogue of cytosine. Capecitabine is actually a prodrug of fluorouracil and is converted to that drug in the liver and other body tissues. Because of its prodrug form, it can be given orally. Gemcitabine inhibits the action of two essential enzymes, DNA polymerase and ribonucleotide reductase. Overall, these drugs act in a way that is very similar to that of the purine antagonists, incorporating themselves into the metabolic pathway for the synthesis of DNA and RNA and thereby interrupting the synthesis of both of these nucleic acids.

## Indications

Antimetabolite antineoplastic drugs are used for the treatment of a variety of solid tumors and some hematologic cancers. They may also be used in combination chemotherapy regimens to enhance the overall cytotoxic effect. Methotrexate is also used to treat severe cases of psoriasis (a skin condition) as well as rheumatoid arthritis (see Chapter 47). Because some of these drugs are available in both oral and topical preparations, they are sometimes used for low-dose maintenance and palliative (noncurative) cancer therapy.

Allopurinol and rasburicase are both indicated for the hyperuricemia associated with tumor lysis syndrome and are usually given in anticipation of this condition during various chemotherapy regimens associated with this syndrome. Allopurinol is also used commonly in oral form to treat gout (see Chapter 44). The commonly used drugs and their common specific therapeutic uses are listed in the Dosages table on p. 733.

## Adverse Effects

Like most antineoplastic drugs, antimetabolites can cause hair loss, nausea, vomiting, diarrhea, and myelosuppression. The relative emetic potentials for some of these drugs are listed in Box 45-1. In addition, other major types of toxicity including neurologic, cardiovascular, pulmonary, hepatobiliary, GI, genitourinary, dermatologic, ocular, otic, and metabolic toxicity. Common manifestations of these various toxicities are listed in Table 45-6, roughly in order of increasing severity. Note that a single drug may not cause all of the specific symptoms that are listed for each toxicity category, and actual symptoms may vary widely in severity among patients. The most common general symptoms are fever and malaise. Metabolic toxicity also includes tumor lysis syndrome, a common postchemotherapy

## TABLE 45-6 COMMON MANIFESTATIONS OF ANTINEOPLASTIC TOXICITY

| TYPE OF TOXICITY | COMMON MANIFESTATIONS |
|---|---|
| Neurologic | Fatigue, weakness, depression, agitation, euphoria, insomnia, sedation, headache, reduced libido, confusion, amnesia, hallucinations (visual and auditory), dizziness, loss of taste or altered taste sensations, dysarthria (joint pain), polyneuropathy (e.g., numbness in extremities), neuritis, paresthesia (abnormal touch sensations), facial paralysis, migraine, tremor, hemiplegia, loss of consciousness, seizures, ataxia, stroke, encephalopathy |
| Cardiovascular | Hot flushes, edema, thrombophlebitis and bleeding (e.g., near infusion site), chest pain, tachycardia, bradycardia, other dysrhythmias, angina, venous or arterial thrombosis, transient ischemic attacks, heart failure, myocardial ischemia, pericarditis, pericardial effusion, pulmonary embolism, aneurysm, cardiomyopathy, myocardial infarction, stroke, cardiac arrest, sudden cardiac death |
| Pulmonary-respiratory | Cough, rhinorrhea (runny nose), sore throat, sinusitis, bronchitis, pharyngitis, laryngitis, epistaxis (nosebleed), abnormal breath sounds, asthma, bronchospasm, atelectasis, pleural effusion, hemoptysis, hypoxia, respiratory distress, pneumothorax, diffuse interstitial pneumonitis, fibrosis, hemorrhage, anaphylaxis and generalized allergic reactions |
| Hepatobiliary | Increased bilirubin and liver enzyme levels, jaundice, cholestasis, acalculic cholecystitis (inflamed gallbladder without stones), hepatitis, sclerosis, fibrosis, fatty liver changes, venoocclusive hepatic disease, cirrhosis, hepatic coma |
| Gastrointestinal (GI) | Dyspepsia (heartburn), hiccups, gingivitis (inflamed gums), glossitis (inflamed tongue), abdominal pain, nausea, vomiting, diarrhea, constipation, gastroenteritis, stomatitis (painful mouth sores), oral candidiasis (thrush), ulcers, proctalgia (rectal pain), hematemesis, GI hemorrhage, melena (blood in stool), toxic intestinal dilation, ileus (bowel paralysis), ascites, necrotizing enterocolitis |
| Genitourinary | Oliguria, nocturia, dysuria, proteinuria, crystalluria, hematuria, urinary retention, abnormal renal function test results, hemorrhagic cystitis, renal failure |
| Dermatologic | Rash, erythema, pruritus, ecchymosis, dryness, edema, photosensitivity, sweating, discoloration (pigmentation changes), freckling, petechiae, purpura, numbness, tingling, hypersensitivity, fissuring, scaling, seborrhea, acne, eczema, psoriasis, skin hypertrophy, subcutaneous nodules, alopecia, nail disorder including onycholysis (loss of nails), dermatitis, cellulitis, excoriation, maceration, ulceration, urticaria, abscesses, benign skin neoplasm, hemorrhage (at injection site), palmar-plantar dysesthesia-paresthesia, toxic epidermal necrolysis, Stevens-Johnson syndrome |
| Ocular | Eye irritation, increased lacrimation, nystagmus, photophobia, visual changes, conjunctivitis, keratitis, dacryostenosis (narrowing of lacrimal duct) |
| Otic | Hearing loss |
| Metabolic | Weight loss or gain, anorexia, dehydration, hypokalemia, hypocalcemia, hypomagnesemia, hypertriglyceridemia, hyperglycemia, syndrome of inappropriate secretion of antidiuretic hormone, hypoadrenalism, protein-losing enteropathy, hyperuricemia, tumor lysis syndrome |
| Musculoskeletal | Back pain, limb pain, bone pain, myalgia, joint stiffness, arthralgia, muscle weakness, fibromyositis |

condition. This syndrome is often associated with induction (initial) chemotherapy for rapidly growing hematologic malignancies. It may include hyperphosphatemia, hyperkalemia, and hypocalcemia. These electrolyte abnormalities are often treated with diuretics such as mannitol, IV calcium supplementation, oral or rectal potassium exchange resin, and oral aluminum hydroxide. Hyperuricemia can lead to nephropathy, and hemodialysis may be required in severe cases of tumor lysis syndrome.

A severe, but usually reversible, form of dermatologic toxicity is known as *palmar-plantar dysesthesia* or paresthesia (also called *hand-foot syndrome*). It can range from mild symptoms such as painless swelling and erythema to painful blistering of the patient's palms and soles. Other severe, but fortunately uncommon, dermatologic syndromes that can similarly affect the skin in more generalized regions include Stevens-Johnson syndrome and toxic epidermal necrolysis.

## Interactions

As is true for cancer drugs in general, the administration of one antimetabolite drug with another that causes similar toxicities may result in additive toxicities. Therefore, the respective risks and benefits must be weighed carefully before therapy is initiated with either another antimetabolite or any other drug possessing a similar toxicity profile. Table 45-7 lists some known common examples of drugs that cause interactions with antimetabolites.

## Dosages

For dosage information on selected antimetabolite chemotherapeutic drugs, see the table on p. 733. It is important to note that dosages of antineoplastics are highly variable based on type of cancer, prior therapy, and planned co-administration of other agents.

## DRUG PROFILES

### FOLATE ANTAGONIST

♦ **methotrexate**

Methotrexate is the prototypical antimetabolite of the folate antagonist group and is currently one of only three antineoplastic folate antagonists used clinically. It has proved useful for the treatment of solid tumors such as breast, head and neck, and lung cancers and for the management of acute lymphocytic leukemia and non-Hodgkin's lymphomas. Methotrexate also has immunosuppressive activity, because it can inhibit lymphocyte multiplication. For this reason, it may be useful in the treatment of rheumatoid arthritis (see Chapter 47). Its combined immunosuppressant and antiinflammatory properties also make it useful for the treatment of psoriasis.

High-dose methotrexate is associated with severe bone marrow suppression and is always given in conjunction with the "rescue" drug leucovorin. Leucovorin is an antidote for folic acid antagonists. The body produces active folic acid via metabolic steps utilizing the enzyme dihydrofolate reductase. Because

## TABLE 45-7   SELECTED ANTIMETABOLITES: COMMON DRUG INTERACTIONS

| ANTIMETABOLITE | INTERACTING DRUG | OBSERVED AND REPORTED EFFECTS* |
|---|---|---|
| capecitabine | warfarin | Altered coagulation test results with potential for fatal bleeding |
| | phenytoin | Reduced phenytoin clearance and toxicity |
| | leucovorin | Potentiation of capecitabine with possible toxicity |
| cladribine | None listed | None listed |
| cytarabine | digoxin | Reduced absorption likely due to cytarabine-induced damage to intestinal mucosa; elixir form may be better absorbed |
| | Aminoglycoside antibiotics | Reduced antibiotic efficacy against *Klebsiella pneumoniae* infections |
| floxuridine | None listed | None listed |
| fludarabine | cytarabine | Increased antitumor activity of cytarabine |
| | pentostatin | Potentially fatal pulmonary toxicity; do not use together |
| fluorouracil | warfarin | Enhanced anticoagulant effects |
| | leucovorin | Same as for capecitabine |
| | cimetidine | Increases toxicity of fluorouracil |
| gemcitabine | None listed | None listed |
| mercaptopurine (6-MP) | allopurinol | Inhibition of 6-MP metabolism by inhibition of xanthine oxidase enzyme, with possible enhanced 6-MP toxicity; reduce dose to one third to one fourth |
| | warfarin | 6-MP reported to both enhance and inhibit effects of warfarin |
| | Hepatotoxic drugs | Increased risk of liver toxicity |
| methotrexate (MTX) | Protein-bound drugs and weak organic acids (e.g., salicylates, sulfonamides, sulfonylureas, phenytoin) | Possible displacement of MTX from protein-binding sites, enhancing its toxicity |
| | Penicillins, NSAIDs | Possible reduced renal elimination of MTX with potentially fatal hematologic and GI toxicity |
| | Live virus vaccines | Viral infection (true for any immunosuppressive drug) |
| | folic acid | Reduced MTX efficacy (theoretical only) |
| | theophylline | Reduced theophylline clearance |
| | Hepatotoxic drugs | Increased risk of liver toxicity |
| pentostatin | fludarabine | Potentially fatal pulmonary toxicity |
| thioguanine | busulfan | Reports of hepatotoxicity, esophageal varices, and portal hypertension |
| | Other cytotoxic drugs in general | Reports of hepatotoxicity |

*GI,* Gastrointestinal; *NSAIDs,* nonsteroidal antiinflammatory drugs.
*Not all mechanisms for these drug interactions have been clearly identified. The information in this table is based on reported clinical observations, with mention of known or theorized mechanisms when available.

## DOSAGES

### Selected Antimetabolites

| DRUG (PREGNANCY CATEGORY) | PHARMACOLOGIC CLASS | USUAL DOSAGE RANGE* | INDICATIONS |
|---|---|---|---|
| capecitabine (Xeloda) (D) | Pyrimidine antagonist (analogue) | PO: 1250 mg/m² bid for 2 wk, followed by 1-wk rest period; this 3-wk cycle repeatable as ordered | Metastatic colorectal and breast cancer |
| cladribine (Leustatin) (D) | Purine antagonist (analogue) | IV: 0.09 mg/kg/day by continuous infusion for 7 consecutive days | Hairy cell leukemia |
| ◆ cytarabine (Cytosar-U) (D) | Pyrimidine antagonist (analogue) | IV: 100 mg/m²/day by continuous infusion for 7 days (other regimens as well) | Leukemias (several varieties), NHL |
| fludarabine (Fludara) (D) | Purine antagonist (analogue) | IV: 25 mg/m²/day for 5 consecutive days; repeatable q28d | Various acute and chronic leukemias, NHL |
| fluorouracil (Adrucil) (D) | Pyrimidine antagonist (analogue) | IV: short infusion: 400 mg/m²; continuous infusion: 2400 mg/m² over 46 hr; dosage varies afterward depending on patient response | Colon, rectal, breast, esophageal, head and neck, cervical, and renal cancer |
| gemcitabine (Gemzar) (D) | Pyrimidine antagonist (analogue) | IV: 1000 mg/m² once weekly or as protocol dictates; cycle may be repeated or modified according to patient tolerance | Pancreatic, non–small cell lung, and bladder cancer |
| ◆ methotrexate (Trexall, tablet form; otherwise generic) (X) | Folate antagonist (analogue) | IV: 30-40 mg/m²/wk<br>PO: 15-30 mg/day for 5 days, repeated q7d for 3-5 courses | Acute lymphocytic† leukemia; gestational choriocarcinoma; breast, head and neck, and many other cancers |

*IV,* Intravenous; *NHL,* non-Hodgkin's lymphoma; *PO,* oral.
*Note: Dosages are highly variable.
†The term *lymphocytic* is synonymous in the literature with the term *lymphoblastic.*

methotrexate inhibits this enzyme, healthy cells die due to lack of folic acid. By giving leucovorin (which is rapidly converted to the active form of folic acid), it provides the body with active folic acid, which prevents death of normal cells. Methotrexate is available in both injectable and oral (tablet) form. A preservative-free injectable formulation is required for intrathecal (into the subarachnoid space) administration, used in the treatment of some cancers. Other folate antagonists are pemetrexed and pralatrexate, which have actions similar to that of methotrexate. However, they are used less commonly than methotrexate because they have limited indications: lung cancer and T cell lymphoma, respectively.

## PURINE ANTAGONISTS

The currently available purine antagonists are cladribine, fludarabine, mercaptopurine, pentostatin, and thioguanine. Mercaptopurine and thioguanine are administered orally, whereas the other three are available only in injectable form. These drugs are used largely in the treatment of leukemia and lymphoma.

### cladribine

Cladribine (Leustatin) is indicated specifically for the treatment of a certain type of leukemia known as *hairy cell leukemia,* so named because of the appearance of its cancerous cells under the microscope.

### fludarabine

Fludarabine (Fludara), like cladribine, also has a very specific single indication—in this case, chronic lymphocytic leukemia. It is also commonly used in the treatment of follicular lymphoma and as part of salvage therapy in acute myelogenous leukemia.

## PYRIMIDINE ANTAGONISTS

The currently available pyrimidine antagonists are capecitabine, cytarabine, floxuridine, fluorouracil, and gemcitabine. These drugs are used more commonly than the purine antagonists. They are available only in parenteral formulations except for capecitabine, which is currently available only in tablet form. Dosage and other information appear in the Dosages table on p. 733.

### capecitabine

Capecitabine (Xeloda) is indicated primarily for the treatment of metastatic breast cancer.

### ♦ cytarabine

Cytarabine (ara-C) (Cytosar) is used primarily for the treatment of leukemias (acute myelocytic and lymphocytic leukemia and meningeal leukemia) and non-Hodgkin's lymphomas. It is available only in injectable form and may be given IV, subcutaneously, or intrathecally. It is also now available in a special encapsulated liposomal form for intrathecal use only in treating meningeal leukemia. Cytarabine has a unique set of adverse reactions, called "cytarabine syndrome." Cytarabine syndrome is characterized by fever, muscle and bone pain, maculopapular rash, conjunctivitis, and malaise. It usually occurs 6 to 12 hours following cytarabine administration. The syndrome may be treated or prevented by the use of corticosteroids.

### fluorouracil

Fluorouracil (5-FU) (Efudex, Adrucil) is used in a variety of treatment regimens, including the palliative treatment of cancers of the colon, rectum, stomach, breast, and pancreas. It also is used in the adjuvant setting in the treatment of breast and colorectal cancer.

### gemcitabine

Gemcitabine (Gemzar) is an antineoplastic drug structurally related to cytarabine. Gemcitabine is believed to have antitumor activity superior to that of cytarabine. It is used as first-line therapy for locally advanced or metastatic cancer of the pancreas and for the treatment of non–small cell lung cancer. Gemcitabine is increasingly used to treat other solid tumors, including breast cancer.

## MITOTIC INHIBITORS

Mitotic inhibitors include natural products obtained from the periwinkle plant and semisynthetic drugs obtained from the mandrake plant (also known as the "may apple"). The periwinkle plant contains antineoplastic alkaloids. These vinca alkaloids include vinblastine, vincristine, and vinorelbine. Two newer plant-derived drugs are the taxanes. These include paclitaxel, once derived from the bark of the slow-growing Western (Pacific) yew tree, and docetaxel, a semisynthetic taxane produced from the needles of the European yew tree. The current process of isolating the starting material for paclitaxel from the needles has made the drug supply more abundant. Docetaxel is pharmacologically similar to paclitaxel. The newest taxanes are cabazitaxel (Jevtana), which is indicated for prostate cancer, and eribulin (Halaven), which is indicated for breast cancer. Dosage and other information appears in the Dosages table on p. 736.

## Mechanism of Action and Drug Effects

Depending on the particular drug, these plant-derived compounds can work in various phases of the cell cycle (late S phase, throughout $G_2$ phase, and M phase), but they all work shortly before or during mitosis and thus retard cell division. Each different subclass inhibits mitosis in a unique way.

The vinca alkaloids (vincristine, vinblastine, and vinorelbine) bind to the protein tubulin during the metaphase of mitosis (M phase). This prevents the assembly of key structures called *microtubules.* This, in turn, results in the dissolution of other important structures known as *mitotic spindles.* Without these mitotic spindles, cells cannot reproduce properly. This results in inhibition of cell division and cell death.

The taxanes paclitaxel, docetaxel, and cabazitaxel act in the late $G_2$ phase and M phase of the cell cycle. They work by causing the formation of nonfunctional microtubules, which halts mitosis during metaphase.

## Indications

Mitotic inhibitors are used to treat a variety of solid tumors and some hematologic malignancies. They are often used in combination chemotherapy regimens to enhance the overall cytotoxic

## TABLE 45-8 MITOTIC INHIBITOR AND ETOPOSIDE EXTRAVASATION: LISTED SPECIFIC ANTIDOTE

| DRUG | ANTIDOTE PREPARATION | METHOD |
|------|----------------------|--------|
| etoposide teniposide vinblastine vincristine | hyaluronidase (Wydase) 150 units/mL: add 1 mL NaCl (150 units/mL) | 1. Inject 1-6 mL into the extravasated site with multiple subcut injections. 2. Repeat subcut dosing over the next few hours. 3. Apply warm compresses.* No total dose established. |

*subcut,* Subcutaneous.
*Important: Administration of corticosteroids and topical cooling appear to worsen toxicity.

effect. Selected drugs and some of their specific therapeutic uses are listed in the Dosages table on p. 736.

## Adverse Effects

Like many of the antineoplastic drugs, mitotic inhibitor antineoplastic drugs can cause hair loss, nausea and vomiting, and myelosuppression (see Table 45-6). The emetic potential of some of these drugs is given in Box 45-1.

## Toxicity and Management of Extravasation

Most of the mitotic inhibitor antineoplastics are administered IV, and extravasation of these drugs is potentially serious. Specific antidotes and additional measures to be taken for the treatment of extravasation of the mitotic inhibitors are given in Table 45-8.

## Interactions

A variety of drug interactions are possible with most antineoplastic drugs, some more significant than others. A few basic principles apply to all antineoplastic drug classes. Any drug that reduces the clearance of an anticancer drug also increases the risk of toxicity, whereas a drug that increases the elimination of an anticancer drug reduces its efficacy. The use of multiple antineoplastic drugs can cause severe neutropenia and infection, due to additive bone marrow suppression. Monitor and treat patients accordingly for hematologic toxicity and infections. Observed drug interactions specific for mitotic inhibitors are summarized in Table 45-9.

## Dosages

For dosage information on selected mitotic inhibitors and alkaloid topoisomerase II inhibitors, see the table on p. 736.

## ALKALOID TOPOISOMERASE II INHIBITORS

Etoposide and teniposide are derivatives of epipodophyllotoxin. They exert their cytotoxic effects by inhibiting the enzyme topoisomerase II, which causes breaks in DNA strands. These drugs work during the late S phase and the $G_2$ phase of the cell cycle.

## TABLE 45-9 SELECTED MITOTIC INHIBITORS AND ETOPOSIDE: COMMON DRUG INTERACTIONS

| DRUG | INTERACTING DRUG | OBSERVED AND REPORTED EFFECTS* |
|------|------------------|-------------------------------|
| etoposide | warfarin | Enhanced anticoagulation |
| | cyclosporine | Reduced etoposide clearance |
| docetaxel | CYP3A4 inhibitors (e.g., azole antifungals, ciprofloxacin, clarithromycin, imatinib, verapamil, many others) | Enhanced docetaxel effect (possible toxicity) |
| | CYP3A4 inducers (e.g., carbamazepine, rifampin, phenytoin) | Reduced docetaxel effect |
| paclitaxel | doxorubicin | Increased cardiotoxicity |
| | CYP3A4 inhibitors and inducers | Same as for docetaxel |
| vincristine | phenytoin | Reduced phenytoin concentrations with consequent enhanced seizure risk |
| | asparaginase | Reduced vincristine clearance and increased neurotoxicity (give vincristine 12 to 24 hours before asparaginase) |
| | mitomycin | Increased risk of pulmonary toxicity |
| | CYP3A4 inhibitors and inducers | Same as for docetaxel |

*CYP3A4,* Cytochrome P-450 liver enzyme 3A4.
*Not all mechanisms for these drug interactions have been clearly identified. The information in this table is based on reported clinical observations, with mention of known or theorized mechanisms when available.

## Dosages

For dosage information on selected mitotic inhibitors and alkaloid topoisomerase II inhibitors, see the table on p. 736.

## DRUG PROFILES

### SELECTED MITOTIC INHIBITORS AND ETOPOSIDE

#### ♦ etoposide

Etoposide (VP-16) (generic) is a topoisomerase II inhibitor. Its structure, mechanism of action, and adverse effect profile are similar to those of teniposide. It is believed to kill cancer cells in the late S phase and the $G_2$ phase of the cell cycle. It is indicated for the treatment of small cell lung cancer and testicular cancer. It is available in both oral and injectable forms. The oral form is poorly absorbed and has fallen out of favor because it produces significant toxicities without therapeutic benefit. The IV drug is formulated in a hydroalcoholic diluent, which can cause toxicity (hypotension) if administered in too high a concentration. A water-soluble form of the drug (Etopophos) can eliminate these administration issues, but it is very expensive compared with the standard preparation.

## DOSAGES

### Selected Mitotic Inhibitors and Etoposide

| DRUG (PREGNANCY CATEGORY) | PHARMACOLOGIC CLASS | USUAL DOSAGE RANGE* | INDICATIONS |
|---|---|---|---|
| **Epipodophyllotoxin Derivative** | | | |
| ◆ etoposide (Toposar, generics) (D) | Topoisomerase II inhibitor | IV: 50-160 mg/m²/day for 4-5 days, then repeated cycles and dosage based on type of cancer | Testicular and small cell lung cancer |
| **Taxane** | | | |
| ◆ paclitaxel (Taxol, Onxol) (D) | Mitotic inhibitor | IV: 135-250 mg/m² q3wk | Ovarian, breast, esophageal, bladder, head and neck, cervical cancer; non–small cell and small cell lung cancer; Kaposi's sarcoma |
| **Vinca Alkaloid** | | | |
| ◆ vincristine (Vincasar PFS, generics) (D) | Mitotic inhibitor | IV: 1.4 mg/m² q1wk; usual max dose 2 mg; fatal if given intrathecally | ALL, AML, HL, NHL, rhabdomyosarcoma, neuroblastoma, Wilms tumor, brain tumors, small cell lung cancer, Kaposi's sarcoma |

*ALL,* Acute lymphocytic leukemia; *AML,* acute myelocytic leukemia; *HL,* Hodgkin's lymphoma; *IV,* intravenous; *NHL,* non-Hodgkin's lymphoma.
*\*NOTE: Dosages may vary widely among treatment protocols.*

### ◆ paclitaxel

Paclitaxel (Taxol) is a natural mitotic inhibitor that was originally isolated from the bark of the Pacific yew tree. The European yew tree is the source for another mitotic inhibitor known as docetaxel (Taxotere). Paclitaxel is currently approved for the treatment of ovarian cancer, breast cancer, non–small cell lung cancer, and Kaposi's sarcoma, among other cancers. Paclitaxel is water-insoluble (hydrophobic), and for this reason it is put into a solution containing oil rather than water. The particular oil used is a type of castor oil called Cremophor EL, the same oil with which cyclosporine is formulated. Many patients tolerate it poorly and show hypersensitivity associated with infusion. For this reason, before patients receive paclitaxel they are premedicated with a steroid (dexamethasone), $H_1$ receptor antagonist (diphenhydramine), and $H_2$ receptor antagonist (ranitidine). Paclitaxel is available only in injectable form. There is an albumin-bound form of the drug (Abraxane) that is not associated with severe infusion reactions.

### ◆ vincristine

Vincristine is an alkaloid isolated from the periwinkle plant that is indicated for the treatment of acute lymphocytic leukemia and other cancers. It is available only in injectable form. It is an M phase–specific drug that inhibits mitotic spindle formation. Vincristine is the most significant neurotoxin of the cytotoxic drug class, but it continues to be used in part because of its relative lack of bone marrow suppression. Special care must be taken not to inadvertently give vincristine via the intrathecal route. Several deaths have been reported due to this error. The World Health Organization and the Institute for Safe Medication Practices suggest that vincristine be diluted in 25 mL of fluid and never dispensed via a syringe to prevent this lethal error from occurring. A special warning is required for all vincristine products dispensed that states "For Intravenous Use Only—Fatal If Given By Other Routes." (See the Safety and Quality Improvement: Preventing Medication Errors box.)

### ⚡ SAFETY AND QUALITY IMPROVEMENT: PREVENTING MEDICATION ERRORS

#### Vincristine: Right Route Is Essential

For several years, the Institute for Safe Medication Practices has recommended changes in procedures to ensure that vincristine and other vinca alkaloids are not given intrathecally (via the spinal route) or by any other route. Administering these drugs through the spinal route is almost always fatal, and the death is slow and excruciating. Mistakes occur when the drug is drawn up in a syringe for intravenous administration and then is inadvertently given via the intrathecal route. These errors are preventable. The World Health Organization has suggested that pharmacies prepare vincristine in a diluted volume, such as in a 50-mL minibag of normal saline, to deter practitioners from giving the drug intrathecally. Drugs given intrathecally are not normally dispensed in a minibag. The nurse, who may be assisting the health care practitioner with intrathecal procedures, needs to be aware of the potential fatal error that may occur if vincristine is given via the wrong route.

Data from Institute for Safe Medication Practices, *Nurse Advise ERR* 9(11):2, 2011, available at www.ismp.org/newsletters/nursing/Issues/NurseAdviseERR201101.pdf. Accessed October 17, 2011.

## TOPOISOMERASE I INHIBITORS

Topoisomerase I inhibitors are a relatively new class of chemotherapy drugs. The two drugs currently available in this class are topotecan and irinotecan. Both are semisynthetic analogues of the compound camptothecin, which was originally isolated in the 1960s from *Camptotheca acuminata*, a Chinese shrub. For this reason, these drugs are also referred to as *camptothecins*.

## Mechanism of Action and Drug Effects

The camptothecins inhibit proper DNA function in the S phase by binding to the DNA–topoisomerase I complex. This complex normally allows DNA strands to be temporarily cleaved and then reattached in a critical step known as *religation*. The binding of the camptothecin drugs to this complex retards this religation process, which results in a DNA strand break.

## Indications

The two currently available topoisomerase I inhibitors are used primarily to treat ovarian and colorectal cancer. Topotecan has been shown to be effective even in cases of metastatic ovarian cancer that have failed to respond to platinum-containing regimens (e.g., cisplatin, carboplatin) and paclitaxel. Topotecan is also used to treat small cell lung cancer. Irinotecan is currently approved for the treatment of metastatic colorectal cancer, small cell lung cancer, and cervical cancer.

## Adverse Effects

The main adverse effect of topotecan is bone marrow suppression. Topotecan is not given to patients with baseline neutrophil counts of less than 1500 cells/mm$^3$. Other adverse effects are relatively minor compared with those of the other antineoplastic drug classes. These include mild to moderate nausea, vomiting, and diarrhea; headache; rash; muscle weakness; and cough.

| TABLE 45-10 | **IRINOTECAN: COMMON DRUG INTERACTIONS** |
|---|---|
| **INTERACTING DRUG** | **OBSERVED AND REPORTED EFFECTS\*** |
| CYP2B6 inhibitors (e.g., paroxetine, sertraline) | Increased effects and toxicity of irinotecan |
| CYP3A4 inhibitors (e.g., azole antifungals, ciprofloxacin, clarithromycin, imatinib, isoniazid, verapamil) | Increased effects and toxicity of irinotecan; concurrent use not recommended |
| CYP2B6 inducers (e.g., carbamazepine, phenytoin, nevirapine) | Reduced effects of irinotecan |
| CYP3A4 inducers (e.g., aminoglutethimide, rifampin, nevirapine, phenytoin) | Reduced effects of irinotecan |
| St. John's wort (CYP3A4 inducer) | Reduced effects of irinotecan; stop St. John's wort 2 wk before initiating irinotecan therapy |

*CYP2B6,* Cytochrome P-450 liver enzyme 2B6; *CYP3A4,* cytochrome P-450 liver enzyme 3A4.
\*Note that not all mechanisms for these drug interactions have been clearly identified. The information in this table is based on reported clinical observations, with mention of known or theorized mechanisms when available.

Irinotecan causes more severe adverse effects than topotecan. In addition to producing similar hematologic adverse effects, it has been associated with severe diarrhea known as *cholinergic diarrhea.* It is recommended that this condition be treated with atropine unless use of that drug is strongly contraindicated. Delayed diarrhea may occur 2 to 10 days after infusion of irinotecan. This diarrhea can be severe and even life-threatening and must be treated aggressively with loperamide. There is a moderate risk of nausea and vomiting with irinotecan, which requires appropriate supportive care such as IV rehydration and antiemetic drug therapy.

## Interactions

Topotecan has a unique drug interaction involving the granulocyte colony-stimulating factor filgrastim (see Chapter 47). Filgrastim is commonly used to enhance WBC recovery after chemotherapy. When topotecan is given along with filgrastim, myelosuppression has actually been shown to be worsened. It is recommended that filgrastim be administered 24 hours after completion of the topotecan infusion. Laxatives and diuretics are not given with irinotecan, because of the potential to worsen the dehydration resulting from the severe diarrhea that this drug can produce. Severe cardiovascular toxicity, including thrombosis, pulmonary embolism, stroke, and acute fatal myocardial infarction, have been reported when irinotecan is given with fluorouracil and leucovorin. The role of irinotecan in this toxicity syndrome is unclear, because fluorouracil is a well-recognized cause of myocardial ischemia, including myocardial infarction and sudden death. Such drug combinations are given with careful monitoring. Several additional recognized drug interactions occur with irinotecan, which are summarized in Table 45-10.

## Dosages

For dosage information on selected topoisomerase I inhibitors, see the table below.

## DRUG PROFILES

### irinotecan

Irinotecan (Camptosar) is often given with both fluorouracil and leucovorin. It is available only in injectable form.

### topotecan

After initial therapy with other antineoplastics, cancer cells commonly become resistant to their effects. The use of topotecan (Hycamtin) to treat ovarian cancer and small cell lung

## DOSAGES

### Selected Topoisomerase I Inhibitors

| DRUG (PREGNANCY CATEGORY) | PHARMACOLOGIC CLASS | USUAL DOSAGE RANGE\* | INDICATIONS |
|---|---|---|---|
| irinotecan (Camptosar) (D) | Synthetic camptothecin | IV: 125-350 mg/m$^2$ on various days depending on protocol | Metastatic colorectal cancer, small cell lung cancer, cervical cancer |
| topotecan (Hycamtin) (D) | Semisynthetic camptothecin | IV: 1.5 mg/m$^2$ once daily for 5 consecutive days on a repeatable 21-day course | Ovarian and small cell lung cancer |

*IV,* Intravenous.
\*Note: Dosages are highly variable.

cancer has been studied extensively. As noted earlier, it produces therapeutic responses even in cases in which powerful drugs such as cisplatin and paclitaxel have failed. Topotecan is available only in injectable form.

## ANTINEOPLASTIC ENZYMES

Two antineoplastic enzymes are commercially available: asparaginase and pegaspargase. A third, *Erwinia* asparaginase, is available only by special request from the National Cancer Institute for patients who have developed allergic reactions to *Escherichia coli*–based asparaginase. All three drugs are synthesized from cultures of certain bacteria using recombinant DNA technology.

| TABLE 45-11 | SELECTED ANTINEOPLASTIC ENZYMES: COMMON DRUG INTERACTIONS | |
| --- | --- | --- |
| **ENZYME** | **INTERACTING DRUG** | **OBSERVED AND REPORTED EFFECTS*** |
| asparaginase | cyclophosphamide, mercaptopurine, vincristine | Interference with efficacy or clearance of asparaginase |
| | mercaptopurine, methotrexate, prednisone | Enhanced liver toxicity of asparaginase |
| | methotrexate | Reduced antineoplastic effect when given concurrently, but possibly enhanced antineoplastic effect when given 9 to 10 days before or shortly after methotrexate |
| | prednisone | Hyperglycemia (give asparaginase after prednisone) |
| | vincristine | Neuropathy (give asparaginase after vincristine) |
| | aspirin, NSAIDs, dipyridamole, heparin, warfarin | Use with caution due to possible coagulation abnormalities |

*NSAIDs,* Nonsteroidal antiinflammatory drugs.
*Note that not all mechanisms for these drug interactions have been clearly identified. The information in this table is based on reported clinical observations, with mention of known or theorized mechanisms when available.

## Indications

The antineoplastic enzymes are currently approved exclusively for the treatment of acute lymphocytic leukemia.

## Adverse Effects

Of particular note for the antineoplastic enzymes is a fairly unique adverse effect of impaired pancreatic function. This can lead to hyperglycemia and severe or fatal pancreatitis. Other types of adverse effects associated with these drugs are dermatologic, hepatic, genitourinary, neurologic, musculoskeletal, GI, and cardiovascular effects.

## Interactions

Commonly reported drug interactions involving the antineoplastic enzymes are summarized in Table 45-11.

## Dosages

For dosage information on antineoplastic enzymes, see the table below.

## DRUG PROFILES

### ♦ asparaginase

Asparaginase (Elspar) is used for the treatment of acute lymphocytic leukemia. Its mechanism of action is slightly different from that of traditional antineoplastic drugs in that it is an enzyme that catalyzes the conversion of the amino acid asparagine to aspartic acid and ammonia. Leukemic cells are then unable to synthesize the asparagine required for the synthesis of DNA and proteins needed for cell survival.

The only commercially available asparaginase product in the United States is Elspar. It is derived from the *E. coli* bacterium, and it is common for patients to develop allergic reactions to it. When this happens, one alternative is to switch to a product synthesized from *Erwinia* bacteria. This product is not sold commercially in the United States but is available by special request from the National Cancer Institute. Another treatment alternative is to use the commercially available pegaspargase product described in the following drug profile. All antineoplastic enzymes are available only in injectable form.

### pegaspargase

Pegaspargase (Oncaspar) has a mechanism of action, indications, and contraindications similar to those of asparaginase. It is essentially the same enzyme that has been formulated so as to

## DOSAGES

### *Selected Antineoplastic Enzymes*

| DRUG (PREGNANCY CATEGORY) | PHARMACOLOGIC CLASS | USUAL DOSAGE RANGE* | INDICATIONS |
| --- | --- | --- | --- |
| ♦ asparaginase (Elspar) (C) | *Escherichia coli*–derived l-asparagine amidohydrolase enzyme | IV/IM: 200 units/kg/day to 40,000 units per dose depending on protocol | Acute lymphocytic leukemia |
| pegaspargase (Oncaspar) (C) | Pegylated version of asparaginase | IV/IM: 2500 IU/m$^2$ q14d (smaller pediatric dosages) | Acute lymphocytic leukemia (usually in patients who have developed an allergy to asparaginase) |

*IM,* Intramuscular; *IV,* intravenous.
*NOTE: Dosages are highly variable.

reduce its allergenic potential. This process involves chemical conjugation of the enzyme with units of a relatively inert compound known as monomethoxypolyethylene glycol. Because polyethylene glycol is abbreviated PEG, this process is known as *pegylation*. It is a process that is increasingly used in formulating various drugs, some of which are described in other chapters (e.g., see Chapter 47). These drugs are recognized by the prefix *peg* in their generic names. Pegaspargase is usually prescribed for patients who have developed an allergy to asparaginase—a common occurrence, as mentioned earlier, especially with repeated treatment.

# NURSING PROCESS

## ASSESSMENT

With antineoplastic therapy, perform the following components of a thorough physical assessment: nursing history; past and present medical history; family history; medication profile with a notation of allergies as well as a listing of all prescription drugs, over-the-counter (OTC) drugs, and herbals; height, weight, and vital signs; and baseline hearing and vision testing (as ordered). Also assess bowel and bladder patterns, neurologic status, heart sounds, heart rhythm, breath sounds, and lung function. Examine the skin and mucosa, giving attention to turgor, hydration, color, and temperature. Note any signs and symptoms of fear and anxiety with attention to complaints of insomnia, irritability, shakiness, restlessness, and/or palpitations. Also complete an assessment of cultural, emotional, spiritual, sexual, and financial influences, concerns, and issues. Assess the patient's ability to perform activities of daily living and the patient's mobility status and gait. Perform a pain assessment using objective methods such as an intensity rating scale (e.g., 0 to 10, where 0 = no pain and 10 = worst pain ever). Note the pattern of pain, focusing on the location, quality, onset, duration, and precipitating or alleviating factors. Document any oral, pharyngeal, esophageal, and/or abdominal pain; painful swallowing; epigastric or gastric pain, especially after eating spicy or acidic foods; achiness in joints or lower extremities; or numbness, tingling, and any burning or sharp pain. Question the patient about past experiences with pain and about any drug, nondrug, or alternative therapies used as well as any previous successes or failures in pain management. Cultural beliefs and background as they relate to pain are important to assess because the individual's culture may affect how pain is perceived, verbalized, and treated (see Chapter 10).

Assess contraindications, cautions, and drug interactions. Document the findings prior to the use of these drugs. Laboratory tests that are usually ordered include levels of electrolytes and minerals, uric acid levels, complete blood count, platelet count, bleeding time, tests of renal and hepatic function, and cardiac enzyme levels (see the Safety: Laboratory Values Related to Drug Therapy box). Assays of tumor markers may also be ordered to establish baseline levels and determine the impact of the disease and subsequent therapeutic effectiveness. For more information about the specific adverse effects associated with the destruction of various populations of normal cells due to chemotherapy, see Box 45-2. Specific areas of assessment related

---

## BOX 45-2   EFFECTS OF ANTINEOPLASTIC DRUGS ON NORMAL CELLS AND RELATED ADVERSE EFFECTS

Antineoplastic drugs are designed to kill rapidly dividing *cancer* cells, but they also kill rapidly dividing *normal* cells. Such normal cells include cells of the oral and gastrointestinal (GI) mucous membranes, hair follicles, reproductive germinal epithelium, and components of bone marrow (e.g., WBCs, RBCs, and platelets). The more common adverse effects of normal cell kill are as follows:

- Killing of normal cells of the GI mucous membranes may result in adverse effects such as *altered nutritional status, stomatitis* with inflammation and/or ulceration of the oral mucosa throughout the GI tract, *altered bowel function, poor appetite, nausea, vomiting* (often intractable and requiring aggressive antiemetic treatment), and *diarrhea*.
- Killing of the normal cells of hair follicles leads to *alopecia* (loss of hair).
- Killing of normal cells in the bone marrow results in dangerously low (life-threatening) blood cell counts. Because of the negative impact on these normal cells, the nurse must carefully assess the patient's WBCs levels (leukocytes, neutrophils, and band neutrophils), RBC counts, hemoglobin level, hematocrit, and platelet counts (see the Safety: Laboratory Values Related to Drug Therapy box). In addition, monitoring of the patient's absolute neutrophil count (ANC) is needed (ANC = % of neutrophils + % bands × WBC). Monitoring ANC values allows the nurse and other health care providers to identify the nadir—the time of the lowest count when the patient is most vulnerable. An ANC of 500 cells/mm$^3$ or lower indicates high risk for infection.
- Killing of germinal epithelial cells (also rapidly dividing) leads to *sterility* (irreversible) in males, damage to the ovaries with subsequent *amenorrhea* in females, and *teratogenic* effects with possible fetal death in pregnant women.

---

to some of the more common adverse effects of chemotherapy on normal, rapidly dividing cells include the following:

- For *altered nutritional status* and *impaired oral mucosa:* Assess signs and symptoms of altered nutrition with a focus on weight loss, abnormal serum protein-albumin and blood urea nitrogen (BUN) levels (a negative nitrogen status due to low protein levels would be indicated by a decreasing BUN level), weakness, fatigue, lethargy, poor skin turgor, and pale conjunctiva. Assess oral mucosa for any signs and symptoms of *stomatitis,* such as pain or burning in the mouth, difficulty swallowing, taste changes, viscous saliva, dryness, cracking, and/or fissures with or without bleeding of the mucosa.
- For *effects on the GI mucosa:* Assess bowel sounds (hyperactive or hypoactive versus normoactive). Assess for signs and symptoms of *diarrhea,* such as frequent, loose stools (more than three stools per day), urgency, and abdominal cramping. Obtain information about the presence of blood in the stool as well as consistency, color, odor, and amount. Assess for *nausea and vomiting* and determine whether symptoms are acute, delayed, or anticipatory; if vomiting occurs, determine the color, amount, consistency, frequency, and odor, and whether blood is present. The severity of nausea and vomiting may be rated using a scale of 1 to 10 (where 10 is the worst symptoms) or using the terms *mild, moderate,* and *severe.*
- For *alopecia:* Assess the patient's views, concerns, and emotions about potential hair loss. Assess the patient's need to prepare for hair loss, either by leaving the hair as it is and

## SAFETY: LABORATORY VALUES RELATED TO DRUG THERAPY

### Rationales for Assessment and Monitoring of Blood Cell Counts with Antineoplastics

Antineoplastic drugs kill both normal and abnormal cells that are rapidly dividing, and thus the bone marrow and its rapidly dividing cellular constituents are negatively impacted. Because of this characteristic of chemotherapeutic drugs, RBCs, WBCs, and platelets are suppressed and therefore their levels require frequent monitoring. This box presents information specifically on RBCs and hemoglobin (Hgb) and hematocrit (Hct) levels as well as platelet levels. Chapter 46 presents more information on WBCs with neutrophil counts and nadir levels.

| LABORATORY TEST | NORMAL RANGES | RATIONALE FOR ASSESSMENT |
|---|---|---|
| RBC count | M: 4.6-6.2 million cells/mm$^3$<br>F: 4.2-5.4 million cells/mm$^3$ | Bone marrow suppression from antineoplastics affects RBC values, leading to severe anemia. RBCs carry oxygen—attached to the hemoglobin—from the lungs to the rest of the body. RBCs also help carry carbon dioxide back to the lungs for exhalation. Therefore, if RBC counts are low (e.g., with anemia), the body does not get the oxygen it needs, which leads to lack of energy, fatigue, intolerance of activity, shortness of breath, and hypoxemia. For the cancer patient who may already be experiencing the effects of bone marrow suppression from the disease and then from the treatment, this loss of oxygen saturation will be exacerbated resulting in a lesser ability to get up and about and perform activities of daily living. |
| Hct | M: 40%-54%<br>F: 37%-47% | Hct measures the amount of space or volume of RBCs in the blood, so if the RBC value is low the Hct is also low. The impact of this low value is discussed above under RBCs. |
| Hgb level | M: 14-18 g/dL<br>F: 12-16 g/dL | Hgb is the major substance in RBCs. It carries oxygen and is responsible for the red color of the blood cell. With low levels of Hgb, the consequence to the patient is as noted with RBCs. |
| Platelet count | 150,000-140,000 platelets/mm$^3$ | Platelets are the smallest type of blood cell and play a large role in the process of blood clotting. When bleeding occurs, the platelets swell, clump, and form a plug that helps stop the bleeding. Therefore, if platelet levels are lower than 100,000 platelets/mm$^3$, the patient is at high risk for uncontrolled bleeding and/or hemorrhage. Some guidelines may use a platelet count of 50,000 platelets/mm$^3$ and above as the criterion. Seek out further information in policies and procedures, or contact the prescriber. |

*F,* Female; *M,* male.

allowing it to fall out on its own; having the hair cut short; or wearing a scarf, hat, bandana, or hair wrap and/or purchasing a wig before the hair is actually lost. Purchasing a wig prior to chemotherapy will allow for a closer match to a patient's pre-chemotherapy hairstyle.

- For *bone marrow suppression:* Assess for signs and symptoms of *anemia* or the decrease in RBCs, hemoglobin level, and hematocrit (e.g., pallor of the skin, oral mucous membranes, and conjunctiva; fatigue; lethargy; loss of interest in activities; shortness of breath; and inability to concentrate). Assess for signs and symptoms of *leukopenia* (decrease in WBCs [see Chapter 46] and/or absolute neutrophil count [ANC; normal range is 1500 cells/mm$^3$, with severe neutropenia being less than 500 cells/mm$^3$]), including fever; chills; tachycardia; abnormal breath sounds; productive cough with purulent, green, or rust-colored sputum; change in the color of the urine; lethargy; fatigue; and/or acute confusion. Assess for signs and symptoms of *thrombocytopenia* (decrease in thrombocytes [usually less than 100,000] and platelet clotting factors), including indications of unusual bleeding such as petechiae; purpura; ecchymosis; gingival (gum) bleeding; excessive or prolonged bleeding from puncture sites (e.g., intramuscular or IV administration sites or blood draw sites); unusual joint pain; blood in the stool, urine, or vomitus; and a decrease in blood pressure with elevated pulse rate (see the Safety: Laboratory Values Related to Drug Therapy box in this chapter as well as Chapters 26 and 27; see also Box 45-2). Always assess for the normal ranges of laboratory values.
- For possible *sterility, teratogenesis,* damage to ovaries with *amenorrhea:* In adult male patients, assess baseline

reproductive history with attention to sexual functioning, fathering of children, and/or past or current reproductive or sexual problems or concerns. In female adult patients, in addition to the relevant aspects already mentioned, inquire about fertility, menstrual and childbearing history, and age of onset of menses and menopause, if applicable.

With *cell cycle–specific drugs,* document all allergies, cautions, contraindications, and drug interactions. Most *antimetabolite drugs* do not produce severe emesis (i.e., in fewer than 10% of cases). Pentostatin and some of the pyrimidine analogues have emetic potential, so perform an assessment of baseline GI functioning. In addition, the folate antagonists are not as likely to cause emesis but may be associated with GI abnormalities, such as ulcers and stomatitis. Because these drugs are generally administered parenterally (IV), assessing peripheral access areas or central venous sites is critical to prevent risk of damage to surrounding tissue, joints, and tendons. Assess IV sites every hour, as needed, or as per facility protocol for redness, swelling, heat, and pain. One specific assessment consideration associated with the use of the antimetabolite cytarabine is monitoring for the occurrence of *cytarabine syndrome.* This syndrome usually occurs within 6 to 12 hours after drug administration and is characterized by fever, muscle and bone pain, maculopapular rash, conjunctivitis, and malaise. Assessment and quick identification of this syndrome can lead to its prevention and appropriate treatment.

In patients receiving *mitotic inhibitors* (e.g., vinblastine, vincristine) and *alkaloid topoisomerase II inhibitors* (e.g., etoposide), perform baseline hepatic and renal function tests, as ordered. Serum uric acid levels are usually ordered because these levels rise with increased cell death from cancer and/or its treatment. The increase in uric acid may precipitate or exacerbate gout, which, if diagnosed accurately, may be managed. Other mitotic inhibitors, docetaxel and paclitaxel, are associated with severe neutropenia and a decrease in platelet counts (see the Safety: Laboratory Values Related to Drug Therapy box on p. 740, as well as Chapter 47); therefore, perform blood counts before, during, and after drug therapy. Constantly assess the patient for severe hypersensitivity reactions characterized by dyspnea, severe hypotension, and angioedema and generalized urticaria (during treatments). Drops in blood cell counts may even occur before any clinical evidence is present. Note baseline neurologic functioning as well as the presence of any peripheral neuropathies. Because these drugs have multiple incompatibilities and are irritants (irritating the IV site and vein) or vesicants (causing cell death with extravasation and necrosis with ulcerations), you must become familiar with potential solution and/or drug interactions. Consulting with the prescriber and pharmacist as well as authoritative resources would be appropriate. Documentation must include initial and frequent follow-up assessments of the IV site.

*Topoisomerase I inhibitors* are associated with hematologic adverse effects; thus, perform baseline WBC counts as ordered. Bone marrow suppression is predictable, noncumulative, reversible, and manageable; therefore, do not give drugs such as topotecan to patients with baseline neutrophil counts of fewer than 1500 cells/mm³. Irinotecan causes more severe adverse effects than topotecan; assess related systems and note the findings. The potential for irinotecan-related *cholinergic diarrhea* requires continual assessment of the GI tract. Diarrhea may appear 2 to 10 days after the irinotecan infusion, and further medical treatment may be required if severe forms of diarrhea occur. The diarrhea may even be life-threatening. There is only moderate risk of nausea and vomiting with irinotecan, which requires immediate and appropriate assessment and care. Drug interactions to assess for include the concurrent administration of topotecan with filgrastim which results in a worsening of myelosuppression. Do not give laxatives or diuretics with irinotecan due to the potential for severe diarrhea, volume loss, and subsequent dehydration. When given with fluorouracil and leucovorin, severe cardiovascular (toxicity including thrombosis), pulmonary embolism, stroke, and acute fatal myocardial infarction may occur. Perform a cautious and skillful assessment of related systems. See Table 45-10 for more drug interactions.

With the use of *natural enzyme* drugs (e.g., asparaginase, pegaspargase), assess pancreatic function because of the potential for severe or even fatal pancreatitis. Because of this risk of pancreatitis, assess the patient closely for moderate to severe abdominal pain (upper left quadrant), nausea, vomiting, and hyperglycemia. Serum alkaline phosphatase and WBC counts, if elevated, may indicate possible pancreatitis if also supported by clinical presentation. Additionally, assessment and documentation of dermatologic, hepatic, genitourinary, neurologic, musculoskeletal, GI, and cardiovascular systems is important due to impact on these systems.

Genetic considerations are an additional area of importance in the treatment of cancer with antineoplastics, as well as with all drug therapy. Assess individuals for the presence of the following characteristics before chemotherapy is initiated: (1) genetic markers for oral cancers, (2) genetic determinants of testosterone or estrogen metabolism, and (3) genetically linked enzyme system abnormalities such as those involving specific cytochrome P-450 enzymes that metabolically convert nicotine to a carcinogenic substance. These genetic factors are very complex; nevertheless, be aware of the possible influence of genetic differences and be forward thinking on the impact of drug research and genetics. See Chapter 8 for more information on genetics as related to drug therapy and the nursing process.

## NURSING DIAGNOSES

1. Diarrhea related to the adverse effects of antineoplastic drugs
2. Acute pain related to the disease process and drug-induced joint pain, stomatitis, GI distress, and other discomforts associated with antineoplastic cell cycle–specific therapy
3. Risk for infection related to drug-induced bone marrow suppression with possible leukopenia and neutropenia

## PLANNING

### GOALS

1. Patient regains as near normal as possible bowel elimination patterns during antineoplastic therapy.
2. Patient achieves improved comfort levels with improved pain control, and symptom and adverse effect management.
3. Patient remains free from infection.

### OUTCOME CRITERIA

1. Patient states measures to minimize diarrhea.
   - Patient states foods and beverages to avoid such as hot, spicy foods and beverages; alcohol; foods high in fiber; gaseous foods such as cruciferous vegetables; and raw seafood.
   - Patient takes antidiarrheal medication, as instructed and if indicated, to avoid dehydration and electrolyte loss.
2. Patient experiences improved pain relief through use of pharmacologic and nonpharmacologic measures to maximize comfort levels associated with chemotherapy-related adverse effects, such as joint pain, stomatitis, and GI distress.
   - Patient requests medication(s) for comfort before pain is uncontrollable and severe.
   - Patient uses a number scale of 0 to 10 for identification of pain level, with 0 being no pain and 10 representing worst pain ever experienced.
   - Patient uses nonpharmacologic measures (such as relaxation, music therapy, pet therapy, biofeedback, massage, therapeutic touch, and diversion) concurrently with drug therapy for increasing comfort levels.
3. Patient states measures to assist in supporting immune system and preventing infection such as frequent handwashing, performance of deep breathing exercises, forcing of fluids, consumption of a well-balanced diet, avoidance of malls and other crowded places, and avoidance of persons with colds, flu, or communicable respiratory illnesses.

- Patient states ways to minimize oral mucosal breakdown and infection, such as frequent mouth care and dental hygiene measures using mild toothpaste, gentle sponge-type toothettes, and non–alcohol-based mouthwash, as well as taking fluids frequently.
- Patient demonstrates the use of various measures to enhance skin integrity, such as keeping skin clean, dry, and lubricated.
- Patient adheres to daily regimen for increasing urinary health, such as forcing fluids and consuming fluids that minimize urinary infections (e.g., cranberry juice).

(Note that the nursing diagnoses, goals, and outcome criteria presented here are appropriate to treatment with many antineoplastic drugs.)

## IMPLEMENTATION

Antineoplastic drugs are some of the most toxic medications given to patients because they cause the death of normal cells along with the death of cancer cells. The high potency of these drugs also places the patient at higher risk for toxicity, serious complications, and adverse effects. The possibility of such adverse effects and toxicities requires skillful nursing care based on cautious and thorough assessment and subsequent critical thinking. General considerations in nursing implementation applicable to most antineoplastic drugs as well as some specific aspects of implementation related to cell cycle–specific drugs are discussed in the following paragraphs. Other nursing process information related to cell cycle–nonspecific drugs is presented in Chapter 46.

For antineoplastic therapy in general, nursing considerations related to *reducing fear and anxiety* include establishing a therapeutic relationship beginning with trust and empathy. Approach the patient in a warm, empathic, and supportive manner while projecting confidence in providing nursing care. Provide individualized explanations and teaching about the patient's illness, care, and treatments that are appropriate to the patient's educational level. Collaborate with all members of the health care team. Encourage patients to consider relaxation techniques such as listening to music, performing meditation, or engaging in guided imagery. It may be necessary to call on all potential sources of support, including social services, counseling services, financial assistance services, Meals On Wheels, and religious-spiritual or belief systems with respect to the patient's needs. Appropriate consults may also be necessary with other practitioners such as a licensed clinical social worker, discharge planner, clinical psychiatrist, mental health nurse, nurse practitioner, and oncology nurse specialist, as well as with support groups for the patient, family, and/or significant others.

A variety of interventions that may be indicated for the management of *stomatitis* or excessive oral mucosa dryness and irritation include the following: (1) Instruct the patient to perform oral hygiene before and after eating or as needed to provide cleanliness and comfort. Advise the patient to avoid lemon, glycerin, undiluted peroxide, or alcohol-containing products because they are drying and irritating to the oral mucosa.

(2) Recommend using a soft-bristle toothbrush or soft-tipped toothette or swab with solutions of diluted warm saline. (3) If dentures are worn, encourage the patient to remove and clean them frequently and, if stomatitis is severe, to insert only at mealtimes. (4) Advise using OTC saliva substitutes, keeping the lips moist, and using sugarless candy or gum to stimulate saliva flow. (5) Stress that spicy, acidic, or hot foods; alcohol; and tobacco must be avoided because they are irritants. (6) Oral antifungal suspensions (e.g., nystatin) may be ordered if white patches are noted on the oral mucosa; use analgesic solutions (e.g., lidocaine swish and swallow), as ordered, to help manage discomfort. Other regimens may be prescribed, as needed.

*Nausea and vomiting* occur commonly with antineoplastic drugs. Emetic potential varies depending on the drug and treatment protocol (see earlier discussion and Box 45-1). Educate the patient on measures to enhance comfort during times of nausea and vomiting, including restricting oral intake as ordered; removing noxious odors or sights to avoid stimulating the vomiting center; performing oral hygiene as needed; promoting relaxation through slow, deep breathing; consuming small, frequent meals and eating slowly; and consuming clear liquids and a bland diet. Use of IV fluids may be indicated if nausea and vomiting are severe for hydration purposes. Antiemetics are also a vital part of antineoplastic therapy (see Chapter 52 for more specific drug-related information). Premedication with antiemetics 30 to 60 minutes before administration of the antineoplastic(s) is the preferred treatment protocol to help reduce nausea and vomiting, prevent dehydration and malnutrition, and promote comfort. Combination antiemetic drug therapy may be more effective than single-drug therapy. An antiemetic may be given with the chemotherapeutic regimen and prescription medication for at home use. Ginger ale and ginger-based teas may be helpful.

*Diarrhea* is also a common adverse effect of antineoplastic therapy. Perform the following nursing interventions: (1) Advise the patient to avoid or limit oral intake of irritating, spicy, and gas-producing foods; caffeine; high-fiber foods; alcohol; very hot or cold foods or beverages; and lactose-containing foods and beverages. (2) Consult appropriate personnel, as ordered, to help the patient and family plan meals and arrange ways to meet the patient's dietary and bowel elimination needs. (3) Administer opioids (e.g., paregoric) or synthetic opioids (e.g., loperamide, diphenoxylate hydrochloride) as prescribed, as antidiarrheals. Adsorbents-protectants and antisecretory drugs may also help reduce GI upset and diarrhea (see Chapter 51).

To address *nutritional concerns,* the following measures may prove beneficial in improving oral intake and nutritional status: (1) Perform a 24-hour recall of food intake, and report the typical week's diet for the patient. (2) Use antiemetic therapy, pain management, mouth care, and hydration, as ordered, to reduce the adverse effects of therapy and improve appetite. (3) To ease taste alterations, advise the patient to consume mild-tasting foods and to use chicken, turkey cheese, or greek yogurt for protein sources as tolerated. (4) Provide plastic rather than metal utensils if the patient complains of a metallic taste. (5) Encourage eating foods that are easy to swallow, such as custards; gelatins; puddings; milkshakes; eggnog; commercially prepared high-protein, high-calorie supplemental shakes; mashed white or sweet potatoes; blended drinks with crushed ice, fruit, and yogurt; nutritional supplement drinks and snacks; frozen popsicles; and lactose-free ice cream. (6) Instruct the patient to avoid sticky or dry foods. (7) Encourage the consumption of small, frequent meals in an environment that is conducive to eating (e.g., free of odors and excess noise). (8) Appetite stimulants such as megestrol acetate or dronabinol may be helpful. (9) Encourage the patient to practice energy conservation, with frequent rest periods before and after meals.

*Alopecia* is a common adverse effect of antineoplastics and is very disturbing regardless of age or gender. Warn the patient and family about the possibility of hair loss, and tell them when it will occur (usually 7 to 10 days after treatment begins but dependent upon the specific drug used) and that it is reversible. Inform the patient that new hair growth is often a different color and/or texture from the hair lost. Provide information about the options of acquiring a wig or hairpiece, or wearing scarves or hats, before the actual hair loss. The American Cancer Society may be a resource for items such as wigs, scarves, and hats.

Antineoplastic-induced bone marrow suppression leads to *anemias, leukopenia, neutropenia,* and *thrombocytopenia* (see previous discussion and Safety: Laboratory Values Related to Drug Therapy boxes in this chapter and Chapter 46). Anemias result in fatigue and loss of energy and are common adverse effects of therapy and the disease process. Anemias may require blood transfusions, peripheral blood stem cell treatment, or treatment with prescribed medications such as iron preparations, folic acid, or erythropoietic growth factors (e.g., epoetin or darbepoetin alfa). These injections may be given at home and may be administered at the first sign of a decrease in RBC counts. Conservation of energy and planning of care is very important in minimizing patient fatigue.

Risk of infection from leukopenia or neutropenia and/or immunosuppression is one of the more significant adverse effects that requires close attention. Inform the patient and family and/or caregivers that when WBC counts are low, the patient is at high risk for infection and that defenses remain low until the counts recover. Following Standard Precautions and using good handwashing technique are most important in preventing transmission of infection in the hospital and home settings. Because fever is a principal early sign of infection, take oral or axillary temperature at least every 4 hours during periods in which the patient is at risk. Avoid taking the temperature rectally to minimize tissue trauma, breaks in skin integrity, and thus loss of the first line of defense and increased risk to infection. Encourage the patient to immediately report to the prescriber a temperature elevation of 100.5° F (38.1° C) or higher so that appropriate treatment may be initiated and complications avoided.

If needed, and as ordered, administration of colony-stimulating factors may be beneficial. Filgrastim, pegfilgrastim, and sargramostim are examples of drugs given to accelerate WBC recovery during antineoplastic drug therapy. Use these drugs, as ordered, to minimize neutropenia. These medications act on the bone marrow to enhance neutrophil production and help decrease the incidence, severity, and duration of neutropenia. You must administer these drugs within a certain time frame (see Chapter 47). Encourage patients with *immune suppression* to be aware of environments and persons to avoid, such as individuals who have recently been vaccinated (who may have a subclinical infection) or who have a cold or flu or other symptoms of an infection. Maintaining a "low-microbe" diet by washing fresh fruits and vegetables and making sure foods are well cooked is also recommended. Educate patients on the importance of performing oral care frequently (see discussion of stomatitis) and to turn, cough, and deep breathe to help prevent stasis of respiratory secretions.

Thrombocytopenia is also an adverse effect of antineoplastic therapy and puts the patient at risk for bleeding. Monitor platelet counts, coagulation studies, RBC counts, hemoglobin levels, and hematocrit values, and report any decreases (see the Safety: Laboratory Values Related to Drug Therapy box). Avoid injections if possible, and utilize alternative routes of administration. If injections or venipunctures are absolutely necessary, always use the smallest gauge needle possible and apply gentle, prolonged pressure to the site afterward. Monitor patients undergoing bone marrow aspiration closely after the procedure for bleeding at the aspiration site. Perform blood pressure monitoring as needed. Be efficient and quick and without overinflating the cuff to avoid bruising. Monitor the patient for bleeding from the mouth, gums, and nose. Check for bleeding after teeth brushing and report excessive bleeding to the prescriber.

Inform the patient that antineoplastics may also have a *negative impact on the reproductive tract,* causing destruction of the germinal epithelium of the testes and damage to the ovaries and to a fetus (teratogenesis). Other problems may include sterility; amenorrhea; premature menopausal symptoms of hot flashes, decreased vaginal secretions, mood changes, or irritability; and decreased libido or sexual dysfunction. Counsel male patients about the risk of sterility which may be irreversible. Discuss with male patients the option and topic of sperm banking before chemotherapy, if deemed appropriate. Stress that female patients of childbearing age who are sexually active need to protect themselves against pregnancy because of the risk of embryonic death. Encourage contraceptive measures during chemotherapy and for up to 8 weeks after discontinuation of therapy; however, some antineoplastic drugs require use of contraception for up to 2 years after completion of treatment because of the long-term risk for genetic abnormalities.

With *antimetabolites,* always follow the prescriber's orders regarding premedication with antiemetics and/or antianxiety drugs. Follow orders or protocol for the use of other symptom-control medications, as prescribed. GI adverse effects are common with antimetabolites and usually occur on about the fourth day and require preplanning for special pharmacologic interventions (e.g., antiemetics, antispasmodics, analgesics) and nonpharmacologic measures (dietary changes, oral care). Antibiotic therapy may also be ordered prophylactically. See earlier discussion of nursing considerations associated with stomatitis, loss of appetite, diarrhea, nausea, nutrition, hydration, vomiting, and anemias. For further discussion of the handling of antimetabolites and other IV antineoplastic drugs, see Box 46-3.

Use extreme caution in handling and administration of cytarabine by the various routes (IV, subcutaneous, or intrathecal). Other major concerns with cytarabine therapy are bone marrow suppression (see earlier discussion) and cytarabine syndrome (see the Assessment section). If high dosages are used, cytarabine may also cause central nervous system, GI, and/or pulmonary toxicity, so closely monitor these systems to ensure patient safety and comfort. For intrathecal administration, the drug may be reconstituted with sodium chloride, or the prescriber may use the patient's spinal fluid. Do not add fluorouracil to any other IV infusions; administer the drug by itself in the appropriate diluent. When an infusion port is not used, do not use IV sites over joints, tendons, or small veins, or in extremities that are edematous. Give IV dosages exactly as ordered, and constantly monitor the IV site, infusion port, and/or infusion solution and equipment. If IV infiltration occurs, follow the protocol for management of infiltration and contact the prescriber. Follow all hospital or infusion protocols without exception because treatment of extravasation is handled differently depending on the specific drug. If extravasation of a vesicant occurs, the drug is usually discontinued immediately; leave the IV cannula in place (for possible use of antidotes through cannula to access affected area), and follow facility protocol. Antidotes and use of other drugs, as well as use of hot or cold packs, is usually outlined in the protocol for managing extravasation (see Box 46-1). If topical forms of the drug are used, inform the patient that it is important to apply the drug exactly as ordered and to the affected area only. Use gloves or a finger cot to apply the topical dosage form.

Gemcitabine another antimetabolite, is dosed based on absolute granulocyte counts and platelet nadirs and is given if the counts exceed $1500 \times 10^6$ cells/L and $100,000 \times 10^6$ platelets/L, respectively. Keep IV solutions at room temperature to avoid crystallization and use within 24 hours. Give infusions as ordered. Antiemetics and antidiarrheals may be needed. Mercaptopurine comes in oral dosage forms; give as ordered. Finally, the antimetabolite methotrexate has numerous toxicities and adverse effects that may be minimized by appropriate medical treatment. For example, there may be orders for boosting the immune status and blood cell counts before aggressive therapy is initiated. Cytoprotective drugs are used. Continue to monitor creatinine clearance, as ordered, to detect any nephrotoxicity. Nutritional status may be enhanced by the intake of foods high in folic acid, including bran, dried beans, nuts, fruits, asparagus, and other fresh vegetables, if tolerated. Consumption of these foods is yet another measure to help minimize the possibility of methotrexate toxicity. If GI upset and/or stomatitis occur, the patient may need to decrease any sources of irritation (e.g., high-fiber food). Methotrexate is usually given orally or IV. Wear gloves when giving the drug. If any of the solution comes in contact with the skin, wash the area immediately and thoroughly with soap and water. (See Box 46-3 for discussion of concerns in the handling and administration of vesicant drugs.)

For the *mitotic inhibitors,* specifically the taxane family of drugs and docetaxel in particular, premedication protocols are usually specified and include administration of oral corticosteroids (e.g., dexamethasone) beginning several days before day 1 of therapy to help decrease the risk of hypersensitivity. Measure vital signs frequently during the infusion, especially in the first hour of the infusion. Closely monitor the patient for the sudden onset of bronchospasm, flushing of the face, and localized skin reactions; these may indicate a hypersensitivity response requiring immediate treatment. Contact the prescriber immediately. These symptoms may occur within just a few minutes of beginning the infusion. In addition, any dyspnea, abdominal distension, crackles in the lungs, or dependent edema during therapy require immediate attention. Cutaneous reactions may also appear during therapy and include rash on the hands and feet; these also need immediate attention and treatment. With paclitaxel, the patient may also be premedicated with diphenhydramine, corticosteroids, and $H_2$ antagonist drugs. Take all measures to minimize tissue trauma (e.g., avoidance of intramuscular injections and rectal temperature taking, if possible) to promote comfort and prevent bleeding and infection.

With the *topoisomerase I inhibitors,* irinotecan and topotecan, monitor blood counts closely with every treatment. A drop in blood counts and/or severe diarrhea may cause a temporary postponement of therapy. Treat any extravasation of the solution immediately, and follow protocol. Ensuring that IV sites remain patent is critical to the prevention of tissue damage secondary to extravasation of antineoplastic drugs that are considered to be irritants and/or vesicants. Nausea and vomiting may lead to dehydration and electrolyte disturbances. Advise patients and family members to report these symptoms immediately before negative consequences occur (see previous discussion for specific interventions). IV incompatibilities are numerous for both these drugs and are of constant concern. With topotecan, IV extravasation is usually accompanied by a mild local reaction such as erythema or bruising. If these symptoms are noted, they must be managed immediately to avoid further trauma and/or risk for loss of skin integrity (the first line of defense against infection). Headaches and difficulty breathing may be more common with topotecan; therefore, closely and frequently monitor the patient for these symptoms.

Handle the *enzyme antineoplastics* asparaginase and pegaspargase with extreme caution and care. The patient may receive an intradermal test dose of asparaginase before therapy begins or when a week or longer has passed between doses. With asparaginase and pegaspargase, if the solution comes in contact with the skin, thoroughly wash or rinse the area with copious amounts of water for a minimum of 15 minutes. During therapy, if there are signs and symptoms of oliguria, anuria (renal failure), or pancreatitis, the drug will most likely be discontinued. The intramuscular route of administration is usually preferred because it carries a lower risk of causing clotting abnormalities, GI disorders, and renal and hepatic toxicity. If solutions are cloudy, do not use them. If more than 2 mL is ordered/required for an intramuscular dosing, use two injections. Pancreatitis is problematic with these drugs and can be serious. Pay close attention to symptoms such as severe abdominal pain with nausea and vomiting. Constantly monitor serum lipase and amylase levels. If any signs or symptoms of pancreatitis occur, the prescriber will usually discontinue the drugs immediately. Use of cytoprotective drugs has been briefly discussed in the Pharmacology section of this chapter, with further discussion provided in Chapter 46.

## ▌EVALUATION

Focus evaluation of nursing care on reviewing whether goals and outcomes are being met as well as monitoring for therapeutic responses and adverse and toxic effects of the antineoplastic therapy. Therapeutic responses may manifest as clinical improvement, decrease in tumor size, and decrease in metastatic spread. Evaluation of nursing care, with reference to goals and outcomes, may reveal improvements related to a decrease in adverse effects and a decrease in the impact of cancer on the patient's well-being. There will be increases in comfort, nutrition, hydration, energy levels, ability to carry out activities of daily living, and improved quality of life with therapeutic effectiveness. Revisit goals and outcomes to identify more specific areas to monitor. In addition, certain laboratory studies such as tumor marker levels, levels of carcinoembryonic antigens, RBC and WBC counts, and platelet counts may be performed to aid in determining how well the treatment protocol has worked and to monitor adverse effects of bone marrow suppression. Also, if absolute neutrophil count (ANC) drops below 500 cells/mm³, the prescriber may discontinue chemotherapy but

then reinitiate when the level is above 1000 cells/mm³ or as facility policy or prescriber dictates. Other blood counts are considered, too. As part of the evaluation, prescribers may also order additional radiographs, computed tomographic scans, magnetic resonance images, tissue analyses, or other studies appropriate to the diagnosis both during and after antineoplastic therapy has been completed, at time intervals related to the anticipated tumor response.

---

### CASE STUDY

#### *Facing Chemotherapy*

Mrs. D., a 48-year-old married mother of two teenage daughters, has been diagnosed with breast cancer. She has undergone lumpectomy to remove the tumor and is about to start adjuvant chemotherapy. She states that she has "faced the facts" about her disease and the threat to her life but says, "I know this is silly, but I hate the thought of losing my hair to this disease."

1. What measures can be taken to help Mrs. D. deal with her hair loss?
2. Ten days after the chemotherapy, Mrs. D.'s neutrophil count drops to 2000 cells/mm³. She has been hospitalized because she has developed a cough, and several of her friends have come in to visit her with a fresh fruit basket. What actions will be taken to protect her from infection?
3. During rounds, the nurse finds Mrs. D. curled up in the bed and sobbing. Mrs. D. says that she feels "so afraid" and is worried about who will care for her family if she dies. What actions will the nurse take at this time?

For answers, see http://evolve.elsevier.com/Lilley.

---

## ▌ PATIENT TEACHING TIPS

- Educate patients that GI adverse effects and irritation to the oral and GI mucosa may be decreased by avoiding intake of alcohol, tobacco, spicy and high-fiber foods, citrus fruit juices or foods, and foods that are too hot or cold or have a rough texture.
- Stress that daily mouth care is needed. Instruct the patient to report mouth sores, pain, or white patches to the prescriber immediately. Headache, fatigue, faintness, shortness of breath (possibly indicative of anemia), bleeding, easy bruising (possibly indicative of a drop in platelet count), sore throat, and fever (possibly indicative of infection) also need to be reported immediately to the appropriate prescriber. Fever and/or chills may be the first sign of an oncoming infection.
- Discuss contraception, sperm banking, and other reproductive issues with male patients and women of childbearing age.
- Emphasize to the patient receiving antineoplastic drugs which OTC medications to avoid (e.g., aspirin, ibuprofen, and any combination products containing these OTC drugs).
- Antineoplastics may cause alopecia (hair loss). Before therapy, provide the patient with the opportunity to discuss options for hair and scalp care. These options may include, but are not limited to, having the hair cut short before treatment; selecting, purchasing, or renting a wig or hairpiece comparable to the patient's existing hair in color, texture,

length, and style; or having bandanas, scarves, or hats on hand before the hair is actually lost. Although hair loss is temporary, inform patients that it will occur and that hair will appear differently upon growing back. The American Cancer Society may be a resource for wigs and hairpieces.
- The following websites are helpful online resources for the patient and significant others: www.fda.gov, http://www.fda.gov/ForHealthProfesionals/default.htm,www.nih.gov, http://www.healthfinder.gov, www.who.int/en, and http://www.oncolink.org/index.cfm.
- With *cytarabine*, encourage the patient to increase fluid intake to help decrease the risk of dehydration and/or hyperuricemia.
- With *fluorouracil* and *gemcitabine,* encourage frequent oral hygiene and for the patient to report to the prescriber immediately any bleeding, bruising, chest pain, diarrhea, nausea, vomiting, heart palpitations, infection, or changes in vision. Instruct patients to protect themselves from the sun while taking fluorouracil, including avoiding overexposure to sun or ultraviolet light and using protective clothing, sunscreen, and sunglasses.
- With *mercaptopurine*, educate the patient that alcohol must be avoided to help minimize drug toxicity.
- With *methotrexate,* inform the patient to notify the prescriber if nausea and vomiting are problematic or uncontrollable, or if fever, sore throat, muscle aches and pains, or

## PATIENT TEACHING TIPS—cont'd

unusual bleeding occurs. Advise the patient to avoid alcohol, salicylates, nonsteroidal antiinflammatory drugs, and exposure to sunlight or ultraviolet light. Instruct both male and female patients to use contraceptive measures for up to 3 months or longer, if appropriate.

• With *taxanes,* specifically paclitaxel, counsel the patient to report to the prescriber immediately any signs or symptoms of neuropathy (e.g., numbness or tingling of the extremities).

• With *etoposide* and *teniposide* as with other antineoplastics, if WBC counts are low, caution the patient to avoid individuals who are ill. Additionally, advise the patient to report to the prescriber immediately any easy bleeding, bruising, difficulty breathing, fever, sore throat, or chills.

• With *asparaginase* and *pegaspargase,* encourage the patient to force fluids and to report any severe nausea or vomiting, bleeding, excessive fatigue, or fever or other signs or symptoms of infection.

## KEY POINTS

• Cancers are diseases that are characterized by uncontrolled cellular growth.

• *Malignancy* refers specifically to a neoplasm that is anaplastic, invasive, and metastatic, as opposed to benign.

• Tumors are generally classified by tissue of origin, as follows: epithelial (carcinoma), connective (sarcoma), lymphatic (lymphoma), and leukocytes (leukemia).

• Antineoplastics are drugs that are used to treat malignancies. They may be either cell cycle–specific or cell cycle–nonspecific drugs or may have miscellaneous actions.

• Cell cycle–specific drugs kill cancer cells during specific phases of the cell growth cycle. Cell cycle–nonspecific drugs kill cancer cells during any phase of the cell growth cycle.

• Chemotherapy, or antineoplastic drug therapy, requires very skillful and perceptive nursing care. It is important to act prudently and think critically when making decisions about the nursing care of patients receiving these drugs.

• Cell cycle–specific drug classes include antimetabolites, mitotic inhibitors, alkaloid topoisomerase II inhibitors, topoisomerase I inhibitors, and antineoplastic enzymes.

• Antineoplastic antimetabolites are cell cycle–specific antagonistic analogues that work by inhibiting the actions of key cellular metabolites.

• Two plant-derived antineoplastic drugs are the taxanes paclitaxel, derived from the bark of the slow-growing Western (Pacific) yew tree, and docetaxel, a semisynthetic taxoid produced from the needles of the European yew tree. Docetaxel is pharmacologically similar to paclitaxel.

• The topoisomerase I inhibitors topotecan and irinotecan compose a relatively new class of chemotherapy drugs.

• Antineoplastic enzymes include asparaginase and pegaspargase.

• Several drugs are available that are classified as cytoprotective and help reduce the toxicity of various antineoplastics.

## NCLEX® EXAMINATION REVIEW QUESTIONS

1 A patient is experiencing stomatitis after a round of chemotherapy. Which intervention by the nurse is correct?
   a Clean the mouth with a soft-bristle toothbrush and warm saline solution.
   b Rinse the mouth with commercial mouthwash twice a day.
   c Use lemon-glycerin swabs to keep the mouth moist.
   d Keep dentures in the mouth between meals.

2 The nurse is caring for a patient who becomes severely nauseated during chemotherapy. Which intervention is most appropriate?
   a Encourage light activity during chemotherapy as a distraction.
   b Provide antiemetic medications 30 to 60 minutes before chemotherapy begins.
   c Provide antiemetic medications only upon the request of the patient.
   d Hold fluids during chemotherapy to avoid vomiting.

3 The nurse monitors a patient who is experiencing thrombocytopenia from severe bone marrow suppression by looking for
   a severe weakness and fatigue.
   b elevated body temperature.
   c decreased skin turgor.
   d excessive bleeding and bruising.

4 A patient receiving chemotherapy is experiencing severe bone marrow suppression. Which nursing diagnosis is most appropriate at this time?
   a Activity intolerance
   b Risk for infection
   c Disturbed body image
   d Impaired physical mobility

5 If extravasation of an antineoplastic medication occurs, which intervention will the nurse perform first?
 a Apply cold compresses to the site while elevating the arm.
 b Inject subcutaneous doses of epinephrine around the IV site every 2 hours.
 c Stop the infusion immediately while leaving the catheter in place.
 d Inject the appropriate antidote through the IV catheter.

6 The nurse is assessing a patient who has experienced severe neutropenia after chemotherapy and will monitor for which possible signs of infection? (Select all that apply.)
 a Elevated WBC count
 b Fever
 c Nausea
 d Sore throat
 e Chills

7 The order for chemotherapy reads: "Give asparaginase (Elspar) IV 200 units/kg/day." The patient weighs 297 lb. The pharmacy department will prepare the medication for intravenous infusion. How much drug will be given per dose? Is this a safe dose?

1. a, 2. b, 3. d, 4. b, 5. c, 6. b, d, e, 7. 27,000 units; yes

For Critical Thinking and Prioritization Questions, see http://evolve.elsevier.com/Lilley.

# Antineoplastic Drugs Part 2: Cell Cycle–Nonspecific and Miscellaneous Drugs

## ⊖volve WEBSITE

- Animations
- Answer Key—Textbook Case Studies
- Critical Thinking and Prioritization Questions

- Key Points—Downloadable
- Review Questions for the NCLEX® Examination
- Unfolding Case Studies

## OBJECTIVES

When you reach the end of this chapter, you will be able to do the following:

1  Review the concepts related to carcinogenesis, the types of malignancies and related terminology, and the different treatment modalities, including the use of cell cycle–nonspecific and miscellaneous antineoplastic drugs.

2  Identify the various drugs that are classified as cell cycle nonspecific or hormonal or are considered to be miscellaneous antineoplastic drugs.

3  Discuss the common adverse effects and toxic effects of the cell cycle–nonspecific and miscellaneous antineoplastic drugs, including the reasons for their occurrence and methods of treatment, such as any antidotes.

4  Describe the mechanisms of action, indications, dosages, routes of administration, cautions, contraindications,

and drug interactions of the cell cycle–nonspecific drugs, hormonal drugs, and miscellaneous antineoplastic drugs.

5  Apply knowledge about the cell cycle–nonspecific, hormonal agonist-antagonist, and other miscellaneous antineoplastic drugs and their characteristics in the development of a comprehensive nursing care plan for patients with cancer who are receiving these drugs.

6  Briefly describe extravasation and other major adverse effects associated with the cell cycle–nonspecific and miscellaneous antineoplastics, including discussion of protocols and antidotes.

## DRUG PROFILES

**bevacizumab, p. 754**
- ♦ **cisplatin, p. 752**
- ♦ **cyclophosphamide, p. 752**
- ♦ **doxorubicin, p. 753**
  **hydroxyurea, p. 755**
  **imatinib, p. 755**

- ♦ **mechlorethamine, p. 752**
  **mitotane, p. 755**
  **mitoxantrone, p. 754**
  **octreotide, p. 755**

- ♦ *Key drug*

## KEY TERMS

**Alkylation** A chemical reaction in which an alkyl group is transferred from one molecule to another. In chemotherapy, alkylation leads to damage of the cancer cell deoxyribonucleic acid (DNA) and cell death. (p. 749)

**Bifunctional** Referring to those alkylating drugs composed of molecules that have two reactive alkyl groups and that are therefore able to alkylate at two sites on the DNA molecule. (p. 750)

**Extravasation** The leakage of any intravenously or intraarterially administered medication into the tissue space surrounding the vein or artery. Such an event can cause serious tissue injury, especially with antineoplastic drugs. (p. 751)

**Mitosis** The process of cell reproduction occurring in somatic (nonsexual) cells and resulting in the formation of two genetically identical daughter cells, each containing the diploid (complete) number of chromosomes characteristic of the species. (p. 750)

**Polyfunctional** Referring to the action of alkylating drugs that can engage in several alkylation reactions with cancer cell DNA molecules per single molecule of drug. (p. 750)

This chapter is a continuation of Chapter 45 and focuses on additional classes of antineoplastic drugs. Chapter 45 describes the various antineoplastic drugs that are effective against cancer cells during specific phases in the cell growth cycle. In contrast, this chapter focuses on drugs that have antineoplastic activity regardless of the phase of the cell cycle. Also discussed in this chapter are drugs that are classified as miscellaneous antineoplastics, either because of their lack of clear cell cycle specificity or their unique or novel (new) mechanisms of action. For a description of the cell growth cycle, see Chapter 45.

## PHARMACOLOGY OVERVIEW

### CELL CYCLE–NONSPECIFIC ANTINEOPLASTIC DRUGS

There are currently two broad classes of cell cycle–nonspecific cancer drugs: alkylating drugs and cytotoxic antibiotics.

### ALKYLATING DRUGS

Records of the use of drugs to treat cancer date back several centuries. However, truly successful systemic cancer chemotherapy treatments are not documented until the 1940s. At this time, the first alkylating drugs were developed from mustard gas agents that were used for chemical warfare before and during World War I. The first drug to be developed was mechlorethamine, which is also known as *nitrogen mustard*. It is the prototypical drug of this class and is still used today for cancer treatment. Since its antineoplastic activity was discovered in the mid-twentieth century, many analogues have been synthesized for use in the treatment of cancer, and they are collectively referred to as nitrogen mustards also.

The alkylating drugs commonly used in clinical practice in the United States today fall into three categories: classic alkylators (the nitrogen mustards); nitrosoureas, which have a different chemical structure than the nitrogen mustards but also work by alkylation; and miscellaneous alkylators, which also have a different chemical structure than the nitrogen mustards but are known to work at least partially by alkylation. These

drugs are used to treat a wide spectrum of malignancies. The drugs in each category are as follows:

**Classic alkylators (nitrogen mustards)**
- chlorambucil
- cyclophosphamide
- ifosfamide
- mechlorethamine
- melphalan

**Nitrosoureas**
- carmustine
- lomustine
- streptozocin

**Miscellaneous alkylators**
- altretamine
- busulfan
- carboplatin
- cisplatin
- dacarbazine
- oxaliplatin
- procarbazine
- temozolomide
- thiotepa

### Mechanism of Action and Drug Effects

The alkylating drugs work by preventing cancer cells from reproducing. Specifically, they alter the chemical structure of the cells' deoxyribonucleic acid (DNA), which is essential to the reproduction of any cell. DNA molecules consist of two adjacent strands, each consisting of alternating sequences of phosphate and sugar molecules (Figure 46-1). These components make up what is called the "backbone" of the DNA strands. These two strands are chemically linked to each other by the third DNA structural element: nitrogen-containing bases (adenine, guanine, thymine, and cytosine, abbreviated A, G, T, and C, respectively). These bases are bound to the sugar molecules of the DNA backbone, and two bases, linked to each other by hydrogen bonds, form the molecular bridges between the two DNA strands that bring them into the double helix structure. A nucleotide, which consists of one molecule each of base, sugar, and phosphate that are bound together, is the structural unit of the molecules of both DNA and ribonucleic

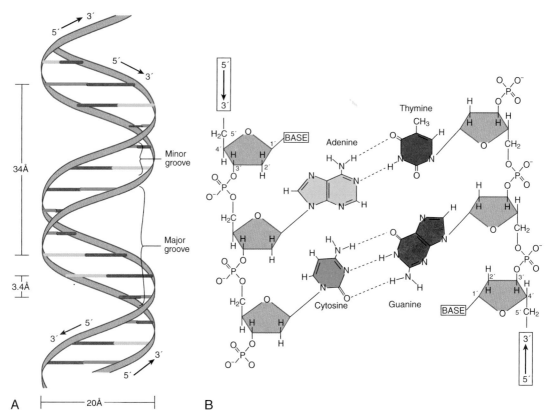

**FIGURE 46-1** Deoxyribonucleic acid (DNA) double helix. **A,** Diagrammatic model of the helical structure, showing its dimensions, the major and minor grooves, the periodicity of the bases, and the antiparallel orientation of the backbone chains (represented by ribbons). The base pairs (represented by rods) are perpendicular to the axis and lie stacked one on another. **B,** The chemical structure of the backbone and bases of DNA, showing the sugar-phosphate linkages of the backbone and the hydrogen bonding between the base pairs. There are two hydrogen bonds between adenine and thymine, and three between cytosine and guanine. (From *Dorland's illustrated medical dictionary,* ed 31, Philadelphia, 2007, Saunders.)

acid (RNA), another nucleic acid that is important in cellular reproduction. Messenger RNA (mRNA) molecules are produced by DNA molecules during the complex process of transcription. These mRNA molecules differ from DNA molecules in at least three ways: they are single stranded (instead of double stranded), the thymine base is replaced by another base known as uracil (U), and the sugar molecule is ribose, which has a slightly different structure from that of the deoxyribose molecules of DNA.

During the normal process of reproduction, the double helix uncoils, and its two strands separate. A strand of RNA is then assembled next to each single DNA strand in a process known as *transcription*. RNA strands, in turn, are involved in both protein synthesis (translation) and replication of the original DNA structure before cell division, or mitosis. These processes ultimately result in the creation of a new cell with the same DNA sequence, and thus the same characteristics, as its parent cell.

Alkyl groups that are part of the structure of antineoplastic alkylating drugs attach to DNA molecules by forming covalent bonds with the bases described earlier. As a result, abnormal chemical bonds form between the adjacent DNA strands, which leads to the formation of defective nucleic acids that are then unable to perform the normal cellular reproductive functions mentioned previously. This leads to cell death.

Alkylating drugs can be characterized by the number of alkylation reactions in which they can participate. Bifunctional alkylating drugs have two reactive alkyl groups that are able to alkylate two sites on the DNA molecule. Polyfunctional alkylating drugs can participate in several alkylation reactions. Figure 46-2 shows the location along the DNA double helix where the alkylating drugs work.

## Indications

The most commonly used alkylating drugs today are effective against a wide spectrum of malignancies, including both solid and hematologic tumors. Common examples of the various types of cancer that different alkylating drugs are used to treat are listed in the Dosages table on p. 752.

## Adverse Effects

Alkylating drugs are capable of causing all of the dose-limiting adverse effects described in Chapter 45. Other adverse effects are described in Table 46-1. The relative emetic potential of the various alkylating drugs is given in Box 45-1. The adverse effects of these drugs are important because of their severity, but they can often be prevented or minimized by prophylactic measures. For instance, nephrotoxicity from cisplatin can often be prevented by adequately hydrating the patient with intravenous fluids.

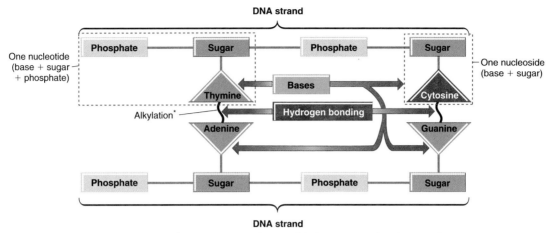

**FIGURE 46-2** Organization of deoxyribonucleic acid (DNA) and site of action (*) of alkylating drugs.

| TABLE 46-1 | COMMONLY USED ALKYLATING DRUGS: SEVERE ADVERSE EFFECTS | |
|---|---|---|
| **DRUG** | **ADVERSE EFFECTS** | |
| busulfan | Pulmonary fibrosis | |
| carboplatin* | Nephrotoxicity, neurotoxicity, bone marrow suppression | |
| cisplatin | Nephrotoxicity, peripheral neuropathy, ototoxicity | |
| cyclophosphamide | Hemorrhagic cystitis | |

*Carboplatin has less nephrotoxicity and neurotoxicity but more bone marrow suppression than cisplatin.

Drug extravasation (Box 46-1) occurs when an intravenous catheter punctures the vein and medication leaks (infiltrates) into the surrounding tissues. With cancer chemotherapeutic drugs, in particular doxorubicin (a cytotoxic antibiotic), extravasation can cause severe tissue damage and necrosis (tissue death). Extravasation antidotes for selected drugs are listed in Table 46-2.

## Interactions

Only a few alkylating drugs are capable of causing significant drug interactions. The most important rule for preventing such drug interactions is to avoid administering an alkylating drug with any other drug capable of causing similar toxicities. For example, a major adverse effect of cisplatin is nephrotoxicity. Therefore, if possible, do not administer it with a drug such as an aminoglycoside antibiotic (gentamicin, tobramycin, or amikacin) because of the resulting additive nephrotoxic effects and hence the increased likelihood of renal failure. Mechlorethamine and cyclophosphamide, both of which have significant bone marrow–suppressing effects, are not to be administered with radiation therapy or with other drugs that suppress the bone marrow. In general, you need to work with available pharmacy and oncology staff to proactively anticipate (and avoid, if possible) undesirable drug and treatment interactions.

## Dosages

For dosage information on selected alkylating drugs, see the table on p. 752. It is important to note that dosages are highly

| BOX 46-1 | EXTRAVASATION OF ANTINEOPLASTICS |
|---|---|

Extravasation is one of the more devastating complications of antineoplastic therapy and may lead to extensive tissue damage, the need for skin grafting, other problems in the surrounding areas, and even loss of limb. Because many cell cycle–specific and cell cycle–nonspecific drugs are given intravenously, there is a constant danger of extravasation of vesicants and subsequent injury, including permanent damage to nerves, tendons, and muscles. Skillful and perceptive nursing care helps to prevent extravasation or to identify it early if it does occur, which may reduce the severity of tissue damage. There are important reasons for the placement of central venous intravenous catheters rather than peripheral catheters when long-term treatment is anticipated. Infiltration may occur with any intravenous catheter; it is the specific drug and its characteristics, such as irritant (irritating the IV site or vein) or vesicant (causing cell death with extravasation and necrosis with ulcerative properties, that poses the concern. Because peripheral veins are small and offer minimal dilution of the intravenous drug with blood, there is a greater risk of severe and irreversible damage if a substance infiltrates and spreads to surrounding areas. If the drug is a vesicant, extravasation may lead to massive tissue injury, whereas extravasation of an irritant results in significantly less damage. Central venous access is needed for administration of vesicants to avoid the problems associated with extravasation. However, extravasation may occur with central lines and PICC lines due to dislodging of the access catheter, venous thrombosis, and catheter breakage. Blood needs to be aspirated prior to administration to check for patency. Extravasation may be suspected if the following occurs at either a central line site, PICC line site, or peripheral IV site: complaints of burning, stinging pain, or any other acute change of sensation at the site or along the chest wall, neck, or shoulder (central line); or leakage, swelling, or induration at the site. If extravasation of a vesicant is suspected, immediate action must be taken and the antidote, if known, must be given following strict guidelines and procedures. Steps to help manage extravasation of an irritant and/or a vesicant include the following: (1) Stop the infusion immediately and contact the prescriber, leaving the intravenous catheter in place. (2) Next, it is usually recommended to aspirate any residual drug and/or blood from the catheter. (3) Consult institutional policy or guidelines or the pharmacist regarding the use of antidotes, application of hot or cold packs and/or sterile occlusive dressings, and elevation and rest of the affected limb. Document the extravasation incident with attention to all phases of the nursing process related to the problem. Remember to always consult facility protocol and guidelines.

Data from National Cancer Institute website, http://www.nci.nih.gov; United States Pharmacopeial Convention: *USP DI volume 1: drug information for the health care professional*, Greenwood Village, CO, 2005, Micromedex. Internet resources for additional information: www.cancer.org, www.oncolink.org/index.cfm, www.hospicenet.org, http://www.acponline.org.

## TABLE 46-2    ALKYLATING DRUG EXTRAVASATION: SPECIFIC ANTIDOTES

| DRUG | ANTIDOTE PREPARATION | METHOD |
|---|---|---|
| carmustine | Mix equal parts 1 mEq/mL sodium bicarbonate (premixed) with sterile NS (1:1 solution); resulting solution is 0.5 mEq/mL. | 1. Inject 2 to 6 mL IV through the existing line along with multiple subcut injections into the extravasated site.<br>2. Apply cold compresses.<br>3. Total dose is not to exceed 10 mL of 0.5-mEq/mL solution. |
| mechlorethamine | Mix 4 mL 10% sodium thiosulfate with 6 mL sterile water for injection. | 1. Inject 5 to 6 mL IV through the existing line with multiple subcut injections into the extravasated site.<br>2. Repeat subcut injections over the next few hours.<br>3. Apply cold compresses.<br>4. No total dose has been established. |

*IV*, Intravenous; *NS*, normal saline; *subcut*, subcutaneous.

## DOSAGES

### Selected Alkylating Drugs

| DRUG (PREGNANCY CATEGORY) | PHARMACOLOGIC SUBCLASS | USUAL DOSAGE RANGE* | INDICATIONS |
|---|---|---|---|
| ◆ cisplatin (Platinol-AQ) (D) | Platinum coordination complex | IV: 50-100 mg/m$^2$ q4wk | Metastatic testicular, ovarian, and bladder cancer; brain tumors; esophageal, head, neck, lung, and cervical cancer |
| ◆ cyclophosphamide (Cytoxan) (D) | Classic alkylator | IV: 3-5 mg/kg 2 × wk **(many other regimens as well)** | HL, NHL, leukemia; breast, ovarian, and testicular cancer; retinoblastoma; almost every solid tumor |
| ◆ mechlorethamine (Mustargen) (D) | Classic alkylator | IV: 6 mg/m$^2$ day 1 and day 28 q4wk | HL, NHL, leukemia, bronchogenic carcinoma, others |

*HL*, Hodgkin's lymphoma; *IV*, intravenous; *NHL*, non-Hodgkin's lymphoma.
*Note: Dosages are highly variable.

variable based on type of cancer, previous drugs used, and concurrent drug administration.

## DRUG PROFILES

The most widely used alkylating drugs, based on standard treatment protocols, are profiled here. Information for these drugs also appears in the Dosages table on this page.

### ◆ cisplatin

Cisplatin (Platinol) is an antineoplastic drug that contains platinum in its chemical structure. It is classified as a probable alkylating drug because it is believed to destroy cancer cells in the same way as the classic alkylating drugs—by forming cross-links with DNA and thereby preventing its replication. It is also considered a bifunctional alkylating drug.

Cisplatin is used for the treatment of many solid tumors, such as bladder, lung, testicular, and ovarian tumors. It is available only in injectable form. Medication errors, resulting in deaths, have occurred when cisplatin was confused for carboplatin. The best practice is to use both trade name and generic name when dealing with chemotherapy drugs.

### ◆ cyclophosphamide

Cyclophosphamide (Cytoxan) is a nitrogen mustard derivative that was discovered during the course of research to improve mechlorethamine. It is a polyfunctional alkylating drug and is a prodrug requiring *in vivo* activation. It is used in the treatment of cancers of the bone and lymph, as well as other solid tumors. Cyclophosphamide is also used in the treatment of leukemias

and multiple myeloma, as well as for non-cancer related illnesses such as prophylaxis for rejection of kidney, heart, liver, and bone marrow transplants and severe rheumatoid disorders. It is available in both oral and injectable dosage forms.

### ◆ mechlorethamine

Mechlorethamine (nitrogen mustard) (Mustargen) is the prototypical alkylating drug. It is a nitrogen analogue of sulfur mustard (mustard gas) that was used for chemical warfare in World War I. Mechlorethamine was the first alkylating antineoplastic drug discovered, and its beneficial effects in the treatment of various cancers were identified after the war. Although its use has declined with the development of newer and better drugs, it continues to be administered in the treatment of Hodgkin's and Non-Hodgkin's lymphoma.

Mechlorethamine is a bifunctional alkylating drug capable of forming cross-links between two DNA nucleotides, which interferes with RNA transcription and prevents cell division and protein synthesis. It is available in parenteral form only, for administration intravenously or by an intracavitary route, such as intrapleurally or intraperitoneally. It can also be used topically for treatment of cutaneous T-cell lymphoma.

## CYTOTOXIC ANTIBIOTICS

The cytotoxic antibiotics consist of natural substances produced by the mold *Streptomyces* as well as semisynthetic substances in which chemical changes are made in the natural molecule. Cytotoxic antibiotics have bone marrow suppression as a common toxicity. The one exception is bleomycin, which instead causes pulmonary toxicity (pulmonary fibrosis and pneumonitis). Other severe toxicities associated with the use of cytotoxic antibiotics are heart failure (daunorubicin) and in rare cases acute left ventricular failure (doxorubicin). The available cytotoxic antibiotics, categorized according to the specific subclass to which they belong, are as follows:

**Anthracyclines**
- daunorubicin
- doxorubicin
- epirubicin
- idarubicin
- valrubicin

**Other cytotoxic antibiotics**
- bleomycin (which is actually a cell cycle–specific drug)
- dactinomycin
- mitomycin
- mitoxantrone
- plicamycin

## Mechanism of Action and Drug Effects

Cytotoxic antibiotic antineoplastic drugs are cell cycle–nonspecific drugs. They interact with DNA through a process called *intercalation,* in which the drug molecule is inserted between the two strands of a DNA molecule, ultimately blocking DNA synthesis. These drugs inhibit the enzyme topoisomerase II, which leads to DNA strand breaks. Many of these drugs are able to generate free radicals, which also leads to DNA strand breaks and programmed cell death.

## Indications

Cytotoxic antibiotics are used to treat a variety of solid tumors and some hematologic malignancies as well. Commonly used examples of these drugs and the malignancies they are used to treat are presented in the Dosages table on p. 754.

## Adverse Effects

As with all of the antineoplastic drugs, cytotoxic antibiotics have the undesirable effects of hair loss, nausea and vomiting, and myelosuppression. The emetic potential of the various drugs in this category is given in Box 45-1. Major adverse effects specific to the cytotoxic antibiotics are listed in Table 46-3.

### Toxicity and Management of Overdose

Severe cases of cardiomyopathy are associated with large cumulative doses of doxorubicin. Routine monitoring of cardiac ejection fraction with multiple-gated acquisition (MUGA) scans, cumulative dose limitations, and the use of cytoprotective drugs such as dexrazoxane can decrease the incidence of this devastating toxicity. Box 46-2 outlines the management of doxorubicin extravasation.

## Interactions

The cytotoxic antibiotics that are used in chemotherapy interact with many drugs. They all tend to produce increased toxicities when used in combination with other chemotherapeutic drugs or with radiation therapy. Some drugs, most notably bleomycin

| TABLE 46-3 | **CYTOTOXIC ANTIBIOTICS: SEVERE ADVERSE EFFECTS** |
|---|---|
| **DRUG** | **ADVERSE EFFECTS** |
| bleomycin | Pulmonary fibrosis, pneumonitis |
| dactinomycin, daunorubicin | Liver toxicity, tissue damage in the event of extravasation, heart failure |
| doxorubicin, idarubicin | Liver and cardiovascular toxicities |
| mitomycin | Liver, kidney, and lung toxicities |
| mitoxantrone | Cardiovascular toxicity |
| plicamycin | Tissue damage in the event of extravasation |

| BOX 46-2 | **TREATMENT OF DOXORUBICIN EXTRAVASATION** |
|---|---|

1. Cool the site to patient tolerance for 24 hours.
2. Elevate and rest the extremity for 24 to 48 hours, and then have the patient resume normal activity as tolerated.
3. If pain, erythema, or swelling persists beyond 48 hours, discuss with the prescriber the need for surgical intervention or other treatment options.

Data from National Cancer Institute website, http://www.nci.hih.gov; United States Pharmacopeial Convention: *USP DI volume 1: drug information for the health care professional,* Greenwood Village, CO, 2005, Micromedex; Internet resources for additional information: www.cancer.org, www.oncolink.org/index.cfm, w; http://www.hospicenet.org; http://www.acponline.org.

and doxorubicin, have been known to cause serum digoxin levels to increase. Observe patients receiving one of these drugs along with digoxin for signs of digoxin toxicity. Dosage reduction or elimination of digoxin therapy may be indicated (see Chapter 24).

## Dosages

For dosage information on selected cytotoxic antibiotics, see the table on p. 754.

## DRUG PROFILES

### ◆ doxorubicin

Doxorubicin (Adriamycin) is used in many combination chemotherapy regimens. The drug is contraindicated in patients with a known hypersensitivity to it, patients with severe myelosuppression, and patients who are at risk for severe cardiotoxicity because they have already received a large cumulative dose of any of the anthracycline antineoplastics. It is available only in injectable form. Doxorubicin is also available in a liposomal drug delivery system (Doxil). In this dosage formulation, the drug is encapsulated in a lipid molecule bilayer called a *liposome.* The advantages of liposomal encapsulation are reduced systemic toxicity and increased duration of action. Liposomal encapsulation extends the biologic half-life of doxorubicin to 50 to 60 hours and increases its affinity for cancer cells. The liposomal dosage formulation is currently indicated for the treatment of ovarian cancer and in combination with bortezomib for the treatment of multiple myeloma.

## DOSAGES

### Selected Cytotoxic Antibiotics

| DRUG (PREGNANCY CATEGORY) | PHARMACOLOGIC SUBCLASS | USUAL DOSAGE RANGE* | INDICATIONS |
|---|---|---|---|
| **Anthracycline Antibiotics** | | | |
| ◆ doxorubicin, conventional (Adriamycin, Rubex) (D) | Anthracycline | IV: 30-75 mg/m2 q7-28d (depending on type of cancer) | Multiple cancers, including breast, bone, and ovarian cancer, and leukemia, neuroblastoma, HL, NHL |
| ◆ doxorubicin, liposomal (Doxil) (D) | Anthracycline | IV: 20-50 mg/m2 q3-4wk for as long as tolerated and tumor is responsive to treatment | AIDS-related Kaposi's sarcoma when other chemotherapy drugs have failed or patient is intolerant of them; recurrent metastatic ovarian cancer |
| **Anthracenedione Antibiotic** | | | |
| mitoxantrone (Novantrone) (D) | Anthracenedione | IV: 12 mg/m2 q3wk (prostate cancer) **(many other regimens as well)** | Prostate cancer, acute myelocytic leukemia |

*AIDS,* Acquired immunodeficiency syndrome; *HL,* Hodgkin's lymphoma; *IV,* intravenous; *NHL,* non-Hodgkin's lymphoma.
*Note: Dosages are highly variable.

## ⚡ SAFETY AND QUALITY IMPROVEMENT: PREVENTING MEDICATION ERRORS

### Sound-Alike Drugs: "Rubicins"

The anthracycline chemotherapy drugs have the same sound-alike suffix and are often nicknamed the "rubicins." These drugs include daunorubicin, doxorubicin, epirubicin, idarubicin, and valrubicin. Even though these drugs are in the same class, their use and drug effects are very different. Medication errors have occurred because one "rubicin" has been mistaken for another. It is important to refer to these drugs by both trade and generic names rather than as a "rubicin."

### mitoxantrone

Mitoxantrone (Novantrone) is indicated for the treatment of acute nonlymphocytic leukemia and prostate cancer as well as the neurologic disorder multiple sclerosis. It is available only in injectable form.

## MISCELLANEOUS ANTINEOPLASTICS

The miscellaneous antineoplastic drugs are those that, because of their unique structure and mechanism of action, cannot be classified into the previously described categories. However, some drugs that are originally classified as miscellaneous drugs are later reclassified as more is learned about their mechanisms of action and other characteristics. Drugs currently in the miscellaneous category include bevacizumab, everolimus, hydroxyurea (which is actually cell-cycle specific), ipilimumab, imatinib, mitotane, ofatumumab, pazopanib, romidepsin, sorafenib, sunitinib, hormonal drugs, and radioactive and related antineoplastic drugs. Selected miscellaneous drugs are profiled in the following sections.

## DRUG PROFILES

The various drugs in the miscellaneous category of antineoplastics are used to treat a wide range of neoplasms. Hydroxyurea and imatinib are administered orally. Bevacizumab and mitotane are available only in injectable form.

### bevacizumab

Bevacizumab (Avastin) was the first antineoplastic drug in a new category—*angiogenesis inhibitors. Angiogenesis* is the creation of new blood vessels that supply oxygen and other blood nutrients to growing tissues. In the case of malignant tumors, angiogenesis that occurs within the tumor mass promotes continued tumor growth. As a tumor enlarges, its central tissues gradually die off *(necrosis).* However, its outer portion continues to grow, often to fatal proportions. Thus, inhibiting this process offers a promising new mechanism for antineoplastic drug action. Bevacizumab is a recombinant "humanized" monoclonal immunoglobulin G1 antibody derived from mouse antibodies. The scientific name for any compound derived from mouse tissue is *murine. Humanization* refers to the use of recombinant DNA techniques to make animal-derived antibody proteins more genetically similar to those of humans. It works by binding to and inhibiting the biologic activity of human vascular endothelial growth factor (VEGF). VEGF is an endogenous protein that normally promotes angiogenesis in the body. Bevacizumab is available only in injectable form. The only recognized contraindication is severe drug allergy or allergy to other murine products. It is approved for the treatment of metastatic colon cancer, rectal cancer in combination with 5-flurouracil (see Chapter 45), non–small cell lung cancer, and malignant glioblastoma. Bevacizumab was approved for treatment of breast cancer; however, the FDA revoked the breast cancer indication in 2011.

Adverse reactions include those affecting the cardiovascular system (hypertension or hypotension, deep vein thrombosis), central nervous system (pain, headache, dizziness, asthenia), skin (alopecia, dry skin), metabolism (weight loss, hypokalemia), gastrointestinal (GI) tract (nausea, vomiting, diarrhea, epistaxis, abdominal pain, constipation, GI hemorrhage), kidneys (nephrotoxicity with proteinuria), hematopoeitic system (leukopenia), and respiratory tract (infection). More severe effects can occur in any of these systems but are much less common than those listed. Drug interactions reported to date are limited but include potentiation of the cardiotoxic effects of the anthracycline antibiotics such as doxorubicin.

### hydroxyurea

Hydroxyurea (Hydrea, Droxia) is an antimetabolite that interferes with the synthesis of DNA by inhibiting the incorporation of thymidine into DNA. More specifically, it inhibits ribonucleotide reductase, which is involved in conversion of ribonucleotides to deoxyribonucleotides. It works primarily in the S and $G_1$ phases of the cell cycle, which makes it a cell cycle–specific drug. It is discussed in this chapter because it is included as a miscellaneous drug.

It is used in the treatment of squamous cell carcinoma in concert with radiation to take advantage of its radiosensitizing activity. It is also used in the treatment of various types of leukemia. The drug is available only in oral form. Adverse reactions include edema, drowsiness, headache, rash, hyperuricemia, nausea, vomiting, dysuria, myelosuppression, elevated liver enzyme levels, muscular weakness, peripheral neuropathy, nephrotoxicity, dyspnea, and pulmonary fibrosis. Hydroxyurea interacts with the anti-HIV drugs zidovudine, zalcitabine, and didanosine (see Chapter 40), all of which can have a synergistic effect with hydroxyurea. Concurrent use with fluorouracil increases the risk of neurotoxic symptoms. Because hydroxyurea can reduce the clearance of cytarabine, dosage reduction of cytarabine is recommended when the two are used concurrently.

### imatinib

Imatinib (Gleevec) is the standard of care for the treatment of chronic myeloid leukemia (CML). It works by inhibiting the action of a key enzyme (bcr-abl tyrosine kinase) responsible for causing CML. Although its name sounds similar to those of various monoclonal antibody drugs, imatinib is not a monoclonal antibody but rather a targeted therapy. It is available only in oral form. Common adverse reactions include fatigue, headache, rash, fluid retention, GI and hematologic effects, musculoskeletal pain, cough, and dyspnea. Potential drug interactions are numerous and involve other drugs metabolized by the cytochrome P-450 hepatic enzymes. Examples include amiodarone, verapamil, warfarin, azole antifungals, antidepressants, and antibiotics. A pharmacist may be needed to review the patient's medication regimen and adjust dosages or delete medications accordingly, in collaboration with the patient's prescriber.

### mitotane

Mitotane (Lysodren) is an adrenal cytotoxic drug that is indicated specifically for the treatment of inoperable adrenal corticoid carcinoma. It is available only in oral form. Adverse reactions include CNS depression, rash, nausea, vomiting, muscle weakness, and headache. Reported drug interactions include enhanced CNS depressive effects when taken concurrently with other CNS depressants (e.g., benzodiazepines). Mitotane may also increase the clearance of both warfarin and phenytoin, reducing their effects. The potassium-sparing diuretic spironolactone may negate the effects of mitotane.

### octreotide

Octreotide (Sandostatin) (see Chapter 30) is a unique medication used for the management of a cancer-related condition called *carcinoid crisis* and treatment of the diarrhea caused by vasoactive intestinal peptide–secreting tumors (VIPomas).

## HORMONAL ANTINEOPLASTICS

Hormonal drugs are used in the treatment of a variety of neoplasms. The rationale is that sex hormones act to accelerate the growth of some common types of malignant tumors, especially certain types of breast and prostate cancer. Therefore, therapy may involve administration of hormones with opposing effects (i.e., male versus female hormones) or drugs that block the body's sex hormone receptors. These drugs are used most commonly as palliative and adjuvant therapy. For certain types of cancer, they may be used as drugs of first choice. Some of the more commonly used hormonal drugs for female-specific neoplasms such as breast cancer are the aromatase inhibitors anastrazole and aminoglutethimide, the selective estrogen receptor modulators tamoxifen and toremifene, the progestins megestrol and medroxyprogesterone, the androgens fluoxymesterone and testolactone, and the estrogen receptor antagonist fulvestrant. For male-specific neoplasms such as prostate cancer, the following drugs are used: the antiandrogens bicalutamide, flutamide, and nilutamide; and the antineoplastic hormone estramustine. The most common adverse effects of these drugs used to treat female and male cancers are listed in Table 46-4.

## RADIOPHARMACEUTICALS AND RELATED ANTINEOPLASTICS

Antineoplastic drugs that are administered by prescribers include porfimer sodium and various radioactive pharmaceuticals

| TABLE 46-4 | HORMONAL ANTINEOPLASTICS: ADVERSE EFFECTS | |
|---|---|---|
| **CLASS** | **DRUG** | **ADVERSE EFFECTS** |
| Aromatase inhibitors | anastrozole, aminoglutethimide | Vasodilation, hypertension, hot flashes, mood disorders, weakness, arthritis |
| Selective estrogen receptor modulators | tamoxifen, toremifene | Hypertension, peripheral edema, mood disorders, depression, hot flushes, nausea, weakness |
| Progestins | megestrol, medroxy-progesterone | Hypertension, chest pain, headache, weight gain, hepatotoxicity, dizziness, abdominal pain |
| Androgens | fluoxymesterone, testolactone | Menstrual irregularities, virilization of female, gynecomastia, hirsutism, acne, anxiety, headache, nausea |
| Estrogen receptor antagonists | fulvestrant | Vasodilation, pain, headache, hot flushes, nausea, vomiting, pharyngitis |
| Antiandrogens | bicalutamide, flutamide, nilutamide | Peripheral edema, pain, hot flushes, gynecomastia, anemia, nausea, diarrhea |
| Gonadotropin-releasing hormone agonists | leuprolide, goserelin | Rash, pain on injection, alopecia, body odor |
| Antineoplastic hormone | estramustine | Edema, dyspnea, leg cramps, breast tenderness, nausea, anorexia, diarrhea |

(radiopharmaceuticals). Porfimer sodium is used to treat esophageal or bronchial tumors that are present on the surface mucosa. The medication is given intravenously, and administration is followed by one or more sessions of laser light therapy to the esophageal or bronchial mucosa for direct tumor lysis and manual débridement. Radiopharmaceuticals are used to treat a variety of cancers or symptoms caused by cancers. Five commonly used radioisotopes are chromic phosphate P 32 (for cancer-induced peritoneal or pleural effusions), samarium SM 153 lexidronam (for bone cancer pain), sodium iodide I 131 (for thyroid cancer and hyperthyroidism), sodium phosphate P 32 (for various leukemias and palliative treatment of bone metastases), and strontium Sr 89 chloride (for bone cancer pain). Two drugs used in the treatment of various forms of non-Hodgkin's lymphoma are iodine I 131 tositumomab (Bexxar) and yttrium Y 90 ibritumomab tiuxetan (yttrium 90–labeled CD20 antibody; Zevalin). These medications are usually administered by nuclear medicine specialists.

## NURSING PROCESS

Antineoplastics are some of the most toxic drugs given to patients (see Chapter 45), and because of these toxicities, serious complications and adverse effects may occur. Nursing care must be based on a thorough knowledge of cancer, its treatment, and the subsequent effects of different treatment modalities. This chapter presents information about cell cycle–nonspecific, hormonal, and miscellaneous antineoplastic drugs, whereas Chapter 45 covers cell cycle–specific antineoplastic drugs.

## ASSESSMENT

Begin the overall assessment of patients taking any of these drugs with a thorough nursing history, medication profile, and past and present medical history. Measure and record vital signs. Document the presence of conditions that represent cautions or contraindications as well as potential drug interactions. Perform a head-to-toe physical assessment that includes attention to the following: skin turgor with level of moisture and integrity of the skin and oral mucosa; baseline level of neurologic functioning including level of consciousness, alertness, motor and sensory intactness, reflexes, and presence of any abnormal sensations; bowel sounds, bowel patterns, and inquiry into any problems such as diarrhea, constipation, nausea, vomiting, or reflux; urinary patterns and color, amount, and odor of urine; breath sounds as well as respiratory rate, rhythm, and depth; and heart sounds. Laboratory tests that may be ordered include fluid and electrolyte levels (sodium, potassium, chloride, magnesium, calcium), RBC and WBC counts, hemoglobin, hematocrit, renal and hepatic function tests, and serum protein-albumin levels.

For patients receiving *alkylating drugs,* bone marrow suppression (carboplatin), pulmonary fibrosis (busulfan), nephrotoxicity and/or neurotoxicity (more with cisplatin than carboplatin), and hemorrhagic cystitis (cyclophosphamide) may occur; thus, perform an appropriate and thorough nursing assessment (see Assessment in Chapter 45). Assess deep tendon reflexes and baseline hearing level. Document

the findings. Assess results of any baseline pulmonary function testing and perform a thorough respiratory assessment. High-dose cyclophosphamide may lead to hemorrhagic cystitis; therefore, document urinary patterns and any abnormal symptoms. Note hydration status before administering cyclophosphamide to avoid hemorrhagic cystitis.

One of the major adverse effects associated with the use of *cytotoxic antibiotics* (e.g., bleomycin) is pulmonary fibrosis. Medical testing (e.g., radiographs, computed tomographic [CT] scans, magnetic resonance imaging [MRI] scans, arterial blood gas levels, and partial pressures of $CO_2$ and $O_2$) may be ordered so assess findings. When dactinomycin or daunorubicin are given intravenously, it is generally administered via a central line indwelling catheter device (e.g., Port-A-Cath or MediPort), because if it is given by peripheral intravenous line and extravasation occurs, there is a risk for necrosis with tissue sloughing that may erode through the layers of skin and underlying supportive structures (e.g., muscles, ligaments). See the pharmacology discussion of extravasation as well as Table 46-2 and Box 46-3. In addition, in patients with documented cardiac disease or a history of thoracic irradiation, administer dactinomycin, daunorubicin, and doxorubicin with extreme caution due to cardiovascular toxicity. CT scans and ultrasound studies may be needed before and during treatment to assess cardiac ejection fraction because of the risk of cardiotoxicity, which is often associated with cumulative doses.

With use of *hormonal antineoplastic drugs,* obtain a thorough medical, nursing, and medication history. Many of the drugs included in this category are presented in depth in Chapters 34 and 35, which also discuss aspects of the nursing process related

---

**BOX 46-3** **CONCERNS IN THE HANDLING AND ADMINISTRATION OF VESICANT DRUGS**

The handling and administration of antineoplastic drugs is of major concern because the nurse mixing and giving the drug may experience negative consequences. The pharmacy department is responsible for mixing these drugs, and preparation must be carried out carefully in an appropriate environment with use of a laminar airflow hood and personal protective equipment (mask, gown, gloves). Many facilities recommend taking special precautions during the care of a patient who is receiving chemotherapy, such as double-flushing the patient's bodily secretions in the commode and using special hampers for the disposal of all items that come into contact with the patient, including used personal protective equipment. Special spill kits are employed to clean up even the smallest chemotherapy spills. These precautions are necessary to protect the health care provider from the cytotoxic effects of these drugs. In addition, proper and up-to-date knowledge about these drugs is important to safe and appropriate nursing care. All nurses giving these drugs must be certified to administer chemotherapy and must remain current in their level of practice and competencies related to this treatment modality. All equipment and containers must be handled appropriately once the infusion is completed. Hands and any exposed areas must be washed to ensure the safety of the health care provider. The Centers for Disease Control and Prevention and the Oncology Nursing Society offer exceptional resources for individuals involved in the care of patients receiving chemotherapy.

to their use. Assessment associated with the use of *estrogen antagonists* such as fulvestrant, tamoxifen, raloxifene, and toremifene citrates often begins with a review of the results of any tumor estrogen receptor assays, CT scans, radiographs, and other diagnostic testing. Perform a neurologic assessment (see previous discussion and Chapters 34 and 45) with attention to baseline complaints of any pain, abnormal sensations, or headaches. Note any menopausal symptoms upon assessment because of the possible adverse effect of vasodilation and hot flashes. In addition, these drugs may cause nausea and vomiting so a thorough GI assessment is beneficial.

With the use of *androgens* (e.g., fluoxymesterone or testosterone), obtain a thorough gynecologic history of the female patient with attention to any menstrual issues or problems because of the adverse effect of menstrual irregularities. It is also important to assess the patient's body image and feelings of self-esteem because of the possible adverse effects of acne, hirsutism, and virilization in female patients as well as gynecomastia in male patients. See Chapter 35 for more information on the side effects of androgens.

Bicalutamide, flutamide, and nilutamide are *antiandrogens* and require thorough assessment of any cardiac diseases due to the potential for peripheral edema. This could exacerbate any pre-existing cardiac disorder. Perform a thorough GI and gynecologic assessment because of the possibility for nausea, diarrhea, and hot flashes. Documentation of the use of a reliable form of birth control is important because of teratogenic effects. Male sperm production may be affected (see Chapter 45), and a decline in sexual functioning and/or desire may occur because of the antiandrogenic effects.

With use of *gonadotropin-releasing hormone agonists,* such as leuprolide and goserelin, assess the patient for allergies to the drugs. Contraceptive history is important because women who are taking these drugs must use a nonhormonal contraceptive. Often the prescriber will order laboratory tests for serum testosterone and prostatic acid phosphatase level for male patients before and during therapy; an increase will be noted during the initial week of therapy, with levels returning to baseline by 4 weeks.

For patients taking *antiadrenal drugs* (e.g., mitotane), in addition to performing a basic assessment, inquire about any GI disturbances because of the common adverse effects of nausea and vomiting. The *miscellaneous antineoplastic drugs* glucocorticoids and mineralocorticoids may be given to prevent adrenal insufficiency and may also play a part in the therapeutic regimen. An understanding of baseline adrenal functioning through examination of laboratory test results is important.

With the *miscellaneous* drug hydroxurea, assessment of liver, renal, neurologic, and pulmonary function with baseline blood cell counts are important due to the adverse reactions associated with this drug. With use of bevacizumab, an *angiogenesis inhibitor,* assess cardiovascular, central nervous system, GI tract, and renal functioning. Assess adverse effects of hypotension or hypertension, headache, pain, dizziness, nausea, vomiting, diarrhea, and nephrotoxicity.

## CASE STUDY

### *Chemotherapy with Alkylating Drugs*

W.S. is receiving cisplatin as part of treatment for ovarian cancer. She is receiving her third treatment today and has just arrived at the cancer treatment center for her outpatient infusion. W.S. says that she felt "okay" during the time between the last treatment and today but is not looking forward to today's treatment because of the side effects.

1. While the nurse prepares to start the infusion, what is important for the nurse to assess before beginning the chemotherapy?
2. What will the nurse do before the infusion to help reduce or prevent adverse effects?
3. During the infusion, W.S. mentions that she is hearing a slight "roaring" sound and that she feels a bit dizzy. What will the nurse do next?
4. After stopping the infusion, the nurse spills some of the chemotherapy solution on her arm and the floor. What is the nurse's priority action at this time?

For answers, see http://evolve.elsevier.com/Lilley.

## NURSING DIAGNOSES

1. Decreased cardiac output related to the adverse effect of cardiotoxicity associated with cytotoxic antibiotics
2. Diarrhea related to the adverse effects of antineoplastic drugs
3. Imbalanced nutrition, less than body requirements, related to loss of appetite, nausea, and vomiting, as a result of antineoplastic therapy

## PLANNING

### GOALS

1. Patient's cardiac output remains within normal limits while the patient is taking antineoplastics.
2. Patient experiences minimal problems with alteration in bowel elimination (e.g., diarrhea).
3. Patient maintains adequate and balanced nutritional status while taking antineoplastics.

### OUTCOME CRITERIA

1. Patient maintains normal blood pressure and heart rate while being monitored during therapy with cytotoxic antibiotics.
   - Patient demonstrates adequate knowledge of self-monitoring of blood pressure and pulse rate daily.
   - Patient understands the importance of daily weights.
   - Patient, family member, or caregiver adheres to a daily heart-healthy regimen of conserving energy, planning activities, and asking for assistance with care and activities as needed.
   - Patient, family member, or caregiver contacts prescribers immediately with the occurrence of shortness of breath, high or low blood pressure or pulse rate, and chest pain.
2. Patient states measures to prevent or decrease the occurrence of diarrhea during antineoplastic therapy such as avoiding

spicy, irritating foods, gas-producing foods, caffeine, high fiber foods, alcohol and very hot or cold foods and beverages.

- Patient has preventative medication, as prescribed, such as synthetic opioids (e.g., loperamide) or adsorbents-protectants, to be taken to help with excess diarrhea.

3. Patient maintains daily regimen for healthy nutritional patterns such as maintaining adequate fluid intake, maintaining a balanced diet as tolerated, avoiding foods that are irritating to the GI tract, and taking nutritional supplements as prescribed.

## IMPLEMENTATION

Before initiating drug therapy with the cell cycle–nonspecific drugs, hormonal antineoplastics and miscellaneous drugs, you must be completely knowledgeable about the drug, its use, and its impact on all rapidly dividing cells, whether normal or malignant (see Chapters 34, 35, and 45 for additional information).

With *alkylating drugs,* always handle these and all other antineoplastics with caution because of their possible carcinogenic, mutagenic, and teratogenic properties (see Box 46-3). The patient receiving alkylating drugs will more than likely experience problems related to bone marrow suppression, such as anemia, leukopenia, and thrombocytopenia (see Chapter 45 for specific interventions). Most nursing interventions are focused on preventing infection, conserving energy, preventing bleeding and injury, and reducing nausea. Other nursing considerations for these drugs include taking vital signs every 1 to 2 hours, or as needed during infusion forcing fluids; monitoring intake and output; following orders for intravenous therapy for hydration; and monitoring any vomiting. Contact the prescriber if vomiting is uncontrolled. Monitor the patient constantly for abnormal peripheral sensations, especially with cisplatin. Report to the prescriber any numbness or tingling of extremities and any ringing or roaring in the ears and/or hearing loss. Encourage the patient experiencing peripheral neuropathies to avoid extremely cold temperatures or the handling of cold objects. Cisplatin is particularly nephrotoxic, so monitor renal function closely throughout therapy. Intravenous hydration is often required at a rate of 100 to 200 mL/hr starting before cisplatin administration with a total of 2000 to 3000 mL/day, depending on the dose of cisplatin and if not contraindicated. Do not use aluminum needles or administration sets with many of these drugs because aluminum can degrade their platinum compounds ensure that the proper infusion equipment is used. Because hemorrhagic cystitis is associated with cyclophosphamide use, make sure the patient's hydration is maintained to minimize this adverse effect. Pulmonary toxicity may occur with some of the alkylating drugs, particularly busulfan; therefore, constantly monitor and be alert to cough, shortness of breath, and abnormal breath sounds. Immediately report these adverse effects to the prescriber. Other drugs in this group may be given by various routes, such as intrapericardial, intratumoral, and intravesical. Be sure you perform appropriate interventions per the manufacturer's guidelines or hospital/facility policy. Reconstitute the parenteral formulations for any of these drugs according to the manufacturer's guidelines and suggestions. Not all diluents are compatible.

One very important component of nursing care with alkylating drugs and their parenteral administration is monitoring the IV site/infusion continually for signs and symptoms of infiltration. Infiltration could lead to extravasation of the medication into the surrounding tissue. To briefly review, IV infiltration is the leakage of fluids or blood from a dislodged catheter or needle cannula from the intima of the vein and into the surrounding tissue. Signs and symptoms of infiltration include inflammation at or near the insertion site with swollen, taut skin with pain, blanching, and coolness of skin around the IV site; slowed or stopped IV infusion; and no backflow of blood into the IV tubing. The reason infiltration is of concern with these drugs is that some of them are irritants and others are vesicants with the potential of severe tissue damage. Therefore, if extravasation occurs with some of these drugs, antidotes are required to try and prevent damage from leakage of the drug into the tissue. Specific antidotes for alkylating drugs are presented in Table 46-2. Always follow hospital/facility policy when treating extravasation of any medication. With IV infusions of antineoplastics, monitoring of the IV site and infusions is usually more frequent, and some guidelines state hourly assessment. It is important to mention that the vast majority of chemotherapeutic drugs are administered via a central line indwelling catheter device (such as Port-A-Cath or MediPort). Check the device and its patency prior to the drug's administration.

Patients receiving *cytotoxic antibiotics* such as bleomycin may require more frequent monitoring of pulmonary function. Baseline chest radiographs may be obtained for comparison with subsequent radiographs if pneumonitis occurs. Monitor results of liver and renal function tests throughout therapy with dactinomycin, daunorubicin, doxorubicin, and mitomycin. Heart sounds, daily weights, blood pressure, pulse rate, and monitoring for signs and symptoms of cardiovascular toxicities (e.g., alterations in vital signs, abnormal heart sounds, dyspnea, chest pain) are especially important with doxorubicin, idarubicin, and mitoxantrone. Additionally, if the patient experiences an increase of 2 pounds or more in 24 hours or 5 pounds or more in 1 week, notify the prescriber, as this may reflect fluid retention related to heart failure. Mitomycin is associated with liver, kidney, and lung toxicities. Close monitoring of these systems during treatment is key to patient safety.

Use of *hormone antagonists* in the treatment of various neoplasms is common, particularly with breast and prostate cancer. Associated nursing interventions and patient education for the use of these hormone antagonists are discussed in depth in Chapters 34 and 35. Corticosteroid therapy and related nursing considerations are presented in Chapter 33.

*Hydroxyurea* is used sparingly but is a component of some treatment protocols. This drug is given orally. Monitor platelet and leukocyte counts due to the adverse effect of bone marrow suppression. Monitoring must be ongoing during therapy. If platelet count falls below 100,000 platelets/mm$^3$ or leukocyte count falls below 2000 cells/mm$^3$, therapy may need to be temporarily halted until counts rise toward the normal values. See earlier discussion and Chapter 45 about nursing considerations associated with anemias, fatigue, weakness, bleeding tendencies, and infection. Additionally, hyperuricemia may precipitate

## SAFETY: LABORATORY VALUES RELATED TO DRUG THERAPY

### Rationales for Assessment and Monitoring of Blood Cell Counts with Antineoplastics

| LABORATORY TEST | NORMAL RANGES | RATIONALE FOR ASSESSMENT |
|---|---|---|
| Leukocytes (WBCs) | 5000 to 10,000 cells/mm³ | WBCs protect against infection and when an infection develops, the WBCs attack and destroy the causative bacteria, virus, or other organism. In response to the infection, WBCs increase in number dramatically. If WBC levels are decreased from antineoplastic treatment and subsequent bone marrow suppression, and if they decrease to levels less than 2000 cells/mm³ (leukopenia), there is a high risk for severe infection and immunosuppression. |
| WBC components:<br>Neutrophils<br><br>Band neutrophils | <br>47% to 77% or above 1500 cells/mm³<br>0% to 3% | The major types of WBCs are neutrophils, lymphocytes, monocytes, eosinophils, and basophils. Immature neutrophils are called *band neutrophils* and their number, along with neutrophil counts, provides a picture of the patient's immune system. If neutrophils are decreased to levels of less than 500 cells/mm³ (neutropenia), then there is risk for severe infection. If band neutrophils are included in the WBC differential count, then an abnormally low value reinforces the risk for severe infection (see Chapter 45). |
| Nadir | See normal range of each blood cell. | *Nadir* refers to the lowest levels of bone marrow cells that are reached. The time to reach this nadir may become shorter and the recovery time longer with successive courses of antineoplastic treatment. A general estimate of the time to nadir is 10 to 28 days. Anticipation of the nadir allows the oncologist and health care team to develop a preventative treatment plan which may include use of biologic response modifiers and antibiotics. |

*WBCs,* White blood cells.
NOTE: Similar information on red blood cell and platelet counts is presented in Chapter 45. Also note that chemotherapy may be discontinued with anemia, leukopenia, neutropenia, and/or thrombocytopenia. Once counts recover (sometimes more quickly with certain drugs), treatment is often reinitiated.

gout-related symptoms (e.g., painful, swollen joints); report these to the prescriber so that the appropriate medication may be ordered. Often a drug such as allopurinol is prescribed to help control the levels of uric acid caused by cell death from the chemotherapy.

In addition to the nursing interventions discussed earlier and in Chapter 45, keep epinephrine, antihistamines, and antiinflammatory drugs available in case of an allergic or anaphylactic reaction. Each antineoplastic drug has its own peculiarities and its own set of cautions, contraindications, nursing implementations, and toxicities. *Cytoprotective drugs* are useful in reducing certain toxicities. For example, use of intravenous amifostine may help to reduce the renal toxicity associated with cisplatin; intravenous or oral allopurinol may be given to reduce hyperuricemia (see Table 45-6 and Box 45-2). Other major concerns related to the care of patients receiving chemotherapy are the oncologic emergencies that arise because of damage occurring to rapidly dividing normal cells as well as rapidly dividing cancerous cells. Some of the complications that are potential emergencies include infections, infusion reactions and allergy, stomatitis with severe ulceration, bleeding, metabolic aberrations, severe diarrhea, renal failure, liver failure, and cardiotoxicity, including dysrhythmia or heart failure (Box 46-4).

## EVALUATION

Focus the evaluation of nursing care upon determining whether goals and outcomes have been met, as well as on monitoring for therapeutic responses and adverse and toxic effects of antineoplastic therapy. Therapeutic responses may manifest as clinical improvement, decrease in tumor size, and decrease in metastatic spread. Evaluation of nursing care with reference

---

### BOX 46-4   INDICATIONS OF AN ONCOLOGIC EMERGENCY

Fever and/or chills with a temperature higher than 100.5° F (38.1° C)
New sores or white patches in the mouth or throat
Swollen tongue with or without cracks and bleeding
Bleeding gums
Dry, burning, "scratchy," or "swollen" throat
A cough that is new and persistent
Changes in bladder function or patterns
Blood in the urine
Changes in GI or bowel patterns, including "heartburn" or nausea, vomiting, constipation, or diarrhea lasting longer than 2 or 3 days
Blood in the stools

NOTE: The patient must contact the prescriber immediately if any of the listed signs or symptoms occurs. If the prescriber is not available, the patient must seek medical treatment at the closest emergency department.

to goals and outcomes may reveal improvements related to a decrease in adverse effects; a decrease in the impact of cancer on the patient's well-being; an increase in comfort, nutrition, and hydration; improved energy levels and ability to carry out the activities of daily living; and improved quality of life. The goals and outcomes may be revisited to identify more specific parameters to monitor. In addition, certain laboratory studies such as measurement of tumor markers, levels of carcinoembryonic antigens, red blood cell, white blood cell, and platelet counts may also be used to determine how well the goals and outcomes have been met. As part of the evaluation, prescribers may also order additional radiographs, CT scans, MRIs, tissue analyses, and other studies appropriate to the diagnosis during and after antineoplastic therapy, at time intervals related to anticipated tumor response.

## PATIENT TEACHING TIPS

- Advise the patient to avoid aspirin, ibuprofen, and products containing these drugs to help prevent excessive bleeding.
- Be open with discussion about the risk of alopecia (a complete discussion is presented in Chapter 45) as an adverse effect of many of the antineoplastic drugs.
- Encourage forcing of fluids up to 3000 mL/day, if not contraindicated, to prevent dehydration and further weakening and, in the case of cyclophosphamide therapy, to prevent or help manage hemorrhagic cystitis.
- Constipation and diarrhea may be problematic, so educate the patient about ways to help manage these alterations in bowel status that may be due to the antineoplastic or due to narcotics used for pain management. To help avoid constipation, forcing of fluids and consumption of a balanced diet are important; however, the oncologist often orders either a stool softener or a mild noncramping laxative to prevent the problem. Diarrhea is generally treated by dietary restrictions and use of antidiarrheals, as ordered.
- The following are helpful online resources for the patient and significant others: www.fda.gov, www.fda.gov/ForHealthPro fessionals/default.htm, www.nih.gov, www.healthfinder.gov, www.who.int/en, and www.oncolink.org/index.cfm.

## KEY POINTS

- Antineoplastics are drugs that are used to treat malignancies and are classified as cell cycle–specific drugs, cell cycle–nonspecific drugs, miscellaneous antineoplastics, and hormonal drugs.
- Cell cycle–specific drugs kill cancer cells during specific phases of the cell growth cycle, whereas the cell cycle–nonspecific drugs discussed in this chapter kill cancer cells during any phase of the growth cycle.
- Chemotherapy, or antineoplastic drug therapy, requires very skillful and perceptive care and you must act prudently and make critical decisions about the nursing care of patients receiving these drugs.
- Knowledge is important to ensure patient and health care provider safety and for protection from the adverse effects of antineoplastics.
- Always exercise extreme caution in the handling and administration of cell cycle–nonspecific (as well as cell cycle–specific) drugs.
- Hormonal drugs, both agonists and antagonists, are used to treat a variety of malignancies.
- Extravasation of strong vesicants (e.g., doxorubicin) may lead to severe tissue injury with complications such as permanent damage to muscles, tendons, and ligaments, and possible loss of limb. Constantly monitor the IV site and infusions to prevent this possible complication. Checking the patency of central venous access devices is also important because the majority of chemotherapy drugs are given via this route.
- Oncologic emergencies occur as a consequence of cell death and may be life-threatening. Skillful assessment and immediate intervention may help to decrease the severity of the problem or even reduce the occurrence of such emergencies.

## NCLEX® EXAMINATION REVIEW QUESTIONS

1 A patient who is receiving chemotherapy with cisplatin (Platinol) has developed pneumonia. The nurse would be concerned about nephrotoxicity if which type of antibiotic was ordered as treatment for the pneumonia at this time?
   a Penicillin
   b Sulfa drug
   c Fluoroquinolone
   d Aminoglycoside
2 During treatment with doxorubicin (Adriamycin), the nurse must monitor closely for which potentially life-threatening adverse effect?
   a Nephrotoxicity
   b Peripheral neuritis
   c Cardiomyopathy
   d Ototoxicity
3 While teaching a patient who is about to receive cyclophosphamide (Cytoxan) chemotherapy, the nurse will instruct the patient to watch for potential adverse effects, such as
   a cholinergic diarrhea.
   b hemorrhagic cystitis.

   c peripheral neuropathy.
   d ototoxicity.
4 When chemotherapy with alkylating drugs is planned, the nurse expects to implement which intervention to prevent nephrotoxicity?
   a Hydrating the patient with intravenous fluids before chemotherapy
   b Limiting fluids before chemotherapy
   c Monitoring drug levels during chemotherapy
   d Assessing creatinine clearance during chemotherapy
5 During therapy with the cytotoxic antibiotic bleomycin, the nurse will assess for a potentially serious adverse effect by monitoring
   a blood urea nitrogen and creatinine levels.
   b cardiac ejection fraction.
   c respiratory function.
   d cranial nerve function.

## NCLEX® EXAMINATION REVIEW QUESTIONS

6  While administering bevacizumab (Avastin), what will the nurse assess to look for drug-related toxicities? (Select all that apply.)
a  Blood pressure
b  Color of the skin and sclera of the eye (for jaundice)
c  Blood glucose level
d  Urine protein level
e  Hearing

7  The nurse is preparing to add a dose of bevacizumab (Avastin) to a patient's intravenous infusion. The dose is 70 mg of bevacizumab in 100 mL of normal saline, and it is to infuse over 90 minutes. The nurse will set the infusion pump to what rate for this dose?

1. d, 2. c, 3. b, 4. a, 5. c, 6. a, d, 7. 67 mL/hour (66.66 rounds to 67)

For Critical Thinking and Prioritization Questions, see http://evolve.elsevier.com/Lilley.

# Biologic Response–Modifying and Antirheumatic Drugs

## evolve WEBSITE

*http://evolve.elsevier.com/Lilley*

- Animations
- Answer Key—Textbook Case Studies
- Critical Thinking and Prioritization Questions

- Key Points—Downloadable
- Review Questions for the NCLEX® Examination
- Unfolding Case Studies

## OBJECTIVES

When you reach the end of this chapter, you will be able to do the following:

1. Describe the basic anatomy, physiology, and functions of the immune system.
2. Compare the two major classes of biologic response–modifying drugs: hematopoietic drugs and immunomodulating drugs.
3. Discuss the mechanisms of action, indications, dosages, routes of administration, adverse effects, cautions, contraindications, and drug interactions of the different biologic response–modifying drugs.
4. Describe the pathology associated with rheumatoid arthritis.
5. Discuss the mechanisms of action, indications, dosages, routes of administration, adverse effects, cautions, contraindications, and drug interactions of the different antirheumatic drugs.
6. Develop a nursing care plan that includes all phases of the nursing process for patients receiving biologic response–modifying drugs and for those receiving antirheumatic drugs.

## DRUG PROFILES

abatacept, p. 778
adalimumab, p. 772
♦ aldesleukin, p. 775
alemtuzumab, p. 772
anakinra, p. 775
belimumab, p. 773
bevacizumab, p. 773
certolizumab, p. 773
cetuximab, p. 773
denileukin diftitox, p. 775
etanercept, p. 777
♦ filgrastim, p. 768
golimumab, p. 773
ibritumomab tiuxetan, p. 773
infliximab, p. 773

♦ interferon alfa-2a, interferon alfa-2b, interferon alfa-n3, interferon alfacon-1, peginterferon alfa-2a, and peginterferon alfa-2b, p. 770
♦ interferon beta-1a, interferon beta-1b, p. 770
interferon gamma-1b, p. 770
leflunomide, p. 777
methotrexate, p. 777
natalizumab, p. 773
♦ oprelvekin, p. 768
♦ rituximab, p. 773
♦ sargramostim, p. 768
tocilizumab, p.775
tositumomab and iodine I 131 tositumomab, p. 774
trastuzumab, p. 774

♦ *Key drug*

## KEY TERMS

**Adjuvant** A nonspecific *immunostimulant* that enhances overall immune function, rather than stimulating the function of a specific immune system cell or cytokine through specific chemical reactions. (p. 776)

**Antibodies** Immunoglobulin molecules (see Chapter 49) that have the ability to bind to and inactivate antigen molecules through formation of an antigen-antibody complex. This process serves to inactivate foreign antigens that enter the body and are capable of causing disease. (p. 765)

**Antigen** A biologic or chemical substance that is recognized as foreign by the body's immune system. (p. 764)

**Arthritis** Inflammation of one or more joints. (p. 777)

**Autoimmune disorder** A disorder that occurs when the body's tissues are attacked by its own immune system. (p. 776)

**B lymphocytes (B cells)** Leukocytes of the humoral immune system that develop into plasma cells, and then produce the antibodies that bind to and inactivate antigens. B cells are one of the two principal types of lymphocytes; T lymphocytes are the other. (p. 765)

**Biologic response–modifying drugs** A broad class of drugs that includes hematopoietic drugs and immunomodulating drugs. Often referred to as *biologic response modifiers (BRMs)*, they alter the body's response to diseases such as cancer as well as autoimmune, inflammatory, and infectious diseases. Examples are cytokines (e.g., interleukin, interferons), monoclonal antibodies, and vaccines. They are also called *biomodulators* or *immunomodulating drugs*. Biologic response–modifying drugs may be adjuvants, immunostimulants, or immunosuppressants. (p. 764)

**Cell-mediated immunity** Collective term for all immune responses that are mediated by T lymphocytes (T cells). Also called *cellular immunity*. Cell-mediated immunity acts in collaboration with humoral immunity. (p. 764)

**Colony-stimulating factors** Cytokines that regulate the growth, differentiation, and function of bone marrow stem cells. (p. 766)

**Complement** Collective term for about 20 different proteins normally present in plasma that assist other immune system components (e.g., B cells and T cells) in mounting an immune response. (p. 774)

**Cytokines** The generic term for nonantibody proteins released by specific cell populations (e.g., activated T cells) on contact with antigens. Cytokines act as intercellular mediators of an immune response. (p. 765)

**Cytotoxic T cells** Differentiated T cells that can recognize and lyse (rupture) target cells that have foreign antigens on their surfaces. These antigens are recognized by the corresponding antigen receptors that are expressed (displayed) on the cytotoxic T-cell surface. Also called *natural killer cells*. (p. 765)

**Differentiation** The process of cellular development from a simplified into a more specialized cellular structure. In hematopoiesis, it refers to the multistep processes involved in the maturation of blood cells. (p. 766)

**Disease-modifying antirheumatic drugs (DMARDs)** Medications used in the treatment of rheumatic diseases that have the potential to arrest or slow the actual disease process instead of providing only antiinflammatory and analgesic effects. (p. 777)

**Hematopoiesis** Collective term for all of the body's processes originating in the bone marrow that result in the formation of various types of blood components (adjective: *hematopoietic*). It includes the three main processes of *differentiation* (see earlier): erythropoiesis (formation of red blood cells, or erythrocytes), leukopoiesis (formation of white blood cells, or leukocytes), and thrombopoiesis (formation of platelets, or thrombocytes). (p. 764)

**Humoral immunity** Collective term for all immune responses that are mediated by B cells, which ultimately work through the production of antibodies against specific antigens. Humoral immunity acts in collaboration with *cell-mediated immunity*. (p. 764)

**Immunoglobulins** Complex immune system glycoproteins that bind to and inactivate foreign antigens. The term is synonymous with *immune globulins*. (p. 765)

**Immunomodulating drugs** Collective term for various subclasses of biologic response–modifying drugs that specifically or nonspecifically enhance or reduce immune responses. The three major types of immunomodulators, based on mechanism of action, are adjuvants, immunostimulants, and immunosuppressants (see Chapter 48). (p. 764)

**Immunostimulant** A drug that enhances immune response through specific chemical interactions with particular immune system components. An example is interleukin-2. (p. 776)

**Immunosuppressant** A drug that reduces immune response through specific chemical interactions with particular immune system components. An example is cyclosporine (see Chapter 48). (p. 769)

**Interferons** One type of cytokine that promotes resistance to viral infection in uninfected cells and can also strengthen the body's immune response to cancer cells. (p. 768)

**Leukocytes** The collective term for all subtypes of white blood cells. Leukocytes include the granulocytes (neutrophils, eosinophils, and basophils), monocytes, and lymphocytes (B cells and T cells). Some monocytes also develop into tissue macrophages. (p. 766)

**Lymphokine-activated killer (LAK) cell** *Cytotoxic T cells* that have been activated by interkeukin-2 and therefore have a stronger and more specific response against cancer cells. (p. 774)

**Lymphokines** Cytokines that are produced by sensitized T lymphocytes on contact with antigen particles. (p. 765)

**Memory cells** Cells involved in the humoral immune system that remember the exact characteristics of a particular foreign invader or antigen for the purpose of expediting immune response in the event of future exposure to this antigen. (p. 765)

**KEY TERMS—cont'd**

**Monoclonal** Denoting a group of identical cells or organisms derived from a single cell. (p. 765)

**Plasma cells** Cells derived from B cells that are found in the bone marrow, connective tissue, and blood. They produce antibodies. (p. 765)

**Rheumatism** General term for any of several disorders characterized by inflammation, degeneration, or metabolic derangement of connective tissue structures, especially joints and related structures. (p. 776)

**T helper cells** Cells that promote and direct the actions of various other cells of the immune system. (p. 765)

**T lymphocytes (T cells)** Leukocytes of the cell-mediated immune system. Unlike B cells, they are not involved in the production of antibodies but instead occur in various cell subtypes (e.g., T helper cells, T suppressor cells, and cytotoxic T cells). They act through direct cell-to-cell contact or through production of cytokines that guide the functions of other immune system components (e.g., B cells, antibodies). (p. 765)

**T suppressor cells** Cells that regulate and limit the immune response, balancing the effects of T helper cells. (p. 766)

**Tumor antigens** Chemical compounds expressed on the surfaces of tumor cells. They signal to the immune system that these cells do not belong in the body, labeling the tumor cells as foreign. (p. 764)

## ANATOMY, PHYSIOLOGY, AND PATHOPHYSIOLOGY OVERVIEW

### OVERVIEW OF IMMUNOMODULATORS

Over the last two decades, medical technology has developed a group of drugs whose primary site of action is the immune system. This has resulted in new additions to the class of drugs known as biologic response–modifying drugs, or biologic response modifiers(s). These drugs alter the body's response to diseases such as cancer and autoimmune, inflammatory, and infectious diseases. These drugs can enhance or restrict the patient's immune response to disease, can stimulate a patient's hematopoietic (blood-forming) function, and can prevent disease. Hematopoiesis is the collective term for all of the blood component–forming processes of the bone marrow. Two broad classes of biologic response–modifying drugs are hematopoietic drugs and immunomodulating drugs. Subclasses of immunomodulating drugs include interferons, monoclonal antibodies, interleukin receptor agonists and antagonists, and miscellaneous drugs. Disease-modifying antirheumatic drugs are drugs that are used to treat rheumatoid arthritis, which is discussed later in the chapter.

Immunomodulating drugs therapeutically alter a patient's immune response. In cancer treatment, they make up the fourth type of cancer therapy, along with surgery, chemotherapy, and radiation. The human immune system is most commonly viewed as the body's natural defense against pathogenic bacteria and viruses. However, it also has effective antitumor capabilities. An intact immune system can identify cells as malignant and destroy them. In contrast to chemotherapeutic drugs, a healthy immune system can distinguish between tumor cells and normal body tissues. Normal cells are recognized as "self" and are not damaged, whereas tumor cells are recognized as "foreign" and are destroyed. People develop cancerous cells in their bodies on a regular basis. Normally the immune system is able to eliminate these cells before they multiply to uncontrollable levels. It is only when the natural immune responses fail to keep pace with these initially microscopic cancer cell growths that a person develops a true "cancer" requiring clinical intervention.

In terms of their activity against cancer cells, biologic response–modifying drugs work by one of three mechanisms: (1) enhancement or restoration of the host's immune system defenses against the tumor; (2) direct toxic effect on the tumor cells, which causes them to lyse, or rupture; or (3) adverse modification of the tumor's biology, which makes it harder for the tumor cells to survive and reproduce.

Some immunomodulating drugs are used to treat autoimmune, inflammatory, and infectious diseases. In these instances, the drug functions either to reduce the patient's inappropriate immune response (in the case of inflammatory and autoimmune diseases such as rheumatoid arthritis) or to strengthen the patient's immune response against microorganisms (especially viruses) and cancer cells. To better understand these complex drugs, a review of immune system physiology is beneficial.

### IMMUNE SYSTEM

The immune system is an intricate biologic defense network of cells that are capable of distinguishing an unlimited variety of substances as either foreign ("nonself") or a natural part of the host's body ("self"). When a foreign substance such as a bacteria or virus enters the body, the immune system recognizes it as being foreign and mounts an immune response to eliminate or neutralize the invader. Tumors are not truly foreign substances because they arise from cells of normal tissues whose genetic material (deoxyribonucleic acid [DNA] and ribonucleic acid [RNA]) has somehow mutated. Tumor cells express chemical compounds on their surfaces that signal the immune system that these cells are a threat. These chemical markers are called tumor antigens or *tumor markers,* and they label the tumor cells as abnormal cells. An antigen is any substance that the body's immune system recognizes as foreign. Recognition of antigens varies among individuals, which is why some people are more prone than others to immune-related diseases such as allergies, inflammatory diseases, and cancer.

The two major components of the body's immune system are humoral immunity, mediated by B-cell functions (primarily *antibody* production), and cell-mediated immunity, which is mediated by T-cell functions. These two systems work together to recognize and destroy foreign particles and cells in the blood or other body tissues. Communication between these two divisions is vital to the success of the immune system as a whole. Attack against tumor cells by antibodies produced by the B lymphocytes (B cells) of the humoral immune system prepares those tumor cells for destruction by the T lymphocytes (T cells) of the cell-mediated immune system. This is just one example of the effective way that the two divisions of the immune system communicate with each other for a collaborative immune response.

## Humoral Immune System

The functional cells of the humoral immune system are the B lymphocytes. They are also called *B cells* because they originate in the bone marrow. The B cells that are capable of generating a particular antibody normally remain dormant until the corresponding antigen is detected. When an antigen binds to receptors located on the B cells, a biochemical signal is sent to the B lymphocytes. These B cells then mature or *differentiate* into plasma cells, which in turn produce antibodies. Antibodies are immunoglobulins (large glycoprotein molecules; *glyco* = sugar; *protein* = amino acid chain) that bind to specific antigens, forming an *antigen-antibody complex* that inactivates disease-causing antigens.

The immune system in a healthy individual is genetically preprogrammed to be able to mount an antibody response against literally millions of different antigens. This ability results from the individual's lifetime antigen exposure and is further developed through exposure to new antigens and passed down through many generations. Antibodies that a single plasma cell makes are all identical. They are therefore called monoclonal antibodies. Since the 1980s, monoclonal antibodies have also been prepared synthetically using recombinant DNA technology, which has resulted in newer drug therapies.

There are five major types of naturally occurring immunoglobulins in the body: immunoglobulins A, D, E, G, and M. These unique types have different structures and functions and are found in various areas of the body. During an immune response, when B lymphocytes differentiate into plasma cells, some of these B cells become memory cells. Memory cells

"remember" the exact characteristics of a particular foreign invader or antigen, which allows a stronger and faster immune response in the event of reexposure to the same antigen. The cells of the humoral immune system are shown in Figure 47-1.

## Cell-Mediated Immune System

The functional cells of the cell-mediated (as opposed to antibody-mediated) immune system are the T lymphocytes. They are also referred to as *T cells* because they mature in the thymus. There are three distinct populations of T cells: cytotoxic T cells, T helper cells, and T suppressor cells (Figure 47-2). They are distinguished by the different functions that they perform. Cytotoxic T cells directly kill their targets by causing cell lysis or rupture. T helper cells are considered the master controllers of the immune system. They direct the actions of many other immune components, such as lymphokines and cytotoxic T cells. Cytokines are nonantibody proteins that serve as chemical mediators of various physiologic functions. Lymphokines are a subset of cytokines. They are released by T lymphocytes upon contact with antigens and serve as chemical mediators

**FIGURE 47-1** Cells of the humoral (antibody-mediated) immune system. *Ig*, Immunoglobulin.

**FIGURE 47-2** Cells of the cellular immune system.

of the immune response. T suppressor cells have an effect on the immune system that is opposite to that of T helper cells and serve to limit or control the immune response. A healthy immune system has about twice as many T helper cells as T suppressor cells at any given time.

The major cells involved in the destruction of cancer cells are part of the cell-mediated immune system (see Figure 47-2). The cancer-killing cells of the cellular immune system are the macrophages (derived from monocytes), natural killer (NK) cells (another type of lymphocyte), and polymorphonuclear leukocytes (not lymphocytes), which are also called *neutrophils.* In contrast, T suppressor cells have an important negative influence on antitumor actions of the immune system. Overactive T suppressor cells may be responsible for clinically significant cancer cases by permitting tumor growth beyond the immune system's control.

## PHARMACOLOGY OVERVIEW

Therapy with biologic response–modifying drugs combines the knowledge of several disciplines, including general biology, genetics, immunology, pharmacology, medicine, and nursing. The general therapeutic effects of these drugs are as follows:
- Enhancement of hematopoietic function
- Regulation or enhancement of the immune response, including cytotoxic or cytostatic activity against cancer cells
- Inhibition of metastases, prevention of cell division, or inhibition of cell maturation

Box 47-1 lists the currently available biologic response–modifying drugs used in the treatment of cancer and other illnesses that have varying levels of immune system–related pathophysiology. The drugs are classified according to their biologic effects.

## HEMATOPOIETIC DRUGS

Hematopoietic drugs include several medications developed over the past 10 to 15 years. Falling into this category are two erythropoietic drugs (epoetin alfa and darbepoetin alfa), three colony-stimulating factors (filgrastim, pegfilgrastim, and sargramostim), and one platelet-promoting drug (oprelvekin). All of these drugs promote the synthesis of various types of major blood components by promoting the growth, differentiation, and function of their corresponding precursor cells in the bone marrow.

### Mechanism of Action and Drug Effects

Although the hematopoietic drugs are not toxic to cancer cells, they do have beneficial effects in the treatment of cancer. All hematopoietic drugs have the same basic mechanism of action. They decrease the duration of chemotherapy-induced anemia, neutropenia, and thrombocytopenia and enable higher dosages of chemotherapy to be given; decrease bone marrow recovery time after bone marrow transplantation or irradiation; and stimulate other cells in the immune system to destroy or inhibit the growth of cancer cells, as well as virus- or fungus-infected cells.

All of these drugs are produced by recombinant DNA technology, which allows them to be essentially identical to their endogenously produced counterparts. These substances work by binding to receptors on the surfaces of specialized progenitor cells in the bone marrow. Progenitor cells are responsible for the production of three particular cell lines: red blood cells (RBCs), white blood cells (WBCs), and platelets. When a hematopoietic drug binds to a progenitor cell surface, the immature progenitor cell is stimulated to mature, proliferate (reproduce itself), differentiate (transform into its respective type of specialized blood component), and become functionally active. Hematopoietic drugs may enhance certain functions of mature cell lines as well.

Epoetin alfa is a synthetic derivative of the human hormone erythropoietin, which is produced primarily by the kidney. It promotes the synthesis of erythrocytes (RBCs) by stimulating RBC progenitor cells in the bone marrow. Darbepoetin alfa is a longer-acting form of epoetin alfa. These drugs

---

**BOX 47-1   BIOLOGIC RESPONSE–MODIFYING DRUGS**

**Hematopoietic Drugs**
*Colony-Stimulating Factors*
filgrastim (G-CSF)
pegfilgrastim
sargramostim (GM-CSF)

*Other*
darbepoetin alfa
epoetin alfa
oprelvekin (IL-11)

**Immunomodulating Drugs**
*Interferons*
interferon alfa-2a
interferon alfa-2b*
peginterferon alfa-2a
peginterferon alfa-2b
interferon alfacon-1
interferon alfa-n3
interferon beta-1a
interferon beta-1b
interferon gamma-1b

*Monoclonal Antibodies*
adalimumab
alemtuzumab
belimumab
bevacixumab
certolizumab
golimumab
ibritumomab tiuxetan
infliximab
rituximab
trastuzumab

*Interleukin Receptor Agonists and Antagonists*
*Agonist*
aldesleukin (IL-2)

*Antagonists*
anakinra
denileukin diftitox
tocilizumab

*Miscellaneous Immunomodulators*
*Tumor Necrosis Factor Receptor Antagonist*
etanercept

*Enzymes*
Pegademase bovine

*Retinoid Receptor Agonists*
tretinoin
bexarotene

*Adjuvants (Nonspecific Immunostimulants)*
Bacille Calmette-Guérin vaccine
leflunomide
levamisole
mitoxantrone
thalidomide
abatacept

*G-CSF,* Granulocyte colony-stimulating factor; *GM-CSF,* granulocyte-macrophage colony-stimulating factor; *IL,* interleukin.
*Also available in combination with the antiviral drug ribavirin.

are discussed in detail in Chapter 54. Filgrastim is a colony-stimulating factor that stimulates progenitor cells for the subset of WBCs (leukocytes) known as *granulocytes* (including basophils, eosinophils, and neutrophils). For this reason, it is also commonly called *granulocyte colony-stimulating factor (G-CSF)*. Pegfilgrastim is a longer-acting form of filgrastim. Sargramostim is also a colony-stimulating factor that works by stimulating the bone marrow precursor cells that synthesize both granulocytes and the phagocytic (cell-eating) cells known as *monocytes*, some of which become macrophages. For this reason, it is also called *granulocyte-macrophage colony-stimulating factor (GM-CSF)*. Oprelvekin is classified as an *interleukin*, namely, interleukin-11 (IL-11). Other interleukins are discussed later in the chapter. Oprelvekin stimulates the bone marrow cells, specifically megakaryocytes that eventually give rise to platelets.

## Indications

Neutrophils are the most important granulocytes for fighting infection. Infections often appear in patients who have experienced destruction of bone marrow cells as a result of chemotherapy. Colony-stimulating factors stimulate neutrophils to grow and mature and thus directly oppose the detrimental bone marrow actions of chemotherapy. Because these drugs reduce the duration of low neutrophil counts, they reduce the incidence and duration of infections. Colony-stimulating factors also enhance the functioning of mature cells of the immune system, such as macrophages and granulocytes. This increases the ability of the body's immune system to kill cancer cells, as well as virus- and fungus-infected cells. Ultimately these properties allow patients to receive higher dosages of chemotherapy. Similar benefits occur with epoetin alfa and oprelvekin with regard to RBC and platelet counts, respectively.

The effect of hematopoietic drugs on the bone marrow cells also reduces the recovery time after bone marrow transplantation and radiation therapy. Dosages of chemotherapy used in bone marrow transplantation are often much higher than those used in conventional chemotherapy. Both the chemotherapy and radiation therapy are toxic to the bone marrow. When one or more colony-stimulating factors are administered as part of the drug therapy for bone marrow transplantation, bone marrow cell counts return to normal in a drastically shortened time. This helps to increase the likelihood of a successful bone marrow transplantation and therefore patient

| TABLE 47-1 | HEMATOPOIETIC DRUGS: COMMON ADVERSE EFFECTS |
|---|---|
| **BODY SYSTEM** | **ADVERSE EFFECTS** |
| Cardiovascular | Edema |
| Gastrointestinal | Anorexia, nausea, vomiting, diarrhea |
| Integumentary | Alopecia, rash |
| Respiratory | Cough, dyspnea, sore throat |
| Other | Fever, blood dyscrasias, headache, bone pain |

survival. Specific drug indications are listed in the Dosages table on this page.

## Contraindications

Contraindications for all these drugs include drug allergy. Use of filgrastim, sargramostim, and pegfilgrastim is contraindicated in the presence of more than 10% myeloid blasts (immature tumor cells in the bone marrow), because colony-stimulating factors may stimulate malignant growth of these myeloid tumor cells.

## Adverse Effects

Adverse effects associated with the use of hematopoietic drugs are mild. The most common are fever, muscle aches, bone pain, and flushing. Table 47-1 lists additional adverse effects.

## Interactions

Filgrastim and sargramostim have significant drug interactions when these two drugs are given with myelosuppressive (bone marrow depressant) antineoplastic drugs. Remember that these two drugs are administered to enhance the production of bone marrow cells; therefore, when myelosuppressive antineoplastics are given with them, the drugs directly antagonize each other. Typically filgrastim and sargramostim are not given within 24 hours of administration of myelosuppressive antineoplastics. However, they are given soon after this time to help prevent the WBC nadir from dropping to dangerous levels and also to speed WBC recovery. It is also recommended that these drugs be used with caution or not be given with other medications that can potentiate their myeloproliferative (bone marrow–stimulating) effects. Two examples are lithium and corticosteroids.

## Dosages

For dosage information on hematopoietic drugs, see the table on this page.

## DOSAGES

### Hematopoietic Drugs

| DRUG (PREGNANCY CATEGORY) | PHARMACOLOGIC CLASS | USUAL DOSAGE RANGE | INDICATIONS |
|---|---|---|---|
| ◆ filgrastim (Neupogen) (C) | Colony-stimulating factor | IV/subcut: 5-10 mcg/kg/day | Chemotherapy-induced leukopenia |
| ◆ oprelvekin (IL-11) (Neumega) (C) | Synthetic human interleukin analogue | **Adult only** Subcut: 50 mcg/kg/day for up to 21 days | Chemotherapy-induced thrombocytopenia |
| ◆ sargramostim (Leukine) (C) | Colony-stimulating factor | IV: 250 mcg/m²/day | Chemotherapy-induced leukopenia |

*IL*, Interleukin; *IV*, intravenous; *subcut*, subcutaneous.

## DRUG PROFILES

### ♦ filgrastim

Filgrastim (Neupogen) is a synthetic analogue of human granulocyte colony-stimulating factor and is commonly referred to as *G-CSF*. Filgrastim promotes the proliferation, differentiation, and activation of the cells that make granulocytes. Granulocytes are the body's primary defense against bacterial and fungal infections. Filgrastim has the same pharmacologic effects as endogenous human G-CSF, which is normally secreted by specialized leukocytes known as *monocytes, macrophages,* and *mature neutrophils.* Filgrastim is indicated to prevent or treat febrile neutropenia in patients receiving myelosuppressive antineoplastics for nonmyeloid (non–bone marrow) malignancies. It must be given *before* a patient develops an infection, but not within 24 hours before or after myelosuppressive chemotherapeutic drugs. Pegfilgrastim (Neulasta) is a long-acting form of filgrastim that reduces the number of injections required. Both drugs are available for injection only. These drugs are usually discontinued when a patient's absolute neutrophil count (ANC) rises above 10,000 cells/mm$^3$. However, some prescribers will stop it when the ANC is between 1000 and 2000 cells/mm$^3$.

### Pharmacokinetics

| Route | Onset of Action | Peak Plasma Concentration | Elimination Half-life | Duration of Action |
|---|---|---|---|---|
| Subcut or IV | 1 hr | 2-6 hr | 3-5 hr | 12-24 hr |

### ♦ sargramostim

Sargramostim (Leukine) is a synthetic analogue of human granulocyte-macrophage colony-stimulating factor and is commonly referred to as *GM-CSF*. There are three major subsets of leukocytes: *granulocytes, monocytes,* and *lymphocytes* (B cells and T cells). Granulocytes are further subdivided into *basophils, eosinophils,* and *neutrophils*. Neutrophils are the most important in fighting infection. Macrophages are tissue-based (as opposed to circulating) cells that are derived from monocytes, which circulate in the blood. Neutrophils, monocytes, and macrophages make up the three main categories of phagocytic (cell-eating) blood cells, and they literally ingest foreign cells and other antigens as part of their immune system function. Sargramostim has the same pharmacologic effects as endogenous human GM-CSF. It stimulates the proliferation, differentiation, and activation of the cells in the bone marrow that eventually become granulocytes, monocytes, and macrophages.

Sargramostim is indicated for promoting bone marrow recovery after autologous (own marrow) or allogenic (donor marrow) bone marrow transplantation in patients with various types of leukemia and lymphoma. This drug is available for injection only.

### Pharmacokinetics

| Route | Onset of Action | Peak Plasma Concentration | Elimination Half-life | Duration of Action |
|---|---|---|---|---|
| Subcut or IV | 4 hr | 2 hr | 2 hr | 10 days |

### ♦ oprelvekin

Oprelvekin (Neumega) is both a hematopoietic drug and one of the interleukins. However, its function is similar to that of the colony-stimulating factors (filgrastim and sargramostim) in that it enhances synthesis of a specific blood component—in this case, the platelets. Oprelvekin is indicated for the prevention of chemotherapy-induced severe thrombocytopenia and avoidance of the need for platelet transfusions. Its use is contraindicated in cases of known drug allergy. It is available for injection only.

### Pharmacokinetics

| Route | Onset of Action | Peak Plasma Concentration | Elimination Half-life | Duration of Action |
|---|---|---|---|---|
| Subcut | 5-9 days* | 3 hr | 7 hr | 14 days |

*Platelet counts begin to increase.

## INTERFERONS

Interferons are proteins that have three basic properties: they are antiviral, antitumor, and immunomodulating. There are three different groups of interferon drugs—the alpha, beta, and gamma interferons—each with its own antigenic and biologic activity. Interferons are most commonly used in the treatment of certain viral infections and certain types of cancer.

## Mechanism of Action and Drug Effects

Interferons are recombinantly manufactured substances that are identical to the interferon cytokines that are naturally present in the human body. In the body, interferons are produced by activated T cells and by other cells in response to viral infection. Interferons protect human cells from virus attack by enabling the human cells to produce enzymes that stop viral replication and prevent viruses from penetrating into healthy cells. Interferons prevent cancer cells from dividing and replicating and also increase the activity of other cells in the immune system, such as macrophages, neutrophils, and natural killer cells. Their effect on cancer cells is caused by a combination of direct inhibition of DNA and protein synthesis within cancer cells (antitumor effects) and multiple immunomodulatory effects on the host's immune system. Interferons increase the cytotoxic activity of natural killer cells and the phagocytic ability of macrophages. Interferons also increase the expression of cancer cell antigens on the cell surface, which enables the immune system to recognize cancer cells more easily, specifically marking them for destruction.

Overall, interferons have three different effects on the immune system. They can (1) restore its function if it is impaired, (2) augment (amplify) the immune system's ability to function as the body's defense, and (3) inhibit the immune system from working. This latter function may be especially useful when the immune system has become dysfunctional, causing an *autoimmune* disease. This is believed to be the case in multiple sclerosis. Two interferons (interferon beta-1a and interferon beta-1b) are specifically indicated for treatment of multiple sclerosis. Inhibiting the dysfunctional immune system prevents further damage to the body from the disease process.

## Indications

The beneficial actions of interferons (antiviral, antineoplastic, and immunomodulatory) make them excellent drugs for the treatment of viral infections, various cancers, and some autoimmune disorders. Currently accepted indications for interferons are listed in the Dosages table on this page.

## Contraindications

Contraindications to the use of interferons include known drug allergy and may include autoimmune disorders, hepatitis or liver failure, concurrent use of immunosuppressant drugs, Kaposi's sarcoma related to acquired immunodeficiency syndrome (AIDS), and severe liver disease.

## Adverse Effects

The most common adverse effects can be broadly described as flulike symptoms: fever, chills, headache, malaise, myalgia, and fatigue. The major dose-limiting adverse effect of interferons is fatigue. Patients taking high dosages become so exhausted that they are often confined to bed. Other adverse effects of interferons are listed in Table 47-2.

## Interactions

Drug interactions are seen with both interferon alfa-2a and interferon alfa-2b when they are used with drugs that are metabolized in the liver via the cytochrome P-450 enzyme system. The combination results in decreased metabolism and increased accumulation of these drugs, which leads to drug toxicity. There is also some evidence that using interferons together with antiviral drugs such as zidovudine enhances the activity of both drugs but may lead to toxic levels of zidovudine. Additive toxic effects to the bone marrow can occur when interferon gamma products are used with other myelosuppressive drugs.

## Dosages

For dosage information on interferons, see the table on this page.

### TABLE 47-2 INTERFERONS: ADVERSE EFFECTS

| BODY SYSTEM | ADVERSE EFFECTS |
| --- | --- |
| General | Flulike syndrome, fatigue |
| Cardiovascular | Tachycardia, cyanosis, ECG changes, orthostatic hypotension |
| Central nervous | Confusion, somnolence, irritability, seizures, hallucinations |
| Gastrointestinal | Nausea, diarrhea, vomiting, anorexia, taste alterations, dry mouth |
| Hematologic | Neutropenia, thrombocytopenia |
| Renal and hepatic | Increased BUN and creatinine levels, proteinuria, abnormal liver function test |

*BUN*, Blood urea nitrogen; *ECG*, electrocardiogram.

## DOSAGES

### Interferons

| DRUG (PREGNANCY CATEGORY) | PHARMACOLOGIC CLASS | USUAL DOSAGE RANGE | INDICATIONS |
| --- | --- | --- | --- |
| ◆ interferon alfa-2a (Roferon-A) (C) | Immunomodulator, antiviral, antineoplastic | IM/subcut: 3 million units 3 × per week, depending on indication | Chronic hepatitis C, hairy cell leukemia, AIDS-related Kaposi's sarcoma, chronic myelogenous leukemia |
| ◆ interferon alfa-2b (Intron-A) (C) | Immunomodulator, antiviral, antineoplastic | IM/subcut: 1-30 million units 3 × per week* | Hairy cell leukemia, malignant melanoma, follicular lymphoma, condylomata acuminata (venereal-genital warts), AIDS-related Kaposi's sarcoma, chronic hepatitis C, chronic hepatitis B |
| ◆ peginterferon alfa-2a (Pegasys) (C) | Immunomodulator, antiviral | Subcut: 180 mcg weekly for 48 wk | Chronic hepatitis C |
| ◆ peginterferon alfa-2b (PEG-Intron) (C) | Immunomodulator, antiviral | Subcut: 1 mcg/kg/wk for 1 yr† | Chronic hepatitis C |
| ◆ interferon alfa-n3 (Alferon-N) (C) | Immunomodulator, antiviral | Intralesional: 250,000 units (0.05 mL) into the base of each wart 2 × per week for up to 8 wk | Condylomata acuminata |
| ◆ interferon alfacon-1 (Infergen) (C) | Immunomodulator, antiviral | Subcut: 9 mcg 3 times per week for 24 wk | Chronic hepatitis C |
| ◆ interferon beta-1a (Avonex, Rebif) (C) | Immunomodulator | IM (Avonex): 30 mcg 1 time per week<br>Subcut (Rebif): 44 mcg 3 × per week | Multiple sclerosis |
| interferon gamma-1b (Actimmune) (C) | Immunomodulator | **BSA more than 0.5 m²**<br>Subcut: 50 mcg/m² 3 × per week<br>**BSA less than 0.5 m²**<br>Subcut: 1.5 mcg/kg 3 × per week | Chronic granulomatous disease, osteopetrosis |

*AIDS*, Acquired immunodeficiency syndrome; *BSA*, body surface area; *IM*, intramuscular; *subcut*, subcutaneous.
*May also be given by intravenous infusion for melanoma. Route and dose vary depending on indication.
†Dose is 1.5 mcg/kg/wk if given with ribavirin capsules (see Chapter 40).

## DRUG PROFILES

The three major classes of interferon drugs are alfa, beta, and gamma, which are sometimes also written using the lowercase Greek letters α, β, and γ, respectively. The "alfa" designation is synonymous with the Greek letter "alpha," but "alfa" is now more commonly used clinically. The interferons vary in their antigenic makeup, biologic actions, and pharmacologic properties. The best known interferon class is interferon alfa. Interferon products are biologic response–modifying drugs that can be broadly classified as cytokines. Cytokines are immune system proteins that serve two essential functions: they direct the actions and communication between the cell-mediated and humoral divisions of the immune system, and they augment or enhance the immune response. Other cytokines include tumor necrosis factor (TNF), interleukins, and colony-stimulating factors.

### INTERFERON ALFA PRODUCTS

♦ **interferon alfa-2a, interferon alfa-2b, interferon alfa-n3, interferon alfacon-1, peginterferon alfa-2a, peginterferon alfa-2b**

The most commonly used interferon products are in the alfa class. They are also referred to as *leukocyte interferons* because they are produced from human leukocytes. Two newer types of interferon alfa include peginterferon alfa-2a and peginterferon alfa-2b. The *peg* refers to the attachment of a polymer chain of the hydrocarbon polyethylene glycol (PEG). This "pegylation" process increases the size of the interferon molecule. This increased size delays drug absorption, increases half-life, and decreases plasma clearance rate, which prolongs the drug's therapeutic effects. In addition, pegylation is believed to reduce the immunogenicity of the interferon and thus delay its recognition and destruction by the immune system. Similarly, peg-filgrastim, mentioned previously in this chapter, is a pegylated form of filgrastim and is also longer-acting. The alfa-2a and alfa-2b interferons share the following indications: chronic hepatitis C, hairy cell leukemia, and AIDS-related Kaposi's sarcoma. Interferon alfa-2a (only) is also indicated for the treatment of chronic myelogenous leukemia. Additional indications unique to interferon alfa-2b are chronic hepatitis B, malignant melanoma (an often fatal form of skin cancer), follicular lymphoma (so named because its malignant cells gather in clumps called *follicles*—not to be confused with hair follicles), and condylomata acuminata (virally induced genital or venereal warts). Peg-interferon alfa-2a and peginterferon alfa-2b are currently indicated only for treatment of chronic hepatitis C.

Interferon alfa-n3 is a polyclonal mixture of all interferon alfa subtypes. It is the product of pooled human leukocytes. Its only current indication is condylomata acuminata. Interferon alfacon-1 is a purely synthetic (i.e., non–naturally occurring) recombinant product that is currently indicated only for treatment of hepatitis C.

Interferons are most commonly given by either intramuscular or subcutaneous injection, but intravenous and intraperitoneal routes have been used as well. It is important to note that some interferons are dosed in millions of units. Although it is unacceptable to use the abbreviation MU for "millions of units," you may see it written as such. It is imperative to double-check the dose, because the prescriber's writing of "MU" may be mistaken for "mg" or "mcg." If there is any question about the dose of any medication, double-check with the prescriber, pharmacist, or other experienced colleague before administering the medication to the patient. Although this is true for all medications, it is a special consideration for interferons and other biologic response–modifying drugs, because of both their potency and their dosage variability.

### INTERFERON BETA PRODUCTS

♦ **interferon beta-1a, interferon beta-1b**

Interferon beta-1a and interferon beta-1b are the currently available beta products. They interact with specific cell receptors found on the surfaces of human cells and possess antiviral and immunomodulatory activity. Both are produced by recombinant DNA techniques and are indicated for the treatment of relapsing multiple sclerosis (to slow the progression of physical disability and decrease the frequency of clinical exacerbations). The only contraindication is drug allergy, including allergy to human albumin. Both drugs are available for injection only.

### INTERFERON GAMMA PRODUCT

**interferon gamma-1b**

Interferon gamma-1b (Actimmune) is a synthetic product produced by recombinant DNA technology. It is indicated for the treatment of serious infections associated with chronic granulomatous disease, a genetic immunodeficiency, and osteopetrosis, a genetic bone disease characterized by abnormally dense bone, anemia, and frequent fractures. Interferon gamma-1b is available for injection only.

## MONOCLONAL ANTIBODIES

Monoclonal antibodies are quickly becoming standards of therapy in many areas of medicine, including treatment of cancer, rheumatoid arthritis and other inflammatory diseases, multiple sclerosis, and organ transplantation. In cancer treatment they have advantages over traditional antineoplastics in that they can specifically target cancer cells and have minimal effect on healthy cells. This reduces many of the adverse effects traditionally associated with antineoplastic drugs. There are several commercially available monoclonal antibodies used to treat cancer and rheumatoid arthritis. The most commonly used ones are listed in the Dosages table on p. 772. The *mab* suffix in a drug name is usually an abbreviation for "monoclonal antibody." Muromonab is used in kidney transplantation and is discussed in Chapter 48.

## Mechanism of Action, Drug Effects, and Indications

Because these drugs are so diverse, specific information for each appears in the individual drug profiles provided later in the chapter.

## Contraindications

The only clear contraindication to the use of monoclonal antibodies reported thus far is drug allergy to a specific product. Their use is usually contraindicated in patients with known active infectious processes due to their immunosuppressive qualities. Although known drug allergy is a contraindication, depending on the urgency of the clinical situation, a given monoclonal antibody may be the only viable treatment option for a seriously ill patient. In such situations, allergic symptoms may be controlled with supportive medications such as diphenhydramine and acetaminophen (for fever control). All of the drugs that are TNF antagonists are contraindicated in patients with active tuberculosis or other infections. Infliximab has been shown to worsen severe cases of heart failure and is dosed at no more than 5 mg/kg and only after considering other treatment options for its indications. Use of alemtuzumab is also contraindicated in patients with active systemic infections and immunodeficiency conditions, including AIDS.

## Adverse Effects

Many, if not most, patients receiving these very potent drugs manifest acute symptoms that are comparable to classic allergy or flulike symptoms, such as fever, dyspnea, and chills. The primary objective is to administer the medication and control such symptoms as well as possible. Because the mechanisms of action of these drugs work through augmentation or inhibition of the human immune response, they can have a variety of adverse effects, some mild, some severe, that affect several body systems. Drug-specific adverse effects with the highest reported incidence (10% to 50% or more) are listed in Table 47-3. The risk of such adverse effects must be weighed against the severity of the patient's underlying illness. Many of these adverse effects may also be associated with the patient's disease process (e.g., infections) and even with life in general (e.g., headache, depression). This is especially true for the milder effects. The risk of acquiring an infection is a serious adverse effect of all of the biologic response–modifying agents, because they alter the normal immune response.

## Interactions

Drug interactions associated with monoclonal antibodies are relatively few, and no major food interactions are listed. Administration of adalimumab with the anti–rheumatoid arthritis drug anakinra (an interleukin) may increase the risk of serious infections secondary to neutropenia. The clearance of natalizumab may be reduced by concurrent administration of interferon beta-1a (both used for multiple sclerosis). Coadministration of anti-TNF drugs (e.g., etanercept, anakinra) with infliximab may also increase the risk of neutropenia and infections. Etanercept is not to be given concurrently with varicella-zoster immune globulin (VZIG) because of undesirable drug interactions. However, etanercept may be resumed after completion of VZIG therapy. Bevacizumab is associated with increased risk of severe diarrhea and neutropenia when given concurrently with another anti–colorectal cancer drug, irinotecan (see Chapter 45). Paclitaxel (see Chapter 45) has been shown to reduce the clearance of trastuzumab when the two are administered concurrently to treat breast cancer.

## Dosages

For dosage information on the monoclonal antibodies, see the table on p. 772.

| TABLE 47-3 | SELECTED IMMUNOMODULATING DRUGS: COMMON ADVERSE EFFECTS |
|---|---|
| **DRUG** | **ADVERSE EFFECTS** |
| adalimumab | Localized inflammatory reaction at the injection site, infectious processes such as upper respiratory tract and urinary tract infections, and higher rates of various malignancies |
| alemtuzumab | Rash, pruritus, nausea, vomiting, diarrhea, dyspnea, cough, muscle spasms, fever, fatigue, skeletal pain, myelosuppression |
| belimumab | Nausea, diarrhea, depression, insomnia, fever, infection, anaphylaxis |
| bevacizumab | Deep vein thrombosis, hypertension, diarrhea, abdominal pain, constipation, vomiting, GI hemorrhage, leukopenia, asthenia, headache, dizziness, dry skin, proteinuria, hypokalemia, epistaxis, weight loss |
| certolizumab | Arthralgia, respiratory tract infection, cardiac dysrhythmia, rash, bowel obstruction |
| cetuximab | Headache, insomnia, skin rash, conjunctivitis, GI discomfort, anemia, leukopenia, dehydration, edema, weight loss, dyspnea, asthenia, back pain, fever |
| golimumab | Hypertension, increased liver function tests, infection |
| ibritumomab tiuxetan | Nausea, myelosuppression, asthenia, infection, chills |
| infliximab | Headache, rash, GI discomfort, dyspnea, upper and lower respiratory tract infection |
| natalizumab | Depression, fatigue, headache, GI discomfort, urinary tract infection, lower respiratory tract infection, joint pain. Of even greater concern are case reports of a rare and potentially fatal brain disorder known as progressive multifocal leukoencephalopathy. |
| rituximab | Fever, chills, headache. Potentially fatal infusion-related events, including severe bronchospasm, dyspnea, hypoxia, pulmonary infiltrates, adult respiratory distress syndrome, hypotension, and angioedema. Tumor lysis syndrome (see Chapter 45) with acute renal failure has also been reported. The drug must be stopped immediately and indicated supportive care provided if such a reaction appears imminent. |
| tocilizumab | Hypertension, rash, diarrhea, dizziness, anaphylaxis, infection, injection site reaction |
| tositumomab and iodine I-131 tositumomab | Headache, rash, GI discomfort, muscle pains, dyspnea, pharyngitis, asthenia, fever, chills, infection |
| trastuzumab | Fever, chills, headache, infection, nausea, vomiting, diarrhea, dizziness, headache, insomnia, rash, GI discomfort, edema, dyspnea, rhinitis, asthenia, back pain, fever, chills, infection |

*GI*, Gastrointestinal.

## DOSAGES

### Monoclonal Antibodies

| DRUG (PREGNANCY CATEGORY) | PHARMACOLOGIC CLASS | USUAL DOSAGE RANGE | INDICATIONS |
|---|---|---|---|
| adalimumab (Humira) (B) | Anti–TNF-alpha monoclonal antibody | **Adult only**<br>Subcut: 40 mg every other week; may advance to 40 mg weekly if indicated | Severe, progressive RA for which other RA therapies have failed |
| alemtuzumab (Campath) (C) | Anti–glycoprotein CD52 | IV: 3-10 mg daily to maximum tolerated dose, then 30 mg 3 × per week (alternate days) for up to 12 wk | B-cell chronic lymphocytic leukemia |
| belimumab (Benlysta) (C) | B-lymphocyte stimulator-specific inhibitor | IV: 10 mg/kg at 2-week intervals | Systemic lupus erythematosus |
| certolizumab (Cimzia) (B) | Anti–TNF | Subcut: 400 mg at 2-week intervals × 2, then monthly | RA, Crohn's disease |
| bevacizumab (Avastin) (C) | Anti–human vascular endothelial growth factor | IV: 5-10 mg/kg every 14 days | Metastatic colorectal cancer |
| cetuximab (Erbitux) (C) | Anti–human epidermal growth factor | IV: 400 mg/m$^2$ loading dose, then 250 mg/m$^2$ weekly | Metastatic colorectal cancer |
| golimumab (Simponi) (B) | Anti–TNF | Subcut: 50 mcg monthly | RA, ankylosing spondylitis |
| ibritumomab tiuxetan (Zevalin) (D) | Chelator immunoconjugate | IV: 250 mg/m$^2$ × 2 doses 7 to 9 days apart | Non-Hodgkin's lymphoma |
| infliximab (Remicade) (B) | Anti–TNF-alpha | IV: 3-5 mg/kg at 0, 2, and 6 wk, then every 6 wk | Ankylosing spondylitis, Crohn's disease, RA |
| natalizumab (Tysabri) (C) | Anti–alpha4 integrin subunit | IV: 300 mg every 4 wk | Multiple sclerosis |
| ♦ rituximab (Rituxan) (C) | Anti–CD20 surface antigen | IV: 375 mg/m$^2$ 1 × per week × 4 doses | Non-Hodgkin's lymphoma |
| tositumomab and iodine I-131 tositumomab (Bexxar) (X) | Radioactive MAB | IV: Complex dosing regimen involving both drug components; follow instructions in package insert as ordered | Non-Hodgkin's lymphoma |
| trastuzumab (Herceptin) (B) | Anti–HER2 protein MAB | IV: Loading dose, 4 mg/kg<br>IV: Maintenance dose, 2 mg/kg/wk | Breast cancer |

*IV,* Intravenous; *MAB,* monoclonal antibody; *RA,* rheumatoid arthritis; *subcut,* subcutaneous; *TNF,* tumor necrosis factor.

## DRUG PROFILES

All of the monoclonal antibodies are synthesized using recombinant DNA technology. Because of the complexities of this technology, these drugs tend to be much more expensive than most other medications, with prices in the hundreds or thousands of dollars per single dose. Many of the monoclonal antibodies are used to treat various forms of cancer. Their advantage is that they offer greater cell-killing specificity aimed at cancer cells instead of all body cells. Nonetheless, these drugs are associated with significant adverse effects and therefore with risk, which must be weighed against the benefit using expert clinical judgment. Severe allergic inflammatory-type infusion reactions can occur, and patients may therefore be premedicated with acetaminophen or diphenhydramine to reduce the occurrence of such reactions. If reactions do occur, they may be treated with diphenhydramine and other drugs such as epinephrine and corticosteroids. Conventional pharmacokinetic data are not listed for the majority of these drugs because they do not follow standard pharmacokinetic models owing to their unique behavior in the body. It is known, however, that they may remain in the affected tissues for many weeks or months. The elimination half-life is given in the following profiles when known.

### adalimumab

Adalimumab (Humira) works through its specificity for human tumor necrosis factor (TNF)-alpha. TNF-alpha is a naturally occurring cytokine that is involved in normal inflammatory and immune responses. Adalimumab is indicated for the treatment of severe cases of rheumatoid arthritis that have failed to respond to other medications, including methotrexate. It can be used either alone or concurrently with such medications. In patients with rheumatoid arthritis, elevated levels of TNF are found in the synovial fluid in the spaces of affected joints. In addition to preventing TNF-alpha molecules from binding to TNF cell surface receptors, adalimumab also modulates the inflammatory biologic responses that are induced or regulated by TNF. Use of adalimumab is contraindicated in patients with any active infectious process, whether localized or systemic, acute or chronic.

### alemtuzumab

Alemtuzumab (Campath) is approved to treat B cell–mediated chronic lymphocytic leukemia. It is classified as a recombinant humanized antibody that is directed against the CD52 glycoprotein that appears on the surfaces of virtually all B and T lymphocytes. Humanization involves the insertion of human DNA sequences during drug production to make the drug better tolerated by human patients. It is used specifically in patients for whom other first-line chemotherapy treatments, including treatment with alkylating drugs and the antimetabolite fludarabine (see Chapter 45), have failed. Its contraindications are known drug allergy, active systemic infection, and documented immunodeficiency disease such as HIV-positive status. The half-life of alemtuzumab is 10 hours to 30 days.

### belimumab

Belimumab (Benlysta) is the first drug approved for the treatment of systemic lupus erythematosus in the past 40 years. It is a B-lymphocyte stimulator-specific inhibitor. The most common side effects include nausea, diarrhea, insomnia, bronchitis, migraine, and pain in the extremities. The most serious adverse effects include infection (sometimes fatal), anaphylaxis, and depression. It is given via IV infusion.

### bevacizumab

Bevacizumab (Avastin) is approved for the treatment of metastatic colon cancer, rectal cancer in combination with 5-flurouracil (see Chapter 45), non–small cell lung cancer, and malignant glioblastoma. It is unique in that it binds to and inhibits vascular endothelial growth factor, a protein that promotes development of new blood vessels in tumors (as well as in normal body tissues). It has no listed contraindications but may complicate surgical wound healing because of its antivascular effects. The half-life of bevacizumab is 11 to 50 days.

### certolizumab

Certolizumab (Cimzia) is a tumor necrosis factor (TNF) antagonist. It is indicated for moderately to severe active Crohn's disease that is unresponsive to other therapy and for severe rheumatoid arthritis. The most common adverse effects include headache, nausea, upper respiratory infection, hypertension, and infections. A patient medication guide must be dispensed with each prescription, warning patients of potential serious infections and possible lymphoma.

### cetuximab

Cetuximab (Erbitux) is approved for the treatment of metastatic colorectal cancer. It is a recombinant monoclonal antibody made from both human and mouse (murine) genetic material and is designed for concurrent use with the second-line antineoplastic drug irinotecan (see Chapter 45). It binds to *epidermal growth factor* on the surface of tumor cells, where it hinders cell growth through interference with cell metabolism. Cetuximab is used either in combination with irinotecan or alone in patients who are intolerant of the latter drug. It has no listed contraindications but is known to cause severe infusion reactions in up to 3% of patients receiving it. The half-life of cetuximab is 97 to 114 hours.

### golimumab

Golimumab (Simponi) is a TNF antagonist approved for the treatment of severe rheumatoid arthritis and ankylosing spondylitis. The most common side effects include hypertension, dizziness, increased liver function tests, and infection. It is not to be given with other TNF antagonists. Patients must be monitored for infection, as with all TNF antagonists. Golimumab is given subcutaneously in a dose of 50 mg once a month. It is given in conjunction with methotrexate for RA.

### ibritumomab tiuxetan

Ibritumomab tiuxetan (Zevalin) is approved for treating B-cell non-Hodgkin's lymphoma. This drug is an immunoconjugate, consisting of ibritumomab conjugated with the metal chelator tiuxetan. This drug comes in kits that also include one of two radioactive metal isotopes (radioisotopes). The antibody binds to the CD20 antigen that occurs on the surfaces of both normal and malignant B lymphocytes. Once the complex is bound to the cells, the tiuxetan component binds the radioisotope, which is administered as another part of the anticancer therapy. Radioactive beta emission from the bound radioisotope, a unique feature of this drug, induces free radical formation and cell damage in both the cell containing the drug complex and neighboring cells.

### infliximab

Infliximab (Remicade) is one of the earliest monoclonal antibodies, approved in 1998. It works through an anti–TNF-alpha action, similar to adalimumab. It is approved for the treatment of ankylosing spondylitis, Crohn's disease, and rheumatoid arthritis. It has the special contraindication of severe heart failure (class III or IV on the New York Heart Association scale) because it may worsen this condition. It also carries an FDA black box warning reporting cases of fatal tuberculosis and/or fungal infections associated with the use of this drug. It is recommended that patients be tested for latent tuberculosis before it is administered. The half-life of infliximab is 8 to 9 days.

### natalizumab

Natalizumab (Tysabri) is approved for the treatment of multiple sclerosis. It is a humanized monoclonal antibody derived from murine myeloma cells. Natalizumab works by binding to the alpha$_4$ subunits of integrins, proteins found on the surfaces of leukocytes (with the exception of neutrophils). These proteins are implicated in the multiple sclerosis disease process, but its exact mechanism of action has not been determined. However, the drug is known to inhibit the leukocyte adhesion that is mediated by these alpha$_4$ protein subunits, and this is also believed to be part of the disease process. Natalizumab has no listed contraindications. The half-life is 11 days. Natalizumab was taken off the market only 1 year after it was originally approved in 2004 due to reports of patients developing multifocal leukoencephalopathy, a rare and serious viral infection of the brain. In 2006, the FDA allowed the marketing of natalizumab to resume under a special distribution program. Only patients who are enrolled in the program are allowed to receive the drug.

### ♦ rituximab

Rituximab (Rituxan) specifically binds to antigen CD20. This antigen is a protein on the membranes of both normal and malignant B cells found in patients with non-Hodgkin's lymphoma. Antigen CD20 is expressed in more than 90% of B-cell non-Hodgkin's lymphomas. Once rituximab binds to these B cells, a host immune response causes lysis of the cells. Rituximab has become a standard drug for the treatment of patients with follicular low-grade non-Hodgkin's lymphoma for whom previous therapy has failed. It is recommended that patients be premedicated with acetaminophen and diphenhydramine before each infusion of the drug to reduce its well-known infusion-related adverse effects.

### tositumomab and iodine I 131 tositumomab

Tositumomab and iodine (I-131) tositumomab (Bexxar) are approved for the treatment of non-Hodgkin's lymphoma. This drug is a murine monoclonal antibody with a dual radioactive and nonradioactive component. Both components bind to the CD20 antigen, a transmembrane protein that, as noted earlier, is expressed on the cell membranes of more than 90% of B-cell non-Hodgkin's lymphoma cells. Theoretical mechanisms of action include induction of apoptosis (programmed cell death), *complement-dependent* cytotoxicity, or antibody-dependent cytotoxicity mediated by the drug itself. Complement is a collective term for about 20 different proteins normally present in plasma that aid other immune system components (e.g., B cells and T cells) in mounting an immune response.

### trastuzumab

Trastuzumab (Herceptin) kills tumor cells by mediating antibody-dependent cellular cytotoxicity. It accomplishes this by inhibiting proliferation of human tumor cells that overexpress the HER2 protein. The HER2 protein is overexpressed in 25% to 30% of primary malignant breast tumors and has been established as an adverse prognostic factor for early-stage breast cancer. Because of the relatively selective expression of HER2 on cancer cells, it has been an appealing target for antineoplastic therapy. Trastuzumab has a special FDA black box warning reporting cases of ventricular dysfunction and heart failure associated with this drug. Monitor for signs and symptoms of heart failure and ventricular dysfunction before and during treatment. In addition, fatal hypersensitivity reactions, infusion reactions, and pulmonary events have occurred in association with its use; therefore, careful clinical judgment, risk evaluation, and informed patient consent are called for in its use. The half-life of trastuzumab is 10 to 30 days.

## INTERLEUKINS AND RELATED DRUGS

Interleukins are a natural part of the immune system and are classified as *lymphokines*. Lymphokines are soluble proteins that are released from activated lymphocytes such as natural killer cells. There are several known interleukins in the body (IL-2, IL-3, IL-4, IL-5, IL-6, and IL-11), and more are being identified as knowledge of the immune system increases.

The pharmaceutical interleukin receptor agonists currently available are aldesleukin (IL-2), oprelvekin (IL-11), denileukin diftitox, tocilizumab (IL-6), and anakinra. Oprelvekin was mentioned with the hematopoietic drugs earlier in the chapter and is used to help patients produce platelets. It has a dual classification as both an interleukin and hematologic drug. All interleukins are prepared via recombinant technology.

**BOX 47-2 INTERLEUKIN-2: DRUG EFFECTS**

**Modulating Effects**
Proliferation of T cells
Synthesis and secretion of cytokines
Increased production of B cells (antibodies)
Proliferation and activation of NK cells
Proliferation and activation of LAK cells

**Enhancing Effects**
Enhancement of killer T cell activity
Amplification of the effects of cytokines
Enhancement of the cytotoxic actions of NK cells and LAK cells

*LAK,* Lymphokine-activated killer; *NK,* natural killer.

## Mechanism of Action and Drug Effects

Interleukins cause multiple effects in the immune system, one of which is antitumor action. IL-2 is produced by activated T cells in response to macrophage-"processed" antigens and secreted interleukin (IL-1). It was formerly called *T-cell growth factor* because, among other actions, it aids in the growth and differentiation of T lymphocytes. The IL-2 derivative aldesleukin acts indirectly to stimulate or restore immune response. Aldesleukin binds to receptor sites on T cells, which stimulates the T cells to multiply. One type of cell that results from this multiplication is the lymphokine-activated killer (LAK) cell. These LAK cells recognize and destroy only cancer cells and ignore normal cells. Aldesleukin is currently the most widely used of the interleukin drugs. A detailed list of its specific immunomodulating effects appears in Box 47-2.

Denileukin diftitox consists of one segment (denileukin) that is patterned after natural human IL-2 and a second segment (diftitox) that is patterned after diphtheria toxin. It is an IL-2 receptor antagonist and binds to cell surface IL-2 receptors that are expressed on both normal and certain malignant cells. It causes cell death upon binding to these receptors through the cytocidal activity of diphtheria toxin, which inhibits intracellular protein synthesis.

Anakinra is a recombinant form of the natural human IL-1 receptor antagonist. It competitively inhibits the binding of IL-1 to its corresponding receptor sites, which are expressed in many different tissues and organs. Tocilizumab is a recombinant form of the natural IL-6 receptor antagonist.

## Indications

Aldesleukin was previously indicated only for the treatment of metastatic renal cell carcinoma, a malignancy that originates in the kidney tissues. It is now also approved for the treatment of metastatic melanoma. Denileukin diftitox is currently indicated only as therapy for a skin-based lymphoma known as *cutaneous T-cell lymphoma,* which often metastasizes to other areas of the body. Anakinra and tocilizumab are indicated for symptom control in patients with rheumatoid arthritis for whom other therapy has failed.

## Contraindications

Contraindications to the administration of aldesleukin include drug allergy, organ transplantation, and abnormal results on thallium cardiac stress tests or pulmonary function tests. For denileukin diftitox, the only usual contraindication is drug allergy, as is also the case for anakinra and tocilizumab.

## Adverse Effects

Therapy with aldesleukin is commonly complicated by severe toxicity. A syndrome known as *capillary leak syndrome* is responsible for the severe toxicities of aldesleukin. As the name implies, capillary leak syndrome refers to a condition induced by interleukin therapy in which the capillaries lose their ability to retain vital colloids such as albumin, protein, and other essential components of blood. Because the capillaries are "leaky," these substances migrate into the surrounding tissues. This results in massive fluid retention (20 to 30 pounds), which can lead to the life-threatening problems of respiratory distress, heart failure, dysrhythmias, and myocardial infarction. Fortunately, these are all reversible after discontinuation of the interleukin therapy. Close patient monitoring and vigorous supportive care are essential in the patient receiving aldesleukin therapy. Other adverse effects that may be associated with aldesleukin therapy are fever, chills, rash, fatigue, hepatotoxicity, myalgias, headaches, and eosinophilia.

The most common adverse effects associated with denileukin diftitox administration are GI upset, hypoalbuminemia, elevated liver enzyme levels, edema, dyspnea, cough, fever, chills, asthenia, generalized pain, chest pain, infection, and headache. Anakinra has a much milder adverse effect profile that includes local reactions at the injection site, various respiratory tract infections, and headache. Tocilizumab has a high risk of causing anaphylaxis.

## Interactions

Aldesleukin, when given with antihypertensives, can produce additive hypotensive effects. Coadministration of corticosteroids with aldesleukin can reduce its antitumor effectiveness and is to be avoided. No particular drug interactions have been reported to date for denileukin diftitox. Anakinra and tocilizumab are not to be used (or used cautiously) with other immune modifiers due to increased risk of serious infections.

## Dosages

For dosage information on the interleukin agonists and antagonists, see the table on this page.

## DRUG PROFILES

The interleukins are a group of naturally occurring cytokines in the body that originally were believed to be produced by and to act primarily on leukocytes (WBCs). They are now recognized as multifunctional cytokines that are produced by a variety of cells but act at least partly within the lymphatic system.

### ♦ aldesleukin

Aldesleukin (Proleukin) is a human IL-2 derivative that is manufactured using recombinant DNA technology. It is a cytokine that is produced by lymphocytes and is therefore classified as a lymphokine. Aldesleukin is currently approved only for the treatment of metastatic renal cell carcinoma and metastatic melanoma, despite its activity against other cancers. Off-label uses include HIV infection and AIDS, and non-Hodgkin's lymphoma. Aldesleukin is contraindicated in patients with known drug allergy, abnormal thallium stress test or pulmonary function tests (due to potential drug effects on cardiopulmonary function), and organ transplants (due to the immunostimulating qualities of the drug, which may cause organ rejection). Aldesleukin is available only for injection.

### denileukin diftitox

Denileukin diftitox (Ontak) is an IL-2 receptor antagonist that is used to treat cutaneous T-cell lymphoma. Its only current contraindication is known drug allergy. Denileukin is available for injection only.

### anakinra

Anakinra (Kineret) is an IL-1 receptor antagonist that is used to help control the symptoms of rheumatoid arthritis. Its only current contraindication is known drug allergy. Anakinra is available for injection only.

### tocilizumab

Tocilizumab (Actemra) is an interleukin-6 antagonist approved for the treatment of severe rheumatoid arthritis. It is approved for patients who have not had an adequate response to other agents. It has a significant risk of anaphylaxis, and premedication must be given. A medication guide must be given to all patients receiving tocilizumab. Serious adverse effects include hepatotoxicity, infections, herpes zoster reactivation, and GI perforation. Tocilizumab is not to be given with other biologic response–modifying agents. It is given as an IV infusion.

## DOSAGES

### Interleukins and Related Drugs

| DRUG (PREGNANCY CATEGORY) | PHARMACOLOGIC CLASS | USUAL DOSAGE RANGE | INDICATIONS |
|---|---|---|---|
| ♦ aldesleukin (IL-2) (Proleukin) (C) | Human recombinant IL-2 analogue | IV: 600,000 IU/kg (0.037 mg/kg) q8h (14 doses) | Metastatic renal cell carcinoma or melanoma |
| anakinra (Kineret) (B) | IL-1 receptor antagonist | Subcut: 100 mg/day | Rheumatoid arthritis |
| denileukin diftitox (Ontak) (C) | Recombinant IL-2 and diphtheria toxin protein | IV: 9 or 18 mcg/kg/day for 5 consecutive days every 21 days | Cutaneous T-cell lymphoma |
| tocilizumab (Actemra) | IL-6 antagonist | IV: 4-8 mg/kg monthly | Rheumatoid arthritis |

*IL,* Interleukin; *IV,* intravenous; *subcut,* subcutaneous.

### TABLE 47-4    MISCELLANEOUS IMMUNOMODULATING DRUGS

| DRUG (TRADE AND OTHER NAMES) | CLASSIFICATION | INDICATIONS | MECHANISM OF ACTION |
|---|---|---|---|
| abatacept (Orencia) | Selective costimulation modulator | RA | Inhibits T-cell activation |
| bexarotene (Targretin) | Retinoid receptor agonist | Cutaneous T-cell lymphoma | Exact mechanism is unknown; binds to and activates retinoid X receptor subtypes; this regulates the expression of genes that control cellular differentiation |
| BCG vaccine (Pacis, TICE BCG, TheraCys) | Live virus vaccine, adjuvant | Localized bladder cancer | Promotes local inflammation and immune response in bladder mucosa |
| etanercept (Enbrel) | TNF receptor antagonist | RA (including juvenile) and psoriatic arthritis | Blocks effects of TNF, a major inflammatory mediator in RA |
| leflunomide (Arava) | Antimetabolite | RA | Exerts antiinflammatory effects via inhibition of cellular DNA synthesis |
| levamisole (Ergamisol) | Immunostimulant, adjuvant | Dukes stage C colon cancer (given with fluorouracil) | Exact mechanism is unknown, but may enhance the therapeutic effects of fluorouracil and have its own immunostimulatory effects |
| mitoxantrone (Novantrone) | Anthracycline antibiotic (also an antineoplastic drug) | MS (secondary chronic type) | Inhibits cellular DNA synthesis, which reduces neurologic disability in MS (exact mechanism unclear) |
| pegademase bovine (Adagen) | Immunostimulant | SCID | Modified enzyme that compensates for deficiency of the enzyme adenosine deaminase, which is associated with SCID |
| thalidomide (Thalomid) | Immunostimulant | Erythremia nodosum* | Exact mechanism is unknown, but may have anti-TNF properties, which counter the disease process |
| tretinoin (Vesanoid) | Retinoid receptor agonist | Acute promyelocytic leukemia | Induces differentiation and maturation of leukemic cells, reducing proliferation of immature, disease-causing cells |

*BCG,* Bacille Calmette-Guérin; *MS,* multiple sclerosis; *RA,* rheumatoid arthritis; *SCID,* severe combined immunodeficiency disease; *TNF,* tumor necrosis factor.

*An inflammatory reaction in the subcutaneous fat, often following a bacterial infection, or in reaction to drugs such as oral contraceptives or sulfonamides.

## MISCELLANEOUS IMMUNOMODULATING DRUGS

In addition to the drugs in the major classes discussed thus far, there are several additional medications that can be broadly classified as miscellaneous immunomodulating drugs. They work by various specific and nonspecific mechanisms. A special term used for immunostimulant drugs that work by a nonspecific mechanism is adjuvant. These miscellaneous medications, including some that are classified as adjuvants, are listed in Table 47-4.

## PATHOPHYSIOLOGY OVERVIEW

### RHEUMATOID ARTHRITIS

Rheumatism is a general term for any of several disorders characterized by inflammation, degeneration, or metabolic derangement of connective tissue structures, especially joints and related structures such as muscles, tendons, bursae, fibrous tissue, and ligaments. Rheumatoid arthritis is a chronic autoimmune disorder that commonly causes inflammation and tissue damage in joints. It can also cause anemia and diffuse inflammation in the lungs, eyes, and pericardium of the heart, and subcutaneous nodules under the skin (Figure 47-3). It is a painful and oftentimes disabling disease. It is diagnosed primarily based on symptoms and the results of a blood test for rheumatoid factor. Symptoms include pain, stiffness, and reduced range of motion. Treatment encompasses both pharmacologic

**FIGURE 47-3** Areas of the body affected by rheumatoid arthritis. Rheumatoid arthritis is most frequently seen in the shoulders, elbows, wrists, knees, and ankles, and it often affects the joints on both sides of the body equally.

and nonpharmacologic modalities, including physical and occupational therapy. There is no known cure for rheumatoid arthritis, and the goal of therapy is to alleviate current symptoms and to prevent further damage of the joints. Rheumatoid arthritis affects over 2 million people in the United States and usually appears between the ages of 25 and 50. Women are two to three times more likely than men to have rheumatoid arthritis. Smokers and those with a family history are also at risk. Osteoarthritis is another type of arthritis that tends to be an age-related degeneration of joint tissues resulting in pain and reduced function. This section focuses on rheumatoid arthritis.

Because rheumatoid arthritis is a disease characterized by inflammation, the nonsteroidal antiinflammatory drugs (NSAIDs) are the most commonly used (see Chapter 44). Full dosages of NSAIDs are tried in the early stages of rheumatoid arthritis. Corticosteroids, also potent antiinflammatory drugs (see Chapter 33), are also used to prevent inflammatory symptoms. These drugs, although they are effective in reducing inflammation, do not actually affect the disease itself. Disease-modifying antirheumatic drugs (DMARDs) not only provide antiinflammatory and analgesic effects, but they can arrest or slow the disease processes associated with arthritis.

## PHARMACOLOGY OVERVIEW

### DISEASE-MODIFYING ANTIRHEUMATIC ARTHRITIS DRUGS

DMARDs are drugs that modify the disease of rheumatoid arthritis. They exhibit antiinflammatory, antiarthritic, and immunomodulating effects and work by inhibiting the movement of various cells into an inflamed, damaged area, such as a joint. These cells (neutrophils, monocytes, and macrophages) are responsible for causing many of the deleterious effects of chronic rheumatoid arthritis. By preventing the accumulation of these inflammatory cells in the area of the diseased joint, antiarthritic drugs prevent progression of the disease. DMARDs often have a slow onset of action of several weeks, versus minutes to hours for NSAIDs. For this reason, DMARDs are sometimes also referred to as *slow-acting antirheumatic drugs (SAARDs).* They were previously thought of as second-line drugs for the treatment of arthritis because they can have much more toxic adverse effects than do the NSAIDs. However, the American College of Rheumatology updated its treatment guidelines in 2008 and now recommends the use of DMARDs as first-line therapy in many patients. The guidelines differentiate the DMARDs into nonbiologic and biologic DMARDs. Nonbiologic DMARDs include methotrexate, leflunomide, hydroxychloroquine, and sulfasalazine. The guidelines recommend starting with methotrexate or leflunomide in most patients. Use of the other drugs, including the biologic DMARDs, is generally reserved for those patients who do not respond to methotrexate or leflunomide. The biologic DMARDs include adalimumab, anakinra, certolizumab, etanercept, golimumab, infliximab, adalimumab, abatacept, rituximab, and tocilizumab. Box 47-3 lists the DMARDs. Etanercept and abatacept are discussed in this section; the others were discussed in the section on monoclonal antibodies.

## Mechanism of Action, Indications, and Adverse Effects

The mechanism of action and adverse effects of the different DMARDs vary. The individual drug profiles provide information on mechanism of action and adverse effects. All of these

---

| BOX 47-3 | **DISEASE-MODIFYING ANTIRHEUMATIC DRUGS** |
|---|---|
| abatacept | leflunomide |
| adalimumab | methotrexate |
| anakinra | rituximab |
| certolizumab | tocilizumab |
| etanercept | hydroxychloroquine |
| golimumab | sulfasalazine |
| infliximab | |

---

drugs are indicated for the treatment of rheumatoid arthritis, and some have other uses as previously mentioned.

## Contraindications

DMARDs are not used in patients with active bacterial infection, active herpes zoster, active or latent tuberculosis, or acute or chronic hepatitis B or C. Etanercept, infliximab, and adalimumab are not to be used in patients with heart failure, lymphoma, or multiple sclerosis. Methotrexate and leflunomide are to be avoided during pregnancy and lactation.

## DRUG PROFILES

### methotrexate

Methotrexate is an anticancer drug that is commonly used for treatment of rheumatoid arthritis in much lower dosages than those used for cancer. It is usually started at dosages of 7.5 to 10 mg/wk but can be increased to 25 mg/wk. It is very important to note that the drug is given once per week, not once per day. Serious medication errors, including deaths, have occurred when an order is mistranscribed and the drug is given daily instead of once a week. It is usually given orally for rheumatoid arthritis, but it can also be given by injection. Bone marrow suppression is the main adverse effect of methotrexate. Most patients are advised to take supplemental folic acid to lessen the likelihood of adverse effects. The onset of antirheumatic action is 3 to 6 weeks. The half-life of the drug is 3 to 10 hours.

### leflunomide

Leflunomide (Arava) is indicated for the treatment of active rheumatoid arthritis. It modulates or alters the response of the immune system to rheumatoid arthritis. It has antiproliferative, antiinflammatory, and immunosuppressive activity. Most common adverse effects are diarrhea, respiratory tract infection, alopecia, elevated liver enzyme levels, and rash. It is contraindicated in women who are or may become pregnant and is not to be used by nursing mothers or those with a hypersensitivity to it. It is classified as a pregnancy category X drug. Aspirin, other NSAIDs, and/or low-dose corticosteroids may be continued during leflunomide therapy. Leflunomide is available only for oral use. The half-life is 14 to 15 days.

### etanercept

Etanercept (Enbrel) is a recombinant DNA–derived TNF-blocking drug. It binds TNF and blocks its interaction with cell surface receptors. It is indicated for the treatment of rheumatoid arthritis (including juvenile rheumatoid arthritis) and moderate to severe chronic plaque psoriasis. It is contraindicated in patients with a known hypersensitivity to it and in those with sepsis and active infections (including chronic or local infections). Use with caution in patients with preexisting demyelinating central nervous system disorders, heart failure, or significant hematologic abnormalities. Some dosage forms may contain latex, so screen patients for latex allergy. Reactivation of hepatitis and tuberculosis have been reported. Live vaccines should not be given with etanercept. Common adverse effects include headache, injection site reaction, upper respiratory tract infection, dizziness, and weakness. The drug is administered subcutaneously. Drugs with which it interacts include anakinra, which may increase the risk of infection, and cyclophosphamide, which may increase the risk of malignancy. Etanercept is classified as a pregnancy category B drug. It is not known if the drug is excreted in breast milk, and its use is not recommended in lactating women. The onset of action is 1 to 2 weeks, and the half-life is 72 to 132 hours.

### abatacept

Abatacept (Orencia) is a selective costimulation modulator; it inhibits T-cell activation. Abatacept is indicated for the treatment of rheumatoid arthritis. It is contraindicated in patients with a known hypersensitivity to it or any of its components. Use with caution in patients with a history of recurrent infections or chronic obstructive pulmonary disease. Bring patients up to date with all current immunizations before starting abatacept therapy. Adverse effects include headache, upper respiratory tract infections, and hypertension. Abatacept may increase the risk of infections associated with live vaccines and may decrease the response to dead and/or live vaccines. Abatacept is not to be given with anakinra or TNF-blocking drugs because of the risk of serious infections, or with the herb echinacea, which has immunostimulant properties. Abatacept is dosed according to body weight and is given at 4-week intervals. It is administered intravenously, and a filter must be used. The half-life is 8 to 25 days.

## NURSING PROCESS

## ASSESSMENT

For *hematopoietic* drugs, assess the medication order thoroughly as well as the specific indication for each of the drugs prescribed. Once you understand the indication, specific laboratory value(s) may be easily determined for further assessment (e.g., WBC counts with sargramostim and filgrastim, and platelets with use of oprelvekin). After initial assessment and monitoring of baseline blood counts, measure drug response against these values. Additionally, prior to administering these medications, document baseline assessment of the following: vital signs, skin turgor/intactness, bowel sounds/bowel patterns, and breath sounds. Assess also for any complaints of pain and rate accordingly (see discussion in Chapter 10). These areas are all very important to assess when giving hematopoietic drugs because of the adverse effects of edema, nausea, vomiting, diarrhea, rash, cough, dyspnea, sore throat, fever,

blood dyscrasias, headache, and bone pain. Assess potential intravenous and subcutaneous sites and, if appropriate, note chemotherapy-induced absolute neutrophil nadir (low point). This is important because timing of the dose is critical in helping to boost blood cell counts. For example, with filgrastim, do *not* give the drug within 24 hours before or after the chemotherapy. With use of filgrastim, assess for any existing joint or bone pain because of the possible adverse effect of mild to severe bone pain with filgrastim. Specific information regarding assessment associated with use of epoetin alfa is found in Chapter 54.

Before administering any of the *biologic response–modifying drugs* (and other drugs included in this chapter), assess your own knowledge about these medications with attention to the drug's action, pharmacokinetic properties, associated cautions, contraindications, drug interactions, adverse effects, and toxicities. Assess the patient for the presence of any conditions that represent contraindications or cautions to their administration as well as possible interacting drugs. Assess for hypersensitivity to the drug, egg proteins, or immunoglobulin G. Furthermore, assess the following systems: (1) respiratory system with attention to rate, rhythm, and depth as well as breath sounds, listening for any adventitious (abnormal) sounds; (2) cardiac system with attention to vital signs, heart sounds, heart rate and rhythm, and oxygen saturation levels, as well as assessment for edema and/or shortness of breath, presence of cyanotic discoloration around the mouth or nail beds, and any chest pain; (3) central nervous system with a focus on baseline mental status, as well as assessment for any seizure-like activity or central nervous system abnormalities; and (4) immune system, noting any history of chronic illnesses, ability to fight off infections, and history of suppressed immunity. Note nutritional status, height, and weight as well as results of any prescribed laboratory tests, such as complete blood count (CBC) and especially hemoglobin and hematocrit levels, serum protein and albumin levels, and immunoglobulin levels (see Nursing Process in Chapters 45 and 46). Also document the presence or absence of underlying diseases, symptoms, and success or failure of medication regimens in the past. Assess the patient's ability to carry out the activities of daily living, emotional and socioeconomic status, educational level, learning needs, desire and ability to learn, past coping strategies, and support systems.

Before *interferons* (e.g., interferon alfa-2a or alfa-2b; interferon gamma-1b) are given, assess the patient's history of drug allergies as well as any history of autoimmune disorders, hepatitis, liver failure, or AIDS. Contraindications include concurrent use of immunosuppressant drugs and Kaposi's sarcoma. Determine baseline WBC and platelets prior to initiation of therapy due to the potential of drug-induced neutropenia and thrombocytopenia. Monitor other serum laboratory values such as blood urea nitrogen, creatinine levels, and ALP and AST levels before and during treatment due to the risk of problems with renal and liver functioning. It is important to document baseline neurologic functioning, bowel status, heart sounds, pulse rate, and blood pressure (including postural readings). Significant drug interactions to assess for include those drugs that are metabolized via the cytochrome P-450 enzyme system in the liver because of the risk of subsequent drug toxicity. Bone marrow suppression may be exacerbated when the interferon gamma products are given with other bone marrow suppressive drugs.

With the use of *monoclonal antibody drugs* (e.g., alemtuzumab, rituximab, trastuzumab), assess and document history of allergic reactions. Assess for ranges of responses with these medications including mild to severe reactions (see Table 47-3). Assessment of baseline vital signs and any signs of infection are important because of the risk of acquiring an infection when these drugs are given. Contraindications to their use include any active infectious process and HIV. With infliximab (Remicade), there is an FDA black box warning stating that fatal tuberculosis and/or fungal infections have been associated with use of this drug, so any infections process needs to be ruled out prior to its use. Trastuzumab has an FDA black box warning for cases of ventricular dysfunction and heart failure. Fatal hypersensitivity and infusion reactions have occurred with this drug, so prior to administration there must be very careful risk evaluation and subsequent prudent clinical judgment-making by the prescriber and you. Perform close monitoring and supervision before, during, and after the infusion of these drugs. Table 47-3 provides a listing of common adverse effects associated with these drugs requiring further areas and systems to be assessed.

With *interleukins,* assess for drug allergy as well as the contraindications of organ transplantation. Review results of various tests such as thallium cardiac stress tests and pulmonary function tests. Assess vital signs, and document any history of respiratory and/or cardiac disorders due to the severe toxicities of capillary leak syndrome with aldesleukin. As mentioned earlier in the chapter, capillary leak syndrome results in massive fluid retention of 20 to 30 pounds leading to potentially life-threatening problems of respiratory distress and heart failure. These are reversible after discontinuation of the interleukin therapy. Assess liver function studies prior to therapy. Drug interactions of significance include antihypertensives which produce additive hypotensive effects. Corticosteroid use is contraindicated because of a reduction in antitumor effectiveness. Tocilizumab is one interleukin drug that is indicated for severe rheumatoid arthritis and is not to be given with other biologic response modifiers.

With *DMARDs,* perform a close assessment of any past or present medical conditions as well a thorough assessment of allergies. Compile a complete and thorough medication profile, listing prescription drugs, herbals, and over-the-counter drugs. Assess the specific type of DMARD prescribed because there are nonbiologic and biologic DMARDS. Nonbiologic DMARDs include methotrexate, leflunomide, hydroxychoroquine, and sulfasalazine. Biologic DMARDs include several of the monoclonal antibodies already discussed. Assess for contraindications to the use of DMARDs such as active bacterial infections, active herpes, active/latent tuberculosis, and acute or chronic hepatitis B or C. Additional contraindications are presented in the pharmacology discussion. Because bone marrow suppression is one of the main adverse effects (e.g., with methotrexate), assess and monitor baseline blood cell and platelet counts before, during, and after therapy. Another important area for

## TEAMWORK AND COLLABORATION: LEGAL AND ETHICAL PRINCIPLES

### The Nurse and Patient Care

Never neglect or deceive a patient, even if a conflict arises with your own cultural, racial-ethnic, spiritual, or personal belief systems. Such a dilemma is often encountered in connection with various treatment modalities for cancer patients or patients needing drugs that alter the body's biologic response. You do have the right to refuse to participate in any treatment or aspect of a patient's care that violates personal ethical principles, but it is important to understand that this refusal of care can in *no* way involve desertion or neglect of the patient. In these situations, inform the appropriate supervisory personnel about the conflict, and transfer the patient to the safe care of another qualified professional. As detailed in the American Nurses Association *Code of Ethics for Nurses,* nurses are bound by the profession always to remain ethical in the provision of care to patients. This may include participation in the care of a patient who needs the nurse's care but who may be receiving treatment or care that is not "acceptable" by the nurse's own standards or ethics.

assessment is the medication order by the prescriber, because serious medication errors have occurred when the order for this drug has been transcribed incorrectly and the drug has been given daily instead of in the recommended once-weekly dosing.

Before initiation of therapy with leflunomide, perform a complete assessment of hepatic functioning as well as baseline blood cell counts. Because of the possible adverse effects of diarrhea and respiratory infections, assess respiratory and gastrointestinal functioning. A thorough respiratory assessment includes obtaining a history of past and present respiratory disorders and infections as well as noting breath sounds, presence of sputum, and baseline respiratory rate, rhythm, and depth. Assess bowel patterns and document findings. Etanercept is to be avoided in those with sepsis and active infections, so conduct a thorough assessment of WBC counts and for any signs and symptoms of infection or a history of infection. Because some dosage forms may contain latex, it is critical to also assess for latex allergy. The DMARD abatacept is given based on weight; thus, there is a need for an accurate, predrug therapy weight. Additionally, assess the patient's immunization record because all immunizations must be current prior to beginning therapy with abatacept. Document the findings of a baseline head-to-toe physical assessment, and note any musculoskeletal changes due to the pathology of arthritis and related changes in activities of daily living and other basic activities before drug therapy is initiated as well as throughout the therapeutic regimen.

## NURSING DIAGNOSES

1. Imbalanced nutrition, less than body requirements, related to the adverse effects of biologic response–modifying drugs
2. Impaired skin integrity (rash) related to the adverse effects of biologic response–modifying drugs
3. Risk for infection related to adverse effect of bone marrow suppression related to DMARDs and immunomodulating drugs

# PLANNING

## GOALS

1. Patient regains nutritional status to predrug or as near normal as possible.
2. Patient's skin and mucous membranes remain intact.
3. Patient remains free from infection and/or decreases the risk for infection during drug therapy.

## OUTCOME CRITERIA

1. Patient describes nutritional needs and daily meal planning reflecting dietary needs, such as consumption of a high-calorie, low-residue, high-protein diet, high-energy foods from protein and complex carbohydrates, and forcing of fluids.
   - Patient performs a 24-hour recall of food intake to report a typical week's menus.
   - Patient understands the importance of consuming small, frequent meals in an environment conducive to eating as well as the use of MyPlate.
   - Patient states measures to minimize gastrointestinal adverse effects, such as eating small, frequent meals and avoiding spicy foods, and uses antiemetics as prescribed.
   - Patient understands the importance of energy consumption with frequent rest periods before and after meals while undergoing treatment.
2. Patient's skin and mucous membranes remain intact and clean with daily bathing, skin care with moisturizing products, and daily oral hygiene with gentle flossing as well as follow-up care with a dental professional.
   - Patient reports breaks in skin, redness, irritation, areas of swelling, drainage, or pain to prescriber.
   - Patient contacts prescriber and/or dental professional with complaints or problems of poor dentition, sores in the mouth, bleeding, and/or swelling of gums.
3. Patient states ways to minimize risk of infection such as proper diet, adequate fluid intake, and identifying early signs and symptoms of infection.
   - Patient understands needed food items (e.g., increase in protein), using MyPlate and advice of a nutritional consult to meet additional nutritional demands in prevention of malnourishment and in boosting nutritional status.
   - Patient knows to take temperature orally or via axillary route every 4 hours during periods of increased risk of infection.
   - Patient states need to report temperature elevations of 100.5° F (38.1° C) to the prescriber for appropriate and immediate treatment.

# IMPLEMENTATION

Administer *biologic response–modifying drugs* exactly as prescribed and in keeping with manufacturer guidelines to minimize adverse effects. It is important to acknowledge that acquiring an infection is a serious adverse effect of these drugs and so the risk must always be weighed against the severity of the patient's underlying illness. Measure vital signs with special attention to temperature. Premedication with acetaminophen and diphenhydramine may be deemed necessary when any of the biologic response–modifying drugs are administered to help minimize any allergic type of reaction. With some of the biologic response–modifying drugs, treatment with opioids, antihistamines, and/or anti-inflammatory drugs may be required for the management of bone pain and chills if treatment with acetaminophen or diphenhydramine is not successful. Antiemetics may also be needed for any drug-related nausea or vomiting and may be administered prior to the administration of the biologic response–modifying drug. Antiemetics may need to be dosed around the clock if nausea and vomiting are problematic. Encourage the patient to rest when tired, not to overexert self during therapy, and to contact the prescriber if he or she experiences profound fatigue or loss of appetite. Encourage forcing fluids up to 3000 mL/day (unless contraindicated) to promote excretion of the by-products of cellular breakdown and maintain cellular hydration. Consultation with a dietitian or nutritionist may be helpful for the patient to learn about a nourishing diet to promote health and wellness (e.g., foods high in protein, complex carbohydrates, and necessary minerals, vitamins, and/or herbals). Discuss menu planning and grocery shopping with specific individualized suggestions. Nowadays, many grocery stores support internet food shopping with car pickup at the store on the same day or home delivery at no or minimal cost to the patient. Inform patients of community resources (e.g., Meals On Wheels, respite care organizations) as deemed appropriate and as needed.

With *hematopoietic drugs,* it is important to administer the drug as ordered. Determine and rotate subcutaneous and IV sites, as specified by facility policy. With filgrastim, administer the drug before a patient receiving myelosuppressive chemotherapy develops an infection, but not within 24 hours before or after a myelosuppressive chemotherapy drug is given. Once a patient's absolute neutrophil count (ANC) reaches 10,000 cells/mm³, discontinue the drug, as ordered and as recommended by the manufacturer. Give filgrastim and use D₅W to dilute the product. With sargramostim, reconstitute the dose with sterile water for injection. Do not use oprelvekin if any discoloration or particulate matter is noted in the vial. Treatment may be ordered to begin within 6 to 24 hours after completion of antineoplastic therapy. Daily subcutaneous dosing for 14 days has been found to produce dose-dependent platelet elevations, with counts increasing within 5 to 9 days of starting injections. Once oprelvekin is discontinued, counts remain increased for about 7 days and return to baseline within 14 days. Subcutaneous sites for oprelvekin administration include the thigh, abdomen, hip, and upper arm. When drugs are given subcutaneously, rotate injection sites. See the Patient Teaching Tips for more information.

When *interferons* are given, be sure to first read the order for correct spelling and be careful not to confuse with any other sound-alike, look-alike drugs. Administer the interferons parenterally by either the subcutaneous, intravenous, or intramuscular route, depending on the drug. For example, give interferon alfa-2a subcutaneously or intramuscularly. Be sure to rotate sites and use accurate technique (see Chapter 9). With concerns of infection, as with many of the biologic response–modifying drugs, monitor the patient's vital signs with attention to temperature and also for the occurrence of chills and headache. An ECG, before and during treatment, is generally prescribed, so monitor the results and report any chest pain, hypotension, hypertension, or dyspnea. Make sure to always check each brand of medication for the dilution directions as each brand has different directions. Read the package insert prior to giving these drugs. Acetaminophen may be prescribed to help with fever and headache. Encourage forcing of fluids.

With *monoclonals*, serious infections are a major concern. With belimumab, the most serious concern is infection, which may sometimes be fatal. Constantly monitor for infection during therapy. Certolizumab, which is used with severe Crohn's disease and severe rheumatoid arthritis, is also associated with the risk of serious infections and possible lymphoma, all of which need to be explained to the patient. Continue to monitor blood counts during and after therapy with these drugs. Monitor the patient for changes in blood pressure and pulse rate and for chest pain. Contact the prescriber immediately if there are significant changes in baseline parameters. Avoid infliximab in patients with severe heart failure. When giving this drug, it is important monitor the patient for heart sounds, blood pressure, pulse rate, pulse oximetry reading, and ECG. If there are signs and symptoms of infection and/or changes in cardiac status, contact the prescriber immediately.

With the the biologic DMARD methotrexate, a test dose is usually administered to see how the patient react to the medication. Be aware of the FDA black box warning about the cautious administration of this drug in those with renal disease, infection, pulmonary disease, and stomatitis. Be sure that if methotrexate is ordered for rheumatoid arthritis, it is administered weekly as ordered. For more information on methotrexate, see Chapter 45. Give etanercept, yet another drug with black box warnings (see the pharmacology discussion), subcutaneously into the thigh, abdomen, or upper arm, rotating injection sites. Give leflunomide very cautiously while monitoring liver and renal functioning; administer it orally with meals or food to minimize gastrointestinal upset. Monitor daily weights due to possible edema.

## CASE STUDY

### Hematopoietic Biologic Response Modifiers

P.S., a 38-year-old surveyor, is receiving a second round of chemotherapy as part of treatment for non-Hodgkin's lymphoma. The oncologist is monitoring for signs of bone marrow suppression of the various blood cell components.

1. What symptoms would the nurse expect to see if P.S. had diminished production of platelets? White blood cells? Explain your answers.

One week after this round of chemotherapy, P.S.'s white blood cell count is 0.8 cells/mm$^3$ (pretherapy value was 6200 cells/mm$^3$), and his absolute neutrophil count is 450 cells/mm$^3$ (pretherapy value was 1600 cells/mm$^3$). The oncologist orders strict neutropenic precautions and filgrastrim (Neupogen), 480 mcg, subcut daily.

2. Explain the purpose of the order for the filgrastim. The nurse will need to assess P.S. for what conditions before beginning the filgrastim?
3. The nurse notices a woman with a baby about to enter P.S.'s room. The baby is fussy, and the woman is wiping the baby's nose after the baby sneezed. What does the nurse need to do at this time?
4. P.S.. asks the nurse, "How long will I need to take these injections? I hate having to have another shot!" What is the answer to his question?

For answers, see http://evolve.elsevier.com/Lilley

## EVALUATION

Therapeutic responses to *biologic response–modifying drugs* include a variety of responses, such as a decrease in the growth of the lesion or mass, decreased tumor size, and an easing of symptoms related to the tumor or disease process. Other therapeutic effects are an improvement in WBC and platelet counts and/or a return of blood counts to normal levels, and absence of infection and hemorrhage. Encourage patient journaling which may help provide health care providers with more data from which to evaluate the patient's response during and after therapy. Possible adverse effects for which to evaluate are presented in Tables 47-1 and 47-2. *DMARDs* are expected to have therapeutic results within a documented time frame (often weeks) with the patient experiencing increased ability to move joints, less discomfort, and an overall increased sense of improvement and well-being. Toxicity of these drugs may be manifested by liver, renal, and respiratory dysfunction and, for methotrexate, bone marrow suppression.

## PATIENT TEACHING TIPS

• Advise the patient to avoid hazardous tasks because of the central nervous system changes noted with several biologic response–modifying drugs. Fatigue is also a common adverse effect; instruct the patient to report any excessive fatigue.

• Instruct the patient to report to the prescriber immediately any signs of infection, such as sore throat, diarrhea, vomiting, and/or fever of 100.5° F (38.1° C) or higher. Advise the patient also to report excessive fatigue, loss of appetite, edema, or bleeding.

• Pregnancy is discouraged while the patient is taking a biologic response–modifying drug. Educate patients of childbearing age about contraceptive choices and the need to use contraception for up to 2 years after completion of therapy.

• Inform the patient that adverse effects associated with biologic response–modifying drugs usually disappear within 72 to 96 hours after therapy is discontinued.

*Continued*

## PATIENT TEACHING TIPS — cont'd

- Interleukins may be self-administered; therefore, teach the patient self-injection technique and proper disposal of equipment (e.g., needles, syringes). Provide the patient with corresponding written instructions. Encourage the daily keeping of a journal to record the site of injection and an overall rating of how the patient feels.
- Bone pain and flulike symptoms often occur with some of the biologic response–modifying drugs, and the use of non-opioid or, in some cases, opioid analgesics may be required. Some patients may find relief with acetaminophen or ibuprofen.
- With DMARDs, the patient will experience improved joint function and decreased pain. Encourage the patient to report any bleeding, excess fatigue, fever, or respiratory symptoms.

## KEY POINTS

- Cancer treatment has traditionally involved surgery, radiation, and chemotherapy. Surgery and radiation are usually local or regional therapies. Chemotherapy is generally systemic, but it often does not completely eliminate all of the cancer cells in the body. Adjuvant therapy is frequently used to destroy undetected distant micrometastases.
- The humoral and cellular immune systems act together to recognize and destroy foreign particles and cells. The humoral immune system is composed of lymphocytes that are known as B cells until they are transformed into plasma cells when they come in contact with an antigen (foreign substance). The plasma cells then manufacture antibodies to that antigen.
- Biologic response–modifying drugs provide another treatment option for patients who have malignancies and/or those who are receiving chemotherapy and have a need to boost blood cell counts. Biologic response–modifying drugs include hematopoietics, interferons, interleukins, monoclonal antibodies, and DMARDs. Use of these drugs may augment, restore, or modify host defenses against the tumor.
- Nursing management associated with the administration of biologic response–modifying drugs focuses on the use of careful aseptic technique and other measures to prevent infection; proper nutrition; oral hygiene; monitoring of blood counts; and management of adverse effects, including joint/bone pain and flulike symptoms.
- Do not administer filgrastim and sargramostim within 24 hours of a myelosuppressive antineoplastic, and follow the timeframe for their use (as prescribed), whether in an inpatient or home setting.
- The recommend therapy with nonbiologic DMARDs usually begins with methotrexate or leflunomide for most patients. Biologic DMARDs are generally reserved for those patients whose disease does not respond to methotrexate or leflunomide. The biologic DMARDs include etanercept, infliximab, adalimumab, abatacept, and rituximab.

## NCLEX® EXAMINATION REVIEW QUESTIONS

1 The nurse is conducting a class on drugs for malignant tumors for a group of new oncology staff members. Which best describes the action of interferons in the management of malignant tumors?
   a Interferons increase the production of specific anticancer enzymes.
   b Interferons have antiviral and antitumor properties and strengthen the immune system.
   c Interferons stimulate the production and activation of T lymphocytes and cytotoxic T cells.
   d Interferons help improve the cell-killing action of T cells because they are retrieved from healthy donors.

2 When planning care for a patient who is receiving interferon therapy, the nurse must keep in mind that the major dose-limiting factor is
   a fatigue.
   b bone marrow suppression.
   c fever.
   d nausea and vomiting.

3 The nurse is administering methotrexate as part of the treatment for rheumatoid arthritis and will monitor for which sign of bone marrow suppression?
   a Edema
   b Tinnitus
   c Increased bleeding tendencies
   d Tingling in the extremities

4 In caring for a patient receiving therapy with a myelosuppressive antineoplastic drug, the nurse notes an order to begin filgrastim after the chemotherapy is completed. Which statement correctly describes when the nurse will begin the filgrastim therapy?
   a It can be started during the chemotherapy.
   b It will begin immediately after the chemotherapy is completed.
   c It will be initiated 24 hours after the chemotherapy is completed.
   d It will not be started until at least 72 hours after the chemotherapy is completed.

5 The nurse is monitoring a patient who has been receiving aldesleukin (IL-2) (Proleukin) for treatment of malignant melanoma. Which adverse effect, if noted on assessment, is of primary concern?

a Chills

b Fatigue

c Headache

d Fluid retention

6 The nurse is reviewing the medical history of a patient who is about to receive therapy with etanercept (Enbrel). Which conditions, if present, would be a contraindication or caution for therapy with this drug? (Select all that apply.)

a Urinary tract infection

b Psoriasis

c Heart failure

d Glaucoma

e Latex allergy

7 A patient is to receive filgrastim (Neupogen) after therapy with carmustine and radiation therapy for treatment of a brain tumor. The patient weighs 132 pounds. The protocol that the oncologist has written states that the filgrastim will be dosed at 5 mcg/kg. Filgrastim comes in a 300-mcg/mL vial. What dose will the patient receive? How many milliliters will the patient be given?

1. b, 2. a, 3. c, 4. c, 5. d, 6. a, c, e, 7. 300 mcg; 1 mL.

For Critical Thinking and Prioritization Questions, see http://evolve.elsevier.com/Lilley.

# 48

# Immunosuppressant Drugs

## ⊝volve WEBSITE

*http://evolve.elsevier.com/Lilley*

- Animations
- Answer Key—Textbook Case Studies
- Critical Thinking and Prioritization Questions

- Key Points—Downloadable
- Review Questions for the NCLEX® Examination
- Unfolding Case Studies

## OBJECTIVES

When you reach the end of this chapter, you will be able to do the following:

1  Discuss the role of immunosuppressive therapy in organ transplantation and in the treatment of autoimmune diseases.
2  Discuss the mechanisms of action, contraindications, cautions, adverse effects, routes of administration, drug interactions, and toxicity of the most commonly used immunosuppressants.

3  Develop a nursing care plan that includes all phases of the nursing process for patients receiving immunosuppressants after organ transplantation or for the treatment of autoimmune disease.

## DRUG PROFILES

- ♦ **azathioprine, p. 787**
  **basiliximab and daclizumab, p. 787**
- ♦ **cyclosporine, p. 788**
  **glatiramer acetate, p. 789**
- ♦ **muromonab-CD3, p. 790**

- ♦ **mycophenolate mofetil, p. 790**
  **sirolimus and tacrolimus, p. 790**

  _____

- ♦ *Key drug*

## KEY TERMS

**Autoimmune diseases** A large group of diseases characterized by the alteration of the function of the immune system so that the immune response is directed against normal tissue(s) of the body, which results in pathologic conditions. (p. 785)

**Grafts** The term used for transplanted tissues or organs. (p. 787)

**Immune-mediated diseases** A large group of diseases that result when the cells of the immune system react to a variety of situations, such as transplanted organ tissue or drug-altered cells. (p. 785)

**Immunosuppressants** Drugs that decrease or prevent an immune response. (p. 785)

**Immunosuppressive therapy** A drug treatment used to suppress the immune system. (p. 785)

# ANATOMY, PHYSIOLOGY, AND PATHOPHYSIOLOGY DISEASE OVERVIEW

## IMMUNE SYSTEM

The purpose of the *immune system* is to distinguish self from nonself and to protect the body from foreign material (antigens). There are three layers of barriers to protect the body (Figure 48-1). There are two types of immunity: humoral immunity, which is mediated by B lymphocytes, and cellular immunity, which is mediated by T lymphocytes. This chapter focuses on drugs that suppress the T lymphocytes.

The immune system defends the body against invading pathogens, foreign antigens, and its own cells that become cancerous, or neoplastic. Besides performing this beneficial function, it can also attack itself and cause what are known as autoimmune diseases or immune-mediated diseases. The immune system also participates in hypersensitivity, or anaphylactic, reactions, which can be life-threatening. The rejection of kidney, liver, and heart (whole organ) transplants is directed by the immune system as well.

Drugs that decrease or prevent an immune response, and hence suppress the immune system, are known as immunosuppressants. Treatment with such drugs is referred to as immunosuppressive therapy. Immunosuppressants are used for many immune-related disorders, including rheumatoid arthritis, systemic lupus erythematosus, Crohn's disease, multiple sclerosis, myasthenia gravis, psoriasis, and others. Examples of these drugs include cyclophosphamide (see Chapter 46), glatiramer acetate, fingolimod, and many immunomodulators, which are discussed in Chapter 47. This chapter focuses on the drugs used in organ transplantation.

Transplantation is one of the most complex areas of modern medicine. Many different types of transplants are routinely done including, but not limited to, kidney, heart, liver, lung, pancreas, small bowel, bone marrow, and cornea transplantation.

The primary concern with transplantation is rejection, which could necessitate the transplanted organ to be removed. Rejection occurs from an immune response targeted against the transplanted organ. Immunosuppressants are used to inhibit the immune system and prevent organ rejection. Transplant patients are on immunosuppressant therapy for their lifetime.

# PHARMACOLOGY OVERVIEW

## IMMUNOSUPPRESSANT DRUGS

### Mechanism of Action and Drug Effects

All immunosuppressants have similar mechanisms of action in that they selectively suppress certain T-lymphocyte cell lines. By suppressing the T-lymphocyte cell lines, they prevent their involvement in the immune response. This results in a pharmacologically immunocompromised state similar to that in a cancer patient or in a patient with acquired immunodeficiency syndrome (AIDS). Each drug differs in the exact way in which it suppresses certain cell lines involved in an immune response. The major classes of immunosuppressant drugs used in preventing organ rejection include glucocorticoids, calcineurin inhibitors, antimetabolites, and biologics. Corticosteroids inhibit all stages of T-cell activation and are used for induction, maintenance immunosuppression, and acute rejection. Corticosteroids are discussed in depth in Chapter 33 and are not discussed further in this chapter. Calcineurin inhibitors (e.g., cyclosporine, tacrolimus, sirolimus) inhibit the phosphate required for interleukin 2 production. Siromilus does not inhibit calcineurin but instead inhibits mTOR, which ultimately inhibits interleukin 2 communication. Antimetabolites (e.g., azathioprine, mycophenolate) inhibit cell proliferation. Biologics (e.g., muromonab-CD3, basiliximab, daclizumab) inhibit cytotoxic T killer cell function. Table 48-1 gives the mechanisms of action and indications of the available immunosuppressant drugs.

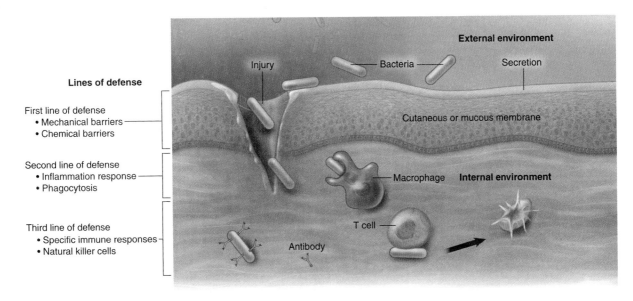

**FIGURE 48-1** A simplified depiction of the complicated immune system. (From Patton KT, Thibodeau GA: *Anatomy and physiology,* ed 7, St Louis, 2010, Mosby.)

## TABLE 48-1  AVAILABLE IMMUNOSUPPRESSANT DRUGS: MECHANISMS OF ACTION AND INDICATIONS

| DRUG NAME, YEAR OF FDA APPROVAL | MECHANISM OF ACTION | INDICATIONS/USES |
|---|---|---|
| azathioprine (Imuran), 1980 | Blocks metabolism of purines, inhibiting the synthesis of T-cell DNA, RNA, and proteins and thereby blocking immune response | Prevention of organ rejection in kidney transplantation; treatment of rheumatoid arthritis |
| basiliximab* (Simulect), 1998 | Suppresses T-cell activity by blocking the binding of the cytokine mediator IL-2 to a specific receptor | Prevention of organ rejection in kidney transplantation |
| cyclosporine (Sandimmune, Neoral, Gengraf), 1983 | Inhibits activation of T cells by blocking the production and release of the cytokine mediator IL-2 | Prevention of organ rejection in kidney, liver, and heart transplantation; treatment of rheumatoid arthritis and psoriasis. Unlabeled uses* include prevention of rejection in pancreas, bone marrow, and heart/lung transplantation. |
| daclizumab* (Zenapax), 1997 | Suppresses T-cell activity by blocking the binding of the cytokine mediator IL-2 to a specific receptor | Prevention of organ rejection in kidney transplantation |
| fingolimod (Gilenya), 2010 | Decreases the amount of lymphocytes available to the central nervous system. | Reduction of relapse frequency in patients with RRMS |
| glatiramer acetate (Copaxone), 1996 | Precise mechanism unknown; believed to somehow modify immune system processes that are associated with MS symptoms | Reduction of relapse frequency in patients with RRMS |
| muromonab-CD3† (Orthoclone OKT3), 1986 | Binds to CD3 glycoprotein on T-cell receptors, which blocks antigen recognition and reverses graft rejection that is already in progress | Treatment of acute organ rejection in kidney, liver, and heart transplantation |
| mycophenolate mofetil (Cell-Cept), 1995 | Prevents proliferation of T cells by inhibiting intracellular purine synthesis | Prevention of organ rejection in kidney, liver, and heart transplantation |
| sirolimus (Rapamune), 1999 | Inhibits T-cell activation by binding to an intracellular protein known as FKBP-12 that subsequently prevents cellular proliferation | Prevention of organ rejection in kidney transplantation |
| tacrolimus (Prograf), 1994 | Inhibits T-cell activation, possibly by binding to an intracellular protein known as FKBP-12 | Prevention of organ rejection in liver, kidney, and heart transplantation. Unlabeled uses† include prevention of rejection in bone marrow, pancreas, pancreatic islet cell, and small intestine transplantation; treatment of autoimmune diseases; and severe psoriasis. |

*FDA*, U.S. Food and Drug Administration; *FKBP-12*, FK-binding protein 12; *IL-2*, interleukin-2; *MS*, multiple sclerosis; *RRMS*, relapsing-remitting multiple sclerosis.
*Non–FDA-approved but under investigation.
†Note that "ab" in any drug name usually indicates that it is a monoclonal antibody synthesized using recombinant DNA technology.

## Indications

The therapeutic uses of immunosuppressants vary from drug to drug, as noted in Table 48-1. They are primarily indicated for the prevention of organ rejection. Three of the immunosuppressants are indicated for both prevention of rejection and treatment of organ rejection; they include muromonab-CD3, mycophenolate, and tacrolimus. Fingolimod and glatiramer acetate are immunosuppressants that are indicated for reduction of the frequency of relapses (exacerbations) in a type of multiple sclerosis known as *relapsing-remitting multiple sclerosis*.

## Contraindications

The main contraindication for all immunosuppressants is known drug allergy. Relative contraindications, depending on the patient's condition, may include renal or hepatic failure, hypertension, and concurrent radiation therapy. Pregnancy is not necessarily a contraindication to the use of these drugs, but immunosuppressants should be given to pregnant women only in clinically urgent situations.

## Adverse Effects

Immunosuppressant drugs have many significant adverse effects, which are listed in Table 48-2. By virtue of their actions, immunosuppressants place patients at increased risk of opportunistic infections. Immunosuppressant drugs may also increase the risk of certain types of cancers, especially skin cancers. Other serious adverse effects are limited to the particular drug. For example, cyclosporine and tacrolimus can cause nephrotoxicity, and corticosteroids, cyclosporine, and tacrolimus can cause posttransplant diabetes mellitus. Patients taking immunosuppressant drugs need to avoid live vaccines.

## Interactions

Because transplant patients are on immunosuppressant drugs for their lifetime and are often on combination therapy, they are at increased risk for drug interactions. Immunosuppressants have narrow therapeutic windows, and drug interactions can be significant. Drugs that cause increased levels of immunosuppressant drugs can cause toxicity, whereas drugs that reduce

## TABLE 48-2   SELECTED IMMUNO-SUPPRESSANT DRUGS: COMMON ADVERSE EFFECTS

| BODY SYSTEM | ADVERSE EFFECTS |
|---|---|
| **Azathioprine** | |
| Hematologic | Leukopenia, thrombocytopenia |
| Hepatic | Hepatotoxicity |
| **Cyclosporine** | |
| Cardiovascular | Moderate hypertension in as many as 50% of patients |
| Central nervous | Neurotoxicity, including tremors, in 20% of patients |
| Hepatic | Hepatotoxicity with cholestasis and hyperbilirubinemia |
| Renal | Nephrotoxicity is common and dose limiting |
| Other | Posttransplant diabetes mellitus, gingival hyperplasia, and hirsutism |
| **Muromonab-CD3** | |
| Cardiovascular | Chest pain |
| Central nervous | Pyrexia (fever), chills, tremors |
| Gastrointestinal | Vomiting, nausea, diarrhea |
| Respiratory | Dyspnea, wheezing, pulmonary edema |
| Other | Flulike symptoms, fluid retention |
| **Tacrolimus** | |
| Central nervous | Agitation, anxiety, confusion, hallucinations, neuropathy |
| Renal | Albuminuria, dysuria, acute renal failure, renal tubular necrosis |
| Other | Posttransplant diabetes mellitus |
| **Antibody Immunosuppressants (basiliximab, daclizumab, and muromonab-CD3)** | |
| Multiple body systems | Cytokine release syndrome, which includes such immune-mediated symptoms as fever, dyspnea, tachycardia, sweating, chills, headache, nausea, vomiting, diarrhea, muscle and joint pain, and general malaise |

immunosuppressant drug levels may lead to organ rejection. The major drug interactions with immunosuppressant drugs are listed in Table 48-3. Many of the immunosuppressant drugs are metabolized by the cytochrome P-450 enzyme system, thus drug interactions are common and can be significant. Grapefruit can inhibit metabolizing enzymes and thus can increase the activity of cyclosporine, tacrolimus, and sirolimus. Grapefruit juice may increase the bioavailability of cyclosporine by 20% to 200% and should be avoided. Foods that are high in potassium, such as bananas and tomatoes, can increase cyclosporine nephrotoxicity. Meals that have high fat content can increase sirolimus levels.

Because the antibodies basiliximab, daclizumab, and muromonab-CD3 are generally given in a relatively short single course of therapy, they have few recognized drug interactions. However, cases of encephalopathy have occurred in patients in whom the antiinflammatory drug indomethacin (see Chapter 44) was used concurrently with muromonab-CD3.

The potential for interactions between immunosuppressant drugs and herbal preparations also should not be overlooked. For example, the enzyme-inducing properties of St. John's wort have been demonstrated to reduce the therapeutic levels of cyclosporine and cause organ rejection. The immunostimulant properties of cat's claw and echinacea may be similarly undesirable in transplant recipients, because they have effects that are opposite those of the immunosuppressants.

## Dosages

For dosage information on selected immunosuppressants, see the table on p. 789. Immunosuppressants must be taken exactly as directed and at the exact times and with the exact foods. Adherence to dosing schedules can be very difficult for patients because they are on multiple medications that must be taken at different times throughout the day. Patients should never stop taking their immunosuppressants without being told to do so by their transplant doctor. Cyclosporine and tacrolimus should not be taken at the same time. Sirolimus should be taken 4 hours after cyclosporine. If a dose is missed, it should be taken as soon as the patient remembers, unless it is close to the time the next dose is due; in this case, the patient must contact the transplant doctor.

## DRUG PROFILES

### ◆ azathioprine
Azathioprine (Imuran) is a chemical analogue of the physiologic purines, such as adenine and guanine. It blocks T-cell proliferation by inhibiting purine synthesis, which in turn prevents synthesis of deoxyribonucleic acid (DNA). Azathioprine is used for prophylaxis of organ rejection concurrently with other immunosuppressant drugs, such as cyclosporine and corticosteroids. It is available in both oral and injectable forms.

### Pharmacokinetics

| Route | Onset of Action | Peak Plasma Concentration | Elimination Half-life | Duration of Action |
|---|---|---|---|---|
| PO | 2-4 days* | 1-2 hr | 5 hr | Unknown |

*6 to 8 weeks for rheumatoid arthritis.

### basiliximab and daclizumab
Basiliximab (Simulect) and daclizumab (Zenapax) are both monoclonal antibodies that work by inhibiting the binding of the cytokine mediator interleukin-2 (IL-2) to the high-affinity IL-2 receptor. These drugs are used to prevent rejection of transplanted kidneys (grafts) and are generally used as part of a multidrug immunosuppressive regimen that includes cyclosporine and corticosteroids. Both basiliximab and daclizumab have a tendency to cause the allergy-like reaction known as *cytokine release syndrome,* which can be severe and even involve anaphylaxis. Patients are often premedicated with corticosteroids (e.g., intravenous methylprednisolone) in an effort to avoid or alleviate this problem. Both basiliximab and daclizumab are available only in injectable form.

## TABLE 48-3　IMMUNOSUPPRESSANT DRUGS: SELECTED DRUG INTERACTIONS

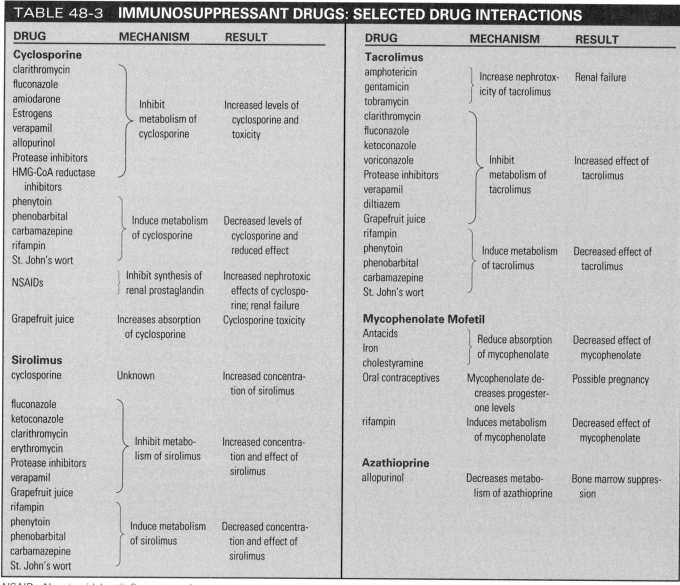

| DRUG | MECHANISM | RESULT |
|------|-----------|--------|
| **Cyclosporine** | | |
| clarithromycin | | |
| fluconazole | | |
| amiodarone | | |
| Estrogens | Inhibit metabolism of cyclosporine | Increased levels of cyclosporine and toxicity |
| verapamil | | |
| allopurinol | | |
| Protease inhibitors | | |
| HMG-CoA reductase inhibitors | | |
| phenytoin | | |
| phenobarbital | | |
| carbamazepine | Induce metabolism of cyclosporine | Decreased levels of cyclosporine and reduced effect |
| rifampin | | |
| St. John's wort | | |
| NSAIDs | Inhibit synthesis of renal prostaglandin | Increased nephrotoxic effects of cyclosporine; renal failure |
| Grapefruit juice | Increases absorption of cyclosporine | Cyclosporine toxicity |
| **Sirolimus** | | |
| cyclosporine | Unknown | Increased concentration of sirolimus |
| fluconazole | | |
| ketoconazole | | |
| clarithromycin | | |
| erythromycin | Inhibit metabolism of sirolimus | Increased concentration and effect of sirolimus |
| Protease inhibitors | | |
| verapamil | | |
| Grapefruit juice | | |
| rifampin | | |
| phenytoin | | |
| phenobarbital | Induce metabolism of sirolimus | Decreased concentration and effect of sirolimus |
| carbamazepine | | |
| St. John's wort | | |

| DRUG | MECHANISM | RESULT |
|------|-----------|--------|
| **Tacrolimus** | | |
| amphotericin | | |
| gentamicin | Increase nephrotoxicity of tacrolimus | Renal failure |
| tobramycin | | |
| clarithromycin | | |
| fluconazole | | |
| ketoconazole | | |
| voriconazole | Inhibit metabolism of tacrolimus | Increased effect of tacrolimus |
| Protease inhibitors | | |
| verapamil | | |
| diltiazem | | |
| Grapefruit juice | | |
| rifampin | | |
| phenytoin | Induce metabolism of tacrolimus | Decreased effect of tacrolimus |
| phenobarbital | | |
| carbamazepine | | |
| St. John's wort | | |
| **Mycophenolate Mofetil** | | |
| Antacids | | |
| Iron | Reduce absorption of mycophenolate | Decreased effect of mycophenolate |
| cholestyramine | | |
| Oral contraceptives | Mycophenolate decreases progesterone levels | Possible pregnancy |
| rifampin | Induces metabolism of mycophenolate | Decreased effect of mycophenolate |
| **Azathioprine** | | |
| allopurinol | Decreases metabolism of azathioprine | Bone marrow suppression |

*NSAIDs,* Nonsteroidal antiinflammatory drugs.

### Pharmacokinetics (basiliximab)

| Route | Onset of Action | Peak Plasma Concentration | Elimination Half-life | Duration of Action |
|-------|-----------------|---------------------------|-----------------------|--------------------|
| IV | 1 day | 3-4 days | 7-9 days | Unknown |

### Pharmacokinetics (daclizumab)

| Route | Onset of Action | Peak Plasma Concentration | Elimination Half-life | Duration of Action |
|-------|-----------------|---------------------------|-----------------------|--------------------|
| IV | 1 day | 3-5 days | 20 days | Unknown |

### ♦ cyclosporine

Cyclosporine (Sandimmune) and cyclosporine-modified (Neoral, Gengraf) are immunosuppressant drugs indicated for the prevention of organ rejection. They are classified as calcineurin inhibitors and work by inhibiting the production and release of IL-2. Like azathioprine, they may also be used for the treatment of other immunologic disorders, such as various forms of arthritis, psoriasis, and irritable bowel disease.

Cyclosporine is available in both oral and injectable forms. Neoral and Gengraf are brand names for cyclosporine-modified and were developed to improve absorption over Sandimmune (cyclosporine). Although these three products contain the same active ingredient (cyclosporine), they cannot be used interchangeably. The nurse must double-check the formulation before giving cyclosporine. Neoral, Gengraf, or generic cyclosporine-modified refer to interchangeable products; however, if the patient is prescribed the aforementioned, Sandimmune or generic cyclosporine must not used. If an error occurs in which product is administered, it is extremely important that the prescribing transplant physician be notified. When a change is made from Neoral or Gengraf to Sandimmune, the starting dose should be a 1:1 mg amount, but dosage adjustments may be necessary to compensate for the greater bioavailability of Neoral and Gengraf. It is recommended that cyclosporine blood concentration be monitored in patients changing from

## DOSAGES

### Selected Immunosuppressant Drugs

| DRUG (PREGNANCY CATEGORY) | PHARMACOLOGIC CLASS | USUAL DOSAGE RANGE | INDICATIONS/USES |
|---|---|---|---|
| ◆ azathioprine (Imuran) (D) | Antimetabolite | **Adult and pediatric**<br>IV/PO: 2-5 mg/kg/day to start, then 1-3 mg/kg/day maintenance | Prevention of rejection of kidney transplants |
| basiliximab (Simulect) (B) | Monoclonal antibody | **Pediatric 2-15 yr, less than 35 kg**<br>IV: 10 mg within 2 hr of transplant surgery, then 4 days afterward<br>**Adult and pediatric 35 kg or more**<br>Use 20-mg doses in same regimen | Prevention of rejection of kidney and liver transplants |
| ◆ cyclosporine (Sandimmune, Neoral, Gengraf) (C) | Calcineurin inhibitor | **Adult and pediatric**<br>PO: 15 mg/kg as a single dose 4-12 hr preoperatively; continue same dose daily postoperatively for 1-2 wk, then reduce by 5%/wk to a maintenance dose of 5-10 mg/kg/day<br>IV: 5-6 mg/kg as a single dose 4-12 hr preoperatively and continued daily postoperatively until patient can be switched to PO dosing | Prevention of rejection of kidney, liver, and heart transplants |
| daclizumab (Zenapax) (C) | Monoclonal antibody | **Adult and pediatric**<br>IV: Bolus injection of 1 mg/kg 24 hr preoperatively and for 4 additional postoperative doses, spaced 14 days apart | Prevention of rejection of kidney transplants |
| glatiramer acetate (Copaxone) (B) | Miscellaneous biologic | **Adult only**<br>Subcut: 20 mg once daily | Treatment of RRMS |
| ◆ muromonab-CD3 (Orthoclone OKT3) (C) | Monoclonal antibody | **Adult and pediatric**<br>IV: 2.5-5 mg/day as a single bolus injection for 10-14 days (pediatric patients often started with 2.5 mg/day) | Treatment of active rejection of kidney transplants; treatment of active rejection of liver, heart, pancreas, and bone marrow transplants that are resistant to conventional treatment |
| mycophenolate mofetil (CellCept, Myfortic) (C) | Antimetabolite | **Adult**<br>IV/PO: 1 g twice daily (delayed-release formulation)<br>**Pediatric**<br>IV/PO: 600 mg/m$^2$ twice daily (maximum daily dose: 400 mg or 720 mg twice daily) | Prevention of rejection of kidney, liver, or heart transplants; treatment of rejection of kidney transplants |
| sirolimus (Rapamune) (C) | mTOR kinase Inhibitor | **Adult and pediatric**<br>IV/PO: 6-mg loading dose on day 1, followed by maintenance dose of 2 mg/day | Prevention of rejection of kidney transplants |
| tacrolimus (Prograf) (C) | Calcineurin inhibitor | **Adult and pediatric**<br>IV: 0.03-0.05 mg/kg/day as continuous IV infusion; then PO: 0.1-0.2 mg/kg/day divided q12h | Prevention and treatment of rejection of liver, kidney, heart, lung, pancreas, and small bowel transplants |

*IV,* Intravenous; *PO,* oral; *RRMS,* relapsing-remitting multiple sclerosis; *subcut,* subcutaneous.

one product to another. Cyclosporine has a narrow therapeutic range, and for this reason laboratory monitoring of drug levels may be used to ensure therapeutic plasma concentrations and to avoid toxicity.

### Pharmacokinetics

| Route | Onset of Action | Peak Plasma Concentration | Elimination Half-life | Duration of Action |
|---|---|---|---|---|
| PO | 1-3 hr | 3.5 hr | 1-2 hr (parent compound) 10-40 hr (metabolites) | Unknown |

### glatiramer acetate

Glatiramer acetate (Copaxone) is a mixture of random polymers of four different amino acids. This mixture results in a compound that is antigenically similar to myelin basic protein. This is a protein that is found on the myelin sheaths of nerves. The drug is believed to work by blocking T-cell autoimmune activity against this protein, which reduces the frequency of the neuromuscular exacerbations associated with multiple sclerosis. This drug is mixed in the sugar known as mannitol; therefore, it is contraindicated in patients who are allergic to that component. It is available only in injectable form.

A new drug, fingolimod (Gilenya), which actually failed as an antirejection drug, was approved in 2010 for multiple sclerosis. It is the only oral drug for relapsing forms of multiple sclerosis. It has significant adverse effects, including headache, hepatotoxicity, flulike symptoms, back pain, AV block, bradycardia, hypertension, and macular edema. For these reasons, the FDA requires a patient medication guide for all patients dispensed fingolimod.

### ♦ muromonab-CD3

Muromonab-CD3 (Orthoclone OKT3) is indicated for the reversal and prevention of graft rejection. It is a monoclonal antibody, synthesized using recombinant DNA technology, and it is very similar to the antibodies produced naturally by the body (immunoglobulins G, M, D, A, and E). It specifically targets the binding sites on the T cells that recognize foreign invaders, such as a transplanted organ. It differs from human antibodies in that it comes from mice. Other monoclonal antibodies used for the prevention of organ rejection are basiliximab and daclizumab. Muromonab-CD3, often called OKT3, is contraindicated in patients with hypersensitivity to murine products and in those who are experiencing fluid overload. Muromonab-CD3 can cause cytokine release syndrome, and patients are often pretreated with a corticosteroid as described previously for basiliximab and daclizumab. This drug is available only in injectable form.

### Pharmacokinetics

| Route | Onset of Action | Peak Plasma Concentration | Elimination Half-life | Duration of Action |
|---|---|---|---|---|
| IV | Rapid | 3 days | 18 hr | Unknown |

### ♦ mycophenolate mofetil

Mycophenolate (CellCept) is an antimetabolite and suppresses T cell proliferation. It is indicated for the prevention of organ rejection as well as the treatment of organ rejection. Mycophenolate has a black box warning from the FDA stating that it is associated with an increased risk of congenital malformations and spontaneous abortions when used during pregnancy. It is available in oral and intravenous forms. Common side effects include hypertension (28% to 77% incidence), hypotension, peripheral edema, tachycardia, pain, headache, hyperglycemia, hyperlipidemia, electrolyte disturbances, abdominal pain, leukopenia, thrombocytopenia, cough, and dyspnea.

### Pharmacokinetics

| Route | Onset of Action | Peak Plasma Concentration | Elimination Half-life | Duration of Action |
|---|---|---|---|---|
| PO | 4 wk | 0.8-1.8 hr | 8-16 hr | Unknown |

### ♦ sirolimus and tacrolimus

Sirolimus (Rapamune) is an immunosuppressant drug, similar in structure to tacrolimus (Prograf). Sirolimus is a macrocyclic immunosuppressive, antifungal, and antitumor drug, and tacrolimus is used to prevent rejection and to treat rejection once it occurs. Sirolimus works by inhibiting T-lymphocyte activation in response to antigenic stimulation and inhibits antibody production, which in turn suppresses cytokine-mediated T-cell proliferation. Sirolimus and tacrolimus are structurally related and act through similar mechanisms. Sirolimus is classified as an mTOR kinase inhibitor, whereas tacrolimus is classified as a calcineurin inhibitor. Sirolimus is available only for oral use, whereas tacrolimus is available in both oral and

injectable forms. Sirolimus levels are increased when taken with high-fat meals.

Everolimus (Certican) originally was approved for the treatment of advanced renal cell carcinoma and recently has been approved for the prevention of rejection in kidney transplant. It is an analogue of sirolimus.

### Pharmacokinetics (sirolimus)

| Route | Onset of Action | Peak Plasma Concentration | Elimination Half-life | Duration of Action |
|---|---|---|---|---|
| PO | Rapid | 1-3 hr | 60-80 hr | Unknown |

### Pharmacokinetics (tacrolimus)

| Route | Onset of Action | Peak Plasma Concentration | Elimination Half-life | Duration of Action |
|---|---|---|---|---|
| PO | Variable | 0.5-4 hr | 21-61 hr | Unknown |

## NURSING PROCESS

## ASSESSMENT

Transplantation is indeed a very complex medical and ethical health care issue. With transplants, the primary concern (as previously discussed) is that of rejection and the possibility of subsequent removal of the transplanted organ. Therefore, immunosuppressants are used to inhibit the patient's immune system to help prevent rejection. It also means that patients are on drug therapy for their entire lifetime. Before administering any of the *immunosuppressants,* perform a thorough patient assessment with baseline measurements of vital signs and weight. Obtain a thorough history of past and present medical conditions, and document the following systems assessment information: (1) preexisting diseases that impact the patient's immune status, such as diabetes, hypertension, and cancer; (2) urinary functioning and patterns; (3) presence of jaundice, edema, and/or ascites; (4) history of cardiac disease and/or dysrhythmias, chest pain, or heart failure; (5) level of central nervous system functioning, with attention to any seizure disorders, alteration of motor or sensory function, paresthesias, or changing levels of consciousness; (6) respiratory status and baseline respiratory functioning, breath sounds, presence of asthma, pulmonary diseases, wheezing, cough, activity intolerance, dyspnea, or sputum production; (7) gastrointestinal (GI) functioning and patterns and bowel disease; (8) musculoskeletal intactness, with attention to ability to perform activities of daily living, range of motion, and appearance of joints and any deformities; and (9) presence and location of any inflammatory reactions as well as any pain, redness, and/or drainage. In addition, the following laboratory and diagnostic tests may be ordered: renal function tests with blood urea nitrogen (BUN) and creatinine levels; hepatic function tests with ALP, AST, ALT, and bilirubin levels; and cardiovascular function with baseline electrocardiogram. See Table 48-2 for information on other systems affected by the *immunosuppressant drugs*. Assess for and document all cautions, contraindications, and drug interactions.

With azathioprine, assess white blood cell and platelet counts, noting any signs and symptoms of infection as well as any bleeding tendencies due to the potential for drug-related leukopenia and thrombocytopenia. Assess liver function prior to administering this drug. A significant drug interaction is with allopurinol. It important to assess for this interaction to avoid the resultant effect of bone marrow suppression. For cyclosporine, specifically assess the functional level of all organs as well as assess for any underlying cardiovascular, central nervous system, hepatic, and/or renal disease because of potential drug-related toxicities involving these systems and the physiologic impact of the organ transplant process on multiple systems. Perform a baseline oral assessment because of the possible adverse effect of drug-induced gingival hyperplasia. Assess and document baseline blood pressures because as many as 50% of patients on this drug suffer from subsequent moderate hypertension. Common drug interactions to assess for include estrogens, protease inhibitors, HMG-CoA reductase inhibitors, clarithromycin, phenytoin, phenobarbital, St. John's wort, NSAIDs, and grapefruit juice (see Table 48-3).

Muromonab-DC3 requires assessment for cardiovascular disorders as well as a history of GI and respiratory disorders. Assess baseline temperature as well as breath sounds and respiratory rate. Fluid retention may also occur, so baseline vital signs and weight are important to note and document.

With tacrolimus, obtain a thorough patient history with attention to medication use, and perform a physical assessment with close attention to renal functioning through monitoring of BUN, serum creatinine, and serum electrolyte levels. When the drug is administered, closely assess the patient for the first 30 minutes with the first dose of the medication. Concern for anaphylactic reaction also continues past this first 30 minutes and first dose. It is important to confirm that resuscitative equipment is accessible and functioning and that appropriate doses of epinephrine and oxygen are also readily available. Drug interactions to assess for are listed in Table 48-3. With basiliximab, daclizumab, and muromonab-CD3 (antibody immunosuppressants), complete a thorough documentation of baseline vital signs and other presenting complaints because of the possible occurrence of cytokine release syndrome with resultant fever, dyspnea, tachycardia, sweating, chills, vomiting, diarrhea, muscle/joint pain, and general malaise.

With the assessment phase, it is also important to be aware of the difference between cyclosporine-modified (Neoral, Gengraf) and cyclopsorine (Sandimmune). Neoral and Gengraf were modified to improve absorption over Sandimmune. If cylcosporine-modified drugs are prescribed, they cannot be interchangeably used with Sandimmune. The nurse must always double-check the medication order against the formulation on hand.

# NURSING DIAGNOSES

1. Acute pain (e.g., joint and muscle aches and pain and flulike symptoms) related to adverse effects of immunosuppressant medications
2. Risk for injury related to the physiologic effects of the disease, overall weakness, and the adverse effects of immunosuppressants
3. Risk for infection related to altered immune status caused by chronic disease, treatment with immunosuppressants, and/or the transplantation process

# PLANNING

## GOALS

1. Patient experiences maximal comfort during drug therapy with immunosuppressants.
2. Patient remains free from injury.
3. Patient remains free from infection during therapy with immunosuppressants.

## OUTCOME CRITERIA

1. Patient states measures to help maximize comfort and minimize unpleasant adverse effects of drug therapy, such as taking acetaminophen for fever and joint pain, reporting unusually high blood pressure readings, and engaging in relaxation therapy, massage, diversional activities, hypnosis, imagery, and biofeedback.
2. Patient states measures to decrease injury to self such as reporting to the prescriber the onset of fever, rash, sore throat, fatigue, or breaks in skin (rash, sores) or other unusual problems or symptoms that may develop during therapy.
3. Patient maintains immune system and prevents infection with healthy diet inclusive of an increase in caloric and protein intake, as deemed necessary by nutritional consult, during drug therapy.
   - Patient reports fever, chills, increased malaise, productive cough, lethargy, fatigue, and/or confusion.
   - Patient minimizes contact with large crowds and those individuals with known bacterial or viral infections while on immunosuppressive therapy.

# IMPLEMENTATION

Oral *immunosuppressants* need to be taken with food to minimize GI upset. It is also important, because of the immunosuppressed state of patients receiving immunosuppressants, that oral forms of the drugs be used whenever possible to decrease the risk for infection associated with parenteral injections and subsequent injury to the first line of defense (skin). An oral antifungal medication may be ordered to treat the oral candidiasis that may occur as a consequence of the treatment and the disease process; however, significant drug interactions may occur between the immunosuppressant and the antifungal drug so always check for drug interactions. It is also important with the use of any of the immunosuppressants to be sure that supportive treatment equipment and related drugs

## CASE STUDY

### *Cyclosporine*

V., a 62-year-old retired orchestra teacher, moved to Florida after her husband died. Over the past few years she has developed renal problems and last year was told that she needed a kidney transplant. After a year of waiting and undergoing hemodialysis, she was told that her niece was a match and was willing to donate a kidney. She has had the transplant, and after 1 week, the transplant seems to be successful so far.

Cyclosporine is one of the immunosuppressants she will be receiving. She was given her first dose of cyclosporine 12 hours before surgery and is now receiving oral doses. The nurse has provided instructions on how to take the oral doses at home.

1. The next day, when another nurse comes in with V.'s morning medications, V. says, "You can't give me the medicine like that. Don't you know how to mix it?" What do you think the nurse did wrong?
2. What important measures will be taken to prevent toxicity?
3. V. tells the nurse that she can't wait to get home and relax by her pool. She is also looking forward to getting her strength back and going shopping with her girlfriends. How will the nurse respond to these statements?
4. After V. gets home, she calls the office to ask about eating grapefruit. "The pill bottle says no grapefruit, but I thought the doctor said I could have a little bit. I have a wonderful grapefruit tree in my backyard, and I love fresh grapefruit juice. What should I do?" What is the nurse's best answer?

For answers, see http://evolve.elsevier.com/Lilley.

are available in case of an anaphylactic or allergic reaction. Be aware of the high risk for such an occurrence, and be constantly prepared. The use of premedication protocols involving various antihistamines and/or antiinflammatory drugs is also common.

Cyclosporine is available in both oral and injectable formulations. As noted previously, Neoral and Gengraf are cyclorpsorine-modified and are not to be used interchangeably with Sandimmune (cyclosporine) which is unmodified. If an error occurs, the prescribing physician must be notified immediately. Do not refrigerate these oral solutions. To safely administer oral liquid dosage forms, use a calibrated liquid measuring device. Oral solutions may be mixed in a glass container with chocolate milk, milk, or orange juice and served at room temperature. Once the solution is mixed, make sure the patient drinks it immediately. Avoid Styrofoam containers or cups because the drug has been found to adhere to the inside wall of such containers. If the prescriber orders a change to be made from Neoral or Gengraf to Sandimmune, there is a dosage adjustment that may be needed (see pharmacology discussion). With intravenous administered cyclosporine, the dose must be diluted as recommended by the manufacturer and given according to standards of care and institutional policy. Cyclosporine is usually diluted with normal saline or 5% dextrose in water and infused using an intravenous infusion pump. Always infuse over the recommended period. Monitor the patient very closely during the infusion, especially during the first 30 minutes, for any allergic reactions manifested by facial flushing, urticaria,

wheezing, dyspnea, and rash. Record vital signs frequently and document. It is also important to closely monitor the patient's levels of BUN, LDH, AST, and ALT during therapy, as ordered, to detect possible renal and hepatic impairment. Oral hygiene may be performed frequently to prevent dry mouth and subsequent infections. The prescriber will also order blood tests to confirm therapeutic serum levels of cyclosporine. These serum drug levels must be closely monitored. Intravenously administered muromonab-CD3 is usually infused over 1 minute. When the dose is prepared, withdraw the medication from the ampule through a low protein-binding 0.22-micron filter, detach the filter, and apply a new sterile needle after withdrawing the medication. Follow the premedication protocol to help minimize reactions. Basiliximab and daclizumab are administered parenterally. Follow manufacturer guidelines regarding the type and amount of dilutional solution. Closely monitor the intravenous drip. Using an intravenous infusion pump may help to ensure that the proper dose is administered.

Sirolimus and tacrolimus need to be administered as ordered by either the intravenous or oral route. If intravenous tacrolimus is to be discontinued and maintenance dosing needed, oral tacrolimus is usually ordered to be given 8 to 12 hours after the discontinuation of the intravenous drug. Do not store intravenous solution in polyvinyl chloride containers. It must be administered in an appropriately designed container and tubing. Oral doses of tacrolimus are given on an empty stomach. As with cyclosporine, the oral dosage forms of tacrolimus are not to be put in Styrofoam cups/containers. Inform the patient to avoid the consumption of grapefruit within 2 hours of taking the drug. Both sirolimus and tacrolimus have long half-lives, so toxicity is an added concern because of possible cumulative effects.

Because immunosuppressant therapy is lifelong, it is important for the patient to receive adequate and appropriate emotional, spiritual, social, and financial support. Additionally, there are other specifics of therapy that must be emphasized with patients, family members, and significant others, such as the need to always have a 1-week supply of medication available so that there is never a risk of running out. There also needs to be discussion about the estimated cost of medication to all involved. Drug regimens are expensive and lifelong, and, as such, constant monitoring of drug serum levels is required. Complexity of dosing must be explained clearly and thoroughly.

Ethical dilemmas are also of a complex nature. Organ transplantation raises a number of complex bioethical issues, including definition of death, consents for transplantation, and payment for transplanted organs. Additionally, transplantation tourism and the broader socioeconomic context in which organ harvesting or transplantation may occur are of concern. Organ trafficking is another bioethical issue. More information about the many ethical concerns associated with transplantation is provided by the World Health Organization and the Universal Declaration of Human Rights. Even within developed countries, there is concern that enthusiasm for increasing the supply of organs may adversely and negatively impact the respect for the right to life.

# EVALUATION

Continually evaluate and reevaluate patient goals and outcome criteria related to the nursing process and administration of *immunosuppressants*. In addition, evaluate therapeutic responses to immunosuppressants, including acceptance of the transplanted organ or graft and improved symptoms in those with autoimmune disorders. Complete blood count; erythrocyte sedimentation rate; C-reactive protein level; liver, kidney, and cardiac function tests; pulmonary function tests; chest radiography; and analysis of T-lymphocyte surface phenotype are a few of the tests performed to evaluate patients during and after drug therapy. Continually evaluate for drug-specific adverse effects and toxicity (see Table 48-2).

# PATIENT TEACHING TIPS

- Educate transplant patients on the need for life-long immunosuppressant therapy with often complex therapeutic regimens.
- Emphasize the importance of avoiding situations that pose an increased risk of exposure to infection, such as being in crowds, malls, or movie theaters.
- Stress the importance of reporting any fever, sore throat, chills, joint pain, or fatigue to the prescriber, as these may indicate infection and require immediate medical attention.
- Educate female patients of childbearing age who are receiving immunosuppressants about the need to use some form of contraception during treatment and for up to 12 weeks after therapy ends.
- Advise patients to take the drug at the same time every day (as with most immunosuppressants) and, if a dose is omitted, to contact the prescriber for further instructions.
- Follow-up appointments are important because of the need to monitor the patient's status through examinations and blood testing.
- Educate patients about the adverse effects of cyclosporine (e.g., headache, tremor), and inform patients to avoid consumption of grapefruit or grapefruit juice because of the potential for an increase in the blood concentration of cyclosporine.
- Inform patients that gelcaps are to be stored in a cool, dry environment and must not be exposed to light. The dosage form must be kept in its original packaging. Also, instruct patients to avoid prolonged exposure to the sun and encourage them to use sunscreen and wear protective clothing when outdoors.

- Inform patients who are to undergo transplant surgery and are receiving cyclosporine about the fact that several days before surgery they may be told to take the cyclosporine with corticosteroids. They may also be given an oral antifungal as prophylaxis for *Candida* infections.
- Encourage patient to inspect the oral cavity frequently for any white patches on the tongue, mucous membranes, and/or oral pharynx. These patches may indicate oral candidiasis.
- Advise patients taking oral forms of cyclosporine to take the medication with meals or mixed with milk to minimize GI upset.
- Inform patients taking azathioprine or muromonab-CD3 that several days before transplant surgery they are to take all of their medication by the oral route if possible and avoid trauma and subcutaneous and intramuscular injections, which increase the risk for infection.
- Provide patients on tacrolimus a list of foods, especially those high in fats and carbohydrates, so that the absorption of the medication will not be negatively impacted. Nutritional counseling would be extremely beneficial in understanding food interactions as well as any concerns related to hyperlipidemia and increased triglycerides associated with many of the immunosuppressive drugs.
- All immunosuppressants taken at home are to be taken exactly as ordered and at the same time every day. Educate patients about the adverse effects of the medication. Instruct them to report problems of particular concern, such as fever, chest pain, dizziness, headache, problems with urination, rash, and respiratory and/or other infections.

# KEY POINTS

- Immunosuppressants decrease or prevent the body's immune response.
- Some of the clinical uses for immunosuppressants are suppression of immune-mediated disorders, malignancies, and improvement of short-term and long-term allograft survival.
- Oral antifungals are generally given with immunosuppressant medications to treat the oral candidiasis that occurs as a result of immunosuppression and fungal overgrowth.

- Monitor the results of prescriber-ordered laboratory studies such as hemoglobin level, hematocrit, and red blood cell, white blood cell, and platelet counts. If the values drop below normal ranges, notify the prescriber.

# NCLEX® EXAMINATION REVIEW QUESTIONS

1 A patient has a new order for glatiramer acetate. The patient has not had an organ transplant. The nurse knows that the patient is receiving this drug for which condition?
   a Psoriasis
   b Rheumatoid arthritis
   c Irritable bowel syndrome
   d Relapse-remitting multiple sclerosis

2 While assessing a patient who is to receive muromonab-CD3, the nurse knows that which condition would be a contraindication for this drug?
   a Acute myalgia
   b Fluid overload
   c Polycythemia
   d Diabetes mellitus

3 During therapy with azathioprine (Imuran), the nurse must monitor for which common adverse effect?
   a Bradycardia
   b Diarrhea
   c Vomiting
   d Thrombocytopenia

4 During a teaching session for a patient receiving an immunosuppressant drug, the nurse will include which statement?
   a "It is better to use oral forms of these drugs to prevent the occurrence of thrush."
   b "You will remain on antibiotics to prevent infections."
   c "It is important to use some form of contraception during treatment and for up to 12 weeks after the end of therapy."
   d "Be sure to take your medications with grapefruit juice to increase absorption."

5 During drug therapy with basiliximab, the nurse monitors for signs of cytokine release syndrome, which results in
   a fever, dyspnea, and general malaise.
   b neurotoxicity and peripheral neuropathy.
   c hepatotoxicity with jaundice.
   d thrombocytopenia with increased bleeding tendencies.

6 When assessing a patient who is to begin therapy with an immunosuppressant drug, the nurse recognizes that such drugs should be used cautiously in patients with which condition(s)? (Select all that apply.)
   a Pregnancy
   b Glaucoma
   c Anemia
   d Myalgia
   e Renal dysfunction
   f Hepatic dysfunction

7 The order reads: "Give tacrolimus IV 0.03 mg/kg/day as a continuous IV infusion." The patient weighs 110 lb. How many milligrams per day will this dose provide?

1. d, 2. b, 3. d, 4. c, 5. a, 6. a, f, d, 7. 1.5 mg/day

For Critical Thinking and Prioritization Questions, see http://evolve.elsevier.com/Lilley.

# Immunizing Drugs and Biochemical Terrorism

## ⓔvolve WEBSITE

*http://evolve.elsevier.com/Lilley*

- Animations
- Answer Key—Textbook Case Studies
- Critical Thinking and Prioritization Questions

- Key Points—Downloadable
- Review Questions for the NCLEX® Examination
- Unfolding Case Studies

## OBJECTIVES

When you reach the end of this chapter, you will be able to do the following:

1  Discuss the importance of immunity as it relates to the various immunizing drugs and their use in patients of all ages.
2  Identify the diseases that are treated or prevented with toxoids or vaccines.
3  Compare the mechanisms of action, indications, cautions, contraindications, adverse effects, toxicity, drug interactions, and routes of administration of various toxoids and vaccines.

4  Develop a nursing care plan that includes all phases of the nursing process related to the administration of immunizing drugs across the life span.
5  Develop a nursing care plan covering aspects of the nursing process related to bioterrorism, with emphasis on the nurse's role.

## DRUG PROFILES

- ◆ **diphtheria and tetanus toxoids and acellular pertussis vaccine tetanus (adsorbed), p. 803**
  *Haemophilus influenzae* type b conjugate vaccine, p. 804
- ◆ **hepatitis B immunoglobulin, p. 806**
- ◆ **hepatitis B virus vaccine (inactivated), p. 804**
  herpes zoster vaccine, p. 806
  human papillomavirus vaccine, p. 806
- ◆ **immunoglobulin, p. 806**
- ◆ **influenza virus vaccine, p. 804**
- ◆ **measles, mumps, and rubella virus vaccine (live), p. 805**
- ◆ **meningococcal vaccine, p. 805**

- ◆ **pneumococcal vaccine, polyvalent and thirteen valent, p. 805**
- ◆ **poliovirus vaccine (inactivated), p. 805**
  rabies immunoglobulin, p. 807
  rabies virus vaccine, p. 805
  $Rh_0(D)$ immunoglobulin, p. 807
  tetanus immunoglobulin, p. 807
- ◆ **varicella virus vaccine, p. 806**
  varicella-zoster immunoglobulin, p. 807

---

◆ *Key drug*

## KEY TERMS

**Active immunization** A type of immunization that causes development of a complete and long-lasting immunity to a certain infection through exposure of the body to the associated disease antigen; it can be natural active immunization (i.e., having the disease) or artificial active immunization (i.e., receiving a vaccine or toxoid). (p. 797)

**Active immunizing drugs** Toxoids or vaccines that are administered to a host to stimulate host production of antibodies. (p. 799)

**Antibodies** Immunoglobulin molecules that have an antigen-specific amino acid sequence and are synthesized by the humoral immune system (B cells) in response to exposure to a specific antigen. Their purpose is to attack and destroy molecules of this antigen. (p. 797)

**Antibody titer** The amount of an antibody needed to react with and neutralize a given volume or amount of a specific antigen. (p. 799)

**Antigens** Substances, usually proteins and foreign to a host, that stimulate the production of antibodies and that react specifically with those antibodies. Examples of antigens include bacterial exotoxins and viruses. An allergen (e.g., dust, pollen, mold) is an antigen that can produce an immediate-type hypersensitivity reaction or allergy. (p. 797)

**Antiserum** A serum that contains antibodies. It is usually obtained from an animal that has been immunized against a specific antigen. (p. 799)

**Antitoxin** An antiserum against a toxin (or toxoid). It is most often a purified antiserum obtained from animals (usually horses) by injection of a toxin or toxoid so that antibodies to the toxin (i.e., antitoxin) can be collected from the animals and used to provide artificial passive immunity to humans exposed to a given toxin (e.g., tetanus immunoglobulin). (p. 799)

**Antivenin** An antiserum against a venom (poison produced by an animal) used to treat humans or other animals that have been envenomed (e.g., by snakebite, spider bite, or scorpion sting). (p. 799)

**Biologic antimicrobial drugs** Substances of biologic origin used to prevent, treat, or cure infectious diseases (e.g., vaccines, toxoids, immunoglobulins). These drugs are often simply referred to as *biologics*. However, *biologics* also refers to drugs of bioterrorism (e.g., anthrax spores, smallpox virus), depending on the context. (p. 797)

**Bioterrorism** The use of infectious biologic or chemical agents as weapons for human destruction. (p. 807)

**Booster shot** A repeat dose of an antigen, such as a vaccine or toxoid, which is usually administered in an amount smaller than that used in the original immunization. It is given to maintain the immune response of a previously immunized patient at, or return the response to, a clinically effective level. (p. 799)

**Cell-mediated immune system** The immune response that is mediated by T cells (as opposed to B cells, which produce antibodies). T cells mount their immune response through activities such as the release of cytokines (chemicals that stimulate other protective immune functions) as well as through direct cytotoxicity (e.g., phagocytosis of an antigen). (p. 799)

**Herd immunity** Resistance to a disease on the part of an entire community or population because a large proportion of its members are immune to the disease. (p. 800)

**Immune response** A cascade of biochemical events that occurs in response to entry of an antigen (foreign substance) into the body; key processes of the immune response include

phagocytosis ("eating of cells") of foreign microorganisms and synthesis of antibodies that react with specific antigens to inactivate them. Immune response centers around the blood but may also involve the lymphatic system and the *reticuloendothelial system* (see later). (p. 797)

**Immunization** The induction of immunity by administration of a vaccine or toxoid (active immunization) or antiserum (passive immunization). (p. 797)

**Immunizing biologics** Toxoids, vaccines, or immunoglobulins that are targeted against specific infectious microorganisms or toxins. (p. 797)

**Immunoglobulins** Glycoproteins synthesized and used by the humoral immune system (B cells) to attack and kill all substances foreign to the body. The term is synonymous with *immune globulins.* (p. 797)

**Passive immunization** A type of immunization in which immunity to infection occurs by injecting a person with antiserum or concentrated antibodies that directly give the host the means to fight off an invading microorganism (artificial passive immunization). The host's immune system therefore does not have to manufacture these antibodies. This process also occurs when antibodies pass from mother to infant during breastfeeding or through the placenta during pregnancy (natural passive immunization). (p. 797)

**Passive immunizing drugs** Drugs containing antibodies or antitoxins that can kill or inactivate pathogens by binding to the associated antigens. These are directly injected into a person (host) and provide that person with the means to fend off infection, bypassing the host's own immune system. (p. 798)

**Recombinant** Relating to or containing a combination of genetic material from two or more organisms. Such genetic recombination is one of the key methods of biotechnology and is often used to manufacture immunizing drugs and various other medications. (p. 799)

**Reticuloendothelial system** Specialized cells located in the liver, spleen, lymphatics, and bone marrow that remove miscellaneous particles from the circulation, such as aging antibody molecules. (p. 800)

**Toxin** Any poison produced by a plant, animal, or microorganism that is highly toxic to other living organisms. (p. 798)

**Toxoids** Bacterial exotoxins that are modified or inactivated (by chemicals or heat) so that they are no longer toxic but can still bind to host B cells to stimulate the formation of antitoxin; toxoids are often used in the same manner as vaccines to promote artificial active immunity in humans. They are one type of active immunizing drug (e.g., tetanus toxoid). (p. 797)

**Vaccines** Suspensions of live, attenuated, or killed microorganisms that can promote an artificially induced active immunity against a particular microorganism. They are another type of active immunizing drug (e.g., tetanus vaccine). (p. 798)

**Venom** A poison that is secreted by an animal (e.g., snake, insect, or spider). (p. 799)

# ANATOMY, PHYSIOLOGY, AND PATHOPHYSIOLOGY OVERVIEW

## IMMUNITY AND IMMUNIZATION

Centuries ago it was noticed that people who contracted certain diseases acquired an immune tolerance to the disease so that, when exposed to it again, they did not experience a second bout of illness. This basic observation prompted scientists to investigate ways of artificially producing this tolerance. Along with this came an understanding of how the normal immune system functions, which is important to an understanding of how immunizing drugs work. Briefly, when the body first comes into contact with antigens (foreign proteins) from an invading organism, specific information is imprinted into a cellular "memory bank" of the immune system. The body can then effectively fight any future invasion by that same organism by mounting an immune response. This cellular memory bank consists of specialized immune cells known as *memory cells*. When an antigen presents itself to a person's humoral immune system (B cells, or B lymphocytes) by binding to B cells, the B cells differentiate into two other types of cells. One type is the memory cells. The second type is plasma cells, which produce large volumes of antibodies against the antigen in question. Antibodies are immunoglobulin molecules that have antigen-specific amino acid sequences. Immunoglobulins, or immune globulins, are glycoprotein molecules synthesized by the humoral immune system for the purpose of destroying all substances that the body recognizes as foreign. Immunoglobulins can be general or specific. A general immunoglobulin lacks a specific amino acid sequence that allows it to recognize a specific antigen. An immunoglobulin with such a specific amino acid sequence is known as an *antibody*. It is because of this process that people rarely suffer twice from certain diseases such as mumps, chickenpox, and measles. Instead they have a complete and long-lasting immunity to those infections.

In contrast to the humoral immune system, which is the focus of this chapter, the cell-mediated immune system is the branch of the immune system that does not synthesize antibodies. Instead, it is driven by T cells (T lymphocytes) and works by the release of cytokines (chemicals that promote other immune system functions, e.g., inflammatory responses, runny nose) and by phagocytosis (engulfing and destruction of the antigens by the T cells). The cell-mediated immune system is discussed in Chapter 47, because it is the target of immunosuppressant drugs. To varying degrees, these two immune system branches work simultaneously or even interdependently. The humoral immune system is also activated and/or driven partly by cytokines from the cell-mediated immune system.

There are two ways of obtaining immunity to certain infections: active immunization and passive immunization. Each can be an artificial or natural process. In artificial active immunization, the body is clinically exposed to a relatively harmless form of an antigen that does not cause an actual infection. Information about the antigen is then imprinted into the memory of the immune system and the body's defenses are stimulated to resist any subsequent exposure (by producing antibodies). In contrast, natural active immunization occurs when a person acquires immunity by surviving the disease itself and producing antibodies to the disease-causing organism. Artificial passive immunization involves administration of serum or concentrated immunoglobulins. This directly gives the inoculated person the substance needed to fight off the invading microorganism. This type of immunization bypasses the host's immune system. Finally, natural passive immunization occurs when antibodies are transferred from the mother to her infant in breast milk or through the bloodstream via the placenta during pregnancy. The major differences between active and passive immunization are summarized in Table 49-1 and are discussed in greater depth in the following sections.

## Active Immunization

In general, biologic antimicrobial drugs (also referred to simply as *biologics*) are substances such as antitoxins, antisera, toxoids, and vaccines that are used to prevent, treat, or cure infectious diseases. Toxoids and vaccines are known as immunizing biologics, and they target a particular infectious microorganism.

### Toxoids

Toxoids are substances that contain antigens, most often in the form of bacterial (usually gram-positive bacterial) exotoxins.

| TABLE 49-1 | ACTIVE VERSUS PASSIVE IMMUNIZATION | |
|---|---|---|
| **CHARACTERISTIC** | **ACTIVE** | **PASSIVE** |
| **Artificial** | | |
| Type of immunizing drug | Toxoid or vaccine | Immunoglobulin or antitoxin |
| Mechanism of action | Results from an antigen-antibody response similar to that after antigen exposure in the natural disease process | Results from direct administration of exogenous antibodies; antibody concentration will decrease over time, so if reexposure is expected, it is wise to continue passive immunizations. |
| Use | To prevent development of active disease in the event of exposure to a given antigen in individuals who have at least a partially functioning immune system | To provide temporary protection against disease in individuals who are immunodeficient, those for whom active immunization is contraindicated, and those who have been exposed to or anticipate exposure to the organism or toxin; an antibody response is not stimulated in the host. |
| **Natural** | | |
| Mechanism of action | Production of one's own antibodies during actual infection | Transmission of antibodies from mother to infant through placenta or during breastfeeding |

These substances have been detoxified or weakened (attenuated) with chemicals or heat, which renders them nontoxic and unable to revert back to a toxic form. Nonetheless, they remain highly antigenic and can stimulate an artificial active immune response (production of antitoxin antibodies) when injected into a host patient. These antibodies can then neutralize the same exotoxin upon any future exposure. Toxoids were first developed in 1923 at the Pasteur Institute by Gaston Ramon and his associates, and modern versions are effective against diseases such as diphtheria and tetanus caused by toxin-producing bacteria.

## Vaccines

Vaccines are suspensions of live, attenuated (weakened), or killed (inactivated) microorganisms that can stimulate production of antibodies against the particular organism. As with toxoids, these slight alterations in the bacteria and viruses prevent the person injected from contracting the disease. They are still able to promote active immunization against the organism, including an antibody response. People vaccinated with live bacteria or viruses (as well as those who recover from an actual infection) enjoy lifelong immunity against that particular disease. However, only partial immunity is conferred on those vaccinated with killed bacteria or viruses, and for this reason they must be given periodic booster shots to maintain immune system protection against infection with the given organism.

Edward Jenner, an English physician born in 1749, noticed that milkmaids who had contracted cowpox infections were rarely victims of smallpox and was the first to study the relationship of cowpox to smallpox immunity. His observation led to the development of the smallpox vaccine. In 1796, Jenner successfully immunized a young boy against smallpox by vaccinating him with cowpox virus obtained from a cowpox vesicle on an infected cow. With the help of the modern version of this vaccine, smallpox was considered to be eradicated as of 1980. However, following the terrorist attacks in the United States on September 11, 2001, fears arose of a large-scale bioterrorism attack using the smallpox virus. By 2003, these fears had subsided somewhat, and the Centers for Disease Control and Prevention (CDC) released guidelines recommending routine early detection surveillance activities on the part of all public health agencies. These guidelines also included a plan for rapid vaccination of local populations in the event of a suspected smallpox outbreak and listed several high-priority high-risk groups, including direct health care personnel, who need to be vaccinated first if a suspected outbreak occurs.

Today there are more than 20 infectious diseases for which vaccines are available. New vaccines appear periodically but not with the rapidity of other types of drugs, because of the complexities of developing a safe and effective vaccine. Most modern vaccines are produced in a laboratory by genetic engineering methods and contain some extract of the pathogen, or a synthetic extract, rather than the microbe itself. Some vaccines, such as influenza vaccine, may contain actual whole or split virus particles. Most, however, contain a smaller fraction of the organism, such as the bacterial capsular polysaccharides that are used to make pneumococcal vaccine. The attenuating or killing agent is usually a chemical such as formaldehyde or a physical mechanism such as heat. Attenuation may also be accomplished by repeated passage of the microbe through some medium such as a fertile hen egg or a special tissue culture. The search for new and better drugs will never end. Current goals include finding vaccines against human immunodeficiency virus infection/acquired immunodeficiency syndrome (HIV/AIDS) and malaria; the ultimate goal is to develop an effective vaccine against all infectious diseases. The currently available immunizing vaccines are listed in Box 49-1. Note that the drug given to prevent respiratory syncytial virus (RSV) infection is not an immunizing drug per se but is a specialized antiviral drug. It is discussed in Chapter 40. The RSV immunoglobulin is listed in Box 49-1. People who travel to different parts of the world may require specific vaccines. This information can be found on the CDC website at http://wwwnc.cdc.gov/travel/page/vaccinations.htm.

The current childhood immunization schedule published by the CDC is available at http://www.cdc.gov/vaccines. This advisory is published annually as a joint effort of the American Academy of Pediatrics, the CDC's Advisory Committee on Immunization Practices, and the American Academy of Family Physicians. The CDC also posts on its website a catch-up schedule for children who may have missed scheduled immunizations. The CDC's current adult immunization schedule can be found online at http://www.cdc.gov/vaccines/recs/schedules/adult-schedule.htm#print.

## Passive Immunization

In passive immunization, the host's immune system is bypassed, and the person is inoculated with serum containing immunoglobulins obtained from other humans or animals. These substances give the person the means to fight off the invading organism. This is known as *artificially acquired passive immunity* and it confers temporary immunity against a particular antigen following exposure to the antigen. It differs from active immunization in that it produces a transitory (short-lived) immune state and the antibodies are already prepared for the host—the host's immune system does not have to synthesize its own antibodies. This allows for more rapid prevention or treatment of disease. Important examples include immunization with tetanus immunoglobulin, hepatitis immunoglobulin, rabies immunoglobulin, and snakebite antivenin.

Passive immunization occurs naturally between a mother and the fetus or the nursing infant when the mother passes maternal antibodies directly, either through the placenta to the fetus or through breast milk to the nursing infant. This is called *naturally acquired passive immunity*.

There are specific populations that can benefit from passive immunization but not from active immunization (see Table 49-1). These are people who have been rendered immunodeficient for one reason or another (e.g., by drugs or disease) and who therefore cannot mount an immune response to a toxoid or vaccine injection because their immune system is suppressed. Passive immunizing drugs are also used in people who already have the given disease, especially those with diseases that are rapidly harmful or fatal, such as rabies, tetanus, and hepatitis. Because these diseases can progress rapidly, the body does not have time to mount an adequate immune defense against them before death occurs. The passive immunization of such

## BOX 49-1   AVAILABLE IMMUNIZING DRUGS

**Passive Immunizing Drugs**

Antivenin, pit viper (Crotalidae), polyvalent

Crotalidae polyvalent immune Fab (for pit viper snakebite; e.g., rattlesnake, water moccasin)

Antivenin, *Latrodectus mactans* (black widow spider)

Antivenin, *Micrurus fulvius* (coral snake)

Botulism immunoglobulin

Cytomegalovirus immunoglobulin (human)

Digoxin immune Fab

Hepatitis B immunoglobulin

Immunoglobulin, intramuscular

Immunoglobulin, intravenous

Lymphocyte immunoglobulin, antithymocyte globulin

Rabies immunoglobulin (human)

Respiratory syncytial virus immunoglobulin, intravenous (human)

$Rh_0$(D) immunoglobulin

Tetanus immunoglobulin

Vaccinia immunoglobulin

Varicella-zoster immunoglobulin (chickenpox/shingles)

**Active Immunizing Drugs**

BCG (bacille Calmette-Guérin) vaccine (tuberculosis)

Diphtheria and tetanus toxoids (adsorbed)

Diphtheria and tetanus toxoids, and acellular pertussis vaccine (adsorbed)

Diphtheria and tetanus toxoids, acellular pertussis, and *Haemophilus influenzae* type b conjugate vaccines

Diphtheria and tetanus toxoids, acellular pertussis (adsorbed), hepatitis b (recombinant), and inactivated poliovirus vaccine combined

*H. Influenzae* type b conjugate vaccine

*H. Influenzae* type b conjugate vaccine with hepatitis b vaccine

Hepatitis a virus vaccine (inactivated)

Hepatitis b virus vaccine (recombinant)

Hepatitis a virus vaccine (inactivated) and hepatitis b virus vaccine (recombinant)

Herpes zoster virus vaccine (live, attenuated)

Human papillomavirus vaccine (attenuated)

Influenza virus vaccine

Japanese encephalitis virus vaccine

Measles virus* vaccine (live, attenuated)

Measles, mumps, and rubella virus vaccine (live)

Meningococcal bacterial vaccine

Mumps virus vaccine (live)

Pneumococcal bacterial vaccine, polyvalent

Pneumococcal thirteen-valent conjugate vaccine

Poliovirus vaccine (inactivated)

Rabies virus vaccine

Rubella virus vaccine (live)

Rubella and mumps virus vaccine (live)

Rubella, measles, and mumps virus vaccine (live)

Smallpox virus vaccine†

Tetanus toxoid (fluid)

Tetanus toxoid (adsorbed)

Typhoid bacterial vaccine

Varicella virus vaccine

Yellow fever virus vaccine

*Also known as *rubeola* virus.

†Not currently on the U.S. market but according to the Centers for Disease Control and Prevention website may be reintroduced because of current bioterrorism threats.

---

individuals confers a temporary protection that is usually sufficient to keep the invading organisms from killing them, even though it does not stimulate an antibody response.

The passive immunizing drugs are divided into three groups: antitoxins, immunoglobulins, and snake and spider antivenins. An antitoxin is a purified antiserum that is usually obtained from horses inoculated with the toxin. An immunoglobulin is a concentrated preparation containing predominantly immunoglobulin G and is harvested from a large pool of blood donors. An antivenin, often referred to as *antivenom*, is an antiserum containing antibodies against a venom, which is a poison secreted by an animal such as a reptile, insect, or other arthropod (e.g., spider). Most antivenins are obtained from animals (usually horses) that have been injected with the particular venom; however, the newer ones are produced by recombinant technology. The serum contains immunoglobulins that can neutralize the toxic effects of the venom.

## PHARMACOLOGY OVERVIEW

### IMMUNIZING DRUGS

#### Mechanism of Action and Drug Effects

Active immunizing drugs consist of vaccines and toxoids that may be given either orally or intramuscularly and work by stimulating the humoral immune system. This system synthesizes substances called *immunoglobulins*, of which there are five distinct types, designated as M, G, A, E, and D. These immunoglobulins attack and kill the foreign substances that invade the body. In this case, these foreign substances are called *antigens*, and the immunoglobulins are called *antibodies*.

Vaccines contain substances that trigger the formation of these antibodies against specific pathogens. They may contain the actual live or attenuated pathogen or a killed pathogen. The antibody titer is a measure of how many antibodies to a given antigen are present in the blood and is used to assess whether enough antibodies are present to protect the body effectively against the particular pathogen. Sometimes the antibody levels decline over time. When this happens, another dose of the vaccine is given to restore the antibody titers to a level that can protect the person against the infection. This repeat dose is referred to as a booster shot. Toxoids are altered forms of bacterial toxins that stimulate the production of antibodies in the same way as vaccines.

Because both toxoids and vaccines rely on the immunized host to mount an immune response, the host's immune system must be intact. Therefore, patients who are immunocompromised (i.e., who cannot mount an immune response) may not benefit from receiving vaccines or toxoids. Instead, their clinical situations may warrant giving them passive immunizing drugs such as immunoglobulins.

Passive immunizing drugs are the actual antibodies (immunoglobulins) that can kill or inactivate the pathogen. The process is called *passive* because the person's immune system does not participate in the synthesis of antibodies; instead, the antibodies are provided by the immunizing drug. Immunity acquired in this way generally lasts for a much shorter time than that produced by active immunization. Passive immunization lasts only until the injected immunoglobulins are removed from the person's immune system by the reticuloendothelial system. The reticuloendothelial system is composed of specialized cells in the liver, spleen, lymphatics, and bone marrow.

## Indications

Vaccines and toxoids are active immunizing drugs that have been developed for the prevention of many illnesses caused by bacteria and their toxins, as well as those caused by various viruses. Antivenins, antitoxins, and immunoglobulins are passive immunizing drugs. Such drugs can inactivate spider and snake venom, bacterial toxins (exotoxins), and potentially lethal viruses. Box 49-1 lists the currently available immunizing drugs. The successful immunization of 95% or more of a population confers protection on the entire population. This is called herd immunity.

Antivenins, also known as *antisera,* are used to prevent or minimize the effects of poisoning by the venoms of crotalids (rattlesnakes, copperheads, cottonmouths, water moccasins), black widow spiders, and coral snakes, some of which can be lethal. Most healthy adults do not die from the bites of spiders or snakes if they receive prompt and appropriate treatment (i.e., administration of the appropriate antivenin). However, very young children and older persons with health problems are particularly susceptible to the effects of the venom of some of these animals. In either situation, an antivenin is needed to neutralize the venom.

## Contraindications

Contraindications to the administration of immunizing drugs include allergy to the immunization itself or allergy to any of its components, such as eggs or yeast. In the case of a potentially fatal illness such as rabies, the drug may still need to be given and any allergic reaction controlled with other medications. Administration of some immunizing drugs is best deferred until after recovery from a febrile illness or temporary immunocompromised state (e.g., following cancer chemotherapy), if possible. However, this is often a matter of clinical judgment, and the individual patient's condition and risk factors for serious illness may be arguments for or against administration of a given immunizing drug at a given time.

## Adverse Effects

The undesirable effects of the various immunizing drugs can range from mild and transient to serious and even life-threatening and are listed in Table 49-2. The overwhelming majority of adverse effects are minor. Minor reactions can be treated with acetaminophen and rest. More severe reactions, such as fever higher than 103° F (39.4° C), can be treated with acetaminophen and sponge baths. Serum sickness sometimes

| TABLE 49-2 | IMMUNIZING DRUGS: MINOR AND SEVERE ADVERSE EFFECTS |
|---|---|
| **BODY SYSTEM** | **ADVERSE EFFECTS** |
| **Minor Effects** | |
| Central nervous | Fever, adenopathy |
| Integumentary | Minor rash, soreness at injection site, urticaria, arthritis |
| **Severe Effects** | |
| Central nervous | Fever higher than 103° F (39.4° C), encephalitis, convulsions, peripheral neuropathy, anaphylactic reaction, shock, unconsciousness |
| Integumentary | Rash |
| Respiratory | Dyspnea |
| Other | Cyanosis |

occurs after repeated injections of equine (horse)–derived immunizing drugs. The signs and symptoms consist of edema of the face, tongue, and throat; rash; urticaria; arthritis; adenopathy; fever; flushing; itching; cough; dyspnea; cyanosis; vomiting; and cardiovascular collapse. Serum sickness is best treated with analgesics, antihistamines, epinephrine, and/or corticosteroids. In these cases, hospitalization may be required.

Any serious or unusual reactions to immunizing drugs need to be reported to the Vaccine Adverse Event Reporting System (VAERS). This is a national vaccine safety surveillance program that is cosponsored by the Food and Drug Administration (FDA) and the CDC. A report can be submitted via the toll-free telephone number 800-822-7967. Alternatively, a reporting form can be printed from the website of either the FDA (http://www.fda.gov) or the CDC (http://www.cdc.gov). These websites have extensive information describing this reporting system and the data collected by it. Such data are used to improve the quality of immunizing drugs and can even be grounds for an FDA recall of biologic drugs whose adverse effects exceed acceptable safety thresholds.

In the early 1980s, in response to vaccine-related injuries, many parents became reluctant to immunize their children against common, and even potentially fatal, childhood illnesses. Increasing numbers of legal actions were also brought by parents of injured children. In 1986, the U.S. Congress passed the Childhood Vaccine Injury Act, which in turn established the National Vaccine Injury Compensation Program (VICP). The purpose was to create a no-fault alternative to the civil tort system, which had driven many vaccine manufacturers out of the field. Serious adverse events following vaccination are very uncommon. The Vaccine Injury Table published by the Health Resources and Services Administration itemizes serious adverse events reported for vaccines that are covered under the VICP, as well as the expected time frame for such events to occur. The first symptom must appear within the listed time frame (Table 49-3) for it to be presumed to be caused by the vaccine. For more information, the reader is referred to www.hrsa.gov/vaccinecompensation/index.html.

## TABLE 49-3   U.S. DEPARTMENT OF HEALTH AND HUMAN SERVICES VACCINE INJURY TABLE

| VACCINE | ADVERSE EVENT | TIME INTERVAL |
|---|---|---|
| Tetanus toxoid–containing vaccines (e.g., DTaP, Tdap, DTP-Hib, DT, Td, TT) | Anaphylaxis or anaphylactic shock | 0-4 hr |
| | Brachial neuritis | 2-28 days |
| | Any acute complication or sequela (including death) of above events | NA |
| Pertussis antigen–containing vaccines (e.g., DTaP, Tdap, DTP, P, DTP-Hib) | Anaphylaxis or anaphylactic shock | 0-4 hr |
| | Encephalopathy (or encephalitis) | 0-72 hr |
| | Any acute complication or sequela (including death) of above events | NA |
| Measles, mumps, and rubella virus–containing vaccines in any combination (e.g., MMR, MR, M, R) | Anaphylaxis or anaphylactic shock | 0-4 hr |
| | Encephalopathy (or encephalitis) | 5-15 days |
| | Any acute complication or sequela (including death) of above events | NA |
| Rubella virus–containing vaccines (e.g., MMR, MR, R) | Chronic arthritis | 7-42 days |
| | Any acute complication or sequela (including death) of above event | NA |
| Measles virus–containing vaccines (e.g., MMR, MR, M) | Thrombocytopenic purpura | 7-30 days |
| | Vaccine-strain measles viral infection in an immunodeficient recipient | 0-6 mo |
| | Any acute complication or sequela (including death) of above events | NA |
| Polio live virus–containing vaccines (OPV) | Paralytic polio | |
| | In a nonimmunodeficient recipient | 0-30 days |
| | In an immunodeficient recipient | 0-6 mo |
| | In a vaccine-associated community case | NA |
| | Vaccine-strain polio viral infection | |
| | In a nonimmunodeficient recipient | 0-30 days |
| | In an immunodeficient recipient | 0-6 mo |
| | In a vaccine-associated community case | NA |
| | Any acute complication or sequela (including death) of above events | NA |
| Polio inactivated virus–containing vaccines (e.g., IPV) | Anaphylaxis or anaphylactic shock | 0-4 hr |
| | Any acute complication or sequela (including death) of above event | NA |
| Hepatitis B antigen–containing vaccines | Anaphylaxis or anaphylactic shock | 0-4 hr |
| | Any acute complication or sequela (including death) of above event | NA |
| Haemophilus influenzae type b polysaccharide conjugate vaccines | No condition specified for compensation | NA |
| Varicella vaccine | No condition specified for compensation | NA |
| Rotavirus vaccine | No condition specified for compensation | NA |
| Vaccines containing live, oral, rhesus-based rotavirus | Intussusception | 0-30 days |
| | Any acute complication or sequela (including death) of above event | NA |
| Pneumococcal conjugate vaccines | No condition specified for compensation | NA |
| Any new vaccine recommended by the Centers for Disease Control and Prevention for routine administration to children, after publication by the Secretary of DHHS of a notice of coverage* | No condition specified for compensation | NA |

*DHHS, Department of Health and Human Services; DT, diphtheria and tetanus vaccine; DTaP, diphtheria, tetanus, and acellular pertussis vaccine; DTP, diphtheria, tetanus, and pertussis vaccine; Hib, Haemophilus influenzae type b conjugate vaccine; IPV, inactivated poliovirus; M, measles vaccine; MMR, measles, mumps, and rubella vaccine; MR, measles and rubella vaccine; NA, not applicable; OPV, oral polio vaccine; P, pertussis vaccine; R, rubella vaccine; Td, tetanus and diphtheria toxoids; Tdap, tetanus and diphtheria toxoids and acellular pertussis vaccine; TT, tetanus toxoid.*
*Refer to the "News & Updates" link on the National Vaccine Injury Compensation Program website (www.hrsa.gov/vaccinecompensation) for more information.

For many years, there was controversy in the national news pertaining to the link between immunizations and autism in children. It was thought that thimerosal (a mercury-containing preservative used in vaccines) may have been a causative link, so since 2001 thimerosal has no longer been used in the preparation of vaccines. In 2011, the medical community declared that the original study suggesting a link to autism was fraudulent. It is suggested that the original author falsified the medical histories of the patients in his study and that he was "hoping to create a vaccine scare." Although there is absolutely no scientific data to support a link between autism and vaccines, many parents are still reluctant to vaccinate their children.

## Interactions

Drug interactions are not generally a problem with the majority of immunizing drugs, because they are normally given in a single dose or a relatively small number of doses. One drug class of note that can potentially reduce the efficacy of immunizing drugs is immunosuppressive drugs, including corticosteroids (see Chapter 33), transplant anti-rejection drugs (see Chapter 48), and cancer chemotherapy drugs (see Chapters 45 and 46). All of these drugs can, to varying degrees, hinder the generation of the active immunity that would normally occur following vaccine or toxoid administration. The bacille Calmette-Guérin vaccine for tuberculosis (used mostly outside the United States in developing countries) can cause false-positive results on the tuberculin skin test (see Chapter 41).

Some vaccines are not to be given close in time to one other. For example, the meningococcal vaccine, whole-cell pertussis vaccine, and typhoid vaccine together have undesirably large bacterial endotoxin content and should not be administered simultaneously. The effectiveness of measles, mumps, and rubella vaccines may be reduced by concurrent interferon therapy (see Chapter 47). Influenza vaccine may also theoretically lose efficacy if given while antiviral influenza drugs are being taken (see Chapter 40). Recommendations are to give the influenza vaccine at least 48 hours after stopping such antiviral drug therapy. In general, immunizations requiring intramuscular injection are given with particular caution (and with appropriate monitoring) to patients receiving anticoagulant drugs such as warfarin (see Chapter 26). Review the package insert for any immunizing drugs given to obtain the latest information and identify other specific drug interactions that may occur. Hepatitis B

## DOSAGES

### Selected Immunizing Drugs

| DRUG (PREGNANCY CATEGORY) | PHARMACOLOGIC CLASS | USUAL DOSAGE RANGE* | INDICATIONS/USES |
|---|---|---|---|
| **Active Immunizing Drugs** | | | |
| diphtheria, tetanus, and acellular pertussis vaccine (DTaP) (Daptacel) | Mixed toxoid/vaccine | **Pediatric only**<br>IM: Series of three 0.5-mL injections; age of first injection 6 wk-7 yr; give second and third doses at 4-8 wk intervals | Prophylaxis against diphtheria, tetanus, and pertussis |
| *Haemophilus influenzae* type b conjugate vaccine (HibTITER) (C) | Bacterial capsular antigenic extract vaccine | **Pediatric**<br>*Infant 2-6 mo*<br>Give three IM injections (0.5 mL each) about 2 mo apart<br>*Previously unvaccinated child 7-11 mo*<br>Give two IM injections about 2 mo apart<br>*Previously unvaccinated child 12-14 mo*<br>Give only one IM injection | *H. influenzae* type b prophylaxis |
| ◆ hepatitis B virus vaccine, inactivated (Recombivax HB) (C) | Viral surface antigen vaccine | **Pediatric to age 10 yr**<br>IM: 5 mcg (0.5 mL) at birth, and then again at 1 mo and 6 mo<br>**Adult**<br>IM: Three 10-mcg (1-mL) doses: day 0, 1 mo, and 6 mo | Hepatitis B virus prophylaxis |
| ◆ influenza virus vaccine (Fluzone, FluShield, Fluvirin) (C) | Viral surface antigen vaccine | **Pediatric 6 mo-9 yr**<br>IM: Single yearly dose (two doses of 0.25 mL at least 1 mo apart if receiving influenza vaccine for first time)<br>**Adult**<br>IM: Single yearly dose (0.5 mL) | Influenza prophylaxis |
| ◆ measles, mumps, and rubella virus vaccine, live (M-M-R II) (C) | Live, attenuated viral vaccine | **Adult and pediatric older than 12 mo**<br>Subcut: 0.5-mL single dose; booster recommended for children entering middle or high school | Prophylaxis against measles, mumps, and rubella |
| ◆ meningococcal vaccine (Menactra, Menveo) (B) | Inactivated | **Menactra: Adult and pediatric 9 mo-55 yr:**<br>0.5 mL IM<br>**Menveo: Adult and pediatric 11-55 yr:** 0.5 mL IM | Prophylaxis against meningococcal disease |
| ◆ pneumococcal vaccine, polyvalent (Pneumovax 23) (C) | Bacterial capsular antigenic extract vaccine | **Adult and pediatric 2 yr and older**<br>Subcut: 0.5 mL × 1 | *Streptococcus pneumoniae* prophylaxis |
| ◆ poliovirus vaccine, inactivated (IPOL) (C) | Inactivated viral vaccine | **Pediatric (infant)**<br>Subcut: Three 0.5-mL doses: 4-8 wk, 2-4 mo, and 6-12 mo<br>**Adult**<br>Subcut: Two 0.5-mL doses 1-2 mo apart, and then a third dose 6-12 mo later | Polio prophylaxis |
| rabies virus vaccine (Imovax, RabAvert) (C) | Inactivated viral vaccine | **Adult and pediatric**<br>*Postexposure prophylaxis*<br>IM: 1 mL on days 3, 7, and 14 (with one dose of rabies immunoglobulin [see later] within 8 days of first vaccine dose)<br>*Preexposure prophylaxis for those at high risk for rabies exposure (e.g., veterinarians)*<br>IM/ID: 1 mL IM or 0.1 mL ID on days 0, 7, and once between days 21 and 28, for a total of three doses; then q2-5yr, depending on antibody titers | Rabies prophylaxis |

## DOSAGES—cont'd

### Selected Immunizing Drugs

| DRUG (PREGNANCY CATEGORY) | PHARMACOLOGIC CLASS | USUAL DOSAGE RANGE* | INDICATIONS/USES |
|---|---|---|---|
| tetanus and diphtheria toxoids, adsorbed (Tdap) (Adacel) | Mixed toxoid | **Adult and pediatric**<br>IM: Doses vary based on age; once initial series has been completed, give 0.5-mL booster shot every 10 years | Prophylaxis against diphtheria, tetanus, and pertussis |
| ◆ varicella virus vaccine (Varivax) (C) | Live, attenuated viral vaccine | **Adult and pediatric older than 12 yr**<br>Subcut: Two 0.5-mL doses given 4-8 wk apart<br>**Pediatric 1-12 yr**<br>Subcut: One 0.5-mL dose | Prophylaxis against varicella virus<br>(causes chickenpox and shingles) |
| **Passive Immunizing Drugs** | | | |
| ◆ hepatitis B immunoglobulin (BayHep B, Nabi-HB) (C) | Pooled human immunoglobulin | **Infant (of mother known to be hepatitis B positive)**<br>IM: 0.5 mL within 12 hr after birth<br>**Adult**<br>IM: 0.06 mg/kg after exposure and 30 days later | Passive hepatitis B prophylaxis |
| ◆ immunoglobulin intravenous (Gammar-P IV, Panglobulin NF, others) (C) | Pooled human immunoglobulin | Dosages vary widely; refer to manufacturer's current dosage information for specific indications | Therapy for many disorders, including primary immune deficiency syndrome, pediatric AIDS, idiopathic thrombocytopenic purpura, B-cell lymphocytic leukemia |
| rabies immunoglobulin (Imogam, Rabies-HT, BayRab) (C) | Pooled human immunoglobulin | **Adult and pediatric**<br>Single dose of 20 IU/kg; infiltrate as much of dose as possible into bite wound area, and give remainder IM in gluteal region; do not give into same site as rabies vaccine | Rabies prophylaxis |
| Rh$_0$(D) immunoglobulin (Rho-GAM, MICRhoGAM) (C) | Immunosuppressant globulin | **Adult female**<br>IM (full dose): Inject total contents of a single vial within 72 hr after delivery<br>IM (microdose): Inject full contents of a single vial after spontaneous or elective abortion of pregnancy of 12 wk gestation or less | Postpartum antibody suppression to prevent hemolytic disease of future newborns |
| tetanus immunoglobulin (BayTet) (C) | Pooled human immunoglobulin | **Adult and pediatric**<br>IM: 250 units as a single dose | Postexposure tetanus prophylaxis |
| | | IM: 3000-6000 units as a single dose | Tetanus treatment |

*AIDS*, Acquired immunodeficiency syndrome; *ID*, intradermal; *IM*, intramuscular; *subcut*, subcutaneous.

*Note: Dosages given are only for brands listed. Dosing amounts and regimens may vary for different brands. Always follow manufacturer's current dosing directions.

immunoglobulin interacts with live vaccines; defer administration of such vaccines until 3 months after the dose of immunoglobulin is given.

## Dosages

For dosage information on selected immunizing drugs, see the table on p. 802.

## DRUG PROFILES

Some of the more commonly used vaccines, toxoids, and immunoglobulins are described in the following sections. The immunizing drugs currently available commercially in the United States, including several combination vaccines for prevention of more than one disease, are listed in Box 49-1. Combination vaccines obviously reduce the number of injections that the patient receives, and thus their use is desirable when possible, especially in children.

## ACTIVE IMMUNIZING DRUGS

### diphtheria and tetanus toxoids and acellular pertussis vaccine (adsorbed)

The active immunizing drugs include diphtheria and tetanus toxoids and the acellular pertussis vaccine (adsorbed) (Tripedia, Daptacel, Infanrix). *Adsorption* refers to the laboratory techniques used to make most vaccines and toxoids. The biologic materials (i.e., virus or toxin particles) are adsorbed (separated out of solution and dried) onto carrier media such as alum, from which they are later removed for packaging into final dosage forms. Diphtheria, tetanus, and pertussis are very different disorders, but an injection that combines all three vaccines (DTP; also commonly called DPT) was routinely given to children since the 1940s. The vaccine combination called *diphtheria and tetanus toxoids with acellular pertussis vaccine (adsorbed) (DTaP [Daptacel])* was approved for the full childhood immunization series and has replaced DPT. Tdap (Adacel, Boostrix) is also a combination vaccine used for teenagers and adults. DTaP (Daptacel) and Tdap use a different form of the pertussis component, known as *acellular pertussis*. Acellular pertussis consists of only a single weakened toxoid, whereas previous pertussis vaccines contained multiple toxoids; this may reduce the number of adverse effects seen from DTP. Pertussis, also known as *whooping cough*, is highly contagious and is spread through contact with respiratory secretions. Its incidence has increased in several states. Currently DTaP is the preferred preparation for primary and booster immunization against these diseases in children from 6 weeks to 6 years of age, unless use of the pertussis component is contraindicated. Tdap (Adacel) is the recommended vaccine for adolescents and adults. See the Safety and Quality Improvement: Preventing Medication Errors box on p. 808.

Tetanus, diphtheria, and pertussis are prevalent in the populations of many developing countries throughout the world. Full immunization against these diseases with Tdap or DTaP is recommended for travelers to these areas and as well as for their inhabitants. A combination product containing only tetanus and diphtheria toxoids (Td) used to be administered to persons 7 years of age and older who require a primary or booster immunization against tetanus for routine wound management. Booster doses were required approximately every 10 years. However, with the recent increase in pertussis cases, Tdap or DTaP are recommended in place of Td. If persons had received Td in the past, it is recommended that they receive another immunization containing pertussis with Tdap or DTaP.

These toxoids (DTP, DTaP, Tdap, and Td) are available only as parenteral preparations, given as deep intramuscular injections. Their use is contraindicated in persons who have had a prior systemic hypersensitivity reaction or a neurologic reaction to one of the ingredients. Some manufacturers state that use is contraindicated in cases of concurrent acute or active infections but not in cases of minor illness. Although there have been very few studies, if any, documenting the safety of their use in pregnant women, it is generally considered safe to give diphtheria, tetanus, and pertussis toxoids after the first trimester.

### *Haemophilus Influenzae* type b conjugate vaccine

*Haemophilus influenzae* type b (Hib) (HibTITER, ActHIB, Liquid PedvaxHIB) vaccine is a noninfectious, bacteria-derived vaccine. It is made by extracting *H. influenzae* particles that are antigenic and then chemically attaching these particles to a protein carrier medium for use in injections. The vaccine is given by injection to adults and children considered at high risk for acquiring *H. influenzae* infection. Conditions that may predispose an individual to Hib infection are septicemia, pneumonia, cellulitis, arthritis, osteomyelitis, pericarditis, sickle cell anemia, an immunodeficiency syndrome, and Hodgkin's disease. Before this vaccine was developed, infections caused by Hib were the leading cause of bacterial meningitis in children 3 months to 5 years of age. This form of bacterial meningitis has a mortality rate of 5% to 10%. Of those who survive, 20% to 45% suffer serious morbidity in the form of neurologic deficits. All Hib vaccine products are parenteral formulations that are administered intramuscularly.

### ◆ hepatitis B virus vaccine (inactivated)

Hepatitis B virus vaccine (inactivated) (Recombivax HB, Engerix-B) is a noninfectious viral vaccine containing hepatitis B surface antigen (HBsAg). It is made from viral particles and yeast using recombinant DNA technology. In this technique, DNA from two or more organisms is combined. Yeast cells then produce this viral antigenic substance in mass quantities. The substance is then attached to a carrier medium (alum) and made into a vaccine injection preparation. This antigenic HBsAg is used to promote active immunity to hepatitis B infection in persons considered at high risk for potential exposure to the hepatitis B virus or HBsAg-positive materials (e.g., blood, plasma, serum). Health care workers, for example, are persons considered at high risk, and many hospitals require this vaccination upon employment. It is recommended that all children receive this vaccine, and it is usually started shortly after birth. It is also recommended that adults with diabetes mellitus receive hepatitis B vaccination.

Use of the vaccine is contraindicated in persons who are hypersensitive to yeast. Pregnancy is not considered a contraindication to use. The vaccine is administered by intramuscular injection and is given as a series of three injections. There are three main formulations designed for three different populations: a pediatric formulation for neonates, infants, children, and adolescents; an adult formulation for persons older than 20 years of age; and a dialysis formulation for predialysis and dialysis patients and for other immunocompromised individuals.

### ◆ influenza virus vaccine

The influenza virus vaccine (Fluzone, Fluvirin, FluMist) is the vaccine used to prevent influenza. It needs to be given each year before the influenza season begins. Such inoculation is the single most important influenza control measure. FluMist is given intranasally, whereas the others are given intramuscularly.

Each year a new influenza vaccine is developed by virology researchers. It usually contains three different influenza virus strains. These strains are chosen from among the hundreds of influenza virus strains in the environment based on the latest epidemiologic data indicating which influenza viruses will most likely circulate in North America in the upcoming winter. The latest influenza vaccine in the United States also included activity against the H1N1 strain. The vaccine is made from highly purified, egg-grown viruses that have been rendered noninfectious (inactivated).

Influenza is characterized by abrupt onset of fever, myalgia, sore throat, and nonproductive cough. Severe malaise may last several days. More severe illness can occur in certain populations. Older individuals, children, and adults with underlying serious health problems (e.g., HIV infection, asthma, cardiopulmonary disease, cancer, diabetes) are at increased risk for complications from influenza infection. Health care personnel are also considered a high-risk group. Increased mortality results not only from influenza but also from other chronic diseases that can be exacerbated by influenza. More than 90% of the deaths attributed to pneumonia and influenza occur among persons 65 years of age or older. Another fairly unusual but important risk group is children and teenagers who are receiving long-term aspirin therapy (e.g., for juvenile arthritis) and who therefore might be at risk for developing Reye's syndrome after influenza (see Chapter 44).

The effectiveness of influenza vaccine varies. Factors that may alter its effectiveness are the age and immunocompetence of the vaccine recipient and the degree of similarity between the virus strains included in the vaccine and those that actually predominate during a given influenza season. Healthy persons younger than 65 years of age have a 70% chance of avoiding illness caused by influenza virus when there is a good match between the vaccine and the circulating viruses.

Older persons, especially those residing in nursing homes, can avoid severe illness, secondary complications, and death by taking the influenza vaccine. In elderly persons, the vaccine can prevent hospitalization and pneumonia up to 50% to 60% of the time and death up to 80% of the time. Achieving a high rate of vaccination among nursing home residents can reduce the spread of infection in a facility, thus preventing disease through herd immunity. The CDC now recommends that all people older than 6 months of age receive the influenza vaccine.

#### ◆ measles, mumps, and rubella virus vaccine (live)
The measles, mumps, and rubella vaccine (M-M-R II) is a virus preparation consisting of live measles, mumps, and rubella viruses that are weakened (attenuated). The vaccine promotes active immunity to these diseases by inducing the production of virus-specific immunoglobulin G and immunoglobulin M antibodies. The antibody response to initial vaccination resembles that caused by primary natural infection.

Administration of the measles vaccine or any of the combination products that includes the measles virus is contraindicated in persons with a history of anaphylactic or anaphylactoid reaction, or some other immediate reaction to egg ingestion. Use of these products is also contraindicated in persons who have had an anaphylactic reaction to topically or systemically administered neomycin, because this antibiotic is used as a preservative in some of the vaccine preparations. These vaccines are not to be administered to pregnant women, and pregnancy needs to be avoided for 3 months after measles virus vaccination and 30 days after vaccination with a rubella-containing (measles-rubella or measles-mumps-rubella [MMR]) measles virus vaccine. This precaution is based on the theoretic risk that the live virus vaccine may cause a fetal infection.

#### ◆ meningococcal vaccine
There are two meningococcal vaccines, Menactra and Menveo. They are indicated for active immunization to prevent invasive meningococcal disease caused by *Neisseria meningitidis*. Menactra is approved for patients 9 months to 55 years of age, and Menveo is approved for persons 11 to 55 years of age. The powder must be diluted with the included liquid conjugate component. Side effects include a 41% incidence of pain at injection site and a 30% incidence of headache. Other side effects include myalgia, malaise, and nausea. Caution must be used to prevent sound-alike errors with Menactra and Menomune. The most current recommendations indicate at a two-dose series be given for adults with asplenia or those who are immunocompromised. All other patients receive a one-time dose.

#### ◆ pneumococcal vaccine, polyvalent and thirteen valent
Two forms of vaccine against pneumococcal pneumonia are available that also protect against any illness caused by *Streptococcus pneumoniae. Pneumococcus* is the common name for the bacterium *S. pneumoniae,* the causative organism of this common bacterial infection. The polyvalent type of vaccine (Pneumovax 23) is used primarily in adults. (The term *polyvalent* refers to the fact that the vaccine is designed to be effective against the 23 strains of pneumococcus most commonly implicated in adult cases of pneumonia.) This vaccine also may sometimes be recommended for pediatric patients at higher risk for pneumonia as a result of serious chronic illnesses, especially those who are immunocompromised. However, the thirteen-valent vaccine is the pneumococcal vaccine that is routinely recommended for children. Its official full name is *thirteen-valent conjugate vaccine (PVC13,* or *Prevnar 13).* The name *thirteen-valent* refers to the fact that the vaccine is designed to immunize against the top thirteen pneumococcal strains found in pediatric pneumonia cases. In 2008, the CDC recommended that all smokers 19 to 64 years of age receive the pneumococcal vaccine. Contraindications to the use of either vaccine include known drug allergy to components of the vaccine itself, as well as the presence of current significant febrile illness or immunosuppressed state as a result of drug therapy (e.g., cancer chemotherapy). The vaccine may sometimes still be given in such cases, if it is felt that withholding the vaccine poses an even greater risk to the patient.

#### ◆ poliovirus vaccine (inactivated)
The use of live oral polio vaccine (OPV) is no longer routine in the United States, due to case reports of vaccine-acquired polio. Since 1979, the only indigenous cases of poliomyelitis reported in the United States (44 cases) have been associated with use of the live OPV. Injected doses of inactivated polio vaccine (brand name, IPOL) are instead recommended for routine use. The use of OPV is reserved for the following groups: populations that are the target of mass vaccination campaigns to control outbreaks of paralytic polio, unvaccinated children who will be traveling in fewer than 4 weeks to areas in which polio is endemic, and children of parents who object to the recommended number of IPV injections.

#### rabies virus vaccine
Although vaccination against the rabies virus is not normally a routine immunization, situations requiring it occur periodically in many practice settings. Rabies virus vaccine (Imovax, RabAvert) is produced using laboratory techniques involving infected human cell cultures and selected antimicrobial drugs. Rabies is a virus that can infect a variety of mammals, including skunks, foxes, raccoons, bats, dogs, and cats. The virus is usually transferred to humans by an animal bite and almost universally causes fatal brain tissue destruction if the patient is not treated with rabies vaccine and immunoglobulin (discussed later). Current recommendations call for a total of five intramuscular injections on days 0, 3, 7, 14, and 28 following an animal bite that raises concern for rabies transmission. This includes a bite by any animal whose rabies immunization status is unknown or which escapes and cannot be observed for signs of rabies. This type of treatment is known as *postexposure prophylaxis. Preexposure prophylaxis* is recommended for persons at high risk for exposure to the rabies virus (e.g., veterinarians). The preexposure course consists of only three injections on day 0, day 7, and

sometime between days 21 and 28. Periodic booster shots are also recommended for such individuals approximately every 2 to 5 years, or based on the levels of the patient's rabies virus antibody titers. Patients who have been previously immunized who have a new bite may need only two booster shots on days 0 and 3. Contraindications to the administration of rabies vaccine include a history of allergic reaction to the vaccine itself or to the drugs neomycin, gentamicin, or amphotericin B. However, given the life-threatening nature of rabies infection, treatment may still be required, with supportive therapy (e.g., epinephrine, diphenhydramine, corticosteroids) provided to minimize allergic reactions. Patients with any kind of febrile illness need to delay occupational preexposure prophylaxis treatment until the illness has subsided.

### human papillomavirus vaccine

Human papillomavirus virus (HPV) is a common cause of genital warts and cervical cancer. Genital HPV is a common virus that is transmitted through genital contact, most often during sex. Most sexually active people will get HPV at some time in their lives, although most will never even know it. It is most common in people in their late teens and early twenties. Every year, about 12,000 women are diagnosed with cervical cancer, and almost 4000 women die from this disease in the United States. The papillomavirus vaccines (Gardasil, Cervarix) are the first and only vaccines known to prevent cancer. Cervarix is a bivalent vaccine, whereas Gardasil is a quadrivalent vaccine. The most current recommendations are that either vaccine is recommended for all girls 11 and 12 years of age and for women 13 to 26 years of age who have not yet been vaccinated. In 2012, the CDC began recommending the HPV vaccine for all boys ages 11 and 12, and for males through age 21, who have not already received all three doses. The vaccine is also recommended for gay and bisexual men (or any man who has sex with men), and men with compromised immune systems (including those with HIV) through age 26 if they did not get fully vaccinated when they were younger.

HPV vaccine protects against four types of HPV: two types known to cause 70% of reported cervical cancers and two types known to cause 90% of genital warts. The vaccine is given in three injections—the first dose, and then two more doses 2 months and 6 months later. It is contraindicated in patients who show hypersensitivity to yeast or to their first injection of the vaccine. The HPV vaccine is not recommended for pregnant patients, because appropriate studies have not been completed. Pain on injection is common.

### herpes zoster vaccine

Zoster vaccine (Zostavax) is a newly released vaccine (first available in 2008) for the prevention of herpes zoster. Herpes zoster, also known as *shingles,* is an extremely painful condition caused by the varicella-zoster virus that also causes chickenpox. The vaccine is recommended for patients 50 years of age or older to prevent reactivation of the zoster virus that causes shingles. It is a one-time vaccine. The vaccine does not prevent postherpetic neuralgia. It can be given to patients who have already had shingles. Herpes zoster virus vaccine is a live attenuated vaccine. Its use is contraindicated in patients with hypersensitivity to neomycin, gelatin, or any component of the vaccine. It is also contraindicated in immunosuppressed patients or those receiving immunosuppressant therapies, as well as in pregnant women. Because it is a live vaccine, there is a risk of transmission of the virus from the person who is vaccinated to other people. The vaccine is not to be used for the prevention of chickenpox and is not given to children. The drug must be stored in the freezer.

### ♦ varicella virus vaccine

The live attenuated varicella virus vaccine (Varivax) is used to prevent varicella (chickenpox). Varicella primarily occurs in children younger than 8 years of age or in individuals with compromised immune systems such as elderly or HIV-infected patients. It is estimated that only 10% of children older than 12 years of age are still susceptible to varicella. Only 2% of adults develop varicella-zoster virus infections. However, 50% of the deaths associated with varicella are in adults. Half of these are in immunocompromised patients.

The virus in varicella vaccine is attenuated by the passage of virus particles through human and embryonic guinea pig cell cultures. Varicella vaccine must be stored in a freezer. It is not to be given to immunodeficient patients or to patients who have received high doses of systemic steroids in the previous month. It is also recommended that salicylates be avoided for 6 weeks after administration of varicella vaccine because of the possibility of Reye's syndrome (see Chapter 44). The varicella vaccine is given at 12 months of age, and then a second dose given at 4 to 6 years of age. All patients need to receive a second dose.

## PASSIVE IMMUNIZING DRUGS

The currently available antivenins, antitoxins, and immunoglobulins that compose the passive immunizing drugs are listed in Box 49-1. Those that are more commonly used are described in the following profiles.

### ♦ hepatitis B immunoglobulin

Hepatitis B immunoglobulin (BayHep B, Nabi-HB) is used to provide passive immunity against hepatitis B infection in the postexposure prophylaxis and treatment of persons exposed to hepatitis B virus or HBsAg-positive materials (e.g., blood, plasma, serum). It is prepared from the plasma of human donors with high titers of antibodies to HBsAg. All donors are tested for HIV antibodies to prevent HIV transmission.

Because of the possible devastating consequences of hepatitis B infection, pregnancy is not considered a contraindication to the use of hepatitis B immunoglobulin when there is a clear need for it.

### ♦ immunoglobulin

Immunoglobulin (BayGam, Octagam) is available in both intramuscular and intravenous dosage forms. It provides passive immunity by increasing antibody titer and antigen-antibody reaction potential. Immunoglobulins are given to help prevent certain infectious diseases in susceptible persons or to ameliorate the diseases in those already infected. Immunoglobulins are pooled from the blood of at least 1000 human donors. This plasma is prepared by cold alcohol fractionation and usually washed with a detergent to destroy any harmful viruses, such as hepatitis virus or HIV. There are many FDA-approved and non–FDA-approved uses for immunoglobulins; the approved uses are listed in Box 49-2. In recent years, there has been a shortage of immunoglobulin products. The supply of these drugs is dependent on donors. Because of fluctuations in supply and the unfavorable risk/benefit ratio of using products derived from human donors, product insurers have restricted reimbursement to force practitioners to administer the drugs for FDA-approved indications only. "Off-label" or non–FDA-approved uses have been severely curtailed because of such restrictions as well as because of product shortages.

### Rh$_0$(D) immunoglobulin

Rh$_0$(D) immunoglobulin (RhoGAM, WinRho) is used to suppress the active antibody response and the formation of anti-Rh$_0$(D) antibodies in an Rh$_0$(D)-negative person exposed to Rh-positive blood. Because an Rh$_0$(D)-negative person reacts to Rh-positive blood as if it were a foreign, "nonself" substance, an immune response develops against it and an antigen-antibody reaction occurs. This reaction can be fatal. The administration of this immunoglobulin helps to prevent the reaction. The most common use of this product is in cases of maternal-fetal Rh incompatibility (postpartum). Only the mother is normally dosed. The objective is to prevent a harmful maternal immune response to a fetus during a future pregnancy if an Rh-negative mother becomes pregnant with an Rh-positive child.

Rh$_0$(D) immunoglobulin is prepared from the plasma or serum of adults with a high titer of anti-Rh$_0$(D) antibody to the red blood cell antigen Rh$_0$(D). Administration of this immunoglobulin is contraindicated in persons who have been previously immunized with this drug and in Rh$_0$(D)-positive/Du-positive patients. It is normally given postpartum but is classified as a pregnancy category C drug.

### rabies immunoglobulin

Rabies immunoglobulin (BayRab, Imogam Rabies-HT) is a passive immunizing drug that is administered concurrently with rabies virus vaccine following suspected exposure to the rabies virus. In humans, this usually occurs after an animal bite. Rabies immunoglobulin is derived from human cells that are harvested from persons who have been immunized with rabies vaccine. The only contraindication to its use is drug allergy, although an

allergic patient may still need to be dosed rather than face infection with the almost universally fatal rabies virus. The decision to dose a patient in such a case is based on the probability of rabies infection given the particular circumstances surrounding the animal bite.

### tetanus immunoglobulin

Tetanus immunoglobulin (BayTet) is a passive immunizing drug effective against tetanus. It contains tetanus antitoxin antibodies that neutralize the bacterial exotoxin produced by *Clostridium tetani,* the bacterium that causes tetanus. Tetanus immunoglobulin is prepared from the plasma of adults who are hyperimmunized with the tetanus toxoid and is given as prophylaxis to persons with tetanus-prone wounds. It may also be used to treat active tetanus.

### varicella-zoster immunoglobulin

Varicella-zoster immunoglobulin (VZIG; available only in generic form from the American Red Cross) can be used to modify or prevent chickenpox in susceptible individuals who have had recent significant exposure to the disease. VZIG is best administered within 96 hours of exposure. Candidates for therapy with VZIG are those at high risk of serious disease or complications if they become infected with the varicella-zoster virus. Two examples are newborn children, including premature infants with significant exposure, and immunocompromised adults. If the infection manifests in a pregnant woman within 5 days of delivery, a dose of VZIG is recommended for the infant. It may also be beneficial to both mother and infant when given to the mother during pregnancy, preferably as soon as possible after diagnosis of infection. Healthy adults, including pregnant women, are evaluated on a case-by-case basis. The duration of protection against infection provided by VZIG is at least 3 weeks. VZIG is prepared from the plasma of normal blood donors with high antibody titers to varicella-zoster virus.

## BIOLOGIC AND CHEMICAL TERRORISM

Because of the terrible tragedy that occurred on September 11, 2001, there is heightened concern regarding the potential use of infectious or otherwise toxic agents as weapons against human populations. A terrorist attack involving the use of pathogenic microorganisms or other biologic agents is referred to as **bioterrorism,** whereas an attack in which harmful chemical agents are used is called *chemical terrorism.* In June 2002, President George W. Bush signed into law the Public Health Security and Bioterrorism Preparedness and Response Act (the Bioterrorism Act). This legislation marked the official beginning of the President's Countering Bioterrorism Initiative, which attempts to address this issue proactively as a matter of public health. The Center for Biologics Evaluation and Research (CBER), a branch of the FDA, is an important participant in this public health initiative. Recent CBER activities include the funding of rapid development by private industry of new vaccines for the prevention of anthrax and smallpox as well as vaccinia immunoglobulin to prepare for possible bioterrorist attack using these infectious organisms. Although smallpox vaccine is no longer routinely administered in the United States, supplies are maintained by the CDC in

## ⚡ SAFETY AND QUALITY IMPROVEMENT: PREVENTING MEDICATION ERRORS

### Tdap and DTaP

The Institute for Safe Medication Practices has reported several errors that involve incorrect use of two vaccines that are used to immunize patients against diphtheria, tetanus, and pertussis (whooping cough). Adacel (Tdap) and Daptacel (DTaP) have similar official names but are used in different situations and for different patients.

DTaP, sold under the trade names Daptacel, Tripedia, and Infanrix, contains toxoids of diphtheria and tetanus as well as the acellular pertussis vaccine. This vaccine is for active immunization of pediatric patients 6 weeks to 6 years of age.

Tdap, sold under the trade names Boostrix and Adacel, contains tetanus toxoid, reduced diphtheria toxoid, and acelluar pertussis vaccine. It is used as a booster vaccine for older children, adolescents, and adults.

The lettering gives a clue as to the contents and strengths of the various vaccines contained in each formulation. In the DTaP vaccine, the uppercase letters correspond with higher amounts of antigens of the diphtheria and pertussis components, as compared to the Tdap (where the *d* and *p* are in lowercase letters). The DTaP, with its larger amount of antigens, is indicated for initial immunizations.

If an adult received the DTaP instead of the Tdap immunization, a higher amount of the antigens is delivered and the patient usually suffers nothing more than a sore arm at the injection site. However, an infant or child who receives Tdap instead of DTaP receives a lower amount of antigen and may not be sufficiently immunized against diphtheria and pertussis.

The similar names and commonly used abbreviations are the main cause of the confusion between the two vaccines. As a result of these medication mix-ups, the manufacturers have taken steps to provide the medications with labels that are clearly marked with the vaccines' purpose. Recommendations include encouraging prescribers to order the vaccines by brand names, not by the vaccine abbreviations. In addition, ensure that parents and caregivers are aware of which vaccine is needed through the use of written information sheets.

Data from ISMP: DTaP-Tdap mix-ups now affecting hundreds of patients, *ISMP Medication Safety Alert,* July 2010, available at www.ismp.org/Newsletters/acutecare/articles/20100701.asp. Accessed October 30, 2011.

the event of a smallpox bioterrorist attack. The Department of Defense currently owns all lots of anthrax vaccine produced in the United States. Although the CDC does not currently recommend public inoculation with the anthrax vaccine, it is administered prophylactically to military personnel considered to be at higher risk of anthrax exposure because of the location and nature of their assigned duties. The Environmental Health Laboratory of the CDC's Division of Laboratory Sciences oversees planned responses to chemical terrorist attacks. One of its newest developments is the Rapid Toxic Screen. This laboratory test is able to analyze the blood and/or urine of multiple patients to detect 150 chemicals that could potentially be used in a terrorist attack to confirm exposure and direct treatment decisions. Tables 49-4 and 49-5 provide examples of microorganisms and chemical agents, respectively, believed potentially likely to be used in a terrorist attack. The chemical agents listed all have a history of prior military use. Because a small-scale attack with anthrax has already occurred in the United States, this disease is also discussed in more detail in the following section.

## ANTHRAX

In October 2001, the month following the September 11 terrorist attacks, six U.S. Postal Service workers were infected with anthrax via contaminated mail. Two of them did not survive. Anthrax is a bacterial infectious disease caused by spores of the bacterium *Bacillus anthracis.* In humans, infection can occur via three routes of exposure: skin (20% mortality), gastrointestinal tract (25% to 75% mortality), and inhalation (80% or higher mortality). Antibiotics such as the fluoroquinolone ciprofloxacin are used to treat more severe cases (i.e., the inhalational form). Milder cases (i.e., cutaneous and gastrointestinal forms) are often treated with the tetracycline antibiotic doxycycline.

## TABLE 49-4 ILLNESSES CAUSED BY CDC CATEGORY "A" POSSIBLE BIOTERRORISM AGENTS*

| NAME OF ILLNESS | CAUSATIVE ORGANISM | CLINICAL PRESENTATION | PREVENTION/TREATMENT |
|---|---|---|---|
| Anthrax | Bacterium: *Bacillus anthracis* | Inhalational form most severe and can lead to potentially fatal bacteremia | Vaccine available; treatable with antibiotics such as ciprofloxacin and dicloxacillin |
| Smallpox | Virus: vaccinia | Flulike symptoms followed by total-body disfiguring rash | Vaccine available and may be effective for up to 3 days after exposure; antiviral drug cidofovir possibly effective |
| Botulism | Bacterium: *Clostridium botulinum* | Visual changes; dry mouth; muscle weakness; progressive downward paralysis, including paralysis of diaphragm | Vaccine available only for highly exposed persons; antitoxin effective if given early in disease; immunoglobulin also now available; antibiotics of no benefit |
| Tularemia | Bacterium: *Francisella tularensis* | Severe, potentially life-threatening respiratory illness | Vaccine still under review by FDA; treatable with antibiotics such as tetracycline and ciprofloxacin |
| Viral hemorrhagic fever | Viruses: several viral causes, including Ebola, Marburg, and Lassa viruses, yellow fever virus, Argentine hemorrhagic fever virus | Bleeding from body orifices and in internal organs in severe cases; possible renal failure and coma | No vaccines except for yellow fever virus and Argentine hemorrhagic fever virus; no current treatment other than supportive care; prevention focuses on rodent control |
| Plague | Bacterium: *Yersinia pestis* | Can occur in lungs (pneumonic plague), skin (bubonic plague—most common), or blood (septicemic plague); death possible from respiratory failure and shock | No vaccine currently available in U.S.; antibiotics best if given within 24 hr and include gentamicin and tetracycline |

*CDC,* Centers for Disease Control and Prevention; *FDA,* Food and Drug Administration.
*Classified as "high-priority" biologic diseases by the CDC.
Data from U.S. Centers for Disease Control and Prevention: Emergency preparedness and response, available at www.bt.cdc.gov/bioterrorism/. Accessed March 20, 2012.

The vaccine is produced from an attenuated strain of *B. anthracis*. It has a calculated efficacy level of 92.5% for protection against anthrax infection. Anthrax vaccination is recommended for selected military personnel and others considered being at higher than average risk for exposure to the bacterium. Included are veterinarians and others who handle potentially infected animals as well as workers who process imported animal hair, which is used to manufacture various commercial products.

# NURSING PROCESS

## ASSESSMENT

Before administering a toxoid or vaccine, gather complete information about the patient's health history, including a list of medications taken (prescription, over-the-counter, and herbal), reactions to drugs, present and past health status, previous allergy test results, use of any immunosuppressants, presence of autoimmune or immunosuppressive diseases or infections, pregnancy and lactation status, and any unusual reaction to any substance. When pediatric patients are to receive a vaccine or toxoid, assess and follow the prescribed immunization schedule and dose. The Department of Health and Human Services, specifically the CDC, provides the latest recommendations for adult and pediatric immunizations in the United States. These recommendations along with cautions and contraindications are easily accessible on the Internet at www.cdc.gov and are available for referral to gain updated information prior to giving vaccines.

Because *passive immunizing drugs* may precipitate serum sickness, carefully assess patients who have chronic illnesses, are debilitated, or are elderly. This includes measuring vital signs, completing a physical assessment, and obtaining a medication history, as well as examining the results of any laboratory testing ordered by the prescriber. Document the patient's general health status with attention overall well-being and any illness. See the pharmacology discussion on passive vaccines as well as Box 49-1 and Table 49-1 for further information.

For the various *active immunizing drugs*, the pharmacology section and Tables 49-1, 49-2, and 49-3, as well as the Dosages table, provides more specific insight and information including contraindications, cautions, and drug interactions. It is also important to note that use of these drugs in the following patient groups must be considered carefully: pregnant patients; those with active infections (especially those caused by the same pathogen or organism producing the same toxin); patients with severe febrile illnesses excluding minor illnesses such as a cold, mild infection, ear infection, or low-grade fever; and patients with a history of reactions or serious adverse effects to the drug. In addition, research has shown that patients who are already immunosuppressed (e.g., those with AIDS, elderly patients, those with chronic diseases or cancer, neonates) are at increased risk for serious adverse effects to toxoids or vaccines; therefore, use these drugs cautiously or not at all in such patients. Many adults assume that the vaccines they received as children will protect them for a lifetime. This is usually the case. Some adults, however, were never vaccinated as children, or newer vaccines were not available at the time they were vaccinated. In addition, immunity may fade over time, and as an individual ages, he or she may become more susceptible to serious diseases caused by common infections, such as *Pneumococcus* infections.

*Tetanus, diphtheria, and pertussis vaccines* are to be used in patients 6 weeks to 6 years of age and are contraindicated in those with previous vaccine reactions. In addition, the use of these toxoids is contraindicated in patients with any type of neurologic reactions to the vaccine. Pertussis, or whooping cough, is very contagious, spread through respiratory secretions, and can certainly become a widespread problem. Assess age of the patient because DTaP is the preferred preparation in children from 6 weeks to 6 years of age unless the pertussis component is contraindicated. In adolescents and adults, Tdap is indicated.

The *H. influenzae* type b vaccine is administered to adults and children considered at high risk for acquiring *H. influenzae* infection, such as individuals with septicemia, pneumonia, cellulitis, arthritis, osteomyelitis, pericarditis, sickle cell anemia,

## TABLE 49-5 POSSIBLE CHEMICAL TERRORISM AGENTS

| AGENT (CLASSIFICATION) | EFFECTS | TREATMENT |
|---|---|---|
| Sarin (nerve gas) | Headache, runny nose, difficulty breathing, seizures | Remove from area; provide supportive care (e.g., mechanical ventilation). Specific antidote drugs include atropine, pralidoxime, and pyridostigmine. FDA approved special pediatric atropine dosage forms in 2003. |
| Mustard (blistering agent) | Skin burns, pulmonary edema, ocular damage | Rinse copiously with water; remove contaminated clothing; provide airway support as needed. FDA approved special skin lotion in 2003. |
| Cyanide (blood agent) | Seizures, gastrointestinal hemorrhage, respiratory arrest | Remove from area; provide airway support. Specific antidote drug therapy includes the chemicals amyl nitrite (by inhalation) and sodium nitrite and sodium thiosulfate (both by injection). |
| Chlorine (choking agent) | Eye and respiratory irritation; pulmonary edema | Remove from area; remove contaminated clothing; provide airway support. |
| Radioactive elements | DNA mutations, tissue fibrosis, vascular insufficiency, bone marrow toxicity, organ failure, pneumonitis, enteritis | Several chelating drugs are used to facilitate bodily excretion of various radioactive elements. For example, in 2004, FDA approved two new drugs (pentetate calcium trisodium and pentetate zinc trisodium) for internal decontamination of various radioactive elements (plutonium, americium, curium). |
| Ricin (by-product of processing of castor beans for production of castor oil) | Respiratory failure, seizures, fever, cough, diarrhea | Remove from area; remove and dispose of contaminated clothing; provide supportive care as needed (e.g., mechanical ventilation, intravenous hydration). |

*FDA,* Food and Drug Administration.

an immunodeficiency syndrome, or Hodgkin's disease. It is important to note that each year a new influenza vaccine is developed (see the pharmacology discussion). The latest one developed in the United States included activity against the H1N1 strain of influenza. Assess whether the patient belongs in a high-risk group for exposure, such as health care personnel. Assessment of age and medical history is important with these vaccines because individuals 65 years of age and older or those with chronic diseases are at risk for increased mortality from the influenza. The influenza virus vaccine is contraindicated in those with a known hypersensitivity to it. *Hepatitis B virus vaccines* are indicated for those at high risk for exposure to the hepatitis B virus or HBsAg-positive materials (e.g., blood, plasma, serum), such as health care workers. This vaccine is contraindicated in those allergic to yeast. Assess the need of the patient receiving the vaccine because there are different formulations for pediatric patients, adults older than 20 years of age, and individuals receiving dialysis or other immunocompromised patients.

The *MMR vaccine* is contraindicated in pregnant women, in persons with a history of anaphylactic reaction or other immediate reaction to egg ingestion, and in those with an anaphylactic reaction to topically or systemically administered neomycin. With the *meningococcal vaccine,* gather data about any history of allergies as well as age because Menactra is indicated for patients who are 9 months to 55 years of age, and Menveo is indicated for those who are 11 to 55 years of age. The *pneumococcal vaccine* is contraindicated in those with known allergy to the drug or its components or in those patients with significant febrile illness or immunosuppressed state as a result of drug therapy (e.g., chemotherapy).

Do not give the *papillomavirus vaccine* (Gardasil, Cervarix) to patients with allergies to yeast or patients who have a documented allergic reaction to the first injection of the vaccine. This vaccine is also contraindicated in pregnancy. The *zoster vaccine* (Zostavax) is for the prevention of herpes zoster. Assessment of age is an important factor in the administration of this vaccine. It is recommended for patients 50 years of age and older to prevent shingles and is not to be given to those patients with allergic reactions to neomycin, gelatin, or any component of the vaccine. Assessment of immune status is also important because it is not to be given to those who are pregnant, immunosuppressed, or receiving immunosuppressant therapies. The *varicella vaccine virus,* Varivax, is used to prevent chickenpox, which occurs mainly in those younger than 8 years of age or in those who are immunocompromised. Assess the patient's medical and medication history because it should not be given to individuals who have received high doses of systemic steroids in the previous month. Advise the patient to avoid salicylates for 6 weeks after its administration because of the risk of Reye's syndrome (see Chapter 44). Age of the patient is important because it is given at 12 months of age and then again at 4 to 6 years of age.

*Bioterrorism* and *chemical terrorism* are unfortunately a reality in today's society. Your role as a nurse may range from contributing significantly during emergency drills to preparation for a biologic terrorist attack after a warning has been issued or performing triage and carrying out the nursing process during such an attack. It may also include assessing individuals, groups, and communities and providing related education to help people understand the benefits of being informed, making plans, and maintaining a state of preparedness at all times as much as it is possible. Cultural background, level of knowledge and education, age, motor skills, cognitive abilities, awareness of extended family members and their level of preparedness, and ability to manage stress and to think during a crisis are just a few of the areas worthy of assessment. Regardless of the situation, maintain a calm, reassuring, compassionate, caring, and empathic manner during the assessment phase and all other phases of the nursing process. Avoid excessively anxiety-provoking comments or actions. Just discussing the topic of terrorism or bioterrorism can evoke fear and other emotions in individuals. Conduct questioning and assessment in a way that is calming and provides a sense of control.

## NURSING DIAGNOSES

1. Acute pain related to local and/or systemic effects of the injection of a toxoid, vaccine, or passive immunizing drug
2. Deficient knowledge related to the use of toxoids, vaccines, or passive immunizing drugs
3. Anxiety related to suspected risk of bioterrorism

## PLANNING

### GOALS

1. Patient experiences minimal pain associated with the injection of toxoid, vaccine, or immunizing drug.
2. Patient demonstrates adequate and updated knowledge regarding the use of toxoids, vaccines, or immunizing drugs.
3. Patient experiences minimal anxiety associated with the daily stress of suspected risk of bioterrorism.

### OUTCOME CRITERIA

1. Patient uses measures to increase comfort associated with injection such as the application of warm packs to the site of injection, as indicated and as ordered by the prescriber, to help relieve localized discomfort or alleviate any localized reactions.
   - Patient uses additional comfort measures such as eating small meals, controlling the environmental temperature, decreasing stimuli, increasing opportunity for rest, and using analgesics and antiinflammatory drugs as prescribed or recommended.
2. Patient states rationale and benefits versus risks of the use of toxoids, vaccines, or immunizing drugs.
   - Patient describes symptoms to report to the prescriber immediately if they occur, such as fever higher than 101° F (38.3° C), infection, wheezing, increasing weakness, or any other unusual reaction.
3. Patient minimizes anxiety by becoming more informed and staying informed about the true risk/possibility of bioterrorism.

- Patient describes full understanding of specific actions for self-protection, including reading reliable sources, staying abreast of local and national news, and even keeping special kits in the home containing items useful in a disaster, such as hurricane preparedness kits and, even more importantly, Homeland Security bioterrorism kits.

## IMPLEMENTATION

When any *immunizing drug* is administered, always check and then recheck the specific protocols and schedules of administration to ensure patient safety and accuracy. Provide individuals receiving any immunizing drug with the proper instructions and updated written materials about the medication, technique and route of administration, adverse effects, and potential complications. Educate the patient receiving the vaccine that he or she will not "get" the disease in question from receiving the attenuated or dead virus. It is also important to follow the manufacturer's recommendations concerning storage and administration of the drug, routes and site of administration, dosage, precautions pertaining to the drug's use, and contraindications to its use. Always provide the patient with a written record of immunization with the date of administration and reminder of when a booster is needed. Encourage and teach parents of young children how to maintain an accurate journal of the child's immunization status, including dates of immunization and any reactions if they occur. Prior to giving the vaccine, always inquire again about any previous reaction. Administer all immunizing drugs, as prescribed, using the route specified. The midlateral muscle of the thigh is the preferred site for infants. The deltoid muscle is preferred for older children and adults. If the patient experiences discomfort at the injection site, apply warm compresses to the site or administer an analgesic, antipyretic, or antiinflammatory medication as ordered. Have epinephrine 1:1000 readily available at the time of injection due to the risk of hypersensitivity reactions. Additionally, if fever (101° F or 38.3° C or higher), convulsions with or without fever, altered consciousness, neurologic symptoms, collapse, or somnolence occur, report them immediately to the prescriber, monitor the patient, and initiate emergency treatment as needed.

With regard to the possibility of *bioterrorism*, keep patients well informed and be aware of the need to minimize anxiety at all times. See the Patient Teaching Tips for more information.

## EVALUATION

The therapeutic response in patients receiving *immunizing drugs* is the prevention or amelioration of the specific disease being targeted. Adverse reactions for which to monitor in patients receiving immunizing drugs are specific to the drug, but there may be a localized reaction including swelling, redness, discomfort, and heat at the site of injection or a more serious reaction that must be reported immediately to the prescriber (e.g., high fever, lymphadenopathy, rash, itching, joint pain, severe flulike symptoms, decreased level of consciousness, and/or shortness of breath). For a complete list of expected reactions or adverse effects, including minor and severe, see Table 49-2. As immunizing drugs improve and newer ones are developed, it is hoped that fewer adverse effects will occur and fewer adverse drug events and complications will be seen. For biologic and chemical terrorism, constantly monitor for individuals, groups, or situations that may require intervention from other health care or governmental officials.

## PATIENT TEACHING TIPS

- A localized reaction to the injection sometimes occurs when toxoids and vaccines are administered. Inform the patient that the discomfort can be relieved by placing warm compresses on the injection site, resting, and taking acetaminophen and/or diphenhydramine, as directed by the prescriber. Instructions for the care of infants or children experiencing such reactions are generally given by the child's prescriber when the immunizing drug is administered.

- Advise the patient or parent/caregiver to notify the prescriber if high or prolonged fever, rash, itching, or shortness of breath occur after the vaccination.
- Stress that the patient or parent/caregiver always keep a double record (two copies stored in separate places) of all of the medications being taken, especially all vaccinations received.
- A vaccine adverse event reporting system is available through the FDA by calling 800-822-7967.

## KEY POINTS

- A foreign substance in the body is termed an *antigen;* the body creates a substance called an *antibody* specifically to bind to it.
- B lymphocytes (B cells), when stimulated by the binding of an antigen molecule, begin to differentiate into memory cells and plasma cells.
- Memory cells remember what that particular antigen looks like in case the body is exposed to the same antigen again in the future. Plasma cells manufacture the antibodies and will mass-produce clones of the antibodies upon reexposure to a particular antigen.
- The two types of immunity are active and passive immunity. Different types of drugs are used to induce each, and these drugs are indicated for different populations, as follows:
  - Active immunization involves administration of a toxoid or a vaccine that exposes the body to a relatively harmless form of the antigen (foreign invader) to imprint cellular memory and stimulate the body's defenses to fight any subsequent exposure. It provides long-lasting or permanent immunity. The recipient must have an active, functioning immune system to benefit.
- Passive immunization involves the administration of immunoglobulins, antitoxins, or antivenins. Serum or concentrated immunoglobulins are obtained from humans or animals and, after screening and testing, are injected into the patient, directly giving the individual the ability to fight off an invading microorganism or inactivate a toxin. Passive immunization provides temporary protection and does not stimulate an antibody response in the host. It is used in patients who are immunocompromised or who have been exposed to, or anticipate exposure to, an organism or toxin.
- Patients who are not to receive immunizing drugs include those with active infections, febrile illnesses, or history of a previous reaction to the drug. Use of these drugs in pregnant women is usually contraindicated.
- Patients who are immunocompromised are at greater risk of experiencing serious adverse effects from immunizing drugs.
- Encourage parents to keep updated records of their children's and their own immunizations with any toxoids or vaccines.

## NCLEX® EXAMINATION REVIEW QUESTIONS

1 When assessing a patient who will be receiving a measles vaccine, the nurse will consider which condition to be a possible contraindication?
   a  Anemia
   b  Pregnancy
   c  Ear infection
   d  Common cold

2 When giving a vaccination to an infant, the nurse should tell the mother to expect which adverse effect?
   a  Fever over 101° F (38.3° C)
   b  Rash
   c  Soreness at the injection site
   d  Chills

3 In the emergency department, several patients have possibly been exposed to anthrax. The nurse will prepare to administer prophylactic doses of
   a  ciprofloxacin.
   b  cidofovir.
   c  immunoglobulin.
   d  antitoxin.

4 During a routine checkup, a 72-year-old patient is advised to receive an influenza vaccine injection. He questions this, saying, "I had one last year. Why do I need another one?" What is an appropriate response from the nurse?
   a  "The effectiveness of the vaccine wears off after 6 months."
   b  "Each year a new vaccine is developed based on the flu strains that are likely to be in circulation."
   c  "When you reach 65 years of age, you need boosters on an annual basis."
   d  "Taking the flu vaccine each year allows you to build your immunity to a higher level each time."

5 A 28-year-old is in the urgent care center after stepping on a rusty tent nail. The nurse evaluates the patient's immunity status and notes that the patient thinks she had her last tetanus booster about 10 years ago, just before starting college. Which immunization would be most appropriate at this time?
   a  Immunoglobulin intravenous (Gammar-P IV)
   b  DTaP (Daptacel) (diphtheria, tetanus, and acellular pertussis)
   c  Tdap (Adacel) (diphtheria, tetanus, and acellular pertussis)
   d  No immunizations are necessary at this time.

6 The nurse is providing teaching after an adult receives a booster immunization. Which adverse reactions should be reported immediately to the health care provider? (Select all that apply.)
   a  Swelling and redness at the injection site
   b  Fever of 100° F (37.8° C)
   c  Joint pain
   d  Heat over the injection site
   e  Rash over the arms, back, and chest
   f  Shortness of breath

7 The order for an adult who needs passive hepatitis B prophylaxis reads: "Give hepatitis B immunoglobulin (Bay-Hep B), 0.06 mg/kg IM now, and then again in 30 days." The patient weighs 176 pounds. How many milligrams will this patient receive per dose?

1. b, 2. c, 3. a, 4. b, 5. c, 6. c, e, f, 7. 4.8 mg per dose

For Critical Thinking and Prioritization Questions, see http://evolve.elsevier.com/Lilley.

# Drugs Affecting the Gastrointestinal System and Nutrition

## ACTIVE QUESTIONING

There is one technique for study that cannot be overemphasized: active questioning. In the PURR study model, it is critical to be able to generate questions in the Plan, Rehearsal, and Review steps. The questions you generate when applying the PURR method are essential in helping you maintain concentration as you study, improving your comprehension as you read assigned material, and developing your long-term memory. Active questioning is a strategy that you must practice continuously. It is a strategy that develops with practice.

## WHAT ARE THE RIGHT QUESTIONS?

Some questions generated during the Plan step will be useful and will focus on exactly the right issues for maximum learning. On the other hand, sometimes the questions generated by looking at the chapter outline or accented material in the body of the text will be inappropriate. These questions seem logical and important when you are working with the limited amount of information available in the Plan step, but as you read the chapter you will find that they miss the mark. Do not worry about whether each question you ask is perfectly focused. As you read, rehearse, and review the material, you can and should revise questions based on your growing understanding of the material. The important point is to ask many questions to help you  maintain active involvement in the learning process and anticipate questions that will appear on exams. The more questions you ask, the more effective you will become, both as an active questioner and as an active learner.

## KINDS OF QUESTIONS

First, you must realize that there is more than one kind of question to be asked. Over the years, many questioning hierarchies have been proposed by educators and scholars. The different kinds of questions identified vary from three or four to as many as seven or eight. The following is a simple approach that focuses on two types of questions.

## Literal Questions

Literal questions are those that are answered directly and specifically by the text. When you were reading a story in elementary school and the teacher asked, "What did Sally do when she lost her movie money?" you were able to answer easily because the question asked for specific information that was stated clearly and directly in the story. If you were reading an American history text and found a topic heading for "The First President," an obvious question would be, "Who was the first president?" The answer is one that would be stated clearly and directly in the body of this topic. These are examples of literal questions. A literal question usually has a single correct response. The answer is stated directly in the text, and every reader will find that same information.

## Interpretive Questions

Interpretive questions are more challenging questions that require the reader to interpret, synthesize, evaluate, and analyze the material. Interpretive questions require knowing the literal information

in addition to understanding the reading material well enough to be able to select several different pieces or bits of data and put them together to formulate a response that demonstrates your understanding. In the American history example about the first president, an interpretive question might be, "Why was George Washington considered to be such an exemplary model as the first president of the new nation?" This question requires not only that you know the literal facts about Washington, but also that you be able to evaluate and judge those facts to reach a conclusion that could be supported by the literal information. Even though a question is interpretive, it is possible that there is only one correct response. However, it is equally possible that there is more than one correct response to an interpretive question. The literal information can be evaluated in a number of different ways in responding to the question, and the answers derived by different readers will vary. This is why it is a good choice to work with a study group when reviewing for interpretive

questions. A study group can develop a variety of responses that result in a more comprehensive understanding of the course material. This depth of learning is what is necessary to pass not only your course test but also the NCLEX Examination, as well as to become a competent nurse. Both literal and interpretive questions are essential in the learning process.

## QUESTIONING APPLICATION

Italicization is used to gain the reader's attention and to indicate that the italicized material is especially noteworthy. Accented material should always be considered as a potential source of questions. Again, the questioning can begin with simple, literal questions, but it is essential that interpretive questions also be asked. Your questions should require that you read for broader general understanding and not just focus on "the facts."

Critical Thinking and Prioritization Questions are available on the Evolve website for your textbook. Even though you may answer these questions as they are stated, you should consider generating additional questions of your own. The first question for Chapter 53 is, "The nurse is about to administer calcium supplemental therapy to a patient with a history of cardiac disease. What is the most important assessment that is needed before the nurse gives the drug?" In answering this question, some additional questions will help you focus your learning. What is calcium supplemental therapy? How does calcium affect cardiac patients? Why? Is calcium supplemental therapy inappropriate for all cardiac patients? If not, what are the circumstances that might rule out supplemental calcium? Of what signs and symptoms should the caregiver be aware if calcium supplemental therapy is being administered to a cardiac patient?

The more active you become as a questioner, the easier it will become to ask the kinds of questions that are necessary for your own learning.

# Acid-Controlling Drugs

## OBJECTIVES

When you reach the end of this chapter, you will be able to do the following:

1. Discuss the physiologic influence of various pathologies, such as peptic ulcer disease, gastritis, spastic colon, gastro-esophageal reflux disease, and hyperacidic states, on the health of patients and their gastrointestinal tracts.

2. Describe the mechanisms of action, indications, cautions, contraindications, drug interactions, adverse effects, dosages, and routes of administration for the following classes of acid-controlling drugs: antacids, histamine 2 ($H_2$)–blocking drugs ($H_2$ receptor antagonists), proton pump inhibitors, and acid suppressants.

3. Develop a nursing care plan that includes all phases of the nursing process for patients receiving acid-controlling drugs.

## DRUG PROFILES

antacids, general, p. 819
♦ cimetidine, p. 821
♦ famotidine, p. 822
lansoprazole, p. 823
misoprostol, p. 824
omeprazole, p. 823

pantoprazole, p. 823
ranitidine, p. 822
simethicone, p. 824
♦ sucralfate, p. 823

_____

♦ *Key drug*

## KEY TERMS

Antacids Basic compounds composed of different combinations of acid-neutralizing ionic salts. (p. 818)

Chief cells Cells in the stomach that secrete the gastric enzyme pepsinogen (a precursor to pepsin). (p. 816)

Gastric glands Secretory glands in the stomach containing the following cell types: parietal, chief, mucous, endocrine, and enterochromaffin. (p. 816)

Gastric hyperacidity The overproduction of stomach acid. (p. 816)

Hydrochloric acid (HCl) An acid secreted by the *parietal cells* in the lining of the stomach that maintains the environment of the stomach at a pH of 1 to 4. (p. 816)

Mucous cells Cells whose function in the stomach is to secrete mucus that serves as a protective mucous coat against the digestive properties of HCl. Also called *surface epithelial cells.* (p. 816)

Parietal cells Cells in the stomach that produce and secrete HCl. These cells are the primary site of action for many of the drugs used to treat acid-related disorders. (p. 816)

Pepsin An enzyme in the stomach that breaks down proteins. (p. 816)

One of the conditions of the stomach requiring drug therapy is hyperacidity, or excessive acid production. Left untreated, hyperacidity can lead to serious conditions such as acid reflux, ulcer disease, esophageal damage, and even esophageal cancer. Overproduction of stomach acid is also referred to as gastric hyperacidity.

## ANATOMY, PHYSIOLOGY, AND PATHOPHYSIOLOGY OVERVIEW

### ACID-RELATED PATHOPHYSIOLOGY

The stomach secretes several substances with various physiologic functions, including the following:

- Hydrochloric acid, an acid that aids digestion and also serves as a barrier to infection
- Bicarbonate, a base that is a natural mechanism to prevent hyperacidity
- Pepsinogen, an enzymatic precursor to pepsin, an enzyme that digests dietary proteins
- Intrinsic factor, a glycoprotein that facilitates gastric absorption of vitamin $B_{12}$
- Mucus, which protects the stomach lining from both hydrochloric acid and digestive enzymes
- Prostaglandins, which have a variety of antiinflammatory and protective functions (see Chapter 44)

The stomach, although one structure, can be divided into three functional areas. Each area is associated with specific glands. These glands are composed of different cells, and these cells secrete different substances. Figure 50-1 shows the three functional areas of the stomach and the distribution of the associated types of stomach glands.

The three primary types of glands in the stomach are the cardiac, pyloric, and gastric glands. These glands are named for their positions in the stomach. The cardiac glands are located around the cardiac sphincter (also known as the *gastroesophageal sphincter*); the gastric glands are in the fundus, also known as the *greater part of the body of the stomach;* and the pyloric glands are in the pyloric region and in the transitional area between the pyloric and the fundic zones.

The gastric glands are highly specialized secretory glands composed of several different types of cells: parietal, chief, mucous, endocrine, and enterochromaffin. Each cell secretes a specific substance. The three most important cell types are parietal cells, chief cells, and mucous cells. These cells are depicted in Figure 50-1.

Parietal cells produce and secrete hydrochloric acid (HCl). They are the primary site of action for many of the drugs used to treat acid-related disorders. Chief cells secrete *pepsinogen*. Pepsinogen is a *proenzyme* (enzyme precursor) that becomes pepsin when activated by exposure to acid. Pepsin breaks down proteins and is therefore referred to as a *proteolytic* enzyme. Mucous cells are mucus-secreting cells that are also called *surface epithelial cells.* The secreted mucus serves as a protective coating against the digestive action of hydrochloric acid and digestive enzymes.

These three cell types play an important role in the digestive process. When the balance of these cells and their secretions is

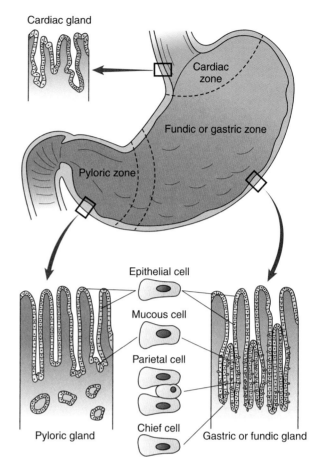

**FIGURE 50-1** The three zones of the stomach and the associated glands.

impaired, acid-related diseases can occur. The most harmful of these involve hypersecretion of acid and include peptic ulcer disease and esophageal cancer. However, the most common condition is mild to moderate hyperacidity. Many lay terms (e.g., indigestion, sour stomach, heartburn, acid stomach) have been used to describe this condition of overproduction of hydrochloric acid by the parietal cells. Hyperacidity is often associated with gastroesophageal reflux disease (GERD). This is the tendency of excessive and acidic stomach contents to back up, or reflux, into the lower (and even upper) esophagus. Over time, this condition can lead to more serious disorders such as erosive esophagitis and Barrett esophagus, a precancerous condition. Therefore, to prevent serious disorders from occurring and to promote patient comfort, GERD is aggressively treated with one or more of the medications described in this section.

Hydrochloric acid is secreted by the parietal cells in the lining of the stomach and maintains the environment of the stomach at a pH of 1 to 4. This acidity aids in the proper digestion of food and also serves as one of the body's defenses against microbial infection via the gastrointestinal (GI) tract. Several substances stimulate hydrochloric acid secretion by the parietal cells, such as food, caffeine, chocolate, and alcohol. In moderation, any of these is usually not problematic. However, excessive consumption of large, fatty meals or alcohol, as well as emotional stress, may result in hyperproduction of hydrochloric acid and lead to hypersecretory disorders such as peptic ulcer disease.

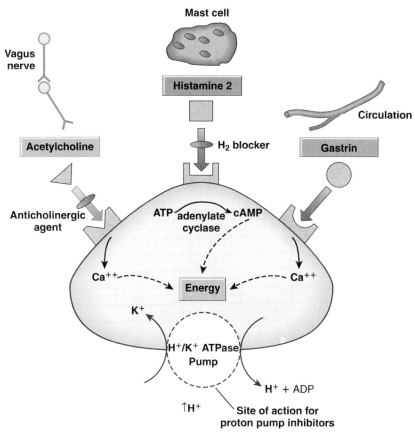

**FIGURE 50-2** Parietal cell stimulation and secretion. *ADP,* Adenosine diphosphate; *ATP,* adenosine triphosphate; *ATPase,* adenosine triphosphatase; *cAMP,* cyclic adenosine monophosphate.

The parietal cell is the primary target for many of the most effective drugs for the treatment of acid-related disorders. A closer look at how the parietal cell receives signals to produce and secrete hydrochloric acid will enhance the understanding of the mechanism of action of many of the drugs used to treat acid-related disorders.

The wall of the parietal cell contains three types of receptors: acetylcholine (ACh), histamine, and gastrin. When any one of these is occupied by its corresponding chemical stimulant (ACh, histamine, or gastrin, which can all be considered *first messengers*), the parietal cell will produce and secrete hydrochloric acid. Figure 50-2 shows the parietal cell with its three receptors. Once these receptors have become occupied, a *second messenger* is sent inside the cell. In the case of histamine receptors, occupation results in the production of adenylate cyclase. Adenylate cyclase converts adenosine triphosphate (ATP) to cyclic adenosine monophosphate (cAMP), which provides energy for the proton pump. The proton pump—or, more precisely, the hydrogen–potassium–adenosine triphosphatase (ATPase) pump—is a pump for the transport of hydrogen ions and is located in the parietal cells. The pump requires energy to work. If energy is present, the proton pump will be activated, and the pump will be able to transport hydrogen ions needed for the production of hydrochloric acid.

In the case of both ACh and gastrin receptors, the second messenger that drives the proton pump is not cAMP but is instead calcium ions. Anticholinergic drugs (see Chapter 21)

such as atropine block ACh receptors, which also results in decreased hydrogen ion secretion from the parietal cells. However, these drugs are no longer used for this purpose and have been superseded by other drug classes discussed in this chapter. There is currently no drug to block the binding of the hormone gastrin to its corresponding receptor on the parietal cell surface.

*Peptic ulcer disease* is a general term for gastric or duodenal ulcers that involve digestion of the GI mucosa by the enzyme pepsin. Pepsin normally breaks down only food proteins and is the activated form of pepsinogen. Pepsinogen is produced by the chief cells of the stomach in response to hydrochloric acid released from the parietal cells. The sight, smell, and taste of food and its presence in the stomach are the primary stimulus for the release of hydrochloric acid from the parietal cells. Because the process of ulceration is driven by the proteolytic (protein breakdown) actions of pepsin together with the caustic effects of hydrochloric acid, peptic ulcer disease and related problems are also referred to by the more general term *acid-peptic disorders.*

In 1983, a gram-negative spiral bacterium, *Campylobacter pylori*, was isolated from several patients with gastritis. Over the next few years this bacterium was studied further, and it became implicated in the pathophysiology of peptic ulcer disease. The official name of the bacterium was changed to *Helicobacter pylori* because it was felt to have more characteristics of the *Helicobacter* genus. The prevalence of *H. pylori* as measured by serum antibody tests is approximately 40% to 60%

for patients older than 60 years of age but only 10% for those younger than 30 years of age. The bacterium is found in the GI tracts of roughly 90% of patients with duodenal ulcers and 70% of those with gastric ulcers. This bacterium is also found in many patients who do not have peptic ulcer disease, and its presence is not associated with acute, perforating ulcers. These latter observations suggest that more than one factor is involved in ulceration. The American College of Gastroenterologists published treatment guidelines in 2007 for *H. pylori* infections. First-line therapy includes a 10- to 14-day course of a proton pump inhibitor (discussed later in the chapter) and the antibiotics clarithromycin and either amoxicillin or metronidazole (see Chapters 38 and 39) or a combination of a proton pump inhibitor, bismuth subsalicylate (see Chapter 51), and the antibiotics tetracycline and metronidazole (see Chapters 38 and 39). Many different combinations are used, but all incorporate the aforementioned key drugs.

Stress-related mucosal damage is an important issue for critically ill patients. Stress ulcer prophylaxis (or therapy to prevent severe GI damage) is undertaken in almost every critically ill patient in an intensive care unit (ICU) and for many patients on general medical surgical units. GI lesions are a common finding in ICU patients, especially within the first 24 hours after admission. The etiology and pathophysiology of stress-related mucosal damage is multifactorial and is not fully understood. Factors include decreased blood flow, mucosal ischemia, hypoperfusion, and reperfusion injury. Procedures performed commonly in critically ill patients, such as passing nasogastric (NG) tubes, placing patients on ventilators, and others, predispose patients to bleeding of the GI tract. Coagulopathy, a history of peptic ulcer or GI bleed, sepsis, use of steroids, ICU stay of longer than 1 week, and occult bleeding are considered to indicate high risk of GI lesions. Guidelines suggest that all such patients receive either a histamine receptor–blocking drug or a proton pump inhibitor, both of which are discussed in detail in this chapter.

## PHARMACOLOGY OVERVIEW

### ANTACIDS

Antacids are basic compounds used to neutralize stomach acid. Most commonly they are nonprescription salts of aluminum, magnesium, calcium, and/or sodium. They have been used for centuries in the treatment of patients with acid-related disorders. The ancient Greeks used crushed coral (calcium carbonate) in the first century AD to treat patients with dyspepsia. Antacids were the principal antiulcer treatment, along with anticholinergic drugs, until the introduction of the *histamine 2 (H₂) receptor antagonists* in the late 1970s. The use of anticholinergic drugs has fallen out of favor; however, the antacids, especially the over-the-counter (OTC) formulations, are still used extensively. They are available in a variety of dosage forms, some including more than one antacid salt. In addition, many antacid preparations also contain the *antiflatulent* (antigas) drug simethicone (see the section on miscellaneous acid-controlling drugs), which reduces gas and bloating.

Many aluminum- and calcium-based formulations also include magnesium, which not only contributes to the acid-neutralizing capacity but also counteracts the constipating effects of aluminum and calcium. There are multiple salts of calcium, with calcium carbonate being used most often. However, calcium antacids may lead to the development of kidney stones and increased gastric acid secretion, so they are not used as frequently as other antacids. Antacids containing magnesium must be avoided in patients with renal failure. Sodium bicarbonate is a highly soluble antacid form with a quick onset but short duration of action.

## Mechanism of Action and Drug Effects

Antacids work primarily by neutralizing gastric acidity. They do not prevent the overproduction of acid but instead help to neutralize acid secretions. It is also believed that antacids promote gastric mucosal defensive mechanisms, especially at lower dosages. They do this by stimulating the secretion of mucus, prostaglandins, and bicarbonate from the cells inside the gastric glands. Mucus serves as a protective barrier against the destructive actions of hydrochloric acid. Bicarbonate helps buffer the acidity of hydrochloric acid. Prostaglandins prevent histamine from binding to its corresponding parietal cell receptors, which inhibits the production of adenylate cyclase. Without adenylate cyclase, no cAMP can be formed and no second messenger is available to activate the proton pump (see Figure 50-2).

The primary drug effect of antacids is the reduction of the symptoms associated with various acid-related disorders, such as pain and reflux ("heartburn"). A dose of antacid that raises the gastric pH from 1.3 to 1.6 (only 0.3 point) reduces gastric acidity by 50%, whereas acidity is reduced by 90% if the pH is raised an entire point (e.g., 1.3 to 2.3). Antacid-associated pain reduction is thought to be a result of base-mediated inhibition of the protein-digesting ability of pepsin, increase in the resistance of the stomach lining to irritation, and increase in the tone of the cardiac sphincter, which reduces reflux from the stomach.

## Indications

Antacids are indicated for the acute relief of symptoms associated with peptic ulcer, gastritis, gastric hyperacidity, and heartburn.

## Contraindications

The only usual contraindication to antacid use is known allergy to a specific drug product. Other contraindications may include severe renal failure or electrolyte disturbances (because of the potential toxic accumulation of electrolytes in the antacids themselves) and GI obstruction (antacids may stimulate GI motility when it is undesirable because of the presence of an obstructive process requiring surgical intervention).

## Adverse Effects

The adverse effects of the antacids are limited. The magnesium preparations, especially milk of magnesia, can cause diarrhea. Both the aluminum- and calcium-containing formulations can result in constipation. Calcium products can also cause kidney

Aluminum, used to reduce gastric acid, binds to phosphate and may lead to hypercalcemia. Early hypercalcemia is characterized by constipation, headache, increased thirst, dry mouth, decreased appetite, irritability, and a metallic taste in the mouth. Later signs and symptoms of hypercalcemia include confusion, drowsiness, increase in blood pressure, irregular heart rate, nausea, vomiting, and increased urination. Use of aluminum-based antacids may also produce hypophosphatemia, which is characterized by loss of appetite, malaise, muscle weakness, and/or bone pain. The use of calcium-containing antacids (e.g., calcium carbonate) may lead to *milk-alkali syndrome,* which is associated with headache, anorexia, nausea, vomiting, and unusual tiredness. Use of sodium bicarbonate may lead to metabolic alkalosis if the drug is abused or used over the long term. Alkalosis is manifested by irritability, muscle twitching, numbness and tingling, cyanosis, slow and shallow respirations, headache, thirst, and nausea. Acid rebound occurs with the discontinuation of antacids that have high acid-neutralizing capacity and with overuse or misuse of antacid therapy. If acid neutralization is sudden and high, the result is an immediate elevation in pH to alkalinity and just as rapid a decline in pH to a more acidic state in the gut.

**TABLE 50-1   ANTACIDS: DRUG INTERACTIONS**

| INTERACTING DRUG | MECHANISM | RESULT |
|---|---|---|
| Benzodiazepines Sulfonylureas Sympathomimetics valproic acid | pH effects | Increased activity of interacting drugs |
| allopurinol tetracycline Thyroid hormones captopril Corticosteroids digoxin Histamine antagonists phenytoin isoniazid ketoconazole methotrexate nitrofurantoin Phenothiazines Salicylates Quinolone antibiotics | Decreased GI absorption | Reduced effects of interacting drugs |

stones. Excessive use of any antacid can theoretically result in systemic alkalosis. This is more common with sodium bicarbonate. Another adverse effect that is more common with the calcium-containing products is rebound hyperacidity, or acid rebound, in which the patient experiences hyperacidity when antacid use is discontinued. Long-term self-medication with antacids may mask symptoms of serious underlying disease such as bleeding ulcer or malignancy. Patients with ongoing symptoms need to undergo regular medical evaluations, because additional medications or other interventions may be needed. Box 50-1 lists several specific nursing concerns for patients taking antacids.

## Interactions

Antacids are capable of causing several interactions when administered with other drugs (see Table 50-1). There are four basic mechanisms by which antacids cause interactions:
- *Adsorption* of other drugs to antacids, which reduces the ability of the other drug to be absorbed into the body
- *Chelation,* which is the chemical inactivation of other drugs that produces insoluble complexes
- *Increased stomach pH,* which increases the absorption of basic drugs and decreases the absorption of acidic drugs
- *Increased urinary pH,* which increases the excretion of acidic drugs and decreases the excretion of basic drugs

Most drugs are either weak acids or weak bases. Therefore, pH conditions in both the GI and urinary tracts will affect the extent to which drug molecules are absorbed. Common examples of drugs whose effects may be chemically enhanced by the presence of antacids (due to pH effects) are benzodiazepines, sulfonylureas (effects may also be reduced, depending on the drugs involved), sympathomimetics, and valproic acid. More commonly, the presence of antacids reduces the efficacy of interacting drugs by interfering with their GI absorption. Such drugs include allopurinol, tetracycline, thyroid hormones, captopril, corticosteroids, digoxin, histamine antagonists, phenytoin,

isoniazid, ketoconazole, methotrexate, nitrofurantoin, phenothiazines, salicylates, and quinolone antibiotics. Advise patients to dose any interacting drugs at least 1 to 2 hours before or after antacids are taken. Significant patient harm may ensue when the quinolone antibiotics (ciprofloxacin, levofloxacin, moxifloxacin) are given with antacids. These antibiotics are administered orally to treat serious infections. Antacids can reduce their absorption by more than 50%. Thus, antacids must be given either 2 hours before or 2 hours after the dose of a quinolone antibiotic.

## Dosages

For dosage information on selected antacid drugs, see the table on p. 820.

## DRUG PROFILES

### antacids, general
Some of the available magnesium, aluminum, calcium, and sodium salts that are used in many of the antacid formulations are listed in Box 50-2. There are far too many individual antacid products on the market to mention all formulations. Briefly, OTC antacid formulations are available as capsules, chewable tablets, effervescent granules and tablets, powders, suspensions, and plain tablets. This allows patients a variety of options for self-medication. Pharmacokinetic parameters are not normally listed for antacids, but these drugs are generally excreted quickly through the GI tract and/or the electrolyte homeostatic mechanisms of the kidneys. Antacids are considered safe for use during pregnancy if prolonged administration and high dosages are avoided. It is recommended that pregnant women consult their health care providers before taking an antacid. Aluminum- and sodium-based antacids are often recommended for patients with renal compromise because they are more easily excreted than

## DOSAGES

### Selected Antacid Drugs*

| DRUG (PREGNANCY CATEGORY) | PHARMACOLOGIC CLASS | USUAL DOSAGE RANGE | INDICATIONS |
|---|---|---|---|
| aluminum hydroxide (Amphojel) (A) | Aluminum-containing antacid | **Adult**<br>PO: 600-1500 mg 3-6 times per day | Hyperacidity |
| aluminum hydroxide and magnesium hydroxide (Maalox, Mylanta) (A) | Combination antacid | **Adult**<br>400-2400 mg 3-6 times per day | Hyperacidity |
| calcium carbonate (Tums) (A) | Calcium-containing antacid | **Adult**<br>PO: 0.5-1.5 g prn | Hyperacidity |
| magnesium hydroxide (milk of magnesia) (A) | Magnesium-containing antacid | **Adult**<br>PO: 0.65-1.3 g prn, up to 4 times per day | Hyperacidity (more commonly used as a laxative) |

*PO*, Oral.

*Many more antacid products are available on the market than appear in this table. Dosages given are approximate dosages of active ingredients; there may be variations among different products and different dosage forms of the same product.

---

### BOX 50-2   ANTACIDS

**Antacids: Salt Content**

| MAGNESIUM SALTS | ALUMINUM SALTS | CALCIUM SALTS | SODIUM SALTS |
|---|---|---|---|
| Carbonate | Carbonate | Carbonate | Bicarbonate |
| Hydroxide | Hydroxide | | Citrate |
| Oxide | | | |
| Trisilicate | | | |

**Commonly Available Antacid Products**

*Magnesium-Containing Antacids*
Carbonate salt: Gaviscon Liquid, Gaviscon Extra Strength Relief Formula Tablets
Hydroxide salt: milk of magnesia
Oxide salt: Mag-Ox (included for information only; used primarily as a magnesium supplement)
Trisilicate salt: Gaviscon Tablets

*Aluminum-Containing Antacids*
Carbonate salt: Basaljel
Hydroxide salt: AlternaGEL, Amphojel
Combination products: Gaviscon, Maalox, Mylanta, Di-Gel

*Calcium-Containing Antacids*
Carbonate salt: Tums, Maalox Antacid Caplets, Extra Strength Alkets Antacid

*Sodium-Containing Antacids*
Bicarbonate salt: Alka-Seltzer
Citrate salt: Citra pH

antacids in other categories. Calcium-containing antacids are currently advertised as an extra source of calcium. Calcium carbonate neutralization will produce gas and possibly belching. For this reason, it may be combined with an antiflatulent drug such as simethicone (see the section on Miscellaneous Acid-Controlling Drugs). Magnesium-containing antacids commonly have a laxative effect, and frequent administration of these antacids alone often cannot be tolerated. Both calcium- and magnesium-based antacids are more likely to accumulate to toxic levels in patients with renal disease and are often avoided in this patient group.

## H₂ RECEPTOR ANTAGONISTS

$H_2$ receptor antagonists, commonly abbreviated as H2RAs and also called *$H_2$ receptor blockers*, are the prototypical acid-secretion antagonists. These drugs reduce but do not completely abolish acid secretion. They have become the most popular drugs for the treatment of many acid-related disorders, including peptic ulcer disease. This can be attributed to their efficacy, patient acceptance, and excellent safety profile. These drugs include cimetidine, ranitidine, famotidine, and nizatidine. There is little difference among the four available $H_2$ receptor antagonists from the standpoint of efficacy. All are available OTC.

### Mechanism of Action and Drug Effects

$H_2$ receptor antagonists competitively block the $H_2$ receptor of acid-producing parietal cells. This makes the parietal cell less responsive not only to histamine but also to the stimulation of ACh and gastrin. This is shown in Figure 50-2. Up to 90% inhibition of vagal- and gastrin-stimulated acid secretion occurs when histamine is blocked. However, complete inhibition has not been shown. The effect of these drugs is reduced hydrogen ion secretion from the parietal cells, which results in an increase in the pH of the stomach and relief of many of the symptoms associated with hyperacidity-related conditions.

### Indications

$H_2$ receptor antagonists have several therapeutic uses, including treatment of GERD, peptic ulcer disease, and erosive esophagitis; adjunct therapy in the control of upper GI tract bleeding; and treatment of pathologic gastric hypersecretory conditions such as Zollinger-Ellison syndrome. The latter is one form of hyperchlorhydria, or excessive gastric acidity. $H_2$ receptor antagonists are commonly used for stress ulcer prophylaxis in critically ill patients.

### Contraindications

The only usual contraindication to the use of $H_2$ receptor antagonists is a known drug allergy. Liver and/or kidney dysfunction are relative contraindications that may warrant dosage adjustment.

| TABLE 50-2 | $H_2$ RECEPTOR ANTAGONISTS: ADVERSE EFFECTS |
|---|---|
| **BODY SYSTEM** | **ADVERSE EFFECTS** |
| Cardiovascular | Hypotension (monitor for this effect with intravenous administration) |
| Central nervous | Headache, lethargy, confusion, depression, hallucinations, slurred speech, agitation |
| Endocrine | Increased prolactin secretion, gynecomastia (with cimetidine) |
| Gastrointestinal | Diarrhea, nausea, abdominal cramps |
| Genitourinary | Impotence; increased blood urea nitrogen, creatinine levels |
| Hepatobiliary | Elevated liver enzyme levels, jaundice |
| Hematologic | Agranulocytosis, thrombocytopenia, neutropenia, aplastic anemia |
| Integumentary | Urticaria, rash, alopecia, sweating, flushing, exfoliative dermatitis |

## Adverse Effects

The $H_2$ receptor antagonists have a remarkably low incidence of adverse effects (less than 3% of cases). The four available $H_2$ receptor antagonists are similar in many respects but have some differences in adverse effect profiles. Table 50-2 lists the adverse effects associated with these drugs. Central nervous system adverse effects occur in less than 1% of patients taking these drugs but are sometimes seen in elderly patients. These adverse effects include confusion and disorientation. Be alert for mental status changes when giving these drugs, especially if they are new to the patient. Cimetidine may induce impotence and gynecomastia. This is the result of cimetidine's inhibition of estradiol metabolism and displacement of dihydrotestosterone from peripheral androgen-binding sites. All four $H_2$ receptor antagonists may increase the secretion of prolactin from the anterior pituitary gland. Thrombocytopenia has been reported with ranitidine and famotidine.

## Interactions

Cimetidine carries a higher risk of drug interactions than the other three drugs, especially in elderly patients. These interactions may be of clinical importance. Cimetidine binds enzymes of the hepatic cytochrome P-450 microsomal oxidase system. This is a group of enzymes in the liver that metabolize many different drugs. By inhibiting the metabolism of drugs metabolized via this pathway, cimetidine may raise the blood concentrations of certain drugs. Ranitidine has only 10% to 20% of the binding action of cimetidine on the P-450 system, and nizatidine and famotidine have essentially no effect. This interaction has little clinical significance for most drugs; however, significant interactions are more likely to arise with medications having a narrow therapeutic range, such as theophylline, warfarin, lidocaine, and phenytoin. All $H_2$ receptor antagonists may inhibit the absorption of certain drugs, such as ketoconazole, that require an acidic GI environment for gastric absorption. Smoking has also been shown to decrease the effectiveness of $H_2$ antagonists. For optimal results, $H_2$ receptor antagonists are taken 1 to 2 hours before antacids.

## DOSAGES

### Selected $H_2$ Receptor Antagonists

| DRUG (PREGNANCY CATEGORY) | USUAL DOSAGE RANGE | INDICATIONS |
|---|---|---|
| ♦ cimetidine (Tagamet, Tagamet HB) (B) | **Adult** PO: 200 mg bid | Dyspepsia, heartburn |
| | PO: 300 mg qid or 400 mg bid and at bedtime or 800 mg at bedtime | Ulcers |
| | PO: 1600 mg/day divided in 2 to 4 doses | GERD |
| | PO/IM/IV: 300 mg tid and at bedtime; do not exceed 2400 mg/day | Pathologic hypersecretion |
| ♦ famotidine (Pepcid, Pepcid AC) (B) | **Adult** PO: 10 mg daily-bid | Dyspepsia, heartburn |
| | PO: 40 mg daily at bedtime or 20 mg bid | Ulcers |
| | PO: 20-160 mg q6h IV: 20 mg q12h | Pathologic hypersecretion |
| | PO: 20 mg bid | GERD |
| ranitidine (Zantac) (B) | **Adult** PO: 75 mg bid | Dyspepsia, heartburn |
| | PO: 150 mg daily-bid or 300 mg at bedtime | Ulcers |
| | PO: 150 mg bid | |
| | PO: 150 mg qid | Erosive esophagitis |

*GERD*, Gastroesophageal reflux disease; *IM*, intramuscular; *IV*, intravenous; *PO*, oral.

## Dosages

For dosage information on the $H_2$ antagonists, see the table above.

## DRUG PROFILES

$H_2$ receptor antagonists are the prototypical acid-secretion antagonists. These drugs reduce acid secretion. They are among the most commonly used drugs in the world, due to their efficacy, OTC availability, and overall excellent safety profile. However, this drug class has been partially replaced by proton pump inhibitors (see the next section).

### ♦ cimetidine

In 1977, cimetidine (Tagamet) became the first drug in this class to be released on the market. It is the prototypical $H_2$ receptor antagonist and was the first major prescription drug to go OTC. Because of its potential to cause drug interactions, its use has been largely replaced by ranitidine and famotidine. Cimetidine is still used to treat certain allergic reactions.

### Pharmacokinetics

| Route | Onset of Action | Peak Plasma Concentration | Elimination Half-life | Duration of Action |
|---|---|---|---|---|
| PO | 15-60 min | 1-2 hr | 2 hr | 4-5 hr |

### ranitidine

Ranitidine (Zantac) was the second $H_2$ receptor antagonist introduced. It does not carry the concerns over drug interactions that cimetidine has and has become the most widely used $H_2$ receptor antagonist. It is available in oral and intravenous forms. Dosing is different for the different forms: oral ranitidine is dosed as 150 mg twice a day or 300 mg at bedtime, whereas the intravenous form is dosed at 50 mg every 8 hours.

#### Pharmacokinetics

| Route | Onset of Action | Peak Plasma Concentration | Elimination Half-life | Duration of Action |
|-------|-----------------|---------------------------|------------------------|--------------------|
| PO    | 1 hr            | 2-4 hr                    | 2-3 hr                 | 4-12 hr            |
| IV    | Immediate       | Less than 15 min          | 2-3 hr                 | 4-12 hr            |

### ◆ famotidine

Famotidine (Pepcid) was the last $H_2$ receptor antagonist introduced and, like ranitidine, has no drug interaction concerns. It is available in oral and injectable forms. The dosing is the same for both forms.

#### Pharmacokinetics

| Route | Onset of Action | Peak Plasma Concentration | Elimination Half-life | Duration of Action |
|-------|-----------------|---------------------------|------------------------|--------------------|
| PO    | 1.4 hr          | 3 hr                      | 2.6-4 hr               | 9-12 hr            |
| IV    | Immediate       | Less than 15 min          | 2.6-4 hr               | 9-12 hr            |

## PROTON PUMP INHIBITORS

The newest drugs introduced for the treatment of acid-related disorders are the proton pump inhibitors (PPIs). These include lansoprazole (Prevacid), omeprazole (Prilosec), rabeprazole (AcipHex), pantoprazole (Protonix), and esomeprazole (Nexium). These drugs are even more powerful than the $H_2$ receptor antagonists. The PPIs bind directly to the hydrogen-potassium-ATPase pump mechanism and irreversibly inhibit the action of this enzyme, which results in a total blockage of hydrogen ion secretion from the parietal cells.

### Mechanism of Action and Drug Effects

The action of the hydrogen-potassium-ATPase pump is the final step in the acid-secretory process of the parietal cell (see Figure 50-2). If chemical energy is present to run the pump, the pump will transport hydrogen ions out of the parietal cell, which increases the acid content of the surrounding gastric lumen and lowers the pH. Because hydrogen ions are protons (positively charged atoms), this ion pump is also called the *proton pump*. PPIs bind irreversibly to the proton pump. This inhibition prevents the movement of hydrogen ions out of the parietal cell into the stomach and thereby blocks all gastric acid secretion. The PPIs stop more than 90% of acid secretion over 24 hours, which makes most patients temporarily achlorhydric (without acid). However, food absorption is not affected. For acid secretion to return to normal after a PPI has been stopped, the parietal cell must synthesize new hydrogen-potassium-ATPase.

Although there are other proton pumps in the body, hydrogen-potassium-ATPase is structurally and mechanically distinct from other hydrogen-transporting enzymes and appears to exist only in the parietal cells. Thus, the action of PPIs is limited to its effects on gastric acid secretion.

### Indications

PPIs are currently indicated as first-line therapy for erosive esophagitis, symptomatic GERD that is poorly responsive to other medical treatment such as therapy with $H_2$ receptor antagonists, short-term treatment of active duodenal ulcers and active benign gastric ulcers, gastric hypersecretory conditions (e.g., Zollinger-Ellison syndrome), nonsteroidal antiinflammatory drug (NSAID)–induced ulcers, and for stress ulcer prophylaxis. Long-term therapeutic uses include maintenance of healing of erosive esophagitis and pathologic hypersecretory conditions, including both GERD and Zollinger-Ellison syndrome. All of the PPIs can be used in combination with antibiotics to treat patients with *H. pylori* infections. The PPIs can be given orally or through an NG or percutaneous enterogastric tube. For example, esomeprazole capsules may be opened, the granules dissolved in 50 mL of water, and the solution given through the tube. Similar tubal administration is also listed by the manufacturer for lansoprazole capsules and omeprazole powder for oral suspension. Consult the drug packaging for drug-specific instructions. Be aware of the particle size of the drug once it is in solution and the tube size being used. For example, pantoprazole granules are to be used with NG tubes that are larger than 16-French, and it may clog the tube if used with small tubes. Several of the PPIs are now also available for intravenous use.

### Contraindications

The only usual contraindication to use of the PPIs is known drug allergy.

### Adverse Effects

PPIs are generally well tolerated. The frequency of adverse effects has been similar to that for placebo or $H_2$ receptor antagonists. There was some early concern that long-term use of PPIs might promote malignant gastric tumors. This has not proved to be the case, however, and this initial concern has subsided. There are some concerns that these drugs may be overprescribed and may predispose patients to GI tract infections because of the reduction of the normal acid-mediated antimicrobial protection. New concerns have arisen over the potential for long-term users of PPIs to develop osteoporosis. This is thought to be due to the inhibition of stomach acid, and it is speculated that PPIs speed up bone mineral loss. The Food and Drug Administration issued a warning in 2010 regarding long-term use of high-dose PPIs, which has been associated with *Clostridium difficile* infections; risk of wrist, hip, and spine fractures; and pneumonia. In 2011, depletion of magnesium was added to the warning.

### Interactions

Few drug interactions occur with the PPIs; however, they may increase serum levels of diazepam and phenytoin. There may be an increased chance of bleeding in patients who are taking both a PPI and warfarin. Other possible interactions include interference with the absorption of ketoconazole, ampicillin, iron salts, and digoxin. When given with clopidogrel, there is some concern of an increased risk of death if the patient has acute coronary syndrome; however, recent studies have not substantiated this concern. Sucralfate may delay the absorption of PPIs. Food may decrease absorption of the PPIs, and it is recommended that they be taken on an empty stomach.

## Dosages

For dosage information on selected PPIs, see the table on this page.

## DRUG PROFILES

### omeprazole

Omeprazole (Prilosec) was the first drug in this breakthrough class of antisecretory drugs. Omeprazole and rabeprazole are not available in injectable form. Other PPIs include lansoprazole (Prevacid), esomeprazole (Nexium), and pantoprazole (Protonix). Orally administered PPIs (and $H_2$ receptor antagonists) often work best when taken 30 to 60 minutes before meals. Omeprazole was the first PPI to become available generically.

Pharmacokinetics

| Route | Onset of Action | Peak Plasma Concentration | Elimination Half-life | Duration of Action |
|-------|-----------------|---------------------------|----------------------|---------------------|
| PO | 2 hr | 5 days | 0.5-1 hr | 1-5 days |

### lansoprazole

Lansoprazole (Prevacid) is available in a delayed-release capsule, granules for oral suspension, and orally disintegrating tablets (Prevacid SoluTab). The capsules can be opened and mixed (not crushed) with apple juice for administration via NG tube, or the SoluTab can be dissolved in water. Lansoprazole is also available as Prevpac, a combination product for the treatment of *H. Pylori* infection.

Pharmacokinetics

| Route | Onset of Action | Peak Plasma Concentration | Elimination Half-life | Duration of Action |
|-------|-----------------|---------------------------|----------------------|---------------------|
| PO | 1.7 hr | 4 wk | 1-2 hr | 24 hr |

### pantoprazole

Pantoprazole (Protonix) was the first PPI available for intravenous use. It was also the first drug to be used as a continuous infusion for the treatment of GI bleeding. It is available as an oral tablet and as delayed-release granules for NG administration. However, the granules are large, and the NG tube must be at least size 16-French or the granules may clog the tube.

Pharmacokinetics

| Route | Onset of Action | Peak Plasma Concentration | Elimination Half-life | Duration of Action |
|-------|-----------------|---------------------------|----------------------|---------------------|
| PO | 2.5 hr | 2-2.5 hr | 1 hr | 7 days |
| IV | End of infusion | End of infusion | 1 hr | 7 days |

## DOSAGES

### Selected Proton Pump Inhibitors

| DRUG (PREGNANCY CATEGORY) | USUAL DOSAGE RANGE | INDICATIONS |
|---------------------------|--------------------|-------------|
| lansoprazole (Prevacid) (B) | **Adult** PO: 30 mg daily | GERD, ulcer, erosive esophagitis |
| omeprazole (Prilosec) (C) | **Adult** PO: 20 mg/day for 4-8 wk PO: 60 mg PO once daily initially, then titrated and given in single or multiple daily doses, with dosage titration up to a maximum of 120 mg PO tid | Esophagitis, duodenal ulcer Hypersecretory conditions |
| pantoprazole (Protonix) (B) | **Adult** PO/IV: 20-80 mg/day depending on indication | GERD, ulcer, stress ulcer prophylaxis |

*GERD*, Gastroesophageal reflux disease; *IV*, intravenous; *PO*, oral.

## MISCELLANEOUS ACID-CONTROLLING DRUGS

There are a few other acid-controlling drugs that are unique in terms of their mechanisms and other features. These include sucralfate, misoprostol, and simethicone. They are profiled individually in the following paragraphs. Other drugs are bismuth subsalicylate (Pepto-Bismol; see Chapter 51) and metoclopramide (see Chapter 52).

## DRUG PROFILES

### ◆ sucralfate

Sucralfate (Carafate) is a drug used as a mucosal protectant in the treatment of active stress ulcerations and in long-term therapy for peptic ulcer disease. Sucralfate acts locally, not systemically, binding directly to the surface of an ulcer. Sucralfate has as its basic structure a sugar, sucrose. Once sucralfate comes into contact with the acid of the stomach, it begins to dissociate into aluminum hydroxide (an antacid) and sulfate anions. The aluminum salt stimulates secretion of both mucus and bicarbonate base. The sulfated sucrose molecules of sucralfate are attracted to and bind to positively charge tissue proteins at the bases of ulcers and erosions, forming a protective barrier that can be thought of as a liquid bandage. By binding to the exposed proteins of ulcers and erosions, sucralfate also limits the access of pepsin. Pepsin is an enzyme that normally breaks down proteins in food but can have the same effect on GI epithelial tissue, either causing ulcers or making them worse. Sucralfate also binds and concentrates epidermal growth factor, present in the gastric tissues, which promotes ulcer healing. In addition, the drug stimulates the gastric secretion of prostaglandin molecules, which serve a mucoprotective function. Despite its many beneficial actions, sucralfate has fallen out of common use because its effects are transient and multiple daily dosing (up to four times daily) is therefore needed. It is indicated for stress ulcers, esophageal erosions, and peptic ulcer disease. The only usual contraindication to sucralfate use is known drug allergy. Adverse effects are uncommon but include nausea, constipation, and dry mouth. Only minimal systemic absorption occurs, and the drug is virtually inert. Sucralfate does not display typical pharmacokinetic parameters, and, as such, no pharmacokinetic table is listed. Drug interactions mainly involve physical interference with the absorption of other drugs. This can be alleviated by taking other drugs at least 2 hours ahead of sucralfate. Sucralfate is also best given 1 hour before meals and at bedtime. It is classified as a pregnancy category B drug that is normally dosed at 1 g orally four times daily.

### misoprostol

Misoprostol (Cytotec), a prostaglandin E analogue, has been shown to effectively reduce the incidence of gastric ulcers in patients taking NSAIDs (see Chapter 44). Prostaglandins have a wide variety of biologic activities. They are thought to inhibit gastric acid secretion. They are also believed to protect the gastric mucosa from injury (cytoprotective function), possibly by enhancing the local production of mucus or bicarbonate, by promoting local cell regeneration, and by helping to maintain mucosal blood flow. Use of misoprostol is contraindicated in patients with known drug allergy and in pregnant women (see later in the chapter). Adverse effects include headache, GI distress, and vaginal bleeding. There are no major drug interactions, although antacids may reduce drug absorption.

Although some studies show that synthetic analogues of prostaglandins promote the healing of duodenal ulcers, the drugs must be used in dosages that usually produce disturbing adverse effects, such as abdominal cramps and diarrhea. Thus, they are not believed to be as effective as $H_2$ receptor antagonists and PPIs for this indication. Misoprostol is also used for its abortifacient properties as discussed in Chapter 34. For this reason, it is classified a pregnancy category X drug. The usual dosage is 200 mcg four times daily with meals for the duration of NSAID therapy in patients at high risk for ulceration.

### Pharmacokinetics

| Route | Onset of Action | Peak Plasma Concentration | Elimination Half-life | Duration of Action |
|-------|-----------------|---------------------------|-----------------------|--------------------|
| PO | 30 min | 12 min | 20-40 min | 1-2 days |

### simethicone

Simethicone (Mylicon) is used to reduce the discomforts of gastric or intestinal gas (flatulence) and aid in its release via the mouth or rectum. It is therefore classified as an antiflatulent drug. Gas commonly appears in the GI tract as a consequence of the swallowing of air as well as normal digestive processes. Gas in the upper GI tract is composed of swallowed air and thus consists largely of nitrogen. It is usually expelled from the body by belching. The composition of flatus, however, is determined largely by the dietary intake of carbohydrates and the metabolic activity of the bacteria in the intestines.

Some foods, including legumes (beans) and cruciferous vegetables (e.g., cauliflower, broccoli), are well known for their gas-producing ability. Gas can also result from disorders such as diverticulitis, dyspepsia (heartburn), peptic ulcers, and spastic or irritable colon; gaseous distention can also occur postoperatively. Simethicone works by altering the elasticity of mucus-coated gas bubbles, which causes them to break into smaller ones. This reduces gas pain and facilitates the expulsion of gas via the mouth or rectum. Simethicone has no listed adverse effects, drug interactions, or pharmacokinetic parameters. It is available only for oral use. The usual simethicone dosage is 1 to 2 tablets four to six times daily as needed. A variety of different simethicone products are available for OTC use.

## NURSING PROCESS

## ASSESSMENT

Before an *acid-controlling drug* is given, perform a thorough patient assessment with attention to past and present medical history with special focus on GI tract–related disorders and signs and symptoms of ulcer disease and GERD. Assess current bowel patterns, any change in bowel patterns or GI tract functioning, and GI tract–related pain. Document the findings. Assess results of baseline serum chemistry laboratory tests, as ordered, with specific attention to hepatic function (e.g., serum ALP, ALT, AST levels) and renal function (serum creatinine and BUN levels). Assess for contraindications, cautions, and drug interactions. The knowledge that acid-controlling drugs have many interactions must spark your close attention to all medications the patient is taking. This underscores the importance of obtaining a medication history that includes information about prescription drugs, OTCs, and herbals. Other components of assessment include performing a physical examination and taking a thorough cardiac history with close attention to a history of heart failure, hypertension, other cardiac diseases, the presence of edema, fluid and electrolyte imbalances and/or or renal disease. One reason it is important to assess for these conditions is that the high sodium content of various antacids may lead to exacerbation of cardiac problems, renal dysfunction, and fluid-electrolyte problems.

When *antacids* containing aluminum and/or magnesium are used, identify all other medications the patient is taking. It is important to note that combination products containing both magnesium and aluminum may have fewer adverse effects than either type of antacid by itself. For example, aluminum-containing antacids are associated with constipation, whereas magnesium-containing antacids may lead to diarrhea. The net effect of a combination of these antacids is a balancing out of both adverse effects and fewer problems with altered bowel patterns. Calcium-based antacids may also be used, especially as a source of calcium; however, they carry the risks of rebound hyperacidity, milk-alkali syndrome, and changes in systemic pH, especially if the patient has abnormal renal functioning (see Box 50-1). Sodium bicarbonate is generally not recommended as an antacid because of the high risk for systemic electrolyte disturbances and alkalosis. The sodium content of sodium bicarbonate is also high, which is very problematic for patients who have hypertension, heart failure, or renal insufficiency.

For patients using $H_2$ receptor antagonist drugs, assess renal and liver function as well as level of consciousness because of possible drug-related adverse effects. Elderly patients are known to react to these drugs with more disorientation and confusion. Do not administer drugs such as cimetidine and famotidine simultaneously with antacids. These drugs may be spaced 1 hour apart if both drugs need to be given. In patients taking nizatidine or ranitidine, assess baseline blood chemistry results with attention to levels of BUN, creatinine, bilirubin, ALP, AST, and ALT to document renal and hepatic functioning before treatment is initiated.

For *PPIs* (e.g., lansoprazole, omeprazole, and pantoprazole), assess swallowing capacity because of the size of some of the oral capsules. Assess of the patient's medical history with an emphasis on any history of GI tract infections due to decreased acid-mediated antimicrobial protection. Since there are documented concerns about the use of PPIs and the development of osteoporosis, thoroughly assess patients for any history of this disorder. Drug interactions have been discussed previously in the pharmacology section, but important to mention are the interactions with diazepam, phenytoin, warfarin, ampicillin, and iron salts. Always check the patient's medication list before these or any other types of medication are given.

*Other GI related drugs* include sucralfate and simethicone. The use of simethicone (an antiflatulent) and sucralfate (an ulcer adherent) requires assessment of the patient's bowel patterns and bowel sounds. Assess for abdominal distention and rigidity, which may indicate a medical emergency. Treatment of peptic ulcer disease has become focused on the use of antibiotics (to attack the *H. pylori* bacteria) with frequent dosing of other drugs. Inquire also about the presence of any unusual signs and symptoms related to the GI tract.

## NURSING DIAGNOSES

1. Constipation related to the adverse effects of aluminum-containing antacids and other drugs used to treat hyperacidity
2. Diarrhea related to the adverse effects of magnesium-containing antacids and other drugs used to treat hyperacidity
3. Deficient knowledge related to lack of information about antacids, H$_2$ receptor antagonists, or PPIs, including their use and potential adverse effects

## PLANNING

### GOALS
1. Patient experiences minimal to no constipation while using antacids and/or other acid-controlling drugs.
2. Patient experiences minimal to no diarrhea during antacid and/or acid-controlling medication regimen.
3. Patient demonstrates adequate knowledge about use of antacid and/or acid-controlling medications and expected adverse effects.

### OUTCOME CRITERIA
1. Patient states measures to help prevent and minimize adverse effect of constipation, such as taking the antacid only as directed and taking combination aluminum/magnesium products.

2. Patient states measures to help prevent and minimize the adverse effect of diarrhea such as avoiding magnesium-only antacids, especially milk of magnesia, and taking combination aluminum/magnesium products.
3. Patient states the purpose of taking antacids, H$_2$ receptor antagonists, and PPIs for management of gastric hyperacidity.
   - Patient describes the various adverse effects associated with antacids such as diarrhea, constipation, and acid rebound.
   - Patient describes the expected adverse effects associated with other acid-controlling drugs such as constipation, diarrhea, headache, and confusion, and seeks advice from the prescriber if adverse effects worsen or are not relieved after several days.

### CASE STUDY
#### *Proton Pump Inhibitors*

A 50-year-old attorney has self-treated for heartburn for years by drinking large amounts of antacids. She finally made an appointment with her family practice physician, who referred her to a gastroenterologist. Her family practice physician instructed her to stop taking the antacids.

1. Why did the physician ask her to stop taking the antacids?

In a few weeks, the attorney had an endoscopy, and it was discovered that she had gastroesophageal reflux disease (GERD) and gastritis secondary to stress-induced hyperacidity. The physician has prescribed the proton pump inhibitor (PPI) omeprazole (Prilosec) 20 mg once a day.

2. What other conditions will the gastroenterologist test for during this diagnostic stage?
3. What is the rationale for the use of PPIs to treat GERD?
4. What patient teaching is important regarding the PPI?

For answers, see http://evolve.elsevier.com/Lilley.

## IMPLEMENTATION

When giving *acid-controlling drugs,* instruct the patient to thoroughly chew the chewable tablets and to thoroughly shake liquid forms before they are taken. *Antacids* need to be given with at least 8 oz of water to enhance absorption of the antacid in the stomach, except for newer forms that are rapidly dissolving drugs. If constipation or diarrhea occurs with single-component drugs, a combination aluminum- and magnesium-based product may be preferred. Educate the patient about the adverse effects of aluminum-only or magnesium-only products. It is also recommended that antacids be given as ordered but not within 1 to 2 hours of other medications because of the effect of antacids on the absorption of oral medications. You may safely implement this dosing schedule without interrupting the safe dosing of other medications. The dosing will differ if the prescriber has ordered the drug to be given with antacids. With quinolone antibiotics, there may be serious harm if given with antacids because of a 50% reduction in antibiotic absorption. Serious infections may then go unsuccessfully treated due to altered absorption. Antacid overuse or misuse or the rapid discontinuation of antacids with high acid-neutralizing capacity may lead to acid rebound. Therefore, antacids are only to be used as prescribed and/or as directed.

Because so many *H₂ receptor antagonists* and other acid-controlling drugs are now available OTC, instruct the patient about proper use (see the Patient Teaching Tips for more information). For example, cimetidine is to be taken with meals, and antacids, if also used, need to be taken 1 to 2 hours after the cimetidine. Intravenous dosing and related mixing and infusing for intravenous cimetidine are similar to those described later for intravenous famotidine. Famotidine may be given orally in tablet or suspension form and without regard to meals or food. Rapid-release forms of famotidine dissolve quickly under the patient's tongue and can be taken without water. Give ranitidine as ordered, and, if administered with antacids, give 1 to 2 hours before the antacid. Dilute intravenous forms of famotidine or ranitidine with appropriate solutions and infuse over the documented time frame. With intravenous H₂ receptor antagonists, hypotension may occur with rapid infusion, so careful monitoring is critical to patient safety. Refer to appropriate sources for information on other specific drugs and their intravenous administration. For all H₂ receptor antagonists, monitor blood pressure readings as needed during intravenous infusion because of the risk of hypotension. Continue to monitor the patient for GI tract bleeding with the diagnosis of ulcers or GI irritation. Report any blood in the stools or the occurrence of black, tarry stools or hematemesis. Listen to bowel sounds and examine the abdomen to monitor for possible complications.

With *PPIs,* give lansoprazole oral dosage forms as ordered. If the patient has difficulty swallowing these capsules, a capsule may be opened and the granules sprinkled over at least a tablespoon of applesauce, which then must be swallowed immediately. Administer omeprazole before meals, and educate the patient that the capsule must be taken whole and not crushed, opened, or chewed. Omeprazole may also be given with antacids, if ordered. Always double-check the names and dosages of these drugs to ensure that they are not confused with similarly named drugs. Pantoprazole may be given orally without crushing or splitting of the tablet form. Give intravenous dosage forms exactly as ordered using the correct dilutional fluids. Infuse over the recommended time period.

*Other GI related drugs,* such as simethicone, may also be added to the oral medication protocol with PPIs. Simethicone is usually well tolerated. It is to be taken after meals and at bedtime. Instruct patients to thoroughly chew the tablets or to shake suspensions well before use. Sucralfate is usually given 1 hour before meals and at bedtime. Tablets may be crushed or dissolved in water, if needed. Antacids are to be avoided for 30 minutes before or after administration of sucralfate. Misoprostol is to be given with food and is usually ordered to be taken with meals and at bedtime. Suggestions for drug-related patient education are presented in the Patient Teaching Tips.

## EVALUATION

Therapeutic response to the administration of *antacids, H₂ receptor antagonists, PPIs,* and *other GI-related drugs* includes the relief of symptoms associated with peptic ulcer, gastritis, esophagitis, gastric hyperacidity, or hiatal hernia (i.e., decrease in epigastric pain, fullness, and abdominal swelling). Adverse effects for which to monitor include all of those listed for each of the drug categories and range from constipation or diarrhea to nausea, vomiting, abdominal pain, and hypotension. Milk-alkali syndrome, acid rebound, hypercalcemia, and metabolic alkalosis are known complications associated with the various antacids; evaluate the patient for these adverse effects and take measures to prevent or resolve them.

## PATIENT TEACHING TIPS

- Medications are not to be taken, unless prescribed, within 1 to 2 hours of taking an antacid because of their impact on the absorption of many medications in the stomach.
- Advise the patient to contact the prescriber immediately if he or she experiences severe or prolonged constipation and/or diarrhea; increase in abdominal pain; abdominal distension; nausea; vomiting; hematemesis; or black, tarry stools (a sign of possible GI tract bleeding).
- If the patient is taking enteric-coated medications, tell the patient that the use of antacids may promote premature dissolution of the enteric coating. Enteric coatings are used to diminish the stomach upset caused by irritating medications, and if the coating is destroyed early in the stomach, gastric upset may occur.

- Encourage the patient to take H₂ receptor antagonists exactly as prescribed. Inform the patient that smoking decreases the drug's effectiveness. Advise that patient that H₂ receptor antagonists are not to be taken within 1 hour of antacids.
- Advise the patient to take omeprazole and other PPIs before meals. Inform the patient that if lansoprazole is being used, the granules may be sprinkled from the capsule into a tablespoon of applesauce if needed.
- Instruct the patient to follow the manufacturer's directions when taking simethicone. Chewable forms must always be chewed thoroughly; liquid preparations need to be shaken thoroughly before administration. Encourage patients experiencing flatulence to avoid problematic foods (e.g., spicy, gas-producing foods) and carbonated beverages.

## PATIENT TEACHING TIPS—cont'd

- Sucralfate must be taken on an empty stomach, and antacids are to be avoided or, if indicated, taken 2 hours before or 1 hour after sucralfate administration.
- For a patient taking the drug regimen for the treatment of *H. pylori* infection–peptic ulcer disease, it is important to emphasize the need to take each drug, including the antibiotics, exactly as prescribed and without fail to guarantee successful treatment. If treatment protocols are not followed appropriately, the condition may likely recur.

## KEY POINTS

- The stomach secretes many substances (hydrochloric acid, pepsinogen, mucus, bicarbonate, intrinsic factor, and prostaglandins).
- The parietal cell is responsible for the production of acid.
- In acid-related disorders, there is an impairment of the balance among the substances secreted by the stomach.
- $H_2$ receptor antagonists are $H_2$ blockers that bind to and block histamine receptors located on parietal cells. This blockade renders these cells less responsive to stimuli and thus decreases their acid secretion. Up to 90% inhibition of acid secretion can be achieved with the $H_2$ receptor antagonists.
- PPIs block the final step in the acid production pathway, the hydrogen-potassium-ATPase pump and they block all acid secretion.
- Sucralfate is used for the treatment of peptic ulcer disease and stress-related ulcers. It binds to tissue proteins in the eroded area and prevents exposure of the ulcerated area to stomach acid.
- Misoprostol is a synthetic prostaglandin analogue that inhibits gastric acid secretion and is used to prevent NSAID-related ulcers.
- Cautious use of antacids is recommended in patients who have heart failure, hypertension, or other cardiac diseases or who require sodium restriction, especially if the antacid is high in sodium.
- Many drug interactions occur with the acid-controlling drugs due to alteration of oral dosage forms, and so other medications are to be avoided within 1 to 2 hours of taking an antacid. Antacids are sometimes to be avoided when other acid-controlling drugs are taken.
- Magnesium-aluminum combination antacids are used to prevent the adverse effects of constipation and diarrhea. Some of the more serious concerns with antacids include acid rebound, hypercalcemia, milk-alkali syndrome, and metabolic alkalosis.

## NCLEX® EXAMINATION REVIEW QUESTIONS

1 A 30-year-old man is taking simethicone for excessive flatus associated with diverticulitis. During a patient teaching session, the nurse explains the mechanism of action of simethicone by saying:
  a "It neutralizes gastric pH, thereby preventing gas."
  b "It buffers the effects of pepsin on the gastric wall."
  c "It decreases gastric acid secretion and thereby minimizes flatus."
  d "It causes mucus-coated gas bubbles to break into smaller ones."

2 When evaluating the medication list of a patient who will be starting therapy with an $H_2$ receptor antagonist, the nurse is aware that which drug may interact with it?
  a codeine
  b penicillin
  c ketoconazole
  d acetaminophen

3 When administering sucralfate, which action by the nurse is most correct?
  a Giving the drug with meals
  b Giving the drug on an empty stomach

  c Instructing the patient to restrict fluids
  d Waiting 30 minutes before administering other drugs

4 A patient with a history of renal problems is asking for advice about which antacid he should use. The nurse will make which recommendation?
  a "Patients with renal problems cannot use antacids."
  b "Aluminum-based antacids are the best choice for you."
  c "Calcium-based antacids are the best choice for you."
  d "Magnesium-based antacids are the best choice for you."

5 A patient who is taking oral tetracycline complains of heartburn and requests an antacid. Which action by the nurse is correct?
  a Give the tetracycline, but delay the antacid for 1 to 2 hours.
  b Give the antacid, but delay the tetracycline for at least 4 hours.
  c Administer both medications together.
  d Explain that the antacid cannot be given while the patient is taking the tetracycline.

6 When the nurse is administering a proton pump inhibitor (PPI), which actions by the nurse are correct? (Select all that apply.)
  a Giving the PPI on an empty stomach
  b Giving the PPI with meals
  c Making sure the patient does not crush or chew the capsules
  d Instructing the patient to open the capsule and chew the contents for best absorption
  e Administering the PPI only when the patient complains of heartburn

7 The order reads: "Give cimetidine (Tagamet) 300 mg in 100 mL normal saline IVPB tid and at bedtime. Infuse over 30 minutes." The infusion pump can only be programmed to deliver over 60 minutes (mL per hour). The nurse will set the pump to deliver how many mL/hour for each IVPB dose?

1. d, 2. c, 3. b, 4. b, 5. a, 6. a, c, 7. 200 mL/hour

For Critical Thinking and Prioritization Questions, see http://evolve.elsevier.com/Lilley.

# Bowel Disorder Drugs

## evolve WEBSITE

*http://evolve.elsevier.com/Lilley*

- Animations
- Answer Key—Textbook Case Studies
- Critical Thinking and Prioritization Questions

- Key Points—Downloadable
- Review Questions for the NCLEX® Examination
- Unfolding Case Studies

## OBJECTIVES

When you reach the end of this chapter, you will be able to do the following:

1 Discuss the anatomy and physiology of the gastrointestinal tract, including the process of peristalsis.
2 Identify the various factors affecting bowel elimination and/or bowel patterns.
3 List the various groups of drugs used to treat alterations in bowel elimination, specifically diarrhea, constipation, and irritable bowel syndrome (IBS).

4 Discuss the mechanisms of action, indications, cautions, contraindications, drug interactions, dosages, routes of administration, and adverse effects of the various antidiarrheals, probiotics, laxatives, and IBS drugs.
5 Develop a nursing care plan that includes all phases of the nursing process for patients taking antidiarrheals, probiotics, laxatives, and IBS drugs.

## DRUG PROFILES

belladonna alkaloid combinations, p. 831
bisacodyl, p. 838
bismuth subsalicylate, p. 831
♦ diphenoxylate with atropine, p. 831
♦ docusate salts, p. 837
♦ glycerin, p. 837
*Lactobacillus*, p. 832
♦ lactulose, p. 838
♦ loperamide, p. 832

magnesium salts, p. 838
methylcellulose, p. 836
mineral oil, p. 837
polyethylene glycol 3350, p. 838
♦ psyllium, p. 837
♦ senna, p. 838

_____

♦ *Key drug*

## KEY TERMS

Antidiarrheal drugs Drugs that counter or combat diarrhea. (p. 830)
Constipation A condition of abnormally infrequent and difficult passage of feces through the lower gastrointestinal tract. (p. 833)
Diarrhea The abnormally frequent passage of loose stools. (p. 830)

Irritable bowel syndrome (IBS) A recurring condition of the intestinal tract characterized by bloating, flatulence, and often periods of diarrhea that alternate with periods of constipation. (p. 838)
Laxatives Drugs that promote bowel evacuation, such as by increasing the bulk of the feces, softening the stool, or lubricating the intestinal wall. (p. 833)

## ANATOMY, PHYSIOLOGY, AND PATHOPHYSIOLOGY OVERVIEW

Diarrhea and the diseases associated with it account for 5 to 8 million deaths per year in infants and small children and are among the leading causes of death and morbidity in underdeveloped nations. The key symptoms of gastrointestinal (GI) disease are abdominal pain, nausea and/or vomiting, and diarrhea. Diarrhea is defined as the passage of stools with abnormally increased frequency, fluidity, and weight, or increased stool water excretion. Acute diarrhea refers to diarrhea of sudden onset in a previously healthy individual. It lasts from 3 days to 2 weeks and is self-limiting, resolving without sequelae. Chronic diarrhea lasts for longer than 3 to 4 weeks and is associated with recurrent passage of diarrheal stools, possible fever, nausea, vomiting, weight reduction, and chronic weakness.

The probable cause of diarrhea needs to be taken into consideration when designing a drug regimen to treat it. Causes of acute diarrhea include drugs, bacteria, viruses, nutritional factors, and protozoa. Causes of chronic diarrhea include tumors, acquired immunodeficiency syndrome (AIDS), diabetes mellitus, hyperthyroidism, Addison's disease, and irritable bowel syndrome (IBS). Treatment is aimed at stopping the stool frequency, alleviating the abdominal cramps, replenishing fluids and electrolytes, and preventing weight loss and nutritional deficits from malabsorption. Often, replacement of fluids is the only treatment needed. Patients with diarrhea associated with a bacterial or parasitic infection must not use antidiarrheal drugs, because this will cause the organism to stay in the body longer and will prolong recovery.

## PHARMACOLOGY OVERVIEW

### ANTIDIARRHEALS

Drugs used to treat diarrhea are called antidiarrheal drugs. Based on the specific mechanism of action, they are divided into different groups: adsorbents, antimotility drugs (anticholinergics and opiates), and probiotics (also known as *intestinal flora modifiers* and *bacterial replacement drugs*). The specific classes and the drugs in each are listed in Table 51-1. Antidiarrheal and laxative drugs do not have the classic pharmacokinetics of other drugs, and thus pharmacokinetics tables such as those presented throughout the book are not included in this chapter.

| TABLE 51-1 | ANTIDIARRHEALS: DRUG CATEGORIES AND SELECTED DRUGS |
|---|---|
| **CATEGORY** | **ANTIDIARRHEAL DRUGS** |
| Adsorbents | Activated charcoal, aluminum hydroxide, bismuth subsalicylate, cholestyramine, polycarbophil |
| Anticholinergics | Atropine, hyoscyamine |
| Opiates | Opium tincture, paregoric, codeine, diphenoxylate, loperamide |
| Probiotics and intestinal flora modifiers | *Lactobacillus acidophilus, Lactobacillus GG, Saccharromyces boulardii* |

## Mechanism of Action and Drug Effects

Antidiarrheal drugs have varying mechanisms of action. Adsorbents act by coating the walls of the GI tract. They bind the causative bacteria or toxin to their adsorbent surface for elimination from the body through the stool. Adsorption is similar to absorption but differs in that it involves the chemical binding of substances (e.g., ions, bacterial toxins) onto the surface of an adsorbent. In contrast, absorption refers to the penetration of a substance into the interior structure of the absorbant or the uptake of a substance across a surface (e.g., the absorption of dietary nutrients into the intestinal villi). The adsorbent bismuth subsalicylate is a form of aspirin, or acetylsalicylic acid, and therefore it also has many of the same drug effects as aspirin (see Chapter 44). Activated charcoal not only is helpful in coating the walls of the GI tract and adsorbing bacteria but also is useful in cases of overdose because of its drug-binding properties. The antilipemic drugs colestipol and cholestyramine (see Chapter 27) are anion exchange resins that are sometimes prescribed as antidiarrheal adsorbents and lipid-lowering drugs. Besides binding to diarrhea-causing toxins, they have the additional benefit of decreasing cholesterol levels.

Anticholinergic drugs work to slow peristalsis by reducing the rhythmic contractions and smooth muscle tone of the GI tract; they also have a drying effect and reduce gastric secretions. They are used in combination with adsorbents and opiates (see later in the chapter). Anticholinergics are discussed in detail in Chapter 21.

Probiotics are products obtained from bacterial cultures, most commonly *Lactobacillus* organisms, which make up the majority of the body's normal bacterial flora. These organisms are commonly destroyed by antibiotics. Probiotics work by replenishing these bacteria, which helps to restore the balance of normal flora and suppress the growth of diarrhea-causing bacteria.

The primary action of *opiates* (see Chapter 10) in diarrhea treatment is to reduce bowel motility. A secondary effect that makes opiates beneficial in the treatment of diarrhea is reduction of the pain associated with diarrhea by relief of rectal spasms. Because they decrease the transit time of food through the GI tract, they permit longer contact of the intestinal contents with the absorptive surface of the bowel, which increases the absorption of water, electrolytes, and other nutrients from the bowel and reduces stool frequency and net volume.

## Indications

Antidiarrheal drugs are indicated for the treatment of diarrhea of various types and levels of severity. Adsorbents are more likely to be used in milder cases, whereas anticholinergics and opiates tend to be used in more severe cases. Probiotics are often helpful in patients with antibiotic-induced diarrhea.

## Contraindications

Contraindications to the use of antidiarrheals include known drug allergy and any major acute GI condition, such as intestinal obstruction or colitis, unless the drug is ordered by the patient's prescriber after careful consideration of the specific case.

## Adverse Effects

The adverse effects of the antidiarrheals are specific to each drug family. Most of these potential effects are minor and are not life threatening. The major adverse effects of specific drugs in each drug class are listed in Table 51-2. Probiotics do not have any listed adverse effects.

## Interactions

Many drugs are absorbed from the intestines into the bloodstream, where they are delivered to their respective sites of action. A number of the antidiarrheals have the potential to alter this normal process, by either increasing or decreasing the absorption of these other drugs.

The adsorbents can decrease the effectiveness of many drugs, primarily by decreasing the absorption of certain drugs. Examples include digoxin, quinidine, and hypoglycemic drugs. The oral anticoagulant warfarin (see Chapter 26) is more likely to cause increased bleeding times or bruising when coadministered with adsorbents. This is thought to be because the adsorbents bind to vitamin K, which is needed to make certain clotting factors. Vitamin K is synthesized by the normal bacterial flora in the bowel. The toxic effects of methotrexate are more likely to occur when it is given with adsorbents.

The therapeutic effects of the anticholinergic antidiarrheals can be decreased by coadministration with antacids. Amantadine, tricyclic antidepressants, monoamine oxidase inhibitors, opiates, and antihistamines, when given with anticholinergics, can result in increased anticholinergic effects. The opiate antidiarrheals have additive central nervous system (CNS) depressant effects if they are given with CNS depressants, alcohol, opioids, sedative-hypnotics, antipsychotics, or skeletal muscle relaxants.

Bismuth subsalicylate can lead to increased bleeding times and bruising when administered with warfarin as well as aspirin and other nonsteroidal antiinflammatory drugs. It can also cause confusion in the elderly. Cholestyramine, when administered with glipizide, can result in decreased hypoglycemic effects. Cholestyramine also decreases the absorption of any drug that is given within 2 hours of it. It is important not to give any drug within 2 hours before or 2 hours after cholestyramine.

## Dosages

For dosage information on the antidiarrheal drugs, see the table on p. 832.

| TABLE 51-2 | SELECTED ANTIDIARRHEALS: ADVERSE EFFECTS |
|---|---|
| **DRUG** | **ADVERSE EFFECTS** |
| bismuth subsalicylate | Increased bleeding time, constipation, dark stools, confusion, tinnitus, metallic taste, blue gums |
| atropine, hyoscyamine | Urinary retention, impotence, headache, dizziness, anxiety, drowsiness, bradycardia, hypotension, dry skin, flushing, blurred vision |
| codeine, diphenoxylate | Drowsiness, dizziness, lethargy, nausea, vomiting, constipation, hypotension, urinary retention, flushing, respiratory depression |

## DRUG PROFILES

Drug therapy for diarrhea depends on the specific cause of the diarrhea (if known). All antidiarrheals are orally administered drugs available as suspensions, tablets, or capsules. Some antidiarrheals are over-the-counter (OTC) medications, whereas others require a prescription.

### ADSORBENTS
#### bismuth subsalicylate

Even though it is available OTC, it should be used with caution in children and teenagers who have or are recovering from chickenpox or influenza because of the risk of Reye's syndrome (see the Patient-Centered Care: Lifespan Considerations for the Pediatric Patient box). It can also cause all of the adverse effects that are associated with an aspirin-based product (see Chapter 44). Two alarming but harmless adverse effects are temporary darkening of the tongue and the stool. Bismuth subsalicylate is available OTC for oral use.

### ANTICHOLINERGICS

The anticholinergics atropine and hyoscyamine are used either alone or in combination with other antidiarrheals because they slow GI tract motility. These drugs are referred to as *belladonna alkaloids* and are discussed in Chapter 21. Their safety margin is not as wide as that of many of the other antidiarrheals, because they can cause serious adverse effects if used inappropriately. For this reason, they are available only by prescription.

#### belladonna alkaloid combinations

Belladonna alkaloids can be used to treat many GI disorders, including diarrhea; however, their use is limited. Donnatal is the most commonly used drug in this class. Use of the belladonna alkaloid preparations is contraindicated in patients who have shown a hypersensitivity to anticholinergics and in patients with narrow-angle glaucoma, GI obstruction, myasthenia gravis, paralytic ileus, and toxic megacolon. Donnatal tablets contain a combination of four different alkaloids: atropine, hyoscyamine, phenobarbital, and scopolamine. Available dosage forms of this combination include elixir, tablets, and extended-release tablets. Donnatal Extentabs contain increased amounts of the aforementioned ingredients. Belladonna alkaloid preparations are classified as pregnancy category C to X drugs, depending on the ingredients of the specific product.

### OPIATES

There are five opiate-related antidiarrheal drugs: codeine, diphenoxylate with atropine, loperamide, paregoric, and tincture of opium. The only opiate-related antidiarrheal that is available as an OTC medication is loperamide; all others are prescription-only drugs because of the risks of respiratory depression and dependency associated with opiate use. Numerous medication errors and deaths have been reported with paregoric and tincture of opium. For those reasons, their use is very limited.

#### ◆ diphenoxylate with atropine

Diphenoxylate (Lomotil, Lonox) is a synthetic opiate agonist that is structurally related to meperidine. It acts on smooth

## DOSAGES

### Selected Antidiarrheal Drugs

| DRUG (PREGNANCY CATEGORY) | PHARMACOLOGIC CLASS/ INDICATION | USUAL DOSAGE RANGE | ONSET OF ACTION |
|---|---|---|---|
| belladonna alkaloids/phenobarbital combinations (Donnatal Elixir, Donnatal capsules and tablets, Donnatal Extentabs) (C to X) | Fixed-combination anticholinergic/diarrhea | **Adult**<br>PO: Donnatal Elixir, 5-10 mL tid-qid<br>Donnatal capsules and tablets, 1-2 caps or tabs tid-qid<br>PO: Donnatal Extentabs, 1 tab q8-12h | 1-2 hr |
| bismuth subsalicylate (Pepto-Bismol) (D) | Antimicrobial, antidiarrheal/diarrhea | Doses repeated q30-60 min, not to exceed 8 per day; all doses PO<br>**Pediatric 3-5 yr***<br>5 mL or ⅓ tab<br>**Pediatric 6-12 yr***<br>10 mL or ⅔ tab<br>**Adult**<br>30 mL or 2 tab | 0.5-2 hr |
| ♦ diphenoxylate with atropine (Lomotil) (C) | Opioid with anticholinergic/diarrhea | **Pediatric 2-12 yr**<br>0.3-0.4 mg/kg/day in 4 divided doses; use oral solution in children.<br>**Adult**<br>Initially 5 mg (2 tabs) 3-4 × per day, then reduce to 2.5 mg (1 tab) 3-4 × per day as needed. (max of 8 tabs/day) | 40-60 min |
| *Lactobacillus acidophilus* (Bacid, Lactinex) (A) | Probiotic/dietary supplementation,† diarrhea, need for bacterial replacement | **Adult**<br>PO (Bacid): 2 caps bid-qid<br>PO (Lactinex): 1 packet granules with liquid or food tid-qid; 4 tabs tid-qid with liquid or food | Unknown |
| ♦ loperamide (Imodium A-D) (B) | Opiate antidiarrheal/diarrhea | **Pediatric 2-5 yr**<br>PO: 1 mg tid (liquid only)<br>**Pediatric 6-8 yr (21.8-26.8 kg)**<br>PO: 2 mg after the first unformed stool, followed by 1 mg PO after each subsequent unformed stool; not to exceed 4 mg/day for 2 days<br>**Pediatric 9-12 yr (27.3-43.2 kg)**<br>PO: 2 mg after the first unformed stool, followed by 1 mg PO after each subsequent unformed stool; not to exceed 6 mg/day for 2 days<br>**Adult**<br>PO: 4 mg followed by 2 mg after each BM (not to exceed 16 mg/day) | 1-3 hr |

*BM,* Bowel movement; *PO,* oral.

*Used with caution in children and teenagers who have or are recovering from chickenpox or influenza because of the risk of Reye's syndrome.

†Often used to treat uncomplicated diarrhea, although this is an off-label (non–U.S. Food and Drug Administration approved) use.

muscle of the intestinal tract, inhibiting GI motility and excessive GI propulsion. It has little or no analgesic activity; however, because it is an opioid, abuse and physical dependence may occur. Diphenoxylate is combined with subtherapeutic quantities of atropine to discourage its use as a recreational opiate drug. The amount of atropine present in the combination is too small to interfere with the conjugated diphenoxylate. When taken in large dosages, however, the combination results in extreme anticholinergic effects (e.g., dry mouth, abdominal pain, tachycardia, blurred vision).

Use of the combination of diphenoxylate and atropine is contraindicated in patients experiencing diarrhea associated with pseudomembranous colitis or toxigenic bacteria. It is available only for oral use.

### ♦ loperamide

Loperamide (Imodium A-D) is a synthetic antidiarrheal that is similar to diphenoxylate. It inhibits both peristalsis in the intestinal wall and intestinal secretion, thereby decreasing the number of stools and their water content. Although the drug exhibits many characteristics of the opiate class, physical dependence on loperamide has not been reported. Because of its safety profile, it is the only opiate antidiarrheal drug that is available as an OTC medication. Loperamide use is contraindicated in patients with severe ulcerative colitis, pseudomembranous colitis, and acute diarrhea associated with *Escherichia coli*.

### PROBIOTICS

Probiotics suppress the growth of diarrhea-causing bacteria and reestablish the flora that normally resides in the intestine. Most commonly, they are bacterial cultures of *Lactobacillus* organisms. Probiotics are often referred to as *intestinal flora modifiers*. Their mechanism of action is not completely understood, but the general benefits are suppression of growth or invasion by pathogenic bacteria, improvement of intestinal barrier function, modulation of the immune system, and modulation of pain perception.

### Lactobacillus

*Lactobacillus acidophilus* (Bacid) and *Lactobacillus GG* (Culturelle) are acid-producing bacteria prepared in a concentrated,

## PATIENT-CENTERED CARE: LIFESPAN CONSIDERATIONS FOR THE PEDIATRIC PATIENT

### Antidiarrheal Preparations

- If diarrhea is accompanied by fever, malaise, or abdominal pain, contact the prescriber immediately because of the possibility of excessive fluid and electrolyte loss. Dehydration and electrolyte loss occur very rapidly in the pediatric patient because of the patient's size and sensitivity to loss of fluid volume and electrolytes through the stool.
- Always contact the prescriber or pharmacist for the proper dosage of antidiarrheals if the child is 6 years of age or younger or if there is any doubt as to proper dosing. Never hesitate to contact the prescriber with any concern or question regarding any medication recommended for the pediatric patient.
- Bismuth subsalicylate is a salicylate by chemical structure; therefore, it is to be used very cautiously in children and teenagers who have been or are recovering from chickenpox or influenza because of the risk for Reye's syndrome (see Chapter 44).
- Immediately report to the prescriber any abdominal distention, firm abdomen, painful abdomen, or worsening of or lack of improvement in diarrhea 24 to 48 hours after medication administration. Measurement of the amount of diarrhea by the number of soiled diapers or number of stools per day provides important information.
- Antidiarrheal preparations are always to be used very cautiously in the pediatric patient. If symptoms persist or dehydration occurs (e.g., no tears and decreased urine output in the child), contact the prescriber.
- If the patient is sluggish, lethargic, or confused or the diarrhea is bloody, contact the prescriber immediately or go to the closest emergency facility.
- Always assess the pediatric patient, including adolescents, for the presence of an eating disorder such as bulimia or anorexia due to the associated use/abuse of laxatives in these conditions.

### TABLE 51-3 CAUSES OF CONSTIPATION

| CAUSE | EXAMPLES |
|---|---|
| Adverse drug effects | Analgesics, anticholinergics, iron supplements, aluminum antacids, calcium antacids, opiates, calcium channel blockers |
| Lifestyle | Poor bowel movement habits: voluntary refusal to defecate resulting in constipation |
| | Diet: poor fluid intake and/or low-residue (low-fiber) diet or excessive consumption of dairy products |
| | Physical inactivity: lack of proper exercise, especially in elderly individuals |
| | Psychological factors: anxiety, stress, hypochondria |
| Metabolic and endocrine disorders | Diabetes mellitus, hypothyroidism, pregnancy, hypercalcemia, hypokalemia |
| Neurogenic disorders | Autonomic neuropathy, intestinal pseudo-obstruction, multiple sclerosis, spinal cord lesions, Parkinson's disease, stroke |

The usual time span between ingestion and defecation is 24 to 36 hours. The last segment of the GI tract, the large intestine (colon), is responsible for (1) forming the stool by removing excess water from the fecal material, (2) temporarily storing the stool until defecation, and (3) extracting essential vitamins from the intestinal bacteria (especially vitamin K). The colon is 120 to 150 cm long and is separated from the small intestine by the ileocecal valve. The colon extends into the rectum, which terminates at the anus. The rectum is the temporary storage site for the stool, which is composed of water and unabsorbed and indigestible material. Evacuation of the rectal contents is accomplished by bowel movements.

A bowel movement (defecation) is a reflex act that involves both smooth and skeletal muscles. The entry of feces into the rectum stimulates mass peristaltic movement that results in a bowel movement. However, voluntary initiation or inhibition of defecation is also possible via skeletal muscle pathways.

Treatment of constipation is individualized, with consideration of the patient's age, concerns, and expectations; duration and severity of constipation; and potential contributing factors. Treatment can be either surgical (in extreme cases) or nonsurgical. Nonsurgical treatments can be separated into three broad approaches: dietary (e.g., fiber supplementation), behavioral (e.g., increased physical activity), and pharmacologic. The focus in this chapter is on pharmacologic treatment.

Laxatives are among the most misused OTC medications. Long-term and often inappropriate use of laxatives may result in laxative dependence, produce damage to the bowel, or lead to previously nonexistent intestinal problems. With the exception of the bulk-forming type, laxatives are not to be used for long periods. Based on their mechanisms of action, laxatives are divided into five major groups: bulk-forming, emollient, hyperosmotic, saline, and stimulant laxatives. Table 51-4 lists the currently available laxative drugs categorized by drug family. The onset of action of laxatives is the most important pharmacokinetic feature of these drugs and is listed in the Dosages table on p. 836.

dried culture for oral administration. They are normal inhabitants of the GI tract where, through the fermentation of carbohydrates (which produces lactic acid), they create an unfavorable environment for the overgrowth of harmful fungi and bacteria. *L. acidophilus* has been used for more than 75 years for the treatment of uncomplicated diarrhea, particularly that caused by antibiotic therapy that destroys normal intestinal flora. Another commonly used probiotic is *Saccharomyces boulardii* (Florastor).

## LAXATIVES

Laxatives are used for the treatment of constipation, which is defined as the abnormally infrequent and difficult passage of feces through the lower GI tract. Constipation is a symptom, not a disease; it is a disorder of movement through the colon and/or rectum that can be caused by a variety of diseases or drugs. Some of the more common causes of constipation are listed in Table 51-3.

The GI tract is responsible for the digestive process, which involves (1) ingestion of dietary intake, (2) digestion of dietary intake into basic nutrients, (3) absorption of basic nutrients, and (4) storage and removal of fecal material via defecation (Figure 51-1).

Ingestion → digestion → absorption → storage & removal

**FIGURE 51-1** The digestive system. (From Patton KT, Thibodeau GA: *Mosby's handbook of anatomy and physiology*, St Louis, 2000, Mosby.)

| TABLE 51-4 | LAXATIVES: DRUG CATEGORIES AND SELECTED DRUGS |
|---|---|
| **CATEGORY** | **LAXATIVE DRUGS** |
| Bulk-forming | psyllium, methylcellulose |
| Emollient | docusate salts, mineral oil |
| Hyperosmotic | polyethylene glycol, lactulose, sorbitol, glycerin |
| Saline | magnesium hydroxide, magnesium sulfate, magnesium citrate |
| Stimulant | senna, bisacodyl |

## Mechanism of Action and Drug Effects

All laxatives promote bowel movements, but each class of laxative has a different mechanism of action. Laxatives may act by (1) affecting fecal consistency, (2) increasing fecal movement through the colon, and/or (3) facilitating defecation through the rectum. Bulk-forming laxatives act in a manner similar to that of the fiber naturally contained in the diet. They absorb water into the intestine, which increases bulk and distends the bowel to initiate reflex bowel activity, thus promoting a bowel movement.

Emollient laxatives are also referred to as *stool softeners* (docusate salts) and *lubricant laxatives* (mineral oil). Fecal softeners work by lowering the surface tension of GI fluids, so that more water and fat are absorbed into the stool and the intestines. The lubricant type of emollient laxatives works by lubricating the fecal material and the intestinal wall and preventing absorption of water from the intestines. Instead of being absorbed, this water in the bowel softens and expands the stool. This promotes

bowel distention and reflex peristaltic actions, which ultimately lead to defecation.

Hyperosmotic laxatives work by increasing fecal water content, which results in distention, increased peristalsis, and evacuation. Their site of action is limited to the large intestine. Saline laxatives increase osmotic pressure in the small intestine by inhibiting water absorption and increasing both water and electrolyte (salt) secretions from the bowel wall into the bowel lumen. This results in a watery stool. The increased distention promotes peristalsis and evacuation. Rectal enemas of sodium phosphate, a saline laxative, produce defecation 2 to 5 minutes after administration.

As the name implies, stimulant laxatives stimulate the nerves that innervate the intestines, which results in increased peristalsis. They also increase fluid in the colon, which increases bulk and softens the stool. Table 51-5 summarizes the specific drug effects of the different classes of laxatives.

In 2008, a new class of drugs was approved for the treatment of very specific types of constipation related to opioid use and bowel resection surgery. These peripherally acting opioid antagonists include methylnaltrexone (Relistor) and alvimopan (Entereg). These drugs block the entrance of an opioid drug into the bowel cells, thus allowing bowels to function normally, even with continued opioid use. Methylnaltrexone is approved only for terminally ill (hospice) patients who have opioid-induced constipation. It is available as an injection only and is given once a day. Alvimopan is indicated to accelerate GI recovery time following partial large or small bowel resection surgery. Patients must be hospitalized and registered to receive Alvimopan.

## TABLE 51-5   LAXATIVES: DRUG EFFECTS

| DRUG EFFECT | BULK | EMOLLIENT | HYPEROSMOTIC | SALINE | STIMULANT |
|---|---|---|---|---|---|
| Increases peristalsis | Yes | Yes | Yes | Yes | Yes |
| Causes increased secretion of water and electrolytes in small bowel | Yes | Yes | No | Yes | Yes |
| Inhibits absorption of water in small bowel | Yes | Yes | No | Yes | Yes |
| Increases wall permeability in small bowel | No | Yes | No | No | Yes |
| Acts only in large bowel | No | No | Yes | No | No |
| Increases water in fecal mass | Yes | Yes | Yes | Yes | Yes |
| Softens fecal mass | Yes | Yes | Yes | Yes | Yes |

## TABLE 51-6   LAXATIVES: INDICATIONS

| CATEGORY | INDICATION |
|---|---|
| Bulk-forming | Acute and chronic constipation, irritable bowel syndrome, diverticulosis |
| Emollient | Acute and chronic constipation, fecal impaction, anorectal conditions requiring facilitation of bowel movements |
| Hyperosmotic | Chronic constipation, bowel preparation for diagnostic and surgical procedures |
| Saline | Constipation, bowel preparation for diagnostic and surgical procedures |
| Stimulant | Acute constipation, bowel preparation for diagnostic and surgical procedures |

## TABLE 51-7   LAXATIVES: ADVERSE EFFECTS

| CATEGORY | ADVERSE EFFECTS |
|---|---|
| Bulk-forming | Impaction above strictures, fluid disturbances, electrolyte imbalances, gas formation, esophageal blockage, allergic reaction |
| Emollient | Skin rashes, decreased absorption of vitamins, lipid pneumonia, electrolyte imbalances |
| Hyperosmotic | Abdominal bloating, rectal irritation, electrolyte imbalances |
| Saline | Magnesium toxicity (with renal insufficiency), electrolyte imbalances, cramping, diarrhea, increased thirst |
| Stimulant | Nutrient malabsorption, skin rashes, gastric irritation, electrolyte imbalances, discolored urine, rectal irritation |

## Indications

The following are some of the more common uses of laxatives:

- Facilitation of bowel movements in patients with inactive colon or anorectal disorders
- Reduction of ammonia absorption in hepatic encephalopathy (lactulose only)
- Treatment of drug-induced constipation
- Treatment of constipation associated with pregnancy and/or postobstetric period
- Treatment of constipation caused by reduced physical activity or poor dietary habits
- Removal of toxic substances from the body
- Facilitation of defecation in megacolon
- Preparation for colonic diagnostic procedures or surgery
  See Table 51-6 for specific therapeutic indications for each laxative drug class.

## Contraindications

All categories of laxatives share the same general contraindications and precautions, including avoidance in cases of drug allergy and the need for cautious use in the presence of the following: acute surgical abdomen; appendicitis symptoms such as abdominal pain, nausea, and vomiting; fecal impaction (mineral oil enemas excepted); intestinal obstruction; and undiagnosed abdominal pain.

## Adverse Effects

The adverse effects of the various drugs are specific to the laxative group. Most of the adverse effects from laxatives are confined to the intestine; however, the overuse and misuse of laxatives lead to many unwanted effects that are not expected or designed to occur with appropriate use. The major adverse effects of the laxative drugs are listed in Table 51-7.

## Interactions

Laxatives alter intestinal function; therefore, they can interact with other drugs, because many drugs are absorbed in the intestines. Bulk-forming laxatives can decrease the absorption of antibiotics, digoxin, salicylates, tetracyclines, and warfarin. Mineral oil can decrease the absorption of fat-soluble vitamins (A, D, E, and K). Hyperosmotic laxatives can cause increased CNS depression if they are given with barbiturates, general anesthetics, opioids, or antipsychotics. Oral antibiotics can decrease the effects of lactulose. Stimulant laxatives decrease the absorption of antibiotics, digoxin, nitrofurantoin, salicylates, tetracyclines, and oral anticoagulants.

## Dosages

For dosage information on selected laxatives, see the table on p. 836.

## DRUG PROFILES

Laxatives are used for the treatment of constipation. Such treatment must involve an understanding of the whole patient. Many drugs in the five major groups of laxatives are available as OTC medications, whereas others require a prescription for use. The following profiles describe the prototypical drugs in each of the laxative groups.

## BULK-FORMING LAXATIVES

Bulk-forming laxatives are composed of water-retaining (hydrophilic) natural and synthetic cellulose derivatives. Psyllium is an example of a natural bulk-forming laxative, and methylcellulose is an example of a synthetic cellulose derivative. Bulk-forming drugs increase water absorption, which results in greater total volume (bulk) of the intestinal contents. Bulk-forming laxatives tend to produce normal, formed stools. Their action is limited to the GI tract, so there are few, if any, systemic effects. However, they need to be taken with liberal amounts of water to prevent esophageal obstruction and/or fecal impaction. The bulk-forming laxatives are all obtainable OTC, are among the safest laxatives available, and are the only ones that are recommended for long-term use.

### methylcellulose

Methylcellulose (Citrucel) is a synthetic bulk-forming laxative that attracts water into the intestine and absorbs excess water into the stool, stimulating the intestines and increasing peristalsis. Specific contraindications include GI obstruction and hepatitis. Methylcellulose is an oral drug available in powdered form that provides approximately 2 g of fiber per heaping tablespoon.

## DOSAGES

### Selected Laxatives

| DRUG (PREGNANCY CATEGORY) | PHARMACOLOGIC CLASS | USUAL DOSAGE RANGE | ONSET OF ACTION |
|---|---|---|---|
| bisacodyl (Dulcolax) (C) | Stimulant laxative | **Pediatric younger than 2 yr**<br>5-mg suppository<br>**Pediatric older than 2 yr**<br>10-mg suppository<br>**Pediatric older than 6 yr**<br>PO: 0.3 mg/kg<br>**Adult**<br>5-15 mg oral or 10 mg-suppository | Oral: 6-12 hr<br>Rectal: 15-60 minutes |
| ♦ docusate sodium (Colace, others) and docusate calcium (Surfak, others) (C) | Fecal softener, emollient laxative | **Pediatric 2-11 yr***<br>PO: 33-120 mg/day divided daily-tid<br>**Pediatric 12 yr and older, and adult***<br>PO: 50-300 mg/day divided daily-qid | 1-3 days |
| ♦ glycerin (Sani-Supp, Colace, Fleet Babylax) (C) | Hyperosmotic laxative | **Adult and pediatric**<br>Rectal only: Insert one adult, child, or infant suppository PR daily-bid prn; attempt to retain 15-30 min; suppository does not have to melt to induce BM | 16-36 min |
| ♦ lactulose (Enulose, others) (B) | Disaccharide, hyper-osmotic laxative | **Pediatric, infant†**<br>PO: 2.5-10 mL/day divided bid-qid<br>**Child and adolescent†**<br>PO: 40-90 mL/day divided bid-qid<br>**Adult†**<br>PO: 30-45 mL tid-qid | 24 hr |
| magnesium citrate (generic only), magnesium sulfate (Epsom salts by various manufacturers) (B) | Saline laxative | ***Citrate, PO***<br>**Pediatric younger than 6 yr**<br>0.5mL/kg (max 200 mL); may repeat q4-6h until stools clear<br>**Pediatric 6-11 yr**<br>100-150 mL × 1 dose<br>**Adult**<br>120-300 mL × 1 dose | 0.5-3 hr |
| methylcellulose (Citrucel, others) (B) | Bulk-forming laxative | **Pediatric 6-11 yr**<br>½ dose of that for pediatric 12 yr and older, and adult<br>**Pediatric 12 yr and older, and adult**<br>PO: 1 heaping tbsp in 8 oz cold water daily-tid | 12-24 hr |
| mineral oil (Kondremul Plain, Fleet Mineral Oil Enema) (B) | Emollient laxative | ***PO***<br>**Pediatric 6-11 yr**<br>5-15 mL oil or 10-25 mL Kondremul Plain emulsion<br>**Pediatric 12 yr and older, and adult**<br>15-45 mL oil or 30-75 mL Kondremul Plain emulsion taken at bedtime<br>***Rectal enema***<br>**Pediatric 2-11 yr**<br>PR: 59 mL × 1<br>**Pediatric 12 yr and older, and adult**<br>PR: 118 mL × 1 | 6-8 hr |

## DOSAGES—cont'd

### Selected Laxatives

| DRUG (PREGNANCY CATEGORY) | PHARMACOLOGIC CLASS | USUAL DOSAGE RANGE | ONSET OF ACTION |
|---|---|---|---|
| polyethylene glycol (Colyte, GoLYTELY, Half-Lytely, MiraLax) (C) | Hyperosmotic laxative | **Adult only**<br>PO: 4 L solution, usually ending before procedure; patient needs to fast at least 4 hr before drinking solution<br>MiraLax: 17 g once daily | 1 hr |
| ◆ psyllium (Metamucil, Fiberall, others) (B) | Bulk-forming laxative | **Pediatric 6-11 yr**<br>PO: ½ rounded tsp in water or juice daily-tid<br>**Pediatric 12 yr and older, and adult**<br>PO: 1 rounded tsp in 8 oz water or juice daily-tid | 12-24 hr |
| ◆ senna (Senokot, others) (C) | Stimulant-irritant laxative | **Pediatric 2-5 yr‡**<br>PO (liquid): 2.5 mL (max: ½ tsp bid)<br>**Pediatric 6-11 yr‡**<br>PO (tabs): 1 tab daily (max: 2 tabs bid)<br>PO (liquid): 7.5-10 mL daily (max: 5 mL bid)<br>**Pediatric 12 yr and older, and adult‡**<br>PO (tabs): Start with 2 tabs daily (max: 4 tabs bid)<br>PO (liquid): 15 mL daily (max: 30 mL bid) | 6-24 hr |

*BM*, Bowel movement; *PO*, oral; *PR*, per rectum.

\*Docusate sodium is available in both capsule and liquid forms. Docusate calcium is available in capsule form only.

†Rectal route is sometimes used to reverse certain types of coma.

‡Many dosage forms; consult product labeling if in doubt. Most common dosage forms are 8.6-mg sennosides in tablet form and 8.8 mg/5 mL of sennosides in liquid form.

#### ◆ psyllium

Psyllium (Metamucil) is a natural bulk-forming laxative obtained from the dried seed of the *Plantago psyllium* plant. It has many of the characteristics of methylcellulose. Psyllium is contraindicated in patients with intestinal obstruction or fecal impaction. Its use is also contraindicated in patients experiencing abdominal pain and/or nausea and vomiting. Psyllium is available for oral use in wafer and powder form.

### EMOLLIENT LAXATIVES

Emollient laxatives either directly lubricate the stool and the intestines, as with mineral oil, or act as fecal softeners. By lubricating the fecal material and the intestinal walls, lubricant emollient laxatives prevent water from moving out of the intestines, which softens and expands the stool. Stool softeners (docusate salts) work by lowering the surface tension of fluids, which allows more water and fat to be absorbed into the stool and the intestines.

#### ◆ docusate salts

Docusate salts (calcium and sodium) (Colace) are stool-softening emollient laxatives that facilitate the passage of water and lipids (fats) into the fecal mass, which softens the stool. These drugs are used to treat constipation, soften fecal impactions, and facilitate bowel movements in patients with hemorrhoids and other painful anorectal conditions. They do not cause patients to defecate; they simply soften the stool to ease its passage. In addition to the docusate salt formulations, combination products are also available. Docusate use is contraindicated in patients with intestinal obstruction, fecal impaction, or nausea and vomiting.

#### mineral oil

Mineral oil eases the passage of stool by lubricating the intestines and preventing water from escaping the stool. Mineral oil is the only lubricant laxative in the emollient category. It is a mixture of liquid hydrocarbons derived from petroleum and is most commonly used to treat constipation associated with hard stools or fecal impaction.

Mineral oil use is contraindicated in patients with intestinal obstruction, abdominal pain, or nausea and vomiting. Mineral oil drugs are available as enemas and in products for oral use. There are also combination products that contain mineral oil, such as Haley's M-O, which includes both mineral oil and milk of magnesia (magnesium hydroxide).

### HYPEROSMOTIC LAXATIVES

The hyperosmotic laxatives glycerin, lactulose, sorbitol, and polyethylene glycol (PEG) relieve constipation by increasing the water content of the feces, which results in distention, peristalsis, and evacuation. They are most commonly used to treat constipation and to evacuate the bowels before diagnostic and surgical procedures.

#### ◆ glycerin

Glycerin promotes bowel movement by increasing osmotic pressure in the intestine, which draws fluid into the colon. Because it is a very mild laxative, it is often used in children. Glycerin has properties similar to those of sorbitol, another hyperosmotic laxative. Glycerin use is contraindicated in patients who have shown a hypersensitivity reaction to it. It is available as a rectal solution and as both adult and pediatric suppositories.

#### ♦ lactulose

Lactulose is a synthetic derivative of the natural sugar lactose, which is not digested in the stomach or absorbed in the small bowel. Instead it passes unchanged into the large intestine, where it is metabolized. Colonic bacteria digest lactulose to produce lactic acid, formic acid, and acetic acid, which creates a hyperosmotic environment that draws water into the colon and produces a laxative effect. This drug-induced acidic environment also reduces blood ammonia levels by converting ammonia to ammonium. Ammonium is a water-soluble cation that is trapped in the intestines and cannot be reabsorbed into the systemic circulation. This effect has proved helpful in reducing serum ammonia levels in patients with hepatic encephalopathy. Lactulose use is contraindicated in patients on a low-galactose diet. It is available as a solution for either oral or rectal use.

#### polyethylene glycol 3350

PEG-3350 is most commonly given before diagnostic or surgical bowel procedures, because it is a very potent laxative that induces total cleansing of the bowel. The 3350 designation refers to the osmolality of the drug. It is usually available in a powdered dosage form that contains mixtures of electrolytes that also help stimulate bowel evacuation (e.g., Colyte, GoLYTELY, MoviPrep, Half-Lytely). The powder is usually reconstituted in a large volume of fluid (1 gal) that is then gradually drunk by the patient on the afternoon of the day before the procedure. Use of PEG is contraindicated in patients with GI obstruction, gastric retention, bowel perforation, toxic colitis, toxic megacolon, or ileus.

An oral solution of PEG-3350 and electrolytes is available for GI lavage. Diarrhea usually occurs within 30 to 60 minutes after ingestion; complete evacuation and cleansing of the bowel is accomplished within 4 hours. MiraLax is a PEG-3350 product that is available OTC and can be used daily for constipation in much smaller amounts than those used for total bowel cleansing.

### SALINE LAXATIVES

Saline laxatives consist of various magnesium or sodium salts. They increase osmotic pressure and draw water into the colon, producing a watery stool, usually within 3 to 6 hours of ingestion. The currently available saline laxatives are listed in Box 51-1. Oral sodium phosphate–containing products used for bowel evacuation, such as Fleet Phospho-Soda, were taken off the market in 2008 because of concerns about acute phosphate nephropathy.

#### magnesium salts

The magnesium saline laxatives, magnesium citrate (Citroma), and magnesium hydroxide (Phillips Milk of Magnesia) are unpleasant-tasting OTC laxative preparations. They are to be used with caution in patients with renal insufficiency, because they can be absorbed enough to cause hypermagnesemia. They are most commonly used to evacuate the bowel rapidly in preparation for endoscopic examination and to help remove unabsorbed poisons from the GI tract.

Use of magnesium salts is contraindicated in patients with renal disease, abdominal pain, nausea and vomiting, obstruction, acute surgical abdomen, or rectal bleeding. Magnesium hydroxide, more commonly referred to as *milk of magnesia*, is available in oral liquid and tablet form. It is also found in a variety of combination products, such as Haley's M-O (see mineral oil profile). Other magnesium products are listed in the discussion of saline laxatives earlier in the chapter. Note that magnesium *oxide* is used as a supplement, not as a laxative (see Chapter 53).

### STIMULANT LAXATIVES

Stimulant laxatives induce intestinal peristalsis. In the past, several different stimulant laxatives were available; however, the U.S. Food and Drug Administration has required that all except bisacodyl (Dulcolax) and senna (Senokot) be removed from the market. Their site of action is the entire GI tract. The action of the stimulant laxatives is proportional to the dose. The stimulant class is the most likely of all laxative classes to cause dependence.

#### bisacodyl

Bisacodyl (Dulcolax) is the most commonly used stimulant laxative. It is available as an oral tablet and rectal suppository. It is used for constipation or for whole bowel evacuation prior to endoscopic examination. It is available OTC.

#### ♦ senna

Senna (Senokot) is a commonly used OTC stimulant laxative. Senna is obtained from the dried leaves of the *Cassia acutifolia* plant. It may be used for relief of acute constipation or bowel preparation for surgery or examination. Because of its stimulating action on the GI tract, it may cause abdominal pain. It can produce complete bowel evacuation in 6 to 12 hours. Senna is available in a variety of dosages as tablets, syrup, and granules. One product, Senokot-S, includes both senna and the stool softener docusate sodium.

### DRUGS FOR IRRITABLE BOWEL SYNDROME

Irritable bowel syndrome (IBS) is a condition of chronic intestinal discomfort characterized by cramps, diarrhea, and/or constipation. Patients usually cope with the symptoms by avoiding irritating foods and/or taking OTC laxatives and antidiarrheal drugs. Women are affected more often than men. In 2009, the American College of Gastroenterology Task Force on Irritable Bowel Syndrome released a position statement on the treatment of IBS. Their conclusions are as follows: psyllium is moderately effective in IBS; the antidiarrheal loperamide is not more effective than placebo at reducing pain or bloating, but it is an effective agent for the treatment of diarrhea,

| BOX 51-1 | SALINE LAXATIVES | |
| --- | --- | --- |
| **Magnesium Laxatives** | *Citrate* | |
| *Sulfate* | Citrate of magnesia | |
| Epsom salts | | |
| | **Sodium Laxatives** | |
| *Hydroxide* | Fleet Enema | |
| Milk of magnesia | | |

reducing stool frequency, and improving stool consistency; the 5-hydroxytryptamine 3 (5-HT$_3$) receptor antagonist alosetron is more effective than placebo; alosetron is most favorable in women with severe IBS and diarrhea who have not responded to conventional therapies; the 5-hydroxytryptamine 4 (5-HT$_4$) receptor agonist tegaserod and the chloride channel activator lubiprostone are more effective than placebo; and tricyclic antidepressants and selective serotonin reuptake inhibitors are more effective than placebo at relieving IBS symptoms, and appear to reduce abdominal pain.

Tegaserod (Zelnorm) is a serotonin 5-HT$_4$ receptor agonist and is approved for treatment of IBS with constipation and chronic idiopathic constipation in women younger than 55 years of age for whom no alternative therapy exists. Tegaserod was approved in 2002, taken off the market in 2007, and then reintroduced under restricted availability in 2008. Tegaserod has been associated with serious adverse events including angina, heart attacks, and stroke. Patients must be registered with the manufacturer. It is categorized as a pregnancy category B drug and is dosed at 6 mg twice a day for 4 to 6 weeks.

Lubiprostone (Amitiza) is a chloride channel activator that is indicated for the treatment of chronic idiopathic constipation and IBS with constipation in women 18 years of age and older. It is dosed at 24 mcg twice a day for idiopathic constipation and 8 mcg twice a day for IBS. The most common adverse effects are nausea, diarrhea, and abdominal pain. It is classified as a pregnancy category C drug. Lubiprostone is contraindicated in patients with known or suspected bowel obstruction.

Alosetron (Lotronex) is a selective serotonin 5-HT$_3$ receptor antagonist that is indicated for the treatment of severe, chronic, diarrhea-predominant IBS in women who have failed conventional therapy. It is dosed at 0.5 mg twice daily for 4 weeks and may be increased to 1 mg twice a day. If response is inadequate after 4 weeks, the drug is to be discontinued. It must be discontinued immediately if constipation or signs of ischemic colitis occur. Only physicians who have enrolled in the manufacturer-sponsored prescribing program can prescribe alosetron.

## NURSING PROCESS

## ASSESSMENT

Before giving *antidiarrheal* preparations, obtain a thorough history and perform an assessment of bowel patterns, general state of health, any recent illness, and any dietary changes. In the abdominal assessment, include auscultation of bowel sounds in all four quadrants *after* inspection of the entire abdomen but *before* percussion and palpation. Performing auscultation and inspection before percussion prevents any possible stimulation of peristalsis or bowel sounds that would not occur otherwise. When the frequency of bowel sounds ranges from 6 to 32 per minute, it is important to describe exactly what is heard and the amount of activity in each of the four quadrants. Terms such as *high-pitched, low-pitched, gurgling,* or *tinkling* may be used to describe the character of the sounds, whereas activity may be described as *hypoactive* (less than 6 sounds per minute), *normoactive* (between 6 and 32 sounds per minute), or *hyperactive*

(more than the normal range). Perform a thorough abdominal assessment for any patient with GI complaints, including altered bowel status. Note the presence of tenderness, rigidity, changes in contour, bulges, and obvious peristaltic waves across the abdomen. Assess frequency, consistency, amount, color, and odor (if present) of stools, and document the findings. In addition, it is critical to patient safety and health to be sure that the possibility of *Clostridium difficile* infection or other infectious diarrhea is ruled out. Assess for and document any contraindications, cautions, and drug interactions for all drugs. Report complaints of abdominal pain, bloody stools, confirmation of hypoactive to no bowel sounds, and/or fever to the prescriber immediately. When administering diphenoxylate with atropine, be wary of overuse because large amounts may result in dry mouth, abdominal pain, tachycardia, and blurred vision. Elderly patients are more susceptible to fluid and electrolyte depletion associated with diarrhea; therefore, closely assess hydration status and age.

*Laxative* use requires further assessment in addition to the abdominal assessment and bowel pattern history described earlier. For example, focus questions on changes in bowel patterns, long-term use of laxatives (because patients may become laxative dependent), and dietary and fluid intake. Assess vital signs, daily weights, intake and output, and fluid and electrolyte levels, and note the presence of any weakness because of the possibility of hypotension and volume or electrolyte depletion (with long-term laxative use). Another important area to assess is that of laxative abuse in the elderly as well as in pediatric and adolescent patients. Specifically, in the pediatric or adolescent patients, assess for eating disorders with concurrent use of laxatives.

The type of laxative and the related mechanism of action dictate specific assessments because of differences in how strongly the patient reacts to the various laxative drugs. The bulk-forming laxatives are often used to treat chronic constipation and have few adverse effects, but a basic abdominal and bowel pattern assessment and related history taking are still needed. Always assess and document contraindications, cautions, and drug interactions. Use docusate salts or emollient laxatives cautiously in the elderly.

With hyperosmotic laxatives (e.g., polytheylene glycol, lactulose, sorbitol, glycerin), assess baseline fluid and electrolyte levels to identify any deficits prior to use. All of the previously mentioned assessment measures regarding abdominal examination and bowel patterns are also appropriate for these drugs, with the additional assessment for the presence of abdominal pain, the degree of peristalsis, and any history of recent abdominal surgery, nausea, vomiting, or weight loss. Elderly patients react more adversely to this class of laxatives, so use in this group is to be avoided.

Saline laxatives (e.g., magnesium hydroxide, magnesium sulfate, and magnesium citrate) are to be used with caution in elderly patients because of possible dehydration and electrolyte loss. They may also cause magnesium toxicity in those with compromised renal status. Renal function studies are important to assess in those at risk. Senna and bisacodyl are examples of stimulant laxatives. They may also cause electrolyte imbalances, so baseline electrolyte levels are important to assess and monitor.

Patients taking *drugs for IBS* need additional assessment of liver functioning as well as assessment for any underlying cardiac disease. The availability of tegaserod is restricted, and patients are registered with the manufacturer because of the risk of severe adverse effects (e.g., angina, heart attack, and stroke). Therefore, thoroughly assess the patient's medical and medication history as well as complete a thorough head-to-toe physical assessment. Do not use lubiprostone in patients with a known or suspected bowel obstruction.

## CASE STUDY

### Long-Term Laxative Use

Mrs. M. is a 66-year-old retired schoolteacher. She enjoys good health and exercises three times a week with a senior citizen group in a supervised arthritis swim class at the local recreation center. She arrives at the family practice office with complaints of "constipation" and says that for the past 3 months she has had only one bowel movement every 3 days instead of one every day. In the assessment of this patient, the nurse discovers that Mrs. M. has been taking a stimulant laxative up to twice a day and is also now feeling "weak." Mrs. M. also says that she is experiencing "a lot of tummy cramping."

1. What are at least five questions the nurse should ask Mrs. M.? Provide reasons for each question.
2. What types of problems are generally related to long-term use of laxatives? Explain your answer.
3. What are some nonpharmacologic ways to help prevent constipation?
4. What over-the-counter drug is the best choice to help prevent constipation? Explain your answer.

For answers, see http://evolve.elsevier.com/Lilley.

## NURSING DIAGNOSES

1. Constipation related to improper and/or inadequate diet
2. Diarrhea related to GI irritation from food, bacteria or viruses, or pathology
3. Deficient fluid volume related to loss of fluids and electrolytes caused by frequent, loose stools

## PLANNING

### GOALS

1. Patient experiences minimal constipation.
2. Patient experiences minimal diarrhea.
3. Patient remains free from fluid and electrolyte disturbances related to changes in bowel patterns and lack of proper management of bowel alterations.

### OUTCOME CRITERIA

1. Patient states measures to manage/prevent constipation such as forcing fluids; increasing intake of bulk and fiber (unless contraindicated); and increasing physical activity.
   - Patient takes recommended bulk-forming laxatives, stool softeners, as well as other approved laxatives, as prescribed and follows directions closely.

2. Patient states measures to manage and prevent diarrhea such as increasing bulk; avoiding spicy, irritating foods and beverages; and avoiding caffeine.
   - Patient takes recommended antidiarrheal preparation as prescribed and instructed, with close attention to following directions on the medication.
3. Patient reports to the prescriber any signs and symptoms of fluid and electrolyte loss, such as weakness, lethargy, decreased urinary output, and dizziness.
   - Patient implements measures to prevent fluid and electrolyte loss such as nonpharmacologic and pharmacologic therapies (see above).

## IMPLEMENTATION

With *antidiarrheals,* educate the patient that the drugs must be taken *exactly* as directions indicate, with strict adherence to the recommended dose, frequency, and duration of treatment. Encourage the patient to be aware of fluid intake and any dietary changes that would impact his or her health status or possibly exacerbate present symptoms. Instruct the patients to be aware of the factors precipitating the diarrhea and, if symptoms persist, to contact his or her health care provider. Document any changes in bowel patterns, weight, fluid volume, intake and output as well as in the mucous membranes during and after treatment—whether for constipation or diarrhea. Inform the patient that bismuth subsalicylate must be taken as directed and that this medication will turn the stool black or gray. If tablets are used, they must be chewed thoroughly before swallowing and with at least 6 oz of fluid. Bismuth subsalicylate is a salicylate-based product and is not to be taken with other salicylates to avoid the risk of toxicity. Encourage parents to check with their children's health care provider before giving bismuth subsalicylate to a child or teenager with a viral infection, such as chickenpox or influenza, because of the risk for Reye's syndrome (see the Patient-Centered Care: Lifespan Considerations for the Pediatric Patient box).

Diphenoxylate hydrochloride and loperamide may be given without regard to food intake but must be given with adequate fluid. Additionally, advise the patient to follow the specific directions (e.g., the specific number of tablets recommended by the manufacturer after the first loose stool and the total number of tablets to be taken within a 24-hour period). Maximum amounts are not to be exceeded, and if diarrhea continues or other symptoms occur (e.g., fever, abdominal pain, bloody stools), instruct the patient to contact the prescriber immediately. See the Patient Teaching Tips for more information.

*Probiotics* may be recommended for a variety of altered bowel elimination patterns, whether diarrhea or constipation. Probiotics are available in foods and dietary supplements and in capsules, tablets, and powder dosage forms. Most of the probiotics are derived from *Lactobacillus* or *Bifidobacterium* bacteria. It is important to educate the patient about probiotics and to emphasize their healthy benefits when administered in the proper amounts. Tell the patient to take probiotics exactly as directed. Foods that contain probiotics include yogurt, fermented milk, miso, empeh, and some juices and soy beverages.

Bulk-forming *laxatives* such as methylcellulose must be administered, as specified by package insert or as ordered. Methylcellulose is to be taken with at least 8 oz or 1 full glass of liquid after the powder form has been thoroughly stirred into it. The fluid must be taken immediately because of a congealing effect that continues to harden with time. To avoid choking or swelling of the product in the throat or esophagus, the patient must swallow or receive the drug immediately upon stirring. The medication must never be taken or administered in its dry form. See the Patient Teaching Tips for more information.

Docusate is available in a variety of oral dosage forms (e.g., capsules, tablets, syrups, elixir), and it is recommended to take it with at least 6 oz of water or other fluid. An additional 6 to 8 glasses of water a day is also suggested to help with stool softening. Bisacodyl, if ordered, is best taken on an empty stomach for faster action, and whole tablets should not be chewed or crushed. Advise the patient not to take milk, antacids, or juices with the dose or within 1 hour of taking the medication. Rectal suppositories, if too soft, may be placed in a medicine cup with ice to harden the suppository before insertion. Once the wrapper is removed, apply a water-soluble lubricant to the suppository prior to insertion into the rectum. Use a gloved hand or finger cot for insertion. Encourage the patient to try and keep the suppository in place by lying still on the left side for at least 15 to 30 minutes to allow the drug to dissolve for maximal effectiveness. Lactulose may be taken with juice, milk, or water to increase palatability. It is important to note that the normal color of the oral solution is pale yellow. Administer rectal dosage forms as a retention enema with dilution as ordered, and instruct the patient to retain for 30 to 60 minutes. For proper insertion of a retention enema, lubricate the tip of the apparatus well, and insert it carefully with the nozzle pointed toward the umbilicus of the patient, with the patient lying on the left side. Release the fluid gradually, and discontinue administration if the patient experiences severe abdominal pain. If long-term use of the drug is indicated, monitoring serum electrolyte levels is needed.

Magnesium-based laxatives are generally used only in certain situations because they are very potent. Force fluids, and follow other instructions per the prescriber's order or the package instructions. Refrigeration may help increase the palatability of the oral solution. Emphasize the importance that this type of drug is to be taken exactly as prescribed for constipation, with consumption of plenty of fluids and careful attention to adverse effects. Instruct the patient to mix the PEG-electrolyte solution with water or flavored sports drink as directed and to shake well before drinking. Chilled solutions are tolerated better. Rapid drinking of each dose is recommended.

*IBS drugs* should be given as ordered and usually on an empty stomach before meals. Tegaserod, only available under restricted guidelines, must also be taken exactly as prescribed and only for up to 4 to 6 weeks. With this drug, monitoring for the serious cardio-cerebrovascular adverse effects is so important to patient safety. Continual observation of complaints of chest pain, lightheadedness, and dizziness as well as frequent monitoring of vital signs and neurologic checks (e.g., LOC, reflexes, pupils for reactivity and size, speech) are all very important. Lubiprostone must also be given as prescribed and is usually ordered for twice-daily dosing. Alosetron (Lotronex) is generally given twice daily. Be sure the patient receives the FDA-approved medication guide with each dispensing of alosetron. Encourage the patient to keep a daily journal to help the prescriber in identifying the effectiveness of therapy.

## ▌EVALUATION

Therapeutic responses to any of these medications include an improvement in the GI-related signs and symptoms reported by the patient (e.g., decrease in diarrhea or constipation), return to normal bowel patterns with normal bowel sounds, and absence of abnormal findings on assessment of the abdomen and bowel patterns. Adverse effects for which to monitor patients vary according to drug. Use goals and outcome criteria as a means to evaluate the nursing care plan related to each problem, whether it is constipation, diarrhea, or both.

## ▌PATIENT TEACHING TIPS

- Instruct the patient that antidiarrheals are to be taken exactly as prescribed, giving close attention to indicated dosages with warnings of overuse!
- Counsel the patient to take antidiarrheal drugs with caution when performing tasks that require mental alertness or motor skills until it is clear how the drug actually affects him or her. Advise the patient to immediately report to the prescriber any abdominal distention or firm/hard abdomen, abdominal pain, worsening (or no improvement) of symptoms, rectal bleeding, unrelieved constipation or diarrhea, fever, nausea, vomiting or other GI-related signs and symptoms, dizziness, muscle weakness, and muscle cramping.
- Encourage frequent mouth care, fluid intake, or use of sugarless gum or candy to help with the adverse effect of dry mouth.

- Bismuth subsalicylate may turn the stool tarry black, so warn the patient that this may happen. Patients must avoid other drugs containing salicylates while taking bismuth. Always check for cautions and contraindications of this drug, especially for pediatric patients.
- Increasing the intake of fluids, preferably water, as well foods high in fiber and whole grain, green leafy vegetables, and fruits may help to minimize constipation. Exercise is also beneficial.
- Educate the patient that what are normal bowel patterns for one person may not be normal for another.
- Keep all antidiarrheals and laxatives out of the reach of children.
- For patients taking powder forms of methylcellulose, emphasize the need to have the powder thoroughly mixed with at

least 6 oz of liquid, which is stirred and drunk immediately to avoid esophageal or throat obstruction.

- Probiotics come in various dosages, under different product names, and OTC. Advise the patient to take them exactly as instructed and to be aware that side effects are generally not of concern. Cultured yogurt and cultured milk products provide probiotics.

- Inform the patient taking senna to avoid other medications within 1 hour of taking it and that it often takes 6 to 12 hours for the laxative effect to occur.

## KEY POINTS

- Diarrhea is a leading cause of morbidity and mortality in underdeveloped countries.
- Drugs used to treat diarrhea include adsorbents, anticholinergics, opiates, and probiotics.
- Most acute diarrhea is self-limiting, subsiding in 3 days to 2 weeks.
- Fluid and electrolyte replacement is vital while a patient is experiencing diarrhea.
- Encourage patients to check and recheck dosage instructions before taking medication and to note any drug-food and drug-drug interactions.
- Anticholinergics work by decreasing GI peristalsis through their parasympathetic blocking effects. Adverse effects include urinary retention, headache, confusion, dry skin, rash, and blurred vision.
- Adsorbents work by coating the walls of the GI tract. They remain in the intestine and bind the causative bacteria or toxin to the adsorbent surface, so that it can be eliminated

from the body through the stool. They may increase bleeding and cause constipation, dark stools, and black tongue.
- Probiotics are also used to manage diarrhea and consist of bacterial cultures of *Lactobacillus*. They reestablish normal intestinal flora destroyed by infection or antibiotics and suppress the growth of diarrhea-causing bacteria.
- Opiates are also used as antidiarrheals and help to decrease bowel motility and thus permit longer contact of intestinal contents with the absorptive surface of the bowel. Opiates also help to reduce the pain associated with rectal spasms.
- Laxatives, especially osmotic medications, may cause fluid and electrolyte loss.
- Alert patients to the abuse potential of laxatives and the problems associated with their misuse as well as laxative dependency issues.
- Stool softeners and bulk-forming drugs are often preferred to other drug classes in the treatment of constipation because they are not as problematic with regard to fluid and electrolyte loss.

## NCLEX® EXAMINATION REVIEW QUESTIONS

1 A patient is being prepared for a colonoscopy. The nurse expects which laxative to be used as preparation for this procedure?
   a methylcellulose
   b docusate sodium
   c PEG-3350
   d glycerin

2 The nurse is administering oral methylcellulose (Citrucel) and keeps in mind that a major potential concern with this drug is
   a dehydration.
   b tarry stools.
   c renal calculi.
   d esophageal obstruction.

3 A 45-year-old woman has been diagnosed with irritable bowel syndrome (IBS) and will be taking lubiprostone (Amitiza). The nurse assesses for conditions that may be contraindications to this drug, such as
   a constipation.
   b bowel obstruction.
   c renal calculi.
   d anemia.

4 When the nurse teaches a patient about taking bisacodyl tablets, which instruction is correct?
   a "Take this medication on an empty stomach."
   b "Chew the tablet for quicker onset of action."
   c "Take this medication with juice or milk."
   d "Take this medication with an antacid if it upsets your stomach."

5 A patient has been receiving long-term antibiotic therapy as part of treatment for an infected leg wound. He tells the nurse that he has had "spells of diarrhea" for the last week. Which medication is most appropriate for him at this time?
   a bismuth subsalicylate
   b *L. acidophilus*
   c diphenoxylate with atropine
   d codeine

6 A parent calls to ask about giving a medication for diarrhea to his child, 12 years of age, who is recovering from the flu. The nurse expects the prescriber to recommend which medication?

a  bismuth subsalicylate (Pepto-Bismol)
b  *Lactobacillus GG* (Culturelle)
c  belladonna alkaloid/phenobarbital combination (Donnatal Elixir)
d  loperamide (Imodium A-D)

7 A patient has been instructed to use an over-the-counter (OTC) form of the bulk-forming laxative methylcellulose (Citrucel) to prevent constipation. The nurse will advise the patient of potential adverse effects, including *(Select all that apply)*

a  fluid and electrolyte disturbances.
b  decreased absorption of vitamins.
c  gas formation.
d  darkened stools.
e  discolored urine.

1. c, 2. d, 3. b, 4. a, 5. b, 6. d, 7. a, c

For Critical Thinking and Prioritization Questions, see http://evolve.elsevier.com/Lilley.

# CHAPTER

# 52

# Antiemetic and Antinausea Drugs

## evolve WEBSITE

*http://evolve.elsevier.com/Lilley*

- Animations
- Answer Key—Textbook Case Studies
- Critical Thinking and Prioritization Questions

- Key Points—Downloadable
- Review Questions for the NCLEX® Examination
- Unfolding Case Studies

## OBJECTIVES

When you reach the end of this chapter, you will be able to do the following:

1  Discuss the pathophysiology of nausea and vomiting, including specific precipitating factors and/or diseases.
2  Identify the various antiemetic and antinausea drugs and their drug classification groupings.
3  Describe the mechanisms of action, indications for use, contraindications, cautions, and drug interactions of the

various categories of antiemetic and antinausea drugs.
4  Develop a nursing care plan that includes all phases of the nursing process for patients taking antiemetic and antinausea drugs.

## DRUG PROFILES

aprepitant, p. 851
dronabinol, p. 850
♦ meclizine, p. 849
♦ metoclopramide, p. 850
♦ ondansetron, p. 850
phosphorated carbohydrate solution, p. 851

♦ prochlorperazine, p. 849
promethazine, p. 849
scopolamine, p. 849

_____

♦  *Key drug*

## KEY TERMS

Antiemetic drugs  Drugs given to relieve nausea and vomiting. (p. 846)

Chemoreceptor trigger zone (CTZ)  The area of the brain that is involved in the sensation of nausea and the action of vomiting. (p. 845)

Emesis  The forcible emptying or expulsion of gastric and, occasionally, intestinal contents through the mouth; also called *vomiting*. (p. 845)

Nausea  Sensation often leading to the urge to vomit. (p. 845)

Vomiting center  The area of the brain that is involved in stimulating the physiologic events that lead to nausea and vomiting. (p. 845)

# ANATOMY, PHYSIOLOGY, AND PATHOPHYSIOLOGY OVERVIEW

## NAUSEA AND VOMITING

Nausea and vomiting are two gastrointestinal (GI) disorders that can be extremely unpleasant but also can lead to more serious complications if not treated promptly. Nausea is an unpleasant feeling that often precedes vomiting. If it does not subside spontaneously or is not relieved by medication, it can lead to vomiting. Vomiting, which is also called emesis, is the forcible emptying or expulsion of gastric and, occasionally, intestinal contents through the mouth. A variety of stimuli can induce nausea and vomiting, including foul odors or tastes, unpleasant sights, irritation of the stomach or intestines, and certain drugs (ipecac or antineoplastic drugs).

The vomiting center is an area in the brain that is responsible for initiating the physiologic events that lead to nausea and vomiting. Neurotransmitter signals are sent to the vomiting center from the chemoreceptor trigger zone (CTZ), another area in the brain involved in the induction of nausea and vomiting. These signals alert those areas of the brain to the existence of nauseating substances (noxious stimuli) that need to be expelled from the body. Once the CTZ and vomiting center are stimulated, they initiate the events that trigger the vomiting reflex. The neurotransmitters involved in this process and their respective receptors are listed in Table 52-1. The various pathways and the areas of the body that send the signals to the vomiting center are illustrated in Figure 52-1. Two specific types of nausea and vomiting, chemotherapy-induced and postoperative, produce much more intense symptoms and are treated much more aggressively than general nausea and vomiting.

| TABLE 52-1 | NEUROTRANSMITTERS INVOLVED IN NAUSEA AND VOMITING |
|---|---|
| **NEUROTRANSMITTER (RECEPTOR)** | **SITE IN THE VOMITING PATHWAY** |
| Acetylcholine (ACh) | VC in brain; vestibular and labyrinthine pathways in inner ear |
| Dopamine ($D_2$) | GI tract and CTZ in brain |
| Histamine ($H_1$) | VC in brain; vestibular and labyrinthine pathways in inner ear |
| Prostaglandins | GI tract |
| Serotonin (5-$HT_3$) | GI tract; CTZ and VC in brain |

*CTZ*, Chemoreceptor trigger zone; *ACh*, acetylcholine receptor; *$D_2$*, dopamine 2 receptor; *GI*, gastrointestinal; *$H_1$*, histamine 1 receptor; *5-$HT_3$*, 5-hydroxytryptamine 3 receptor; *VC*, vomiting center.

### PATIENT-CENTERED CARE: LIFESPAN CONSIDERATIONS FOR THE PEDIATRIC PATIENT

#### *Syrup of Ipecac and Poisioning*

- Since November 2003, the American Academy of Pediatrics (AAP) has strongly advised *against* the use of syrup of ipecac as an emetic when children swallow a poisonous substance. In a statement published in the November 2003 issue of *Pediatrics*, the AAP recommended that syrup of ipecac no longer be used as a home treatment for poisoning. Syrup of ipecac is still not recommended for use at this time. See http://www.healthychildren.org for more information.
- If a child has been exposed to a toxic substance, the caregiver must call the national poison control hotline at 800-222-1222. Calls are routed to the local poison control center or take to the nearest emergency department.
- Steps to follow to prevent accidental poisoning, as identified by the AAP, include the following: (1) Keep potential poisons out of sight and out of reach. (2) Always check to make sure containers are securely closed and the cabinets where they are stored are securely shut and locked after poisonous substances are used. (3) Never transfer a substance from its original to an alternate container. (4) Safely dispose of all unused and unneeded medications. (5) *Never* refer to medicines as "candy."
- The AAP specifies that the following steps be implemented for the treatment of poisoning in young children: (1) If the poison has been ingested, *first* call the national poison control hotline at 800-222-1222. (2) If the poison has touched the skin or eyes, run tap water over the skin or eyes for 15 to 20 minutes. (3) If the poison has been inhaled, remove the child from the hazardous environment. (4) In *all* cases of poisoning, *if the victim is conscious and alert, call the local poison control center. If the victim has collapsed or stopped breathing, call 911* for emergency transport to a hospital.
- There remains no indication for use of syrup of ipecac in any setting including health care settings.

Modified from American Academy of Pediatrics: Poison treatment in the home, *Pediatrics* 112:1061-1064, 2003; Tips for poison prevention and treatment, available at http://www.healthychildren.org.

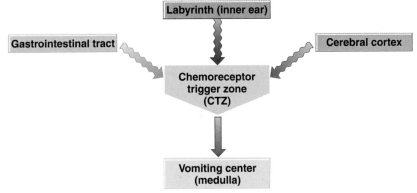

**FIGURE 52-1** Various pathways and areas in the body sending signals to the vomiting center.

## PHARMACOLOGY OVERVIEW

### ANTIEMETIC DRUGS

Drugs used to relieve nausea and vomiting are called antiemetic drugs. All antiemetic drugs work at some site in the vomiting pathways. There are six categories of such drugs with varying mechanisms of action. When drugs from different categories are combined, the antiemetic effectiveness is increased because more than one pathway becomes blocked. Some of the more commonly used antiemetics in the various categories are listed in Table 52-2. The sites at which antiemetics work in the vomiting pathway are shown in Figure 52-2.

### Mechanism of Action and Drug Effects

Drugs used to prevent or treat nausea and vomiting have many different mechanisms of action. Most work by blocking one of the vomiting pathways, as shown in Figure 52-2. In doing so, they block the neurologic stimulus that induces vomiting. The mechanisms of action of the drugs in the six antiemetic drug categories are summarized in Table 52-3.

Anticholinergic drugs (see Chapter 21) have several uses. As antiemetics, they act by binding to and blocking acetylcholine (ACh) receptors in the vestibular nuclei, which are located deep

| TABLE 52-2 | ANTIEMETIC DRUGS: COMMON DRUG CATEGORIES AND INDICATIONS | |
|---|---|---|
| CATEGORY | ANTIEMETIC DRUGS | INDICATIONS |
| Anticholinergics (acetylcholine blockers) | scopolamine | Motion sickness, secretion reduction before surgery, nausea and vomiting |
| Antihistamines (H₁ receptor blockers) | dimenhydrinate, diphenhydramine, meclizine | Motion sickness, nonproductive cough, sedation, rhinitis, allergy symptoms, nausea and vomiting |
| Antidopaminergics | prochlorperazine, promethazine, droperidol | Psychotic disorders (mania, schizophrenia, anxiety), intractable hiccups, nausea and vomiting |
| Prokinetics | metoclopramide | Delayed gastric emptying, gastroesophageal reflux, nausea and vomiting |
| Serotonin blockers | dolasetron, granisetron, ondansetron, palonosetron | Nausea and vomiting associated with chemotherapy, postoperative nausea and vomiting |
| Tetrahydrocannabinoids | dronabinol | Nausea and vomiting associated with chemotherapy, anorexia associated with weight loss in patients with AIDS and cancer |

| TABLE 52-3 | ANTIEMETIC DRUGS: MECHANISMS OF ACTION |
|---|---|
| CATEGORY | MECHANISM OF ACTION |
| Anticholinergics | Block ACh receptors in the vestibular nuclei and reticular formation |
| Antihistamines | Block H₁ receptors, thereby preventing ACh from binding to receptors in the vestibular nuclei |
| Antidopaminergics | Block dopamine in the CTZ and may also block ACh |
| Prokinetics | Block dopamine in the CTZ or stimulate ACh receptors in the GI tract |
| Serotonin blockers | Block serotonin receptors in the GI tract, CTZ, and VC |
| Tetrahydrocannabinoids | Have inhibitory effects on the reticular formation, thalamus, and cerebral cortex |

*ACh*, Acetylcholine; *CTZ*, chemoreceptor trigger zone; *GI*, gastrointestinal; *VC*, vomiting center.

**FIGURE 52-2** Sites of action of selected antinausea drugs. *THC,* Tetrahydrocannabinol.

within the brain. When ACh is prevented from binding to these receptors, nausea-inducing signals originating in this area cannot be transmitted to the chemoreceptor trigger zone (CTZ). Anticholinergics also block receptors located in the reticular formation so that nausea-inducing signals originating in this area cannot be transmitted to the vomiting center. Anticholinergics also tend to dry GI secretions and reduce smooth muscle spasms, both of which effects are often helpful in reducing acute GI symptoms, including nausea and vomiting.

Antihistamines (histamine 1 [$H_1$] receptor blockers) act by inhibiting vestibular stimulation in a manner that is very similar to that of the anticholinergics. Although they bind primarily to $H_1$ receptors, they also have potent anticholinergic activity, including antisecretory and antispasmodic effects. Thus, the antihistamines (see Chapter 36) prevent cholinergic stimulation in both the vestibular and reticular systems. Nausea and vomiting occur when these systems are stimulated. Note that these drugs are not to be confused with histamine 2 [$H_2$] receptor blockers used for gastric acid control (see Chapter 50).

Antidopaminergic drugs, although they are traditionally used for their antipsychotic effects (see Chapter 16), also prevent nausea and vomiting by blocking dopamine receptors in the CTZ. Many of the antidopaminergics also have anticholinergic actions similar to those of anticholinergic drugs. In addition, antidopaminergic drugs calm the central nervous system (CNS).

Prokinetic drugs, in particular metoclopramide, act as antiemetics by blocking dopamine receptors in the CTZ, which desensitizes the CTZ to impulses it receives from the GI tract. Their primary action, however, is to stimulate peristalsis in the GI tract. This enhances the emptying of stomach contents into the duodenum, as well as intestinal movements.

Serotonin blockers work by blocking serotonin receptors located in the GI tract, CTZ, and vomiting center. There are many subtypes of serotonin receptors, and they are located throughout the body (CNS, smooth muscle, platelets, and GI tract). The receptor subtype involved in the mediation of nausea and vomiting is the 5-hydroxytryptamine 3 (5-$HT_3$) receptor. These receptors are the site of action of the serotonin blockers such as ondansetron, granisetron, dolasetron, and palonosetron.

Tetrahydrocannabinol (THC), in a drug class by itself, is the major psychoactive substance in marijuana. Nonintoxicating doses in the form of the drug dronabinol are occasionally used as an antiemetic because of the drug's inhibitory effects on the reticular formation, thalamus, and cerebral cortex. These effects cause an alteration in mood and in the body's perception of its surroundings, which may be beneficial in relieving nausea and vomiting. Although this particular category of antiemetics is less commonly prescribed, there are occasionally patients who respond well to THC. Examples are patients being treated for cancer or acquired immunodeficiency syndrome (AIDS) who experience nausea and vomiting. In such patients, dronabinol may also stimulate the appetite, and nutritional wasting syndromes are common in both diseases. The drug also demonstrates some benefit in controlling the symptoms of glaucoma. There is a large, but highly controversial, political movement with participation of many cancer, AIDS, and glaucoma patients in favor of legalization of the marijuana plant for these uses.

## Indications

The therapeutic uses of the antiemetic drugs vary depending on the drug category. There are several indications for the drugs in each class. These are listed in Table 52-2.

## Contraindications

The primary contraindication for all antiemetics is known drug allergy. Other contraindications for various specific drugs are mentioned in the drug profiles.

## Adverse Effects

Most of the adverse effects of the antiemetics stem from their nonselective blockade of various receptors. Some of the more common adverse effects associated with the various categories of antinausea drugs are listed in Table 52-4.

| TABLE 52-4 | ANTINAUSEA DRUGS: ADVERSE EFFECTS |
|---|---|
| **BODY SYSTEM** | **ADVERSE EFFECTS** |
| **Anticholinergics** | |
| Central nervous | Dizziness, drowsiness, disorientation |
| Cardiovascular | Tachycardia |
| Ears, eyes, nose, throat | Blurred vision, dilated pupils, dry mouth |
| Genitourinary | Difficult urination, constipation |
| Integumentary | Rash, erythema |
| **Antihistamines** | |
| Central nervous | Dizziness, drowsiness, confusion |
| Ears, eyes, nose, throat | Blurred vision, dilated pupils, dry mouth |
| Genitourinary | Urinary retention |
| **Antidopaminergics** | |
| Cardiovascular | Orthostatic hypotension, tachycardia |
| Central nervous | Extrapyramidal symptoms, tardive dyskinesia, headache |
| Ears, eyes, nose, throat | Blurred vision, dry eyes |
| Genitourinary | Urinary retention |
| Gastrointestinal | Dry mouth, nausea and vomiting, anorexia, constipation |
| **Prokinetics** | |
| Cardiovascular | Hypotension, supraventricular tachycardia |
| Central nervous | Sedation, fatigue, restlessness, headache, dystonia |
| Gastrointestinal | Dry mouth, nausea and vomiting, diarrhea |
| **Serotonin Blockers** | |
| Central nervous | Headache |
| Gastrointestinal | Diarrhea |
| Other | Rash, bronchospasm, prolonged QT interval |
| **Tetrahydrocannabinoids** | |
| Central nervous | Drowsiness, dizziness, anxiety, confusion, euphoria |
| Ears, eyes, nose, throat | Visual disturbances |
| Gastrointestinal | Dry mouth |

## Interactions

The drug interactions associated with the antiemetic drugs are specific to the individual drug categories. Anticholinergics have additive drying effects when given with antihistamines and antidepressants. Increased CNS depressant effects are seen when antihistamine antiemetics are administered with barbiturates, opioids, hypnotics, tricyclic antidepressants, or alcohol. Increased CNS depression also occurs when alcohol or other CNS depressants are given together with antidopaminergic drugs. Combining metoclopramide with alcohol can result in additive CNS depression. Anticholinergics and analgesics can block the motility effects of metoclopramide. Serotonin blockers and THC have no significant drug interactions.

## Dosages

For dosage information on selected antiemetic drugs, see the table on this page.

## DRUG PROFILES

Antiemetics are used to treat nausea and vomiting in a variety of clinical situations, including chemotherapy-induced and postoperative nausea and vomiting, both of which can be especially difficult to treat. The ultimate goals of antiemetic therapy are minimizing or preventing fluid and electrolyte disturbances and minimizing deterioration of the patient's nutritional status. Most of the antiemetics act by blocking receptors in the CNS, but some work directly in the GI tract. There are six major classes of antiemetic drugs, although there are other drugs that may also be used to treat nausea and vomiting, including corticosteroids such as dexamethasone (see Chapter 33) and anxiolytics such as lorazepam (see Chapter 16). Lorazepam is often used in the treatment and prevention of chemotherapy-induced nausea and vomiting. In addition to an antiemetic effect, it also helps to blunt the memory of the nausea and vomiting experience (especially with cancer chemotherapy). Dexamethasone,

## DOSAGES

### Selected Antiemetic and Antinausea Drugs

| DRUG (PREGNANCY CATEGORY) | PHARMACOLOGIC CLASS | USUAL DOSAGE RANGE | INDICATIONS/USES |
|---|---|---|---|
| **Anticholinergics** | | | |
| scopolamine (Transderm-Scōp) (C) | Anticholinergic, belladonna alkaloid | Apply 1 patch to hairless area behind ear every 3 days (starting at least 4 hr before travel) | Motion sickness prophylaxis |
| **Antihistamines** | | | |
| ♦ meclizine (Antivert, Bonine) (B) | Anticholinergic, antihistamine | **Adult** PO: 25-50 mg 1 hr before travel and repeated daily during travel | Motion sickness prophylaxis |
| | | PO: 25-100 mg/day, divided 1-4 times daily | Treatment of vertigo |
| **Antidopaminergics** | | | |
| ♦ prochlorperazine (Compazine) (C) | Phenothiazine | **Pediatric\*** Doses vary based on weight and age **Adult** PO: 5-10 mg 3-4 times daily IM: 5-10 mg q3-4h (max 40 mg/day) PR: 25 mg twice daily IV: 5-10 mg q6h | Antiemetic |
| promethazine (Phenergan) (C) | Phenothiazine | **Pediatric older than 2 yr** IV, IM, PO, PR: 0.25-0.5 mg/kg/dose 4-6 times daily **Adult** IV, IM, PO, PR: 12.5-25 mg q4-6h | Antiemetic |
| **Prokinetics** | | | |
| ♦ metoclopramide (Reglan) (B) | Dopamine antagonist | **Adult** IV: 1-2 mg/kg (30 min before chemotherapy; repeat q2h × 2 doses, then q3h × 3 doses) | Chemotherapy antiemetic |
| | | IM: 10-20 mg × 1 dose near end of surgery; repeat q4-6h as needed | Prevention of postoperative nausea and vomiting |
| **Serotonin Blockers** | | | |
| ♦ ondansetron (Zofran) (B) | Antiserotonergic | **Pediatric\*** Doses vary based on age and weight **Adult** PO: 8 mg tid **Adult** IV: 24-32 mg once daily | Chemotherapy antiemetic |

## DOSAGES

### Selected Antiemetic and Antinausea Drugs—cont'd

| DRUG (PREGNANCY CATEGORY) | PHARMACOLOGIC CLASS | USUAL DOSAGE RANGE | INDICATIONS/USES |
|---|---|---|---|
| | | **Pediatric: 1 mo-12 yr**<br>Less than 40 kg: 0.1 mg/kg<br>More than 40 kg: 4 mg as single dose<br>**Adult**<br>4 mg as single dose 30 min before surgery ends | Prevention and treatment of postoperative nausea |
| **Tetrahydrocannabinoids**<br>dronabinol (Marinol) (C) | Marijuana-derived antiemetic | **Adult**<br>PO: Initially, 5 mg/m² 1-3 hr before chemotherapy, then q2-4h after chemotherapy up to 6 times daily for 3 days; this dose may, if needed, be increased in 2.5-mg/m² increments to a max dose of 15 mg/m² | Chemotherapy antiemetic |
| | | PO: 2.5 mg twice daily before lunch and before or after dinner to a maximum dose of 20 mg/day in divided doses. Adverse effects increase greatly in doses above 20 mg/day. | Appetite stimulation in HIV/AIDS and cancer patients |

*AIDS,* Acquired immunodeficiency syndrome; *HIV,* human immunodeficiency virus (infection); *IM,* intramuscular; *IV,* intravenous; *PO,* oral; *PR,* per rectum.
*There are optional dosage regimens for chemotherapy-induced nausea and vomiting; the reader is referred to a drug information handbook.

lorazepam, and dronabinol are beneficial in preventing nausea and vomiting caused by chemotherapy, especially when used in combination with the serotonin blockers.

## ANTICHOLINERGIC

### scopolamine

Scopolamine (Transderm-Scōp, Scopace) is the primary anticholinergic drug used as an antiemetic. It has potent effects on the vestibular nuclei, which are located in the area of the brain that controls balance. Scopolamine works by blocking the binding of ACh to the cholinergic receptors in this region and thereby correcting an imbalance between the two neurotransmitters ACh and norepinephrine. These effects make scopolamine one of the most commonly used drugs for the treatment and prevention of the nausea and vomiting associated with motion sickness. Scopolamine is also used to treat postoperative nausea and vomiting. Use of the drug is contraindicated in patients with glaucoma. Scopolamine is available in oral, injectable, transdermal, and even ocular forms (see Chapter 57). The most commonly used formulation for nausea is the 72-hour transdermal patch, which releases a total of 1 mg of the drug.

### Pharmacokinetics

| Route | Onset of Action | Peak Plasma Concentration | Elimination Half-life | Duration of Action |
|---|---|---|---|---|
| Transdermal | 1-2 hr | 6-8 hr | 8-9.5 hr | 72 hr |

## ANTIHISTAMINES

Antihistamine antiemetics are some of the most commonly used and safest antiemetics. Some of the popular antihistamines are meclizine (Antivert), dimenhydrinate (Dramamine), and diphenhydramine (Benadryl). Many of the antihistamines are available over the counter. Hydroxyzine (Vistaril) is used for antiemetic purposes and is available in oral and intramuscular formulations. Hydroxyzine must never be given by the intravenous route (see the Safety and Quality Improvement: Preventing Medication Errors Box on p. xxx).

### ♦ meclizine

Meclizine (Antivert) is commonly used to treat the dizziness, vertigo, and nausea and vomiting associated with motion sickness. Contraindications include shock and lactation. It is available for oral use only.

### Pharmacokinetics

| Route | Onset of Action | Peak Plasma Concentration | Elimination Half-life | Duration of Action |
|---|---|---|---|---|
| PO | 1 hr | Variable | 6 hr | 8-24 hr |

## ANTIDOPAMINERGICS

Prochlorperazine (Compazine) and promethazine (Phenergan) are the most commonly used antiemetics in the antidopaminergic class. These drugs have antidopaminergic as well as antihistaminergic and anticholinergic properties. Droperidol was one of the most commonly used drugs to treat and prevent postoperative nausea and vomiting for several decades until the U.S. Food and Drug Administration (FDA) called for a black box warning and required continuous electrocardiographic monitoring with its use. These restrictions were in response to concerns over QT widening and possible ventricular dysrhythmias. Some institutions still use droperidol, whereas others have banned its use.

### ♦ prochlorperazine

Prochlorperazine (Compazine), especially in the injectable form, is used frequently in the hospital setting. The drug is contraindicated in patients with hypersensitivity to phenothiazines, those in a coma, and those who have seizures, encephalopathy, or bone marrow suppression. It is available for both injection and oral use.

#### Pharmacokinetics

| Route | Onset of Action | Peak Plasma Concentration | Elimination Half-life | Duration of Action |
|-------|-----------------|---------------------------|-----------------------|--------------------|
| IM | 30-40 min | 2-4 hr | 6-8 hr | 3-4 hr |

### promethazine

Promethazine (Phenergan) is commonly used in hospitalized patients as an antiemetic. The preferred route is oral or intramuscular. The intravenous route is not the preferred route but is commonly used. However, extreme care must be taken to avoid accidental intraarterial injection. If promethazine is inadvertently given intraarterially instead of intravenously, severe tissue damage, often requiring amputation, can occur. Promethazine is best diluted in at least 10 mL of fluid (the more dilute the better) and given in a running intravenous line at the port furthest from the patient's vein or through a large-bore vein (not hand or wrist vein). Therapy must be discontinued immediately if burning or pain occurs with administration. Promethazine is contraindicated in children younger than 2 years of age. Sedation is the most common adverse effect and actually may be beneficial. The drug is also available as a rectal suppository. It is not to be given subcutaneously. For more information, see the Safety and Quality Improvement: Preventing Medication Errors Box on p. 851.

#### Pharmacokinetics

| Route | Onset of Action | Peak Plasma Concentration | Elimination Half-life | Duration of Action |
|-------|-----------------|---------------------------|-----------------------|--------------------|
| IM | 20 min | 4.4 hr | 9-16 hr | 2-6 hr |

### PROKINETIC

Prokinetic drugs promote the movement of substances through the GI tract and increase GI motility. The only prokinetic drug that is also used to prevent nausea and vomiting is metoclopramide.

### ♦ metoclopramide

Metoclopramide (Reglan) is available only by prescription because it can cause some severe adverse effects if not used correctly. Metoclopramide is used for the treatment of delayed gastric emptying and gastroesophageal reflux and also as an antiemetic. Its use is contraindicated in patients with seizure disorder, pheochromocytoma, breast cancer, or GI obstruction and also in patients with a hypersensitivity to it or to procaine or procainamide. Metoclopramide is available in both oral and parenteral formulations. Extrapyramidal adverse effects can occur with its use, especially in young adults. In 2009, the FDA posted a public health advisory regarding the potential of developing tardive dyskinesia with long-term use of metoclopramide.

#### Pharmacokinetics

| Route | Onset of Action | Peak Plasma Concentration | Elimination Half-life | Duration of Action |
|-------|-----------------|---------------------------|-----------------------|--------------------|
| PO | 20-60 min | 1-2.5 hr | 2.5-6 hr | 3-4 hr |

### SEROTONIN BLOCKERS

The serotonin blockers are also called *5-HT3 receptor blockers* because they block the 5-HT$_3$ receptors in the GI tract, the CTZ, and the vomiting center. (The chemical name for serotonin is 5-hydroxytryptamine, or 5-HT.) Drugs in this class have very specific actions, and as a result they have very few adverse effects. No significant drug interactions are known to occur. These drugs are indicated for the prevention of nausea and vomiting associated with cancer chemotherapy and also for the prevention of postoperative or radiation-induced nausea and vomiting. Currently there are four drugs in this category: dolasetron (Anzemet), granisetron (Kytril), ondansetron (Zofran), and palonosetron (Aloxi). This class of drugs revolutionized the treatment of nausea and vomiting, especially in cancer patients and postoperative patients. When used to prevent postoperative nausea and vomiting, a dose is usually given approximately 30 minutes before the end of the surgical procedure. When used to prevent or treat nausea and vomiting associated with cancer treatment, the drug is given in the first 24 to 48 hours of chemotherapy. All drugs in this class are classified as pregnancy category B drugs. In 2010, the FDA issued a warning regarding dolasetron and the risk of cardiac dysrhythmias. In 2011, the FDA added the same warning for ondansetron. The FDA no longer recommends dolasetron to be used for chemotherapy-induced nausea and vomiting.

### ♦ ondansetron

Ondansetron (Zofran) is the prototypical drug in this class. Approved in 1992, it represented a major breakthrough in treating chemotherapy-induced nausea and vomiting and, later, postoperative nausea and vomiting. It is also used for the treatment of hyperemesis gravidarum (nausea and vomiting associated with pregnancy). Its only listed contraindication is known drug allergy. It is available in both oral and injectable forms and as orally disintegrating tablets. Doses up to 8 mg can be given by intravenous push over 2 to 5 minutes. Ondansetron was the first of the class to become available as a generic formulation, which significantly increased its use.

#### Pharmacokinetics

| Route | Onset of Action | Peak Plasma Concentration | Elimination Half-life | Duration of Action |
|-------|-----------------|---------------------------|-----------------------|--------------------|
| IV | 15-30 min | 1-1.5 hr | 3.5-5 hr | 6-12 hr |

### TETRAHYDROCANNABINOID

#### dronabinol

Dronabinol (Marinol) is the only commercially available tetrahydrocannabinoid. It is a synthetic derivative of THC, the major active substance in marijuana. Dronabinol was approved by the FDA in 1985 for the treatment of nausea and vomiting associated with cancer chemotherapy. It is generally used as a second-line drug after treatment with other antiemetics has failed. It is also used to stimulate appetite and weight gain in patients with AIDS and chemotherapy patients. Its only listed contraindication is known drug allergy. It is available for oral use only.

## Pharmacokinetics

| Route | Onset of Action | Peak Plasma Concentration | Elimination Half-life | Duration of Action |
|---|---|---|---|---|
| PO | 30-60 min | 1-3 hr | 19-36 hr | 4-6 hr |

## MISCELLANEOUS ANTINAUSEA DRUGS
### phosphorated carbohydrate solution

Phosphorated carbohydrate solution (Emetrol) is a mint-flavored, pleasant-tasting oral solution used to relieve nausea. It works by direct local action on the walls of the GI tract, where it reduces cramping caused by excessive smooth muscle contraction. It can be used to control mild cases of nausea and vomiting. It does not have a pregnancy category rating, but one of its listed unlabeled (non–FDA-approved) uses is for treatment of morning sickness during pregnancy. Phosphorated carbohydrate solution is not sufficient for treatment of more severe nausea symptoms such as those associated with cancer chemotherapy. Its only contraindication is known drug allergy. It is available for oral use only.

### aprepitant

Aprepitant (Emend) is the first in a new class of antiemetic drugs and was approved in 2003. It is an antagonist of substance P–neurokinin 1 receptors in the brain. In contrast to other antiemetics, this drug has little affinity for 5-HT$_3$ (serotonin) and dopamine receptors. Studies show that aprepitant augments the antiemetic actions of both ondansetron and the corticosteroid dexamethasone. This drug is specifically indicated for the prevention of nausea and vomiting associated with highly emetogenic cancer chemotherapy regimens, including high-dose cisplatin, as well as postoperative nausea and vomiting. Common adverse effects include dizziness, headache, insomnia, and GI discomfort, but these are generally no more common than with other standard antiemetic regimens. Aprepitant may induce the metabolism of warfarin, and international normalized ratio (INR) needs to be checked before each cycle of aprepitant. The drug may reduce the effectiveness of oral contraceptives. Because aprepitant is a major inhibitor of the cytochrome P-450 enzyme system, caution must be used in giving it together with drugs that are primarily metabolized by cytochrome P-450 enzyme 3A4, including azole antifungals, clarithromycin, diltiazem, nicardipine, protease inhibitors, and verapamil. It may increase the bioavailability of corticosteroids, including dexamethasone and methylprednisolone, and dosages of these drugs may need to be adjusted by 25% to 50%. Aprepitant is classified as a pregnancy category B drug.

## NURSING PROCESS

## ASSESSMENT

Before any antinausea or antiemetic drug is administered, obtain a complete nursing history and perform a thorough

## SAFETY AND QUALITY IMPROVEMENT: PREVENTING MEDICATION ERRORS
### Right Route Is Essential

Two commonly used antiemetic drugs may have serious consequences for the patient if they are given via the wrong route.

Hydroxyzine (Vistaril) is an antihistamine-class antiemetic that is only to be given either by oral or intramuscular routes. However, when so many other antiemetics are given by the intravenous route, it may be easy to make the mistake of giving hydroxyzine intravenously. It is important to note that intravenous, intraarterial, or subcutaneous administration of hydroxyzine may result in significant tissue damage, thrombosis, and gangrene.

Promethazine (Phenergan) is another commonly used antiemetic. The oral and intramuscular routes are the preferred routes of administration; the intravenous route, while commonly used, is not the preferred route. If this drug is given intraarterially, severe tissue damage, possibly leading to amputation, may occur.

These are just two examples that illustrate the importance of the "right route" with drug administration.

physical assessment with attention to the following: history of the symptoms of nausea and vomiting; medical history and current medical status; medication history and drugs currently taken including over-the-counter drugs, herbals, prescription drugs, and social drugs (e.g., cigarettes, alcohol); and any alternative therapies used. Identify any factors precipitating nausea or vomiting; note any weight loss; measure baseline vital signs; assess intake and output; examine the skin and mucous membranes, noting turgor and color; and assess and document capillary refill (normal is less than 5 seconds). If laboratory tests are ordered (e.g., serum sodium, potassium, and chloride levels; hemoglobin level and hematocrit; red and white blood cell counts; urinalysis), assess and document the findings to establish baseline levels. Assess for any contraindications or cautions to the use of these drugs and for drug interactions, as well as any allergies.

Only give the *anticholinergic drug* scopolamine after careful assessment of the patient's health history and medication history. One very important concern to emphasize with scopolamine, which is commonly administered in patch form to prevent motion sickness, is the contraindication to its use in patients with narrow-angle glaucoma. If the patient has a history of this disorder, use another antiemetic or antinausea drug. The same concern regarding use in patients with narrow-angle glaucoma applies to *antihistamines* (e.g., meclizine); in addition, use antihistamines cautiously in pediatric patients, who may have severe paradoxical reactions. Elderly patients may develop agitation, mental confusion, hypotension, and even psychotic-type reactions in response to these drugs. Other medications need to be considered for patients if these reactions occur.

*Antidopaminergic drugs*, such as promethazine, are to be used only after cautious assessment for signs and symptoms of dehydration and electrolyte imbalance by evaluating skin turgor and examining the tongue for the presence of longitudinal furrows. Monitor vital signs, especially blood pressure and pulse rate, due to adverse effects of orthostatic hypotension and tachycardia. CNS concerns to assess for include any abnormal movements at baseline functioning because these drugs can lead to adverse effects of extrapyramidal symptoms. Contraindications, cautions, and drug interactions for these drugs have been discussed earlier. Double-checking the name and mechanism of action is also important *prochlorperazine* may be confused with *promethazine*) to prevent sound-alike medication errors.

The *prokinetic drug* metoclopramide is often reserved for the treatment of nausea and vomiting associated with antineoplastic drug therapy or radiation therapy and for the treatment of GI motility disturbances. The action of this drug is decreased when it is taken with anticholinergics or opiates; therefore, assess for this interaction. Remember the FDA public health advisory regarding untoward reactions with long-term use (see the pharmacology section).

Only give the *serotonin blocker* granisetron after assessment of baseline vital signs and age (its safety in those younger than 2 years of age has not been established). Ondansetron use requires assessment for the signs and symptoms of dehydration and electrolyte disturbances. Assess skin turgor and examine mucous membranes for dryness and/or longitudinal furrows in the tongue.

With the *tetrahydrocannabinoid* dronabinol, assess patients for signs and symptoms of dehydration, with attention to low urine output, dry mucous membranes, poor skin turgor, and lethargy. Perform a thorough assessment of hydration status because treatment of volume and electrolyte imbalances may be required in addition to treatment with antinausea or antiemetic drugs. Assess motor and cognitive abilities.

 **SAFETY: HERBAL THERAPIES AND DIETARY SUPPLEMENTS**

### *Ginger* (Zingiber officinale)

**Overview**
Found naturally in the Asian tropics; now cultivated in other continents, including part of the United States; plant parts utilized are the rhizome and root; active ingredients include gingerols and gingerdione

**Common Uses**
Used as an antioxidant; also used for relief of such varied symptoms as sore throat, migraine headache, and nausea and vomiting (including that induced by cancer chemotherapy, morning sickness, and motion sickness); many other varied uses

**Adverse Effects**
Skin reactions, anorexia, nausea, vomiting

**Potential Drug Interactions**
Can increase absorption of all oral medications; may theoretically increase bleeding risk with anticoagulants (e.g., warfarin [Coumadin]) or antiplatelet drugs (e.g., clopidogrel [Plavix])

**Contraindications**
Contraindicated in cases of known product allergy; may worsen cholelithiasis (gallstones); anecdotal evidence of abortifacient properties—some clinicians recommend not using during pregnancy

## NURSING DIAGNOSES

1. Nausea related to disease pathology and adverse effects of specific groups of medications
2. Impaired physical mobility related to adverse effects (e.g., sedation, lethargy, confusion) of antiemetics
3. Risk for injury (falls) related to the adverse effects of antiemetic medications (e.g., sedation and dizziness)
4. Risk for deficient fluid volume related to nausea and vomiting and limited oral intake

## PLANNING

### GOALS

1. Patient remains free from nausea and vomiting with use of pharmacologic and nonpharmacologic therapies.
2. Patient regains mobility status and/or remains with stable mobility during drug therapy.
3. Patient remains free from injury during drug therapy with antiemetic.
4. Patient maintains/regains fluid volume balance while undergoing treatment.

### OUTCOME CRITERIA

1. Patient states specific rationales for reducing nausea and vomiting through use of antiemetic drug therapy as well as specific nondrug measures.
   - Patient states action of specific antiemetic drug, specific dosage, and best time to take the drug, and identifies related adverse effects such as sedation, dizziness, and dry mouth.
   - Patient states specific measures to decrease nausea and vomiting, such as avoiding irritating, spicy foods and beverages, and possibly avoiding fluids and food until nausea and vomiting subsides (but prior to becoming dehydrated).
   - Patient states signs and symptoms of dehydration to report to the prescriber if they occur, such as dry mouth, decrease in urinary output, decreased to no intake of fluids, lethargy, weakness, and dizziness.
2. Patient increases physical mobility and activity, with assistance if needed, by 10 to 15 minutes per day with cautious movements, changing of positions, rising, walking, and performing activities of daily living.
3. Patient states measures to implement to prevent injury, such as obtaining assistance while ill, rising slowly, changing positions slowly, taking medications as ordered, and initiating fluid intake once nausea and/or vomiting subside.
4. Patient states measures to implement to prevent further fluid volume deficits, such as consumption of oral fluids (e.g., clear liquids) or chilled gelatin along with medications.

## IMPLEMENTATION

Undiluted forms of diphenhydramine, an *antihistamine,* must be cautiously administered intravenously at the recommended rate of 25 mg/min as ordered. Administer intramuscular forms

### Nausea and Chemotherapy

Mr. S., a 68-year-old retired bus driver, has begun outpatient chemotherapy after a recent diagnosis of lung cancer. He has recovered well from a right lung lobectomy, the incisions are well healed, and he is now physically and emotionally ready for a 3-month regimen of chemotherapy. The premedication orders call for a variety of drugs, including granisetron (Kytril). Mr. S. has a prescription for oral ondansetron (Zofran) for use at home.

1. What is the mechanism of action of granisetron that makes it effective in the management of chemotherapy-induced nausea and vomiting?
2. What important patient teaching points should you emphasize to Mr. S. about the ondansetron?
3. After 2 weeks of therapy, the oncologist discontinues the ondansetron because Mr. S. complains that it does nothing to help the nausea and vomiting. Mr. S. receives a prescription for dronabinol but expresses concern, exclaiming, "There's marijuana in that pill!" What would you explain to Mr. S.?

For answers, see http://evolve.elsevier.com/Lilley.

into large muscles (e.g., ventral gluteal), and rotate sites if repeated injections are necessary. Promethazine may be given orally without regard to meals, and suppository forms are available, if needed. Keep suppository dosage forms in their foil covering until use and, once the wrap is removed, you may moisten them with water or water-soluble lubricating gel before being inserted well into the rectum. Place the patient on the left side for suppository insertion and keep the patient there for several minutes (see Chapter 9). Tell the patient to hold in the suppository for as long as possible to increase its absorption. Measure vital signs and monitor the patient for extrapyramidal symptoms throughout therapy. Encourage the patient to avoid other CNS depressants and alcohol as well as limit caffeine when this drug is used. Instruct the patient to avoid driving and other activities that require mental alertness or motor coordination.

Frequently monitor blood pressure in patients taking meclizine, especially if they are elderly. Be aware of the concern sedation poses for patient safety and emphasize the need for cautious movement at all times. Dry mouth, another adverse effect, produced by any of these medications may be alleviated by using sugarless gum or hard candy. Metoclopramide given orally is best taken 30 minutes before meals and at bedtime. Infuse intravenous dosage forms over the recommended time period. In addition, keep solutions for parenteral dosing for only 48 hours, and protect them from light. Do not give metoclopramide in combination with any other medications, such as phenothiazines, that would lead to exacerbation of extrapyramidal reactions. The occurrence of extrapyramidal reactions needs to be reported to the prescriber immediately. The development of tardive dyskinesia, an involuntary neurologic movement, has been associated with the long-term use of metoclopramide. The FDA issued a public health advisory on the topic in 2009. Monitor for and educate patients about this potential problem.

The scopolamine transdermal patch is applied behind the ear as directed. The area behind the ear needs to be cleansed and dried before the patch is applied. If the patch becomes dislodged, the residual drug must be washed off and a fresh patch put in place. Remind the patient to avoid tasks requiring mental clarity or motor skills while taking the medication. Granisetron may be given intravenously or orally. Infuse intravenous doses over the recommended time period, and dilute as appropriate. A transient taste disorder may occur, especially if the drug is taken with antineoplastic medications, but will diminish with continued therapy. Encourage the use of various relaxation techniques as complementary therapies. Ondansetron may be given orally, intramuscularly, or intravenously. Inject intramuscular doses into a large muscle mass. Intravenous push is usually given over 2 to 5 minutes and infusions over 15 minutes as ordered and as per manufacturer guidelines. Oral forms are well tolerated regardless of the relation of dosing to meals. Encourage the patient to avoid alcohol and other CNS depressants during this therapy and to avoid any activities requiring mental alertness or motor skill. *Antiemetics* are usually given 30 to 60 minutes before chemotherapy (depending on the specific drug). Ondansetron is usually given 30 minutes before chemotrherapy. Dronabinol is to be administered 1 to 3 hours before antineoplastic therapy and may be taken at home before the scheduled treatment appointment. Relief of nausea and vomiting usually occurs within approximately 15 minutes of oral drug administration. Aprepitant is often used in combination with other medications to prevent nausea and vomiting associated with chemotherapy and is given, as ordered, for postoperative nausea and vomiting. The prescriber's orders may indicate other drugs to be administered as well as the timing of the dosage. Oral dosage forms are to be given as ordered.

## EVALUATION

The therapeutic effects of *antiemetic* and *antinausea drugs* include a decrease in or elimination of nausea and vomiting, and avoidance or elimination of complications such as fluid and electrolyte imbalances and weight loss. Monitor the patient for adverse effects such as GI upset, drowsiness, lethargy, weakness, extrapyramidal reactions, and orthostatic hypotension during antiemetic therapy. Laboratory testing (e.g., electrolyte levels, blood urea nitrogen level, urinalysis with specific gravity) may be ordered for evaluation purposes. Defined goals and outcomes may also be used to evaluate therapeutic effectiveness.

## PATIENT TEACHING TIPS

- Warn the patient using an antiemetic or antinausea drug about the adverse effect of drowsiness, and instruct the patient to use caution while performing hazardous tasks or driving (while taking these drugs). Caution the patient about taking antiemetic or antinausea drugs with alcohol and other CNS depressants because of the possible toxicity and exacerbation of CNS depression.
- Educate the patient about the possible adverse effects of ondansetron, including headache, which may be relieved by taking a simple analgesic (e.g., acetaminophen).
- Remind the patient taking dronabinol to change positions slowly to prevent syncope or dizziness resulting from the hypotensive effects of the drug. Advise the patient to be cautious when engaging in activities that require mental alertness while taking this medication.
- Rotate the application sites for transdermal scopolamine patches, and apply the patches to nonirritated areas behind the ear; wash the hands thoroughly before and after application.

## KEY POINTS

- Antiemetics help to control vomiting, or emesis, and are also useful in relieving or preventing nausea. Antiemetics are used to prevent motion sickness, reduce secretions before surgery, treat delayed gastric emptying, and prevent postoperative nausea and vomiting. Most of these drugs can cause drowsiness.
- Anticholinergics work by blocking ACh receptors in the vestibular nuclei and reticular formation. This blockade prevents areas in the brain from being activated by nauseous stimuli.
- Antihistamines work by blocking H$_1$ receptors, which produces the same effect as the anticholinergics. Antidopaminergic antiemetics block dopamine receptors in the CTZ and may also block ACh receptors. Prokinetic drugs also block dopamine receptors in the CTZ.
- The serotonin-blocking drugs (granisetron and ondansetron) may be highly effective antiemetics. They are most commonly used for the prevention of chemotherapy-induced nausea and vomiting.
- Antiemetics are often given 30 to 60 minutes before a chemotherapy drug is administered (time may vary depending on the specific drug) and may also be given during the chemotherapeutic treatment.
- Dronabinol therapy is used to prevent chemotherapy-induced nausea and vomiting and is associated with postural hypotension.
- Caution patients taking antiemetic or antinausea drugs that drowsiness and hypotension may occur and to avoid driving and using heavy machinery while taking these medications.

## NCLEX® EXAMINATION REVIEW QUESTIONS

1  The nurse is providing patient teaching regarding scopolamine transdermal patches (Transderm-Scōp) to a patient who is planning an ocean cruise. Which instruction is most appropriate?
   a  "Apply the patch the day before traveling."
   b  "Apply the patch at least 4 hours before traveling."
   c  "Apply the patch to the shoulder area."
   d  "Apply the patch to the temple just above the ear."

2  A middle-aged woman is experiencing severe vertigo. The nurse expects this patient will receive which drug, which is considered the most appropriate drug treatment for vertigo?
   a  meclizine (Antivert)
   b  prochlorperazine (Compazine)
   c  metoclopramide (Reglan)
   d  dronabinol (Marinol)

3  A 33-year-old patient is in the outpatient cancer center for his first round of chemotherapy. The nurse knows that which schedule is the most appropriate timing for the intravenous antiemetic drug?
   a  Four hours before the chemotherapy begins
   b  Thirty minutes before the chemotherapy begins
   c  At the same time as the chemotherapy drugs
   d  At the first sign of nausea

4  When reviewing the various types of antinausea medications, the nurse recognizes that prokinetic drugs are also used for
   a  motion sickness.
   b  vertigo.
   c  delayed gastric emptying.
   d  GI obstruction.

5  A patient who has been receiving chemotherapy tells the nurse that he has been searching the Internet for antinausea remedies and that he found a reference to a product called Emetrol (phosphorated carbohydrate solution). He wants to know if this drug would help him. What is the nurse's best answer?
   a  "This may be a good remedy for you. Let's talk to your physician."
   b  "This drug is used only after other drugs have not worked."
   c  "This drug is used only to treat severe nausea and vomiting caused by chemotherapy."
   d  "This drug may not help the more severe nausea symptoms associated with chemotherapy."

## NCLEX® EXAMINATION REVIEW QUESTIONS — cont'd

6  The nurse is preparing to administer dronabinol (Marinol) to a patient. Which statements about dronabinol therapy are true? (Select all that apply.)

a  It is approved for nausea and vomiting related to cancer chemotherapy.

b  It is approved for use with hyperemesis gravidarum (nausea and vomiting associated with pregnancy).

c  It is approved to help stimulate the appetite in patients with nutritional wasting due to cancer or AIDS.

d  It may cause extrapyramidal symptoms.

e  It may cause drowsiness or euphoria.

7  The order reads: "Give promethazine (Phenergan) 12.5 mg IM q4h prn nausea/vomiting." The medication is available in 25-mg/mL vials. How many milliliters will the nurse draw up for this dose?

1. b, 2. a, 3. b, 4. c, 5. d, 6. a, c, e, 7. 0.5 mL.

For Critical Thinking and Prioritization Questions, see http://evolve.elsevier.com/Lilley.

# CHAPTER

# 53

# Vitamins and Minerals

## ⊖volve WEBSITE

*http://evolve.elsevier.com/Lilley*

- Animations
- Answer Key—Textbook Case Studies
- Critical Thinking and Prioritization Questions

- Key Points—Downloadable
- Review Questions for the NCLEX® Examination
- Unfolding Case Studies

## OBJECTIVES

When you reach the end of this chapter, you will be able to do the following:

1 Discuss the importance of the various vitamins and minerals to the normal functioning of the human body.
2 Briefly describe the various acute and chronic disease states and conditions that may lead to various imbalances in vitamin and mineral levels.
3 Discuss the pathologies that result from vitamin and mineral imbalances.
4 Describe the treatment of these vitamin and mineral imbalances.

5 Identify mechanisms of action, indications, cautions, contraindications, drug interactions, dosages, recommended daily allowances, and routes of administration of each of the vitamins and minerals.
6 Develop a nursing care plan related to the use of vitamins and minerals that includes all phases of the nursing process.

## DRUG PROFILES

ascorbic acid (vitamin C), p. 869
calcifediol (vitamin D), p. 862
calcitriol (vitamin D), p. 862
calcium, p. 871
cyanocobalamin (vitamin $B_{12}$), p. 868
dihydrotachysterol (vitamin D), p. 862
ergocalciferol (vitamin D), p. 862
magnesium, p. 872

niacin (vitamin $B_3$), p. 866
phosphorus, p. 873
pyridoxine (vitamin $B_6$), p. 867
riboflavin (vitamin $B_2$), p. 866
thiamine (vitamin $B_1$), p. 865
vitamin A, p. 861
vitamin E, p. 863
vitamin $K_1$, p. 864

## KEY TERMS

Beriberi A disease of the peripheral nerves caused by a dietary deficiency of thiamine (vitamin $B_1$). Symptoms include fatigue, diarrhea, weight loss, edema, heart failure, and disturbed nerve function. (p. 865)
Coenzyme A nonprotein substance that combines with a protein molecule to form an active enzyme. (p. 857)

Enzymes Specialized proteins that catalyze biochemical reactions. (p. 857)
Fat-soluble vitamins Vitamins that can be dissolved (i.e., are soluble) in fat. (p. 857)
Minerals Inorganic substances that are ingested and attach to enzymes or other organic molecules. (p. 857)

**Pellagra** A disease resulting from a deficiency of niacin or a metabolic defect that interferes with the conversion of tryptophan to niacin (vitamin $B_3$). (p. 865)

**Rhodopsin** The purple pigment in the rods of the retina, formed by a protein, opsin, and a derivative of retinol (vitamin A). (p. 859)

**Rickets** A condition caused by a deficiency of vitamin D. (p. 862)

**Scurvy** A condition resulting from a deficiency of ascorbic acid (vitamin C). (p. 869)

**Tocopherols** Biologically active chemicals that make up vitamin E compounds. (p. 863)

**Vitamins** Organic compounds essential in small quantities for normal physiologic and metabolic functioning of the body. (p. 857)

**Water-soluble vitamins** Vitamins that can be dissolved (i.e., are soluble) in water. (p. 857)

## ANATOMY, PHYSIOLOGY AND PATHOPHYSIOLOGY OVERVIEW

For the body to grow and maintain itself, it needs the essential building blocks provided by carbohydrates, fats, and proteins. Vitamins and minerals are needed to efficiently utilize these nutrients. Vitamins are organic molecules needed in small quantities for normal metabolism and other biochemical functions, such as growth or repair of tissue. Equally important are minerals, inorganic elements found naturally in the earth. Enzymes are proteins secreted by cells; they act as catalysts to induce chemical changes in other substances. A coenzyme is a substance that enhances or is necessary for the action of enzymes. Many enzymes are useless without the appropriate vitamins and/or minerals that cause them to function properly. Both vitamins and minerals act primarily as coenzymes, binding to enzymes (or other organic molecules) to activate anabolic (tissue-building) processes in the body. For example, coenzyme A is an important carrier molecule associated with the citric acid cycle, one of the body's major energy-producing metabolic reactions. However, it requires pantothenic acid (vitamin $B_5$) to complete its function in the citric acid cycle.

Vitamins and minerals are essential in our lives, whether or not we are conscientious in our food choices. Under most circumstances, daily requirements of vitamins and minerals are met by ingestion of fluids and balanced meals. Ingesting food maintains adequate stores of essential vitamins and minerals, serves to preserve intestinal structure, provides chemicals for hormones and enzymes, and prevents harmful overgrowth of bacteria.

Various illnesses can cause acute or chronic deficiencies of vitamins, minerals, electrolytes, and fluids. These conditions require replacement or supplementation of these nutrients. Common examples include extensive burn injuries and acquired immunodeficiency syndrome (AIDS). Excessive loss of vitamins and minerals may also be the result of poor dietary intake, an inability to swallow after cancer chemotherapy or radiation, or mental disorders such as anorexia nervosa. Poor dietary absorption can also be caused by various gastrointestinal (GI) malabsorption syndromes. In addition, drug and alcohol abuse are frequently associated with inadequate nutritional intake that warrants vitamin and mineral supplementation.

Deficiencies in dietary protein, fat, and carbohydrates are also common. These nutrients are discussed in Chapter 55. Because of some of their distinct properties and functions in the body related to blood formation, iron and the vitamin folic acid (vitamin $B_9$) are discussed separately in Chapter 54.

## PHARMACOLOGY OVERVIEW

The human body requires vitamins in specific minimum amounts on a daily basis, and these can be obtained from both plant and animal food sources. In some cases, the body synthesizes some of its own vitamin supply. Supplemental amounts of vitamin B complex and vitamin K are synthesized by normal bacterial flora in the GI tract. Vitamin D can be synthesized by the skin when the skin is exposed to sunlight.

An inadequate diet will cause various nutrition-related vitamin deficiencies. In 1941, the Food and Nutrition Board of the National Academy of Sciences published its first list of recommended daily allowances (RDAs) of essential nutrients. A newer published standard is the list of dietary reference intakes (DRIs). Whereas the RDAs represented minimum nutrient requirements, the DRIs are designed to represent optimal nutrient amounts for good health. The United States requires that detailed nutritional information be listed on any packaged food product. The values that appear on the labels are the percentage daily values and indicate what percentage of the DRI for a specific nutrient is met by a single serving of the food product. Information regarding DRIs is available from the following sources:

1. Federal Food and Nutrition Information Center: http://fnic.nal.usda.gov/nal_display/index.php?info_center=4&tax_level=1
2. Institute of Medicine: Dietary Reference Intakes (DRIs): recommended intakes for individuals available at www.iom.edu/

Vitamins are classified as either fat-soluble or water-soluble. Water-soluble vitamins can be dissolved in water and are easily excreted in the urine. Fat-soluble vitamins are dissolvable in fat and tend to be stored longer in the liver and fatty tissues. Because water-soluble vitamins (B-complex group and vitamin C) cannot be stored in the body in large amounts, daily intake is required to prevent the development of deficiencies. Conversely, fat-soluble vitamins (vitamins A, D, E, and K) do not

## TABLE 53-1    FAT-SOLUBLE AND WATER-SOLUBLE VITAMINS

| FAT-SOLUBLE | | WATER-SOLUBLE | |
| --- | --- | --- | --- |
| DESIGNATION | NAME | DESIGNATION | NAME |
| vitamin A | retinol | vitamin $B_1$ | thiamine |
| vitamin D | $D_3$, cholecalciferol; $D_2$, ergocalciferol, dihydrotachysterol | vitamin $B_2$ | riboflavin |
| vitamin E | tocopherols | vitamin $B_3$ | niacin |
| vitamin K | $K_1$, phytonadione | vitamin $B_5$ | pantothenic acid |
| | $K_2$, menaquinone | vitamin $B_6$ | pyridoxine |
| | | vitamin $B_9$ | folic acid |
| | | vitamin $B_{12}$ | cyanocobalamin |
| | | vitamin $B_7$ | biotin |
| | | vitamin C | ascorbic acid |

need to be taken daily unless one is deficient, because substantial amounts are stored in the liver and fatty tissues. Deficiencies of these vitamins occur only after prolonged deprivation from an adequate supply or from disorders that prevent their absorption. Table 53-1 lists the fat-soluble and water-soluble vitamins.

One controversial topic related to vitamins is that of nutrient "megadosing," as a strategy both for health promotion and maintenance and for treatment of various illnesses. Some cancer patients elect to use supplemental megadosing of specific nutrients in hopes of strengthening their body's response to more conventional cancer treatments. The American Dietetic Association defines megadosing as "doses of a nutrient that are 10 or more times the recommended amount." A related term was coined in 1968 by the Nobel Prize–winning chemist Linus Pauling. He defined *orthomolecular medicine* to be "the preventive or therapeutic use of high-dose vitamins to treat disease." The best-known claim of Dr. Pauling was that megadoses of vitamin C (at more than 100 times the U.S. RDA) could prevent or cure the common cold and cancer. Many studies since have not substantiated this claim. However, there are some situations in which nutrient megadosing are known to be helpful, including the following:

- When concurrent long-term drug therapy depletes vitamin stores or otherwise interferes with the function of a vitamin. A common clinical example is the use of vitamin $B_6$ (pyridoxine) supplementation in patients receiving the drug isoniazid for treatment of tuberculosis (see Chapter 41).
- In GI malabsorption syndromes such as those seen in patients with severe colitis and cystic fibrosis (all major nutrient classes, including protein, fat, carbohydrates, vitamins, and minerals).
- For the treatment of pernicious anemia, which results from cyanocobalamin (vitamin $B_{12}$) deficiency. The GI tract uses a fairly complex mechanism to drive cyanocobalamin absorption. Specifically, a glycoprotein known as *intrinsic factor* is secreted by the parietal cells of the gastric glands (see Chapter 50). Intrinsic factor facilitates absorption of cyanocobalamin in the intestine. When this process is compromised (e.g., by disease), administration of megadoses of cyanocobalamin can bypass this absorption mechanism by allowing a small amount of the vitamin to diffuse on its own through the intestinal mucosa.

- When the vitamin acts as a drug when megadosed. The most common example is niacin (vitamin $B_3$, also called *nicotinic acid*). At dosages of up to 20 mg daily, it functions as a vitamin, but at dosages 50 to 100 times higher, it reduces blood levels of both triglycerides and low-density lipoprotein cholesterol (see Chapter 27).

In contrast with the aforementioned examples, there are some situations in which nutrient megadosing is known to be harmful. For example, any excess of one or more nutrients can result in deficiencies of other nutrients due to their chemical competition for sites of absorption in the intestinal mucosa. This is likely to be the case with megadosing of minerals, such as calcium, copper, iron, and zinc, and is less likely to result from vitamin megadosing. Vitamin megadosing can lead to toxic accumulations known as *hypervitaminosis,* especially with the fat-soluble vitamins A, D, and K. Vitamin E appears safer, however, even at doses 10 to 20 times the recommended DRI. Hypervitaminosis is less likely to occur with the water-soluble vitamins (B complex and C) because they are readily excreted through the urinary system. Nevertheless, it is known that megadosing with vitamin $B_6$ (pyridoxine) at 50 to 100 times the DRI can cause nerve damage.

Persons with an illness may be less tolerant of nutrient megadosing, although megadosing regimens are often prescribed for them. For example, megadosing may be more of a strain for a GI tract that is already weakened by illness. Megadosing can even interfere with chemotherapy drugs as well as radiation treatments, because these therapies work to destroy cancer cells through oxidation processes. Nutritional supplementation with antioxidants may impede such treatment mechanisms. Patients need to tell their health care providers any unusual nutritional regimens that they plan to try, especially if they have a serious illness.

## FAT-SOLUBLE VITAMINS

Fat-soluble vitamins are not readily excreted in the urine and are stored in the body. Thus, daily ingestion of these vitamins is not necessary to maintain good health and, in fact, is more likely to result in hypervitaminosis.

The fat-soluble vitamins are A, D, E, and K. As a group, they share the following characteristics:

- They are present in both plant and animal foods.
- They are stored primarily in the liver.

- They exhibit slow metabolism or breakdown.
- They are excreted via the feces.
- They can reach toxic levels (*hypervitaminosis*) if excessive amounts are consumed.

## VITAMIN A

Vitamin A (retinol) is derived from animal fats such as those found in dairy products, eggs, meat, liver, and fish liver oils. Vitamin A is also derived from carotenes, which are found in plants (e.g., green and yellow vegetables, yellow fruits). Therefore, vitamin A is an exogenous substance for humans because it must be obtained from either plant or animal foods. There are more than 600 naturally occurring carotenoid compounds in plant-based foods. Of these, 40 to 50 occur commonly in the human diet. Beta carotene is the most prevalent of these, followed by alpha carotene and cryptoxanthin. These are known as *provitamin A carotenoids*, because they are all metabolized to various forms of vitamin A in the body. Table 53-2 lists the food sources for several nutrients.

### Mechanism of Action and Drug Effects

Vitamin A is essential for night vision and for normal vision, because it is part of one of the major retinal pigments called rhodopsin. Beta carotene is metabolized in the body to retinal (retinaldehyde), and some of this retinal is reduced to the alcohol compound known as *retinol*. The remainder of the retinal may be oxidized to the carboxylic acid compound retinoic acid. Unlike retinal, retinoic acid has no direct role in vision, but it is essential for normal cell growth and differentiation and for the development of the physical shapes of the body's many parts—a process known as *morphogenesis*. It is also involved in the growth and development of bones and teeth and in other body processes, including reproduction, maintenance of the integrity of mucosal and epithelial surfaces, and cholesterol and steroid synthesis.

### Indications

Supplements of vitamin A may be used to satisfy normal body requirements or an increased demand, such as in infants and pregnant and nursing women. A normal diet usually provides adequate amounts of vitamin A, but in cases of excessive need or inadequate dietary intake, vitamin A supplementation is indicated. Symptoms of vitamin A deficiency include night blindness, xerophthalmia, keratomalacia (softening of the cornea), hyperkeratosis of both the stratum corneum (outermost layer) of the skin and the sclera (outermost layer of eyeball), retarded infant growth, generalized weakness, and increased susceptibility of mucous membranes to infection. Vitamin A–related compounds, such as isotretinoin, are also used to treat various skin conditions, including acne, psoriasis, and keratosis follicularis.

### Contraindications

Contraindications to vitamin A supplementation include known allergy to the individual vitamin product; known current state of hypervitaminosis; and excessive supplementation beyond recommended guidelines, especially during pregnancy or in oral malabsorption syndromes.

### TABLE 53-2   FOOD SOURCES FOR SELECTED NUTRIENTS

| VITAMINS/ MINERALS | FOOD SOURCES |
|---|---|
| vitamin A | Liver; fish; dairy products; egg yolks; dark green, leafy, yellow-orange vegetables and fruits |
| vitamin D | Dairy products, fortified cereals and fortified orange juice, liver, fish liver oils, saltwater fish, butter, eggs |
| vitamin E | Fish, egg yolks, meats, vegetable oils, nuts, fruits, wheat germ, grains, fortified cereals |
| vitamin K | Cheese, spinach, broccoli, brussels sprouts, kale, cabbage, turnip greens, soybean oils |
| vitamin $B_1$ (thiamine) | Yeast, liver, enriched whole-grain products, beans |
| vitamin $B_2$ (riboflavin) | Meats, liver, dairy products, eggs, legumes, nuts, enriched whole-grain products, green leafy vegetables, yeast |
| vitamin $B_3$ (niacin) | Liver, turkey, tuna, peanuts, beans, yeast, enriched whole-grain breads and cereals, wheat germ |
| vitamin $B_6$ (pyridoxine) | Organ meats, meats, poultry, fish, eggs, peanuts, whole grain products, vegetables, nuts, wheat germ, bananas, fortified cereals |
| vitamin $B_{12}$ (cyanocobalamin) | Liver, kidney, shellfish, poultry, fish, eggs, milk, blue cheese, fortified cereals |
| vitamin C (ascorbic acid) | Broccoli, green peppers, spinach, Brussels sprouts, citrus fruits, tomatoes, potatoes, strawberries, cabbage, liver |
| calcium | Dairy products, fortified cereals and calcium-fortified orange juice, sardines, salmon |
| magnesium | Meats, seafood, milk, cheese, yogurt, green leafy vegetables, bran cereal, nuts |
| phosphorus | Milk, yogurt, cheese, peas, meat, fish, eggs |
| zinc | Red meats, liver, oysters, certain seafood, milk products, eggs, beans, nuts, whole grains, fortified cereals |

Adapted from USDA: Dietary guidelines for Americans, 2010, available at http://www.health.gov/dietaryguidelines/dga2010/DietaryGuidelines 2010.pdf, accessed March, 2012.

### Adverse Effects

There are very few acute adverse effects associated with normal vitamin A ingestion. Only after long-term excessive ingestion of vitamin A do symptoms appear. Adverse effects are usually noticed in bones, mucous membranes, the liver, and the skin. Table 53-3 lists some of the symptoms of long-term excessive ingestion of vitamin A.

### Toxicity and Management of Overdose

The major toxic effects of vitamin A result from ingestion of excessive amounts, which occurs most commonly in children. A few hours after administration of an excess dose of vitamin A, irritability, drowsiness, vertigo, delirium, coma, vomiting, and/or diarrhea may occur. In infants, excessive amounts of vitamin A can cause an increase in cranial pressure, resulting in symptoms such as bulging fontanelles, headache, papilledema, exophthalmos (bulging eyeballs), and visual disturbances. Papilledema is the presence of edematous fluid, often including blood, in the optic disc. This is the portion of the eye in the

## TABLE 53-3 VITAMIN A: ADVERSE EFFECTS

| BODY SYSTEM | ADVERSE EFFECTS |
|---|---|
| Central nervous | Headache, increased intracranial pressure, lethargy, malaise |
| Gastrointestinal | Nausea, vomiting, anorexia, abdominal pain, jaundice |
| Integumentary | Dry skin, pruritus, increased pigmentation, night sweats |
| Metabolic | Hypomenorrhea, hypercalcemia |
| Musculoskeletal | Arthralgia, retarded growth |

back of the retina, where nerve fibers converge to form the optic nerve. Over several weeks, a generalized peeling of the skin and erythema (skin reddening) may occur. These symptoms seem to disappear a few days after discontinuation of the drug, which is the only treatment necessary in situations of overdose.

## Interactions

Vitamin A is absorbed less when used together with lubricant laxatives and cholestyramine. In addition, the concurrent use of isotretinoin and vitamin A supplementation can result in additive effects and possible toxicity.

## Dosages

For dosage information on vitamin A, see the table below.

## DOSAGES

### Selected Vitamins

| DRUG | PHARMACOLOGIC CLASS | USUAL DOSAGE RANGE | INDICATIONS/USES |
|---|---|---|---|
| **Vitamin D–Active Compounds** | | | |
| calcifediol (hydroxyvitamin D$_3$) (Calderol) | Fat-soluble | **Adult and pediatric 2-10 yr**<br>PO: 50 mcg once daily | Hypocalcemia in hemodialysis patients |
| calcitriol (dihydroxyvitamin D$_3$) (Rocaltrol, Calcijex) | Fat-soluble | **Adult and pediatric 6 yr and older**<br>PO/IV: 0.5-2 mcg/day | Hypoparathyroidism; hypocalcemia in patients receiving regular hemodialysis |
| dihydrotachysterol (DHT, Hytakerol) | Fat-soluble (a form of vitamin D) | **Adult and pediatric 12 yr and older**<br>PO: 0.75-2.5 mg/day × 4 days, then 0.2-1 mg/day | Hypoparathyroidism |
| ergocalciferol (vitamin D$_2$) (Drisdol, Calciferol) | Fat-soluble | **Pediatric/Adult\***<br>PO: 300-12,500 mcg/day (equals 12,000-500,000 units/day) | Rickets, hypoparathyroidism, renal failure |
| **Vitamin B–Active Compounds** | | | |
| vitamin B$_1$ (thiamine) (Thiamilate) | Water-soluble, B-complex group | **Adult**<br>100 mg/day until normal dietary intake is established<br>5-30 mg/day × 30 days | Alcohol-induced deficiency<br>Beriberi |
| vitamin B$_2$ (riboflavin) (Lactoflavin) | Water-soluble, B-complex group | **Adult**<br>PO: 5-30 mg/day<br>**Pediatric**<br>3-10 mg/day | Deficiency |
| vitamin B$_3$ (niacin, nicotinic acid) (Nicotinex) | Water-soluble, B-complex group | **Adult**<br>PO: 1-6 g/day<br>**Adult**<br>PO: Up to 500 mg/day<br>**Pediatric**<br>IV: Up to 300 mg/day | Hyperlipidemia<br><br>Pellagra (deficiency) |
| vitamin B$_6$ (pyridoxine) (Aminoxin, Vitelle) | Water-soluble, B-complex group | **Adult**<br>PO/IV: 2.5-10 mg/day<br>**Pediatric**<br>PO/IV: 5-25 mg/day × 3 wk, then give multivitamin product<br>**Adult**<br>PO/IV: 100-200 mg/day<br>**Pediatric**<br>10-50 mg/day | Deficiency<br><br><br>Drug-induced neuritis (e.g., isoniazid for tuberculosis) |
| vitamin B$_{12}$ (cyanocobalamin) (Nascobal) | Water-soluble, B-complex group | **Adult and pediatric**<br>IM/subcut: 100 mcg/mo<br>**Adult and pediatric**<br>PO: 50-100 mcg/day<br>**Adult only**<br>Intranasal gel: 500 mcg/wk | Deficiency; anemia |

## DOSAGES—cont'd
### Selected Vitamins

| DRUG | PHARMACOLOGIC CLASS | USUAL DOSAGE RANGE | INDICATIONS/USES |
|---|---|---|---|
| **Vitamins A, C, E, and K** | | | |
| vitamin A (Aquasol A, others) | Fat-soluble | **Adult and pediatric older than 8 yr** PO: 100,000 units/day × 3 days, then 50,000 units/day for 14 days | Deficiency |
| vitamin C (ascorbic acid) (Vita-C, Dull-C, others) | Water-soluble | **Adult and pediatric** PO/IV/IM/subcut: 100-250 mg 1-2 times daily | Deficiency; scurvy |
| vitamin E (d-alpha tocopherol) (Aquavit E, others) | Fat-soluble | **Adult** PO: 60-75 units/day **Pediatric** 1 unit/kg/day | Nutritional supplementation |
| vitamin K (phytonadione) (Mephyton, AquaMEPHYTON) | Fat-soluble | **Adult** PO: 2.5-10 mg/day IM/IV: 1-10 mg single dose | Warfarin-induced hypoprothrombinemia |
| | | **Infant and pediatric** PO: 2.5-5 mg/day IM/IV: 1-2 mg single dose | Deficiency; hemorrhagic disease of newborn infant |

*IM,* Intramuscular; *IV,* intravenous; *PO,* oral; *subcut,* subcutaneous; *mo,* month.
*Dosages are individualized. Higher doses may be required based on response to therapy.

## DRUG PROFILE

There are three forms of vitamin A: retinol, retinyl palmitate, and retinyl acetate. Medications containing vitamin A may require a prescription, but many over-the-counter (OTC) products, such as vitamin A–containing multivitamins, are also available. All vitamin A products are classified as pregnancy category A.

### vitamin A

Vitamin A (Aquasol A), also known as *retinol, retinyl palmitate,* and *retinyl acetate,* is available in a variety of oral forms as well as an injectable form. Doses for vitamin A are expressed as *retinol activity equivalents (RAEs).* One RAE is approximately equal to the following:

- 1 mcg of retinol (either dietary or supplemental)
- 2 mcg of supplemental beta carotene
- 12 mcg of dietary beta carotene
- 24 mcg of dietary carotenoids

### Pharmacokinetics

| Route | Onset of Action | Peak Plasma Concentration | Elimination Half-life | Duration of Action |
|---|---|---|---|---|
| PO | N/A | 4 hr | 50-100 days | Unknown |

## VITAMIN D

Vitamin D, also called the *sunshine vitamin,* is responsible for the proper utilization of calcium and phosphorus in the body. The two most important members of the vitamin D family are vitamin $D_2$ (ergocalciferol) and vitamin $D_3$ (cholecalciferol). They have different sites of origin but similar functions in the body. Ergocalciferol (vitamin $D_2$) is plant derived and is therefore obtained through dietary sources. The natural form of vitamin D produced in the skin by ultraviolet irradiation (sun) is chemically known as *7-dehydrocholesterol.* It is more commonly referred to as *cholecalciferol* (vitamin $D_3$). This endogenous synthesis of vitamin $D_3$ usually produces sufficient amounts to meet daily requirements. Vitamin D is obtained through both endogenous synthesis and consumption of vitamin $D_2$–containing foods such as fish oils, salmon, sardines, and herring; fortified milk, bread, and cereals; and animal livers, tuna fish, eggs, and butter. Normal serum levels are 12 to 50 ng/mL.

## Mechanism of Action and Drug Effects

The basic function of vitamin D is to regulate the absorption and subsequent utilization of calcium and phosphorus. It is also necessary for the normal calcification of bone. Vitamin D in coordination with parathyroid hormone and calcitonin regulates serum calcium levels by increasing calcium absorption from the small intestine and extracting calcium from the bone. Ergocalciferol and cholecalciferol are inactive and require transformation into active metabolites for biologic activity. Both vitamin $D_2$ and vitamin $D_3$ are biotransformed in the liver by the actions of parathyroid hormone. The resulting compound, calcifediol, is then transported to the kidney, where it is converted to calcitriol, which is believed to be the most physiologically active form of vitamin D. Calcitriol promotes the intestinal absorption of calcium and phosphorus and the deposition of calcium and phosphorus into the structure of teeth and bones.

The drug effects of vitamin D are very similar to those of vitamin A and essentially all vitamin and mineral compounds. It is used as a supplement to satisfy normal daily requirements or an increased demand, as in infants and pregnant and nursing women.

## Indications

Vitamin D can be used either to supplement dietary intake or to treat a deficiency of vitamin D. In the case of supplementation, it is given as a prophylactic measure to prevent deficiency-related problems, and it is recommended for breastfed infants. Vitamin D may also be used to treat and correct the result of a long-term deficiency that leads to such conditions as infantile rickets, tetany (involuntary sustained muscular contractions), and osteomalacia (softening of the bones). Rickets is specifically a vitamin D deficiency state. Symptoms include soft, pliable bones, which causes deformities such as bowlegs and knock knees; nodular enlargement on the ends and sides of the bones; muscle pain; enlarged skull; chest deformities; spinal curvature; enlargement of the liver and spleen; profuse sweating; and general tenderness of the body when touched. Vitamin D can also help promote the absorption of phosphorus and calcium. For this reason, its use is important in preventing osteoporosis. Because of the role of vitamin D in the regulation of calcium and phosphorus, it may be used to correct deficiencies of these two elements. Other uses include dietary supplementation and treatment of osteodystrophy, hypocalcemia, hypoparathyroidism, pseudohypoparathyroidism, and hypophosphatemia. Many patients have low vitamin D levels, and it is common to see doses of 1000 to 2000 units daily prescribed.

## Contraindications

Contraindications to vitamin D products include known allergy to the product, hypercalcemia, renal dysfunction, kidney stones, and hyperphosphatemia.

## Adverse Effects

Very few acute adverse effects are associated with normal vitamin D ingestion. Only after long-term excessive ingestion of vitamin D do symptoms appear. Such effects are usually noticed in the GI tract or the central nervous system (CNS) and are listed in Table 53-4.

## Toxicity and Management of Overdose

The major toxic effects from ingesting excessive amounts of vitamin D occur most commonly in children. Discontinuation of vitamin D and reduced calcium intake reverse the toxic state. The amount of vitamin D considered to be toxic varies considerably among individuals but is generally thought to be 1.25 to 2.5 mg of ergocalciferol daily in adults and 25 mcg daily in infants and children.

The toxic effects of vitamin D are those associated with hypertension, such as weakness, fatigue, headache, anorexia, dry mouth, metallic taste, nausea, vomiting, abdominal cramps, ataxia, and bone pain. If not recognized and treated, these symptoms can progress to impairment of renal function and osteoporosis.

## Interactions

Reduced absorption of vitamin D occurs with the concurrent use of lubricant laxatives and cholestyramine.

## Dosages

For dosage information on vitamin D, see the table on p. 860.

---

| TABLE 53-4 | VITAMIN D: ADVERSE EFFECTS |
|---|---|
| **BODY SYSTEM** | **ADVERSE EFFECTS** |
| Cardiovascular | Hypertension, dysrhythmias |
| Central nervous | Fatigue, weakness, drowsiness, headache |
| Gastrointestinal | Nausea, vomiting, anorexia, cramps, metallic taste, dry mouth, constipation |
| Genitourinary | Polyuria, albuminuria, increased blood urea nitrogen level |
| Musculoskeletal | Decreased bone growth, bone and muscle pain |

## DRUG PROFILES

There are four forms of vitamin D: calcifediol, calcitriol, dihydrotachysterol, and ergocalciferol. Vitamin D is available in OTC medications, such as multivitamin products, or by prescription. Although various pharmaceutical manufacturers may list their individual vitamin D products as pregnancy category C, these products are generally considered to be category A or B as long as the patient is not dosed at higher levels than recommended.

### calcifediol

Calcifediol (Calderol) is the 25-hydroxylated form of cholecalciferol (vitamin $D_3$). It is a vitamin D analogue used primarily for the management of hypocalcemia in patients with chronic renal failure who are undergoing hemodialysis. Calcifediol is also used for signs of hyperparathyroid disease. It is available only for oral use.

### calcitriol

Calcitriol (Rocaltrol) is the 1,25-dihydroxylated form of cholecalciferol (vitamin $D_3$). It is a vitamin D analogue used for the management of hypocalcemia in patients with chronic renal failure who are undergoing hemodialysis. Calcitriol is also used in the treatment of hypoparathyroidism and pseudohypoparathyroidism, vitamin D–dependent rickets, hypophosphatemia, and hypocalcemia in premature infants. It is available in both oral and injectable forms.

#### Pharmacokinetics

| Route | Onset of Action | Peak Plasma Concentration | Elimination Half-life | Duration of Action |
|---|---|---|---|---|
| PO | Less than 3 hr | 3-6 hr | 3-6 hr | 3-5 days |

### dihydrotachysterol

Dihydrotachysterol (Hytakerol) is a vitamin D analogue that is administered orally once daily for the treatment of any of the previously mentioned conditions. Intramuscular use is indicated for patients with GI, liver, or biliary disease associated with malabsorption of vitamin D analogues. It is available orally and parenterally.

### ergocalciferol

Ergocalciferol (Drisdol) is vitamin $D_2$. It is indicated for use in patients with GI, liver, or biliary disease associated with malabsorption of vitamin D analogues. It is available orally and parenterally.

**Pharmacokinetics (ergocalciferol, vitamin D$_2$)**

| Route | Onset of Action | Peak Plasma Concentration | Elimination Half-life | Duration of Action |
|---|---|---|---|---|
| PO | 30 days | Unknown | 19 days | Months to years |

## VITAMIN E

Four biologically active chemicals called tocopherols (alpha, beta, gamma, and delta) make up the vitamin E compounds. Alpha tocopherol is the most biologically active natural form of vitamin E and can come from plant and animal sources.

### Mechanism of Action and Drug Effects

Vitamin E is a powerful biologic antioxidant and an essential component of the diet. Its exact nutritional function has not been fully demonstrated. The only recognized significant deficiency syndrome for vitamin E occurs in premature infants. In this situation, vitamin E deficiency may result in irritability, edema, thrombosis, and hemolytic anemia.

The drug effects of vitamin E are not as well defined as those of the other fat-soluble vitamins. It is believed to protect polyunsaturated fatty acids, a component of cellular membranes. It has also been shown to hinder the deterioration of substances such as vitamin A and ascorbic acid (vitamin C), two substances that are highly oxygen sensitive and readily oxidized; thus it acts as an antioxidant.

### Indications

Vitamin E is most commonly used as a dietary supplement to augment current daily intake or to treat a deficiency. Premature infants are those at greatest risk for complications from vitamin E deficiency. Vitamin E has received much attention as an antioxidant. Preventing the oxidation of various substances prevents the formation of toxic chemicals within the body, some of which are believed to cause cancer. There is a popular but unproved theory that vitamin E has beneficial effects for patients with cancer, heart disease, premenstrual syndrome, and sexual dysfunction. However, the American Heart Association no longer recommends the use of high-dose vitamin E to prevent heart disease. In fact, recent studies have shown no benefit and possible harm.

### Contraindications

Contraindications for vitamin E include known allergy to a specific vitamin E product. There are currently no approved injectable forms of this vitamin.

### Adverse Effects

Very few acute adverse effects are associated with normal vitamin E ingestion, because it is relatively nontoxic. Adverse effects are usually noticed in the GI tract or CNS and are listed in Table 53-5.

### Dosages

For the dosage information on vitamin E, see the table on p. 860.

**TABLE 53-5  VITAMIN E: ADVERSE EFFECTS**

| BODY SYSTEM | ADVERSE EFFECTS |
|---|---|
| Central nervous | Fatigue, headache, blurred vision |
| Gastrointestinal | Nausea, diarrhea, flatulence |
| Genitourinary | Increased blood urea nitrogen level |
| Musculoskeletal | Weakness |

### DRUG PROFILE

Vitamin E is available as an OTC medication. It has four forms: alpha, beta, gamma, and delta tocopherol. It is available in many multivitamin preparations and is also available by prescription. Vitamin E products are usually contraindicated only in cases of known drug allergy.

**vitamin E**

Vitamin E (Aquasol E) activity is generally expressed in U.S. Pharmacopeia (USP) or international units. It is available for oral and topical use.

## VITAMIN K

Vitamin K is the last of the four fat-soluble vitamins (A, D, E, and K). There are three types of vitamin K: phytonadione (vitamin K$_1$), menaquinone (vitamin K$_2$), and menadione (vitamin K$_3$). The body does not store large amounts of vitamin K; however, vitamin K$_2$ is synthesized by the intestinal flora, which provides an endogenous supply.

Vitamin K is essential for the synthesis of blood coagulation factors, which takes place in the liver. Vitamin K–dependent blood coagulation factors are factors II, VII, IX, and X. Other names for these clotting factors are as follows: factor II (prothrombin); factor VII (proconvertin); factor IX (Christmas factor); and factor X (Stuart-Prower factor). Normal serum levels are 0.1 to 2.2 ng/mL.

### Mechanism of Action and Drug Effects

Vitamin K activity is essential for effective blood clotting because, as noted earlier, it facilitates the hepatic biosynthesis of factors II, VII, IX and X. Vitamin K deficiency results in coagulation disorders caused by hypoprothrombinemia. Coagulation defects affecting these clotting factors can be corrected with administration of vitamin K. Vitamin K deficiency is rare because intestinal flora are normally able to synthesize sufficient amounts. If a deficiency develops, it can be corrected with vitamin K supplementation.

### Indications

Vitamin K is indicated for dietary supplementation and for treatment of deficiency states. Although rare, deficiency states can develop with inadequate dietary intake or inhibition of the intestinal flora resulting from the administration of broad-spectrum antibiotics. Deficiency states can also be seen in newborns because of malabsorption attributable to inadequate amounts of bile. For this reason, infants born in hospitals are

## TABLE 53-6 VITAMIN K: ADVERSE EFFECTS

| BODY SYSTEM | ADVERSE EFFECTS |
|---|---|
| Central nervous | Headache, brain damage (large doses) |
| Gastrointestinal | Nausea, decreased liver enzyme levels |
| Hematologic | Hemolytic anemia, hemoglobinuria, hyperbili-rubinemia |
| Integumentary | Rash, urticaria |

often given a prophylactic intramuscular dose of vitamin K on arrival to the nursery. Vitamin K deficiency can also result from the administration and pharmacologic action of the oral anticoagulant warfarin (see Chapter 26). Warfarin's anticoagulant effects occur by inhibiting vitamin K–dependent clotting factors II, VII, IX, and X in the liver. Administration of vitamin K overrides the mechanism by which the anticoagulant inhibits production of vitamin K–dependent clotting factors. Thus vitamin K can be used to reverse the effects of warfarin. It is important to note that when vitamin K is used in this manner, the patient becomes unresponsive to warfarin for approximately 1 week after vitamin K administration.

## Contraindications

The only usual contraindication to treatment with vitamin K is known drug allergy.

## Adverse Effects

Vitamin K is relatively nontoxic and thus causes very few adverse effects. Severe reactions limited to hypersensitivity or anaphylaxis have occurred rarely during or immediately after intravenous administration. Adverse effects are usually related to injection-site reactions and hypersensitivity. See Table 53-6 for a list of such major effects by body system.

## Toxicity and Management of Overdose

Toxicity is primarily limited to use in the newborn. Hemolysis of red blood cells (RBCs) can occur, especially in infants with low levels of glucose-6-phosphate dehydrogenase. In severe cases, replacement with blood products may be indicated.

## Dosages

For the dosage information on vitamin K, see the table on p. 860.

## DRUG PROFILE

The most commonly used form of vitamin K is phytonadione (vitamin $K_1$). Both phytonadione and menadione (vitamin $K_3$) are available by prescription only in oral and parenteral forms. Menadione is classified as a pregnancy category X drug, whereas phytonadione is a category C drug. Both are contraindicated in patients with a known hypersensitivity to them. Their use is also contraindicated in patients who are in the last few weeks of pregnancy and in patients with severe hepatic disease. Vitamin K must be used with caution in patients taking warfarin.

## BOX 53-1 WATER-SOLUBLE VITAMINS: ALTERNATE NAMES

| DESIGNATION | ALTERNATE NAME |
|---|---|
| vitamin B complex | |
| vitamin $B_1$ | thiamine |
| vitamin $B_2$ | riboflavin |
| vitamin $B_3$ | niacin |
| vitamin $B_5$ | pantothenic acid |
| vitamin $B_6$ | pyridoxine |
| vitamin $B_9$ | folic acid |
| vitamin $B_{12}$ | cyanocobalamin |
| vitamin C | ascorbic acid |

### vitamin $K_1$

Vitamin $K_1$ (phytonadione) (AquaMEPHYTON) is available in both oral and injectable forms. Because of its potential to cause anaphylaxis (due to the formulation), for intravenous use it is usually diluted and given over 30 to 60 minutes. Vitamin K is given IV or subcutaneously and not intramuscularly when used to reverse warfarin effects.

### Pharmacokinetics

| Route | Onset of Action | Peak Plasma Concentration | Elimination Half-life | Duration of Action |
|---|---|---|---|---|
| PO | 6-12 hr | 24-48 hr | 1.2 hr | 24 hr |
| IV | 1-2 hr | 12-14 hr | 1.2 hr | 24 hr |

## WATER-SOLUBLE VITAMINS

The water-soluble vitamins include the vitamin B complex and vitamin C (ascorbic acid). They are present in a variety of plant and animal food sources. The vitamin B complex is a group of 10 vitamins that are often found together in food, although they are chemically dissimilar and have different metabolic functions. Because the B vitamins were originally isolated from the same sources, they were grouped together as B-complex vitamins. Vitamin C (ascorbic acid), the other principal water-soluble vitamin, is concentrated in citrus fruits and is not classified as part of the B complex. The numeric subscripts associated with various B vitamins reflect the order in which they were discovered. In clinical practice, some B vitamins are more often referred to by their common name, whereas others are more often referred to by their numeric designation. For example, "vitamin $B_{12}$" is used more often in clinical practice than the corresponding common name "cyanocobalamin." However, "folic acid" is rarely referred to as "vitamin $B_9$." The most commonly used B-complex vitamins, as well as vitamin C, are listed in Box 53-1. Folic acid (vitamin $B_9$) has a special role in hematopoiesis and therefore is described further in Chapter 54.

Water-soluble vitamins are a chemically diverse group sharing only the characteristic of being dissolvable in water. Like fat-soluble vitamins, they act primarily as coenzymes or oxidation-reduction agents in important metabolic pathways. Unlike fat-soluble vitamins, water-soluble vitamins are not stored in the body in appreciable amounts. Their water-soluble properties promote urinary excretion and reduce their half-life in the body. Therefore, dietary intake must be adequate and regular or else deficiency states will develop. The body excretes what it does not need, which makes toxic reactions to water-soluble vitamins very rare.

## VITAMIN B₁

A deficiency of vitamin B₁ (thiamine) results in the classic disease beriberi or Wernicke's encephalopathy (cerebral beriberi). Common findings in beriberi include brain lesions, polyneuropathy of peripheral nerves, serous effusions (abnormal collections of fluids in body tissues), and cardiac anatomic changes. Vitamin deficiency can result from poor diet, extended fever, hyperthyroidism, liver disease, alcoholism, malabsorption, and pregnancy and breastfeeding. Normal serum levels are 66 to 200 nmol/L.

### Mechanism of Action and Drug Effects

Vitamin B₁ (thiamine) is an essential precursor for the formation of thiamine pyrophosphate. When thiamine combines with adenosine triphosphate (ATP), the result is thiamine pyrophosphate coenzyme. This is required for the citric acid cycle (Krebs cycle), a major part of carbohydrate metabolism, as well as several other metabolic pathways. In addition, thiamine plays a key role in the integrity of the peripheral nervous system, cardiovascular system, and GI tract.

### Indications

The essential role of thiamine in many metabolic pathways makes it useful in treating a variety of metabolic disorders. These include subacute necrotizing encephalomyelopathy, maple syrup urine disease, and lactic acidosis associated with pyruvate carboxylase enzyme deficiency and hyper-beta-alaninemia. Some of the deficiency states treated by thiamine are beriberi, Wernicke's encephalopathy, peripheral neuritis associated with pellagra (niacin deficiency), and neuritis of pregnancy. Thiamine is used as a dietary supplement to prevent or treat deficiency in cases of malabsorption such as that induced by alcoholism, cirrhosis, or GI disease. Other situations in which thiamine may have therapeutic value are the management of poor appetite, ulcerative colitis, chronic diarrhea, and cerebellar syndrome or ataxia (impaired muscular coordination). It is also used as an oral insect repellent.

### Contraindications

The only usual contraindication to any of the B-complex vitamins is known allergy to a specific vitamin product.

### Adverse Effects

Adverse effects are rare but include hypersensitivity reactions, nausea, restlessness, pulmonary edema, pruritus, urticaria, weakness, sweating, angioedema, cyanosis, and cardiovascular collapse. Administration by intramuscular injection can produce local tenderness, and intravenous injections can produce anaphylaxis.

### Interactions

Thiamine is incompatible with alkaline- and sulfite-containing solutions.

### Dosages

For the dosage information on vitamin B₁, see the table on p. 860.

### DRUG PROFILE

**thiamine**

Thiamine is contraindicated only in individuals with a known hypersensitivity to it. Thiamine is available for both oral use and injection. It is classified as a pregnancy category A drug.

#### Pharmacokinetics

| Route | Onset of Action | Peak Plasma Concentration | Elimination Half-life | Duration of Action |
|---|---|---|---|---|
| PO | Unknown | 1-2 hr | 1.2 hr | 24 hr |

## VITAMIN B₂

A deficiency of vitamin B₂ (riboflavin) results in cutaneous, oral, and corneal changes that include cheilosis (chapped or fissured lips), seborrheic dermatitis, and keratitis.

### Mechanism of Action and Drug Effects

Riboflavin serves several important functions in the body. Riboflavin is converted into two coenzymes (flavin mononucleotide and flavin adenine dinucleotide) that are essential for tissue respiration. Riboflavin also plays an important part in carbohydrate catabolism. Another B vitamin, vitamin B₆ (pyridoxine), requires riboflavin for activation. Riboflavin is also needed to convert tryptophan into niacin and to maintain erythrocyte integrity. Deficiency is rare and does not usually occur in healthy people.

### Indications

Riboflavin is primarily used as a dietary supplement and for treatment of deficiency states. Patients who may experience riboflavin deficiency include those with long-standing infections, liver disease, alcoholism, or malignancy, and those taking probenecid. Riboflavin supplementation may also be beneficial in the treatment of microcytic anemia; acne; migraine headache; congenital methemoglobinemia (presence in the blood of an abnormal, nonfunctional hemoglobin pigment); muscle cramps; and Gopalan's syndrome, a symptom of suspected riboflavin (and possibly pantothenic acid [vitamin B₅]) deficiency that involves a sensation of tingling in the extremities (for this reason, it is also called *burning feet syndrome*).

### Contraindications

The only usual contraindication to riboflavin is known allergy to a given vitamin product.

### Adverse Effects

Riboflavin is a very safe and effective vitamin; to date, no adverse effects or toxic effects have been reported. In large dosages, riboflavin will discolor urine to a yellow-orange.

**FIGURE 53-1** Niacin, once in the body, is converted to nicotinamide adenosine dinucleotide (NAD) and nicotinamide adenosine dinucleotide (NADP), which are coenzymes needed for many metabolic processes.

## Dosages

For dosage information on riboflavin, see the table on p. 860.

## DRUG PROFILE

### riboflavin

Riboflavin (vitamin $B_2$) is needed for normal respiratory functions. It is a safe, nontoxic water-soluble vitamin with almost no adverse effects. Riboflavin is available only for oral use. It is classified as a pregnancy category A drug.

### Pharmacokinetics

| Route | Onset of Action | Peak Plasma Concentration | Elimination Half-life | Duration of Action |
|---|---|---|---|---|
| PO | Unknown | Unknown | 66-84 min | 24 hr |

## VITAMIN $B_3$

The body is able to produce a small amount of vitamin $B_3$ (niacin) from dietary tryptophan, an essential amino acid occurring in dietary proteins and some commercially available nutritional supplements. A dietary deficiency of niacin (vitamin $B_3$) will produce the classic symptoms known as *pellagra*. Symptoms of pellagra include various psychotic disorders; neurasthenic syndrome; crusting, erythema, and desquamation of the skin; scaly dermatitis; inflammation of the oral, vaginal, and urethral mucosa, including glossitis (inflamed tongue); and diarrhea or bloody diarrhea.

## Mechanism of Action and Drug Effects

The metabolic actions of niacin (vitamin $B_3$) are not due to niacin in the ingested form but rather to its metabolic product, nicotinamide. Nicotinamide is required for numerous metabolic reactions, including those involved in carbohydrate, protein, purine, and lipid metabolism, as well as tissue respiration (Figure 53-1). A key example involves two compounds, nicotinamide adenosine dinucleotide (NAD) and nicotinamide adenosine dinucleotide phosphate (NADP), both of which are necessary for the carbohydrate pathway known as *glycogenolysis* (the breakdown of stored glycogen into usable glucose). The parent compound, niacin itself, also has a pharmacologic role as an antilipemic drug (see Chapter 27). The doses of niacin required for its antilipemic effect are substantially higher than those required for the nutritional and metabolic effects.

| TABLE 53-7 | NIACIN (VITAMIN $B_3$): ADVERSE EFFECTS |
|---|---|
| **BODY SYSTEM** | **ADVERSE EFFECTS** |
| Cardiovascular | Postural hypotension, dysrhythmias |
| Central nervous | Headache, dizziness, anxiety |
| Gastrointestinal | Nausea, vomiting, diarrhea, peptic ulcer |
| Genitourinary | Hyperuricemia |
| Hepatic | Abnormal liver function test results, hepatitis |
| Integumentary | Flushing, dry skin, rash, pruritus, keratosis |
| Metabolic | Decreased glucose tolerance |

## Indications

Niacin is indicated for the prevention and treatment of pellagra, a condition caused by a deficiency of vitamin $B_3$ that is most commonly the result of malabsorption. It is also used for management of certain types of hyperlipidemia (see Chapter 27). Niacin also has a beneficial effect in peripheral vascular disease.

## Contraindications

Niacin, unlike certain other B-complex vitamins, has additional contraindications besides drug allergy. These include liver disease, severe hypotension, arterial hemorrhage, and active peptic ulcer disease.

## Adverse Effects

The most frequent adverse effects associated with the use of niacin are flushing, pruritus, and GI distress. These usually subside with continued use and are most frequently seen when larger doses of niacin are used in the treatment of hyperlipidemia. Table 53-7 lists adverse effects by body system.

## Dosages

For dosage information on niacin, see the table on p. 860.

## DRUG PROFILE

### niacin

Niacin is used to treat pellagra, hyperlipidemias, and peripheral vascular disease. Its use must be monitored closely in patients who have a history of coronary artery disease, gallbladder disease, jaundice, liver disease, or arterial bleeding. Niacin is available only for oral use. It is classified as a pregnancy category A drug.

**Pharmacokinetics (niacin, vitamin B$_3$)**

| Route | Onset of Action | Peak Plasma Concentration | Elimination Half-life | Duration of Action |
|---|---|---|---|---|
| PO | 30-60 min | 45 min | 45 min | Variable |

## VITAMIN B$_6$

Vitamin B$_6$ (pyridoxine) is composed of three compounds: pyridoxine, pyridoxal, and pyridoxamine. Deficiency of vitamin B$_6$ can lead to a type of anemia known as *sideroblastic anemia,* neurologic disturbances, seborrheic dermatitis, cheilosis, and xanthurenic aciduria (formation of xanthine crystals or "stones" in urine). It may also result in convulsions, especially in neonates and infants; hypochromic microcytic anemia; and glossitis (inflamed tongue) and stomatitis (inflamed oral mucosa). Pyridoxine deficiency also affects the peripheral nerves, skin, and mucous membranes. Inadequate intake or poor absorption of pyridoxine causes the development of these conditions. Vitamin B$_6$ deficiency may occur as a result of uremia, alcoholism, cirrhosis, hyperthyroidism, malabsorption syndromes, and heart failure. It may also be induced by various drugs, such as isoniazid and hydralazine.

### Mechanism of Action and Drug Effects

Pyridoxine, pyridoxal, and pyridoxamine are all converted in erythrocytes to the active coenzyme forms of vitamin B$_6$: pyridoxal phosphate and pyridoxamine phosphate. These compounds are necessary for many metabolic functions, such as protein, carbohydrate, and lipid utilization in the body. They also play an important part in the conversion of the amino acid tryptophan to niacin (vitamin B$_3$) and the neurotransmitter serotonin. They are also essential in the synthesis of gamma-aminobutyric acid, an inhibitory neurotransmitter in the CNS. They are important in the synthesis of heme and the maintenance of the hematopoietic system. In addition, these substances are necessary for the integrity of the peripheral nerves, skin, and mucous membranes.

### Indications

Pyridoxine is used to prevent and treat vitamin B$_6$ deficiency. This includes deficiency that can result from therapy with certain medications, including isoniazid (for tuberculosis) and hydralazine (for hypertension). Although vitamin B$_6$ deficiency is rare, it can occur in conditions of inadequate intake or poor absorption of pyridoxine. Seizures that are unresponsive to usual therapy, morning sickness during pregnancy, and various metabolic disorders may respond to pyridoxine therapy.

### Contraindications

The only usual contraindication to pyridoxine use is known drug allergy.

### Adverse Effects

Adverse effects with pyridoxine use are rare and usually do not occur at normal dosages; high dosages and long-term use may produce the adverse effects listed in Table 53-8. Toxic effects are

| TABLE 53-8 | PYRIDOXINE (VITAMIN B$_6$): ADVERSE EFFECTS |
|---|---|
| **BODY SYSTEM** | **ADVERSE EFFECTS** |
| Central nervous | Paresthesias, flushing, warmth, headache, lethargy |
| Integumentary | Pain at injection site |

a result of very large dosages sustained for several months. Neurotoxicity is the most likely result, but this will subside upon discontinuation of the pyridoxine.

### Interactions

Pyridoxine will reduce the activity of levodopa; therefore, vitamin formulations containing B$_6$ must be avoided in patients taking levodopa alone. However, the overwhelming majority of patients with Parkinson's disease take a combination of levodopa and carbidopa, and this interaction does not occur with combination therapy.

### Dosages

For dosage information on vitamin B$_6$, see the table on p. 860.

### DRUG PROFILE

**pyridoxine**

Pyridoxine is a water-soluble B-complex vitamin composed of three components: pyridoxine, pyridoxal, and pyridoxamine. It has several vital roles in the body but is primarily responsible for the integrity of peripheral nerves, skin, mucous membranes, and the hematopoietic system. Pyridoxine is available only for oral use. It is classified as a pregnancy category A drug.

**Pharmacokinetics**

| Route | Onset of Action | Peak Plasma Concentration | Elimination Half-life | Duration of Action |
|---|---|---|---|---|
| PO | Unknown | 30-60 min | 15-20 days | Unknown |

## VITAMIN B$_{12}$

Vitamin B$_{12}$ (cyanocobalamin) is a water-soluble B-complex vitamin that contains cobalt (hence, its name; and *cyano-* means "blue"). It is synthesized by microorganisms and is present in the body as two different coenzymes: adenosylcobalamin and methylcobalamin. Cyanocobalamin is a required coenzyme for many metabolic pathways, including fat and carbohydrate metabolism and protein synthesis. It is also required for growth, cell replication, hematopoiesis, and nucleoprotein and myelin synthesis (Figure 53-2).

Vitamin B$_{12}$ deficiency results in GI lesions, neurologic changes that can result in degenerative CNS lesions, and megaloblastic anemia. The major cause of cyanocobalamin deficiency is malabsorption. Other possible but less likely causes are poor diet, chronic alcoholism, and chronic hemorrhage. Normal serum levels are 200 to 900 pg/mL.

### Mechanism of Action and Drug Effects

Humans must have an exogenous source of cyanocobalamin, because it is required for nucleoprotein and myelin synthesis,

FIGURE 53-2 Cyanocobalamin is a required coenzyme for many body processes.

FIGURE 53-3 Oral absorption of cyanocobalamin requires the presence of intrinsic factor, which is secreted by gastric parietal cells.

| TABLE 53-9 | CYANOCOBALAMIN (VITAMIN B$_{12}$): ADVERSE EFFECTS |
|---|---|
| **BODY SYSTEM** | **ADVERSE EFFECTS** |
| Cardiovascular | Heart failure, vascular thrombosis, pulmonary edema |
| Central nervous | Flushing, optic nerve atrophy |
| Gastrointestinal | Diarrhea |
| Integumentary | Pruritus, rash, pain at injection site |
| Metabolic | Hypokalemia |

cell reproduction, normal growth, and the maintenance of normal erythropoiesis. The cells that have the greatest requirement for vitamin B$_{12}$ are those that divide rapidly, such as epithelial cells, bone marrow, and myeloid cells.

Reduced sulfhydryl (−5H) groups are required to metabolize fats and carbohydrates and to synthesize protein. Cyanocobalamin is involved in maintaining sulfhydryl groups in the reduced form. Cyanocobalamin deficiency can lead to neurologic damage that begins with an inability to produce myelin and is followed by gradual degeneration of the axon and nerve head.

Cyanocobalamin activity is identical to the activity of the anti–pernicious anemia factor present in liver extract called *extrinsic factor* or *Castle factor*. The oral absorption of cyanocobalamin (extrinsic factor) requires the presence of intrinsic factor, which is a glycoprotein secreted by gastric parietal cells. A complex is formed between the two factors, which is then absorbed by the intestines. This is depicted in Figure 53-3.

## Indications

Cyanocobalamin is used to treat deficiency states that develop because of an insufficient intake of the vitamin. It is also included in multivitamin formulations that are used as dietary supplements. Deficiency states are most often the result of malabsorption or poor dietary intake, including consumption of a strict vegetarian diet, because the primary source of cyanocobalamin is foods of animal origin.

The most common manifestation of untreated cyanocobalamin deficiency is pernicious anemia. The use of vitamin B$_{12}$ to treat pernicious anemia and other megaloblastic anemias results in the rapid conversion of a megaloblastic bone marrow to a normoblastic bone marrow. The preferred route of administration of vitamin B$_{12}$ in treating megaloblastic anemias is deep intramuscular injection. If not treated, deficiency states can lead to megaloblastic anemia and irreversible neurologic damage. Cyanocobalamin is also useful in the treatment of pernicious anemia caused by an endogenous lack of intrinsic factor.

## Contraindications

The only usual contraindication to cyanocobalamin (vitamin B$_{12}$) is known drug product allergy. This may include sensitivity to the chemical element cobalt, which is part of the structure of cyanocobalamin. Another contraindication is hereditary optic nerve atrophy (Leber's disease).

## Adverse Effects

Vitamin B$_{12}$ is nontoxic, and large doses must be ingested to produce adverse effects, which include itching, transitory diarrhea, and fever. Other adverse effects are listed by body system in Table 53-9.

## Interactions

Concurrent use with anticonvulsants, aminoglycoside antibiotics, or long-acting potassium preparations decreases the oral absorption of vitamin B$_{12}$.

## Dosages

For dosage information on vitamin B$_{12}$, see the table on p. 860.

## DRUG PROFILE

### cyanocobalamin

Cyanocobalamin is a water-soluble B-complex vitamin required for maintenance of body fat and carbohydrate metabolism and protein synthesis. It is also needed for growth, cell replication, blood cell production, and the integrity of normal nerve function. Cyanocobalamin (vitamin B$_{12}$) is available both as OTC preparations and by prescription. Most of the OTC cyanocobalamin-containing products are oral multivitamin preparations, whereas many of the cyanocobalamin-only products contain large doses for parenteral injection and are available by prescription only. Other available dosage forms are an intranasal gel and a sublingual tablet. It is classified as a pregnancy category A drug.

**Pharmacokinetics (cyanocobalamin, vitamin B$_{12}$)**

| Route | Onset of Action | Peak Plasma Concentration | Elimination Half-life | Duration of Action |
|-------|----------------|---------------------------|----------------------|--------------------|
| PO | Unknown | 8-12 hr | 6 days | Unknown |

## VITAMIN C

Vitamin C (ascorbic acid) can be used in many therapeutic situations. Prolonged ascorbic acid deficiency results in the nutritional disease scurvy, which is characterized by weakness, edema, gingivitis and bleeding gums, loss of teeth, anemia, subcutaneous hemorrhage, bone lesions, delayed healing of soft tissues and bones, and hardening of leg muscles. Scurvy has been recognized for several centuries, especially among sailors. In 1795, the British navy ordered the consumption of limes to prevent the disease.

### Mechanism of Action and Drug Effects

Vitamin C is reversibly oxidized to dehydroascorbic acid and acts in oxidation-reduction reactions. It is required for several important metabolic activities, including collagen synthesis and the maintenance of connective tissue; tissue repair; maintenance of bone, teeth, and capillaries; and folic acid metabolism (specifically, the conversion of folic acid into its active metabolite). It is also essential for erythropoiesis. Vitamin C enhances the absorption of iron and is required for the synthesis of lipids, proteins, and steroids. It has also been shown to aid in cellular respiration and resistance to infections.

### Indications

Vitamin C is used to treat diseases associated with vitamin C deficiency and as a dietary supplement. It is most beneficial in patients who have larger daily requirements because of pregnancy, lactation, hyperthyroidism, fever, stress, infection, trauma, burns, smoking, and the use of certain drugs (e.g., estrogens, oral contraceptives, barbiturates, tetracyclines, and salicylates). Because vitamin C is an acid, it can also be used as a urinary acidifier. The benefits of other uses of vitamin C are undocumented. For example, taking vitamin C to prevent or treat the common cold is common practice. However, most large controlled studies have shown that ascorbic acid has little or no value as a prophylactic for the common cold.

### Contraindications

The only usual contraindication for vitamin C use is known allergy to a specific vitamin product.

### Adverse Effects

Vitamin C is usually nontoxic unless excessive dosages are consumed. Megadoses can produce nausea, vomiting, headache, and abdominal cramps and will acidify the urine, which can result in the formation of cystine, oxalate, and urate renal stones. Furthermore, individuals who discontinue taking excessive daily doses of ascorbic acid can experience scurvy-like symptoms.

### Interactions

Ascorbic acid has the potential to interact with many classes of drugs. However, clinical experience concerning many interactions is inconclusive. Coadministration with acid-labile drugs such as penicillin G or erythromycin must be avoided. Large doses of vitamin C can acidify the urine and may enhance the excretion of basic drugs and delay the excretion of acidic drugs.

### Dosages

For dosage information on vitamin C, see the table on p. 860.

### DRUG PROFILE

**ascorbic acid**

Ascorbic acid is a water-soluble vitamin required for the prevention and treatment of scurvy. It is also required for erythropoiesis and the synthesis of lipids, protein, and steroids. It is available both in OTC preparations such as multivitamin products and by prescription. Ascorbic acid is available in many oral dosage forms as well as an injectable form. It is classified as a pregnancy category A drug.

## MINERALS

Minerals are essential nutrients that are classified as inorganic compounds. They act as building blocks for many body structures and thus are necessary for a variety of physiologic functions. They are also needed for intracellular and extracellular body fluid electrolytes. Iron is essential for the production of hemoglobin, which is required for transport of oxygen throughout the body (see Chapter 54). Minerals are necessary for muscle contraction and nerve transmission, and are required components of essential enzymes.

Mineral compounds are composed of various metallic and nonmetallic elements that are chemically combined with ionic bonds. When these compounds are dissolved in water, they separate (dissociate) into positively charged metallic cations and electrolytes or negatively charged nonmetallic anions (Figure 53-4). Ingestion of minerals provides essential elements necessary for vital bodily functions. Elements that are required in larger amounts are called *macrominerals;* those required in smaller amounts are called *microminerals* or *trace elements*. Table 53-10 classifies these nutrient elements as either *macrominerals* or *microminerals* and as *metal* or *nonmetal*.

### CALCIUM

Calcium is the most abundant mineral element in the human body, accounting for approximately 2% of the total body weight. The highest concentration of calcium is in bones and teeth. The efficient absorption of calcium requires adequate amounts of vitamin D.

Calcium deficiency results in hypocalcemia and can affect many bodily functions. Causes of calcium deficiency include inadequate calcium intake and/or insufficient vitamin D to facilitate absorption; hypoparathyroidism; and malabsorption syndrome, especially in older individuals. Calcium deficiency–related disorders include infantile rickets, adult osteomalacia, muscle cramps, osteoporosis (especially in postmenopausal

**FIGURE 53-4** When mineral compounds are dissolved in water, they separate into positively charged metallic cations or negatively charged nonmetallic anions.

| TABLE 53-10 | MINERAL ELEMENTS | | |
|---|---|---|---|
| **ELEMENT** | **SYMBOL** | **TYPE** | **IONIC/ ELECTROLYTE FORM** |
| **Macrominerals** | | | |
| calcium* | Ca | Metal | $Ca^{2+}$ calcium cation |
| chlorine | Cl | Nonmetal | $Cl^-$ chloride anion |
| magnesium* | Mg | Metal | $Mg^{2+}$ magnesium cation |
| phosphorous* | P | Nonmetal | $PO_4{}^{3-}$ phosphate anion |
| potassium | K | Metal | $K^+$ potassium cation |
| sodium | Na | Metal | $Na^+$ sodium cation |
| sulfur | S | Nonmetal | $SO_4{}^{2-}$ sulfate anion |
| **Microminerals** | | | |
| chromium | Cr | Metal | $Cr^{3+}$ chromium cation |
| cobalt | Co | Metal | $Co^{2+}$ cobalt cation |
| copper | Cu | Metal | $Cu^{2+}$ copper cation |
| fluorine | F | Nonmetal | $F^+$ fluoride anion |
| iodine* | I | Nonmetal | $I^+$ iodide anion |
| iron* | Fe | Metal | $Fe^{2+}$ ferrous cation |
| manganese | Mn | Metal | $Mn^{2+}$ manganese cation |
| molybdenum | Mo | Metal | $Mo^{6+}$ molybdenum cation |
| selenium* | Se | Metal | $Se^{2-}$ selenium cation |
| zinc* | Zn | Metal | $Zn^{2+}$ zinc cation |

*Mineral elements that have a current recommended daily allowance (RDA).

females), hypoparathyroidism, and renal dysfunction. Table 53-11 lists the possible causes of calcium deficiency and the resulting disorders. Normal serum levels are 9 to 10.5 mg/dL.

## Mechanism of Action and Drug Effects

Calcium participates in a variety of essential physiologic functions and is a building block for body structures. Specifically, calcium is involved in the proper development and maintenance of teeth and skeletal bones. It is an important catalyst in many of the coagulation pathways in the blood. Calcium acts as a cofactor in clotting reactions involving the intrinsic and extrinsic pathways of thromboplastin. It is also a cofactor in the conversion of prothrombin to thrombin by thromboplastin and the conversion of fibrinogen to fibrin. Calcium is essential for the normal maintenance and function of the nervous,

| TABLE 53-11 | CALCIUM DEFICIENCY: CAUSES AND DISORDERS |
|---|---|
| **CAUSE** | **DISORDER** |
| Inadequate intake | Infantile rickets |
| Insufficient vitamin D | Adult osteomalacia |
| Hypoparathyroidism | Muscle cramps |
| Malabsorption syndrome | Osteoporosis |

muscular, and skeletal systems and for cell membrane and capillary permeability. It is an important catalyst in many enzymatic reactions, including transmission of nerve impulses; contraction of cardiac, smooth, and skeletal muscles; renal function; respiration; and, as noted earlier, blood coagulation. Calcium also plays a regulatory role in the release and storage of neurotransmitters and hormones, in white blood cell (WBC) and hormone activity, in the uptake and binding of amino acids, and in intestinal absorption of cyanocobalamin (vitamin $B_{12}$) and gastrin secretion.

## Indications

Calcium salts are used for the treatment or prevention of calcium depletion in patients for whom dietary measures are inadequate. Calcium requirements are also high for growing children and for women who are pregnant or breastfeeding. Many conditions may be associated with calcium deficiency, including the following:
- Achlorhydria
- Alkalosis
- Chronic diarrhea
- Hyperphosphatemia
- Hypoparathyroidism
- Menopause
- Pancreatitis
- Pregnancy and lactation
- Premenstrual syndrome
- Renal failure
- Sprue
- Steatorrhea
- Vitamin D deficiency

Calcium is also used to treat various manifestations of established deficiency states, including adult osteomalacia, hypoparathyroidism, infantile rickets or tetany, muscle cramps, osteoporosis, and renal insufficiency. In addition, calcium is used as a dietary supplement for women during pregnancy and lactation.

More than 12 different selected calcium salts are available for treatment or nutritional supplementation. Each calcium salt contains a different amount of elemental calcium per gram of calcium salt. Table 53-12 lists the available salts and their associated calcium content.

## Contraindications

Contraindications for administration of exogenous calcium include hypercalcemia, ventricular fibrillation of the heart, and known allergy to a specific calcium drug product.

## TABLE 53-12 CALCIUM SALTS: CALCIUM CONTENT

| CALCIUM SALT | ELEMENTAL CALCIUM CONTENT (PER GRAM) |
|---|---|
| phosphate tribasic | 400 mg (20 mEq) |
| carbonate* | 400 mg (20 mEq) |
| phosphate dibasic anhydrous | 290 mg (14.5 mEq) |
| chloride | 270 mg (13.5 mEq) |
| acetate | 253 mg (12.7 mEq) |
| phosphate dibasic dihydrate | 230 mg (11.5 mEq) |
| citrate* | 211 mg (10.6 mEq) |
| glycerophosphate | 191 mg (9.6 mEq) |
| lactate | 130 mg (6.5 mEq) |
| gluconate* | 90 mg (4.5 mEq) |
| gluceptate | 82 mg (4.1 mEq) |
| glubionate | 64 mg (3.2 mEq) |

*Most commonly used forms for the prevention of osteoporosis.

## Adverse Effects

Although adverse effects and toxicity are rare, hypercalcemia can occur. Symptoms include anorexia, nausea, vomiting, and constipation. In addition, when calcium salts are administered by intramuscular or subcutaneous injection, mild to severe local reactions, including burning, necrosis and sloughing of tissue, cellulitis, and soft tissue calcification, may occur. Venous irritation may occur with intravenous administration. Other adverse effects associated with both oral and parenteral use of calcium salts are listed in Table 53-13.

### Toxicity and Management of Overdose

Long-term excessive calcium intake can result in severe hypercalcemia, which can cause cardiac irregularities, delirium, and coma. Management of acute hypercalcemia may require hemodialysis, whereas milder cases will respond to discontinuation of calcium intake.

## Interactions

Calcium salts will chelate (bind with) tetracyclines and quinolones to produce an insoluble complex. If hypercalcemia is present in patients taking digoxin, serious cardiac dysrhythmias can occur.

## Dosages

For dosage information on calcium and other selected minerals, see the table below.

## TABLE 53-13 CALCIUM SALTS: ADVERSE EFFECTS

| BODY SYSTEM | ADVERSE EFFECTS |
|---|---|
| Cardiovascular | Hemorrhage, rebound hypertension |
| Gastrointestinal | Constipation, nausea, vomiting, flatulence |
| Genitourinary | Renal dysfunction, renal stones, renal failure |
| Metabolic | Hypercalcemia, metabolic alkalosis |

## DRUG PROFILE

### calcium

Calcium salts are primarily used in the treatment or prevention of calcium depletion in patients in whom dietary measures are inadequate. Many calcium salts are available, all with a different content of elemental calcium per gram of salt. Calcium is available in both oral and parenteral forms. Numerous calcium preparations are available that have different names and provide different doses. Consult manufacturer instructions for recommended dosages. The pharmacokinetics of calcium is highly variable and depends on individual patient physiology and the characteristics of the specific drug product used. Medication errors and confusion are common with calcium products, because the amount of the salt is not the same as the amount of elemental calcium. For example, calcium carbonate 1250 mg is equal to 500 mg of elemental calcium. Depending on the institution, the drug may be profiled as 1250 mg, but the tablet is labeled as 500 mg. Additional confusion occurs with the injectable forms, calcium chloride and calcium gluconate. Calcium chloride provides about three times as much elemental calcium as calcium gluconate, but they are both ordered as 1 g or 1 ampule. Calcium chloride can cause severe problems if it infiltrates from the intravenous line. For that reason, it is recommended that it be diluted or given through a central line if it is given by intravenous push. Adding to the confusion is calcium acetate (PhosLo), which is used not for calcium replacement but to bind phosphate in renal patients. Calcium products are classified as pregnancy category C drugs.

## MAGNESIUM

Magnesium is one of the principal cations present in the intracellular fluid. It is an essential part of many enzyme systems associated with energy metabolism. Magnesium deficiency (hypomagnesemia) is usually caused by (1) malabsorption, especially in the presence of high calcium intake;

## DOSAGES

### Selected Minerals

| DRUG | PHARMACOLOGIC CLASS | USUAL DOSAGE RANGE | INDICATIONS/USES |
|---|---|---|---|
| calcium carbonate (Tums, others) | Mineral salt | PO: 500 mg 2-4 times daily | Antacid, nutritional-calcium supplementation, hyperphosphatemia associated with chronic renal failure |
| magnesium oxide (Max-Ox 400, others) | Mineral salt | PO: 400 mg 1-2 times daily | Magnesium supplementation, hypomagnesemia |

*PO*, Oral.

(2) alcoholism; (3) long-term intravenous feeding; (4) diuretic use; and (5) metabolic disorders, including hyperthyroidism and diabetic ketoacidosis. Symptoms associated with hypomagnesemia include cardiovascular disturbances, neuromuscular impairment, and mental disturbances. Dietary intake from vegetables and other foods will usually prevent magnesium deficiency. However, magnesium is required in greater amounts in individuals with diets high in protein-rich foods, calcium, and phosphorus. Normal serum levels are 1.7 to 2.2 mg/dL.

## Mechanism of Action and Drug Effects

The precise mechanism for the effects of magnesium has not been fully determined. Magnesium is a known cofactor for many enzyme systems. It is required for muscle contraction and nerve function. Magnesium produces an anticonvulsant effect by inhibiting neuromuscular transmission in selected convulsive states.

## Indications

Magnesium is used for treatment of magnesium deficiency and as a nutritional supplement in total parenteral nutrition and multivitamin preparations. It is used as an anticonvulsant in magnesium deficiency–induced seizure states; to manage complications of pregnancy, including preeclampsia and eclampsia; as a tocolytic drug for inhibition of uterine contractions in premature labor; for treatment of pediatric acute nephropathy; for management of various cardiac dysrhythmias; and for short-term treatment of constipation.

## Contraindications

Contraindications to magnesium administration include known drug product allergy, heart block, renal failure, adrenal gland failure (Addison's disease), and hepatitis.

## Adverse Effects

Adverse effects of magnesium are due to hypermagnesemia, which results in tendon reflex loss, difficult bowel movements, CNS depression, respiratory distress and heart block, and hypothermia.

### Toxicity and Management of Overdose

Toxic effects are extensions of symptoms caused by hypermagnesemia, a major cause of which is the long-term use of magnesium products (especially antacids in patients with renal dysfunction). Severe hypermagnesemia is treated with intravenous calcium and possibly the diuretic furosemide.

## Interactions

The use of magnesium with neuromuscular blocking drugs and CNS depressants produces additive effects.

## DRUG PROFILE

**magnesium**
Magnesium is a mineral that has a variety of dosage forms and uses. It is an essential part of many enzyme systems. When it is absent or diminished in the body, cardiovascular, neuromuscular, and mental disturbances can occur. Magnesium sulfate is the most common form of magnesium used as a mineral replacement. It is available in both oral and injectable forms. It is classified as a pregnancy category B drug.

## PHOSPHORUS

Phosphorus is widely distributed in foods, and thus a dietary deficiency is rare. Deficiency states are primarily due to malabsorption, extensive diarrhea or vomiting, hyperthyroidism, hepatic disease, and long-term use of aluminum or calcium antacids. Normal serum levels are 2.8 to 4.2 mg/dL.

## Mechanism of Action and Drug Effects

Phosphorus in the form of the phosphate group and/or anion $(PO_4^{3-})$ is a required precursor for the synthesis of essential body chemicals and an important building block for body structures. Phosphorus is required as a structural unit for the synthesis of nucleic acid and the adenosine phosphate compounds (adenosine monophosphate [AMP], adenosine diphosphate [ADP], and adenosine triphosphate [ATP]) responsible for cellular energy transfer. It is also necessary for the development and maintenance of the skeletal system and teeth. The skeletal bones contain up to 85% of the phosphorus content of the body. In addition, phosphorus is required for the proper utilization of many B-complex vitamins, and it is an essential component of physiologic buffering systems.

## Indications

Phosphorus is used for treatment of deficiency states and as a dietary supplement in many multivitamin formulations.

## Contraindications

Contraindications to phosphorous or phosphate administration include hyperphosphatemia and hypocalcemia.

## Adverse Effects

Adverse effects are usually associated with the use of phosphorus replacement products. These effects include diarrhea, nausea, vomiting, and other GI disturbances. Other adverse effects include confusion, weakness, and breathing difficulties.

### Toxicity and Management of Overdose

Toxic reactions to phosphorus are extremely rare and usually occur only after ingestion of the pure element.

## Interactions

Antacids can reduce the oral absorption of phosphorus.

### DRUG PROFILE

#### phosphorus

Phosphorus is a mineral that is essential to our well-being. It is needed to make energy in the form of ADP and ATP for all bodily processes. Phosphorus is present in a large number of drug formulations and appears as a phosphate salt ($PO_4$). Phosphorus is to be used with caution in patients with renal impairment. It is available in both oral and parenteral formulations.

## ZINC

The metallic element zinc is often taken orally in the form of the sulfate salt as a mineral supplement. Normally a dietary trace element, zinc plays a crucial role in the enzymatic metabolic reactions involving both proteins and carbohydrates. This makes it especially important for normal tissue growth and repair. It therefore also has a major role in wound healing.

## NURSING PROCESS

## ASSESSMENT

Before administering *vitamins*, assess the patient for nutritional disorders by reviewing the results of various laboratory tests, such as hemoglobin, hematocrit, WBC and RBC counts, serum albumin, and total protein levels. Assess the patient's dietary intake, dietary patterns, menu planning, grocery shopping/food practices and habits, and cultural influences before giving any supplemental therapy. For vitamin A deficiencies, perform a baseline vision assessment, including night vision, and conduct a thorough examination of the skin and mucous membranes, and document the findings. Assess for contraindications to vitamin A such as known allergy as well as a current state of excessive supplementation and/or hypervitaminosis. Additionally, assess for drug interactions with laxatives and cholestyramine leading to possible decreased absorption of the vitamin. Baseline assessment and documentation of level of consciousness, GI functioning and complaints, vision, condition of the skin, and musculoskeletal status is also important due to the adverse effects and signs and symptoms of toxicity associated with overdosage of vitamin A (see the pharmacology discussion and Table 53-3).

For patients who are deficient in *vitamin D,* perform a baseline assessment of skeletal formation with attention to any deformities. Serum vitamin D (12 to 50 ng/mL) and calcium levels are usually ordered as baseline and then during therapy. It is also important to assess for known contraindications such as renal dysfunction and hypercalcemia or hyperphosphatemia. Assess for drug interactions with laxatives and cholestyramine leading to possible decreased absorption of the vitamin. Before *vitamin E* is administered, assess patients for hypoprothrombinemia because this condition may occur secondary to vitamin E deficiency. Document any baseline bleeding or hematologic problems and conduct a thorough skin assessment with attention to skin integrity, presence of any edema, muscle weakness, easy bruising, and/or bleeding.

The last of the fat-soluble vitamins, *vitamin K,* is associated with clotting function; therefore, prior to its use, measure and document the patient's prothrombin time, international normalized ratio, and platelet counts. Assess the skin for bruises, petechiae, and erythema. Examine the gums for gingival bleeding. Assess urine and stool for the presence of blood. Also assess vital signs with attention to blood pressure and pulse rate. If intravenous dosage forms are prescribed, baseline assessment must include vital signs because of the risk of anaphylactic reactions. This is particularly important with vitamin $K_1$ (phytonadione or AquaMEPHYTON) because of an associated higher risk of anaphylaxis. Assessment of liver function is also important. It is critical to patient safety to remember that the fat-soluble vitamins are all stored in the body tissue when excessive quantities are consumed and may become toxic if taken in large dosages. Assess and document baseline values of vitamin K; normal ranges are 0.1 to 2.2 ng/mL.

*Vitamin $B_1$* (thiamine) hypersensitivity may cause skin rash and wheezing; therefore, document the presence of any allergic reactions to vitamin B compounds. Also document baseline assessment of vital signs. Because it is rare for a deficiency of only one B-complex vitamin to occur, rule out deficiencies of all the B vitamins before treatment begins. Vitamin $B_1$ (thiamine) levels range from 66 to 200 nmol/L, and vitamin $B_{12}$ (cyanocolbalamin) levels range from 200 to 900 pg/mL. Urinary thiamine levels may also be ordered (in adults, urinary thiamine levels of less than 27 mcg/dL indicate deficiency). Vitamin $B_1$ deficiency may result in Wernicke's encephalopathy (see the pharmacology discussion); thus, there is a need for a thorough mental status assessment. Thoroughly assess the medication order for accuracy and for route of administration. Drug interactions include alkaline and sulfite-containing solutions, so be sure to assess for drugs being administered at the same time. *Vitamin $B_2$* (riboflavin) has no major toxic effects or drug interactions, but assessing for any known allergy to any vitamin product is important. *Vitamin $B_3$* (niacin) has several important indications. Assess for contraindications such as liver disease, severe hypotension, and active peptic ulcer disease. With *vitamin $B_6$* (pyridoxine), perform a thorough neurologic assessment due to associated neurotoxicity with large dosages. Levodopa is a significant drug interaction to assess for with pyridoxine because the vitamin reduces the action of levodopa. *Vitamin $B_{12}$* (cyanocobalamin) requires thorough assessment of the medication order. Note the route of administration because the preferred route is deep IM injection. Drug interactions to assess for include anticonvulsants, aminoglycoside antibiotics, and long-acting potassium supplements because they decrease the oral absorption of vitamin $B_{12}$.

*Vitamin C* (ascorbic acid) is usually well tolerated; however, assess the patient for any history of nutritional deficits or problems with dietary intake as well as any allergies to a specific vitamin product. Assess for drug interactions that include acid-labile drugs such as penicillin G or erythromycin. Additionally, it is important to note that large doses of vitamin C may increase the excretion of many basic (opposite of acidic) drugs and delay the excretion of acidic drugs.

With the minerals *calcium* and *magnesium,* include allergies, nutritional status, use of medications, medical history, contraindications, cautions, and drug interactions in the baseline assessment. Laboratory studies that may be prescribed include serum calcium (9 to 10.5 mg/dL), magnesium (1.7 to 2.2 mg/dL), hemoglobin, hematocrit, and RBC and WBC counts. Calcium interacts with many medications, as described previously, so a thorough assessment of the patient's medication history is important to patient safety. The specific interaction of calcium is that of chelation or binding with the drug and, in this case, it is with tetracycline and quinolone antibiotics. The chelation then forms an insoluble complex rendering the antibiotic inactive. Another significant interaction occurs when a patient is hypercalcemic and takes digitalis with the result of serious cardiac dysrhythmias. If there is a history of cardiac disease, a baseline electrocardiogram (ECG) recording may be ordered prior to calcium therapy. Because of the various calcium preparations with different names and doses, always thoroughly assess the medication order and be certain that the right product is being given. Also note that the injectable forms of calcium (i.e., calcium chloride, calcium gluconate) may be easily confused, so be cautious. Assess patency of the IV site, if intravenous dosage forms are ordered, because infiltrates may lead to severe irritation of the vein and surrounding tissue.

Magnesium is also associated with several drug interactions. Review for potential interactions before drug therapy is initiated, such as with CNS depressants and neuromuscular blocking drugs. Assess the patient's renal, cardiac, and hepatic functioning. Important to document prior to giving magnesium is neurologic functioning and grading of deep tendon reflexes. Hyporeflexia may indicate toxicity. It is also important to assess the prescriber's order for completeness and reason for use so that it is fully understood why the drug is being given (e.g., replacement, antacid, or laxative purposes). In addition, thoroughly assess any order for the use of calcium, magnesium, and/or zinc within total parenteral nutritional infusions.

## NURSING DIAGNOSES

1. Impaired physical mobility related to poorly developed muscles from vitamin D and/or vitamin E deficiency and/or from fatigue related to poor nutrition and vitamin B deficiency
2. Impaired tissue integrity related to vitamin C deficiency and subsequent decreased healing
3. Risk for injury related to possible night blindness or altered vision due to vitamin A deficiency

## PLANNING

### GOALS

1. Patient regains or maintains normal or near-normal physical mobility and musculoskeletal functioning.
2. Patient maintains intact skin and tissue integrity.
3. Patient remains free from injury.

## CASE STUDY

### Vitamin Supplements

S.C., 49 years of age, was found unconscious in a vacant house and was brought to the emergency department. He had an elevated blood alcohol level and eventually manifested delirium tremens. Now, a week later, he is in stable condition on a medical-surgical unit. He is weak and malnourished, and he cannot remember how he got to the hospital. The nurse is reviewing his medication list and notes that several vitamin supplements are ordered.

1. Based on S.C.'s history, what vitamin deficiencies are possible?
2. Which vitamin supplement is especially used to treat complications associated with alcoholism? Explain your answer.
3. S.C. is receiving large doses of several vitamins, and the nurse is concerned about vitamin toxicities. Which type of vitamin, water-soluble or fat-soluble, carries the risk of toxicities? Explain your answer.
4. Because of S.C.'s long-term malnourished state, the physician is concerned about the condition of his bones and starts S.C. on phosphorus and calcium supplementation, along with vitamin D. Explain the rationale behind the addition of vitamin D.

For answers, see http://evolve.elsevier.com/Lilley.

## OUTCOME CRITERIA

1. Patient increases mobility daily with performance of ADLs and usual exercise regimen or as prescribed.
   - Patient states measures to increase energy, stamina, and strength such as increase in dietary consumption of well-balanced diet and fluids with vitamin or mineral supplementation.
2. Patient states measures to minimize injury and maximize intactness of skin and mucous membranes, such as performing frequent mouth care, keeping skin clean and dry and applying moisturizers as needed, as well as drinking at least 6 to 8 glasses of water per day.
3. Patient states measures to prevent injury such as minimizing obstacles in the home setting, removing area or throw rugs, and adding night lights.
   - Patient states measures to replace vitamin A deficiencies through replacement therapy and dietary intake such as increased intake of liver, fish, dairy products, egg yolks, and yellow-orange vegetables/fruits.

## IMPLEMENTATION

Before administering *vitamin A* or any vitamin or supplement, document the patient's dietary intake for the preceding 24 hours. Document any signs and symptoms of hypervitaminosis or hypercarotenemia (excess vitamin A).; *Vitamin D* is available in OTC products (e.g., multivitamins) or by prescription but attention to the product prescribed is important to patient safety. Oral dosage forms are available with IM dosage forms for those with GI, liver, biliary and/or malabsorptive syndromes. During therapy, advise the patient to report any palpitations, unresolved nausea, vomiting, constipation, or muscle pain. Instruct the patient to take *vitamin B₁* (thiamine) as directed. *Vitamin B₂* (riboflavin) is not associated with any adverse or toxic effects but it is important to note that in large doses it may turn the urine yellowish-orange. Tell patients to take *vitamin B₃* (niacin) with milk or food to decrease GI upset. Niacin is often used for hyperlipidemia (see Chapter 27) and in much larger doses. *Vitamin B₆* (pyridoxine) is more commonly used to treat drug-induced B₆ deficiencies. Two examples of this are with the antituberculin drug isoniazid (INH) and antihypertensive drug hydralazine. *Vitamin B₁₂* (cyanocobalamin) is administered orally with meals to increase its absorption. Intranasal gel and sublingual tablets are other dosage forms available. If given for megaloblastic anemia, deep IM injection is the preferred route of administration. Give *vitamin C* (ascorbic acid) orally, and if oral effervescent forms are used, instruct the patient to dissolve it in at least 6 oz of water or juice. If vitamin C is administered for acidification of urine, it is important to frequently monitor the patient's urinary pH.

Various oral *calcium* products are available and, because of the differences in the amount of elemental calcium they provide (e.g., calcium carbonate 1250 mg is equal to only 500 mg of elemental calcium), medication errors may occur and confusion may arise about the various dosages available OTC. A list of the various calcium salts available is found in Table 53-12. Instruct the patient to take oral dosage forms of calcium 1 to 3 hours after meals. Injectable dosage forms of calcium may also be confusing. Follow the medication order carefully and check policy and standards regarding infusions (see previous discussion in the pharmacology section and the Safety and Quality Improvement: Preventing Medication Errors box on p. 875). Because of problems with venous irritation, give intravenous calcium via an intravenous infusion pump and with proper dilution. Giving intravenous calcium too rapidly may precipitate severe hypercalcemia with subsequent cardiac irregularities, delirium, and coma. Administer intravenous calcium slowly, as ordered, and within the manufacturer guidelines (e.g., usually less than 1 mL/min). Patients need to remain recumbent for 15 minutes after the infusion to prevent further problems. Should extravasation of the intravenous calcium solution occur, discontinue the infusion immediately but leave the intravenous catheter in place for antidote administration. The prescriber may then order an injection of 1% procaine and/or other antidotes or fluids to reduce vasospasm at the site and dilute the irritating effects of calcium on surrounding tissue. However, follow all facility policies and procedural guidelines and/or manufacturer insert information as is deemed appropriate. In addition, include the appearance of the intravenous site (e.g., erythema, swelling, and any drainage) in the documentation.

Administer *magnesium* according to manufacturer guidelines and as ordered. Always give intravenous magnesium sulfate very cautiously; use an infusion pump, and follow manufacturer guidelines for dosage and dilutional concentration. During intravenous magnesium infusion, monitor the patient's ECG and vital signs, and rate patellar or knee-jerk reflexes. Impaired reflexes are used as an indication of drug-related CNS depressant effects. CNS depression may quickly lead to respiratory and/or cardiac depression; thus perform frequent monitoring. Document IV calcium infusion and record each set of vital sign measurements with ratings of reflexes. If there is a decrease in the strength of reflexes and/or a decrease in respirations to less than 12 breaths/min, contact the prescriber immediately, stop the infusion, and monitor the patient. Other signs that require immediate attention are confusion, irregular heart rhythm, cramping, unusual fatigue, lightheadedness, and dizziness. Calcium gluconate must be readily accessible for use as an antidote to magnesium toxicity. Administer oral dosage forms of magnesium as ordered and in the exact dosage prescribed. See the Patient Teaching Tips for more information related to the use of vitamins, minerals, and trace elements.

## EVALUATION

In the patient's evaluation, always review whether goals and outcome criteria have been met. Monitor for therapeutic responses and adverse effects of each vitamin or mineral. Therapeutic responses to *vitamin A* include restoration of normal vision and intact skin; adverse effects include lethargy, headache, nausea, and vomiting (see Table 53-3). Therapeutic responses to *vitamin D* include improved bone growth and formation and an intact skeleton with decreased or no pain compared with baseline musculoskeletal deformity, weakness, and discomfort; adverse effects include hypertension, dysrhythmias, fatigue, weakness, headache, and decreased bone growth (see Table 53-4). Therapeutic responses to *vitamin E* include improved muscle strength, improved skin integrity, and alpha tocopherol levels within normal limits; adverse effects are listed in Table 53-5. Therapeutic responses to *vitamin K* include return to normal clotting; adverse effects include headache, nausea, and hemolytic anemia (see Table 53-6). Therapeutic responses to *vitamin B₁* (thiamine) include improved mental status and less confusion. Therapeutic responses include improved skin integrity, normal vision, improved mental status, and normal RBC count, hemoglobin level, and hematocrit. Adverse effects from vitamin B are rare, but *vitamin B₃* (niacin) is associated with postural hypotension, dysrhythmias, headache, and nausea (see Table 53-7 for complete listing). *Vitamin B₆* (pyridoxine) adverse effects include flushing, paresthesias, lethargy, and headache. *Vitamin B₁₂* (cyanocobalamin) has adverse effects of heart failure, flushing, diarrhea, itching, and hypokalemia. Therapeutic responses to *vitamin C* include improvements in capillary intactness, integrity of the skin and mucous membranes, healing, energy level, and mental state. Therapeutic responses to *calcium* include improved deficiency states. Adverse effects are listed in Table 53-13. Therapeutic effects of *magnesium* include bolstering of many enzymatic functions in the body with other uses as an anticonvulsant, treatment of preeclampsia and eclampsia, and management of various dysrhythmias. Adverse effects include loss of deep tendon reflexes, CNS depression, constipation, respiratory distress, and heart block.

## PATIENT TEACHING TIPS

- Educate the patient about the best dietary sources of both water- and fat-soluble vitamins (vitamins A, B, C, D, E, and K), as well as about the best sources of elements and minerals. See Table 53-2 for the nutrient content of various food items.
- Monitor any patient taking vitamins or minerals closely for therapeutic and adverse effects. Encourage the patient to monitor his or her own progress in how well he or she feels and to note any improvement in the related condition or health status. Encourage intake of fluids with all vitamin and mineral therapy.
- Inform patients who have had a gastrectomy or ileal resection and those with pernicious anemia of the necessity for vitamin $B_{12}$ injections.

- Educate the patient taking up to 600 mg/day of vitamin C that there may be a slight increase in daily urination and that diarrhea is associated with intake of more than 1 g/day.
- Stress that patients taking calcium and/or magnesium (see Table 53-10) must take the medication as prescribed and with adequate amounts of fluids.
- Educate the patient about calcium therapy and about food items and drugs that will chelate (or bind) with calcium. For example, calcium binds with tetracycline antibiotics and decreases or negates the effect of the antibiotic.

## KEY POINTS

- OTC use of vitamins and minerals may lead to serious problems and adverse effects and requires careful consideration prior to self-medication. A prescriber may be consulted prior to use if there are any questions or concerns.
- Incorporate the nutritional status of the patient into the nursing care plan to provide comprehensive care during vitamin or mineral therapy.
- Provide information about dietary needs and the body's need for vitamins and minerals as part of the patient's health promotion.

- Focus patient education related to vitamin and mineral replacement on dietary sources of the specific nutrient, drug and food interactions, and adverse effects. Instruct the patient on when it is necessary to contact the prescriber.
- Vitamins and minerals can be dangerous to the patient if given without concern or caution for the patient's overall condition and underlying disease processes.
- Never assume that because the drug is a vitamin or a mineral it does not have adverse reactions or toxicity.

## NCLEX® EXAMINATION REVIEW QUESTIONS

1 When giving calcium intravenously, the nurse needs to administer it slowly, keeping in mind that rapid intravenous administration of calcium may cause which problem?
   a Ototoxicity
   b Renal damage
   c Tetany
   d Cardiac dysrhythmias
2 The nurse will assess which laboratory test results before administration of vitamin K?
   a Prothrombin time and international normalized ratio
   b Red blood cell and white blood cell counts
   c Phosphorous and calcium levels
   d Total protein and albumin levels
3 A patient has GI malabsorption due to severe intestinal damage from a gastrointestinal infection. The nurse will need to assess for signs of a deficiency of which vitamin?
   a Vitamin A (retinol)
   b Vitamin $B_{12}$ (cyanocobalamin)
   c Vitamin $B_6$ (pyridoxine)
   d Vitamin E (tocopherols)
4 The nurse is providing wound care for a patient with a stage IV pressure ulcer and expects that the patient will receive which supplement to assist in wound healing?
   a Vitamin K
   b Vitamin $B_1$
   c Zinc
   d Calcium

5 While caring for a newly admitted patient who has a long history of alcoholism, the nurse anticipates that part of the patient's medication regimen will include which vitamin?
   a Vitamin $B_1$ (thiamine)
   b Vitamin $B_6$ (pyridoxine)
   c Vitamin C (ascorbic acid)
   d Vitamin A (retinol)
6 When administering vitamin and mineral supplements, the nurse implements which appropriate interventions? (Select all that apply.)
   a Not administering oral calcium tablets along with oral tetracyclines
   b Administering intravenous calcium via a rapid intravenous push infusion
   c Monitoring the heart rhythm (ECG) of a patient receiving an intravenous magnesium infusion
   d Giving oral niacin with milk or food to decrease gastrointestinal upset
   e Monitoring for the formation of renal stones in patients taking large doses of vitamin C
7 The order reads: "Give vitamin K (AquaMEPHYTON) 0.5 mg IM within 1 hour of birth." The medication is available in a vial that contains 1 mg/0.5 mL. How many milliliters will the nurse draw up for the injection?

1. d, 2. a, 3. b, 4. c, 5. a, 6. a, c, d, e, 7. 0.25 mL.

For Critical Thinking and Prioritization Questions, see http://evolve.elsevier.com/Lilley.

# Anemia Drugs

## OBJECTIVES

When you reach the end of this chapter, you will be able to do the following:

1. Discuss the importance of iron, vitamin $B_{12}$, and folic acid in the formation of blood cells.
2. Describe the various types of anemia-related drug treatments.
3. Discuss the mechanisms of action, cautions, contraindications, drug interactions, uses, dosages, and special administration techniques of the various drugs used to treat

anemia, as well as measures to enhance the effectiveness and decrease the adverse effects of these drugs.

4. Develop a nursing care plan that includes all phases of the nursing process for patients taking drugs used to treat anemia.

## DRUG PROFILES

- ♦ **epoetin alfa, p. 880**
  **ferric gluconate, p. 883**
  **ferrous fumarate, p. 882**
- ♦ **ferrous sulfate, p. 882**

- ♦ **folic acid, p. 884**
  **iron dextran, p. 883**
  **iron sucrose, p. 883**

  _____

- ♦ *Key drug*

## KEY TERMS

**Erythrocytes** Another name for red blood cells (RBCs). (p. 878)

**Erythropoiesis** The process of erythrocyte production. (p. 878)

**Globin** The protein part of the *hemoglobin* molecule (see later); the four different structural globin chains most often found in adults are the alpha$_1$, alpha$_2$, beta$_1$, and beta$_2$ chains. (p. 878)

**Hematopoiesis** The normal formation and development of all blood cell types in the bone marrow. (p. 878)

**Heme** Part of the *hemoglobin* molecule; a nonprotein, iron-containing pigment. (p. 878)

**Hemoglobin** A complex protein-iron compound in the blood that carries oxygen to the cells from the lungs and carbon dioxide away from the cells to the lungs. (p. 878)

**Hemolytic anemias** Anemias resulting from excessive destruction of erythrocytes. (p. 879)

**Hypochromic** Pertaining to less than normal color. The term usually describes an RBC with decreased hemoglobin content and helps further characterize anemias associated with reduced synthesis of hemoglobin. (p. 878)

**Microcytic** Pertaining to or characterized by smaller than normal cells. (p. 878)

**Pernicious anemia** A type of megaloblastic anemia usually seen in older adults and caused by impaired intestinal absorption of vitamin $B_{12}$ (cyanocobalamin) due to lack of availability of intrinsic factor. (p. 879)

**Reticulocytes** An immature erythrocyte characterized by a meshlike pattern of threads and particles at the former site of the nucleus. (p. 878)

**Spherocytes** Small, globular, completely hemoglobinated erythrocytes without the usual central concavity or pallor. (p. 879)

## ANATOMY, PHYSIOLOGY, AND PATHOPHYSIOLOGY OVERVIEW

### ERYTHROPOIESIS

The formation of new blood cells is one of the primary functions of bones. This process is known as hematopoiesis, and it includes the production of erythrocytes (red blood cells, or RBCs), as well as leukocytes (white blood cells) and thrombocytes (platelets). This process takes place in the myeloid tissue or bone marrow. This specialized tissue is located primarily in the ends, or *epiphyses,* of certain long bones and also in the flat bones of the skull, pelvis, sternum, scapulae, and ribs.

Erythropoiesis, the process of erythrocyte formation, is the focus of this chapter. This involves the maturation of a nucleated RBC precursor into a hemoglobin-filled, nucleus-free erythrocyte. This process is driven by the hormone erythropoietin, which is produced by the kidneys. Erythropoietin is also produced commercially and is used to treat anemia in certain specific circumstances and is discussed in detail later in the chapter.

When RBCs are manufactured in the bone marrow by myeloid tissue, they are released into the circulation as immature RBCs called reticulocytes. Once in the circulation, reticulocytes undergo a 24- to 36-hour maturation process to become mature, fully functional RBCs. After this, they have a lifespan of about 120 days.

More than one third of an RBC is composed of hemoglobin. Hemoglobin (abbreviated *Hgb*) is composed of two parts: heme and globin. Heme is a red pigment. Each heme group contains one atom of iron. Globin is a protein chain. The four different structural globin chains most often found in adults are the $alpha_1$, $alpha_2$, $beta_1$, and $beta_2$ chains. Together, four heme groups, each linked to one protein chain of globin, make up one hemoglobin molecule (Figure 54-1).

### TYPES OF ANEMIA

Anemias are classified into four main types based on the underlying causes (Figure 54-2). Anemia of chronic disease is another common type of anemia. Anemias can be caused by maturation defects, or they can be secondary to excessive RBC destruction. Two types of maturation defects lead to anemias, categorized by the location of the defect within the cell: cytoplasmic maturation defects occur in the cell cytoplasm, and nuclear maturation defects occur in the cell nucleus. Factors responsible for excessive RBC destruction can be either intrinsic or extrinsic.

Figure 54-3 summarizes the types of anemias arising from cytoplasmic maturation defects. Major examples include iron-deficiency anemia and genetic disorders such as thalassemia, which result in defective globin synthesis. For each of these anemias, the RBCs appear hypochromic (lighter red than normal) and microcytic (smaller than normal) on blood smear. Cytoplasmic maturation anemias occur as a result of reduced or abnormal hemoglobin synthesis. Because hemoglobin is synthesized from both iron and globin, a deficiency in either one can lead to a hemoglobin deficiency. Some common

**FIGURE 54-1** Schematic structure of a hemoglobin molecule.

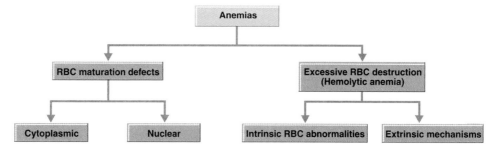

**FIGURE 54-2** Underlying causes of anemia are red blood cell (RBC) maturation defects and factors secondary to excessive RBC destruction.

causes of iron-deficiency anemia are blood loss, surgery, childbirth, gastrointestinal bleeding (which can be caused by NSAID ingestion; see Chapter 44), menstrual blood loss, and hemorrhoids.

Figure 54-4 summarizes the types of anemias arising from nuclear maturation defects. These occur because of defects in deoxyribonucleic acid (DNA) or protein synthesis. Both DNA and protein synthesis require vitamin $B_{12}$ and folic acid ($B_9$) to be present in normal amounts for their proper production. If either of these two vitamins is absent or deficient, anemias secondary to nuclear maturation defects may develop. In such anemias, RBCs actually appear to be *normochromic* (normal in color) but are commonly *macrocytic* (larger than normal) on blood smear. One example is *pernicious anemia*. This type of anemia results from deficiency of vitamin $B_{12}$, which is used in the formation of new RBCs. The usual underlying cause is the failure of the stomach lining to produce intrinsic factor. Intrinsic factor is a gastric glycoprotein that allows vitamin $B_{12}$ to be absorbed in the intestine (see Chapter 53). Another example is the anemia caused by folic acid deficiency. Both pernicious anemia and folic acid deficiency anemia are also known as types of *megaloblastic*

anemia, because they are both characterized by large, immature RBCs. Megaloblastic anemias not caused from a lack of intrinsic factor are usually related to poor dietary intake and are most commonly seen in infancy, childhood, and pregnancy.

Figure 54-5 summarizes the types of anemias arising from excessive RBC destruction, or *hemolytic anemias.* These can occur because of abnormalities within the RBCs themselves (intrinsic factors) or as a result of factors outside of (extrinsic to) the RBCs. In both cases, the erythrocytes appear on blood smear as *spherocytes.* RBC abnormalities caused by intrinsic factors are usually the result of a genetic defect. Examples include sickle cell anemia, hereditary spherocytosis, glucose-6-phosphate dehydrogenase (G6PD) deficiency, and paroxysmal nocturnal hemoglobinuria. Examples of extrinsic mechanisms for excessive RBC destruction include drug-induced antibodies that target and destroy RBCs, septic shock that produces disseminated intravascular coagulation, and mechanical forces such as those created by intraaortic balloon pumps, ventricular assist devices, and continuous venovenous hemodialysis (CVVHD), commonly used in intensive care units.

**FIGURE 54-3** Schematic showing common causes and results of red blood cell (RBC) cytoplasmic maturation defects. ↓, Decreased.

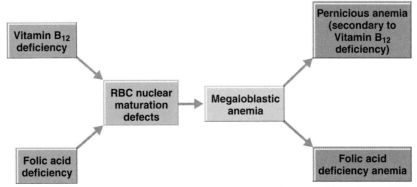

**FIGURE 54-4** Schematic showing common causes and results of red blood cell (RBC) nuclear maturation defects.

**FIGURE 54-5** Increased red blood cell (RBC) destruction occurs as a result of intrinsic and extrinsic factors. ↑, Increased; *DIC*, disseminated intravascular coagulation; *G6PD*, glucose-6-phosphate dehydrogenase.

## PHARMACOLOGY OVERVIEW

### ERYTHROPOIESIS STIMULATING AGENTS

#### ◆ epoetin alfa

Epoetin alfa (Epogen) is a biosynthetic form of the natural hormone erythropoietin, which is normally secreted by the kidneys in response to a decrease in RBCs. It promotes the synthesis of erythrocytes (RBCs) by stimulating RBC progenitor cells in the bone marrow. Epoetin alfa is used to treat anemia that is associated with end-stage renal disease, chemotherapy-induced anemia, and for anemia associated with zidovudine therapy (see Chapter 40). Epoetin causes the progenitor cells in the bone marrow to manufacture large numbers of immature RBCs and to greatly speed up their maturation. This medication is ineffective without adequate body iron stores and bone marrow function. Most patients receiving epoetin alfa need to also receive an oral iron preparation. A longer-acting form of epoetin called *darbepoetin (Aranesp)* is available that reduces the required number of injections, although one cost study found that there is no significant difference in overall cost between the two. Both drugs are available for injection only and can be given intravenously or subcutaneously. When the drugs are given by the subcutaneous route, the onset of action is slower, and lower dosages can be used.

Contraindications for erythropoiesis-stimulating agents (ESAs) include known drug allergy. Use of epoetin and darbepoetin is contraindicated in cases of uncontrolled hypertension and when hemoglobin levels are above 10 g/dL for cancer patients and 12 g/dL for renal patients. Use in patients with head or neck cancers or patients at risk for thrombosis is controversial as these medications increase tumor growth and risk for thrombosis. The most frequent adverse effects include hypertension, fever, headache, pruritus, rash, nausea, vomiting, arthralgia, and injection site reaction.

In 2010, the U.S. Food and Drug Administration (FDA) issued a public health advisory regarding the overzealous use of epoetin. It was found that when hemoglobin levels are above 12 g/dL and the drug is continued, patients experienced serious adverse events, including heart attack, stroke, and death. Based on these findings, the FDA now requires that any patient receiving epoetin for chemotherapy-induced anemia must be registered in a risk mitigation program called ESA Apprise Oncology. Only physicians and hospitals that are registered in this program may dispense epoetin for cancer patients. The FDA has not yet required the same for its use in chronic kidney disease; however, it is not to be given to renal patients unless their hemoglobin level is less than 12 g/dL. More information can be found at www.esa-apprise.com/ESAAppriseUI/ESAAppriseUI/default.jsp. Abuse of erythropoietin by athletes hoping to increase oxygen-carrying capacity and improve performance places the athlete at risk for diseases caused by increased blood viscosity (stroke, myocardial infarction).

### Pharmacokinetics

| Route | Onset of Action | Peak Plasma Concentration | Elimination Half-life | Duration of Action |
|---|---|---|---|---|
| Subcut or IV | 7-10 days | 5-24 hr | 4-13 hr | Variable |

## IRON

Iron is a mineral that is essential for the proper function of all biologic systems in the body. It is stored in many sites throughout the body (liver, spleen, and bone marrow). Deficiency of this mineral is the principal nutritional deficiency resulting in anemia. Individuals who require the highest amount of iron are

| TABLE 54-1 | FERROUS SALTS: IRON CONTENT | |
|---|---|---|
| **FERROUS SALT\*** | **IRON CONTENT** | **NUMBER OF TABLETS TAKEN PER DAY (ADULTS)** |
| Ferrous fumarate | 33% iron or 330 mg/g | 6-8 of 100-mg tablets or 2-3 of 325-mg tablets |
| Ferric gluconate | 12% iron or 120 mg/g | 3-4 |
| Ferrous sulfate | 20% iron or 200 mg/g | 3-4 |
| Ferrous sulfate (desiccated or dried) | 30% iron or 300 mg/g | 3-4 |

\*Some patients may tolerate different formulations better; however, the number of tablets that must be consumed may decrease patient adherence.

| TABLE 54-2 | IRON PREPARATIONS: ADVERSE EFFECTS |
|---|---|
| **BODY SYSTEM** | **ADVERSE EFFECTS** |
| Gastrointestinal | Nausea, constipation, epigastric pain, black and tarry stools, vomiting, diarrhea |
| Integumentary | Temporarily discolored tooth enamel and eyes, pain on injection |

women (especially pregnant women) and children, and they are the groups most likely to develop iron-deficiency anemia. For women, this is partly due to ongoing menstrual blood losses. Most vitamin supplements for men contain little or no iron, because men are much less likely to develop iron-deficiency anemia. Nonetheless, dietary iron is usually sufficient for both men and women in developed countries.

Dietary sources of iron include meats and certain vegetables and grains. These forms of iron must be broken down by gastric juices before the iron can be absorbed. Other foods such as orange juice, veal, fish, and ascorbic acid may help with iron absorption. Conversely, eggs, corn, beans, and many cereal products containing chemicals known as *phytates* may impair iron absorption. Beans and eggs are common dietary sources of iron. Oral iron preparations are available as ferrous salts. See Table 54-1 for a list of the currently available oral iron salts and their respective iron content. When a patient cannot tolerate oral iron, intravenous iron may be administered. There are four injectable iron products available: iron dextran (INFeD), iron sucrose (Venofer), ferric gluconate (Ferrlecit, Nulecit), and ferumoxytol (Feraheme).

## Mechanism of Action and Drug Effects

Iron is an oxygen carrier in both hemoglobin and *myoglobin* (oxygen-carrying molecule in muscle tissue) and is critical for tissue respiration. Iron is also a required component of a number of enzyme systems in the body and is necessary for energy transfer in the *cytochrome oxidase* and *xanthine oxidase* enzyme systems. Administration of iron corrects iron-deficiency symptoms such as anemia, dysphagia, dystrophy of the nails and skin, and fissuring of the angles of the lips, and also maintains the bodily functions described earlier.

## Indications

Supplemental iron contained in multivitamins plus iron or iron supplements alone are indicated for the prevention or treatment of iron-deficiency anemia. In all cases, an underlying cause needs to be identified. After identification of the cause, treatment is aimed at attempting to correct the cause (e.g., chronic blood loss, such as from a peptic or duodenal ulcer, cancerous colon lesion, or Crohn's disease) rather than simply alleviating the symptoms. Iron supplementation is also used in erythropoietin therapy because it is essential for the production of RBCs.

## Contraindications

Contraindications to the use of iron products include known drug allergy, *hemochromatosis* (iron overload), hemolytic anemia, and any other anemia not associated with iron deficiency.

## Adverse Effects

The most common adverse effects associated with oral iron preparations are nausea, vomiting, diarrhea, constipation, stomach cramps, and stomach pain. Excess iron intake can lead to accumulation and iron toxicity. See Table 54-2 for a more complete listing of the undesirable effects associated with iron preparations. Elderly patients tend to respond to lower doses of iron supplementation, and lower doses tend to decrease the rate of adverse effects.

### Toxicity and Management of Overdose

Iron overdose is the most common cause of pediatric poisoning deaths reported to U.S. poison control centers. Many iron supplements are enteric coated and resemble candy. Toxicity from iron ingestion results from a combination of the corrosive effects on the gastrointestinal mucosa and the metabolic and hemodynamic effects caused by the presence of excessive elemental iron.

Treatment is based on symptomatic and supportive measures, including suction and maintenance of the airway, correction of acidosis, and control of shock and dehydration with intravenous fluids or blood, oxygen, and vasopressors. Abdominal radiographs may be helpful, because iron preparations are radiopaque and may be visualized on x-ray film. Serum iron concentrations may be helpful in establishing the amount ingested. A serum iron concentration of more than 300 mcg/dL places the patient at serious risk for toxicity. The GI tract is decontaminated via whole bowel irrigation. In patients with severe symptoms of iron intoxication, such as coma, shock, or seizures, chelation therapy with deferoxamine is initiated. In 2011, the FDA approved deferiprone, which can also be used in iron overload.

## Interactions

The absorption of iron can be enhanced when it is given with ascorbic acid and decreased when it is given with antacids and calcium. Iron preparations can decrease the absorption of certain antibiotics, including tetracyclines and quinolones.

## DOSAGES

### Selected Anemia Drugs

| DRUG (PREGNANCY CATEGORY) | PHARMACOLOGIC CLASS | USUAL DOSAGE RANGE | INDICATIONS/USES |
|---|---|---|---|
| ♦ epoetin alfa (Epogen, Procrit) (C) | Human recombinant hormone (erythropoietin) analogue | IV/subcut: 2000-40,000 units 1-3 times per week, depending on weight and indication | Chemotherapy-induced anemia; anemia associated with chronic renal failure |
| ferric gluconate (Ferrlecit) (B) | Parenteral iron salt | **Pediatric\* older than 6 yr** 1.5 mg/kg/dose for 8 doses **Adult** 125 mg/dose for 8 doses | Iron deficiency associated with hemo-dialysis |
| ferrous fumarate (Feostat) (A) | Oral iron salt | **Pediatric\*** 4-6 mg/kg/day 3 mg/kg/day 1-2 mg/kg/day **Adult\*** 100-200 mg given 1-3 times daily | Severe iron-deficiency anemia Mild to moderate iron-deficiency anemia Prophylaxis Prophylaxis |
| ♦ ferrous sulfate (A) | Oral iron salt | **Pediatric\*** 4-6 mg/kg/day in 3 divided doses **Adult\*** 300 mg 2 × daily, up to 300 mg 4 × daily | Iron deficiency |
| ♦ folic acid (A) | Water-soluble B-complex vitamin | **Pediatric†** PO/IV/IM/subcut: 0.1-0.4 mg/day **Adult†** PO/IV/IM/subcut: Up to 1 mg/day | Folate deficiency; tropical sprue; nutri-tional supplementation; pregnancy-related supplementation |
| iron dextran (INFeD, Dexferrum) (C) | Parenteral iron salt | **Pediatric†** IM/IV: 5-10 kg: 25 mg/day (0.5 mL/day); greater than 10 kg: 50 mg/day (1 mL/day) **Adult†** IM/IV: 100 mg/day (2 mL/day) | Iron deficiency when oral iron therapy is unsatisfactory |
| iron sucrose (Venofer) (B) | Parenteral iron salt | IV: 100 mg 1-3 times weekly to a cumulative dose of 1000 mg; may give up to 500 mg as single dose on days 1 and 14 | Iron deficiency in patients with chronic renal failure |

*IM*, Intramuscular; *IV*, intravenous; *PO*, oral; *subcut*, subcutaneous.
\*Doses are expressed in terms of elemental iron, not the salt itself.
†Expressed in milligrams of elemental iron. Dosages are calculated for each patient's weight according to manufacturer's label. Doses are approximate.

## Dosages

For dosage information on iron preparations, see the table on this page.

## DRUG PROFILES

Iron preparations are available by prescription and as over-the-counter (OTC) medications. They are contraindicated in patients with ulcerative colitis and regional enteritis, conditions of excessive body iron stores (e.g., hemosiderosis, hemochromatosis), peptic ulcer disease, hemolytic anemia, cirrhosis, gastritis, and esophagitis. Goals of therapy include maintenance of normal hemoglobin and hematocrit levels, and improved energy level.

### ferrous fumarate

The ferrous fumarate iron salts (Femiron) contain the largest amount of iron per gram of salt consumed. Ferrous sulfate and ferric gluconate are two other forms of iron that are commonly used. Ferrous fumarate is 33% elemental iron; therefore, a 325-mg tablet of ferrous fumarate provides 107 mg of elemental iron. Ferrous fumarate is available only for oral use.

### Pharmacokinetics

| Route | Onset of Action | Peak Plasma Concentration | Elimination Half-life | Duration of Action |
|---|---|---|---|---|
| PO | 3-10 days | Unknown | 6 hr | Variable |

### ♦ ferrous sulfate

Ferrous sulfate is the most frequently used form of oral iron. Ferrous sulfate ($FeSO_4$) is dosed as 300 mg two to three times a day for most adult patients. Confusion arises with ferrous sulfate, because the dose is 300 mg, but many commercially available products are 324 mg. The two doses are used interchangeably. To add to the confusion, each 324-mg tablet contains 65 mg of elemental iron. The adult dose of elemental iron is 50 to 100 mg given two to three times daily. Pediatric dosing is based on elemental iron.

### Pharmacokinetics

| Route | Onset of Action | Peak Plasma Concentration | Elimination Half-life | Duration of Action |
|---|---|---|---|---|
| PO | 1 wk | 2 hr | 6 hr | Variable |

### iron dextran

Iron dextran (INFeD, Dexferrum) is a colloidal solution of iron (as ferric hydroxide) and dextran. It is intended for intravenous or intramuscular use for treatment of iron deficiency. Anaphylactic reactions to iron dextran, including major orthostatic hypotension and fatal anaphylaxis, have been reported in 0.3% of patients. Because of this, a test dose of 25 mg of iron dextran is administered before injection of the full dose. Although anaphylactic reactions usually occur within a few moments after the test dose, it is recommended that a period of at least 1 hour elapse before the remaining portion of the initial dose is given. Because of the potential of iron dextran to cause anaphylaxis, its use has been replaced by use of the newer products, ferric gluconate and iron sucrose. Iron dextran is available only for injection.

#### Pharmacokinetics

| Route | Onset of Action | Peak Plasma Concentration | Elimination Half-life | Duration of Action |
|-------|-----------------|---------------------------|-----------------------|---------------------|
| IM | Unknown | 24-48 hr | 5-20 hr | 3 wk |

### ferric gluconate

Ferric gluconate (Ferrlecit) is an injectable iron product that is indicated for repletion of total body iron content in patients with iron-deficiency anemia who are undergoing hemodialysis. The risk of anaphylaxis is much less than with iron dextran, and a test dose is not required. Doses higher than 125 mg are associated with increased adverse events, including abdominal pain, dyspnea, cramps, and itching.

#### Pharmacokinetics

| Route | Onset of Action | Peak Plasma Concentration | Elimination Half-life | Duration of Action |
|-------|-----------------|---------------------------|-----------------------|---------------------|
| IV | End of infusion | 7 min | 1 hr | 4 days |

### iron sucrose

Iron sucrose (Venofer) is another injectable iron product indicated for the treatment of iron-deficiency anemia in patients with chronic renal disease. It is also used for patients without kidney disease. Its risk of precipitating anaphylaxis is much less than that of iron dextran, and a test dose is not required. Hypotension is the most common adverse effect and appears to be related to infusion rate. Large doses of iron sucrose are infused over 2.5 to 3.5 hours. Low-weight elderly patients appear to be at greatest risk of hypotension. The newest injectable iron product is ferumoxytol (Feraheme). It offers the advantage of being given undiluted as IV push in 1 minute.

#### Pharmacokinetics

| Route | Onset of Action | Peak Plasma Concentration | Elimination Half-life | Duration of Action |
|-------|-----------------|---------------------------|-----------------------|---------------------|
| IV | End of infusion | Unknown | 6 hr | Unknown |

## FOLIC ACID

Folic acid is a water-soluble B-complex vitamin. It is also referred to as *folate,* the name of its anionic form. The human body requires oral intake of folic acid. Dietary sources of folic acid include dried beans, peas, oranges, and green vegetables. Several conditions can lead to folic acid deficiency. However, because folic acid is absorbed in the upper duodenum, malabsorption syndromes are the most common cause of deficiency.

### Mechanism of Action and Drug Effects

Folic acid is converted in the body to *tetrahydrofolic acid,* which is used for erythropoiesis and for synthesis of nucleic acids (DNA and ribonucleic acid [RNA]). Dietary ingestion of folate is required for the production of DNA and RNA. It is also essential for normal erythropoiesis. Folic acid is not active in the ingested form. It must first be converted to tetrahydrofolic acid, which is a cofactor for reactions in the biosynthesis of nucleic acids.

### Indications

Folic acid is primarily used to prevent and treat folic acid deficiency. Anemias caused by folic acid deficiency can be treated by exogenous supplementation of folic acid. There is also much evidence to support the use of folic acid in the prevention of neural tube defects such as spina bifida, anencephaly, and encephalocele. It is recommended that administration begin at least 1 month before pregnancy and continue through early pregnancy to reduce the risk for fetal neural tube defects. Folic acid is also indicated for the treatment of tropical sprue, a malabsorption syndrome.

### Contraindications

Contraindications to the use of folic acid include known allergy to a specific drug product and any anemia not related to folic acid deficiency (e.g., pernicious anemia). Folic acid is not to be used to treat anemias until the underlying cause and type of anemia have been determined. For example, administering folic acid to a patient with pernicious anemia may correct the hematologic changes of anemia (making the CBC normal), while deceptively masking neurologic and other symptoms of pernicious anemia that result from $B_{12}$ deficiency.

### Adverse Effects

Adverse effects associated with folic acid use are rare. Allergic reaction or yellow discoloration of urine may occur.

### Interactions

No significant drug interactions occur with folic acid. However, oral contraceptives (see Chapter 34), corticosteroids (see Chapter 33), sulfonamides (see Chapter 38), and dihydrofolate reductase inhibitors (including the antineoplastic drug methotrexate [see Chapter 45] and the antibiotic trimethoprim [see Chapter 38]) can all cause signs of folic acid deficiency, but are not affected by folic acid administration.

### Dosages

For dosage information on folic acid, see the table on p. 882.

## DRUG PROFILE

### ♦ folic acid

Folic acid is a water-soluble B-complex vitamin that is used primarily in the treatment and prevention of folic acid deficiency and anemias caused by folic acid deficiency. Folic acid is available as an OTC medication in multivitamin preparations and by prescription as a single drug. It is contraindicated in patients with anemias other than megaloblastic or macrocytic anemia. The conditions representing contraindications include vitamin $B_{12}$ deficiency anemia and uncorrected pernicious anemia. Folic acid is available for both oral and injectable use.

### Pharmacokinetics

| Route | Onset of Action | Peak Plasma Concentration | Elimination Half-life | Duration of Action |
|-------|-----------------|---------------------------|-----------------------|--------------------|
| PO | Unknown | 60-90 min | Unknown | Unknown |

## OTHER ANEMIA DRUGS

Cyanocobalamin (vitamin $B_{12}$), which is discussed in Chapter 53, is used to treat pernicious anemia and other megaloblastic anemias. It can be given orally or intranasally to treat vitamin $B_{12}$ deficiency but is usually given by deep intramuscular injection to treat pernicious anemia. Once remission of the anemia is seen, cyanocobalamin can be dosed once a month.

## NURSING PROCESS

## ASSESSMENT

Before any drug is given to treat an anemia, assess the patient's past and present medical history; compile a medication

### TEAMWORK AND COLLABORATION: PHARMACOKINETIC BRIDGE TO NURSING PRACTICE

Iron preparations provide a perfect example of how pharmacokinetic properties can impact drug dosing and efficacy. Oral iron is available in a variety of salt forms, such as ferrous fumarate, ferrous sulfate, and ferric gluconate. Although very similar in mechanism of action, the specific salt form is associated with different pharmacokinetics and offers varying amounts of elemental iron. The ferrous fumarate iron salts contain some of the largest amount of iron per gram of salt consumed. For example, each 100 mg of ferrous fumarate provides 33 mg of elemental iron, whereas each 324-mg tablet of ferrous sulfate contains 65 mg of elemental iron. Even though the pharmacokinetics of the different oral iron salts are similar, the amount of elemental iron varies significantly per 100 mg. Because of these varying amounts of elemental iron, the iron salts must not be exchanged for one another and must be given with caution to avoid medication errors. Other similar pharmacokinetic properties of oral iron products, such as absorption and excretion, must be understood because unabsorbed iron—though harmless—turns the stool black and may possibly mask melena (blood in the stools). It is recommended to take oral iron with juice (orange juice is preferred) or water but not with milk or antacids because of subsequent decreased drug absorption.

profile, including all prescription, OTC, and herbal medications the patient is taking; and also assess for drug allergies. It is important to assess for and document any signs and symptoms of anemia, such as fatigue, changes in nails and skin, and fissuring/cracking of the angles of the lip. It is also necessary to assess the patient for contraindications, cautions, and drug interactions prior to beginning treatment with any of these medications. *Erythropoiesis-stimulating agents* (epoetin alfa and darbepoetin) are used to treat anemia associated with end-stage renal disease and/or chemotherapy-induced anemia. Assessment of adequate body iron stores and bone marrow function is needed prior to administration of the drug. Document baseline vital signs because blood pressure may elevate as hematocrit rises; medical intervention may be needed. Assess for allergies to these drugs as well as for other contraindications, such as uncontrolled hypertension and hemoglobin levels of greater than 10g/dL for cancer patients and greater than 12g/dL for renal patients. Discussion of the 2010 FDA requirements and use of epoetin in those with chemotherapy-induced anemia is further clarified in the pharmacology section.

With *iron products*, significant contraindications include hemochromatosis, hemolytic anemia, and any other anemia that is not iron-deficiency related. Drug interactions affecting the absorption of iron preparations include ascorbic acid (increased absorption), antacids (decreased absorption), as well as decreased absorption of other drugs such as tetracyclines and quinolones. Some laboratory studies that may be ordered before, during, and after therapy include RBC count, hemoglobin level, hematocrit, reticulocyte count, bilirubin level, and baseline levels of folate and/or B-complex vitamins. Perform a nutritional assessment with a focus on the amount of iron in the patient's diet. A 24-hour recall of all food intake with serving sizes may prove to be beneficial. A nutritional and dietary consult may also be ordered. In addition, asking questions about the patient's energy levels, ability to carry out activities of daily living, overall immunity to illnesses, and state of health may also provide valuable information.

## NURSING DIAGNOSES

1. Activity intolerance related to fatigue and lethargy associated with anemias
2. Imbalanced nutrition, less than body requirements, related to the disease process
3. Constipation related to adverse effects of iron products

## PLANNING

### GOALS

1. Patient maintains/regains normal level of activity, as ordered.
2. Patient attains adequate nutrition status through use of non-pharmacologic and/or pharmacologic measures.
3. Patient remains free from or experiences minimal constipation as an adverse effect of iron products.

## CASE STUDY

### *Hematopoietic Biologic Response Modifiers*

J.T., a 37-year-old homemaker, is receiving a second round of chemotherapy as part of treatment for ovarian cancer. Chemotherapeutic drugs may lead to the adverse effect of bone marrow suppression of various blood cell components.

Two weeks after this round of chemotherapy, J.T.'s hemoglobin level is 7.9 g/dL (pretherapy value was 11 g/dL), and the hematocrit is 28.5% (pretherapy value was 34%). The following orders are received: epoetin alfa (Epogen) 150 units/kg subcutaneously three times a week; ferrous sulfate, 300 mg by mouth daily.

1. What is the purpose of the order for ferrous sulfate?
2. The nurse will assess for what conditions before beginning the epoetin therapy?
3. The nurse needs to monitor J.T. closely. What assessment findings would be of the most concern during this therapy?
4. After 5 weeks, J.T.'s hemoglobin level is 11.4 g/dL and her hematocrit is 33%. The next dose of epoetin is due today. What action will the nurse take?

For answers, see http://evolve.elsevier.com/Lilley.

### ▌OUTCOME CRITERIA

1. Patient is able to tolerate a gradual increase in activity as ordered (e.g., performing activities of daily living, walking 10 minutes a day with increases as tolerated) while on drug therapy for anemia.
   - Patient reports improved energy levels and less shortness of breath and/or activity intolerance during drug therapy.
2. Patient improves dietary intake as recommended with use of MyPlate (www.choosemyplate.gov/index.html) with recommended amounts of fruits/vegetables, grains/starches, and meat/proteins.
   - Patient increases daily intake of iron such as green leafy vegetables, eggs, and beans.
3. Patient implements measures to minimize constipation, such as dietary intake of increased roughage, fiber, fruits, and vegetables and increase in fluids.
   - Patient reports unresolved constipation to prescriber once above measures have been implemented.
   - Patient takes medication, as prescribed, for management of constipation such as bulk-forming laxatives.

### ▌IMPLEMENTATION

With *erythropoiesis-stimulating agents,* do not administer with any other product and do not shake the vial. During treatment, always monitor blood pressure and give vitamin $B_{12}$ supplements orally as prescribed. Instruct the patient to dilute oral liquid dosage forms of *iron products* per manufacturer instructions and to sip through a plastic straw to avoid discoloration of tooth enamel. Other oral forms of iron need to be given with plenty of fluids but not with antacids or milk, and preferably not with meals, because of the risk for decreased absorption of the drug. However, most individuals find that they do need to take oral iron products with

## PATIENT-CENTERED CARE: LIFESPAN CONSIDERATIONS FOR THE ELDERLY PATIENT

### *Iron Products*

- Instructions on how to take oral forms of iron are crucial to safe administration. Implement all types of teaching strategies to reinforce all verbal and/or written instructions. Make sure education is individualized and geared to patients with alterations in sensory perception. Caution patients not to make changes in their medication regimen, such as doubling doses or discontinuing a drug, without the prescriber's order.
- Provide elderly patients and their spouses and/or caregivers with instructions about food sources that are high in iron and how to include these foods in their menu planning. Instruct patients to steam vegetables and not to overcook them through excessive boiling. Advise patients that to preserve the content of vitamins and minerals, including iron, it is important to avoid overcooking or boiling vegetables.
- Remind elderly patients that gastrointestinal upset may occur with many drugs, including vitamins and iron. Iron products are to be taken with food or a snack to help decrease GI upset.
- Always educate elderly patients, as well as their spouses, other family members or significant others, and/or caregivers, about appropriate community resources (e.g., Meals on Wheels, senior citizen community centers, public recreation centers). A list of these community resources is often made available through a city web page, social services department, and other outlets.

meals or food because of the commonly encountered adverse effect of gastrointestinal upset. If antacids or milk products are used, schedule them at least 1 to 2 hours before or after the oral dosage of iron. Iron products are generally packaged in a light-resistant, airtight container. Instruct patients to remain in an upright or sitting position for up to 30 minutes after taking oral dosage forms of iron, ferrous products, and related drugs to help minimize esophageal irritation or corrosion. Warn patients that the use of iron products will turn the stools from brown to a black, tarry color. Patients taking epoetin alfa may also be taking oral iron preparations (see the pharmacology discussion for specific information on FDA restrictions). See the Patient Teaching Tips for more information.

If a patient cannot tolerate oral iron, intravenous iron (e.g., iron dextran, iron sucrose, or ferric gluconate) may be prescribed. A test dose of iron dextran may be ordered, with the remaining dose given an hour later if no adverse reaction occurs. Intramuscularly administered iron must be given deep in a large muscle mass using the Z-track method (see Chapter 9). Intravenous iron dextran must be given after the intravenous line is flushed with 10 mL of normal saline and administered with the recommended amount of diluent and at the recommended drip rate. Keep epinephrine and resuscitative equipment available in case of anaphylactic reaction (to iron or any drug that has an increased risk of causing anaphylaxis). In addition, it may be necessary for the patient to remain recumbent for 30 minutes after the intravenous injection to prevent drug-induced orthostatic hypotension. Encourage the patient to move slowly and purposefully during this time.

## EVALUATION

Focus the evaluation of therapeutic responses to drugs used for anemia on ensuring that goals and outcome criteria have been met as well as monitoring for therapeutic and adverse effects. Therapeutic responses to *erythropoiesis-stimulating agents* may take 2 to 6 weeks, so monitor for increased energy, appetite, and sense of well-being. Adverse effects of *erythropoiesis stimulating agents* may include heart attack, stroke and possible death if used in patients with Hgb > 12g/dl. Therapeutic responses to *iron products* include improved nutritional status, increased weight, increased activity tolerance and well-being, and absence of fatigue. Adverse effects of *iron products* include nausea, constipation, epigastric pain, black and tarry stools, and vomiting. Signs of toxicity include nausea, diarrhea, hematemesis, pallor, cyanosis, shock, and coma.

## PATIENT TEACHING TIPS

- Epoetin alfa (Epogen) is indicated for anemias associated with end-stage renal disease and chemotherapy and requires very careful use. Always check for route of administration with the subcutaneous route having a slower onset of action as compared to the intravenous route.
- Educate the patient about taking oral iron supplements with the erythropoeisis-stimulating agents. These supplements are often needed to ensure adequate body iron stores, which are needed for the drug therapy to be effective.
- Encourage the patient to take iron products cautiously and to be aware of the potential for poisoning if these drugs are taken in greater than the recommended amounts. Oral iron products need to be taken in their original dosage form and without alteration; for example, without crushing.

- It is recommended that oral dosage forms of iron be taken with at least 4 to 6 oz of water or other fluid to help minimize gastrointestinal upset and increase absorption.
- Oral dosage forms of iron are not interchangeable, and prescription forms of these products may be very different from one another. Each product contains different forms of the iron salt and also comes in different dose amounts. (One exception is that the 300-mg and 324-mg dosage forms of ferrous sulfate are used interchangeably.)
- Instruct the patient to remain upright for up to 30 minutes after taking an oral iron product to prevent esophageal irritation or corrosion. Remind the patient that iron products may turn the stools a black, tarry color.
- Encourage the patient to maintain a diet high in iron including foods such as meat; dark green, leafy vegetables; dried beans; dried fruits; and eggs.

## KEY POINTS

- Erythropoiesis-stimulating agents are ineffective without adequate body iron stores.
- Iron and folic acid are very important in the treatment of many disorders and diseases (e.g., malignancies) to achieve RBC and hemoglobin formation that is as adequate as possible and to help prevent nutritional deficits that can affect all body systems, especially the immune system.

- Blood-forming drugs are often used in the treatment of pernicious anemia, malabsorption syndromes, hemolytic anemias, hemorrhage, and renal and liver diseases.
- Instruct patients to take iron products exactly as ordered. Parenteral dosage forms may cause anaphylaxis and orthostatic hypotension.

## NCLEX® EXAMINATION REVIEW QUESTIONS

1 When administering oral iron tablets, the nurse should keep in mind that the most appropriate substance, other than water, to give with these tablets is
  a pudding.
  b an antacid.
  c milk.
  d orange juice.

2 The nurse is teaching a patient about oral iron supplements. Which statement is correct?
  a "You need to take this medication on an empty stomach or else it won't be absorbed."
  b "It is better absorbed on an empty stomach, but if that causes your stomach to be upset, you can take it with food."
  c "Take this medication with a sip of water, and then lie down to avoid problems with low blood pressure."
  d "If you have trouble swallowing the tablet, you may crush it."

# NCLEX® EXAMINATION REVIEW QUESTIONS

3 The nurse is administering an intravenous dose of iron dextran. For which potential adverse effect is it most important for the nurse to monitor at this time?
  a Anaphylaxis
  b Gastrointestinal distress
  c Black, tarry stools
  d Bradycardia

4 The nurse is assessing a patient who is to receive folic acid supplements. It is important to rule out which condition before giving the folic acid?
  a Malabsorption syndromes
  b Pernicious anemia
  c Tropical sprue
  d Pregnancy

5 A patient with renal failure has severe anemia, and there is an order for darbepoetin (Aranesp). As the nurse assesses the patient, which condition listed will the nurse consider a contraindication to use of this medication?
  a Uncontrolled hypertension
  b Diabetes mellitus
  c Hypothyroidism
  d Angina

6 When iron sucrose is administered, which nursing interventions are correct? (Select all that apply.)
  a Administer a test dose before giving the full dose.
  b Give via deep intramuscular injection into a large muscle mass using the Z-track method.
  c Administer large doses over 2.5 to 3.5 hours, intravenously.
  d Monitor the patient for hypertension.
  e Monitor the patient for hypotension.

7 The order reads: "Give epoetin alfa (Epogen), 3500 units subcut, three times a week." The medication is available in a vial that contains 4000 units/mL. How many milliliters will the nurse draw up for the ordered dose? Round to hundredths.

1. d, 2. b, 3. a, 4. b, 5. a, 6. c, e, 7. 0.88 mL (rounded from 0.875)

For Critical Thinking and Prioritization Questions, see http://evolve.elsevier.com/Lilley.

## OBJECTIVES

When you reach the end of this chapter, you will be able to do the following:

1. Describe the various pathophysiologic processes and/or disease states that may lead to nutritional deficiencies and require nutritional supplemental support.
2. Discuss the various enteral and parenteral nutritional supplements used to treat the various deficiencies, including specific ingredients.
3. Describe the nurse's role in the process of initiating and maintaining continuous or intermittent enteral feedings, total parenteral nutrition, and other forms of nutritional supplementation.
4. Compare the various enteral feeding tubes, including specific uses, and detail the special needs of patients requiring this nutritional support.

5. Discuss the mechanisms of action, cautions, contraindications, routes of administration, drug interactions, adverse effects, and complications associated with enteral and parenteral nutritional supplementation.
6. Develop a nursing care plan that includes all phases of the nursing process for patients receiving enteral and parenteral supplemental feedings.
7. Discuss the various laboratory values related to nutritional deficits or altered nutritional status and their impact on monitoring the therapeutic effects of the therapy.

## DRUG PROFILES

amino acids, p. 894
carbohydrate formulation, p. 892
carbohydrates, p. 894

fat formulation, p. 892
lipid emulsions, p. 895
protein formulation, p. 892

## KEY TERMS

**Anabolism**  Metabolism characterized by the conversion of simple substances into the more complex compounds; tissue building. (p. 889)

**Casein**  The principal protein of milk and the basis for curd and cheese. (p. 892)

**Catabolism**  A complex metabolic process in which energy is liberated for use in work, energy storage, or heat production by the destruction of complex substances to form simple compounds. (p. 894)

**Dumping syndrome**  A complex reaction to the rapid entry of concentrated nutrients into the jejunum of the small intestine. The patient may experience nausea, weakness, sweating, palpitations, syncope, sensations of warmth, and diarrhea. Most commonly occurs with eating following partial gastrectomy or with enteral feedings that are administered too rapidly into the stomach or jejunum via a feeding tube. (p. 891)

**Enteral nutrition**  The provision of food or nutrients via the gastrointestinal tract, either naturally by eating or through a feeding tube in patients who are unable to eat. (p. 889)

**Essential amino acids**  Those amino acids that cannot be manufactured by the body. (p. 894)

**Essential fatty acid deficiency**  A condition that develops if fatty acids that the body cannot produce are not present in dietary or nutritional supplements. (p. 894)

**Hyperalimentation**  An older term for parenteral nutrition; its use is now discouraged because it may be misinterpreted to mean overfeeding; now referred to as *total parenteral nutrition (TPN)*. (p. 892)

**Malnutrition**  Any disorder of undernutrition. (p. 889)

**Multivitamin infusion (MVI)**  A concentrated solution that contains several water- and fat-soluble vitamins and is used as part of an intravenous (parenteral) nutrition source. (p. 895)

**Nonessential amino acids**  Those amino acids that the body can produce without extracting them from dietary intake. (p. 894)

**Nutrients**  Substances that provide nourishment and affect the nutritive and metabolic processes of the body. (p. 889)

**Nutritional supplements**  Oral, enteral, or intravenous nutritional preparations used to provide optimal nutrients to meet the body's nutritional needs. (p. 889)

**Nutritional support**  The provision of nutrients orally, enterally, or parenterally for therapeutic reasons. (p. 889)

**Parenteral nutrition**  The administration of nutrients by a route other than through the alimentary canal, such as intravenously. (p. 889)

**Semiessential amino acids**  Those amino acids that can be produced by the body but not in sufficient amounts in infants and children. (p. 894)

**Total parenteral nutrition (TPN)**  The intravenous administration of the total nutrient requirements of the patient with gastrointestinal dysfunction, accomplished via peripheral or central venous catheter. (p. 892)

**Whey**  The thin serum of milk remaining after the casein and fat have been removed. It contains proteins, lactose, water-soluble vitamins, and minerals. (p. 892)

## ANATOMY, PHYSIOLOGY, AND PATHOPHYSIOLOGY OVERVIEW

**Nutrients** are dietary products that undergo chemical changes when ingested (and metabolized) that cause tissue to be enhanced and energy to be liberated. Nutrients are required for cell growth and division; enzyme activity; protein, carbohydrate, and fat synthesis; muscle contraction; secretion of hormones (e.g., vasopressin, gastrin); wound repair; immune competence; gut integrity; and numerous other essential cellular functions. Providing for these nutritional needs is known as **nutritional support.** Adequate nutritional support is needed to prevent the breakdown of tissue proteins for use as an energy supply to sustain essential organ systems, which is what occurs during starvation. Malnutrition can decrease organ size and impair the function of organ systems (e.g., cardiac, respiratory, gastrointestinal, hepatic, renal). Nutritional supplements are a means of providing adequate nutritional support to meet the body's nutritional needs.

**Malnutrition** is a condition in which the body's essential need for nutrients is not met by nutrient intake. The purpose of nutritional support is the successful prevention, recognition, and management of malnutrition. **Nutritional supplements** are dietary products used to provide nutritional support. Nutritional supplement products can be administered to patients in a variety of ways. They vary in the amount and chemical complexity of the carbohydrates, proteins, fats, electrolytes, vitamins, and minerals that compose them, as well as in their osmolality. These nutrients may be given in a digested form, a partially digested form, or an undigested form. Nutritional supplements can also be tailored for specific disease states.

Patients' nutrient requirements vary according to age, gender, size or weight, physical activity, preexisting medical conditions, nutritional status, and current medical or surgical treatment. Nutritional supplements are classified according to the method of administration as either enteral or parenteral. **Enteral nutrition** is the provision of food or nutrients via the gastrointestinal tract. Nutritional supplements may also be administered parenterally. **Parenteral nutrition** is the intravenous administration of nutrients. Its purpose is to promote **anabolism** (tissue building), nitrogen balance, and maintenance or improvement of body weight. It is used when the oral or enteral feeding routes cannot be used (e.g., in postoperative patients or patients who are cachectic from advanced cancer or acquired immunodeficiency syndrome [AIDS]). The selection of either enteral nutrition or parenteral nutrition and the specific nutritional composition of the product used depend on the specific patient and the clinical situation. Enteral nutrition is used when the patient has a functioning gastrointestinal tract.

## PHARMACOLOGY OVERVIEW

### ENTERAL NUTRITION

Enteral nutrition is the provision of food or nutrients through the gastrointestinal tract. The most common and least invasive route of administration is oral consumption. A feeding tube is used in the other five enteral routes (Figure 55-1). The six routes of enteral nutrition delivery are listed in Table 55-1.

Patients who may benefit from feeding tube delivery of nutritional supplements include those with abnormal esophageal or stomach peristalsis, altered anatomy secondary to surgery, depressed consciousness, or impaired digestive capacity. The enteral route is considered to be the superior route of administration of nutritional supplements.

Approximately 100 different enteral supplement formulations are available. The enteral supplements have been divided into groups according to the basic characteristics of the individual formulations. The enteral formulation groups are elemental, polymeric, modular, altered amino acid, and impaired glucose tolerance. These are described in Box 55-1.

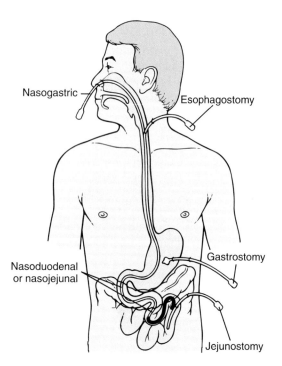

**FIGURE 55-1** Tube feeding routes. (From Lewis SM et al: *Medical-surgical nursing: assessment and management of clinical problems,* ed 8, St Louis, 2011, Mosby.)

| TABLE 55-1 | ROUTES OF ENTERAL NUTRITION DELIVERY |
|---|---|
| **ROUTE** | **DESCRIPTION** |
| Esophagostomy | Feeding tube surgically inserted into the esophagus |
| Gastrostomy | Feeding tube surgically inserted directly into the stomach |
| Jejunostomy | Feeding tube surgically inserted into the jejunum |
| Nasoduodenal | Feeding tube placed from the nose to the duodenum |
| Nasojejunal | Feeding tube placed from the nose to the jejunum |
| Nasogastric | Feeding tube placed from the nose to the stomach |
| Oral | Nutritional supplements delivered by mouth |

### BOX 55-1    ENTERAL FORMULATIONS

**Elemental Formulations**

Peptamen
Vital HN
Vivonex Plus
Vivonex TEN

**Contents:** dipeptides, tripeptides, or crystalline amino acids; glucose oligosaccharides; and vegetable oil or medium-chain triglycerides (MCTs)

**Comments:** minimal digestion; minimal residue

**Indications:** malabsorption, partial bowel obstruction, irritable bowel disease, radiation enteritis, bowel fistula, short bowel syndrome

**Polymeric Formulations**

Complete
Ensure
Ensure Plus
Isocal
Osmolite
Portagen
Jevity
Sustacal

**Contents:** complex nutrients (proteins, carbohydrates, and fat)

**Indications:** preferred over elemental formulations for patients with fully functional gastrointestinal tracts and few specialized nutrient requirements

**Modular Formulations**

*Carbohydrate*
Moducal
Polycose

**Contents:** single-nutrient formulas (protein, carbohydrate, or fat)

**Indications:** can be added to a monomeric or polymeric formulation to provide a more individualized nutrient formulation

*Fat*
MCT Oil
Microlipid

*Protein*
Casec
ProMod
Propac
Stresstein

**Altered Amino Acid Formulations**

Amin-Aid
Hepatic-Aid
Travasorb Renal
Traum-Aid HBC

**Contents:** varying amounts of specific amino acids

**Indications:** for use in patients with diseases associated with altered metabolic capacities

**Formulation for Impaired Glucose Tolerance**

Glucerna

**Contents:** protein, carbohydrate, fat, sodium, potassium

**Indications:** for use in patients with impaired glucose tolerance (e.g., diabetic patients)

## Mechanism of Action and Drug Effects

The enteral formula groups provide the basic building blocks for anabolism. Different combinations and amounts of these nutrients are used based on the individual patient's anabolic needs. Enteral nutrition supplies complete dietary needs through the gastrointestinal tract by the normal oral route or by feeding tube.

## Indications

Enteral nutrition can be used to supplement an oral diet that is currently insufficient for a patient's nutrient needs or used alone to meet all of the patient's nutrient needs. Box 55-2 lists the main types of enteral nutritional supplements and their indications.

## Contraindications

The usual contraindication to nutritional supplements of any kind is known allergy to a specific product or genetic disease that renders a patient unable to metabolize certain types of nutrients.

## Adverse Effects

The most common adverse effect of nutritional supplements is gastrointestinal intolerance, manifesting as diarrhea. Infant nutritional formulations are most commonly associated with allergies and digestive intolerance. The other nutritional supplements are commonly associated with osmotic diarrhea. Rapid feeding or bolus doses can result in dumping syndrome, which produces intestinal disturbances. In addition, tube feeding places the patient at significant risk for aspiration pneumonia. This is especially true in patients in whom mental status, gag reflexes, and general mobility are compromised.

## Interactions

Various nutrients can interact with drugs to produce significant food-drug interactions. With some exceptions, food usually delays the absorption of drugs when administered simultaneously. High gastric acid content or prolonged emptying time can result in decreased effects of certain antibiotics (cephalosporins, erythromycin, and penicillins). An increased absorption rate resulting in increased therapeutic effects can be seen when corticosteroids or vitamins A and D are given with nutritional supplements. The antibiotic effects of tetracyclines and quinolones are decreased when they are given with nutritional supplements as a result of chemical inactivation. These drugs must be given at least 2 hours before or after tube feedings.

Tube feedings can also reduce the absorption of phenytoin, which may result in seizures. It is recommended that tube feedings be held for at least 2 hours before and after the administration of phenytoin. This can be problematic, because the patient may not receive adequate nutrition due to withholding of feedings. This issue is somewhat controversial, and some suggest that the interaction is more theoretical than actual. Thus, some institutions have decided to ignore this possible interaction and to monitor phenytoin levels and patient status, rather than holding the tube feedings, whereas others continue to hold the tube feedings. Often the patient requires intravenous phenytoin when continuous tube feedings are necessary.

## Dosages

Because nutrient requirements vary greatly, dosages are individualized according to patient needs.

## DRUG PROFILES

Enteral nutrition can be provided by a variety of supplements. Individual patient characteristics determine the appropriate enteral supplement. The four most commonly used enteral formulations are elemental, polymeric, modular, and altered amino acid.

### ELEMENTAL FORMULATIONS

Elemental formulations are enteral supplements that contain dipeptides, tripeptides, or crystalline amino acids. Minimal digestion is required with elemental formulations. These supplements are indicated for patients with pancreatitis, partial bowel obstruction, irritable bowel disease, radiation enteritis, bowel fistulas, and short bowel syndrome. They are contraindicated in patients who have had hypersensitivity reactions to them. Elemental formulation supplements are available without a prescription and have no pregnancy category.

### POLYMERIC FORMULATIONS

Polymeric formulations are enteral supplements that contain complex nutrients derived from proteins, carbohydrates, and fat. The polymeric formulations are some of the most commonly used enteral formulations because they most closely resemble normal dietary intake. They are preferred over elemental formulations in patients who have fully functional gastrointestinal tracts and have no specialized nutrient needs. Polymeric formulations are less hyperosmolar than elemental formulations and therefore cause fewer gastrointestinal problems. They are contraindicated in patients who have had hypersensitivity reactions to them. They are available without a prescription and have no pregnancy category classification.

---

| BOX 55-2 | ENTERAL NUTRITIONAL SUPPLEMENTS: INDICATIONS |
|---|---|

**Complete Nutritional Formulations
(i.e., for General Nutritional Deficiencies)**
- Inability to consume or digest normal foods
- Accelerated catabolic status
- Undernourishment because of disease

**Incomplete Nutritional Formulations
(i.e., for Specific Nutritional Deficiencies)**
- Genetic metabolic enzyme deficiency
- Hepatic or renal impairment

**Infant Nutritional Formulations**
- Sole nutritional intake for premature and full-term infants
- Supplemental nutritional intake for older infants receiving solid foods
- Supplemental nutritional intake for breast-fed infants

The most commonly used enteral supplement in the polymeric formulation category of enteral nutrition products is Ensure. It is lactose free and is also available in a higher-calorie formula called Ensure Plus. Other polymeric formulations are listed in Box 55-1. These drugs contain complex nutrients such as casein and soy protein for protein, corn syrup, and maltodextrins for carbohydrates, and vegetable oil or milk fat for fat. They are available in liquid formulations only.

## MODULAR FORMULATIONS

### carbohydrate formulation

Modual and Polycose are examples of commonly used enteral supplements in the carbohydrate modular formulation category. Both are carbohydrate supplements that supply carbohydrates only. They are intended to be used in addition to monomeric or polymeric formulations to provide a more individual specialized nutrient mix. They are available in liquid formulations only. These products are obtainable without a prescription, have no pregnancy category classification, and are contraindicated only in patients who have had hypersensitivity reactions to them.

### fat formulation

Microlipid and MCT Oil are the formulations available in the fat category. Microlipid is a fat supplement supplying only fats. It is a concentrated source of calories and contains 4.5 kcal/mL. These drugs are given to help individualize nutrient formulations. They may be used in patients with malabsorption and other gastrointestinal disorders and in patients with pancreatitis. They are available in liquid formulations only. These products are obtainable without a prescription, have no pregnancy category classification, and are contraindicated only in patients who have had hypersensitivity reactions to them.

### protein formulation

Casec, ProMod, and Propac are examples of protein modular formulations. They are used to increase patients' protein intake and provide additional proteins. They are derived from a variety of sources such as whey, casein, egg whites, and amino acids. All of the available products are dried powders that must be reconstituted with water. They may sometimes be reconstituted by placing them in enteral feedings that are already in liquid form. They are indicated for patients with increased protein needs. They are contraindicated in patients who have had hypersensitivity reactions to them. Protein formulation supplements are available without a prescription and have no pregnancy category classification.

## ALTERED AMINO ACID FORMULATIONS

Amin-Aid is one of the many amino acid formulation nutritional supplements available. Many of the nutritional supplements in this category are also listed as modular formulations because they can be used as both single-nutrient formulas and as nutritional formulations for patients with genetic errors of metabolism. Specialized amino acid formulations are used most commonly in patients who have metabolic disorders

| TABLE 55-2 | **PERIPHERAL AND CENTRAL PARENTERAL NUTRITION: CHARACTERISTICS** | |
|---|---|---|
| **CHARACTERISTIC** | **PERIPHERAL** | **CENTRAL** |
| Goal of nutritional therapy (total versus supplemental) | Supplemental (total if moderate to low needs) | Total |
| Length of therapy | Short (fewer than 14 days) | Long (7 days or longer) |
| Osmolarity | Hyperosmolar (600-900 mOsm/L) | Hyperosmolar (600-900 mOsm/L) |
| Fluid tolerance | Must be high | Can be fluid restricted |
| Dextrose | Less than 10%* | 10%-35% |
| Amino acids | Less than 3% | More than 3%-7% |
| Fats | 10%-20% | 10%-20% |
| Calories per day | Less than 2000 kcal/day | More than 2000 kcal/day |

*Many institutions use a maximum of 12.5% dextrose.

such as phenylketonuria, homocystinuria, and maple syrup urine disease. They are also used to supply nutritional support to patients with illnesses such as renal impairment, eclampsia, heart failure, or liver failure.

## PARENTERAL NUTRITION

Parenteral nutritional supplementation (intravenous administration) is the preferred method for patients who are unable to tolerate and/or maintain adequate enteral or oral intake. Instead of administration of partially digested nutrients into the gastrointestinal tract (as in enteral nutrition), vitamins, minerals, amino acids, dextrose, and lipids are administered intravenously directly into the circulatory system. This effectively bypasses the entire gastrointestinal system, which eliminates the need for absorption, metabolism, and excretion. Parenteral nutrition is also called total parenteral nutrition (TPN) or hyperalimentation.

TPN can supply all of the calories, carbohydrates, amino acids, fats, trace elements, vitamins, and minerals needed for growth, weight gain, wound healing, convalescence, immunocompetence, and other health-sustaining functions.

TPN can be administered through either a peripheral vein or a central vein. Each route of delivery of TPN has specific requirements and limitations. It is generally accepted that TPN is used only when oral or enteral support is impossible or when the gastrointestinal absorptive or functional capacity is not sufficient to meet the nutritional needs of the patient. Some of the factors that must be considered in deciding whether to use peripheral or central TPN for a given patient are listed in Table 55-2.

## PERIPHERAL TOTAL PARENTERAL NUTRITION

Peripheral TPN (PPN) is one route of administration of TPN. A peripheral vein is used to deliver nutrients to the patient's circulatory system. PPN is usually a temporary method of administration. The long-term administration of nutritional supplements via a peripheral vein may lead to phlebitis. It is considered a temporary measure to provide adequate nutrients in patients who have mild deficits or who are restricted from oral intake and have slightly elevated metabolic rates.

PPN is valuable in patients who do not have large nutritional needs, can tolerate moderately large fluid loads, and need nutritional supplements only temporarily. PPN may be used alone or in combination with oral nutritional supplements to provide the necessary fat, carbohydrate, and protein needed by the patient to maintain health.

## Mechanism of Action and Drug Effects

PPN provides the basic nutrient building blocks for anabolism. Different combinations and amounts of these nutrients are used based on the individual patient's anabolic needs.

## Indications

PPN is used to administer nutrients to patients who need more nutrients than their current oral intake can supply or to provide complete daily nutrition. It is meant only as a temporary means (less than 2 weeks) of delivering TPN.

Circumstances under which patients may benefit from the delivery of PPN are as follows:
- The patient must undergo a procedure that restricts oral feedings.
- The patient has anorexia caused by radiation or cancer chemotherapy.
- The patient has a gastrointestinal illness that prevents oral food ingestion.
- The patient has just undergone surgery of any type.
- The patient's nutritional deficits are minimal, but oral nutrition will not be started for longer than 5 days

## Contraindications

As mentioned previously for the enteral nutritional products, the only usual contraindication to nutritional supplementation of any kind is known drug allergy to a specific product or a genetic disease that renders a patient unable to assimilate certain types of nutrients.

## Adverse Effects

The most devastating adverse effect of PPN is phlebitis, which is vein irritation or inflammation of a vein. If phlebitis is severe and is not treated appropriately, it can lead to the loss of a limb, although this is rare. Another potential adverse effect is fluid overload. PPN is limited to solutions with a lower dextrose concentration, generally less than 10%, to avoid sclerosing of the vein. Thus, large volumes are needed to meet a patient's daily nutritional requirements. Some patients, such as those with renal failure or heart failure, cannot tolerate large fluid volumes. In these patients, fluid restrictions may make it impossible to provide adequate calories through PPN.

## CENTRAL TOTAL PARENTERAL NUTRITION

In central TPN, a large central vein is used to deliver nutrients directly into the patient's circulation. Usually, the subclavian or internal jugular vein is used. Central TPN is generally indicated for patients who require nutritional supplements for a prolonged period, usually longer than 7 to 10 days. It can also be used in the home care setting. There are a variety of indications for central TPN. The disadvantages of central TPN are the risks associated with venous catheter insertion and the use and maintenance of the central vein. There is a greater potential for infection, more serious catheter-induced trauma and related events, metabolic alterations, and other technical or mechanical problems than with peripheral parenteral nutrition (PPN).

## Mechanism of Action and Drug Effects

Central TPN is used to supply nutrients to patients who cannot ingest nutrients by mouth and cannot meet required daily nutritional needs by the enteral or peripheral parenteral routes. Like PPN, central TPN supplies the basic building blocks for anabolism. It provides the necessary fat, carbohydrate, and protein that the patient needs to maintain health.

## Indications

TPN delivers total dietary nutrients to patients who require nutritional supplementation. Patients who may benefit from the delivery of TPN include the following:
- Patients who have large nutritional requirements (metabolic stress or hypermetabolism)
- Patients who need nutritional support for prolonged periods (longer than 7 to 10 days)
- Patients who are unable to tolerate large fluid loads

## Contraindications

TPN is contraindicated in patients with allergy to any of its components. Rarely, a patient who is allergic to eggs may have cross-sensitivity to lipid formulations. TPN is used only when the gastrointestinal tract cannot be used (e.g., in postoperative patients or those who are otherwise unable to eat or digest and absorb nutrients).

## Adverse Effects

The most common adverse effects of central TPN are those associated with the use of the central vein for delivery of the TPN. The risks associated with insertion of the infusion line, as well as the use and maintenance of the central vein for administration of TPN, can create some complications. There is a greater potential for infection, serious catheter-induced trauma and related events, and other technical or mechanical problems than with PPN. Larger and more concentrated volumes of nutritional supplements are being delivered with central TPN, and therefore there is a greater chance for metabolic complications such as hyperglycemia.

## Dosages

Dosage requirements vary from patient to patient. Age, gender, weight, and numerous other factors must be considered for proper administration of TPN. Guidelines for amino acids appear in Table 55-3.

| TABLE 55-3 | AMINO ACIDS: RECOMMENDED DAILY DOSAGE GUIDELINES | |
|---|---|---|
| **HEALTHY** | | **MALNOURISHED OR TRAUMA/BURN** |
| ADULT | INFANT/CHILD | ADULT |
| 0.9 g/kg | 1.5-3 g/kg | Up to 2 g/kg |

## DRUG PROFILES

The individual components of peripheral and central TPN are the same. The difference lies in the concentrations and amounts of the components delivered per volume of nutritional supplement. The basic components of peripheral or central TPN are amino acids, carbohydrates, lipids, trace elements, vitamins, fluids, and electrolytes. Most of the electrolyte components are discussed in Chapter 29.

### AMINO ACIDS

Amino acids have many roles in the maintenance of normal nutritional status. The primary role is protein synthesis, or anabolism. Provision of adequate amino acids in nutritional supplements reduces the breakdown of proteins (catabolism) and also helps to promote normal growth and wound healing.

Amino acids are commonly classified as essential or nonessential according to whether they can or cannot be produced by the body. Nonessential amino acids are those that the body produces and therefore need not be present in dietary intake. The body is able to manufacture, from nutritional nitrogen sources, all but eight of the available amino acids. Essential amino acids are those amino acids that cannot be produced by the body. Therefore, they must be included in daily dietary intake. Amino acids are used as building blocks for the protein that is needed for normal growth and development. Two amino acids, histidine and arginine, are not manufactured by the body in large enough quantities during rapid growth periods such as infancy or childhood. Thus, they are referred to as semiessential amino acids. Box 55-3 lists the amino acids according to their categories.

### amino acids

Amino acid crystalline solutions (Aminosyn 3%, 5%, and 10%, and FreAmine III 8.5% and 10%) can be used in either peripheral or central TPN. Amino acids are a source of both protein and calories. They provide 4 kcal/g. The two currently available brands of amino acid solutions differ only in their respective concentrations. The dosage of these solutions varies depending on the patient's weight and requirements. These drugs have no restrictions regarding pregnancy and have no contraindications to use.

### CARBOHYDRATES

In nutritional support, carbohydrates are usually supplied to patients through dextrose. Dextrose is normally the greatest source of calories and provides 3.4 kcal/g. However, protein

| BOX 55-3 | AMINO ACIDS: CLASSIFICATION |

**Essential**
- Isoleucine
- Leucine
- Lysine
- Methionine
- Phenylalanine
- Threonine
- Tryptophan
- Valine

**Semiessential**
- Arginine
- Histidine

**Nonessential**
- Alanine
- Asparagine
- Aspartic acid
- Cysteine
- Glutamine
- Glutamic acid
- Glycine
- Proline
- Serine
- Tyrosine

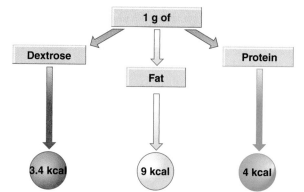

**FIGURE 55-2** One gram of dextrose, fat, or protein will provide varying amounts of energy as calories.

(amino acids) and lipids are also used as calorie sources (Figure 55-2). The concentration of dextrose in TPN is an important consideration. In PPN, dextrose concentrations are kept below 10% to decrease the possibility of phlebitis. In central TPN, dextrose concentrations can range from 10% to 50%, but they are commonly 25% to 35%. Because dextrose is a sugar, supplemental insulin may be given simultaneously in nutritional supplements. Use of a balanced nutritional supplement that contains dextrose and lipids as caloric sources decreases the need for large amounts of insulin.

### FAT

The average North American diet contains 40% fat. This means that of the total calories supplied, 40% to 50% of the calories are obtained through fat grams. The ideal diet contains no more than 30% fat. Intravenous fat emulsions serve two functions: they supply essential fatty acids, and they are a source of energy or calories. As with the amino acids, certain fatty acids are essential because the body cannot produce them. Linoleic acid cannot be synthesized by the body. It is needed to produce linolenic and arachidonic acid. If these fatty acids are not present in dietary or nutritional supplements, an essential fatty acid deficiency may develop. Clinical signs of essential fatty acid deficiency are hair loss, scaly dermatitis, growth retardation, reduced wound healing, decreased platelet levels, and fatty liver (Figure 55-3).

**FIGURE 55-3** Lipid emulsions supply essential fatty acids and energy.

### lipid emulsions

The currently marketed lipid emulsions, Intralipid and Liposyn, are available as 10%, 20%, or 30% emulsions. They differ in fat origin. Liposyn is made from safflower oil, and Intralipid is made from soybean oil.

Lipid emulsions normally deliver 20% to 30% of the total daily calories and must not exceed 60% of daily caloric intake. Fat emulsions are most beneficial when combined with dextrose solutions. The use of fat to meet caloric needs prevents potentially harmful conditions—such as hyperglycemia, hyperinsulinemia, and hyperosmolarity—that can occur when a patient's entire caloric needs are being met solely by dextrose.

## TRACE ELEMENTS

Trace elements are available in individual solutions and in many different combinations. The following are considered trace elements:

- Chromium
- Copper
- Iodine
- Manganese
- Molybdenum
- Selenium
- Zinc

Specific dosages and frequencies depend on the individual patient's requirements. Vitamins and other minerals may also be added accordingly. A common multivitamin combination is multivitamin infusion (MVI).

## NURSING PROCESS

## ASSESSMENT

Perform a thorough nutritional assessment with attention to dietary history, weekly and daily food intake, weight, and height before initiating any *nutritional supplements*. Conduct a thorough nursing history and survey of all systems, including questions about any unusual symptoms, possible nutritional concerns, nausea, vomiting, loss of appetite, and weight gain or loss. Focus other questions on past and present medical and health history; history of any difficulties with nutrition, gastrointestinal absorption, or food intolerance; stressors; and a complete medication profile, including a listing of all prescription drugs, over-the-counter drugs, herbals, and supplements. Consultation with a registered dietitian is crucial to identify the nutrients that are missing in a particular patient's diet. Total body metabolic rate, body mass index, muscle mass, and other variables linked to nutritional status will most likely be assessed and are data that a nutritional consult may provide. Laboratory findings that may need to be assessed include the following: total protein level, albumin level, blood urea nitrogen (BUN) level, red blood cell (RBC) count, white blood cell (WBC) count, vitamin $B_{12}$ level, hemoglobin level, and hematocrit. Other laboratory studies may include cholesterol level, electrolyte levels, total lymphocyte count, serum transferrin level, iron level, urine creatinine clearance, lipid profile, and urinalysis. All of these objective and subjective data will help the prescriber, nutritionist/dietitian, and other members of the health care team to select the appropriate nutritional supplements for the patient.

Before administering an *enteral nutrition* supplement that is an elemental formulation, determine if the patient has a history of allergic reaction to any of the contents of the solution. Assess for contraindications, cautions, and drug interactions, and document the findings. Of most concern is assessing the patient's cardiac and renal status and ensuring that the ingredients and the amount of solution are not too taxing on these systems. In addition, because these solutions are given orally, either by mouth or via tube feedings (see Chapter 9), it is most important to assess ability to swallow, gag reflex, and bowel sounds, and to note any nausea or vomiting. Remember that protein-based formulations are to be avoided in patients with allergies to egg whites and whey.

With *parenteral nutrition,* assess for allergies to any of the ordered components of the intravenous solution, and pay attention to age and metabolic needs. There are usually multiple combinations of products available; thus, it is important to assess the patient carefully for allergies to essential proteins, amino acids, carbohydrates, trace elements, minerals, vitamins, lipids, high concentrations of dextrose, and any other ingredients. Assess your knowledge base about parenteral nutrition and the need for infusions through a central line, peripherally inserted central line, or peripherally inserted midline catheter. Some of the complications of parenteral nutrition include pneumothorax, infection, air emboli or emboli related to protein or lipid aggregation (associated with central catheter intravenous lines), septicemia related to the nutrient-rich solutions with invasive intravenous route of administration, and metabolic imbalances due to the solution ingredients and vomiting (seen with lipid administration in the parenteral nutrition). Also perform a complete baseline assessment and continuously monitor the following: (1) central line site, including patency, intactness, and appearance, (2) WBC and RBC counts as well as other laboratory values and parameters (listed earlier), (3) vital signs, (4) serum glucose levels, and (5) cardiac rhythm with electrocardiogram readings (as prescribed).

## NURSING DIAGNOSES

1. Nutrition, less than body requirements, related to inability to take in sufficient nutrients
2. Diarrhea related to a decreased tolerance to enteral feedings and their ingredients
3. Risk for infection (sepsis) related to parenteral infusions and use of central venous access line

## CASE STUDY

### Total Parenteral Nutrition

Mrs C., a 28-year-old florist, has been unable to eat due to severe vomiting related to her pregnancy. She is at 13 weeks' gestation and has been admitted to the hospital because of dehydration and inability to eat due to her severe nausea and vomiting. The decision has been made to give her total parenteral nutrition (TPN) for at least 1 week. After 1 week of therapy, her obstetrician will then decide whether to continue or stop the infusion, based on her response. She will be receiving the TPN infusion via a peripheral intravenous catheter with infusion bags that will be changed every 24 hours.

1. Mrs. C. is anxious about this infusion and asks the nurse, "Why is that bag so large? What is in the bag?" How will the nurse answer these questions?
2. The nurse explains to Mrs. C. that her blood glucose levels will need to be monitored while she is receiving the TPN. Mrs. C. begins to cry, saying, "This morning sickness is bad enough, but now I have diabetes too? How can that be?" What is the nurse's best response?
3. The nurse will monitor for what potential complication that can occur with peripherally administered TPN?
4. Before beginning the infusion, the nurse checks the ingredients of the TPN bag. The nurse notices that one of the contents is listed as 20% dextrose. Will the nurse add this bag to the patient's infusion? Explain your answer.

For answers, see http://evolve.elsevier.com/Lilley.

## PLANNING

### GOALS

1. Patient regains normal nutritional status through adequate dietary intake and supplemental feedings or nutrients.
2. Patient remains free from diarrhea as related to enteral supplementation.
3. Patient remains free from infection during parenteral nutritional supplementation.

### OUTCOME CRITERIA

1. Patient's nutritional status improves with enteral/parenteral nutritional supplement as prescribed, as evidenced by proportional weight gain, adequate fluid volume status with improved skin turgor, improved urinary output to at least 30 mL/hr, and laboratory values such as total protein, albumin, iron, Hct, and Hgb that return to normal.
2. Patient identifies measures to decrease diarrhea while receiving enteral feedings, such as use of prescribed drugs to decrease motility and/or use of over-the-counter drugs or herbal products, as ordered.
3. Patient states measures to minimize risk for infection at total parenteral nutrition site (peripheral or central), such as checking the site frequently for redness, swelling, drainage, or abnormal warmth, fever, or chills, and reporting these to the prescriber or home health care nurse immediately.

## IMPLEMENTATION

A prescriber's order must be complete and dated before *enteral* or *parenteral* (peripheral or central) *nutrition supplementation*

is begun. In general, monitoring the status of the patient during and after *enteral feedings* is crucial to safe and prudent nursing care. With nasogastric tube feeding solutions, check for proper placement (and detect gastric residuals so as to avoid aspiration and other complications. Checking for placement ensures that the tube is within the stomach and has not passed through the larynx, into the trachea and down into the bronchi of the lungs. Aspirating fluid from the tube with a syringe with testing of the pH to determine the acidity of the fluid aspirate is one method of placement checking. With a pH of 5.5 or lower, the tube is in the correct position. If these are not possible, a chest radiograph must be used. Measure gastric residual volumes and document before each feeding as well as before administration of each medication. When checking gastric residual volumes, stop the tube feeding and then aspirate stomach contents using a syringe connected to the particular tube. If the volume aspirated is more than the volume delivered over the previous 2 hours (of continuous feeding), return the aspirate, hold the feeding, and contact the prescriber while keeping the head of the patient's bed elevated. For intermittent bolus feedings, if the residual amount is more than 50% of the volume previously infused, it is the standard of care to return the aspirate, withhold the feeding, and contact the prescriber. A reduction in the tube feeding volume will probably then be ordered. Always check hospital/facility policy or protocol before use of enteral feedings, while also checking and managing residuals.

Newer tubes for nasogastric and other enteral feeding have smaller diameters and are thinner (5 French to 10 French) and more pliable for better patient tolerance. However, the smaller-diameter tubes make checking for gastric aspiration more difficult. To prevent clogging of the feeding tube, it is often helpful to flush the tube with 30 mL of cranberry juice or other designated solution (per institutional policy) followed by 10 mL of water. The juice may help break up the formula residue and unclog certain types of feeding tubes; the water helps to keep the tube clean and free of residue. Percutaneous enteral gastrostomy (PEG) tubes are also commonly used in many situations but do require surgical insertion by a gastroenterologist and are often procedurally done under moderate sedation. Their care includes performing dressing changes during the initial period and then checking for residuals. Placement need not be checked, but if it appears that the tube has come out of the opening and is longer than previously noted, stop the infusion and contact the prescriber.

Follow prescriber-ordered enteral feeding infusion rates and concentrations carefully. Usually the initial rate is 50 mL/hr at one-half strength, but this may be increased per patient tolerance to a rate ordered by the physician or appropriate health care provider. More rapid feeding increases the risk for hyperglycemia, dumping syndrome and diarrhea. Infusion rates of enteral feedings may be adjusted by the prescriber as per the patient's tolerance (of the feeding). Keep tube feeding formulas at room temperature and never administer cold or warm. If all the necessary steps to decrease or prevent diarrhea have been taken and have failed, antidiarrheal medications may be needed. Lactose-free solutions are available and are recommended for patients who are lactose intolerant. Patients who have lactose intolerance may experience cramping, diarrhea, abdominal bloating, and flatulence with the ingestion of milk-based enteral feedings.

Assess *parenteral nutrition infusions* every hour or per the facility's policies and procedures. Document the status of the entire infusion system and equipment as well as the condition of the patient. It is the standard of care to examine the patient first and then check the insertion site, tubing, infusion pump, and solution. To prevent infection, change the parenteral nutrition tubing every time a new bag is added to the infusion, or as per facility policy. It is also recommended that tubing changes occur daily with the beginning of each new infusion. A 1.2-micron filter is used to trap bacteria, including *Pseudomonas* species. Record the patient's temperature every 4 hours, or as prescribed, during the infusion, and report any increase in temperature over 100° F (37.8° C) to the prescriber immediately. Check the patient frequently for signs and symptoms of hyperglycemia such as polydipsia (excessive thirst), polyuria (excessive urination), polyphagia (excessive hunger), headache, dehydration, nausea, vomiting, and weakness. Never accelerate these infusion rates to increase plasma volume because the rapid increase in the amount of dextrose solution may precipitate hyperglycemia and other related complications. Insulin replacement may be needed with the increase in dextrose; therefore, measure serum glucose levels by glucometer so that hyperglycemia may be immediately recognized and treated.

Hypoglycemia is manifested by cold, clammy skin; dizziness; tachycardia; and tingling of the extremities. Hypoglycemia associated with parenteral nutrition may be prevented by gradual reduction of the intravenous feeding rate to allow the pancreas time to adapt to the changing blood glucose levels. If parenteral nutrition is discontinued abruptly, rebound hypoglycemia may occur. This can be prevented by providing infusions of 5% to 10% glucose in situations in which parenteral nutrition must be discontinued immediately. Fluid overload may also occur with parenteral nutrition, manifested by weak pulse, hypertension, tachycardia, confusion, decreased urine output, and pitting edema. This may be prevented by maintaining infusion rates as ordered. If signs of fluid overload occur, slow the infusion rate, measure vital signs, contact the prescriber, and remain with the patient until the patient's condition has stabilized. Include auscultation of breath and heart sounds in the patient assessment, especially if additional therapies are administered that may precipitate fluid overload. Measurement of intake and output is usually indicated when parenteral nutrition is administered (and with enteral supplementation as well). See the Patient Teaching Tips for more information on the use of nutritional supplements.

## ▌EVALUATION

Therapeutic responses to *nutritional supplementation* include improved well-being, energy, strength, and performance of activities of daily living; an increase in weight; and laboratory test results that reflect an improved nutritional status. Specific laboratory values may include some of the following: albumin level, total protein level, hematocrit level, hemoglobin level, RBC and WBC counts, BUN level, electrolyte levels, blood glucose and insulin levels, and iron values. Perform ongoing evaluation for adverse effects associated with all *enteral* and/or *parenteral nutrition* infusions during and after therapy, and complete nutritional reevaluation periodically so that the patient's nutritional needs are met. This may require frequent prescriber appointments or monitoring by a home health care nurse. Always refer to goals and outcome criteria to evaluate the effectiveness of therapy.

## ▌PATIENT TEACHING TIPS

- Because patients are often discharged with the need for various types of tube feedings, provide the patient, family, and/or caregiver with education, instructions, and demonstrations about the daily care of the tube, preparation of tube feedings, and related procedures. Present the education in a way that reflects the learning needs of the patient and/or those involved in the patient's care.
- Instruct the patient, family, and/or caregiver about the need for correct placement of the tube, which should be checked before each tube feeding if a nasogastric tube is used. Incorrect placement of a nasogastric tube would be manifested by coughing, choking, difficulty in speaking, cyanosis, and subsequent respiratory distress. The head of the bed must remain elevated during infusions; this is more critical with nasogastric tube feedings than with gastrostomy tube feedings.
- Provide contact names and phone numbers for the prescriber, home health care nurse, and other resources to the patient, family, and/or caregiver so that therapy can be monitored and problems and complications averted as related to the feeding.

A fever, difficulty breathing, sounds of lung congestion, high residual amounts, resistance to the flow of the feeding solution, and resistance in checking for residual are all causes for concern. Appropriate interventions must be implemented, including seeking emergency medical care if needed.
- Patients who are homebound and are receiving parenteral nutrition will need individualized education as well as support from home health care or related health care services. Practice is critical to acquisition of skill by the patient, family, and/or caregiver and must be an integral part of patient education. Before the patient is discharged, explain and demonstrate all procedures for storage, cleansing and care of the site, dressing changes, irrigation of the catheter, pump function and care, and changing of the bag, filters, and tubing, with a return demonstration by the patient. Advise the patient that parenteral nutrition in the home setting requires home health care services by a registered nurse to help prevent the complications of infection at the site, sepsis, fever, and pneumonia.
- Educate the patient about the need to check serum glucose levels at home as ordered by the prescriber if parenteral

## PATIENT TEACHING TIPS—cont'd

nutrition or other infused solutions high in dextrose are administered. Thoroughly explain the operation of a glucometer, with specific steps for its use included in a demonstration to the patient, family, and/or caregiver. In addition, include and reinforce instructions in self-administration of insulin, if needed.

• Instruct the patient to report to the prescriber immediately any signs and symptoms of potential complications of parenteral nutrition, including fever, cough, chest pains, dyspnea, and chills, (all of which are indicative of adverse reactions to lipid infusions). Restlessness, nervousness, fainting, and tachycardia are associated with hypoglycemia and must also be reported, as must the occurrence of polyuria, polydipsia, polyphagia, nausea, vomiting, dehydration, headache, and/or weakness (indicating hyperglycemia).

## KEY POINTS

• A thorough nutritional assessment and possible consultation with a registered dietitian or nutritionist are essential for adequate intervention for the malnourished patient.
• Various enteral feeding formulations with different nutritional content are available, including some that are lactose free.
• Enteral feedings may result in complications such as hyperglycemia, dumping syndrome, and aspiration of the nutritional supplement.
• Parenteral nutrition supplementation (intravenously administered) is total parenteral nutrition (TPN) or hyperalimentation. PN or TPN may be administered through a central vein or through a peripheral vein (PPN).
• TPN is administered through a central venous catheter because of the hyperosmolarity of the substances used and the need for dilution provided by a larger-diameter vein to prevent damage to the vein. Parenteral nutrition given through a peripherally inserted central catheter (PPN) line is another option but uses a solution with a lower concentration of dextrose and other ingredients.
• Parenteral feedings may result in air embolism, fever, infection, fluid volume overload, hyperglycemia, or hypoglycemia. If they are discontinued abruptly, rebound hypoglycemia may result.
• Cautious and skillful nursing care may prevent or decrease the occurrence of complications associated with enteral or parenteral nutritional supplementation.

## NCLEX® EXAMINATION REVIEW QUESTIONS

1 The nurse is assessing an enteral feeding that is infusing via a nasogastric feeding tube. Which statement about this tube is accurate?
   a It is surgically inserted into the stomach.
   b It is inserted through the nose into the jejunum.
   c It is surgically inserted directly into the jejunum.
   d It is inserted through the nose into the stomach.
2 When administering total parenteral nutrition (TPN), the nurse is aware that one purpose of intravenous fat (lipid) emulsions is to provide which nutrient?
   a Calories
   b Amino acids
   c Minerals
   d Immunoglobulins
3 The nurse is monitoring a patient who is receiving a total parenteral nutrition (TPN) infusion and notes that the patient has cold clammy skin, shows tachycardia, and is complaining of feeling dizzy. What is the immediate action of the nurse?
   a Stop the TPN infusion.
   b Check the patient's blood glucose level.
   c Order a stat (immediate) electrocardiogram.
   d Obtain an order for blood cultures.
4 A patient has new orders for administration of peripheral parenteral nutrition (PPN). The nurse knows that PPN is most appropriate in which situation?
   a Therapy is expected to last longer than 2 weeks.
   b Therapy is expected to last fewer than 14 days.

   c A dextrose concentration of 20% is needed.
   d Nutritional needs are 3000 kcal/day.
5 During the night shift, a patient's total parenteral nutrition (TPN) infusion runs out, the pharmacy is closed, and a new TPN bag will not be available for about 6 hours. The nurse's most appropriate action at this time would be to
   a hang a bottle of lipid solution.
   b hang a bag of normal saline.
   c hang a bag of 10% dextrose.
   d call the prescriber for stat TPN orders.
6 The nurse is assessing a patient who is receiving an enteral tube feeding. Which are possible adverse effects associated with enteral feedings? (Select all that apply.)
   a Hypoglycemia
   b Air embolism
   c Aspiration
   d Diarrhea
   e Infection
7 A patient is receiving a tube feeding via a percutaneous enteral gastrostomy (PEG) tube of Glucerna at 50 mL/hr. The orders also read to check the residual and flush the tubing every 4 hours with 30 mL of water. Calculate the total intake of fluid at the end of a 12-hour shift.

1. d, 2. a, 3. b, 4. b, 5. c, 6. c, d, 7. 690 mL.

For Critical Thinking and Prioritization Questions, see http://evolve.elsevier.com/Lilley.

# Dermatologic, Ophthalmic, and Otic Drugs

## STUDY SKILLS TIPS

Time Management • PURR • Repeat the Steps

### TIME MANAGEMENT

As you plan your study time for Part 10, it should be very clear that Chapter 57 will take significantly more time to complete than the other chapters. Do not let the length of the chapter overwhelm you. Apply the principles of time management to this chapter and you will succeed. The most important aspect of time management to apply to this chapter is the use of clear goal statements and action plan steps to help you achieve the goals.

### Goal Statements

Remember the criteria for goal statements. First, they must be realistic; the statements must be things you know you can accomplish. Second, they must be specific to the task. "I will study the chapter" is not a very specific goal. Specify what you expect to accomplish. "I will master the 31 key terms" is a more specific goal statement. Third, there must be a time limit. How long will you spend in achieving this goal? Set a time limit for completion of each learning activity, specifying the quantity of time to be spent in that activity. Finally, goal statements must be measurable. In the example about studying the key terms, including the number of terms contained in Chapter 57 helps clarify the goal.

### Action Planning

The second segment of time management is the use of action planning. An action plan is a series of smaller, specific activities that you will accomplish to meet your goal statements. Your goal is to master the 31 terms. What will you do to meet that goal?

### Action Steps Example

1. I will spend 1 hour from 3:00 to 4:00 PM on Monday making vocabulary drill cards for the key terms found in Chapter 57.
2. I will spend 15 minutes in rehearsal and review of these cards every day until the exam on this chapter is over.
3. Each time I cannot define and explain a term, I will put an X on the card to identify it as a term needing more review.

4. I will spend 1 hour the night before the exam doing a comprehensive review of the terms in Chapter 57, with special emphasis on those cards that have one or more *X* marks.

Action steps help ensure that you are spending your study time actively focusing on what you need to learn.

## PURR

### Prepare Example

Chapter 57, Objective 3 reads, "Discuss the mechanisms of action, indications, dosage forms with application techniques, adverse effects, cautions, contraindications, and drug interactions of the various ophthalmic drugs."

Question 1: What does *ophthalmic* mean? (literal question [LQ])

Question 2: What are ophthalmic drugs? (LQ)

Question 3: What is the mechanism of action of ophthalmic drugs? (LQ)

Question 4: Is there more than one mechanism of action? (LQ)

Question 5: If there is more than one mechanism of action, how are the mechanisms similar and how are they different? (interpretive question)

These questions are only suggestions for generated questions based on the chapter objectives. Many more questions can be asked about Objective 3. These questions are an essential part of the study process. Questions help make you an active reader and an active learner. The more questions you generate, the easier it will be to understand the chapter.

### Outline Example

1. *Looking through the chapter, decide how much material is appropriate.* The section that begins with Antiglaucoma Drugs is probably too much material. Based on the chapter headings, this section could be broken down into six blocks of material. Block 1 would cover the material under the heading Cholinergic Drugs (Miotics). Block 2 would be the material under the heading Sympathomimetics (Mydriatics). The next four blocks would be Beta-Adrenergic Blockers, Carbonic Anhydrase Inhibitors, Osmotic Diuretics, and Prostaglandin Agonists.

2. *Apply the Prepare step to each block.* Beginning with Cholinergic Drugs (Miotics), generate some questions to guide your reading. Remember that it is important to ask both questions that will focus on literal information and questions that will help you interpret, evaluate, and analyze when you read.

3. *Read the material.* As soon as you have completed the self-questioning on the first block of material, read the material in the chapter. It is important that the reading be done immediately. Read for understanding, and as you read remember the questions you generated. This approach will help your concentration and comprehension.

4. *Take a short break.* Once you have completed the reading of this section of the chapter, give your mind a chance to reflect and consolidate the learning. Limit the time you allow for a break and use the time for something pleasurable. Give yourself 5 or 10 minutes to read the newspaper, get a snack, or just take a short walk.

5. *Rehearse.* Before going on to the next section of the chapter it is important to spend a few minutes in rehearsal. Using the questions from step 2, go back over the material you read and try to respond to those questions. When you find yourself unable to answer a question, put a mark in the text beside the heading that caused the difficulty and move on. The mark will serve as a reminder for future review. At this point, the objective is not complete mastery of the material. The objective is to see what you have learned so that you can move smoothly into the next section. Breaking a chapter into blocks is useful, but it is imperative that the links between sections be made as you study.

6. *Review.* After you have completed two or three major sections of the chapter, it is time to review. Start at the beginning of the chapter. Ask your questions. Try to answer them. If you cannot formulate a clear answer, then some rereading is necessary. Also, pay attention to the marks made during the rehearsal step. Those marks indicate areas that you have already identified as needing review. When rereading, remember that the object is to read only as much of the material as needed to be able to respond to self-generated questions. There simply is not enough time to read the entire chapter a second or third time.

## REPEAT THE STEPS

Prepare, read for understanding, take a short break, and then rehearse the material you've just read. It may seem that this process takes an excessive amount of time and involves a lot of repetition, but in the long run this process will produce better learning. The time spent in Prepare, Understand, and Rehearse will reduce the time needed to review. Frequent review as you move through the chapter will make the final review at exam time proceed more quickly and enable you to achieve mastery of the material.

**e**volve WEBSITE

*http://evolve.elsevier.com/Lilley*
- Animations
- Answer Key—Textbook Case Studies
- Critical Thinking and Prioritization Questions

- Key Points—Downloadable
- Review Questions for the NCLEX® Examination
- Unfolding Case Studies

## OBJECTIVES

When you reach the end of this chapter, you will be able to do the following:

1 Discuss the normal anatomy, physiology, and functions of the skin.
2 Describe the different disorders, infections, and other conditions commonly affecting the skin.
3 Identify the various dermatologic drugs used to treat these disorders, infections, and other conditions, and describe the various classifications of these drugs.

4 Discuss the mechanisms of action, indications, contraindications, cautions, other drug interactions, application techniques, and adverse effects of the various topical dermatologic drugs.
5 Develop a nursing care plan that includes all phases of the nursing process for patients using topical dermatologic drugs.

## DRUG PROFILES

anthralin, p. 909
♦ bacitracin, p. 904
♦ benzoyl peroxide, p. 905
calcipotriene, p. 909
clindamycin, p. 905
♦ clotrimazole, p. 907
fluorouracil, p. 911
imiquimod, p. 911
♦ isotretinoin, p. 905
♦ lindane, p. 910
miconazole, p. 907

minoxidil, p. 910
mupirocin, p. 905
neomycin and polymyxin B, p. 905
♦ pimecrolimus, p. 911
♦ silver sulfadiazine, p. 905
tar-containing products, p. 909
tazarotene, p. 909
tretinoin, p. 906

---

♦ *Key drug*

## KEY TERMS

**Acne vulgaris** A chronic inflammatory disease of the *pilosebaceous* glands of the skin, involving lesions such as *papules* and *pustules* ("pimples" or "comedones"); referred to in this chapter as *acne*. (p. 905)

**Actinic keratosis** A slowly developing, localized thickening of the outer layers of the skin resulting from long-term, prolonged exposure to the sun; also called *solar keratosis*. (p. 911)

**Atopic dermatitis** A chronic skin inflammation seen in patients with hereditary susceptibility. (p. 903)

**Basal cell carcinoma** The most common form of skin cancer; it arises from epidermal cells known as *basal cells* and is rarely metastatic. (p. 903)

## KEY TERMS—cont'd

**Carbuncles** Necrotizing infections of skin and subcutaneous tissue caused by multiple furuncles (boils). They are usually caused by the bacterium *Staphylococcus aureus.* (p. 904)

**Cellulitis** An acute, diffuse, spreading infection involving the skin, subcutaneous tissue, and sometimes muscle as well. It is usually caused by infection of a wound with *Streptococcus* or *Staphylococcus* species. (p. 904)

**Dermatitis** Any inflammation of the skin. (p. 903)

**Dermatophytes** Any of the common groups of fungi that infect skin, hair, and nails. These fungi are most commonly from the genera *Microsporum, Epidermophyton,* and *Trichophyton.* (p. 906)

**Dermatosis** The general term for any abnormal skin condition. (p. 903)

**Dermis** The layer of the skin just below the epidermis, consisting of papillary and reticular layers and containing blood and lymphatic vessels, nerves and nerve endings, glands, and hair follicles. (p. 902)

**Eczema** A pruritic, papulovesicular dermatitis occurring as a reaction to many endogenous and exogenous agents, and characterized by erythema, edema, and an inflammatory infiltrate of the dermis accompanied by oozing, crusting, and scaling. (p. 903)

**Epidermis** The superficial, avascular layers of the skin, made up of an outer dead, cornified portion and a deeper living, cellular portion. (p. 902)

**Folliculitis** Inflammation of a follicle, usually a hair follicle. A follicle is defined as any sac or pouchlike cavity. (p. 904)

**Furuncles** Painful skin nodules caused by *Staphylococcus* organisms that enter the skin through the hair follicles; also called a *boil.* (p. 904)

**Impetigo** A pus-generating, contagious superficial skin infection, usually caused by *Staphylococci* or *Streptococci.* It generally occurs on the face and is most commonly seen in children; may be recognized by honey-colored crusts. (p. 904)

**Papules** Small, circumscribed, superficial, solid elevations of the skin that are usually pink and less than 0.5 to 1 cm in diameter. (p. 904)

**Pediculosis** An infestation with lice of the family Pediculidae. (p. 910)

**Pruritus** An unpleasant cutaneous sensation that provokes the desire to rub or scratch the skin to obtain relief. (p. 907)

**Psoriasis** A common, chronic squamous cell dermatosis with polygenic (multigene) inheritance and a fluctuating pattern of recurrence and remission. (p. 903)

**Pustules** Visible collections of pus within or beneath the epidermis. (p. 904)

**Scabies** A contagious disease caused by *Sarcoptes scabiei,* the itch mite, characterized by intense itching of the skin and injury to the skin (excoriation) resulting from scratching. (p. 910)

**Tinea** A fungal skin disease caused by a dermatophyte and characterized by itching, scaling, and, sometimes, painful lesions. *Tinea* is a general term for an infection with any of various dermatophytes that occur at several sites; also called *ringworm.* (p. 906)

**Topical antimicrobials** Substances applied to any surface that either kill microorganisms or inhibit their growth or replication. (p. 904)

**Vesicles** Small sacs containing liquid; also called *cysts.* (p. 904)

## ANATOMY, PHYSIOLOGY, AND PATHOPHYSIOLOGY OVERVIEW

The skin is the largest organ of the body. It covers the body and serves several functions, including protection, sensation, temperature regulation, excretion, absorption, and metabolism. It acts as a protective barrier for the internal organs. Without skin, harmful external agents such as microorganisms and chemicals would gain access to and damage or destroy many of our delicate internal organs. Part of this protection includes the skin's ability to maintain a surface pH of 4.5 to 5.5. This weakly acidic environment discourages the growth of microorganisms that thrive at a more alkaline pH. The skin also has the ability to sense changes in temperature (heat or cold), pressure, or pain—information that is then transmitted along nerve endings. The temperature of the environment changes continually; despite this, the body maintains an almost constant internal temperature due in large part to the skin, which plays a major role in the regulation of body temperature. Heat loss and conservation are regulated in coordination with the blood vessels that supply blood to the skin and by means of perspiration. The skin is also able to excrete fluid and electrolytes through sweat glands. In addition, it stores fat, synthesizes vitamin D, and provides a site for drug absorption.

The skin is made up of two layers: the dermis and the epidermis (Figure 56-1). The outer skin layer, or epidermis, is itself composed of four layers. From the outermost to innermost, these are the stratum corneum, stratum lucidum, stratum granulosum, and stratum germinativum. The respective functions of these layers are described in Table 56-1.

None of these layers has a direct blood supply of its own. Instead, nourishment is provided through diffusion from the dermis below. The dermis lies between the epidermis and subcutaneous fat and differs from the epidermis in many ways. It is approximately 40 times thicker than the epidermis. Traversing the dermis is a rich supply of blood vessels, nerves, lymphatic tissue, elastic tissue, and connective tissue, which provide extra support and nourishment to the skin. Also contained in the dermis are the exocrine glands—the eccrine, apocrine, and sebaceous glands—and the hair follicles. The functions of the various types of exocrine glands are explained in Table 56-2.

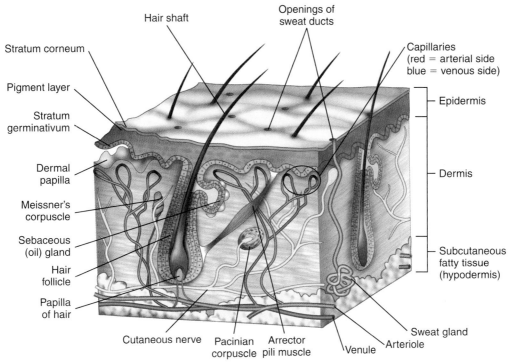

Hair shaft
Openings of
sweat ducts
Stratum corneum
Pigment layer
Stratum
germinativum
Dermal
papilla
Meissner's
corpuscle
Sebaceous
(oil) gland
Hair
follicle
Papilla
of hair
Capillaries
(red = arterial side
blue = venous side)
Epidermis
Dermis
Subcutaneous
fatty tissue
(hypodermis)
Cutaneous nerve  Pacinian
corpuscle  Arrector
pili muscle  Venule  Arteriole  Sweat gland

**FIGURE 56-1** Microscopic view of the skin. The epidermis, shown in longitudinal section, is raised at one corner to reveal the ridges in the dermis. (Modified from Thibodeau GA, Patton KT: *Anatomy and physiology,* ed 5, St Louis, 2003, Mosby.)

| TABLE 56-1 | EPIDERMAL LAYERS |
|---|---|
| **LAYER** | **DESCRIPTION** |
| Stratum corneum ("horny layer," so named because keratin is the same protein that makes up the horns of animals) | Outermost layer consisting of dead skin cells that are made of a converted water-repellant protein known as *keratin;* it is the protective layer for the entire body. After it is desquamated or shed, it is replaced by new cells from below. |
| Stratum lucidum ("clear layer") | Layer where keratin is formed; it is translucent and contains flat cells. |
| Stratum granulosum ("granular layer") | Cells die in this layer; granulated cells are located here, which gives this layer the appearance for which it is named. |
| Stratum germinativum ("germinative layer") | New skin cells are made in this layer; it contains melanocytes, which produce melanin, the skin color pigment. |

| TABLE 56-2 | EXOCRINE GLANDS OF THE SKIN |
|---|---|
| **GLAND** | **FUNCTION** |
| Sebaceous | Large lipid-containing cells that produce oil or film that covers the epidermis, protects and lubricates the skin, and is water repellent and antiseptic |
| Eccrine | Sweat glands that are located throughout the skin surface; help regulate body temperature and prevent skin dryness |
| Apocrine | Mainly in axilla, genital organs, and breast areas; emit an odor; believed to be scent or sex glands |

cancers, including basal cell carcinoma, squamous cell carcinoma, and melanoma.

## PHARMACOLOGY OVERVIEW

Drugs that are administered directly to a skin site are called *topical dermatologic drugs.* These drugs are available in a variety of formulations that are suitable for specific indications. Each formulation has certain characteristics that make it beneficial for certain uses. For example, ointments have an oil base that makes them stickier than creams and better for smaller areas, whereas creams have a water base that makes them better for larger surfaces. Gels tend to enhance penetration of the active ingredient. Lotions are similar to creams but are lighter. More information on the formulations, their characteristics, and examples are provided in Table 56-3. Note that the focus of this chapter is topically administered medications. Because so many

Below the dermis is a layer of loose connective tissue called the *hypodermis.* It helps make the skin flexible. It is also here that the subcutaneous fat tissue is located, which provides thermal insulation and cushioning or padding. It is also the source of nutrition for the skin.

Reactions or disorders of the skin are common and numerous. A dermatosis is any abnormal skin condition. Dermatoses include a variety of types of dermatitis (skin inflammation). Among these are conditions such as atopic dermatitis, eczema, and psoriasis. In addition, there are also a variety of skin

## TABLE 56-3 DERMATOLOGIC FORMULATIONS: CHARACTERISTICS AND EXAMPLES

| FORMULATION | CHARACTERISTICS | EXAMPLES |
|---|---|---|
| Aerosol foam | Can cover large area; useful for drug delivery into a body cavity (e.g., vagina, rectum) or hair areas | ProctoFoam, Epifoam, contraceptive foams |
| Aerosol spray | Spreads thin liquid or powder film; covers large areas; useful when skin is tender to touch (e.g., burns) | Solarcaine, Desenex, Kenalog |
| Bar | Similar to a bar of soap; useful as a wash with water | PanOxyl (benzoyl peroxide) |
| Cleanser | Nongreasy; used as an astringent (oil remover) and/or wash with water | ZoDerm |
| Cream | Contains water and can be removed with water; not greasy or occlusive; usually white semisolid; good for moist areas | Hydrocortisone cream (Cortaid), Benadryl cream |
| Gel/jelly | Contains water and possibly alcohol; easily removed and good lubricator; usually clear, semisolid substance; useful when lubricant properties are desirable | K-Y Jelly, Saligel, Surgilube |
| Lotion | Contains water, alcohol, and solvents; may be a suspension, emulsion, or solution; good for large or hairy areas | Calamine lotion, Lubriderm lotion, Kwell lotion |
| Oil | Contains very little if any water; occlusive, liquid; not removable with water | Lubriderm bath oil |
| Ointment | Contains no water; not removable with water; occlusive, greasy, and semisolid; desirable for dry lesions because of occlusiveness | Vaseline (petrolatum), zinc oxide ointment, A & D ointment |
| Paste | Similar properties to those of ointments; contains more powder than ointments; excellent protectant properties | Zinc oxide paste (Balmex) |
| Pledget (pad) | Moistened pad that is applied to or wiped over affected area | EryPads (erythromycin) |
| Powder | Slight lubricating properties; may be shaken on affected area; promotes drying of area where applied | Tinactin powder, Desenex powder |
| Shampoo | Soapy liquid for washing hair and/or skin | Nizoral (ketoconazole) |
| Solution | Nongreasy liquid; dries quickly | Erythromycin topical solution (Eryderm) |
| Stick | Spreads thin chalky or viscous liquid film; often better for smaller areas | Benadryl Itch Relief |
| Tape | Most occlusive formulation; consistent topical drug delivery; useful when small, straight areas require drug application | Cordran tape |

topical drugs are available, the scope of this chapter is limited to some of the more commonly used medications. Systemically administered drugs (transdermal) are also used to treat several skin disorders (see Part 7) and are cross-referenced throughout this chapter.

There are many therapeutic categories of dermatologic drugs. Some of the most common ones are the following:

- Antibacterial drugs
- Antifungal drugs
- Antiinflammatory drugs
- Antineoplastic drugs
- Antipruritic drugs (for itching)
- Antiviral drugs
- Burn drugs
- Débriding drugs (promote wound healing)
- Emollients (skin softeners)
- Keratolytics (cause softening and peeling of the stratum corneum)
- Local anesthetics
- Sunscreens
- Topical vasodilators

## ANTIMICROBIALS

Topical antimicrobials are antibacterial, antifungal, and antiviral drugs that, as the name implies, are applied topically. Although topical antimicrobials have many of the same properties as the systemic forms, there are differences in terms of their absorption, distribution, toxicities, and adverse effects.

## GENERAL ANTIBACTERIAL DRUGS

Common skin disorders caused by various bacteria are folliculitis, impetigo, furuncles, carbuncles, papules, pustules, vesicles, and cellulitis. The bacteria responsible are most commonly *Streptococcus pyogenes* and *Staphylococcus aureus*. Dermatologic antibacterial drugs are used to treat or prevent these skin infections. The most commonly used drugs are bacitracin, polymyxin, and neomycin. Unfortunately, due to the high incidence of infection with methicillin-resistant *S. aureus* (MRSA), mupirocin is now also commonly used.

## DRUG PROFILES

### ♦ bacitracin

Bacitracin is a polypeptide antibiotic that is applied topically for the treatment or prevention of local skin infections caused by susceptible aerobic and anaerobic gram-positive organisms such as staphylococci, streptococci, anaerobic cocci, corynebacteria, and clostridia. It works by inhibiting bacterial cell wall synthesis, which leads to cell death. It can be either bactericidal or bacteriostatic, depending on the causative organism. Its antimicrobial spectrum is broadened in several available combination drug products. Most of these also contain neomycin and/or polymyxin B (see later in the chapter).

Adverse reactions are usually minimal; however, reactions ranging from skin rash to allergic anaphylactoid reactions have occurred. If itching, burning, inflammation, or other signs of sensitivity occur, discontinue bacitracin. This drug is available in ointment form and is usually applied to the affected area one to three times daily. It is also available in systemic and ophthalmic (see Chapter 57) formulations.

### neomycin and polymyxin B

Neomycin and polymyxin B are two additional broad-spectrum antibiotics that are available as the nonprescription product known as Neosporin. Neosporin cream is a combination of these two drugs alone, whereas Neosporin ointment also contains bacitracin. Several brand name and generic combinations of these three topical antibiotics are available, and all are commonly used as topical antiseptics for minor skin wounds. Although neomycin/polymyxin B is still a very popular over-the-counter (OTC) product, there is evidence that use of the drug can increase the likelihood of future allergic reactions of the skin.

### mupirocin

Mupirocin (Bactroban) is an antibacterial product available only by prescription. It is used on the skin for treatment of staphylococcal and streptococcal impetigo. It is used topically and intranasally to treat nasal colonization with MRSA. The drug is applied topically three times daily and intranasally twice daily to treat MRSA colonization. Adverse reactions are usually limited to local burning, itching, or minor pain.

### ◆ silver sulfadiazine

Silver sulfadiazine (Silvadene) has proved both effective and safe in the prevention and treatment of infections in burns. A major concern for burn victims is infection at the burn site. However, because increased systemic absorption of a drug can occur in compromised skin areas, topical burn drugs must not be too potent or toxic to avoid causing dangerous systemic effects. This is especially true when larger burned areas must be treated, because the drug may be applied over a large surface area of skin and therefore may be absorbed in greater quantities. On the other hand, the blood supply to burned areas is often drastically reduced, so that systemically administered antibiotics either cannot reach the site or do so only in quantities too low to be effective. Therefore, the only way of applying these drugs to ensure that they reach the burn site is to do so topically.

Silver sulfadiazine is a synthetic antimicrobial drug produced when silver nitrate reacts with the chemical sulfadiazine. It appears to act on the cell membrane and cell wall of susceptible bacteria and is used as an adjunct in the prevention and treatment of infection in second- and third-degree burns and less frequently in cellulitic or eczematous extremities. The adverse effects of silver sulfadiazine are similar to those of other topical drugs and include pain, burning, and itching. This drug should not be used in patients who are allergic to sulfonamide drugs. It is available only as a 1% cream and is applied topically to cleansed and débrided burned areas once or twice daily using a sterile-gloved hand.

## ANTIACNE DRUGS

Acne vulgaris is the most common skin infection. Its precise cause is unknown and somewhat controversial. Likely causative factors include heredity, stress, drug reactions, hormones, and

bacterial infections. Common bacterial causes include *Staphylococcus* species (spp.) and *Propionibacterium acnes*. Some of the most commonly used antiacne drugs are benzoyl peroxide, clindamycin, erythromycin, tetracycline, isotretinoin, and the vitamin A acid known as *retinoic acid*. Many other drugs are also used in the treatment and prevention of acne, including systemic formulations of the antibiotics minocycline, doxycycline, and tetracycline (see Chapter 38). Some practitioners also prescribe oral contraceptives (see Chapter 34) for female acne patients, because in some controlled studies estrogen has been shown to have beneficial effects against acne, especially hormone-driven acne.

## DRUG PROFILES

### ◆ benzoyl peroxide

The microorganism that most commonly causes acne, *P. acnes*, is an anaerobic bacterium; that is, it needs an environment that is poor in oxygen to grow. Benzoyl peroxide is effective in combating such infection because it slowly and continuously liberates active oxygen in the skin, resulting in antibacterial, antiseptic, drying, and keratolytic actions. These actions create an environment that is unfavorable for the continued growth of the *P. acnes* bacteria, and they soon die. Drugs such as benzoyl peroxide that soften scales and loosen the outer horny layer of the skin are referred to as *keratolytics*.

Benzoyl peroxide generally produces signs of improvement within 4 to 6 weeks. Adverse effects tend to be related to dose (including overuse) and include peeling skin, red skin, or a sensation of warmth. Blistering or swelling of the skin is generally considered an allergic reaction to the product and is an indication to stop treatment. Overuse of this drug and also of tretinoin is common in teenage patients who are attempting to cure their acne quickly. The result can be painful, reddened skin, which usually resolves on return to use of these medications as prescribed.

Benzoyl peroxide is available in multiple topical dosage forms, including a cleansing bar, liquid, lotion, mask, cream, gel, and cleanser. It is also available in various combination drug products. It is usually applied topically one to four times daily, depending on the dosage form and prescriber's instructions. Benzoyl peroxide is classified as a pregnancy category C drug.

### clindamycin

Clindamycin (Cleocin T) is a topical form of the systemic antibiotic described in Chapter 39. Adverse reactions are usually limited to minor local skin reactions, including burning, itching, dryness, oiliness, and peeling. The drug is available in gel, lotion, suspension, pledgettes, and foam. Clindamycin is usually applied once or twice daily. It is classified as a pregnancy category B drug.

### ◆ isotretinoin

Isotretinoin (Amnesteem, Claravis, Sotret) is an oral product indicated for the treatment of severe recalcitrant cystic acne. Isotretinoin inhibits sebaceous gland activity and has antikeratinizing (anti–skin hardening) and antiinflammatory effects.

Isotretinoin is one of relatively few medications that are classified as pregnancy category X drugs. This means that it is a proven human *teratogen,* or a chemical that is known to induce birth defects. It is imperative that female patients of childbearing age be counseled and agree not to become pregnant during use of the drug. For these reasons, in 2005, the U.S. Food and Drug Administration (FDA) approved stringent guidelines regarding the prescription and use of this medication. It is now officially required that at least two reliable contraceptive methods be used by sexually active women during therapy with isotretinoin and for 1 month after completion of therapy. A risk management program of unprecedented size and scope has been designed and approved by the FDA especially for this drug. It is known as *iPLEDGE* and was fully implemented as of March 1, 2006. As a result, federal law now requires that any health care provider who prescribes this drug be a registered and active member of this program, and patients must also be qualified and registered. Further information is available at the iPLEDGE call center at 866-495-0654 or online at https://www.ipledgeprogram.com/default.aspx. In addition, there have been case reports of suicide and suicide attempts in patients receiving this medication. It has not been determined if the drug increases the risk for suicide or if psychosocial sequelae from severe acne are to blame for increased suicide risk. Educate patients to report any signs of depression immediately to their prescribers. Follow-up treatment may be needed, and simply stopping the drug may be insufficient. The company that produced the brand name Accutane has withdrawn it from the market. Despite these rather strong concerns, this drug does prove to be very helpful in treating severe acne cases. Isotretinoin is available only for oral use.

### tretinoin

Tretinoin (retinoic acid, vitamin A acid) (Renova, Retin-A) is a derivative of vitamin A that is used to treat acne and ameliorate the dermatologic changes (e.g., fine wrinkling, mottled hyperpigmentation, roughness) associated with photodamage (sun damage). The drug appears to act as an irritant to the skin, in particular to the follicular epithelium. Specifically, it stimulates the turnover of epidermal cells, which results in skin peeling. While this is occurring, the free fatty acid levels of the skin are reduced, and horny cells of the outer epidermis cannot then adhere to one another. Without fatty acids and horny cells, acne and its comedo, or pimple, cannot exist.

Topically administered tretinoin has been shown to enhance the repair of skin damaged by ultraviolet (UV) radiation, or sunlight. It does this by increasing the formation of fibroblasts and collagen, both of which are needed to rebuild skin. The drug also may reduce collagen degradation by inhibiting the enzyme collagenase that breaks down collagen.

Tretinoin's main adverse effects are local inflammatory reactions, which are reversible when therapy is discontinued. Common adverse effects are excessively red and edematous blisters, crusted skin, and temporary alterations in skin pigmentation. Tretinoin is available in many topical formulations, including creams, gels, and a liquid. Because of its potential to cause severe irritation and peeling, it may initially be applied once every 2 or 3 days, and treatment often starts with a lower-strength product.

Retin-A Micro has been approved for the treatment of acne vulgaris. This particular acne product contains tretinoin formulated inside a synthetic polymer called a *Microsponge system.* This system is made of round microscopic particles of synthetic polymer. These microspheres act as reservoirs for tretinoin, allowing the skin to absorb small amounts of the drug over time. Retin-A Micro is currently available only in gel form. All topical forms of tretinoin are classified as pregnancy category C drugs. They are not to be confused with the oral capsule form of tretinoin that is used to treat leukemia and is classified as a pregnancy category D drug. Another antiacne retinoid is adapalene, a topical solution.

## ANTIFUNGAL DRUGS

A few fungi produce keratinolytic enzymes, which allow them to live on the skin. Topical fungal infections are primarily caused by *Candida* spp. (candidiasis), dermatophytes, and *Malassezia furfur* (tinea versicolor). These fungi are found in moist, warm environments, especially in dark areas such as the feet or groin.

Candidal infections are most commonly caused by *Candida albicans,* a yeastlike opportunistic fungus present in the normal flora of the mouth, vagina, and intestinal tract. Two significant factors that commonly predispose a person to a candidal infection are broad-spectrum antibiotic therapy, which promotes an overgrowth of nonsusceptible organisms in the natural body flora, and immunodeficiency disorders. Because these infections favor warm, moist areas of the skin and mucous membranes, they most commonly occur orally (e.g., thrush in infants), vaginally, and cutaneously in sites such as beneath the breasts and in diapered areas. They may also cause nail infections.

Dermatophytes are a group of three closely related genera consisting of *Epidermophyton* spp., *Microsporum* spp., and *Trichophyton* spp. that use the keratin found on the skin to feed their growth. They produce superficial mycotic (fungal) infections of keratinized tissue (hair, skin, and nails). Infections caused by dermatophytes are called tinea, or *ringworm,* infections. The name *ringworm* comes from the fact that the infection sometimes assumes a circular pattern at the site of infection. Tinea infections are further identified by the body location where they occur: tinea pedis (foot), tinea cruris (groin), tinea corporis (body), and tinea capitis (scalp). Tinea infections of the foot are also known as *athlete's foot* and those of the groin as *jock itch.*

Fungi usually invade the stratum corneum, which is the dead layer of desquamated (shed) cells. Inflammation occurs when the fungi invade this layer; sensitivity (e.g., itching) occurs when they penetrate the epidermis and dermis.

Many of the fungi that cause topical infections are very difficult to eradicate. The organisms are very slow growing, and antifungal therapy may be required for periods ranging from several weeks to as long as 1 year. However, many topical antifungal drugs are available for the treatment of both dermatophytic infections and those caused by yeast and yeastlike fungi. Some of these drugs, their dosage forms, and their uses are

## TABLE 56-4   TOPICAL ANTIFUNGAL DRUGS

| DRUG | TRADE NAME | DOSAGE FORM | INDICATIONS | LEGAL STATUS |
|------|-----------|-------------|-------------|--------------|
| butenafine | Mentax, Lotrimin Ultra | 1% cream | Tinea pedis | Rx |
| butoconazole | Femstat 3 | 2% vaginal cream | Candidiasis | OTC |
| ciclopiroxolamine | Loprox | 0.77% cream and lotion, 8% solution (for nails) | Candidiasis, dermatophytoses, tinea versicolor | Rx |
| clotrimazole | Gyne-Lotrimin 3 | 2% vaginal cream, 100- and 200-mg vaginal tabs | Candidiasis | OTC |
| | Lotrimin | 2% cream, 1% lotion and solution | Candidiasis, tinea versicolor | Rx |
| | Lotrimin AF | 1% cream, lotion, and solution | Dermatophytoses | OTC |
| | Mycelex | 1% cream and solution | Dermatophytoses | Rx |
| | Mycelex | 10-mg troches | Oropharyngeal candidiasis | Rx |
| | Mycelex-7 | 1% vaginal cream, 100-mg vaginal tabs | Candidiasis | OTC |
| ketoconazole | Nizoral | 2% cream and shampoo | Candidiasis, dermatophytoses, tinea versicolor | Rx |
| miconazole | Micatin | 2% cream, powder, and spray | Dermatophytoses | OTC |
| | Monistat-Derm | 2% cream | Candidiasis, dermatophytoses, tinea versicolor | Rx |
| nystatin | Nilstat, Mycostatin | Cream, ointment, powder | Candidiasis | Rx |
| terbinafine | Lamisil | 1% cream and spray | Dermatophytoses | OTC |
| tolnaftate | Tinactin | 1% cream, solution, gel, powder, and spray | Dermatophytoses | OTC |
| undecylenic acid | Cruex, Desenex | Powder, cream, solution, soap | Dermatophytoses | OTC |

*OTC,* Available over the counter without prescription; *Rx,* currently available by prescription only.

listed in Table 56-4. Systemically administered antifungal drugs are sometimes used to treat skin conditions as well. These drugs are discussed in Chapter 42.

The most commonly reported adverse effects of topical antifungals are local irritation, pruritus, a burning sensation, and scaling. Ciclopirox and clotrimazole are classified as pregnancy category B drugs, and econazole, ketoconazole, and miconazole are classified as pregnancy category C drugs. Hypersensitivity is the one contraindication to the use of any of these drugs.

## DRUG PROFILES

### ♦ clotrimazole

Clotrimazole (Lotrimin, Mycelex-G) is available both OTC and by prescription. It is available as a lozenge for the treatment of oropharyngeal candidiasis, commonly known as *thrush*. It is also available as a cream, lotion, or solution for the treatment of dermatophytoses (e.g., athlete's foot), superficial mycoses, and cutaneous candidiasis. Similar topical preparations are available for intravaginal administration in the treatment of vulvovaginal candidiasis, commonly called a *yeast infection,* and vaginal trichomoniasis. Clotrimazole is available in many topical formulations: a powder; a 10-mg oral topical lozenge; a 1% cream, lotion, and solution; 1% and 2% vaginal creams; and 100- and 500-mg vaginal tablets. Different dosages and dosage forms are used for the treatment of different fungal infections. Clotrimazole is classified as a pregnancy category B drug.

### miconazole

Miconazole (Monistat) is a topical antifungal drug that is available in several OTC and prescription products. It inhibits the growth of several fungi, including dermatophytes and yeast, as well as gram-positive bacteria, and is commonly used to treat dermatophytoses, superficial mycoses, cutaneous candidiasis,

and vulvovaginal candidiasis. It is present in many OTC remedies for athlete's foot, jock itch, and yeast infections.

For the treatment of athlete's foot, jock itch, ringworm, and other susceptible fungal infections, miconazole is applied sparingly to the cleansed, dry, infected area twice daily in the morning and evening. For the treatment of yeast infections, one 200-mg suppository is inserted in the vagina once daily at bedtime for 3 consecutive days or 100 mg (one suppository or 5 g of the 2% cream) is administered intravaginally once daily at bedtime for 7 days. The most common adverse effects of topically administered miconazole are vulvovaginal burning and itching, pelvic cramps and rash, urticaria, stinging, and contact dermatitis. Miconazole is available in a variety of topical formulations: as a 2% aerosol spray and powder, a 2% powder, a 2% cream, a 2% vaginal cream, and a 100- and 200-mg vaginal suppository. It is also available as a 1200-mg vaginal suppository for one-time dosing. It is classified as a pregnancy category C drug.

## ANTIVIRAL DRUGS

Topical antivirals are now used less frequently than before, because systemic antiviral drug therapy has generally been shown to be superior for controlling such viral skin conditions. Nevertheless, two antiviral ointments are described here. As is the case with systemic drug therapy, these products are best used early in a viral skin lesion outbreak. Topical antivirals are more likely to be used for acute outbreaks, whereas systemic drugs are used for acute outbreaks as well as ongoing prophylaxis against outbreaks. Viral infections are very difficult to treat because they live in the body's own healthy cells and use their cell mechanisms to reproduce. The same holds true for topical viral infections. Infections caused by herpes simplex virus types 1 and 2 and human papillomavirus (which causes anogenital warts) are particularly serious and are becoming more common.

The only topical antiviral drugs currently available to treat such viral infections are acyclovir (Zovirax) and penciclovir (Denavir). They work by comparable mechanisms as described for similar antiviral drugs in Chapter 40. Acyclovir and penciclovir are available as topical ointments (5% and 1%, respectively). Acyclovir is applied every 3 hours, or six times daily, for 1 week. Penciclovir is applied every 2 hours while awake for 4 days. A finger cot or rubber glove is to be worn for the application of the ointment to prevent the spread of infection. The most common adverse effects are stinging, itching, and rash. Acyclovir is classified as a pregnancy category C drug and penciclovir as a pregnancy category B drug.

## ANESTHETIC, ANTIPRURITIC, AND ANTIPSORIATIC DRUGS

### TOPICAL ANESTHETICS

Topical anesthetics are drugs that are used to numb the skin. They accomplish this by inhibiting the conduction of nerve impulses from sensory nerves, thereby reducing or eliminating the pain or pruritus associated with insect bites, sunburn, and allergic reactions to plants such as poison ivy, as well as many other uncomfortable skin disorders. They are also used to numb the skin before a painful injection (e.g., insertion of an intravenous line in a pediatric patient). Topical anesthetics are available as ointments, creams, sprays, liquids, and jellies, and are discussed in Chapter 11. A lidocaine/prilocaine combination drug (EMLA) and lidocaine alone (Elamax) are topical anesthetic drugs that are used frequently, especially in pediatric patients. EMLA is applied 1 hour before the procedure, whereas Ela-max is effective within 30 minutes.

### TOPICAL ANTIPRURITICS AND ANTIINFLAMMATORIES

Topical antipruritic (anti-itching) drugs contain antihistamines or corticosteroids. Many exert a combined anesthetic and antipruritic action when applied topically. The antihistamines and their therapeutic effects are covered in Chapter 36. New recommendations for the use of topical antihistamines state that these drugs are not to be used to treat the following conditions because of systemic absorption and subsequent toxicity: chickenpox, widespread poison ivy lesions, and other lesions involving large body surface areas.

The most commonly used topical antiinflammatory drugs are the corticosteroids (see Chapter 33). They are generally indicated for the relief of inflammatory and pruritic dermatoses. When topically administered corticosteroids are used, many of the undesirable systemic adverse effects associated with the use of the systemically administered corticosteroids are avoided. The beneficial drug effects of topically administered corticosteroids are their antiinflammatory, antipruritic, and vasoconstrictive actions.

| TABLE 56-5 | COMMONLY USED TOPICAL CORTICOSTEROIDS (IN ORDER OF DECREASING POTENCY) |
|---|---|
| **RANGE OF POTENCY*** | **CORTICOSTEROID** |
| 1. Higher potency | Betamethasone dipropionate (cream and ointment), clobetasol propionate, halobetasol propionate, diflorasone diacetate |
| 2. Moderate potency | Amcinonide, betamethasone dipropionate (cream), betamethasone benzoate, betamethasone valerate (0.1% cream, ointment, and lotion), desoximetasone (0.05% cream), desoximetasone, fluocinolone, halcinonide, fluocinolone (cream and ointment), flurandrenolide, mometasone, triamcinolone acetonide (0.5% cream and ointment) |
| 3. Lower potency | Alclometasone, desonide, fluocinolone (0.01% solution), triamcinolone (0.1% cream, lotion), hydrocortisone, dexamethasone |

*Skin penetration and thus potency is enhanced by the vehicle (dosage form) containing the steroid. In decreasing order of effectiveness are ointments, gels, creams, and lotions.

The many different available dosage forms of the various corticosteroids vary in their relative potency, and this often guides their selection for treating various conditions. For instance, corticosteroids that are fluorinated (which increases the potency) are used for the treatment of dermatologic disorders such as psoriasis. The vehicle in which the corticosteroid is contained also may alter its vasoconstrictor properties and therapeutic efficacy. Ointments are generally the most penetrating, followed next by gels, creams, and lotions. Propylene glycol also enhances the penetration of the corticosteroid and its vasoconstrictor effects. Most corticosteroids are available in many topical formulations, which provide a variety of options. The currently available topical corticosteroids, along with their respective potencies, are listed in Table 56-5.

Adverse effects of these drugs include skin reactions such as acne eruptions, allergic contact dermatitis, burning sensations, dryness, itching, skin fragility, hypopigmentation, purpura, hirsutism (usually facial), folliculitis, round and swollen face, and alopecia (usually of the scalp). Another adverse effect is the opportunistic overgrowth of bacteria, fungi, or viruses as a result of the immunosuppressive effects of this class of drugs. *Tachyphylaxis* (weakening of drug effect over time) may also occur with these drugs, especially with long-term use or overuse. The usual adult dosage of these drugs is one or two applications daily as a thin layer over the affected area. Less potent topical corticosteroids are used in children, following the same dosing schedule. Corticosteroids are classified as pregnancy category C drugs and are contraindicated in patients with a known hypersensitivity to them. Because many of these products are available orally as well as topically, the potential exists for both to be administered simultaneously. This is not recommended and is potentially harmful. The combined use of topical and oral preparations of the same drug can lead to toxicity.

## ANTIPSORIATIC DRUGS

Psoriasis is a common skin condition in which areas of the skin become thick, reddened, and covered with silvery scales. Psoriasis is actually a result of a disordered immune system, although it is generally referred to as a skin condition. It is believed to involve *polygenic* (multigene) inheritance. Psoriasis has fluctuating patterns of recurrence and remission. Flare-ups can be triggered by changes in climate, infection, stress, excessive alcohol intake, or dry skin. Although there are many subtypes, the most classic one is known as *plaque psoriasis* and typically manifests as large, dry, erythematous scaling patches of the skin that are often white or silver on top. Commonly affected skin areas include nails, scalp, genitals, and lower back. Treatment usually begins with a topical corticosteroid for mild to moderate cases. When this therapy is not successful, topical antipsoriatic drugs are used. In addition to these topical drugs, there are also newer systemically administered antipsoriatic drugs. A thorough discussion of these drugs is beyond the scope of this chapter on topical medications, but those given by injection include etanercept (Enbrel), which is given subcutaneously, and alefacept (Amevive), which is given intramuscularly. Another drug, efalizumab (Raptiva), was withdrawn from the U.S. market in 2009. Etanercept is discussed in more detail in Chapter 47 on biologic response modifiers. In addition, the antineoplastic drug methotrexate (see Chapter 45) is also used for its antipsoriatic properties. The newest injectable drug, ustekinumab (Stelara), is an interleukin 12 inhibitor and is indicated for plaque psoriasis. It is given subcutaneously. Patients must receive an FDA-approved patient medication guide when receiving ustekinumab. The most serious side effect is increased risk of infection.

## DRUG PROFILES

### tazarotene

Tazarotene is a receptor-selective retinoid. It is thought to normalize epidermal differentiation, reducing the influx of inflammatory cells into the skin. Synthetic retinoids are vitamin A analogues and are thought to play a role in skin cell differentiation and proliferation. Tazarotene is available in gel form and is approved for the treatment of stable plaque psoriasis and mild to moderately severe facial acne. Like isotretinoin, tazarotene is classified as a pregnancy category X drug, and a negative pregnancy test 2 weeks before starting therapy is required for female patients.

### tar-containing products

Drug products containing coal tar derivatives were among the first medications used to treat psoriasis and are still used today for this purpose. Tar derivatives are known to have antiseptic, antibacterial, and antiseborrheic properties, and they work to soften and loosen scaly or crusty areas of the skin. *Seborrhea* is excessive secretion of *sebum*, a normal skin secretion containing fat and epithelial cell debris. Tar-containing products are available in a variety of shampoo forms (for scalp psoriasis), as well as solution, oil, ointment, cream, lotion, gel, and even soap forms for bathing. These products typically contain 1% to 10% coal tar. Adverse reactions usually include minor skin burning, photosensitivity, and other irritations. These products may be applied from one to four times daily or once or twice weekly as prescribed.

### anthralin

Anthralin (Anthra-Derm) is a unique drug that is thought to work by inhibition of deoxyribonucleic acid (DNA) synthesis and mitosis within the epidermis to reduce psoriatic lesions. It is available in ointment and cream form and is usually applied once daily. Adverse reactions are generally limited to minor skin irritation. Anthralin is classified as a pregnancy category C drug.

### calcipotriene

Calcipotriene (Dovonex) is a synthetic vitamin $D_3$ analogue that works by binding to vitamin $D_3$ receptors in skin cells known as *keratinocytes,* the abnormal growth of which contributes to psoriatic lesions. Calcipotriene helps to regulate the growth and reproduction of keratinocytes. The most common adverse reaction is minor skin irritation. However, more serious reactions can occur in some cases, including worsening of psoriasis, dermatitis, skin atrophy, and folliculitis. Calcipotriene is usually applied twice daily. It is classified as a pregnancy category C drug. Taclonex is a combination product containing calcipotriene and betamethasone, a topical steroid.

## MISCELLANEOUS DERMATOLOGIC DRUGS

There are many other topically applied drugs. Those discussed in this section are the topical ectoparasiticides (scabicides and pediculicides), hair growth drugs, sunscreens, antineoplastics, and immunomodulating drugs. Many of these drugs are available both OTC and by prescription. Aloe vera herbal preparations (see the Safety: Herbal Therapies and Dietary Supplements box) are also available OTC.

 **SAFETY: HERBAL THERAPIES AND DIETARY SUPPLEMENTS**

### *Aloe* (Aloe vera L.)

**Overview**
The dried juice of the leaves of the aloe plant contains anthranoids, which give aloe a laxative effect when taken orally. The topical application of the plant juice has been known for years to help aid in wound healing.

**Common Uses**
Wound healing, constipation

**Adverse Effects**
Diarrhea, nephritis, abdominal pain, dermatitis when used topically

**Potential Drug Interactions**
Digoxin, antidysrhythmics, diuretics, corticosteroids

**Contraindications**
Contraindicated in patients who are menstruating or have renal disease; can increase menstrual blood flow and also cause acute renal failure

# DRUG PROFILES

## ECTOPARASITICIDAL DRUGS

Ectoparasites are insects that live on the outer surface of the body, and the drugs that are used to kill them are called *ectoparasiticidal drugs*. Lice are transmitted from person to person by close contact with infested individuals, clothing, combs, or towels. A parasitic infestation on the skin with lice is called pediculosis, and such infestations go by one of the following three names, depending on the location of the infestation:

- Pediculosis pubis—pubic louse or "crabs"; infestation by *Phthirus pubis*
- Pediculosis corporis—body louse; infestation by *Pediculus humanus corporis*
- Pediculosis capitis—head louse; infestation by *Pediculus humanus capitis*

Common findings in infested persons include itching; eggs of the lice attached to hair shafts (called *nits*); lice on the skin or clothes; and, in the case of pubic lice, sky blue macules (discolored skin patches) on the inner thighs or lower abdomen. Pediculoses are treated with a class of drugs called pediculicides. A second common parasitic skin infection known as scabies is that caused by the itch mite *Sarcoptes scabiei*. Scabies is transmitted from person to person by close contact, such as by sleeping next to an infested person. The scabies mite causes irritation and itching by boring into the horny layers of skin located in cracks and folds. Itching seems to occur most commonly in the evening. The drugs used to treat these infestations are called *scabicides*.

Treatment of these parasitic infestations begins with identification of the source of infestation to prevent re-infestation. Next, the clothing and personal articles of the infested person must be decontaminated. This is best accomplished by washing them in hot, soapy water or by dry cleaning them. All close contacts of the person also need to be treated to prevent re-infestation.

In addition to lindane (see profile), malathion (Ovide) and crotamiton (Eurax) are also ectoparasiticidal drugs. The newest drugs approved for lice treatment are benzyl alcohol 5% (Ulesfia), which works by suffocating the lice, and spinosad (Natroba). Natroba is indicated for children 4 years of age and older and offers the benefit of not requiring nit combing as do the other treatments.

### ◆ lindane

Lindane (Kwell) is a chlorinated hydrocarbon originally developed as an agricultural insecticide. It is both a scabicide and a pediculicide because it is effective in treating both scabies and pediculosis. High resistance rates to lindane and malathion have limited its use. It is available in two topical formulations: a 1% lotion and a 1% shampoo.

For the treatment of pubic or body lice, the cream or lotion is applied in a sufficient quantity to cover the skin and hair of the infested and surrounding areas. It is left on for 12 hours and then thoroughly washed off. A second application is seldom needed. Head lice can be treated with lindane shampoo, which is worked into the hair and left on for 4 minutes. The hair is then rinsed and dried, after which the nits (eggs) are combed

from the hair shafts. The treatment for scabies is similar. It involves the application of lindane over the entire body, from the neck down. It is left on for 8 to 12 hours and then washed off. A similar second application 1 week later is often recommended. The OTC products are applied in similar fashion, although details may vary among individual products. Adverse effects of lindane are an eczematous skin rash and central nervous system toxicity. The latter is more common in young children and in cases of overuse. For many years, lindane was the most widely used pediculicide, but it has been superseded to some degree by permethrin. This is because of case reports of neurotoxicity, including dizziness, seizures, and deaths, caused by lindane. Most of the adverse events occurred due to product misuse (e.g., ingestion) or overuse. Children are at higher risk of neurotoxicity because their skin surface area is larger in relation to body weight. Lindane is still recommended as second-line therapy for lice and scabies after failure of one of the OTC preparations. However, the FDA has recommended that it be sold in smaller containers (1 to 2 oz) with definitive patient instructions on proper use.

## HAIR GROWTH DRUGS

### minoxidil

Minoxidil (Rogaine) is a vasodilating drug that is administered systemically to control hypertension (see Chapter 22). Topically it has the same vasodilating effect, but when used in this way it is applied to the scalp to stimulate hair growth. The vasodilation it causes is one possible explanation for how it promotes hair growth. It may also act at the level of the hair follicle, possibly stimulating hair follicle growth directly.

Minoxidil can be used by both men and women who experience baldness or hair thinning. Treatment involves administering the drug to the affected areas (those with balding and anticipated balding) twice daily, usually morning and evening. It generally takes 4 months before results are seen. Systemic absorption of topically applied minoxidil may occur with possible adverse effects, including tachycardia, fluid retention, and weight gain. Local effects may include skin irritation, and the drug is not to be applied to skin that is already irritated, nor used concurrently with other topical medications applied to the same site. Minoxidil is classified as a pregnancy category C drug. Note that the beneficial effects of this drug can be reduced by heat, including the use of a blow dryer.

The systemically administered drug finasteride (Proscar, 5 mg) is used to treat benign prostatic hyperplasia, as discussed in Chapter 35. A lower-strength version known as Propecia (1 mg) is also used to treat male pattern alopecia. Finasteride is classified as a pregnancy category X drug, and women are not to handle this drug without gloves or crush this drug, thereby making it airborne.

## SUNSCREENS

Sunscreens are topical products used to protect the skin from damage caused by the UV radiation of sunlight. There are currently nearly 160 specific sunscreen products on the market. None requires a prescription for use. Each is composed of typically three to five various chemical ingredients that work together to provide UV protection and, usually, a moisturizing effect as well. Common examples of these ingredients are titanium dioxide, octyl methoxycinnamate, homosalate, and parabens. Sunscreens are given a sun protection factor (SPF) rating, which is a number ranging from 2 to 50 (and even higher in some newer products) in order of increasing potency of UV protection. In 2011, the FDA stated that only those with SPF of 15 or greater may state they reduce the risk of skin cancer and early skin aging. Most sunscreens come in lotion, cream, or gel form. A smaller number of lip balms are also available. It is important for sunscreens to have both UVA and UVB protection. Sunscreen is not to be used on infants.

## ANTINEOPLASTIC DRUGS

Skin cancer is the most common form of cancer. There are two types of nonmelanoma skin cancer: basal cell carcinoma and squamous cell carcinoma. Basal cell carcinoma is the most common and is rarely fatal, but it can be highly disfiguring. Squamous cell carcinoma, on the other hand, can be fatal, with 2500 deaths reported annually. The most aggressive skin cancer is melanoma and accounts for only 3% of all skin cancers but is responsible for 75% of deaths associated with skin cancer. The most common cause of skin cancer is exposure to the sun and tanning beds. Early detection and prevention (with the use of sunscreen) are of the utmost importance.

### fluorouracil

Various premalignant skin lesions and basal cell carcinomas may be treated with the topically applied antineoplastic drug fluorouracil (Efudex). As noted in Chapter 45, this drug is an antimetabolite that acts by interfering with key cellular metabolic reactions, destroying rapidly growing cells, such as premalignant and malignant cells. It is also used topically in the treatment of solar or actinic keratosis and superficial basal cell carcinomas of the skin—often in addition to local surgical excision. More aggressive skin cancers *(squamous cell carcinoma and malignant melanoma)* are not treated with fluorouracil but are usually treated with more aggressive interventions, such as surgery, radiation therapy, and/or systemic chemotherapy (see Chapters 45 and 46).

The adverse effects associated with the topical use of this antineoplastic drug are generally limited to local inflammatory reactions such as dermatitis, stomatitis, and photosensitivity. More serious effects include swelling, scaling, pain, pruritus, burning, soreness, tenderness, suppuration, scarring, and hyperpigmentation.

Fluorouracil is available in both cream and solution form. It can be applied with a nonmetallic applicator, clean fingertips, or gloved fingers. If the fingers are used, they need to be washed thoroughly immediately after application. Either a 1% or 2% fluorouracil solution is used for the treatment of multiple actinic keratoses of the head and neck. The solution is applied twice daily to the lesions. Superficial basal cell carcinoma may be treated with 5% fluorouracil, administered twice daily for at least 2 to 6 weeks. Another topical drug also used for the treatment of actinic keratoses and basal cell carcinomas is the immunomodulator imiquimod, discussed in the following section.

## IMMUNOMODULATORS

### ◆ pimecrolimus

Pimecrolimus (Elidel) is available in a cream form for use in treating atopic dermatitis. Atopic dermatitis is caused by a hereditary susceptibility to pruritus and is often associated with allergic rhinitis, hay fever, and asthma. This drug works through a mechanism similar to that of the anti–transplant-rejection drug tacrolimus (Prograf), which was discussed in Chapter 48. A topical form of tacrolimus (Protopic) is also used and has similar actions and indications. Adverse reactions to both drugs are usually limited to minor skin irritations.

### imiquimod

Imiquimod (Aldara) is an immunomodulating drug that has demonstrated efficacy in treating actinic keratosis, superficial basal cell carcinoma, and anogenital warts. Its exact mechanism of action is unknown, but it is believed somehow to enhance the body's immune response to these conditions. It is applied two to five times per week, as prescribed, depending on the condition being treated. Adverse reactions include mild skin reactions such as burning, induration (hardness), irritation, pain, and bleeding, which can occur both locally (at the site of medication administration) and at skin areas remote from the site of administration. More severe adverse skin reactions include edema, erosion or ulceration, scaling, scabbing, exudation, and vesicle formation. Systemic reactions, likely related to systemic immunomodulating effects, include cough, upper respiratory tract infection, musculoskeletal reactions (e.g., back pain), and lymphadenopathy. This drug is available only in cream form.

## WOUND CARE DRUGS

Although superficial skin wounds usually require minimal interventions, deeper skin wounds often require more definitive care for optimal healing. Such care includes addressing the systemic issues (e.g., body nutritional status) that are critical to tissue repair. Vitamin C (ascorbic acid) and zinc have been shown to improve wound healing when they are given orally. Topical wound care medications are one of the fundamental steps of wound care, referred to in the literature as *preparation of the wound bed*. Wound *débridement* is removal of nonviable tissue and elimination of bacteria by suitable cleansing or surgical intervention. Until 2009, drugs containing papain or papain/urea were commonly used as topical débriding drugs. However, the FDA no longer allows these drugs to be manufactured, because they never received FDA approval. Table 56-6 provides information regarding selected currently available wound care medications.

## SKIN PREPARATION DRUGS

The skin must be disinfected before any invasive procedure. Isopropyl alcohol (70%) is most commonly used to prepare the skin before minor procedures such as drawing blood or giving injections. Isopropyl alcohol has been shown to lower the bacterial count for 20 to 40 minutes after application. Other drugs that are used to prepare the skin include povidone-iodine (Betadine), chlorhexidine (Hibiclens), and benzalkonium chloride (Zephiran). Benzalkonium chloride is a surface-active

## TABLE 56-6 SELECTED WOUND CARE PRODUCTS

| PRODUCT NAME | ADVANTAGES | DISADVANTAGES | CONTRAINDICATIONS |
|---|---|---|---|
| acetic acid (vinegar) | Low cost | Cytotoxic | Allergy |
| sodium hypochlorite (Dakin's bleach solution, ¼%, ½%, 1%) | Aids débridement; reduces microbial count | Partly toxic and irritating to healing tissue | Clean, noninfected wounds |
| cadexomer iodine (Iodosorb, others) | Slow release; safe for viable cells; absorbs exudates; promotes wound healing | Partly toxic to fibroblast cells; stains tissue | Iodine allergy |
| collagenase (Santyl) | Good for patients taking anticoagulants or in whom surgery is contraindicated; selectively removes necrotic tissue; does not harm normal tissue; Okay for infected wounds | Requires prescriber's order; not for use with other common wound products such as silver sulfadiazine (Silvadene) or Dakin's solution; expensive | Clean wounds with granulation tissue and signs of healing but with limited areas of necrosis; product allergy |
| biafine topical emulsion | Can be used for "tunneling" wounds as well as full-thickness wounds and radiation dermatitis | Must not be applied within 4 hr of radiation therapy | Bleeding wounds, skin rashes related to food or drug allergies |

## TABLE 56-7 SKIN PREPARATION DRUGS

| DRUG | EFFECTIVE AGAINST | ADVERSE EFFECTS |
|---|---|---|
| isopropyl alcohol | Bacteria, fungi, virus | Excessive dryness of skin |
| chlorhexidine (Hibiclens) | Bacteria, fungi | Central nervous system toxicity in neonates and burn patients |
| povidone-iodine (Betadine) | Bacteria, fungi, virus | Staining of skin, irritation and pain at wound sites; retards or reverses the granulation process |
| benzalkonium chloride (Zephiran) | Bacteria, fungi | Chemical burns if left in contact with skin for too long |

drug that works by denaturing the microorganism or essentially destroying its protein. Chlorhexidine acts by disrupting bacterial membranes and inhibiting cell wall synthesis. It is used primarily as a surgical scrub or hand-washing agent by health care professionals. Povidone-iodine is an antiseptic that kills bacteria, fungi, and viruses. It is used for the prevention or treatment of topical infections associated with surgery, burns, and minor cuts and scrapes, and for relief of minor vaginal infections. It is the most widely used antiseptic, but patients should be screened for iodine or shellfish allergies before using it. It is available in many different dosage forms. See Table 56-7 for more information on selected skin preparation drugs.

## NURSING PROCESS

### ASSESSMENT

Before administering any *dermatologic preparation,* assess the patient for any allergies (including allergies to all drug ingredients), contraindications, cautions, and drug interaction. Topical antibacterials are associated with a wide range of reactions because of the generalized sensitivity of patients to antibiotics, even when in a different dosage form; therefore, if a patient is allergic to a systemic antibacterial, he or she will also be allergic to topical dosage forms. Assess the results of any culture and sensitivity testing that was ordered before giving the antibacterial to ensure appropriate identification of effective drugs. Before administering any type of topical medication (e.g., antimicrobial, corticosteroid, antiacne drug), always consider the concentration of the medication, length of exposure to the skin, condition of the skin, size of the affected area, and hydration of the skin. All of these factors have a significant influence on the action of the medication. Additionally, assess the medication order for not only the correct drug but also the prescribed route. Inspect the skin or affected area thoroughly under an adequate light source. Palpate the area with a gloved hand. In dark-skinned patients, an erythematous area may not be visible but may be palpated as an area of warmth. Accompany physical assessment of the skin with an assessment and documentation of surrounding structures, including lymph nodes.

Assess the patient's overall health status and hygiene practices, including whether the patient has experienced any trauma and whether there is any history of immunosuppression. Remember that the skin of very young and elderly patients is more fragile and permeable to certain topical dermatologic preparations. These characteristics also lead to a higher risk for systemic absorption from the skin. It is also important to note other possible situations that may result in a drug effect that is less than therapeutic, such as the use of topical drugs over an area that is full of pus or debris. The use of herbal products, such as topical aloe vera, also requires thorough assessment and notation of any allergies, contraindications, cautions, and drug interactions (see the Safety: Herbal Therapies and Dietary Supplements box on p. 909).

### NURSING DIAGNOSES

1. Impaired skin integrity related to specific diseases, reactions, conditions, or breaks in the skin barrier
2. Deficient knowledge related to lack of experience with and exposure to use of topical drugs

3. Noncompliance related to lack of experience taking or applying medication and maintaining frequent dosing

## PLANNING

### GOALS

1. Patient's skin remains intact and healed in appearance, and skin integrity is maintained.
2. Patient demonstrates adequate knowledge about the use of the medication.
3. Patient remains compliant as related to the drug regimen.

### OUTCOME CRITERIA

1. Patient's skin improves daily as stated by the patient, with less redness, drainage, discomfort, itching, and/or rash.
2. Patient states the rationale for treatment, adverse effects of the specific dermatologic preparation, and symptoms associated with the dermatologic therapy that are to be reported to the prescriber.
   - Patient demonstrates how to apply the medication in keeping with the prescriber's orders, with specific attention to the requirements for emollient, lotion, solution, spray, cream, and ointment dosage forms.

3. Patient experiences improvement in the condition of affected area(s) with continued compliance to the medication regimen.
   - Patient applies or self-administers the medication regimen with frequent dosing, as prescribed or directed.

## IMPLEMENTATION

Generally speaking, before any *topical medication* is applied, cleanse the affected area of any debris, drainage, and/or residual medication, taking care to follow any specific directions such as removing water- or alcohol-based topical preparations with soap and water. Always begin (and end) by performing hand hygiene and maintain Standard Precautions (see Box 9-1). Store all dosage forms of medication as recommended. Wear gloves, not only to prevent contamination from secretions but also to prevent absorption of the medication through the skin. Applying topical drug using a gloved hand, tongue depressor, or cotton-tipped applicator is recommended. Shake or mix lotions and solutions thoroughly before use, and apply evenly (see Chapter 9). Wash hands before and after application of the medication. Apply any dressings as ordered, paying special attention to directions concerning occlusive, wet, or wet-to-dry dressing changes. It is important to note, however, that most topical dermatologic drugs do not require use of a dressing once the medication is applied. The medication order may also state that any type of dressing or coverage of the affected area is to be avoided. When medications are used for wound care, there is usually a step-by-step protocol for application of a cleansing agent, possible débridement drug, and rinsing solution, as well as final application of an antibacterial, antifungal, burn, antiseptic, or other solution that may have been ordered. Provide comprehensive patient education regarding wound care and/or use of topical dermatologic drugs to ensure effective and safe treatment. If home health care is needed after discharge, arrangements need to be in place before the patient returns home. Document information about the site of drug application, including drainage (color and amount), swelling, temperature, odor, color, and pain or other sensations, as well as the type of treatment rendered and the response, with each treatment or application, and record a comparative before-and-after assessment.

Follow the manufacturer's guidelines regarding the use of any of the dermatologic preparations because each medication has a different type of base solution. Specific application procedures may be required for different dosage forms. It is also important to follow any instructions or orders regarding other treatments to the affected area, such as the use of an occlusive or wet dressing (see earlier in the chapter). Medicated areas may also need to be protected from exposure to air or sunlight. Strict adherence to the proper method of application and dosage of any dermatologic preparation is important to its effectiveness. Doubling up of a missed dose is not recommended. After the medication administration process is complete, dispose of all contaminated dressings, gloves, or equipment properly. Maintain safety, comfort, and privacy of the patient at all times. See the Patient Teaching Tips for more information. Also see

Table 56-6 for information about specific drugs for wound care and their advantages and disadvantages.

# EVALUATION

Begin the evaluation by monitoring to ensure that goals and outcome criteria are being met. Therapeutic responses to the various *dermatologic preparations* include improved condition of the skin and healing of lesions or wounds; a decrease in the size of lesions with eventual resolution; and a decrease in swelling, redness, weeping, itching, and burning of the area.

Notify the prescriber if a therapeutic response is not observed within an appropriate time (anywhere from 48 to 72 hours or longer, depending on the drug, disorder or skin problem, and acute or chronic nature of the condition) or if signs and symptoms worsen or new ones appear. Adverse effects for which to evaluate include increased severity of symptoms—for example, increased redness, swelling, pain, and drainage; fever; or any other unusual problems at the affected area. Adverse effects may range from slight irritation of the site where the topical drug has been applied to an allergic reaction to toxic systemic effects.

# PATIENT TEACHING TIPS

- Advise the patient to keep the skin clean and dry or clean and moist as prescribed. Provide instructions to the patient and caregivers about maintaining adequate general hygiene, cleanliness, adequate hydration, and proper nutrition during drug therapy.
- Ensure that the patient has a full understanding on how to prepare the skin for application of the medication and any other instructions.
- Apply dressings to the affected area as directed, if indicated or ordered. Perform dressing application after medication use, and properly dispose of contaminated dressings or equipment. Emphasize the need for thorough hand washing before and after application of medication with a gloved hand, cotton-tipped applicator, or tongue depressor. Demonstrate to all individuals involved in the care of the patient. Always emphasize the importance of compliance with the drug regimen.
- Encourage the patient to notify the prescriber if any unusual or adverse reactions occur or if the original condition worsens or fails to improve within a designated period of time.
- Counsel all female patients of childbearing age regarding the birth defect hazards associated with exposure to certain dermatologic drugs. All sexually active women must use contraception during treatment with any teratogenic medication and for at least 1 month after its discontinuation.
- Educate the patient about ways to prevent exposure to the sun through the use of sunscreen and protective clothing, and avoidance of overexposure. Tanning beds create risk for skin cancer as well, so share with the patient appropriate and accurate information regarding their use and risk. Sunscreen must also be used with tanning beds.
- Vitamin D deficiency may be an issue for some sunscreen users and those who live at higher latitudes or are not exposed to sunlight. As adequate oral intake is difficult to achieve without supplementation, many people with minimal exposure to sunlight do not activate vitamin D and are deficient.
- Assess all skin moles or lesions, and monitor for any unusual changes in color, size, texture, and/or shape.
- Adverse effects of lindane (for lice) include skin rash and, rarely, central nervous system toxicity. Lindane's use has been surpassed to some degree by perethrin because of case reports of neurotoxicity, including dizziness, seizures, and deaths. Make sure parents or caregivers understand all instructions regarding this drug's use, application, and cautions/concerns.

# KEY POINTS

- Dermatologic drugs are used to treat topical infections.
- Common skin disorders caused by bacteria are folliculitis, impetigo, furuncles, carbuncles, and cellulitis.
- The bacterium most commonly responsible for acne is *P. acnes.*
- The fungi that are responsible for causing topical fungal infections are *Candida,* dermatophytes, and *M. furfur.*
- The most common topical fungal infections are *Candida* infections; for example, yeast infections.
- One of the most common topical viral infections is infection with herpes simplex virus types 1 and 2.
- Topical anesthetics are used therapeutically to numb the skin. Indications for topical anesthetics include insect bites, sunburn, poison ivy, and prevention of pain from injections.
- Corticosteroids are some of the most widely used topical drugs and are indicated for relief of topical inflammatory and pruritic disorders.
- Beneficial effects of corticosteroids include antiinflammatory, antipruritic, and vasoconstrictor actions. Some of the negative effects of potent corticosteroid use or prolonged use of weaker corticosteroids include dermal atrophy and adrenal insufficiency.
- Adverse and toxic reactions to dermatologic drugs can and do occur; therefore, administer these drugs cautiously, and follow the prescriber's orders and manufacturer's guidelines. This is critical to ensure safe and effective treatment.
- Patient education about the medication, its administration, and its effectiveness are important to ensure compliance with the treatment regimen.

# NCLEX® EXAMINATION REVIEW QUESTIONS

1 The nurse is assessing the skin of a teenage patient who has been using a benzoyl peroxide product for 2 weeks as part of treatment for acne. Which assessment findings indicate that the patient is having an allergic reaction and will need to stop treatment?
   a Reddened skin over the treatment area
   b Blistering skin over the treatment area
   c Peeling skin over the treatment area
   d Sensation of warmth when the product is applied

2 When considering the variety of OTC topical corticosteroid products, the nurse is aware that which type of preparation is generally most penetrating and effective?
   a Gel
   b Lotion
   c Spray
   d Ointment

3 The nurse is monitoring for an allergic reaction to topical bacitracin, which would be evident by presence of
   a petechia.
   b thickened skin.
   c itching and burning.
   d purulent drainage.

4 When the nurse is teaching a patient about the mechanism of action of tretinoin, which statement by the nurse is correct?
   a "This medication acts by killing the bacteria that cause acne."
   b "This medication actually causes skin peeling."
   c "This medication acts by protecting your skin from UV sunlight."
   d "This medication has antiinflammatory actions."

5 When the nurse is providing wound care with Dakin's solution for a patient who has a stage III pressure ulcer, the patient exclaims, "I smell bleach! Why are you putting bleach on me?" The nurse's best explanation is:
   a "This is a very dilute solution and acts to reduce the bacteria in the wound so that it can heal."
   b "This solution is used instead of medication to promote wound healing."
   c "This solution is used to dissolve the dead tissue in your wound."
   d "Don't worry; we would never use bleach on a patient!"

6 The nurse is instructing a parent on the use of lindane (Kwell) shampoo for treatment of a child's head lice. Which statement by the parent indicates a need for further education?
   a "I will wash his hair, then rinse out the shampoo immediately."
   b "I will leave the shampoo on his hair for 4 minutes before rinsing."
   c "After shampooing, I will rinse and dry his hair."
   d "When the hair is dry, I will comb the hair to remove the nits."

7 The nurse is performing wound care on a burned area using silver sulfadiazine cream in a patient with an arm wound. Which actions by the nurse are correct? (Select all that apply.)
   a Applying the cream over the previous layer to avoid disturbing the wound bed
   b Gently cleansing the wound to remove the previous layer of cream and wound debris
   c Using clean gloves to apply the ointment
   d Using sterile gloves to apply the ointment
   e Always covering the wound with a dressing after applying the cream
   f Washing hands before and after the procedure

1. b, 2. d, 3. c, 4. b, 5. a, 6. a, 7. b, d, f

For Critical Thinking and Prioritization Questions, see http://evolve.elsevier.com/Lilley.

- Animations
- Answer Key—Textbook Case Studies
- Critical Thinking and Prioritization Questions
- Key Points—Downloadable
- Review Questions for the NCLEX® Examination
- Unfolding Case Studies

## OBJECTIVES

When you reach the end of this chapter, you will be able to do the following:

1. Discuss the anatomy and physiology of the structures of the eye and the impact of glaucoma and other disorders and disease processes on these structures.
2. List the various classifications of ophthalmic drugs, with examples of specific drugs in each class.
3. Discuss the mechanisms of action, indications, dosage forms with application techniques, adverse effects, cautions, contraindications, and drug interactions of the various ophthalmic drugs.
4. Develop a nursing care plan that includes all phases of the nursing process for patients receiving ophthalmic drugs.

## DRUG PROFILES

acetylcholine, p. 923
apraclonidine, p. 924
- artificial tears, p. 933
- atropine sulfate, p. 933
- bacitracin, p. 930
- betaxolol, p. 925
- ciprofloxacin, p. 930
cromolyn, p. 933
cyclopentolate, p. 933
- dexamethasone, p. 932
- dipivefrin, p. 925
- dorzolamide, p. 926
- echothiophate p. 923
- erythromycin, p. 929
fluorescein, p. 933
flurbiprofen, p. 932

- gentamicin, p. 929
glycerin, p. 927
ketorolac, p. 932
- latanoprost, p. 928
mannitol, p. 927
natamycin, p. 931
olopatadine, p. 933
- pilocarpine, p. 923
- sulfacetamide, p. 931
tetracaine, p. 933
tetrahydrozoline, p. 933
- timolol, p. 926
trifluridine p. 931

---

- *Key drug*

# KEY TERMS

**Accommodation** The adjustment of the lens of the eye for variations in distance. (p. 919)

**Angle-closure glaucoma** Glaucoma that occurs as a result of a narrowed anatomic angle between the lens and cornea. Also called *closed-angle glaucoma, narrow-angle glaucoma, congestive glaucoma,* and *pupillary closure glaucoma.* (p. 920)

**Anterior chamber** The bubble-like portion of the front of the eye between the iris and the cornea. (p. 919)

**Aqueous humor** The clear, watery fluid circulating in the *anterior* and *posterior chambers* of the eye. (p. 919)

**Canal of Schlemm** A tiny circular vein at the angle of the anterior chamber of the eye through which the aqueous humor is drained and ultimately funneled into the bloodstream. Also called *Schlemm canal.* (p. 919)

**Cataract** An abnormal progressive condition of the lens of the eye, characterized by loss of transparency with resultant blurred vision. (p. 919)

**Ciliary muscle** The circular muscle between the anterior and posterior chambers of the eye behind the iris. It is connected to the suspensory ligaments that control the curvature of the lens. (p. 919)

**Cones** Photoreceptive (light-receiving) cells in the retina of the eye that enable a person to perceive colors and play a large role in central (straight-ahead) vision. (p. 920)

**Cornea** The convex, transparent anterior part of the eye. (p. 919)

**Cycloplegia** Paralysis of the ciliary muscles, which prevents the accommodation of the lens for variations in distance. (p. 919)

**Cycloplegics** Drugs that paralyze the ciliary muscles of the eye. (p. 919)

**Dilator muscle** A muscle that constricts the iris of the eye but dilates the pupil. Also called *dilator pupillae.* (p. 919)

**Glaucoma** An abnormal condition of elevated pressure within an eye because of obstruction of the outflow of aqueous humor. (p. 920)

**Intraocular pressure** The pressure of the fluids of the eye against the tunics (retina, choroid, and sclera). (p. 919)

**Iris** The round, muscular portion of the eye that gives the eye its color and serves as an aperture controlling the amount of light passing through the pupil. (p. 919)

**Lacrimal ducts** Small tubes that drain tears from the lacrimal glands into the nasal cavity. (p. 919)

**Lacrimal glands** Glands located at the medial corners of the eyelids that produce tears. (p. 919)

**Lens** The transparent, curved structure of the eye that is located directly behind the iris and the pupil and is attached to the ciliary body by ligaments. (p. 919)

**Lysozyme** An enzyme with antiseptic actions that destroys some foreign organisms. It is normally present in tears, saliva, sweat, and breast milk. (p. 919)

**Miotics** Drugs that constrict the pupil. (p. 919)

**Mydriatics** Drugs that dilate the pupil. (p. 919)

**Open-angle glaucoma** A type of glaucoma that is often bilateral, develops slowly, is genetically determined, and does not involve a narrowing of the angle between the iris and the cornea. (Also called *chronic glaucoma, wide-angle glaucoma,* and *simple glaucoma.*) (p. 920)

**Optic nerve** A major nerve that connects the posterior end of each eye to the brain, to which it transmits visual signals. (p. 920)

**Pupil** A circular opening in the iris of the eye, located slightly to the nasal side of the center of the iris. The pupil lies behind the anterior chamber of the eye and the cornea and in front of the lens. (p. 919)

**Retina** The innermost layer of the eye, containing both rods and cones that receive visual stimuli and transmit them to the optic nerve. (p. 920)

**Rods** The photoreceptive elements arranged perpendicularly to the surface of the retina. Rods are especially sensitive to low-intensity light and are responsible for black-and-white and peripheral ("off-to-the-side") vision. (p. 920)

**Sphincter pupillae** A muscle that expands the iris while constricting or narrowing the diameter of the pupil. (p. 919)

**Tears** Watery saline or alkaline fluid secreted by the lacrimal glands to moisten the conjunctiva (see Figure 57-1). (p. 919)

**Uvea** The fibrous tunic beneath the sclera that includes the iris, the ciliary body, and the choroid of the eye (see Figure 57-1). Also called *tunica vasculosa bulbi* or *uveal tract.* (p. 919)

**Vitreous body** A transparent, semigelatinous substance contained in a thin membrane filling the cavity behind the lens. Also called the *corpus vitreum.* (p. 919)

**Vitreous humor** The fluid component of the vitreous body. (p. 919)

## ANATOMY, PHYSIOLOGY, AND PATHOPHYSIOLOGY OVERVIEW

The eye is the organ responsible for the sense of sight. The structures of the eye are illustrated in Figure 57-1. Each eyeball is nearly spherical and approximately 1 inch in diameter. Each eye is recessed into a small frontal skull cavity known as an *orbit.* The exposed anterior (front) portion of the eye is covered by three layers: the protective external layer (cornea and sclera), a vascular middle layer known as the *uvea* (includes the choroid, iris, and ciliary body), and the internal layer, known as the *retina.* All of these layers are protected by the eyelid, which serves as an external protective tissue.

Each eye is held in place and moved by six muscles that are controlled by cranial nerves. These muscles include the rectus and oblique muscles. There are four types of rectus

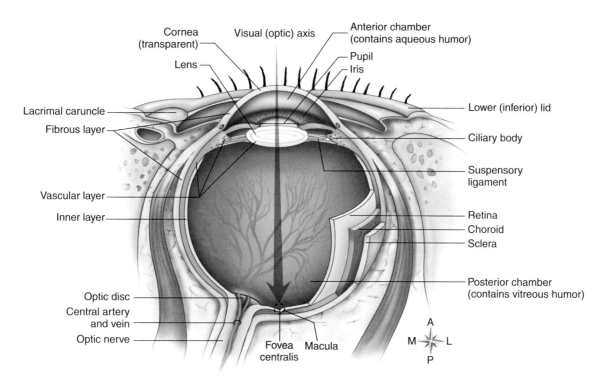

**FIGURE 57-1** Horizontal section through the left eyeball, looking from the top down. (Modified from Patton KT, Thibodeau GA: *Anatomy and physiology*, ed 7, St Louis, 2010, Mosby.)

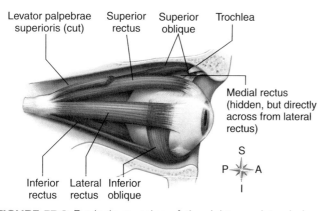

**FIGURE 57-2** Extrinsic muscles of the right eye, lateral view. (Modified from Patton KT, Thibodeau GA: *Anatomy and physiology*, ed 7, St Louis, 2010, Mosby.)

muscles: *inferior, superior, medial,* and *lateral.* There are two types of oblique muscles: *inferior* and *superior.* These muscles are shown in Figure 57-2. (The medial rectus muscle is hidden from view in this figure but is directly across from the lateral rectus muscle.) The levator palpebrae superioris muscle opens the eyelid (see later in the chapter). This muscle rests on top of the superior rectus muscle. There are several other important structures that are either part of or adjacent to the eye. The structures and the purpose of each are as follows:

- *Eyebrow:* Rows of short hair above (superior to) the upper eyelids. The eyebrow protects the eye from direct light, falling dust or other small particles, and perspiration coming from the forehead.

- *Eyelid:* The layer of muscle and skin lined interiorly by the conjunctiva. The conjunctiva also covers the outer anterior surface of the eye, which includes the cornea. The eyelid is moveable and can open or close. It protects the eye when closed and allows vision when open. The eyelid is raised by contraction of the levator palpebrae superioris muscle and is lowered by relaxation of this muscle (see Figure 57-2).

- *Cornea:* The convex (outward-projecting; opposite of concave), transparent, anterior portion of the eye. It can be thought of as a window that sits in front of the lens and allows the passage of light.

- *Eyelashes:* Two or three rows of hairs that are located on the edge (margin) of the eyelids. They help prevent small particles from falling into the eye when it is open.

- *Palpebral fissure:* The space between the upper and lower eyelids when the eyelids are open but relaxed.

- *Sclera:* A tough, white coat of fibrous tissue that surrounds the entire eyeball except for the cornea. It helps maintain the shape of the eye. Commonly called the *white* of the eye, the sclera is nonvascular and allows light to pass through it to the lens.

- *Choroid:* One of the middle-layer structures of the eyeball that contains blood vessels that supply the eye; it also absorbs light.

- *Ciliary body:* The structure that supports the ciliary muscles that control the curvature of the lens via attached suspensory ligaments.

- *Conjunctiva:* The mucous membrane that lines the eyelids and also covers the exposed anterior surface of the eyeball.

- *Iris:* The colored (pigmented) muscular apparatus behind the cornea.

**FIGURE 57-3** Different nervous systems control pupil size.

- *Pupil:* The variable-sized opening in the center of the iris that allows light to enter into the eyeball when the eyelids are open. The pupil is the rear portion of the window of the eye through which light passes to the lens and the retina (the cornea is the front part of this window).
- *Medial canthus:* The site of union of the upper and lower eyelids near the nose.
- *Lacrimal caruncle:* A small, red, rounded elevation covered by modified skin at the medial angle of the eye; the site of the lacrimal glands (see later in the chapter).
- *Lateral canthus:* The site of union of the upper and lower eyelids away from the nose.

## LACRIMAL GLANDS

The eye is kept moist and healthy by an intricate network of connected canals, ducts, and sacs that work together. The lacrimal glands produce tears that bathe and cleanse the exposed anterior portion of the eye. Tears are composed of an isotonic, aqueous solution that contains an enzyme called lysozyme, which acts as an antibacterial to help prevent eye infections. Tears drain into the nasal cavity through the lacrimal ducts.

## LAYERS OF THE EYE

Overall, the eye can be thought of as having three separate anatomic layers. The fibrous outer layer of the eye has two parts that are continuous with each other: the sclera and the cornea. The sclera is a tough, fibrous layer that protects and maintains the shape of the eye. The cornea is a nonvascular transparent portion of the outer layer that allows light to enter the eye. It is located at the very front of the eye and is continuous with the sclera. It is pain-sensitive (a protective function) and obtains nutrition from the aqueous humor, the clear watery fluid that circulates in the anterior and posterior chambers of the eye.

The vascular middle layer of the eye is composed of the iris (to the anterior), ciliary body, and choroid (to the posterior). These three structures are collectively called the uvea. The iris gives color to the eye and has an adjustable opening in the center called the pupil. The main function of the iris is to regulate the amount of light that enters the eye by causing the size of the pupil to vary. Pupil size is controlled by two smooth muscles. The sphincter pupillae muscle is controlled by the parasympathetic nervous system and constricts the diameter of the pupil (called *miosis*) (Figure 57-3). In contrast, the pupil is opened (called *mydriasis*) by a radial smooth muscle called the dilator muscle. It is composed of radiating fibers, like spokes of a wheel, which converge from the circumference of the iris

**FIGURE 57-4** Drug classes and their effects on pupil size.

toward its center. Sympathetic nervous system impulses control this muscle (see Figure 57-3).

The anterior portions of both the retina and choroid merge to become the ciliary body, which produces aqueous humor. This is the clear, watery fluid that circulates in both the anterior and posterior chambers, not to be confused with tears. Aqueous humor contributes, along with vitreous humor to the intraocular pressure of the eye. This is the internal pressure of all fluids against the tunics (retina, choroid, sclera) of the eye. Given the small space of the eye, any change in the volume of aqueous humor present can lead to increased or reduced intraocular pressure. Normally, the aqueous humor is removed from the anterior chamber via the canal of Schlemm at a rate that balances out its production by the ciliary body. The ciliary body also provides a support for the suspensory ligaments to which the lens is attached. The lens is the transparent crystalline structure of the eye, located directly behind the iris and the pupil. It has a biconvex (oval-spherical) shape and is held in place by suspensory ligaments that are attached to the ciliary muscle. Contraction of the ciliary muscle changes the shape of the lens. This function is important for visual accommodation as well as the focusing of light (and visual images) onto the retina. The ciliary muscle is controlled by the parasympathetic nervous system through the oculomotor cranial nerve (cranial nerve III). The lens divides the interior of the eyeball into posterior (rear) and anterior (forward) chambers. The larger chamber behind the lens is filled with a jellylike fluid called the vitreous body. The lens is transparent to allow light to pass through easily. A loss of lens transparency results in a visual condition called a cataract. A cataract is a gray-white opacity that can be seen within the lens. If cataracts are untreated, sight may eventually be completely lost. At the onset of a cataract, vision is blurred and may be further worsened by the glare of bright lights. *Diplopia* or double vision may also develop.

Before light rays reach the retina, they are focused into a sharp image by the lens of the eye. The elasticity of the lens enables it to change its shape and focusing power. This process is called accommodation and is facilitated by the ciliary body. Paralysis of accommodation is called cycloplegia. Mydriatics are drugs that dilate the pupil (e.g., apraclonidine). Drugs that constrict the pupil are called miotics (e.g., acetylcholine, pilocarpine). Drugs that paralyze the ciliary body are called cycloplegics, but they also have mydriatic properties (e.g., atropine, cyclopentolate) (Figure 57-4).

FIGURE 57-5 Function of rods and cones in relation to color vision.

FIGURE 57-6 How increased aqueous humor can result in impaired vision. *IOP*, Intraocular pressure.

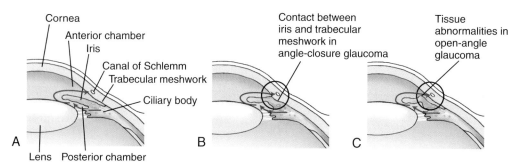

FIGURE 57-7 Main structures of the eye and an enlargement of the canal of Schlemm showing the flow of aqueous humor. **A,** Flow in a normal eye. **B,** In angle-closure glaucoma, the closure of the anterior angle due to contact between the iris and the trabecular meshwork prevents aqueous humor from exiting through the canal of Schlemm, which leads to increased intraocular pressure. **C,** In open-angle glaucoma, the anterior angle remains open, but the canal of Schlemm is obstructed by tissue abnormalities. (Modified from McKenry LM, Tessier E, Hogan MA: *Mosby's pharmacology in nursing*, ed 22, St Louis, 2006, Mosby.)

All of these medications are used to facilitate visualization of the inner eye during ophthalmic examinations.

The third and inner layer of the eye is a thin delicate layer known as the retina. It contains light-sensitive photoreceptors called rods and cones. The basic function of the retina is to receive the light image formed by the lens and to convert it via the rods and cones into the neural signals that support vision. Rods produce black-and-white vision, including shades of gray, and are especially sensitive in low light; cones are responsible for color vision (Figure 57-5). In addition, rods are more active in providing peripheral (to-the-side) vision, whereas cones are more active in central (straight-ahead) vision. In the posterior central part of the retina, the nerve fibers of retinal cells join to form the optic nerve. The function of this nerve is to connect the retina with the visual center of the brain, located within the occipital lobe that extends above and behind the cerebellum. It is this portion of the brain that interprets incoming visual stimuli.

## PATHOPHYSIOLOGY OF GLAUCOMA

Glaucoma is a group of eye disorders that damages the optic nerve. In most cases, this is due to increased intraocular pressure that is caused by abnormally elevated levels of aqueous humor. Glaucoma occurs when the aqueous humor is not drained through the canal of Schlemm as quickly as it is formed by the ciliary body. The accumulated aqueous humor creates a backward pressure that pushes the vitreous humor against the retina. Continued pressure on the retina destroys its neurons, which leads to impaired vision and eventual blindness (Figure 57-6). Unfortunately, glaucoma is often without early symptoms, and many patients are not diagnosed until some permanent sight loss has occurred.

Two major types of glaucoma are discussed in this chapter: angle-closure glaucoma and open-angle glaucoma. Figure 57-7 shows the pathophysiology of each and provides an enlarged view of the involved eye structures. Table 57-1 lists additional characteristic features of each type. Glaucoma can be a primary illness (occurring on its own), or it can be secondary to another eye condition or injury (e.g., posttraumatic glaucoma). Congenital glaucoma can also occur in infants. The visual and optic nerve changes typical of glaucoma can also occur in the absence of increased intraocular pressure (normotensive glaucoma). There are a few other less common forms of glaucoma (e.g., pigmentary glaucoma, pseudoexfoliative glaucoma) that are beyond the scope of this chapter.

## TABLE 57-1 GLAUCOMA: TYPES AND CHARACTERISTICS

| | ANGLE-CLOSURE GLAUCOMA | OPEN-ANGLE GLAUCOMA |
|---|---|---|
| Synonyms | Closed-angle glaucoma, narrow-angle glaucoma, congestive glaucoma, pupillary closure glaucoma | Chronic glaucoma, wide-angle glaucoma, simple glaucoma |
| Chronicity | Acute (can cause rapid vision loss) | Chronic |
| Relative incidence | Less common | More common |
| Nature of angle | Narrow | Larger |
| Most common age of onset and race | 30 yr or older, white | 30 yr or older, African American |
| Major symptoms | Blurred vision, severe headaches, eye pain | Blurred vision, occasional headaches |
| Treatment | Topical or systemic drugs, surgery | Topical or systemic drugs, surgery |

## TABLE 57-2 ANTIGLAUCOMA DRUGS: EFFECTS ON AQUEOUS HUMOR

| DRUG CLASS | INCREASED DRAINAGE | DECREASED PRODUCTION | COLOR-CODED EYEDROPPER |
|---|---|---|---|
| **Miotics** | | | |
| Direct-acting cholinergics | +++ | 0 | Green |
| Indirect-acting cholinergics (cholinesterase inhibitors) | +++ | 0 | Green |
| **Mydriatics** | | | |
| Sympathomimetics | ++ | +++ | Purple |
| **Others** | | | |
| Beta blockers | + | +++ | Yellow, blue |
| Carbonic anhydrase inhibitors | 0 | +++ | Orange |
| Osmotic diuretics | +++ | 0 | |
| Prostaglandin agonists | +++ | 0 | Clear, teal |

0, No effect; +, minor effect; ++, moderate effect; ++, pronounced effect.

## PHARMACOLOGY OVERVIEW

Medications used to treat disorders of the eye can be divided into several major drug groups: antiglaucoma drugs, antimicrobials, antiinflammatory drugs, topical anesthetics, diagnostic drugs, antiallergic drugs, and lubricants and moisturizers. There are also a variety of combination drug products that include two or more medications from different subclasses. The reader can assume the same therapeutic indications and drug effects for these combination products as for the single-ingredient drug products corresponding to their individual components. The focus of this chapter is on commonly used therapeutic medications.

A multitude of various products are also available for use in the care of contact lenses, including contact lens–cleaning enzymes, irrigating solutions, and eye washes. Their use is fairly straightforward, and they carry limited risk. More complicated surgical drugs are beyond the scope of this chapter. The reader is advised to refer to the manufacturer's packaging information for details about any unfamiliar product encountered in clinical practice.

## ANTIGLAUCOMA DRUGS

Treatment of glaucoma involves reducing intraocular pressure by either increasing the drainage of aqueous humor or decreasing its production. Some drugs may do both. Drug therapy can delay and possibly even prevent the development of glaucoma. Glaucoma eyedrops are color-coded according to medication class to aid the patient in identification, and they are listed in Table 57-2. Drug classes used to reduce intraocular pressure include the following:

- Direct-acting cholinergics (also called *miotics* and *parasympathomimetic drugs*)
- Indirect-acting cholinergics (also called *miotics, cholinesterase inhibitors,* and *parasympathomimetic drugs*)
- Adrenergics (also called *mydriatics* and *sympathomimetic drugs*)
- Antiadrenergics (beta blockers; also called *sympatholytic drugs*)
- Carbonic anhydrase inhibitors
- Osmotic diuretics
- Prostaglandin agonists

See Table 57-2 for a comparison of the effects of these drugs on aqueous humor.

## CHOLINERGIC DRUGS (MIOTICS)

There are two categories of ocular parasympathetic drugs, more concisely referred to as cholinergic drugs: direct acting and indirect acting. Directing-acting cholinergics include acetylcholine, carbachol, and pilocarpine. Indirect-acting drugs, which are also called *cholinesterase inhibitors,* include echothiophate, currently the only available drug in this class. Because the primary drug effect of these drugs is pupillary constriction, or *miosis* (see later), they are also commonly called *miotics.*

**FIGURE 57-8** Cholinergic response of miosis to parasympathomimetic drugs. *ACh*, Acetylcholine; *PSNS*, parasympathetic nervous system.

**FIGURE 57-9** Therapeutic effects of direct- and indirect-acting miotics on glaucoma. *IOP*, Intraocular pressure.

## Mechanism of Action and Drug Effects

Acetylcholine is the neurochemical mediator of nerve impulses in the parasympathetic nervous system. It stimulates parasympathetic or cholinergic receptors located in the brain and throughout the body along parasympathetic nerve branches. This results in several effects on the eye: miosis (pupillary constriction), vasodilation of blood vessels in and around the eye, contraction of ciliary muscles, drainage of aqueous humor, and reduced intraocular pressure. Ciliary muscle contraction promotes aqueous humor drainage by widening the space where the drainage occurs. Miosis promotes aqueous humor drainage by causing the iris to stretch, which also serves to widen this space.

Both direct- and indirect-acting miotics have effects similar to those of acetylcholine, but their actions are more prolonged (Figure 57-8). The direct-acting miotics are able to directly stimulate ocular cholinergic receptors and mimic acetylcholine. Indirect-acting miotics work by binding to and inactivating the cholinesterases acetylcholinesterase and pseudocholinesterase, the enzymes that break down acetylcholine. As a result, acetylcholine accumulates and acts longer at the cholinergic receptor sites. This leads to drug effects that include miosis, ciliary muscle contraction, enhanced aqueous humor drainage, and reduced intraocular pressure by an average of 20% to 30% (Figure 57-9). Drug-induced miotic effects may be less pronounced in individuals with dark eyes (e.g., brown or hazel) than in those with lighter eyes (e.g., blue). This is because the pigment of the iris also absorbs the drug (which reduces its therapeutic effects), and dark eyes have more pigment.

## Indications

The direct- and indirect-acting miotics are used for treatment of open-angle glaucoma, angle-closure glaucoma, and convergent strabismus (a condition in which one eye points toward the other, or "cross-eye") and in ocular surgery. They are also used to reverse the effect of mydriatic (pupil-dilating) drugs after ophthalmic examination. Specific indications may vary for different drugs, as shown in Table 57-3.

| TABLE 57-3 | MIOTICS: INDICATIONS |
|---|---|
| **DRUG** | **INDICATIONS** |
| acetylcholine | Need for complete and rapid miosis after cataract lens extraction, iridectomy |
| carbachol | Open-angle glaucoma |
| echothiophate | Accommodative esotropia, obstructive aqueous humor outflow, open- and angle-closure glaucoma after iridectomy |
| pilocarpine | Open-angle glaucoma, secondary glaucoma after iridectomy, reversal of cycloplegia |

## Contraindications

Contraindications to the use of miotics include known drug allergy and any serious active eye disorder in which induction of miosis might be harmful.

## Adverse Effects

Most of the adverse effects from the use of cholinergic and cholinergic inhibitors (miotics) are local and limited to the eye. Adverse effects are more likely to occur with indirect-acting miotics because they have longer-lasting effects. Effects include blurred vision, drug-induced myopia (nearsightedness), and accommodative spasms. Such effects are secondary to contraction of the ciliary muscle. Miotic drugs also cause vasodilation of blood vessels supplying the conjunctiva, iris, and ciliary body, which may lead to vascular congestion and ocular inflammation. Other undesirable effects include temporary stinging upon drug instillation, reduced nighttime or low-light vision, conjunctivitis, lacrimation (tearing), twitching of the eyelids (blepharospasm), and eye or brow pain. Prolonged use can result in iris cysts, lens opacities, and, rarely, retinal detachment. Systemic effects are uncommon but are more likely to occur with cholinesterase inhibitors (indirect-acting miotics). See Chapters 20 and 21 for more information on the systemic effects of these drugs.

## Interactions

Drug interactions are unlikely because of the local actions of these drugs. When miotic drugs are given with topical

## DOSAGES

### *Selected Miotics*

| DRUG (PREGNANCY CATEGORY) | PHARMACOLOGIC CLASS | USUAL DOSAGE RANGE | INDICATIONS |
|---|---|---|---|
| acetylcholine (Miochol-E) (C) | Direct-acting cholinergic | 0.5 to 2 mL preoperatively | Need for surgical miosis |
| ◆ echothiophate (Phospholine Iodide) (C) | Indirect-acting cholinergic | 1 drop 1-2 times daily | Early and advanced chronic open-angle glaucoma; glaucoma secondary to cataract surgery; accommodative esotropia |
| ◆ pilocarpine (Pilocar, Isopto Carpine, Akarpine, Pilopine HS) (C) | Direct-acting cholinergic | Solution: 1-2 drops 3-4 times daily Gel: 0.5-inch ribbon into lower conjunctival sac at bedtime (use any other eyedrops at least 5 min before gel) | Chronic open-angle and angle-closure glaucoma; acute angle-closure glaucoma; preoperative and postoperative intraocular hypertension; need for reversal of drug-induced mydriasis |

adrenergics, antiadrenergics (e.g., beta blockers), or carbonic anhydrase inhibitors, additive lowering effects on intraocular pressure can be seen. Systemic cholinergic drugs can theoretically have additive cholinergic effects when given with miotics. Indirect-acting miotics (cholinesterase inhibitors) may also potentiate the effects of the neuromuscular blocker succinylcholine (see Chapter 11).

## Dosages

For dosage information on selected miotic drugs, see the table on this page.

## DRUG PROFILES

Direct-acting ocular cholinergics include acetylcholine (Miochol-E), carbachol (Carboptic), and pilocarpine (Pilocar). Indirect-acting drugs, which are also called *cholinesterase inhibitors,* include echothiophate (Phospholine Iodide). These drugs are used for management of glaucoma, as adjuncts for ocular surgery, and for treatment of various other ophthalmic conditions.

### DIRECT-ACTING MIOTICS

#### acetylcholine

Acetylcholine (Miochol-E) is a direct-acting cholinergic drug that is used to produce miosis during ophthalmic surgery. It is a pharmaceutical form of the naturally occurring neurotransmitter in the body. It has very quick onset and may begin to work almost immediately. It is administered directly into the anterior chamber of the eye before and after securing one or more sutures.

#### Pharmacokinetics

| Route | Onset of Action | Peak Plasma Concentration | Elimination Half-life | Duration of Action |
|---|---|---|---|---|
| Ocular | Instant | Instant | 3 min | 10 min |

#### ◆ pilocarpine

Pilocarpine (Pilocar) is a direct-acting cholinergic drug that is used as a miotic in the treatment of glaucoma. Pilocarpine is available in different strengths as an ocular gel and solution. One special formulation is the pilocarpine ocular insert system (Ocusert Pilo-20), which is applied once weekly by the patient.

#### Pharmacokinetics (Immediate-Release Formulation)

| Route | Onset of Action | Peak Plasma Concentration | Elimination Half-life | Duration of Action |
|---|---|---|---|---|
| Ocular | 10-30 min | 75 min | Unknown | 4-8 hr |

### INDIRECT-ACTING MIOTIC

#### ◆ echothiophate

Echothiophate (Phospholine Iodide) is an indirect-acting cholinergic that has an organophosphate structure and acts by phosphorylating cholinesterase enzymes. This effect is normally irreversible until new enzymes are synthesized by the body, which may take days or even weeks. For these reasons, this drug is considered to be long acting.

#### Pharmacokinetics

| Route | Onset of Action | Peak Plasma Concentration | Elimination Half-life | Duration of Action |
|---|---|---|---|---|
| Ocular | 10-30 min | 24 hr | Long | 7-28 days |

## SYMPATHOMIMETICS (MYDRIATICS)

Sympathomimetic drugs are used for the treatment of glaucoma and ocular hypertension. These drugs include the alpha receptor agonists brimonidine (Alphagan P) and apraclonidine (Iopidine), as well as the alpha and beta receptor agonists epinephryl (Epinal) and dipivefrin (Propine).

## Mechanism of Action and Drug Effects

Sympathomimetic drugs mimic the sympathetic neurotransmitters norepinephrine and epinephrine. They stimulate the dilator muscle to contract by means of alpha and/or beta receptor interaction. This stimulation results in increased pupil size or *mydriasis* (Figure 57-10). Dilation is seen within minutes of instillation of the ophthalmic drops and lasts for several hours, during which time the intraocular pressure is reduced (Figure 57-11). Alpha receptor stimulation reduces intraocular pressure by enhancing aqueous humor outflow through the canal of Schlemm. Production of aqueous humor by the ciliary body is also reduced. Both of these effects appear to be dose dependent.

FIGURE 57-10 Mechanism of mydriasis.

FIGURE 57-11 Ocular effects of alpha (α) and beta (β) stimulation. *IOP*, Intraocular pressure.

## DOSAGES

### *Selected Ocular Sympathomimetics*

| DRUG (PREGNANCY CATEGORY) | PHARMACOLOGIC CLASS | USUAL DOSAGE RANGE | INDICATIONS/USES |
|---|---|---|---|
| apraclonidine (Iopidine) (C) | Direct acting | 0.5% solution: 1-2 drops 3 times daily | Short-term adjunctive therapy for glaucoma not controlled by other drugs |
| ♦ dipivefrin (Propine) (C) | Direct acting | 1 drop q12h | Chronic open-angle glaucoma |

## Indications

Both epinephrine and dipivefrin are used to reduce elevated intraocular pressure in the treatment of chronic open-angle glaucoma, either as initial therapy or as long-term therapy. Increases in intraocular pressure during ophthalmic surgery are usually mediated via increased catecholamine stimulation of the sympathetic nervous system. Apraclonidine stimulates the alpha$_2$ receptors, which oppose those effects, and thus corrects the surgery-induced elevation in intraocular pressure. Brimonidine also has primarily alpha$_2$ activity but is used to lower intraocular pressure in patients with open-angle glaucoma or ocular hypertension.

## Contraindications

Contraindications for the sympathomimetic ophthalmics include known drug allergy.

## Adverse Effects

Adverse effects of the sympathomimetic mydriatics are primarily limited to ocular effects and include burning, eye pain, and lacrimation. Such effects are usually temporary and may subside as the patient grows accustomed to the medication. Other ocular effects may include conjunctival hyperemia, localized melanin deposits in the conjunctiva, and release of pigment granules from the iris. Although systemic effects associated with the use of sympathomimetic mydriatics are uncommon, they are theoretically possible, especially with the use of larger doses or prolonged drug therapy. They include cardiovascular effects such as extrasystoles, tachycardia, and hypertension. Other effects that may be noticed are headache and faintness.

## Interactions

With sufficient topical absorption, sympathomimetic mydriatics have the potential to react with other drugs. Cardiac dysrhythmias are potentiated when mydriatic drugs are given with halogenated anesthetics, cardiac glycosides, thyroid hormones, or tricyclic antidepressants.

## Dosages

For dosage information on sympathomimetic drugs, see the table on this page.

## DRUG PROFILES

Sympathomimetic ophthalmic drugs include dipivefrin (Propine), epinephryl (Epinal), apraclonidine (Iopidine), and brimonidine (Alphagan P). These drugs are used for management of glaucoma and ocular hypertension, and for ocular surgery.

### apraclonidine

Apraclonidine (Iopidine) is structurally and pharmacologically related to the alpha$_2$ stimulant clonidine. It reduces intraocular pressure 23% to 39% by stimulating alpha$_2$ and beta$_2$ receptors. It also prevents ocular vasoconstriction, which reduces ocular blood pressure as well as aqueous humor formation. Apraclonidine is primarily used to inhibit perioperative intraocular pressure increases, rather than to treat glaucoma. Brimonidine (Alphagan P) is a similar drug but is used primarily for glaucoma.

## Pharmacokinetics (apraclonidine)

| Route | Onset of Action | Peak Plasma Concentration | Elimination Half-life | Duration of Action |
|-------|-----------------|---------------------------|-----------------------|--------------------|
| Ocular | 1 hr | 3-5 hr | 8 hr | 12 hr |

### ◆ dipivefrin

Dipivefrin (Propine) is a synthetic sympathomimetic miotic drug. It is a prodrug of epinephrine that has little or no pharmacologic activity until hydrolyzed in the eye to two chemically modified forms of epinephrine. These chemical alterations account for the main advantage of this drug over epinephrine: it has enhanced lipophilicity (fat solubility) and can better penetrate into the tissues of the anterior chamber of the eye. This quality also reduces the likelihood of any systemic adverse effects. Dipivefrin typically reduces mean intraocular pressure approximately 15% to 25%. On a weight basis, dipivefrin is 4 to 11 times as potent as epinephrine in reducing intraocular pressure and 5 to 12 times as potent as epinephrine in terms of its mydriatic effects. Epinephryl (Epinal) is a newer drug with similar properties and uses.

## Pharmacokinetics

| Route | Onset of Action | Peak Plasma Concentration | Elimination Half-life | Duration of Action |
|-------|-----------------|---------------------------|-----------------------|--------------------|
| Ocular | 30 min | 1 hr | 1-3 hr | 12 hr |

## BETA-ADRENERGIC BLOCKERS

The antiglaucoma beta-adrenergic blockers that reduce intraocular pressure include the $beta_1$-selective drugs betaxolol and levobetaxolol.

## Mechanism of Action and Drug Effects

The ophthalmic beta blockers reduce both elevated and normal intraocular pressure. They reduce intraocular pressure by reducing aqueous humor formation. In addition, timolol may produce a minimal increase in aqueous outflow.

## Indications

Ophthalmic beta blockers are used to reduce elevated intraocular pressure in various conditions, including chronic open-angle glaucoma and ocular hypertension. They may also be used alone or in combination with a topical miotic (e.g., echothiophate iodide, pilocarpine), topical dipivefrin, and/or systemic carbonic anhydrase inhibitors. When used in combination, these drugs may have an additive intraocular pressure-lowering effect. They may also be used to treat some forms of angle-closure glaucoma.

## Contraindications

Contraindications for ophthalmic beta blockers include known drug allergy and any ocular condition for which beta-receptor blockade might be harmful.

## Adverse Effects

The adverse effects of antiglaucoma beta blockers are primarily limited to ocular effects. The most common ocular effects are transient burning and discomfort. Other effects include blurred vision, pain, photophobia, lacrimation, blepharitis, keratitis (inflammation of the cornea), and decreased corneal sensitivity. Because these drugs are administered topically, few, if any, systemic effects are expected. Theoretical systemic effects include bradycardia, bronchospasm, headache, and dizziness as described for systemic beta blockers in Chapter 19. However, ocular beta blockers have not been shown to affect glucose metabolism.

## Interactions

Drug interactions with systemic drugs are unlikely due to the primarily localized nature of ophthalmically administered drugs. Theoretically, ophthalmic beta blockers can have additive therapeutic and/or adverse effects when given with systemically administered beta blockers or other cardiovascular drugs (e.g., calcium channel blockers).

## Dosages

For dosage information on beta-adrenergic blockers, see the table on this page.

## DRUG PROFILES

The currently available ophthalmic beta-blocking drugs are betaxolol (Betoptic), carteolol (Ocupress), levobunolol (Betagan), levobetaxolol (Betaxon), metipranolol (OptiPranolol), and timolol (Timoptic). These drugs are used to treat glaucoma and ocular hypertension.

### ◆ betaxolol

Betaxolol (Betoptic) is a $beta_1$-selective beta blocker. It is one of the most potent and selective beta-blocking drugs. Its ability to decrease aqueous humor formation and reduce

## DOSAGES

### Selected Ocular Beta Blockers

| DRUG (PREGNANCY CATEGORY) | PHARMACOLOGIC CLASS | USUAL DOSAGE RANGE | INDICATIONS |
|---------------------------|---------------------|---------------------|-------------|
| ◆ betaxolol (Betoptic, Betoptic S) (C) | Direct acting | 1-2 drops twice daily | Chronic open-angle glaucoma; ocular hypertension |
| ◆ timolol (Betimol, Timoptic, Timoptic-XE) (C) | Direct acting | Solution: 1 drop twice daily<br>Gel-forming solution: 1 drop daily | Open-angle glaucoma; ocular hypertension |

intraocular pressure has made it an excellent drug for the treatment of ocular disorders such as open-angle glaucoma and ocular hypertension.

### Pharmacokinetics

| Route | Onset of Action | Peak Plasma Concentration | Elimination Half-life | Duration of Action |
|---|---|---|---|---|
| Ocular | 0.5-1 hr | 2 hr | Unknown | More than 12 hr |

### ◆ timolol

Timolol (Timoptic) differs slightly from the other ophthalmic beta blockers in that it may increase the outflow of aqueous humor as well as decrease its formation. The drug acts at both beta$_1$ and beta$_2$ receptors and is indicated for the treatment of open-angle glaucoma and ocular hypertension. It is available in various liquid forms, both with and without preservatives. Preservative-free products were developed because of patient allergies to benzalkonium chloride, a commonly used preservative. Timolol is also available in a gel-forming solution (with preservatives). The gel-forming products are longer acting and allow for once-daily dosing, a convenience over the twice-daily dosing that many patients require of the other timolol formulations.

### Pharmacokinetics

| Route | Onset of Action | Peak Plasma Concentration | Elimination Half-life | Duration of Action |
|---|---|---|---|---|
| Ocular | 15-30 min | 1-2 hr | Unknown | 12-24 hr |

## CARBONIC ANHYDRASE INHIBITORS

Ophthalmic carbonic anhydrase inhibitors include brinzolamide (Azopt) and dorzolamide (Trusopt). These two drugs are available only in topical ophthalmic form. Systemic carbonic anhydrase inhibitors for oral use are sometimes also used as adjunct drug therapy for glaucoma and are described in Chapter 28. Both drugs are also sulfonamides and are chemically related to the sulfonamide antibiotics (see Chapter 38). They are to be used with caution in patients who are allergic to sulfa antibiotics.

## Mechanism of Action and Drug Effects

Carbonic anhydrase inhibitors work by inhibiting the enzyme carbonic anhydrase, which results in decreased intraocular pressure by reduction of aqueous humor formation.

## Indications

Ocular carbonic anhydrase inhibitors are used primarily for management of glaucoma, including both open-angle and angle-closure glaucoma; they may also be used preoperatively to control intraocular pressure.

## Contraindications

Contraindications include known drug allergy and any ocular condition for which their use might be harmful in the judgment of an ophthalmologist. Allergy to sulfonamide antibiotics is a precaution, not a contraindication; however, patients need to be educated on the possibility of cross-reaction.

## Adverse Effects

Systemic absorption of these drugs occurs, although systemic adverse effects are unlikely. The same adverse effects listed for sulfonamide antibiotics in Chapter 38 can theoretically occur with these drugs. Patients with sulfa allergies may develop cross-sensitivities to the carbonic anhydrase inhibitors.

## Interactions

The systemic use of carbonic anhydrase inhibitors can result in several significant drug interactions, and the ocular carbonic anhydrase inhibitors have a theoretical (but less likely) potential for these interactions. See Chapter 28 for information on systemic drug interactions.

## Dosages

For dosage information on the carbonic anhydrase inhibitor dorzolamide, see the table on this page.

## DRUG PROFILE

There are currently two ocular carbonic anhydrase inhibitors: brinzolamide (Azopt) and dorzolamide (Trusopt).

### ◆ dorzolamide

Dorzolamide (Trusopt) is indicated for treatment of elevated intraocular pressure associated with either ocular hypertension or open-angle glaucoma. It is available only as an ophthalmic solution. The other drug in this class, brinzolamide, has comparable indications, dosages, and pharmacokinetics.

### Pharmacokinetics

| Route | Onset of Action | Peak Plasma Concentration | Elimination Half-life | Duration of Action |
|---|---|---|---|---|
| Ocular | Rapid | Variable | 3-4 mo | Variable |

## DOSAGES

### *Ocular Carbonic Anhydrase Inhibitor*

| DRUG (PREGNANCY CATEGORY) | PHARMACOLOGIC CLASS | USUAL DOSAGE RANGE | INDICATIONS |
|---|---|---|---|
| ◆ dorzolamide (Trusopt) (C) | Carbonic anhydrase inhibitor | 1 drop 3 times daily | Open-angle glaucoma; ocular hypertension |

FIGURE 57-12 Mechanism and ocular effects of osmotic diuretics. *IOP,* Intraocular pressure.

| TABLE 57-4 | OSMOTIC DIURETICS: ADVERSE EFFECTS |
|---|---|
| **BODY SYSTEM** | **ADVERSE EFFECTS** |
| Cardiovascular | Edema, thrombophlebitis, hypotension, hypertension, tachycardia, angina-like chest pains, fever, chills |
| Central nervous | Dizziness, headache, convulsions, rebound increased intracranial pressure, confusion |
| Electrolytes | Fluid electrolyte imbalances, acidosis, dehydration |
| Eyes, ears, nose, throat | Loss of hearing, blurred vision, nasal congestion |
| Gastrointestinal | Nausea, vomiting, dry mouth, diarrhea |
| Genitourinary | Marked diuresis, urinary retention, thirst |

## OSMOTIC DIURETICS

Osmotic drugs may be administered either intravenously, orally, or topically to reduce intraocular pressure. The osmotic diuretics that are most commonly used for this purpose are glycerin and mannitol.

## Mechanism of Action and Drug Effects

Osmotic diuretics reduce ocular hypertension by causing the blood to become hypertonic in relation to both intraocular and spinal fluids. This creates an osmotic gradient that draws water from the aqueous and vitreous humors into the bloodstream, which causes a reduction in the volume of intraocular fluid; the result is a decrease in intraocular pressure (Figure 57-12). Systemic (nonocular) effects of these drugs are discussed in Chapter 28.

## Indications

Ocular uses for osmotic diuretics include treatment of acute glaucoma episodes and reduction of intraocular pressure before or after ocular surgery. Typically, glycerin is used first; if the treatment is unsuccessful, mannitol is tried. Isosorbide and urea are two other osmotic drugs that may also be used in similar situations. They are usually administered after glycerin or mannitol has failed.

## Contraindications

Osmotic diuretics are contraindicated in patients with known drug allergy, pronounced anuria, acute pulmonary edema, cardiac decompensation, and severe dehydration, because they can worsen all of these conditions.

## Adverse Effects

The most frequent reactions to osmotic diuretics are nausea, vomiting, and headache. The most significant adverse effects are fluid and electrolyte imbalances. Other effects are possible irritation and thrombosis at the injection site. Other potential adverse effects are listed in Table 57-4.

## Interactions

The only significant drug interaction is increased lithium excretion associated with mannitol and urea.

## Dosages

For dosage information on osmotic drugs, see the table on p. 928.

## DRUG PROFILES

Osmotic diuretics include mannitol, glycerin, urea, and isosorbide. These drugs are normally reserved for acute reduction of intraocular pressure during glaucoma crises and perioperative reduction of intraocular pressure in ophthalmic surgery.

### glycerin

Glycerin is an osmotic drug given orally to lower intraocular pressure or topically to reduce superficial corneal edema. Another use is before iridectomy in individuals with acute narrow-angle glaucoma. It is also used preoperatively and/or postoperatively in procedures such as treatment of congenital glaucoma, repair of retinal detachment, cataract extraction, and keratoplasty (corneal transplant). It may also be used in the management of secondary glaucoma.

Pharmacokinetics

| Route | Onset of Action | Peak Plasma Concentration | Elimination Half-life | Duration of Action |
|---|---|---|---|---|
| Ocular | 10-30 min | 1-1.5 hr | 30-45 min | 4-5 hr |

### mannitol

Mannitol (Osmitrol) is administered by intravenous infusion to reduce elevated intraocular pressure when the pressure cannot be lowered by other methods. Mannitol is effective in treating acute episodes of angle-closure, absolute, or secondary glaucoma and in lowering intraocular pressure before intraocular surgery. Mannitol does not penetrate the eye and may be used when irritation is present, unlike some of the other osmotic drugs, such as urea.

Pharmacokinetics

| Route | Onset of Action | Peak Plasma Concentration | Elimination Half-life | Duration of Action |
|---|---|---|---|---|
| IV | 30-60 min | 1 hr | 15-100 min | 6-8 hr |

## PROSTAGLANDIN AGONISTS

The newest class of drugs used to treat glaucoma is the prostaglandin agonists. There are currently three drugs in this class: latanoprost (Xalatan), travoprost (Travatan-Z), and bimatoprost (Lumigan).

## DOSAGES

### Osmotic Diuretics

| DRUG (PREGNANCY CATEGORY) | PHARMACOLOGIC CLASS | USUAL DOSAGE RANGE | INDICATIONS/USES |
|---|---|---|---|
| glycerin (Ophthalgan) (C) | Organic alcohol | 1-2 drops before eye exam as lubricant; more if needed during exam | Gonioscopy of edematous cornea |
| mannitol (Osmitrol) (C) | Organic alcohol | IV: 1.5-2 g/kg infused over at least 30 min; for preoperative use, give 1-1.5 hr before surgery | Acute reduction of elevated intraocular pressure |

*IV*, Intravenous.

## DOSAGES

### Ocular Prostaglandin Agonist

| DRUG (PREGNANCY CATEGORY) | PHARMACOLOGIC CLASS | USUAL DOSAGE RANGE | INDICATIONS |
|---|---|---|---|
| ♦ latanoprost (Xalatan) (C) | Prostaglandin | 1 drop every day in evening | Open-angle glaucoma and ocular hypertension in patients who are intolerant of or whose condition is uncontrolled by other drugs |

## Mechanism of Action and Drug Effects

Prostaglandins reduce intraocular pressure by increasing the outflow of aqueous humor between the uvea and sclera as well as via the usual exit through the trabecular meshwork (see Figure 57-7). A single dose of a prostaglandin agonist lowers intraocular pressure for 20 to 24 hours, which allows a single daily dosing regimen. The drug effects are primarily limited to these ocular effects.

## Indications

Prostaglandin agonists are used in the treatment of glaucoma.

## Contraindications

The only usual contraindication is known drug allergy.

## Adverse Effects

Prostaglandin agonists are generally well tolerated. Adverse effects include foreign body sensation, punctate epithelial keratopathy (dotted appearance of the cornea), stinging, conjunctival hyperemia ("bloodshot" eyes), blurred vision, itching, and burning. Systemic effects occur in a small percentage of patients and include skin reactions, upper respiratory tract infections, and headache. There is one unique adverse effect associated with all prostaglandin agonists: in some people with hazel, green, or bluish-brown eye color, eye color will turn permanently brown, even if the medication is discontinued. This adverse effect appears to be cosmetic only with no known ill effects on the eye.

## Interactions

Concurrent administration of prostaglandin agonists with any other eyedrops containing the preservative thimerosal may result in precipitation. It is recommended that the two medications be administered at least 5 minutes apart.

## Dosages

For dosage information on the prostaglandin agonist latanoprost, see the table on this page.

## DRUG PROFILE

### ♦ latanoprost

Latanoprost is a prodrug of a naturally occurring prostaglandin known as *prostaglandin F₂-alpha*. When it is administered, it is converted by hydrolysis (with water from ocular fluids) to prostaglandin $F_2$-alpha, which in turn reduces intraocular pressure. Latanoprost is available only in eyedrop form. About 3% to 10% of patients treated with latanoprost (Xalatan) have shown increased iris pigmentation after 3 to 4½ months of treatment.

### Pharmacokinetics

| Route | Onset of Action | Peak Plasma Concentration | Elimination Half-life | Duration of Action |
|---|---|---|---|---|
| Ocular | 30-60 min | 2 hr | 17 min | 24 hr |

## ANTIMICROBIAL DRUGS

A variety of infections can occur in the eye; many are self-limiting. However, some infections require the use of ocular antimicrobials to be eliminated. Topical antimicrobials used to treat ocular infections include antibacterial, antifungal, and antiviral drugs. All require a prescription. Many of these drugs are also available for systemic administration for treatment of infections elsewhere in the body. The most commonly used antimicrobials from the main antimicrobial drug classes are discussed in this chapter. Some common eye infections may require antibiotic therapy and are listed in Table 57-5. The choice of a particular ophthalmic antimicrobial drug is based on the following:

- Clinical experience
- Sensitivity and characteristics of the organisms most likely to have caused the infection
- Characteristics of the disease itself
- Sensitivity and response of the patient
- Laboratory results (cultures and sensitivity testing)

## TABLE 57-5   COMMON OCULAR INFECTIONS

| INFECTION | DESCRIPTION |
|---|---|
| Blepharitis | Inflammation of the eyelids. |
| Conjunctivitis | Inflammation of the conjunctiva (the mucous membrane lining the back of the eyelids and the front of the eye except the cornea). It may be bacterial or viral and is often associated with common colds. When caused by *Haemophilus* organisms, it is commonly called *pink eye*. It is highly contagious but usually self-limiting. |
| Hordeolum (sty) | Acute localized infection of the eyelash follicles and the glands of the anterior lid. It results in the formation of a small abscess or cyst. |
| Keratitis | Inflammation of the cornea caused by bacterial infection. Herpes simplex keratitis is caused by viral infection. |
| Uveitis | Infection of the uveal tract or the vascular layer of the eye, which includes the iris, ciliary body, and choroid. |
| Endophthalmitis | Inflammation of the inner eye structure caused by bacteria. |

## Mechanism of Action and Drug Effects

Topical antimicrobials used to treat infections of the eye work to destroy the invading organism. Their specific antimicrobial actions are similar to those described for systemically administered drugs, which are discussed in Chapters 38, 39, 40, and 42. Some antimicrobials destroy the causative organism, whereas others simply inhibit the organism's growth, allowing the body's immune system to fight the infection.

## Indications

The indication for ocular antimicrobials is known or suspected infection with one or more specific microorganisms. Empirical treatment is based on reasonable clinical evaluation of presenting signs and symptoms. Topical use of antimicrobials helps prevent the antimicrobial drug resistance that could arise from unnecessary systemic use. However, systemic antimicrobials may be administered to treat more severe ocular infections.

## Contraindications

Contraindications to the use of antimicrobials include known drug allergy or other severe previous adverse drug reaction.

## Adverse Effects

The most common adverse effects of ocular antibiotics are local and transient inflammation, burning, stinging, urticaria, dermatitis, angioedema, and drug hypersensitivity. Topical application of antimicrobial drugs may also interfere with growth of the normal bacterial flora of the eye, which may encourage the growth of other, more harmful organisms. If large doses are given, systemic side effects are possible.

## Interactions

Systemic drug interactions are unlikely due to the primarily local effects of ocular antimicrobials. One possible interaction involves the concurrent use of antibiotics and corticosteroids (e.g., dexamethasone). Corticosteroids have immunosuppressive effects that may impede the therapeutic effects of ocular antimicrobials.

## Dosages

For dosage information on ocular antimicrobials, see the table on p. 930.

## DRUG PROFILES

### AMINOGLYCOSIDES

Aminoglycosides (see Chapter 39) are antimicrobials that destroy bacteria by interfering with protein synthesis in bacterial cells, which leads to bacteria death. Aminoglycosides used to treat ocular infections include gentamicin (Garamycin) and tobramycin (Tobrex). Adverse effects include swollen eyelids, mydriasis, and local erythema. Systemic reactions are rare because of poor topical absorption. Overgrowth of nonsusceptible organisms, which can lead to eye infections that are resistant to treatment, is a possibility.

#### ◆ gentamicin

Gentamicin (Garamycin) is effective against a wide variety of gram-negative and gram-positive organisms. It is particularly useful against *Pseudomonas, Proteus,* and *Klebsiella* organisms. Gram-positive organisms that are effectively destroyed by gentamicin include staphylococci and streptococci that have developed resistance to other antibiotics. Gentamicin is available as an ophthalmic ointment and a solution.

### Pharmacokinetics

| Route | Onset of Action | Peak Plasma Concentration | Elimination Half-life | Duration of Action |
|---|---|---|---|---|
| Ocular | Variable | Immediate | Unknown | 6-12 hr |

### MACROLIDE ANTIBIOTICS

Macrolide antibiotics include erythromycin, azithromycin, and other drugs (see Chapter 38). Erythromycin is the most commonly used macrolide for ophthalmic use.

#### ◆ erythromycin

Erythromycin is a macrolide antibiotic indicated for the treatment of various ophthalmic infections, as well as other infections. It is available in oral and intravenous forms and as an ophthalmic ointment. Erythromycin eye ointment is indicated for the treatment of neonatal conjunctivitis caused by *Chlamydia trachomatis* and for the prevention of eye infections in newborns that may be caused by *Neisseria gonorrhoeae* or other susceptible organisms.

### Pharmacokinetics

| Route | Onset of Action | Peak Plasma Concentration | Elimination Half-life | Duration of Action |
|---|---|---|---|---|
| Ocular | Variable | Immediate | Unknown | Variable |

## DOSAGES

### Selected Ocular Antimicrobials

| DRUG (PREGNANCY CATEGORY) | PHARMACOLOGIC CLASS | USUAL DOSAGE RANGE | INDICATIONS |
|---|---|---|---|
| **Antibacterial Drugs** | | | |
| ◆ bacitracin (AK-Tracin) (C) | Miscellaneous antibiotic | Solution: 1-2 drops q1-4h | |
| | | Ointment: 0.5-inch ribbon into lower conjunctival sac 3-4 times daily | |
| ◆ ciprofloxacin (Ciloxan) (C) | Quinolone | Solution: 1-2 drops every 2 hr for 2 days, and then 2 drops every 4 hr for 5 days | |
| | | Ointment: 0.5-inch ribbon tid for 2 days, then 0.5-inch ribbon daily for 5 days | Bacterial ocular infections |
| ◆ erythromycin (Ilotycin) (C) | Macrolide | Ointment: 0.5-inch ribbon 2-6 times/day | |
| ◆ gentamicin (Genoptic, others) (C) | Aminoglycoside | Solution: 1-2 drops every 2-4 hr | |
| | | Ointment: 0.5-inch ribbon 2-3 times/day | |
| ◆ sulfacetamide (Bleph-10, others) (C) | Sulfonamide | Solution: 1-2 drops every 2-3 hr | |
| | | Ointment: Apply 1-4 times/day | |
| **Antifungal Drug** | | | |
| natamycin (Natacyn) (C) | Antifungal | 1 drop into conjunctival sac q1-2h, and then usually reduce after first 3-4 days to 6-8 drops/day; therapy usually continues for 14-21 days | Fungal ocular infections |
| **Antiviral Drug** | | | |
| trifluridine (Viroptic) (C) | Antiviral | Initially 1 drop q2h while awake (max 9 drops/day); may later decrease to 5 drops/day | Viral ocular infections: keratitis and keratoconjunctivitis due to HSV types 1 and 2 |

*HSV,* Herpes simplex virus.
NOTE: Dosages vary based on the type and severity of infection.

## POLYPEPTIDE ANTIBIOTICS

Bacitracin and polymyxin B are polypeptide antibiotics. These drugs are rarely used systemically because of their nephrotoxic effects. They are bactericidal antimicrobials that inhibit protein synthesis in susceptible organisms, which leads to cell death. They are most commonly used in the treatment of superficial infections caused by gram-positive bacteria.

### ◆ bacitracin

Bacitracin (AK-Tracin) is an ophthalmic antimicrobial drug used to treat various eye infections. It is available as a single-ingredient product and as a combination product with polymyxin or neomycin and polymyxin. The combination products have a broader spectrum of activity. Bacitracin is available in ointment form.

### Pharmacokinetics

| Route | Onset of Action | Peak Plasma Concentration | Elimination Half-life | Duration of Action |
|---|---|---|---|---|
| Ocular | Variable | Immediate | Unknown | Variable |

## QUINOLONE ANTIBIOTICS

Quinolone antibiotics are very effective broad-spectrum antibiotics. They are discussed in detail in Chapter 39. They are bactericidal, destroying a wide spectrum of organisms that are often very difficult to treat. Currently five ophthalmic quinolones

are available: ciprofloxacin (Ciloxan), gatifloxacin (Zymar), moxifloxacin (Vigamox), levofloxacin (Quixin), and ofloxacin (Ocuflox).

Significant adverse effects include formation of corneal precipitates during treatment for bacterial keratitis. Other reactions include corneal staining and infiltrates. Systemic reactions are limited because of poor topical absorption. Those that occur are usually taste disorders and nausea. There are no significant drug interactions.

### ◆ ciprofloxacin

Ciprofloxacin (Ciloxan) is a synthetic quinolone antibiotic. It is available in ointment and solution form. Ciprofloxacin is indicated for the treatment of bacterial keratitis and conjunctivitis caused by susceptible gram-positive and gram-negative bacteria. One notable adverse reaction to ophthalmic ciprofloxacin is the appearance of white, crystalline precipitates occurring within any corneal lesions. This has occurred in approximately 17% of patients, and within 1 to 7 days of starting therapy. In all cases to date, the condition has been self-limiting, has not required drug discontinuation, and has not adversely affected clinical outcome.

### Pharmacokinetics

| Route | Onset of Action | Peak Plasma Concentration | Elimination Half-life | Duration of Action |
|---|---|---|---|---|
| Ocular | Variable | Immediate | 1-2 hr | Variable |

## SULFONAMIDES

Sulfonamides are synthetic bacteriostatic antibiotics that work by blocking the synthesis of folic acid in susceptible bacteria. Sulfacetamide sodium (Bleph-10) and sulfisoxazole (Gantrisin) are used to treat conjunctivitis and other ocular infections caused by susceptible bacteria.

The adverse effects are primarily limited to local reactions and include local irritation and stinging. Sulfonamide use can result in the overgrowth of nonsusceptible organisms. No significant topical toxic effects have been reported with the use of ophthalmic sulfonamides.

### ◆ sulfacetamide

Sulfacetamide (Bleph-10) is the most commonly used ophthalmic sulfonamide antibacterial drug. It is available in solution and ointment form.

### Pharmacokinetics

| Route | Onset of Action | Peak Plasma Concentration | Elimination Half-life | Duration of Action |
|---|---|---|---|---|
| Ocular | Variable | Immediate | Unknown | Variable |

## ANTIFUNGAL DRUG
### natamycin

Natamycin (Natacyn) is a polyene antifungal drug. It destroys fungi in the eye by binding to sterols in the fungal cell membrane, which disrupts the protective capabilities of the cell and results in cell death. Natamycin is used topically in the treatment of blepharitis, conjunctivitis, and keratitis caused by susceptible fungi (*Candida* and *Aspergillus* species). It is available only in suspension form.

### Pharmacokinetics

| Route | Onset of Action | Peak Plasma Concentration | Elimination Half-life | Duration of Action |
|---|---|---|---|---|
| Ocular | Variable | Immediate | Unknown | Variable |

## ANTIVIRAL DRUGS

Three antiviral ophthalmic drugs are currently available: fomivirsen (Vitravene), ganciclovir (Vitrasert), and trifluridine (Viroptic). Fomivirsen and ganciclovir are used to treat cytomegalovirus infections; they are implanted in the eye by an ophthalmologist and are beyond the scope of this chapter.

### trifluridine

Trifluridine (Viroptic, 1% ophthalmic drops) is a pyrimidine nucleoside. It inhibits viral replication by blocking the synthesis of viral deoxyribonucleic acid (DNA) by inhibiting viral DNA polymerase, an enzyme needed for DNA synthesis. It is used for ocular infections (keratitis and keratoconjunctivitis) caused by types 1 and 2 of the herpes simplex virus. Significant adverse effects include secondary glaucoma, corneal punctate defects, uveitis, and stromal edema (edema in the tough, fibrous, transparent portion of the cornea known as the *stroma*). The drugs exhibit no appreciable topical absorption, and no significant drug interactions have been reported.

## ANTIINFLAMMATORY DRUGS

Many of the same antiinflammatory drugs used systemically may also be used ophthalmically to treat various ocular inflammatory disorders and ocular surgery-related pain and inflammation. These drugs include both nonsteroidal antiinflammatory drugs (NSAIDs) and corticosteroids and are listed in Box 57-1.

## Mechanism of Action and Drug Effects

Corticosteroids and NSAIDs, as discussed in Chapters 33 and 44, respectively, both act to reduce inflammatory responses. When tissues are damaged, the membranes of affected cells release phospholipids, which are broken down by several different enzymes within the arachidonic acid metabolic pathway. Phospholipase is one of the first enzymes involved, and its activity is inhibited by corticosteroids. A second enzyme, cyclooxygenase, is the site of action of the NSAIDs. Both drug actions reduce the production of various inflammatory mediators. This in turn reduces pain, erythema, and other inflammatory processes.

## Indications

Corticosteroids and NSAIDs are applied topically for the symptomatic relief of many ophthalmic inflammatory conditions. They may be used to treat corneal, conjunctival, and scleral injuries from chemical, radiation, or thermal burns or from penetration of foreign bodies. They are used during the acute phase of the injury process to prevent fibrosis and scarring, which result in visual impairment. Corticosteroids produce a greater immunosuppressant effect than the NSAIDs. Consequently, NSAIDs are often preferred as initial topical therapy for such injuries. NSAIDs are also used in the symptomatic treatment of seasonal allergic conjunctivitis.

Corticosteroids and NSAIDs are used prophylactically before ocular surgery to prevent or reduce the intraoperative miosis. They are also used prophylactically after ocular surgery, such as cataract extraction, glaucoma surgery, and corneal transplantation, to prevent inflammation and scarring.

## Contraindications

These drugs are contraindicated in cases of known drug allergy. In addition, they are not used for minor abrasions or wounds because they may suppress the ability of the eye to resist bacterial, viral, or fungal infections. This is especially true of corticosteroids, which have stronger immunosuppressant effects.

## Adverse Effects

The most common adverse effect of corticosteroids is transient burning or stinging on application. The extended use of corticosteroids may result in cataracts, increased intraocular pressure, and optic nerve damage. If large doses are given, systemic absorption is possible. Systemic side effects of corticosteroids and NSAIDs are discussed in Chapters 33 and 44.

## DRUG PROFILES

Corticosteroids and NSAIDs used to treat ophthalmic inflammatory disorders are listed in Box 57-1. The ophthalmic formulations share many of the same characteristics as their systemic drug counterparts. However, the ophthalmic derivatives have limited systemic absorption. Therefore, most therapeutic and toxic effects are restricted to the eye. These drugs are pregnancy category C.

### CORTICOSTEROID

#### ♦ dexamethasone

Dexamethasone (Decadron) is a synthetic corticosteroid that is available in many systemic and ophthalmic formulations. It is used to treat inflammation of the eye, eyelids, conjunctiva, and cornea, and it may also be used in the treatment of uveitis, iridocyclitis, allergic conditions, and burns and in the removal of foreign bodies. Dexamethasone is available in ointment, suspension, and solution form.

Pharmacokinetics

| Route | Onset of Action | Peak Plasma Concentration | Elimination Half-life | Duration of Action |
|-------|-----------------|---------------------------|----------------------|--------------------|
| Ocular | Variable | Immediate | Unknown | Variable |

### NONSTEROIDAL ANTIINFLAMMATORY DRUGS
#### flurbiprofen

Flurbiprofen (Ocufen) is an NSAID used to treat inflammatory ophthalmic conditions, such as postoperative inflammation after a cataract extraction. It is also used to inhibit intraoperative miosis that may be induced by operative trauma and tissue injury. Flurbiprofen is available in solution form.

Pharmacokinetics

| Route | Onset of Action | Peak Plasma Concentration | Elimination Half-life | Duration of Action |
|-------|-----------------|---------------------------|----------------------|--------------------|
| Ocular | 30 min | 90 min | Unknown | 3 hr |

#### ketorolac

Ketorolac (Acular) is an NSAID that is available in both oral and injectable formulations for systemic use. The ophthalmic formulation is used to reduce ocular inflammation caused by trauma, such as ocular surgery, and inflammation secondary to external agents, such as allergens and bacteria. Ketorolac is contraindicated in patients with known drug allergy. It is available in solution form. It is important to know that this drug may delay eye wound healing and lead to corneal epithelial breakdown; therefore, constantly monitor the eye through the duration of therapy.

Pharmacokinetics

| Route | Onset of Action | Peak Plasma Concentration | Elimination Half-life | Duration of Action |
|-------|-----------------|---------------------------|----------------------|--------------------|
| Ocular | Rapid | Immediate | Unknown | 4-6 hr |

## TOPICAL ANESTHETICS

Topical anesthetic ophthalmic drugs are local anesthetics that are used to alleviate eye pain. The two currently available topical anesthetics used for ophthalmic purposes are proparacaine and tetracaine.

## Mechanism of Action and Drug Effects

As described in Chapter 11, local anesthetics stabilize the membranes of nerves, which results in a decrease in the movement of ions into and out of the nerve endings. When nerves are stabilized in this way, they cannot transmit signals about painful stimuli to the brain. Usually, the application of topical anesthetic drugs to the eye results in local anesthesia in less than 30 seconds.

## Indications

Ophthalmic topical anesthetic drugs are used to produce ocular anesthesia for short corneal and conjunctival procedures. They prevent pain during surgical procedures and certain painful ophthalmic examinations, including removal of imbedded foreign objects. They are recommended only for short-term use and are not recommended for self-administration.

## Contraindications

Contraindications to local ophthalmic anesthetics include known drug allergy.

## Adverse Effects

Adverse effects are rare with ophthalmic anesthetic drugs and are limited to local effects such as stinging, burning, redness, lacrimation, and blurred vision. Systemic toxicity is rare but can theoretically lead to central nervous system (CNS) stimulation and/or CNS or cardiovascular depression.

## Interactions

Because of limited systemic absorption and short duration of action, ophthalmic anesthetic drugs have no significant drug interactions.

## DRUG PROFILE

Currently available topical ophthalmic anesthetic drugs are proparacaine (Alcaine) and tetracaine (generic only). They are very similar in their indications and dosing regimens.

## tetracaine

Tetracaine is a local anesthetic of the ester type (see Chapter 11). It is applied as an eyedrop to numb the eye for various ophthalmic procedures. Tetracaine begins to work in about 25 seconds and lasts for about 15 to 20 minutes. Additional drops are applied as needed. It is currently available only in solution form. Pregnancy category C.

### Pharmacokinetics

| Route | Onset of Action | Peak Plasma Concentration | Elimination Half-life | Duration of Action |
|-------|-----------------|---------------------------|----------------------|--------------------|
| Ocular | Less than 30 sec | 1-5 min | Short | 15-20 min |

# DIAGNOSTIC DRUGS

## DRUG PROFILES

### CYCLOPLEGIC MYDRIATICS

#### ◆ atropine sulfate

Atropine sulfate (Isopto Atropine) solution and ointment are used as mydriatic and cycloplegic drugs. The drug dilates the pupil (mydriasis) and paralyzes the ciliary muscle (cycloplegic refraction), which prevents accommodation. It is used to assist in eye examination or to treat uveal tract inflammatory states. The usual dosage for uveitis (inflammation of the choroid, iris, or ciliary body) in children and adults is 1 to 2 drops of the solution, or 0.3 to 0.5 cm of ointment, 2 to 3 times daily. The dosage for eye examination is 1 drop of solution, ideally 1 hour before the procedure. Pregnancy category C.

#### cyclopentolate

Cyclopentolate solution (Cyclogyl) is used primarily as a diagnostic mydriatic and cycloplegic drug. Unlike atropine, it is not used to treat uveitis. The usual adult dose is 1 to 2 drops (0.5%, 1%, or 2%). This is repeated in 5 to 10 minutes if needed. The dose for children is the same as that for adults. The drug effects usually subside within 24 hours. Other cycloplegic mydriatics are scopolamine (Isopto Hyoscine), homatropine (Isopto Homatropine), and tropicamide (Mydriacyl). All three are topical ophthalmic solutions with indications similar to those of atropine and cyclopentolate, except that tropicamide, like cyclopentolate, is generally used for diagnostic purposes only and not for treatment of inflammatory states. Pregnancy category C.

### OPHTHALMIC DYE

#### fluorescein

Fluorescein (AK-Fluor) is an ophthalmic diagnostic dye used to identify corneal defects and to locate foreign objects in the eye. It is also used in fitting hard contact lenses. After the instillation of fluorescein, various defects are highlighted in either bright green or yellow-orange, and foreign objects have a green halo around them. Fluorescein is available for use as an ophthalmic injection, solution, and diagnostic applicator strips. Dose determination and drug administration are usually carried out by an ophthalmologist. Pregnancy category C.

# ANTIALLERGIC DRUGS

## DRUG PROFILES

### ANTIHISTAMINES

#### olopatadine

Olopatadine (Patanol) is an ocular antihistamine used to treat symptoms of allergic conjunctivitis (hay fever), which can be seasonal or nonseasonal. It works by competing at the receptor sites for histamine. Histamine normally produces ocular symptoms such as itching and tearing. Other ocular antihistamines include azelastine (Optivar), emedastine (Emadine), ketotifen (Zaditor), and epinastine (Elestat). These drugs have mechanisms of action, therapeutic and adverse effects, and drug interactions similar to those of the systemic antihistamines described in Chapter 36, although systemic effects are less likely with ophthalmic administration. Recommended dosages for olopatadine are given in the Dosages table on p. 934. Pregnancy category C.

### MAST CELL STABILIZERS

#### cromolyn

Cromolyn sodium (Crolom) is an antiallergic drug that inhibits the release of inflammation-producing mediators from sensitized inflammatory cells called *mast cells.* It is used in the treatment of vernal keratoconjunctivitis (springtime inflammation of the cornea and conjunctiva). Other mast cell stabilizers with similar effects are pemirolast (Alamast), nedocromil (Alocril), and lodoxamide (Alomide). Recommended dosages for cromolyn are given in the Dosages table on p. 934. Pregnancy category B.

### DECONGESTANTS

#### tetrahydrozoline

Tetrahydrozoline is an ocular decongestant. It works by promoting vasoconstriction of blood vessels in and around the eye. This reduces the edema associated with allergic and inflammatory processes. It is specifically indicated to control redness, burning, and other minor irritations. Other ocular decongestants include phenylephrine (Neo-Synephrine), oxymetazoline (Visine LR), and naphazoline (Clear Eyes). Recommended dosages for tetrahydrozoline are given in the Dosages table on p. 934. Pregnancy category C.

### LUBRICANTS AND MOISTURIZERS

#### ◆ artificial tears

An array of products is available over the counter to provide lubrication or moisture for the eyes. This is helpful to patients with dry or otherwise irritated eyes. Artificial tears are isotonic and contain buffers to adjust pH. In addition, they contain preservatives for microbial control and may contain viscosity agents for extension of ocular activity. Selected over-the-counter brand names include Moisture Drops, Murine, Nu-Tears, Akwa Tears, and Tears Plus. Many similar products are available on the market both as solutions (eyedrops) and as lubrication ointments. They are often dosed to patient comfort as needed. Restasis is an ophthalmic form of the immunosuppressant drug cyclosporine (see Chapter 48). It is also used to promote tear production in the condition technically known as *keratoconjunctivitis sicca* (dry eyes). It can be used together with artificial tears, if the drugs are given 15 minutes apart. Pregnancy category B.

## DOSAGES

### Ocular Antiallergics

| DRUG (PREGNANCY CATEGORY) | PHARMACOLOGIC CLASS | USUAL DOSAGE RANGE | INDICATIONS |
|---|---|---|---|
| cromolyn (Crolom) (C) | Mast cell stabilizer | 1-2 drops in affected eye(s) 4-6 times daily | Vernal (springtime) conjunctivitis and/or keratitis (corneal inflammation) |
| olopatadine (Patanol 0.1%) (C) | Antihistamine | 1-2 drops in affected eye(s) 2 times per day at an interval of 6-8 hours | Allergic conjunctivitis |
| olopatadine (Patanol 0.2%) (C) | Antihistamine | 1 drop in affected eye(s) once a day | Allergic conjunctivitis |
| tetrahydrozoline (Murine Plus, others) (C) | Decongestant | 1-2 drops in affected eye(s) up to 4 times daily | Redness, burning, or other minor irritation |

## NURSING PROCESS

## ASSESSMENT

Before administering any *ophthalmic drug* per the prescriber's orders, perform a baseline assessment of the eye and its structures, documenting normal and abnormal findings. It is also important to document any redness, swelling, pain, excessive tearing, eye drainage or discharge, decrease in visual acuity, or other unusual symptoms. Assess the patient for hypersensitivity to any medications or chemicals and for any drug- or disorder-related contraindications, cautions, and drug interactions. You may need to perform a visual acuity test (e.g., Snellen chart test), if indicated, noting the findings before, during, and after drug treatment. Focus the nursing history on past or present systemic disease processes and exposure to any chemicals that could be topical irritants to the eye, skin, or mucous membranes, including past or present occupational and environmental exposures.

## NURSING DIAGNOSES

1. Acute pain related to the eye disorder, infection, and/or inflammatory eye condition
2. Deficient knowledge related to lack of information about the eye disorder and associated medication therapy
3. Risk for injury (to eye) related to improper use of medication and improper instillation procedures

## PLANNING

### GOALS

1. Patient remains free from eye pain.
2. Patient demonstrates adequate knowledge related to the use of the medication, its application, and side effects.
3. Patient remains free from injury (to eye) related to therapy.

### OUTCOME CRITERIA

1. Patient minimizes eye pain related to the eye disorder by applying warm or cold compresses as prescribed, using non-aspirin analgesics as directed, and properly applying prescribed ophthalmic medication.
2. Patient identifies rationale for use of ophthalmic medication, adverse effects associated with each medication, as well

## CASE STUDY

### Medications for Eye Trauma

P.L., a construction worker, is being seen in the emergency department because of a possible eye injury. He was working without eye protection, and a gust of wind sprayed metal shavings into his face. The physician has instilled fluorescein sodium and has noted areas in the eyeball with green halos around them.

1. What is the purpose of the fluorescein sodium, and what is indicated by the green halos?
2. P.L. is sent to an ophthalmologist for further treatment. What eye medication do you expect will be used for the next procedure?
3. After the procedure, P.L. receives a prescription for dexamethasone ocular ointment, to be administered three times a day. What specific patient teaching information will the nurse share with P.L.?
4. How could this have been prevented?

For answers, see http://evolve.elsevier.com/Lilley.

as signs and symptoms to report to the prescriber such as increase in eye pain, drainage, redness, and decreased visual acuity.
3. Patient minimizes self-injury related to the adverse effects of therapy by creating a safe environment at home, including reducing clutter and moving out any unused rugs or furniture; putting in more lighting, especially night lights; and using assistive devices as needed, if vision is altered.

## IMPLEMENTATION

Always inspect the solution, and administer only clear, unexpired products (e.g., drops, ointments, solutions) to the eye. Shake all solutions, and mix contents thoroughly. Do not use solutions with any particulate matter. One of the most important standards to follow during instillation of drops or ointment is to avoid touching the eye with the tip of the dropper or container to prevent contamination of the product. Remove any excess medication promptly and apply pressure to the inner canthus for 1 minute (or other specified time frame). Applying pressure to the inner canthus after instillation of medication is needed to prevent or decrease systemic absorption and subsequent systemic adverse effects. Apply ointments and any other ophthalmic topical drug dosage form to the conjunctival sac and never directly onto the eye itself (cornea). To facilitate the instillation of ophthalmic medication, tilt the patient's head back and have him or her look up at the ceiling. Several ophthalmic drugs with different actions may be ordered; give each drug exactly as prescribed and within the specified time period. This is particularly important when surgical procedures are being performed on the eye because several drugs with different actions may be ordered and must be given at specific times. Ointments may cause a temporary blurring of vision because of the film that bathes the eye. This film will decrease once the drug is absorbed, and vision will then become clearer. Always refer to the medication order, as well as an authoritative drug source for specific instructions and guidelines regarding application technique, length of time to apply pressure to the inner canthus, and any other special directions. See Chapter 9 for opthalmic drug administration.

Follow directions for the use of *antiviral ophthalmic preparations* closely. Administer *topical anesthetics,* as ordered, for use in removal of a foreign body or treatment of eye injury. Repeated and continuous use is not recommended because of the risk for delayed wound healing, corneal perforation, permanent corneal opacification, and vision loss. When there is an abrasion or other injury to the eye and appropriate medications are ordered, patching of the affected eye is recommended. This helps prevent further injury resulting from loss of the blink reflex due to overuse of topical anesthetic. Include education regarding any change in eye color caused by the medication.

For example, latanoprost actually changes the eye color permanently from hazel, green, or bluish-brown to brown. See the Patient Teaching Tips for more information regarding ophthalmic medications.

## EVALUATION

Therapeutic responses to *miotics* include decreased aqueous humor of the eye with resultant decreased intraocular pressure and decreased signs, symptoms, and long-term effects associated with glaucoma. *Beta-adrenergic blockers* are therapeutic if there is a resultant decrease in intraocular pressure. Possible adverse effects for which to evaluate include weakness, eye irritation, rash, bradycardia, hypotension, and dysrhythmias (see Chapter 19). Therapeutic responses to *antibiotic, antifungal,* and *antiviral ophthalmic drugs* include elimination of the infection or condition and resolution of symptoms, and prevention of complications. Therapeutic responses to *ophthalmic anesthetics* include prevention/relief of pain associated with the injury. Adverse effects may include CNS excitation (e.g., dizziness, tremors, restlessness, nervousness) if the drug is systemically absorbed. *Antiinflammatory ophthalmic solutions result* in a decrease in allergic reactions with a decrease in itching, tearing, redness, and eye discharge. Potential complications of these solutions include swelling of the conjunctiva (chemosis). Further monitoring includes reevaluation of goals and outcome criteria.

## PATIENT TEACHING TIPS

- Educate the patient about correct administration technique. A demonstration with return demonstrations by the patient is a recommended teaching strategy.
- Encourage the patient to use only solutions that are clear and unexpired. Keep eyedroppers and solutions in containers for direct application sterile by avoiding touching the tip of the eyedropper or container to the surface of the eye.
- Educate patients receiving indirect cholinergics about adverse effects such as blurred vision, bronchospasm, nausea, vomiting, bradycardia, hypotension, and sweating.
- With any ophthalmic drug, instruct the patient to report to the prescriber any severe stinging, burning, itching, or redness of the eye; excessive tearing or excessive dryness of the eye; puffiness of the eye/eyelids; discharge from the eye; fever; eye pain, or loss of or change in vision.
- Instill sympatholytic drugs as ordered. Once these drugs (and many other drugs used in the eye) are instilled, instruct the patient to apply pressure to the inner canthus with a tissue or 2-inch by 2-inch gauze pad for 1 full minute or as directed. Application of pressure to the inner canthus helps to minimize absorption and decrease the risk of systemic adverse effects. Advise the patient to report to the prescriber immediately any blurred vision, difficulty breathing, wheezing, sweating, flushing, or loss of sight.

- Photosensitivity is an expected adverse effect of mydriatics; therefore, when these drugs are administered, encourage the patient to wear sunglasses to help minimize eye discomfort and/or headaches while in sunlight.
- With topical anesthetics, advise the patient to avoid rubbing or touching the eye while it is numb, because eye damage may result. An eye patch may be worn, if prescribed, to protect the eye because of loss of the blink reflex.
- Instruct the patient to use ophthalmic medications as prescribed and never to overuse. Stress that products with expiration dates that have passed are not to be used and are to be discarded appropriately. Advise the patient never to stop medications without consulting the prescriber first because of the possibility of adverse reactions.
- Inform the patient not to wear contact lenses while ophthalmic drugs are being instilled and for the duration of therapy, because the lenses may lead to further irritation.
- Ophthalmic ketorolac, an antiinflammatory drug, may delay eye wound healing and lead to corneal epithelial breakdown. Instruct the patient to report these problems if present or suspected.

## KEY POINTS

- Glaucoma is a disorder of the eye caused by inhibition of the normal flow and drainage of aqueous humor, and treatment helps to reduce intraocular pressure either by increasing the drainage of aqueous humor or decreasing its production.
- Drugs that increase aqueous humor drainage are direct cholinergics, indirect cholinergics, sympathomimetics, and beta blockers.
- A large proportion of the inflammatory diseases of the eye are caused by viruses, and many ocular antimicrobials are available to treat bacterial, viral, and fungal infections of the eye. Common ocular infections include conjunctivitis, hordeolum (sty), keratitis, uveitis, and endophthalmitis.

- Antiinflammatory ophthalmic drugs include corticosteroids and are used to inhibit inflammatory responses to mechanical forces, chemicals, and immunologic reactions.
- Topical anesthetics are used to prevent pain to the eye and are beneficial during surgery, ophthalmic examinations, and removal of foreign bodies.
- Administer all ophthalmic preparations exactly as ordered. Always apply into the conjunctival sac. Safe and accurate application or instillation technique also includes avoiding contact of the eyedropper or tube to the eye to prevent contamination of the drug.
- Patients need to report to the prescriber immediately any increase in symptoms, such as eye pain or drainage and fever.

## NCLEX® EXAMINATION REVIEW QUESTIONS

1 The ophthalmologist has given a patient a dose of ocular atropine drops before an eye examination. Which statement by the nurse accurately explains to the patient the reason for these drops?
   a "These drops will cause the surface of your eye to become numb so that the doctor can do the examination."
   b "These drops are used to check for any possible foreign bodies or corneal defects that may be in your eye."
   c "These drops will reduce your tear production for the eye examination."
   d "These drops will cause your pupils to dilate, which makes the eye examination easier."

2 When assessing a patient who is receiving a direct-acting cholinergic eyedrop as part of treatment for glaucoma, the nurse anticipates that the drug affects the pupil in which way?
   a It causes mydriasis, or pupil dilation.
   b It causes miosis, or pupil constriction.
   c It changes the color of the pupil.
   d It causes no change in pupil size.

3 During patient teaching regarding self-administration of ophthalmic drops, which statement by the nurse is correct?
   a "Hold the eyedrops over the cornea, and squeeze out the drop."
   b "Apply pressure to the lacrimal duct area for 5 minutes after administration."
   c "Be sure to place the drop in the conjunctival sac of the lower eyelid."
   d "Squeeze your eyelid closed tightly after placing the drop into your eye."

4 When the nurse is providing teaching about eye medications for glaucoma, the nurse tells the patient that miotics help glaucoma by which mechanism of action?
   a Decreasing intracranial pressure
   b Decreasing intraocular pressure
   c Increasing tear production
   d Causing pupillary dilation

5 During the assessment of a glaucoma patient who has newly prescribed carbonic anhydrase inhibitor eyedrops, the nurse would report a history of which condition?
   a Allergy to sulfa drugs
   b Decreased renal function
   c Diabetes mellitus
   d Hypertension

6 The nurse is preparing to administer ketorolac (Acular) eyedrops. The patient asks, "Why am I getting these eyedrops?" Which is the correct answer by the nurse?
   a "These drops will reduce the pressure inside your eye as part of treatment for glaucoma."
   b "These drops are for a bacterial eye infection."
   c "These drops will relieve your dry eyes."
   d "These drops work to reduce the inflammation in your eyes."

7 A patient has undergone an eye procedure during which ophthalmic mydriatics and anesthetic drops were used. The nurse gives which instructions to the patient prior to discharge? (Select all that apply.)
   a "Do not rub or touch the numb eye."
   b "You may reinsert your contact lenses before you leave."
   c "Be sure to wear sunglasses when you go outside."
   d "Your pupils will appear very tiny until the medication wears off."
   e "Report any increase in eye pain or drainage to the ophthalmologist immediately."

1. d, 2. b, 3. c, 4. b, 5. a, 6. d, 7. a, c, e.

For Critical Thinking and Prioritization Questions, see http://evolve.elsevier.com/Lilley.

# Otic Drugs

## OBJECTIVES

When you reach the end of this chapter, you will be able to do the following:

1 Describe the anatomy of the ear including external, middle, and inner ear.
2 Cite the various categories of ear disorders, and describe their causes and signs and symptoms.
3 List the various types of otic preparations and their indications.
4 Discuss the mechanisms of action, dosage, cautions, contraindications, drug interactions, and specific application techniques of each of the otic drugs.
5 Develop a nursing care plan that includes all phases of the nursing process for patients taking otic drugs.

## DRUG PROFILES

♦ **carbamide peroxide, p. 939**

---

♦ *Key drug*

## KEY TERMS

**Cerumen** A yellowish or brownish waxy excretion produced by modified sweat glands in the external ear canal. Also called *earwax*. (p. 939)

**Otitis externa** Inflammation or infection of the external auditory canal. (p. 938)

**Otitis media (OM)** Inflammation or infection of the middle ear. (p. 938)

## ANATOMY, PHYSIOLOGY, AND PATHOPHYSIOLOGY OVERVIEW

The ear is made up of four parts: the external, outer, middle, and inner ears. The external ear is composed of the pinna (outer projecting part of the ear) and the external auditory meatus or opening of the ear canal. Synonyms for the pinna are *auricle* and *ala*. The term *outer ear* refers primarily to the external auditory canal. This is the space between the external auditory meatus and the tympanic membrane (eardrum). The middle ear is composed of the tympanic cavity, which is the space that begins with the tympanic membrane and ends with the oval window. Included in the middle ear are three bony structures of the mastoid bone—the malleus ("hammer"), incus ("anvil"), and

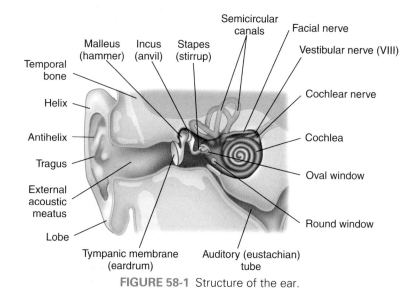

**FIGURE 58-1** Structure of the ear.

stapes ("stirrup")—as well as the auditory or eustachian tube. The inner ear includes the cochlea and semicircular canals. The ear and its associated structures are illustrated in Figure 58-1.

Disorders of the ear can be categorized according to the portion of the ear affected. External ear (pinna) disorders are generally the result of physical trauma to the ear and consist of lacerations or scrapes to the skin and localized infection of the hair follicles, which often causes the development of a boil. These disorders also tend to be self-limiting and heal with time. Other examples of external ear disorders are contact dermatitis, seborrhea, and psoriasis, as evidenced by itching, local redness, inflammation, weeping, or drainage. These conditions usually respond to the same topical medications used for any other local skin disorders, as discussed in Chapter 56. However, symptoms such as drainage, pain, and dizziness are sometimes also the first signs of a more serious underlying condition (e.g., head trauma, meningitis) and warrant prompt medical evaluation. Medications for disorders affecting the outer ear (ear canal) and middle ear are the focus of this chapter. Diseases of the inner ear involve highly specialized medical practices that are beyond the scope of this book.

The most common disorders affecting the outer and middle ear are bacterial and fungal infections, inflammation, and earwax accumulation. Such disorders are often self-limiting, and treatments are usually successful. If problems persist or are left untreated, however, more serious problems such as hearing loss may result. Infections affecting the ear canal are known as *otitis externa,* whereas those affecting the middle ear are known as *otitis media (OM).* OM is a common disease of infancy and early childhood. It is often preceded by an upper respiratory tract infection. It may also occur in adults, but it is then generally associated with trauma to the tympanic membrane. Foreign objects and infection or inflammation associated with water sports are the usual sources of such trauma. In adults, the condition is also more likely to manifest as otitis externa, involving the ear canal and/or external tympanic membrane. Common symptoms of both otitis media and otitis externa are pain, fever, malaise, pressure, a sensation of fullness in the ears, and impaired hearing. If the condition is left untreated, tinnitus (ringing in the ears), nausea, vertigo, mastoiditis, and even temporary or permanent hearing deficits may occur.

OM is the second most common infection in children, accounting for more than 20 million physician visits annually. Medical management of OM is debated among the medical community, primarily due to the increased incidence of antibiotic resistance. Because of these concerns, treatment of OM has significantly changed over the last decade. In 2004, the American Academy of Pediatrics published guidelines based on expert opinion and a thorough review of the literature. A growing number of physicians do not recommend antibiotic treatment in children with mild OM without a fever (or with minimal fever). More emphasis is now given to observation and close follow-up. Many parents have concerns regarding this option. If a decision is made to treat with an antibiotic, amoxicillin should be the first-line drug for most children. If the patient fails to respond within 48 to 72 hours, the patient must be reassessed. If no antibiotics were given initially, they should be started or the initial antibiotic may need to be changed. Antibiotics are discussed in Chapters 38 and 39.

## PHARMACOLOGY OVERVIEW

## TREATMENT OF EAR DISORDERS

Some of the minor ailments that affect the outer or middle ear can be treated with over-the-counter medications, but persistent, painful conditions generally require prescription medications. Drugs used to treat ear conditions are known as *otic drugs,* and most are applied topically to the ear canal. Because of this, they generally are not involved in drug interactions. Adverse effects are uncommon and usually do not extend beyond localized irritation, and otic drugs are normally contraindicated only in cases of known drug allergy. Pertinent classes of otic drugs include the following:

- Antibacterials (antibiotics)
- Antifungals
- Antiinflammatory drugs
- Local analgesics

## TABLE 58-1   COMMON ANTIBACTERIAL OTIC PRODUCTS

| STEROID COMPONENT | ANTIBIOTIC COMPONENT | TRADE NAME |
|---|---|---|
| hydrocortisone (1%) | 5 mg of neomycin and 10,000 units of polymyxin B per 10-mL bottle | Cortisporin Otic, others |
| hydrocortisone (1%) | ciprofloxacin 2 mg/mL | Cipro HT Otic |
| dexamethasone (0.1%) | ciprofloxacin 3 mg/mL | Ciprodex |
| None | ofloxacin 3 mg/mL | Floxin Otic |

## TABLE 58-2   COMMON ANTIFUNGAL OTIC PRODUCTS

| INGREDIENTS | TRADE NAME |
|---|---|
| hydrocortisone, 1%; pramoxine, 1%; chloroxylenol, 0.1%; propylene glycol diacetate, 3%; benzalkonium chloride (amount not specified) | Cortic, Otomar, Aero Otic HC, Mediotic HC |
| hydrocortisone, 1%; acetic acid, 2%; propylene glycol diacetate, 3%; sodium acetate, 0.015%; benzethonium chloride, 0.02% | Acetasol HC |

Neopmycin, polymixin B, and hydrocortisone otic preparations are contraindicated in patients with a perforated eardrum.

- Local anesthetics
- Corticosteroids
- Wax emulsifiers

More serious cases of ear disorders may require treatment with systemic drugs such as antimicrobial drugs, analgesics, antiinflammatory drugs, and antihistamines. These medications are discussed in detail in previous chapters dealing with the respective drug classes.

## ANTIBACTERIAL AND ANTIFUNGAL OTIC DRUGS

Antibacterial and antifungal otic drugs are often combined with steroids to take advantage of the antiinflammatory, antipruritic, and antiallergic effects of the latter drugs. These drugs are used to treat outer and middle ear infections. Because they all work and are dosed very similarly, four products are profiled together here. Systemic antibiotics are also commonly prescribed for these conditions (e.g., amoxicillin; see Chapter 38), either alone or in addition to the otic drugs described in the following sections. Tables 58-1 and 58-2 list several commonly used products and their component amounts. These drugs are pregnancy category C.

## DRUG PROFILES

### ANTIBACTERIAL PRODUCTS

Cortisporin (and other brands) is a three-drug combination that includes hydrocortisone and two antimicrobials, neomycin (an *aminoglycoside*; see Chapter 39) and polymyxin B. Hydrocortisone is the corticosteroid most commonly used in otic drugs, although there is one preparation (Ciprodex) that contains ciprofloxacin (a *fluoroquinolone*; see Chapter 39) and

dexamethasone. In either case, the purpose of the steroid component is to reduce the inflammation and itching associated with ear infections. Ciprofloxacin is also available in combination with hydrocortisone (Cipro HC Otic). Ofloxacin (Floxin Otic) is another fluoroquinolone available only as a single-drug product. All of these products are used for the treatment of bacterial otitis externa or otitis media caused by susceptible bacteria such as *Staphylococcus aureus*, *Escherichia coli*, *Klebsiella* species, and others. Neomycin, polymyxin B, and hydrocortisone otic preparations are contraindicated in patients with a perforated eardrum; ciprofloxacin and ofloxacin can be used with perforated eardrums. Their usual dosage is 4 drops three to four times daily, except for ofloxacin, which is dosed at 5 to 10 drops twice daily (5-drop dose for children younger than 12 years of age). With some otic drugs, it is recommended to saturate a retrievable cotton or tissue wick and let this wick soak inside the ear canal, as a means of dosing the drug. The wick can be periodically remoistened with additional drug or removed and further eardrops inserted directly into the ear canal. Follow the specific instructions on the drug package or the method recommended by the prescriber or pharmacist.

### ANTIFUNGAL PRODUCTS

Fungal infections account for about 4% of ear infections. Antifungal otic drugs are used primarily for otitis externa. These drugs may also have antibacterial and antiviral properties. Two commonly used preparations are Cortic and Acetasol HC. Cortic, also available as Otomar, Aero Otic HC, and Mediotic HC, is composed of hydrocortisone (a steroid), pramoxine (a local anesthetic), chloroxylenol (an antiseptic antifungal), propylene glycol diacetate (an emulsifying drug), and benzalkonium chloride (an antiseptic preservative). Acetasol HC consists of hydrocortisone, acetic acid (an antifungal), propylene glycol diacetate, sodium acetate (a preservative), and benzethonium chloride (an antiseptic preservative). The local anesthetic components help ease both the pain and itching common in ear infections.

## EARWAX EMULSIFIERS

An additional common ear problem is the accumulation and eventual impaction (hardening) of earwax, or cerumen, which can also contribute to or complicate the infectious and inflammatory conditions described earlier. Products that soften and help to eliminate earwax are referred to as *earwax emulsifiers*. Wax, or cerumen, is a natural product of the ear and is produced by modified sweat glands in the ear canal. However, it can occasionally build up and become impacted, which results in pain and partial temporary deafness. From chemistry, a nonpolar substance is one that is not water-soluble. Such a substance is said to be emulsified when it is chemically and/or physically converted to a more water-soluble form. *Earwax emulsifiers* loosen impacted cerumen, which allows it to be flushed out of the ear canal through irrigation (with water).

## DRUG PROFILE

### ♦ carbamide peroxide

Carbamide peroxide (Debrox) is a commonly used earwax emulsifier. It is combined with other components (e.g., glycerin, a lubricant) that help soften and lubricate cerumen prior to irrigation. Carbamide peroxide slowly releases hydrogen peroxide and oxygen when exposed to moisture. This release of oxygen imparts a weak antibacterial action to this otic drug. In addition, the *effervescence* (foaming) resulting from the release of oxygen has the mechanical effect of emulsifying impacted cerumen to release it from the walls of the ear canal. Earwax emulsifiers are not to be used without physician recommendation when ear drainage, tympanic membrane rupture, or significant pain or other irritation is present. After allowing the drug to dissolve the earwax, one can remove it by gentle flushing the ear canal with warm water from a bulb syringe. Some earwax removal products include such a syringe in the package. This drug is pregnancy category C.

---

### ⚡ SAFETY AND QUALITY IMPROVEMENT: PREVENTING MEDICATION ERRORS

#### *Eardrops Do NOT Go into the Eyes!*

The Institute for Safe Medication Practices (ISMP) reports that painful medication errors have occurred when eardrops have been mistakenly used in the eyes. The tissues of the eye are more sensitive than ear tissue, and eye medications are specially formulated for ophthalmic use. Patients who receive eardrops in the eyes will immediately complain of burning and stinging; redness and swelling may develop later.

It may seem to be common sense that eardrops should not be used in the eyes, but the ISMP has reported several instances of this occurrence. Some errors are blamed on the similarities between the words "otic" (meaning ear) and "optic" (meaning eye).

The ISMP recommends several actions to reduce the risk of harming patients due to administration of eardrops into the eyes, including:

- Placing an extra label on the dropper bottle that specifies "eye" or "ear"
- Keep medications in their original cartons as these often have drawings of an eye or an ear on the carton, unlike the actual vials.
- In the pharmacy, separate eardrop and eyedrop vials. Storing them together increases the chance of a mix-up between medications that have similar names.
- Nurses should confirm the medication route with the patient before administering the drops.
- If a patient is receiving both eardrops and eyedrops, administer them on different time schedules if possible.

Data from ISMP: "And the 'eyes' have it": eardrops, that is..., *ISMP Medication Safety Alert,* October 19, 2006, available at http://www.ismp.org/Newsletters/acutecare/articles/Oct06.asp#19. Accessed November 2, 2011.

---

## NURSING PROCESS

### ASSESSMENT

Before administering any of the *otic preparations,* assess baseline hearing or auditory status, if deemed appropriate, and document the findings. Assess the patient's symptoms, past and present medical history, and use of prescription drugs, over-the-counter drugs, and herbals. Document any drug or food allergies. A basic understanding of the anatomy of the ear, especially anatomic variations in patients of different age groups, is needed to ensure proper application technique. Contraindications, cautions, and drug interactions for the otic drugs, chemicals, and/or solutions have been discussed previously in the pharmacology section; always assess the patient for these and document the findings. In addition, if the patient has a perforated eardrum, this is a contraindication to the use of otic drugs.

### NURSING DIAGNOSES

1. Acute pain related to ear infection or ear disorder
2. Deficient knowledge related to lack of experience with otic drugs and their method of administration
3. Noncompliance related to a lack of motivation and or lack of understanding for the need of frequent eardrop instillation, as ordered

### PLANNING

#### GOALS

1. Patient is free from pain and other symptoms related to the ear disorder.
2. Patient demonstrates adequate knowledge about the treatment regimen, its use, application, and adverse effects.
3. Patient remains compliant and adheres to medication regimen as prescribed.

#### OUTCOME CRITERIA

1. Patient experiences minimal to no discomfort with use of prescribed medication.
   - Patient uses measures to enhance comfort such as use of warm compresses, as prescribed, as well as non-narcotic analgesics, as directed.
   - Patient reports immediately to the prescriber the increase in ear pain and other symptoms once therapy is initiated.
2. Patient states rationale for the use of otic medication and ways to increase the drug's effectiveness, such as accurate application or instillation and remaining supine or sitting with the affected ear upward for a short period.
3. Patient instills medication as prescribed as related to dosage, frequency, and duration of therapy.

### IMPLEMENTATION

Instill *otic preparations* only after the ear has been thoroughly cleansed, all cerumen (earwax) has been removed (by irrigation if necessary, or as ordered). Eardrops, solutions, and ointments need to be stored at room temperature before instillation. Administration of solutions that are too cold may cause a vestibular type of reaction with vomiting and dizziness. If the solution has been refrigerated, allow it to warm to room temperature. Higher temperatures may affect the potency of these solutions, and storage at room temperature is recommended. When administering eardrops to adults, hold the pinna *up* and back. In children younger than 3 years of age, hold the pinna *down* and back. Allow a period of time for adequate coverage of the ear by the medication. Gentle massage to the tragus area of the ear may also help to increase coverage of the medication after the solution is given. See the Patient Teaching Tips and also Chapter 9 for more information on eardrop instillation.

## CASE STUDY

### *Ear Medications*

T.E. is 8 years old and loves to swim in the neighborhood pool. Lately she has had a feeling of fullness in her left ear, and today she tells her mother that her ear is hurting and itching and that she feels "awful." Her mother takes her temperature and finds that it is 101° F (38.3° C). She calls the pediatrician's office for an appointment, and T.E. is seen the next morning. After examining T.E., the pediatrician says that T.E. has otitis media in the left ear and some earwax buildup in both ears. The pediatrician removes some of the earwax manually, writes prescriptions for oral antibiotics for T.E., and gives instructions to use an earwax emulsifier. The nurse meets with them to review the instructions.

1. T.E.'s mother asks, "Why is the antibiotic a pill? It seems to me that if she has an ear infection, she should take eardrops!" What is the nurse's best response?

2. T.E.'s mother has another question: "What will happen if this ear infection does not get better?"

3. T.E. complains that her ear "really hurts and itches." What can be given to her for this problem? How will it be given?

For answers, see http://evolve.elsevier.com/Lilley.

## EVALUATION

The therapeutic effects of *otic drugs,* as with all drugs, are gauged by evaluating whether goals and objectives have been met. Therapeutic effects of otic drugs include less pain, redness, and swelling in the ear; a reduction in fever; and resolution of any other signs and symptoms associated with the ear disorder. Improvement in hearing may also be an anticipated therapeutic effect. Monitor the ear canal for the occurrence of rash and/or any signs of local irritation, such as redness and heat at the site. Evaluate the patient for adverse effects with each application or instillation, and report any unusual appearance of the outer ear and ear canal immediately to the prescriber.

## PATIENT TEACHING TIPS

- Provide thorough instructions to the patient about the proper use of eardrops or instillation of any medication into the ear. Warn the patient that dizziness may occur after application of the medication, requiring the patient to remain supine or sitting during instillation and for a few minutes thereafter.

- Medication to be applied to the ear must be at room temperature. This may be achieved by running warm water over the medication bottle, but care must be taken to prevent water from getting into the container, damaging the label so that the directions are unreadable, or making the solution too warm to use. Advise the patient not to heat the medication; for example, a microwave oven must not be used for warming—because eardrops that are overheated may lose potency. If the pharmacy indicates that the drug should be kept in a refrigerator, instruct the patient to take the drug out of the refrigerator up to 1 hour before it is to be instilled so that it may warm up to room temperature. Most medications for the ear are stored at room temperature.

- Instruct patient to lie on the side opposite to that of the affected ear for about 5 minutes after instillation of the drug. If the patient prefers, a small cotton ball may be inserted gently into the ear canal to keep the drug in place, but avoid forcing it into the ear or jamming it down into the ear canal.

## KEY POINTS

- Otic drugs may include the following ingredients, either by themselves or mixed together (depending on the prescriber's order): steroids, antibacterials, antifungals, antiinflammatories, and wax-emulsifying compounds. Many of the antiinfective drugs are combined with steroids (in solution) to take advantage of the additional antiinflammatory, antipruritic, and antiallergic drug effects of the steroids.

- Some ear infections require additional drug therapy with systemic dosage forms of corticosteroids, antibiotics, antifungals, and antiinflammatory drugs, so remind the patient of oral and other dosage forms.

- Some disorders of the ear are self-limiting to a degree, but appropriate treatment is important to prevent complications to the ear and/or systemic complications. If left untreated, ear infections or disorders may lead to a decrease in or loss of hearing.

- Wax, or cerumen, is a natural product of the ear and is normally produced by modified sweat glands in the auditory canal; emulsifying otic drugs (such as carbamide peroxide) loosen and help remove this wax.

- Single drugs and combination drug products are used to treat many ear conditions, and it is important to know the indications for and specific information about these drugs to ensure their safe use.

# NCLEX® EXAMINATION REVIEW QUESTIONS

1 While teaching a patient about treatment of otitis media, the nurse should mention that untreated otitis media may lead to
   a  mastoiditis.
   b  throat infections.
   c  fungal ear infection.
   d  decreased cerumen production.

2 During a teaching session about eardrops, the patient tells the nurse, "I know why an antibiotic is in this medicine, but why do I need to take a steroid?" Which is the nurse's best answer?
   a  "The steroid will help to soften the cerumen."
   b  "The steroid reduces itching and inflammation."
   c  "The steroid also has antifungal effects."
   d  "This medication helps to anesthetize the area to decrease pain."

3 The nurse is preparing to administer eardrops. Which technique for administering eardrops is correct?
   a  Warm the solution to 100° F (37.7° C) before using.
   b  Position the patient so that the unaffected ear is accessible.
   c  Massage the tragus before administering the eardrops.
   d  Gently insert a cotton ball into the outer ear canal after the drops are given.

4 The nurse is discussing treatment of earwax buildup with a patient. Which statement about earwax emulsifiers is true? These drugs:
   a  are useful for treatment of ear infections.
   b  loosen impacted cerumen so that it may be removed by irrigation.
   c  are used to rinse out excessive earwax.
   d  enhance the secretion of earwax.

5 During an examination, the nurse notes that a patient has a perforated tympanic membrane. There is an order for eardrops. Which action by the nurse is most appropriate?
   a  Give the medication as ordered.
   b  Check the patient's hearing, and then give the drops.
   c  Hold the medication, and check with the prescriber.
   d  Administer the drops with a cotton wick.

6 The nurse is preparing to administer eardrops and finds that the bottle has been stored in the medication room refrigerator. Which is the best action by the nurse?
   a  Remove the bottle from the refrigerator, and administer the drops.
   b  Heat the bottle for 5 seconds in the microwave oven before administering the drops.
   c  Let the bottle sit in a cup of hot water for 15 minutes before administering the drops.
   d  Remove the bottle from the refrigerator 1 hour before the drops are due to be given.

7 The nurse is preparing to administer carbamide peroxide (Debrox) to an adult patient with impacted cerumen. Which actions by the nurse are correct? (Select all that apply.)
   a  Have the patient lie on his side with the affected ear up.
   b  Chill the medication before administering it.
   c  Pull the pinna of the ear down and back.
   d  Pull the pinna of the ear up and back.
   e  Gently irrigate the ear with warm water to remove the softened earwax.

1. a, 2. b, 3. d, 4. b, 5. c, 6. d, 7. a, d, e

For Critical Thinking and Prioritization Questions, see http://evolve.elsevier.com/Lilley.

# Pharmaceutical Abbreviations

| ABBREVIATION | TRANSLATION |
|---|---|
| **Drug Dosage** | |
| cc*† | Cubic centimeter (equivalent to 1 mL) |
| g or gm | Gram |
| gr | Grain |
| gtt | Drop |
| IU*† | International unit |
| L | Liter |
| Lb | Pound |
| mEq | Milliequivalent |
| min | Minute |
| ml or mL | Milliliter |
| no or # | Number |
| os† | Quantity sufficient, as much as needed |
| ss† | One half |
| oz | Ounce |
| tbsp | Tablespoon |
| tsp | Teaspoon |
| u or U* | Unit |
| μg*† or mcg | Microgram |
| **Drug Route** | |
| AD† | Right ear |
| AS† | Left ear |
| AU† | Both ears |
| ID | Intradermal |
| IM | Intramuscular |
| IV | Intravenous |
| NG | Nasogastric |
| OD† | Right eye |
| OS† | Left eye |
| OU† | Both eyes |
| PO | By mouth |
| SC†, SQ†, subcut | Subcutaneous |
| SL | Sublingual |

| | |
|---|---|
| **Drug Administration** | |
| aa | Of each |
| ac | Before meals |
| ad lib | As desired, freely |
| bid | Twice a day |
| h or hr | Hour |
| hs† | Hour of sleep, at bedtime |
| HS† | Half-strength |
| NPO | Nothing by mouth |
| pc | After meals |
| prn | When needed |
| qd*† | Every day, once a day |
| qh | Every hour |
| qid | Four times a day |
| qod*† | Every other day |
| Rx | Prescribe, take |
| stat | Immediately |
| tid | Three times a day |

*As part of its 2004 National Patient Safety Goals, the Joint Commission announced that all accredited organizations must discontinue using the following abbreviations, acronyms, and symbols: U, IU, qd, qod, MS, $MSO_4$, and $MgSO_4$. Trailing zeros and lack of leading zeros were also discontinued. In other words, a zero should never appear by itself *after* a decimal point (1 mg instead of 1.0 mg), and a zero should always be used *before* a decimal point (0.1 mg instead of .1 mg). In addition, abbreviations for drug names should not be used because they can be misinterpreted. Other items are being considered for future inclusion on the official "do not use" list, such as the @ sign (write out the word at) and the symbols > and < (write out as *greater than* and *less than*). The abbreviations "cc" and "μg" should also be avoided and are being considered for inclusion on future lists. This National Patient Safety Goal was incorporated into the Information Management standards in 2010.

†These abbreviations are on the *List of Error Prone Abbreviations, Symbols, and Dose Designations* of the Institute for Safe Medication Practices (ISMP). These abbreviations have been reported to the ISMP as being frequently involved in medication errors. The ISMP recommends not ever using these abbreviations when communicating medical information, including medication orders and medication administration records.

Data from The Joint Commission: Official "do not use" abbreviation list, February 27, 2012, available at http://www.jointcommission.org/assets/1/18/Official_Do_Not_Use_List_6_111.PDF. Accessed March 28, 2012; Institute for Safe Medication Practices (ISMP): ISMP's list of error-prone abbreviations, symbols, and dose designations, 2012, available at http://www.ismp.org/tools/errorproneabbreviations.pdf. Accessed April 13, 2012.

**Chapter 1**
© Jose AS Reyes

**Chapter 2**
© forestpath

**Chapter 3**
© Katrina Brown

**Chapter 4**
© Andrew Gentry

**Chapter 5**
© Oliver Hoffmann

**Chapter 6**
© Supri Suharjoto

**Chapter 7**
© David Gilder

**Chapter 8**
© Felix Mizioznikov

**Chapter 10**
© Gpalmer

**Chapter 11**
© Vgstudio

**Chapter 12**
© Rohit Seth

**Chapter 13**
© Michael Jung

**Chapter 14**
© ZanyZeus

**Chapter 15**
© Jeff Banke

**Chapter 16**
© Ostill

**Chapter 17**
© Carme Balcells

**Chapter 18**
© Andi Berger

**Chapter 19**
© Sophie Louise Asselin

**Chapter 20**
© Gina Smith

**Chapter 21**
© Simone van den Berg

**Chapter 22**
© Flashon Studio

**Chapter 23**
© Rohit Seth

**Chapter 24**
© Steve Carroll

**Chapter 25**
© YellowCrest Media

**Chapter 26**
© Martin Allinger

**Chapter 27**
© William Casey

**Chapter 28**
© Monkey Business Images

**Chapter 29**
© Dundanim

**Chapter 30**
© Junial Enterprises

**Chapter 31**
© Felix Mizioznikov

**Chapter 32**
© Rob Marmion

**Chapter 33**
© Konstantin Sutyagin

**Chapter 34**
© Martina Ebel

**Chapter 35**
© Olga OSA

**Chapter 36**
© Perkus

**Chapter 37**
© Ragne Kabanova

**Chapter 38**
© Arvind Balaraman

**Chapter 39**
© Monkey Business Images

**Chapter 40**
© William Casey

**Chapter 41**
© Justin Paget

**Chapter 42**
© Monkey Business Images

**Chapter 43**
© Matt Antonino

**Chapter 44**
© Monkey Business Images

**Chapter 45**
© Monkey Business Images

**Chapter 46**
© Lisa F. Young

**Chapter 47**
© Jacques PALUT

**Chapter 48**
© Iofoto

**Chapter 49**
© Monkey Business Images

**Chapter 50**
© Rob Marmion

**Chapter 51**
© Layland Masuda

**Chapter 52**
© Brocreative

**Chapter 53**
© Wrangler

**Chapter 54**
© Brian Chase

**Chapter 55**
© Andry Starostin

**Chapter 56**
© Mona Makela

**Chapter 57**
© CURAphotography

**Chapter 58**
© Juriah Mosin

## A

A fibers, 143, 144t
**Abatacept** (Orencia), 776t, 778–779
Abbreviations, 68b
Ablation, 504–505
Abortifacients, 556
Absolute neutrophil count, 730
Absorption
  cold effects on, 23
  drug interactions effect on, 33t
  in elderly patients, 43b, 44
  process of, 22–26
  route of administration effects on
    enteral, 22–23
    inhalation, 25–26
    intramuscular, 23
    parenteral, 23
    subcutaneous, 23
    sublingual, 23
    topical, 25–26
    transdermal, 25
**Acamprosate**, 288–289
**Acarbose** (Precose), 521t, 522–523
Accelerated Drug Review Regulations, 55t
Accommodation, 917, 919–920
**Acebutolol** (Sectral), 315t, 406t
Acellular pertussis, 803–804
Acetaldehyde syndrome, 288, 288t
Acetaminophen
  administration of, 161
  adverse effects of, 156
  contraindications, 156
  dosing of, 156
  indications, 156
  interactions, 156
  mechanism of action, 156
  overdose of, 156
  poisoning, 35t
  profile of, 157
**Acetazolamide**, 461–462
Acetic acid, 912t
Acetic acid derivatives, 712
Acetylation, 677
Acetylcholine, 246, 324–325, 335, 817, 845t
**Acetylcholine** (Miochol-E), 923, 923t
Acetylcholine receptors, 817
Acetylcholinesterase, 324–326
**Acetylcysteine**, 161
**Acetylsalicylic acid**, 708
Acid, 475–476
Acid-base balance
  importance of, 475–476
  regulation of, 476
Acid-controlling drugs
  antacids. *See* Antacids.
  assessments before using, 824
  $H_2$ receptor antagonists, 818, 820–822, 824–826
  misoprostol, 824
  nursing process for, 824–826
  patient teaching about, 826–827
  proton pump inhibitors, 822–823, 823t, 825–826
  sucralfate, 823–827

Acidosis, 476
Acne vulgaris, 901, 905–906
Acquired disease, 94–96
Acquired immunodeficiency syndrome. *See also*
  Human immunodeficiency virus.
  definition of, 650–652
  indicator diseases of, 662b
  opportunistic infections, 624, 651, 661, 662b
  pathophysiology of, 658–662
Acrocyanosis, 312–313
Actinic keratosis, 901, 911
Action potential
  in cardiac tissue, 400t
  definition of, 397–398
  phases of, 398–399, 398f–399f
  Purkinje fiber, 399f
Action potential duration, 397, 399–400, 400f
Activated charcoal, 830
Activated partial thromboplastin time, 440b
Active immunization
  characteristics of, 797, 797t
  definition of, 795
  toxoids, 797–798
  vaccines, 798–799
Active immunizing drugs. *See also* Immunizing
  drugs.
  assessments before using, 809
  definition of, 795, 799
  dosages of, 802t–803t
  profiles of, 803–806
  types of, 799b
Active transport, 300
  definition of, 37
  in pregnancy, 38
Acute diarrhea, 830
Acute pain, 140, 142, 143t
Acute therapy, 31
**Acyclovir** (Zovirax), 655t–656t, 657–658, 659b, 667–669, 908
AD, 68b
**Adalimumab** (Humira), 771t–772t, 772
Addiction, 140, 144–145, 147–148, 281
Addisonian crisis, 598, 605
Addison's disease, 533, 535
**Adenosine** (Adenocard), 407t–408t, 413
Adenosine deaminase, 98f
Adenosine triphosphate, 397, 460
Adherence versus compliance, 8
Adjunctive anesthetics, 169–171, 171t
Adjunctive drugs, 237
Adjuvants, 140, 763, 776
Administration of drugs
  checking of, 13–14
  computer-controlled dispensing system, 102, 102f
  enteral
    absorption affected by, 22–23
    description of, 21t
  gastrostomy tube for, 108, 108f
  inhalation
    absorption effects, 25–26
    environment considerations, 603b
    metered-dose inhalers, 130, 130f, 378–379, 602

Administration of drugs *(Continued)*
    metered-dose inhalers for, 130, 130f
    nursing considerations for, 24t–25t
    small-volume nebulizers, 131, 131f
  nasogastric tube, 108, 108f
  preparations for, 102–103, 102f
  rectal, 109, 109f
  sublingual, 23
    absorption effects of, 23, 24t–25t, 25
    nursing considerations for, 24t–25t
    procedure for, 104, 105f
  transdermal
    absorption effects, 25
    contraceptives, 552t
    estrogen, 548t
    fentanyl, 148b, 152t–153t, 163
    nitroglycerin, 378–379
    nursing considerations for, 24t–25t
    opioid analgesics, 148b, 163
    procedure for, 132, 133f
    testosterone, 568t
  vaginal, 135, 135f–136f
Adrenal cortex, 533–534, 535t
Adrenal crisis, 533, 540
Adrenal drugs
  adverse effects of, 536–537, 537t
  assessments before using, 539
  contraindications, 536
  dosages of, 537, 537t, 540
  drug effects of, 535–536
  indications, 536
  interactions, 537
  mechanism of action, 535–536
  nursing process for, 539–541
  overview of, 535–537
  patient teaching about, 541
Adrenal gland
  anatomy of, 534–535
  characteristics of, 539b
  hormones produced by, 535b
Adrenal medulla, 533–534, 535t
Adrenal suppression, 538
Adrenergic agonists
  beta-. *See* Beta agonists.
  definition of, 298–299
Adrenergic drugs, 300–304
  administration of, 308
  adverse effects of, 303–304, 310, 352
  assessments, 306–307
  cardiovascular indications for, 303
  centrally acting, 348, 351–352, 360, 362
  in chronic lung disease patients, 309
  classification of, 301–302
  contraindications, 303, 352
  definition of, 300, 575
  dosages of, 352
  drug effects of, 302, 350–352
  in elderly patients, 307
  hypertension treated with, 350–353
  indications, 302–303, 352
  interactions, 304, 352, 352t
  mechanism of action, 301f, 302, 350–352
  monoamine oxidase inhibitors and, 304

Page numbers followed by *b, t,* and *f* indicate boxes, tables, and figures, respectively. Blue entries indicate disorders. Boldface entries indicate generic drug names.

Adrenergic drugs *(Continued)*
 nasal decongestant use of, 302
 noncatecholamine, 301
 nursing process for, 306–310
 ophthalmic indications for, 302–303, 309
 overdose of, 303–304
 patient teaching about, 308–310
 in pediatric patients, 307
 profiles of, 304–306
 respiratory indications for, 302
 therapeutic effects of, 310
 toxicity of, 303–304
 types of, 304t, 350b
 vasoactive, 304t, 305–306
Adrenergic receptors
 definition of, 298, 312, 350
 responses of, to stimulation, 300t
Adrenergic-blocking drugs
 alpha. *See* Alpha-adrenergic blockers
 beta. *See* Beta blockers
 nursing process for, 319–322
 overview of, 313
 patient teaching about, 322
 types of, 315t
Adrenocorticotropic hormone, 495t, 534
Adsorbents, 830t, 831
Adverse drug events, 17, 33, 64–65
Adverse drug reactions, 17, 34, 64–65
Adverse drug withdrawal events, 33
Adverse effects, 17, 31–32
Aerobic, 672–673
Aerosol foam, 904t
Aerosol spray, 904t
Affective disorders
 definition of, 253, 255
 dysregulation hypothesis of, 254, 260
 permissive hypothesis of, 254, 260, 261f
Affective domain, 74–75
Afferent arterioles, 459–460
Affinity, 30
African-Americans
 cultural practices of, 52b
 drug responses in, 53b
 health beliefs of, 52b, 53
 pain management practices, 141b
Agonist(s)
 beta. *See* Beta agonists.
 definition of, 17, 140, 147, 312
 opioid, 163
 partial, 140, 147–148
Agonist–antagonist
 definition of, 140, 155
 opioid, 147, 160, 164
Agoraphobia, 253, 255
Agranulocytes, 598t
AIDS. *See* Acquired immunodeficiency
 syndrome.
AIDS-related complex, 661
Air-lock technique, 114, 114f
Akathisia, 253, 268
Akinesia, 237, 239t
Albendazole, 701t–702t
Albumin, 478–479, 478t, 485
Albuterol (Proventil, Ventolin), 592t–593t, 593–594
Alcohol
 adverse effects of, 287–288
 barbiturates and, 287
 benzodiazepines and, 286–287

Alcohol *(Continued)*
 CAGE Questionnaire for, 291
 description of, 180–181
 disulfiram for, 288, 288t
 drug effects of, 287
 in elderly patients, 293b
 indications, 287
 interactions, 288–289
 mechanism of action, 287
 overdose of, 288–289
 toxicity, 288–289
 withdrawal, 288–289, 288b, 291
Aldesleukin, 774–775, 775t
Aldosterone, 355t, 384, 459–461, 533–534
Aldosterone antagonists, 385, 391
Alefacept (Amevive), 909
Alemtuzumab (Campath), 771t–772t, 772–773
Alendronate (Fosamax), 553–554, 553t
Alfentanil (Alfenta), 171t
Alfuzosin (Uroxatral), 315t, 566
Alkaloid topoisomerase II inhibitors, 735–736, 736b,
 736t, 740–741
Alkaloids
 belladonna, 337, 831, 832t
 description of, 35
 ergot, 203, 209, 212, 214–215, 556, 559
 vinca, 734
Alkylamines, 578t
Alkylating drugs
 adverse effects of, 750–751, 751t, 758
 drug effects of, 749–750
 extravasation of, 752t
 indications, 750
 mechanism of action, 749–750
 overview of, 749–752
Alkylation, 749
Allele, 94–96
Allergen, 588–590
Allergic asthma, 588
Allergic reactions, 34
 definition of, 17
 description of, 64–65
 to local anesthetics, 176
Allergies, 102–103
Allodynia, 146
Allopurinol (Zyloprim), 713–714, 731
Aloe, 909b
Alopecia, 729, 743, 745
Alosetron (Lotronex), 839, 841
Alpha$_1$ blockers, 348, 351, 353
Alpha$_2$ receptor agonists, 350–353, 353t
5-Alpha reductase inhibitors, 566, 568t
Alpha-adrenergic blockers
 adverse effects of, 314, 315t, 568t
 assessments, 319–320, 360
 benign prostatic hyperplasia treated with, 313,
 566
 contraindications, 314
 dosages, 314, 315t
 drug effects of, 313
 indications, 313–314
 interactions, 314, 315t, 568
 mechanism of action, 313, 314f
 nursing interventions for, 321, 362
 nursing process for, 319–322
 overdose of, 314
 patient teaching about, 322, 366
 phentolamine, 315t, 316

Alpha-adrenergic blockers *(Continued)*
 profiles of, 316
 tamsulosin, 315t, 316
 toxicity of, 314
Alpha-adrenergic receptors, 298–299, 313
Alpha-glucosidase, 522
Alpha-glucosidase inhibitors, 522–523
Alprazolam, 256t–257t, 257–258
Alprostadil (Caverject), 566
Alteplase (Activase), 432, 432t
Alternative medicine
 categories of, 87–88
 definition of, 84, 87–88
Aluminum hydroxide (Amphojel), 820t
Aluminum hydroxide and magnesium hydroxide
 (Maalox, Mylanta), 820t
Alveoli, 588–589
Alvimopan (Entereg), 834
Alzheimer's disease
 cholinergic drugs for, 329, 329b, 331
 definition of, 324
 description of, 47b
 donepezil for, 327–328, 328t, 329b
Amantadine (Symmetrel)
 adverse effects of, 655, 656t
 antiviral uses of, 655t
 contraindications, 655
 dopaminergic uses, 240, 240t–242t, 243
 patient teaching about, 669
 profile of, 656–658
Ambrisentan (Letairis), 359–360
Amebiasis, 698, 698t
American Medical Association, 67–68
American Nurses Association, 59, 75
Amifostine, 759
Amikacin (Amikin), 635, 635t–637t, 638, 676t
Amiloride (Midamor), 466, 466t
Amin-Aid, 892
Amino acids, 894, 894b
Aminocaproic acid (Amicar), 422, 432–434, 439
Aminoglutethimide, 537t, 538–539
Aminoglycosides
 administration of, 646
 adverse effects of, 637
 assessments before using, 644
 contraindications, 637
 definition of, 635
 drug effects of, 636
 indications, 636–637
 interactions, 637
 mechanism of action, 636
 ophthalmic, 929
 patient teaching about, 646
 in pediatric patients, 636–637
 profiles of, 638
 spectrum of activity, 636t
 types of, 635t
Aminopenicillins, 617t, 618–619
4-Aminoquinoline derivatives, 694–695
Amiodarone (Cordarone, Pacerone), 375t, 404b,
 405t–408t, 411, 411t, 413b, 414–415, 415b
Amitriptyline, 262–264, 263t
Amlodipine (Norvasc), 357, 374t–375t, 376
Amoxicillin (Amoxil), 619, 619t
Amphetamine(s)
 abuse of, 284–285
 attention-deficit/hyperactivity disorder treated
 with, 206–208

Amphetamine(s) (Continued)
definition of, 203, 281, 284
interactions, 207t
narcolepsy treated with, 206–208
profile of, 207–208
treatment uses of, 206, 207t
types of, 284t
**Amphetamine/dextroamphetamine** (Adderall), 211t
**Amphotericin B** (Fungizone), 684–686, 685t–687t, 688, 690
**Ampicillin**, 619, 619t
Ampules
illustration of, 111f
medication removal from, 112, 112f
Amylin agonists, 524, 526
Anabolic activity, 564–565
Anabolic steroids, 565
Anabolism, 889–890
**Anakinra** (Kineret), 774–775, 775t
Analeptics, 203, 212–214
Analgesia, patient-controlled, 124, 125f, 144
Analgesic(s)
definition of, 140
nonopioid, 140, 143
nursing diagnoses for, 160
nursing process for, 157–166
opioid
abuse of, 283–284, 291
administration of, 163t
adverse effects of, 147b, 149–151, 283–284
agonist–antagonist, 160
antagonists, 152t–153t, 155, 160, 163–164
antitussives, 583
assessments, 159–160
central nervous system depression caused by, 150
chemical classification of, 148t
chemical structure of, 147
codeine sulfate, 152t–153t, 153, 163t
contraindications, 149, 283
definition of, 140, 147, 281, 283
diarrhea treated with, 830–832, 834
dosage of, 149b, 151, 152t–153t
drug effects of, 147–148, 283
in elderly patients, 162b
gastrointestinal tract effects, 150
heroin, 283
histamine release caused by, 150
indications, 148–149, 283
interactions, 151
laboratory tests, 151b
mechanism of action, 147–148, 283
meperidine hydrochloride, 152t–153t, 154, 163t
methadone, 152t–153t, 154, 283, 284b
morphine sulfate, 151–153, 152t–153t, 163t
overdose of, 150–151, 283–284
oxycodone, 152t–153t, 163t, 283
oxymorphone, 163t
in pediatric patients, 158b
physical dependence on, 150
poisoning, 35t
reversal of, 150t
subacute overdose, 147b
toxicity of, 150–151, 283–284
transdermal administration of, 148b, 163
withdrawal from, 140, 151, 283–284, 283b–284b
outcome criteria for, 160

Analgesic ceiling effect, 140
Analogue, 723, 730
Anaphylactic shock, 613–614
Anaplasia, 723
**Anastrozole**, 755
Androgen(s)
adverse effects of, 567–568, 568t, 755t
antineoplastic uses of, 755t, 757
contraindications, 567
definition of, 564–565
drug effects of, 565–567
indications, 567, 567t
inhibitors of, 566
mechanism of action, 565–567
Androgenic activity, 564
Anemia
causes of, 878f
of chronic disease, 878
classification of, 878
hemolytic, 877, 879
iron-deficiency, 881
megaloblastic, 879
nursing process for, 884–886
patient teaching about, 886
pernicious, 868, 879
types of, 879f
Anesthesia
balanced, 169–171, 190–191
definition of, 169–170
elderly patients, 172b
epidural, 175b
general. See General anesthesia.
home health care considerations, 183
local. See Local anesthesia.
nursing process for
assessment, 180–182
evaluation, 185
implementation, 183–185
nursing diagnoses, 182
outcome criteria, 182–183
planning, 182–183
pediatric considerations, 172b
Anesthetics
adjunctive, 169–171, 171t
definition of, 169
intravenous, 172t
parenteral, 170, 170t, 174, 175t
topical, 174, 908, 932–933, 935
Angina pectoris
beta blockers for, 317
causes of, 369
chronic stable, 368–369
definition of, 312, 368–369
Prinzmetal, 369
unstable, 369
vasospastic, 369
Angioedema, 355
Angiotensin II, 351, 355t, 384
Angiotensin II receptor blockers
administration of, 363
adverse effects of, 356
contraindications, 356
description of, 349, 356
dosages of, 355t, 357
drug effects of, 356
heart failure treated with, 385
indications, 356

Angiotensin II receptor blockers (Continued)
interactions, 357, 357t
mechanism of action, 356
overdose of, 356
profile of, 357
toxicity of, 356
Angiotensin-converting enzyme, 354
Angiotensin-converting enzyme inhibitors
adverse effects of, 355
assessments, 361, 390
cardioprotective effect of, 354–355
cardiovascular effects of, 354
contraindications, 355
definition of, 353–354, 384
dosages of, 355, 355t
drug effects of, 354
heart failure treated with, 383–385
hemodynamic effects of, 354–355
indications, 354–355
interactions, 355, 466
mechanism of action, 354
monitoring of, 363
nonsteroidal antiinflammatory drugs and, 355, 357t
overdose of, 355
pregnancy contraindications, 354
renal effects of, 354
toxicity of, 355
types of, 350b, 354t, 384
Angle-closure glaucoma, 917, 920, 921t
Anisoylated plasminogen streptokinase activator complex, 431
Anorexiants, 204, 207t, 208–209, 215–216
Antacids
adverse effects of, 818–819
assessments before using, 824
contraindications, 818
definition of, 815, 818
dosages of, 819, 820t
drug effects of, 818
indications, 818
interactions, 819, 819t
mechanism of action, 818
nursing concerns, 819b
overview of, 818–819
profiles of, 819–820, 820b
Antagonist(s)
competitive, 147–148
definition of, 17, 140, 147–148, 312, 575
neuromuscular blocking agents, 177
opioid, 152t–153t, 160, 163–164
Antagonistic effect, 17, 33
Anterior chamber, 917, 919
Anterior pituitary gland, 494b, 495t
Anthelmintic drugs, 692, 701–704, 701t, 703t
Anthracycline antibiotics, 754t
**Anthralin** (Anthra-Derm), 909
Anthrax, 808–809, 808t
Antiacne drugs, 905–906
Antiadrenal drugs, 538–539
Antiallergic drugs, 933, 934t
Antiandrogens, 755t
Antianginal drugs
administration of, 378–379
beta blockers, 372–374, 374t
calcium channel blockers, 374–376
nitrates/nitrites, 370–371, 371t, 376, 378–379
nursing process for, 377–379
overview of, 369

Antianginal drugs *(Continued)*
  patient teaching about, 379–380
  ranolazine, 376
  summary of, 376–377
  therapeutic effects of, 369, 370t
Antianxiety drugs
  adverse effects of, 256–257, 257t
  benzodiazepines, 256–258. *See also*
      Benzodiazepines
  description of, 256
  drug effects of, 256
  hydroxyzine, 256t
  indications, 256
  interactions, 257
  mechanism of action, 256
Antibacterial drugs, 904–905, 939, 939t
Antibiotics
  allergic reaction to, 613–614
  aminoglycosides. *See* Aminoglycosides
  beta-lactam. *See* Beta-lactam antibiotics
  broad-spectrum, 612
  carbapenems, 623, 628
  cephalosporins. *See* Cephalosporins
  classification of, 614
  clindamycin, 640–646, 641t, 648
  colistimethate, 641t, 643–644
  daptomycin, 641t, 643, 645
  definition of, 610
  food interactions with, 613
  host factors that affect, 613–614
  interactions, 613
  ketolides, 626
  linezolid, 641–642, 641t, 645–648
  macrolides, 623–628, 625t, 630–631, 929–930
  mechanism of action, 614
  metronidazole, 641t, 642, 645, 647–648
  monopenems, 623–625
  nitrofurantoin, 641t, 642, 645, 647–648
  nursing process for, 628–630, 644–647
  overprescribing of, 613
  overview of, 612–614
  patient teaching about, 631, 648
  penicillins. *See* Penicillin(s).
  prophylactic uses of, 612
  quinolones, 638–640, 639b, 639t–640t, 644–646,
      648, 930–931, 930t
  quinupristin/dalfopristin, 641t, 642–643, 647
  resistance to, 613
  sites of activity, 614f
  sulfonamides, 614–616, 615t, 628, 630, 931
  telavancin, 641t, 644, 647
  tetracyclines, 39, 626–631, 626b
  therapeutic efficacy monitoring, 612–613
  vancomycin, 641t, 643, 645, 647–648
Antibodies, 588–590, 650, 652–653, 763, 765,
    795–797, 799
Antibody titer, 796, 799
Anticholinergics. *See also* Cholinergic-blocking drugs
  administration of, 603
  adverse effects of, 336, 337t, 847t
  antidiarrheal uses of, 830–831
  antiemetic uses of, 846–847, 846t
  assessments before using, 601
  asthma treated with, 591t, 594, 600–602
  cardiovascular effects of, 336, 336t
  definition of, 246, 575
  dosage of, 338t
  in elderly patients, 336

Anticholinergics *(Continued)*
  gastrointestinal disorders treated with, 336
  nursing process for, 339–341
  patient teaching about, 604
  sites of action, 335–336
Anticholinesterase drugs, 537
Anticoagulants
  adverse effects of, 423–424, 423t, 439
  antidotes for, 438
  assessments before using, 434
  contraindications, 423
  definition of, 419, 421–422
  dosages of, 424, 426t
  drug effects of, 422–423
  function of, 421, 422t
  indications, 423
  interactions, 424
  laboratory tests for, 440b
  mechanism of action, 422–423
  monitoring of, 438
  overdose of, 423–424, 439
  patient teaching about, 440–441
  profiles of, 424–427
  toxicity of, 423–424
Anticonvulsants, 219
Antidepressants
  administration of, 276
  assessments, 273–274
  description of, 259–261
  monoamine oxidase inhibitors
    adverse effects of, 262t, 264
    barbiturates and, 195
    food interactions, 264t
    interactions, 262t, 264t
    overdose of, 264
    Parkinson's disease treated with, 238, 240–243
    types of, 264
  second-generation, 263t, 265–267
  tricyclic
    administration of, 276
    adverse effects of, 261–262, 262t
    amitriptyline, 262–264, 263t
    assessments, 274
    characteristics of, 261–262
    contraindications, 261
    interactions, 262, 262t
    list of, 260t
    overdose of, 262
    poisoning, 35t
    profile of, 262–264
  types of, 260t
Antidiabetic drugs
  alpha-glucosidase inhibitors, 522–523
  amylin agonists, 524, 526
  biguanides, 520, 521t, 523
  dipeptidyl peptidase IV inhibitors, 523–524
  glinides, 521–522, 524
  incretin mimetics, 524–525
  injectable, 524
  insulin. *See* Insulin
  nursing process for, 525–530
  sulfonylureas, 521, 526
  thiazolidinediones, 522, 526
Antidiarrheal drugs
  adsorbents, 830t, 831
  adverse effects of, 831
  assessments before using, 839–840
  contraindications, 830

Antidiarrheal drugs *(Continued)*
  definition of, 829–830
  dosages of, 831, 832t
  drug effects of, 830
  indications, 830
  interactions, 831
  mechanism of action, 830
  nursing process for, 839–841
  overview of, 830–831
  patient teaching about, 840–842
  in pediatric patients, 833b
  probiotics, 830, 832–833, 840, 842
  profiles of, 831–833
  types of, 830t
Antidiuretic hormone, 495, 495t, 555
Antidopaminergic drugs, 847, 847t, 849–852
Antidotes, 35t
Antidysrhythmic drugs
  adverse effects of, 405–406, 405t
  assessments before using, 413–414
  class Ia, 403–404, 404b, 405t, 406–408, 407t–408t
  class Ib, 403–404, 404b, 405t, 408–409
  class Ic, 403–404, 404b, 405t, 409–410
  class II, 404, 404b, 405t, 407t–408t, 410
  class III, 404, 404b, 405t, 407t–408t, 410–412. *See
      also* Beta blockers.
  class IV, 404, 404b, 405t, 407t–408t, 412–413. *See
      also* Calcium channel blockers.
  contraindications, 404–405
  dosages of, 406, 407t–408t
  drug effects of, 403–404
  indications, 404, 405t
  interactions, 406
  mechanism of action, 403–404, 404t
  monitoring of, 414
  nursing process for, 413–416
  overdose of, 405–406, 406t
  overview of, 403
  patient teaching about, 416
  profiles of, 406–413, 407t–408t
  therapeutic response to, 417
  toxicity of, 405–406
  Vaughn Williams classification of, 397, 403,
      403t–404t, 417
Antiemetic drugs
  adverse effects of, 847, 847t
  anticholinergics, 846–847, 846t
  antidopaminergic drugs, 847, 847t, 849–850
  antihistamines, 846t, 847, 849
  contraindications, 847
  definition of, 844, 846
  dosages of, 848, 848t–849t
  drug effects of, 846–847
  indications, 847–849
  interactions, 848
  mechanism of action, 846–847, 846t
  nursing process for, 851–853
  overview of, 846–848
  patient teaching about, 854
  profiles of, 848–851
  prokinetics, 846t–847t, 847, 850, 852
  serotonin blockers, 846t–847t, 847, 850
  sites of action, 846f
Antiepileptic drugs
  administration of, 233
  adverse effects of, 224, 224t
  benzodiazepines, 226
  carbamazepine, 225t–228t, 229, 232, 234

Antiepileptic drugs (Continued)
 clonazepam, 226
 clorazepate dipotassium, 226
 contraindications, 224
 definition of, 219
 description of, 221
 divalproex, 225t–226t
 dosages of, 224, 226t–228t
 effectiveness evaluations, 222
 effects of, 221
 ethosuximide, 227t–228t, 229
 felbamate, 226
 fosphenytoin, 222t, 224t, 227t–229t, 228–229
 gabapentin, 224t, 227t–228t, 229–230, 232, 234
 goal of, 221
 hydantoins, 225t–226t, 232, 234
 indications, 223
 interactions, 224, 225t–226t
 lamotrigine, 224t, 227t–228t, 230, 232, 234
 levetiracetam, 225t–228t, 230, 234
 mechanism of action, 222–223
 monitoring of, 233
 nursing process for, 231–235
 oral administration of, 234
 oxcarbazepine, 227t–228t, 229, 234
 patient teaching about, 235
 pediatric patients, 223b
 phenobarbital, 222t, 226–228, 227t–228t
 phenytoin, 222t, 227t–229t, 228–229
 primidone, 226–228, 227t–228t
 profile of, 226–231
 single, 221–222
 succinimides, 225t–226t, 229
 therapeutic levels of, 226t
 therapeutic ranges for, 222
 tiagabine, 227t–228t, 230, 235
 topiramate, 227t–228t, 230–232
 types of, 222t
 valproic acid, 226, 227t–228t, 231–232, 235
 zonisamide, 227t–228t, 231
Antifibrinolytic drugs
 adverse effects of, 433, 433t
 assessments before using, 436
 contraindications, 433
 definition of, 419, 432
 dosages of, 433, 433t
 drug effects of, 432–433
 function of, 421, 422t, 439
 indications, 433
 interactions, 433
 mechanism of action, 432–433, 433t
 profiles of, 433–434
 therapeutic effects of, 440
Antifungal drugs
 adverse effects of, 685, 685t–686t
 contraindications, 685
 dermatologic applications of, 905–907, 907t
 dosages of, 686, 687t
 drug effects of, 684
 indications, 684–685
 interactions, 685
 mechanism of action, 684
 nursing process for, 688–689
 ophthalmic, 931
 otic, 939, 939t
 overview of, 683–686
 patient teaching about, 690
 profiles of, 686–688
 topical, 684, 905–907, 907t

Antigens, 575, 588, 650, 763–764, 796–797, 799
Antiglaucoma drugs
 miotics, 921–923, 921t–923t
 overview of, 921
Antigout drugs, 713–716, 718
Antihistamines
 adverse effects of, 578f, 579, 847t
 antiemetic uses of, 846t, 846–847
 assessments before using, 584
 contraindications, 579
 definition of, 575, 577
 description of, 240t
 dosages of, 579–580, 579t
 drug effects of, 577–578, 578t
 indications, 578–579
 interactions, 579
 mechanism of action, 577–578
 nonsedating, 576, 580, 584
 nursing process for, 584–586
 ophthalmic, 933
 over-the-counter, 576
 overview of, 576–580
 patient teaching about, 586–587
 peripherally acting, 580
Antihypertensive drugs
 adrenergic drugs, 350–353. See also Adrenergic
  drugs
 adverse effects of, 362
 alpha$_1$ blockers, 348, 351, 353
 angiotensin II receptor blockers. See Angiotensin
  II receptor blockers
 angiotensin-converting enzyme inhibitors. See
  Angiotensin-converting enzyme inhibitors
 beta blockers. See Beta blockers
 bosentan, 359–360, 359t
 calcium channel blockers, 357
 categories of, 349, 350b
 cultural considerations, 361b
 definition of, 348
 diuretics, 357. See also Diuretics
 eplerenone, 359, 359t, 385
 goals of, 349
 mechanism of action, 351f
 nursing process for, 360–365
 overview of, 348–349
 patient teaching about, 365–366
 site of action, 351f
 treprostinil, 359t, 360
 vasodilators. See Vasodilators
 vasodilatory effects of, 349
Antiinflammatory drugs, 931–932
Antilipemic drugs
 assessments before using, 454
 bile acid sequestrants, 450–451, 451t, 454–457
 definition of, 443, 446
 fibric acid derivatives, 452–454, 453t
 HMG-CoA reductase inhibitors, 443, 448–451,
  449t, 454–455, 457
 niacin, 450t, 451–452, 452t, 456–457
 nursing process for, 454–456
 patient teaching about, 457
Antimalarial drugs
 adverse effects of, 695, 695t
 assessments before using, 702–703
 contraindications, 695
 definition of, 692
 dosages of, 696, 696t–697t
 drug effects of, 694–695
 indications, 695

Antimalarial drugs (Continued)
 interactions, 696, 696t
 mechanism of action, 694–695
 overview of, 693–696
 patient teaching about, 704
 profiles of, 696–698
Antimanic drugs, 259
Antimetabolites, 682, 684, 730–734, 732t, 740,
 743–744
Antimicrobials
 ophthalmic, 928–932
 topical, 902, 904
Antineoplastic drugs
 adverse effects of, 729, 739b, 742–743
 alkaloid topoisomerase II inhibitors, 735–736,
  736b, 736t, 740–741
 alkylating drugs. See Alkylating drugs
 antimetabolites, 682, 684, 730–734, 732t, 740,
  743–744
 assessments before using, 739–741, 756–757
 bevacizumab, 754
 blood cell count assessments, 740b, 759b
 contraindications, 730
 definition of, 723, 728
 dose-limiting adverse effects of, 723, 729
 efficacy of, 729
 emetic potential of, 723, 729, 730b
 extravasation of, 751, 751b
 handling of, 756b
 hormonal, 755–758
 hydroxyurea, 755, 757–759
 imatinib, 755
 indications, 729–730
 mitotane, 755
 mitotic inhibitors, 734–735, 735t, 740–741, 744
 nursing considerations for, 742
 nursing process for, 739–745, 756–759
 octreotide, 755
 patient teaching about, 745–746, 760
 topical, 911
 topoisomerase I inhibitors, 736–738, 737t, 741,
  744
 toxicity of, 742
 vinca alkaloids, 735t–736t, 736, 736b
Antineoplastic enzymes, 738–739, 738t, 741
Antiparkinsonian drugs
 adverse effects of, 241t
 anticholinergics, 246
 catechol O-methyltransferase inhibitors, 240t,
  243–244
 in elderly patients, 248b
 monoamine oxidase inhibitors, 240–243
 types of, 240t
Antiplatelet drugs
 adverse effects of, 429, 429t
 aspirin, 427–430, 429t–430t, 438
 assessments before using, 435
 contraindications, 429
 definition of, 419
 description of, 427
 drug effects of, 427–429
 function of, 421, 422t
 indications, 429
 interactions, 429–430
 mechanism of action, 427–429
 monitoring of, 438
Antiprotozoal drugs, 692, 698–700, 699t, 703–704
Antipruritics, topical, 908
Antipsoriatic drugs, 909

Antipsychotic drugs
administration of, 276–277
adverse effects of, 268–269, 268t–269t
atypical, 268, 270–271, 270t, 274–275
butyrophenones, 269–271, 269t
contraindications, 268
description of, 267–269
drug effects of, 268
haloperidol, 269–270, 269t, 274, 277
indications, 268
interactions, 269
mechanism of action, 268
nursing process for, 274–275
phenothiazines
chlorpromazine, 267
description of, 267
schizophrenia treated with, 268
types of, 267t
Antiretroviral drugs
administration of, 669–670
adverse effects of, 664
assessments before using, 668
contraindications, 664
definition of, 650, 659
dosages of, 664, 665t
drug effects of, 663
highly active antiretroviral therapy, 661–663
indications, 664
interactions, 664
mechanism of action, 663
nonnucleoside reverse transcriptase inhibitors, 662–663, 663t
nucleoside reverse transcriptase inhibitors, 662–663, 663t, 665t
nursing process for, 667–670
overview of, 662–664
patient teaching about, 670
profiles of, 664–666
therapeutic effects of, 670
Antiseptics, 610, 612, 612t, 629b
Antiserum, 796, 799
**Antithrombin III** (Thrombate), 419, 422–423
Antithrombotic drugs. *See* Anticoagulants
Antithyroid drugs, 504–508, 505t
Antitoxin, 796, 799
Antitubercular drugs
administration of, 679–680
adverse effects of, 675, 676t
assessments before using, 678–679
contraindications, 675
definition of, 672
dosages of, 675
drug effects of, 674
ethambutol, 676t–677t, 677
first-line, 674b
indications, 674–675, 676t
interactions, 675, 676t
isoniazid, 672, 674, 676t–677t, 677–678
mechanism of action, 674, 675t
nursing process for, 678–680
overview of, 674–675
patient teaching about, 680–681
profiles of, 677–678
rifabutin, 676t–677t, 678, 680
rifapentine, 676t–677t, 678
second-line, 674b
streptomycin, 636–637, 636t, 676t–677t, 678

Antitussives, 575–576, 582–586, 582t
Antivenin, 796, 800
Antiviral drugs
adverse effects of, 655, 656t–657t
amantadine, 240t–242t
contraindications, 655
definition of, 651, 653
drug effects of, 655
indications, 655
mechanism of action, 653, 655
topical, 907–908
types of, 655t
Anxiety
characteristics of, 255
definition of, 253, 255
depression and, 261
disorders of, 255
drug therapy for. *See* Antianxiety drugs.
Anxiolytics, 190
administration of, 276
characteristics of, 256–257
nursing process for, 272–273
Apical pulse, 104, 105f, 321
**Apixaban** (Eliquis), 423
Apnea, neonatal, 205–206
Apocrine glands, 903t
Apolipoproteins, 443–445
**Apraclonidine** (Iopidine), 924–925, 924t
Aqueous humor, 917, 919, 920f
Arachidonic acid, 707, 707f
Arachidonic acid pathway, 427
**Arformoterol**, 592t
**Argatroban** (Argatroban), 423, 426t, 427
Arginine vasopressin, 483
Aromatase inhibitors, 755, 755t
Arrhythmia, 397
Arthritis
definition of, 763
osteoarthritis, 776–777
rheumatoid. *See* Rheumatoid arthritis
Artificial tears, 933
Artificially acquired passive immunization, 798
AS, 68b
Ascariasis, 701t
Ascites, 459
Ascorbic acid, 859t–861t, 869, 873–875
Asian Americans
cultural practices of, 52b
drug responses in, 53b
health beliefs of, 53
**Asparaginase** (Elspar), 738, 738t, 746
Aspergillosis, 683t
Aspiration, 104
**Aspirin** (ASA), 427–430, 429t–430t, 438, 708, 711t, 712, 715–718
Aspirin triad, 715–716
Assessments
description of, 7–9
herbal products, 90
neuromuscular blocking agents, 181
over-the-counter drugs, 89–90
pain, 157–160
substance abuse, 290–292
Asthma
allergic, 588
anticholinergics for, 591t, 594, 600–601
beta blocker contraindications in, 352

Asthma (Continued)
beta-adrenergic agonists for, 591–594, 591t
bronchial, 588–589
corticosteroids for, 591t, 597–600
drug therapy for, 590b, 592f
drug-induced, 590
extrinsic, 589–590
intrinsic, 589–590
leukotriene receptor antagonists for, 591t, 596–597, 597t, 601, 603–604
management steps for, 590t
monoclonal antibody antiasthmatic drugs for, 605
triggers of, 589–590
Asthma attack, 588–589, 590b
**Atenolol** (Tenormin), 315t, 318, 318t, 374, 374t, 410
Atherosclerosis, 368–369
Atherosclerotic plaque, 446
Athlete's foot, 906–907
**Atomoxetine**, 206, 207t, 211t
Atonic seizures, 220–221
Atony, 324, 326
Atopic dermatitis, 901, 903
**Atorvastatin** (Lipitor), 450, 450t
**Atovaquone** (Mepron), 699t–700t, 700
Atrial fibrillation, 382, 387–390, 401–403, 401t–402t, 411–412, 415b
Atrial flutter, 401t–402t, 411–412
Atrioventricular. *See* AV
**Atropine**, 171t, 246, 337, 338t, 339–341, 831t
diphenoxylate with, 831t–832t, 831t–832t
**Atropine sulfate** (Isopto Atropine), 933
Attention-deficit disorder, 203
Attention-deficit/hyperactivity disorder, 203, 205, 215–216
Atypical antipsychotics, 268, 270–271, 270t, 274–275
AU, 68b
Autoimmune diseases/disorders, 763, 768–769, 776–777, 784–785
Autoinduction, 219, 229
Automaticity, 382, 385, 398, 400
Autonomic functions, 298–299
Autonomic nervous system, 299
anatomy of, 313
definition of, 298–299
divisions of, 350
transmission in, 350
Autonomy, 58b
AV block, 403
AV cells, 399
AV nodal reentrant tachycardia, 403
Avian influenza, 667
**Azathioprine** (Imuran), 786t, 787, 789t, 791, 793
**Azithromycin** (Zithromax), 624–626, 625t
Azole antifungals, 684–685
interactions, 375t
**Aztreonam** (Azactam), 623, 624t

**B**

B lymphocytes, 763–765, 785, 797
Bachmann bundle, 397, 400
Bacille Calmette-Guérin, 674b, 776t
Bacillus, 672–673
**Bacitracin** (AK-Tracin), 904–905, 930t
**Baclofen**, 197, 197t
Bacteria, 611, 611f

Bactericidal antibiotics, 610, 616
Bacteriostatic antibiotics, 610, 614–615
Balanced anesthesia, 148, 169–171, 190–191
Bar, 904t
Barbiturates
    adverse effects of, 194, 194t, 286–287
    alcohol and, 287
    antiepileptic uses of, 234
    central nervous system effects, 194
    contraindications, 194
    definition of, 188
    dosage of, 195t
    drug effects of, 193–194, 286
    duration of, 195t
    history of, 193
    indications, 194, 286
    interactions, 194–195
    mechanism of action, 193–194, 286
    monoamine oxidase inhibitors and, 195
    onset of action, 195t, 199–200
    overdose of, 194, 286–287
    pentobarbital, 171t, 195, 195t
    profile of, 195–196
    sedative properties of, 194
    side effects of, 224t
    therapeutic index of, 193
    withdrawal, 286–287
Basal cell carcinoma, 901, 911
Basal ganglia, 238
Basal-bolus insulin regimen, 519–520, 528
Base, 475–476
Basiliximab (Simulect), 786t, 787–788, 789t
Basophils, 598t
Beers Criteria, 47b
Belimumab (Benlysta), 771t–772t, 773
Belladonna alkaloids, 337, 831, 832t
Benazepril (Lotensin), 354t
Beneficence, 58b
Benign, 723–724, 724t
Benign prostatic hyperplasia, 313, 564, 566
Benzalkonium chloride (Zephiran), 912t
Benzocaine, 175t
Benzodiazepines
    adverse effects of, 191, 257t, 286–287
    alcohol and, 286–287
    alprazolam, 256t–257t, 257–258
    antagonists, 191t
    antianxiety uses of, 256–258
    antiepileptic uses of, 226
    assessments, 273
    central nervous system effects of, 190
    chlordiazepoxide, 256t
    clonazepam, 226
    clorazepate dipotassium, 226
    contraindications, 191
    definition of, 188, 190
    diazepam, 192, 192t
    dosages of, 191, 192t
    drug effects of, 190, 286
    eszopiclone, 192t, 193
    flumazenil reversal of, 191, 191t, 257, 286–287
    indications, 190–191, 256, 286
    interactions, 191t
    lorazepam, 256t–257t, 258
    mechanism of action, 190, 286
    midazolam, 192–193
    moderate sedation uses of, 174
    onset of action, 199

Benzodiazepines (Continued)
    overdose of, 191, 257, 286–287
    poisoning, 35t
    profiles of, 192–193, 257–259
    ramelteon, 192t, 193, 198
    sedative–hypnotic, 190t
    temazepam, 192t, 193
    toxicities, 257, 286–287
    withdrawal, 286–287
    zaleplon, 192t, 193, 198–199
    zolpidem, 192t, 193, 199
Benzonatate (Tessalon Perles), 582t, 583
Benzothiazepines, 374t, 376
Benzoyl peroxide, 905
Benztropine mesylate, 240t, 242t, 246
Beriberi, 856, 865
Beta agonists
    administration of, 603
    adverse effects of, 303, 593, 603
    assessments before using, 601
    asthma treated with, 591–594, 591t
    contraindications, 593
    dosages of, 593, 593t
    in elderly patients, 303b
    indications, 593
    interactions, 593
    mechanism of action, 591–593, 591t
    overview of, 591–594
    patient teaching about, 604
    poisoning, 35t
    profiles of, 593–594
    types of, 592t
Beta blockers
    administration of, 379
    adverse effects of, 317, 317t, 362–363, 373, 373t,
        405t
    angina treated with, 317, 372–374, 374t
    antidysrhythmic uses of, 404b, 405t
    assessments, 319–320, 361, 377
    cardioprotective effects of, 317, 385
    cardioselective, 316, 362–363
    contraindications, 317, 373
    dosages of, 318, 318t
    drug effects of, 316–317, 372–373
    heart failure treated with, 385
    hypertension treated with, 317
    indications, 317, 372–373, 415
    interactions, 317–318, 318t, 373, 373t, 375t
    mechanism of action, 316–317, 372–373,
        410
    nonselective, 316, 593
    nursing process for, 319–322, 361, 377, 379
    ophthalmic uses of, 925–926, 925t
    overdose of, 317
    patient teaching about, 322, 366
    poisoning, 35t
    profiles of, 318–319, 373–374, 374t, 410
    therapeutic effects of, 373
    toxicity of, 317
    types of, 318t
Beta₁ receptors, 373
Beta-adrenergic receptors
    definition of, 298–299
    description of, 372
    site of, 300
    stimulation of, 306
    types of, 302
Beta-hemolytic streptococci, 431

Beta-lactam antibiotics
    carbapenems, 623, 628
    cephalosporins. See Cephalosporins
    definition of, 610
    overview of, 616
    penicillins. See Penicillin(s)
Beta-lactamase, 610, 616
Beta-lactamase inhibitors, 610, 616
Betamethasone, 536, 536t
Betaxolol (Betoptic, Betoptic S, Kerlone), 315t,
    925–926, 925t
Bethanechol (Urecholine), 326–328, 328t, 330
Bevacizumab (Avastin), 754, 771t, 773
Bexarotene (Targretin), 776t
Bias, 50
Bicalutamide (Casodex), 566, 757
Bicarbonate, 816
Bifunctional, 749–750
Biguanides, 520, 521t, 523
Bile acid sequestrants, 450–451, 451t, 454–457
Bile acid-binding resins, 450–451
Biliary excretion, 29
Bioavailability, 17, 22
Biogenic amine hypothesis of depression, 253, 259, 260f
Biogenic amines, 285
Biologic antimicrobial drugs, 796–797
Biologic response–modifying drugs
    administration of, 780
    assessments before using, 778
    definition of, 763–764
    hematopoietic drugs, 766–768, 766b, 767t, 778,
        780
    interferons. See Interferon(s)
    interleukins, 767, 774–775, 774b, 775t, 779, 782
    monoclonal antibodies. See Monoclonal
        antibodies
    nursing process for, 778–781
    patient teaching about, 781–782
    therapeutic responses to, 781
Biologic terrorism, 807–809, 808t
Bioterrorism, 796, 807–808, 808t, 810
Biotransformation, 17
    drug-induced changes in, 28t
    hepatic, 27
    principles of, 27, 27t
Bipolar disorder
    antimanic drugs for, 259
    definition of, 253, 255
    prevalence of, 255
Bisacodyl (Dulcolax), 836t–837t, 838
Bismuth subsalicylate (Pepto-Bismol), 831,
    831t–832t, 841
Bisoprolol (Zebeta), 315t
Bisphosphonates, 552–553, 559–560, 562
Bitolterol (Tornalate), 593
Bivalirudin (Angiomax), 423
Black box warning, 50
Blastomycosis, 683t
Blepharitis, 929t
Blinded investigational drug study, 50, 56–57
Blood, 473
Blood pressure
    classification of, 348
    determinants of, 348
    elevated. See Hypertension
    fundal changes, 364–365
    goals for, 364
    regulation of, 349f

Blood products, 479–480, 479t–480t, 485, 487–488
Blood-brain barrier, 18, 27
Body mass index, 205
Body surface area nomogram, 40f
Bone marrow suppression, 729, 740, 743
Booster shot, 796
**Bosentan** (Tracleer), 359–360, 359t
Botulism, 808t
Bowel sounds, 839
Bradykinesia, 237, 239t, 246
Bradykinin, 354, 355t
Braxton Hicks contractions, 555–556
*BRCA1*, 726
*BRCA2*, 726
Breach of duty, 59b
Breakthrough pain, 140, 146
Breast feeding, 38
Breast milk, 38
Bridge therapy, 423
**Bromocriptine**, 240t, 242t, 244–245
**Brompheniramine**, 578t
Bronchial asthma, 588–589
Bronchioles, 316–317
Bronchodilators, 302, 588, 591, 602
Bronchopulmonary dysplasia, 205–206
B-type natriuretic peptides, 386–387, 386t, 391
Buccal administration, 23
Buccal medications, 104, 105f
Bulk-forming laxatives, 834, 834t–837t, 836–837, 841
Bundle branch blocks, 403
**Buprenorphine**, 163t
**Bupropion** (Wellbutrin, Zyban), 263t, 266, 289, 290t
Burkitt's lymphoma, 726
**Buspirone** (BuSpar), 256t–257t, 258–259, 273
**Busulfan**, 751t
**Butenafine** (Mentax, Lotrimin Ultra), 907t
**Butoconazole** (Femstat 3), 907t
**Butorphanol**, 163t

## C

**C** fibers, 143, 144t
**Cabazitaxel** (Jevtana), 734
Cachexia, 725
**Cadexomer iodine** (Iodosorb), 912t
Caffeine, 211t, 212–213, 213t, 594–595
CAGE Questionnaire, 291
**Calcifediol** (Calderol), 860t–861t, 862
Calcineurin inhibitors, 785
**Calcipotriene** (Dovonex), 909
**Calcitonin** (Calcimar, Miacalcin), 552–554, 553t
**Calcitriol** (Rocaltrol, Calcijex), 860t–861t, 861–862
Calcium, 859t, 869–871, 870t–871t, 874–875
**Calcium carbonate** (Tums), 820t, 871t
Calcium channel blockers
  administration of, 379
  adverse effects of, 375, 375t, 405t
  angina treated with, 374–376
  antidysrhythmic uses of, 404, 404b, 405t, 412–413
  antihypertensive use of, 357
  assessments, 377
  cardiovascular effects of, 374–375
  classification of, 374, 374t
  contraindications, 375
  description of, 349
  dosages of, 375, 375t
  drug effects of, 374–375

Calcium channel blockers *(Continued)*
  indications, 375
  interactions, 375, 375t
  mechanism of action, 374–376, 412
  nursing considerations for, 364
  poisoning, 35t
  types of, 350b
**Camptothecin**, 736
*Campylobacter pylori*, 817–818
Canal of Schlemm, 917, 919–920
Cancer
  age-related differences in, 725–726
  definition of, 723–724
  drug therapy for
    antineoplastic drugs. *See* Antineoplastic drugs
    overview of, 728–730
  ethnic factors, 726
  etiology of, 725–728, 725t
  gender-related differences in, 725–726
  genetic factors, 726
  immunologic factors, 726
  lung, 725–726
  nasopharyngeal, 726
  nursing process for, 739–745
  during pregnancy, 730
  radiation as cause of, 726
Cancer pain, 140, 143, 164–166, 165t
*Candida albicans*, 683, 906
Candidiasis, 683, 683t
Cannabinoids, 286
**Capecitabine** (Xeloda), 731, 733t, 734
**Capreomycin**, 676t
Capsaicin, 155–156
**Captopril** (Capoten), 354, 354t–355t, 356
**Carbamazepine**, 225t–228t, 229, 232, 234
**Carbamide peroxide** (Debrox), 939–940
Carbapenems, 623, 628
**Carbidopa-levodopa**, 240t–242t
Carbohydrates, 891, 894
Carbon dioxide, 476
Carbon monoxide poisoning, 35t
Carbonic anhydrase inhibitors
  diuretics, 461–462, 461t, 466, 468
  ophthalmic, 926–927
**Carboplatin**, 751t
Carbuncles, 902, 904
Carcinogenesis, 724f
Carcinogens, 35, 35b, 723, 726
Carcinomas, 723–724, 725t
Cardiac Arrhythmia Suppression Trial (CAST), 397, 409
Cardiac glycosides
  adverse effects of, 388–389, 388t
  contraindications, 388
  description of, 387–388
  digoxin. *See* Digoxin (Lanoxin)
  drug effects of, 388
  indications, 388
  mechanism of action, 388
  nursing considerations for, 392
  overdose of, 388–389
  toxicity of, 388–389
Cardiac output, 348
Cardiac rhythm disturbances, 397
Cardiovascular disease, 348
**Carvedilol** (Coreg, Coreg CR), 315t, 318–319, 318t, 351–353, 353t, 385

Casec, 892
Casein, 673, 889
**Caspofungin** (Cancidas), 685t–687t, 686–688, 690
Castle factor, 868
Catabolism, 564, 889
Cataplexy, 203, 205
Cataract, 917, 919
Catechol *O*-methyltransferase
  catecholamine metabolism by, 300
  inhibitors of, 240t, 243–244
Catecholamines
  definition of, 298, 300
  endogenous, 300
  metabolism of, 300
  types of, 302t
Causation, 59b
cc, 68b
CD4 T cells, 658, 661
**Cefazolin** (Ancef, Kefzol), 620–621, 621t
**Cefepime** (Maxipime), 621t, 622
**Cefoxitin** (Mefoxin), 621–622, 621t
**Ceftaroline** (Teflaro), 620, 622
**Ceftazidime** (Ceptaz, Fortaz, Tazidime), 621t, 622
**Ceftriaxone** (Rocephin), 621t, 622
**Cefuroxime** (Kefurox, Zinacef), 621t, 622
**Celecoxib** (Celebrex), 711t, 713, 717–718
Cell cycle, 727f, 727t
Cell cycle–nonspecific antineoplastic drugs
  alkylating drugs. *See* Alkylating drugs
  cytotoxic antibiotics, 752–754, 753b, 753t, 756, 758
  definition of, 723, 728–729
Cell cycle–specific antineoplastic drugs
  alkaloid topoisomerase II inhibitors, 735–736, 736b, 736t, 740–741
  antimetabolites, 682, 684, 730–734, 732t, 740, 743–744
  antineoplastic enzymes, 738–739, 738t, 741, 744–745
  assessments before using, 740
  definition of, 723, 728–729
  mitotic inhibitors, 734–735, 735t, 740–741, 744
  nursing process for, 739–745
  topoisomerase I inhibitors, 736–738, 737t, 741, 744
Cell growth cycle, 726–728, 727f, 727t
Cell-mediated immunity, 651–653, 763–766, 785, 796–797
Cellulitis, 902, 904
Central nervous system
  barbiturates effect on, 194
  benzodiazepines effect on, 190
  cholinergic blockers effect on, 336
  description of, 299
  general anesthetics effect on, 171
  muscle relaxants effect on, 196
Central nervous system stimulants. *See also* Stimulant(s)
  amphetamines. *See* Amphetamine(s)
  analeptics, 203, 212–214
  anorexiants, 203–204, 207t, 208–209, 216
  caffeine, 211t, 212–213, 213t
  classification of, 204, 204t
  contraindications, 206
  definition of, 203–204
  doxapram, 211t, 213, 215

Central nervous system stimulants (Continued)
  drug effects of, 206
  indications, 206
  interactions, 207, 207t
  mechanism of action, 206
  methylphenidate, 207–208, 207t, 211t
  modafinil, 206, 211t
  nursing process for, 213–216
  orlistat, 208–209, 211t
  profile of, 207–209, 211–213
  sibutramine, 207t, 211–212
  site of action, 204t
  sumatriptan, 211–212, 211t
Central pain, 140, 143
Centrally acting adrenergic drugs, 348, 351–352,
    360, 362
Cephalosporins
  assessments before using, 628
  definition of, 619
  dosages of, 621t
  fifth-generation, 620t
  first-generation, 620–621, 620t–621t
  fourth-generation, 620t, 622
  interactions, 620t
  nursing considerations for, 630
  overview of, 619–620
  patient teaching about, 630–631
  penicillins and, cross-reactivity between, 617–618,
    620
  profiles of, 620–622
  second-generation, 620t, 621–622
  spectrum of activity, 620
  third-generation, 620t, 622
Certolizumab (Cimzia), 771t–772t, 773, 781
Cerumen
  definition of, 937
  removal of, 129, 939–940
Cetuximab (Erbitux), 771t–772t, 773
Chamomile, 89t
Charting guidelines, 15b
Cheese effect, 240–241
Chemical name, 18–19
Chemical terrorism, 807–810, 809t
Chemoreceptor trigger zone, 844, 847
Chemotherapy, 728
Chickenpox, 654–655
Chief cells, 815–816
Childhood Vaccine Injury Act, 800
Children. See Pediatric patients
Chlamydia trachomatis, 929
Chloasma, 543
Chlordiazepoxide, 256t
Chlorhexidine (Hibiclens), 911–912, 912t
Chlorine, 809t
Chloroquine (Aralen), 695–698, 695t–697t, 704
Chlorothiazide, 466
Chlorpheniramine, 578t
Chlorpromazine, 267
Cholecalciferol, 861
Cholesterol
  coronary heart disease and, 446
  definition of, 443–444, 534
  functions of, 444–445
  homeostasis of, 445–446, 445f
Cholesterol absorption inhibitor. See Ezetimibe
Cholestyramine (Questran), 450–451, 450t,
    455–456, 553
Cholinergic crisis, 324, 327

Cholinergic diarrhea, 737
Cholinergic drugs
  adverse effects of, 327, 327t, 331
  contraindications, 327
  description of, 325–326
  direct-acting, 325–326
  dosages of, 327, 328t, 331
  drug effects of, 326
  indications, 326–327
  indirect-acting, 325–327
  interactions, 327
  mechanism of action, 326
  monitoring of, 331
  nursing interventions for, 330
  nursing process for, 329–331
  overdose of, 327
  patient teaching about, 332
  profiles of, 327–329
  toxicity of, 327
  types of, 326b
Cholinergic receptors, 324–325, 350
Cholinergic-blocking drugs. See also
    Anticholinergics.
  adverse effects of, 336, 337t
  as competitive antagonists, 335
  benztropine mesylate, 240t, 242t, 246
  cardiovascular effects of, 335–336, 336t
  contraindications, 336
  definition of, 334
  dosages of, 337, 338t
  drug effects of, 335–336, 336t
  gastrointestinal effects of, 335–336, 336t
  indications, 336–337
  mechanism of action, 335–336
  nursing process for, 339–341
  overdose of, 337
  patient teaching about, 341–342
  profiles of, 337–339
  toxicity of, 337
  types of, 335b
Cholinesterase inhibitors, 325–327, 921
Chondroitin, 716b
Chorea, 237
Choriogonadotropin alfa, 554–555
Choroid, 918
Chromatin, 94, 96
Chromosomes, 94
Chronic bronchitis, 589–591
Chronic diarrhea, 830
Chronic myeloid leukemia, 755
Chronic obstructive pulmonary disease, 205–206,
    589
Chronic pain, 140, 143t, 145b–146b
Chronic stable angina, 368–369
Chronotropic drugs
  definition of, 383–384
  description of, 394
  negative, 384
Chylomicrons, 443
Ciclopiroxolamine (Loprox), 907t
Cidofovir, 655, 655t, 667
Ciliary body, 918
Ciliary muscle, 917
Cilostazol, 429
Cimetidine (Tagamet, Tagamet HB), 821–822, 821t
Ciprofloxacin (Cipro, Ciloxan), 638–640, 640t,
    930–931, 930t, 939
Cisplatin (Platinol), 751t–752t, 752

Cladribine (Leustatin), 731, 733t
Clarithromycin (Biaxin), 624–626
Cleanser, 904t
Clemastine, 578t
Clindamycin (Cleocin), 640–646, 641t, 648, 905
Clomiphene (Clomid, Serophene), 554–555, 555t,
    559
Clonazepam, 226
Clone, 723–724
Clonidine (Catapres), 284b, 351–353, 353t
Clopidogrel (Plavix), 428–430, 429t–430t, 439–440
Clorazepate dipotassium, 226
Clostridium difficile infection, 613
Clot, 419–420, 431
Clotrimazole (Gyne-Lotrimin 3, Lotrimin, Mycelex),
    907, 907t
Clozapine, 269t, 271, 277
Coagulation
  definition of, 419–420
  extrinsic pathway of, 420–421, 420f
  intrinsic pathway of, 420f
  pathways of, 420–421, 420f
  substances that promote, 419–420
Coagulation cascade
  definition of, 419–421
  platelets in, 428f
Coagulation modifiers
  anticoagulants. See Anticoagulants
  antifibrinolytic drugs. See Antifibrinolytic drugs
  antiplatelet drugs. See Antiplatelet drugs
  assessments before using, 434–436
  comparison of, 422t
  nursing process for, 434–440
  overview of, 421
  patient teaching about, 440–441
Cocaine, 175t, 284–285, 284t
Coccidioidomycosis, 683t
Cochleovestibular nerve, 637
Code of Ethics
  American Nurses Association, 59, 330–331
  International Council of Nurses, 59, 59b
Codeine (antitussive), 582t, 583
Codeine sulfate, 152t–153t, 153, 163t, 831t
Coenzyme, 856
Cognition, 332b
Cognitive domain, 74
"Cogwheel" rigidity, 239t
Colchicine, 714–715, 718
Colesevelam, 450–451
Colestipol, 450–451, 455–456
Colistimethate (Colistin, Coly-Mycin), 641t,
    643–644
Collaborative nursing practice, 78b
Collagen, 427
Collagenase (Santyl), 912t
Collecting duct, 459–461
Colloid oncotic pressure, 473, 475, 475f
Colloids, 473, 478t, 478–479
Colonization, 610
Colony-stimulating factors, 743, 763, 766
Commission E monographs, 87–88
Community-associated infection, 610–611
Competitive antagonists, 335
Complement, 763
Complementary medicine, 84
Compliance
  adherence versus, 8
  definition of, 6

Computer-controlled dispensing system, 102, 102f
Computerized physician order entry, 66–67
Concentration-dependent killing, 633
Conduction blocks, 401
Cones, 917, 920, 920f
Confidentiality, 58b
  genetic testing, 100
**Conivaptan** (Vaprisol), 483–484, 487
Conjugated estrogens, 545–546, 548t, 562
Conjunctiva, 918
Conjunctivitis, 929t
Conscious sedation, 173–174, 174b, 184b
Constipation
  causes of, 833t
  definition of, 829
  laxatives for. *See* Laxatives
  opioid-related, 147b, 149
Contraceptives, 550–551, 551t–552t, 560, 562
Contraindication, 18, 31
Controlled Substance Act of 1970, 55t
Controlled substances
  categories of, 56t
  classification of, 55t
  definition of, 50
  dispensing restrictions for, 56t
  opioids as, 162b. *See also* Opioid analgesics
Conventional medicine, 84, 87–88
Convulsion, 219–220
Cornea, 917–919
Coronary arteries, 368–370
Coronary artery disease
  definition of, 368–369
  hypertension and, 348
Coronary artery spasms, 375
Coronary heart disease
  cholesterol and, 446
  laboratory tests, 457b
  risk for, 447b
Corpus luteum, 543
Cortex, 533
Corticosteroids. *See also* Glucocorticoids
  adrenal, 534
  adverse effects of, 598, 603
  antiinflammatory uses of, 931
  assessments before using, 601
  asthma treated with, 591t, 597–600, 603
  contraindications, 598
  definition of, 533–534, 576
  drug effects of, 598–599
  indications, 598
  inhaled, 591t, 597–600, 603–605
  interactions, 599
  mechanism of action, 597–598
  patient teaching about, 604–605
  profiles of, 537–538, 599–600
  synthetic, 535t
  systemic, 536t, 537–538
  topical, 908, 908t
Corticotropin, 534
Cortisol, 536
Cortisone, 536t
**Cosyntropin**, 495–496
**Coumarin**, 424
COX-2 inhibitors, 708, 713
Crack, 285
Cranberry, 89t
Creams, 132, 904t
**Cremophor EL**, 736

Cretinism, 502
**Cromolyn sodium** (Crolom), 933, 934t
Cross-matching tests, 479
Crushing of tablets, 104, 105f
Cryoprecipitate, 479t
Cryptococcal meningitis, 685
Cryptococcosis, 683t
Crystal meth, 284
Crystalloids, 473, 476–478, 476t–477t
Culture
  antihypertensive drugs and, 361b
  assessment of, 60, 60b
  communication affected by, 54
  definition of, 50
  description of, 51
  diversity of, 51
  drug responses and, 90b
  drug therapy considerations, 53–54
  genetic considerations, 90b
  health care barriers, 53
  pain management and, 141b
  patient education affected by, 80b
  psychotherapeutic drugs and, 276b
Curare, 177
Cushing's syndrome, 533–535, 538
Cyanide, 809t
Cyanocobalamin, 859t, 867–869, 868f, 868t,
  873–875, 884
Cyclic adenosine monophosphate,
  594–595, 817
**Cyclobenzaprine**, 197, 197t
Cyclooxygenase, 708, 931
Cyclooxygenase-1, 708
Cyclooxygenase-2, 708
Cyclooxygenase pathway, 428f
**Cyclopentolate** (Cyclogyl), 933
**Cyclophosphamide** (Cytoxan), 751t–752t, 752
Cycloplegia, 917, 919–920
Cycloplegic mydriatics, 933
Cycloplegics, 917, 919–920
**Cycloserine**, 676t
**Cyclosporine** (Sandimmune, Neoral, Gengraf), 375t,
  786t, 788–789, 789t, 792–793
**Cyproheptadine**, 578t
Cystic fibrosis, 589
**Cytarabine** (Ara-C, Cytosar-U), 733t, 734, 740,
  744–745
Cytochrome enzymes, 98
Cytochrome oxidase, 881
Cytochrome P-450, 18, 27, 27t, 52, 265, 685
Cytokines, 652–653, 763, 765–766
Cytomegalovirus, 654, 658
Cytosine deaminase, 684
Cytotoxic antibiotics, 752–754, 753b, 753t, 756, 758
Cytotoxic T cells, 763, 765–766

**D**

**Dabigatran** (Pradaxa), 423, 427, 435, 438, 441
**Daclizumab** (Zenapax), 786t, 787–788, 789t
**Dalteparin** (Fragmin), 422–423
**Danazol** (Danocrine), 565
**Dantrolene**, 196–197
**Daptomycin** (Cubicin), 641t, 643, 645
Data analysis, 9
D/C, 68b
Decongestants
  administration of, 580–581
  adverse effects of, 581

Decongestants (*Continued*)
  assessments before using, 585
  contraindications, 581
  definition of, 576
  drug effects of, 581
  indications, 581
  interactions, 581
  intranasal, 581
  mechanism of action, 581
  nursing process for, 585–586
  ocular, 933
  over-the-counter, 576
  profile of, 582, 582t
  topical, 302
Deep brain stimulation, 239–240
Deep pain, 140, 143
Deep vein thrombosis, 419, 422–423, 426
Defecation, 833
Definitive therapy, 610, 612
Dehydration
  conditions that cause, 476t
  definition of, 474
  fluid disturbances caused by, 475
  hypertonic, 476t
  hypotonic, 476t
  isotonic, 476t
  types of, 476t
7-Dehydrocholesterol, 861
Delirium tremens, 288b
Delta receptor, 148t
Deltoid, intramuscular injections in, 121, 121f
**Demeclocycline** (Declomycin), 627, 627t
**Denileukin diftitox** (Ontak), 774–775, 775t
**Denosumab** (Prolia), 552–553
Deoxyribonucleic acid, 651, 654, 749–750,
  750f–751f
Dependence, 18, 32, 291b
Depolarization, 397–399
Depot drugs, 23
Depressants
  alcohol. *See* Alcohol
  barbiturates. *See* Barbiturates
  benzodiazepines. *See* Benzodiazepines
  definition of, 285
  withdrawal, 286–287
Depression
  anxiety and, 261
  biogenic amine hypothesis of, 253, 259, 260f
  definition of, 254–255
  prevalence of, 255
  tools for assessing, 260
  treatment-resistant, 261
Dermatitis, 902–903
Dermatologic drugs
  anesthetics, 174, 908
  antibacterial drugs, 904–905
  antipruritics, 908
  antipsoriatic drugs, 909
  antiviral drugs, 907–908
  assessments before using, 912
  corticosteroids, 908, 908t
  ectoparasiticidal drugs, 910
  formulations of, 904t
  hair growth drugs, 910
  nursing process for, 912–914
  overview of, 903–904
  patient teaching about, 914
  topical antimicrobials, 903–904

Dermatomes, 654–655
Dermatophytes, 682–683, 902, 906
Dermatophytosis, 683t
Dermatosis, 902–903
Dermis, 902, 903f
Desiccated thyroid, 502–503
Desiccation, 502–503
Desmopressin (DDAVP), 434, 495, 496t, 498–499
Desvenlafaxine (Pristiq), 265
Detoxification, 281, 283–284
Development, 76b
Dexamethasone (Decadron), 536t, 932
Dexchlorpheniramine, 578t
Dextran 40, 478t, 479
Dextran 70, 478t, 479
Dextromethorphan, 582t, 583–584
Diabetes ketoacidosis, 510, 513–514, 514t
Diabetes mellitus
    complications of, 512–514
    definition of, 510, 512
    diagnostic criteria for, 512b, 530
    foot care, 531
    glycemic goals, 515–516
    hyperglycemia caused by, 512–513
    nonpharmacologic interventions for, 515
    nursing process for, 525–530
    pathophysiology of, 512–516
    patient teaching about, 530–531
    prevention of, 515
    screening for, 515
    type 1, 511, 512t–513t, 513–514
    type 2, 511, 512t–513t, 513–515
Diaminopyrimidines, 695, 697
Diarrhea
    acute, 830
    chronic, 830
    definition of, 829–830
    description of, 742
Diazepam, 192, 192t
    antiepileptic uses of, 222t, 224t
    general anesthetic uses of, 171t
    profile of, 258
Diazoxide, 358
Dibucaine, 175t
Dicyclomine (Bentyl), 337–338, 338t
Didanosine, 656t
Dietary reference intakes, 857
Dietary Supplement Act of 2010, 88
Dietary Supplement and Health Education Act, 54–55, 88
Dietary supplements
    consumer use of, 88
    definition of, 84, 87
    FDA approval of, 88
    legend drugs versus, 88
    level of use, 89
    safety of, 88–89
Diethylstilbestrol, 38, 545, 546b
Differentiation, 723–724, 728, 763
Diffusion
    definition of, 37
    in pregnancy, 38
Digestive system, 834f
Digoxin immune Fab, 388–390, 393
Digoxin (Lanoxin)
    adverse effects of, 388, 388t
    assessments, 391
    contraindications, 388

Digoxin (Continued)
    dosage of, 390b, 392
    indications, 388
    interactions, 389, 389t
    mechanism of action, 388
    monitoring of, 393
    nursing considerations for, 392
    overdose of, 388–389, 406t
    patient teaching about, 394
    profile of, 386t, 389–390
    toxicity of, 35t, 388, 389t, 393
Dihydrotachysterol (Hytakerol), 860t–861t, 862
Dihydrotestosterone, 566
Dilator muscle, 917, 919
Diltiazem (Cardizem, Dilacor, Tiazac, Dilacor XR, Cartia XT, Matzim LA, Taztia XT, Dilita XT), 374t–375t, 376, 404b, 405t, 407t–408t, 412–413, 415
Dimenhydrinate, 578t
Dinoprostone (Prostin E2, Prepidil, Cervidil), 556, 557t, 561
Dipeptidyl peptidase IV inhibitors, 523–524
Diphenhydramine (Benadryl), 578t–579t, 580, 849
Diphenoxylate with atropine (Lomotil, Lonox), 831–832, 831t–832t, 840
Diphtheria, tetanus, and acellular (DTaP) vaccine, 802t–803t, 803–804, 808b
Diphyllobothriasis, 701t
Dipivefrin (Propine), 924t, 925
Dipyridamole, 428–429
Direct thrombin inhibitors, 424
Direct vasodilators, 349
Direct-acting cholinergic drugs, 325–326
Direct-acting miotics, 923, 923t
Direct-acting sympathomimetics, 300–301, 301f
Discharge teaching, 81b
Disease-modifying antirheumatic drugs, 763, 777–779, 777b, 781–782
Disinfectants, 610, 612, 612t, 629b
Disopyramide, 404b, 405t–406t
Dissolution, 18
Distal convoluted tubule, 459–461
Distribution, 26–27
    definition of, 26–27
    drug interactions effect, 33t
    in elderly patients, 43b, 44
Disulfiram (Antabuse), 288, 288t
Diuretics
    assessments before using, 468–469
    carbonic anhydrase inhibitors, 461–462, 461t, 468
    classification of, 461t
    definition of, 459–460
    in elderly patients, 464b, 469b
    loop. See Loop diuretics.
    nursing process for, 468–471
    osmotic, 464–465
    patient teaching about, 471
    potassium-sparing, 465–466, 465t–466t, 469–470
    thiazide, 460, 466–468, 467t–468t
    types of, 350b
Divalproex, 225t–226t
DNA microarray technology, 99
Dobutamine (Dobutrex), 302t, 304t, 305, 385–386
Docetaxel, 734, 735t
Documentation, 14
Docusate calcium (Surfak), 836t–837t, 837, 841
Docusate sodium (Colace), 836t–837t, 837, 841
Dofetilide (Tikosyn), 404b, 405t, 407t–408t, 412, 415

Done nomogram, 706, 710
Donepezil (Aricept), 327–328, 328t, 329b
Dopamine agonists, 247–248
Dopamine hypothesis, 254–256
Dopamine (Intropin), 204, 238, 302t, 304t, 305, 845t
Dopaminergic drugs
    adverse effects of, 241t
    amantadine, 240t–242t
    assessments before using, 247–248
    bromocriptine, 240t, 242t, 244–245
    carbidopa-levodopa, 240t–242t, 245–246
    description of, 243
    drug effects of, 244
    entacapone, 240t–242t, 242–244
    interactions, 242t
    levodopa, 240t
    mechanism of action, 244
    patient education regarding, 250–251
    pramipexole, 240t
    ropinirole, 240t–242t, 244, 247
    tolcapone, 240t, 243–244
Dopaminergic receptors, 299–300
Doripenem (Doribax), 623
Dorzolamide (Trusopt), 926–927, 926t
Dosage
    checking of, 13, 13b
    forms of, 21–22, 21t
    parenteral, 23
Dose-limiting adverse effects, 723, 729
Double-blind investigational drug study, 50, 56–57
Doxapram, 211t, 213, 215
Doxazosin (Cardura), 315t, 353, 353t, 360, 566
Doxorubicin (Adriamycin, Rubex), 753
Doxycycline (Vibramycin), 627, 627t
Dreaming sleep, 194
Dromotropic drugs
    definition of, 383
    description of, 394
    positive, 384
Dronabinol (Marinol), 850–852, 854
Dronedarone (Multaq), 404b, 405t, 411, 415b
Drop attacks, 220–221
Drug(s)
    checking of, 11–13
    definition of, 18
    names of, 19
    protein binding of, 26f
    sources of, 35
Drug actions, 18
Drug activity, 20f
Drug administration
    checking of, 13–14
    computer-controlled dispensing system, 102, 102f
    enteral
        absorption affected by, 22–23
        description of, 21t
    gastrostomy tube for, 108, 108f
    inhalation
        absorption effects, 25–26
        environment considerations, 603b
        metered-dose inhalers, 130, 130f, 378–379, 602
        nursing considerations for, 24t–25t
        small-volume nebulizers, 131, 131f
    nasogastric tube, 108, 108f
    preparations for, 102–103, 102f
    rectal, 109, 109f
    standard precautions, 103b

Drug administration *(Continued)*
  sublingual, 23
    absorption effects of, 23, 25, 24t–25t
    nursing considerations for, 24t–25t
    procedure for, 104, 105f
  transdermal
    absorption effects, 25
    contraceptives, 552t
    estrogen, 548t
    fentanyl, 148b, 152t–153t, 163
    nitroglycerin, 378–379
    nursing considerations for, 24t–25t
    opioid analgesics, 148b, 163
    procedure for, 132, 133f
    testosterone, 568t
  vaginal, 135, 135f–136f
Drug approval
  expedited, 55
  FDA process for, 55–56, 85
Drug classification, 18, 20
Drug concentration, 32
Drug development
  description of, 54–57
  informed consent, 56
  investigational drug studies
    phases of, 56–57
    preclinical, 56
  investigational new drug, 56
  new, 54–57
  new drug application, 57
Drug effects
  definition of, 18, 29
  teratogenic, 35
Drug handbooks, 69b
Drug history, 7
Drug holidays, 249
Drug interactions
  definition of, 18
  description of, 27
  herbal products, 89t
  polypharmacy risks, 42, 43t
  types of, 32–33, 33t
Drug misadventure, 33
Drug polymorphism, 50–52
Drug transport, 26f
Drug-induced teratogenesis, 18, 35
D-tubocurarine, 177
**Duloxetine**, 263t, 265, 267
Dumping syndrome, 889
Duration of action, 18, 29
Durham-Humphrey Amendment of 1951, 55t
**Dutasteride** (Avodart), 566, 568
Duty, 59b
**Dyclonine**, 175t
Dye, ophthalmic, 933
Dyskinesia, 237, 239, 254
Dysregulation hypothesis, 254
Dysrhythmias
  atrial fibrillation, 382, 387–390, 401–403, 401t–402t
  classification of, 401
  definition of, 312, 317, 397, 417
  types of, 401–403, 401t–402t
Dystonia, 237, 239, 254, 268

**E**

Ear
  anatomy of, 937–938, 938f
  disorders of, 938–939

Eardrops, 129, 129f, 940
Earwax emulsifiers, 939–940
Eccrine glands, 903t
Echinacea, 89t, 577b
Echinocandins, 684
**Echothiophate** (Phospholine Iodide), 923, 923t
Ectasy. *See* Methylenedioxymethamphetamine
Ectoparasiticidal drugs, 910
Ectopic foci, 401
Eczema, 902–903
Edema, 474–475
**Edrophonium** (Tensilon), 329
Effective refractory period, 397, 399–400, 400f
Efferent arterioles, 459–460
Effervescence, 939–940
Ejection fraction, 383
Elderly patients
  adrenergic drugs in, 307
  alcohol abuse in, 293b
  anesthesia considerations for, 172b
  anticholinergics in, 336
  antiparkinsonian drugs in, 248b
  Beers Criteria on drug use in, 47b
  beta-adrenergic agonists in, 303b
  definition of, 37, 42
  description of, 42–44
  diuretics in, 464b, 469b
  iron products in, 885b
  kidney functioning in, 43
  life expectancy of, 42
  noncompliance by, 42–43
  nonsteroidal antiinflammatory drugs in, 717b
  nursing diagnoses for, 46
  nursing process for, 44–49
  opioid analgesics in, 162b
  overactive bladder in, 340b
  over-the-counter medications used by, 42
  pharmacokinetic changes in
    absorption, 43b, 44
    distribution, 43b, 44
    excretion, 43b, 44
    metabolism, 43b, 44
    overview of, 43–44
  physiologic changes in, 43, 43t
  polypharmacy in, 42
  problematic drugs in, 44, 45t
  psychotherapeutic drugs in, 272b
  statistics regarding, 42
  substance abuse in, 293b
  thyroid hormones in, 506b
  warfarin sodium in, 424
  xanthine derivatives in, 601b
Electrocardiography, 400–401, 401f
Electroconvulsive therapy, 261
Electroencephalogram, 219–220
Electrolytes
  balance of, 480
  monitoring of, 486
  nursing process for, 484–488
  patient teaching about, 488–489
  potassium, 480–482, 484, 485b, 489
  sodium, 482–485, 487
Embolus, 419–420, 422
Emesis, 844–845
Emetic potential, 723, 729, 730b
Emollient laxatives, 834, 834t–835t, 837
Emphysema, 589, 591

Empiric therapy, 31, 576, 610, 612
Empty stomach, 23b
**Enalapril** (Vasotec), 354, 354t–355t, 356, 364
Endocrine glands, 543–544
Endocrine system, 494, 494b, 494f
Endometrial cancer, 559b
Endometrium, 545
Endophthalmitis, 929t
Endorphins, 143–144
Endothelin receptors, 359
**Enfuvirtide** (Fuzeon), 664–666, 665t
Enkephalins, 143–144
Enolic acid derivatives, 713
**Enoxaparin** (Lovenox), 422–423, 425–426, 426t
**Entacapone**, 240t–242t, 242–244
Enteral administration
  absorption affected by, 23
  description of, 21t
Enteral nutrition
  adverse effects of, 891
  contraindications, 891
  definition of, 889–890
  dosages of, 891
  drug effects of, 891
  feeding routes for, 890f, 890t
  formulations, 890b, 891–892
  indications, 891, 891b
  interactions, 891
  mechanism of action, 891
  nursing process for, 895–897
  patient teaching about, 897–898
Enteric-coated tablets, 21, 105f, 438
Enterobiasis, 700–701, 701t
Enterohepatic recirculation, 29
Entry inhibitor–CCR5 coreceptor antagonists, 662, 663t, 665–666, 665t
Enuresis, 281, 285
Enzyme, 419
  definition of, 18, 856–857
  interactions, 30
Enzyme induction, 195
Enzyme inhibitors, 27
Eosinophils, 598t
Ephedrine, 592t
Epidermis, 902, 903f, 903t
Epidural anesthesia, 175b, 185
Epilepsy
  definition of, 220
  diagnosis of, 220
  electroencephalography for, 219–220
  etiology of, 220
  idiopathic, 220
  primary, 220
  secondary, 220
**Epinephrine** (Adrenalin, EpiPen), 302t, 304t, 305, 534, 591, 592t, 600
Epiphyses, 878
**Eplerenone** (Inspra), 359, 359t, 385
**Epoetin alfa** (Epogen), 766–767, 880, 882t, 886
**Eptifibatide** (Integrilin), 430, 430t
Equianalgesia, 148
Erectile dysfunction, 567b, 569b, 570–571
**Ergocalciferol** (Drisol, Calciferol), 860t–861t, 861–863
Ergosterol, 682, 684
Ergot alkaloids, 203, 209, 212, 214–215, 556, 559
**Eribulin** (Halaven), 734

Erikson's stages of development, 76b
Erythrocytes, 877–878
Erythroid cells, 536
**Erythromycin** (E-mycin, EryPed, Eryc, E.E.S.), 624, 627
Erythropoiesis, 877–878
Erythropoiesis-stimulating agents, 880, 884–885
Erythropoietic effect, 564–565
Erythropoietin, 878
**Esmolol** (Brevibloc), 315t, 318t, 319, 406t, 410
Esophagostomy tube, 890f
Essential amino acids, 889, 894
Essential fatty acid deficiency, 889, 894
Essential hypertension, 348, 359
**Estradiol** (Estrace), 544–545, 548t
Estrogen receptor antagonists, 755t
Estrogen-progestin combination products, 548–549, 560
**Estrogens** (Cenestin, Premarin)
    adverse effects of, 547, 548t, 561
    assessments before using, 558
    conjugated, 545–546, 548t, 562
    contraindications, 547
    definition of, 543–544
    dosages of, 547
    drug effects of, 546–547, 561
    endogenous, 545
    exogenous, 545
    functions of, 544
    indications, 547, 547b
    interactions, 547
    mechanism of action, 546–547
    ovarian production of, 544–545
    patient teaching about, 562
    profile of, 547–549, 551
**Eszopiclone** (Lunesta), 192t, 193
**Etanercept** (Enbrel), 776t, 777–779, 909
**Ethambutol** (Myambutol), 676t–677t, 677
Ethanol. *See* Alcohol.
Ethics
    American Nurses Association code of, 59
    definition of, 51
    description of, 59
    gene therapy, 98
**Ethionamide**, 676t
Ethnicity
    definition of, 51
    drug response affected by, 51–53
    genetics effect, 51–53
    influences of, 51–53
Ethnopharmacology, 51
**Ethosuximide**, 227t–228t, 229
**Ethyl chloride**, 175t
Ethylene glycol poisoning, 35t
**Etonogestrel–ethinyl estradiol vaginal ring** (NuvaRing), 552t
**Etoposide** (VP-16, Etopophos), 735, 735t–736t, 746
Eugenics, 98
Eustachian tube, 938f
Euthyroid, 501, 503
Evaluation phase of nursing process, 15
Evening primrose, 89t
**Everolimus** (Certican), 790
Excretion
    definition of, 27–28
    drug interactions effect on, 33t
    in elderly patients, 43b, 44
    renal, 27–28, 28f

**Exenatide** (Byetta), 525–526
Exercise, 332b
Exogenous, 237, 245
Exogenous lipids, 443, 445
Expectorants, 576, 582t, 584–585
Expedited drug approval, 51, 55
Expiration date of medications, 102
Extended-spectrum beta-lactamases, 633–634
Extended-spectrum penicillins, 617, 617t, 619
Extensively drug-resistant tuberculosis, 673
External ear, 937–938
Extracellular fluid, 474–475, 475t
Extraocular muscles, 917–918, 918f
Extrapyramidal symptoms, 254, 268
Extravasation, 312–314, 723, 729–730, 749, 751b, 753b
Extravascular fluid, 474–475, 475t
Extrinsic asthma, 589–590
Extrinsic factor, 868, 880f
Eye
    anatomy of, 917, 918f
    infections of, 929t
    layers of, 919–920
    muscles of, 917–918, 918f
Eye medications
    eye ointment, 128, 129f
    eyedrops, 128, 128f
Eye ointment, 129f
Eyebrow, 918
Eyedrops, 128, 128f
Eyelashes, 918
Eyelid, 918
**Ezetimibe** (Zetia), 447, 450t, 453–454, 456

**F**

Fallopian tubes, 543–544
**Famotidine** (Pepcid, Pepcid AC), 821t, 822, 826
Fast channels, 398–399
Fast-channel cells, 399
Fast-response cells, 399
Fat, 894–895
Fat-soluble vitamins
    characteristics of, 858
    definition of, 856–858
    excretion of, 858
    overview of, 858–859
    types of, 858t
    vitamin A, 859–861, 859t–861t, 873–875
    vitamin D, 859t, 861–863, 862t, 873–875, 914
    vitamin E, 859t–861t, 863, 863t, 875
    vitamin K, 424, 435, 859t–861t, 863–864, 864t, 873, 875
Febrile seizures, 220
**Febuxostat** (Uloric), 714
Federal Food, Drug, and Cosmetic Act of 1938, 55t
Federal Food and Drug Act of 1906, 55t
Felbamate, 226
**Felodipine** (Plendil), 374t
Female reproductive system, 544–545
Female sex hormones
    contraceptives. *See* Contraceptives
    estrogens. *See* Estrogens
Feminization, 546–547
**Fenofibrate**, 452–453
**Fenoldopam** (Corlopam), 304t, 305
**Fentanyl**
    administration of, 163t
    characteristics of, 153–154

**Fentanyl** (*Continued*)
    general anesthetic uses of, 171t
    in pediatric patients, 174b
    transdermal delivery of, 148b, 152t–153t, 163
**Fentanyl citrate**, 174b
**Ferric gluconate** (Ferrlecit), 882t, 883
**Ferrous fumarate** (Femiron), 882, 882t
**Ferrous salts**, 881t
**Ferrous sulfate**, 882–883, 882t
Fertility drugs, 554–555, 555t, 560–561
Fetal alcohol syndrome, 288
Fetus, 38
Feverfew, 161b
**Fexofenadine**, 578t–579t
Fibrates, 452
Fibric acid derivatives, 452–454, 453t
Fibrin, 419–421, 439
Fibrin plug, 427
Fibrin specificity, 419
Fibrinogen, 419, 428–429
Fibrinolysis, 419, 421
Fibrinolytic system, 419, 421, 421f, 431
Fibromyalgia, 155–156
**Filgrastim** (Neupogen), 737, 766–768, 767t, 780
Filter needle, 111f–112f
Filtrate, 459
Fimbriae, 544
**Finasteride** (Propecia, Proscar), 566, 568–571, 568t, 910
**Fingolimod** (Gilenya), 786, 786t, 789
First-dose phenomenon, 312, 314
First-dose syncope, 352, 360
First-pass effect, 18, 22, 25b, 372
Fixed-combination insulins, 519
Flax, 444b
**Flecainide** (Tambocor), 404b, 405t–406t, 409
**Floxuridine**, 733t
**Fluconazole** (Diflucan), 684–685, 685t–687t, 687–689
**Flucytosine**, 684–685
**Fludarabine** (Fludara), 731, 733t, 734
**Fludrocortisone** (Florinef), 537t, 538, 540
Fluids
    administration of, 486
    assessments before using, 484–485
    blood products, 479–480, 479t–480t, 485, 487–488
    colloids, 473, 478–479, 478t
    crystalloids, 473, 476–478, 476t–477t
    extracellular, 474–475, 475t
    extravascular, 474–475, 475t
    intracellular, 474, 475t
    intravascular, 474–475, 475t
    location of, 475t
    nursing process for, 484–488
    overview of, 474–476
    patient teaching about, 488–489
**Flumazenil**, 191, 191t, 257, 286–287
**Flunitrazepam**, 286
Fluorescein, 933
Fluoroquinolones. *See* Quinolones
**5-Fluorouracil** (Efudex, Adrucil), 684, 733t, 734, 742, 911
**Fluoxetine** (Prozac), 266
**Fluoxymesterone** (Halotestin), 565
**Flurbiprofen** (Ocufen), 932

**Flutamide** (Eulexin), 566, 757
**Fluticasone propionate** (Flovent, Flonase), 599, 599t
Foam cells, 443
Folate, 883
Folate antagonists, 732–734
Folic acid, 731, 882t, 883–884
Folic acid deficiency, 879
Follicle-stimulating hormone, 495t, 544
Folliculitis, 902
**Fondaparinux** (Arixtra), 423, 427
Food and Drug Administration drug approval
    process, 55–56
**Formoterol**, 592t
**Foscarnet**, 655t–656t
**Fosinopril** (Monopril), 354t
**Fosphenytoin**, 222t, 224t,
    227t–229t, 228–229
Frailty, 730
Fresh frozen plasma, 479t, 480
Fungal infections
    overview of, 683
    types of, 683t
Fungi, 682–683
**Furosemide** (Lasix), 463–464, 463t
Furuncles, 902, 904
Fusion, 651
Fusion inhibitor, 663, 663t, 665t

**G**

**Gabapentin**, 224t, 227t–228t, 229–230, 232, 234
**Galantamine** (Razadyne), 327
Gamma-aminobutyric acid
    definition of, 188, 194, 254–255
    mental illness and, 256
    muscle relaxant effects on, 196
Gamma-hydroxybutyric acid, 286
**Ganciclovir** (Cytovene), 656t, 658, 669
Garlic, 89t, 444b
Gastric dumping, 22–23
Gastric glands, 815–816
Gastric hyperacidity, 815
Gastric inhibitory peptide, 524–525
Gastrin receptors, 817
Gastroesophageal reflux disease, 816
Gastrointestinal tract
    age-related changes in, 44
    cholinergic-blocking drugs effect on, 335–336, 336t
    in elderly patients, 44
    functions of, 833
    opioid analgesics effect on, 150
Gastrostomy tube, 108, 108f
Gate theory of pain, 140, 143, 144f
Gels, 904t
**Gemcitabine** (Gemzar), 731, 733t, 734, 744–745
**Gemfibrozil** (Lopid), 450t, 453
Gene, 94
Gene expression, 723
Gene therapy, 94, 97–98
General anesthesia
    definition of, 170
    historical perspective of, 170b
    nursing process for
        assessment, 180–182
        evaluation, 185
        implementation, 183–185
        nursing diagnoses, 182
        outcome criteria, 182–183
        planning, 182–183

General anesthetics
    adverse effects of, 172–173
    central nervous system effects, 171
    contraindications, 171
    definition of, 170
    drug effects of, 171, 172t
    indications, 171
    inhalational, 171t–172t
    injectable, 170
    interactions, 173
    intravenous, 172t
    isoflurane, 173
    ketamine, 173
    mechanism of action, 171
    nitrous oxide, 173
    overdose of, 173
    propofol, 173–174
    sevoflurane, 173
Generic name, 18–19, 728
Genetic disease, 94–96
Genetic inheritance, 95–96
Genetic material, 94–96
Genetic polymorphisms, 94, 98
Genetic predisposition, 94
Genetic testing, 100
Genetics, 99–100
    definition of, 95
    drug response affected by, 51–53
Genital herpes, 654
Genome, 95–96, 651
Genomics, 95–96
Genotype, 95–96
**Gentamicin** (Garamycin), 635, 635t–637t, 638, 929
Gestational age, 38
Gestational diabetes, 510, 515, 517–518
Giardiasis, 698, 698t
Ginger, 89t, 852b
Gingival hyperplasia, 220
Ginkgo biloba, 89t, 214b, 330b
Ginseng, 214b, 274b
**Glatiramer acetate** (Copaxone), 786, 786t, 789
Glaucoma
    angle-closure, 917, 920, 921t
    definition of, 917, 920
    open-angle, 460–461, 920, 921t
    pathophysiology of, 920
**Glimepiride** (Amaryl), 521t
Glinides, 521–522, 524
**Glipizide** (Glucotrol, Glucotrol XL), 517t, 521t, 523
**Glipizide/metformin** (Metaglip), 521t
Glitazones, 522
Globin, 877–878
Globus pallidus, 238
Glomerular capsule, 460
Glomerular filtration rate, 460
Glomerulus, 460
Glucagon, 511
Glucagon-like peptide 1, 524–525
Glucocorticoids. *See also* Corticosteroids.
    assessments before using, 540
    definition of, 534
    description of, 534–535, 535t
    inhalers of, 540–541
    interactions, 537
    nasal administration of, 536, 540
    patient teaching about, 541
    therapeutic response to, 541
Glucosamine, 716b

Glucose
    blood, 526
    description of, 511
    drugs that elevate, 525–526
Glucose-6-phosphate dehydrogenase deficiency,
    18, 610, 614
Glucose-6-phosphate hydrogenase deficiency
    cultural considerations, 34b
    description of, 156
    drug interactions, 34b
**Glycerin** (Sani-Supp, Colace, Fleet Babylax,
    Ophthalgan), 836t–837t, 837, 927
Glycogen, 511
Glycogenolysis, 511
Glycoprotein IIb/IIIa, 427
Glycoprotein IIb/IIIa inhibitors, 429, 429t, 435,
    438–439
**Glycopyrrolate** (Robinul), 171t, 338–341, 338t
Glycosylated hemoglobin, 531t
**Glycylcycline**, 627
Goals, 6, 11
Goiter, 502
Goldenseal, 577b
**Golimumab** (Simponi), 771t–772t, 773
Gonadotropin, 544
Gonadotropin-releasing hormone, 554
Gonadotropin-releasing hormone agonists, 755t,
    757
Gonadotropin-releasing hormone analogues, 566
**Goserelin** (Zoladex), 566
Gout
    antigout drugs for, 713–716, 718
    definition of, 706
Gradient, 474, 476
Grafts, 784, 787
Gram stain, 611
Gram-negative, 611
Gram-positive, 611
**Granisetron**, 852
Granulocyte colony-stimulating factor, 766–767
Granulocyte-macrophage colony-stimulating factor,
    766–767
Granulocytes, 598t, 766–768
Granulomas, 672–673
Grapefruit, 89t
Graves' disease, 505
**Griseofulvin**, 684–685
Growth fraction, 723, 728
Growth hormone, 495t
Growth hormone analogues, 496t
**Guaifenesin** (Guiatuss, Humibid, Robitussin,
    Mucinex), 582t, 584
Guarana, 214b

**H**

H₂ receptor antagonists, 818, 820–822, 824–826
Habitrol, 290t
Habituation, 281
*Haemophilus influenzae*, 624
*Haemophilus influenzae* type b conjugate vaccine,
    802t–803t, 804, 809–810
Hair growth drugs, 910
Half-life, 18, 29, 29t
**Haloperidol**, 269–270, 269t, 274, 277
Hand-foot syndrome, 732
Handwashing, 611–612, 647
Harrison Narcotic Act of 1914, 55t
Hawthorn, 89t

**Headaches**
migraine. *See* Migraine headaches
spinal, 184, 184b
Health care-associated infections, 610–612
Health Insurance Portability and Accountability Act
(HIPAA), 51, 54
Health literacy
definition of, 74
facts regarding, 76b
Heart
conduction system of, 384f, 397
electrocardiography of, 400–401, 401f
functions of, 369
Heart failure
defects that cause, 383
definition of, 383
incidence of, 383
New York Heart Association functional
classification of, 383–384
nursing process for, 390–393
pathophysiology of, 383
patient teaching about, 394
in pediatric patients, 391b
treatment of
aldosterone antagonists, 385, 391
angiotensin II receptor blockers, 385
angiotensin-converting enzyme inhibitors,
384–385
beta blockers, 385, 390–391
B-type natriuretic peptides, 386–387, 386t, 391
dobutamine, 385–386
hydralazine/isosorbide dinitrate, 385, 391–392
phosphodiesterase inhibitors, 387, 391–392
Heartburn, 818
*Helicobacter pylori*, 817–818
Helminthic infections, 692, 700–701, 701t
Helper T cells, 661, 764
Hematopoiesis, 763–764, 877
Hematopoietic drugs, 766–768, 766b, 778, 780
Hematopoietic growth factors, 729
Hematopoietic stem cells, 728
Heme, 877–878
Hemoglobin, 877–878, 878f
Hemoglobin A1C, 511–512, 515–516, 530–531
Hemolysis, 614
Hemolytic anemias, 877, 879
Hemophilia, 419, 421, 432
Hemorheologic drugs
definition of, 419, 429
function of, 421
Hemostasis, 419–420
Hemostatic drugs
definition of, 419
functions of, 421
**Heparin**
administration of, 436–437
assessments before using, 434–435
conversion of, to warfarin, 438
deep vein thrombosis prophylaxis using, 426
dosage of, 426, 426t
effects of, 422–423
intravenous administration of, 437b
low molecular weight, 422–423, 425, 434–437
oral administration of, 437b
parenteral, 435
patient teaching about, 440–441
pharmacokinetics of, 426t
profile of, 426–427

**Heparin** *(Continued)*
protamine sulfate reversal of, 423–424, 437–438
sources of, 35
subcutaneous injection of, 437b
toxicity of, 423–424
Heparin-induced thrombocytopenia, 423
**Hepatitis B immunoglobulin** (BayHep B, Nabi-HB),
802t–803t, 806
Hepatitis B virus vaccine, 802t–803t, 804
Hepatitis C virus, 664
Herb(s)
consumer uses of, 88
definition of, 84
drug interactions, 89t
ginkgo biloba, 89t, 214b, 330b
ginseng, 214b, 274b
guarana, 214b
history of, 87–88
kava, 89t, 192b
patient education regarding, 92
safety of, 88–89
St. John's wort, 89t, 262, 264b
valerian, 192b
Herbal medicine
definition of, 84, 87
level of use, 89
managed care reimbursement for, 89
nursing process for, 89–92
Herd immunity, 796, 800
Heredity, 95
Heroin, 283
Herpes simplex viruses, 654
Herpes zoster
description of, 654–655
vaccine against, 806
Herpesviruses, 651, 654, 655t, 726
Hetastarch, 478t
High-density lipoprotein, 317, 445
Highly active antiretroviral therapy, 661–663
Hispanics
cultural practices of, 52b
drug responses in, 53b
health belief practices of, 52b, 53
pain management practices, 141b
His-Purkinje system, 403
Histamine, 576, 845t
Histamine antagonists, 576–577
Histamine receptors, 576, 578, 817
Histoplasmosis, 683t
HIV. *See* Human immunodeficiency virus
HIV integrase strand transfer inhibitor, 663, 663t
HIV wasting syndrome, 661
HMG-CoA reductase inhibitors, 443, 448–451, 449t,
454–455, 457
H1N1, 667
H5N1, 667
Hordeolum, 929t
Hormonal antineoplastic drugs, 755–758
Hormone replacement therapy, 544, 547
Host, 651
Host factors, 610, 613–614
HS, 68b
Huffing, 293b
Human chorionic gonadotropin, 554–555
Human Genome Project, 95, 97
Human herpesvirus 3, 654
Human immunodeficiency virus. *See also* Acquired
immunodeficiency syndrome

Human immunodeficiency virus *(Continued)*
antiretroviral drugs for
administration of, 669–670
adverse effects of, 664
assessments before using, 668
contraindications, 664
dosages of, 664, 665t
drug effects of, 663
highly active antiretroviral therapy,
661–663
indications, 664
interactions, 664
mechanism of action, 663
nonnucleoside reverse transcriptase inhibitors,
662–663, 663t
nucleoside reverse transcriptase inhibitors,
662–663, 663t, 665t
nursing process for, 667–670
overview of, 662–664
patient teaching about, 670
profiles of, 664–666
therapeutic effects of, 670
antiretrovirals for, 659
definition of, 651–652
epidemiology of, 660b
hepatitis C virus and, 664
high-risk populations for, 660
life cycle of, 660f
occupational exposure chemoprophylaxis, 664t
pathophysiology of, 658–662, 659f
stages of, 661, 662f
transmission of, 659–660
**Human papillomavirus vaccine** (Gardasil,
Cervarix), 806, 810
Humanization, 754, 772–773
Humoral immune system, 765
Humoral immunity, 651, 763–765, 785
Hydantoins, 225t–226t, 232, 234
**Hydralazine** (Apresoline), 349, 358t, 359, 874–875
**Hydralazine/isosorbide dinitrate** (BiDil), 385,
391–392
Hydrochloric acid, 815–816, 818
**Hydrochlorothiazide** (HydroDIURIL), 466–468,
468t
**Hydrocodone**, 149, 583
**Hydrocortisone** (Solu-Cortef), 536, 536t, 539b
**Hydromorphone**, 163t, 174b
Hydrostatic pressure, 474–475
**Hydroxychloroquine** (Plaquenil), 695–698,
695t–697t, 704
Hydroxymethylglutaryl-coenzyme A reductase
inhibitors. *See* HMG-CoA reductase inhibitors
**5-Hydroxytryptamine**, 209, 838–839, 850
**Hydroxyurea** (Hydrea, Droxia), 755, 757–759
**Hydroxyzine**, 171t, 256t, 578t
Hymenolepiasis, 701t
**Hyoscyamine**, 831t
Hyperacidity, 816
Hyperalimentation, 889, 892
Hypercapnia, 205–206
Hypercholesterolemia, 444–446
Hyperglycemia, 511–513
Hyperkalemia, 389, 389t, 465–466, 474, 480,
486–487
Hyperlipidemias, 446–447, 447t
Hypernatremia, 474, 482–483, 485, 488
Hyperosmolar nonketotic syndrome, 511, 513–514,
514t

Hyperosmotic laxatives, 834–835, 834t–835t, 837–839

Hypersensitivity reactions, 34

Hypertension
advances in, 349
antihypertensive drugs for. *See* Antihypertensive drugs
beta blockers for, 317
coronary artery disease and, 348
definition of, 348
essential, 348, 359
prevalence of, 348
primary, 349
rebound, 352
secondary, 348–349
stages of, 348

Hyperthermia, malignant, 181

Hyperthyroidism, 501–502, 508

Hypertonic dehydration, 476t

Hypertonic saline, 476t, 477, 483, 487

Hypervitaminosis, 858

Hypnotics, 189

Hypochromic, 877–879

Hypodermis, 903

Hypoglycemia, 511, 521, 525, 897

Hypokalemia, 462–463, 470–471, 474, 480–481, 481b, 486

Hypomania, 254–255

Hyponatremia, 474, 482, 487

Hypothalamic-pituitary-adrenal axis, 534, 538

Hypothalamus, 493

Hypothyroidism, 501–502, 508

Hypotonic dehydration, 476t

**I**

Iatrogenic effects, 84, 87–88

**Ibritumomab tiuxetan** (Zevalin), 771t–772t, 773

**Ibuprofen** (Motrin, Advil), 20f, 210b, 711t, 712–713

**Ibutilide** (Corvert), 404b, 405t, 411–412

Identification bracelet, 102–103, 103f

Idiosyncratic reaction, 18, 34, 64

Illicit drug use
definition of, 281
prevalence of, 282

**Imatinib** (Gleevec), 755

Imidazoles, 684

Iminostilbenes, 227t–228t, 229

**Imipenem/cilastatin** (Primaxin), 623, 624t

**Imiquimod** (Aldara), 911

Immediate-release dosage forms, 21

Immune responses, 652–653, 796–797

Immune system
cell-mediated, 765–766, 765f
cells of, 765f
components of, 764–765
humoral, 765
overview of, 764–766
purpose of, 785
schematic diagram of, 785f

Immune-mediated diseases, 784–785

Immunity
cell-mediated, 651–653, 763–766, 785, 796–797
description of, 797–799
herd, 796, 800
humoral, 651, 763–765, 785

Immunization
active. *See* Active immunization. *See also* Active immunizing drugs

Immunization *(Continued)*
childhood schedule of, 798
definition of, 796
passive. *See* Passive immunization. *See also* Passive immunizing drugs

Immunizing biologics, 796–797, 799b

Immunizing drugs
active. *See* Active immunizing drugs
administration of, 811
adverse effects of, 800–801, 800t
assessments before using, 809–810
contraindications, 800
dosages of, 802t–803t, 803
drug effects of, 799–800
indications, 800
interactions, 801–803
mechanism of action, 799–800
nursing process for, 809–811
passive. *See* Passive immunizing drugs
patient teaching about, 811
therapeutic response of, 811

Immunoglobulin
endogenous, 589–590, 651, 653, 763, 765
immunization uses of, 796–797, 799, 802t–803t, 807b

**Immunoglobulin** (BayGam, Octagam), 806–807, 807b

Immunomodulating drugs
adverse effects of, 771t
definition of, 763–764
interferons. *See* Interferon(s)
monoclonal antibodies. *See* Monoclonal antibodies
overview of, 764
topical, 911
types of, 766b

Immunostimulants, 763, 776

Immunosuppressant drugs
administration of, 791–792
adverse effects of, 786, 787t
contraindications, 786
definition of, 763, 769, 784–785
dosages of, 787, 789t
drug effects of, 785
indications, 786
interactions, 786–787, 788t
mechanism of action, 785
nursing process for, 790–793
patient teaching about, 793

Immunosuppressive therapy, 784–785

Impaired fasting glucose level, 511, 515

Impetigo, 902, 904

Implantation, 544–545

Implementation phase of nursing process, 11–15

Incompatibility, 18, 33

Incretin mimetics, 524–525

**Indinavir** (Crixivan), 656t, 665, 665t

Indirect-acting cholinergic drugs, 325–327

Indirect-acting dopamine receptor agonists, 240, 248

Indirect-acting miotics, 923

Indirect-acting sympathomimetics, 300–301, 301f

**Indomethacin** (Indocin), 557, 560, 711t, 712

Infants, 107, 107f. *See also* Pediatric patients

Infections
definition of, 610
health care-associated, 610–612
superinfections, 610, 613, 644

Infertility, 554–555, 555t, 560–561

Inflammation
definition of, 706–707
signs and symptoms of, 707

**Infliximab** (Remicade), 770–771, 771t–772t, 773, 779, 781

Influenza, 576, 651, 804

**Influenza vaccine** (Fluzone, FluShield, Fluvirin), 802t–803t, 804–805

Information collection, 7–8

Informed consent, 51, 56

Inhalation administration
absorption effects, 25–26
environment considerations, 603b
metered-dose inhalers, 130, 130f, 378–379, 602
nursing considerations for, 24t–25t
small-volume nebulizers, 131, 131f

Inhalers, 130, 130f

Inherited disease, 95

Injections
in children, 120b
intradermal, 115, 115f
intramuscular
deltoid, 121, 121f
needle insertion angle for, 114f
overview of, 118–121
vastus lateralis site for, 120, 120f
ventrogluteal site for, 119, 119f
Z-track method for, 118–121, 118f
intravenous
infusion bag for, 123f
piggyback admixtures, 122, 122f–123f, 124–126, 125f
preparations for, 122
push medications, 126, 127f
needle insertion angles for, 114f
in pediatric patients, 120b
subcutaneous
insulin administration, 116, 117f
needle insertion angle for, 114
procedure for, 116, 116f–117f

Inotropic drugs
definition of, 383–384
description of, 394
positive, 384

Institute for Safe Medication Practices, 81–82, 372b

Institute of medicine, 65

Insulin
administration of, 528b
adverse effects of, 516
basal-bolus dosing of, 519–520, 528
contraindications, 516
definition of, 511
dosages of, 517, 517t
drug effects of, 516
fixed-combination, 519
hypoglycemic effect of, 317–318
indications, 516
interactions, 516, 517t
intermediate-acting, 519
long-acting, 517t, 519
mechanism of action, 516
metabolic functions of, 511–512
mixing of, 117f, 516t, 528b
in pediatric patients, 517
pharmacokinetics of, 518f
in pregnancy, 517–518
profiles of, 518–520
rapid-acting, 517t, 518

**Insulin** (*Continued*)
short-acting, 517t, 518–519
sliding-scale dosing of, 519–520
sources of, 35, 516
storage of, 528b
subcutaneous administration of, 527
syringes for, 116, 117f
**Insulin, regular** (Humulin R, Novolin R), 517t, 518–519
**Insulin detemir**, 519
**Insulin glargine** (Lantus), 517t, 519
**Insulin isophane suspension** (NPH), 519, 527
**Insulin lispro** (Humalog), 517t, 518
Insulin pump therapy, 529b
Insulin resistance, 515
Insulin-resistance syndrome, 515
Insulin-sensitizing drugs, 522
Integrase inhibitors, 663, 665t, 666
Integrative medicine, 87–88
Intercalation, 753
Interferon(s)
administration of, 780–781
adverse effects of, 769, 769t
assessments before using, 778–779
contraindications, 769
definition of, 763, 768
dosages of, 769, 769t
drug effects of, 768–769
indications, 769
interactions, 769
mechanism of action, 768–769
**Interferon alfa-2a** (Roferon-A), 769t, 770
**Interferon alfa-2b** (Intron-A), 769t, 770
**Interferon alfacon-1** (Infergen), 769t, 770
**Interferon alfa-n3** (Alferon-N), 769t, 770
**Interferon beta-1a** (Avonex, Rebif), 769t, 770
**Interferon beta-1b**, 770
**Interferon gamma-1b** (Actimmune), 769t, 770
Interleukins, 767, 774–775, 774b, 775t, 779, 782
International Council of Nurses Code of Ethics for Nurses, 59, 59b
International League Against Epilepsy, 220, 221b
International normalized ratio, 406, 440b
International Society of Nurses in Genetics, 95
Internodal pathways, 397, 400
Interstitial fluid, 474
Interview of patient, 7–8
Intoxication, 281
Intraarterial, 18, 23
Intraarticular, 18, 23
Intracellular fluid, 474, 475t
Intradermal injections
needle insertion angle for, 114
procedure for, 115, 115f
Intramuscular administration
absorption effects, 23
injections
air-lock technique for, 114, 114f
deltoid, 121, 121f
needle insertion angle for, 114
overview of, 118–121
vastus lateralis site for, 120, 120f
ventrogluteal site for, 119, 119f
Z-track method for, 118–121, 118f
nursing considerations for, 24t–25t
Intraocular pressure, 917, 919
Intrathecal, 18, 23, 723, 732–734
Intravascular fluid, 474–475, 475t
Intravenous infusions, 309b

Intravenous injections
heparin, 437b
infusion bag for, 123f
nursing considerations for, 24t–25t
piggyback admixtures, 122, 122f–123f, 124–126, 125f
preparations for, 122
push medications, 126, 127f
Intravenous lock, 126, 127f
Intrinsic asthma, 589–590
Intrinsic factor, 816, 879, 880f
Intrinsic sympathomimetic activity, 312, 316
Investigation, new drug, 51
Investigation, new drug application, 51, 55–56
Investigational new drug
definition of, 56
process of, 56–57
**Iodoquinol**, 699t
**Ipratropium** (Atrovent), 594–595
**Irinotecan** (Camptosar), 737, 737t
Iris, 917–918
**Iron dextran** (Dexferrum), 882t, 883
Iron products, 884b
administration of, 885
adverse effects of, 881, 881t
contraindications, 881, 884
deficiency of, 880–881
definition of, 880–881
dietary sources of, 881
dosages of, 882, 882t
drug effects of, 881
in elderly patients, 885b
indications, 881
interactions, 881
mechanism of action, 881
overdose of, 881
patient teaching about, 886
profiles of, 882–883
toxicity of, 881
**Iron sucrose** (Venofer), 882t, 883
Irreversible cholinesterase inhibitors, 325–326
Irritable bowel syndrome, 829, 838–841
Ischemia, 368–369
Ischemic heart disease, 368–369
Islets of Langerhans, 511, 513
**Isoflurane**, 173
**Isoniazid** (INH), 672, 674, 676t–677t, 677–678, 874–875
**Isopropyl alcohol**, 912t
**Isosorbide dinitrate** (Isordil, Dilatrate), 371, 371t, 379–380
**Isosorbide mononitrate** (Imdur, Monoket), 371–372, 371t, 379–380
Isotonic, 474–475
Isotonic dehydration, 476t
**Isotretinoin** (Amnesteem, Claravis, Sotret), 905–906, 909
**Isradipine** (DynaCirc), 374t
**Itraconazole**, 684–685, 686t
**Ivermectin**, 701t–702t

**J**

Jejunostomy, 890f, 890t
Jelly, 904t
Jenner, Edward, 798
Jock itch, 906–907
Justice, 58b

**K**

**Kanamycin**, 676t
Kaposi's sarcoma, 654, 658–659, 661–662
Kappa receptor, 148t
Kava, 89t, 192b
Kefauver-Harris Amendment of 1962, 55t
Kefir, 630
Keratitis, 929t
Keratolytics, 904
Keratomalacia, 859
Kernicterus, 613
**Ketamine**, 173
**Ketoconazole** (Nizoral), 684–685, 907t
Ketolides, 626
Ketones, 511
**Ketorolac** (Toradol, Acular), 711t, 712, 716–718, 932
Kidneys
drug excretion by, 27–28, 28f
functions of, 460
*Klebsiella pneumoniae* carbapenemase, 634
Korsakoff's psychosis, 281, 287

**L**

**Labetalol** (Normodyne, Trandate), 315t, 318t, 319, 351–352
Lacrimal caruncle, 919
Lacrimal ducts, 917
Lacrimal glands, 917, 919
Lactated Ringer's solution, 476t
Lactic acid, 369
*Lactobacillus acidophilus* (Bacid, Lactinex), 832–833, 832t
**Lactulose** (Enulose), 836t–837t, 838
**Lamotrigine**, 224t, 227t–228t, 230, 232, 234
**Lansoprazole** (Prevacid), 823, 823t, 826
**Latanoprost** (Xalatan), 928t, 928t
Lateral canthus, 919
Laxatives
adverse effects of, 835, 835t
assessments before using, 839
bulk-forming, 834, 834t–837t, 836–837, 841
categories of, 834t
contraindications, 835
definition of, 829
dosages of, 835, 836t–837t
drug effects of, 834, 835t
emollient, 834, 834t–835t, 837
hyperosmotic, 834–835, 834t–835t, 837–839
indications, 833, 835, 835t
mechanism of action, 834
misuse of, 833
profiles of, 835–838, 836t–837t
saline, 838–839, 838b
stimulant, 834, 834t–835t, 838
Learning
aging-related changes in, 79t
barriers to, 76b
definition of, 74–75
evaluation of, 81
principles of, 79b
teaching-learning sessions, 77–78, 80
Learning needs
assessment of, 75–77
implementation and, 77–81
nursing diagnoses related to, 77
planning and, 77
**Leflunomide** (Arava), 776t, 777, 779

Left ventricular end-diastolic volume, 383
Legal nursing considerations, 57–59
Legend drugs, 51, 55t, 84, 88
Legislation, 54
    Controlled Substance Act of 1970, 55t
    Durham-Humphrey Amendment of 1951, 55t
    Federal Food, Drug, and Cosmetic Act of 1938,
        55t
    Federal Food and Drug Act of 1906, 55t
    Harrison Narcotic Act of 1914, 55t
    Kefauver-Harris Amendment of 1962, 55t
    Orphan Drug Act of 1983, 55t
    overview of, 54
    Sherley Amendment of 1912, 55t
Lens, 917
**Lepirudin** (Refludan), 423
**Leucovorin**, 732–734
Leukemias, 723–725
Leukocytes, 598t, 763, 878
Leukopenia, 740, 743
Leukotriene receptor antagonists, 591t, 596–597,
    597t, 601, 603–604
**Leuprolide** (Lupron), 566
**Levalbuterol** (Xopenex), 592t, 594
**Levamisole** (Ergamisol), 776t
**Levetiracetam**, 225t–228t, 230, 234
**Levodopa**, 240t
**Levofloxacin** (Levaquin), 638–640,
    639t–640t
**Levonorgestrel and ethinyl estradiol** (Seasonale,
    Yaz, Lybrel), 552t
**Levorphanol**, 163t
**Levothyroxine** (Synthroid, Levoxyl), 502–504,
    503t–504t, 504b
Liability, 59b
**Lidocaine** (Xylocaine)
    administration of, 414
    adverse effects of, 409
    antidysrhythmic uses of, 404b, 405t–406t
    assessments before using, 413
    dosage of, 407t–408t
    interactions, 407t
    overdose of, 406t
    parenteral uses of, 175t
    profile of, 409
    properties of, 176–177
    topical uses of, 175t
    transdermal, 157, 159
Life expectancy, 42
**Lindane** (Kwell), 910, 914
**Linezolid** (Zyvox), 641–642, 641t, 645–648
**Liothyronine**, 502–503, 503t
**Liotrix** (Thyrolar), 502–503, 503t
Lipid emulsions, 895, 895f
Lipids
    description of, 444–446
    exogenous, 443, 445
    hepatic metabolism of, 445
Lipopeptides, 643
Lipophilicity, 313, 317
Lipoproteins
    classification of, 445t
    definition of, 444–445
    functions of, 444–445
Liposomes, 97, 753
Liquid medications, 107, 107f
**Lisinopril** (Prinivil, Zestril), 354, 354t, 385
Listening, 80

**Lithium carbonate**, 259, 357t
**Lithium citrate**, 259, 357t
Liver
    functions of, 445–446
    lipid metabolism by, 445
Local anesthesia
    definition of, 170
    infiltration, 175b
    nursing process for
        assessment, 180–182
        evaluation, 185
        implementation, 183–185
        nursing diagnoses, 182
        outcome criteria, 182–183
        planning, 182–183
    types of, 175b
Local anesthetics
    adverse effects of, 176
    allergic reactions to, 176
    chemical groups of, 176b
    contraindications, 176
    description of, 174–175
    drug effects of, 175–176
    indications, 176
    interactions, 176
    mechanism of action, 175–176
    overdose of, 176
    routes of administration, 175b
    systemic effects of, 176
Long-acting beta agonist inhalers, 591
Loop diuretics
    adverse effects of, 463, 463t
    assessments before using, 468–469
    contraindications, 462–463
    description of, 349
    drug effects of, 462
    indications, 462
    mechanism of action, 462
    monitoring of, 470
    nursing process for, 468–469
    overdose of, 463
    profiles of, 464
    toxicity of, 463
Loop of Henle, 460
**Loperamide** (Imodium A-D), 832t, 840
**Loratadine** (Claritin), 578t–579t, 580
**Lorazepam**
    antianxiety uses of, 222t, 256t–257t, 258
    status epilepticus treated with, 224t
**Losartan** (Cozaar), 355t, 357
Lotions, 132, 132f, 904
**Lovastatin**, 448
Low molecular weight heparin, 422–423, 425,
    434–437
Low-density lipoprotein, 445, 448t
Lower respiratory tract, 589, 591
**Lubiprostone** (Amitiza), 839
Luteinizing hormone, 495t, 544
Lymphocytes, 598t
Lymphokine-activated killer cells,
    763, 774
Lymphokines, 763, 765–766
Lymphomas
    Burkitt's, 726
    definition of, 723–725
    types of, 725
Lysosomes, 536
Lysozyme, 917, 919

**M**

Macrolides, 623–628, 625t, 630–631, 929–930
Macrominerals, 869
Macrophages, 768
Magnesium, 859t, 871–872, 874–875
**Magnesium citrate**, 836t–837t, 838, 841
**Magnesium hydroxide** (Milk of Magnesia), 820t,
    838, 841
**Magnesium oxide** (Max-Ox 400), 871t
**Magnesium sulfate**, 557
Maintenance therapy, 31
Major depressive disorder, 255
Malabsorption syndromes, 858
Malaria, 693, 694f. See also Antimalarial drugs
*Malassezia furfur*, 906
Male reproductive system, 565
Malignant, 723–724, 724t
Malignant hyperthermia, 170, 172, 181
Malnutrition, 889
Malpractice, 51, 59b
Mania, 254–255
**Mannitol** (Osmitrol), 463t, 464–465, 927, 928t
**Maraviroc** (Selzentry), 665–666, 665t, 668
Marijuana, 285–286, 291
Mast cell stabilizers, 591t, 596, 933
mcg, 68b
MCT Oil, 892
MDMA. *See* Methylenedioxymethamphetamine
Measles, mumps, rubella vaccine, 801t–803t, 805, 810
**Mechlorethamine** (Mustargen), 752, 752t
**Meclizine** (Antivert, Bonine), 848t–849t, 849
Medial canthus, 919
Medical error, 64
Medicare Prescription Drug Improvement and
    Modernization Act, 55t
Medication administration
    rights of, 11–15, 58–59
    routes of. *See* Route of administration.
Medication administration record, 102, 103f, 106f
Medication errors
    abbreviations that cause, 68b
    computer systems for detecting, 66–67
    consequences of, 71–72
    definition of, 6, 15, 18, 33, 64
    documenting of, 68–70
    drugs commonly confused, 65, 66b
    educational system issues and, 67
    "high-alert" medications for, 65, 66b
    nursing considerations, 71–72
    nursing measures to prevent, 68–71
    organizational issues and, 66–67
    patient effects of, 65
    patient notification regarding, 71
    in pediatric patients, 69b
    prevention of, 68, 69b
    reporting of, 68–70
    responding to, 68–70
    sociologic factors associated with, 67–68
    technologies used to reduce, 66–67
Medication order, 13
Medication reconciliation, 64, 70–71
Medication use process, 18, 33
Medication use system, 65
**Medroxyprogesterone acetate** (Provera, Depo-
    Provera), 549–550, 550t, 552t
Medulla, 534
MedWatch, 70, 89

Mefloquine (Lariam), 695, 695t–697t, 697
Megadosing, 858
Megaloblastic anemia, 879
Megestrol (Megace), 549–550, 550t
Melena, 423–424
Meloxicam, 713
Memantine (Namenda), 328–329, 328t
Membrane fluidization, 287
Memory cells, 763, 797
Menadione, 863–864
Menaquinone, 863
Menarche, 544–545
Meningococcal vaccine (Menactra, Menveo), 802t–803t, 805
Menopause, 544–545
Menotropins, 554–555
Men's health drugs
    androgens. See Androgen(s)
    indications, 567, 567t
    list of, 567b
    nursing process for, 569–571
    patient teaching about, 571
Menses, 544
Menstrual cycle, 544–545, 545t, 546f
Mental illness, 255
Meperidine hydrochloride, 152t–153t, 154, 163t, 171t, 174b
Mephobarbital, 194
Meprobamate, 256t
Mercaptopurine, 731, 733t, 744–745
Meropenem (Merrem), 623
Messenger RNA, 749–750
Metabolic syndrome, 254, 447, 448b, 515
Metabolism
    drug interactions effect on, 33t
    in elderly patients, 43b, 44
    principles of, 27
Metabolite, 18
Metaproterenol, 592t
Metastasis, 723–724
Metered-dose inhalers, 130, 130f, 378–379, 602
Metformin (Glucophage, Glucophage XL), 517t, 520, 521t, 523
Methadone, 152t–153t, 154, 283, 284b
Methamphetamine, 284
Methicillin-resistant Staphylococcus aureus, 611, 615, 622, 634–635, 643
Methimazole (Tapazole), 505, 505t
Methotrexate (Trexall), 731–734, 733t, 744–746, 777
Methylcellulose (Citrucel), 836, 836t–837t, 841–842
Methyldopa, 351
Methylenedioxymethamphetamine, 285
Methylergonovine maleate (Methergine), 556–557, 557t, 559
Methylnaltrexone (Relistor), 834
Methylphenidate, 206–208, 207t, 211t
Methylprednisolone (Solu-Medrol), 23, 536, 536t–537t, 538, 539b, 540, 599–600, 599t
Methyltestosterone (Android), 565
Metoclopramide (Reglan), 848t–849t, 850, 852
Metolazone (Zaroxolyn), 466, 468
Metoprolol (Lopressor, Toprol XR), 315t, 318t, 319, 320b, 374, 374t, 390–391, 407t–408t, 410
Metronidazole (Flagyl), 641t, 642, 645, 647–648, 699t–700t, 700, 703–704
Miconazole (Micatin, Monistat-Derm), 907, 907t
Microbial infection, 610–612
Microcytic, 878–879

Microgram, 634
Microlipid, 892
Microminerals, 869
Microorganisms, 610–611
Microtubules, 684
Micturition, 281, 285
Midazolam, 171t, 174, 192–193
Midodrine (ProAmatine), 304t, 305–306, 309–310
Mifepristone (RU-486), 555–556
Miglitol (Glyset), 522
Migraine headaches
    definition of, 204–205
    description of, 205
    ibuprofen for, 210b
    serotonin receptor agonists for. See Serotonin receptor agonists
Military time, 13t
Milnacipran (Savella), 155–156
Milrinone (Primacor), 386t, 387, 391–393
Mineral(s)
    calcium, 859t, 869–871, 870t–871t, 874–875
    definition of, 856–857
    description of, 869
    magnesium, 859t, 871–872, 874–875
    patient teaching about, 876
    phosphorus, 872–873
    zinc, 873
Mineral oil (Kondremul Plain, Fleet Oil-Retention Enema), 836t–837t, 837
Mineralocorticoids, 534, 535t
Minimum inhibitory concentration, 634
Minority groups, 51
Minoxidil (Rogaine), 357–358, 910
Miosis, 324, 919
Miotics, 917, 921–923, 921t–923t
Mirtazapine, 266–267
Misoprostol (Cytotec), 556, 709, 824
Mitomycin, 758
Mitosis, 723, 749–750
Mitotane (Lysodren), 755, 757
Mitotic index, 723, 728
Mitotic inhibitors, 734–735, 735t, 740–741, 744
Mitotic spindles, 734
Mitoxantrone (Novantrone), 754, 754t, 776t
Mixed-acting sympathomimetics, 300–301, 301f
Modafinil, 206, 211t
Moderate sedation
    assessments, 182
    benzodiazepines for, 174
    definition of, 170
    drugs for, 173–174
    monitoring of, 183
    patient education about, 184b
    in pediatric patients, 174b
Moducal, 892
Moexipril (Univasc), 354t
Molds, 682
Monoamine oxidase, 300
Monoamine oxidase inhibitors
    administration of, 276
    adrenergic drugs and, 304
    adverse effects of, 262t, 264
    barbiturates and, 195
    food interactions, 264t
    interactions, 262t, 264t
    monitoring of, 274
    overdose of, 264
    Parkinson's disease treated with, 240–243

Monoclonal, 764
Monoclonal antibodies
    adverse effects of, 771, 771t
    assessments before using, 779
    contraindications, 770–771, 779
    description of, 730, 770
    dosages of, 771, 772t
    interactions, 771
    nursing considerations for, 781
    profiles of, 772–774
    types of, 766b
Monoclonal antibody antiasthmatic drugs, 605
Monocytes, 598t
Monopenems, 623–625
Montelukast (Singular), 596–597, 597t
Mood-stabilizing drugs, 259, 260t, 263t, 273, 276
Moricizine, 406t
Morphine sulfate
    description of, 151–153, 152t–153t, 163t, 171t
    in pediatric patients, 174b
Morphogenesis, 859
Moxifloxacin (Avelox), 638–639, 639t
Mu receptor, 148t
Mucous cells, 815–816
Mucus, 816, 818
Multidrug-resistant organisms, 634
Multidrug-resistant tuberculosis, 672–673
Multivitamin infusion, 889
Mupirocin (Bactroban), 905
Muronomab-CD3 (Orthoclone, OKT3), 770, 786t, 789t, 790–791
Muscarinic receptors, 324–325, 325f, 350
Muscle relaxants
    adverse effects of, 196
    baclofen, 197, 197t
    central nervous system effects of, 196
    central-acting, 196
    contraindications, 196
    cyclobenzaprine, 197, 197t
    definition of, 196
    dosages of, 196, 197t
    drug effects of, 196, 199
    indications, 196
    interactions, 196
    mechanism of action, 196
    overdose of, 196
    profile of, 197
    toxicities of, 196
Mustard gas, 809t
Mutagen, 35, 723, 726
Mutation, 723–724
Mycobacterium avium-intracellular complex infections, 624, 661, 678
Mycobacterium bovis, 673
Mycobacterium tuberculosis, 673
Mycophenolate mofetil (CellCept), 786t, 789t, 790
Mycosis, 682
Mycotic infections, 683t
Mydriasis, 299, 303, 334–336, 919, 923
Mydriatics
    cycloplegic, 933
    definition of, 917, 919–920, 921t
Myelosuppression, 723, 729
Myocardial deficiency, 384b
Myocardial infarction, 317
    definition of, 368–369
    sudden cardiac death after, 410
Myoclonic seizures, 220–221

Myometrium, 545, 555–556
Myopathy, 449

## N

Nabumetone (Relafen), 713
Nadir, 723
Nadolol (Corgard), 315t
Nafcillin, 618, 619t
Nalbuphine, 163t
Naloxone hydrochloride, 150, 152t–153t, 155, 161
Naltrexone, 150, 152t–153t, 155, 284, 288–289
Nandrolone (Deca-Durabolin), 565
Naphazoline (Privine), 582, 582t
Narcolepsy
    amphetamines for, 206–208, 285
    definition of, 204–205, 281
Narcosis, 283
Narcotics, 51, 55t, 140
Narrow therapeutic index, 226t
Nasal decongestants. See Decongestants
Nasal drops, 134, 134f
Nasal medications, 134, 134f
Nasal spray, 134, 134f
Nasoduodenal tube, 890f, 890t
Nasogastric tube, 108, 108f, 890f, 890t
Nasojejunal tube, 890f, 890t
Nasopharyngeal cancer, 726
Natalizumab (Tysabri), 771t, 773
Nateglinide (Starlix), 521
National Alliance on Mental Illness, 255
National Center for Complementary and Alternative
    Medicine, 54–55, 87–88
National Cholesterol Education Program Adult
    Treatment Panel III, 446
National Coalition for Health Professional Education
    in Genetics, 95
National Coordinating Council for Medication Error
    Reporting and Prevention, 15
National Council on Patient Information and
    Education, 82, 82b
National Vaccine Injury Compensation Program, 800
Native Americans, 52b, 53
Naturally acquired passive immunization, 798
Nausea and vomiting
    antineoplastic drugs as cause of, 742
    definition of, 844
    neurotransmitters involved in, 845t
    opioid-related, 147b
    physiology of, 845–846, 845f
Nebivolol (Bystolic), 315t, 353
Nebulizers, small-volume, 131, 131f
Needles
    illustration of, 110f–111f
    medication removal from vial using, 113f
Needlestick prevention, 110f
Negative chronotropic drugs, 384
Negative chronotropic effect, 393
Negative dromotropic effect, 388, 393
Negative feedback loop, 493–494
Negligence, 51
Neisseria gonorrhoeae, 929
Neomycin, 636t–637t, 638
Neomycin and polymyxin B, 905
Neonatal apnea, 205–206
Neonates
    definition of, 37
    pharmacokinetic changes in, 39, 39b
    physiology of, 39

Neoplasm, 723–724
Nephrolithiasis, 665
Nephron, 460, 461f
Nephrotoxicity, 634–635
Nerve block, 175b
Nesiritide (Natrecor), 386–387, 386t
Neural tube defects, 883
Neuraminidase inhibitors, 658
Neuroendocrine system, 493–494
Neuroleptic malignant syndrome, 254, 268
Neuromuscular blocking agents
    adverse effects of, 178–179
    antagonists, 177
    assessments, 180–182
    classification of, 177, 179b
    conditions that affect, 178, 178b
    contraindications, 178
    curare, 177
    depolarizing, 177, 179–180
    description of, 177
    dosages of, 179t
    drug effects of, 177–178
    d-tubocurarine, 177
    ganglionic blockade by, 178t
    hyperkalemia caused by, 178
    indications, 178
    interactions, 179, 179b, 181
    intermediate-acting, 179b
    long-acting, 179b
    mechanism of action, 177–178
    monitoring of, 183
    nondepolarizing, 177, 180
    overdose of, 178–179
    pancuronium, 179t, 180
    short-acting, 179b
    succinylcholine, 178–180, 179t
    vecuronium, 179t, 180
Neuropathic pain, 140, 143, 146
Neurotransmission, 254–255
Neurotransmitters, 254–255, 845t
Neutrophils, 598t, 767
Nevirapine (Viramune), 656t, 665t, 666
New drug application, 57
New York Heart Association functional classification
    of heart failure, 383–384
Niacin (nicotinic acid, Nicotinex), 450t, 451–452,
    452t, 456–457, 858, 859t, 866f, 873–875. See also
    Vitamin B3 (Nicotinex)
Nicardipine (Cardene), 374t
Nicoderm, 290t
Nicotinamide adenosine dinucleoside, 866
Nicotinamide adenosine dinucleoside phosphate,
    866
Nicotine
    adverse effects of, 289–290, 292
    description of, 180–181
    drug effects of, 289
    indications, 289
    mechanism of action, 289
    replacement therapies, 86b
    transdermal systems for, 86b, 289, 290t
    withdrawal from, 289–290, 290t
Nicotinic acid, 447
Nicotinic receptors, 324–325, 325f, 350f
Nicotrol, 290t
Nifedipine (Adalat, Procardia), 374t, 375, 557, 560
Nigrostriatal cells, 238
Nilutamide (Nilandron), 566, 757

Nimodipine (Nimotop), 357, 374t, 375
Nitrates/nitrites, 370–371, 371t, 376, 378–379
Nitrofurantoin (Macrodantin, Furadantin), 641t,
    642, 645, 647–648
Nitrogen, 565–566
Nitrogen mustard, 749
Nitroglycerin (Nitro-Bid, Nitrostat, Nitrol), 25,
    371t, 372, 376b, 378b, 379–380
Nitrous oxide, 173
N-methyl-D-aspartate receptor, 328
Nociception, 140, 142–143, 142f
Nociceptors, 140, 142–143
Nomogram, 37
Nonbronchodilating respiratory drugs, 596
Noncompliance
    definition of, 6
    description of, 77
Nondopamine dopamine receptor agonists, 244
Non–English-speaking patients, 78–80
Nonessential amino acids, 889, 894
Nonmaleficence, 58b
Nonnucleoside reverse transcriptase inhibitors,
    662–663, 665t
Nonopioid analgesics
    adverse effects of, 156
    contraindications, 156
    definition of, 140, 143
    indications, 156
    interactions, 156
    mechanism of action, 156
    overdose of, 156
Non–rapid eye movement sleep, 189, 189t
Nonsedating antihistamines, 576, 580, 584
Nonspecific immune responses, 652–653
Nonsteroidal antiinflammatory drugs
    acetic acid derivatives, 712
    administration of, 717–718
    adverse effects of, 709–710, 709t
    angiotensin-converting enzyme inhibitors and,
        355, 357t
    antiinflammatory uses of, 931
    chemical categories of, 708b
    contraindications, 709
    definition of, 140, 706
    dosages of, 711, 711t
    drug effects of, 708
    in elderly patients, 717b
    enolic acid derivatives, 713
    FDA warnings for, 710b
    indications, 708–709, 708b, 709t
    interactions, 710–711, 711t
    mechanism of action, 708
    nursing process for, 715–718
    ophthalmic, 932
    overdose of, 710
    overview of, 707–711
    patient teaching about, 718–719
    profiles of, 712–713
    propionic acid derivatives, 712–713
    therapeutic responses to, 718
    toxicity of, 86, 710
Nonsustained ventricular tachycardia, 401t–402t
Norelgestromin and ethinyl estradiol, 552t
Norepinephrine (Levophed), 303, 304t, 306, 534
Norethindrone and ethinyl estradiol (Ortho-
    Novum, Necon, Jenest, Loestrin, Modicon,
    Estrostep, Tri-Norinyl), 552t
Norfloxacin (Noroxin), 638–639, 639t

Normal saline, 476t, 477
North American Nursing Diagnosis Association, 9
Nosocomial infection, 611
Nucleic acids, 95–96, 544, 546–547, 651–652, 723, 726
Nucleoside, 96, 651
Nucleoside reverse transcriptase inhibitors, 662–663
Nucleotide, 96, 651
Nursing diagnoses
    description of, 9–10
    for elderly patients, 46
    formulation of, 9–10
    learning needs, 77
    NANDA, 9, 10b
    for pediatric patients, 46
Nursing process
    acid-controlling drugs, 824–826
    adrenal drugs, 539–541
    adrenergic drugs, 306–310
    adrenergic-blocking drugs, 319–322
    alpha-adrenergic blockers, 319–322
    analgesics, 157–166
    anemia, 884–886
    anesthesia, 180–185
    antianginal drugs, 377–379
    anticholinergics, 339–341
    antidiabetic drugs, 525–530
    antidiarrheal drugs, 839–841
    antidysrhythmic drugs, 413–416
    antiemetic drugs, 851–853
    antiepileptic drugs, 231–235
    antifungal drugs, 688–689
    antihistamines, 584–586
    antihypertensive drugs, 360–365
    antilipemic drugs, 454–456
    antineoplastic drugs, 739–745, 756–759
    antipsychotic drugs, 274–275
    antiretroviral drugs, 667–670
    antitubercular drugs, 678–680
    anxiolytics, 272–273
    assessment phase of, 7–9
    beta blockers, 319–322, 361, 377, 379
    biologic response–modifying drugs, 778–781
    cancer, 739–745
    cell cycle–specific antineoplastic drugs, 739–745
    central nervous system stimulants, 213–216
    cholinergic drugs, 329–331
    cholinergic-blocking drugs, 339–341
    coagulation modifiers, 434–440
    culturally competent nursing, 61–62
    decongestants, 585–586
    definition of, 6
    dermatologic drugs, 912–914
    diabetes mellitus, 525–530
    diuretics, 468–471
    elderly patients, 44–49
    electrolytes, 484–488
    enteral nutrition, 895–897
    evaluation phase of, 15
    fluids, 484–488
    general anesthesia, 180–185
    heart failure, 390–393
    herbal medicine, 84, 89–92
    immunizing drugs, 809–811
    immunosuppressant drugs, 790–793
    implementation phase of, 11–15
    local anesthesia, 180–185
    loop diuretics, 468–469

Nursing process (Continued)
    men's health drugs, 569–571
    nonsteroidal antiinflammatory drugs, 715–718
    nursing diagnoses, 9–10
    nutritional supplements, 895–897
    ophthalmic drugs, 934–935
    otic drugs, 940–941
    over-the-counter drugs, 89–92
    overview of, 8b
    pain, 157–166
    parenteral nutrition, 895–897
    Parkinson's disease, 246–250
    pediatric patients, 44–49
    pituitary drugs, 498–499
    planning phase of, 10–11
    psychotherapeutic drugs, 271–278
    respiratory drugs, 600–603
    sedative–hypnotics, 197–200
    substance abuse, 290–294
    thyroid gland, 506–508
    tuberculosis, 678–680
    vitamins, 873–875
    women's health drugs, 558–561
Nutrients, 889
Nutritional supplements
    definition of, 889
    enteral nutrition. See Enteral nutrition
    nursing process for, 895–897
    parenteral nutrition. See Parenteral nutrition
    patient teaching about, 897–898
    therapeutic responses to, 897
Nutritional support, 889
Nystatin (Nilstat, Mycostatin, Nystex), 684–685, 685t–687t, 688, 907t

O

Obesity, 205
Objective data, 7
Octreotide (Sandostatin), 495–498, 496t–497t, 755
Ocular infections, 929t
Off-label prescribing, 20
Oil, 904t
Ointments, 132, 133f, 904t
Oligonucleotide, 96
Olopatadine (Patanol), 933, 934t
Omalizumab, 605
Omega-3 fatty acids, 446b
Omeprazole (Prilosec), 823, 823t, 826
Oncogenic, 723, 726
Oncologic emergency, 759b
Ondansetron (Zofran), 848t–849t, 850, 853
On-off phenomenon, 237
Onset of action, 18, 29–30
Open-angle glaucoma, 460–461, 917, 920, 921t
Ophthalmic drugs
    aminoglycosides, 929
    anesthetics, 174, 908, 932–933, 935
    antiallergic, 933, 934t
    antifungal, 931
    antihistamines, 933
    antiinflammatory, 931–932
    antimicrobial drugs, 928–932
    beta blockers, 925–926, 925t
    carbonic anhydrase inhibitors, 926–927
    decongestants, 933
    description of, 299, 302–303, 309
    dye, 933
    lubricants, 933

Ophthalmic drugs (Continued)
    macrolide antibiotics, 929–930
    mast cell stabilizers, 933
    miotics, 921–923, 921t–923t
    moisturizers, 933
    nonsteroidal antiinflammatory drugs, 932
    nursing process for, 934–935
    osmotic diuretics, 927, 927f, 927t
    prostaglandin agonists, 927–929, 928t
    sympathomimetics. See Sympathomimetics
Opioid abstinence syndrome, 150
Opioid analgesics
    abuse of, 283–284, 291
    administration of, 163t
    adverse effects of, 147b, 149–151, 283–284
    agonist–antagonist, 160
    antagonists, 152t–153t, 155, 160, 163–164
    antitussives, 583
    assessments, 159–160
    central nervous system depression caused by, 150
    chemical classification of, 148t
    chemical structure of, 147
    codeine sulfate, 152t–153t, 153, 163t
    contraindications, 149, 283
    definition of, 140, 147, 281, 283
    diarrhea treated with, 830–832, 834
    dosage of, 149b, 151, 152t–153t
    drug effects of, 147–148, 283
    in elderly patients, 162b
    gastrointestinal tract effects, 150
    heroin, 283
    histamine release caused by, 150
    indications, 148–149, 283
    interactions, 151
    laboratory tests, 151b
    mechanism of action, 147–148, 283
    meperidine hydrochloride, 152t–153t, 154, 163t
    methadone, 152t–153t, 154, 283, 284b
    morphine sulfate, 151–153, 152t–153t, 163t
    overdose of, 150–151, 283–284
    oxycodone, 152t–153t, 163t, 283
    oxymorphone, 163t
    in pediatric patients, 158b
    physical dependence on, 150
    poisoning, 35t
    reversal of, 150t
    subacute overdose, 147b
    toxicity of, 150–151, 283–284
    transdermal administration of, 148b, 163
    withdrawal from, 140, 151, 283–284, 283b–284b
Opioid naïve, 140, 150
Opioid receptors, 148–150, 148t, 283
Opioid tolerance, 140, 144–145, 150
Opioid tolerant, 140, 145
Opportunistic infections, 624, 651, 661, 662b
Oprelvekin (Neumega), 766–768, 767t, 780
Optic nerve, 917, 920
Oral administration
    aspiration prevention, 104
    buccal medications, 104, 105f
    crushing of tablets, 104, 105f
    heparin, 437b
    in infants, 107, 107f
    liquid medications, 107, 107f
    nursing considerations for, 24t–25t
    oral medications, 104, 105f
    orally disintegrating medications, 104–105
    PO medications, 104

Oral administration (Continued)
    standard precautions for, 103b
    sublingual medications, 104, 105f
Oral contraceptives, 550–551, 551t–552t, 560, 562
Oral medications, 104, 105f
Orally disintegrating medications, 104–105
Organophosphates, 35t
Orlistat, 208–209, 211t
Orphan Drug Act of 1983, 55t
Orphan drugs, 51, 55t
Orthomolecular medicine, 858
Orthostatic hypotension, 313, 348, 352, 362
Oseltamivir (Tamiflu), 655t–656t, 658
Osmotic demyelination syndrome, 477
Osmotic diuretics, 464–465, 927, 927f, 927t
Osmotic pressure, 474
Osteoarthritis, 776–777
Osteoclasts, 552
Osteoporosis
    bisphosphonates for, 552–553, 559–560, 562
    definition of, 544, 551
    drug therapy for, 551–554, 559
    prevalence of, 551
    selective estrogen receptor modulators for,
        551–553, 559, 561
OTC Drug Review, 85
Otic drugs
    antibacterial, 939t
    antifungal, 939t
    classes of, 938
    earwax emulsifiers, 939–940
    nursing process for, 940–941
    patient teaching about, 941
Otitis externa, 937–939
Otitis media, 937–938
Ototoxicity, 634–635
Outcome criteria, 11
    definition of, 6, 11
    for elderly patients, 47
    herbal products, 91–92
    over-the-counter drugs, 91–92
    for pediatric patients, 47
Ova, 544
Ovarian follicles, 544
Ovaries, 544
Overactive bladder, 340b
Over-the-counter drugs
    abuse of, 86–87, 293b
    adolescent use of, 293b
    annual use of, 85–87
    assessments, 89–90
    cough and cold products, 576
    definition of, 51, 84
    elderly patient use of, 42
    hazards associated with, 86
    label for, 86f
    nursing process for, 89–92
    patient education regarding, 85
    prescription drugs vs., 85
    reclassification as, 85, 86b
    types of, 87t
Overton-Meyer theory, 170–171
Ovulation, 544
Oxandrolone (Oxandrin), 565
Oxcarbazepine, 227t–228t, 229, 234
Oxybutynin (Ditropan, Ditropan XL, Oxytrol), 338t,
    339, 341
Oxycodone, 152t–153t, 163t, 283

OxyContin, 148
Oxymetholone (Anadrol-50), 565
Oxymorphone, 163t
Oxytocics, 555–556
Oxytocin (Pitocin, Syntocinon), 495t, 555, 557, 557t,
    559–561

**P**

Packed red blood cells, 479t, 480
Paclitaxel (Taxol, Onxol), 734, 735t–736t
Pain
    acute, 142, 143t
    breakthrough, 140, 146
    cancer, 140, 143, 164–166, 165t
    central, 140, 143
    chronic, 140, 142, 143t, 145b–146b
    cultural considerations, 141b
    deep, 143
    definition of, 140
    gate theory of, 140, 143, 144f
    herbal therapies for, 161b
    neuropathic, 140, 143, 146
    nursing process for
        assessment, 157–160
        description of, 157
        implementation, 160–166
        planning, 160
    overview of, 141–144
    phantom, 140, 143
    physiology of, 141–144
    referred, 140, 143
    somatic, 143
    in special situations, 144–146, 165–166
    superficial, 143
    vascular, 141, 143
    visceral, 143
Pain fibers, 143, 144t
Pain perception, 142
Pain threshold, 140, 142, 143t
Pain tolerance, 142
    conditions that affect, 143t
    definition of, 140, 142
Palliative therapy, 31
Palmar-plantar dysesthesia, 732
Palpebral fissure, 918
Pancreas
    anatomy of, 511–512, 514f
    hormones produced by, 511
Pancuronium, 179t, 180
Pantoprazole (Protonix), 823, 823t, 826
Papules, 902, 904
Para-aminobenzoic acid, 176, 614–615
Para-aminosalicylic acid, 676t
Paraneoplastic syndromes, 723, 725, 725t
Parasite, 693
Parasitic protozoans, 693
Parasympathetic nervous system
    anatomy of, 325f
    description of, 325, 335, 594
Parasympatholytics, 334–335
Parasympathomimetics, 324–326. See also
    Cholinergic drugs
Parent drug, 18
Parenteral administration
    absorption effects, 23
    ampules
        illustration of, 111f
        medication removal from, 112, 112f

Parenteral administration (Continued)
    description of, 21t
    needles for, 110f–111f
    vials, 112–113, 113f
Parenteral anesthetics, 170, 170t, 174, 175t
Parenteral nutrition
    assessments before, 895
    definition of, 889–890, 892
    monitoring of, 897
    nursing process for, 895–897
    patient teaching about, 897–898
    total. See Total parenteral nutrition
Parietal cells, 815–817, 817f
Parkinson's disease
    cause of, 238
    definition of, 238
    dyskinesia associated with, 239
    epidemiology of, 238–239
    history of, 238
    nursing process for, 246–250
    pathophysiology of, 238–239
    patient teaching about, 250–251
    symptoms of, 239, 239t
    treatment of, 239–240
Parkinson's disease-associated dementia, 239
Paromomycin, 699t
Paroxysm, 693
Paroxysmal supraventricular tachycardia, 401t–402t,
    403
Partial agonists, 140, 147–148
Partial thromboplastin time, 440b
Passive immunization
    artificially acquired, 798
    characteristics of, 797–799, 797t
    definition of, 796
    naturally acquired, 798
Passive immunizing drugs. See also Immunizing
    drugs.
    assessments before using, 809
    definition of, 796
    description of, 798–800, 799b
    dosages of, 802t–803t
    profiles of, 806–807
Paste, 904t
Pathologic fungi, 682–683
Patient(s)
    checking of, 14
    interview of, 7–8
    medication errors, 71
Patient teaching
    acid-controlling drugs, 826–827
    alpha-adrenergic blockers, 322, 360
    anorexiants, 216
    antianginal drugs, 379–380
    antibiotics, 631, 648
    anticoagulants, 440–441
    antidiarrheal drugs, 840–842
    antiemetic drugs, 854
    antiepileptic drugs, 235
    antihypertensive drugs, 365–366
    antilipemic drugs, 457
    antimalarial drugs, 704
    antineoplastic drugs, 745–746, 760
    antiretroviral drugs, 670
    antitubercular drugs, 680–681
    beta blockers, 322, 366
    cholinergic drugs, 332
    cholinergic-blocking drugs, 341–342

Patient teaching (Continued)
   coagulation modifiers, 440–441
   corticosteroids, 604–605
   cultural considerations, 80b
   dermatologic drugs, 914
   diuretics, 471
   dopaminergic agents, 250–251
   effectiveness of, 75
   enteral nutrition, 897–898
   heparin, 440–441
   herbs, 92
   immunizing drugs, 811
   immunosuppressant drugs, 793
   iron products, 886
   isosorbide dinitrate, 380
   isosorbide mononitrate, 380
   men's health drugs, 571
   minerals, 876
   moderate sedation, 184b
   nitroglycerin, 379–380
   nonsteroidal antiinflammatory drugs, 718–719
   nutritional supplements, 897–898
   otic drugs, 941
   over-the-counter drugs, 85
   parenteral nutrition, 897–898
   Parkinson's disease, 250–251
   psychotherapeutic agents, 278–279
   respiratory drugs, 604–605
   serotonin receptor agonists, 216
   substance abuse, 294
   testosterone, 571
   vitamins, 876
   women's health drugs, 562
Patient-controlled analgesia, 124, 125f, 144
Peak effect, 18, 29
Peak level, 18, 30
Pediatric patients
   adrenergic drugs in, 307
   age-based classification of, 39t
   aminoglycosides in, 636–637
   anesthesia in, 172b
   antidiarrheal drugs in, 833b
   antiepileptic drugs in, 223b
   antiviral drugs in, 656t
   body surface area calculations, 40f
   classification of, 39t
   definition of, 37
   dose calculations for, 39–42
   heart failure in, 391b
   injections in, 120b
   insulin use in, 517
   medication administration in, 41b
   medication errors in, 69b
   moderate sedation in, 174b
   nursing diagnoses for, 46
   nursing process for, 44–49
   opioid analgesics in, 158b
   oral medication administration in, 107
   pharmacodynamics in, 39
   pharmacokinetic changes in, 39, 39b
   psychotherapeutic agents in, 272b
   Reye's syndrome in, 714b
   syrup of Ipecac in, 845b
Pediculosis, 902, 910
Pegademase bovine (Adagen), 776t
Pegaspargase (Oncaspar), 738–739, 738t, 746
Peginterferon alfa-2a (Pegasys), 769t, 770
Peginterferon alfa-2b (PEG-Intron), 769t, 770

Peliosis of the liver, 567
Pellagra, 857, 865–866
Penbutolol (Levatol), 315t
Penciclovir (Denavir), 908
Penicillin(s)
   adverse effects of, 617–618, 618t
   aminopenicillins, 617t, 618–619
   anaphylactic reactions to, 617–618
   assessments before using, 628
   cephalosporins and, cross-reactivity between,
      617–618, 620
   chemical structure of, 616f
   classification of, 617t
   contraindications, 617
   definition of, 616
   dosages of, 618, 619t
   drug effects of, 617
   extended-spectrum, 617, 617t, 619
   indications, 617
   interactions, 618, 618t
   mechanism of action, 617
   nursing considerations for, 630
   patient teaching about, 630–631
Penicillin G, 618, 628
Penicillin V potassium, 618, 619t
Penicillinase-resistant penicillins, 617t, 618
Penicillin-binding proteins, 617
Pentamidine (NebuPent, Pentam 300), 699t–700t,
      700
Pentazocine, 163t
Pentobarbital, 171t, 195, 195t
Pentostatin, 733t, 740
Pentoxifylline, 429
Pepsin, 815
Pepsinogen, 816–817
Peptic ulcer disease, 817
Perimetrium, 545
Perindopril (Aceon), 354t
Peripheral nervous system, 299
Peripheral total parenteral nutrition, 892–893
Peripherally acting antihistamines, 580
Permissive hypothesis, 254, 261f
Pernicious anemia, 868, 878–879
Personalized medicine, 95
Pertussis, 803–804
pH, 475–476
Phantom pain, 140, 143
Pharmaceutics, 18
   definition of, 20
   description of, 21–22
   elements of, 21–22
Pharmacodynamics, 18
   definition of, 20, 30
   genetic effects on, 52
   mechanism of action, 30–31
Pharmacoeconomics, 18, 20, 35
Pharmacogenetics
   definition of, 95, 98
   description of, 98–99
Pharmacogenomics, 19, 98–99, 256
   clinical applications of, 99t
   definition of, 34, 95
Pharmacognosy, 19–20, 35
Pharmacokinetics
   in children, 39, 39b
   definition of, 19–20
   distribution, 26–27, 33t
   drug interactions effect on, 33t

Pharmacokinetics (Continued)
   excretion, 27–29
   genetic effects on, 52
   half-life, 29, 29t
   metabolism, 27, 33t
Pharmacology, 19
   definition of, 19
   sciences involved in, 19
Pharmacotherapeutics, 19
   assessment, 31
   definition of, 20, 31
   monitoring, 31–35
Phencyclidine, 293b
Phenobarbital
   anesthetic uses of, 195, 195t
   antiepileptic uses of, 222t, 226–228,
      227t–228t
   status epilepticus treated with, 224t
Phenothiazines
   chlorpromazine, 267
   description of, 267
Phenotype, 95
Phenotyping, 447
Phenoxybenzamine (Dibenzyline), 315t
Phentermine, 209
Phentolamine (Regitine), 315t
Phenylephrine (Neo-Synephrine), 303, 304t, 306
Phenytoin, 222, 222t, 227t–229t, 228–229, 404b,
      405t–406t
Phenytoin equivalents, 228–229
Pheochromocytoma, 313, 316
Phonophobia, 205
Phosphodiesterase inhibitors, 387, 391–392, 566,
      600–603, 605
Phosphorus, 859t, 861, 872–873
Physical dependence, 32
   definition of, 140, 142, 281
   to opioid analgesics, 150
Physostigmine (Antilirium), 326–327, 328t
Phytochemicals, 84, 89
Phytonadione, 863–864
Piggyback admixtures, for intravenous injections,
      122, 122f–123f, 124–126, 125f
Pilocarpine (Pilocar), 923, 923t
Pimecrolimus (Elidel), 911
Pindolol (Visken), 315t
Pioglitazone (Actos), 521t, 522–524
Pioglitazone/metformin (ACTOplus Met),
      521t
Piperacillin, 619
Piperacillin/tazobactam (Zosyn), 619
Piperazine, 701t
Pirbuterol (Maxair), 592t, 594
Piroxicam, 713
Pituitary drugs. see also specific drug
   adverse effects of, 496, 496t
   contraindications, 496
   dosages of, 496, 497t
   drug effects of, 495
   indications, 495–496
   interactions, 496, 496t
   mechanism of action, 495
   nursing process for, 498–499
   overview of, 494–496
   patient teaching about, 499
   profiles of, 496–498
Pituitary gland, 493–494, 494b
Pituitary hormones, 494b, 494f, 495t

Placebo
  administering of, 60
  definition of, 51, 56–57, 60
Placebo effect, 145
Plague, 808t
Planning phase of nursing process, 10–11
Plant-derived drugs, 35, 87t
Plaque psoriasis, 909
Plasma, 474
Plasma cells, 764–765
Plasma protein fraction, 479t
Plasmids, 97
Plasmin, 419, 421, 431
Plasminogen, 419, 421
*Plasmodium* spp., 693, 695, 697
Pledget, 904t
Pneumococcal conjugate vaccine, 801t–803t
Pneumococcal vaccine, 805
*Pneumocystis jiroveci*, 615, 661, 698
Pneumocystosis, 698–699, 698t
Poison control centers, 35
Polarization, 397
Poliovirus vaccine, 801t–803t, 805
Polycose, 892
Polydipsia, 511–512
Polyenes, 684
**Polyethylene glycol** (Colyte, GoLYTELY, Half-
  Lytely, Miralax), 770, 836t–837t, 837–838
Polyfunctional, 749–750
Polypeptide antibiotics, 930
Polyphagia, 511–512
Polypharmacy, 37, 42
Polyuria, 511–512
**Porfimer sodium**, 755–756
Porphyria, 226
Positive chronotropic effect, 299, 302
Positive dromotropic effect, 299, 302
Positive inotropic effect, 299, 302, 388
Postanesthetic respiratory depression,
  205–206
Postantibiotic effect, 634
Posterior pituitary gland, 494b, 495t
Postherpetic neuralgias, 654–655
Postural hypotension, 352
Postural instability, 238, 239t
Potassium, 480–482, 484, 485b, 489
Potassium chloride, 487
Potassium-sparing diuretics, 465–466, 465t–466t,
  469–470, 537
Potassium-wasting diuretics, 349
**Povidone-iodine** (Betadine), 911–912, 912t
Powders, 132, 904t
**Pramipexole**, 240t
**Pramlintide** (Symlin), 524, 526
**Prasugrel** (Effient), 428–429
**Praziquantel**, 701t–703t, 702
**Prazosin** (Minipress), 315t
Prediabetes, 515
**Prednisolone** (Deltasone, Sterapred, Liquid PRED),
  536t–537t, 538
**Prednisone**, 536t, 538, 540
**Prefilgrastim** (Neulasta), 766–768
**Pregabalin**, 227t–228t, 230, 234–235
Pregnancy
  antiepileptic drug contraindications, 224
  cancer during, 730
  drug therapy during, 38
  gestational diabetes during, 510, 515, 517–518

Pregnancy *(Continued)*
  insulin administration during, 517–518
  safety categories for, 39t
Prehypertension, 364
Premature ventricular contractions, 401t–402t, 403
Prescriber, 6, 8
Prescription drugs
  handling of, 216b
  over-the-counter drugs vs., 85
Presynaptic, 238, 243
Preterm labor management, 557–558
**Prilocaine**, 175t
**Primaquine**, 695, 695t–697t, 697
Primary lesion, 723–724
**Primidone**, 226–228, 227t–228t
Prinzmetal angina, 369
Privacy, 100
prn, 13
**Probenecid**, 715
Probiotics, 830, 832–833, 840, 842
**Procainamide** (Pronestyl), 404b, 405t, 406–408
**Procaine**, 175t
**Prochlorperazine** (Compazine), 848t–849t, 849–850
Prodrug, 19, 348, 354
Prodysrhythmic, 405
Progenitor cells, 766
Progesterone, 544–545, 562
Progestins, 544, 549–551, 549t–550t, 558–560, 755t
Prokinetics, 846t–847t, 847, 850, 852
Prolactin, 495t
**Promethazine** (Phenergan), 171t, 578t, 848t–849t,
  849–853
ProMod, 892
Propac, 892
**Propafenone** (Rythmol), 404b, 405t–408t,
  409–410
**Proparacaine**, 175t
Prophylactic therapy, 31, 610, 612
*Propionibacterium acnes*, 905
Propionic acid derivatives, 712–713
**Propofol**, 173–174
**Propranolol** (Inderal), 315t, 318t, 319
**Propylthiouracil**, 505–506, 505t
**Prostacyclin**, 428
Prostaglandin agonists, 927–929, 928t
Prostaglandin E$_2$, 560–561
Prostaglandin F$_2$-alpha, 928
Prostaglandins, 556, 709, 816, 845t
Prostate cancer, 564, 566, 566b
**Protamine sulfate**, 423–424, 437–438
Protease, 651, 659
Protease inhibitors, 663t, 664–665, 665t
Protein synthesis, 96–97
Proteolytic enzyme, 816
Proteome, 95, 97
Proteomics, 95, 97
Prothrombin time, 440b
Proton pump, 817
Proton pump inhibitors, 822–823, 823t, 825–826
Protozoal infections
  pathophysiology of, 698
  types of, 698t
Protozoans, 693
Proximal convoluted tubule, 460
Pruritus, 902, 907
**Pseudoephedrine**, 284
Pseudomembranous colitis, 610, 613, 634,
  641, 645

Psoriasis
  antipsoriatic drugs for, 909
  definition of, 902–903, 909
  plaque, 909
Psychoactive properties, 282, 284
Psychological dependence, 32, 140, 282
Psychomotor domain, 74–75
Psychosis, 254–256
Psychotherapeutic agents
  culture and, 276b
  in elderly patients, 272b
  nursing process for
    assessment, 271–275
    evaluation, 277–278
    implementation, 276–277
    nursing diagnoses, 275
    outcome criteria, 275
    planning, 275
  patient education regarding, 278–279
  in pediatric patients, 272b
Psychotherapeutics, 254–255
Psychotropic drugs
  definition of, 254, 256
  description of, 256
**Psyllium** (Metamucil), 451, 836t–837t, 836t–837t
Puberty, 544
Public Health Security and Bioterrorism
  Preparedness and Response Act, 807–808
Pulmonary embolism, 419, 422–423
Pulse, apical, 104, 105f
Pupil, 917, 919
Purified protein derivative, 674b, 678
Purine antagonists, 731, 734
Purkinje fiber action potential, 399f
Push medications, intravenous, 126, 127f
Pustules, 902, 904
**Pyrantel**, 701–702, 701t–703t
**Pyrazinamide** (PZA), 676t–677t, 678
**Pyridostigmine** (Mestinon), 328t, 329
Pyridoxine, 859t, 867, 867t, 873–875
**Pyrimethamine** (Daraprim), 695, 695t, 697–698
Pyrimidine antagonists, 731, 734

**Q**

Q.D., 68b
Q.O.D., 68b
QRS complex, 400–401
QT interval, 400–401
QTc interval, 409b
**Quinapril** (Accupril), 354t
**Quinidine**, 404b, 405t–408t, 408, 414
**Quinine**, 695, 695t
Quinolones, 638–640, 639b, 639t–640t, 644–646,
  648, 930–931, 930t
**Quinupristin/dalfopristin** (Synercid), 641t,
  642–643, 647

**R**

**Rabies immunoglobulin** (BayRab, Imogam
  Rabies-HT), 807
**Rabies virus vaccine** (Imovax, RabAvert), 802t–803t,
  805–806
Race, 51
Radiation, 726
Radiopharmaceuticals, 755–756
**Raloxifene** (Evista), 552–554, 553t
**Raltegravir** (Isentress), 665t, 666, 668
**Ramelteon** (Rozerem), 192t, 193, 198

**Ramipril** (Altace), 354t
**Ranitidine** (Zantac), 821–822, 821t, 826
**Ranolazine** (Ranexa), 376–377
Rapid eye movement sleep, 189, 189t
**Rasagiline** (Azilect), 240t, 241
**Rasburicase**, 731
Raves, 282, 285
Raynaud's disease, 313, 357
Rebound hypertension, 352
Receptor(s)
    acetylcholine, 817
    beta1, 373
    beta-adrenergic. *See* Beta-adrenergic receptors
    cholinergic, 324–325, 350
    definition of, 19, 30
    delta, 148t
    dopaminergic, 299–300
    endothelin, 359
    gastrin, 817
    histamine, 576, 578, 817
    interactions, 30
    muscarinic receptors, 324–325, 325f, 350
    nicotinic, 324–325, 325f, 350f
    opioid, 148–150, 148t, 283
Recombinant, 796, 799
Recombinant DNA, 35, 95, 97–98
Recommended daily allowances, 857
Rectal administration, 24t–25t, 109, 109f
Rectal suppositories, 109, 109f
Red blood cells, 878
Red man syndrome, 643
Referred pain, 140, 143
Reflex stimulation, 576, 583
Reflex tachycardia, 369, 371
Refractory period, 383
Regional anesthesia, 185
Relapse, 282
Relative refractory period, 397, 399–400, 400f
REM interference, 189
REM rebound, 189
Remodeling, 465
Renin, 351, 373
Renin-angiotensin-aldosterone system, 384
**Repaglinide** (Prandin), 521, 521t, 524
Replication, 651–652, 652f
Respiratory depression
    analeptic-responsive syndromes, 205–206
    opioid-related, 147b, 150
    postanesthetic, 205–206
Respiratory diseases
    asthma. *See* Asthma
    chronic bronchitis, 589–591
    chronic obstructive pulmonary disease, 589
    emphysema, 589, 591
    pathophysiology of, 589–591
Respiratory drugs
    anticholinergics, 591t, 594
    beta agonists. *See* Beta agonists
    beta-adrenergic agonists, 591–594, 591t
    bronchodilators, 591
    leukotriene receptor antagonists, 591t, 596–597,
        597t, 601, 603–604
    mast cell stabilizers, 591t, 596
    nonbronchodilating, 596
    nursing process for, 600–603
    patient teaching about, 604–605
    phosphodiesterase-4 inhibitors, 600–601, 603, 605
    xanthine derivatives, 595–596, 595t, 601–604, 601b

Respiratory system, 576, 589
Resting membrane potential, 397–400, 399f
Restless legs syndrome, 244
Reticulocytes, 878
Reticuloendothelial system, 796
Retina, 917, 920
**Retinoic acid**, 905
Retrograde transmission, 10024#p0140
Retroviruses, 651, 653, 659
Reverse transcriptase, 651, 659
Reverse transcriptase inhibitors, 662
Reversible cholinesterase inhibitors, 325–326
Reye's syndrome, 654–655, 714b
Rhabdomyolysis, 449, 666
Rheumatism, 764, 776–777
Rheumatoid arthritis
    disease-modifying antirheumatic drugs for, 763,
        777–779, 777b, 781–782
    overview of, 776–777, 776f
Rhinovirus, 576
**Rh$_O$(D) immunoglobulin** (RhoGAM,
    MICRhoGAM), 802t–803t, 807
Rhodopsin, 857, 859
**Ribavirin** (Virazole), 655t–656t, 658, 667
Riboflavin, 859t, 865–866, 874–875
Ribonucleic acid, 95–96, 651, 654
Ribosomal RNA, 96–97
Ricin, 809t
Rickets, 857
**Rifabutin** (Mycobutin), 676t–677t, 678
**Rifamate**, 678
**Rifampin** (Rifadin, Rimactane), 357t, 595, 674,
    676t–677t, 678, 680
**Rifapentine** (Priftin), 676t–677t, 678
Rifater, 677
Rigidity, 238, 239t
**Rimantadine**, 655t–656t, 656–658
**Risperidone**, 269t, 271, 277
**Rituximab** (Rituxan), 771t–772t, 773–774
**Rivastigmine** (Exelon), 327
Robotripping, 86–87
Rods, 917, 920, 920f
**Roflumilast** (Daliresp), 600
Roofies, 282, 286
**Ropinirole**, 240t–242t, 244, 247
Rotavirus vaccine, 801t
Route of administration
    buccal, 23
    checking of, 13–14
    computer-controlled dispensing system,
        102, 102f
    enteral, 21t
        absorption affected by, 22–23
        description of, 21t
    gastrostomy tube for, 108, 108f
    inhalation
        absorption effects, 25–26
        environment considerations, 603b
        metered-dose inhalers, 130, 130f, 378–379,
            602
        metered-dose inhalers for, 130, 130f
        nursing considerations for, 24t–25t
        small-volume nebulizers, 131, 131f
    local anesthetics, 175b
    nasogastric tube, 108, 108f
    preparations for, 102–103, 102f
    rectal, 109, 109f
    standard precautions, 103b

Route of administration *(Continued)*
    sublingual, 23
        absorption effects of, 23, 24t–25t, 25
        nursing considerations for, 24t–25t
        procedure for, 104, 105f
    transdermal
        absorption effects, 25
        contraceptives, 552t
        estrogen, 548t
        fentanyl, 148b, 152t–153t, 163
        nitroglycerin, 378–379
        nursing considerations for, 24t–25t
        opioid analgesics, 148b, 163
        procedure for, 132, 133f
        testosterone, 568t
    vaginal, 135, 135f–136f
Rubella vaccine, 801t

**S**

**Salagen**, 243b
Salicylates
    profiles of, 712
    toxicity caused by, 710
Salicylism, 706, 710
Saline laxatives, 838–839, 838b
**Salmeterol** (Serevent, Advair), 309, 592t, 594
Sarcomas
    definition of, 723–724
    types of, 725t
*Sarcoptes scabiei*, 910
**Sargramostim** (Leukine), 767–768, 767t
Sarin, 809t
Saw palmetto, 89t, 570b
**Saxagliptin/metformin** (Kombiglyze), 521t
Scabicides, 910
Scabies, 902, 910
Schizophrenia, 255–256, 268
Sclera, 918–919
**Scopolamine** (Transderm-Scop patch, Scopace),
    171t, 246, 338t, 339, 341, 341b, 848t–849t, 851, 853
Scurvy, 857, 869
Sebaceous glands, 903t
Seborrhea, 909
Secobarbital, 171t
Secondary hypertension, 348–349
Second-generation antidepressants,
    263t, 265–267
Sedative–hypnotics
    definition of, 189
    nursing process for, 197–200
    properties of, 192t
Seizures
    atonic, 220–221
    definition of, 220
    febrile, 220
    generalized, 223t
    generalized onset, 220–221
    International League Against Epilepsy
        classification of, 220, 221b
    myoclonic, 220–221
    partial, 223t
    partial onset, 220
    tonic-clonic, 220–221
    unclassified, 220–221
Selective aldosterone blockers, 359
Selective estrogen receptor modulators, 551–553,
    559, 561, 755t
Selective serotonin receptor agonists, 209–210, 215

Selective serotonin reuptake inhibitors
 advantages of, 265
 adverse effects of, 265
 contraindications, 265
 drug effects of, 265
 fluoxetine, 266
 indications, 265
 interactions, 262t–263t
 mechanism of action, 265
**Selegiline**, 240–241, 240t–242t, 243b
 transdermal patch, 264–265
Semicircular canals, 937–938
Semiessential amino acids, 889
Seminiferous tubules, 565
**Senna** (Senokot), 836t–837t, 838
Sequential nephron blockade, 463
Serotonin, 204, 845t
Serotonin blockers, 846t–847t, 847, 850
Serotonin receptor agonists
 adverse effects of, 210
 considerations for, 214
 contraindications, 210
 definition of, 204
 drug effects of, 209
 indications, 209–210
 mechanism of action, 209
 patient teaching about, 216
 profile of, 211–212
 selective, 209–210, 215
 therapeutic responses to, 215–216
 types of, 209
Serotonin syndrome, 254, 265, 265b, 642
Serotonin-norepinephrine reuptake inhibitors, 265
Serum, 474
Severe acute respiratory syndrome, 667
**Sevoflurane**, 173
Shampoo, 904t
Sherley Amendment of 1912, 55t
Shingles, 655
Short bowel syndrome, 22–23
Short-acting beta agonist inhalers, 591
**Sibutramine**, 211–212
Sideroblastic anemia, 867
**Sildenafil** (Viagra, Revatio), 359–360, 566–569, 567b, 568t, 572
**Silodosin** (Rapaflo), 566
**Silver sulfadiazine** (Silvadene), 905
**Simethicone** (Mylicon), 824–826
**Simvastatin** (Zocor), 450, 450t, 455
Sinoatrial node, 399
**Sirolimus** (Rapamune), 786t, 789t, 790, 792
**Sitagliptin** (Januvia), 521t, 524
**Sitagliptin/metformin** (Janumet), 521t
Sjögren's syndrome, 326
Skin
 anatomy of, 902, 903f
 blood supply to, 902
 exocrine glands of, 903t
Skin preparation drugs, 132, 133f, 911–912, 912t
Sleep
 definition of, 189
 non–rapid eye movement, 189, 189t
 physiology of, 189–190
 rapid eye movement, 189, 189t
 stages of, 189t
Sleep architecture, 189
Sliding-scale insulin regimen, 519–520, 528

Slow acetylation, 610, 614
Slow acetylator, 672, 677
Slow channels, 398–399
Slow-acting antirheumatic drugs, 777
Small intestine, 22–23
Smallpox, 798, 808t
Small-volume nebulizers, 131, 131f
Smoking cessation, 289
Sodium, 482–485, 487
Sodium channels, 398–399
Sodium chloride, 477–478, 483
**Sodium hypochlorite** (Dakin's bleach solution), 912t
**Sodium nitroprusside** (Nipride, Nitropress), 358–359, 358t, 363, 363b
**Sodium polystyrene sulfonate** (Kayexalate), 481–482, 486–487
Sodium-potassium adenosine triphosphatase pump, 397
Solution, 904t
Somatic pain, 140, 143
**Somatostatin**, 495
**Somatrem**, 495–496
**Somatropin** (Humatrope), 495–497, 496t–497t
**Sotalol** (Betapace), 315t, 318t, 319, 404b, 405t, 407t–408t, 412
Soy, 547b
Special pain situations, 140, 144–146, 165–166
Spherocytes, 878–879
Sphincter pupillae, 917, 919
Spinal anesthesia, 175b
 assessments, 182
 definition of, 170, 174–175
 monitoring of, 183–184
Spinal headaches, 184, 184b
**Spironolactone** (Aldactone), 385, 465–466, 466t
Squamous cell carcinoma, 911
St. John's wort, 89t, 262, 264b
ST segment, 400–401
Standard precautions, 103b
Standard time, 13t
Statins, 375t, 444, 448, 456b. See also HMG-CoA reductase inhibitors
Status asthmaticus, 589
Status epilepticus, 220–221, 223, 224t
Steady state, 19, 29
*Stenotrophomonas maltophilia*, 615
Steroid psychosis, 538
Sterols, 682, 684
Steven Johnsons syndrome, 468–469
Stick, 904t
Stigma, 254–255
Stimulant(s)
 abuse of, 284–285, 291
 adverse effects of, 285
 amphetamines
  attention-deficit/hyperactivity disorder treated with, 206–208
  definition of, 203
  interactions, 207t
  narcolepsy treated with, 206–208
  treatment uses of, 206, 207t
 contraindications, 285
 drug effects of, 285
 indications, 285
 mechanism of action, 285
 withdrawal from, 285, 285b

Stimulant laxatives, 834, 834t–835t, 838
Stomach, 816, 816f
Stomatitis, 742
Storytelling, 364b
Stratum corneum, 903t, 906
Stratum germinativum, 903t
Stratum granulosum, 903t
Stratum lucidum, 903t
*Streptococcus pyogenes*, 624
**Streptokinase**, 431
**Streptomycin**, 636–637, 636t, 676t–677t, 678
Stress ulcers, 818
Stroke, 419, 422, 455
Subcutaneous administration
 absorption effects, 23
 heparin, 437b
 injections
  insulin administration, 116, 117f
  needle insertion angle for, 114
  procedure for, 116, 116f–117f
Subjective data, 7
Sublingual administration, 23
 absorption effects of, 24t–25t, 25
 nursing considerations for, 24t–25t
 procedure for, 104, 105f
Substance abuse
 alcohol. See Alcohol
 assessment of, 290–292
 definition of, 282
 in elderly patients, 293b
 family effects of, 294
 nicotine. See Nicotine
 nursing process for, 290–294
 opioid analgesics, 283–284. See also Opioid analgesics
 organizations and agencies concerned with, 294b
 patient teaching about, 294
 stimulants, 284–285
 substances commonly abused, 282b
 treatment of, 294
Substance P, 155–156
Substantia nigra, 238
Substrates, 19, 27, 27t
Subtherapeutic, 610, 612–613
Succinimides, 225t–226t, 229
**Succinylcholine**, 178–180, 179t
**Sucralfate** (Carafate), 823–827
Sudden cardiac death, 397, 410
**Sufentanil**, 171t
"Sulfa allergy", 615
**Sulfacetamide** (Bleph-10), 931
**Sulfamethoxazole/trimethoprim** (Bactrim, Septra), 615–616, 616t, 695
Sulfites, 615
Sulfonamides, 614–616, 615t, 628, 630, 931
Sulfonylureas, 317–318, 521, 526
**Sumatriptan**, 211–212, 211t
Sunscreens, 910–912
Superficial pain, 140, 143
Superinfections, 610, 613, 644
Supplemental therapy, 31
Supportive therapy, 31
Suppositories
 rectal, 109, 109f
 vaginal, 135, 135f–136f
Surface epithelial cells, 816

Sustained ventricular tachycardia, 401t–402t
Sympathetic nervous system, 299–300, 299f, 325f
Sympatholytics, 313
Sympathomimetics
    adverse effects of, 924
    bronchodilators, 591
    contraindications, 924
    definition of, 204, 299, 576, 581
    description of, 204
    direct-acting, 300–301, 301f
    drug effects of, 923
    indications, 924
    indirect-acting, 300–301, 301f
    interactions, 581, 924
    mechanism of action, 923
    mixed-acting, 300–301, 301f
    ophthalmic applications of, 923–925
    profiles of, 924–925
Synaptic cleft, 299
Syndrome X, 515
Synergistic effects, 19, 33, 141, 146, 634, 636
Syringes
    illustration of, 111f
    insulin, 116, 117f
Syrup of Ipecac, 845b
Systemic vascular resistance, 348, 354

**T**

T3. *See* Triiodothyronine
T4. *See* Thyroxine
T helper cells, 661, 764–766
T lymphocytes, 764–765, 785
T suppressor cells, 764–766
Tablets
    crushing of, 104, 105f
    enteric-coated, 105f
Tacrolimus (Prograf), 786t, 789t, 790–793
Tadalafil (Cialis), 359–360, 566–568
Taeniasis, 701t
Tamsulosin (Flomax), 315t, 316, 566
Tape, 904t
Tar-containing products, 909
Tardive dyskinesia, 254, 268
Taxanes, 736t, 746
Tazarotene, 909
Teaching
    definition of, 74–75
    principles of, 79b
Teaching-learning sessions, 77–78, 80
Tears, 917, 919
Tegaserod (Zelnorm), 839, 841
Tegretol, 320b
Telavancin (Vibativ), 641t, 644, 647
Temazepam, 192t, 193
Tenecteplase (TNKase), 432
Teniposide, 735t, 746
Tenofovir (Viread), 665t, 666
Teratogen, 35, 610, 614, 905–906
Teratogenic effects, 35
Terazosin (Hytrin), 315t, 566
Terbinafine (Lamisil), 684, 685t–687t, 688–689, 907t
Terbutaline (Brethine), 557, 559, 592t, 594
Teriparatide, 552–553
Terrorism, 807–810, 808t–809t
Testes, 565
**Testosterone**
    administration of, 570
    assessments before using, 569

Testosterone (*Continued*)
    deficiency of, 565
    definition of, 564–565
    patient teaching about, 571
**Testosterone, transdermal** (Testoderm, Androderm, AndroGel), 568t, 569
**Testosterone cypionate** (Depo-Testosterone), 568t
**Tetanus and diphtheria toxoids** (Decavac), 802t–803t, 808b, 809
**Tetanus immunoglobulin** (BayTet), 802t–803t, 807
Tetanus toxoid-containing vaccines, 801t
**Tetracaine**, 175t, 933
Tetracyclines, 39, 626–631, 626b
**Tetrahydrocannabinol** (Marinol), 286, 846t–849t, 847, 850–852
**Tetrahydrofolate**, 695
**Tetrahydrozoline** (Murine Plus), 933, 934t
**Thalidomide** (Thalomid), 776t
The Joint Commission, 14, 57, 75
    coagulation modifiers and, 421
    medication error prevention efforts by, 66
    medication reconciliation, 71
**Theophylline** (Elixophyllin, Theo-Dur, Uniphyl), 596, 595t
Therapeutic, 610
Therapeutic drug monitoring, 19, 30, 634–635
Therapeutic effect, 19, 30
Therapeutic equivalence, 19–20
Therapeutic index, 19
    of barbiturates, 193
    definition of, 32, 189
    low, 337
    narrow, 226t
Therapy
    acute, 31
    empiric, 31
    maintenance, 31
    palliative, 31
    prophylactic, 31
    supplemental, 31
    supportive, 31
**Thiabendazole**, 702t
Thiamine, 859t, 865, 873, 875
Thiazide diuretics, 466–468, 467t–468t
Thiazolidinediones, 522, 526
**Thimerosal**, 928
**Thioguanine**, 733t
Thionamide derivatives, 504–505
Threshold potential, 397, 400
Thrombin, 422–423
Thrombocytopenia, 740, 743
Thromboembolic events, 419, 422
Thrombolytic drugs
    advantages of, 431–432
    assessments before using, 436
    contraindications, 431
    definition of, 419, 430
    dosage of, 432, 432t
    drug effects of, 431
    function of, 421, 422t
    indications, 431
    interactions, 432
    mechanism of action, 431
    nursing considerations for, 439
    overdose of, 431–432
    profile of, 432, 432t
    toxicity of, 431–432
Thromboplastin, 420–421

Thromboprevention, 429
Thrombosis, 422–423
Thromboxane A$_2$, 427–428
Thrombus, 419–420
Thyroid gland
    anatomy of, 502
    nursing process for, 506–508
Thyroid replacement drugs, 502–504, 503t, 506, 506b, 508
Thyroid storm, 506
Thyroid-stimulating hormone, 495t, 501–502
Thyroxine, 501–502
**Tiagabine**, 227t–228t, 230, 235
**Ticarcillin** (Timentin), 619
**Tigecycline** (Tygacil), 627, 627t
Time, 13t
Time-dependent killing, 634
Timing of administration, 13–14
**Timolol** (Blocadren, Betimol, Timoptic, Timoptic-XE), 315t, 925t, 926
Tinea, 902, 906
Tinea versicolor, 683t
**Tiotropium** (Spiriva), 594
**Tissue plasminogen activator**, 419–420, 431
**Tobramycin**, 635, 635t–637t, 638
**Tocilizumab** (Actemra), 775, 775t
Tocolytics, 557, 560–561
Tocopherols, 857
**Tolcapone**, 240t, 243–244
Tolerance, 19, 32, 141–142
**Tolnaftate** (Tinactin), 907t
**Tolterodine** (Detrol, Detrol XL), 338t, 339, 341
**Tolvaptan** (Samsca), 483
Tonic-clonic seizure, 220–221
Topical administration
    absorption effects, 25–26
    anesthetics, 174, 908, 932–933
    antifungal drugs, 905–907, 907t
    antineoplastic drugs, 911
    antipruritics, 908
    antipsoriatic drugs, 909
    antiviral drugs, 907–908
    corticosteroids, 908, 908t
    description of, 21t, 25–26
    eardrops, 129, 129f
    eye medications, 128, 128f–129f
    immunomodulators, 911
    nasal medications, 134, 134f
    nursing considerations for, 24t–25t
    skin preparations, 132, 133f
Topical antimicrobials, 902, 904
**Topiramate**, 227t–228t, 230–232
Topoisomerase I inhibitors, 736–738, 737t, 741, 744
**Topotecan** (Hycamtin), 737–738, 737t
Torsades de pointes, 397, 401t–402t, 403
**Tositumomab and iodine tositumomab** (Bexxar), 771t, 774
Total body water, 474, 474f
Total parenteral nutrition
    central, 893–895
    definition of, 889
    peripheral, 892–893
Toxic, 19–20
Toxicity, 19, 30
Toxicology, 19–20, 35
Toxin, 796
Toxoids, 796–798, 800

Toxoplasmosis, 698t
Trace elements, 895
Trade name, 19, 728
**Tramadol hydrochloride**, 152t–153t, 155–157, 161
**Trandolapril** (Mavik), 354t
**Tranexamic acid** (Cyklokapron), 433t, 439
Transcription, 96–97, 750
Transdermal administration
  absorption effects, 25
  contraceptives, 552t
  estrogen, 548t
  fentanyl, 148b, 152t–153t, 163
  nitroglycerin, 378–379
  nursing considerations for, 24t–25t
  opioid analgesics, 148b, 163
  procedure for, 132, 133f
  testosterone, 568t
Transfer RNA, 96–97
Translators, 78–80
Transplantation, 785, 790–792. *See also* Immunosuppressant drugs
Transurethral resection of the prostate, 566
TRAP, 238–239
**Trastuzumab** (Herceptin), 771t–772t, 774
**Trazodone**, 263t, 265–266
Trematodes, 701
Tremor
  definition of, 238
  in Parkinson's disease, 238, 239t
**Treprostinil** (Remodulin), 359t, 360
**Tretinoin** (Renova, Retin-A, Vesanoid), 776t, 906
**Triamcinolone**, 536t
**Triamterene** (Dyrenium), 465–466, 466t
Triazoles, 684
Trichomoniasis, 698t
Tricyclic antidepressants
  administration of, 276
  adverse effects of, 261–262, 262t
  amitriptyline, 262–264, 263t
  assessments, 274
  characteristics of, 261–262
  contraindications, 261
  interactions, 262, 262t
  list of, 260t
  overdose of, 262
  poisoning, 35t
  profile of, 262–264
**Trifluridine** (Viroptic), 655t, 931
Triglycerides, 444–445
**Trihexyphenidyl**, 240t
Triiodothyronine, 501–502
Triptans, 209–210
**Triptorelin** (Trelstar), 566
Trough level, 19
Tubercle, 672
Tubercle bacilli, 672–673
Tuberculosis
  antitubercular drugs for. *See* Antitubercular drugs
  definition of, 672
  diagnosis of, 673b
  extensively drug-resistant, 673
  incidence of, 673
  multidrug-resistant, 672–673
  nursing process for, 678–680
  pathophysiology of, 673–674
  ~lence of, 673
  673

Tularemia, 808t
Tumor
  benign, 723–724, 724t
  classification of, 725t
  definition of, 723–724
  malignant, 723–724, 724t
Tumor antigens, 764
Tumor lysis syndrome, 723, 731
Tympanic membrane, 937–938, 938f
Type 1 diabetes mellitus, 511, 512t–513t, 513–514
Type 2 diabetes mellitus, 511, 512t–513t, 513–515

## U

U, 68b
Ultraviolet light, 726
**Undecylenic acid** (Cruex, Desenex), 907t
United States Pharmacopeia Medication Errors Reporting Program, 70
Unstable angina, 369
Upper respiratory tract, 589
Upper respiratory tract infection, 576
Uric acid, 714f
**Urokinase**, 431
U.S. Pharmacopeia, 7, 80–82
U.S. Pharmacopeia Medication Errors Reporting Program, 70
**Ustekinumab** (Stelara), 909
Uterine stimulants, 555–557, 556t–557t, 559, 561
Uterus, 544–545
Uvea, 917, 919
Uveitis, 929t

## V

Vaccine(s)
  adverse effects of, 800–801, 800t
  definition of, 796, 798
  description of, 798–799
  dosages of, 802t–803t, 803
  indications, 800
  interactions, 801–803
Vaccine Adverse Event Reporting System, 800
Vaccine Injury Table, 800, 801t
Vagina
  anatomy of, 544–545
  drug administration in, 135, 135f–136f
Vaginal suppositories, 135, 135f–136f
**Valacyclovir**, 655t
Valerian, 89t, 192b
**Valganciclovir** (Valcyte), 658
**Valproic acid**, 226, 227t–228t, 231–232, 235
**Valsartan** (Diovan), 385
**Vancomycin** (Vancocin, Vancoled), 641t, 643, 645, 647–648
Vancomycin-resistant *Enterococcus*, 634–635, 641
**Vardenafil** (Levitra), 566–568
**Varenicline** (Chantix), 289–290, 290t
**Varicella virus vaccine** (Varivax), 801t–803t, 806
Varicella zoster immunoglobulin (VZIG), 807
Varicella zoster virus, 654–655
Vascular endothelial growth factor, 754
Vascular pain, 141, 143
Vasodilators
  adverse effects of, 358
  baseline testing before using, 361
  contraindications, 358
  direct, 349
  dosages of, 358t
  drug effects of, 357

Vasodilators *(Continued)*
  indications, 357–358
  mechanism of action, 357
  nursing considerations for, 363, 379
  overdose of, 358
  profiles of, 358t, 359
  toxicity of, 358
  types of, 350b
**Vasopressin** (Pitressin), 495–499, 496t–497t
Vasospastic angina, 369
Vastus lateralis site, for intramuscular injections, 120, 120f
Vaughn Williams classification, 397, 403, 403t–404t, 417
Vectors, 97
**Vecuronium**, 179t, 180
Venom, 796, 799
Ventricular fibrillation, 401t–402t
Ventricular remodeling, 354–355
Ventricular tachycardia, 401t–402t
Ventrogluteal site, for intramuscular injections, 119, 119f
Veracity, 58b
**Verapamil** (Calan, Isoptin, Verelan), 376, 404b, 405t–408t, 413, 415
Very-low-density lipoprotein, 445
Vesicles, 902, 904
Vials, 112–113, 113f
**Vidarabine**, 656t
**Vinblastine**, 735t
Vinca alkaloids, 734
**Vincristine** (Vincasar PFS), 735t–736t, 736, 736b
VIPoma, 495, 498b
Viral capsid, 651–652
Viral hemorrhagic fever, 808t
Viral illnesses
  herpes simplex viruses, 654
  overview of, 653–654
  treatment of, 653–654
  varicella-zoster virus, 654–655
Viral infections, 652–653
Virion, 651
Virology, 651–653
Viruses
  definition of, 651
  replication of, 652, 652f
  structure of, 651–652
  transmission of, 652
Visceral pain, 141, 143
Vital signs, 160
Vitamin(s)
  definition of, 857
  fat-soluble. *See* Fat-soluble vitamins
  nursing process for, 873–875
  patient teaching about, 876
  water-soluble. *See* Water-soluble vitamins
Vitamin A (Aquasol A, Retinol), 859–861, 859t–861t, 873–875
Vitamin B$_1$ (Thiamilate), 859t, 865, 873, 875
Vitamin B$_2$ (Lactoflavin), 859t, 865–866, 873–875
Vitamin B$_3$ (Nicotinex), 857, 859t, 866–867, 866t, 873–875. *See also* Niacin.
Vitamin B$_6$ (Aminoxin, Vitelle), 859t, 867, 867t, 873–875
Vitamin B$_{12}$ (Nascobal), 859t, 867–869, 868f, 868t, 873–875, 884
Vitamin C, 859t–861t, 869, 873–875, 911
Vitamin D, 859t, 861–863, 862t, 873–875, 914

Vitamin E, 859t–861t, 863, 863t, 875
Vitamin K (Metaphyton, AquaMEPHYTON), 424, 435, 859t–861t, 863–864, 864t, 873, 875
Vitamin K–dependent clotting factors, 423
Vitreous body, 917, 919
Vitreous humor, 917, 919
Volume of distribution, 27
Vomiting center, 844–845
von Willebrand factor, 434
**Voriconazole** (Vfend), 684, 685t–687t, 688

## W

**Warfarin sodium** (Coumadin)
    administration of, 437
    assessments before using, 435
    in elderly patients, 424
    food interactions, 424–425
    genetic conditions that affect, 98
    heparin conversion to, 438
    interactions, 424–425, 425t, 615, 863–864
    international normalized ratio of, 406, 424
    mechanism of action, 423
    overdose of, 424
    profile of, 424–425
    toxicity of, 424
Water-soluble vitamins
    definition of, 857–858
    description of, 864–865
    types of, 858t, 864b
    vitamin $B_1$, 859t, 865, 873, 875
    vitamin $B_2$, 859t, 865–866, 873–875
    vitamin $B_3$, 857, 859t, 866–867, 866t, 873–875

Water-soluble vitamins (Continued)
    vitamin $B_6$, 859t, 867, 867t, 873–875
    vitamin $B_{12}$, 859t, 867–869, 868f, 868t, 873–875, 884
    vitamin C, 859t–861t, 869, 873–875
Wearing-off phenomenon, 238–239
Wernicke's encephalopathy, 282, 287
West Nile virus, 666–667
West nomogram, 40, 40f
Whey, 889, 892
White blood cells, 598t
Whooping cough, 803–804
Withdrawal
    alcohol, 288–289, 288b, 291
    definition of, 282
    depressants, 286–287
    ethanol, 288–289, 288b
    nicotine, 289–290, 290t
    opioid, 140, 151, 283–284, 283b–284b
    stimulants, 285, 285b
Wolff-Parkinson-White syndrome, 403
Women's health drugs
    contraceptives, 550–551, 551t–552t, 560, 562
    estrogens. See Estrogens
    fertility drugs, 554–555, 555t, 560–561
    nursing process for, 558–561
    osteoporosis. See Osteoporosis
    patient teaching about, 562
    preterm labor management, 557–558
    progestins, 549–551, 549t–550t, 558–560
    uterine stimulants, 555–557, 556t–557t, 559, 561
Women's Health Initiative, 547–548

World Health Organization
    analgesic ladder, 146
    definition of, 141
    patient safety information from, 67b
Wound care drugs, 911, 912t
Wound debridement, 911

## X

Xanthine derivatives, 595–596, 595t, 601–604, 601b
Xanthine oxidase, 714f

## Y

Yeasts, 682–683
Yin-yang, 53

## Z

**Zafirlukast** (Accolate), 596, 597t
**Zalcitabine**, 656t
**Zaleplon**, 192t, 193, 198–199
**Zanamivir** (Relenza), 655t–656t, 658
**Zidovudine** (AZT, ZDV, Retrovir), 656t, 666
**Zileuton** (Zyflo), 596, 597t
Zinc, 859t, 873
Zollinger-Ellison syndrome, 822
**Zolpidem**, 192t, 193, 198–199
Zona fasciculata, 534
Zona reticularis, 534
**Zonisamide**, 227t–228t, 231
**Zostavax**, 806
Zostrix, 659b
Z-track method, for intramuscular injections, 118–121, 118f

# SPECIAL FEATURES

**Note:** Case Studies, Patient Teaching Tips, Key Points, and NCLEX® Examination Review Questions are provided in each chapter (except the Photo Atlas of Drug Administration, Chapter 9). Teamwork and Collaboration: Pharmacokinetic Bridge to Nursing Practice boxes are provided in several chapters.

## EVIDENCE-BASED PRACTICE

Improving Retention, Confidence, and Competence of New Graduate Nurses: A 10-Year Longitudinal Study (Chapter 1), p. 12

Update on Application of the Beers Criteria for Prevention of Adverse Drug Events in Older Adults (Chapter 3), p. 45

Building a Collaborative Nursing Practice to Promote Patient Education: An Inpatient and Outpatient Partnership (Chapter 6), p. 78

Student Nurses' Misconceptions of Adults with Chronic Non-malignant Pain (Chapter 10), p. 145

Ibuprofen May Help Relieve Acute Migraine Headaches (Chapter 13), p. 210

Exercise and Improved Cognition (Chapter 20), p. 332

Storytelling to Improve Blood Pressure (Chapter 22), p. 364

A Short-Term, Randomized, Double-Blind, Parallel-Group Study to Evaluate the Efficacy and Safety of Dronedarone Versus Amiodarone in Patients with Persistent Atrial Fibrillation: The DIONYSOS Study (Chapter 25), p. 415

Post-Stroke Statins Improve Patient Outcomes (Chapter 27), p. 456

Sensor-Augmented Insulin Pump Therapy Trumps Multiple Daily Injections (Chapter 32), p. 529

## PATIENT-CENTERED CARE: CULTURAL IMPLICATIONS

Glucose-6-Phosphate Dehydrogenase Deficiency (Chapter 2), p. 34

A Brief Review of Common Practices among Selected Cultural Groups (Chapter 4), p. 52

Examples of Varying Drug Responses in Different Racial or Ethnic Groups (Chapter 4), p. 53

Patient Education (Chapter 6), p. 80

Drug Responses and Cultural Factors (Chapter 7), p. 90

The Patient Experiencing Pain (Chapter 10), p. 141

Understanding Your Patient's Sleep Needs (Chapter 12), p. 190

Psychotherapeutic Drugs (Chapter 16), p. 276

Antihypertensive Drug Therapy (Chapter 22), p. 361

Racial Disparities between Black Women and White Women in the Incidence, Treatment, and Prognosis of Endometrial Cancer (Chapter 34), p. 559

's Health Concerns: Prostate Cancer and Its Occurrence Mortality (Chapter 35), p. 566

## PATIENT-CENTERED CARE: LIFESPAN CONSIDERATIONS FOR THE ELDERLY PATIENT

Percentage of Population Older than Age 65 (Chapter 3), p. 42

Pharmacokinetic Changes (Chapter 3), p. 43

A Brief Look at the Sixth Leading Cause of Death in the United States: Alzheimer's Disease (Chapter 3), p. 47

Opioid Use (Chapter 10), p. 162

Anesthesia (Chapter 11), p. 172

Antiparkinson Drugs (Chapter 15), p. 248

Psychotherapeutic Drugs (Chapter 16), p. 272

Alcohol and Substance Abuse (Chapter 17), p. 293

Use of Beta-Adrenergic Agonists (Chapter 18), p. 303

Overactive Bladder (Chapter 21), p. 340

Diuretic Therapy (Chapter 28), p. 469

Thyroid Hormones (Chapter 31), p. 506

Sildenafil: Use and Concerns (Chapter 35), p. 567

Xanthine Derivatives (Chapter 37), p. 601

NSAIDs (Chapter 44), p. 717

Iron Products (Chapter 54), p. 885

## PATIENT-CENTERED CARE: LIFESPAN CONSIDERATIONS FOR THE PEDIATRIC PATIENT

Pharmacokinetic Changes in the Neonate and Pediatric Patient (Chapter 3), p. 39

Age-Related Considerations for Medication Administration from Infancy to Adolescence (Chapter 3), p. 41

Medication Errors (Chapter 5), p. 69

Opioid Use (Chapter 10), p. 158

Anesthesia (Chapter 11), p. 172

Moderate or Conscious Anesthesia (Chapter 11), p. 174

Antiepileptic Drugs (Chapter 14), p. 223

Psychotherapeutic Drugs (Chapter 16), p. 272

Abuse of Over-the-Counter Drugs and Huffing Practices in Adolescents (Chapter 17), p. 293

Heart Failure (Chapter 24), p. 391

Diuretics (Chapter 28), p. 464

Reye's Syndrome (Chapter 44), p. 714

Antidiarrheal Preparations (Chapter 51), p. 833

Syrup of Ipecac and Poisoning (Chapter 52), p. 845

## SAFETY: HERBAL THERAPIES AND DIETARY SUPPLEMENTS

Feverfew (*Chrysanthemum parthenium*) (Chapter 10), p. 161

Possible Effects of Popular Herbal Products When Combined with Anesthetics (Chapter 11), p. 182

Kava (*Piper methysticum*) (Chapter 12), p. 192

Valerian (*Valeriana officinalis*) (Chapter 12), p. 192